Pediatric Surgery and Urology

This highly regarded textbook provides a unique clinical reference for all pediatric surgeons. This new edition analyzes and updates what is known about long-term outcomes in pediatric surgery and urology. The editors have succeeded in bringing together critical reviews written by leading international experts in pediatric surgery and urology. The second edition of this successful and popular textbook has been completely revised and updated with new chapters on urolithiasis, small bowel transplantation, pancreatitis, breast disorders, and a completely new section on trauma.

An understanding of long-term outcomes is critical if individual surgeons and health policy-makers are to achieve optimum results in current clinical practice. This is an essential reference source for pediatric surgeons and urologists, pediatricians, adult specialists, and others dealing with the sequelae of childhood surgical problems.

Reviews of the First Edition

"It is an excellent book, well written by a host of experienced surgeons reviewing the results of the surgery of their particular subspecialties and interests . . . This book should not only be bought by departments of pediatric surgery and pediatric urology, but should also be read by all surgeons and trainees who operate on infants and children."
British Journal of Urology

" . . . institutional experience and expert clinical review of the literature make the text current and applicable to daily practice . . . A book that emphasizes outcome rather than diagnosis and procedures has become essential, as health care moves to measures of efficacy, safety, acceptability, and cost effectiveness . . . I heartily endorse this work to my colleagues." Robert J. Touloukian, M. D., review in *JAMA*.

Pediatric Surgery and Urology

Long-term Outcomes

Second Edition

Edited by

Mark D. Stringer, M.S., F.R.C.S., F.R.C.P.C.H.

Professor of Paediatric Surgery, Department of Paediatric Surgery, St James's University Hospital Leeds, UK

Keith T. Oldham, M.D., F.A.C.S.

Professor and Chief, Division of Pediatric Surgery, Medical College of Wisconsin
Marie Z Uihlein Chair and Surgeon-in-Chief, Children's Hospital of Wisconsin, Milwaukee, Wisconsin, USA

Pierre D. E. Mouriquand, M.D., F.R.C.S. (Eng.), F.A.P.U.

Professor of Pediatric Urology and Head of Pediatric Surgery, Department of Pediatric Urology, Debrousse Hospital, Claude Bernard University Lyon I, Lyon, France

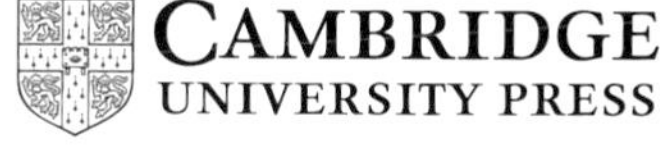

CAMBRIDGE UNIVERSITY PRESS
Cambridge, New York, Melbourne, Madrid, Cape Town, Singapore, São Paulo

Cambridge University Press
The Edinburgh Building, Cambridge CB2 2RU, UK

Published in the United States of America by Cambridge University Press, New York

www.cambridge.org
Information on this title: www.cambridge.org/9780521839020

First published 2006

Printed in the United Kingdom at the University Press, Cambridge

A catalog record for this publication is available from the British Library

ISBN-13 978-0-521-83902-0 hardback
ISBN-10 0-521-83902-5 hardback

We dedicate this book to our patients and their families.

Contents

† deceased.

Part V Urology

† deceased.

Part VI Oncology

Part VII Transplantation

Part VIII Trauma

Part IX Miscellaneous

Contributors

P. David Adelson
Department of Pediatric Neurosurgery
Children's Hospital of Pittsburgh and
The University of Pittsburgh
3705 Fifth Avenue
Pittsburgh, PA 15213-2583, USA

Craig T. Albanese
Lucile Packard Children's Hospital
Stanford Medical Center
780 Welch Road, Suite 206
Stanford, CA 94305-5733, USA

Jennifer H. Aldrint
Division of Pediatric Surgery
PO Box 3815
Duke University Medical Center
Durham, NC 27710, USA

Frederick Alexander
Department of Pediatric Surgery
Cleveland Clinic
Children's Hospital
9500 Euclid Avenue M14
Cleveland, OH 44195, USA

Nikki Almendinger
Department of Surgery
Children's Hospital
300 Longwood Avenue
Fegan 3
Boston, MA 02115, USA

Maria H. Alonso
Department of Pediatric General and Thoracic Surgery
Transplantation Division
Cincinnati Children's Hospital Medical Center
3333 Burnet Avenue
Cincinnati, OH 45229, USA

Richard Appleton
The Roald Dahl EEG Unit
Department of Paediatric Neurology
Royal Liverpool Children's Hospital
Alder Hey, Eaton Road
Liverpool L12 2AP, UK

A. Martin Barrett
Department of Paediatric Surgery
Royal Victoria Infirmary
Queen Victoria Road
Newcastle upon Tyne NE1 4LP, UK

Laurence S. Baskin
Department of Urology
University of California
400 Parnassus Avenue, A640, Box 0738
San Francisco, CA 94143, USA

Spencer W. Beasley
Department of Paediatric Surgery
Christchurch Hospital
Private Bag 4710
Christchurch, New Zealand

Geoffrey Bond
Department of Pediatric Neurosurgery
Children's Hospital of Pittsburgh and
The University of Pittsburgh
3705 Fifth Avenue
Pittsburgh, PA 15213-2583, USA

Sophie Branchereau
Division of Surgery
Federation of Paediatrics
78 rue du Général Leclerc
Centre Hospitalier Universitaire Bicêtre
Le Kremlin Bicêtre, France

Mark F. H. Brougham
Department of Paediatric Haematology and Oncology
Royal Hospital for Sick Children
17 Millerfield Place
Edinburgh EH9 1LW, UK

Steven W. Bruch
University of Michigan Medical School
C. S. Mott Children's Hospital
Section of Pediatric Surgery F3970
1500 E. Medical Center Drive
Ann Arbor, Mi 48109-0245, USA

Neil Buxton
Department of Paediatric Neurosurgery
Royal Liverpool Children's Hospital
Alder Hey, Eaton Road
Liverpool L12 2AP, UK

Anthony A. Caldamone
Division of Pediatric Urology
Hasbro Children's Hospital
Brown University School of Medicine
Providence, RI, USA

Philip A. J. Chetcuti
Clarendon Wing
Leeds General Infirmary
Leeds LS2 9NS, UK

Younghoon R. Cho
Department of Plastic Surgery
Medical College of Wisconsin
9200 West Wisconsin Avenue
Milwaukee, WI 53226, USA

Bartley G. Cilento, Jr.
Department of Pediatric Urology
The Children's Hospital
300 Longwood Avenue
Boston, MA 02115-5737, USA

Arnold G. Coran
University of Michigan Medical School
C. S. Mott Children's Hospital
Section of Pediatric Surgery F3970
1500 E. Medical Center Drive
Ann Arbor, MI 48109-0245, USA

Robin T. Cotton
Department of Pediatric Otolaryngology
Cincinnati Children's Hospital Medical Center
3333 Burnet Avenue
Cincinnati, OH 45229, USA

David C. G. Crabbe
Department of Paediatric Surgery
Clarendon Wing
Leeds General Infirmary
Leeds LS2 9NS, UK

Peter M. Cuckow
Department of Paediatric Urology
Institute for Child Health and
Great Ormond Street Hospital
for Children NHS Trust
30 Guilford Street
London WC1N 3JH, UK

Mark Davenport
Department of Paediatric Surgery
King's College Hospital
Denmark Hill
London SE5 9RS, UK

Andrew M. Davidoff
St. Jude Children's Research Hospital
332 N Lauderdale
Memphis TN 38105, USA

Pascale de Lonlay
Département de Pédiatrie
Hôpital Necker-Enfants Malades
149 rue de Sèvres
75743 Paris Cedex 15, France

Jean de Ville de Goyet
Transplant and Paediatric Surgery
St. Luc University Hospital
10 Avenue Hippocrate
B-1200 Brussels, Belgium

Nadeem N. Dhanani
Department of Urology
University of Texas
Houston Medical School
6431 Fannin Street, Suite 6018
Houston
Texas 77030, USA

Maria Di Lorenzo[†]
(formerly) Department of Surgery
University of Montreal
Hôpital Sainte-Justine
3175 Côte Ste-Catherine
Montreal
Quebec
Canada H3T 1C5

Patrick G. Duffy
Department of Paediatric Urology
Institute of Child Health and Great Ormond Street Hospital
for Children NHS Trust
30 Guilford Street
London WC1N 3JH, UK

Peter F. Ehrlich
University of Michigan Medical School
C. S. Mott Children's Hospital
Section of Pediatric Surgery F3970
1500 E. Medical Center Drive
Ann Arbor, MI 48104, USA

Rui Fernandes
Department of Oral and Maxillofacial Surgery
University of Maryland
666 W Baltimore Street
Baltimore, MD 21201, USA

Steven J. Fishman
Department of Surgery
Children's Hospital
300 Longwood Avenue
Fegan 3
Boston, MA 02115, USA

Henri R. Ford
Children's Hospital of Los Angeles
University of Southern California
Los Angeles, CA, USA

Julie R. Fuchs
Department of Pediatric Surgery
J. W. Riley Hospital for Children
Indianapolis, IN, USA

[†] deceased.

Stephanie M. P. Fuller
Division of Cardiothoracic Surgery
Heart, Lung, and Heart Transplant Services
Children's Hospital of Philadelphia
34th Street and Civic Center Blvd.
Suite 8527, Main Building
Philadelphia, PA 19104, USA

Frédéric Gauthier
Division of Surgery
Federation of Paediatrics
Centre Hospitalier Universitaire Bicêtre
78 rue du Général Leclerc
Le Kremlin Bicêtre, France

John P. Gearhart
Brady Urological Institute
The Johns Hopkins Hospital
600 North Wolfe Street
Baltimore, MD 21287-2101, USA

Prasad Godbole
Department of Paediatric Urology
Sheffield Children's NHS Trust,
Sheffield, UK

Adam Goldin
Division of Pediatric Surgery
Department of Surgery
University of Washington
Seattle, WA, USA

Arun K. Gosain
Department of Plastic Surgery
Medical College of Wisconsin
9200 W. Wisconsin Avenue
Milwaukee, WI 53226, USA

†David Gough
Department of Paediatric Urology
Royal Manchester Children's Hospital
Pendlebury
Manchester M27 4HA, UK

Nigel D. Heaton
Liver Transplant Surgical Service
King's College Hospital
Denmark Hill
London SE5 9RS, UK

† deceased.

W. Hardy Hendren
Children's Hospital
300 Longwood Avenue
Boston, MA 02115, USA

Marion C. W. Henry
Section of Pediatric Surgery
Yale University School of Medicine
333 Cedar Street, FMB 132
PO Box 208062
New Haven, CT 06520-8062, USA

Edward R. Howard
(formerly) Department of Surgery
King's College Hospital
Denmark Hill
London SE5 9RS, UK

John M. Hutson
Department of General Surgery
Royal Children's Hospital
Flemington Road
Parkville, VIC 3052, Australia

Paul E. Hyman
Department of Pediatrics
University of Kansas Hospital
3901 Rainbow Boulevard
Kansas City, KS 66160, USA

Venkata R. Jayanthi
Division of Urology
Children's Hospital
Room ED343, Ed Building
700 Children's Drive
Columbus, OH 43205-2696, USA

Bruce A. Kaufman
Department of Neurosurgery
Children's Hospital of Wisconsin
9000 W Wisconsin Avenue
MS 405
Milwaukee, WI 53226, USA

Brigid K Killelea
In-CHOIR (International Center for Health Outcomes and Innovation Research)
600W. 168th Street, 7th Floor,
New York, NY10032, USA

Stephen A. Koff
Division of Urology
Children's Hospital
Room ED343, Ed Building
700 Children's Drive
Columbus, OH 43205-2696, USA

Göran Läckgren
Department of Paediatric Urology
Uppsala University
Akademiska Sjukhuset Ing 95
S-75185 Uppsala, Sweden

Dave R. Lal
(formerly) Department of Surgery and Pediatrics
Memorial Sloan-Kettering Cancer Center
C-1176, 1275 York Avenue
New York
New York 10021, USA

John D. Langdon
(formerly) Department of Oral and Maxillofacial Surgery
King's College London
London, UK

Jacob C. Langer
Room 1526
Department of Surgery
Hospital for Sick Children
University of Toronto
555 University Avenue
Toronto ON M5G 1X8, Canada

Michael P. LaQuaglia
Department of Surgery and Pediatrics
Memorial Sloan-Kettering Cancer Center
C-1176, 1275 York Avenue
New York
NY 10021, USA

Eric L. Lazar
Children's Hospital of New York
3959 Broadway
Room 201 South
New York
NY 10032, USA

Claude Le Coultre
Paediatric Surgery Department
Children's Hospital
6 rue Willy Donze-HUG
CH-1211 Geneva 14, Switzerland

Gill A. Levitt
Department of Paediatric Urology
Great Ormond Street Hospital
for Children NHS Trust
30 Guilford Street
London WC1N 3JH, UK

Marc A. Levitt
Colorectal Center for Children Cincinnati
Children's Hospital for Pediatric
Surgery
3333 Bunet Avenue, ML 2023
Cincinnati, OH 46229, USA

Lorraine Ludman
Institute of Child Health
Great Ormond Street Hospital for Children NHS Trust
30 Guilford Street 46229, USA
London WCIN 3JH, UK

David K. Magnuson
University Hospital Health System
Rainbow Babies & Childrens Hospital
1100 Euclid Ave, Room RBC 122
Cleveland, OH 44106, USA

Preeti Malladi
Stanford University Pediatric Surgery
780 Welch Rd., Ste. 206
Stanford, CA 94305-5733, USA

Padraig S. J. Malone
Southampton University Hospitals
Tremona Road
Southampton SO16 6YD, UK

Gianantonio M. Manzoni
Sezione Urologia Pediatrica, Divisione di Urologia
Ospedale di Circolo e Fondazione Macchi
Varese
Italy

Anthony J. Michalski
Department of Paediatric Urology
Great Ormond Street Hospital
London WC1N 3JH, UK

Gerald C. Mingin
Department of Urology
Denver Children's Hospital
Colorado, CO, USA

Takeshi Miyano
Department of Pediatric General and Urogenital Surgery
Juntendo University School of Medicine
2-1-1 Hongo
Bunkyo-ku
Tokyo 113-8421, Japan

Alan Mortell
Children's Research Centre
Our Lady's Hospital for Sick Children
Crumlin
Dublin 12, Ireland

R. Lawrence Moss
Section of Pediatric Surgery
Yale University School of Medicine
333 Cedar Street, FMB 132
PO Box 208062
New Haven, CT 06520-8062, USA

Pierre D. E. Mouriquand
Department of Paediatric Urology/Surgery
Debrousse Hospital
29 rue Soeur Bouvier
69322 Lyon Cedex 05, France

Paolo Muiesan
Liver Transplant Surgical Services
King's College Hospital,
Denmark Hill
London SE5 9RS, UK

Evan P. Nadler
New York University School of Medicine
530 First Avenue, Suite 10 W
New York, NY 10016, USA

Jaimie D. Nathan
Division of Pediatric Surgery
Duke University Medical Center
PO Box 3815
Durham, NC, 27710, USA

Tryggve Nevéus
Department of Paediatrics
Uppsala University
Akademiska Sjukhuset Ing 95
S-75185 Uppsala, Sweden

Hiep T. Nguyen
Department of Pediatric Urology
The Children's Hospital
300 Longwood Avenue
Boston, MA 02115-5737, USA

Thomas E. Novak
Brady Urological Institute
The Johns Hopkins Hospital
600 North Wolfe Street
Baltimore, MD 21287-2101, USA

Donald Nuss
Pediatric Surgery
Children's Hospital of the King's Daughters
601 Children's Lane, Suite 5A
Norfolk, VA 23507, USA

Barry O'Donnell
28 Merlyn Road,
Ballsbridge
Dublin 4, Ireland

Keith T. Oldham
Children's Hospital of Wisconsin
9000 W Wisconsin Avenue
PO Box 1997
Milwaukee, WI 53201, USA

Robert Ord
Department of Oral and Maxillofacial Surgery
University of Maryland
666 W Baltimore Street
Baltimore, MD 21201, USA

Jean-Bernard Otte
Transplant and Paediatric Surgery
St. Luc University Hospital
10 Avenue Hippocrate
B-1200 Brussels, Belgium

Mikko Pakarinen
Children's Hospital
University of Helsinki
PO Box 281
FIN-00029 HUS, Finland

Danièle Pariente
Division of Radiology
Federation of Paediatrics
Centre Hospitalier Universitaire Bicêtre
78 rue du Général Leclerc
Le Kremlin Bicêtre, France

Emma J. Parkinson
Department of Paediatric Surgery
Institute of Child Health
30 Guilford Street
London WC1N 1EH, UK

Alberto Peña
Colorectal Center for Children
Cincinnati Children's Hospital for Pediatric Surgery
3333 Bunet Avenue ML 2023
Cincinnati, OH 46229, USA

Agostino Pierro
Department of Paediatric Surgery
Institute of Child Health and Great Ormond Street Hospital NHS Trust
30 Guilford Street
London WC1N 1EH, UK

John W. L. Puntis
Clarendon Wing
Leeds General Infirmary
Leeds LS2 9NS, UK

Prem Puri
Children's Research Centre
Our Lady's Hospital for Sick Children
Crumlin
Dublin 12, Ireland

Faisal G. Qureshi
University of Pittsburgh Medical Center
300 Halket Street, Suite 5500
Pittsburgh, PA 15213, USA

Ashok Rajimwale
Southampton University Hospitals
Tremona Road
Southampton SO16 6YD, UK

Janet M. Rennie
Department of Neonatal Medicine
Elizabeth Garrett Anderson Obstetric Hospital
University College London Hospitals
Huntley Street
London WCIE 6 DH, UK

Yann Revillon
Service de Chirurgie Pediatrique
149 rue de Sevres
75743 Paris Cedex 15, France

Jorge Reyes
Transplant Surgery
University of Washington
Seattle, USA

Henry E. Rice
Division of Pediatric Surgery
PO Box 3815
Duke University Medical Center
Durham, NC 27710, USA

Risto J. Rintala
Department of Pediatric Surgery
Children's Hospital
University of Helsinki
PO Box 281
FIN-00029 HUS, Finland

Michael L. Ritchey
Department of Surgery and Pediatrics
Division of Urology
University of Texas
Houston Medical School
6431 Fannin Street, Suite 6018
Houston
Texas 77030, USA

Jean-Jacques Robert
Département de Pédiatrie
Hôpital Necker – Enfants Malades
149 rue de Sèvres
75743 Paris Cedex 15, France

Frederick C. Ryckman
Department of Pediatric General and Thoracic Surgery
Transplantation Division
Cincinnati Children's Hospital Medical Center
3333 Burnet Avenue
Cincinnati, OH 45229, USA

Jacqueline Saito
Division of Pediatric Surgery
University of Alabama
Birmingham, AL, USA

Thomas T. Sato
Children's Hospital of Wisconsin
9000 W Wisconsin Avenue
C320
Milwaukee, WI 53226, USA

Frédérique Sauvat
Service de Chirurgie Pediatrique
149 rue de Sevres
75743 Paris Cedex 15, France

Justine M. Schober
333 State Street, Suite 201
Erie, PA 16506
USA
and
Department of Urology
Hamot Medical Center
Erie, PA, USA

Joel Shilyansky
Children's Hospital of Wisconsin
9000 W. Wisconsin Avenue
C320
Milwaukee, WI 53226, USA

Michael A. Skinner
Division of Pediatric Surgery
Duke University Medical Center
PO Box 3815
Durham, NC 27710, USA

Charles A. Sklar
Department of Surgery and Pediatrics
Memorial Sloan-Kettering Cancer Center
C-1176, 1275 York Avenue
New York
New York 10021, USA

Alistair G. Smyth
Northern and Yorkshire Cleft Lip and Palate Service
Clarendon Wing
The General Infirmary at Leeds
Gt. George Street
Leeds LS2 9NS, UK

Manu R. Sood
Department of Pediatric Gastroent erology
Children's Hospital of Wisconsin
9000 W. Wisconsin Avenue Milwaukee,
WI 53226, USA

Lewis Spitz
Department of Paediatric Surgery
Institute of Child Health and Great Ormond Street Hospital NHS Trust
30 Guilford Street
London WC1N 1EH, UK

Thomas Spray
Division of Cardiothoracic Surgery
Heart, Lung, and Heart Transplant Services
Children's Hospital of Philadelphia
34th Street and Civic Center Blvd.
Suite 8527, Main Building
Philadelphia, PA 19104
USA

Roly Squire
Department of Paediatric Surgery
Gledhow Wing
St. James's University Hospital
Beckett Street
Leeds LS9 7TH, UK

Christian J. Streck
St. Jude Children's Research Hospital
332 N Lauderdale
Memphis TN 38105, USA

Mark D. Stringer
Children's Liver and GI Unit
Gledhow Wing
St. James's University Hospital
Leeds, LS9 7TF, UK

Steven Stylianos
Department of Pediatric Surgery
Miami Children's Hospital
3200 SW 60th CT-Suite 201
Miami, FL 33155, USA

Karl Sylvester
Stanford University Pediatric Surgery
780 Welch Rd., Ste. 206
Stanford, CA 94305-5733
USA

Dana Mara Thompson
Department of Pediatric Otolaryngology and the Aerodigestive and Sleep Center
Cincinnati Children's Hospital Medical Center
3333 Burnet Avenue
Cincinnati, OH 45229, USA

Greg Tiao
Department of Pediatric General and Thoracic Surgery
Transplantation Division
Cincinnati Children's Hospital Medical Center
3333 Burnet Avenue
Cincinnati, OH 45229, USA

Pierre Tissières
Multidisciplinary Paediatric Intensive Care Unit
Bicêtre Hospital
78 rue de Genberal Leclerc
92475 Le Kremlin-Bicêtre, France

J. S. Valla
Service de Chirurgie Pediatrique
Hôpital Lenval
56 avenue de Californie
06200 Nice, France

Judith van der Voort
KRUF Children's Kidney Centre for Wales
University Hospital of Wales
Heath Park
Cardiff CF14 4XW, UK

Kate Verrier Jones
KRUF Children's Kidney Centre for Wales
University Hospital of Wales
Heath Park
Cardiff CF14 4XW, UK

Michael G. Vitale
Children's Hospital of New York
3959 Broadway, 8 North
New York, NY 10032, USA

Adam M. Vogel
Department of Surgery
Children's Hospital
300 Longwood Avenue
Fegan 3
Boston, MA 02115, USA

W. Hamish B. Wallace
Department of Paediatric Haematology and Oncology
Royal Hospital for Sick Children
17 Millerfield Place
Edinburgh EH9 1LW, UK

Son Lee West
Department of Surgery
Children's Hospital
300 Longwood Avenue, Fegan 3
Boston, MA 02115, USA

Duncan T. Wilcox
Department of Pediatric Urology
The University of Texas
Southwestern Medical Center at Dallas
Dallas, Texas, USA

Jay Wilson
Department of Surgery
Children's Hospital
300 Longwood Avenue
Fegan 3
Boston, MA 02115, USA

Christopher R. J. Woodhouse
Institute of Urology
Gower Street Campus
48 Riding House Street
London W1W 7EY, UK

Adrian S. Woolf
Nephro-Urology Unit, UCL
Institute of Child Health
30 Guilford Street
London WC1N 1EH, UK

Hilary Wyatt
Department of Child Health
King's College Hospital
Denmark Hill
London SE5 9RS, UK

Salam Yazbeck
Department of Surgery
University of Montreal
Hôpital Sainte-Justine
3175 Côte Ste-Catherine
Montreal
Quebec H3T 1C5, Canada

Acknowledgments

We are indebted to our partners, Emma, Karen, and Jessica, and to our children, Paul, Stephen, Catherine, Christian, Brian, David, and Caroline. Without their support and encouragement, our endeavors as pediatric surgeons would not be possible.

We also wish to thank Peter Silver, Senior Editor at Cambridge University Press, for his steadfast support and encouragement throughout the project and Joseph Bottrill, Production Editor, and Mary Sanders (Copyeditor), for their expertise in collating the material for this second edition.

Preface

The second edition of this book attempts to bring together and analyze what we currently know about the long-term effects of conditions and operative procedures in pediatric surgery and urology. The subject of long-term outcomes has been relatively neglected in the past. However, the realization that there is an ever-expanding cohort of children reaching maturity with a variable legacy from childhood surgical problems has prompted a more critical and detailed study of outcomes with the aim of optimizing current surgical practice. Encouragingly, all major international pediatric surgical meetings now include data on long-term outcomes. Furthermore, in the decade since the first edition of this text was conceived, the quality and relevance of the data are substantially more robust. Much more is now known about long-term function and quality of life. Data on outcomes provide a barometer for healthcare, indicating its efficacy, safety, acceptability, and sometimes its cost-effectiveness. Such data will be used increasingly to shape public policy and guide surgical practice. Perhaps, more than in any other field of surgery, it is necessary for pediatric surgeons and urologists to look critically at long-term outcomes and the effect these have on the quality of life of their patients and their families.

By inviting contributions from leading experts around the world including the USA, Europe, Australia, and Japan, we have collected together critical analyses of the literature, framed within the context of a wealth of institutional and personal experience. We are grateful to our many authors for their outstanding efforts. We hope that the second edition of this text is reasonably comprehensive, but it is not intended to be encyclopedic. A completely new section on trauma has been added, together with new chapters on the organization and delivery of pediatric surgical care, urolithiasis, pancreatitis, intestinal motility disorders, small bowel transplantation, and pediatric breast disorders.

Since the first edition was published, Professor Ted Howard has retired and stepped down from the editorial team. He was a major influence in the initiation of this project and a keen advocate of the importance of long-term follow-up. We are much indebted to him and wish him a long and happy retirement.

This book is intended to be a unique reference work for pediatric surgeons and urologists, but it should also be of value to pediatricians, adult specialists, and others who are involved in the long-term follow-up of patients with congenital malformations. We hope that clinicians will continue to be stimulated to look critically and honestly at their long-term results so that we can better inform our patients and their families in the future.

Part I

General issues

1a

Introduction and historical overview: North American perspective

W. Hardy Hendren

Children's Hospital, Boston, MA, USA

William E. Ladd (1880–1967) is considered to be the father of pediatric surgery in North America. However, delving into records from the Massachusetts General Hospital (MGH), founded in 1821, discloses pediatric surgical cases cared for by surgeons 60 years before Ladd's time. A book published in 1839 by John C. Warren,[1] who performed the first publicly demonstrated operation under general anesthesia at the MGH in 1846, included pediatric cases. A generation later, his son, J. Mason Warren, wrote a book after anesthesia was well established in which many more pediatric cases were described.[2] When the Children's Hospital in Boston was founded in 1869 (Philadelphia Children's Hospital predated it in 1855), Benjamin Shaw, resident physician at the MGH wrote to the press, "Our existing institutions public and private provide adequately for hospital treatment of children." He stated that 190 of 1264 (14%) admissions to the MGH in 1868 were children.

A recent book, *The Children's Hospital of Boston, Built Better Than They Knew*, by Clement A. Smith,[3] describes a century of history at Children's. From 1882 to 1914 the most frequent surgical admission was for bone and joint tuberculosis. Early on there were no recognized cases of appendicitis, because Reginald Fitz at the MGH had not yet described that entity. In contrast there were 113 admissions for appendicitis from 1911 to 1913. When the present Children's Hospital was built in 1914, next to Harvard Medical School, a herd of cows was maintained across the street to provide tuberculosis-free milk for the patients. Ladd graduated from the Harvard Medical School in 1906. He trained as a general surgeon at the Boston City Hospital. He held an appointment as a Volunteer Assistant Surgeon at Children's in 1910, but maintained a private practice of general surgery and gynecology. On December 6, 1917, during World War I, a munitions ship exploded in the harbor at Halifax, Nova Scotia. There were hundreds of deaths and injuries. A plea for help was made to physicians from Boston. Ladd was among those who responded. Many of the patients were children. His career path changed soon thereafter to concentrate on pediatric surgery, succeeding James Stone as Chief of Surgery in 1927. He became the first geographic full-time surgeon for children and soon established a link with the Peter Bent Brigham Hospital, recognizing that pediatric surgeons should have strong ties with general surgery.

Another surgeon who responded to the call from Nova Scotia was Ernest Armory Codman (1869–1940). This textbook, which stresses long-term outcomes of pediatric surgery, would be incomplete without mention of Codman. He was a classmate of Harvey Cushing. Codman developed the anesthesia chart, with name, diagnosis, operation, vital signs, and remarks. When he wrote a paper on ether anesthesia and presented it for review, a senior surgeon at MGH described it as "too frank for the good of the hospital, for it described in detail the cases which I lost." When X-ray diagnosis was introduced in 1896, Codman became interested in that new tool. Although he was a surgeon, he became the first radiologist at the Children's Hospital in 1899. It was established as the first Pediatric Radiology Department in America. Although contemporary literature for the past decade has emphasized the importance of long-term follow-up and quality improvement, *Codman preached that philosophy almost a century ago.* He introduced the "end result idea." His approach was methodical, complete, and precise. When the Clinical Congress of Surgeons of North America met in 1912, Codman was made chairman of a committee on hospital standardization to

Pediatric Surgery and Urology: Long-term Outcomes, Mark Stringer, Keith Oldham, Pierre Mouriquand.
Published by Cambridge University Press.

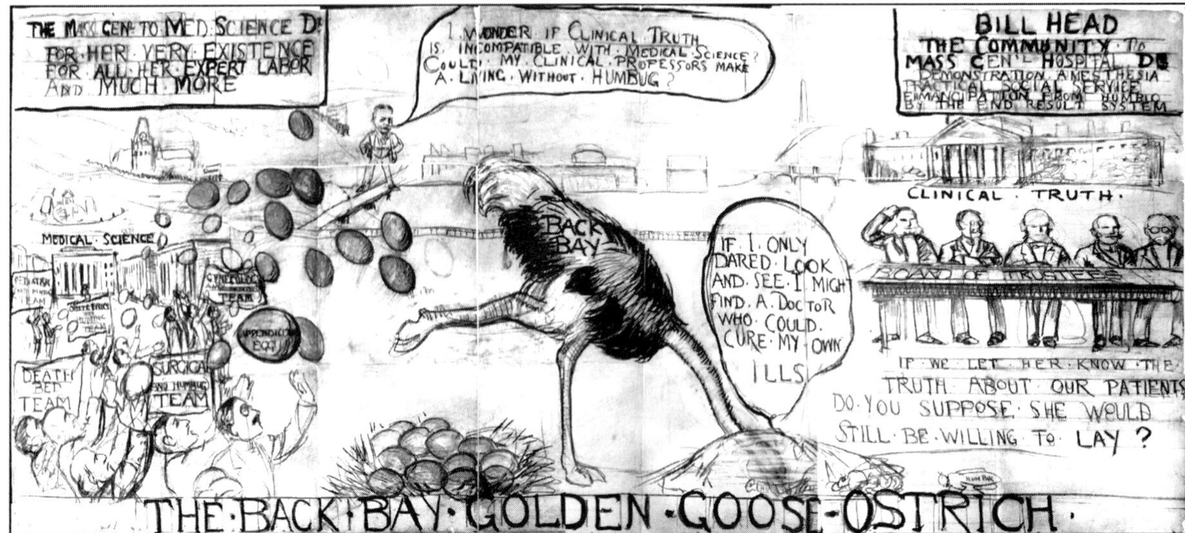

Fig. 1a.1. Cartoon shown by Ernest A. Codman on January 8, 1915, to a meeting of surgeons at the Boston Medical Library. It created a storm of resentment. The ostrich is kicking golden eggs into the outstretched hands of MGH staff who are labeled: Surgical, Gynecologic, Obstetric, and Pediatric (and humbug) Teams, and a Death Bed Team. President Lowell of Harvard stands above, straddling a bridge across the Charles River and saying, "I wonder if clinical truth is incompatible with medical science? Could my clinical professors make a living without humbug?" The ostrich is eating humbugs, and muses "If I only dared look and see, I might find a doctor who could cure my own ills." At the Clinical Truth Table are the Board of Trustees of the MGH. They are commenting, "If we let her know the truth about our patients do you suppose she would still be willing to lay?" At the top right is a Bill Head crediting the Massachusetts General Hospital with the first demonstration of Anesthesia, Practical Social Service, and Emancipation from Humbug by the End Result System. On the left, above the clinical teams, stands Harvard Medical School. Harvard College, Massachusetts Institute of Technology and Bunker Hill Monument are seen in the background across the river.

improve the quality of patient care. His zeal, together with his overt criticism of surgical practices of that time, created great animosity from other surgeons. In 1914, at a meeting in Philadelphia, he said, "Hospitals are responsible for the care given by their staff and should carefully note the results of each surgeon, and all of that should be made public." His most famous attack on the establishment occurred on January 8, 1915, at a meeting of surgeons in the Boston Medical Library. He unveiled a large cartoon, shown in Fig. 1a.1. He was virtually ostracized by colleagues in Boston Surgery. Indeed, Codman emphasized the need for long-term outcome research almost a century ago. It is a fascinating chapter in surgery. A recent biography of Codman, by William J. Mallon[4] described that saga. Codman's contributions were enormous. His book on the shoulder is a classic. He started the bone sarcoma registry, which still exists. He wrote many scholarly papers on a wide range of general surgical and orthopedic subjects. The cartoon resides today in the Boston Medical Library, Achieve Room, in the Countway Library of Medicine at Harvard Medical School.

Returning to Ladd, he was a founding member of the Board of Surgery and the American Association for

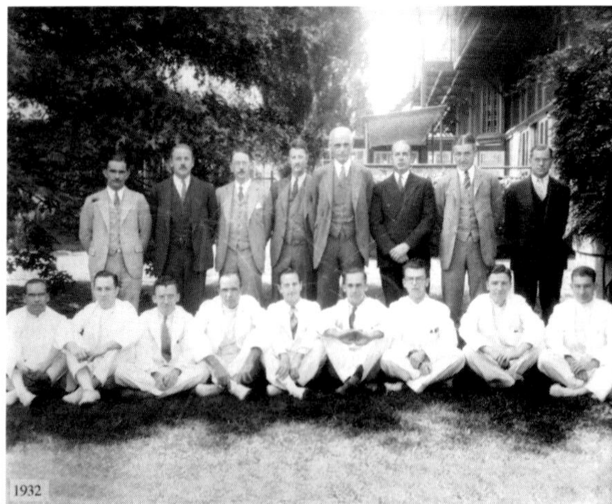

Fig. 1a.2. Department of Surgery under William E. Ladd, 1932. In back row, Ladd is the tallest figure fifth from the left; Thomas Lanman is the seventh. In the front row, Robert Gross, an intern, is seated second from the left. Note cottage-type buildings for patients.

Plastic Surgery (Fig. 1a.2). He wrote about many subjects, including pyloric stenosis, intussusception, biliary atresia, cleft lip, exstrophy of the bladder, Wilms' tumor, and malrotation of the intestine. He devised the treatment for malrotation of the intestine with midgut volvulus. The operation today is still termed "The Ladd's Procedure." In 1939 he saved a newborn with esophageal atresia,[5] a day after the same event occurred in Minneapolis by Dr. Logan Leven.[6] The early cases had division of the tracheoesophageal fistula, marsupialization of the upper pouch in the neck, and insertion of a gastrostomy. Later an antethoracic esophagus was constructed; the lower two-thirds was a Roux-en-Y loop of jejunum placed beneath the skin anterior to the sternum; the gap between the cervical esophagus and the jejunal loop was constructed from a skin tube, performed in stages. His associate Dr. Thomas Lanman, published in 1940 a series of 32 esophageal atresia failures,[7] predicting that, "Given a suitable case in which the patient is seen early I feel that with greater experience, improved technique, and good luck, the successful outcome of a direct anastomosis can and will be reported in the near future".[7] That came true in 1941, when Cameron Haight of Ann Arbor, Michigan reported such a case.[8]

A published genealogy of North American Pediatric Surgery[9] documents a direct line of descent from Ladd to 66% of all pediatric surgeons and 73% of training directors in North America. Reminiscences about Ladd by Orvar Swenson,[9] William Clatworthy,[9] and Alexander Bill,[10] describe Ladd's eminent position in surgery and the great respect that he enjoyed from those associated with him. The William E. Ladd Chair in Surgery was established at Harvard Medical School in 1941. Ladd was the first incumbent, followed by Robert Gross, Aldo Castaneda, and Richard Jonas. It was my privilege as a medical student in 1951 to meet Dr. Ladd. He gave us an informal talk about scrofula. Ten years later, Dr. Edward D. Churchill, Chief of Surgery at the MGH, appointed me to the staff of the MGH, with the charge to develop a Pediatric Surgical Division. An early successful case was a 3 lb infant with esophageal atresia. Dr. Ladd, accompanied by Dr. Lanman, although both long retired, came to the MGH to discuss the case at Surgical Grand Rounds. Imagine what that meant to a young surgeon just getting started! Churchill gave me a cartoon showing a family of birds on a tree limb, in descending order of size, the big birds next to the trunk. At the end of the branch was a tiny bird with one foot on the limb flapping furiously to stay there! That cartoon might well have applied also to other of my surgical colleagues who were introducing pediatric surgery as a specialty in various places. Uniformly there was apprehension and a cool reception by established surgeons. In 1967, while walking down the operating room corridor one evening I chanced to look into an induction room. There was Dr. Ladd about to be anesthetized for surgery on a hip. It was a privilege to hold his hand as he went to sleep. He died that year, at age 87, ending a distinguished career in surgery.

Edward D. Churchill (1894–1972), Chief of Surgery at MGH, also contributed importantly to North American Pediatric Surgery. He developed the "rectangular" Surgical Residency,[11] in which smaller numbers of residents start but most finish a full 5-year program. This contrasted with the steep pyramid system extant at Johns Hopkins, Yale, Peter Bent Brigham Hospital, and Duke. The pyramid system was similar to surgical training in Germany. It graduated a superb and experienced surgeon, but many fell at the wayside who did not reach the top of the pyramid. A rectangular system is most common today. It assures full training for most who start such a program, although there may be an additional year or more for those destined for an academic career or a specialty like pediatric surgery. Churchill developed segmental resection of the lung;[12] some of his patients were children with bronchiectasis. Churchill's establishing a division of pediatric surgery at MGH resulted eventually in entry to pediatric surgery by 41 members of the MGH surgical residency staff. Some became program heads in North America: Scott Adzick, Philadelphia; Jay Vacanti, Boston, MGH; Robert Shamberger, Boston, Children's; Michael Harrison, San Francisco; Michael LaQuaglia, Sloan-Kettering Hospital, New York; Dennis Lund, Madison, Wisconsin; Lucien Leape, Boston, Floating Hospital; Dale Johnson, Salt Lake City; Judson Randolph, Washington D.C.; Willis Williams, Atlanta; Timothy Canty, Louisville; Michael Mitchell, Seattle; Terry Hensle, New York; Kenneth Crooks, Columbus; Jens Rosenkrantz, Los Angeles; and Judah Folkman and Hardy Hendren, each now Emeritus Chiefs in Boston.

Robert E. Gross (1905–1988) (Fig. 1a.3) was the most outstanding of those who trained under Ladd. He graduated from Harvard Medical School in 1931. Charles F. McKhann, Professor of Pediatrics, wrote a letter of recommendation about Gross to Ladd. Quoting from this letter given to me by his son, Charles McKhann Jr.: "Mr. R. E. Gross, a member of the fourth year class of Harvard Medical School, has asked me to write you concerning his qualifications for the position of House Officer in the Children's Hospital. Mr. Gross is an interested, eager and accurate student, somewhat above average, has a pleasant personality, and a good appearance. He should make a satisfactory House Officer." This understated letter did not portend what Gross would accomplish. His training included first a residency in Pathology under S. Burt Wolbach. He trained in general surgery under Elliot Cutler at the Peter Bent Brigham, and in Pediatric Surgery

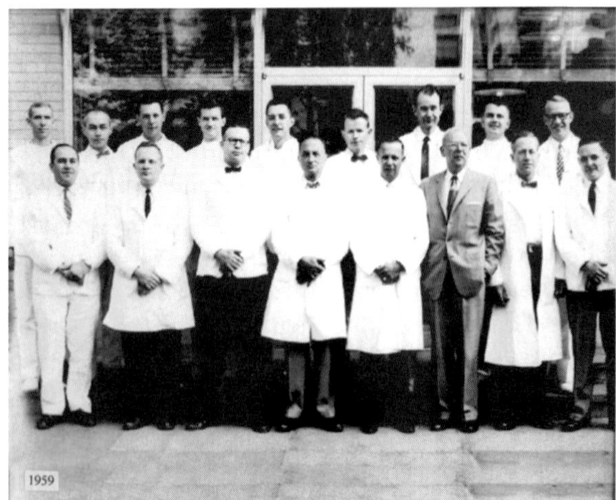

Fig. 1a.3. Department of Surgery in 1959 under Robert E. Gross. Front row, left to right: Ernest Barsamian, Samuel Schuster, Thomas Holder, Robert Gross, Luther Longino, Donald MacCollum, Robert Smith, and Hardy Hendren. Second row, left to right: Lawrence Hill, Arnold Colodny, Donald Brief, John Crowe, Judson Randolph, David Collins, Morton Wooley, Lon Curtis, and Mayo Johnson.

under Ladd. Seven years after McKhann's letter, while he was Chief Surgical Resident, Gross successfully divided a patent ductus arteriosus.[13] The operation was performed when Ladd was out of town. Ladd never forgave Gross for that professional sleight. Gross later confided that he did not think Ladd would have allowed the operation if he had been present. The patient, Lorraine Sweeny, then 8 years old, is alive and well today, 66 years later. This underscores how pediatric surgeons strive to attain a long and productive life for their patients, often not possible in adults. Ladd retired in 1945. Franc Ingraham, Chief of Neurosurgery, was appointed as interim Chief while an *ad hoc* committee deliberated for 2 years (not uncommon at Harvard). Gross was appointed Chief in 1947. Churchill was chairman of the *ad hoc* committee!

Visitors who came to Boston to observe or work with Ladd and Gross included several who became very distinguished pediatric surgeons and mentors. C. Everett Koop, sent by his Chief, Isadore Ravdin, returned to Philadelphia to be the first Surgeon in Chief at that Children's Hospital.[14] Willis J. Potts returned to the Children's Memorial Hospital in Chicago. Robert Zachary returned to Sheffield, England and trained many registrars in pediatric surgery. Jesus Lozoya-Solis returned to Mexico City to become the dominant figure in pediatric surgery there. Alberto Peña was one of his many pupils. Lozoya believed pediatric surgeons should be first a pediatrician and secondarily a surgeon, differing from the opinion of Ladd and Gross. That pattern became prevalent in many Spanish-speaking countries of Central and South America.

Clarence Crafoord of Stockholm, Sweden reported successful resection of coarctation of the aorta in 1944.[15] Gross soon followed with his own important contributions to coarctation.[16] From his laboratory came also the use of human cadaver aortic grafts to replace the narrow aortic segment in coarctation cases which are too long for excision and primary anastomosis.[17] The grafts were freeze-dried and radiated for sterilization. This was a landmark contribution to the field of vascular surgery. Perchance I was recently contacted by an 88-year-old man who is Dr. Gross's first homograft coarctation repair. He is in good health, and had just returned from competitive bowling!

Ladd and Gross published a book in 1941 on *Abdominal Surgery of Childhood*.[18] It presented experience and statistics of follow-up in pediatric surgery at Children's, from 1915 to 1941. The book is a classic. Recently a copy was given to me which was given to Wolbach in 1941 by Gross. An inscription acknowledges Gross' gratitude for Wolbach's mentoring and guidance, expressing his high regard for Wolbach as his primary teacher and advocate.

In 1953 Gross published his own single author book, *The Surgery of Infancy and Childhood*.[19] It was dedicated to Wolbach. The copy given to Wolbach by Gross, which was recently given to me, bears the inscription: "Dear Uncle Burt, With this book come my deepest thanks for all you've done in so many ways. Devotedly, Bob." The book remains a classic today. It should be read by all pediatric surgeons. Many thousands of copies were published in multiple printings, in several different languages. Therefore, it can usually be found and purchased (for 15–20 times its original cost!).

Gross described repair of anomalies of the great vessels, which constrict the trachea, esophagus or both.[20] Little has been added concerning vascular rings in the past 50 years. He described treating omphalocele by wide undermining of the skin, and temporary closure over the viscera, leaving a huge abdominal wall hernia to repair later.[21] An interim technique used by some for several years was painting the sac with mercurochrome, awaiting its gradual epithelialization and contracture. His pupil, Samuel R. Schuster, later introduced temporary silastic covering of the protruding viscera, with staged closure soon thereafter.[22] This has endured.

Willis Potts authored a unique book in 1959[23] describing some of the more common entities in pediatric surgery. He wrote, "I want to dedicate this book to the infant who has the great misfortune of being born with a serious deformity. All life is before him and what is done during the first few days may decide whether life will be a joy or a burden. If this infant could speak it would beg imploringly of the surgeon, 'Please exercise the greatest gentleness with my miniature tissues and try to correct the deformity in the first operation. Give me blood and the proper amount of fluids and electrolytes; add plenty of oxygen to the anesthesia and I will show you that I can tolerate a terrific amount of surgery. You will be surprised at the speed of my recovery and I shall always be grateful to you'." Regarding imperforate anus, Potts wrote, "In general, atresia of the rectum is more poorly handled than any other congenital anomaly of the newborn. A properly functioning rectum is an unappreciated gift of greatest price. The child who is so unfortunate as to be born with an imperforate anus may be saved a lifetime of misery and social seclusion by the surgeon who with skill, diligence and judgment performs the first operation on the malformed rectum". Pediatric surgeons continue to strive to correct the difficult entity of imperforate anus, most espousing the posterior sagittal approach introduced by DeVries and Peña.[24]

Although Gross opened the field of congenital heart surgery, others soon followed him. Alfred Blalock at Johns Hopkins advanced treatment of blue babies by introducing the Blalock–Taussig subclavian–pulmonary artery shunt.[25] Gross regretted that he had not paid heed to Helen Taussig who had visited him earlier from Hopkins and suggested "making a ductus" as treatment for blue babies. Willis Potts devised a direct aorta to pulmonary artery shunt.[26] Other surgeons worked to perfect a heart–lung machine. First was John Gibbon, of Jefferson Medical College in Philadelphia. He successfully closed an atrial septal defect for a child using a cardiopulmonary bypass but did not venture further into more complex defects. His research had started in the laboratory of Edward Churchill in Boston, who did not think there was much merit in that idea! In 1952 John Lewis showed that simple atrial defects could be closed with brief inflow occlusion and hypothermia, but this did not give enough time to repair complex malformations. Gross employed a rubber well sewn to the right atrium to access and close atrial septal defects.[27] Results of that were imperfect. It was C. Walton Lillehei in Minneapolis who focused the spotlight on congenital heart surgery. On April 25, 1954, he closed a large interventricular septal defect in a 4-year-old girl, with the father providing cardiopulmonary support by cross-circulation between parent and child, despite vigorous outcry by members of the medical department. His surgical chief, Owen Wangansteen, stood by him. He then demonstrated repair of complex anomalies, such as Tetralogy of Fallot.[28] This interesting surgical history was recently reported in riveting detail in a book entitled, *King of Hearts* by G. Wayne Miller, in 2000.[29] Thereafter a practical cardiopulmonary bypass machine was introduced by Lillehei and soon adopted by many surgeons, a key development in bringing congenital heart surgery to its current advanced state.

Gross stepped down as Surgeon in Chief in 1967, to concentrate on cardiac surgery. He retired in 1972. Gross revealed later that, during his entire career, he had operated with good vision in only one eye. This was told to one of his former residents who was facing loss of vision in one eye from a melanoma. Gross in retirement underwent surgery for his congenital cataract. That gave him binocular vision he had lacked during his brilliant surgical career. A Harvard Chair was named in his honor in 1985, on the occasion of his 80th birthday. The author was its first incumbent. Gross died with Alzheimer's disease on October 11, 1988, closing the career of a giant in American Surgery.

Ladd and Gross were both accomplished and imaginative surgeons. Their department of surgery trained a multitude of pediatric surgeons in North America. This heritage has been self-perpetuating. Recognition of pediatric surgery as a specialty did not come easily. Randolph outlined the genesis of other early programs in the United States:[30] Willis Potts in Chicago, 1947; Everett Koop in Philadelphia, 1950; Ovar Swenson at Boston Floating Hospital, 1952; William Clatworthy in Columbus, 1955; William Kiesewetter in Pittsburgh, 1958; Thomas Santulli, in New York. There were also Canadian programs in Montreal, Toronto, Winnipeg, Ottawa, and Vancouver.

The first full-time pediatric surgeon in North America was Herbert Coe in Seattle; he had visited Children's Hospital in Boston when Ladd had not yet limited his work to children. Coe was the driving force in establishing in 1948 the Surgical Section of the American Academy of Pediatrics. *The Journal of Pediatric Surgery* began in 1965 through the efforts of Everett Koop and Stephen Gans. The American Pediatric Surgical Association was founded in 1970. Recognition of special competence in pediatric surgery by the American Board of Surgery was finally accomplished in 1975 through the efforts of Harvey Beardmore and others. The British Association of Pediatric Surgeons which formed in 1953, has promoted interchange of knowledge among surgeons the world over. It has been fascinating to be privy to all of these developments spanning more than half a century.

The field of pediatric surgery has been virtually transformed in the past 50 years. Space does not permit mentioning all of the contributions and all of the contributors, but some deserve to be highlighted. Douglas Stephens of Melbourne, Australia, and later Chicago, taught us much about the embryology and classification of anorectal and genitourinary malformation.[31] Jonathan Rhodes of

Philadelphia reported the first primary pullthrough in the neonate with imperforate anus.[32] Cloacal malformations, once a no-man's land of pediatric surgery, have become reparable.[33,34] Infants with cloacal exstrophy always died, until a survivor was reported in 1960 by Peter Rickham, then in Liverpool.[35] Today, most of these infants can be repaired in a satisfactory fashion to lead useful lives. Key to development of much major pediatric surgery was the emergence of pediatric anesthesiology, which can support even small babies through a prolonged surgery as well as help surgeons care for them postoperatively. It is now appreciated that fluid loss and necessary replacement are much greater than we practiced 50 years ago to maintain metabolic hemostasis in the pediatric surgical patient.

Orvar Swenson, another protégé of Ladd, pioneered the enormous contribution of unlocking the mystery of Hirschsprung's disease. With Alexander Bill, he proved the pathology to be the aganglionic distal segment and described an effective operation for it.[36] Originally, the clinical picture of Hirschsprung's disease was an older child with lifelong constipation. Soon it was recognized that the most common presentation is a newborn with intestinal obstruction. It accounts for one-third of neonatal cases of bowel obstruction. To be sure, Duhamel, Soave, Rehbein, and others made modifications, but Swenson's carefully documented clinical research remains the basis for treatment of this problem half a century later. Swenson recently described the long-term result of his experience with Hirschsprung's.[37] Martin described a practical surgical solution for the infant with total colonic aganglionosis.[38]

Judah Folkman succeeded Gross as Surgeon in Chief at Children's Hospital in 1968. Twenty-three years earlier Koop had learned pediatric surgery from Ladd and Gross. In 1968 Folkman went to Philadelphia for a "cram course" in pediatric surgery by Koop, a successful *quid pro quo* for both institutions! For 14 years Folkman carried the Herculean load of that office plus overseeing a large surgical research laboratory, mentoring many postdoctoral research fellows. He chose in 1982 to concentrate his enormous productivity on the ever-expanding research laboratory program, devoted in large part to the field of angiogenesis research. This had begun with Folkman's astute observation that tumors grow by attracting new blood vessels. He reasoned that control of angiogenesis might control growth of tumors, as well as other non-malignant conditions characterized by vascular ingrowth, such as diabetic retinopathy. Alpha interferon, an angiogenic inhibitor, was shown to reduce dramatically the mortality of life-threatening giant hemangiomas in infants.[39] Like many spectacular advances, Folkman's work provoked derisive commentary and skepticism initially. However, his vision was amply vindicated by many other scientists who joined in this investigative effort around the world. Many clinical trials are in progress today at many major hospitals. The author succeeded Folkman as Chief of the Department of Surgery in 1982.

Joseph Murray opened the field of organ transplantation in Dec. 1954 when he transplanted a kidney from one identical twin to his brother in end-stage renal failure.[40] Later in 1962, he demonstrated successful cadaver renal transplantation using immunosuppression. For the seminal advance of transplantation, Murray was awarded The Nobel Prize in 1990.[41] Soon Starzl opened the field of liver transplantation.[42] Now half a century later heart, lung, pancreas, intestine, and even multivisceral organ transplantation have been added to the surgeons' repertoire. Organ availability has been a problem since transplantation began. Joseph Vacanti started the field of tissue engineering to solve this dilemma.[43]

Dudrick's introduction of total parenteral nutrition[44] has saved countless lives of children, and adults, where nutritional needs cannot be met otherwise. This began with a long struggle to save a baby with gangrenous bowel from malrotation and midgut volvulus at Philadelphia Children's Hospital. Another boon to mankind!

Neonatal physiology and nutrition[45] advanced greatly as pediatric surgery grew in scope and stature.[45]

Patricia Donahoe made great strides in developmental biology, starting with investigation of the Mullerian Inhibiting Substance.[46] Her investigations broadened to study mechanisms of fetal growth and differentiation.[47]

Robert Bartlett conceived the idea of extracorporeal membrane oxygenation while working as a resident under Robert Gross.[48] This saved countless lives in children and adults with cardiopulmonary failure. Ancillary to that was vast improvement in treatment of neonates with severe diaphragmatic hernia.

Michael Harrison and Alfred deLormier imaginatively introduced the field of fetal surgery.[49] Harrison's pupils, Adzick, Jennings, Flake, and Longaker and others carried this new field further forward, making it possible to salvage infants with once fatal problems.

Burn treatment was pushed to the forefront by the Coconut Grove Nightclub fire on Nov. 28, 1942 in Boston.[50] Much was learned about burns in caring for victims of that well known tragedy. Ultimately, expeditious excision and grafting of extensive deep burns was developed,[51,52] and the use of artificial skin to close large burn wounds after excision.[53,54] Burn mortality dropped remarkably through early excision and grafting.[55]

Limb replantation began in 1963 when Ronald Malt at Massachusetts General Hospital reunited the severed arm of a young boy after traumatic amputation,[56] sparking worldwide salvage of many digits and limbs.

Tracheal resection in children was made possible by the pioneering work of Hermes Grillo at MGH, who developed segmental tracheal and bronchial resection for benign and malignant conditions in adults. This soon became equally useful in children.[57,58]

Cancer chemotherapy was another seminal advance for pediatric surgery, greatly improving the cure rate of many malignancies. It was my privilege as a surgical resident to witness introduction of this in 1955 in Wilms' tumor cases by Sidney Farber, Chief of Pathology at Children's. Like Gross, Farber was a pupil of S. Burt Wolbach. Farber began with the premise that some types of cancer might be controlled by chemical agents. At the Fourth Annual Internal Cancer Research Conference in St. Louis, MO, in September, 1947, a case was presented of a patient who had a remarkable clinical response to a new experimental chemotherapeutic agent, Teropterin (teryl-triglutamic acid). This was the result of the keen observation by Brian L. Hutchings of the Lederle Laboratories. In 1942 Hutchings was trying to produce folic acid in large quantities and noted that one of the vats contained a filtrate that stimulated growth of a certain microorganism, whereas other vats produced no such growth. This filtrate, initially thought to be folic acid turned out to be a folic acid analog, Teropterin. It was shown subsequently that sarcomatous tumors transplanted into mice disappeared with the addition of this drug.

The anonymous patient presented at the conference was "Babe" Ruth, the celebrated slugger of the New York Yankees. In 1946 he presented with hoarseness, left retroorbital pain, and a neck mass. The neck mass was partially excised. The primary tumor was not laryngeal in origin as generally believed but a primary nasopharyngeal cancer at the base of the skull. He had a remarkable temporary relief from pain and regression of the tumor on treatment with teropterin.[59] Sidney Farber investigated the role of this agent and other folic acid agonists and antagonists. Farber's early work led to saving the lives of many children with leukemia,[60] which was once uniformly fatal. He organized the laboratory and clinical facility for chemotherapy, named the Jimmy Fund, in honor of one of the early tumor successes, a patient with an intestinal lymphoma. That patient is alive today. It was the beginning of a new era. The impact of chemotherapy for pediatric malignancies is now well established after nearly half a century of close collaboration between medical oncologists, radiotherapists, and surgeons. The Jimmy Fund Building was joined to the Charles A. Dana Cancer Center for adults, and was designated a comprehensive cancer center in 1973. Today, it is called the Dana-Farber Cancer Center.

Pediatric urology as a recognized field was virtually nonexistent 50 years ago. On my arrival at Children's Hospital, the resident just finishing gave the news that one duty would be to conduct the Urology Clinic every Monday afternoon. When professing to have no knowledge about pediatric urology, he was reassuring by saying "Don't worry, nobody else does either!" The clinic had many children with various tubes to be changed: nephrostomy, cystostomy, or urethral. There was no senior supervision of the clinic. That sparked an interest to learn something about urologic problems. Looking back through half a century, pediatric urology became a robust and recognized surgical specialty.[61] It began with a few general urologists who founded the Society for Pediatric Urology in 1951. On the 50th Anniversary, there were 437 members and 9 honorary members. Dr. Meredith Campbell of New York was the standard bearer. He was President for 5 years. His two volume *Pediatric Urology*[62] described the anomalies and diseases of the child's urinary tract. It was a scholarly work and illustrated routine operations of that era. All present pediatric urologists should read the book to appreciate the great advances in the past 50 years. Pediatric urology has paralleled the development of pediatric general surgery, although one generation later. As a specialty it was accepted slowly, just as occurred in pediatric surgery in 1975. The American Board of Urology recently approved certification of special competence, 30 years after that was achieved for pediatric general surgery. The Urology Section of the American Academy of Pediatrics, founded in 1971 currently has 462 members. Its annual meeting became the premier forum for those interested in this field. To illustrate progress in the specialty, several areas deserve mention.

Exstrophy of the bladder was managed mainly by ureterosigmoidostomy diversion and cystectomy until Jeffs,[63] and Chisholm[64] and others showed that primary repair is feasible although not always successful. This concept was advanced further with bladder augmentation, continent diversion, and even total repair in the newborn (bladder closure, ureteral reimplantation, and epispadias repair simultaneously).

Cloacal exstrophy was deemed insoluble until Rickham reported a survivor in 1960.[35] From this beginning extensive repair became feasible, with urinary continence in most and pull through of the colon in some of those with contractile muscle of the pelvis and perineum.[65]

Ureterocele was treated largely by wide unroofing; this relieved obstruction but produced massive reflux which furthered renal damage and often produced incontinence in those with ectopic ureteroceles which require repair of the cleft bladder neck and urethra. Superior results were achieved by total repair of the sometimes complex anatomy in one stage.[66]

Urinary tract imaging was formerly limited to intravenous pyelogram, retrograde pyelogram and static cystogram (often under anesthesia). Cine radiography taught much about both function and anatomy, but at the price of excessive radiation exposure. Development of more advanced techniques, such as "spot films," ultrasound study, nuclear contrast, magnetic resonance technique, and computerized tomography improved enormously the accuracy of urodiagnosis.

Endoscopic visualization of the urinary tract 50 years ago using battery powered incandescent light bulbs for illumination was crude to say the least, especially in infants for whom small caliber endoscopes were not available. Fiberoptic endoscopy revolutionized that modality, especially when flexible technique developed. Each training department should retain an old incandescent cystoscope to give trainees an appreciation for the blessings of new technology!

Urethral valves were described accurately in 1919 by Hugh Hampton Young, the father of North American Urology, at Johns Hopkins Hospital.[67] They were destroyed by blindly inserting a cold punch, which did not allow much accuracy. Open cystotomy carried down into the prostate urethra afforded better valve excision but sometimes produced incontinence.[19] Accurate valve surgery resulted from voiding cystourethrography and the improved vision with fiberoptic scopes. The result was recognition that urethral valves, like most pathology, occur in a spectrum of severity[68] from grade 4 with severe obstruction and hydroureteronephrosis, to grade 1 "mini valves," which show only subtle radiographic findings and have no upper tract dilatation.

Vesicoureteral reflux came to the forefront in the late 1950s and early 1960s, as dynamic urography developed. Wyland Leadbetter and his associate Victor Politano described the most often used technique of abolishing reflux by tunneling reimplantation of the ureter:[69] many variations followed. This work not only focused clinical awareness on the importance of reflux, but also served as a starting wedge for much of reconstructive urology.

Ileal loop introduced by Bricker in 1950[70] for drainage after anterior pelvic exenteration became an important method of drainage for both adults and children. It lessened greatly use of ostomy tubes of various sorts, often reducing incidence of urinary infection which always accompanies long standing tube drainage. However, after a decade of ileal loops, it became apparent that upper tracts often deteriorated, secondary to non- sterile reflux.[71] This was prevented by use of the colon conduit in which non-refluxing tunnels can be made.[72]

Megaureter was largely ignored in the literature, but its repair was a logical next step after ureteral reimplantation became well established. A book devoted exclusively to the ureter published in 1967 largely omitted this condition, with conclusion that it lacked importance and was not repairable.[73] However, after Bischoff in Germany described shortening and tapering the ureter,[74] operation was introduced in North America to shorten, taper, and tunnel reimplant the ureter with a high success rate.[75] Clinical experience and urodynamic study proved that a dilated ureter does not propel urine effectively because the walls cannot coapt.

Tubeless ureterostomy became popular, using end, loop, Roux-en-Y and even circle technique, as well as pyelostomy. That phase was short lived after the high complication rate of those diversions was reported,[76] and it was shown that the infant urinary tract can be primarily reconstructed without prior drainage.[77] Evaluation of the changes in urologic surgery described above evolved to reconstruction of previously diverted urinary tracts.[78,79] This led to the conclusions that (i) most diversions can be undiverted and (ii) most diversions are not necessary in the first place!

Hypospadias repair was vastly different at Boston Children's Hospital in 1953[19] from what surgeons practice today. Mild cases were not repaired. Severe cases were done in three stages, and were delayed until pubertal years. At that time MacCollum described 40 patients who had undergone satisfactory chordee release, but only 18 had completed stage 3. He stated, "The results have been exceedingly satisfactory and we see little need for improvement or change in operative technique, with the possible exception that earlier repair might have been desirable in some of the boys, a consideration which we did not find to be of great importance in many cases." From that viewpoint much changed, most recognizing that early repair is both feasible and desirable, and that there are many ways this can be accomplished, giving a penis which looks normal and has satisfactory function for both micturition and procreation!

Conclusions

A retrospective view of both pediatric surgery and pediatric urology in the 20th century shows monumental changes and enormous benefits for pediatric patients. This evokes speculation about what lies ahead as the efforts of many surgeons introduce solutions to many of the problems which still exist. A symposium on Pediatric Surgery was published in 1938.[80] The editor was William E. Ladd. His introduction stated, "Undoubtedly great strides have been made in this field of surgery in the last few years and I have confidence that greater advances are soon to follow." That prophesy was correct. It will surely prove true again when we look back in the distant future to our care of children at the beginning of this century.

REFERENCES

1. Warren, J. C. *Surgical Observations on Tumors with Cases and Operations*. Boston: Crocker and Brewster; London: John Churchill, Princes St., Soho, 1839.
2. Warren, J. M. *Surgical Observations with Cases*. Boston: Ticknor and Fields, 1867.
3. Smith, C. A. *The Children's Hospital of Boston "Built Better Than They Knew."* Boston: Little Brown, 1983.
4. Mallon, W. J. *Ernest Amory Codman: The End Result of a Life in Medicine*. Philadelphia: W. B. Saunders, 2000.
5. Ladd, W. E. The surgical treatment of esophageal atresia and tracheoesophageal fistulas. *N. Engl. J. Med.* 1944; **230**:625.
6. Leven, N. L. Congenital atresia of the esophagus with tracheoesophageal fistula. *J. Thorac. Surg.* 1941; **10**:648.
7. Lanman, T. H. Congenital atresia of the esophagus: a study of thirty-two cases. *Arch. Surg.* 1940; **41**:1060.
8. Haight, C. & Towsley, H. A. Congenital atresia of the esophagus with tracheoesophageal fistula; extrapleural ligation of fistula and end-to-end anastomosis of esophageal segments. *Surg. Gynecol. Obstet.* 1943; **76**:672–688.
9. Glick, P. H. & Azizkhan, R. G. *A Genealogy of North American Pediatric Surgery From Ladd Until Now*. St. Louis, MO: Quality Medical Publishing, 1997.
10. Bill, H. William E. Ladd, M. D., *Great Pioneer of North American Pediatric Surgery. Progr. Pediatr. Surg.* 1986; **20**:52–59.
11. Grillo, H. C. Edward D Churchill and the "rectangular" surgical residency. *Surgery* 2004; **136**:947–952.
12. Churchill, E. D. The segmental and lobular physiology and pathology of the lung. *J. Thorac. Surg.* 1949; **18**:279.
13. Gross, R. E. & Hubbard, J. P. Surgical ligation of a patent ductus arteriosus: report of first successful case. *J. Am. Med. Assoc.*, 1939; **112**:729.
14. Koop, C. E. A perspective on the early days of pediatric surgery. *J. Pediatr. Surg.* 1998; **33**:953–960.
15. Crafoord, C. & Nylin, G. Congenital coarctation of the aorta and its surgical treatment. *J. Thorac. Surg.* 1945; **14**:347.
16. Gross, R. E., Hufnagel, C. A. Coarctation of the aorta. Experimental studies regarding its surgical correction. *N. Engl. J. Med.* 1945; **233**:287.
17. Gross, R. E. Treatment of certain coarctations by homologous grafts: a report of 19 cases. *Ann. Surg.* 1951; **134**:753.
18. Ladd, W. E. & Gross, R. E. *Abdominal Surgery of Infancy and Childhood*. Philadelphia: W.B. Saunders, 1941.
19. Gross, R. E. *The Surgery of Infancy and Childhood*. Philadelphia: W. B. Saunders. 1953.
20. Gross, R. E. & Newhauser, E. B. D. Compression of the trachea or esophagus by vascular anomalies, surgical therapy in 40 cases. *Pediatrics* 1951; **7**:69.
21. Gross, R. E. A new method for surgical treatment of large omphaloceles. *Surgery* 1948; **24**:277.
22. Schuster, S. R. A new method for the staged repair of large omphaloceles. *Surg. Gynecol. Obstet.* 1967; **125**:837–850.
23. Potts, W. J. *The Surgeon and The Children*. Philadelphia: WB Saunders, 1959.
24. DeVries, P. A. & Pena, A. Posterior sagittal anorectoplasty. *J. Pediar. Surg.* 1982; **17**:638–643.
25. Taussig, H. B. Analysis of malformations of the heart amenable to a Blalock–Taussig operation. *Am. Heart. J.* 1943; **36**:321.
26. Potts, W. J., Smith, S., & Gibson, S. Anastomosis of aorta to a pulmonary artery. *J. Am. Med. Assoc.* 1945; **132**:627.
27. Gross, R. E., Pomeranz, A. A., Watkins, E. *et al.* Surgical closure of defects of the interauricular septum by use of an atrial well. *N. Engl. J. Med.* 1952; **247**:455.
28. Lillehei, C. W., Cohen, M., Warden, H. E. *et al.* Direct vision intracardiac surgical correction of the tetralogy of Fallot, pentology of Fallot, and pulmonary atresia: report of first 10 cases. *Ann. Surg.* 1955; **142**:418.
29. Miller, G. W. *King of Hearts*. New York: Random House 2000.
30. Randolph, J. G. The first of the best. *J. Pediatr. Surg.* 1985; **20**:580–591.
31. Stephens, F. D. *Congenital Malformations of the Rectum, Anus and Genito-urinary Tract*. London: Livingstone, 1963.
32. Rhodes, J. E., Pipes, R. L., & Randall, J. P. Simultaneous abdominal and perineal approach in operations for imperforate anus with atresia of rectum and rectosigmoid. *Ann. Surg.* 1948, **127**:552.
33. Hendren, W. H. Cloacal malformations: experience with 105 cases. *J. Pediatr. Surg.* 1992; **27**:890–901.
34. Hendren, W. H. Cloaca, the most severe degree of imperforate anus: experience with 195 cases. *Ann. Surg.* 1998; **228**:331–346.
35. Rickham, P. P. Vesico-intestinal fissure. *Arch. Dis. Child.* 1960; **35**:97–102.
36. Swenson, O. & Bill, A. H. Resection of rectum and rectosigmoid with preservation of the sphincter for benign spastic lesions producing megacolon: an experimental study. *Surgery* 1948; **24**:212.
37. Swenson, O. Early history of the therapy of Hirschsprung's disease: facts and personal observations over 50 years. *J. Pediatr. Surg.* 1996; **31**:1003–1008.
38. Martin, L. Surgical management of total colonic aganglionosis. *Ann. Surg.* 1972; **176**:343.
39. Ezekowitz, R. A., Mulliken, J. B., & Folkman, J. Interferon alpha 2A therapy of "life-threatening" hemangiomas in infancy. *N. Engl. J. Med.* 1992; **326**:1456–1463.

40. Merrill, J. P., Bartlett, J. E., Harrison, J. H. *et al.* Successful homotransplantations of the human kidney between identical twins. *J. Am. Med. Assoc.* 1956; **160**:277–282.
41. Murray, J. E. The first successful organ transplantation in man. *Scand. J. Immunol.* 1994; **39**:1–11.
42. Starzl, T. E. & Demetris, A. J. *Liver Transplantation*. Chicago: Yearbook Medical Publ., 1990.
43. Choi, R. S. & Vacanti, J. P. Preliminary studies of tissue-engineered intestine using isolated epithelial organoid units on tubular synthetic biodegradable scaffolds. *Transpl. Proc.* 1997; **29**:848–851.
44. Dudrick, S. J., Wilmore, D. W., Vars, H. M. *et al.* Long-term total parenteral nutrition with growth, development and positive nitrogen balance. *Surgery* 1968; **64**:134.
45. Coran, A. G. Parenteral nutrition in infants and children. *Surg. Clin. North. Am.* 1981; **61**:1089–1100.
46. Donahoe, P. K., Ito, Y., & Hendren, W. H. A graded organ culture assay for the detection of Mullerian inhibiting substance. *J. Surg. Res.* 1877; **23**:141–148.
47. Teixera, J., He, W. W., Shah, P. C. *et al.* Developmental expression of a candidate Mullerian inhibiting substance type II receptor. *Endocrinology* 1996; **137**:160–165.
48. Bartlett, R. H., Gazzaniga, A. B., Jeffries, M. R. *et al.* Extracorporeal membrane oxygenation (ECMO) cardiopulmonary support in infancy. *Trans. Am. Soc. Artif. Intern. Organs* 1976; **22**:80–93.
49. Harrison, M. R., Golbus, M. S., & Filly, R. A. *The Unborn Patient*, 2nd edn. Philadelphia, PA, 1990.
50. Symposium on the Management of the Coconut Grove Burns at the Massachusetts General Hospital. *Ann. Surg.* 1943; **117**:801–965.
51. Cope, O., Langohr, J. L., Moore, F. D. *et al.* Expeditious care of full-thickness burn wounds by surgical excisions and grafting. *Ann. Surg.* 1947; **125**:1–22.
52. Hendren, W. H., Constable, J. D., & Zawacki, B. E. Early partial excision of major burns in children. *J. Pediatr. Surg.* 1968; **3**:445–464.
53. Burke, J. F., Yannas, I. V., Quinby, W. C. Jr *et al.* Successful use of a physiologically acceptable artificial skin in the treatment of extensive burn injury. *Ann. Surg.* 1981; **194**:413–428.
54. Burke, J. F. From Desperation to skin regeneration: progress in burn treatment. *J. Trauma* 1990; **30**:S36–S40 (suppl 12).
55. Tompkins, R. G., Remensyder, J. P., Burke, J. F. *et al.* Significant reductions in mortality for children with burn injuries through the use of prompt eschar excision. *Ann. Surg.* 1988; **208**:33–41.
56. Malt, R. A. & McKhann, C. F. Replantation of severed arms. *J. Am. Med. Assoc.* 1964; **189**:716–722.
57. Grillo, H. C. & Zannini, P. Management of obstructive tracheal disease in children. *J. Pediatr. Surg.* 1984; **19**:414–416.
58. Grillo, H. C. Pediatric tracheal problems. *Chest Surg. Clin. North. Am.* 1996; **6**:693–700.
59. Bikhazi, N. B., Kramer, A. M., Spiegel, J. H. *et al.* "Babe" Ruth's illness and its impact on medical history. *Laryngoscope* 1999; **109**:1–2.
60. Frei, E. 3rd, Jaffe, N., & Farber, S. Treatment of acute leukemia. *N. Engl. J. Med.* 1971; **287**:1357.
61. Hendren, W. H. From an acorn to an oak. *J. Pediatr. Surg.* 1999; **34**:46–58.
62. Campbell, M. F. *Pediatric Urology*, 2 vol. New York: The MacMillan Co. 1937.
63. Jeffs, R. D. Exstrophy of the urinary bladder. In *Pediatric Surgery*, Chicago, Il: Year Book Medical Publ., 1986.
64. Chisholm, T. C. & McPharland, F. A. Exstrophy of the urinary bladder. In *Pediatric Surgery*, Chicago, Il: Year Book Medical Publ, 1982.
65. Lund, D. P. & Hendren, W. H. Cloacal exstrophy: a 25 year experience with 50 cases. *J. Pediatr. Surg.* 2001; **36**:68–75.
66. Hendren, W. H. & Michael, M. E. Surgical correction of ureteroceles. *J. Urol.* 1979; **121**:590–597.
67. Young, H. H., Frontz, W. A., & Baldwin, J. C. Congenital obstruction of the posterior urethra. *J. Urol.* 1919; **3**:289.
68. Hendren, W. H. Posterior urethral valves in boys: a broad clinical spectrum. *J. Urol.* 1971; **106**:298–307.
69. Politano, V. A. & Leadbetter, W. F. An operative technique for the correction of vesicoureteral reflux. *J. Urol.* 1958; **79**:932–941.
70. Bricker, E. M. Bladder substitution after pelvic evisceration. *Surg. Clin. North Am.* 1950; **30**:1511.
71. Middleton, A. W. & Hendren, W. H. Ileal conduits in children at Massachusetts General Hospital from 1955 to 1970. *J. Urol.* 1976; **115**:591–595.
72. Althausen, A. F., Hagen-Cook, K., & Hendren, W. H. Non-refluxing colon conduit: experience with 70 cases. *J. Urol.* 1978; **120**:35–39.
73. Bergman, H. (ed) *The Ureter*. New York: Harper & Row, 1967.
74. Bischoff, P. Megaureter. *Br. J. Urol.* 1957; **29**:416.
75. Hendren, W. H. Operative repair of megaureter in children. *J. Urol.* 1969; **101**:491–507.
76. Hendren, W. H. Complications of ureterostomy. *J. Urol.* 1978; **120**:269–281.
77. Hendren, W. H. A new approach to infants with severe obstructive uropathy: early complete reconstruction. *J. Pediatr. Surg.* 1970; **5**:184–199.
78. Hendren, W. H. Reconstruction of previously diverted urinary tracts in children. *J. Pediatr. Surg.* 1973; **8**:135–150.
79. Hendren, W. H. Urinary tract refunctionalization after long-term diversion: a 20 year experience with 177 patients. *Ann. Surg.* 1990; **212**:478–495.
80. Ladd, W. E. (Ed) Surgery in Children. Symposium. *Am. J. Surg.* 1938; **39**:227–475.

1b

Introduction and historical overview: European perspective

Barry O'Donnell

Ballsbridge, Dublin, Ireland

'One man can make a difference'

John Fitzgerald Kennedy (1917–1963)

Each country has its own history of pediatric surgery. Each tale is usually short because, although many children's hospitals are more than 100 years old, the growth of pediatric surgery as a specialty in Europe dates from after the Second World War. Before that, surgical services were provided by general surgeons, many of whom saw their appointment to the children's hospital as an exotic and seldom-visited outpost of a far-flung empire. One man changed that. His name was "D.B." – Denis John Walko (Aboriginal for "big man") Browne (1892–1967) – surgeon at The Hospital for Sick Children, Great Ormond Street, London, from 1928 to 1957. An Australian who had served at Gallipoli, he was in the trenches of the First World War. The upright military majestic figure (6ft 3in) with, as he put it, the "long, thin, Irish upper lip," was truly the mainspring of the subject in western Europe. His original mind and wide knowledge of logic and philosophy enabled him to produce "surprise" – the touchstone of genius – solutions to such varied problems as club-foot, cleft lip, and hypospadias. For all his ingenious techniques and specially designed instruments ("the combined mousetrap and can-opener is rarely a success as either"), his most important contribution was to encourage others, not just in the United Kingdom but all over Europe, to concentrate their efforts on the surgery of the child. He promoted his loyal lieutenants, David Waterston (1910–1985) and Harold (Nicky) Nixon (1917–1990), as well as encouraging David Innes Williams (born 1919) the founder of pediatric urology. He performed every form of surgery from hydrocephalus to club-foot, and in-between he would repair an esophageal atresia. Everything he did and touched was irresistibly logical. Most important of all, he was a warm, generous spirit who always put the child first. In Britain, Hunterian Professorships are awarded for innovation. It is a comment on Denis Browne that he was given this award four times. Another apostle of his, Peter Rickham (1918–2003), went to Liverpool where, with the encouragement of the much-loved Isobella Forshall (1900–1989), he built Liverpool into England's second biggest unit.

One overlooks Scotland at one's peril. Glasgow had the Royal Hospital for Sick Children since 1883, and a dedicated surgeon, Matthew White, was a near-contemporary of D.B.'s – and he in turn encouraged his young people such as Wallace Dennison and Sam Davidson.

The founding of the British Association of Paediatric Surgeons (BAPS) in 1953 was a further catalyst to the growth of the specialty in Europe. Although run from the UK, members were enrolled from all over the world and it became the organization outside the Americas. D.B. was its first president, from 1953 to 1957. But from the continent of Europe came David Vervat (Rotterdam), Fritz Rehbein (Bremen), Franco Soave (Genoa), G. Winkel Smith (Copenhagen), Bernard Duhamel (Paris), John Shanley (Dublin), Mattai Sulumma (Helsinki), Max Grob (Zurich) and Theodor Ehrenpreis (Stockholm). These were the principal national representatives in those early years. Bob Zachary of Sheffield was at these early meetings, as was the indefatigable Douglas Stephens of Melbourne.

Most early units were established in the teeth of opposition from professors of surgery and the system specialists who, with some notable exceptions (and this reservation is put in only for legal purposes and has no basis in fact), flatly denied the necessity for the new discipline. "What will you people do?" was the question. At that time the main

Pediatric Surgery and Urology: Long-term Outcomes, Mark Stringer, Keith Oldham, Pierre Mouriquand.
Published by Cambridge University Press.

arguments in favor of the neophytes were neonatal surgery and Hirschsprung's disease, the cure and cause of which had been discovered by Orvar Swenson in Boston. Superior results and shorter bed stay soon became apparent in common problems such as pyloric stenosis (which still had a 3% mortality in the 1950s), daycare of infant hernia, the abandonment of drainage in appendicitis, and orchidopexy based on Denis Browne's anatomical classification.

There were some false dawns. The natural, rare enigmatic regression of some neuroblastomas in patients under 1 year was not appreciated at that time, and its "cure" was mistakenly attributed to repeated injections of vitamin B_{12}; but there were many advances based on reclassification. Perhaps the most striking of these was in Wilms' tumor which was then thought by the pathologists to be a single entity without any concept of an anaplastic, uniformly lethal group. It is chastening to realize now that there are at least 13 subgroups of Wilms' tumor, and this figure seems to be added to every year or so.

The concept of the controlled trial, one of the biggest medical advances of the past 50 years, has never had much allure for surgeons. This has led us into a number of misconceptions. Vesicoureteric reflux was a growth industry in the 1960s; it was looked on then as a progressive rather then regressive disease, and its association with kidney damage was ill-understood. It was assumed that the cause of the reflux was the radiologically impressive but unmeasurable bladder-neck obstruction. This meant that the valuable operation of antireflux ureteric reimplant was often combined with a rarely useful revision of the bladder neck. We were slow learners; we frequently disbelieve our own research. Open spina bifida, which was for many decades an epidemic in western Europe, seemed an appropriate subject for pediatric surgeons, particularly as they would treat the whole child rather than a collection of systems. Indeed, at one stage in the 1970s it almost looked as if the issue of spina bifida was set to dominate the entire subject of pediatric surgery. Evangelical reports of really good outcomes following emergency newborn closure quickly appeared, and controlled trials were felt by the prophets and the promoters to be unnecessary.

However, the results were not really influenced by early operation. When there was a report that 60% of people with spina bifida in a certain area "led normal lives," H. H. Nixon of London was moved to murmur "This is what I have long suspected, normal life in Xville is bloody awful."

Changes in disease

Neonatal surgery has been the flagship of the specialty, never more so than in the early years. But the pattern of disease has changed. Intestinal malrotation and duodenal obstruction have been replaced as the commonest problems by two conditions that did not exist in the 1950s.

Neonatal necrotizing enterocolitis surfaced as a problem for surgeons in the 1960s as smaller and smaller premature infants needing more and more care survived to develop this "survivor's" disease. Most were under 1000 g and many were under 750 g. As with so many new conditions, the early reports were received with bafflement until they began turning up in everyone's practice.

The other entirely "new" condition was gastroschisis. This was thought of in the late 1960s to be a variant of "ruptured exomphalos," but aggregate figures showed many differences, particularly the rarity of associated malformations in the "new" condition. The youth of the mothers – few are over 23 years – remains perplexing in this late-occurring malformation.

Forty years ago, Hirschsprung's disease (HD) was rarely if ever diagnosed in the newborn, but it has become one of the commonest causes of neonatal intestinal obstruction. It took years to discover that, unless there was rapid decompression of the distended bowel, the dreaded "enterocolitis" supervened, increasing the mortality and long-term morbidity of a condition that was thought to be eminently curable. I asked Dr Orvar Swenson in 1965: "What is the biggest problem in Hirschprung's disease?" He said: "enterocolitis." I had never heard of it until then.

Hirschsprung's disease was on every scientific program, and still is. Mattai Sulumma of Helsinki said in 1977: "In the year 2000 you will still be talking about HD." We felt we had an ingenious but basically simple solution to this fascinating problem. "Skip segments" were totally discredited and intestinal neuronal dysplasia was seen as a great rarity of little practical importance. We now know otherwise. Then we were more concerned with the often heated debates about the "best" operation. The rectosigmoidectomy of Swenson, the retrorectal pull-through of Duhamel, and the endorectal pull-through of Soave, all gave "excellent" results in expert hands. If you were getting less than perfect results, then you were not doing the operation properly. We believed this and it took some time to show that there were other factors. That's what long-term results are all about.

Up to 1970, almost all intussusceptions were reduced by surgery before it was shown first that a barium enema and then an air enema was the treatment of choice. The introduction of metronidazole into the management of appendicitis, and with it the great reduction in anaerobic infection, reduced morbidity and reduced the incidence of wound infection in this common condition from over 10% to less than 2%.

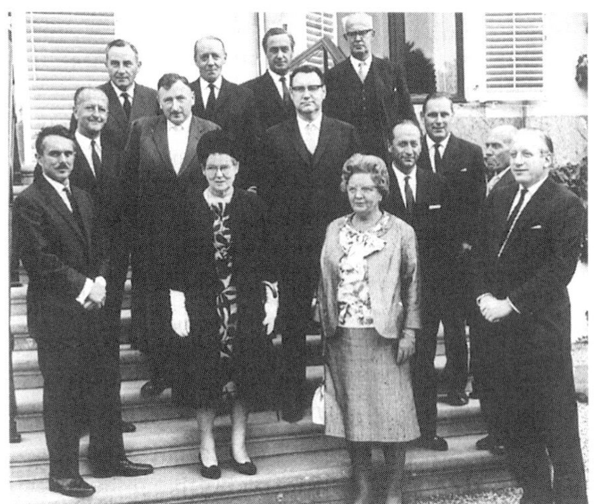

Fig. 1b.1. The British Association of Paediatric Surgeons (BAPS) Annual Meeting, Rotterdam, the Netherlands, July 1964. (Left to right) Front, standing: Queen Juliana of the Netherlands (Patron of the meeting), Peter Rickham (Liverpool); First step: M. E. Muller (Hamburg), Isabella Forshall (Liverpool), Carlo Montagnani (Rome), V. Kafka (Prague). Second step: Theodor Ehrenpreis (Stockholm), C.E. Koop (Philadelphia), David Vervat (Rotterdam). Third step: Bob Zachary (Sheffield). Back row: Fritz Rehbein (Bremen), David Waterston (London), A.G. Brom (St Gallen, Switzerland), Sir Denis Browne (London). This selected group who were presented to the Queen typifies the international nature of the BAPS.

The really big advances

In my view, two of the most important developments in that 40 years were, on the one hand, the advances in anesthesia and intensive care (including intravenous nutrition), and on the other hand the technological advances, particularly radiologic imaging.

Intensive care began by keeping the sick postoperative patients in the hopefully named "recovery rooms" overnight, and the high nursing ratios made the difference between life and death to many. Some patients who had complicated surgery lasting more than 6 hours never came round in those days. In or about 1952, Peter Rickham of Liverpool – whose energy could be measured only on the Richter scale – moved a child with a repaired esophageal atresia into a side-room off the main ward and slept beside his patient for 10 days, feeding and giving him one-to-one care for those vital early days and nights. Was this the beginning of neonatal intensive care? Long intravenous (IV) lines were unknown, and at the beginning of IV feeding in the 1970s peripheral lines were resited daily to reduce venous thrombosis. The concept of empowering the nurses was slow to develop and "intravenous teams" were unknown. There is now a world shortage of intensive care nurses owing to the "burnout" of caring for large numbers of marginal "life or death" patients. Intensive care is said to consume 20% of the entire US medical expenditure. Who could have predicted this?

Technology drives progress, and although the heart–lung machine captured the public imagination, it was the spectrum of advances in what was "radiology" and is now "imaging" that has benefited a far greater number of patients. Ultrasound came into use in the early 1970s, and babies – before and after birth – were studied as never before. The fact that ultrasound interpretation was highly personal (the most important part of any X-ray report is the initials at the bottom) put a premium on old-fashioned talent, and recruitment into the specialty flourished. Computerized axial tomography (CT) in the early 1980s and magnetic resonance imaging (MRI) in the mid-decade opened our eyes still further. Nuclear medical imaging made a big impact, particularly in pediatric urology, where it made us revise our views in many areas (especially kidney function). Scarred kidneys that looked "not too bad" on the intravenous urogram were often shown to have poor function and to be not worth preserving.

But there were so many subtle changes. Improved cannulae meant no more "cutdowns." As a resident my first 1000 IVs were cutdowns. Surgeons got better instruments, especially vascular clamps, needle-holders, and even scissors. Better sutures and needles accelerated the trend towards finer and finer materials, which in turn encouraged us to use magnification for at least part of many operations. Better lighting came with fiberoptic lenses in the early 1970s, and for those who remember this change from the filament bulb it was like the jet engine succeeding the propeller, particularly in all forms of endoscopy. The cardiac surgeons led the way with the use of headlights, although Denis Browne had always worn one from the 1940s on and so had many of his followers. One disappointment was that the laser had a much more limited role than we had expected; and another was the failure of glues to replace sutured anastomoses.

Are surgeons any better? Well, they have produced better results. Good craftsmanship takes time and surgeons no longer have to operate against the clock. The new breed are better taught and many have honed their skills in animal laboratories. I have a lasting and affectionate memory of Dr. Orvar Swenson standing on the other side of the table from "skin to skin" as I divided my first patent ductus arteriosus. He sweated the most, and not without reason.

Time is the touchstone

It has been said that up to 1900 a patient had only a 50% chance of benefiting from an encounter with a doctor, and it is only since about 1950 that we have been able to prove that this ratio has dramatically improved. Statistically validated drug trials are a vital part of modern medicine, but surgery has trodden a more pragmatic and less defensible path. This is one reason why long-term follow-up is so valuable. It often allows a reclassification of a disease possibly into a group that does well and a group that does badly. The differences in outcome between high and low imperforate anus is a classic example. Even classification by birthweight and associated anomalies allowed us better to predict the outcome. Large numbers are important to get reliable reproducible data, but many of the most acceptable figures have come from smaller countries where stable populations cared for under comparable conditions give valuable information. Ilmo Louhimo's long-term follow-up of a variety of conditions in Finland is a good example for us all.

Hospital notes are now preserved because the law and the lawyers insist, but many invaluable records have been destroyed in the past as a false economy because there was "no space" for storage. Computerized records and the paperless revolution have been slow to come to hospitals. To anyone interested in a condition, I would still say get two boxes of 6 by 4 (15 cm by 10 cm) record cards and put the diagnoses and patients' names in one box and the patients' details and diagnoses in the other, and enter the follow-up data into each. The ability to put symbols in sequence has been one of man's greatest achievements, and this simple system is not subject to meltdown or viruses. Reliable long-term results are the cornerstones of our professional achievements.

2

Principles of outcomes analysis

Brigid K. Killelea, Eric L. Lazar, and Michael G. Vitale

Children's Hospital of New York, NY, USA

Outcomes research differs in many ways from more traditionally performed clinical research. Whereas conventional "bench laboratory" experiments are designed to quantify short-term biological parameters for a given number of subjects, outcomes research employs strategies and methods to determine how disease and clinical interventions affect patient populations over time. Often, these studies are carried out in hopes of affecting public policy. In order to do so, study design must be rigorous, satisfying several criteria to ensure successful execution and valid results. For example, groups of equally distributed patients must be carefully selected, ethical and disease appropriate interventions must be implemented, and endpoints must be identified to accurately reflect how these study subjects are affected. At the same time, critical interpretation of results requires that potential biases be acknowledged and accounted for. Furthermore, as we will see, the assessment of children undergoing surgical treatment carries with it certain challenges unique to this population.

A brief history of outcomes research

From the earliest days of contemporary medical practice, observers have questioned the effects of various medical therapies. In fact, the ability to judge and assess the effects of clinical intervention is a necessary prerequisite to gauge the evolution of medical treatment. Codman was among the first physicians to stress the importance of formally assessing the results of clinical intervention. As a result, he is considered the father of Outcomes Research. An orthopedic surgeon in Boston during the 1920s and 1930s, Codman espoused his "End Result Idea."[1]

Thus in the year, 1910, at the age of forty, began the great and still unsuccessful interest of my life, over which I have toiled harder and suppressed more regrets than over any other star gazing period of my career . . .

I had become interested in what I have called the *END RESULT IDEA*, which was merely the common sense notion that every hospital should follow every patient it treats, long enough to determine whether or not the treatment has been successful, and then to inquire "if not, why not?" with a view to preventing similar failures in the future.' (AE Codman in *The Shoulder*, 1934)

Neither Boston nor the broader healthcare community was ready for Codman's idea in 1934, but change was not far off.

The federal government markedly expanded after World War II, leading to unprecedented growth in the US healthcare system and in federal funding for biomedical research and education. The research budget of the National Institutes of Health (NIH) grew from approximately $26 million in 1945 to almost $7 billion in 1990 (both in 1988 inflation-adjusted dollars).[2,3] Subspecialization, academic medicine, and medical innovation flourished in this expansionist environment. Under this system, hospital bills were generated based on tests and services rendered. Charts were reviewed after patients were discharged, and payments were made retrospectively. Likewise, physicians were reimbursed by insurance companies and individuals on a fee-for-service basis; doctors were free to order diagnostic tests, medications, etc. as they deemed appropriate, without present-day worries of cost containment.

Not surprisingly, this growth was followed by an era of increasing concern about cost. Beginning in the 1970s, the diffusion of technology into medical practice was suddenly a target. Big ticket items like CT scanners, renal dialysis machines (and a federal mandate for universal coverage

Pediatric Surgery and Urology: Long-term Outcomes, Mark Stringer, Keith Oldham, Pierre Mouriquand.

for end-stage renal disease patients) were commonly cited examples of technologies that far exceeded initial estimates of cost.[4] The government responded with the creation of several organizations dedicated to the study and regulation of this boom in technological advancement: in 1976 the Medical Device Amendments to the Food, Drug, and Cosmetic Act were introduced to assess the impact of applied biomedical advances and emerging medical interventions; the NIH created the consensus development conferences in 1977, to organize evidence-based assessments of medical practice and controversial issues for both providers and the public;[5] and the National Information Center on Health Services Research and Health Care Technology (NICHSR) was created in 1978 to coordinate the federal government's assessment activities.[6]

Not long after, in the 1980s payers began to take a serious interest in controlling costs. For the first time, payments became fixed. The prospective payment system (PPS), based on diagnosis-related groups (DRGs), was introduced for Medicare recipients. Under this system, hospitals received a fixed amount of reimbursement based not on actual services rendered, but rather on predetermined payment schedules based on diagnoses. The PPS system encouraged fewer diagnostic tests, shorter lengths of hospital stay, greater emphasis on outpatient care, and decreased technology expenditures. During this same period, third-party payers like health maintenance organizations (HMOs) and preferred provider organizations (PPOs), saw an explosion in membership. In the current healthcare environment, HMO coverage has been extended to both Medicaid and Medicare recipients. By the end of 2003, approximately 4.6 million people, 11% of Medicare beneficiaries, were covered by managed health care plans. By employing utilization controls, HMOs have kept costs down. Hospitals and individual practitioners have started competing with other providers for managed care contracts in order to sustain adequate patient loads. But do they offer the same quality of care; are the plans accessible to all who need them, and what is the overall cost to the federal government? To answer these questions there has been an increase in demand for better information about both the quality and cost of current health care. This demand transcends national borders and health system design.

Utilization review, done either retrospectively or prospectively, has also helped shape the development of outcomes research by ensuring that the delivery of health care and related services is clinically appropriate and medically necessary.[7] Beginning in the 1980s, utilization review has been increasingly performed on a prospective basis. Based on physicians' requests for treatment, designated organizations are charged with determining whether or not treatment is medically necessary. After explicit disease-specific criteria are reviewed for each case, treatment is either approved or denied. Utilization review is used to control costs for everything from diagnostic tests and imaging, length of hospital stay, to requests for ambulatory surgery. Data from this activity allows nationwide trends in health care utilization to be identified.

For example, recent evidence has suggested a geographic disparity in the utilization of surgical procedures across the country.[8] Significant differences in rates of prostatectomy, lower back surgery, and carotid endarterectomy have all been well documented for different regions in the United States.[9,10] These regional differences (often up to 20-fold) have not been explained by parallel differences in disease prevalence. Rather, they appear to be based largely on major variations in practice styles among physicians[11] and surgeon availability and experience.

In light of these differences, the importance of a defined standard of care becomes evident. But this standard of care must be applicable under real life situations, not idealized settings. Furthermore, this definition ought to be based not on individual experience, but on carefully designed research generalizable to large groups of patients. In 1962 the Food and Drug Administration (FDA) expanded its mission to include the assessment not only of drug safety but *efficacy*. Defined as "... the effect of a health care intervention on the outcome of care under "ideal" or experimental conditions," it was not long until measurements of efficacy were expected in outcomes research as well. In the past, carefully controlled outcomes studies were carried out by highly skilled specialists under ideal conditions to determine an intervention's *efficacy*. But in everyday practice, few patients and physicians are able to abide by such controlled environments. Furthermore, the practical application of these therapeutic interventions under real life conditions may also reveal unanticipated risks and benefits. Therefore, researchers and practitioners have become increasingly interested in defining outcomes under general or routine conditions to define its *effectiveness*.

These developments highlight the introduction of what was commonly referred to by Relman as the era of assessment and accountability.[13] In 1988 he proposed that the time had come for the medical community to ". . . provide a basis for decisions on the future funding and organization of health care, . . ." and ". . . the relative costs, safety, and effectiveness of all the things physicians do or employ in the diagnosis, treatment, and prevention of disease."[12] It appears that we are now well within this era, and that the science of clinical outcomes research, its design, and related methodologies have emerged as the tools of navigation. The spectrum of what constitutes clinical research has broadened; we are asking questions that relate not only to short-term biological endpoints like mortality, but we are also interested in measuring physiological and socio-economic parameters that affect morbidity, functional status, and access to care. Advances in psychometrics have established a range of reliable and valid instruments for measuring quality of life.[13–15] Hence, we now have the ability to quantify these outcomes and make comparisons across different patient populations. As emphasis has shifted toward less dramatic and often non-lifesaving interventions, we are faced with new ethical considerations; can we afford the sometimes marginal improvements in health status? The inclusion of cost data and cost-effectiveness analyses are of the utmost importance in answering these questions. At the same time that technological and pharmaceutical advances have broadened our capacity to treat, so must our ability to measure their effectiveness and costs.

Foundations of clinical research and clinical evidence

Thus, the merger of a number of cultural, technological and economic forces led to the development of a more rigorous "systematic assessment of clinical intervention" now referred to as "Outcomes Research." New methodological techniques of study design and evaluation have evolved to address questions about the demographics of disease and the applicability of interventions to larger populations. In order to derive clinical evidence to answer such questions, new ideas and treatments need to be tested, and patients observed. To avoid ambiguity in the interpretation of results, study design must control for confounding variables that may affect patient groups. In an effort to accommodate these concerns, various types of studies have evolved, including randomized controlled clinical trials, registries, cohort studies, observational studies, and meta-analyses, to name a few.

Surgical innovation

Despite methodological advances of clinical investigation made in the second half of the twentieth century, evaluation of surgical procedures and devices has lagged. In 2000, the FDA approved 30 new molecular therapies and 90 pharmaceuticals. Prior to this approval, stringent FDA regulations require that new drugs undergo three phases of clinical trials to monitor for adverse and potential side effects. No such regulations exist for surgical procedures. Since there is no formal governmental regulatory system for the development and evaluation of clinical procedures, clinical evaluation has traditionally been far less formal.[9]

Surgical innovation poses unique challenges to traditional models of clinical evaluation. Acceptance of a new surgical technique begins with performance of radical procedures, usually upon animals, followed by technical refinement along a learning curve over time. These procedures are often pioneered by a handful of specialists, usually at large academic centers and then undergo a decentralized period of incremental modification in everyday clinical practice until they become established.[9] Following early clinical experience in a series of patients, many procedures do not undergo randomized controlled clinical trials before their diffusion into more widespread use. However, it is important to keep in mind that there exist several ethical and practical considerations which preclude RCTs from being used in the development of new surgical procedures. For example, double blinding is practically impossible in the operating room, and controls may include standard accepted surgery or alternative treatments involving drugs or devices, which may themselves be in the process of improvement and development. Furthermore, technical expertise may still be evolving over the course of the study, rendering comparisons between procedures performed several months apart fraught with bias. In addition, patient and family bias to obtain particular procedure contribute to difficulty in organizing surgical RCTs. Faced with these issues, observational studies may be particularly useful in this arena, as they permit monitoring of clinical practice and changes in health outcomes. In addition, they are well suited to document incremental changes that typically take place as a procedure finds its way into the surgical armamentarium.

The challenge in pediatric assessment

We have made dramatic strides in our ability to provide treatment for children with a wide range of health problems. However, our understanding of the true effects of our interventions has not evolved at an equal pace. New pressures of accountability brought on by a rapidly evolving system of healthcare financing have underscored the need for standardized, valid measures of outcome, which are appropriately designed to reflect changes in health status for specific areas of clinical intervention. Responding to this need, there has been a burgeoning interest in the area of outcomes assessment and measuring quality of life following surgical intervention in adults. However, much less attention has been focused on pediatric outcomes assessment.

The evaluation of broadly defined outcomes, including general health status and quality of life, has several inherent difficulties in a pediatric population. First, any assessment of functional status must be performed in a developmental context. Key aspects of quality of life such as physical, emotional, and social function develop rapidly as the child ages. Therefore, there is a need for age-adjusted normative values, which allow for the comparison of children with various problems to healthy children of the same age. Secondly, the validity of information attained directly from children is suspect; such data can only be collected on relatively older children. Therefore, parents or caretakers are often proxies for direct patient-based responses. Lastly, unlike adult populations, there is a relatively low prevalence of serious disease in children; often, long periods of follow up are needed to identify the natural history of a disease and the effect of treatment. Given the diversity and relative rarity of significant pediatric problems, the collection of adequate numbers of patients can be a challenge. Multi-center studies and research using large administrative datasets are effective strategies to pursue clinical questions in these patient groups. By pooling data from different sources, more powerful studies can be designed, but again, critical interpretation of these results necessitates acknowledgement of increased opportunity for bias as compared to RCTs.

Despite some difficulties, the development of valid methods of assessing outcomes in this unique pediatric population is necessary in the evolution of surgical practice and innovation in this area. Fortunately, measures to assess functional status and quality of life in children have recently become widely available. The Child Health Questionnaire (CHQ)[16] is perhaps the best validated measure for the assessment of general health status in children. Akin to the Short Form-36 (SF-36) which has been widely used in the adult literature[17] the CHQ consists of a short questionnaire which can be scored, and generates multiple domains which span the spectrum of physical, psychosocial, and social health in injured children. Age-adjusted normative values are available and play an important role for the comparison of health status in children after trauma, for which pre-morbid scores are not available. The Pediatric Orthopedic Society of North America has developed another health status questionnaire, which also exhibits good validity and reliability across a range of pediatric musculoskeletal conditions.[14]

The governmental mandate

The challenges inherent in pediatric evaluation of this type and the shortage of work in this area have not gone unnoticed. Recently, there has been a strong societal push, and subsequent governmental mandate, to stimulate pediatric clinical research. Congress passed legislation to foster clinical research in children (the Pediatric Research Initiative Act), and Federal agencies have responded in turn. In particular, the National Institutes of Health (NIH) has put into place several new initiatives to support pediatric clinical trials. For example, the National Institute of Child Health and Human Development has created a network initiative to support more than 50 industry trials of non-psychiatric drugs, the NIMH has set up a clinical research network to support pediatric psychopharmacology, and the NHBLI is establishing a clinical trials network for testing emerging treatments for pediatric heart disease. Moreover, the FDA has created financial incentives for pharmaceutical and device companies to test their products in children (1997 FDA Modernization Act and April 1999 FDA rule requiring companies that seek approval for new drugs to run trials that include children).

Issues of design and methods

The challenges facing investigators who wish to assess a new device or novel therapy in children influence the design phase of a study. Does one plan an RCT or review a database for clinical outcomes before and after a certain intervention? As we shall see, in pediatrics especially, there are many issues, both ethical and biological which must be taken into consideration. For example, one must take into account available data and resources, issues of time and cost, and ethical considerations related to forming a control or no-treatment group. We discuss several of the more common types of study design, and consider the strengths and weaknesses of each in the context of pediatric surgery.

Randomized controlled clinical trials

It has been routinely asserted that the RCT is the gold standard by which evidence for any change in clinical practice must be gathered. The head-to-head competition of two therapies while controlling for important confounding factors has an irresistible intellectual appeal, well-grounded in the scientific method. In fact, graphically illustrating the hierarchy of clinical evidence, the double blind, randomized clinical trial sits atop a pyramid, towering over all other forms of evidence. The RCT, therefore, is a logical first choice as a study design when considering a new therapy. In it, the results of a treatment are evaluated by comparing a group of patients who received no treatment, i.e., a control group, to a group of patients equally matched for age, sex, ethnicity, etc. who received the therapeutic intervention under investigation. The control group gives the expected rate of the study outcome under the null hypothesis of no effect, and the intervention group gives the observed rate of this outcome under the investigational treatment.

Randomization is crucial in the design of an RCT. Groups that are well matched have less chance of introducing biases that may affect outcome; sample sizes and costs can thus be reduced. The result is a relatively homogeneous sample population. However, this very strategy makes the results only narrowly applicable to patients at large. Extrapolation to individuals or groups outside the inclusion/exclusion criteria is not, strictly speaking, valid. For example, trial results of an oral anticoagulant in males aged 20–40 may not be applicable to post-menopausal females. The designers of such a trial might have strategically excluded this group because of the peri-menopausal hormonal changes that can affect coagulation. This latter group may behave quite differently, obscuring clear results in such a trial. Moreover, physiologic flux and uncertainty in this group could make participation unsafe. Nonetheless, excluding "all-comers" limits the generalizability of the results. In essence, many RCTs demonstrate efficacy, but not effectiveness.

Some trialists have addressed this concern about restrictive entry criteria by advocating large, simple RCTs with few inclusion or exclusion criteria. Typically, these studies require tens of thousands of participants to overcome the issue of variability and garner sufficient statistical power. Surgical trials, however, cannot easily be done on this scale and in children such accrual is impossible, even in multicenter trials.

The key feature of RCTs, the randomization of patient groups, is designed to distribute known and unknown factors that might affect outcome. Randomization can also be difficult in surgical trials because of the perceived magnitude and finality of the decisions. Suppose, for example, we were trialing a life-sparing new cardiac procedure for a congenital cardiac anomaly. In this example, the control group might receive current medical management. Few people would be willing to be randomized to the medical arm of this trial if death was very likely, given the opportunity for survival with surgery. The case is considerably different from enrolling patients in a drug trial where differences in outcome are not so dramatic.

How then, could such a trial ever be executed? Zelen proposed a strategy to account for potential participant aversion to one of the arms of a randomized trial.[18] In his scheme, participants are randomized to either a consented or an unconsented arm of the study. Those randomized to the consented arm are permitted to choose which of the two therapies they wish to receive. The participants randomized to the unconsented arm of the study receive the standard therapy and serve as controls. Despite barriers to acceptability, there is a rational basis for this allocation scheme. If, at the start of the trial, people in both groups have an equal chance of developing the outcome of interest, conclusions about the intervention can be drawn. Final comparisons in outcome are made not between treatment groups, but between consented and unconsented arms. Ultimately, the statistical power of the study depends upon the number of participants that choose the experimental therapy. Clearly, this strategy clearly has drawbacks; the two groups may not be matched with regard to demographic characteristics, and the consented groups may very well be biased for one reason or another. There is also an ethical issue in that randomization occurs without consent in the control group since they never know *a priori* that they are part of a trial. In the end, while it is not an altogether unsound practice, the Zelen strategy is not widely accepted; a trial designed on this basis would be carefully scrutinized by those who seek to use the intervention.

Randomization also requires that the clinician have equipoise concerning the two therapies being compared. A surgeon who believes that surgery should always be attempted prior to medical therapy could hardly convince his patients to be randomized to the latter group. The proclivity to surgery may rest only on anecdote and be greater for the treatment of a skewed population (perhaps patients with severe disease), but without the clinician's acknowledgment of the lack of confirmatory data, a trial simply will not work.

A second feature of the RCT is blinding. In the example of a drug trial, patients who are blinded do not know whether they are in the treatment group or the control group. In a double-blind study, observers who administer the drug or collect patient data have no knowledge of what group patients are in either. Blinding poses a challenge in surgical trials. All would agree that a surgeon needs to see what is being done in the operating room and when comparing two surgical therapies, it is unlikely that we would ever be able to successfully blind the surgeon. Consider the previous example of laparoscopic cholecystectomy. We could not even theoretically propose a method to blind the surgeon. One could blind the patient by the use of large dressings but we would anticipate an early break to the blind in such cases. In surgery, we must usually settle for an appraisal of the functional outcomes by an individual blind to the allocation.

Related to blinding is the placebo effect. Patients who are blinded don't know whether they are receiving the pharmacologically active drug under investigation, or a placebo; these groups are used as controls. While the expectation is that control groups will report no change, sometimes this is not the case. The placebo effect, therefore, is the measurable, observable, or felt improvement in health not attributable to treatment. In place of a placebo, in surgery we could consider a sham operation. The risks here are great, however. In drug trials, the risk of placebo is that active treatment is not being pursued. In sham surgery, the added risk of the surgery itself must be considered. This is ethically thin ice – performing sham surgery for the sole purpose of blinding and controlling for the placebo effect. Hence, these trials are rare in surgery. Sham surgery is occasionally used, however, as was demonstrated in the cranial implantation of fetal cells to treat Parkinson's disease.[19] Because of the concern that one could not accurately compare a group getting fetal cell implants to any group other than a sham craniotomy group, sham operations were performed to account for the effect of surgery itself. The results in this trial debunked the therapy and prevented widespread adaptation of an ineffective therapy, but the data could not have been convincingly obtained without the contribution of participants willing to undergo sham surgery. In general, however, sham surgery has limited practical applicability and is not often used.

Another shortcoming of the RCT, particularly where surgery is concerned, relates to its time course. Well-executed RCTs take considerable time to plan, recruit, accrue, and analyze. The time course for most trials is about 5 years. Unfortunately, some surgical therapies, especially those that are market driven, gain wide acceptance faster than we can trial them.[9] Laparoscopic cholecystectomy was never subjected to the scrutiny of a trial and within 5 years of its introduction, the practice was already widespread. Most would agree that initiating a trial now would have little impact on current practice patterns. Furthermore, accrual of patients in the laparotomy arm would be impossible, given laparoscopy's now apparent benefits. In sum, in certain instances, RCTs risk being viewed as irrelevant.

The proposal of an RCT in surgery must account for two related features not seen in drug trials. The first concerns surgical skill and technique. In a drug trial, a medication is given (or not) and efficacy is evaluated. Drug administration is a fairly straightforward event, with little room for variance in its execution. In surgery, administration of the "intervention" is not quite as straightforward – there can be profound differences among surgeons with regard to skill and technique. This increased variability adds uncertainty to the outcome of a surgical trial. A surgical approach may work when done a certain way, with attention to certain details and nuances, but less well or not at all without the scrutiny of a trial. Variability is introduced into a surgical trial because of these differences. Next, new techniques require a run-in period to approach the plateau of the learning curve prior to the start of a trial. If a participant center enrols patients without such a run-in period, the outcome will be biased toward the null as there will be early technical failures contributing to the analysis. These related features, variable skill and technique and the learning curve, require that the surgical trialist insure, as nearly as is possible, the techniques and skills of the participating surgeons. While neither impossible nor prohibitive, such requirements add considerable time and expense to preparing a surgical trial. In pediatric surgery especially, most areas of clinical inquiry involve fewer patients, many of whom would be used during standardization and run-in periods, leaving fewer cases for randomization in the trial itself.

In a perfect world, all existing therapies would be subjected to RCT methodology to prove their presumed merit and new therapies would only be adopted after rigorous evaluation. Indeed, there are many clinical research authorities who feel that virtually no new therapy should be adopted prior to establishing its superiority in an RCT.[20] Such a clean sweep of all of clinical medicine, however, is unlikely and the cost would be prohibitive. Even if the cost and chaos were tolerable, is the RCT the most desirable assessment tool in general? In surgery? In children? In point of fact, we have seen some of the limitations of RCTs that merit consideration before embarking on a trial destined to fail or be misinterpreted in a broader application.

In sum, trialing a new surgical procedure prematurely places everyone on the upslope of the learning curve, and trialing too late risks making the results irrelevant. Accepting randomization (on the part of the clinician) requires equipoise which is often lacking despite the lack of sound evidence to support a particular approach. Blinding and controlling for the placebo effect in surgical trials add considerable expense and are ethically dubious under some circumstances. How then do we proceed and meet the goals of evidence-based medicine in an era of assessment and accountability given these challenges? How do we plan to study a new device or therapy?

First, we must remember that, today, many surgical trials are not focused on crude outcomes, such as survival. Rather, we are becoming increasingly interested in metrics related either to the economic sequelae of illness (lost work days or length of stay) or non-biologic attributes of illness (health-related quality of life). The traditional trial design is ideal to study an intervention in which the medical outcome is clear and the goal is to establish the superior approach. Perhaps, however, the rigid approach of an RCT is excessive in the setting of these alternate economic or quality of life outcomes.

Observational studies

It is important to recognize the strengths inherent in forms of evidence gathered elsewhere on the clinical outcomes pyramid. Observational data contained in large, administrative databases, for example, can provide a wealth of information about practice patterns evident in a variety of geographic or payer/provider specific situations. While such databases are limited by data points defined by administrative needs, usable information is nonetheless contained therein. Such databases can be used to gauge the performance of a given region, institution, or provider with regard to outcome. These "report cards" are increasingly common in our consumer driven models of health care delivery. So, while we might hesitate to conduct an RCT assigning a patient to one hospital or another to see which had better outcomes for a given surgical diagnosis, we can make such a comparison using an administrative database and surrogate outcome, such as length of stay (LOS) or the occurrence of complications, to gauge performance. Adjustments can easily be made for severity of illness, patient socioeconomic and educational status, volume/outcome relationships, or any other important confounders.

These adjustments may not have the crisp appeal of an RCT, but they are no less rigorous or reliable. The key to making successful inferences lies in understanding the meaning, limitations, and reliability of the data points. By way of simple example, many admission databases code infants and children as unemployed. Any inference about socioeconomic status that is based upon occupation would be wrong unless the investigator is thoroughly familiar with such nuances. In order to avoid problems associated with surrogate endpoints, many centers are developing their own databases. These "homegrown" databases include, *a priori*, demographic data and endpoints of clinical relevance thereby increasing the sophistication of potential analyses.

Observational studies can be done prospectively, retrospectively, or as a cross-sectional study. In a study of risk factors, for example, patient characteristics can be analyzed retrospectively to see if they are related to the disease. In prospective cohort studies the degree of exposure, risk of occurrence, and effect of treatment can all be followed months or years into the future.

Cohort studies

After the RCT, the next best study design for evaluating disease and the effect of treatment is the prospective, matched, controlled cohort study. A cohort is a group of individuals who share common characteristics, and are usually about the same age.[21] Ideally, this group is assembled at a synchronous point in time and observed until a particular endpoint is reached, usually either the conclusion of the study period, or death. As time passes and the group ages, changes in health status are observed reflected in morbidity and mortality of the cohort.[23]

Cohort studies are useful in determining the risk of developing disease. To do this, we must know the incidence of a disease – simply the number of new cases that develop in a cohort over the study period. Incidence is expressed as the number of new cases per person at risk for developing the disease. Generally, epidemiologists refer to two kinds of risk: attributable risk and relative risk. Both compare the incidence of disease in two or more cohorts that have had different exposures to some possible risk factor. Attributable risk is calculated by subtracting the incidence of disease in the unexposed cohort from the incidence of disease in the exposed cohort. This measure gives an absolute increase in the incidence of disease among those exposed to the risk factor. Relative risk designates how many times more likely it is that an exposed person will become diseased than a non-exposed person. This number, expressed as a ratio, is calculated by dividing the number of people who develop the disease by those who do not for a given cohort.

In addition to defining prevalence and studying risk, cohort studies are useful for observing the natural history of a disease, and patients' response to treatment. Since the sample sizes are usually quite large, findings are credible and cause and effect relationships can be established. They are not, however appropriate for disease with long latency periods or diseases that are very uncommon. In addition, they are more vulnerable to bias than RCTs. Without randomization, in order to assemble comparable groups of patients, attempts are made to match patients in the control group with characteristics of patients in the case group except for the exposure or disease. If differences between the groups do exist that are themselves predictive of outcome, then there is a selection bias. Any observed difference in incidence between the two groups may just be reflective of the differences between the two groups.[17] In addition, cohort studies are also subject to patient drop-out and cross-over between groups.

Case control studies

Another type of observational study, the case-control study, uses observational data to investigate potential relationships between exposure to one or more risk factors and the development of disease.[22,23] By selecting a group of patients with a disease (cases) and a comparable group of patients without disease (controls), researchers can then look back in time to try and establish a relationship between exposure and disease in the two groups. Although they are less expensive and quicker to conduct than prospective cohort studies or RCTs, there are limitations to case control studies, and they are susceptible to bias. When choosing a control group, the investigator must be careful not to overmatch. Groups that are overmatched may be so similar that a disease's association with another characteristic of interest becomes masked.[24] For example, suppose we are studying a disease associated with over consumption of meat. Choosing controls based on level of education or income would be overmatching since these characteristics are not independently associated with development of the disease. People who are more educated and/or have higher incomes generally tend to eat more meat and may erroneously lead us to infer a relationship between socioeconomic status and disease.

Case reports and case series

As we have seen, there are a variety of methodologies and strategies that produce valid inferences and permit evidence-based decision making, and the circumstances vary under which each of these various methods is most effective. For the sake of completeness, case reports and case series remain publishable and have an important role in stimulating inquiry, but we cannot infer anything about incidence, or risk from them. Furthermore, outcomes cannot be assessed nor adopted for widespread use based on these more primitive forms of evidence. They are useful ways of describing an unusual presentation or response to treatment, or a novel type of therapy or procedure.

Meta-analysis

Newer to the outcomes tool kit is the meta-analysis. Meta-analysis is a useful way to combine results from multiple studies by calculating a weighted average of study-specific results.[25,26] In pediatric surgery, where cases are often few and far between, meta-analyses hold special promise, but there are limitations. Multiple trials in different clinical settings, perhaps each with different inclusion/exclusion criteria, will generate different effect sizes. The more variability within a trial, the greater the tendency will be toward the null. It may also be difficult to reconcile trial data from that yielded by observational methods. Furthermore, the reader of clinical science may not have access to trials that were not reported. It is important, therefore, to keep in mind the potential for *publication bias*: negative studies (those that affirm the null hypothesis) are either not reported or not published. Very recently, medical journal editors have proposed registering all trials so as to make available these studies for inclusion into the overall assessment of any given therapy. Meta-analysis can synthesize diverse results arising from many types of investigational strategies and yield a statistically powerful estimate of risk. Using clinical trials databases can broaden the pool of studies to include those published in languages other than English. Of greatest value is the ability to increase statistical power for secondary outcomes by combining many well-done studies.

What is newer is the inclusion of patient-centered outcomes. In addition to a biologic endpoint, marker, or mortality, there is new interest in assessing the quality of life of our patients that reflects the impact of their disease and our treatments. Quality of life certainly has different meanings for different individuals but we would all agree that the central elements must account for the ability to complete activities of daily living in a variety of domains – functional, social, and emotional. In the next section, we will focus on some of the endpoints for analysis in outcomes research, namely health related quality of life (HRQOL) and cost.

End-points for analysis

Focusing intense effort solely on cure, disease-free survival, and lowering or eliminating a biologic marker ignores other important attributes of patients' "outcomes." HRQOL includes global assessments of well-being and functional status; as such they are becoming the new currency in outcomes research. These additional domains add depth to our understanding of the effects of our interventions. Interpretation of the outcome of a therapeutic intervention requires more than assessment of the biologic endpoint. So, while we may fail to cure some of our patients whose disease is simply not amenable to treatment, some patients may have a better quality of life as a result of treatment – a joint replacement patient may walk with less pain or an oncology patient may beat the fatigue of anemia, for example. On the other hand, we may extend life by many months with a given intervention, but at some price – being ventilator dependent may not be an acceptable or desirable outcome for many patients. HRQOL data enhances our understanding of the therapeutic intervention in ways not previously appreciated.

Quality of life

Scientific rigor demands objective, quantitative data. The very word *quality* in the phrase "quality of life" (QOL) evokes a qualitative process and in the minds of some, subordinates such research. As have been briefly introduced, contemporary instruments for the measurement of quality of life are vigorously validated and highly reliable. This section examines the background to quantitative measurement of the health-related quality of life.

Illness and the treatments that we offer have an impact on the life of the patient beyond the biophysical parameters that constitute the usual health assessments. Classically, QOL instruments encompass multiple aspects of life – physical, psychological, and emotional functioning. Each of these aspects, known as domains, can be sub-divided into various dimensions. The physical, for example, can be viewed as a composite of objective physical ability, restriction of activity, physical symptoms, beliefs and feelings about physical health, and specific disorders. Each of these dimensions can be quantified on an ordinal scale, generating an overall domain score. Separate domain scores can be combined for a global or overall score. The greatest utility of such an instrument lies in its sensitivity over time for a given individual. Usually, higher scores correlate with a better QOL and even small changes in QOL are reflected in corresponding changes in score. An excellent review of the general principles of measuring quality of life is offered by Testa.[27]

QOL instruments come in two varieties – generic and disease specific. The classic Short Form (SF-36) is one of several widely used generic instruments which assesses HRQOL. The Short Form was derived from the longer Medical Outcomes Study (MOS) questionnaire which contained 100 items. The 36-item version has been well validated and assesses seven domains. Numerous disease specific instruments have been validated for patients living with renal disease, epilepsy, asthma, heart failure, rheumatologic disease, and most recently, obesity, among many others.

One of the greatest challenges in assessing HRQOL in children relates to their ever-changing developmental background, particularly in the youngest children. That is, normative values for children are really a moving target. Instruments, such as the SF-36, are simply not valid in children or adolescents. Perhaps the most widely used child health instrument in the United States is the Child Health Questionnaire (CHQ), which comes in several forms. The self-administered version is an 87-item form that has 11 dimensions and is useful in the older child and adolescent (10–18 years of age). There are three parental versions available, denoted by the suffix PF (parental form) which contain 28, 50, and 98 items. The CHQ-PF28, CHQ-PF50 and the CHQ-PF87 allow the parent to answer as a surrogate for children as young as five years of age (as well as the older children to age 18). Of course, whenever a surrogate is involved, there is always the potential for loss of signal or bias. It is important to remember, however, that the greatest value is these instruments lies in change over time, not necessarily the absolute value of an isolated score.

Another US instrument is the Pediatric Quality of Life Inventory (PedsQL) which has three self-administered versions for the age groups 5–7, 8–12, and 13–18. This 23-item instrument measures function in four domains and takes about 10 minutes to complete. A unique feature of the PedsQL, is that in addition to a module of disease-specific items, it contains a core group of items that constitutes the generic health-related quality of life. This feature is particularly useful in that it allows for comparison of quality of life between groups of patients with different diseases. In addition, there are many other disease specific instruments, including those for children with orthopedic problems, asthma, obesity, and even those who have suffered traumatic injury.

The science of constructing, validating, and using the various available instruments is well covered in other texts.[28] It is important to remember, however, that it is a scientific process and not for the novice. One cannot sit with pen and paper and jot down a good questionnaire for use in a study and expect to have a valid, reliable instrument. Items must be tested, refined, and re-tested. This iterative process can take months to years before normative values can be obtained. Specific items must map strongly to one domain, rather than weakly to several. The response scale must be chosen and then tested. Several questions of design and age-appropriate measures must be considered. Should there be a visual analog scale, an ordinal scale, or pictures? Which items provide for internal validation and is there external validation? There is no question that, in general, one is better off using an established instrument and accepting its flaws rather than creating one *de novo*.

Instruments that are selected for use must also be culturally appropriate. Instruments originating in the US should not be administered elsewhere until an item-by-item evaluation has been made to change whatever culturally based items may exist. Even in the US, an instrument may need to be modified for a particular cultural enclave or region under study. Simple translations from one language to another are not sufficient if the culturally based concepts remain foreign to the subject. Changes to any of the items may change the instrument's sensitivity, specificity, reliability, and/or validity. Hence, the vetting process often has to be done for each country or region where the instrument is intended for use. Since some pediatric illnesses and conditions are not very common, this may mean, particularly for the disease-specific instruments, exhausting the pool of available patients for study in simply validating the instrument.

These admonishments aside, the endeavor of trying to measure child health outcomes is of obvious importance and worth the time and effort to do properly.[29] Biologic outcomes will always remain important, but as our healthcare delivery evolves, uniformly good outcomes will be expected and even demanded. It will be in the improvement of quality of life that will differentiate one treatment option from another rather than survival.

Utility

Utility is a central component to formal decision analysis and policy making. Utility is measured on a scale of zero to one and is best thought of as preference for a given health state. Clearly, it is value-based and is entirely dependent on the person who determines its value. Utility has its basis in game theory and is understood as a standard gamble. For example, suppose we were to ask a subject whether they preferred living with their disease and accepting its eventual outcome (paralysis or death), vs. trying a treatment that could improve their health, but possibly risk hastening the outcome. Clearly, the person making the choice has to understand the chance of the treatment helping vs. making things worse. Furthermore, much of this decision depends upon the time remaining until the inevitable, untreated outcome. For example, for a near event, we accept a lower probability of success to go forward. The patient with a ruptured abdominal aortic aneurysm will accept surgery despite low likelihood of success. To undergo scoliosis surgery with all of its attendant risks, however, is more difficult to rationalize since the event that is being aborted is many years in the future. The essential problem is that few people understand game theory (witness the many who play away their salary in casinos), and children require a surrogate to make the judgment calls. In essence, however, if someone is experiencing a good quality of life, that person is unlikely to risk very much in order to improve their lot.

Perhaps a more accessible concept is known as time trade-off.[30] Rather than giving the subject a choice of a certainty vs. a probability – time trade-off asks the subject to choose between two certainties. The choice comes down to how much time one is willing to give up to live in a desired health state rather than an alternative health state. Hence, a subject might tell us that to live without the effects of chemotherapy might be worth 2 years of life.

Utility scores may be obtained from specially designed questionnaires, not unlike those used for scoring quality of life. More often, however, a face-to-face interview is required to make sure that the subject understands exactly what is being asked by way of assigning a weighted value to their current health state. This can be an intrusive process and again, for children, it can be most difficult, particularly since concepts of end of life are involved. In the end, however, the goal is to provide a modifier to measured survival as a result of a given treatment. Perhaps liver transplant extends the life of a patient with an inborn error of metabolism. This patient, however, may be plagued with hospitalizations, taking multiple daily medications, and opportunistic infections as a result of the therapy (transplant). Further, travel is restricted because of frequent drug level testing and doctors' appointments. This person might live an additional 10 years compared to a conventionally treated patient, an outcome which we would traditionally define as a great success. The utility of the treatment might be low, however, as a result of all of the above conditions and the patient might rate it 0.4. The quality adjusted life years (QALYs) are thus 4 (10×0.4). As noted, the judge can greatly affect the utility score. This individual's spouse or child or parent might rate the utility closer to 0.9 since none of the conditions bother them and the value of having their loved one around is very high. Thus, the QALYs are 9, much higher and indicative of a true success. The endeavor to link quality of life with a weighted value can help make individual decisions where therapeutic choice is involved. Furthermore, health policy can be based on patient experience and favor treatments that not only work but enhance living.

Cost

Most of the clinical science of outcomes research has its basis in cost. It is the competition for third-party payment that drives clinicians to demonstrate a superior product (better outcomes) at lower cost. Health care costs are complex and in many cases, difficult to ascertain. First, there is the charge for services and therapies. The charge is sometimes not rationally related to the cost and the actual and true cost may not be easy to specify. Second, agreements with vendors and suppliers may alter costs dramatically. To illustrate, some drug companies make suture material and other supplies. They might lower the cost of these items if a hospital agrees to purchase their drug products on an exclusive basis at a premium. The hospital might agree to such an arrangement because, overall, they are saving money. However, the charges for a given patient who received no sutures and used few supplies but who received 20 doses of premium priced third-generation drug are high. The patient taking no drug and having multiple dressing changes with special supplies and sutures is having his costs shifted to the first patient. This makes analyzing the real cost of care in a given case very difficult and variable from hospital to hospital. Hence, *resource costs* are difficult to obtain yet they are more accurate then using payer information (altered by contractual adjustments).

Traditionally, one thinks of cost–benefit analyses in which the cost of delivering care is balanced against the benefit gained. The costs are not always dollars spent in achieving the goal, however. If a patient experiences a complication and can no longer perform a vital function (like work) then the cost must include the pain and suffering as well as the lost work life. Likewise, the benefits are not always just the immediate health benefits, but may involve future productive life gained. These extended concepts are very important but very hard to place value on, and so traditional cost–benefit analyses are actually rather limited. In pediatric surgery, the benefits are even more difficult to score – what is the value of repairing a congenital heart anomaly with a low likelihood of survival to a productive work life? From a cold balance sheet, we would never endeavor to undertake such a repair – but what of advances that have come from this surgical boldness. What is the value to our society in terms of other patients in the future? How is the cost and value of future, unknown benefits calculated? The endeavor of inquiry and investigation has value that is simply not accounted for in these traditional models.

An alternative, cost–utility analysis uses the utility measures just described. Now, alternative therapies can be compared by the common QALYs measure. So, comparing a therapy that enhances the QOL but decreases survival with one that decreases QOL but increases survival is possible. By dividing the total cost in dollars of both options by the QALYs, one can get a sense of the cost effectiveness of each therapy.

However one calculates cost, it is a clear mandate that cost-effectiveness is perhaps the single most important aspect of any therapy. Gone are the days when the monies needed to achieve a health-related goal were limitless. With available healthcare resources, it now becomes the burden of every clinician to spend and invest wisely in therapies that work, have value, and that lead to enhanced quality-adjusted survival.

Conclusions

The science of outcomes research has come a long way since the days of Codman. Throughout this evolution, we have seen the progression of different methodologies, and the refinement of more appropriate end-points of evaluation. These developments have not only accelerated the pace of clinical research, but have improved the quality and applicability of resulting data. Looking ahead to the future, the emergence of new technologies, including the internet, will continue to shape this process and make the results accessible to a larger audience. Now more than ever, it is evident that rigorous evaluation of clinical and surgical practice is an important tool in the ongoing quest to best meet the needs of our patients.

REFERENCES

1. Codman, E. A. *The Shoulder*. Boston, MA: Thomas Todd; 1934.
2. Bloom, F. E. & Randolph, M. A. *Funding Health Sciences Research: A Strategy to Restore Balance*. Washington, DC: National Academy Press; 1990.
3. Finneray, K. (ed.) *The Federal Role in Research and Development: Report of a Workshop*. Washington, DC: National Academy Press; 1986.
4. Rettig, R. A. Health policy in radiology: technology assessment – an update. *Invest. Radiol.* 1991; **26**:165.
5. NIH Consensus Development Program. About the Consensus Program. Available at: http://www.consensus.nih.gov/about/about.htm. Accessed August 31, 2004.
6. United States National Library of Medicine, National Institutes of Health. National Information Center on Health Services Research and Health Care Technology (NICHSR). Available at: http://www.nom.nih.gov/nichsr/nichsr.html. Accessed August 31, 2004.
7. Gray, B. H. & Field, M. J. *Controlling and Changing Patient Care? The Role of Utilization Management*. Washington, DC: National Academy Press; 1989.
8. Gelijns, A. C. *Innovation in Clinical Practice: The Dynamics of Medical Technology Development*. Washington, DC: National Academy Press; 1991. p. 82.
9. Roos, L. L. Nonexperimental data systems in surgery. *Int. J. Technol. Assess. Health Care* 1989; **5**(3):341–356.
10. Wennberg, J. E., Roos, N. P., Sola, L., Schor, A., & Jaffe, R. Use of claims data systems to evaluate health care outcomes: mortality and reoperation following prostatectomy. *J. Am. Med. Assoc.*, 1987; **257**(7):933–936.
11. Eddy, D. M. Variations in physician practice: the role of uncertainty. *Health Aff.* (Millwood), 1984; **3**(2):74–89.
12. Relman, A. S. Assessment and accountability: the third revolution in medical care. *N. Engl. J. Med.* 1988; **319**(18):1220–1222.

13. Doltroy, L. H. *et al.* The POSNA pediatric musculoskeletal functional health questionnaire: report on reliability, validity, and sensitivity to change. Pediatric Outcomes Instrument Development Group. Pediatric Orthopaedic Society of North America. *J. Pediatr. Orthop.* 1998; **18**(5):561–571.
14. Landgraf, J. M., Canadian–French, German and UK versions of the Child Health Questionnaire: methodology and preliminary item scaling results. *Quality Life Res.* 1998; **7**(5):433–445.
15. Bukstein, D. A., McGrath, M. M., Buchner, D. A., Landgraf, J., & Gross, T. F. Evaluation of a short form for measuring health-related quality of life among pediatric asthma patients. *J. Allergy Clin. Immunol.* 2000; **105**(2 Pt 1):245–251.
16. Landgraf, J. M., Abetz, L., & Ware, J. E. *The CHQ User's Manual.* 1st edn. Boston, MA: The Health Institute, New England Medical Center, 1996.
17. Hays, R. D., Sherbourne, C. D., & Mazel, R. M. The RAND 36-item health survey 1.0. *Health Econ.* 1993; **2**(3):217–227.
18. Zelen, M. Alternatives to classic randomized trials. *Surg. Clin. North. Am.* 1981; **61**(6):1425–1432.
19. Trott, C. T., Fahn, S., Greene, P. *et al.* Cognition following bilateral implants of embryonic dopamine neurons in PD: a double blind study. *Neurology* 2003; **60**(12):1938–1943.
20. Green, S. B. Using observational data from registries to compare treatments: the fallacy of omnimetrics. *Stat. Med.* 1984; **3**(4):361–373.
21. Timmreck, T. C. *An Introduction to Epidemiology.* 3rd edn. Sudbury, MA: Jones and Bartlett Publishers, 2002.
22. Schlesselman, J. J. *Case-control Studies: Design, Conduct, Analysis.* New York, NY: Oxford University Press, 1982.
23. Fletcher, R. H., Fletcher, S. W., & Wagner, E. H. *Clinical Epidemiology: The Essentials.* Baltimore, MD: Williams and Wilkins, 1988.
24. Friedman, G. D. *Primer of Epidemiology.* 5th edn. New York, NY: McGraw Hill; 2004.
25. Dickersin, K. & Berlin, J. A. Meta-analysis: state of the science. *Epidemiol. Rev.* 1986; **14**:154.
26. Sacks, H. S., Berrier, J., Rietman, D., Ancona-Berk, V. A., Chalmers, T. C. Meta-analyses of randomized controlled trials. *N. Engl. J. Med.* 1987; **316**:450.
27. Testa, M. A. & Simonson, D. C. Assessment of quality-of-life outcomes. *N. Engl. J. Med.* 1996; **334**(13):835–840.
28. Streiner, D. L. & Norman, G. R. *Health Measurement Scales: A Practical Guide to their Development and Use.* 2nd edn. Oxford: Oxford University Press, 1995.
29. Dougherty, D. & Simpson, L. A. Measuring the quality of children's health care: a prerequisite to action. *Pediatrics* 2004; **113**(1)185–198.
30. Torrance, G. W. Measurement of health state utilities for economic appraisal. A review. *J. Health. Econ.* 1986; **5**:1–30.

3

Outcomes analysis and systems of children's surgical care

Keith T. Oldham[1] Mark D. Stringer[2] and Pierre D. E. Mouriquand[3]

[1]Children's Hospital of Wisconsin, Milwaukee, WI, USA
[2]Children's Liver and GI Unit, St James's University Hospital, Leeds, UK
[3]Department of Paediatric Urology/Surgery, Debrousse Hospital, Lyon, France

Institutions which provide the basis for contemporary children's specialty units and pediatric clinical care first developed in the nineteenth and early twentieth centuries. These reflected efforts to care for urban populations of children brought together by the forces of industrialization and were often the work of altruistic individuals, typically but not exclusively, well-to-do women, who were motivated by compassion for children. Their primary mission was often to provide an acceptable level of charity care to poor children in their communities. This is, in fact, still the case for many major children's hospitals worldwide.

The concept that children are unique patients with particular developmental, physiological and psychological needs, for whom a demonstrably better outcome could be obtained with specialized medical care came more recently. With particular regard to children's surgical care, events detailed in Chapter 1 by Dr. Hendren (North America) and Dr. O'Donnell (Europe/UK) gave rise to what we recognize as contemporary pediatric surgery by the mid twentieth century. Specialization and credentialing were progressively driven by the view that the quality of care for children was improved by having practitioners fully dedicated to children, by providing focused professional training for individuals interested in childhood disease, and by creating a children's specific environment for the delivery of that care. The wider medical community has not been free of controversy over these points. Perceived economic threat and fear of professional or institutional loss remain powerful forces even today when we discuss issues like regionalization or consolidation of certain services. Although certifying bodies in much of the world differentiate pediatric from adult practice and training, the lines of distinction between certain patient groups, particular providers and competing institutions remain a source of controversy. As we begin the twenty-first century, many active discussions continue around questions such as: how to best design pediatric trauma systems; where to perform congenital heart surgery; who is best able to do childhood transplants or provide pediatric anesthesia; what is general (adult) as opposed to pediatric urology or surgery; and indeed, within pediatric surgery or urology, should everyone repair a cloaca or perform a portoenterostomy for biliary atresia? These types of questions are currently answered differently around the world, driven by unique local history, available resources and needs.

It is the view of the authors of this chapter and the editors of this text, that policy decisions about providers and venue of care are best driven by relevant, risk-adjusted and accurate outcomes data. What are the best outcomes that can be achieved in correcting a particular anomaly or treating a childhood surgical condition? What are the institutional characteristics and what is the background and training of the individuals who achieve these best outcomes? Where are healthcare system boundaries best drawn to improve quality of care and deliver value? How can optimal outcomes be achieved within the economic constraints of a particular healthcare system and with the least disruption for children and their families? These questions are the fundamental reason to publish this text, an effort to assemble the most critical contemporary analysis of outcomes from international experts in children's surgical care.

Each individual chapter provides relevant data with regard to long-term outcomes in a specific area. Even when they are considered collectively, the reader will recognize that some of the questions posed above will remain

Pediatric Surgery and Urology: Long-term Outcomes, Mark Stringer, Keith Oldham, Pierre Mouriquand.
Published by Cambridge University Press.

unanswered. In the following pages, the authors examine three areas of pediatric surgical practice in some detail: childhood trauma, hepatobiliary surgery (specifically biliary atresia), and pediatric urology. We have chosen these particular areas to illustrate the types of data and analyses that are becoming available to children's surgeons and policy makers in various countries. We have made no attempt to be encyclopedic, rather to use these examples in an illustrative manner. Other examples can be found in other chapters in this book (*e.g., Chapter 6: Cleft Lip and Palate*). Both the potential power of these data, as well as some of the obstacles impeding reform of current practices, will become apparent. The areas selected for discussion are chosen because they involve complex systems of care with multiple specialists dealing with critically ill children, as well as highly complex technical procedures where individual surgical skills are relevant. Thus issues of both individual experience and institutional structure and volume enter into the discussion.

Whilst there is considerable variation among particular types of surgical procedures and in the quality of comparative data, it appears increasingly clear that there is an inverse relationship between hospital and surgeon case volume and surgical mortality and morbidity.[1–5] This general relationship extends beyond the world of surgery.[6] The challenge is to match particular patients with appropriate caregivers, delineating relevant procedures and volume thresholds that are both meaningful and practical. In the sections that follow, we attempt to model types of data available which enable rational policy decisions yielding optimal care for pediatric patients.

Trauma

Trauma is a major pediatric health issue worldwide and it is the leading cause of childhood death in the developed world after the age of 1 year. For children and adolescents between 1 and 20 years of age in the United States in 2001, unintentional injury accounted for 12 916 deaths and intentional injury accounted for approximately 3300 additional deaths.[7] Approximately two-thirds of these deaths in the United States are related to motor vehicles. In 2000, approximately 228 000 children were hospitalized and 10.9 million were treated in an emergency department for injury related problems.[8] The estimated direct cost in 2004 for injury related medical care in the United States was 117 billion USD and approximately one-third of this was expended upon children and adolescents. Despite the number of pediatric patients involved (both generally and within particular subsets) and the obvious scope of the problem, consolidation of pediatric trauma care into specific children's hospitals or programs is not the norm in the United States; indeed, the majority of injured children receive their care in adult oriented environments. There are a number of reasons for this. One important issue is simply that current pediatric systems and centers are not staffed or equipped to handle such a large number of trauma patients. Because specific pediatric systems have not been developed in many regions, more than half of pediatric trauma patients in the United States receive their care in adult centers or general hospitals, even in large urban areas. Access to pediatric specialty care in rural environments is a particular challenge in trauma as well as in many other areas of health care.

In the early 1990s, several authors suggested that outcome following pediatric trauma, as measured by survival, was equivalent in adult trauma centers which cared for children.[9–11] These reports were based generally on retrospective, single institution reviews using TRISS methodology which allows comparison of individual program or institutional survival rates with national norms extrapolated from a largely adult cohort (the Major Trauma Outcomes Study). These comparisons have been criticized for both this flawed methodology (incorrect reference sampling frame) and for the fact that their reported results do not compare favorably with best practice benchmarks, that is, survival in dedicated pediatric trauma centers. The point is also made that survival is a relatively crude measure of pediatric trauma care quality[12–14] since fatalities are relatively uncommon.

More recently, Potoka *et al.*[15] reported a statistically significant survival advantage for the most severely injured children who had head, spleen and liver injuries, when treated at pediatric trauma centers in the state of Pennsylvania in 2000, in comparison to those managed in adult trauma centers in the State over the same time period. These data were derived from a mandatory and uniform statewide trauma reporting system which has produced a uniquely detailed database.

Because overall mortality rates for pediatric trauma are generally low, 1.7–8.9%,[3,6–9,11] functional outcome and quality of life should be considered to be relevant measures of the quality of childhood trauma care. Head injury is the principal cause of both death and disability in pediatric trauma patients. In a follow-up study in 2001 using the same Pennsylvania state database, Potoka *et al.* analyzed functional outcome, i.e., disability, in severely injured children (Injury Severity Score (ISS) > 15 and age 0–16 years).[14] The analysis was complex, taking into account different types of certification among trauma centers, and including age-specific evaluation of feeding, locomotion, expression,

Table 3.1. Pennsylvania trauma outcomes study. Patient demographics (ISS > 15)[14]

	Pediatric trauma center	Adult trauma center (with added qualifications)	Adult trauma center Level I	Adult trauma center Level II
Number of patients treated	553	782	206	546
Mean age (y)	8.7 ± 4.2	10.8 ± 4.8[a]	15.1 ± 1.8[a]	12.0 ± 4.0[a]
Sex (% male)	71.4	68.9	71.4	71.6
Mechanism (% blunt injury)	94.8	95.0	75.2[b]	94.5
Mean ISS	21.5 ± 7.2	23.5 ± 8.4	25.4 ± 10.4	23.1 ± 8.8
Mean GCS	12.0 ± 4.5	11.3 ± 4.8	11.2 ± 5.0	11.8 ± 4.6

[a] $P < 0.05$ vs. PTC by Student's test.
[b] $P < 0.005$ vs. PTC by x^2.
ISS, Injury Severity Score.
GCS, Glasgow Coma Score.

Table 3.2. Pennsylvania trauma outcome study. Functional outcome (ISS > 15)[14]

	Number of dependent patients at discharge (%)			
Functional category	Pediatric trauma center	Adult trauma center (with added qualifications)	Adult trauma center Level I	Adult trauma center Level II
Feeding	80/550 (14.6)	167/781 (21.4)[a]	44/206 (21.4)[a]	84/545 (15.4)
Locomotion	138/550 (25.1)	247/780 (31.7)[a]	61/206 (29.6)[a]	152/546 (27.8)
Transfer	141/549 (25.7)	234/779 (30.0)	65/206 (31.6)[a]	144/546 (26.4)
Social Interaction	59/545 (10.8)	157/779 (20.2)[a]	28/198 (14.1)	67/541 (12.4)
Expression	61/548 (11.1)	148/779 (19.0)[a]	29/199 (14.6)	73/543 (13.4)

[a] $P < 0.05$ vs. PTC by x^2.
ISS, Injury Severity Score.

mobility and social interaction. Key findings are summarized in Tables 3.1 and 3.2.

The data in Table 3.2 show number (percentage) of dependent patients specifically identified within 48 hours of hospital discharge using the five noted functional domains (feeding, locomotion, transfer mobility, social interaction, and expression). Each domain was given a numerical score (1–4): complete independence (4); independent with device (3); modified dependence (2); complete dependence (1); and age < 24 months excluded. Scores of 3 or 4 were considered "independent" while 1 or 2 were considered "dependent", and patients with age < 24 months were excluded as this analysis is not relevant to this age group.

The data in Table 3.1 show that patients treated at pediatric trauma centers and adult centers were similar except for age and mechanism of injury. Adult trauma centers managed an older cohort of children and penetrating injuries were more frequent; however, ISS and GCS were not statistically different. The data in Table 3.2 show significantly fewer dependent patients at the time of hospital discharge from pediatric trauma centers in a number of categories. This is particularly apparent when comparing pediatric trauma centers to adult trauma centers with added qualifications in the domains of feeding, locomotion, social interaction and expression. These differences are not explicable by differences in age. In a somewhat modified additional analysis, stratifying by body region of injury, patients with an ISS > 15 (severe injury) and head injury had the lowest probability of dependency in all domains when treated in a pediatric trauma center (Table 3.3).

One of the authors (KTO) has taken a similar approach to examine the same general question of whether there is a differential outcome for injured children treated in different types of facilities. Like the previous reports, the reference data are derived from an increasingly available and useful tool, a very large, audited database. The KID 2000 database is a government maintained tool containing 2 516 833 hospital discharge records for patients ≤ 20 years of age from 27 of the 50 United States for the year 2000. This represents more than 70% of the entire US pediatric population at that time. The data set contains E-codes, a system of descriptive numerical codes that specifically

Table 3.3. Pennsylvania trauma outcome study. Functional outcome by body region of injury (ISS > 15 and head injury)

	Number of dependent patients at discharge (%)			
Functional category	Pediatric trauma center	Adult trauma center (with added qualifications)	Adult trauma center Level I	Adult trauma center Level II
Feeding	61/374 (16.3)	121/479 (25.3)[a]	22/82 (26.8)[a]	45/270 (16.7)
Locomotion	98/374 (26.2)	156/479 (32.6)[a]	26/82 (31.7)	69/271 (25.5)
Transfer	96/374 (25.7)	152/478 (31.8)[a]	27/82 (32.9)	69/271 (25.1)
Social Interaction	48/370 (13.0)	121/478 (25.3)[a]	20/76 (26.3)[a]	37/269 (13.8)
Expression	50/373 (13.4)	114/477 (23.9)[a]	21/77 (27.3)[a]	44/270 (16.3)

[a] $P < 0.05$ vs. PTC by x^2.
ISS, Injury Severity Score.

provide information about emergency care and injury. Analysis of this large data set using E-codes identified 210 895 cases of pediatric injury. These cases were then coded using ICDMAP-90® (Trianalytics, Inc., Baltimore, MD), a validated software tool which provides an injury severity score (ISS) for each record using ICD-9 codes, the latter being a uniform and detailed numerical system of identifying specific diagnoses. This cross-linkage allows stratification of patients from these many hospitals by injury severity. The ISS stratified records were then limited to only those cases coded for an urgent or emergent admission to the hospital; records with ICD-9 codes representing cases of poisoning, medical errors, adverse drug reactions or late effects of injury were excluded. The resulting records were weighted using the proprietary KID 2000 weighting factor to produce a national estimate, yielding 176 348 evaluable cases. Cases were grouped by age (0–10 and 11–20 years), injury severity (ISS ≤ 15 vs. ISS > 15), and site of care (NACHRI-National Association of Children's Hospitals and Related Institutions defined hospital type). This latter categorization allows comparison of children's and adult hospitals. Measured outcomes included mortality, length of stay (<8 d vs. ≥8 d) and total charges (<USD 15 000 vs. ≥ USD 15 000). Statistical analysis was done using chi square or *t*-test where appropriate.

Among the 176 342 cases, mean age was 12.3 (SD = 8.9) years and ISS was 7.0 (SD = 10.9). Of these patients, 10.7% received care in a Children's Hospital (CH), while Children's Units (CU) in an adult general hospital and Adult Hospitals (AH) cared for the remaining 23% and 67%, respectively. Comparing younger children (≤10 years of age) to older children (between 11 and 20 years of age), and grouped by ISS scores of ≤15 and >15, significant differences were observed in where these children were hospitalized after injury (Table 3.4). It is clear that even for younger children who have severe injuries (ISS > 15), most receive their care in adult oriented institutions.

Table 3.4. Types of institutions where injured children/adolescents received care in the United States in the year 2000, stratified by injury severity

	Age 0–10 years		Age 11–20 years	
	ISS ≤ 15	ISS >15	ISS ≤ 15	ISS > 15
Children's hospital	20%	28%	5%	5%
Children's unit in an adult hospital	23%	38%	20%	29%
Adult hospital	56%	34%	75%	66%

Table 3.5 summarizes survival data which show a significantly higher probability of death for seriously injured children less than 11 years of age when treated in an adult general hospital, as compared to those treated in a children's hospital.[16] There was no apparent difference in hospital length of stay or charges.

Taken together, the preceding data highlight a major problem with regard to the design of trauma systems in the United States. However, this is not unique. All around the world, a large number of injured children are cared for in institutions with an adult focus, either of necessity or because of historical referral practices. This is in spite of the fact that data from several different large databases make it clear that risk-adjusted survival for seriously injured young patients is higher in pediatric specific trauma centers and that functional outcomes are improved.

A similar point can be documented with regard to splenic injuries. Splenic preservation was first proposed in pediatric patients in 1968.[17] Over the ensuing years, it became clear that most children, and indeed many adults, with blunt splenic injury could be safely managed non-operatively, yielding a very high probability of splenic salvage. Guidelines have been published detailing this non-operative approach.[18,19] Generally, the overall splenic

Table 3.5. Outcomes of patients aged 0–10 years with an ISS > 15: comparison of children's and adult hospitals

	Age 0–10 years, ISS >15 (n = 46 002)			
	Mean ISS	Percent mortality	Percent LOS ≥ 8d	Percent charges ≥$ 15K
Children's hospital	18.9 ± 9.1	5.3	45	36
Adult general hospital	19.4 ± 9.3	7.6	45	35
* Chi square, †t-test	P = 0.08†	P = 0.002*	P = 0.84*	P = 0.26*

LOS, length of stay.

salvage rate in children with blunt abdominal trauma should be well over 90%. In the light of these published data, what actually happens in the United States at present? Given the perspective detailed above, that most injured children are cared for in adult trauma systems, we and others examined the incidence of splenic surgery following childhood trauma. Rothstein *et al.*,[20] used the KID 2000 database (referenced above) to explore the question of whether the type of institution in which treatment was provided influenced the type of care with specific regard to the probability of splenectomy in injured children. They found that the crude rate of splenectomy in the USA was 3% (11/338) at dedicated (freestanding) children's hospitals, 9% (45/525) in children's units within adult general hospitals, and 15% (197/1327) in adult general hospitals. Adjusted for severity of injury, children treated at an adult hospital had a 2.8 times higher probability of splenectomy than if treated in a children's hospital, and this likelihood was 2.6 times higher in a children's unit within a general hospital (P = 0.003 and 0.013, respectively). Using similar analytic techniques, Densmore *et al.*[21] found that the probability of operative management for pediatric splenic injury was 17% in a general hospital, 2% in a children's hospital, and 4% in a children's unit in a general hospital. This variance in practice could not be explained by injury severity. Stylianos *et al.*[22] examined the issue of the management of pediatric splenic injury in administrative data sets obtained from California, Florida, New Jersey and New York, and Mooney *et al.*[23] did so for New England. Both reports show substantial variation in practice with regard to the likelihood of operative management for splenic injury, indicating that published "best practice" benchmarks are not routinely achieved in institutions treating injured children. Once again, small scale studies indicate that these findings are not unique to the USA.[24]

In aggregate, these data make clear a clinical care issue that is not satisfactorily resolved at present by policy makers either in government or in medicine. The data summarized here indicate that injured children have a significantly better outcome when cared for in designated pediatric trauma centers. This is demonstrably true with respect to overall survival, functional outcomes, and the likelihood of splenic preservation in the specific case of pediatric blunt splenic injury. One would hope that these observations would become the basis for changes in trauma system design and practice.

Dr. Arnold Epstein writing on this general subject offered several principles for such change in a thoughtful essay entitled "Volume and outcome – it is time to move ahead".[25]

1. The least intrusive action is education . . . Public dissemination of performance reports can lead to improvements in quality . . . Efforts to decrease the proportion of procedures performed in low volume hospitals seem appropriate.
2. Use financial incentives or even regulatory means to promote the use of high-volume centers for certain types of care. Initial restrictions should be confined to metropolitan areas and focused on surgical procedures for which the differences are greatest, with (volume) thresholds set very conservatively.
3. The notion of regulating the broad-scale regionalization of medical care prompts worries about the details and unintended consequences (who and how will this be done?). Demonstration and evaluation should precede broad-scale policy changes.
4. Better measures of quality, such as risk-adjusted mortality, should be used when available.
5. Finally, increasing the proportion of care provided in high-risk centers is only one step toward improving quality of care. Efforts at improvement by individual hospitals will be critical.

Biliary atresia

Biliary atresia (BA) is a rare congenital obliterative cholangiopathy of unknown etiology (see Chapter 35). Reliable incidence figures are available from France (1 in 19 500 live births), the UK and Eire (1 in 16 700 live births), Georgia (United States) and Sweden (1 in 14 000 live births).[26–29] Untreated infants succumb to liver failure within a year or two. In the late 1950s, Morio Kasai, a Japanese surgeon, reported the presence of patent microscopic biliary channels at the porta hepatis in young infants with BA. Exposure of these channels by radical excision of atretic extrahepatic biliary remnants could result in effective drainage of bile, especially if the operation was performed before 8 weeks of age. The Kasai portoenterostomy operation is now accepted as the standard operation for BA. The success of the operation as determined by clearance of jaundice (plasma bilirubin < 20 μmol/l) is related to several factors including age at presentation, type of BA, and the presence of associated anomalies. Children who clear their jaundice and remain anicteric for the first 3 years of life have about an 80% chance of reaching adulthood with their native liver, i.e., without a liver transplant.

Infants who fail to clear their jaundice after portoenterostomy and those who develop complicated or end-stage chronic liver disease despite an initially successful Kasai procedure require liver transplantation. Biliary atresia is the commonest indication for liver transplantation in children. Most of these cases require their transplant in the first few years of life. Techniques such as split-liver grafting and living-related liver transplantation have minimized the risk of these small children dying on the waiting list (see Chapter 65). The combination of Kasai portoenterostomy and liver transplantation has transformed a disease that was almost invariably fatal in the 1960s into one with a current overall 5-year survival of about 90%. Furthermore, long-term studies have shown a relatively good quality of life in BA survivors after portoenterostomy alone[30] and after liver transplantation.[31]

Initial clearance of jaundice is thus an important step in avoiding the need for liver transplantation and its attendant risks. In the UK, a series of three national studies have demonstrated that the outcome of infants with BA is markedly affected by the experience of the center.[27,32,33] This organizational dimension to the delivery of surgical care is an important additional factor in determining the long-term outcome of BA and prompted a major change in the management of affected infants in the UK.

The first of these UK surveys was conducted between 1980 and 1982 (Table 3.6).[32] There was a significant difference in jaundice-free survival between the highest volume center treating more than five cases per year and the 15 low volume centers treating fewer cases. A similar survey of all infants with BA in UK and Eire conducted between 1993 and 1995 again demonstrated that outcome was related to center volume and experience.[27] In this second study, survival without liver transplantation and overall survival were both significantly greater in the two centers managing more than five cases per year than in the 13 centers treating fewer cases. After taking into account age at surgery, sex, gestational age, and presence of the biliary atresia splenic malformation syndrome, stepwise multivariate regression showed that center size was the only significant independent factor predictive of overall survival.

There was much debate within the profession and the media about the dissemination and interpretation of these findings.[34] However, in 1999 the Department of Health decided that the management of BA in England and Wales would be centralized and limited to three supra-regional pediatric liver units in the south (London), midlands (Birmingham) and north (Leeds) of England. Scotland has an independent body regulating these matters. Within pediatric surgery in the UK, there was understandable opposition to this decision.[35] Nevertheless, the decision was implemented, and, most importantly, the subsequent outcome was critically audited. Thus, the third national survey of infants with BA was published (Table 3.6).[33] This showed that, within the three centers, 57% of infants cleared their jaundice after Kasai portoenterostomy. Significantly, there was no difference in outcome between the three centers – all three had uniformly good results equivalent to those previously reported from centers treating five or more cases annually. Estimated actuarial 4-year survival was 89%. Another measure of success after Kasai portoenterostomy is survival with the native liver; this was estimated to be 51% at 4 years in this recent UK survey in comparison to an overall 5-year actuarial survival without liver transplantation of around 44% in the 1993–1995 survey.

It is likely that small improvements soon after Kasai portoenterostomy will progressively translate into larger more significant benefits with the passage of time. Thus, in a recent follow-up of the 1993–1995 cohort of BA patients reassessed at a median age of 8 years, actuarial native liver survival without liver transplantation was statistically significantly more likely in centers treating more than five cases annually (56% vs. 27%, $P = 0.004$).[36]

The advantages of centralizing the management of BA into specialized hepatobiliary units, each dealing with the whole spectrum of liver disease including liver transplantation, are numerous. They include seamless care from rapid evaluation of neonatal obstructive jaundice through to prompt Kasai portoenterostomy and long-term management of the sequelae of chronic liver disease (metabolic, nutritional, infective, etc.); concentration of medical and surgical expertise into a multidisciplinary team with facilities for supporting patients and their families; parental education and advice in a center familiar with the whole

Table 3.6. Summary of three consecutive national surveys of biliary atresia in the United Kingdom

Author	Survey period (duration)	Number of infants with BA	Number of infants undergoing a portoenterostomy-type procedure	Median age at operation (days)	Duration of follow-up (months)	Center/volume effect and jaundice-free outcome
McClement *et al.* 1985[32]	1980–1982 (UK, 3 y)	114	107	63	Mean 27	$>$ 5 cases/yr $(n = 1)$: 43% 2–5 cases/yr $(n = 15)$: 29% $\leq$ 1 case/yr : 11%
McKiernan *et al.* 2000[27]	1993–1995 (UK and Eire, 2 y)	93	91	54	Median 42	$>$ 5 cases/yr $(n = 2)$: 62% 2–5 cases/yr $(n = 5)$: 58% $\leq$1 case/yr $(n = 8)$: 17%
Davenport *et al.* 2004[33]	1999–2002 (England and Wales, 3.5 y)	148	142	54	Median 25	$>$ 5 cases/yr $(n = 3)$: 57%

spectrum of the disorder; optimal timing of liver transplantation (the majority of children with BA will eventually need a new liver); and potential opportunities for better scientific and clinical research. However, there are disadvantages such as the travelling for families and its social and economic burden, the potential deskilling of referring pediatric specialists, and the loss of training opportunities in regional units. Some of these problems are surmountable by good communication, shared care (including outreach clinics) and by arranging for trainees to visit specialist units.

As with the trauma debate, the issues surrounding the management of BA are not unique. For example, in France the situation has been comparable to that in the UK before 1999. Thus, between 1986 and 1996, 472 infants with BA were recorded. The Kasai procedure was performed in 32 centers (nine of which offered pediatric liver transplantation) and overall 5-year survival and native liver survival were 70% and 32%, respectively.[26] Univariate analysis showed significantly better 5-year survival with or without liver transplantation in the single center which performed 20 or more portoenterostomies per year compared with centers treating up to five cases per year. Thus, 5-year survival with the native liver was 39% in the center treating 20 or more new infants with BA each year, 31% in centers treating three to five cases annually and 24% in centers treating no more than two new cases each year.[26]

Pediatric surgeons in the UK were understandably concerned about the centralisation of BA but the carefully audited results of this change in practice have helped to recognize the advantages of this approach (category IIa evidence). Such a model of care for BA is unlikely to be appropriate for all healthcare systems because of variations in population density, geography, socioeconomic factors, healthcare resources, etc. The perceived benefits in the management of BA in the UK are not simply related to surgical volume although, as with many other conditions with a major surgical component, this is undoubtedly an important factor. The situation is much more complex, involving the whole package of long-term multidisciplinary care for these complex patients. It is not known within pediatric surgery how many conditions will benefit from this type of approach. Generally, these are rare and complex disorders where there is evidence that concentrating medical and surgical expertise into designated units is beneficial to the outcome of the patient.

Pediatric urology

Urogenital surgery in children represents between 50% and 75% of the activity of most European units dealing with general pediatric surgery and urology. Fewer and fewer adult surgeons operate on children, especially infants, mainly because regulations for anesthetizing these patients have become more restrictive. This explains the decreasing number of children operated on in district general hospitals (DGH) and small institutions, and the increasing flow of so-called "minor cases" to large university hospitals. Clinical practice in France has also been significantly affected by the new financing system for the National Health Service which was adopted in January 2004. In short, these new arrangements strongly encourage hospitals to operate on as many cases as possible to ensure an increased income. Hence, minor cases which used to be referred to private hospitals or DGHs are now retained in major institutions to increase income. This system is rather perverse since the number of doctors and nurses has not changed appreciably but the number of health administrators has increased dramatically. The most obvious failure of this system is that health authorities wrongly equate the number of patients seen and the quality of care.

With the huge increase of hypospadias cases in Western countries, operations for this condition have become one of the commonest procedures in pediatric urology. Contrary to an old statement, there is no minor hypospadias and this type of surgery should be performed by very experienced surgeons. Testicular surgery is also extremely common and should only be performed after adequate, supervised training in order to avoid relatively high rates of morbidity. Surgery for ambiguous genitalia needs to be concentrated in a few centers with relevant multidisciplinary expertise (including pediatric endocrinologists, geneticists, biologists, psychiatrists, etc.). A country of 60 million inhabitants should require no more than four or five expert centers in this field.

A large part of pediatric urology is made up of patients with prenatally detected congenital impairment of urine flow. Most of these cases (80–85%) will not require any surgical intervention but they do need close urological follow-up involving imaging and isotope departments. Here again, close collaboration between specialties (radiology, obstetrics, nephrology) is required. Another growing area of pediatric urology is represented by all aspects of bladder dysfunction including the challenging problems of neurogenic incontinence and the far more frequent non-neurogenic bladder dysfunction. These highly specialized fields have fostered the development of non-surgical pediatric urology where urodynamics and consultations by clinical nurse specialists are essential.

Finally, specific, rare, major congenital malformations such as bladder exstrophy and cloacal malformations ought to be concentrated in specific centers. The UK now has two centers dealing with bladder exstrophy (London and Manchester). France is not so well organized but most of these malformations are currently referred to Paris or Lyon. Here again, it is multidisciplinary teamwork and the clinical nurse specialist that are essential.

After this brief review of the organizational aspects of pediatric urology which may affect the long-term outcomes of our patients, the question of training in pediatric urology must be considered. In most Western countries there are two main avenues – via urology and pediatric surgery. Efforts are gradually being made to develop a specific career pathway to pediatric urology. At present, there is no consensus about this route but European institutions are working toward a designated pathway with accredited centers and, subsequently, accredited specialists. It will take time and much effort. The Joint Committee for Pediatric Urology, which brings together urologists, pediatric surgeons and pediatric urologists, is a first step in coordinating the actions of different countries. This will not be an easy task since training schemes and standards of practice vary widely between countries. How many pediatric urologists do we need? The answer is extremely variable from one country to another and it will be the task of these institutions to regulate the number of specialists to avoid saturation.

There is an increasingly apparent trend in many countries that pediatric urology is becoming relatively independent from adult urology and from pediatric surgery. This is a controversial issue because both pediatric urology and pediatric surgery are small disciplines and, for many, they need to stay together to have a stronger political voice. Each cannot survive without the other. Most countries have a national pediatric surgical association that includes pediatric surgeons, pediatric urologists, pediatric orthopedic surgeons, and other pediatric subspecialists. However, the two dominant forums for pediatric urology are the urology section of the American Academy of Pediatrics and the European Society for Pediatric Urologists, attended largely by pediatric urologists. There are parallels in pediatric orthopedic surgery. So, how long will pediatric urology and pediatric surgery remain so closely linked? Probably for quite a long time, not just for political reasons but also because children need a special environment to receive the best care. There is the common denominator between the pediatric subspecialties and it is important to preserve it.

Conclusions

To summarize, this brief review highlights the importance of systems of care in affecting outcomes in pediatric surgery and urology. Organizational aspects at different levels influence outcome. Thus, in the case of pediatric trauma, injured children have a significantly better outcome when cared for in designated pediatric trauma centers rather than within adult care facilities. In pediatric urology, there is the need for broad subspecialist care by trained pediatric urologists. Finally, for certain rare, complex conditions such as biliary atresia, centralization within pediatric surgery may have advantages. We conclude that systems of care that recognize the needs of the child; that consolidate particular types of patients into regional centers; that provide and then require specialized training; and that offer comprehensive multidisciplinary access to children's specific providers in all surgical, medical and allied health areas, yield the best outcomes for our patients.[37] While data are still limited at present, we are increasingly able to organize pediatric health care on the basis of demonstrable quality, that is clinically relevant outcomes. Our challenge now is to continue to generate relevant data and to have the wisdom and the will to use these outcomes to provide a rational system of care that is optimal for our patients and their families.

REFERENCES

1. Luft, H. S., Bunker, J. P., & Enthoven, A. C. Should operations be regionalized? The empirical relation between surgical volume and mortality. *N. Engl. J. Med.* 1979.1; **301**:1364–1369.
2. Hughes, R. G., Hunt, S. S., & Luft, H. S. Effects of surgeon volume and hospital volume on quality of care in hospitals. *Med Care* 1987; **29**:1094–1107.
3. Birkmeyer, J. D. High-risk surgery – follow the crowd. *J. Am. Med. Assoc.* 2000; **283**(9): 1191–1193.
4. Birkmeyer, J. D., Siewers, A. E., Finlayson, E. V. *et al.* Hospital volume and surgical mortality in the United States. *N. Engl. J. Med.* 2002; **346**(15) :1128–1137.
5. Birkmeyer, J. D., Stukel, T. A., Siewers, A. E., Goodney, P. P., Wennberg, D. E., & Lucas, F. L. Surgeon volume and operative mortality in the United States. *N. Engl. J. Med.* 2005; **349**(22): 2117–2127.
6. Halm, E. A., Lee, C., Chassin, M. R. Is volume related to outcome in health care? A systemic review and methodologic critique of the literature. *Ann. Intern. Med.* 2002; **137**:511–520.
7. Center for Disease Control and Prevention, Epidemiology Program Office, Division of Public Health Surveillance; available online at: http://www.epo.cdc.gov/wonder.
8. Center for Disease Control and Prevention. Web-based injury statistics query and reporting system (WISQARS) [Online]. (2003) National Center for Injury Prevention and Control, Centers for Disease Control and Prevention (producer). Available from URL: www.cdc.gov/ncipc/wisqars.
9. Knudson, M. M., Shagoury, C., & Lewis, F. R. Can adult trauma surgeons care for injured children? *J. Trauma.* 1992; **32**(6):729–739.
10. Fortune, J. B., Sanchez, J., Graca, L. *et al.* A pediatric trauma center without a pediatric surgeon: a four-year outcome analysis. *J. Trauma.* 1992; **33**(1):130–139.
11. Bensard, D. D., McIntyre, R. C., Moore, E. E., & Moore, F. A. A critical analysis of acutely injured children managed in an adult level I trauma center. *J. Pediatr. Surg.* 1994; **29**(1): 11–18.
12. Hall, J. R., Reyes, H. M., Meller, J. L., Loeff, D. S., & Dembek, R. The outcome for children with blunt trauma is best at a pediatric trauma center. *J. Pediatr. Surg.* 1996; **31**(1):72–77.
13. Nakayama, D. K., Copes, W. S., Sacco, W. Differences in trauma care among pediatric and nonpediatric trauma centers. *J. Pediatr. Surg.* 1992; **27**(4):427–431.
14. Potoka, D. A., Schall, L. C., & Ford, H. R. Improved functional outcome for severely injured children treated at pediatric trauma centers. *J. Trauma. – Injury Infect. Crit. Care.* 2001; **51**(5):824–832; discussion 832–4.
15. Potoka, D. A., Schall, L. C., Gardner, M. J. *et al.* Impact of pediatric trauma centers on morality in a statewide system. *J. Trauma* 2000; **49**:237–245.
16. Densmore, J. S., Oldham, K. T., & Guice, K. S. Relationship of pediatric trauma mortality rates to type of institution providing care. *J. Pediatr. Surg.* 2006; **41**(1):92–98.
17. Upadhyaya, P. & Simpson, J. S. Splenic trauma in children. *Surg, Gynecol. Obstet.* 1968; **126**:781–790.
18. Stylianos, S. and the APSA Trauma Committee. Evidence-based guidelines for resource utilization in children with isolated spleen or liver injury. *J. Pediatr. Surg.* 2000; **35**:164–169.
19. Stylianos, S. and the APSA Liver/Spleen Trauma Study Group. Compliance with evidence-based guidelines in children with isolated spleen or liver injury: a prospective study. *J. Pediatr. Surg.* 2002; **37**:453–456.
20. Rothstein, D. H., Forbes, P. W., & Mooney, D. P. Variation in the management of pediatric splenic injuries in the United States (unpublished data).
21. Densmore, J. S., Oldham, K. T., & Guice, K. S. Splenic surgery rates following pediatric trauma in the United States (unpublished data).
22. Stylianos, S. Variation in practice for splenic injury (unpublished data).
23. Mooney, D. P. & Forbes, P. W. Variation in the management of pediatric splenic injuries in New England. *J. Trauma.* 2004; **56**: 328–333.
24. Godbole, P. & Stringer, M. D. Splenectomy after paediatric trauma: could more spleens be saved? *Ann. R. Coll. Surg. Engl.* 2002; **84**:106–108.
25. Epstein, A. M. Volume and outcome – it is time to move ahead. *N. Eng. J. Med.* 2002; **346**(15):1161–1164.
26. Chardot, C., Carton, M., Spire-Bendelac, N. *et al.* Prognosis of biliary atresia in the era of liver transplantation: French national study from 1986 to 1996. *Hepatology* 1999; **30**:606–611.
27. McKiernan, P. J., Baker, A. J., & Kelly, D. A. The frequency and outcome of biliary atresia in the UK and Ireland. *Lancet* 2000; **355**: 25–29.
28. Yoon, P. W., Bresee, J. S., Olney, R. S., James, L. M., & Khoury, M. J. Epidemiology of biliary atresia: a population-based study. *Pediatrics* 1997; **99**:376–382.
29. Fischler, B., Haglund, B., & Hjern, A. A population-based study on the incidence and possible pre- and perinatal etiologic risk factors of biliary atresia. *J. Pediatr.* 2002; **141**:217–222.
30. Howard, E. R., MacClean, G., Nio, M., Donaldson, N., Singer, J., & Ohi, R. Biliary atresia: survival patterns after portoenterostomy and comparison of a Japanese with a UK cohort of long-term survivors. *J. Pediatr. Surg.* 2001; **36**:892–897.
31. Bucuvalas, J. C., Britto, M., Krug, S. *et al.* Health-related quality of life in pediatric liver transplant recipients: a single-center study. *Liver Transpl.* 2003; **9**:62–71.
32. McClement, J. W., Howard, E. R., & Mowat, A. P. Results of surgical treatment for extrahepatic biliary atresia in United Kingdom 1980–2. *Br. Med. J.* 1985; **290**:345–347.

33. Davenport, M., De Ville de Goyet, J., Stringer, M. D. *et al.* Seamless management of biliary atresia in England and Wales (1999–2002). *Lancet* 2004; **363**:1354–1357.
34. Davison, S., Miller, V., Thomas, A., Bowen, J., & Bruce, J. The profession, not the media, should assess where Kasai portoenterostomy should be performed. *Br. Med. J.* 1999; **318**: 1013.
35. Lloyd, D., Jones, M., & Dalzell, M. Surgery for biliary atresia. *Lancet* 2000; **355**:1099–1100.
36. McKiernan, P., Baker, A., Mieli-Vergani, G., & Kelly, D. The BPSU study of biliary atresia – outcome after 8 years. *J. Pediatr. Gastroenterol. Nutr.* 2003; **36**:529 (abstract) 26.
37. Arul, G. S. & Spicer, R. D. Where should paediatric surgery be performed? *Arch. Dis. Child.* 1998; **79**:65–72.

4

Perinatal mortality and morbidity: outcome of neonatal intensive care

Janet M. Rennie

Department of Neonatal Medicine, University College London Hospitals, UK

Introduction: historical aspects

Perinatal mortality

Perhaps no other medical subspecialty has achieved such a dramatic improvement in survival as that documented in neonatal medicine over the last 40 years. Since the 1960s the survival rate for infants born weighing less than 1500 g (very low birthweight, VLBW) has increased from 45% to over 80%. For the small group born weighing less than 1 kg (extremely low birthweight, ELBW) the increase in survival has been from 20% to almost 70%. These changes have occurred against a background of improving perinatal, infant and childhood mortality in the United Kingdom and elsewhere, although it remains true that a VLBW infant is 100 times more likely to be stillborn or die during the first month of life than an infant born weighing 3000 g or more (Table 4.1). The UK definition of a stillbirth was changed to include all fetuses delivered dead after 24 complete weeks of pregnancy in October 1992. This caused a step up of about 1 per 1000 in the UK perinatal mortality rate, which at 8.0 per 1000 total births remains similar to that in other European countries and the USA (Fig. 4.1). Whilst prematurity remains the leading cause of perinatal and neonatal death, significant contributions continue to be made from perinatal asphyxia, sepsis and congenital malformations. Group B streptococcal infection and chorioamnionitis, where the organism is rarely isolated, are important causes of fetal and neonatal deaths.

Congenital malformations

As the number of deaths from infection has declined dramatically in the last 50 years, the proportion of deaths due to congenital anomalies has increased. In 1998 28% of UK infant deaths were coded as due to congenital anomaly, compared to 13% in 1948. Exactly the same effect has been seen in the USA. This has occurred in spite of the fact that termination of pregnancy, when a malformation which is known to carry a substantial risk of handicap is diagnosed antenatally, has been a legal option in England, Scotland and Wales for some years, although this is still not the case in Eire or many other countries in Europe. English law was amended in 1990 to allow such terminations to be carried out at any stage of pregnancy, and 1813 such terminations were notified in 1999; 449 for CNS malformations and 596 for chromosomal anomalies (data from the Office for National Statistics, www.statistics.gov.uk). Liveborn anencephalic babies are now rarely seen in England, Wales or Scotland unless they are the product of a twin pregnancy, and only 12 were reported in 2001. Periconceptional folate supplementation has the potential to prevent the conception of infants with neural tube defects and is used increasingly by women who are planning to become pregnant. Dietary supplementation is particularly important for epileptic women on treatment. An unlooked-for benefit of dietary supplements has been a reduction in infants with cleft palate, and a protective effect against acute lymphoblastic leukemia in childhood has also been reported.

The reported rate of congenital malformations in the UK in 2001 was 114/10 000 births, which is an increase from 81/10 000 reported in 1994 (Table 4.2). The current monitoring system provides the most comprehensive data yet, and has been in place since 1964 when it was introduced after the thalidomide epidemic in order to recognize any similar hazard. It is a voluntary system,

Pediatric Surgery and Urology: Long-term Outcomes, Mark Stringer, Keith Oldham, Pierre Mouriquand.
Published by Cambridge University Press.

Table 4.1. Perinatal mortality rates in the UK 2002

Birthweight	Stillbirth rate per 1000 total births	Neonatal mortality rate per 1000 live births	Postneonatal mortality rate per 1000 live births	Infant mortality rate per 1000 live births
<1000 g	278.2*	360.6	57.3	417.9
1000–1499 g	83.6*	47.4	12.7	60.2
<1500 g	172.3*	173.2	30.6	203.9
1500–1999 g	38.4*	14.2	8.5	22.7
2000–2499 g	12.4*	4.8	4.5	9.3
<2500 g	48.4*	34.6	9.6	44.2
>2500 g	1.8*	1.0	1.0	2.0
All weights	5.3	3.6	1.7	5.3

Source: Office of National Statistics, www.statistics.gov.uk.
* data from birth counts, for 1996.

Table 4.2. Numbers and rates of congenital malformations per 10 000 births in the UK

	Number of congenital anomalies notified		Rates per 10 000 total livebirths	Rates per 10 000 total stillbirths
	Live	Still	Live	Still
1989	12 191	200	177.4	618.8
1990	7 941	213	112.5	655.8
1991	6 889	186	98.6	572.4
1992	5 909	145	85.7	461.0
1993	5 565	156	82.7	406.7
1994	5 394	180	81.2	474.7
1995	5 657	171	87.3	477.5
1996	5 784	175	89.1	497.6
1997	5 756	171	89.7	499.1
1998	6 035	204	95.0	599.8
1999	7 179	232	115.5	706.7
2000	7 575	301	125.4	948.3
2001	6 776	305	114.0	969.5

Source: Office of National Statistics, www.statistics.gov.uk.

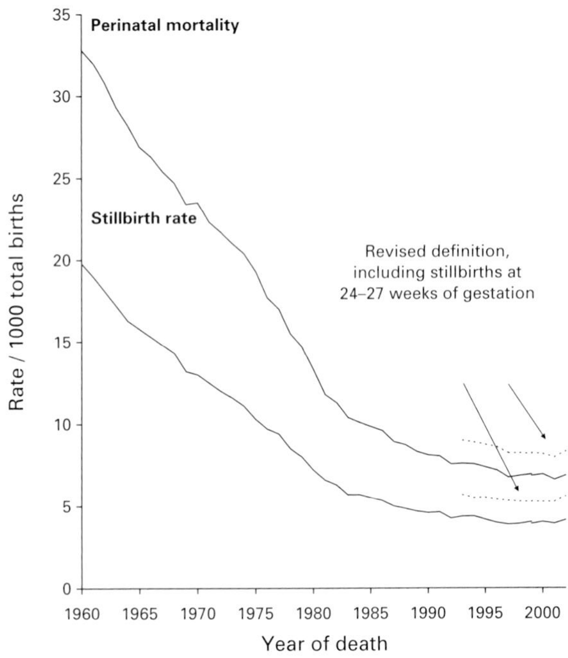

Fig. 4.1. Stillbirth and perinatal mortality rates for England and Wales 1960–2002 (Office for National Statistics).

and from January 1, 1995 anomalies diagnosed at any age can be reported to the National Congenital Anomaly System in the UK. This should improve the accuracy of the data because ascertainment is inevitably incomplete in infancy. However, direct electronic notification from Wales and Trent produces much higher rates than for England and Wales overall, showing that the information is still incomplete. Minor anomalies such as congenital umbilical hernia, undescended testicle, and skin tags are specifically excluded. The commonest malformations notified are those of the musculoskeletal system, particularly deformities of the feet and congenital heart disorders, perhaps because the latter is still difficult to diagnose antenatally. Of interest to pediatric surgeons, there were 563 liveborn cases of hypospadias, 76 cases of diaphragmatic defects, 102 cases of gastroschisis and 547 of cleft lip and/or palate notified in 2001. In contrast, there were only 47 babies notified with spina bifida and 21 with esophageal atresia. Anyone can complete a form, and perhaps pediatric surgeons and others should make every effort to ensure that data are returned to the Office for National Statistics rather than relying on midwives and health visitors to carry out this task.

Prematurity

The World Health Organization recognized prematurity, defined as birth before 37 completed weeks of gestation or birthweight less than 2500 g, as the leading cause of perinatal mortality in 1950. In the UK 7% of births occur before 37 weeks, and about 7.7% of babies are born weighing less than 2500 g. Only 1.25% of babies are VLBW (less than 1500 g at birth). Infants who are below the tenth, third or 2.3rd centile of birthweight (definitions vary) are termed small for gestational age; an infant of 2500 g can therefore be small for gestational age at term, or appropriate for gestational age and preterm if he or she was born at 36 weeks. It is possible to be both preterm and small for gestational age, and this high-risk group is increasingly recognized antenatally. Intrauterine growth restriction (IUGR) often poses a difficult management decision for perinatologists regarding the optimum time of delivery. The condition is an important one for surgeons because many of their patients suffer from IUGR, and because the outcome is worse than for normal weight babies (see below). Mechanical ventilation, antenatal steroid therapy and postnatal surfactant have revolutionized the outcome for the preterm infant by reducing the mortality from respiratory distress syndrome. Better techniques of neonatal ventilation have reduced the risk of air leak from the high rates of 50% recorded in the 1980s to around 11% now. Ensuring a good quality of life for the survivors is the main challenge for the future. Whilst 80% of surviving VLBW infants are neurologically normal, concern centers around the high incidence of cerebral palsy, impaired vision, and hearing reported in these children. School failure, poor attention span, and behavior problems are reported in older preterm survivors. Chronic lung disease with prolonged oxygen requirement and risk of death from infection remains a problem for a few.

Perinatal asphyxia

Perinatal death and morbidity from perinatal asphyxia is reducing, and is less than that for prematurity or congenital malformations but is nevertheless important because it may be preventable (Fig. 4.2). The term should be used to describe a constellation of events, which includes cardiotocographic evidence of fetal distress, depression at birth (low Apgar scores), evidence of metabolic acidosis, and a neonatal encephalopathic illness characterized by seizures and with evidence of other organ system damage such as renal impairment. This complex is difficult to recognize in preterm infants, in whom there is no agreed definition of hypoxic–ischemic encephalopathy. Low Apgar scores alone are insufficient to make a diagnosis of hypoxic–ischemic encephalopathy. Older studies often adopted a less precise definition but trends over time would support a reduction in incidence. The UK Confidential Enquiry into Stillbirths and Deaths in Infancy ascribed some 9% of deaths to intrapartum asphyxia in 1999 (Fig. 4.2).

Short-term outcomes

Mortality by birthweight and gestation

A normally formed infant born weighing more than 2500 g in the developed world has a chance of dying in the neonatal period, which is less than 1 in 1000. For appropriately grown infants of birthweight between 1500 and 2500 g, the mortality remains less than 10%. Below this weight mortality rates gradually increase (Fig. 4.3), and survival below 500 g birthweight is still very rare.[1] The wide availability of dating ultrasound examinations in pregnancy has led to more reliable information on survival by gestation and these data are invaluable when counseling women faced with the prospect of an early delivery. The gestational age at which there is a roughly evens chance of survival has declined to 25 weeks over the last decade, although the margin of viability remains 22–23 weeks. There are only a few claims of survival at 22 weeks and very few intact survivors at 23 weeks.[2] Figure 4.3 shows the outcome for each week of gestation from 22 to 32 weeks, after which survival is above 95%. When compared to previous cohorts, summarized by Rennie (1996), there is a continuing trend to improved survival.[3] Some units achieve better survival figures than this, and if local data are available then women should be counseled using the appropriate information. Figure 4.4 shows the dramatic difference which even a few days can make to the percentage chance of survival at low gestations.

Factors affecting mortality

Gestational age is the predominant factor influencing survival. Survival is enhanced in infants who are of appropriate weight for their gestational age (Fig. 4.3). Most studies have shown a U-shaped curve for survival within each gestational age band when considering weight-for-gestation.[4] Nearly every published report that has examined gender

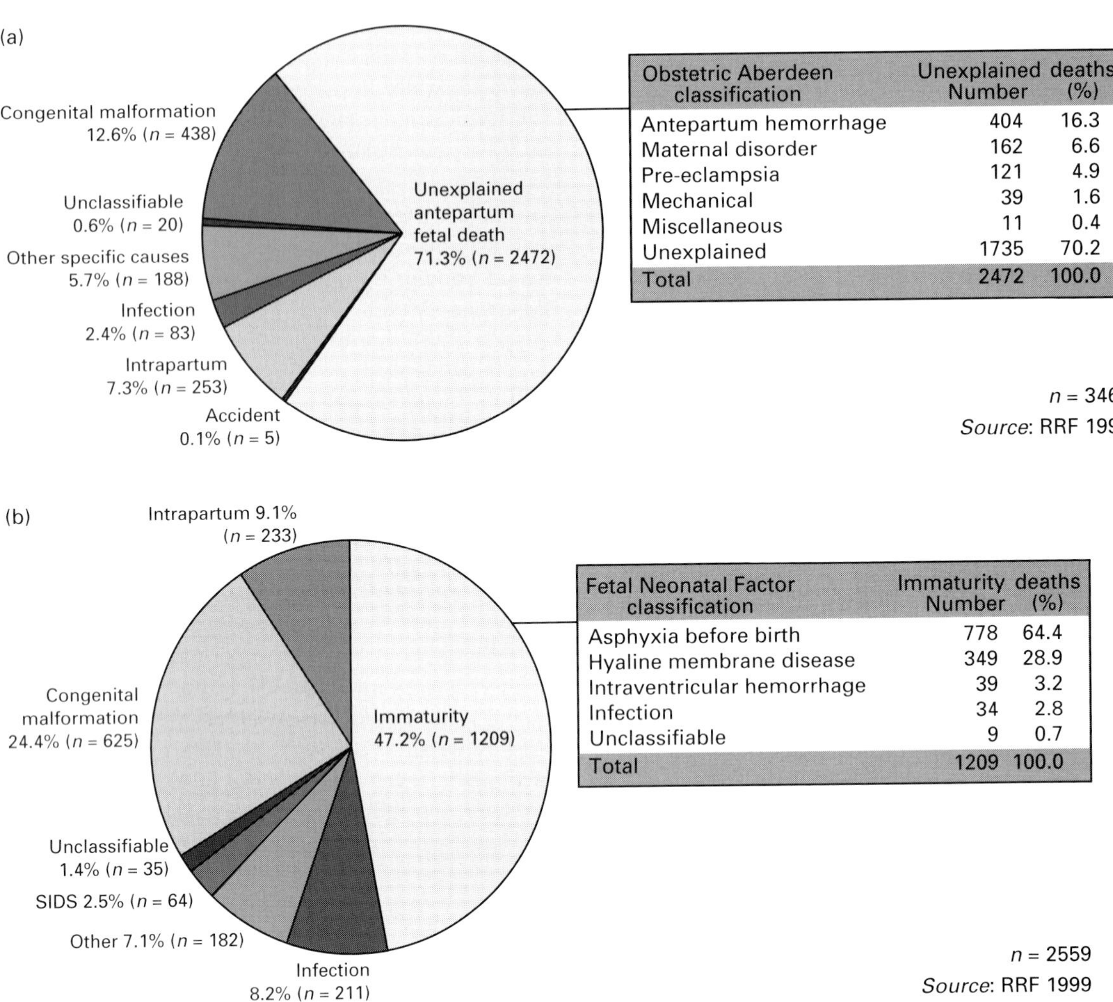

Fig. 4.2. (a) Stillbirths and (b) neonatal deaths in England, Wales, and Northern Ireland 1999 grouped by cause according to the Wigglesworth classification (CESDI).

as a factor has reported an advantage for female infants over males, an effect sometimes as high as a doubling of survival. An effect of similar magnitude can be obtained by the use of antenatal steroids. The American Neonatal Network has also produced survival curves which take into account weight, gestation and gender.[5]

Illness severity can be assessed using the Clinical Risk Index for Babies (CRIB) score.[6] This score has recently been updated and simplified, and has proved a robust tool for predicting mortality.[7] The score is useful in comparative audit, comparing results between neonatal intensive care units and different countries. There is very little evidence to suggest that cesarean section delivery has any advantage for the very preterm baby although no randomized trials have ever been done, nor is it likely that such trials will be possible. Poor condition at delivery certainly influences outcome, and a low Apgar score is predictive of mortality. The results of full cardiopulmonary resuscitation in the delivery room for preterm babies remain very poor in most centers[8,9] although mature babies who respond to cardiopulmonary resuscitation (CPR) within 10–15 minutes have a reasonable chance of intact survival.[10]

Respiratory distress syndrome

Respiratory distress syndrome (RDS) is the main cause of death in preterm infants. Antenatal steroids and postnatal surfactant have reduced the mortality and morbidity, contributing much to the improved prognosis for preterm

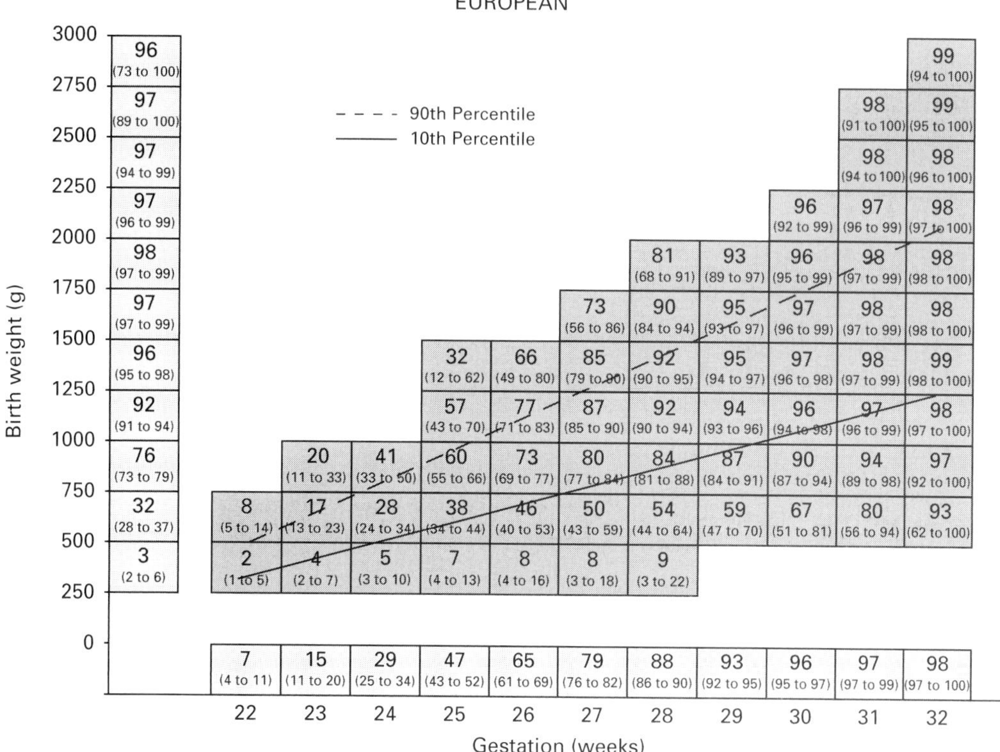

Fig. 4.3. Predicted survival for European infants known to be alive at the start of labor, by birthweight and gestation. From Draper *et al.* *BMJ* 2003 with permission.[1]

infants. The incidence of RDS is strongly related to gestational age, and RDS occurs in the majority of babies under 30 weeks' gestation. It can be helpful to have an idea of how likely it is that a baby will require ventilation at any given gestation, and for how long: Fig. 4.5 shows the percentage of babies who require ventilation at each week of gestation, with the median number of days of ventilation from a large UK cohort. More mature infants are not immune to RDS, which occurs in about 2 per 1000 births at 37 weeks' gestation and above.[11] At term, RDS is most common after elective cesarean section because of the lack of the usual stimuli for clearing lung liquid. The risk of respiratory morbidity is halved with each successive week of gestation between 37 and 39 weeks (Fig. 4.6).[11] These data have important implications when planning elective cesarean sections at term.

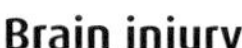

Brain injury

Imaging of the neonatal brain with ultrasound has been possible for over 20 years, and improved technology has

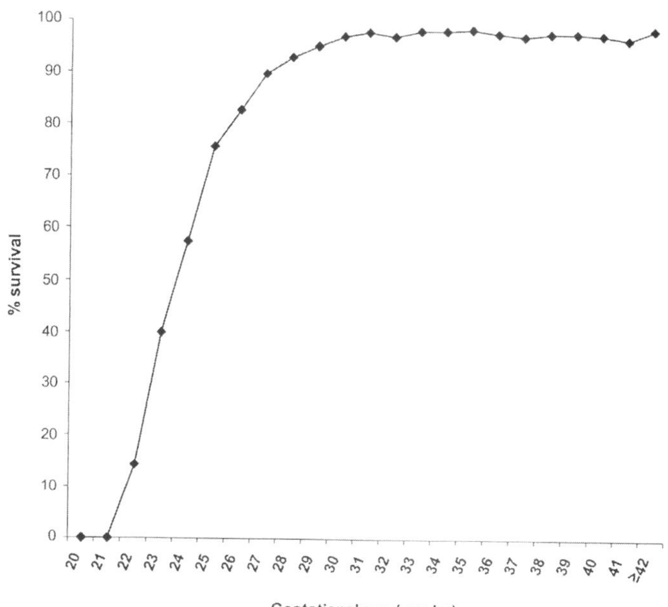

Fig. 4.4. Graph showing increase in percentage survival by each week of gestation. Redrawn from various sources.

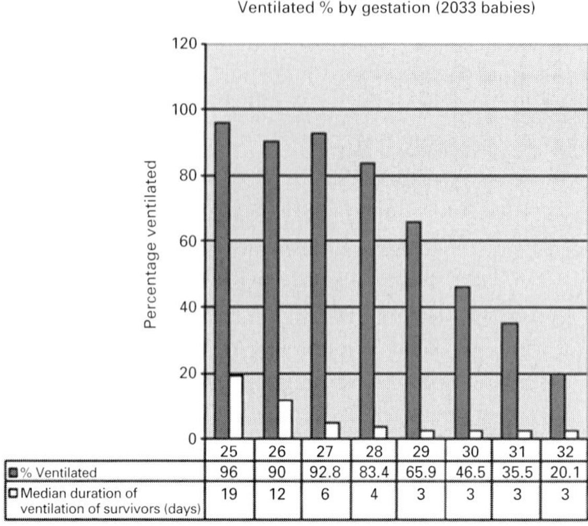

Fig. 4.5. Histogram showing the percentage of babies requiring artificial ventilation for respiratory distress syndrome at each week of gestation between 26 and 32 weeks, with the median number of days of ventilation. From CESDI with permission.

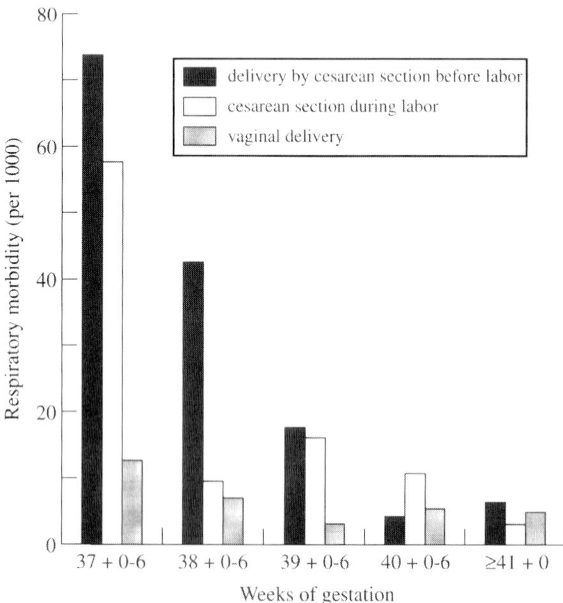

Fig. 4.6. Incidence of respiratory morbidity at term by each week of gestation and mode of delivery. (From Morrison, Rennie & Milton, 1995 with permission.)[11]

increased our ability to recognize subtle and transient abnormalities in the neonatal period. It is now realized that not all the lesions imaged in the parenchyma of the brain are the same, and most ultrasonographers would distinguish between a unilateral parenchymal echodensity on the same side as, and abutting onto, a ventricle which contained blood, and bilateral symmetrical lesions which are separate from the ventricular cavity. The former are largely considered to represent venous infarction secondary to intraventricular hemorrhage and the latter early white matter damage which will evolve into cystic periventricular leukomalacia. Atlases of ultrasound images exist for those who wish to know more.[12]

There are serious limitations in using ultrasound evidence of brain injury as a proxy for neurodevelopmental outcome, and brain imaging will never replace follow-up studies.[13] The significance of transient parenchymal abnormalities remains to be defined. Ultrasound fails to detect all cases of later white matter injury (periventricular leukomalacia), although repeated studies that continue until term equivalence improve the detection rates. Ultrasound is used widely as a screening tool, providing a rapid result which is attractive to parents and doctors alike. The ability to time and document injury can help in research. Trends in incidence are valuable in giving early warning of effects of changes in practice. The efforts of many groups, such as those in New Jersey, Utrecht, Liverpool, and London who have imaged large cohorts of preterm neonates and carefully followed them up have led to the following broad conclusions[14,15] – see also ref.[12]

- A preterm baby who is discharged from a neonatal unit with a consistently normal cranial ultrasound scan is at low risk (less than 10%) of subsequent neurodevelopmental problems;
- The risk of adverse neurodevelopmental outcome is not increased in the presence of an uncomplicated germinal matrix hemorrhage (GMH) or bleeding into the ventricles (intraventricular hemorrhage, IVH) which is not followed by ventricular enlargement;
- Non-progressive ventriculomegaly carries a risk of about 34% of an adverse outcome, and shunted hydrocephalus 50% or more;
- Bilateral cystic change in the occipital cortex, corresponding to the pathological lesion of periventricular leukomalacia, is associated with a very high probability (more than 90%) of cerebral palsy.

The realization that bilateral occipital cystic periventricular leukomalacia diagnosed with ultrasound scanning (Fig. 4.7) carries such a poor prognosis has led to a change in emphasis in research into the causes of neonatal brain injury and strategies for prevention. Fortunately, the complication is rare, although MRI cohort studies reveal more cases than ultrasound does, with about 8% of VLBW infants being diagnosed with cystic periventricular leukomalacia on MRI compared to about 3% with ultrasound (Fig. 4.8).[16,17] MRI also reveals subtle white matter lesions

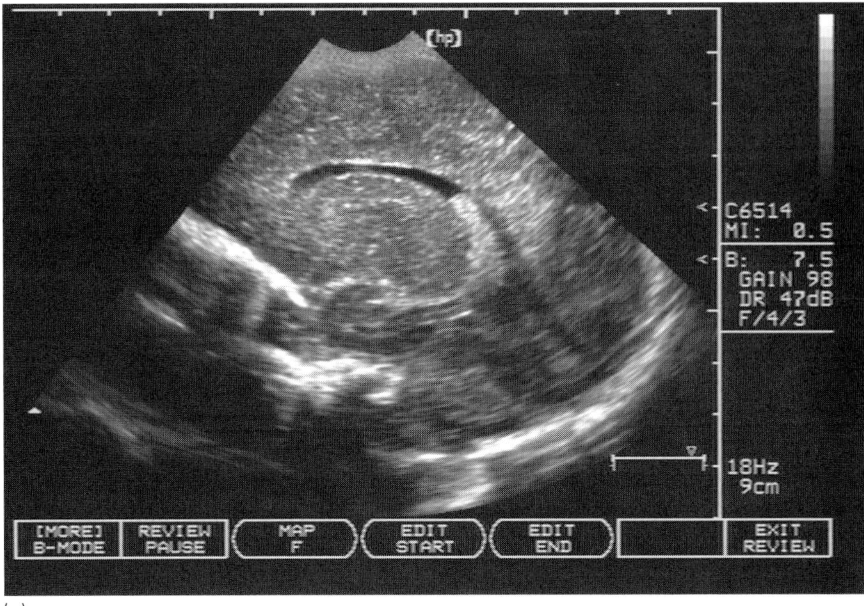

(a)

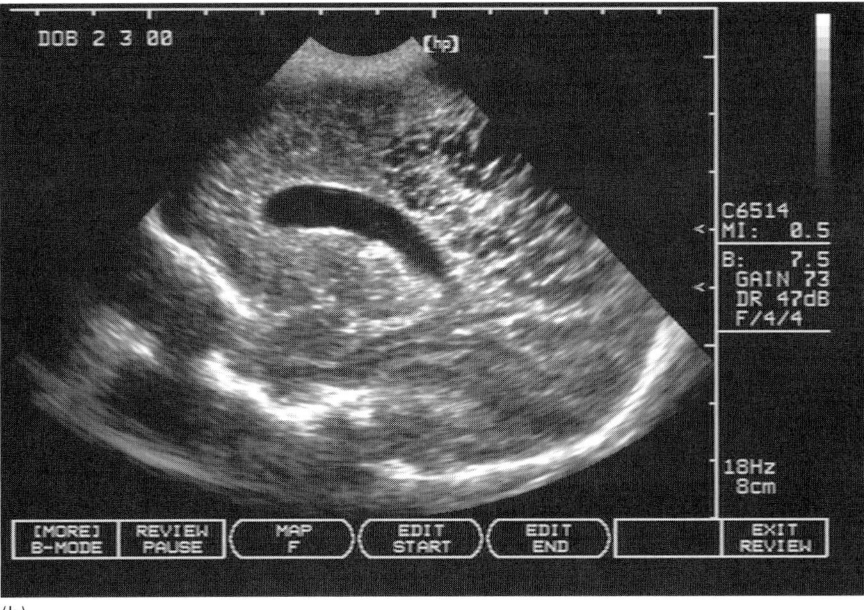

(b)

Fig. 4.7. (a) A normal cranial ultrasound scan in the parasagittal plane. (b) A scan in the same plane showing bilateral cystic periventricular leukomalacia.

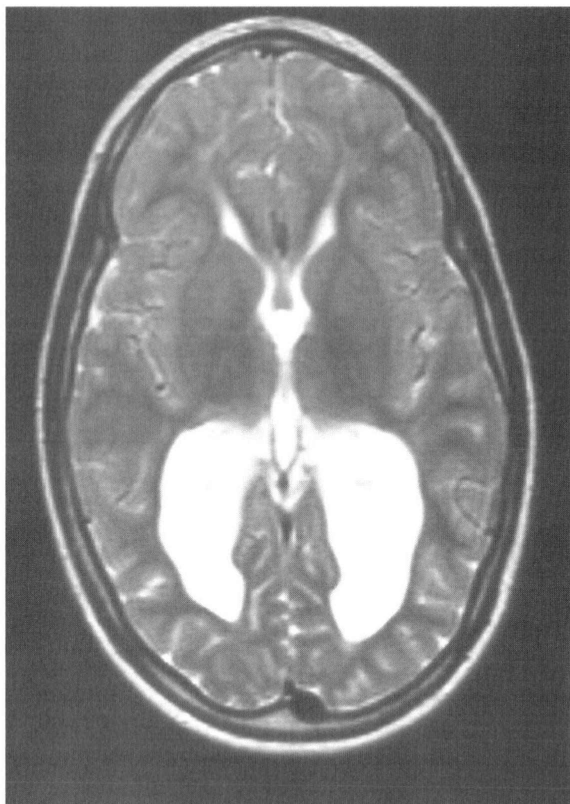

Fig. 4.8. Axial T_2-weighted MRI showing loss of periventricular white matter, with scalloping of the ventricular margin in a child with cerebral palsy.

such as punctate white matter abnormalities, which so far are of uncertain significance.[18,19]

Periventricular leukomalacia is not related so tightly to gestational age as GMH–IVH, and the underlying mechanism of damage to the myelin precursor cells is likely to be different.[20] Recently, several groups have observed that preterm prolonged rupture of membranes and chorioamnionitis increase the risk of cystic lesions appearing during the neonatal period and subsequent cerebral palsy.[21] Much periventricular leukomalacia is acquired postnatally, although perinatal hypoxia–ischemia is undoubtedly a risk factor. Recent studies attest to the protective effect of antenatal steroids, and the adverse effect of postnatal hypocarbia. Intuitively, hypotension has long been thought to be important, and although there is surprisingly little hard evidence some support for this logical hypothesis has emerged.[22] Neonatal intensive care should aim to support blood pressure, avoid acidosis and maintain blood gases, electrolyte levels, and glucose within the normal range.

Early neonatal encephalopathy

The neonatal brain is remarkably resistant to hypoxia ischemia; 10–20 minutes of total circulatory arrest or more than an hour of partial hypoxia are required for damage to occur.[23] Resuscitation of infants who are fresh stillbirths at term can be followed by normal survival, although this becomes unlikely if the circulation is not restored by 10 minutes and/or spontaneous respiration does not occur after 20 minutes. Seizures are the hallmark of encephalopathy, and are seen in the reperfusion phase, 12–48 hours after birth. There are other causes of neonatal seizures apart from hypoxic ischemia, including drug withdrawal, arterial infarction (stroke) and meningitis.[24] Hypoxic–ischemic encephalopathy is the most common cause of seizure in term infants, and this diagnosis is likely if there is a combination of fetal distress, birth depression, cerebral edema on cranial imaging, and evidence of renal or cardiac dysfunction. Grading systems for encephalopathy are helpful in determining prognosis, but basically the presence of seizures means that hypoxic–ischemic encephalopathy is at least moderate (grade II). The risk of sequelae following grade II hypoxic–ischemic encephalopathy is 25%; if the baby becomes comatose, the risk of death or handicap is almost 100%. The adverse prognosis of moderate or severe hypoxic–ischemic encephalopathy has led to the exclusion of such infants, and sometimes those who have required CPR, from many ECMO programs. EEG and MRI are useful in assessing the risk of disability and counselling parents, and can be invaluable when difficult decisions have to be faced regarding the likely prognosis in a complex case where perinatal hypoxia–ischemia was present.

Long-term outcomes

Overview of disabilities in children

When considering the long-term prognosis of cohorts of children, be it ex-preterm babies, those who have suffered from hypoxic–ischemic encephalopathy, or surgically operated newborns, it is important to compare their situation to groups of children who did not have any neonatal problems. Unfortunately, definitions of which children should be classified as disabled varies enormously, and this makes summarizing the outcome literature very difficult. The World Health Organization has tried to reduce confusion by introducing definitions for the terms impairment, disability and handicap (Table 4.3). Recently, several committees have tried to define a standard minimum national/European dataset for outcome at 2 years, and if

Table 4.3. World Health Organisation definitions of impairment, disability and handicap

Impairment

- any loss or abnormality of psychological, physiological or anatomical structure, or function: in principle, impairments represent disturbances at organ level.

Disability

- any restriction or lack (resulting from an impairment) of ability to perform an activity in the manner or within the range considered normal for a human being. A disability thus reflects the consequence of an impairment in terms of functional performance and activity by an individual.

Handicap

- a disadvantage for a given individual resulting from an impairment or disability that limits or prevents the fulfilment of a role that is normal (depending on age, sex, and social and cultural factors). Handicap thus reflects interaction with the surroundings and is a difficult outcome to use for comparison as it depends on attitudes within the family and society to disability.

one of these systems is eventually adopted interpretation of outcome studies will be considerably improved. Suggested examples of severe disabilities at two years of age include being unable to sit unsupported, being unable to use the hands for feeding, responding to light only, requiring hearing aids, and requiring special feeding provision such as total parenteral nutrition or gastrostomy feeds. The number of children who are dependent on technology (ventilators, home oxygen, overnight pump feeds) in the long term has increased considerably in recent years.

The burden of disability and illness in childhood is surprisingly high. The prevalence of disability is not measured regularly at a national level in the UK, so it is not possible to monitor trends. The Office of National Statistics has produced several reports on the health of children and young people, the most recent of which is available as a web publication from the ONS website. This report analyzed the census data of 1991 and 2001, together with the results of the General Household Survey: the previous study reported on a survey of disability conducted between 1985 and 1986. Seventeen percent of children are now reported to have "long standing illness or disability," with around 1 per 1000 "severely disabled". In 2002, 5% of boys aged 0–4 years and 3% of girls were reported as having a "limiting long-standing illness." There are quite wide ethnic variations in childhood disability rates, from around 1.5% in the Black African and Black Caribbean groups to 0.6% in the white population. The most common reported severe disability is autistic spectrum disorder, with cerebral palsy in second place (asthma is the commonest mild disability).

Outcomes for ex-preterm children by each week of gestation from recent studies are presented in Fig. 4.9. Increasing numbers of VLBW infants are now offered intensive care and, whilst there has been a large net gain of normal survivors, there has also been an increase in the absolute number of disabled survivors. Low birthweight infants now comprise about 50% of all cases of cerebral palsy,[25] an alarming trend which gives no room for complacency about the results of neonatal intensive care.

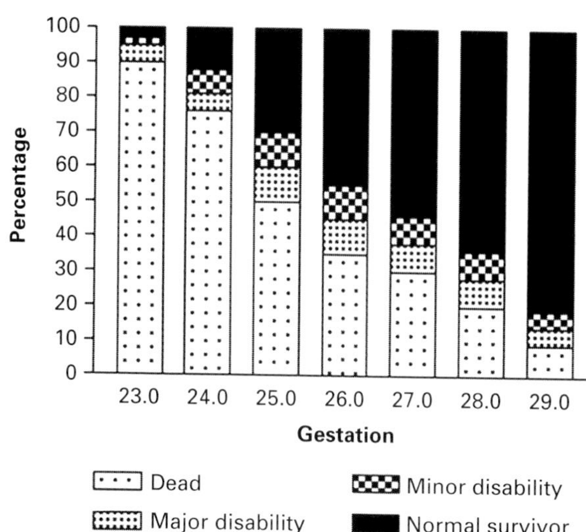

Fig. 4.9. Histogram of disability rates by each week of gestation, compiled from various sources.

Cerebral palsy

Definition and types

Cerebral palsy is usually defined as a non-progressive permanent impairment of voluntary movement or posture due to damage to the developing brain. Cerebral palsy can involve one limb (monoplegia) or all four (quadriplegia). When both lower limbs are involved, the term diplegia is used. Cerebral palsy was diagnosed at the age of 2 years in 7.9% of a geographical cohort of over a thousand

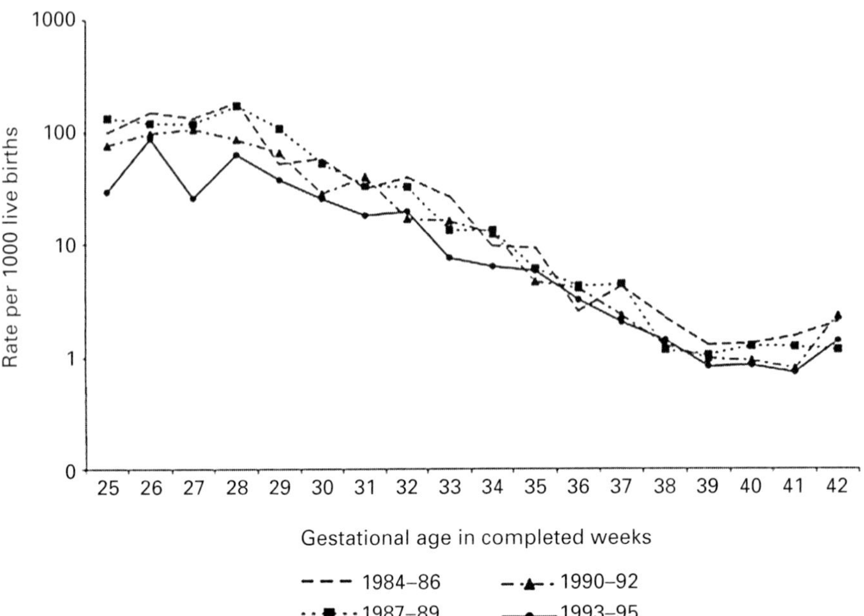

Fig. 4.10. Graph showing the incidence of cerebral palsy by gestational age and year of birth. With permission from Surman *et al.*[32]

children whose birthweight was less than 2 kg,[26] and the figure remains around 10% in most ex-preterm cohorts.[27]

Birthweight specific prevalence

There are several ongoing registers of cerebral palsy around the world, which make it possible to examine trends over time for this condition, and there is now a European collaboration as well as a network for the UK registers (UKCP; website address www.liv.ac.uk/PublicHealth/ukcp/UKCP.html). Time trends show that the prevalence of cerebral palsy is increasing,[25,28] and is currently about 2 per 1000 in Europe. The prevalence of cerebral palsy amongst survivors of birthweight >2500 g born in England and Scotland between 1984 and 1989 was 1.1 per 1000, but 10.2 per 1000 live births amongst those born weighing between 1500 and 2500 g, and 78.1 per 1000 in survivors of birthweight less than 1 kg.[28] These figures are in remarkable agreement with those from the Western Australia register of cerebral palsy, a large geographical cerebral palsy register in California, and a population-based register in Atlanta.[29–31] Recent studies show a welcome fall in the incidence in the smallest babies, and UK regional data show that after the peak prevalence of 90 per 1000 was reached for the group weighing less than 1 kg at birth (in 1987), the rate was 57 per 1000 by 1993–95, and 40 per 1000 for the 1–1.5 kg group, representing a fall in incidence at each week of gestation (Fig. 4.10).[32]

Risk factors

Perinatal asphyxia, mode of delivery

Amongst normal birthweight survivors, the incidence of cerebral palsy remains constant at 1–2 per 1000. In this group about 10%–15% have evidence of intrapartum asphyxia. Children with cerebral palsy were more likely to have multiple late decelerations or loss of beat to beat variability on a cardiotocograph in labour than those who did not, but the false positive rate for this finding was 99.8%.[33] Cesarean section without labor (elective cesarean section) is associated with a reduced incidence of cerebral palsy, but there may be unidentified differences between the babies of mothers who labor and those who do not. The dramatic rise in cesarean section delivery since the 1970s has not resulted in any fall in the overall incidence of cerebral palsy (Fig. 4.11).[34] Breech presentation is associated with an increased risk of cerebral palsy whether or not a cesarean section delivery is carried out, but few obstetricians now conduct vaginal breech delivery if this malpresentation is diagnosed antenatally, following the results of the Term Breech Trial.[35]

Multiple births

There is an increased incidence of cerebral palsy in twins and higher order multiple pregnancies. The risk for twins is 8–12 per 1000 with a risk of 44–71 per 1000 for triplets.[36] A particularly high risk (up to 100 in 1000) exists for a sole twin survivor, and there is a great deal of interest in the

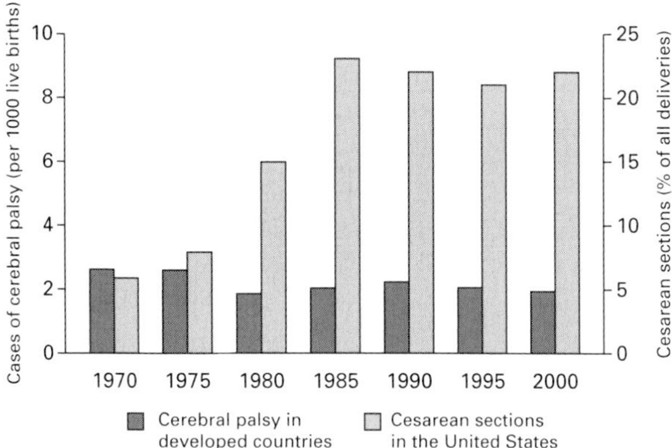

Fig. 4.11. The cesarean section rate related to the prevalence of cerebral palsy. From Nelson[34] with permission.

possibility that "vanishing twins" are important in the etiology of cerebral palsy.[37,38] Following the introduction of legislation in the UK, which limited the number of eggs or embryos which could be transferred during a single cycle to a maximum of two to women under 40 years, there has been a dramatic and welcome reduction in the incidence of triplet and higher-order births in England and Wales, a decline of one quarter.[39] The number of twins continues to rise. About 40% of IVF babies are born as twins compared to about 2% of all births, and twins contribute about 25% of cases to VLBW infant cohorts. An IVF twin's chance of adverse neurological sequelae is the same as their naturally conceived twin peers; in other words, higher than for singletons but with no extra risk conferred by the mode of conception.[40]

IUGR

There does not appear to be an increased risk of cerebral palsy in very preterm infants (less than 31 weeks) who were small for gestational age, although IUGR is known to be a risk factor for this condition in more mature infants.[41]

Perinatal sepsis

Cytokine damage from the inflammatory cascade associated with perinatal sepsis is a current "hot" theory for perinatal brain damage both in term and preterm babies, with support from epidemiologic and basic scientific studies.[21,42–44] This pathway may explain the long-observed link between surgery, particularly for necrotizing enterocolitis, and adverse outcome in preterm babies.[45]

In summary, the risk factors for cerebral palsy are:

- prematurity, especially with ultrasound evidence of periventricular leukomalacia
- prolonged rupture of membranes and chorioamnionitis, perinatal and postnatal sepsis
- hypotension, hypocarbia in preterms
- twinning and higher multiple pregnancies, especially death of a co-twin and twin-to-twin transfusion syndrome *in utero*
- IUGR in infants above 32 weeks' gestation
- intrapartum asphyxia
- breech presentation persisting at term.

Visual handicap

VLBW survivors are at increased risk of long-term visual impairment. The risk is particularly great in those who develop retinopathy of prematurity. An accurate figure for severe visual loss is difficult to ascertain but a rough calculation would suggest that some 5% of infants of birthweight below 1 kg are blind. Perhaps a similar percentage have severely impaired vision. Retinopathy of prematurity is not the only cause of poor visual outcome; cortical blindness can result from damage to the occipital cortex associated with periventricular leukomalacia or optic atrophy due to hydrocephalus. Many surviving ex-preterm children have severe myopia or other refractive errors. Cryotherapy or laser coagulation for retinopathy of prematurity is a proven, effective treatment, reducing the chance of severe visual loss by a half. This means that all neonatal units must have a robust system in place for screening for the disease, because the window of opportunity for treatment is very tight.[46]

Hearing loss

Sensorineural hearing loss seems to be a particular problem in survivors of persistent pulmonary hypertension (PPHN), and high incidences (4–21%) are widely reported in this group whether or not ECMO was used.[47] Hearing aids were being worn by 14/40 term survivors of PPHN.[48] Deafness is the commonest disability in this group of children; perhaps the auditory nerve is particularly sensitive to hypoxia.

Risk factors for deafness also include low birthweight, ototoxic medications, hypoxic–ischemic encephalopathy, meningitis, hyperbilirubinemia requiring exchange transfusion, and a family history of childhood deafness.[49,50] Babies with any of these complications should be screened for hearing loss before they leave the nursery as early aiding and appropriate support can dramatically improve speech later on. Recently, it has been found that the risk of gentamicin toxicity is limited to certain individuals who carry a particular genetic mutation, and in fact huge strides have been made in the genetics of deafness. Mutations in the gene that codes for the connexin protein can now be identified as the cause of deafness in many individuals – about half of the cases with severe congenital hearing impairment.[51]

School performance

Cognitive impairment is a more common adverse outcome than cerebral palsy after preterm birth.[27,52] School failure is likely when a child has language delay, poor concentration, borderline intelligence, parents of low social class, and/or a specific learning deficit. The IQ in 10-year-old ex-VLBW children is shifted down about one standard deviation, or around 10–15 IQ points, when compared to controls.[27,52] An effect of this magnitude is also seen between social class I and social class V and these differences act as confounders in any such study. Even with an IQ in the normal range, the VLBW survivor is more likely to require special educational provision. The chief factors predicting a need for special education resources in VLBW survivors are neonatal sepsis, low socioeconomic status and non-white race. Being small for dates (SFD) also has a significant impact on school performance, and a quarter of a cohort of such babies born in 1985 were failing at school aged 10, compared to 14% of children who had been appropriate for gestational age.[53] The effect of being small for gestational age on later cognitive outcome has been known and debated for years; the SFD survivors of the British Birth cohort (1970) were less likely to have professional or managerial jobs but were mostly married and pronounced themselves satisfied with life.[54] The same good self-esteem ratings are reported for teenage ex-preterm children (see below). Increasingly, long-term outcome studies will include assessments of quality of life made by the individuals affected.

Psychiatric outcomes

More low birthweight children are described as fidgety at school, and formal psychiatric assessment reveals a higher incidence of attention deficit/hyperactivity disorder than in controls.[52] Poor motor coordination, manual dexterity and balance, short attention span, and visual impairment all tend to be present in the same individual and together significantly impair the child's ability to function in school. Problems with "executive functioning" are reported and these affect an individual's ability to organize their life. Clumsiness may contribute to low self-esteem and bad behaviour; it remains to be seen whether early identification and intervention can improve the rather dismal outlook and achievements for this group. Having drawn attention to the many problems faced by ex-preterm children, Hack points out that their self-rated quality of life scores are better than might be expected, and as teenagers the cohort are less likely to run into trouble with the law than their peers.[52]

Cognitive deficits in term infants who required neonatal intensive care

There is much less information available on the school performance and later outcome of term born children who were ill enough to require intensive care than for those born preterm. Most of the studies are limited to specific diagnoses. For example, amongst one of the very sickest groups (ECMO treated infants with congenital diaphragmatic hernia), about a quarter have significant neurodevelopmental problems. More information on this topic is badly needed in order to counsel parents appropriately about expected outcomes of neonatal intensive care.

Chronic lung disease

Gentler ventilation strategies and the increased use of surfactant have not abolished chronic lung disease in ex-preterm babies. Indeed, as the percentage who survive has increased, the absolute number with chronic lung disease has also risen, although the rate remained the same in the 1990s.[56] Chronic lung disease in this population is probably best defined as a requirement for oxygen beyond 36 weeks' gestational age equivalent, and these rates are currently around 30%. Most of these babies eventually do well, even if they are discharged home in oxygen. Abnormal lung function can persist for years, but usually resolves by 8–10 years. Death can occur from cardiac or respiratory failure, or infection. In this respect, the annual winter epidemics of respiratory syncytial virus pose a real threat to the group discharged home on oxygen, and for these babies prophylaxis with palivizumab is justified. Palivizumab is a monoclonal antibody preparation directed against the F glycoprotein of RSV and has been the subject of intense research. It is expensive, has to be given as a course of five injections, and is moderately but not completely effective (55% reduction in hospital admissions).

A very small number of babies are discharged home not only on oxygen, but also requiring artificial ventilation or with a tracheotomy. These children contribute to the growing population of children who are dependent on technology worldwide. There are few UK (or international) data on the size of this population, but UK Government statistics show that respiratory disorders are responsible for 50% of this group. Wallis identified 136 children who were dependent on long-term ventilation in the UK in 1999, 93 of whom were at home and 43 of whom were attending mainstream school.[57] Worldwide, the diagnoses in this group are myopathy, the effects of hypoxic–ischemic encephalopathy, spinal muscular atrophy type 1 (Werdnig–Hoffman disease), chronic lung disease of prematurity, and Ondine's curse. Babies with congenital diaphragmatic hernia or an abdominal wall defect occasionally have non-lethal but nevertheless limiting pulmonary hypoplasia and can contribute to this group.

Economic aspects

There have been numerous publications relating to the cost of neonatal intensive care, many of the most useful emerging from Australia.[58] Doyle has found that neonatal intensive care in Australia has become more efficient over time. The total costs of care to age 9 for a surviving low birthweight child are five times those for a larger child.[59] For those with disability, the costs were much higher, and these authors predicted that the costs of long-term care and special education will far outweigh the cost of the initial neonatal intensive care for this group.[60] By 9 years the cost of special education and care for the 52 disabled children (over £1 million in 1979 prices) represented 52% of the total medical costs for this cohort of 944 children of birthweight <2 kg.

Saigal and his colleagues in Ontario have tackled the enormously difficult problem of scoring quality of life for children, demonstrating that ELBW survivors have a worse score than those of normal birthweight.[61,62] Examples from these studies illustrate the complexity but also the importance of this type of utility analysis: a child with limited ambulation because of hemiplegia who was generally happy and had normal self-care abilities scored 0.82 (1.0 = perfect health); 14% of the index children and half the controls had a perfect score of 1; and a child who was blind, had spastic quadriplegia, was totally dependent, and often fretful and irritable scored 0.09 (0 = death). This utility score requires further validation before it can be used to compare the outcome of neonatal intensive care to other treatment programs. Attempts so far, using quality-adjusted-life-years rather than full cost-utility analysis, place neonatal intensive care on an equivalent cost basis to coronary artery bypass grafting and antepartum anti-D prophylaxis, all of which are considerably cheaper than hemodialysis.

Medico-legal aspects

The last decade has seen an explosion in personal injury litigation, a great number of the cases being brought by parents on behalf of their children. All children in the UK are entitled to legal aid, so that a second opinion on the standard of treatment offered to their child is free to parents. The stakes are very high because the lifetime costs of care for disabled people are so great (see above), and health service provision is often poor. Typical cerebral palsy settlements are of the order of £4 million. The UK NHS Litigation Authority paid out £446 million in 2001/2, of which 60% was in settlement of cerebral palsy claims, although these formed only 6% of the number of claims. The Litigation Authority handles about 400 new cerebral palsy claims each year.

Adult patients of sound mind must issue their writs in respect of personal injuries within 3 years. This time span starts to run when an adult realizes that they have sustained a significant injury and they think they know that it was caused by the person they wish to sue; they do not need to know that the injury was caused by negligence. The difficulty for the pediatrician, or pediatric surgeon, is that time does not run against the child under 18 years, or any patient with a disability at all. Thus, the survivor of a neonatal disaster has the right to issue a writ at any time prior to their twenty-first birthday. Even where an individual has failed to sue promptly on achieving his or her majority, the Court may still (and usually does) exercise discretion to extend the time. If an individual never becomes capable of managing their own affairs, and therefore is regarded by law as laboring under a disability, that individual's right to sue continues throughout their life and endures for the benefit of their estate until 3 years after their death. This means that neonatal notes should be kept for a very long time, perhaps 80 years.

Although the largest settlements are for cerebral palsy in mature infants, with negligence usually alleged against their mother's obstetrician, an increasing number of ex-preterm children with cerebral palsy are also pursuing litigation. These cases are often complex and involve assessing the standard of intensive care delivered over many months. The best, and only, line of defence is a good and meticulous standard of notekeeping. Frequently the problem is not one of the standard of care, but of communication. Smaller claims are frequently sought and settled out of court for scars and other cosmetic defects. Extravasation of infusions is inevitable, but careful observation of infusion and drain sites can limit the damage.

REFERENCES

1. Draper, E. S., Manktelow, B., Field, D. J., & James, D. Tables for predicting survival for preterm births are updated. *Br. Med. J.* 2003; **327**:872.

2. Wood, N. S., Marlow, N., Costeloe, K., Gibson, A. T., & Wilkinson, A. R. Neurologic and developmental disability after extremely preterm birth. *N. Engl. J. Med.* 2000; **343**(6):378–384.
3. Rennie, J. M. Perinatal management at the lower margin of viability. *Arch. Dis. Child.* 1996; **74**:214–218.
4. Synnes, A. R., Ling, E. W., Whitfield, M. F. *et al.* Perinatal outcomes of a large cohort of extremely low gestational age infants (23–28 completed weeks of gestation). *J. Pediatr.* 1994; **125**:952–960.
5. Lemons, J. A., Bauer, C. R., Oh, W. *et al.* Very low birth weight outcomes of the national institute of child health and human development neonatal research network, January 1995 through December 1996. *Pediatrics* 2001; **107**(1):e1–e8.
6. International Neonatal Network. The CRIB (clinical risk index for babies) score: a tool for assessing initial neonatal risk and comparing performance of neonatal intensive care units. *Lancet* 1993; **342**:193–198.
7. Parry, G., Tucker, J., & Tarnow-Mordi, W. Crib II: an update of the clinical risk index for babies score. *Lancet* 2003; **361**:1789–1791.
8. O'Donnell, A. L., Gray, P. H., & Rogers, Y. M. Mortality and neurodevelopmental outcome for infants receiving adrenaline in neonatal resuscitation. *J. Paediatr. Child. Health* 1998; **34**:551–556.
9. Sims, D. G., Heal, C. A., & Bartle, S. M. Use of adrenaline and atropine in neonatal resuscitation. *Arch. Dis. Child.* 1994; **70**:f3–f10.
10. Jain, L., Ferre, C., Vidyasagar, D., Nath, S., & Sheffel, D. Cardiopulmonary resuscitation of apparently stillborn infants. *J. Pediatr.* 1991; **118**:778–782.
11. Morrison, J. J., Rennie, J. M., & Milton, P. J. Neonatal respiratory morbidity and mode of delivery at term: influence of timing of elective caesarean section. *Br. J. Obstet. Gynaecol.* 1995; **102**:101–106.
12. Rennie, J. M. *Neonatal Cerebral Ultrasound.* 1st edn. Cambridge: Cambridge University Press; 1997.
13. Debillon, T., N'Guyen, S., Quere, M. P., Moussaly, F., & Roze, J. C. Limitations of ultrasonography for diagnosing white matter damage in preterm infants. *Arch. Dis. Child.* 2003; **88**(4):275–279.
14. de Vries, L. S., van Haastert, I. L., Rademaker, K. J., Koopman, C., & Groenendaal, F. Ultrasound abnormalities preceding cerebral palsy in high risk preterm infants. *J. Pediatr.* 2004; **144**:815–820.
15. Vollmer, B., Roth, S., Baudin, J., Stewart, A. L., Neville, B. G. R., & Wyatt, J. S. Predictors of long-term outcome in very preterm infants: gestational age versus neonatal cranial ultrasound. *Pediatrics* 2003; **112**:1108–1114.
16. Fujimoto, S., Togari, H., Takashima, S. *et al.* National survey of periventricular leukomalacia in Japan. *Acta. Paediatr. Jpn* 1998; **40**:239–243.
17. Resch, B., Vollaard, E., Maurer, U., Haas, J., Rosegger, H., & Muller, W. Risk factors and determinants of neurodevelopmental outcome in cystic periventricular leucomalacia. *Eur. J. Pediatr.* 2000; **159**:663–670.
18. Counsell, S. J., Allsop, J. M., Harrison, M. C. *et al.* Diffusion-weighted imaging of the brain in preterm infants with focal and diffuse white matter abnormality. *Pediatrics* 2003; **112**(1):1–7.
19. Cornette, L. G., Tanner, S. F., Ramenghi, L. A. *et al.* Magnetic resonance imaging of the infant brain: anatomical characteristics and clinical significance of punctate lesions. *Arch. Dis. Child.* 2002; **86**(3):171–177.
20. Volpe, J. J. Neurobiology of periventricular leukomalacia in the premature infant. *Pediatr. Res.* 2001; **50**:553–562.
21. Nelson, K. B., Grether, J. K., Damabrosia, J. M. *et al.* Neonatal cytokines and cerebral palsy in very preterm infants. *Pediatr. Res.* 2003; **53**:600–607.
22. Dammann, O., Allred, E. N., Kuban, K. C. K. *et al.* Systemic hypotension and white-matter damage in preterm infants. *Dev. Med. Child. Neurol.* 2002; **44**:82–90.
23. Myers, R. E. Four patterns of perinatal brain damage and their occurrence in primates. *Adv. Neurol.* 1975; **10**:223–224.
24. Rennie, J. M. Seizures in the newborn. In *Textbook of Neonatology*, 3rd edn. ed. J. M. Rennie and N. R. C. Robertson, Edinburgh: Churchill Livingstone; 1999. pp. 1213–1223.
25. Colver, A. F., Gibson, M., Hey, E. N., Jarvis, S. N., Mackie, P. C., & Richmond, S. Increasing rates of cerebral palsy across the severity spectrum in north-east England 1964–1993. *Arch. Dis. Child.* 2000; **83**(1):F7–F12.
26. Pinto-Martin, J. A., Riolo, S., Cnaan, A., Holzman, C., Susser, M. W., & Paneth, N. Cranial ultrasound prediction of disabling and nondisabling cerebral palsy at age two in a low birth weight population. *Pediatrics* 1995; **95**:249–254.
27. Marlow, N. Neurocognitive outcome after very preterm birth. *Arch. Dis. Child* 2004; **89**(3):224–228.
28. Pharoah, P. O. D., Cooke, T., Johnson, M. A., King, R., & Mutch, L. Epidemiology of cerebral palsy in England and Scotland 1984–1989. *Arch. Dis. Child.* 1998; **79**:F21–F25.
29. Stanley, F. J. & Watson, F. Trends in perinatal mortality and cerebral palsy in Western Australia 1967–1985. *Br. Med. J.* 1992; **304**:1658–1663.
30. Cummins, S. K., Nelson, K. B., Grether, J. K., & Velie, E. M. Cerebral palsy in four northern Californian counties: births 1983 through 1985. *J. Pediatr.* 1993; **123**:230–237.
31. Winter, S., Autry, A., Boyle, C., & Yeargin-Allsopp, M. Trends in the prevalence of cerebral palsy in a population-based study. *Pediatrics* 2002; **110**:1220–1225.
32. Surman, G., Newdick, H., & Johnson, A. Cerebral palsy rates among low-birthweight infants fell in the 1990s. *Dev. Med. Child. Neurol.* 2003; **45**:456–462.
33. Nelson, K. B., Dambrosia, J. M., Ting, T. Y., & Grether, J. K. Uncertain value of electronic fetal monitoring in predicting cerebral palsy. *N. Engl. J. Med.* 1996; **334**:613–618.
34. Nelson, K. B. Can we prevent cerebral palsy? *N. Engl. J. Med.* 2003; **349**:1765–1770.
35. Hannah, M. E., Hannah, W. J., Hewson, S. A., Hodnett, E. D., Saigal, S., & Willian, A. R. Planned caesarean section versus planned vaginal birth for breech presentation at term: a randomised mulicentre trial. *Lancet* 2000; **356**:1375–1383.

36. Petterson, B., Nelson, K. B., Watson, L., & Stanley, F. Twins, triplets, and cerebral palsy in Western Australia in the 1980s. *Br. Med. J.* 1993; **307**:1239–1243.
37. Pharoah, P. O. D., Price, T. S., & Plomin, R. Cerebral palsy in twins: a national study. *Arch. Dis. Child.* 2002; **87**(2):122–124.
38. Pharoah, P. O. D. Cerebral palsy in the surviving twin associated with infant death of the co-twin. *Arch. Dis. Child.* 2001; **84**:f111–f116.
39. Simmons, R., Doyle, P., Maconochie, N. Dramatic reduction in triplet and higher order births in England and Wales. *Br. J. Obstet. Gyn.* 2004; **111**:856–858.
40. Pinborg, A., Loft, A., Greisen, G., Rasmussen, S., & Andersen, A. N. Neurological sequelae in twins born after assisted conception: controlled national cohort study. *Br. Med. J.* 2004; **329**:311–314.
41. Blair, E. & Stanley, F. Intrauterine growth and spastic cerebral palsy. *Am. J. Obstet. Gynecol.* 1990; **162**:229–237.
42. Nelson, K. B. & Willoughby, R. E. Infection, inflammation and the risk of cerebral palsy. *Curr. Opin. Neurol.* 2000; **13**:133–139.
43. Wu, Y. W. & Colford, J. M. Chorioamnionitis as a risk factor for cerebral palsy. *J. Am. Med. Assoc.* 2000; **284**(11):1417–1424.
44. Damman, O., Kuban, K. C. K., & Leviton, A. Perinatal infection, fetal infllammatory response, white matter damage, and cognitive limitations in children born preterm. *Ment. Retard. Dev. Disabil. Res. Rev.* 2002; 46–50.
45. Perrott, S., Dodds, L., & Vincer, M. A population-based study of prognostic factors related to major disability in very preterm survivors. *J. Perinatol.* 2003; **23**:111–116.
46. Fleck, B. W. Therapy for retinopathy of prematurity. *Lancet* 1999; **353**:166–168.
47. Cheung, P.-Y., Haluschak, M. M., Finer, N. N., & Robertson, C. M. T. Sensorineural hearing loss in survivors of neonatal extracorporeal membrane oxygenation. *Early Hum. Dev.* 1996; **44**:225–233.
48. Hendricks-Munoz, K. D. Hearing loss in infants with persistent fetal circulation. *Pediatrics* 1988; **81**:650–656.
49. Newton, V. Adverse perinatal conditions and the inner ear. *Semin. Neonatol.* 2001; **6**:543–541.
50. Marlow, E. S., Hunt, L. P., & Marlow, N. Sensorineural hearing loss and prematurity. *Arch. Dis. Child.* 2000; **82**(2):F141–F144.
51. Tekin, M., Arnos, K. S., & Pandya, A. Advances in hereditary deafness. *Lancet* 2001; **358**:1082–1090.
52. Bhutta, A. T., Cleves, M. A., Casey, P. H., Cradock, M. M., & Anand, K. J. S. Cognitive and behavioral outcomes of school age children who were born preterm. *J. Am. Med. Assoc.* 2002; **288**(728):737.
53. Hollo, O., Rautavana, P., Korhonen, T., Helenius, H., Kero, P., & Sillanpaa, M. Academic achievement of small for gestational age children at age 10 years. *Arch. Pediat. Adolesc. Med.* 2002; **156**:179–187.
54. Strauss, R. S. Adult functional outcome of those born small for gestational age. *J. Am. Med. Assoc.* 2000; **283**:625–632.
55. Hack, M. Outcomes in young adulthood for very low birth weight infants. *N. Engl. J. Med.* 2002; **346**:149–157.
56. Manktelow, B. N., Draper, E. S., Annamalai, S., & Field, D. Factors affecting the incidence of chronic lung disease of prematurity in 1987, 1992, and 1997. *Arch. Dis. Child.* 2001; **85**(1):f33–f35.
57. Jardine, E., O'Toole, M., paton, J. Y., & Wallis, C. Current status of long term ventilation of children in the United Kingdom: questionnaire survey. *Br. Med. J.* 1999; **318**:295–299.
58. Doyle, L. W. Evaluation of neonatal intensive care for extremely low birth weight infants in Victoria over two decades: I. effectiveness. *Pediatrics* 2004; **113**(3):505–509.
59. Stevenson, R. C., McCabe, C. J., & Pharoah, P. O. D. Cost of care for a geographically determined population of low birth weight infants to age 8–9 years. I. Children without disability. *Arch. Dis. Child.* 1996; **74**:F114–F117.
60. Stevenson, R. C., Pharoah, P. O. D., Stevenson, C. J., Cooke, R. W. I. cost of care for a geographically determined population of low birthweight infants to age 8–9 years. II: Children with disability. *Arch. Dis. Child.* 1996; **74**:F118–F121.
61. Saigal, S. Comprehensive assesment of the health status of elbw children at 8 years: comparison with a reference group. *J. Pediatr.* 1994; **125**:411–424.
62. Saigal, S., Feeny, D., Rosenbaum, P., Furlong, W., Burrows, E., & Stoskopf, B. Self-perceived health status and health-related quality of life of extremely low birth weight infants at adolescence. *J. Am. Med. Assoc.* 1996; **276**:453–459.

5

Psychological aspects of pediatric surgery

Lorraine Ludman

Institute of Child Health and Great Ormond Street Hospital for Children, London, UK

Introduction

As a result of major advances in all branches of pediatric care there have been considerable improvements in survival and physical health of children following pediatric surgery. Follow-up of pediatric surgical patients has, understandably, concentrated on physical or functional outcome, whereas interest in psychological and social sequelae is relatively recent. Conditions requiring pediatric surgery vary along a continuum from acute short-term problems requiring minor surgery, to those requiring major life-threatening surgery. This chapter is primarily concerned with the long-term psychological and social sequelae of conditions requiring major surgery.

The chapter is divided into four sections. The first focuses briefly on methodological issues in psychological research. The second addresses the effects of hospitalization and children's responses to hospitalization. The third section reviews studies of long-term psychological outcomes and the relationship to chronic health problems. Finally, issues arising from the previous sections are discussed.

Methodological issues

Study design

Good psychosocial adjustment in children has been described as being "reflected in behavior that is age-appropriate, normative and healthy and that follows a trajectory towards positive adult functioning".[1] The ideal way to assess long-term psychosocial outcomes is by prospective longitudinal studies. They are unique in their ability to determine the best causal relationship between early and later behavior, and they offer the possibility of studying whether specific risk factors lead to different outcomes, whether the effects are immediate or delayed, whether the effects persist over time and whether they are modified by intervening variables. Another advantage of prospective research is the avoidance of retrospective data. However, longitudinal studies are difficult to conduct for many reasons. They are immensely time consuming and costly, and require the continuing commitment of the patients, their families and the researcher. Consequently, most follow-up studies assessing long-term outcomes use a cross-sectional design.

Assessment measures

In-depth semi-structured interviews using well-validated interview schedules, and carried out by an experienced psychologist, trained in the techniques of obtaining information from children and adults without intimidating them, provide the most relevant data. Where possible, parents and children should be interviewed separately. The addition of standardized self-report questionnaires allows comparisons with population norms and between groups of children with different health problems. The measures most often used are the Achenbach Child Behaviour Checklists.[2–5] These questionnaires have parallel forms for completion by the child, parents, and teachers, thereby providing information about how the patient is perceived within different settings and from different viewpoints. There are also sound standardized psychometric measures for the assessment of self-esteem and depressive symptoms.

Assessments of quality of life (QoL) are an important development in the study of the link between physical and

Pediatric Surgery and Urology: Long-term Outcomes, Mark Stringer, Keith Oldham, Pierre Mouriquand.

psychological health. They allow greater emphasis on the effects on the "whole child" rather than focusing on behavioral outcomes. Unfortunately, those currently available are limited, and few fulfil basic psychometric criteria.[6]

Many potentially intervening variables in the child's environment must also be assessed. These include family circumstances (SES), parental mental health, marital/family adjustment or conflict, family support or cohesiveness and quality and style of parenting behaviors.

Problems with assessment measurements

- Patients' self-reports may be influenced by social desirability.
- Responses during interviews may be colored in order to please the medical staff.
- Children and parents do not necessarily share views about the impact of illness on their lives.
- A child's ability to use self-report rating scales may be limited by age and cognitive development.
- Parental ratings of child adjustment and QoL may be as much a measure of the parent–child relationship as an objective measure of behavior in the child. Parents' responses may be influenced by their mental health, their educational levels and any stress factors.

Effects of hospitalization and separation

Historical background

Towards the end of the 19th century, possibly influenced by the new understanding of the spread of infectious disease, parental access to children in hospital was restricted, and sometimes no physical contact was permitted. Distress was initially categorized as an unavoidable feature of hospitalization, and it was not until the 1930s and 1940s that newer appreciation of the emotional development and needs in childhood fueled concern about this problem. The publication in 1951 of John Bowlby's WHO Monograph on "maternal deprivation" and his later writings on the importance of the attachment relationship between mother and child (1958, 1969) were key milestones in the debate on hospital visiting regimes, which eventually led to major improvements in the care of young children in hospital. Others, for example, Levy (1945) in the USA, also contributed to worries about the adverse effects of hospitalization and surgery on children. A British governmental enquiry into conditions for children in hospital led to the publication of the Platt report in 1959, which formed the basis for changes in the British health system, and subsequently in other countries. Recommendations included allowing parents to stay with their children, and the provision of school and recreational play during admission.[7]

Research data

Early studies on the effects of hospitalization on young children showed that, between 6 months and 4 years of age, children were most likely to demonstrate short-term emotional and behavioral problems during admission. Separation from parents and family, combined with the strange environment and a lack of opportunity to form new attachments, seemed to be the cause of the children's acute distress.[8] Short-term post-hospital behavioral disturbances, especially in children under 5 or 6 years of age, were also reported. Evidence for long-term effects of hospitalization came from two longitudinal cohort studies, which showed that preschool hospitalization was associated with behavioral difficulties and poor educational attainment in later childhood and adolescence.[9,10] Both studies suggested that later disturbance was associated with admissions lasting for more than a week and with repeat hospital admissions. The association was shown to be especially marked among children from disadvantaged homes. Support for these findings came from the 1970 British Births Cohort study, which found an association between the length of preschool hospitalization and educational attainment, and also behavior at 10 years of age.[11]

Hospitalization's effects during the first 6 months of life became controversial with the publication, in the 1970s and 1980s, of studies of premature babies (the most frequently hospitalized newborns) cared for in the newly set-up SCBUs or NICUs. These suggested that early separation could be harmful to the mother–infant bond. Fall out from this misleading application of Bowlby's attachment theory[12] had a powerful effect on those caring for sick newborns (and on the media, and the parents) and was, occasionally, the cause of delays in transferring infants to specialist units.

Prospective longitudinal surgical study

Babies requiring surgery were never included in these studies, and there were no data available about the effects of major neonatal surgery and newborn hospitalization. In 1982 at Great Ormond Street Hospital for Children (GOSH) in London, we began a prospective longitudinal study, which examined the psychological effects of major neonatal surgery on infants and their families.[13] The data from this research, presented below, illustrate how the study of risk factors such as very early hospitalization and/or multiple early admissions, benefits from a prospective longitudinal research design. All the "surgical" children described in the study were born at term and all needed major surgery soon after birth. A carefully matched group of healthy newborns formed the main control group.

Based on a validated observational method, and on interview data, my findings were that very early hospitalization and periods of separation did not differentiate between the case-control pairs, when the babies were 12 months old. However, by 3 years of age, difficulties in the "surgical" mother–child relationships became apparent. This was shown by the fact that the rate of behavioral disturbance was approximately two and a half times greater among the surgical children than among the control group (30% vs. 11.5%). Similarly, a higher proportion of the "surgical" mothers had an overall rating of poor parenting (again based on well-validated observational and interview methods) when compared with the control mothers (27% vs. 12%). Among the surgical group, just over a fifth of the mother–child relationships which were "secure" at the 12-month stage were problematic at 3 years – compared with 4% among the control group. The two factors associated with difficulties in the mother–child relationships were a lengthy first admission (≥25 days) and repeat hospital admissions. When a lengthy first admission was not followed by repeat admissions, none of the children had behavior problems and only one mother was rated as having poor parenting skills. It is also important to note that, at this stage, family factors such as the young age and lower educational levels of the mother, and whether the baby was her first child, contributed to the outcomes.[14] In the longer term, between 11 and 13 years of age, emotional and behavioral problems were more frequent among the surgical group than among the controls based on parent (30% vs. 17%) and teacher (21% vs. 11%) reports; and it was only in the surgical group that behavior problems at 3 years of age were significantly associated with behavior problems in early adolescence. Two-thirds of the youngsters with high scores had had repeat admissions before the age of 3 years. At this stage, family factors were no longer associated with outcomes. This suggests that, within this small heterogeneous sample of patients, surgery and repeat admissions in early childhood had long-term effects on emotional and behavioral adjustment. It could be argued that it is difficult to differentiate between the chronic nature of some medical conditions and the direct impact of repeat admissions itself. However, the design of the study enabled me to follow in detail, the health problems of each child from birth to early adolescence. Although just under a third of the children (30%) were affected by the chronic nature of their condition in their preschool years, at early adolescence only a small proportion of those included in the data analysis were regarded as having a "chronic" condition. It is interesting to note that the youngsters all rated themselves as well adjusted and, in addition, there were no differences between the groups on self-esteem and depression self-report scales. Nonetheless, they appeared to be aware that they were less competent at school than were the controls.

Surgery, hospitalization and repeat admissions also appeared to impair cognitive development over time. At 6 months of age, despite a stormy postoperative period for many of the babies, the overall development (GQ) of the surgical infants was similar to that of the healthy babies. Within the surgical group, maternal depression and total number of operations contributed significantly to outcome. At 12 months, although the surgical group's overall mean score was within the normal range, it was significantly behind that of matched controls. The main predictor of outcome was the total length of hospitalization.[15,16] At 3 years of age, based on a composite IQ score, the surgical group was again significantly behind the controls. However, within the surgical group, the children whose condition was resolved within the first few months of life were doing well and their abilities were comparable with their matched controls, while those undergoing repeat admissions and repeat operative procedures were functioning at a lower level than the other surgical children.[17] At 11 years of age the children in the surgical group were performing significantly less well than their peers by all measures of academic performance. At this age, length of hospitalization, repeat admissions and total number of operative procedures were not associated with outcome. Only one medical factor – mechanical ventilation in the neonatal period for ≥4 days – and one psychosocial measure – behavior scores at 3 years – were independent predictors of outcome for all measures of academic ability.[18]

In summary, surgery and repeat admissions in early childhood may have long term effects on emotional and behavioral adjustment. Although hospitalization and repeat admissions adversely affected cognitive development in the preschool years, this was no longer the case in early adolescence, since factors relating to the length and invasiveness of neonatal treatment procedures appeared to be more influential.

Other evidence

The psychological effects of lengthy (>3 days) or repeated hospital admissions during the so-called "sensitive" period of 6 to 36 months of age, was investigated several years after the children's last discharge from hospital ($n = 40$, mean age 36 months). Compared with children who had a single short admission ($n = 73$, mean age 58 months), the children who had a long-term single admission (4–79 days) and/or multiple admissions were reported to have a higher prevalence of behavior problems, and those who had surgery were significantly more disturbed than the rest of the group. Although the methodology of this study has its limitations, the findings offer further evidence for long-term adverse effects of early hospitalization and surgery.[19]

The only other evidence comes from studies of NICU or SCBU graduates. For the purposes of comparison with surgical neonates, these data are contaminated by the presence of a high proportion of low birth-weight and very low birth-weight babies that are now treated in these units.

Children's psychological responses to hospitalization

Developmental considerations – early stages of emotional development

Newborn period and later infancy

In the early months of life, babies will not necessarily be distressed by separation from a parent, since the emotional needs of a baby can be met by someone else (such as a pediatric nurse), who can interpret the baby's signals and respond appropriately. By 6 to 8 months, babies can discriminate familiar people from strangers, and they develop specific attachments to some – usually the parents and particularly the mother – and a strong need for proximity to the attachment figures especially in times of stress. They become fearful of strangers, especially in an unfamiliar setting. Around 15 months, babies show a peak reaction to separation from their mothers. Between 15 and 22 months, the senses of self and self-esteem are developing, and this stage of development is critical for healthy emotional development.

Second and third years

Around 2 years of age, language development advances dramatically. Recognition of the self is well established, and self-awareness becomes a central part of emotional and social life. Self-consciousness – feelings of shame, embarrassment and pride – emerge now. Children become aware of gender differences, can distinguish between right and wrong, and learn to control bodily functions. Memory, which enables a child to respond to the fear of bodily injury, develops at this stage.

End of preschool period

At this stage in development children should be able to understand simple concrete explanations of their treatment and what they might experience in hospital. Around the age of 4 or 5 years, children may be able to accept reassurance from people other than their parents, making coping with unavoidable separations from their parents somewhat easier.

Developmental considerations – timing of surgery

During the first 6 to 8 months of life a child is unlikely to be distressed, or to recall any distress associated with hospitalization and surgery. This can be extended to around 15 months if a parent can accompany the child. These developmental factors were encapsulated in the new guidelines, proposed by an action committee of the American Academy of Pediatrics Section of Urology, for the timing of urogenital surgery.[20] They recommended that, in circumstances where there is a highly skilled surgeon using child-adapted surgical techniques, and if a parent can accompany the child, the most appropriate age for any corrective surgery is between 6 and 12 months of age.

During later preschool years, reactions to hospitalization, invasive procedures, anesthesia and surgery may be especially stressful, and any verbal explanation of the treatment will be difficult. If a parent is unable to stay in hospital with the child, a surrogate attachment figure such as a personal nurse should be assigned to care for the child regularly. This is crucial. During a prolonged stay, if a child becomes familiar with a dedicated substitute carer, it may not be necessary for a parent to be present all the time. After the age of 5 or 6 years, children can usually understand that the need for surgery and hospitalization is to help them recover, and is not a punishment.

To summarize, the period between 6 and 48 months is the developmental stage most vulnerable to adverse effects of hospitalization, without implying that at other ages it is harmless.

Other factors associated with a child's responses to hospitalization and surgery

Previous medical experiences, temperament and intelligence, and ability and style of coping probably influence both the short- and long-term effects of hospitalization. A child's relationship with his or her parents, before and throughout the course of the treatment, has an important mediating effect on vulnerability to the stress of hospitalization. Children respond to parental attitudes and anxieties as much as anything that actually occurs in hospital.[21] How parents respond to a child's illness and need for hospitalization is inextricably linked with their own physical and emotional health, social circumstances and educational levels, child-rearing practices and experience of hospitals. Finally, the character of the pediatric environment is another important variable. Pediatric hospital procedures should be planned with sensitivity towards the emotional, developmental, and social needs of children; there should be no restrictions on parental access to the child; and every effort should be made to encourage collaboration between health professionals and parents to ensure the best interests of the child.

Long-term psychological effects of major pediatric surgery

Chronic physical illness

Much empirical data on the effects of chronic illness on children's development supports the belief that a disorder that makes a child "different" from other children, and persists for a significant period of time, places that child at an increased risk for behavioral and social problems, psychiatric disturbance and impaired emotional adjustment. Even mild chronic disorders have been shown to increase a child's vulnerability, and an association between physical and psychological disorders has been demonstrated.[1,22–24] Children with chronic disorders (but without brain involvement) have a two to three times greater risk for psychiatric disorder than healthy children. Various theoretical models of psychosocial adjustment have been described to try to make sense of the multiple supposed influences on adjustment in children with chronic physical conditions, but there is no simple or direct relationship between chronic physical illness and psychosocial adjustment (for a review, see Wallander 1995).[1] The psychosocial adjustment of a child is a complex phenomenon and is influenced by a multifaceted interrelationship between child and family factors.

Following surgical repair of life-threatening congenital anomalies, many children may be left with inadequately functioning internal organs and chronic physical health problems. Since repair of anomalies generally begins in the early days or months of life, these children are perceived to be "different" from birth, and, in common with children with chronic illness, this places them at an increased risk for psychosocial maladjustment. For many of these children, the primary chronic physical health problem is "hidden," and from a psychological point of view this may increase the negative impact on psychological adjustment.

Review of studies exploring the long term effects of major pediatric surgery

Well-designed outcome studies, using well-validated standardized methods of assessment, are relatively recent and few in number. Table 5.1 summarizes studies that have examined the long-term psychosocial effects of pediatric surgery for congenital abnormalities of the alimentary tract.

Anorectal malformations

A brief glance at the table will show that a significant proportion of children who require pediatric surgery are at increased risk for psychosocial dysfunction. For example, in our study at GOSH, of children with anorectal malformations (ARM) – the first to examine in detail the long-term psychosocial outcome of a large sample of such children ($n = 160$) – we found that a high proportion of the children had clinically significant emotional problems. Based on psychiatric diagnostic interviews, 29% of the children were shown to have a psychiatric disorder, with 19% having a disorder severe enough to influence their daily lives. Although one might expect a similar proportion in children with chronic illness, the prevalence of 19% was significantly higher when compared with the rate of 10% in the general child population (UK data). The parental assessment identified 27% with significant emotional and behavioral problems and 30% with high internalizing symptom scores; a high proportion of the children (24%) reported depressive symptoms, but the teachers' assessments revealed no maladjustment.[25,26] A very high proportion of the patients were found to have psychiatric disorder and psychosocial dysfunction in the two studies reported by Diseth *et al.*[27,28] However, the samples in both studies were small ($n = 10$ and $n = 33$). Contradictory findings came from the study by Hassink *et al.*, who found no evidence of behavioral maladjustment among their sample of children with ARM.[29]

All of the above studies examined the relationship between the main chronic physical health problem, fecal incontinence (FIC), and psychological disorder. In our GOSH study, for the study group overall, there was no association between psychosocial adjustment and FIC in the longer term. The psychiatric interview revealed a relatively high level of psychological disturbance among the incontinent adolescents (12–17 years) of both sexes (boys 32%; girls 21%), but it was not significantly different from the level of disturbance among the continent adolescents (boys 30%; girls 18%). The parents' and teachers' assessments agreed with these findings. In fact, the teachers and parents tended to rate the continent adolescents as more disturbed than those who were incontinent. Hassink *et al.* also found no association between the parents' and teachers' assessments of psychological disorder and FIC. These patients were still quite young (median age 5.9 years) with approximately one-third under 4 years of age. In contrast, Diseth *et al.* and Bai *et al.*[30] found that FIC correlated significantly with impairment of psychosocial function.

Hirschsprung's disease

Studies examining the relationship between FIC and psychological wellbeing among children with Hirschsprung's

Table 5.1. Summary of studies exploring long term psychological effects following surgery for congenital abnormalities

Date	Reference	Disorder	Sample size	Age range	Psychosocial outcome measures	Findings (% proportion in clinical range)
1987	Ditesheim *et al.*[43]	High anorectal malformations	61	2–24	QOL	QOL directly related to fecal continence/age
1991	Ginn-Pease *et al.*[44]	ARM and abdominal wall defects (AWD)	ARM $n = 34$ AWD $n = 22$	6–16	CBCL TFR	*18% vs. norms 10% (*29% internalizing *25% externalizing) comparable with CBCL
1994	Rintala *et al.*[45]	ARM (high and intermediate)	33 35 Age/sex-matched controls	Mean 35 ± 4.8	QOL	85% with social problems 30% sexual dysfunction
1994	Ludman *et al.*[26]	ARM	160	6–17	Psychiatric interview CBCL TRF DSRS #Self-perception profile	*29% with disorder *27% (norms 18%) 17% (norms 18%) 24% (C vs. IC: ns) (IC boys vs. C boys p. 06)
1994	Diseth *et al.*[27]	Low ARM	10	12–16	CAS CBCL YSR CGAS	60%* 30%* (norms 10%) 10% (norms 10%) 30% severe impairment/social functioning
1996	Diseth *et al.*[28]	ARM	33	12–20	CAS CBCL YSR CGAS	*58% with psychiatric disorder WNR WNR *73% impaired/correlated with FIC
1998	Hassink *et al.*[29]	ARM	109	1–18 median 5.9 yrs	CBCL ($n = 62$) TRF ($n = 54$)	6% (norms 5%) 2% (norms 5%)
2000	Bai *et al.*[30]	ARM	71	8–16	CBCL QOL	18% (norms 10%) (FIC = 66.7%; C = 8.6%) Significantly lower than controls
1995	Catto-Smith *et al.*[33]	Hirschsprung's disease	60	5–16 (+ 1 = 25 years)	CBCL	Overall 15%; IC = 19% C = 20% (norms 10%)
1997	Diseth *et al.*[32]	Hirschsprung's disease	19 control group $n = 33$	10–20	CAS CBCL YSR CGAS	16% v 12% WNR WNR only FIC patients poorer psychosocial functioning
2002	Ludman *et al.*[31]	Hirschsprung's disease: Total colonic aganglionosis (TCA) compared with rectosigmoid aganglionosis (RSA)	15 TCA 15 RSA-age/sex-matched controls	7–18	CBCL TRF YSR DSRS #Self-perception profile	TCA: 27%* vs. RSA: 13% (norms 10%) TCA: 8% vs. RSA: 23% (norms 10%) TCA higher than RSA p. 04* TCA worse than RSA ns TCA lower than RSA p. 03*

(*cont.*)

Table 5.1. *(cont.)*

Date	Reference	Disorder	Sample size	Age range	Psychosocial outcome measures	Findings (% proportion in clinical range)
2000	Bouman *et al.*[46]	Congenital diaphragmatic hernia	11	8–12	IQ Semi-structured interview CBCL TRF DQ #Self-perception profile	mean 85 (range 54–106) 54% doing well 45%* 54%* More symptoms than expected WNR
1999	Bouman *et al.*[35]	Esophageal atresia	36	8–12	IQ CBCL TRF DQ #Self-perception profile	Mean 90 *28.6% vs. 14.5% *34.5% vs. 14.5% WNR WNR
1998	Ure *et al.*[36]	Esophageal atresia	58	20–31	QOL measures: (i) GIQLI; (ii) Spitzer index; (iii) visual analog scale	Unimpaired: primary anastomosis ($n = 50$) Acceptable: colon interposition: ($n = 8$)
2003	Ludman *et al.*[37]	Gastric transposition for pure or long-gap esophageal atresia	28: Group 1 $n = 13$ Group 2 $n = 15$	2–22	QOL: GIQLI (modified) CBCL $n = 22$ TRF $n = 14$ YSR $n = 12$	Generally unimpaired Gp 1: 10% Gp 2: *25% (norms 10%) Gp 1: *29% (*43% internalizing) Gp 2: *29% (*43% externalizing) WNR

Abbreviations: *significantly different from norms; WNR: within normal range; ARM: anorectal malformations; QOL: quality of life; FIC: fecal incontinence; C: continent; CBCL: Achenbach Child Behavior Checklists' parent report; TRF: teacher report form; YSR: youth self-report; DSRS: depression self-report scale (Birleson); CAS: psychiatric interview; CGAS: measure of psychosocial functioning; DQ: depression questionnaire; #Harter: self-perception profile for children; GIQLI: gastrointestinal quality of life index.

disease (HD) are less contradictory. For example, in a recent study at GOSH, we assessed the relationship between functional and psychological outcomes in 15 patients with total colonic aganglionosis (TCA) compared with an age and gender matched group of 15 patients with aganglionosis confined to the rectosigmoid colon (RSA). The proportion of patients with fecal incontinence 7–17 years after definitive surgery was high in both groups, but there was no association between incontinence and behavioral adjustment or depressed mood or self-esteem in either group.[31] Diseth *et al.*[32] and Catto-Smith *et al.*[33] also reported no association between incontinence and the parents' perception of behavioral adjustment (CBCL) in their studies. It is difficult to compare the outcomes from these three studies. In our study, the patients were examined clinically by a surgeon not involved in the patient's surgery or subsequent care, and we attempted to assess sphincter function by endosonography. Patients and parents were interviewed, and a full battery of psychometric assessment measures were used. A comprehensive study design was employed by Diseth *et al.* and although 19 patients were examined and interviewed, only 13 parents were interviewed and completed questionnaires, and teachers were not approached. Catto-Smith *et al.*'s sample was larger but some children were still quite young, and all the data collected were based on responses to postal questionnaires, which have disadvantages as discussed below.

Comparisons between studies looking at psychosocial outcomes or the QoL of patients with FIC are hampered by the fact that the methods used to assess continence vary: some rely solely on parental answers to questionnaires – which vary both in the number and type of items, as well as scoring methods – while the Kelly continence score, for example, requires a physical examination as part of the assessment of FIC.[34] Moreover, postoperative functional problems may be underreported, especially to medical staff. In our study of HD, there was a discrepancy between the surgeon and the psychologist's evaluation of continence, which may reflect the fact that patients are reluctant to admit to bowel control problems when questioned by surgeons – since this may result in further investigations or surgical procedures – while a psychosocial interview provides opportunities to inquire more deeply into difficulties with bowel control. Some researchers have argued that the use of postal questionnaires helps to negate the problem of underreporting to healthcare professionals, but I believe it has the disadvantage of not allowing face-to-face detailed probing questioning.

Esophageal atresia

There is a paucity of studies that have examined the long-term psychological outcome of children with esophageal atresia (EA). Bouman *et al.*'s follow-up study of 36 children with EA revealed that, based on parents' and teachers' reports, more than twice as many children had clinically significant emotional and behavioral problems compared with normative populations.[35] In the main, the children's self-report ratings of self-esteem and depressive symptoms were similar to population norms, but children with lower IQs and chronic physical problems viewed themselves less positively.

Ure *et al.* assessed the long-term quality of life (QoL) of patients with EA who were in their 20s and early 30s, using the Gastrointestinal Quality of Life Index (GIQLI) questionnaire. With the exception of the colon interposition patients, the QoL scores of the patients were comparable with those of healthy controls.[36] In a recent study, using a modified version of the GIQLI questionnaire, we compared the health-related quality of life and the psychosocial adjustment of two groups of patients (28 patients aged 2–22 years) who had undergone gastric transposition. The mean interval since gastric transposition was just under 11 years.[37] The overall QoL of both groups of patients (excluding the young children), was generally unimpaired by any side effects of gastric transposition, although patients who had had the procedure as a primary reconstructive operation (Group 1) experienced fewer disease specific symptoms compared with patients who had undergone previous unsuccessful attempts at reconstruction or replacement of their esophagus (Group 2). Psychosocial adjustment scores are summarized in Table 5.1. The total problem scores of the 12 patients who were able to complete the youth self-report (YSR) questionnaire were no different from the normal population, but clinically significant problems were identified on the CBCL in Group 2 and in both groups on the teachers' ratings. So, patients perceived their QoL and psychosocial adjustment to be comparable to their healthy peers, which contrasted with the views of the parents and teachers. However, our sample size was unavoidably small, and a high proportion of the patients had associated anomalies.

Urogenital surgery

Early studies examining long-term psychosocial adaptation for hypospadias patients were biased by the then current psychoanalytic theories emphasizing castration anxieties and the phallic–oedipal stage of a boy's development, and they also relied on retrospective data. Studies in the last decade have used modern psychological methodology. A recently published report, which compared the psychosocial adaptation of a large sample of boys who had undergone hypospadias repair (between 1985 and 1987) with a community sample of the same age range, found few differences between the groups on emotional and behavioral outcomes.[38] Hypospadias severity was not associated with greater levels of behavioral problems, but boys who had required further surgical procedures and hospitalizations were rated by their parents as having more internalizing symptoms. Additionally, poorer cosmetic appearance of the genitals after surgery – the parent's perception (primarily mother's) – was associated with poorer school performance. However, the children in this study were still young, and emotional and behavioral outcomes (CBCL) were based on one individual's perception (primarily the mother).

In a more comprehensive study, a large sample of boys (n = 116 aged 9–18 years) and adults (n = 73, aged 18–38 years) operated on for hypospadias was compared with an age-matched group of boys (n = 88) and adults (n = 50) who had been treated for an inguinal hernia.[39] The authors found that the hypospadias patients did not have more behavioral or emotional problems than comparison subjects, during adolescence or adulthood. No differences were found between the groups, and there was no significant relationship between the severity of hypospadias and psychosocial functioning, nor with the number of operations or the age at which surgery was completed. The authors were able to conclude that, "in general, males who were treated for hypospadias can expect to have normal psychosexual and psychosocial development." Similar positive findings have been reported in two studies of patients with exstrophy, despite the fact that the abnormality had a great impact on the children and on the lives of their families.[40,41]

Summary

Reports on the prevalence of psychosocial maladjustment are mixed: some studies have reported a significant proportion of children/adolescents with clinically significant problems yet others have revealed no increase in levels of emotional and behavioral problems compared with healthy controls. Similarly, some studies have found significant associations between chronic health problems and psychosocial maladjustment whilst others have not. The reasons for this are not clear but may arise because:

- of small sample sizes, often with a wide age range; this also precludes the use of multivariate analyses to account for the effects of associated anomalies and other confounding variables, such as parental and family factors;
- the standardized psychometric measures used are not suitable for measuring outcome among children with chronic physical health problems;
- the timing of the assessment sessions may coincide with an exacerbation in the child's symptoms or conversely during a period when symptoms are minimal;
- parents and teachers (if they are aware of a child's health problem) may not wish to reveal behavioral disorders in the 'sick' child;
- of faulty methodology.

Despite inconsistencies, the evidence suggests that, irrespective of the presence of chronic health problems, children who require major pediatric surgery are at a two to three times greater risk for psychiatric disorder than healthy children. The reasons for this are not clear but the evidence from my own experience and that derived from the literature suggests that the birth of a child with life-threatening congenital anomalies, together with the subsequent surgery and hospitalizations, can have long-term effects on parent–child relationships and the subsequent development of the child. For many parents, this child is special and "vulnerable", and this affects their responses to the child: many parents found it difficult to treat their child "as normal" and to deal consistently, firmly, and effectively with their child's behavior. There are mediating factors. For example, as we found in our large-scale study of patients with ARM, better parental educational levels were associated with lower levels of behavioral disturbance, and girls were less at risk of psychological disturbance and deviant behavior than boys. It was also apparent that parental (primarily maternal) parenting skills and coping strategies influenced the children's behavior and coping strategies, which in turn varied with age and gender.[42]

Conclusions and future directions

- We need to gain a better understanding of the mechanisms that may be contributing to emotional well-being in children who have major surgery for life-threatening congenital abnormalities.
- We should press for the establishment of long-term, focused, psychological support for the children and their families, to help ameliorate the longer term sequelae of early surgery, hospital admissions and chronic health problems. This should focus on promoting protective factors (such as positive parent–child interactions) and reducing the impact of adverse family factors (such as maternal depression and poor parenting skills).
- This psychological support should be an essential part of the clinical care of the child. A member of the surgical team should introduce the psychologist to the family, during the first admission, and inform the family that psychological support is an essential part of the care of the child. In this way, the parents should become accustomed to the fact that a pediatric psychologist is an intrinsic member of the team caring for the child, negating parental suspicions that a psychologist's help is sought only because they or the child is thought to be psychiatrically disturbed.
- It is essential to evaluate the long-term benefits of this form of focused, psychological support, preferably by longitudinal studies. With the current emphasis on cost containment, research should identify children who are at most risk for difficulty in coping with the stress of surgery and hospitalization and chronic health problems.
- Research should inform practice – clinical work has generally guided research questions, but there has been a failure to put findings from research into practice.

Finally, the psychological approach is one that stresses the complexity of the individual, recognising the complex interactions of biological, interpersonal, familial, and cultural influences that contribute to the psychological development of children.

REFERENCES

1. Wallander, J. L. & Thompson, R. J. Jr. Psychosocial adjustment of children with chronic physical conditions. In Roberts, M. C. (ed) *Handbook of Pediatric Psychology*. 2nd edn. NY: Guilford Press; 1995: 124–141.
2. Achenbach, T. M. *Manual for the Child Behaviour Checklist/4–18 and 1991 Profile*. Burlington, VT: University of Vermont, Department of Psychiatry; 1991.
3. Achenbach, T. M. *Manual for the Teacher's Report Form and 1991 Profile*. Burlington, VT: University of Vermont, Department of Psychiatry; 1991.
4. Achenbach, T. M. *Manual for the Youth Self-Report and 1991 Profile*. Burlington, VT: University of Vermont Department of Psychiatry; 1991.

5. Achenbach, T. M. *Manual for the Child Behaviour Checklist/2–3 and 1992 Profile.* Burlington, VT: University of Vermont Department of Psychiatry; 1992.
6. Eiser, C. & Morse, R. A review of measures of quality of life for children with chronic illness. *Arch. Dis. Child.* 2001; **84**:205–211.
7. Alsop-Shields, L., Mohay, H., Bowlby, J., & Robertson, J. Theorists, scientists and crusaders for improvements in the care of children in hospital. *J. Adv. Nursing* 2001; **35**:50–58.
8. Rutter, M. *Maternal Deprivation Reassessed.* 2nd edn. Harmondsworth: Penguin Books Ltd; 1981.
9. Douglas, J. W. B. Early hospital admissions and later disturbances of behaviour and learning. *Dev. Med. Child. Neurol.* 1975; **17**:456–480.
10. Quinton, D. & Rutter, M. Early hospital admissions and later disturbances of behaviour: an attempted replication of Douglas's findings. *Dev. Med. Child. Neurol.* 1976; **18**:447–457.
11. Haslum, M. N. Length of preschool hospitalization, multiple admissions and later educational attainment and behaviour. *Child Care, health Dev.* 1988; **14**:275–291.
12. Rutter, M. Clinical implications of attachment concepts: retrospect and prospect. *J. Child Psychol. Psychiatry* 1995; **36**:549–572.
13. Ludman, L. The psychological effects of major neonatal surgery on infants and their families [Ph.D.]: University of London; 1990.
14. Ludman, L., Lansdown, R., & Spitz, L. Effects of early hospitalization and surgery on the emotional development of 3 year olds: an exploratory study. *Eur. Child Adolesc. Psychiatry* 1992; **1**:186–195.
15. Ludman, L., Lansdown, R., & Spitz, L. Factors associated with developmental progress of full term neonates who required intensive care. *Arch. Dis. Child.* 1989; **64**:333–337.
16. Ludman, L., Spitz, L., & Lansdown, R. Developmental progress of newborns undergoing neonatal surgery. *J. Pediatr. Surg.* 1990; **25**:469–471.
17. Ludman, L., Spitz, L., & Lansdown, R. Intellectual development at 3 years of age of children who underwent major neonatal surgery. *J. Pediatr. Surg.* 1993; **28**:130–134.
18. Ludman, L., Spitz, L., & Wade, A. Educational attainments in early adolescence of infants who required major neonatal surgery. *J. Pediatr. Surg.* 2001; **36**:858–862.
19. Fahrenfort, J. J., Jacobs, E. A., Miedema, S., & Schweizer, A. T. Signs of emotional disturbance three years after early hospitalization. *J. Pediatr. Psychol.* 1996; **21**:353–366.
20. Timing of elective surgery on the genitalia of male children with particular reference to the risks, benefits, and psychological effects of surgery and anesthesia. American Academy of Pediatrics. *Pediatrics* 1996; **97**:590–594.
21. Rutter, M. Stress, coping and development: some issues and questions. In Garmezy, N., Rutter, M., ed. *Stress, Coping and Development in Children.* New York: McGraw-Hill; 1983:1–42.
22. Cadman, D., Boyle, M., Szatmari, P., & Offord, D. R. Chronic illness, disability, and mental and social well-being: findings of the Ontario Child Health Study. *Pediatrics* 1987; **79**:805–813.
23. Eiser, C. Psychological effects of chronic disease. *J. Child Psychol. Psychiatry* 1990; **31**:85–98.
24. Nolan, T. & Pless, I. B. Emotional correlates and consequences of birth defects. *J. Pediatr.* 1986; **109**:210–216.
25. Ludman, L. & Spitz, L. Psychosocial adjustment of children treated for anorectal anomalies. *J. Pediatr. Surg.* 1995; **30**:495–499.
26. Ludman, L., Spitz, L., & Kiely, E. M. Social and emotional impact of faecal incontinence following surgery for anorectal anomalies. *Arch. Dis. Child.* 1994; **71**:194–200.
27. Diseth, T., Emblem, R., Solbraa, I., & Vandvik, I. A psychosocial follow-up of ten adolescents with low anorectal malformation. *Acta Paediatr.* 1994; **83**:216–221.
28. Diseth, T. H., Emblem, R. Somatic function, mental health, and psychosocial adjustment of adolescents with anorectal anomalies. *J. Pediatr. Surg.* 1996; **31**:638–643.
29. Hassink, E. A., Brugman-Boezeman, A. T., Robbroeckx, L. M. *et al.* Parenting children with anorectal malformations: implications and experiences. *Pediatr. Surg. Int.* 1998; **13**:377–383.
30. Bai, Y., Yuan, Z., Wang, W., Zhao, Y., & Wang, H. Quality of life for children with fecal incontinence after surgically corrected anorectal malformation. *J. Pediatr. Surg.* 2000; **35**:462–464.
31. Ludman, L., Spitz, L., Tsuji, H., & Pierro, A. Hirschsprung's disease: functional and psychological follow up comparing total colonic and rectosigmoid aganglionosis. *Arch. Dis. Child.* 2002; **86**:348–351.
32. Diseth, T. H., Bjornland, K., Novik, T. S., & Emblem, R. Bowel function, mental health, and psychosocial function in adolescents with Hirschsprung's disease. *Arch. Dis. Child.* 1997; **76**:100–106.
33. Catto-Smith, A. G., Coffey, C., Nolan, T., & Hutson, J. Fecal incontinence after the surgical treatment of Hirschsprung's disease. *J. Pediatr.* 1995; **127**:954–957.
34. Kelly, J. H. The clinical and radiological assessment of anal continence in childhood. *Aust. N. Z. J. Surg.* 1972; **42**:62–63.
35. Bouman, N. H., Koot, H. M., & Hazebroek, F. W. Long-term physical, psychological, and social functioning of children with esophageal atresia. *J. Pediatr. Surg.* 1999; **34**:399–404.
36. Ure, B. M., Slany, E., Eypasch, E. P., Gharib, M., Holschneider, A. M., & Troidl, H. Long-term functional results and quality of life after colon interposition for long-gap oesophageal atresia. *Eur. J. Pediatr. Surg.* 1995; **5**:206–210.
37. Ludman, L. & Spitz, L. Quality of life after gastric transposition for oesophageal atresia. *J. Pediatr. Surg.* 2003; **38**:53–57.
38. Sandberg, D. E., Meyer-Bahlburg, H. F., Hensle, T. W., Levitt, S. B., Kogan, S. J., & Reda, E. F. Psychosocial adaptation of middle childhood boys with hypospadias after genital surgery. *J. Pediatr. Psychol.* 2001; **26**:465–475.
39. Mureau, M. A., Slijper, F. M., Slob, A. K., & Verhulst, F. C. Psychosocial functioning of children, adolescents, and adults following hypospadias surgery: a comparative study. *J. Pediatr. Psychol.* 1997; **22**:371–387.
40. Montagnino, B., Czyzewski, D. I., Runyan, R. D., Berkman, S., Roth, D. R., & Gonzales, E. T, Jr. Long-term adjustment issues in patients with exstrophy. *J. Urol.* 1998; **160**:1471–1474.

41. Stjernqvist, K. & Kockum, C. C. Bladder exstrophy: psychological impact during childhood. *J. Urol.* 1999; **162**:2125–2129.
42. Ludman, L. & Spitz, L. Coping strategies of children with faecal incontinence. *J. Pediatr. Surg.* 1996; **31**:563–567.
43. Ditesheim, J. A. & Templeton, J. M. Jr. Short-term v long-term quality of life in children following repair of high imperforate anus. *J. Pediatr. Surg.* 1987; **22**:581–587.
44. Ginn-Pease, M. E., King, D. R., Tarnowski, K. J., Green, L., Young, G., & Linscheid, T. R. Psychosocial adjustment and physical growth in children with imperforate anus or abdominal wall defects. *J. Pediatr. Surg.* 1991; **26**:1129–1135.
45. Rintala, R., Mildh, L., & Lindahl, H. Fecal continence and quality of life for adult patients with an operated high or intermediate anorectal malformation. *J. Pediatr. Surg.* 1994; **29**:777–780.
46. Bouman, N. H., Koot, H. M., Tibboel, D., & Hazebroek, F. W. Children with congenital diaphragmatic hernia are at risk for lower levels of cognitive functioning and increased emotional and behavioral problems. *Eur. J. Pediatr. Surg.* 2000; **10**:3–7.

Part II

Head and neck

6

Cleft lip and palate

Alistair G. Smyth

Northern and Yorkshire Cleft Lip and Palate Service, The General Infirmary at Leeds, UK

Introduction

Cleft lip and palate is a complex congenital anomaly affecting the development of the face, oro-pharynx and nose, resulting in a disturbance of appearance and function. Often multiple treatment outcomes need to be considered for an individual patient due to the wide range of severity of clefts and the nature of the special structures involved. In general, long-term outcomes from cleft lip and palate surgery include an assessment of facial appearance, speech, facial growth, dental development, hearing and psychological well-being. Consequently, final outcomes may need to be assessed many years after the original surgery, usually during early adult life.

It is well recognized that different surgical protocols for primary cleft repair can have a major influence on long-term outcomes. Protocols may differ with regard to technique used, timing of surgery, the sequence of repair, or the possible use of presurgical orthopedic alignment of the maxillary segments. Whilst the severity of the cleft and the effectiveness of the surgery undoubtedly have a major influence on outcomes, other important factors may complicate the picture further, such as general developmental variations, syndromal associations, and socio-economic factors. Non-surgical interventions such as speech and language therapy, orthodontics and audiologic input also influence the final "surgical" outcomes. The technical skill of the surgeon is a further compounding influence – a skilled surgeon can partially compensate for a mediocre technique of repair achieving good results, whereas a poor surgeon may produce unacceptable results despite the application of an otherwise sound reconstructive technique. Such factors make it very difficult to assess long-term outcomes from different protocols of management.

Outcomes in cleft surgery may also be conflicting. For example, early repair of a cleft palate (within the first year) is considered important for normal speech development but this early approach may result in greater problems with facial growth. Conversely, later palatal surgery may favor better facial growth but at the expense of worse speech outcomes. Such controversies in cleft management have yet to be fully resolved. When assessing long-term outcomes, it is also important to consider them in the context of the number and nature of interventions applied. For example, repeated surgical interventions may marginally improve lip or nasal appearance but at what cost to the child and carers in terms of multiple hospital admissions, missed schooling, and potential further psychological trauma, possibly resulting in treatment "burn-out" in early adolescence.

Organization of cleft lip and palate services

Whilst comparative clinical audits such as the Eurocleft study[1] have highlighted the often broad range in quality of outcomes between different centers and generally poor outcomes in the UK when compared with other European centers, the reason why some units have better outcomes is more difficult to define. One outcome measure from the Eurocleft study showed that almost half of the cases of unilateral cleft lip and palate treated in the North West of England required future corrective mid-facial bony surgery (orthognathic surgery) to correct mid-facial retrusion. This contrasts with cases from Norway and Denmark where only 6% of children were thought to require corrective orthognathic surgery. Evaluation of protocols at

Pediatric Surgery and Urology: Long-term Outcomes, Mark Stringer, Keith Oldham, Pierre Mouriquand.
Published by Cambridge University Press.

each center showed minor differences in operative technique with most surgeons adopting a fairly traditional approach. However, major differences in surgical caseload were apparent with Scandinavian surgeons treating more cases with a greater concentration of specialists into a small number of teams.

A further survey of cleft centers in the UK found that the concerns raised by the Eurocleft study were widespread and represented the findings in most centers.[2] Not only was there concern in the UK with low-volume operators[3] but concerns were also raised regarding the lack of rationalization of other ancillary treatments such as orthodontics.[4] Subsequently, a multidisciplinary steering group under the auspices of the Royal College of Surgeons of England carried out a national survey in England and Wales. This revealed widespread involvement of low-volume operators in cleft care, a tendency for low-volume operators to have an incomplete network of associated professionals and non-standardized record keeping protocols. This culminated in recommendations for minimum standards of care for children born with cleft lip and palate[5] and the subsequent appointment of a Clinical Standards Advisory Committee for cleft lip and palate. This committee commissioned an ambitious audit of the outcomes of treatment received by 5-year-old and 12-year-old children with cleft lip and palate throughout the UK. This audit was carried out between 1996 and 1997. The results from the study highlighted concerns in almost all areas of cleft care, including the national reporting of new cases, the process of care, and the standards of outcome. The methods, results and conclusions of the study were published in a comprehensive Clinical Standards Advisory Group (CSAG) report.[6] The study failed to conclusively establish a relationship between outcomes and volume of surgery, except for an influence of the surgeon's experience on speech outcomes.[7] However, the recommendations of the CSAG report were accepted in full by the UK government and subsequently implemented with a major reconfiguration of cleft services into a small number of regional specialist centres.

Subsequent studies in Western Australia raised similar concerns with cleft lip and palate outcomes leading to an examination of healthcare for low incidence congenital anomalies.[8,9] Similarly, in the USA, recommendations were published in 1993 by the American Cleft Palate–Craniofacial Association[10] containing parameters for the evaluation and treatment of patients with cleft lip and palate. One of the key principles in this document was the need for the management of these patients to be carried out by an interdisciplinary team of specialists. In 1984, Bardach *et al.*[11] reported the long term results of the management of unilateral cleft lip and palate patients at the University of Iowa, USA. The lack of other similar long-term outcome studies, however, does not allow any comparison of these results with other American centers. Bardach also emphasized that the best outcomes were not only dependent upon treatment provision within a multidisciplinary team, but that the members of the team must have well-defined roles with excellent cooperation and communication between team members.

Problems with evidence-based care in cleft lip and palate

The quality of published evidence promoting a particular treatment protocol is generally lacking in cleft lip and palate surgery. Treatment protocols and techniques have often developed over generations of surgeons reflecting significant clinical experience over many years, which may be handed down from surgeon to apprentice. These practices are then frequently continued without question and often without scientific justification. The gold standard of medical research remains the randomized controlled trial. Roberts *et al.*,[12] in their review of 25 years of the *Cleft Palate Journal*, identified only five controlled clinical trials, only one of which involved more than 4 years of surgical follow-up. Much of the scientific basis for the surgical management of cleft lip and palate is derived from uncontrolled comparative data, case series and anecdotal case reports. Regrettably, evidence-based care for children with cleft lip and palate is scarcely available.[13] Many reasons may account for the paucity of reliable evidence-based care in cleft lip and palate. These include the need to follow patients up for many years, the diversity of severity and type of the cleft deformity, changing surgical practices within a surgeon's career, small-volume caseload, poor record keeping and research bias. However, the development of methods which may allow an earlier assessment of outcomes and the centralization of cleft surgery with high-volume operators does offer the opportunity for earlier and reliable assessment of outcomes from different protocols.

Randomized controlled trials on primary surgery are currently under way, comparing the outcomes from three parallel trials, in which cleft teams assess their traditional local protocol against a common protocol.[14] It is hoped that the results from these trials will inform clinical practice with regard to the choice of technique, timing, and sequence of primary repair for cleft lip and palate.

Historical aspects and current surgical techniques

Primary cleft lip and palate surgery

The techniques of cleft surgery have evolved over many centuries, since the first documented case of a cleft lip repair on an 18-year-old farm boy, by an unknown Chinese surgeon in the 4th century AD.[15] The farm boy went on to become the Governor General of six Chinese provinces – surely testimony of a good surgical outcome. The evolutionary process has led to a diversification of management, with many different descriptions of technique for the repair of cleft lip and palate, each with the aim of improving outcomes. Virtually no other branch of surgery has such a wide range of different treatment protocols varying in technique, timing, and sequence and consequently few centers carry out exactly the same treatments. In 2000, a survey of European cleft centers found 194 different protocols among a total of 201 teams.[16]

Cleft lip

Early cleft lip repair consisted of simple paring of the cleft margin and re-approximation of the wound edges, right up until the 19th century when Von Graefe[17] proposed the use of curved incisions to achieve lip lengthening. Mirault[18] in 1844 described the use of a local flap from the lateral aspect of the cleft and modifications of this technique were subsequently introduced by Blair and Brown.[19] These methods provided reliable results and remained popular up to the 1950s. The triangular flap technique, introduced by Tennison[20] in 1952, was one of the first procedures that preserved the normal Cupid's bow of the lip. The geometry and design of this method were later described by Randall,[21] providing a reproducible pattern for lip repair. This technique remains popular in many parts of the world today. The technique also has disadvantages – the main flap is taken from the already deficient lateral element of the lip, the unnatural appearance of a zigzag scar, and little correction of the nasal deformity.

The rotation–advancement technique introduced by Millard[22] in 1955 overcame many of the disadvantages of earlier techniques and is still the most popular method of repair for a unilateral cleft lip. The principle of repair is based on a downward rotation of the Cupid's bow and philtrum using a curved incision on the medial side of the cleft. This downward rotation opens up a gap in the superior aspect of the lip, which is filled by an advancement flap brought across from the lateral lip element of the cleft. Modifications to the technique have been introduced to achieve further lip lengthening or to adjust the position of the philtral ridge on the cleft side.[23] Careful repair of the muscles of the upper lip and mid face is an essential part of the repair and Delaire[24] emphasized the importance of a functional lip repair.

Primary nasal correction

Primary correction of the corresponding nasal deformity is now considered an essential part of cleft lip repair and is undertaken at the same time. In complete cleft lip, the nasal floor is interrupted by the cleft and the lack of muscle continuity around the nose and across the upper lip, results in a substantial displacement of the alar base of the nose in an inferior, lateral and posterior direction. Consequently, the cartilage within the nose on the cleft side is deformed and, in particular, the lower lateral cartilage is flattened, elongated and rotated. The unopposed action of the normally inserted muscles on the non-cleft side pull the nasal septum and columella away from the cleft side. Initially, nasal surgery was restricted to reconstruction of the anterior nasal floor, due to concerns that further dissection within and around the nose could impair future growth of the nose. These concerns were subsequently found to be incorrect, so long as the dissection did not transgress the cartilages themselves. McComb[25] described his results with primary nasal correction, consisting of a wide subcutaneous dissection of the nose and the placement of suspensory sutures. McComb subsequently published a longitudinal study of his good nasal outcomes in unilateral cleft lip and palate.[26] Others have described more radical procedures,[27,28] but it remains to be seen whether their long term results are any better.

Cleft palate repair

The aims of cleft palate repair are the complete closure of the cleft with normal speech development through velopharyngeal competence, a primary function of the soft palate. Additional aims of surgery are to promote normal facial growth and dental development.

Von Langenbeck[29] described an approach to cleft palate repair using lateral incisions within the palate to allow medial mobilization of the palatal tissue. This provided a safe and reliable technique, which has stood the test of time and modifications of this technique are still widely used today. In an attempt to improve speech outcomes Veau[30], Wardill[31] and Kilner[32] described a V–Y pushback procedure to lengthen the soft palate, with detachment of the soft palate muscles from their abnormal insertion on the posterior edge of the hard palate. Although speech outcomes were improved by the "push-back" procedure, facial growth was significantly impaired due to large areas of exposed anterior palatal bone, which heals with scar tissue. Studies have shown that young adults with unoperated clefts have normal facial growth and it is widely accepted that the primary surgery can have a major impact on facial growth and, in particular, can inhibit the forward growth of the maxilla.[33–35] Consequently, most centers have now abandoned the "push-back" procedure and surgeons try to avoid leaving large raw areas in the palate, often preferring methods based on the Von Langenbeck procedure.

In 1978, Furlow presented an operation which also had the intention of lengthening the soft palate by transposing soft tissue musculo-mucosal flaps – the Furlow double-reversing Z-palatoplasty.[36] This procedure also lengthened the soft palate and improved muscle alignment, as the soft palate muscles are re-orientated with the transposed mucosal flaps. The Furlow procedure within the soft palate is usually performed in conjunction with a Von Langenbeck repair of the hard palate. These procedures provide a one-stage repair of the palate. However, other surgeons repair the palate in two separate stages. This can reduce the need for lateral palatal incisions and excessive undermining of palatal mucoperiosteum, which favors better facial growth. The hard palate may be repaired initially with a flap of mucosal tissue overlying the vomer of the nasal septum. This vomer flap, first described by Pichler[37] was popularised by Abyholm[38] in Oslo, Norway. Closure of the hard palate with the vomer flap is usually carried out at the same time as the initial lip repair, around 3 months of age. The remaining cleft within the posterior palate is then repaired at a second operation, often around 6–9 months of age. Other surgeons prefer to repair the soft palate first, usually at the time of lip repair, and then close the hard palate at a second operation. The aim of this approach is to allow some maxillary growth and development to occur prior to any hard palate surgery. Schweckendiek[39] proposed delaying hard palate closure until 12 to 16 years of age. Although this technique favored more normal facial growth, studies have shown that speech outcomes are unacceptably poor. Delaire[24] proposed leaving the hard palate closure until 12 to 18 months of age to allow some narrowing of the residual hard palate cleft. Proponents of this method claim good speech outcomes and favorable facial growth.[40,41]

Attention has also focused on the importance of creating a normal muscle sling within the soft palate and formal muscle dissection during soft palate repair is increasingly popular. Veau[42] in 1926 described the abnormal muscular anatomy within a cleft palate and recommended the suture repair of this "cleft-muscle." Kriens[43] developed this further and in 1969 proposed a realignment of the muscle to create a levator muscle sling, coining the term "intra-velar veloplasty." In this procedure, the muscles of the soft palate are detached from their abnormal insertion and realigned transversely within the posterior soft palate.

Presurgical orthopedics

Presurgical orthopedics is the passive or active alignment of the lip and/or palatal segments prior to operative repair. The premise is to facilitate the surgery by generally moving the segments on either side of the cleft closer together. This requires the use of facial strapping with adhesive tapes and the fitting and adjustment of appliances within the mouth, usually by the cleft team orthodontist. These measures are not uniformly applied and many centers prefer to avoid presurgical orthopedic treatment.

Timing of primary cleft surgery

Most surgeons agree that the best time to carry out cleft lip repair is between 2 and 6 months of age. If possible, primary repair of the cleft palate is performed before 18 months of age as this provides better speech outcomes. Many centers now perform cleft palate repair between 6 and 12 months of age. Other factors influence the timing of primary cleft surgery such as significant coexisting congenital cardiac defects or respiratory compromise as in Pierre–Robin sequence.

Fetal surgery, following antenatal diagnosis of cleft lip, was considered by some to offer advantages in terms of "scarless" healing. However, there are no grounds for advocating cleft lip repair at this time due to the high risk of major complications for the mother and baby.

Neonatal repair also has its advocates, claiming a fetal-like tendency to less scarring and less psychological trauma for the mother and family. The appearance and function of neonatal cleft lip repairs are generally inferior and many require further revisional surgery. The majority of cleft centers therefore do not perform cleft lip repair in the neonatal period.

Secondary cleft lip and palate surgery

Secondary speech surgery

Velopharyngeal insufficiency (VPI) following cleft palate repair is the inability to completely close the velopharyngeal sphincter during speech, resulting in an escape of air into the nasal cavity. The resulting hypernasal resonance and nasal emission with consequent abnormal articulations and loss of volume can markedly impair the intelligibility of speech. The CSAG study[6] in the UK reported a 15% prevalence of appreciable hypernasality in 177 5-year-old children with repaired cleft lip and palate. The treatment of significant VPI is usually surgical and aims to reduce the size of the nasopharyngeal port. Popular procedures include the posterior pharyngeal flap[44] and the sphincter pharyngoplasty.[45–47] The posterior pharyngeal flap procedure attaches a midline, often superiorly-based musculomucosal flap to the nasal side of the soft palate. A sphincter pharyngoplasty raises flaps from the lateral pharyngeal walls, which are then inset into the posterior pharyngeal wall. Re-repair of cleft palate with intra-velar veloplasty can also be effective in selected cases.[48] Other causes of VPI include submucous cleft palate[49] and velocardiofacial syndrome.[50]

Alveolar bone grafting

A complete unilateral or bilateral cleft of the lip and palate also involves the alveolus (tooth-bearing area) of the upper jaw. Alveolar bone grafting is an important operation in the reconstruction of the orofacial cleft deformity. The term primary bone grafting is used when this surgery is carried out before 2 years of age. Results with primary bone grafting of alveolar clefts have generally been disappointing with problems of mid-facial growth impairment, poor dental arch form and inadequate alveolar bone for subsequent tooth eruption and support. Secondary alveolar bone grafting[51] with surgery carried out in the mixed dentition, often between 9 and 11 years of age, is a much more successful procedure and provides reliable and predictable results. The grafting material of choice is autogenous cancellous bone, most often harvested from the iliac crest. Successful grafting permits the eruption of the permanent canine tooth and provides bony support for the teeth on either side of the cleft site.

Long-term outcomes in primary and secondary cleft lip and palate surgery

As discussed previously, the long-term outcomes in the UK and other countries have been generally disappointing. In addition, the numerous surgical techniques, multiple protocols of care, variable record keeping and frequent low-volume operators, has hindered the scientific evaluation of which protocols produce the best results in terms of surgical technique, sequence of repair, and the timing of surgery. Notwithstanding this, the following is a distillation of the outcomes from cleft surgery supported by available published evidence.

Outcomes from primary cleft lip surgery

Long-term outcomes from cleft lip repair are based on the final appearance of the reconstructed lip and the range of functional activity. Determinants of satisfactory appearance such as the frequency of the need for secondary lip revisional surgery are rather crude and inaccurate. The current basis of assessment is standardized photographs taken at 5 years of age with the lips at rest and in function. Other methods of assessing appearance, such as 3-D imaging are being currently evaluated. It is likely, however, that the standardized photograph will remain the audit record for some time to come, even though the use of photographs has potential problems, such as technical differences in quality and the influence of surrounding features.[52] Video imaging provides more information regarding the functional outcomes from cleft lip surgery. However, Morrant and Shaw found that while the dynamic view may be more valid, the interexaminer agreement was generally worse than that achieved from a static image.[53] Children with repaired isolated cleft lip will develop normal speech even in the presence of a poor lip repair with shortening or inadequate muscle repair.

Surgical outcomes from complete cleft lip are generally not as good as with an incomplete cleft lip, as the complete cleft presents with greater displacement of the lip segments, total discontinuity of the muscles on the cleft side, more severe nasal deformity and frequent involvement of the underlying bony alveolus. An independent audit of cleft outcomes in the UK[6] which included 218 12-year-old children with repaired unilateral cleft lip and palate found that 20% of the children were considered to have a poor lip appearance and 42% poor nasal appearance.

Long term outcomes in bilateral clefts are usually not as good as in the unilateral cleft. Lack of muscle continuity on both sides allows the central segment of the upper lip and jaw (prolabium and premaxilla) to grow forwards in an unrestrained manner. Adequate soft tissue control of the premaxilla can also be a problem after bilateral lip repair with the premaxilla escaping from lip control in a forward and inferior direction. Such problems following primary lip repair in the bilateral case are difficult to manage and often require a combination of secondary surgery and specialist orthodontic treatment. Techniques of cleft lip repair undoubtedly influence the outcomes from surgery and it is widely accepted that those based on a rotation/advancement method such as Millard[22] and Delaire[24] produce better results than other more geometric forms of repair, such as the triangular flap method of Tennison[20] and Randall.[21] Traditionally, surgeons have concentrated their attention on methods of skin lengthening in cleft lip repair and have introduced numerous modifications of the original rotation/advancement method to achieve further lengthening of the lip or columella of the nose and improved nasal symmetry.

A significant development within the last 30 years has been a gradual acceptance of the importance of a complete muscle repair as part of the overall reconstruction. All cleft surgeons recognize the untoward problem of shortening of the lip in the first few months after surgery. However, beneficial changes in appearance after lip surgery may also occur in response to normal functional use following a complete muscle repair. The initial lip repair should be of a high standard with subsequent good outcomes and minimal subsequent need for revisional surgery. In addition, surgeons need to resist the temptation to reoperate at an early stage for minor irregularities. Revisional lip surgery can often be delayed until it can be combined with another planned procedure, such as an alveolar bone graft. No single technique will provide good outcomes every time and the thoughtful surgeon learns how to assess an individual case and apply combinations of techniques, where appropriate, and to limit the extent of the surgery to that which is compatible with the best overall outcome.

Outcomes from primary cleft palate surgery

Oronasal fistula

This is an abnormal communication between the mouth and nose due to a partial breakdown of the palatal repair. Fistulae are a recognized complication of cleft palate repair and the reported incidence of fistulae varies widely from 0% to 34%.[54] Fistulae within the palate may be small and insignificant but others may be larger and cause problems with nasal regurgitation of food or fluids and nasal emission of air during speech. Very large fistulae can cause hypernasality of speech. Clinically significant fistulae are usually closed surgically. Sommerlad[55] presented his results from a 5-year period between 1993 and 1997 and reported a fistula rate of 14% in unilateral cleft lip and palate, 35% in bilateral cleft lip and palate, and 12% in clefts of the secondary palate alone. It should be noted, however, that only those fistulae that required surgical repair were included.

Speech outcomes

About 20% of children who undergo cleft palate repair will demonstrate velopharyngeal insufficiency.[56] As previously noted, velopharyngeal closure is a primary function of the soft palate and inadequate closure may result from a soft palate that is too short, elevates and/or lengthens poorly, or a combination of these factors. Following the decline in popularity of the "push-back" operation due to excessive palatal scarring, concentration has now focused largely on the nature of the muscle repair within the soft palate.

The muscles within a cleft soft palate consist of the interwoven fibers of levator palati, palatopharyngeus, palatoglossus, and musculus uvulae. No muscle fibers of tensor palati enter the soft palate but the tensor aponeurosis is present as a definite tendinous band located laterally in the soft palate. Intravelar veloplasty (IVV) releases the soft palate muscles from their abnormal insertion on the posterior edge of the hard palate and allows the muscle to be transposed posteriorly within the soft palate, especially after the division of the lateral tensor tendon. Dreyer and Trier[57] compared their results of Von Langenbeck palatal repair with intravelar veloplasty, with historical control data and concluded that intravelar veloplasty was of significant value in providing velopharyngeal competency. They reported that 89% of patients in the IVV group had acceptable or normal speech in comparison with 62% in the historical non-IVV control group. Marsh *et al.*[58] subsequently performed a quasi-randomized controlled trial to investigate the effect of IVV on velopharyngeal function. In this prospective trial, patients were assigned to IVV and non-IVV groups alternately rather than being truly randomized. From a sample of 51 patients they found no difference in speech outcomes between the two groups, but the IVV group required a significantly longer operating time and proved more costly than the non-IVV group. Radical muscle dissection with retropositioning in the soft palate has been shown to be effective in treating velopharyngeal insufficiency in secondary palatal surgery (re-repairs) with significant improvements in hypernasality and nasal emission and improved soft palate function on lateral videofluoroscopy.[59]

Sommerlad[55] reported his incidence of secondary speech surgery as 9 out of 192 palatal repairs (4.6%), following primary cleft palate repair with radical muscle dissection between 1988 and 1992. Evidence is accumulating, which supports the speech benefits of radical muscle dissection but the results of prospective randomized controlled trials are still awaited. Comparable results are achieved with the Furlow double-reversing Z-plasty with long-term results showing an improvement in velopharyngeal competence and a reduced need for secondary pharyngoplasty compared to historic data from other types of repair.[60,61] A randomized controlled trial is currently under way in São Paulo, Brazil, comparing the velopharyngeal competence outcomes in unilateral cleft lip and palate between a Von Langenbeck repair with intravelar veloplasty and the Furlow procedure.[62]

The timing of palatal surgery influences the long-term speech outcomes. The speech is better and fewer compensatory articulation disorders develop when the palate is repaired before 12 months of age. In a randomized controlled trial, Ysunza[63] demonstrated significantly better phonological development when the palate was repaired at 6 months in comparison with surgery at 12 months of age.

Generally, patients with cleft palate and an underlying syndrome, such as velocardiofacial syndrome, have worse speech outcomes as the combination of aberrant anatomic and physiologic characteristics seem to diminish the probability of normal velopharyngeal closure.[64]

Facial growth

Impaired facial growth, particularly affecting the maxilla, can be a consequence of cleft palate surgery (Figs. 6.1 and 6.2). The abnormal facial growth gradually becomes more apparent during adolescence and the additional burden for the child can be considerable. Although this can usually be

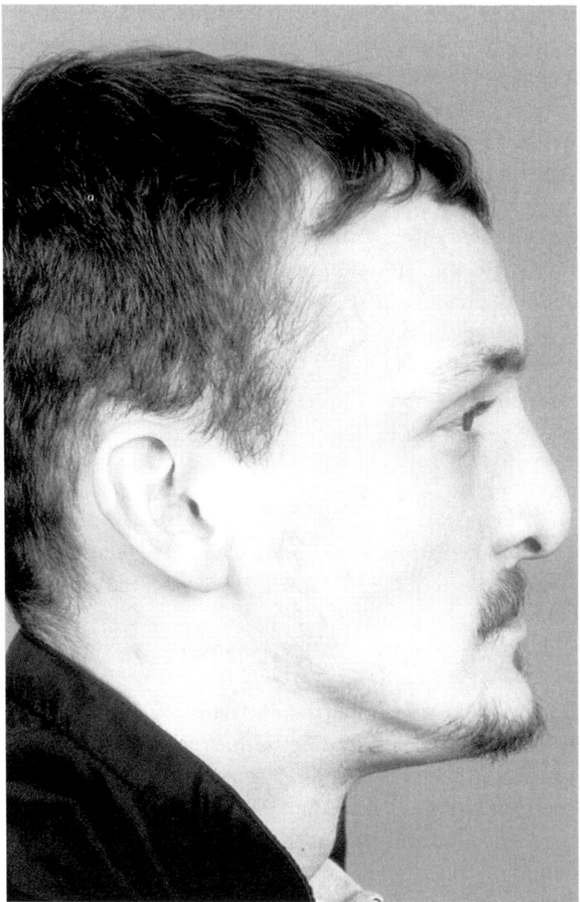

Fig. 6.1. Young adult patient with impaired forward growth of the mid-face as a consequence of excessive scarring in the palate following previous cleft lip and palate surgery.

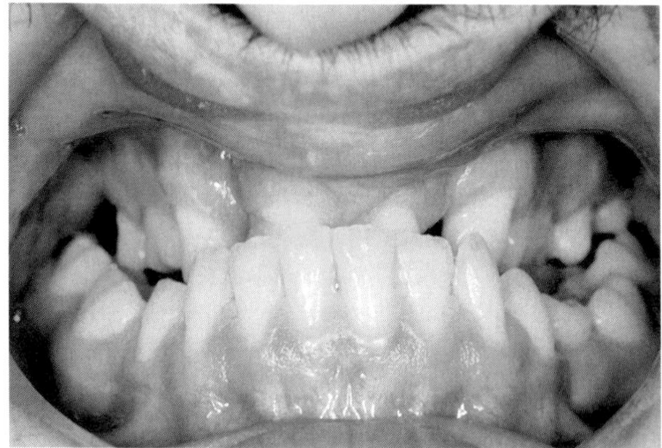

Fig. 6.2. Associated abnormal bite relationship of the jaws and teeth with the upper teeth well behind the lower teeth.

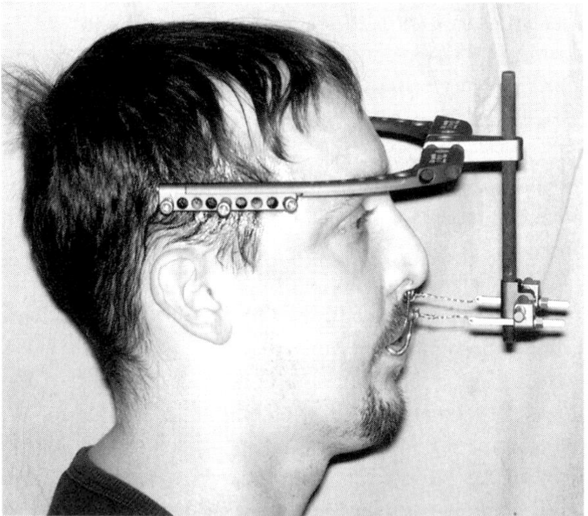

Fig. 6.3. Surgical correction of the retruded upper jaw with anterior distraction of the maxilla following surgical osteotomy of the maxilla.

corrected in early adult life with mid facial skeletal advancement, the surgery is a major undertaking for the patient (Fig. 6.3). Although maxillary retrusion does not occur in every case, the need for maxillary advancement surgery has been reported to be as high as 50%[65] and varies considerably between centers. This was demonstrated in the Eurocleft study,[1] which found that almost half of the unilateral cleft lip and palate cases treated in the North West of England were likely to need maxillary advancement. This compares with only 6% of cases treated in Denmark and Norway.

Facial growth is often assessed from a standardized lateral radiograph of the face – a lateral cephalogram. Detailed angular and linear measurements taken from the radiograph allow a comparison with normal values and ratios, providing a reproducible method of assessing facial growth. Comparison of dental arch relationships, between the upper and lower jaw, also provides a valid method of clinical assessment. The Goslon Yardstick[65] is a method of analysis of the relationship of the dental arches in the permanent dentition, using dental study casts. The five categories described correlate closely with cephalometric X-ray analyses and provide a simple method of predicting facial growth outcome. A similar grading system using study casts of the deciduous dentition has been introduced which allows an even earlier assessment of facial growth outcomes at 5 years of age.[66]

Proponents of delayed hard palate closure have suggested that this can encourage more normal facial growth. Studies of growth outcomes following delayed hard palate repair are conflicting. Robertson and Jolleys[67] studied two groups of 20 cases, one group having had the hard palate closure delayed until 5 years of age. They reported no benefit for facial growth from a delayed hard palate repair. Schweckendiek,[39] however, closed the soft palate at 6 months but delayed hard palate closure until 12 to 16 years of age. Although this approach resulted in near normal facial growth, follow-up studies showed that a majority of the patients had unacceptably poor speech outcomes.[68]

Closure of the hard palate with a vomer flap at the time of lip repair is gaining in popularity. The possible impact of dissection of the vomerine tissue on facial growth remains controversial. Some surgeons believe that the vomerine tissue should not be disturbed,[40] whilst advocates of this method have produced long-term evidence that it does not significantly impair facial growth.[69]

Outcomes from presurgical orthopedic treatment

Improved alignment of the maxillary arch either side of a unilateral or bilateral complete cleft lip and palate with presurgical orthopedics (PSO) is considered advantageous by some authors.[70,71] Protagonists of these pre-surgical techniques claim that the improved alignment facilitates the subsequent cleft repair and that it improves the esthetic outcome. Methods of PSO vary from passive techniques such as simple elasticated strapping over the lip or removable acrylic appliances within the mouth, to appliances which require surgical placement of pins into the maxilla and use active forces to achieve movement of the maxillary segments (Latham technique). There is concern that these methods can disturb the subsequent growth of the maxilla,[72] and treatments which have included these methods have been associated with poor facial growth outcomes.[73]

A recent study reported a higher proportion of abnormal cross-bite in cleft lip and palate patients treated with a protocol, which included the presurgical use of the Latham appliance.[74] PSO requires considerable time and resources and significantly increases the overall treatment costs. Similar improvement in the alignment of the maxillary segments occurs after lip repair without the need for PSO, particularly if a complete muscle repair is performed. Whilst the use of PSO in bilateral complete cleft lip and palate can assist bilateral lip repair and reduce the likelihood of wound dehiscence, the overall benefit of PSO in cleft surgery remains debatable and probably minimal.

Outcomes from alveolar bone grafting

Secondary alveolar bone grafting (ABG) using autogenous cancellous bone in the mixed dentition stage (usually 9–11 years of age) is a highly successful procedure as confirmed by case studies.[75,76] It is generally agreed that the optimum timing for ABG is just before the eruption of the permanent canine tooth; the success rate declines if ABG is carried out after canine eruption, especially in the bilateral case.[77]

Primary bone grafting (within the first 2 years) has yielded generally poor results with unfavorable subsequent facial growth,[78] although some have reported less impact on facial growth.[79] However, the potential for mid-facial growth inhibition, the need for rib-graft harvest and the occasional need to repeat the grafting procedure later on, discourages the use of primary bone grafting which is generally not recommended. Secondary ABG remains the most common approach.

Gingivoperiosteoplasty with advancement of mucoperiosteal flaps over the alveolar cleft at the time of cleft palate repair can result in "boneless bone grafting" as described by Skoog.[80] Whilst good bone formation can occur with this procedure,[81] concerns remain regarding possible impairment of facial growth, inadequate bone formation, and the lack of long term outcome data. At present, the majority of cleft surgeons do not perform primary or early gingivoperiosteoplasty.

Outcomes from secondary speech surgery

Secondary speech surgery for the management of velopharyngeal insufficiency (VPI) mainly consists of either palatal re-repair, posterior pharyngeal flap or sphincter pharyngoplasty. Palatal re-repair can be effective in treating VPI following cleft palate repair and this may have a lower morbidity and be more physiologic than either a pharyngoplasty or pharyngeal flap.[59] The success rate of both pharyngoplasty and pharyngeal flap is similar in both procedures with abolition of VPI in around 70% of cases. Success rates for pharyngoplasty vary between 50% and 85% and those for pharyngeal flap between 66% and 88%.[82–84]

Causes of failure following pharyngeal speech surgery include poor case selection, poor surgical design, and/or technique.[85] Snoring during sleep is a frequent finding (80%) after effective surgery using either technique, although obstructive sleep apnea is an uncommon complication. A 10-year retrospective study[86] of perioperative complications in pharyngeal flap surgery reported a low complication rate (6% overall) and emphasized the importance of experienced surgical, anesthetic and nursing care, provided within an appropriate environment. It is currently popular to try to tailor the operation for an individual patient according to the characteristics of the velopharyngeal dysfunction as assessed on videofluoroscopy and nasendoscopy. However, as yet, studies have not confirmed superior results when such a management protocol is adopted. Indeed, a multicenter randomized controlled trial of pharyngoplasty and pharyngeal flap carried out between

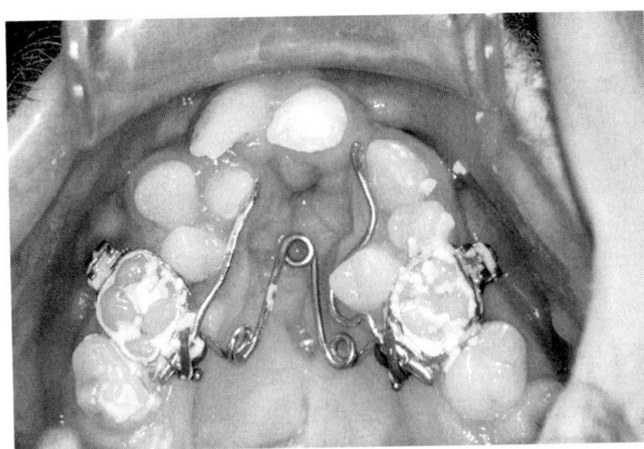

Fig. 6.4. Severe crowding of the upper teeth and collapse of the dental arches. A cemented orthodontic appliance is in place to expand the upper dental arch and improve tooth alignment (same patient as in Fig. 6.1).

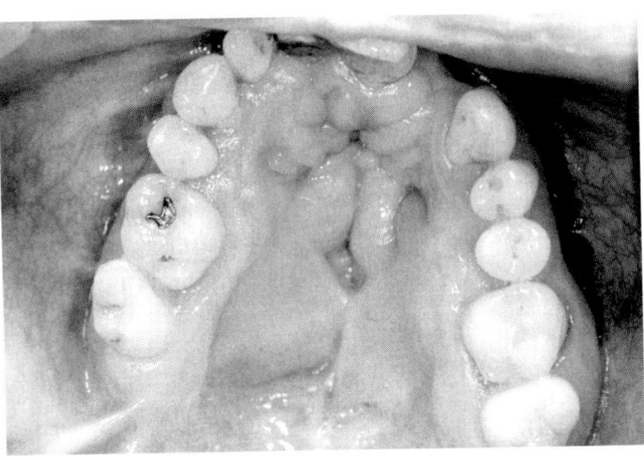

Fig. 6.5. Position of the teeth following orthodontic expansion and alignment. Note scarring in palate from previous surgery.

1993 and 2000 found no statistical difference in speech outcomes for the correction of VPI and no statistical difference in the incidence of perioperative complications.[87]

Other long-term outcomes from cleft lip and palate surgery

Although many children with craniofacial conditions such as cleft lip and palate develop normally and do not experience psychological problems, studies report that a significant number of children (between 30% and 40%) have learning disabilities, lower self-esteem and difficulties with social interaction.[88,89] Other problems include dental anomalies (Figs. 6.4 and 6.5) and hearing impairment, as well as other difficulties due to syndromic associations such as ophthalmic, cardiac and limb defects. The early involvement of a pediatrician is essential to ensure that a global approach is provided for the management of a child with cleft lip and/or palate.[90]

Long-term population-based studies in adults have suggested several other associations with cleft lip and palate. These include an increased prevalence of structural brain anomalies associated with mild cognitive impairment,[91] a higher incidence of psychiatric disorders in adults,[92] and an increased risk of mortality from various causes (including epilepsy) up to the age of 55 years.[93]

Finally, the long-term outcomes of cleft lip and palate would not be complete without considering the possible genetic implications. Cleft lip and palate is frequently associated with other congenital anomalies such as malformations of the upper and lower limbs, vertebral column and the cardiovascular system. Occasionally, multiple congenital anomalies form a recognized syndrome. Isolated clefts with no associated syndrome or other birth defect may also have a genetic etiology. A history may reveal a familial pattern of inheritance and even if this is not present, individuals with cleft lip and palate have a higher recurrence risk than the general population. Isolated cleft palate is associated with a recurrence risk of 2%, whereas cleft lip and palate is 4% overall. In familial cases the risk rises to one in ten when two siblings are affected or one sibling and a parent. The incidence of associated anomalies with cleft lip and palate has been reported to be as high as 38%.[94] One of the commonest syndromes associated with cleft lip and palate is van der Woude syndrome.[95] This autosomal dominant condition is characterized by bilateral pits of the lower lip in conjunction with a cleft of the lip and/or palate. The recurrence risks in van der Woude syndrome are therefore high and approach 50%. A further common syndrome associated with cleft palate, in particular, is velocardiofacial syndrome,[96] which is associated with a microdeletion of chromosome 22q11. Inheritance is autosomal dominant with wide variability in phenotypic expression and features may include facial dysmorphism, structural cardiac defects, cleft palate and velopharyngeal insufficiency. Currently, over 400 syndromes are recognized which include cleft lip and/or palate as a feature.[97]

Conclusions and future directions

Improvement in the long-term outcomes of treatment for cleft lip and/or palate is dependent on:

(i) surgical subspecialization and high-volume skilled operators;
(ii) an effectively working complete multidisciplinary team;

(iii) Protocols of management based on the best currently available evidence;
(iv) centralization of cleft care;
(v) provision of appropriate resources;
(vi) good record keeping and audit review;
(vii) Multicenter randomized control trials to determine the best treatments.

Centralization of cleft care within the UK is now complete with nine established regional cleft centers in England and Wales and a managed clinical network in Scotland. This followed the UK government acceptance in full of the CSAG report[6] and its subsequent implementation. A training interface group (under the auspices of the Royal Colleges of Surgeons) was established in 2000 to oversee the training of future cleft surgeons from the specialties of oral and maxillofacial surgery and plastic surgery. In the USA, centralization and sub-specialization of cleft care has not occurred to the same extent. Several factors may account for this such as commercial pressures within the medical environment, managed clinical care systems and occasional rivalry between surgical specialties. Such difficulties need to be overcome in the UK as well as the USA, so that we can look forward to a new era of centralized high-volume care, provided by expert, effective and highly trained multidisciplinary cleft teams using protocols derived from robust medical evidence. If we can achieve this, then along with the provision of appropriate resources, long-term outcomes in cleft lip and palate care will improve to the high levels that our patients deserve and expect.

REFERENCES

1. Shaw, W. C., Dahl, E., Asher-McDade, C. *et al.* A six-centre international study of treatment outcome in patients with clefts of the lip and palate. Part 5. General discussion and conclusions. *Cleft Palate Craniofac. J.* 1992; **29**:413–418.
2. Asher-McDade, C. M. & Shaw, W. C. Current cleft lip and palate management in the United Kingdom. *Br. J. Plast. Surg.* 1990; **43**:318–321.
3. Williams, A. C., Shaw, W. C., Sandy, J. R. *et al.* The surgical care of cleft lip and palate patients in England and Wales. *Br. J. Plast. Surg.* 1996; **49**:150–155.
4. Williams, A. C., Sandy, J. R., Shaw, W. C. *et al.* Consultant orthodontic services for cleft patients in England and Wales. *Br. J. Orthop.* 1996; **23**:165–171.
5. Shaw, W. C., Sandy, J. R., Williams, A. C. *et al.* Minimum standards for the management of cleft lip and palate: efforts to close the audit loop. *Ann. R. Coll. Surg. Engl.* 1996; **78**:110–114.
6. Clinical Standards Advisory Group – Cleft Lip and/or Palate HMSO. ISBN 0 11 321596 7. 1998:1–119.
7. Williams, A. C., Sandy, J. R., Thomas, S. *et al.* Influence of surgeon's experience on speech outcome in cleft lip and palate. *Lancet* 1999; **354**:1697–1698.
8. Sandy, J. R., Singer, S. L., & Williams, A. C. Healthcare services for low incidence anomalies. *Med. J. Aust.* 2000; **172**:201–202.
9. Williams, A. C., Johnson, N., Singer, S. *et al.* Outcomes of cleft care in Western Australia. *Aust. Dent. J.* 2000; **46**:32–36.
10. American Cleft Palate-Craniofacial Association. Parameters for evaluation and treatment of patients with cleft lip/palate or other craniofacial anomalies. *Cleft Palate Craniofac. J.* 1993; **30** (Suppl.): 1–16.
11. Bardach, J., Morris, H., Olin, W. *et al.* Late results of multidisciplinary management of unilateral cleft lip and palate. *Ann. Plast. Surg.* 1984; **12**:235–242.
12. Roberts, C. T., Semb, G., & Shaw, W. C. Strategies for the advancement of surgical methods in cleft lip and palate. *Cleft Palate Craniofac. J.* 1991; **28**:141–149.
13. Shaw, W. C. & Semb, G. Evidence-based care for children with cleft lip and palate. In Wyszynski, D. F., ed. *Cleft Lip and Palate From Origin to Treatment*, New York: Oxford University Press, Inc., 2002: 428–439.
14. Semb, G. & Shaw, W. C. Facial growth after different methods of surgical intervention in patients with cleft lip and palate. *Acta Odotol. Scand.* 1998; **56**:352–355.
15. Wong, K. C. & Wu, L. T. *History of Chinese Medicine*. Tientsin: Tientsin Press, 1932.
16. Shaw, W. C., Semb, G., Nelson, P. A. *et al. The Eurocleft Project 1996–2000*. Amsterdam: IOS Press.
17. Millard, D. R. Jr. *Cleft Craft: The Evolution of Its Surgery*, vol 1. Boston: Little Brown, 1976.
18. Mirault, G. Deux lettres sur l'operation du bec-de-lievre consideré dans ses divers états de simplicité et de complication. *J. Chir. (Paris)* 1844; **2**:257.
19. Blair, V. P. & Brown, J. B. Mirault operation for single harelip. *Surg. Gynecol. Obstet.* 1930; **51**:81–98.
20. Tennison, C. W. The repair of unilateral cleft lip by the stencil method. *Plast. Reconstr. Surg.* 1952; **9**:115–120.
21. Randall, P. A triangular flap operation for the primary repair of unilateral clefts of the lip. *Plast. Reconstr. Surg.* 1959; **23**:331–347.
22. Millard, D. R. Jr. A primary camouflage of the unilateral harelip. In Skoog, T., ed. *Transactions of the First International Congress of Plastic Surgery*. Baltimore: Williams and Wilkins, 1955: 160–166.
23. Mohler, L. R. Unilateral cleft lip repair. *Plast. Reconstr. Surg.* 1987; **80**:511–516.
24. Delaire, J. Theoretical principles and technique of functional closure of the lip and nasal aperture. *J. MaxFac. Surg.* 1978; **6**:109–116.
25. McComb, H. Treatment of the unilateral cleft lip nose. *Plast. Reconstr. Surg.* 1975; **55**:596–601.
26. McComb, H. K. & Coghlan, B. A. Primary repair of the unilateral cleft lip nose: completion of a longitudinal study. *Cleft Palate Craniofac. J.* 1996; **33**:23–30.
27. Anderl, H. K. (1985). Simultaneous repair of lip and nose in the unilateral cleft (a long term report). In Jackson, I. T. &

Sommerlad, B. *Recent Advances in Plastic Surgery* (3), Edinburgh: Churchill Livingstone, 1985: 1–11.
28. Cutting, C., Grayson, B., Brecht, L. *et al.* Presurgical columellar elongation and primary retrograde nasal reconstruction in one-stage bilateral cleft lip and nose repair. *Plast. Reconstr. Surg.* 1998; **101**:630–639.
29. Von Langenbeck, B. Die uranoplastik Mittels Ablosung des mukos-periostalen Gaumen uberzuges. *Arch. Klin. Chir.* 1861; **2**:205–287.
30. Veau, V. *Division palatine 1931*. Paris:Masson et Cie.
31. Wardill, W. E. M. The technique of operation for cleft palate. *Br. J. Surg.* 1937; **25**:117–130.
32. Kilner, T. P. Cleft lip and palate repair technique. In Maingot, R., ed. *Postgraduate Surgery*, Vol 3. New York/London: D. Appleton-Century Co., 1936.
33. Ortiz-Monasterio, F., Rebeil, A. S., Valderrama, M. *et al.* Cephalometric measurements on adult patients with non-operated cleft palates. *Plast. Reconstr. Surg.* 1959; **24**:53–61.
34. Ross, R. B. Treatment variables affecting facial growth in complete unilateral cleft lip and palate. Part 7: an overview of treatment and facial growth. *Cleft Palate J.* 1987; **24**:71–77.
35. Mars, M. & Houston, W. J. B. A preliminary study of facial growth and morphology in unoperated male unilateral cleft lip and palate subjects over 13 years of age. *Cleft Palate J.* 1990; **27**:7–15.
36. Furlow, L. T. Cleft palate repair by double opposing Z-plasty. *Plast. Reconstr. Surg.* 1986; **78**:724–736.
37. Pichler, H. Zur Operation der doppelten Lippengaumenspalten. *Dtsch. Z. Cir.* 1926; **195**:104.
38. Abyholm, F. E., Borchgrevink, H., & Eskeland, G. Cleft lip and palate in Norway III. Surgical treatment of CLP patients in Oslo 1954–75. *Scand. J. Plast. Reconstr. Surg.* 1981; **15**:15–28.
39. Schweckendiek, W. Primary veloplasty: long-term results without maxillary deformity. A twenty-five year report. *Cleft Palate J.* 1978; **15(3)**: 268–274.
40. Delaire, J. & Precious, D. Avoidance of the use of vomerine mucosa in primary surgical management of velopalatine clefts. *Oral Surg. Oral Med. Oral Path.* 1985; **60**:589–597.
41. Markus, A. F. & Precious, D. S. Effect of primary surgery for cleft lip and palate on mid-facial growth. *Br. J. Oral Maxillofac. Surg.* 1997; **35**:6–10.
42. Veau, V. Discussion on the treatment of cleft palate by operation. *Proc. R. Soc. Med.* 1926–27; **20(2)**:1916–1926.
43. Kriens, O. B. An anatomical approach to veloplasty. *Plast. Reconstr. Surg.* 1969; **43**:29–41.
44. Schoenborn, K. Vorstellung eines falle von Staphyloplastik. *Verh. Dtsch. Ges. Chir.* 1886; **15**:57–68.
45. Hynes, W. Pharyngoplasty by muscle transplantation. *Br. J. Plast. Surg.* 1950; **3**:128–135.
46. Orticochea, M. Construction of a dynamic muscle sphincter in cleft palates. *Plast. Reconstr. Surg.* 1968; **41**:323–327.
47. Jackson, I. T. & Silverton, J. S. The sphincter pharyngoplasty as a secondary procedure in cleft palates. *Plast. Reconstr. Surg.* 1977; **59**:518–524.
48. Sommerlad, B. C., Henley, M., Birch, M. *et al.* Cleft palate re-repair – a clinical and radiographic study of 32 consecutive cases. *Br. J. Plast. Surg.* 1994; **47**:406–410.
49. Calnan, J. Submucous cleft palate. *Br. J. Plast. Surg.* 1954; **6**:264–282.
50. Shprintzen, R. J., Goldberg, R. B., Lewis, M. L. *et al.* A new syndrome involving cleft palate, cardiac anomalies, typical facies, and learning disabilities: velo-cardio-facial syndrome. *Cleft Palate J.* 1978; **15**:56–62.
51. Boyne, P. J. & Sands, N. R. Secondary bone grafting of residual alveolar and palatal clefts. *J. Oral Surg.* 1972; **30**:87–92.
52. Asher-McDade, C., Roberts, C., Shaw, W. C. *et al.* Development of a method for rating nasolabial appearance in patients with clefts of the lip and palate. *Cleft Palate Craniofac. J.* 1991; **28**:385–390.
53. Morrant, D. G. & Shaw, W. C. Use of standardized video recordings to assess cleft surgery outcome. *Cleft Palate Craniofac. J.* 1996; **33**:134–142.
54. Cohen, S. R., Kalinowski, J., La Rossa, D. *et al.* Cleft palate fistulas: a multivariate statistical analysis of prevalence, etiology and surgical management. *Plast. Reconstr. Surg.* 1991; **87**:1041.
55. Sommerlad, B. C. A technique for cleft palate repair. *Plast. Reconstr. Surg.* 2003; **112**:1542–1548.
56. Witt, P. D. & D'Antonio, L. L. Velopharyngeal insufficiency and secondary palatal management: a new look at an old problem. *Clin. Plast. Surg.* 1993; **20**:707–721.
57. Dreyer, T. M. & Trier, W. C. A comparison of palatoplasty techniques. *Cleft Palate J.* 1984; **21**:251–253.
58. Marsh, J. L., Grames, L. M., & Holtman, B. Intravelar veloplasty: a prospective study. *Cleft Palate J.* 1989; **26**:46–50.
59. Sommerlad, B. C., Mehendale, F. V., Birch, M. J. *et al.* Palate re-repair revisited. *Cleft Palate Craniofac. J.* 2002; **39**:295–307.
60. Randall, P., LaRossa, D., Solomon, M. *et al.* Experience with the Furlow double-reversing Z-plasty for cleft palate repair. *Plast. Reconstr. Surg.* 1986; **77**:569–576.
61. McWilliams, B. J., Randall, P., LaRossa, D. *et al.* Speech characteristics associated with the Furlow palatoplasty as compared with other surgical techniques. *Plast. Reconstr. Surg.* 1996; **98**:610–619.
62. Williams, W. N., Seagle, M. B., Nackashi, A. J. *et al.* A methodology report of a randomised prospective clinical trial to assess velopharyngeal function for speech following palatal surgery. *Control Clin. Trials* 1998; **19**:297–312.
63. Ysunza, A., Pamplona, M. C., Mendoza, M. *et al.* Speech outcome and maxillary growth in patients with unilateral complete cleft lip/palate operated on at 6 versus 12 months of age. *Plast. Reconstr. Surg.* 1998; **102**:675–679.
64. Witt, P., Cohen, D., Grames, L. M *et al.* Sphincter pharyngoplasty for the surgical management of speech dysfunction associated with velocardiofacial syndrome. *Br. J. Plast. Surg.* 1999; **52**:613–618.
65. Mars, M., Plint, D. A., Houston, W. J. B. *et al.* The Goslon Yardstick: a new system of assessing dental arch relationships in children with unilateral clefts of the lip and palate. *Cleft Palate J.* 1987; **24**:314–322.

66. Atack, N., Hathorn, I., Mars, M. *et al.* Study models of 5 year old children as predictors of surgical outcome in unilateral cleft lip and palate. *Eur. J. Orthod.* 1997; **19**:165–170.
67. Robertson, N. R. & Jolleys, A. The timing of hard palate repair. *Scand. J. Plast. Reconstr. Surg.* 1974; **8**:49–51.
68. Bardach, J., Morris, H. L., & Olin, W. H. Late results of primary veloplasty: The Marburg Project. *Plast. Reconstr. Surg.* 1984; **73(2)**:207–215.
69. Semb, G. A study of facial growth in patients with unilateral cleft lip and palate treated by the Oslo CLP Team. *Cleft Palate Craniofac. J.* 1991; **28**:1–21.
70. Ross, R. B. & MacNamera, M. C. Effect of pre-surgical infant orthopaedics on facial esthetics in complete bilateral cleft lip and palate. *Cleft Palate Craniofac. J.* 1994; **31**:68–73.
71. Rutrick, R. E., Cohen, S. R., Brack, P. W. *et al.* Presurgical orthopaedic management of the unilateral cleft lip and palate newborn patient. *Oper Tech. Plast. Reconstr. Surg.* 1995; **2**:159–163.
72. Henkel, K. O. & Gundlach, K. K. H. Analysis of primary gingivoperiosteoplasty in alveolar cleft repair. Part 1: Facial Growth. *J. Craniomaxillofac. Surg.* 1997; **25**:266–269.
73. Mars, M., Asher-McDade, C., Brattstrom, V. *et al.* A six centre international study of treatment outcome in patients with clefts of the lip and palate: Part 3. Dental Arch Relationships. *Cleft Palate Craniofac. J.* 1992; **29**:405–408.
74. Berkowitz, S., Mejia, M., & Bystrik, A. A comparison of the effects of the Latham–Millard procedure with those of a conservative treatment approach for dental occlusion and facial aesthetics in unilateral and bilateral complete cleft lip and palate: part 1. Dental Occlusion. *Plast. Reconstr. Surg.* 2004; **113**:1.
75. Bergland, O., Semb, G., & Abyholm, F. E. Elimination of the residual alveolar cleft by secondary bone grafting and subsequent orthodontic treatment. *Cleft Palate J.* 1986; **23**:175–205.
76. Amanat, N. & Langdon, J. D. Secondary alveolar bone grafting in clefts of the lip and palate. *J. Craniomaxillofac. Surg.* 1991; **19**:7–14.
77. Abyholm, F. E., Bergland, O., & Semb, G. Secondary bone grafting of alveolar clefts. *Scand. J. Plast. Reconstr. Surg.* 1981; **15**:127–140.
78. Jolleys, A. & Robertson, N. R. E. A study of the effects of early bone-grafting in complete clefts of the lip and palate – five year study. *Br. J. Plast. Surg.* 1972; **25**:229–237.
79. Rosenstein, S. W., Monroe, C. W., Kernahan, D. A. *et al.* The case for early bone grafting in cleft lip and cleft palate. *Plast. Reconstr. Surg.* 1982; **70**:297–307.
80. Skoog, T. The use of periosteal flaps in the repair of clefts of the primary palate. *Cleft Palate J.* 1965; **2**:332–339.
81. Brusati, R. & Mannucci, N. The early gingivoalveoloplasty. *Scand. J. Plast. Reconstr. Hand Surg.* 1992; **26**:65–70.
82. Albery, E. H., Bennett, J. A., Pigott, R. W. *et al.* The results of 100 operations for velopharyngeal incompetence – selected on the findings of endoscopic and radiological examination. *Br. J. Plast. Surg.* 1982; **35**:118–126.
83. Riski, J. E., Ruff, G. L., Georgiade, G. S. *et al.* Evaluation of failed sphincter pharyngoplasties. *Ann. Plast. Surg.* 1992; **28**:545–553.
84. Schmelzeisen, R., Harsamen, J. E., Loebell, E. *et al.* Long-term results following velopharyngoplasty with a cranially based pharyngeal flap. *Plast. Reconstr. Surg.* 1992; **90**:774–778.
85. Ma, L., James, D. R., & Sell, D. A. Failed pharyngoplasty and subsequent management. *Br. J. Oral Maxillofac. Surg.* 1996; **34**:348–356.
86. Hofer, S. O., Krish Dhar, B., Robinson, P. H. *et al.* A 10-year review of perioperative complications in pharyngeal flap surgery. *Plast. Reconstr. Surg.* 2002; **110**:1393–1397.
87. Abyholm, F., Whitby, D., Skatvedt, O. *et al.* Pharyngeal surgery. Presentation at *The 9th International Congress on cleft palate and related craniofacial anomalies* 2001; Gothenburg, Sweden.
88. Turner, S. R., Rumsey, N., & Sandy, J. R. Psychological aspects of cleft lip and palate. *Eur. J. Orthod.* 1998; **20**:407–415.
89. Endriga, M. C. & Kapp-Simon, K. A. Psychological issues in craniofacial care: state of the art. *Cleft Palate Craniofac. J.* 1999; **36**:3–11.
90. Habel, A., Sell, D., & Mars, M. Management of cleft lip and palate. *Arch. Dis. Child.* 1996; **74**:360–366.
91. Nopoulos, P., Berg, S., Canady, J *et al.* Structural brain anomalies in adult males with clefts of the lip and/or palate. *Genet. Med.* 2002; **4**:1–9.
92. Ramstad, T., Ottem, E., & Shaw, W. C. Psychosocial adjustment in Norweigian adults who had undergone standardised treatment of complete cleft lip and palate. II. Self-reported problems and concerns with appearance. *Scand. J. Plast. Reconstr. Surg. Hand Surg.* 1995; **29**:329–336.
93. Christensen, K., Juel, K., Herskind, A. M., & Murray, J. C. Long term follow up study of survival associated with cleft lip and palate at birth. *Br. Med. J.* 2004; **328**:1405–1406.
94. Tolarova, M. & Cervenka, J. Classification and birth prevalence of orofacial clefts. *Am. J. Med. Genet.* 1998; **75**:126–137.
95. Van der Woude, A. Fistula labii inferioris congenita and its association with cleft lip and palate. *Am. J. Hum. Genet.* 1954; **6**:244–256.
96. Shprintzen, R. J., Goldberg, R. B., Lewin, M. L. *et al.* A new syndrome involving cleft palate, cardiac anomalies, typical facies and learning difficulties: velo-cardio-facial syndrome. *Cleft Palate J.* 1978; **15**:56–62.
97. Winter, R. & Baraitser, M. *London Dysmorphology Database.* Oxford: Oxford University Press, 1998.

7

Lymphangiomas

Salam Yazbeck and Maria Di Lorenzo[†]

Department of Surgery, University of Montreal, Canada

Lymphangiomas are benign abnormal collections of lymphatic vessels forming a mass composed of cystic spaces of variable size, which have the potential for local extension, thereby infiltrating surrounding structures. Lymphangiomas, cystic hygromas, and lymphangiomatosis can affect almost any area of the body where lymphatics are present, but predominate in the head, neck and axilla.[1,2] Constituting 5.6% of all benign lesions of infancy and childhood, lymphangiomas have no predilection for sex or race. Lymphangiomas can also occur in the lung, gastrointestinal tract, spleen, liver and bone, and may be a manifestation of multifocal disease if found in these last three organs.[3] Abdominal lymphangiomas are rare.

Lymphangiomas should not be confused with primary lymphedema, a disorder in children and adolescents causing swelling in an extremity. This condition is associated with several genetic syndromes and in contrast to lymphangiomas has the potential for malignant transformation with time.[4]

Gross observed that 65% of lymphangiomas were apparent at birth, and that 90% appeared by the end of the second year of life.[5] The principal mode of presentation is that of a disfiguring, usually slow growing mass. Rapid enlargement, sometimes overnight, may occur following systemic infection or bleeding into the tumor.

Etiology and pathogenesis

The etiology of lymphangiomatous malformations is believed to be a developmental defect in lymphatic pathways which develop from the sixth week of gestation onwards, resulting in obstructed or inadequate efferent channels and proximal dilatation of afferent channels.[6] The lymphatic system develops from five primitive sacs originating from the venous system. Lymphatic development has been divided into five phases extending between the sixth and tenth weeks of gestation. Lymphangiomas have been traditionally classified into three groups:[7] lymphangioma simplex consists of small capillary-sized channels; cavernous lymphangioma is composed of dilated lymphatic channels frequently covered by a fibrous adventitia; and cystic lymphangiomas or hygromas. Micro-and macrocystic forms may co-exist in different areas of the same lymphangioma.[1]

The pathogenesis and radiologic appearance of lymphatic malformations can be explained by lymphatic embryology as proposed by Zadvinskis *et al.*[8] The authors propose that a descriptive classification of lymphangiomas should not be based merely on size of lymphatic channels but rather that these lesions should be considered as a spectrum of the same pathologic process. Thus, cystic hygromas occur due to failure of embryonic lymph sacs to re-establish communication with the venous system. They may also result from aberrant primordial lymph sac budding. These lesions can reach considerable size due to growth in loose connective tissue. The smaller capillary and cavernous lymphangiomas develop later from abnormal sequestration of lymphatic mesenchyme buds, which have lost their connection with lymphatic primordia which branch peripherally. Growth is inhibited in these tough dermal and epidermal elements, resulting in the capillary form. Subcutaneous cavernous forms occur in less resistant tissues such as muscles or glands. Because they originate from a more peripheral branched network of developing lymphatics than cystic hygromas, their size is smaller,

[†] Dr. Di Lorenzo sadly died in 2003 but made a major contribution to this chapter in the first edition of this text.

Pediatric Surgery and Urology: Long-term Outcomes, Mark Stringer, Keith Oldham, Pierre Mouriquand.

and lymphatic spaces smaller. Lymphangiohemangiomas form when aberrant lymphatic buds maintain connections with the venous system from which they arise and are thus unable to fully differentiate into lymphatics.

Because of the wide spectrum of abnormalities that occur in the lymphatic system and their different modes of presentation, a new classification based on presentation of the disease has been proposed by Hilliard, McKendry and Phillips.[9] This clinical classification of congenital abnormalities of the lymphatics seems to provide a more useful guide to the diagnosis and management of the problem and is summarized as follows: (i) masses; (ii) bone lesions; (iii) presentation due to a single abnormal lymphatic function (e.g., lymphedema, ascites, or pleural effusions); (iv) presentation due to a combination of abnormal lymphatic functions; (v) associated abnormalities (e.g., lymphopenia, hypogammaglobulinemia); and (vi) symptoms related to mixed angiomatosis (blood and lymphatic vessels).

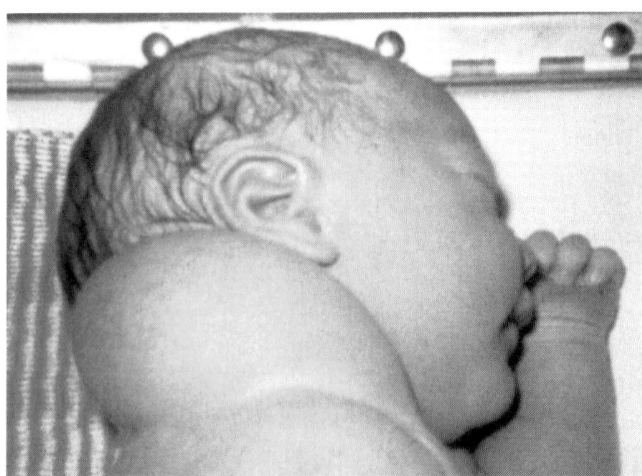

Fig. 7.1. Supraclavicular lymphangioma.

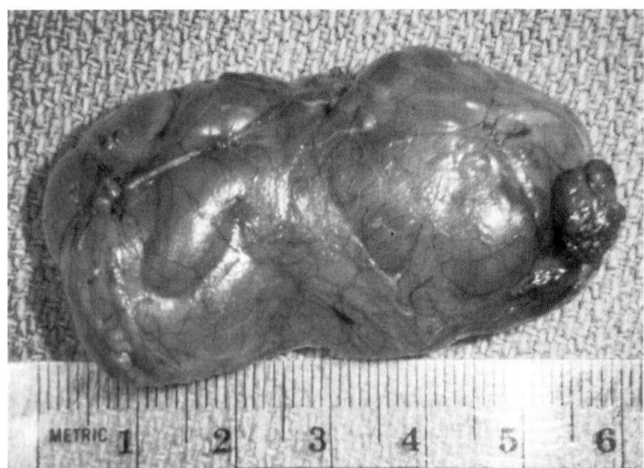

Fig. 7.2. Surgical specimen demonstrating multicystic lesion.

Presentation

Signs and symptoms of lymphangiomas vary according to anatomical location. Two-thirds of cervical lymphangiomas are asymptomatic. They present as a multilobular swelling, which is cystic on palpation. The mass may be circumscribed but most often infiltrating. The posterior triangle of the neck and the submandibular region are the most common sites of presentation (Figs. 7.1 and 7.2). Symptoms presenting in the neonatal period are related to feeding and breathing disturbances. Stridor and progressive respiratory difficulty may occur with extensive infiltrating lesions of the glottis and supraglottic area soon after birth.[10] Macroglossia resulting from lymphangiomatous infiltration and sublingual components are responsible for feeding problems. Thoracic lymphangiomas can also cause respiratory failure in infancy due to compression of mediastinal structures.

Sudden and sometimes painful enlargement of a lymphangioma in older children may be due to infection, hemorrhage and/or fluid accumulation. Acute upper respiratory tract infection has been associated with sudden enlargement of the mass.[11] Fluctuation in size with straining, coughing or respiration in a lymphangioma of the lower neck may be a manifestation of a mediastinal component, observed in 10% of such cases. Although respiratory symptoms here are generally less alarming than those seen in supraglottic lesions, acute respiratory distress has been reported in mediastinal lymphangiomas requiring urgent treatment.[12] Superior vena canal obstruction, chylothorax and chylopericardium have all been associated with intrathoracic lymphangioma.[11]

Lymphangiomatosis of bone is extremely rare, usually involving multiple sites.[13] The bones of the shoulder girdle are most often affected although lesions have been described in any bone. Lymphangiomas of the bone may present as incidental findings on an X-ray or as pathologic fractures. Pain and neurologic dysfunction result from compression. Bone lysis and replacement by fibrous cords (Gorham–Stout disease) can also occur.[14] Lytic lesions with fine sclerotic borders giving a "soap bubble" appearance are characteristic radiologic findings. These lesions have also been associated with chylothorax, chylopericardium or chylous ascites.[3] In a review of 16 cases by Canil *et al.*,[3] most presented with chylothorax. Bone pain was the presenting feature in only three patients. The time from detection of bone lesions to the development of chylothorax ranged from 6 months to 5 years.

Algorithm 1. Outcome after prenatal ultrasound diagnosis of lymphangiomas*

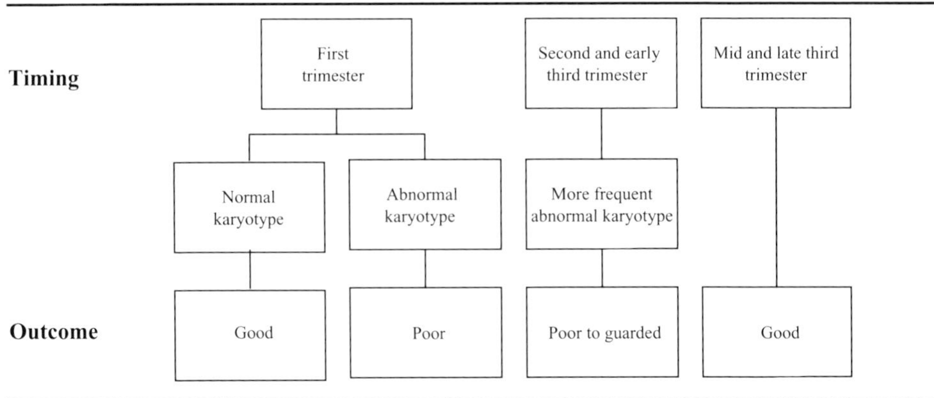

* If hydrops fetalis develops, fetal demise is almost certain.

In our series of 193 patients presenting with lymphangioma, symptoms were present in 17.8% of patients – primarily gastrointestinal, respiratory distress or infection, and local pain or tenderness. Physical signs included an isolated mass in half of the cases. The mass was expanding in an additional one-third of patients. Elephantiasis or gigantism was present in 5%. Intra-abdominal lymphangiomas produced abdominal distension or a palpable mass in 4%. Finally, proptosis, exophthalmos or ocular muscle paralysis occurred in 1.6% and cutaneous vesicles in 1.6% of our patients.[15]

Diagnosis

The diagnostic modalities most commonly used to investigate lymphangiomas and their effects are ultrasound, Doppler ultrasound, computed tomography (CT scan) and magnetic resonance imaging. Ultrasound demonstrates superficial hypoechogenic multilocular cystic masses but fails to demonstrate retropharyngeal, axillary or mediastinal extensions. With CT, it may be difficult to distinguish a mass from soft tissue structures. Recently, magnetic resonance imaging has been shown to be better at delineating tumor extent and can more accurately characterize tissues.[16]

Outcomes

Prenatal

There is much literature and controversy regarding the prenatal ultrasound diagnosis and outcome of lymphangiomas.[17–26] Outcome is essentially dependent on genetic associations and the timing of discovery of the lesion. Between 30% and 70% of fetuses with cystic hygromas are reported to have chromosomal aberrations, particularly Turner or Down syndrome.[26] The presence of these lymphatic abnormalities in such fetuses during the second trimester has been associated with a poor outcome.[27–29] Gallagher *et al.*[26] reports, like others, that progressive hydrops fetalis develops in up to 75% of cases and usually results in fetal death. If the karyotype is abnormal and there is a second significant malformation, the associated mortality is close to 100%. Resolution of nuchal edema or cystic hygromas has been reported in the first trimester fetus with subsequent good outcomes.[28,29,30–34] In a review of 100 consecutive fetuses with nuchal thickening or cystic hygromas detected sonographically at 10–15 weeks' gestation, Nadel *et al.*[21] concluded that, if the karyotype is normal and septations in the mass and hydrops are absent, the prognosis is good.

Axillary lymphangiomas seem to be less frequently associated with chromosomal anomalies.[35]

In a review of the literature, Thomas[24] concluded that fetuses whose lymphangiomas are detected on ultrasound in the first trimester should undergo karyotyping. Those with a normal karyotype have a good prognosis whereas those with an abnormal karyotype have a poor prognosis. Lymphangiomas detected in the second and early third trimester have a poor to guarded outcome due to a stronger link with chromosomal abnormalities. Mid to late third trimester detection is associated with a good outcome (Algorithm 1).

Postnatal

Postnatally, the majority of lymphangiomas present before 2 years of age, but they may present at any time and, in fact, have even been reported in the geriatric population.[36–39] These primary disorders of the lymphatic system represent a spectrum of conditions ranging from developmental defects in peripheral lymphatics to malformations of the thoracic duct, cysterna chyli and mesenteric nodes. Thus, multiple and delayed manifestations may occur in the same patient.[2] The common denominator in these patients is an abnormality in lymphatic channels resulting in dilatation of proximal channels, lymphostasis and lymphatic leakage.

Outcomes in postnatal lymphangiomas are directly related to the site of involvement and the treatment modality used. In their 20-year review of 52 children with cervical, cervicomediastinal and intrathoracic lymphangioma, Glasson and Taylor[11] observed that two-thirds of patients were asymptomatic. Enlargement, inflammation, infection, feeding difficulties, and respiratory symptoms occurred in the remainder. Acute airway obstruction was associated with pharyngeal and laryngeal involvement, seen commonly with large infiltrating lesions. They also observed that mediastinal extension led to less dramatic respiratory symptoms. Approximately 75% of these patients required only one surgical procedure.[11,15] The goal of surgery is complete non-disfiguring excision whenever possible without sacrificing vital structures or function. The most common complication of surgical treatment is excessive fluid accumulation.[11,15] In our series of 263 operations for lymphangiomas over a ten-year period, the overall complication rate was 31.3% with a local complication rate of 50%, mostly consisting of seromas or hematomas.[15] The second most frequent complication is damage to important nerves, in particular, the cervical branch of the facial nerve, accessory nerve, phrenic, recurrent laryngeal and vagus nerves and the sympathetic chain (resulting in Horner's syndrome), particularly after surgery for cervicomediastinal lesions. These neurologic complications accounted for 17% of the total complications in our series.[15] In order to decrease the incidence of these specific complications, the intraoperative use of nerve stimulators is strongly recommended. Lesions requiring thoracotomy may be complicated by chylothorax. Thoracic complications were responsible for 13.4% of all complications in our series.[15]

Very large cervical lesions may be life threatening and may require early tracheostomy in order to secure the airway; the tracheostomy must remain until the lesion has been completely excised. Carbon dioxide (CO_2) laser delivered with the microlaryngoscope facilitates excision of lesions at this site.[11] Neodymium: YAG laser treatment of oral cavity lesions has also been reported to be successful.[40] Both these modalities require repeated treatments for control.

In comparing supra- and infrahyoid cervicofacial lymphangiomas, Ricciardelli and Richardson[41] found that none of 13 children with infrahyoid lesions demonstrated feeding or respiratory difficulties while eight of 21 with suprahyoid involvement presented with dysphagia or airway compromise. Using a combined surgical and CO_2 laser approach, the recurrence rates for infrahyoid and suprahyoid lesions were 15% and 81%, respectively. There were no postoperative complications in the infrahyoid group, but eight of 21 patients with suprahyoid lesions suffered postoperative complications requiring repeated surgical procedures or hospitalization. The importance of the site of the lesion in predicting outcome has been further documented.[42,43] Most authors concur that recurrences are most common after excision of suprahyoid, submandibular and oral lesions. Until recently, conservative surgical management, sparing all important anatomical structures has been the treatment of choice for cervicofacial lymphangiomas. This has been substantiated by the fact that spontaneous regression is rare, although possible[44,45] and that persistent swelling with rapid intermittent enlargement is the rule.

Long-standing oral and mandibulofacial cystic hygromas lead to deformities requiring surgical correction. Osborne *et al.*[46] describe their experience with orthognathic surgical correction of mandibular prognathism and dental malocclusion associated with recurrent, long standing cystic hygromas. Based on their results in three cases and a review of the literature, the authors concluded that patients with large tumors which have not been adequately debulked should not have mandibular surgery at an early age due to the likelihood of recurrence. Stabilization of tumor size and completion of mandibular growth prior to orthognathic surgery led to an improved correction of the resultant deformities.

Chylothorax is associated with mediastinal and bone lymphangiomatosis. Thoracocentesis alone is not successful in any of the reported cases.[3] Dietary manipulation with a low fat diet, medium chain triglyceride enteral feeding, or total parenteral nutrition is transiently effective in slowing lymph flow in a small minority of patients. Thoracotomy with pleurectomy, with or without thoracic duct ligation, achieved the best results. Thoracic duct ligation alone was unsuccessful in all cases. Fourteen of 16 patients presenting with lymphangiomatosis of bone had intrathoracic lesions consistent with lymphangioma, suggesting that bone lesions may just be a manifestation of a more generalized process which may include mediastinal lesions. The authors recommend early thoracotomy and pleurectomy on the affected side. Any mediastinal lesion should be excised if possible. Application of fibrin glue to exposed surfaces after these procedures may decrease the incidence of postoperative fluid accumulation. Keeping the lung expanded with postoperative mechanical ventilation may obliterate the pleural space and favor healing.

In a recent excellent review of the literature, Alvarez *et al.* identified young age and both pleural and pulmonary involvement as poor prognostic factors with thoracic lymphangiomatosis.[47] Although the age distribution in this series was 0 to 76 years, no patient over 11 years old died.

Intra-abdominal lymphangiomas are rare. They are included in the 5–9% of cases located outside the head, neck, trunk, and extremities.[48,49] In our experience two forms exist: localized and diffuse. The localized form is easily amenable to total excision but the diffuse form is refractory to conventional surgical excision. The importance of the abdominal site lies in reports indicating that intra-abdominal lymphangiomas present more commonly in children, with up to 88% being symptomatic,[50,51] and that the localized form frequently presents as an acute abdomen.[50] Symptoms include abdominal pain, vomiting, increasing abdominal girth, and nausea. Approximately two-thirds occur in the mesentery of the small bowel, and one-third in the retroperitoneum.[48,50,52] Stomach and colon involvement have been observed. Ultrasound and CT are the imaging modalities which lead to a prompt diagnosis, thereby helping to avoid potentially catastrophic complications, such as obstruction, hemorrhage, volvulus and rupture.[51] Complete excision is the treatment of choice. Up to 61% of patients may require bowel resection.[50] Invasion of other organs such as the spleen or tail of the pancreas requires excision of the involved part of the organ.[53] However, recurrence is not invariable after incomplete resection of large lesions.[50,53] Postoperatively, ultrasound is recommended for monitoring. After failure of conventional surgical and medical therapy, life-threatening, diffuse abdominal lymphangiomatosis has been treated with argon beam ablation, scoring all peritoneal and serosal surfaces, with acceptable outcome at 6 months postoperatively.[54]

Esophageal and intestinal lymphangioma are rare in children. Most cases are diagnosed in adulthood, usually by endoscopy.[55–57] An association between abdominal cavernous lymphangioma and T-cell lymphoma has been reported.[58] Lymphangiomas causing protein-losing enteropathy are relatively large with intramuscular and subserosal cysts. Smaller mucosal and submucosal cysts do not cause protein-losing enteropathy, and half of them are pedunculated. Electrocautery excision is the preferred treatment. Larger cysts require intestinal resection.[55]

Recurrence

Based on our institutional experience, we agree with Fonkalsrud,[1] that the potential for recurrence exists with all lymphangiomas, regardless of site. Most recurrences are apparent within the first few months after surgery but delayed recurrences can be observed, sometimes after several years. In one of the few long-term follow-up studies of lymphangiomas which extended over 8–41 years, Saijo *et al.*[59] noted a 50% recurrence rate after first excision; recurrences were seen within 4 years of surgery in all cases. Charabi *et al.*[60] reported a long term follow-up of 44 cases of cystic hygroma of the head and neck treated by surgery only. Residual or recurrent lesions were noticed in 50% of cases while 44% had some functional disability and 36% had bad cosmesis. In this series, no histologically confirmed cases of lymphangioma underwent spontaneous regression.

Adjunctive therapies

The success of adjunctive therapies in the treatment of lymphangiomas is variable and controversial. Radiotherapy has been used in the past. It is no longer recommended due to the disappointing results obtained and the potential long term sequelae of growth retardation and induction of neoplastic changes.[46]

Primary treatment of cystic lymphangioma using intralesional bleomycin injection has been used successfully. Okada *et al.*[61] reported their ten-year experience with this approach in 29 pediatric patients. Significant reduction of the mass was observed in 86% and total regression in 55% of cases. The recurrence rate was approximately 10%. Although some authors believe that subsequent surgical dissection is rendered more difficult because of extensive scarring, the 13 patients requiring surgical resection in this series had the extent of their surgery minimized by prior bleomycin therapy. No serious side effects were reported with a total dose of 5 mg/kg administered at intervals of not less than 2 weeks. Minor transient side effects including fever, vomiting, cellulitis, and skin discoloration have been observed in a small number of patients.[62] Orford *et al.*[62] reported complete resolution in 44% and a greater than 50% decrease in size in another 44%, after a mean follow-up of 6 months. Bleomycin injection is more likely to produce a good response in cystic lesions.[62–64] It is contraindicated in cervicomediastinal lesions due to the risk of swelling following injection.

OK-432 is a lyophilized mixture of a low-virulence Su strain of Streptococcus pyogenes of human origin incubated with penicillin G. It has been used for the primary intralesional treatment of lymphangiomas and in the treatment of recurrences. Ogita *et al.* report[65] involving 64 patients treated between 1986 and 1992, demonstrated its efficacy in primary therapy, following incomplete surgical removal, and after failure of bleomycin sclerotherapy. Again, the majority of cystic lesions (22 of 24) responded with significant shrinkage. Only 9 of 22 cavernous lesions improved after treatment. Among responders, no recurrence was noted during a follow-up period ranging from 6 to 87 months. Transient fever and local inflammation lasting only a few days were the only side effects noted. The authors concluded that the intralesional injection of OK-432 should be considered the primary treatment of choice in lymphangiomas. Satisfactory sclerosis of recurrent cervicofacial lymphangiomas using OK-432 has been reported in North America for surgically challenging lesions. Mikhail *et al.*[66] reported its use in two cases with no local or systemic complications, and with definite reduction in the size of the lesion and improvement in cosmetic appearance. Some authors have reported disappointing results[67] while others have been very enthusiastic about its use.[68,69] OK-432 has been used for prenatal treatment of fetuses with cystic hygroma but the results are disappointing.[25] The mechanism of action of OK-432 may relate more to the induction of fibrotic changes in the wall of the lesion(s) than to a direct cytotoxic effect on endothelial cells within the lymphangioma.[70] The treatment with OK-432 may necessitate repeated injections every 4–6 weeks.

Other intralesional agents have been used successfully in the treatment of invasive lymphangiomas. These have included sodium morrhuate,[71] fibrin glue,[72] doxycycline,[73] and triamcinolone.[74] We have not found sclerotherapy with 50% dextrose to be beneficial in the management of recurrent disease or postoperative seromas.[15] Although the numbers of patients treated in these series are small and follow-up periods short, compared to the Japanese series using OK-432 and bleomycin, all forms of sclerotherapy have demonstrated some efficacy in the treatment of lymphangiomas, either primarily or as an adjunct to surgery, more particularly in macrocystic lesions.

Percutaneous embolization of lymphangiomas with Ethibloc® has been used successfully for a number of years by the French.[75] Ethibloc® (Ethicon, GmbH & Co. KG, Norderstedt, Germany) is a non-toxic, sterile sclerosing solution. Each milliliter of sterile solution contains 210 mg of Zein (a yellowish protein derived from corn), 162 mg of sodium-amidotrizoate-tetrahydrate, which is a radio-opaque marker, 145 mg of "Oleum Papaveris" which gives the solution viscosity, 316 mg of ethanol 96%, and 248 mg of aqua ad iniectabilia. This agent polymerizes on contact with blood or any other ionic substance to produce semiliquid biodegradable emboli which will resolve within 4 to 6 weeks after injection, subsequent to causing an inflammatory reaction necessary to collapse the cysts.

In a large series of 70 patients treated over nine years, Herbreteau *et al.*[75] demonstrated the efficacy of percutaneous Ethibloc® embolization under fluoroscopic control in a wide variety of lymphangiomas. Patients require prior opacification of their lesion by direct injection of contrast agent in order to assess size, compartmentation and communications among cysts. Fifty five percent of patients were under 5 years of age and 80% of lesions were located in the maxillofacial region. Results were good to excellent in 62% of patients, 15% required surgery, 5% of lesions remained unchanged, and 20% continued to progress. Failures (24%) occurred in mixed forms of lymphangiomas. Complications were minor and included ulceration with Ethibloc® extrusion treated topically with good results (3), transient hyperthermia, and residual inflammatory nodules (4) requiring excision.

Based on the favorable results of treating a variety of lymphangiomas with Ethibloc®, and the fact that it is a non-toxic, biodegradable substance, we elected to use this form of therapy in our institution. Since 1992, we have been using percutaneous embolization with Ethibloc® in cases of macrocystic or mixed lymphangiomas in order to improve outcome and to decrease the risk of surgically related complications. In a series of ten lymphangiomas (eight cervicofacial and two axillary), we observed good results with complete regression in six macrocystic lesions and partial regression in four mixed lesions (Figs. 7.3, 7.4, 7.5, 7.6).[76] In the four cases with intraoral lesions, tongue position returned to normal. Skin ulceration with Ethibloc® expulsion was noted in 70% of cases but was followed by healing without sequelae (Fig. 7.5) and seemed to predict a good clinical outcome. No other complications have been noted. No recurrences have been documented during follow-up periods ranging from 17 to 36 months. This approach has now been used in 123 patients with no major complications. However, it is important to state that some lesions have necessitated multiple injections of sclerosant. Based on these findings, we recommend percutaneous embolization with Ethibloc® and thus refer all head, neck, trunk and extremity lymphangiomas to our interventional radiologist for evaluation, treatment, and follow-up. Ultrasound and CT scan are used to assess the lesions in all cases. Surgical treatment is reserved for those lesions not responding to embolization and for intrathoracic or intra-abdominal lesions.

To evaluate the potential efficacy of intralesional therapy in lymphangiomas, lymphoscintigraphy using Tc-99m colloid particles to assess lymph flow in these masses has been recommended.[77–79] The pattern of retention and drainage of isotope by the lesion helps to predict the risk of organ toxicity. Those lymphangiomas demonstrating satisfactory

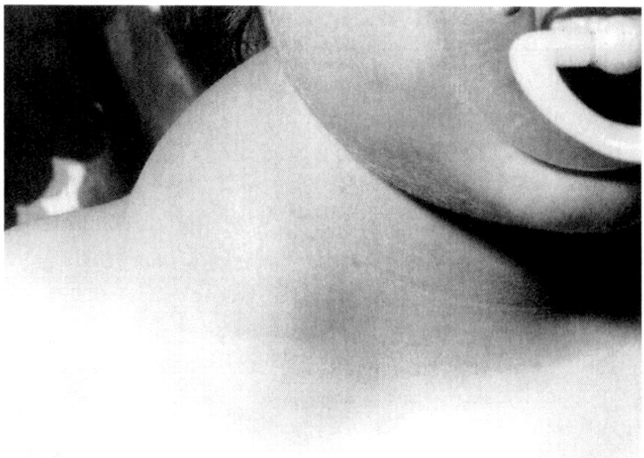

Fig. 7.3. Cervico-mediastinal lymphangioma.

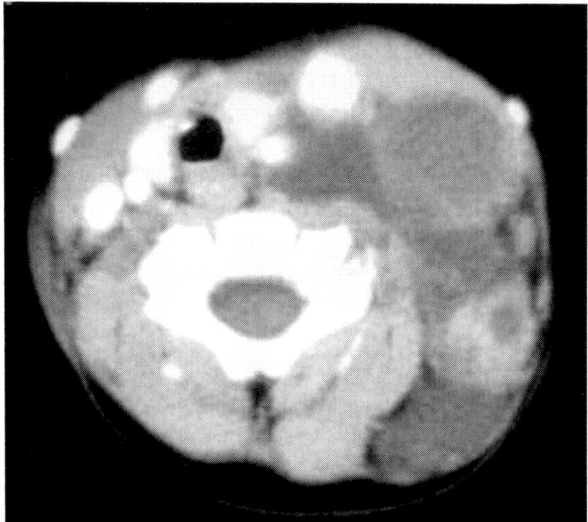

Fig. 7.4. CT scan of patient with cervical lymphangioma.

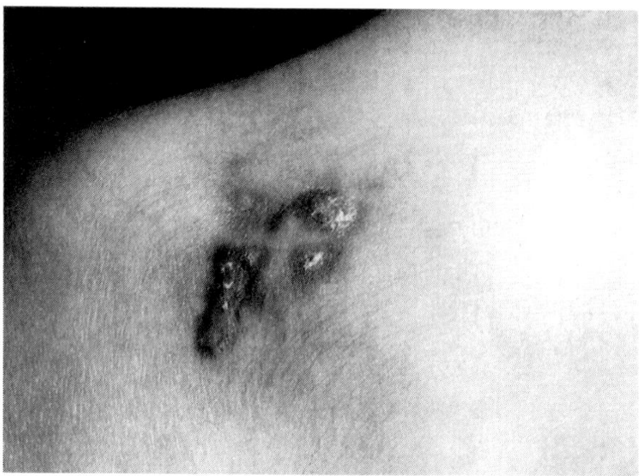

Fig. 7.5. Appearance of lesion in Fig. 7.3, 1 year after intralesional Ethibloc® treatment. Note healing skin ulcerations where expulsion of Ethibloc® occurred.

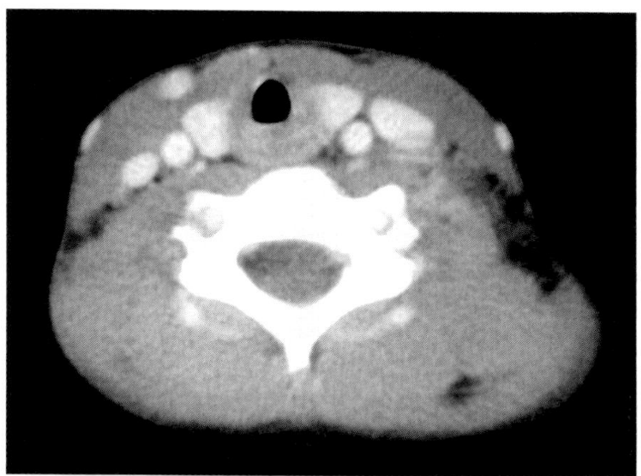

Fig. 7.6. CT scan of the lesion in Fig. 7.4 showing regression of lymphangioma 1 year after Ethibloc® treatment.

retention and slow outflow are also likely to show a better response.

Economic and medicolegal aspects

The economic implications of lymphatic system malformations are far-reaching and touch on all aspects of healthcare. The more extensive the lesion, the more labor intensive and costly is the treatment. A multidisciplinary approach is necessary regardless of the form of therapy undertaken, be it surgical or intralesional. Invasive cervicofacial lesions with the potential for airway obstruction require in-hospital care. The need for tracheostomy necessitates initial observation in an intensive care setting, with subsequent training of the care-giver and, upon discharge, home nursing visits. Although mortality is uncommon, the morbidity associated with lymphangiomas is significant. In addition to complications related to the pathology itself, complications resulting from treatment must be dealt with. Some patients will require long-term hospitalization due to complications related to their specific type of lymphangioma, such as ascites, protein-losing enteropathy, and chylothorax. Surgical complications relating to nerve damage, infection, and local wound seroma also place an economic burden on health care resources. However, prenatal ultrasound diagnosis and counselling have allowed the identification of infants with grim prognoses. In

Algorithm 2. Outcome of postnatal lymphangiomas

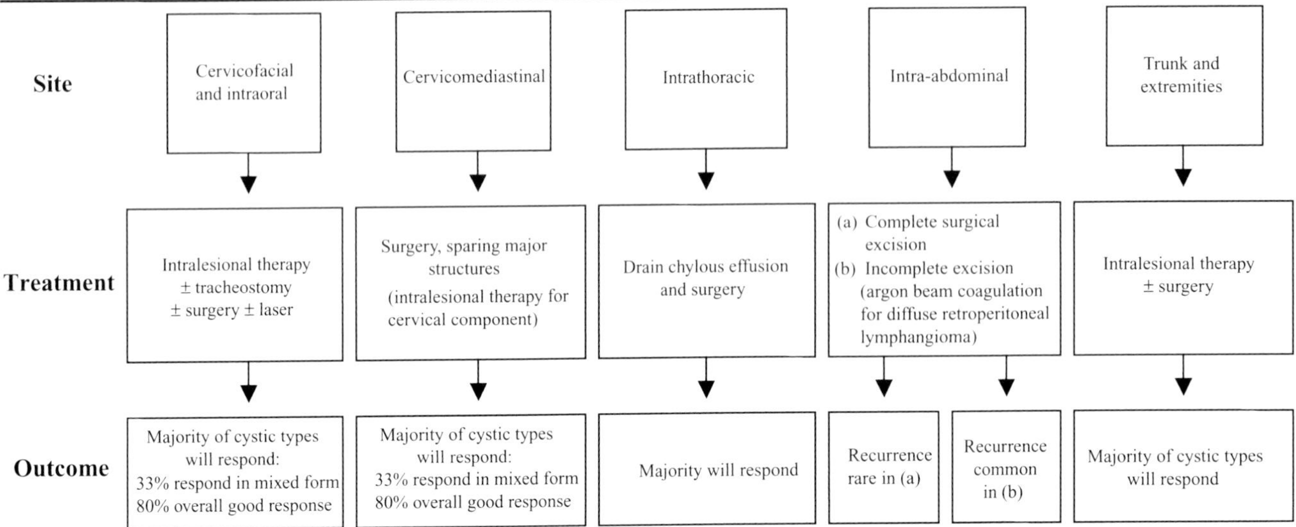

reserving surgery for those cases not responding or only showing a partial response to intralesional therapy, we believe that the economic impact of large invasive masses, and the unavoidable complications resulting from extensive, challenging surgery are diminished.

The ethical as well as the medicolegal implications of prenatal counselling in cases of lymphangioma are of particular interest to the ultrasonographer, perinatologist, and pediatric surgeon. Expert advice and familiarity with recent literature on the subject are of paramount importance when presented with a prenatal diagnosis of lymphangioma. Finally, effective communication is important in order to clearly explain potential complications and the probability of recurrence, such that the child's parents or legal guardian can truly give informed consent to any proposed conventional or experimental treatment modality.

Conclusions

Lymphangiomas are benign lesions which are associated with significant morbidity when treated by standard surgical techniques. Overall mortality rates vary between 3.4 and 5.7%.[15,59,79] The outcome of treatment of lymphangiomas is related to their site and extent, and to the morphology of the cysts in the lesion. In addition, the timing of diagnosis also affects outcome, as does the presence of an abnormal karyotype (Algorithm 1). It is important to note that suprahyoid lesions with mediastinal extension carry the potential for acute airway obstruction and may require tracheostomy. CO_2 and neodymium: YAG laser treatment are valuable adjuncts to surgery and intralesional therapy for airway and oral cavity lesions.

Treatment specific outcomes relate to the use of intralesional and surgical therapies. Regardless of the treatment modality used, an average of one-third of all lesions will recur. The recurrence rate after total excision in our series was 12%, and after partial excision was more than 50% up to 10 years after surgery.[15] With OK-432 sclerotherapy and Ethibloc® embolization, the majority of macrocystic lesions will regress. However, only one-third of mixed lymphangiomas will respond to local intralesional treatment. Cervicomediastinal and intra-abdominal lymphangiomas, as well as chylothorax associated with lymphangioma, require surgery for cure.

Finally, management should be tailored to the anatomical site and nature of the cystic lesion as proposed in Algorithm 2. The results of long-term follow-up are varied due to the diverse methods of treatment advocated for these lesions and the scarcity of publications documenting truly long-term results. We therefore advocate mandatory long-term follow-up of all cases of lymphangioma, regardless of treatment modality, in order to more accurately determine outcome. The poor functional and cosmetic outcomes observed after traditional surgical treatment of extensive lymphangiomas has influenced our current practice. Primary intralesional therapy combined with excision in selected cases only has become our preferred therapeutic modality.

REFERENCES

1. Fonkalsrud, E. W. Congenital malformations of the lymphatic system. *Semin. Pediatr. Surg.* 1994; **3**:62–69.
2. Levine, C. Primary disorders of the lymphatic vessels – a unified concept. *J. Pediatr. Surg.* 1983; **24**:233–240.
3. Canil, K., Fitzgerald, P., & Lau, G. Massive chylothorax associated with lymphangiomatosis of the bone. *J. Pediatr. Surg.* 1994; **29**:1186–1888.
4. Smeltzer, D. M., Stickler, G. B., & Schirger, A. Primary lymphedema in children and adolescents: a follow-up study and review. *Pediatrics* 1985; **76**:206–218.
5. Gross, R. E. *The Surgery of Infancy and Childhood.* Philadelphia, PA: Saunders, 1953.
6. Rhekhi, B. M. & Esselstyn, C. B. Retroperitoneal cystic lymphangioma. *Cleve Clin. Q.* 1972; **39**:125–128.
7. Landing, B. H. & Farber, S. *Tumors of the cardiovascular system.* In *Atlas of Tumor Pathology,* Washington, DC: Armed Forces Institute of Pathology, 1956.
8. Zadvinskis, D. P., Benson, M. T., & Kerr, H. H. Congenital malformations of the cervicothoracic lymphatic system: embryology and pathogenesis. *Radiographics* 1992; **12**:1175–1189.
9. Hilliard, R. I., McKendry, J. B. J., & Phillips, M. J. Congenital abnormalities of the lymphatic system: a new clinical classification. *Pediatrics* 1990; **86**:988–994.
10. Kenton, A., Duncan, N., Bhakta, K., & Fernandes, C. J. Laryngeal lymphatic malformation in a newborn. *J. Perinatol.* 2003; **23**:567–571.
11. Glasson, M. J. & Taylor, S. F. Cervical, cervicomediastinal and intrathoracic lymphangioma. *Prog. Pediatr. Surg.* 1991; **27**:62–83.
12. Grosfeld, J. L. & Weber, T. R. One-stage resection for massive cervicomediastinal hygroma. *Surgery* 1982; **92**:693–699.
13. Kittredge, R. D. & Finby, N. The many facets of lymphangioma. *Am. J. Radiol.* 1965; **95**:56–66.
14. Gorham, L. W., Wright, A. W., & Shultz, H. H. Disappearing bones: a rare form of massive osteolysis. *Am. J. Med.* 1989; **17**:674–682.
15. Hancock, B. J., St-Vil, D., & Di Lorenzo, M. Complications of lymphangiomas in children. *J. Pediatr. Surg.* 1992; **27**:220–226.
16. Borecky, N., Gudinchet, F., & Laurini, R. Imaging of cervicothoracic lymphangiomas in children. *Pediatr. Radiol.* 1995; **25**:127–130.
17. Bernard, P., Chabaud, J. J., & Le Guern, H. Hygroma kystique du cou. *J Gynecol. Obstet. Biol. Reprod.* 1991; **20**:487–495.
18. Langer, J. C., Fitzgerald, P. G., & Desa, D. Cervical cystic hygroma in the fetus: clinical spectrum and outcome. *J. Pediatr. Surg.* 1990; **25**:58–62.
19. Johnson, M. P., Johnson, A., & Holzgreve, W. First-trimester simple hygroma: cause and outcome. *Am. J. Obstet. Gynecol.* 1993; **168**:156–161.
20. Giacalone, P. L., Boulot, P., & Deschamps, F. Prenatal diagnosis of a multifocal lymphangioma. *Prenatal Diagnosis* 1993; **13**:1133–1137.
21. Nadel, A., Bromley, B., Benacerraf, B. R. Nuchal thickening or cystic hygromas in first- and early second-trimester fetuses: prognosis and outcome. *Obstet. Gynecol.* 1993; **82**:43–48.
22. Bronshtein, M., Bar-Hava, I., & Blumenfeld, I. The difference between septated and nonseptated nuchal cystic hygroma in the early second trimester. *Obstet. Gynecol.* 1993; **81**:683–687.
23. van Zalen-Sprock, R. M., van Vugt, J. M. G., & van Geijn, H. P. First-trimester diagnosis of cystic hygroma – course and outcome. *Am. J. Obstet. Gynecol.* 1992; **167**:94–98.
24. Thomas, R. L. Prenatal diagnosis of giant cystic hygroma: prognosis, counselling, and management; case presentation and review of the recent literature. *Prenatal Diagnosis* 1992; **12**:919–923.
25. Ogita, K., Suita, S., & Taguchi, T. Outcome of fetal cystic hygroma and experience of intrauterine treatment. *Fetal Diagn. Ther.* 2001; **16**:105–110.
26. Gallagher, P. G., Mahoney, M. J., & Gosche, J. R. Cystic hygroma in the fetus and newborn. *Semin. Perinatol.* 1999; **23(4)**:341–356.
27. Ville, Y., Lalondrelle, C., & Doumerc, S. First-trimester diagnosis of nuchal anomalies: significance and fetal outcome. *Ultrasound Obstet. Gynecol.* 1992; **2**:314–316.
28. Cullen, M. T., Gabrielli, S., & Green, J. J. Diagnosis and significance of cystic hygroma in the first trimester. *Prenat. Diagn.* 1990; **10**:643–651.
29. Shulman, L. P., Emerson, D. S., & Felker, R. E. High frequency of cytogenetic abnormalities in fetuses with cystic hygroma diagnosed in the first trimester. *Obstet. Gynecol.* 1992; **80**:80–82.
30. Chervenak, F. A., Isaswcson, G., & Blakemore, K. J. Fetal cystic hygroma: Cause and natural history. *N. Engl. J. Med.* 1993; **309**:822–825.
31. Bronshtein, M., Rottem, S., & Yoffe, N. First-trimester and early second-trimester diagnosis of nuchal cystic hygroma by transvaginal sonography: diverse prognosis of the septated from the nonseptated lesion. *Am. J. Obstet. Gynecol.* 1989; **161**:78–82.
32. van Zalen-Sprock, R. M., van Vugt, J. M. G., & van Geijn, H. P. First-trimester diagnosis of cystic hygroma – course and outcome. *Am. J. Obstet. Gynecol.* 1992; **167**:94–98.
33. Bernstein, H. S., Filly, R. A., & Goldberg, J. D. Prognosis of fetuses with a cystic hygroma. *Prenat. Diagn.* 1991; **11**:349–355.
34. Distell, B. M., Hertzberg, B. S., & Bowie, J. D. Spontaneous resolution of a cystic neck mass in a fetus with normal karyotype. *Am. J. Radiol.* 1989; **153**:380–382.
35. Zanotti, S., LaRusso, S., & Coulson, C. Prenatal sonographic diagnosis of axillary cystic lymphangioma. *J. Clin. Ultrasound* 2001; **29**:112–115.
36. Shaffer, K., Rosado-de-Christenson, M. L., Patz, E. F. Thoracic lymphangioma in adults: CT and MR imaging feature. *Am. J. Radiol.* 1994; **162**:283–289.

37. Bhattacharyya, A. K. & Balogh, K. Retroperitoneal lymphangioleiomyomatosis. *Cancer* 1985; **56**:1144–1146.
38. Baer, S. & Davis, J. Cystic hygroma presenting in adulthood. *J. Laryngol Otol.* 1989; **103**:976–977.
39. Schefter, R. P., Olsen, K. D., & Gaffey, T. A. Cervical lymphangioma in the adult. *Otolaryngol. Head Neck Surg.* 1985; **93**:65–69.
40. Suen, J. Y. & Waner, M. Treatment of oral cavity vascular malformations using the neodymiun: YAG laser. *Arch. Otolaryngol. Head Neck Surg.* 1989; **115**:1329–1333.
41. Ricciardelli, E. J. & Richardson, M. A. Cervicofacial cystic hygroma. *Arch. Otolaryngol. Head Neck Surg.* 1991; **117**:546–553.
42. Cohen, S. R. & Thompson, J. W. Lymphangiomas of the larynx in infants and children: a survey of pediatric lymphangioma. *Ann. Otol. Rhinol. Laryngol.* 1986; **127(suppl)**:1–20.
43. Emory, P. J., Bailey, C. M., & Evans, J. M. Cystic hygroma of the head and neck: a review of 37 cases. *J. Laryngol. Otol.* 1984; **98**:613–619.
44. Gross, R. E. & Goeringer, C. F. Cystic hygroma of the neck. *Surg. Gynecol. Obstet.* 1939; **69**:48–60.
45. Broomhead, I. W. Cystic hygroma of the neck. *Br. J. Plast. Surg.* 1964; **17**:225–244.
46. Osborne, T. E., Levin, L. S., Tilghman, D. M., & Haller, J. A. Surgical correction of mandibulofacial deformities secondary to large cervical cystic hygromas *J. Oral Maxillofac. Surg.* 1987; **45**:1015–1021.
47. Alvarez, O. A., Kjellin, I., & Zuppan, C. Thoracic lymphangiomatosis in a child. *J. Pediatr. Hematol. Oncol.* 2004; **26**:136–141.
48. Galifer, R. B., Pous, J. G., & Juskeiwenski, S. Intra-abdominal cystic lymphangioma in childhood. *Prog. Pediatr. Surg.* 1978; **11**:173–238.
49. Enzinger, F. M. & Weiss, S. W. Tumors of lymph vessels. In *Soft Tissue Tumors.* St Louis, MO: Mosby, 1983:485–491.
50. Kosir, M. A., Sonnino, R. E., Gauderer, M. W. L. Pediatric abdominal lymphangiomas: a plea for early recognition. *J. Pediatr. Surg.* 1991; **26**:1309–1313.
51. Takiff, H., Calabria, R., & Vin, L. Mesenteric cysts and intra-abdominal cystic lymphangiomas. *Arch. Surg.* 1985; **120**:1266–1269.
52. Kurtz, R. J., Heimann, T. M., & Holt, J. Mesenteric and retroperitoneal cysts. *Ann. Surg.* 1986; **203**:109–111.
53. Roisman, I., Manny, J., & Fields, S. Intra-abdominal lymphangioma. *Br. J. Surg.* 1989; **76**:485–489.
54. Rothenberg, S. S. & Pokorny, W. J. Use of Argon beam ablation and sclerotherapy in the treatment of a case of life-threatening total abdominal lymphangiomatosis. *J. Pediatr. Surg.* 1994; **29**:322–323.
55. Kuramoto, S., Sakai, S., & Tsuda, K. Lymphangioma of the large intestine. *Dis. Colon Rectum* 1988; **31**:900–905.
56. Yoshida, Y., Okamura, T., & Ezaki, T. Lymphangioma of the oesophagus: a case report and review of the literature. *Thorax* 1994; **49**:1267–1268.
57. Castellanos, D., Sebastian, J. J., & Larrad, A. Esophageal lymphangioma: case report and review of the literature. *Surgery* 1990; **108**:593–594.
58. Valenti, V., Echeveste, J. I., & Hernandez Lizoain, J. L. Intestinal T-cell lymphoma associated with celiac disease masked by cavernous lymphangioma. *Rev. Esp. Enferm. Dig.* 2003; **95**:654–657.
59. Saijo, M., Munro, I. R., & Mancer, K. Lymphangioma – a long term follow-up study. *Plast. Reconstr. Surg.* 1975; **56**:642–651.
60. Charabi, B., Bretlau, P., Bille, M., & Holmelund, M. Cystic hygroma of the head and neck – A long-term follow-up of 44 cases. *Acta Otolaryngol.* 2000; **543**:248–250.
61. Okada, A., Kubota, A., & Fukuzawa, M. Injection of bleomycin as a primary therapy of cystic lymphangioma. *J. Pediatr. Surg.* 1992; **27**:440–443.
62. Orford, J., Barker, A., & Thonell, S. Bleomycin therapy for cystic hygroma. *J. Pediatr. Surg.* 1995; **30**:1282–1287.
63. Tanaka, K., Inomata, Y., & Utsunomiya, H. Sclerosing therapy with bleomycin emulsion for lymphangioma in children. *Pediatr. Surg. Int.* 1990; **5**:270–273.
64. Tanigawa, N., Shimomatsuyz, T., & Takatrashi, K. Treatment of cystic hygroma and lymphangioma with the use of bleomycin fat emulsion. *Cancer* 1987; **60**:741–749.
65. Ogita, S., Tsuto, T., & Nakamura, K. OK-432 therapy in 64 patients with lymphangioma. *J. Pediatr. Surg.* 1994; **29**:784–785.
66. Mikhail, M., Kennedy, R., Cramer, B. *et al.* Sclerosing of recurrent lymphangioma using OK-432. *J. Pediatr. Surg.* 1995; **30**:1159–1160.
67. Hall, N., Ade-Ajayi, N., & Brewis, C. Is intralesional injection of OK-432 effective in the treatment of lymphangioma in children? *Surgery* 2003; **133(3)**:238–242.
68. Giguère, C. M., Bauman, N. M., & Sato, Y. Treatment of lynphangiomas with OK-432 (Picibanil) sclerotherapy. *Arch. Otolaryngol. Head Neck Surg.* 2002; **128**:1137–1144.
69. Claesson, G. & Kuylenstierna, R. OK-432 therapy for lymphatic malformation in 32 patients (28 children). *Int. J. Pediatr. Otorhinolaryngol.* 2002; **65**:1–6.
70. Fujino, A., & Moriya, Y., & Morikawa, Y. A role of cytokines in OK-432 injection therapy for cystic lymphangioma: an approach to the mechanism. *J. Pediatr. Surg.* 2003; **38**:1806–1809.
71. Harrower, G. Treatment of cystic hygroma of the neck by sodium morrhuate. *Br. Med. J.* 1993; **2**:148–149.
72. Gutierrez San Roman, C., Barrios, J., & Lluna, J. Treatment of cervical lymphangioma using fibrin adhesive. *Eur. J. Pediatr. Surg.* 1993; **3**:356–358.
73. Molitch, H. I., Unger, E. C., & Witte, C. L. Percutaneous sclerotherapy of lymphangiomas. *Radiology* 1995; **194**:343–347.
74. Farmand, M. & Kuttenberger, J. J. A new therapeutic concept for the treatment of cystic hygroma. *Oral Surg. Oral Med. Oral Pathol. Oral Radiol. Endocrinol.* 1996; **81**:389–395.
75. Herbreteau, D., Riche, M. C., & Enjolras, O. Percutaneous embolization with Ethibloc® of lymphatic cystic malformations with a review of the experience in 70 patients. *Int. Angiol.* 1993; **12**:34–39.

76. Dubois, J., Garel, L., Abela, A., Laberge, L., & Yazbeck, S. Lymphangiomas in children: percutaneous sclerotherapy with an alcoholic solution of zein. *Radiology* 1997; **204**:651–654.
77. Boxen, I., Zhan, Z. M., & Filler, R. M. Lymphoscintigraphy for cystic hygroma. *J. Nucl. Med.* 1990; **31**:516–518.
78. Takes, R. P., Valdes Olmos, R. A., & Hilgers, F. J. M. Intracystic administration of Tc-99m colloid particles to study retention and drainage in lymphangioma of the neck. *Clin. Nucl. Med.* 1994; **19**:792–794.
79. Bhattacharyya, N. C., Yadav, K., & Mitra, S. K. Lymphangiomas in children. *Aust. N Z J. Surg.* 1981; **51**:296–300.

8

Thyroid and parathyroid (including thyroglossal disorders)

Jaimie D. Nathan and Michael A. Skinner

Duke University Medical Center, Durham, NC, USA

Since the first thyroidectomy was reportedly performed by the Moorish surgeon Albucasis in AD 330, the surgical treatment of thyroid and parathyroid disorders has been approached with trepidation. Even with modern technical advances, many regard pathology in this anatomic location only operable by those with significant experience. This notion is especially true in children. The technical difficulties are more pronounced in younger individuals, and these children must survive a lifetime with the end result of their surgeon's work.

In this chapter, the long-term outcome of surgical diseases of the thyroid and parathyroid glands, including thyroglossal disorders, in children is discussed. Graves' disease, the most common of these disorders, is the first entity considered. Malignancies of the thyroid gland are then considered with a discussion of papillary and follicular carcinoma, followed by a review of medullary carcinoma of the thyroid. Next, childhood disorders of the parathyroid glands are discussed, with emphasis on hyperparathyroidism. Finally, we consider the management and long term outcome of thyroglossal disorders, including cysts and sinuses.

Graves' disease

Toxic diffuse goiter or Graves' disease is the most common cause of hyperthyroidism in children. It is more common in girls than boys, with a ratio of approximately 4:1 to 5:1, and the incidence increases throughout childhood with a peak in the adolescent years.

Graves' disease is an autoimmune process mediated by circulating autoantibodies to the thyroid stimulating hormone (TSH) receptor present on the follicular cells of the thyroid gland. Binding of the antibody to the TSH receptor stimulates the follicular cells via cyclic adenosine monophosphate (cAMP), resulting in thyroid hyperactivity. A number of other autoimmune processes are associated with Graves' disease, including diabetes mellitus, Hashimoto's thyroiditis, Addison's disease, and pernicious anemia.

Clinical manifestations and diagnosis

The onset of Graves' disease is usually insidious and symptoms may be subtle, gradually appearing over several months. There may be minimal changes in behavior in its initial phase, with nervousness, hyperactivity, irritability, disturbed sleep, or a gradual decline in school performance. Eventually, symptoms may become more obvious, with weight loss despite an increased appetite, increased sweating, heat intolerance, or muscle weakness.

On physical examination, the majority of patients with Graves' disease have a goiter, which typically is a firm, smooth, symmetrically enlarged, non-tender mass. The mass slides with swallowing and may have a bruit on auscultation. Whereas exophthalmos is unusual in pediatric Graves' disease, most children have prominent eyes and a conspicuous stare. Other physical findings include tachycardia, a widened pulse pressure, exaggerated deep tendon reflexes, and growth acceleration.

Diagnosis is usually relatively clear once the signs and symptoms have been recognized. Laboratory confirmation usually yields elevated T_4 and T_3 levels and a decreased TSH level. In a minority of patients with Graves' disease, only T_3 is elevated; this condition is known as T_3 thyrotoxicosis.

Pediatric Surgery and Urology: Long-term Outcomes, Mark Stringer, Keith Oldham, Pierre Mouriquand.
Published by Cambridge University Press.

Further diagnostic confirmation of Graves' disease can be achieved by detecting the presence of TSH-stimulating autoantibodies.

Treatment

Although the ideal treatment of pediatric Graves' disease remains controversial, the basic principle of management in children consists of decreasing the production of thyroid hormones or blocking their peripheral effects. This goal may be achieved with medical treatment or by ablation of the thyroid mass with radioiodine or surgery.

A trial of medical management should probably be attempted in children before thyroid gland ablation. Medical treatment can be divided into generalized relief of symptoms or interfering with thyroid hormone synthesis. Symptomatic treatment usually involves the beta-blocker propranolol for management of tachycardia and hypertension in daily doses of 2.5 to 10 mg/kg given orally every 6 to 8 hours. Specific medical treatment to decrease thyroid hormone production and secretion consists of the thioamide drugs propylthiouracil (5 to 10 mg/kg in three divided doses) and methimazole (0.5 to 1 mg/kg as one daily dose). These medications inhibit the incorporation of oxidized iodine into thyroglobulin and block the coupling of iodotyrosine to form T_4 and T_3. Propylthiouracil also inhibits the peripheral conversion of T_4 to T_3.

After the initiation of medical management, patients are followed closely, and upon achieving clinical improvement or euthyroidism, dosages of the medications may be reduced. Medical therapy with the thioamides is usually carried out for several years. Remission rates in children treated with propylthiouracil or methimazole range from 30% to 60%. Most relapses occur within 6 months of ceasing medical therapy, and are more likely to occur if TSH receptor autoantibodies are present before and after treatment. Children with large goiters, a history of prior relapse, or T_3-predominant Graves' disease are at high risk for failure with medical management.

Ablation of the goiter with radioiodine treatment is an option for patients who do not respond to medical therapy, for patients who relapse after medical therapy has been discontinued, or in children who are non-compliant with medications. Historically, because of concerns over the development of malignancies and germline mutations, this mode of treatment has been avoided in children.[1,2] However, studies have failed to demonstrate an increased incidence of malignancies or adverse genetic effects following radioiodine therapy. In addition, there have been very few reports of acute adverse effects of radioiodine treatment in children with Graves' disease. Recent reports have concluded that radioiodine is a safe and effective treatment modality for children and adolescents with Graves' disease.[3,4] Due to the theoretical risk of thyroid carcinoma in patients less than 20 years of age who are treated with radioiodine, most authors recommend high-dose administration in order to reduce the amount of residual thyroid tissue which has potential for neoplastic degeneration.[5]

Surgical management may be required in the management of Graves' disease in the pediatric population. Subtotal thyroidectomy is often utilized in children who initially fail medical therapy or relapse following discontinuation of medical treatment. Surgical management is also indicated in children who have symptoms of airway compression and in those who experience toxic side effects from medical treatment.[6] Prior to subtotal thyroidectomy, the patient is rendered euthyroid by the use of methimazole or propylthiouracil. Preoperative therapy also consists of the administration of iodine in the form of Lugol's solution for 10 to 14 days prior to surgery to decrease the vascularity of the thyroid gland, as well as the management of symptoms with propranolol.

Short-term outcomes

The greatest concern in the immediate postoperative period following subtotal thyroidectomy for Graves' disease is the occurrence of operative complications. The most common complications include vocal cord paralysis due to injury to the recurrent laryngeal nerve and hypoparathyroidism due to disruption of the vascular supply to the parathyroid glands. In the study by Rauh *et al.*, 12 children between the ages of 10 and 18 years underwent subtotal thyroidectomy with no episodes of recurrent laryngeal nerve injury or hypoparathyroidism.[7] In a series of 60 pediatric patients who underwent subtotal thyroidectomy, Csaky *et al.* reported one child with unilateral recurrent laryngeal nerve injury and no instances of hypoparathyroidism.[6] More recently, Bergman *et al.* reported no permanent recurrent laryngeal nerve injury or hypoparathyroidism in a series of ten pediatric patients who underwent subtotal thyroidectomy for Graves' disease.[8] There were no hemorrhagic complications in any of these studies. The critical operative principles include identification of the recurrent laryngeal nerves and preservation of the vascular supply to the parathyroid glands.

Long-term outcomes

The long-term outcome of children operated on for Graves' disease has not been studied extensively. In the series with the longest follow-up, Csaky *et al.* performed a subtotal

Table 8.1. Clinical features of Grave's disease in children in three published series

Clinical series	A[6]	B[7]	C[8]
Patients (n)	60	12	10
Surgical procedure	Subtotal thyroidectomy	Subtotal thyroidectomy	Subtotal thyroidectomy
Follow-up results:			
Euthyroid	18 (30%)	4 (33%)	3 (30%)
Hypothyroid	37 (61.7%)	6 (50%)	4 (40%)
Recurrent hyperthyroidism	5 (8.3%)	2 (12%)	3 (30%)
Median follow-up (years)	13.7	NA	1.7
Postoperative complications	1[a]	0	0

[a] Unilateral recurrent laryngeal nerve injury. NA, data not available.

thyroidectomy in 60 pediatric patients and followed them for a mean period of 13.7 years after surgery.[6] In all cases, the retained portion of thyroid tissue had a mass of approximately 6 to 10 grams. As shown in Table 8.1, the likelihood of achieving a euthyroid state following the surgical treatment of Graves' disease in the pediatric population is approximately 30%. The majority of patients are rendered hypothyroid following subtotal thyroidectomy, but this is not considered a failure by all authors, as it can be managed relatively easily with thyroid hormone replacement. In the current literature, approximately 8% to 30% of patients with Graves' disease managed by subtotal thyroidectomy developed recurrent hyperthyroidism.[6–8]

These studies emphasize the importance of following thyroid function profiles to detect those patients with subclinical hypothyroidism, so that appropriate thyroid replacement can be instituted. Also evident is that, while the hypothyroid and euthyroid patients can be managed with thyroid replacement and serial follow-up, the subgroup with recurrent hyperthyroidism is more difficult to manage. Some authors feel that radioiodine is indicated in these patients *in lieu* of repeated thyroid resection, which carries a very high risk of complication. Further studies are needed to determine the optimal treatment for pediatric patients who have persistent or recurrent hyperthyroidism after subtotal thyroidectomy for Graves' disease.

Malignancies of the thyroid gland

Carcinoma of the thyroid gland can be divided into two types based on tissue of origin: epithelial and non-epithelial. Epithelial-derived thyroid cancers consist of papillary carcinoma and follicular carcinoma, which are well differentiated and constitute approximately 80% and 10% of thyroid malignancies, respectively. Anaplastic thyroid cancer also originates from the thyroid follicular epithelium, is an undifferentiated carcinoma, and is extremely rare in children. The remainder of thyroid malignancies consist of medullary thyroid carcinoma (MTC), which accounts for approximately 10% of cases.

Well-differentiated thyroid carcinoma

Malignancies of the thyroid gland are rare in children, accounting for approximately 3% of all childhood cancers in the USA.[9] This represents an incidence of between one and two cases per million children per year. Girls usually outnumber boys by a ratio of 2:1, and the majority of children afflicted are between 10 and 18 years of age. Thyroid carcinoma in children constitutes approximately 3.5% of all cases of thyroid malignancies in the general population. Studies have demonstrated that the most significant risk factor associated with thyroid carcinoma in children is a history of radiation exposure (especially before the age of 10 years), from either therapeutic or incidental environmental exposures.[10] Therapeutic radiation exposure has historically been given for the treatment of various benign diseases, such as thymic enlargement, tonsillar hypertrophy, keloids, and acne. Environmental radiation exposure has occurred after nuclear testing, from the use of weapons in Hiroshima and Nagasaki, and after the Chernobyl accident in the Republic of Belarus in 1986. Other important risk factors for the development of thyroid carcinoma in children include iodine deficiency, prolonged elevation of plasma TSH, and autoimmune thyroiditis.

Carcinoma of the thyroid gland also occurs as a second malignancy in children who previously have had cancer. In one study, 9% of second malignancies developing after the treatment of childhood tumors were thyroid carcinomas.[11] Approximately 71% of the children with thyroid cancers had undergone prior radiation to the neck as part of their treatment. Hodgkin's disease was the most common primary malignancy associated with the subsequent development of thyroid carcinoma.

Genetic factors are also known to be associated with the development of well-differentiated thyroid carcinoma. The most common genetic abnormality associated with well-differentiated thyroid cancer is a rearrangement involving the *RET* proto-oncogene, which encodes for a tyrosine kinase receptor protein.[12] The *RAS* proto-oncogene has also been shown to be involved in some thyroid carcinomas, especially those of the follicular histological subtype.[13] Patients with some inheritable syndromes are at an increased risk for thyroid carcinoma. Gardner's syndrome, for example, is an autosomal dominant disorder that predisposes patients to develop well-differentiated thyroid cancer, as well as colon carcinoma, lipomas, sarcomas and intestinal polyposis.[14] In addition, a syndrome of familial non-medullary thyroid carcinoma associated with colon cancer alone has been reported.

Histologically, well-differentiated carcinoma of the thyroid consists of papillary and follicular tissue types. The majority of these tumors in children are of the papillary subtype, but both histological subtypes are occasionally found in the same surgical specimen. Despite the difference in histological architecture, papillary and follicular thyroid carcinomas tend to behave similarly, and thus, treatment is similar for these two tumor types.

Clinical manifestations and diagnosis

Children with well-differentiated thyroid carcinomas typically present with a thyroid mass, enlarged cervical lymph nodes, or both. In the series by Harness *et al.* children who presented prior to 1971 had a thyroid mass in 37% of cases, while 63% had palpable cervical adenopathy.[15] In contrast, those children diagnosed between 1971 and 1990 had a thyroid mass on initial presentation in 73% of cases and cervical adenopathy in 36%. The reason for this shift in presentation is unclear, although earlier recognition of the disease by primary care providers may be a factor.

Pathologic diagnosis is generally established preoperatively by fine-needle aspiration (FNA) cytology, although the accurate cytological interpretation of thyroid aspirates is highly dependent on the skill of the cytopathologist. It should also be noted that, while adolescent patients with thyroid nodules may be evaluated safely and effectively by FNA, the effectiveness of FNA cytology in children is not completely defined. Factors that make FNA more difficult in children include the smaller size of the nodule, the need for sedation, and the paucity of experienced pediatric cytopathologists. Moreover, because a thyroid nodule in a child is more likely to be malignant, there is a slightly higher probability of a false-negative result, causing a delay in diagnosis and treatment.

Additional studies that may be performed prior to surgery include a thyroid scan to determine whether the mass comprises functioning thyroid tissue, as well as a thyroid hormone profile in order to exclude hyperthyroidism requiring preoperative management. A preoperative chest radiograph or computed tomography scan of the chest should be performed, as the incidence of pulmonary metastasis in pediatric thyroid carcinomas may be as high as 20%.[16]

Treatment

The surgical management of well-differentiated thyroid carcinoma in children remains controversial, as there are no clinical trials comparing the techniques of thyroid lobectomy, subtotal or near-total thyroidectomy, and total thyroidectomy. Some surgeons advocate aggressive surgical treatment with total thyroidectomy and cervical lymph node dissection. The argument favoring this approach is based on the tendency of well-differentiated thyroid carcinoma to be multifocal or bilateral in as high as 81% of cases.[17] In addition, removal of the entire thyroid makes postoperative ablation with radioiodine more efficacious, as there is less residual normal thyroid tissue, which concentrates the radioiodine more efficiently. Other surgeons take a more conservative approach, and advocating a subtotal thyroidectomy or a thyroid lobectomy. This group contends that the current literature does not provide sufficient support that total thyroidectomy results in improved survival, compared to subtotal thyroidectomy. They also make the argument that a more aggressive thyroid resection is more likely to be associated with serious operative complications.

At the time of surgery, lymph nodes should be examined, and those that are suspicious for regional metastasis should be excised. The rate of regional nodal involvement in children with epithelial thyroid cancer is approximately 88%.[15,17] This incidence is significantly higher than the 35% reported in the adult literature.

Approximately 6 weeks postoperatively, patients should undergo a total body ^{131}I scan to detect any residual tumor in the neck or disseminated disease. Radioiodine treatment is indicated to ablate any residual tumor, and this therapy should be repeated as necessary for metastatic disease. The prophylactic use of radioiodine in the absence of documented residual disease remains controversial.

All patients with well-differentiated thyroid carcinoma should be treated with long term thyroid hormone replacement. While total thyroidectomy mandates this treatment, it is also used in patients with residual thyroid tissue to suppress TSH stimulation of possible malignant thyroid cells. Finally, thyroglobulin has been shown to be a useful marker of residual or metastatic thyroid carcinoma, and should be measured yearly. It should be noted, however, that the diagnostic accuracy of this test is reduced in children having residual thyroid tissue and in patients who are taking thyroid hormone replacement.

Short-term outcomes

As with all operative procedures on the thyroid and parathyroid glands, the immediate concerns after the surgical

Table 8.2. Complications of surgery for well-differentiated thyroid carcinoma

Clinical series	A[17]	B[18]	C[19]	D[20]	E[21]	F[15]	G[22]	H[23]	I[24]
RLN injury[a]	18 (25%)	12 (24%)	14 (14%)	0	NA	6 (6.7%)	4 (8.3%)	7 (2%)	0
Hypoparathyroidism	5 (6.9%)	5 (10.2%)	15 (15%)	14 (24%)	7 (12%)	6 (6.7%)	10 (21%)	39 (12%)	2 (4%)
Tracheostomy needed	1 (1.4%)	5 (10.2%)	11 (11%)	0	NA	0	0	15 (4.6%)	0
Postoperative deaths	0	0	0	0	0	0	0	0	0
Postoperative bleeding	0	0	1 (1%)	0	NA	0	0	1 (0.003%)	0
Surgical procedure									
Total thyroidectomy	29	0	46	21	59	79	44	178	48
Subtotal thyroidectomy	0	49	[b]	22	[b]	5	0	55	[b]
Lobectomy or other	43	0	54	15	0	5	4	96	0

[a] RLN, recurrent laryngeal nerve.
[b] In these studies, the patients who underwent total or subtotal thyroidectomies were not subgrouped.
NA, data not available.

treatment of well-differentiated thyroid carcinoma are the complication rate and the presence of residual disease. Because the optimal surgical management of this disease remains controversial, it is important to determine whether the extent of surgical resection alters either of these two factors.

The most common complications following thyroid surgery include hypoparathyroidism and recurrent laryngeal nerve injury. Other complications reported in the literature include bleeding, the need for tracheostomy, and death. The rates of these complications in various clinical series are shown in Table 8.2.[15,17–24] Of note is that, while deaths and postoperative bleeding were almost uniformly absent, recurrent laryngeal nerve injury and hypoparathyroidism were significant causes of morbidity. Also evident is the lack of correlation between the extent of surgical resection and the rate of operative complications. It should be emphasized that the majority of these complications occurred in children who were operated on in the 1960s and the 1970s, and surgical techniques have improved considerably since that period. It is critical to identify the recurrent laryngeal nerve in each case, and the nerve should not be sacrificed if involved by tumor. In such cases, postoperative radioiodine can be used to ablate residual malignant cells. Management of the parathyroid glands has also improved, and if their vascularity is in question, they may either be implanted into the sternocleidomastoid muscle or autotransplanted into the non-dominant forearm.[25–27]

Long-term outcomes

Despite the fact that well-differentiated thyroid carcinoma is more advanced in children at the time of diagnosis, with a higher incidence of lymph node metastases, the long term outcome of this malignancy in children is more favorable than in adults. Recurrence of well-differentiated thyroid carcinoma in the studies reviewed varied from 2% to 54%, with recurrence occurring either locally or at distant sites. La Quaglia *et al.* noted that while approximately 50% of recurrences occurred between 1 and 6 years after treatment, some patients recurred as many as 25 years following initial treatment.[19] Harness *et al.* contend that their relatively low rates of postoperative persistence of tumor and recurrence are the result of a more aggressive initial operation, consisting of a total or near total thyroidectomy with nodal dissection of involved areas.[15]

The reported cancer mortality rates in children with well-differentiated thyroid carcinomas range from 0% to 17%. The results from several large clinical series are presented in Table 8.3.[15,17–24] The highest mortality rate was seen in the study with the highest rate of limited resection.[17] The cause of death in these children was usually related to lung metastases. However, in the study by Zimmerman *et al.*,[20] the one child who died had lung metastases, but six other children with pulmonary involvement remained long-term survivors at the time of follow-up. This is in contrast to the 74.8% of adults in the study who died within 15 years of diagnosis of lung metastases. Thus, although death from childhood well-differentiated thyroid carcinoma is likely to result from pulmonary metastases and the associated restrictive lung disease, distant metastases do not predict a poor prognosis in children.[28]

In a recent large retrospective review, Newman *et al.* performed a multivariate analysis to determine what factors are predictive of disease progression in well-differentiated thyroid carcinoma in children.[23] Overall, progress-free survival in 329 children followed up for a median of 11.3 years was 67% with only two cancer-related deaths. The two factors that were predictive of disease progression were a lower age at initial diagnosis and the presence of residual cervical

Table 8.3. Clinical features of well-differentiated thyroid carcinoma in children in nine published series

Clinical series	A[17]	B[18]	C[19]	D[20]	E[21]	F[15]	G[22]	H[23]	I[24]
Patients (*n*)	71	48	94	58	56	89	47	329	48
Median age (years)	11.0	14.0	13.3	11.9	NA	12.8	18.0	15.2	18.1
Histology									
Papillary	50	44	87	58	37	83	41	297	40
Follicular	21	4	7	0	19	6	6	32	8
Surgical procedure									
Total thyroidectomy	28	0	40	21	56	79	43	178	48
Subtotal thyroidectomy	0	48	*a*	22	*a*	5	0	55	*a*
Lobectomy or other	43	0	54	15	0	5	4	96	0
Median follow-up (years)	13	7.7	20	28	11	NA	NA	11.3	6.1
Cancer mortality rate (%)	17	2.0	0	3.4	3.4	2.2	0	0.7	0

a In these studies, the patients who underwent total or subtotal thyroidectomies were not subgrouped.
NA, data not available.

disease after thyroid surgery. The extensiveness of thyroid resection did not affect the rate of progression-free survival, although the study was confounded by the application of more aggressive operations in children with more extensive disease. Also of note was the finding that the rate of surgical complications was associated with the aggressiveness of the operation.

In the absence of controlled clinical trials, the optimal surgical management of well-differentiated thyroid carcinoma in children remains controversial. However, it seems reasonable to remove as large a portion of the thyroid gland as possible because of the multicentricity and bilaterality of these cancers. The added advantage of this practice is that it makes postoperative radioiodine therapy more effective and makes following serial thyroglobulin levels more meaningful. After appropriate surgical intervention has been made and radioiodine has been administered if needed for persistent disease, many would agree that suppression therapy be carried out as well. The long-term management of these patients requires lifelong surveillance, as studies have shown that recurrence may occur well into adulthood.

Medullary carcinoma of the thyroid gland

Medullary carcinoma of the thyroid gland (MTC) is a malignancy of the parafollicular or C cells and makes up approximately 5 to 10% of thyroid malignancies. MTC occurs in a sporadic form as well as an autosomal dominant hereditary form.[29] The hereditary form can exist as an isolated entity, as with familial medullary thyroid carcinoma (FMTC), or as a part of the multiple endocrine neoplasia (MEN) syndromes, MEN 2A and 2B. Features of MEN 2A include MTC in greater than 90% of patients, pheochromocytoma in 50%, and hyperparathyroidism in approximately 30% of patients. MEN 2B is characterized by MTC, pheochromocytoma, mucosal and intestinal neuromas, and a marfanoid habitus. Patients with MEN 2B also have characteristic facies, including prominent lips and jaw, pigmented spots, and widespread teeth. In MEN 2A and 2B, MTC develops from the malignant transformation of C-cell hyperplasia. MTC is usually the first tumor to develop in MEN patients, and is the most common cause of death in this cohort. The MTC associated with MEN 2B is especially aggressive and typically presents earlier during childhood and with more widespread disease than in MEN 2A.[30]

Physiology

The parafollicular or C cells of the thyroid migrate from the neural crest during development and are derived from the APUD (amine precursor uptake and decarboxylation) cells. The distribution of C cells within the thyroid gland has its greatest concentration at the junction of the upper one-third and lower two-thirds of each thyroid lobe. The C cells do not produce thyroid hormone and do not respond to any regulatory factors that affect the follicular cells. The C cells produce calcitonin, which is a peptide hormone of 32 amino acids and a useful marker for both MTC as well as C cell hyperplasia. This is especially so following the administration of the secretagogues calcium and pentagastrin which stimulate the release of calcitonin.

Clinical presentation

MTC in the sporadic setting typically presents as a solitary thyroid mass detected by the patient or on physical examination. Patients are usually in their fourth or fifth decade, and females outnumber males by a ratio of 1.4 to 1. As many as one-half of patients may have metastases to cervical and mediastinal lymph nodes at the time of diagnosis. Distant metastases typically occur late in the disease and involve spread to lung, liver, bone, and adrenal glands.

In hereditary MTC, the presentation is typically earlier with the average age of diagnosis two to three decades younger than with sporadic MTC. As previously mentioned, MTC in the hereditary form can exist as FMTC or as MEN 2A or 2B. In MEN 2A patients, MTC generally does not occur prior to 6 years of age, and FMTC is rare before 9 years of age. MTC in MEN 2B has been reported within the first year of life. Genetic or biochemical screening of predisposed families allows for early diagnosis of hereditary disease, as most of these patients are asymptomatic at diagnosis in the current era.

Diagnosis

The diagnosis of sporadic MTC is usually established by fine-needle aspiration cytology during the evaluation of a neck mass. Diagnosis can also be achieved by documenting an elevated serum calcitonin level in the basal state or following administration of calcium and pentagastrin.

While the diagnosis of hereditary MTC can also be made by either of the above methods, direct genetic testing has recently been used to establish the diagnosis of MEN 2A or 2B before the development of clinically detectable MTC.[31] This evaluation consists of utilizing a DNA test based on polymerase chain reaction (PCR) for mutations of the *RET* proto-oncogene in kindred members of families with MEN 2A and 2B. This method of diagnosis has led to the use of prophylactic thyroidectomy in affected patients, with the hope that the gland can be removed while the disease is confined to the thyroid. In MEN 2B, the diagnosis can also be established by identifying the characteristic phenotype associated with the syndrome. However, genetic testing offers the opportunity for earlier diagnosis and management, within the first year of life. This provides a significant advance in the management of MTC, as the clinical diagnosis of MTC has often been made after significant spread of the tumor to adjacent lymph nodes or to distant sites.

Treatment

Surgical resection is the only effective treatment modality for MTC, highlighting the significance of early diagnosis. It is important to remove the entire thyroid gland, especially in the setting of MEN 2A and 2B, because MTC in these syndromes is almost always multicentric and bilateral. In addition, the nodes in the central compartment of the neck (between the carotid sheaths and from the hyoid bone to the sternal notch) should be removed. Ipsilateral lymph node dissection should also be performed whenever macroscopic regional lymph node metastases are identified. Patients should be followed postoperatively with serial calcium levels due to the risk of hypoparathyroidism. In addition, plasma calcitonin levels should be measured following calcium or pentagastrin stimulation in order to detect the presence of residual or recurrent MTC.

If the thyroid gland can be removed in its entirety without compromising the vascular supply of the parathyroid glands, then some surgeons advocate leaving the glands *in situ*. If during the procedure it becomes questionable whether the vascular supply has become impaired, then one should consider autotransplantation of parathyroid tissue into the sternocleidomastoid muscle or the non-dominant brachioradialis muscle. In patients with MEN 2A, the risk of hyperparathyroidism is approximately 35%.[32] In these patients, total parathyroidectomy with autotransplantation of tissue into the non-dominant brachioradialis muscle may be the procedure of choice. Thus, the risks of a repeat neck exploration can be avoided if subsequent resection of parathyroid tissue becomes necessary to manage hyperparathyroidism.

Short-term outcomes

The literature regarding the treatment of children with MTC consists of small clinical series. The principal risks following thyroidectomy for MTC include injury to the recurrent laryngeal nerve and hypoparathyroidism. In several published reports,[33–35] there were no instances of recurrent laryngeal nerve injury, and one study reported a 6% rate of postoperative hypoparathyroidism.[33] However, in this study, the parathyroid glands were preserved in their original site. Although the most effective method of preventing this complication is unknown, heterotopic autotransplantation of parathyroid tissue into either the non-dominant brachioradialis or the sternocleidomastoid muscle has been utilized with success in avoiding hyperparathyroidism.[27] This technique typically results in a period of postoperative hypocalcemia that is transient and easily manageable with temporary vitamin D and calcium supplementation. Prospective studies are needed to validate these techniques.

Long-term outcomes

MTC associated with MEN 2A carries a more favorable prognosis, since it is less aggressive than MTC associated with MEN 2B. Better long-term outcomes are achieved in the management of this form of MTC when diagnosis and treatment are carried out prior to the development of clinical manifestations. Studies have generally demonstrated that a favorable outcome is associated with the absence of a neck mass on presentation, a relatively young age at the time of diagnosis, and a normal basal calcitonin level preoperatively.

In a study reported in 1996 from Washington University, 24 children with MEN 2A underwent thyroidectomy for the management of MTC before the advent of routine genetic testing.[35] Seventeen of these patients had increased stimulated calcitonin levels preoperatively, and the remaining seven patients had a strong family history of MTC. The mean age at the time of surgery was 10.6 years, and patients had been followed for a mean of 9.3 years postoperatively. Of these 24 children, 20 had MTC and four had C cell hyperplasia on pathologic evaluation. One patient had documented metastatic disease to regional lymph nodes. During the follow-up period, five patients had either persistent or recurrent disease. The relative indolence of the MTC associated with MEN 2A is demonstrated by the fact that, in the four patients who developed recurrent MTC, their disease was discovered at a mean of 10.5 years after thyroidectomy. These results underscore the importance of early treatment and long follow-up for the management of MTC associated with the MEN 2A syndrome.

It has long been thought that the development of genetic testing for MEN 2A and 2B could both obviate the need for yearly calcitonin determination, as well as allow early diagnosis of the syndromes with a single blood draw. Thus, thyroidectomy could be offered at a very early age, theoretically removing C cells prior to malignant transformation. Recently, to allow earlier detection of children with MEN 2A, such a DNA test for the mutated *RET* proto-oncogene has been developed and is currently in use to diagnose patients in families at risk.

Recent studies have attempted to define the optimal timing of prophylactic thyroidectomy in children determined to be carriers of the mutated *RET* proto-oncogene (Table 8.4). In the Washington University study, 14 patients were diagnosed with MEN 2A based on genetic testing.[35] Thyroidectomy was performed at a mean age of 10.5 years, and 11 of these patients had MTC and 3 had C cell hyperplasia. There were no instances of metastatic disease in this group. While mean follow-up for this group was only 1.3 years, there were no cases of recurrent MTC in these children diagnosed and treated based on genetic testing. In a more recent study, Kahraman *et al.* performed a prophylactic total thyroidectomy in five children (mean age 8.2 years; range 4 to 14) with MEN 2A based on genetic testing.[36] All five patients had MTC on pathologic evaluation, but there were no cases of recurrent disease at median follow-up of 6.5 years. Despite the absence of studies demonstrating improved long term outcome following prophylactic thyroidectomy in children with MEN 2A, it is recommended that children in kindreds with MEN 2A undergo genetic testing early in childhood. Those found to have the responsible *RET* gene mutations should undergo thyroidectomy at approximately 5 years of age, although the recommended age for prophylactic thyroidectomy also remains debatable. It is also the authors' practice to perform a central neck node dissection, and to remove the parathyroid glands with heterotopic autotransplantation of parathyroid tissue.

Table 8.4. Prophylactic thyroidectomy in children with MEN 2A based on genetic testing

Clinical series	A[35]	B[36]
Patients (n)	14	5
Surgical procedure	Total thyroidectomy	Total thyroidectomy
Pathology		
C cell hyperplasia	3	0
Medullary thyroid carcinoma	11	5
Metastatic disease at operation	0	1
Mean follow-up (years)	1.3	6.5[a]
Recurrent disease	0	0

[a] Median follow-up (years).

MTC associated with MEN 2B is usually more aggressive than that associated with MEN 2A. The MTC usually presents at an earlier age and is more likely to be metastatic at the time of diagnosis. This is evident from the follow-up of 11 patients with MEN 2B from the Washington University study.[35] Diagnosis was made by the presence of the typical MEN 2B phenotype in five patients, the presence of a neck mass in four patients, and an elevated stimulated plasma calcitonin in two patients. Thyroidectomy was performed at a mean age of 8.4 years, and five (45%) of these children had metastases noted at surgery. With a mean follow-up of 11 years, only three (27%) of these 11 patients were disease free. One patient died 13 years after initial surgery, and seven are alive with disease, five with disease in the neck and two with distant metastases.

Because of the young age at which MTC develops in children with MEN 2B, it is important to establish the diagnosis and initiate treatment at an early age. While the MEN 2B phenotype may be obvious in some cases, it is not uniformly evident in infancy. Therefore, genetic testing is recommended to establish the diagnosis of MEN 2B. Because of the aggressive nature of this disease, thyroidectomy should

Table 8.5. Classification of hyperparathyroidism in children

Sporadic hyperparathyroidism
Neonatal (infantile)
Primary
Secondary
Tertiary
Familial hyperparathyroidism
MEN 1
MEN 2A
Isolated

be performed at approximately one year of age. As with MEN 2A, the lymph nodes in the central compartment of the neck should be removed, between the carotid sheaths and from the hyoid bone to the sternal notch. Longer-term studies demonstrating the effectiveness of prophylactic thyroidectomy in children with MEN 2 syndromes are needed.

Hyperparathyroidism

Disease of the parathyroid glands is extremely rare in the pediatric population. However, surgical therapy is the mainstay of treatment for the majority of cases of hyperparathyroidism. The classification of hyperparathyroidism in children is listed in Table 8.5.

Physiology

The primary function of parathyroid hormone (PTH) is to regulate calcium concentration in the extracellular fluid. This is accomplished by the direct effect of PTH on bone to increase calcium mobilization from the skeleton and on the kidneys to stimulate calcium absorption. In addition, PTH exerts indirect effects on the intestine via vitamin D effects. PTH potentiates the formation of 1,25-dihydroxyvitamin D in the kidney, which enhances the absorption of calcium from the gut.[37]

Three pathophysiological classes of hyperparathyroidism have been described. In primary hyperparathyroidism, parathyroid gland hyperfunction occurs independently of the physiologic state of the individual resulting in hypercalcemia. Secondary hyperparathyroidism usually results from physiologic parathyroid overactivity in response to a primary hypocalcemic state that often coexists with chronic renal insufficiency. If the parathyroid glands continue to function in this accelerated state, they can develop autonomous hyperactivity even if the renal insufficiency is corrected (as with renal transplantation), and this is referred to as tertiary hyperparathyroidism.

Diagnosis

The clinical manifestations of hyperparathyroidism in the pediatric population can be very subtle and non-specific.[38] Infants can present with hypotonicity, failure to thrive, respiratory distress, polyuria, or irritability, while older children may have weight loss, fatigue, malaise, weakness, anorexia, nausea, or a decrease in school performance.[39]

Diagnosis is usually made by documenting an elevated PTH level in the setting of hypercalcemia. Confirmation of hyperparathyroidism may be obtained by calculating an elevated chloride-to-phosphate ratio.[40] Once the diagnosis is established, it is helpful to determine whether the hyperparathyroidism is sporadic or familial. Family history of either isolated hyperparathyroidism or MEN 1 or 2A will indicate a hereditary component, although germline mutations arising *de novo* can give rise to these disease entities as well.

Hyperparathyroidism is usually the first abnormality to present in the MEN 1 syndrome, and over 95% of patients with MEN 1 eventually develop hyperparathyroidism due to parathyroid hyperplasia. The other pathologic entities that are commonly found in patients with MEN 1 are gastrinomas of the pancreas or duodenum, producing Zollinger–Ellison syndrome, and adenomas of the pituitary gland. The routine use of potential tumor markers in screening patients with primary hyperparathyroidism for these associated diseases is not indicated due to their low yield. Since the standard management of hyperparathyroidism in MEN 1 requires bilateral neck exploration and identification and evaluation of all four parathyroid glands, preoperative imaging studies are generally not utilized, except in cases of reoperation.

The use of preoperative imaging studies in patients with sporadic primary hyperparathyroidism is controversial. The ^{99m}Tc-sestamibi scan is the non-invasive localization study of choice, although ultrasonography has also been used to identify abnormal parathyroid glands preoperatively. Studies have demonstrated that preoperative localization of parathyroid tumors prior to initial operation for primary hyperparathyroidism is not cost effective.[41–43] However, with the advent of minimally invasive parathyroidectomy techniques, the role of preoperative imaging studies is being redefined. Prospective studies are needed to validate this approach. In the setting of reoperation for persistent or recurrent hyperparathyroidism, preoperative localization studies are critical due to the high frequency of ectopic parathyroid glands.

One particularly severe form of parathyroid hyperfunction is neonatal primary hyperparathyroidism, which presents in the first 3 months of life and usually shortly after birth.[39] Afflicted infants uniformly have four-gland hyperplasia, and therefore, the operative treatment consists of total parathyroidectomy with autotransplantation or subtotal parathyroidectomy.[44]

Treatment

Because medical management has no role in the treatment of primary hyperparathyroidism, surgery should be planned soon after the diagnosis is made. The most likely cause of non-familial primary hyperparathyroidism is a solitary adenoma. Traditionally, treatment has been carried out by exploratory neck surgery in which all four parathyroid glands are identified and examined.[45] In most instances, the solitary adenoma is obvious, and it can be removed. Although gross examination of the normal-appearing glands has been standard, whether to biopsy these glands depends on the individual surgeon's expertise. Non-absorbable suture tags are placed adjacent to the remaining glands in case future neck re-exploration for persistent hyperparathyroidism is required. It should be emphasized that both recurrent laryngeal nerves be identified as well.

Surgery for sporadic primary hyperparathyroidism is evolving with the advent of minimally invasive techniques, which have been developed in adults with hyperparathyroidism. Patients with biochemically proven primary hyperparathyroidism who have undergone a preoperative ^{99m}Tc-sestamibi scan with identification of a solitary adenoma may be offered minimally invasive parathyroidectomy.[46] With preoperative identification of a parathyroid adenoma, a unilateral neck dissection via a small incision may be performed under cervical block analgesia. The use of intraoperative PTH monitoring provides feedback for the surgeon regarding whether an adequate resection has been performed.

The surgical treatment of hyperparathyroidism in the familial setting is unique because in virtually all cases, it involves hyperplasia of multiple glands. The surgical approach is similar whether the hyperparathyroidism is part of MEN 1 or 2A or familial isolated hyperparathyroidism. The most commonly utilized surgical techniques consist of total (four-gland) parathyroidectomy with heterotopic autotransplantation of parathyroid tissue, or the three-and-one-half gland parathyroidectomy sparing 30 to 50 mg of parathyroid tissue.

The confounding factor with subtotal parathyroidectomy is that a significant number of these patients may require neck re-exploration, which significantly increases the likelihood of recurrent laryngeal nerve injury. This potential complication can be avoided by performing a total parathyroidectomy with autotransplantation of parathyroid tissue into the non-dominant brachioradialis muscle.

Operative technique

The operative principles for the management of hyperparathyroidism depend upon whether the hyperfunction is due to single- or multigland disease. Traditionally, most surgeons advocate bilateral exploration with identification of all four parathyroid glands as described by Cady.[47] If a single adenoma is present, it can be removed after confirmation of abnormal histology, as well as at least gross documentation that the remaining glands appear normal. Studies of pathological interpretation have suggested that histological examination can be misleading and that the most reliable indicator of gland abnormality is based upon an experienced surgeon's visual interpretation of gland size.[48]

The technique of minimally invasive parathyroidectomy for treatment of parathyroid adenoma has been developed in the adult population. After performing a cervical block, directed exploration is performed via a small incision guided by preoperative localization by ^{99m}Tc-sestamibi scanning. The recurrent laryngeal nerve is identified and protected from injury, and the adenoma is removed. A rapid intraoperative PTH assay is performed 5 minutes after excision of the adenoma to confirm the adequacy of resection. Due to its very short half-life, a 50% reduction in the circulating PTH level is expected. If the PTH level is higher than expected, additional exploration is indicated, and conversion to general anesthesia may be performed if a bilateral neck exploration is required. The applicability of the minimally invasive parathyroidectomy in the pediatric population requires elucidation.

As mentioned previously, the usual operative management for four-gland hyperplasia is to perform a three-and-one-half-gland parathyroidectomy or a total parathyroidectomy with heterotopic autotransplantation of parathyroid tissue into the non-dominant brachioradialis muscle.[49] If hyperparathyroidism is persistent or recurrent after subtotal parathyroidectomy, the necessary re-exploration carries with it an increased risk of postoperative hypocalcemia and recurrent laryngeal nerve injury. Thus, a significant advantage of heterotopically autotransplanting parathyroid tissue is the prevention of a repeat neck dissection should hyperparathyroidism recur. Rather, it is usually a simple matter of removing parathyroid tissue from the forearm under local anesthesia. To perform the technique of heterotopic autotransplantation into the forearm, the excised parathyroid tissue is placed in chilled

Table 8.6. Neonatal primary hyperparathyroidism: outcomes based on management[39,44]

Treatment (*n*)	Alive (no medication)	Alive (with medication)	Deceased
Subtotal parathyroidectomy (14)[a]	1	6	5
Total parathyroidectomy (5)	0	5	0
Total parathyroidectomy with autotransplantation (2)	2	0	0
Medical management (8)	0	1	7

[a] Two patients who had subtotal parathyroidectomy were known to have survived their operation but were then lost to follow-up.

saline at 4 °C. After the tissue is chilled, it is cut into 1 to 3 mm slices, which are then transplanted into the muscle bed which has been prepared. In most cases, the tissue should be placed into the non-dominant brachioradialis muscle. If normal parathyroid tissue is being autotransplanted because of a total thyroidectomy, and the risk of developing hyperparathyroidism is low, the sternocleidomastoid muscle can be used as re-exploration would be unlikely. Several parathyroid fragments are placed into each muscle pocket and the overlying fascia is sutured with a non-absorbable suture. This will both maintain the position of the transplanted tissue, as well as act as a marker for tissue localization should re-exploration for parathyroid tissue removal become necessary.

Short-term outcomes

Due to the rarity of hyperparathyroidism in the pediatric population, there are few studies describing outcomes following surgical management. In a study by Allo *et al.*, 53 patients from the age of infancy to 30 years underwent neck exploration for primary hyperparathyroidism.[50] The authors reported no deaths and no instances of recurrent laryngeal nerve injury in this cohort. However, six patients (11%) manifested postoperative hypocalcemia. All of these patients had undergone subtotal parathyroidectomy. Another patient had persistent hypercalcemia despite the identification and biopsy of four normal parathyroid glands and was felt to have an unidentified adenomatous fifth gland.

Long-term outcomes

In the study performed by Allo *et al.*, 51 of the 53 patients who underwent parathyroidectomy for hyperparathyroidism were rendered normocalcemic and in no need of further treatment at the time of follow-up.[50] In 35 patients, excision of a single enlarged gland consistent with adenoma was performed. The remaining patients underwent three-and-one-half gland parathyroidectomy for the management of parathyroid hyperplasia. One patient had persistent hypercalcemia postoperatively, and at the time of the publishing of their study, was to undergo evaluation for a mediastinal adenoma. Five of six patients who were hypocalcemic postoperatively no longer require supplemental calcium treatment. Additionally, there were no deaths and no episodes of recurrent laryngeal nerve injury.

More recently, Hsu and Levine described their experience in treating hyperparathyroidism at the Johns Hopkins Children's Center from 1984 to 2001.[51] Twelve patients underwent excision of a parathyroid adenoma, and four patients underwent three-and-one-half gland parathyroidectomy for hyperplasia (three with renal failure, and one with MEN 2A) with either preservation of one-half gland or heterotopic autotransplantation. Although two patients were lost to follow-up and follow-up interval was not stated, only one patient had persistent postoperative hyperparathyroidism (secondary hyperparathyroidism in one of the renal failure patients), and another renal failure patient had persistent hypocalcemia.

The long-term outcome of neonatal primary hyperparathyroidism reveals the remarkable severity of this illness (Table 8.6). Of the 29 infants in the study by Ross *et al.*, there were 17 long-term survivors.[39] Only one of the eight infants treated medically survived, and this infant remained hypercalcemic and exhibited poor growth. Sixteen (76%) of the 21 infants treated surgically in this study survived long term. Although only two patients had operative management consisting of parathyroidectomy with autotransplantation, follow-up (at 2 and at 3.5 years, respectively) revealed that both had survived and were on no medications. Although they were both slightly hypercalcemic and hypocalciuric, their growth and development were normal.

The results discussed are limited because of the rarity of hyperparathyroidism in children. Further studies need to be performed, and these children should be followed well into adulthood to assess the long-term effects of hyperparathyroidism in the pediatric population. However, some conclusions may be drawn despite the paucity of affected children. As in adults, hyperparathyroidism is a surgical disease, and in children, it is best managed by pediatric surgeons experienced in parathyroid surgery. Neonatal primary hyperparathyroidism is a disease with high mortality that must be recognized early so that effective treatment can be offered. Four-gland hyperplasia is the rule with this entity, and medical management has no curative role. Total parathyroidectomy with autotransplantation to a site remote from the neck seems to be superior to subtotal or total parathyroidectomy alone, by simplifying the management of persistent or recurrent hypercalcemia in the setting of four gland hyperplasia.

Thyroglossal duct disorders

Thyroglossal duct cysts are the most common congenital midline neck masses in the pediatric population, and account for approximately 75% of such disorders. The cysts are ectodermal remnants, and there are several indications for their excision, including recurrent infections, sinus formation, risk of malignancy and cosmetic concerns.

Embryology

Thyroglossal duct cysts may develop anywhere along the line of embryological descent of the thyroid gland in the neck. Therefore, knowledge of the embryogenesis of the thyroid gland is critical to the successful management of thyroglossal duct cysts. Between the fourth and seventh weeks of embryological development, the thyroid gland descends from the foramen cecum at the base of the tongue along the midline to its final position in the anterior neck. During this time period, the hyoid bone also develops from the second branchial arch, and therefore, the thyroglossal duct becomes intimately related to the central portion of the hyoid bone. Under normal circumstances, the thyroglossal duct is obliterated; however, its persistence gives rise to the development of cysts and sinuses.

Diagnosis

Because of its distinct embryological basis, the thyroglossal duct cyst has a classic presentation. Thyroglossal duct cysts are most commonly noted in children between 2 and 10 years old, and rarely manifest during the newborn period. On physical examination, the cysts present as a midline mass at or below the hyoid bone. They are usually soft and non-tender, and move with deglutition due to their communication with the foramen cecum. Also as a result of this communication, thyroglossal duct cysts may become infected with oropharyngeal flora. In such circumstances, the cysts may be warm and erythematous, and they may develop an external opening with drainage. Some surgeons confirm the presence of a normal thyroid gland separate from the mass by preoperative ultrasound scanning, thereby avoiding potential resection of an ectopic thyroid which may be the patient's only functioning thyroid tissue. Alternatively, thyroid scintigraphy may also be utilized to demonstrate normal thyroid tissue preoperatively.

Treatment

Walter Sistrunk at the Mayo Clinic described the classic operation for the management of thyroglossal duct cysts in 1920.[52] The operation consists of complete excision of the thyroglossal cyst, removal of the central portion of the hyoid bone, and excision of a core of normal tissue around the thyroglossal duct from the hyoid bone to the foramen cecum. The thyroglossal duct cyst is approached via a horizontal incision in a neck crease, but if a cutaneous fistula is identified, an elliptical incision is made to resect the core of tissue containing the fistula as part of the specimen. In most cases, the thyroglossal duct is located anterior and almost adherent to the central portion of the hyoid bone. However, it must be remembered that in approximately 30% of cases, the duct lies posterior to the hyoid.

An infected thyroglossal duct cyst is usually treated initially with antibiotics and warm compresses, and incision and drainage is performed if necessary. Following the resolution of the infection, the thyroglossal duct cyst may be excised by the Sistrunk procedure.

Short-term outcomes

There are few studies in the literature that review the potential complications associated with the Sistrunk procedure for the treatment of thyroglossal duct cysts. A recent series by Maddalozzo *et al.* reviewed the early postoperative complications in 35 pediatric patients who underwent the Sistrunk procedure.[53] The mean age of the cohort was 4 years, and the length of follow-up was 1.4 months. The authors reported that 29% of patients had minor complications following the Sistrunk procedure. These events included six patients with seromas, three patients with stitch abscesses, and one patient with a local wound infection. However, there were no major complications, which included abscess or hematoma requiring surgical drainage, inadvertent entry into the trachea, intraoperative hemorrhage, hypoglossal nerve injury, and death.

Long-term outcomes

Recurrence remains a treatment challenge of the Sistrunk procedure, and may occur at a rate of approximately 6% to 10%. Inadequate excision of the thyroglossal duct epithelium leads to recurrence. However, even when the procedure is performed properly by skilled surgeons, recurrence may result due to the presence of multiple tracts in the suprahyoid region.[54] The results of two recent series are demonstrated in Table 8.7.

Table 8.7. Clinical features of thyroglossal duct cysts in children in two published series

Clinical series	A[55]	B[56]
Patients (n)	94[a]	41
Surgical procedure	Sistrunk	Sistrunk
Mean age (years)	5.6	4.0
Mean follow-up (years)	9.7	6.7
Recurrence rate (%)	7.4	12.2

[a] Fifteen patients had undergone prior surgical treatment.

Nicollas *et al.* reported on a series of 94 children with mean age of 5.6 years who underwent the Sistrunk procedure for management of thyroglossal duct cysts.[55] It must be noted that 16% of children had undergone previous surgical treatment, and thus, were being managed for recurrence. In this series, seven patients presented with recurrence over a mean follow-up of 9.7 years. The authors did not describe what percentage of their recurrences involved patients who had undergone previous operation. They postulated that their recurrences resulted from the inadequate excision of branches of the thyroglossal duct.

More recently, Marianowski *et al.* published their series of pediatric patients who had undergone the Sistrunk procedure for management of thyroglossal duct cysts.[56] Of the 41 patients who underwent their initial Sistrunk procedure, the recurrence rate was 12.2% over a mean follow-up of 6.7 years. The recurrence rate in the cohort that had undergone a prior surgical procedure was significantly higher (31.3%). This is likely due to the difficulty in identifying residual tracts following prior operation. In addition to a prior surgical procedure, the authors identified three other risk factors for recurrence of thyroglossal duct cysts. Age at operation was a significant factor predicting recurrence, with a recurrence rate of 39.4% for patients younger than 2 years of age and a rate of only 8.3% for patients older than 2 years of age. A history of more than two episodes of thyroglossal duct cyst infection was associated with a significantly higher recurrence rate. The presence of multicystic findings on histological examination was also associated with a higher rate of recurrence, suggesting that in such patients, a branching thyroglossal duct makes complete excision difficult. Thus, it appears likely that recurrence rates following the Sistrunk procedure are lowest in children older than 2 years who have not undergone prior operation, are without a previous infection of their thyroglossal duct cyst, and who demonstrate no branching of the duct on histological examination.

REFERENCES

1. Becker, D. V. & Hurley, J. R. Current status of radioiodine (^{131}I) treatment of hyperthyroidism. In *Nuclear Medicine Annual*. New York: Raven Press, 1990: 265–290.
2. Becker, D. V. Choice of therapy for Graves' hyperthyroidism. *N. Engl. J. Med.* 1984; **311**:464–466.
3. Foley, T. P. & Charron, M. Radioiodine treatment of juvenile Graves' disease. *Exp. Clin. Endocrinol. Diabetes* 1997; **105**:61–65.
4. Rivkees, S. A. The use of radioactive iodine in the management of hyperthyroidism in children. *Curr. Drug Targets Immune Endocrinol. Metab. Disord.* 2001; **1**:255–264.
5. Rivkees, S. A., Sklar, C., & Freemark, M. The management of Graves' disease in children, with special emphasis on radioiodine treatment. *J. Clin. Endocrinol. Metab.* 1998; **83**:3767–3776.
6. Csaky, G., Balazs, G., Bako, G. *et al.* Late results of thyroid surgery for hyperthyroidism performed in childhood. *Prog. Pediatr. Surg.* 1991; **26**:31–40.
7. Rauh, V., Kujath, H. P., Reimers, C. *et al.* Indications, surgical treatment and after-care in juvenile hyperthyroidism. *Prog. Pediatr. Surg.* 1991; **26**:28–30.
8. Bergman, P., Auldist, A. W., & Cameron, F. Review of the outcome of management of Graves' disease in children and adolescents. *J. Paediatr. Child Health* 2001; **37**:176–182.
9. Viswanathan, K., Gierlowski, T. C., Schneider, A. B. *et al.* Childhood thyroid cancer. *Arch. Pediatr. Adolesc. Med.* 1994; **148**:260–265.
10. Nikiforov, Y. & Gnepp, D. R. Pediatric thyroid cancer after the Chernobyl disaster. *Cancer* 1994; **74**:748–766.
11. Smith, M. B., Xue, H., Strong, L. *et al.* Forty-year experience with second malignancies after treatment of childhood cancer: analysis of outcome following the development of the second malignancy. *J. Pediatr. Surg.* 1993; **28**:1342–1349.
12. Bongarzone, I., Butti, M. G., Coronelli, S. *et al.* Frequent activation of ret protooncogene by fusion with a new activating gene in papillary thyroid carcinomas. *Cancer Res.* 1994; **54**:2979.
13. Lemoine, N. R., Mayall, E. S., Wyllie, F. S. *et al.* Activated ras mutations in human thyroid cancers. *Cancer Res.* 1988; **48**: 4459.
14. Gorlin, J. B. & Sallan, S. E. Thyroid cancer in childhood. *Endocrinol. Metab. Clin. North Am.* 1990; **19**:649–662.
15. Harness, J. K., Thompson, N. W., McLeod, M. K. *et al.* Differentiated thyroid carcinoma in children and young adults. *World J. Surg.* 1992; **16**:547–554.
16. Vassilopoulou-Sellin, R., Klein, M. J., Smith, T. H. *et al.* Pulmonary metastases in children and young adults with differentiated thyroid cancer. *Cancer* 1993; **71**:1348–1352.
17. Schlumberger, M., DeVathaire, F., Travagli, J. P. *et al.* Differentiated thyroid carcinoma in childhood: long term follow-up in 72 patients. *J. Clin. Endocrinol. Metab.* 1987; **65**:1088–1094.
18. Ceccarelli, C., Pacini, F., Lippi, F. *et al.* Thyroid cancer in children and adolescents. *Surgery* 1988; **104**:1143–1148.
19. La Quaglia, M. P., Corbally, M. T., Heller, G. *et al.* Recurrence and morbidity in differentiated thyroid carcinoma in children. *Surgery* 1988; **104**:1149–1156.

20. Zimmerman, D., Hay, I. D., Gough, I. R. *et al.* Papillary thyroid carcinoma in children and adults: long term follow up of 1039 patients conservatively treated at one institution during three decades. *Surgery* 1988; **104**:1157–1166.
21. Samuel, A. M. & Sharma, S. M. Differentiated thyroid carcinomas in children and adolescents. *Cancer* 1991; **67**:2186–2190.
22. Danese, D., Gardini, A., Farsetti, A. *et al.* Thyroid carcinoma in children and adolescents. *Eur. J. Pediatr.* 1997; **156**:190–194.
23. Newman, K. D., Black, T., Heller, G. *et al.* Differentiated thyroid cancer: determinants of disease progression in patients <21 years of age at diagnosis. *Ann. Surg.* 1998; **227**:533–541.
24. Giuffrida, D., Scollo, C., Pellegriti, *et al.* Differentiated thyroid cancer in children and adolescents. *J. Endocrinol. Invest.* 2002; **25**:18–24.
25. de Roy van Zuidewijn, D. B. W., Songun, I., Kievit, J. *et al.* Complications of thyroid surgery. *Ann. Surg. Oncol.* 1995; **2**:56–60.
26. Olson, J. A., DeBenedetti, M. K., Baumann, D. S., & Wells, S. A. Parathyroid autotransplantation during thyroidectomy: results of long term follow up. *Ann. Surg.* 1996; **223**:472–480.
27. Skinner, M. A., Norton, J. A., Moley, J. F., DeBenedetti, M. K., & Wells, S. A. Heterotopic autotransplantation of parathyroid tissue in children undergoing total thyroidectomy. *J. Pediatr. Surg.* 1997; **32**:510–513.
28. Vassilopoulou-Sellin, R., Goepfer, H., Raney, B., & Schultz, P. N. Differentiated thyroid cancer in children and adolescents: clinical outcome and mortality after long-term follow-up. *Head Neck* 1998; **20**:549–555.
29. Grauer, A., Raue, F., & Gagel, R. F. Changing concepts in the management of hereditary and sporadic medullary thyroid carcinoma. *Endocrinol. Metab. Clin. North Am.* 1990; **19**: 613–635.
30. O'Riordain, D. S., O'Brien, T., Crotty, T. B. *et al.* Multiple endocrine neoplasia type IIb: more than an endocrine disorder. *Surgery* 1995; **118**:936–942.
31. Wells, S. A., Chi, D. D., Toshima, K. *et al.* Predictive DNA testing and prophylactic thyroidectomy in patients at risk for multiple endocrine neoplasia IIa. *Ann. Surg.* 1994; **220**:237–250.
32. Howe, J. R., Norton, J. A., & Wells, S. A. Prevalence of pheochromocytoma and hyperparathyroidism in multiple endocrine neoplasia type 2a: results of long-term follow-up. *Surgery* 1993; **114**:1070–1077.
33. Telander, R. L., Zimmerman, D., Sizemore, G. W. *et al.* Medullary carcinoma in children. *Arch. Surg.* 1989; **124**:841–843.
34. Barry, R., Pelser, H. H., Nel, C. J. C. *et al.* Early thyroidectomy for medullary thyroid carcinoma in children and young adults with the multiple endocrine neoplasia type 2a (MEN2a) syndrome. *S. Africa Med. J.* 1991; **80**:90–92.
35. Skinner, M. A., DeBenedetti, M. K., Moley, J. F. *et al.* Medullary thyroid carcinoma in children with multiple endocrine neoplasia types 2a and 2b. *J. Pediatr. Surg.* 1996; **31**:177–182.
36. Kahraman, T., de Groot, J. W. B., Rouwe, C. *et al.* Acceptable age for prophylactic surgery in children with multiple endocrine neoplasia type 2a. *Eur. J. Surg. Oncol.* 2003; **29**:331–335.
37. Mallette, L. E. Regulation of blood calcium in humans. *Endocrinol. Metab. Clin. North Am.* 1989; **18**:601–610.
38. Allen, D. B., Friedman, A. L., & Hendricks, S. A. Asymptomatic primary hyperparathyroidism in children. *AJDC* 1986; **140**:819–821.
39. Ross, A. J., Cooper, A., Attie, M. F. *et al.* Primary hyperparathyroidism in infancy. *J. Pediatr. Surg.* 1986; **21**:493–499.
40. Palmer, F. J., Nelson, J. C., & Bucchus, H. The chloride–phosphate ratio in hypercalcemia. *Ann. Intern. Med.* 1974; **80**:200–204.
41. Serpell, J. W., Campbell, P. R., & Young, A. E. Preoperative localization of parathyroid tumours does not reduce operating time. *Br. J. Surg.* 1991; **78**:589–590.
42. Wei, J. P. & Burke, G. J. Cost utility of routine imaging with Tc-99m-sestamibi in primary hyperparathyroidism before initial surgery. *Am. Surg.* 1997; **63**:1097–1100.
43. Pattou, F., Torres, G., Mondragon-Sanchez, A. *et al.* Correlation of parathyroid scanning and anatomy in 261 unselected patients with sporadic primary hyperparathyroidism. *Surgery* 1999; **126**:1123–1131.
44. Kulczycka, H., Kaminski, W., Woziewicz, B. *et al.* Primary hyperparathyroidism in infants: diagnostic and therapeutic difficulties. *Klin. Pediat.* 1991; **203**:116–118.
45. Ross, A. J. Parathyroid surgery in children. *Prog. Pediatr. Surg.* 1991; **6**:48–59.
46. Sosa, J. A. & Udelsman, R. Minimally invasive parathyroidectomy. *Surg. Oncol.* 2003; **12**:125–134.
47. Cady, B. Neck exploration for hyperparathyroidism. *Surg. Clin. North Am.* 1973; **53**:301–306.
48. Saxe, A., Baier, R., Tesluk, H. *et al.* The role of the pathologist in the surgical treatment of hyperparathyroidism. *Surg. Gynecol. Obstet.* 1985; **161**:101–105.
49. Wells, S. A., Ross, A. J., Dale, J. K. *et al.* Transplantation of the parathyroid glands: current status. *Surg. Clin. North Am.* 1979; **59**:167–177.
50. Allo, M., Thompson, N. W., Harness, J. K. *et al.* Primary hyperparathyroidism in children, adolescents, and young adults. *World J. Surg.* 1982; **6**:771–776.
51. Hsu, S. C. & Levine, M. A. Primary hyperparathyroidism in children and adolescents: the Johns Hopkins Children's Center experience 1984–2001. *J. Bone Min. Res.* 2002; **17**:N44–N50.
52. Sistrunk, W. E. The surgical treatment of cysts of the thyroglossal tract. *Ann. Surg.* 1920; **71**:121–122.
53. Maddalozzo, J., Venkatesan, T. K., & Gupta, P. Complications associated with the Sistrunk procedure. *Laryngoscope* 2001; **111**:119–123.
54. Hoffman, M. A. & Schuster, S. R. Thyroglossal duct remnants in infants and children: reevaluation of histopathology and methods from resection. *Ann. Otol. Rhinol. Laryngol.* 1988; **97**:483–486.
55. Nicollas, R., Guelfucci, B., Roman, S., & Triglia, J. M. Congenital cysts and fistulas of the neck. *Int. J. Pediatr. Otorhinolaryngol.* 2000; **55**:117–124.
56. Marianowski, R., Ait Amer, J. L., Morisseau-Durand, M. P., Manach, Y., & Rassi, S. Risk factors for thyroglossal duct remnants after Sistrunk procedure in a pediatric population. *Int. J. Pediatr. Otorhinolaryngol.* 2003; **67**:19–23.

9

Salivary glands disorders

John D. Langdon

(formerly), Department of Oral and Maxillofacial Surgery, King's College London, UK

Introduction

With the exception of mumps, salivary gland disease is relatively uncommon in childhood. However, the range of conditions that can occur are the same as in the adult population, although the relative incidence is very different.

Careful history-taking and detailed examination are critical. Details of onset, duration, periodicity, size, and location of any swelling and the character of any salivary secretions must be recorded. The child must be examined both intraorally and extraorally. Deep lobe parotid tumors may present with swelling in the tonsillar fossa and no external swelling. Swellings of the tail of the parotid or of the submandibular glands are easily confused with cervical lymphadenopathy.

In the majority of salivary diseases in children, imaging of the affected gland is an essential supplement to the history and examination. Bearing in mind that patient compliance cannot be relied upon, and that radiation exposure should be reduced as far as possible, ultrasonography (US) is the method of choice for the initial imaging of most conditions, including inflammatory diseases, obstruction due to calculi, and masses within the glands.[1] Although sialography is the preferred technique for the evaluation of chronic or recurrent inflammation, it is difficult to undertake in the young child. Computed tomography (CT) or magnetic resonance imaging (MRI) are essential in the evaluation of neoplastic disease, although the child may require sedation or even general anesthesia in order to obtain good images.[2]

Whenever bacterial sialadenitis is suspected, it is good practice to obtain a swab from the affected gland orifice, although the infection is usually successfully treated with antibiotics before the results of culture are obtained. Routine hematology supplemented by viral antibody titers or autoantibody screening are sometimes indicated.

Because of the risks of disseminating malignant disease, open biopsy of suspected neoplasms arising in the parotid or submandibular glands should be avoided. Some authors advocate the use of fine-needle aspiration (FNA) biopsy in this situation, but in general sampling error negates the value of FNA, particularly when a negative biopsy is obtained from a clinically obvious mass. Furthermore, the histopathologic diagnosis in this situation rarely influences the management of the condition.[3]

Congenital and developmental conditions

Agenesis of the major salivary glands can occur.[4] Sometimes both parotid and submandibular glands fail to develop, or alternatively just one gland may be absent. When the diagnosis is suspected, it may be confirmed by CT or MRI. Invariably the minor salivary glands are unaffected and speech, mastication and swallowing are not a major problem. However, rampant caries is a major problem and long-term care for caries prevention and periodontal health is important.[5]

Duct atresia rarely occurs. It usually affects the submandibular (Wharton's) duct. It presents with progressive swelling of the involved gland during the first week of life. In effect, a retention cyst forms in the gland and should be surgically excised.

Ectopic salivary tissue is relatively common but only rarely results in disease. Accessory parotid lobes occur in 20% of normal subjects.[6] Their significance lies in the diagnostic confusion which may occur when inflammation or tumor occurs in an unexpected anatomic location.

Pediatric Surgery and Urology: Long-term Outcomes, Mark Stringer, Keith Oldham, Pierre Mouriquand.
Published by Cambridge University Press.

Aberrant salivary tissue may also be found in the lateral part of the neck, in the middle ear, on the gingiva, in the pituitary gland and cerebellopontine region, in the base of the tongue and in the tonsillar fossa.[7] The significance of such tissue is that both benign and malignant tumors may occur within this tissue.[8,9]

The Stafne bone cavity is seen as a clearly demarcated rounded or oval radiolucency in the mandible below the inferior dental canal in the premolar, molar or angle regions. It is a concavity on the lingual aspect of the mandible containing accessory lobes of the submandibular salivary gland. Occasionally neoplasms may arise and these are usually mucoepidermoid carcinomas.[10]

Congenital salivary gland cysts commonly occur in the parotid region. They may be dermoid, branchial, or congenital ductal cysts.[11,12] The dermoid cyst occurs as a mass within the substance of the parotid gland. It contains elements of all three germinal layers, including hair follicles, sweat glands and sebaceous glands. Complete excision with preservation of the facial nerve is curative. Patients with branchial cleft anomalies usually present with a unilateral painless swelling in the region of the parotid. Rarely, there is bilateral involvement. Type 1 branchial cleft cysts result from duplication anomalies of the external auditory canal. They form sinus tracts and swellings either in the crease immediately behind the pinna or in front of the tragus (Fig. 9.1). The lesion must be completely excised. The sinus tract may be very extensive and full dissection of the facial nerve may be required.

Type II cysts are less common. They are the result of a duplication anomaly of the external auditory canal and the pinna. Thus the cysts are composed of both ectodermal elements and mesoderm-cartilage. They present in the upper neck with a sinus tract or fistula which discharges intermittently. Abscess formation due to secondary infection may occur. The sinus tract often extends into the external meatus or middle ear cavity. Meticulous surgical excision is curative and requires careful dissection of the facial nerve.

Branchial pouch cysts arise in the tail of the parotid in the retromandibular region. Complete surgical excision is curative. Congenital duct cysts are true retention cysts and appear in infancy as parotid swellings. Sialography (with sedation) confirms the diagnosis. They are managed conservatively and ultimately resolve spontaneously.[13]

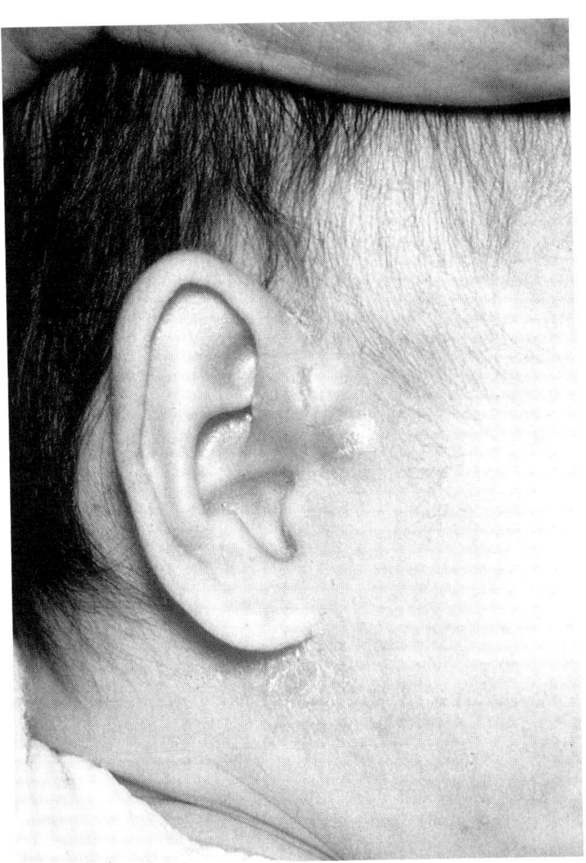

Fig. 9.1. Type 1 branchial cyst in the parotid region presenting as a preauricular sinus.

Inflammatory conditions

Acute viral sialadenitis

Mumps is the most common cause of acute painful parotid swelling. Mumps is endemic in urban areas and spreads via airborne droplet infection of infected saliva. The disease starts with a prodromal period of 1 or 2 days during which the child experiences feverishness, chills, nausea, anorexia and headache. This is typically followed by pain and swelling of one or both parotid glands. The parotid pain can be very severe and is exacerbated by any gustatory stimulus, such as eating. Symptoms resolve over 5–10 days. In a typical case of mumps, the diagnosis is made by clinical examination. A history of recent contact with an affected patient and bilateral painful parotid swelling is sufficient. However, the presentation may be atypical as a sporadic case or with predominantly unilateral or submandibular salivary gland involvement. In this situation, paired blood specimens may be required to confirm the diagnosis. The first specimen is obtained when the diagnosis is first suspected and another specimen is obtained 10–14 days later. Antibodies to mumps S and V antigens are measured and a steep rise in titers between the two samples indicates recent acute infection. One episode of mumps confers lifelong immunity.

The treatment of mumps is symptomatic. Regular paracetamol and maintainenance of fluid intake are helpful. Fortunately, complications such as orchitis, meningoencephalitis, pancreatitis and sensorineural deafness are rare in children. The incidence of mumps has diminished in recent years with the use of mumps, measles and rubella vaccine, but it is important to bear it in mind whenever a febrile fretful child presents with salivary gland enlargement.[11] Rarely, acute suppurative parotitis may occur in a gland already infected by mumps, presumably due to ascending bacterial infection from the oral cavity.[12]

A number of other viruses (Coxsackie A and B, influenza A, parainfluenza 1 and 3, ECHO and lymphocytic choriomeningitis) can all cause identical clinical signs and symptoms. Cytomegalic inclusion disease affects mainly newborn infants and children. It is believed to be an intrauterine infection which becomes manifest after birth.[14]

In recent years it has become apparent that almost invariably the salivary glands harbor the active replication of other viruses. Using *in situ* hybridization and reassociation kinetics, Wolf *et al.*[15] have shown that Epstein–Barr virus (EBV) is present in all parotid specimens examined, and they suggest that the parotids may be the source of virus found in the oropharynx. Similarly, there is evidence that human herpes virus 6 (HHV-6) is latent in salivary glands.[16,17] HHV-6 appears to be linked causally to exanthema subitum, a common febrile disease of infants, but it is uncertain whether HHV-6 is of pathogenic significance for other diseases.

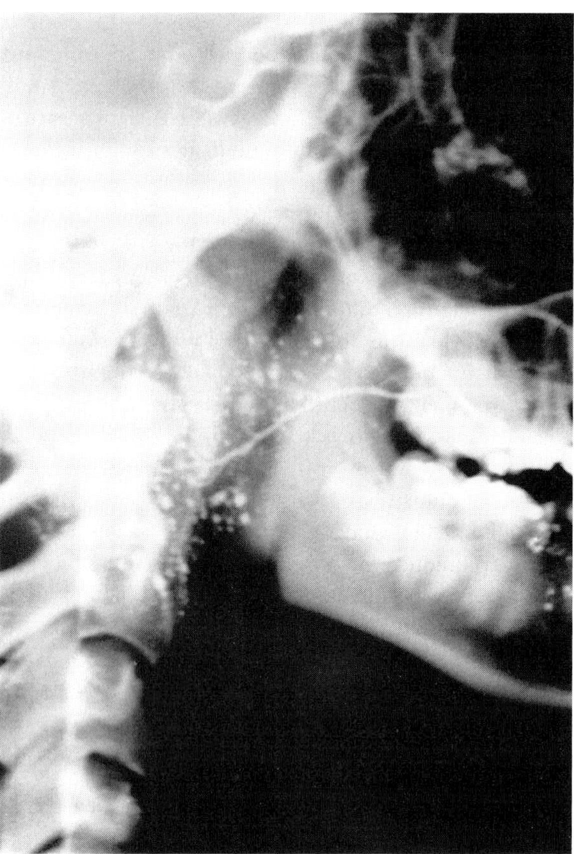

Fig. 9.2. Parotid sialogram of a child with recurrent sialadenitis of childhood, showing the characteristic snowstorm sialectasis.

Recurrent sialadenitis of childhood

This condition undoubtedly exists as a distinct clinical entity, but considerable doubt remains regarding its etiology, management and ultimate prognosis. Recurrent sialadenitis of childhood is characterized by rapid swelling of one parotid gland, accompanied by pain and difficulty in chewing as well as systemic symptoms such as fever and malaise. Rarely the swelling is bilateral, or may involve the submandibular glands. Although each episode of parotid swelling is frequently unilateral, alternate sides may be affected in subsequent episodes. Each episode of pain and swelling lasts for 3–7 days and is followed by a quiescent period of a few weeks to several months. Occasionally, frequent episodes cause the child to lose a considerable amount of schooling. The condition has been reviewed by Galili and Marmary[19] and Grevers.[20] Onset is usually between 3 and 6 years of age, although it has been reported in infants between 4 and 5 months old.[21,22] There is some evidence of a familial predisposition.[23]

Apart from a characteristic clinical history, the diagnosis is confirmed by the presence of characteristic punctate sialectasis on sialography (Fig. 9.2).[24,25] The radiographic appearance is quite different from that of sialectasis seen in autoimmune destruction. In recurrent sialadenitis of childhood, each sialectatic cavity differs in size and there is gross destruction of the proximal ducts, resulting in the classical "snowstorm" appearance. If sialography is not available or the child is not cooperative, ultrasound will reveal multiple small hypoechoic areas within the affected glands.[26–28]

The etiology remains obscure. Heredity, immunology, infection (bacterial or viral), allergy and congenital duct malformation have been implicated. Although allergic mechanisms have been suggested on the basis of sporadic reports of seasonal incidence or drug association, this has not been supported by more detailed investigations.[23,29,30]

Evidence of bacterial infection is based on the isolation of *Streptococcus viridans* from the parotid saliva. As this organism is a normal oral commensal, its presence in parotid saliva suggests ascending infection.[31] Ericson *et al.*[29] have suggested that an underlying congenital malformation of the duct system and infections ascending from the mouth following dehydration are the etiological factors.

In one recent study, autoantibodies reacting with the cytoplasm of acinar cells were found in 17 cases out of 20, and autoantibodies reacting with the cytoplasm of ductal cells were found in another eight.[32] It was suggested that the autoantibodies were produced in response to the primary damage and that they were not causing an autoimmune disease. In another study, immunologic evaluations were performed in 59 children with a history of recurrent sialadenitis and autoantibodies were found in only 20% (12 patients), three of whom were diagnosed as having Sjögren's syndrome.[33]

A viral etiology has also been suggested for recurrent sialadenitis of childhood. Using indirect immunofluorescence techniques for antibody levels, Akaboshi *et al.*[34] found evidence of EBV infection in 85% of a series of sufferers. They suggested that the recurrent episodes of sialadenitis were due to reactivation of EBV replication within the gland. More recently, mumps virus has been implicated,[35] although earlier this had been rejected as a cause.[23]

Traditionally, recurrent sialadenitis in childhood has been managed with antibiotics, as *Strep. viridans* is isolated from the parotid saliva in most cases. Symptoms settle after 3–5 days on this regimen. Galili and Marmary[19] have suggested that diagnostic sialography has a profound effect of reducing the frequency of attacks, even in the absence of antibiotics. This might be a result of mechanical flushing of the duct system, or the antibacterial effect of the iodine in the contrast medium. Occasionally, a child experiences so many attacks that their schooling is affected. In this situation, it has been the author's practice to prescribe long term prophylactic antibiotics, and on an anecdotal basis this has proved effective. In one patient, this regimen failed after a 2-year remission and the patient subsequently required bilateral parotidectomies at the ages of 7 and 9 years.

In their study of 22 children with long term follow-up, some for as long as 28 years, Galili and Mamary demonstrated conclusive evidence of parotid recovery in 86% based on sialographic evidence.[19] In contrast, Geterud *et al.*, in a series of 25 children followed up to age 22 years reported that although 23 became symptom free, the majority of cases continued to have abnormal sialography.[36,37] These findings support the observation that in recurrent sialadenitis of childhood, spontaneous resolution usually takes place. However, if a careful history is taken from patients presenting in adulthood with recurrent bacterial parotitis, many will admit to a history of recurrent parotid swelling during childhood. It is the author's opinion that the structural changes seen in recurrent parotitis of childhood frequently persist and that in later life many patients experience further episodes of parotitis.

Acute bacterial sialadenitis

Bacterial infection is relatively uncommon in childhood, largely because obstruction due to calculi is rare. Predisposing factors include dehydration, duct strictures, autoimmune disease, and occasionally calculi. The parotid gland is affected more frequently than the submandibular gland. Signs and symptoms of acute bacterial sialadenitis include pain, redness and swelling of the affected glands and surrounding soft tissues. Saliva milked from the affected gland is cloudy and floculant. The organisms most commonly cultured are *Staphylococcus aureus* or *Streptococcus viridans*.[38,39]

Sialography must never be attempted in the acute phase. Not only is it extremely painful, but it may result in a bacteremia as the back-pressure in the gland readily ruptures the inflamed acinae. If there is any doubt, ultrasound will confirm the diagnosis.

Treatment consists of a broad-spectrum penicillinase-resistant antibiotic which is started empirically before the results of culture and sensitivity are available. Fluids must be encouraged to increase salivary secretion, which mechanically flushes out the affected gland. Paracetamol is prescribed for pain. This regimen will control the acute infection in most cases, but occasionally an abscess will form, in which case open surgical drainage is essential. In the case of the parotid, a preauricular or retromandibular skin incision is made and the parotid fascia opened by blunt dissection using sinus forceps so as to avoid damage to branches of the facial nerve. Once the abscess cavity has been drained, a small corrugated drain is inserted for up to 48 hours. Following removal of the drain, the tissues heal spontaneously – a salivary fistula does not form. Alternatively, the abscess may be aspirated using a large gauge hypodermic needle introduced into the abscess cavity under ultrasound control.

Approximately 4–6 weeks after resolution of the acute infection, sialography should be undertaken to assess the residual function of the gland. Bacterial sialadenitis in children results in duct metaplasia with an increase in mucous secreting glands.[38] This results in thicker, more viscous saliva and an increased risk of recurrent ascending infection. If, on the emptying film of the sialographic series, there is failure of the gland to completely clear the contrast medium within two minutes following the withdrawal of the catheter, then the gland will be at risk of chronic

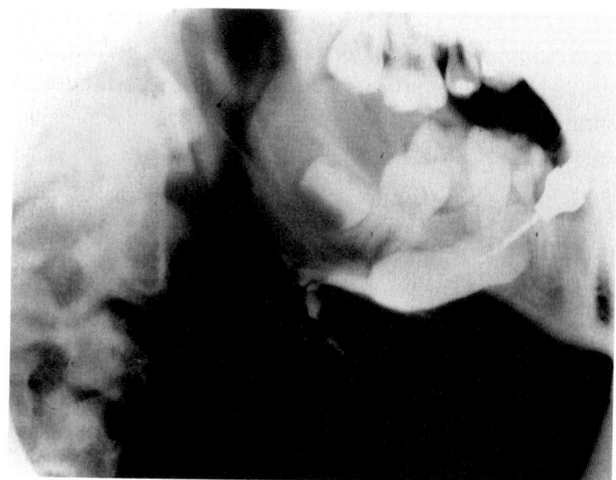

Fig. 9.3. Radiograph showing direct injection of contrast medium into the dilated submandibular duct in a child with a post-traumatic stricture.

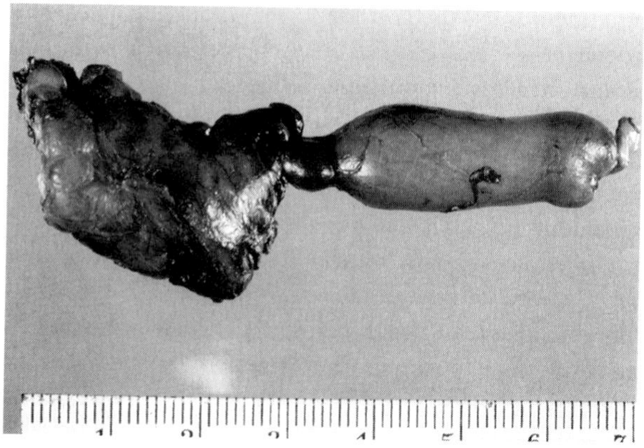

Fig. 9.4. Surgical specimen of the child in Fig. 9.3. The duct stricture is seen anterior to the grossly dilated duct.

or recurrent infection. In this situation, the affected gland should be excised if symptoms persist.

Neonatal sialadenitis

Bacterial sialadenitis may occur in infants up to 1 year of age, but occurs mostly in premature infants in the first week of life. It is more common in the parotid gland but can involve the submandibular gland. The bacteriostatic effect of the mucus in the submandibular gland secretions is thought to be protective.[40] *Staph. aureus* is the most common organism cultured in these infants. Appropriate antibiotic therapy and hydration are effective and the condition resolves rapidly without recurrence.

Obstructive sialadenitis

Inflammatory change secondary to obstruction is more commonly due to stricture formation than calculi. Repeated trauma from biting the parotid duct, or irritation by an orthodontic appliance, can result in fibrosis and stricture formation. Similarly, children who trip and fall with a pencil or stick in their mouth may traumatize the floor of the mouth, resulting in stricture formation at the submandibular papilla (Figs. 9.3 and 9.4).

The child may present with pain and swelling at mealtimes in response to a gustatory stimulus. However, many patients present with a chronically enlarged gland and relatively little discomfort. Strictures are diagnosed on sialography with proximal duct dilatation and delayed emptying.

If the stricture is accessible intraorally, then a linear incision along the duct or papilla at the site of the obstruction lays open the duct and allows saliva to drain freely. If the obstruction has been longstanding, back-pressure within the affected gland will have resulted in permanent atrophy and fibrosis and this renders the gland subject to chronic infection. A sialogram should always be performed some weeks following release of the stricture, and if the gland fails to empty then the gland should be excised. When the stricture is not readily accessible posteriorly in the floor of the mouth where the submandibular duct is related to the lingual nerve, or lateral to the masseter muscle in the parotid, then excision of the gland is necessary. More recently, duct strictures in adults have been successfully dilated using angioplasty balloons positioned under direct fluoroscopic control. It may be that this technique will be applied to children although a degree of cooperation is required. The long-term results of sticture dilatation are not known.

Sialolithiasis

Calculi are seen infrequently in childhood. The average age of presentation is 10 years and males are affected more commonly than females; the reasons for this are not known.[41] The submandibular gland is involved in 90% of cases.[42] The stones usually impact at the orifice of the submandibular duct but may be found anywhere in the duct system or in the gland. In the parotid gland, stones impact most commonly at the parotid papilla.

Salivary gland stones form as a result of the deposition of calcium salts around a central organic nidus such as an epithelial cast, bacteria, or foreign body. The major crystalline component is calcium phosphate with smaller amounts of magnesium, carbonate and ammonia. It is not known why some patients are prone to develop salivary stones, but in these patients recurrent stones, or stones involving more than one gland, occur. Despite their abnormal saliva, patients with cystic fibrosis are not prone to develop salivary stones.[43]

Children with salivary gland stones often present with pain and swelling of the affected gland at mealtimes, and the stone may be palpable in the floor of the mouth. However, in some patients the stone is discovered incidentally during a radiographic examination. The majority (90%) of submandibular stones are radio-opaque and can be seen on dental occlusal films or oblique lateral mandibular films. However, 90% of parotid stones are radiolucent and sialography is needed to confirm the diagnosis.[35] On sialography, the contrast material may pass around the stone and reveal duct dilatation and delayed emptying.[41]

When a stone is located at the orifice of the submandibular or parotid duct, it can be removed by probing or by slitting the duct or papilla but when a stone is located within the parenchyma of the submandibular gland, excision of the gland is required. Gland removal should include as much of the duct as possible, as a remnant may be the site of chronic infection. Stones in the intraglandular ducts of the parotid can be removed through a formal parotidectomy approach without removing the gland, but often it is simpler to perform a formal parotidectomy with preservation of the facial nerve.

Extracorporeal shockwave lithotripsy has been advocated.[44] Although it is possible to shatter most stones, the debris may not be eliminated from the ducts and there is therefore a high risk of recurrence. Under fluoroscopic control, salivary calculi can often be retrieved following cannulation of the duct and the use of a Dormier basket or micro-forceps.

Following removal of the salivary stone, the patient should undergo sialography 4–6 weeks later to assess gland function. If the gland fails to empty it should be excised in order to avoid chronic infection.

Autoimmune salivary disease (Sjögren's syndrome)

Although uncommon in childhood, Sjögren's syndrome may present as recurrent parotitis.[45–47] Careful investigation including minor salivary gland biopsy reveals the classical focal lymphocytic infiltration. Primary Sjögren's syndrome (in the absence of a connective tissue disorder) and secondary Sjögren's syndrome (in association with other autoimmune disorders) can occur. In children, sicca symptoms (xerostomia, xerophthalmia and keratoconjunctivitis sicca) are less marked and often the initial manifestations are fever, exanthema, arthralgia, butterfly rash, Raynaud's phenomenon, muscle weakness, and parotid swelling.[48] Laboratory studies reveal elevated levels of IgG, antinuclear antibody, rheumatoid factor, anti SS-A antibody (anti-Ro) and anti SS-B antibody (anti-La).

Children with Sjögren's syndrome have an increased incidence of bronchitis, pneumonia, otitis media, pancreatitis, atrophic gastritis, and B-cell non-Hodgkin's lymphoma. Any underlying connective tissue disorder must be treated on its merits. Meticulous dental supervision is essential as the dry mouth can result in mucosal ulceration and rampant caries. Artificial tears may be needed to lubricate and hydrate the cornea.

Interestingly, mothers whose sera are positive for the anti SS-A antibody (anti-Ro) are at increased risk of giving birth to infants with neonatal lupus erythematosus.[49]

Granulomatous sialadenitis

This type of inflammation rarely affects children. Possible causes are tuberculosis, sarcoidosis, cat scratch disease, atypical mycobacterial infections, and actinomycosis.[38,50] These conditions present as painless, slowly progressive swellings with little associated inflammation. Sialography reveals extrinsic pressure distorting the duct system. Salivary gland excision is often required to confirm the diagnosis and is also curative. Tuberculous involvement is often part of a systemic illness and requires appropriate antituberculous chemotherapy.

Allergic parotitis

Parotitis may follow the ingestion of some foods (usually shellfish or strawberries), chloramphenicol, oxytetracycline, pollens, and heavy metals. The presence of eosinophilia in the saliva and blood supports the diagnosis.[10] Resolution of symptoms occurs once the allergen is eliminated. Urticaria or bronchospasm may accompany the parotid enlargement.

HIV-associated disease

HIV salivary disease is more common among children than adults.[51] Indeed, chronic parotitis in children is said by Prose to be pathognomonic of HIV infection.[52] Patients present with symptoms similar to Sjögren's syndrome (see above) or with bilateral salivary gland enlargement. Biopsy of the affected glands demonstrates a focal lymphocytic infiltrate similar to that of Sjögren's syndrome, except that the predominant cell is the CD8-positive T-cell as opposed to the CD4-positive T-cell seen in Sjögren's syndrome.

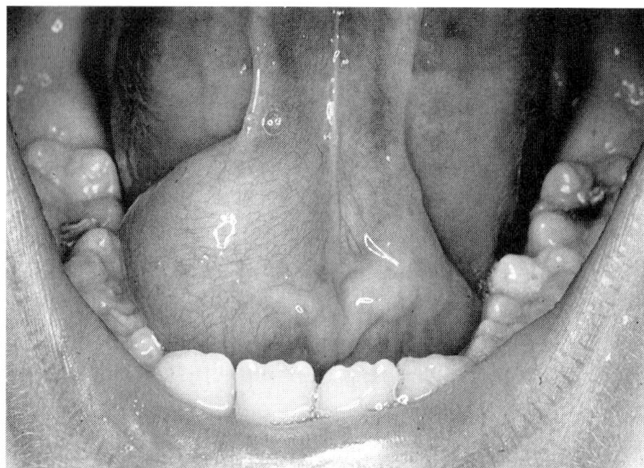

Fig. 9.5. Ranula arising from the right sublingual gland.

HIV-associated salivary gland disease includes lymphoepithelial lesions and cysts involving the salivary gland tissue and/or intraglandular lymph nodes, Sjögren's syndrome-like conditions, and diffuse interstitial lymphocytosis syndrome.[52,53] This latter condition is associated with an increased risk of salivary gland B-cell lymphoma.[49] No specific therapy is available, although salivary gland excision may be required for cosmetic purposes. It has been suggested that HIV-associated salivary gland disease has a more favorable prognosis, with delayed development of AIDS, in HIV-positive patients.[54]

Retention and extravasation cysts

Cystic lesions of the minor salivary glands are relatively common in childhood. They occur mostly on the mucosal aspect of the lower lip or on the cheek mucosa, and arise as a result of chronic irritation and fibrosis which obstructs the drainage of the underlying mucous gland. They present as tense bluish swellings up to 10 mm in diameter arising on the oral mucosa. Often they rupture spontaneously only to recur again some weeks later. Treatment is by excision of the underlying minor salivary gland. Attempts to remove only the cyst result in recurrence.

A ranula is a retention cyst in the floor of the mouth arising from the sublingual salivary gland (Fig. 9.5). It is usually unilateral and lies deep to the mucosa of the floor of the mouth above the mylohyoid muscle. It has a bluish translucent appearance and may be sufficiently large to displace the tongue. A plunging ranula presents as a swelling in the submental region and arises when a simple ranula extends into the neck through a developmental dehiscence in the mylohyoid. In either case, excision of the sublingual salivary gland is curative.[55]

Systemic and metabolic disorders

Progressive salivary gland enlargement in children may result from a number of systemic disorders. Endocrine disorders such as hypothyroidism, diabetes and diseases of the pituitary–adrenal axis are associated with parotid swelling. Cystic fibrosis involves the submandibular glands more frequently than the parotids. Obesity, malnutrition, hyperlipoproteinemia, cirrhosis, uremia and some vitamin deficiencies (B6 and C) may also cause symptomless salivary gland enlargement.

Ingestion of lead, iodide or copper may cause acute toxic parotitis.[56] Several drugs are known occasionally to cause parotid enlargement, but most of them are now rarely prescribed, particularly in pediatric practice. They include thiourea, methimazole, isoproterenol, phenylbutazone, phenothiazine and thiocyanate.[38,56] Management consists of avoiding the offending drug, or treatment of the underlying condition.

Neoplastic conditions

Salivary gland neoplasms in children are rare and in most reviews less than 5% of all salivary tumors occur in children under 16 years of age.[57–61] As in adults, the parotid is the commonest site for a neoplasm.[62,63] However, the pathologic spectrum is quite different, children having a much higher incidence of tumors arising from vasoformative tissues. Also, when a child does develop a solid salivary gland tumor, it is far more likely to be malignant than in an adult.[64–66]

An analysis by Jacques *et al.*[67] of 124 parotid tumors arising in children under 15 years revealed that 32% were endothelial tumors (hemangiomas and lymphangiomas), 40% were benign epithelial tumors (36% pleomorphic adenoma), and 27% were malignant epithelial cell tumors (15% mucoepidermoid carcinoma). In a series of 80 children with epithelial salivary gland tumors analysed by Seifert *et al.*,[62] 71% arose within the parotid, 8% in the submandibular gland, and the remainder from the minor glands. In this series of epithelial tumors, 66% were benign pleomorphic adenomas and 34% were malignant tumors, most of which were mucoepidermoid carcinomas. Broadly similar distributions have been noted by other authors.[58,64,65,68–71]

Benign neoplasms

The majority of benign tumors of the salivary glands arising in children are either hemangiomas or lymphangiomas.

Together, these account for 60% of all pediatric salivary gland tumors.[57,65]

Parotid hemangiomas
Hemangiomas appear shortly after birth and grow progressively over several months. The majority undergo spontaneous regression by 2 years of age. The tumor is usually confined to the intracapsular parotid, but occasionally the overlying skin may be involved. Females are more frequently affected and, in 50% of cases, other cutaneous hemangiomas are present.[57]

The majority of these neoplasms are capillary, but cavernous, mixed, and hypertrophic tumors do occur. The tumor is soft to rubbery in consistency and painless. The treatment of choice is masterly inactivity, as most will undergo spontaneous regression. It is important to reassure the family, as the lesion continues to grow for some months. If ulceration, hemorrhage or infection occur, surgical intervention may be necessary. If the hemangioma does not regress totally, surgery will be needed to remove persistent remnants. Subtotal parotidectomy with preservation of the facial nerve is undertaken. The technique for parotidectomy is in principle the same as for adults, except that the facial nerve has a more superficial position because the mastoid air cells are not fully developed.

Lymphangiomas (cystic hygromas)
Lymphangiomas affecting the salivary glands are less common than hemangiomas. When they do occur, they form sponge-like multi-cystic lesions. Histologically, capillary, cavernous and cystic types are recognized, but most lesions are mixed. Approximately 50% are manifest by 12 months of age, and 90% will be evident by the end of the second year. Unlike hemangiomas, they do not undergo spontaneous involution.[11,57]

Lymphangiomas affect any of the salivary glands and present as soft, painless, compressible swellings. They undergo gradual enlargement interspersed with periods of dramatically rapid growth, perhaps precipitated by infection.[72] Commonly they extend into the neck and mediastinum.

The surgical treatment of a lymphangioma is complete excision. An incomplete excision often results in local recurrence. However, as the lesion is entirely benign, normal structures should not be sacrificed to facilitate total removal.[16] Ideally, surgery is delayed for several years to make surgical dissection easier, but if a lymphangioma involving the submandibular or sublingual gland undergoes rapid growth, the airway can be compromised, and urgent surgery and tracheostomy may be necessary. There have been reports of the successful resolution of these tumors following intralesional injection of OK-432 (see *Chapter on Lymphangiomas*). This initiates a brisk inflammatory response leading to complete regression.[73,74,76]

Rarely, other benign non-epithelial tumors can occur in children, such as neurofibroma, neurilemoma or lipoma.[18,75] Complete excision is curative. The facial nerve should be preserved wherever possible.

Pleomorphic adenoma
This is the most frequently encountered benign epithelial tumor in childhood. It occurs at a later age than hemangiomas and lymphangiomas, with a peak incidence at 10 years.[11,57,69,77] There is some evidence of a male predominance.[11,57] The parotid gland is the most common site[58,59,64,70] but they can occur in the submandibular salivary gland and in the minor palatal glands (Fig. 9.6).[78] Evans and Rubin described two cases of benign pleomorphic adenomas in childhood arising in ectopic salivary tissue in the neck.[8] They present as a slow-growing, firm, discrete nodule within the affected gland. Pain and facial paralysis are extremely unlikely.

Although the tumors appear encapsulated they are lobulated and rupture easily at the time of surgery. For this reason enucleation should never be attempted. The minimal surgery for a parotid tumor is superficial lobectomy, if the tumor lies superficial to the facial nerve, or total parotidectomy for a deep lobe tumor. The facial nerve is always preserved. For a submandibular gland lesion, the entire gland is excised. In the palate, the tumor must be resected in the subperiosteal plane with a 5 mm mucosal margin. Recurrence is unusual with such a policy.[57,64,65] Inadequate surgery inevitably leads to local recurrence.[58,67]

Other benign salivary gland tumors in children are rare. Warthin's tumour[11,57,67] and basal cell adenoma[79] have been reported. Following surgical excision these lesions do not recur.

Malignant neoplasms

Approximately 25% of salivary gland tumors in adults are malignant, whereas in the pediatric population no less than 60% are malignant.[80] Malignant salivary gland tumors are more likely to be symptomatic at presentation. Local pain and facial paralysis or rapid growth suggest malignancy. Metastatic disease can be present in either the regional lymph nodes or at distant sites. The majority of malignant tumors arise in the parotid.[81,82] Tumors arising in the submandibular or sublingual glands, however, are more likely to be malignant than those in the parotid.

The mucoepidermoid carcinoma is the most common of the malignant salivary tumors seen in

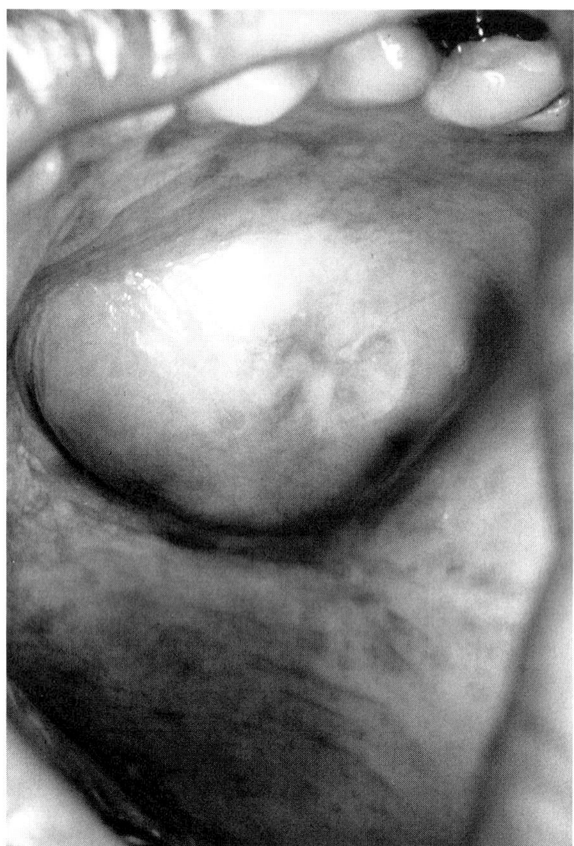

Fig. 9.6. Large palatal pleomorphic adenoma arising in a child of 15 years.

children.[11,63–65,67,81,83] Both high-grade and low-grade tumors occur. High-grade tumors have widely infiltrating margins. Acinic cell carcinoma, adenocarcinoma and adenoid cystic carcinoma are all less common.[63–65,67,83–86]

Malignancies of the parotid gland should be treated by total parotidectomy. The facial nerve should only be sacrificed when it is macroscopically invaded by tumor.[11,63,64] For malignant tumors of the submandibular gland, complete clearance of the submandibular triangle is indicated. For malignant tumors arising in the minor salivary glands, radical excision with clear margins according to the anatomical location of the tumor is needed. If there is local extension of disease into the mandible, maxilla, skin, or pharyngeal wall, radical surgical resection with immediate reconstruction should be undertaken.

Whenever there is clinical or imaging evidence of regional lymph node metastasis, a therapeutic neck dissection must be undertaken. In the absence of such evidence, the author undertakes a supraomohyoid neck dissection for all clinically obvious malignant parotid and submandibular gland tumors as a node sampling procedure.

Radical postoperative radiotherapy is given to those patients with high or intermediate grade histology, inadequate or positive surgical margins, evidence of perineural or perivascular invasion, or involvement of regional nodes.[63–65,87]

Survival of children with malignant salivary tumors tends to be better than that of adults.[84] This is largely due to a higher proportion of low-grade mucoepidermoid and acinic cell tumors and a higher proportion of stage I and II presentations in children. Spiro *et al.*[84] report actuarial 5-year and 10-year survival (of 155 patients) of 80% and 65% in patients treated between 1966 and 1982, compared with 60% and 50% (of 319 patients) treated before 1966. They consider this improvement to result from better surgical resections and postoperative radiotherapy. Callender *et al.*,[64] reporting on 21 children with malignant salivary tumors, quote absolute 2-year and 5-year survival rates of 100% and 90%. Many authors have demonstrated that inadequate primary surgery leads to recurrence, dissemination of disease, and ultimately death.[58,63,65,67,83]

Congenital parotid salivary carcinoma has been described.[58,65,88] In each case the infants were born with large lobulated masses in the parotid region overlying the angle of the mandible. Histologically, the tumors resembled the epithelial–myoepithelial carcinoma seen in adults. Of the two cases described in 1988 by Lack and Upton,[65] one was alive 11 years after surgery having had two local recurrences despite postoperative radiotherapy, and the other was tumor-free 21 years after postoperative radiotherapy and chemotherapy.

Rogers *et al.*[63] reported five mucoepidermoid carcinomas, which arose as second malignancies in patients with acute lymphoblastic leukemia. They had received cranial irradiation 3–14 years prior to the development of the salivary gland malignancy. The association of salivary gland malignancy with previous head and neck irradiation has been reported by others.[89–92]

Rhabdomyosarcoma

This tumor very rarely affects salivary glands.[57,63,65,93–96] Children commonly present with advanced disease with evidence of trigeminal nerve, facial nerve and other cranial nerve deficits, as well as regional or distant metastases.[63] Despite aggressive treatment with a combination of surgery, radiotherapy and chemotherapy, only two patients out of nine reported by Rogers *et al.* survived.[63] One of these underwent thoracotomy and pulmonary resection for metastatic disease 2 years after initial therapy, but nevertheless was tumor-free 6 years later.

Salivary incontinence

Drooling can be a major problem for some children with neurologic or physical disability, particularly cerebral palsy. A variety of management strategies have been advocated. Oral glycopyrrolate[97,98] and benzhexol hydrochloride[99] have been reported to control drooling by reducing salivary flow.

Irradiation of the salivary glands, and excision of the parotid and submandibular glands have also been described. Transposition of the submandibular ducts to the posterior floor of the mouth is simple and very effective.[100–102] This avoids the complications of drug therapy, irradiation and external scarring.[103,104]

There have been several reports of the successful use of the intraglandular injection of botulinum toxin into the submandibular glands to control drooling.[105,106] The author has tried this treatment in a prospective series of 12 patients using ultrasound guidance to ensure that the botulinum toxin was deposited into the glands. Although dramatically effective in a few patients, the overall results were disappointing.

Wong *et al.* have reported a series of six children on whom they undertook intraductal neodymium:yttrium aluminium garnet (Nd:YAG) laser photocoagulation of the parotid ducts.[107] Five of these children had a remarkable reduction in drooling when assessed at 1 month following treatment. However, it is difficult to understand how ablation of the parotid ducts could control drooling as it is widely accepted that it is the submandibular secretions which are the major contribution to drooling.

Complications of salivary gland surgery

In children, the trunk of the facial nerve is relatively superficial as the mastoid bone will not be fully developed. However, the other anatomical landmarks remain constant.[108] Permanent facial nerve paralysis following parotidectomy is rare except when branches of the facial nerve have been deliberately sacrificed. Temporary weakness due to neuropraxia occurs in approximately 30% of operations but recovers rapidly, usually within 6 weeks. Anesthesia of the skin flap slowly resolves as the sensory nerves regenerate from the periphery over a four month period. Anesthesia of the ear lobe due to sectioning of the great auricular nerve takes up to eighteen months to recover and is often never complete.

Gustatory sweating (Frey's syndrome) is a regular sequel to parotid surgery occurring in up to 54% of cases. Surgical manouvers to treat it are not successful and most patients either live with the symptoms or use an antiperspirant containing aluminium chloride. Intractable cases respond well to subcutaneous injection of botulinum toxin into the affected area but this must be repeated at regular intervals.

Tumor spillage from a benign pleomorphic adenoma should not occur but if it does, the wound must be carefully inspected and the area thoroughly irrigated. In such cases, postoperative radiotherapy should be considered even in children in order to avoid multiple recurrences due to tumor seeding. Other rare complications such as sialocele or salivary fistula occasionally follow parotidectomy. Both are managed conservatively and resolve spontaneously after a period.

Three cranial nerves are at risk during removal of the submandibular gland: the mandibular branch of the facial nerve, the lingual nerve (a branch of the third division of the trigeminal nerve) and the hypoglossal nerve. A low neck incision and careful surgical technique will avoid damage to the facial nerve. When chronic infection and subsequent fibrosis have occurred, it may be difficult to identify the lingual nerve and the deep aspect of the deep lobe may be attached to the hypoglossal nerve. The surgeon must be convinced that these structures have been identified before undertaking sharp dissection in the area and meticulous hemostasis is essential.

REFERENCES

1. Diederich, S., Roos, N., Bick, U., Hidding, J., & Birke, D. Diagnostic imaging of the salivary glands in children and adolescents. *Radiologe* 1991; **31**:550–557.
2. White, A. K. Salivary gland disease in infancy and childhood: non-malignant lesions. *J. Otolaryngol.* 1992; **21**:422–428.
3. Spiro, R. H. Salivary neoplasms: overview of a 35-year experience with 2807 patients. *Head Neck Surg.* 1986; **8**:177–184.
4. Sucupira, M. S., Weinseb, J. W., & Carmargo, E. E. Salivary gland imaging and radionuclide dacrocystography in agenesis of salivary glands. *Arch. Otolaryngol.* 1983; **109**:197–198.
5. Gelbier, M. J. & Winter, G. B. Absence of salivary glands in children with rampant dental caries:report of seven cases. *Int. J. Paediatr. Dentistry* 1995; **5**:253–257.
6. Polayes, I. M. & Rankow, R. M. Cysts, masses and tumours of the accessory parotid gland. *Plast. Reconst. Surg.* 1979; **64**:17.
7. Seifert, G., Miehike, A., Haubrich, J., & Chilla, R. *Diseases of the Salivary Glands.* Stuttgart: Georg Thieme, 1986: 63–70.

8. Evans, M. C. & Rubin, S. Z. Pleomorphic adenoma arising in a salivary rest in childhood. *J. Pediatr. Surg.* 1991; **26**:1314–1315.
9. Surana, R., Moloney, R., & Fitzgerald, R. J. Tumours of heterotopic salivary tissue in the upper cervical region in children. *Surg. Oncol.* 1993; **2**:133–136.
10. Cawson, R. A., Langdon, J. D., Eveson, J. W. *Surgical Pathology of the Mouth and Jaws*. Oxford: Wright, 1996:259.
11. Myer, C. & Cotton, R. T. Salivary gland disease in children: a review. *Clin. Pediatr. (Phila)* 1986; **25**:314–322 and 353–357.
12. Pershall, K. E., Koopmann, C. F., & Coulthard, S. W. Sialadenitis in children. *Int. J. Pediatr. Otorhinolaryngol.* 1986; **11**:199–203.
13. Work, W. P. Cysts and congenital lesions of the parotid gland. *Otolaryngol. Clin. North Am.* 1977; **10**:339–343.
14. Epker, B. N. Obstructive and inflammatory diseases of the major salivary glands. *Oral Surg. Oral Med. Oral Pathol.* 1972; **33**:2–27.
15. Wolf, H., Haus, M., & Wilmes, E. Persistence of Epstein–Barr virus in the parotid gland. *J. Virol.* 1984; **51**:795–798.
16. Bagg, J. Human herpesvirus-6: the latest human herpes virus. *J. Oral Pathol. Med.* 1991; **20**:465–468.
17. Birkebaek, N. H., & Halse, H. Human herpesvirus-6: the etiological agent in exanthema sibitum. *Ugeskr. Laeger* 1993; **155**:533–535.
18. Cohen, F. I. A., Gross, S., Nussinovitch, M., Frydman, M., & Varsano, I. Recurrent parotitis. *Arch. Dis. Child.* 1992; **67**:1036–1037.
19. Galili, D. & Marmary, Y. Juvenile recurrent parotitis: clinicoradiologic follow-up study and the beneficial effect of sialography. *Oral Surg. Oral Med. Oral Pathol.* 1986; **61**:550–556.
20. Grevers, G. Chronic recurrent parotitis in childhood. *Laryngorhinootologie* 1992; **71**:649–652.
21. Blatt, I. M. Chronic and recurrent inflammations about the salivary glands with special reference to children. *Laryngoscope* 1966; **76**:917–923.
22. Vichi, C. F. & Pampaloni, A. La sialographie dans les affections inflammatoire et neoplastiques des glandes salivaires de l'enfant. *Ann. Radiol.* 1971; **14**:481–490.
23. Konno, A. & Ito, E. A study on the pathogenesis of recurrent parotitis in childhood. *Ann. Otol. Rhinol. Laryngol.* 1979; **88**:1–20.
24. Cesnek, M. Chronic recurrent parotitis in children: diagnosis and therapy. *Cesk-Pediatr.* 1993; **48**:326–327.
25. Tabernero, C. M., Conzalez, G. M. T., Bueon, C. M., & Torreblanca, P. J. Chronic recurrent parotitis in children: apropos of 25 cases. *Ann. Esp. Pediatr.* 1991; **34**:133–136.
26. Nozaki, H., Harasawa, A., Hara, H., Kohno, A., & Shigeta, A. Ultrasonographic features of recurrent parotitis in childhood. *Pediatr. Radiol.* 1994; **24**:98–100.
27. Shimizu, M., Ussmuller, J., Donath, K. *et al.* Sonographic analysis of recurrent parotitis in children: a comparative study with sialographic findings. *Oral Surg., Oral Med., Oral Pathol., Oral Radiol. Endodont.* 1998; **86**:606–615.
28. Mandel, L. & Kaynar, A. Recurrent parotitis in children. *NY State Dent.* 1995; **61**:22–25.
29. Ericson, S., Zetterlund, B., & Ohman, J. Recurrent parotitis and sialectasis in childhood: clinical, radiologic, immunologic, bacteriologic and histologic study. *Ann. Otol. Rhinol. Laryngol.* 1991; **100**:527–535.
30. Zou, Z. J., Wang, S. L., Zhu, J. R., Yu, S. F., Ma, D. Q., & Wu, Y. T. Recurrent parotitis in children. A report of 102 cases. *Chin. Med. J.* 1990; **103**:575–582.
31. Kaban, L. B., Mulliken, J. B., & Marray, J. E. Sialadenitis in childhood. *Am. J. Surg.* 1978; **135**:570–576.
32. Babal, P. & Capova, L. Serum autoantibodies in recurrent parotitis in children. *Bratisl. Lek. Listy.* 1995; **96**:384–388.
33. Hara, T., Nagata, M., Mizurto, Y., Ura, Y., Matsuo, M., & Ueda, K. Recurrent parotid swelling in children: clinical features useful for differential diagnosis of Sjogren's syndrome. *Acta Paediatr.* 1992; **81**:547–549.
34. Akaboshi, I., Katsuki, T., Jamamoto, J., & Matsuda, I. Unique pattern of Epstein–Barr virus specific antibodies in recurrent parotitis. *Lancet* 1983, **ii**:1049–1051.
35. Zou, Z. J. Recurrent parotitis in childhood (report of 102 cases). *Chung-Hua-Kou-Chiang Hsueh Tsa Chih.* 1991; **26**:208–211.
36. Geterud, A., Lindvall, A. M., & Nylen, O. Follow-up study of recurrent parotitis in children. *Ann. Otol., Rhinol. Laryngol.* 1988; **97**:341–346.
37. Maynard, J. D. Sialectasis, Sjogren's, Mikulicz and HIV-associated salivary gland disease. In Norman, J. E. de, B., & McGurk, M. eds, *Color Atlas and Text of the Salivary Glands*. London: Mosby-Wolfe, 1995: 267–282.
38. Rice, D. H. Non-neoplastic salivary gland disorders. In Gates, C. A., ed, *Current Therapy in Otolaryngology: Head and Neck Surgery*. Trenton: Decker, 1982: 178–183.
39. Wilson, W. R., Eavey, R. D., & Lang, D. W. Recurrent parotitis during childhood. *Clin. Pediatr. (Phila)* 1980; **19**:235–236.
40. Banks, W. W., Handler, S. K., Glade, G. B. *et al.* Neonatal submandibular sialadenitis. *Am. J. Otolaryngol.* 1980; **1**:261–263.
41. Bodner, L. & Azaz, B. Submandibular sialolithiasis in children. *J. Oral Maxillofac. Surg.* 1982; **40**:551–554.
42. Sugiura, N., Kubo, I., Negoro, M. *et al.*. A case of sialolithiasis in a two year old girl. *Jap. J. Pedodontics* 1990; **28**:741–746.
43. Bullock, K. N. Salivary duct calculi presenting as trismus in a child. *Br. Med. J.* 1980; **280**:1357–1358.
44. Iro, H. & McCurk, M. Extracorporeal piezoelectric shockwave lithotripsy of salivary duct stones. In Norman, J. E. de, B., & McGurk, M., eds, *Color Atlas and Text of the Salivary Glands*. London: Mosby-Wolfe, 1995: 263–266.
45. Hearth, H. M., Baethge, B. A., Abreo, F., & Wolf, R. E. Autoimmune exocrinopathy presenting as recurrent parotitis of childhood. *Arch. Otolaryngol. Head Neck Surg.* 1993; **119**:347–349.
46. Stiller, M., Golder, W., Doring, E., & Biedermann, T. Primary and secondary Sjogren's syndrome in children. *Clin. Oral Invest.* 2000; **4**:176–182.
47. Zhang, Z., Zou, Z., & Ma, X. Clinical and radiographic study of Sjogren syndrome in children. *Chin. J. Stomatol.* 1996; **31**:25–27.

48. Tornfita, M., Kohno, Y., Honma, K. *et al.* The clinical manifestations of Sjogren's syndrome in children. *Ryumachi* 1994; **34**:863–870.
49. Nitta, Y., Ohashi, M., Morikawa, M., & Ueki, H. Significance of tubuloreticular structures forming in Daudi cells cultured with sera from mother bearing infants with neonatal lupus erythematosus. *Br. J. Dermatol.* 1994; **131**:525–531.
50. Work, W. P., Hecht, D. W. Inflammatory diseases of the major salivary glands. In Paparella, M. M. & Shumrick, D. A. eds, *Otolaryngology*. Philadelphia: WB Saunders, 1980: 2235–2243.
51. Schiodt, M. HIV-associated salivary gland disease: a review. *Oral Surg. Oral Med. Oral Path.* 1992; **73**:164–167.
52. Prose, N. S. HIV infection in children. *J. Am. Acad. Dermatol.* 1990; **22**:1223–1231.
53. Itescu, S. Diffuse infiltrative lymphocytosis syndrome in children and adults infected with HIV-1: a model of rheumatic illness caused by acquired viral infection. *Am. J. Reprod. Immunol.* 1992; **28**:247–250.
54. Challacombe, S. J. & Schiodt, M. HIV-associated salivary gland disease. In Norman, J. E. de, B., McGurk, M., eds. *Color Atlas and Text of the Salivary Glands*. London: Mosby-Wolfe, 1995; 279–283.
55. Parekh, D., Stewart, M., Joseph, C., & Lawson, H. H. Plunging ranula: a report of three cases and review of the literature. *Br. J. Surg.* 1987; **74**:307–309.
56. Strome, M. Neoplastic salivary gland diseases in children. *Otolaryngol. Clin. North Am.* 1977; **10**:391–398.
57. Schuller, D. E. & McCabe, B. F. Salivary gland neoplasms in children. *Otolaryngol. Clin. North Am.* 1977; **10**:399–412.
58. Bianchi, A. & Cudmore, R. E. Salivary gland tumours in children. *J. Pediatr. Surg.* 1978; **13**:519–521.
59. Nagao, K., Matsuzaki, O., Saiga, H. *et al.* Histopathological studies on parotid gland tumours in Japanese children. *Virchow's Arch. Pathol. Anat. Histol.* 1980; **388**:263–272.
60. Luna, M. A., Batsakis, J. G., & el-Naggar, A. K. Salivary gland tumours in children. *Ann. Otol. Rhinol. Laryngol.* 1991; **100**:869–871.
61. Ethunandam, M., Ethunandam, A., Macpherson, D., Conroy, B., & Pratt, C. Parotid neoplasms in children: experience of diagnosis and management in a district general hospital. *Int. J. Oral Maxillofac. Surg.* 2003; **32**:373–377.
62. Seifert, C., Okabe, H., & Caselitz, J. Epithelial salivary gland tumours in children and adolescents. *Otorhinolaryngology* 1986; **48**:137–149.
63. Rogers, D. A., Rao, B. N., Bowman, L. *et al.* Primary malignancy of the salivary gland in children. *J. Pediatr. Surg.* 1994; **29**:44–47.
64. Callender, D. L., Frankenthaler, R. A., Luna, M. A., Lee, S. S., & Goepfert, H. Salivary gland neoplasms in children. *Arch. Otolaryngol. Head Neck Surg.* 1992; **118**:472–476.
65. Lack, E. E. & Upton, M. P. Histopathologic review of salivary gland tumours in childhood. *Arch. Otolaryngol. Head Neck Surg.* 1988; **114**:898–906.
66. Kessler, A. & Handler, S. D. Salivary gland neoplasms in children: a 10-year survey at the Children's Hospital of Philadelphia. *Int. J. Pediatr. Otorhinolaryngol.* 1994; **29**:195–202.
67. Jacques, D. A., Krolls, S. O., & Chambers, R. G. Parotid tumours in children. *Am. J. Surg.* 1976; **132**:469–471.
68. Fonsceca, L., Martins, A. C., & Soares, J. Epithelial salivary gland tumours of children and adolescents in southern Portugal: a clinicopathologic study of twenty four cases. *Oral Surg. Oral Med. Oral Pathol.* 1991; **72**:696–701.
69. Krolls, S. O., Trodahl, J. N., & Boyers, R. C. Salivary gland lesions in children *Cancer* 1972; **30**:459–469.
70. Gallich, R. Salivary gland neoplasms in childhood. *Arch. Otolaryngol.* 1969; **89**:100–104.
71. Byars, L. T., Ackerman, L. V., & Peacock, E. Tumors of salivary gland origin in children. *Ann. Surg.* 1957; **146**:40–51.
72. Leipzig, B. & Rabuzza, D. D. Recurrent massive cystic lymphangioma. *Otolaryngol.* 1978; **86**:758–760.
73. Mikhail, M., Kennedy, R., Cramer, B., & Smith, T. Sclerosing of recurrent lymphangioma using OK-432. *J. Pediatr. Surg.* 1995; **30**:1159–1160.
74. Banieghbal, B. & Davies, M. R. Guidelines for the succesful treatment of lymphangioma with OK-432. *Eur. J. Pediatr. Surg.* 2003; **13**:103–107.
75. Weitzner, S. Plexiform neurofibroma of major salivary glands in children. *Oral Surg., Oral Med., Oral Pathol.* 1980; **50**:53–57.
76. Karmody, C. S., Fortson, J. K., & Calcaterra, V. E. Lymphangiomas of the head and neck in adults. *Otolaryngol. Head Neck Surg.* 1982; **90**:283–288.
77. Touloukian, R. J. Salivary gland diseases in infancy and childhood. In Rankow, R. M., ed. *Diseases of the Salivary Glands*. Philadelphia: WB Saunders, 1976:284–303.
78. de Courten, A., Lombardi, T., & Samson, J. Pleomorphic adenorna of the palate in a child: 9-year follow-up. *Int. J. Oral Maxfac. Surg.* 1996; **25**:293–295.
79. Canalis, R. F., Mok, M. W., Fishman, S. M. *et al.* Congenital basal cell adenoma of the submandibular gland. *Arch. Otolaryngol.* 1980; **106**:284–286.
80. Biorkland, A. & Eneroth, C. M. Management of parotid gland neoplasms. *Am. J. Otolaryngol.* 1980; **1**:155–167.
81. Rasp, G. & Permanetter, W. Malignant salivary gland tumors: squamous cell carcinoma of the submandibular gland in a child. *Am. J. Otolaryngol.* 1992, **13**:109–112.
82. Taylor, R. E., Cattamaneni, H. R., & Spooner, D. Salivary gland carcinomas in children: a review of 15 cases. *Med. Pediatr. Oncol.* 1993; **21**:429–432.
83. Byers, R. M., Pierkowski, K., & Luna, M. A. Malignant parotid tumours in patients under 20 years of age. *Arch. Otolaryngol.* 1984; **110**:232–235.
84. Spiro, R. H., Armstrong, J., Harrison, L., Geller, N. L., Lin, S.-Y., & Strong, E. W. Carcinoma of major salivary glands. *Arch. Otolaryngol. Head Neck Surg.* 1989; **115**:316–321.
85. Jones, D. C. & Bainton, R. Adenoid cystic carcinoma of the palate in a 9-year-old boy. *Oral Surg., Oral Med., Oral Pathol.* 1990; **69**:483–486.
86. Ustundag, E., Iseri, M., Aydin, O. *et al.* Adenoid cystic carcinoma of the tongue. *J. Laryngol. Otol.* 2000; **114**:477–480.

87. Harrison, L. B., Armstrong, J. G., Spiro, R. H. *et al.* Postoperative. radiation therapy for major salivary gland malignancies. *J. Surg. Oncol.* 1990; **45**:52–55.
88. Vawter, C. F. & Tefft, M. Congenital tumors of the parotid gland. *Arch. Pathol. Lab. Med.* 1966; **82**:242–245.
89. Katz, A. D. Thyroid and associated polyglandular neoplasms in patients who received head and neck irradiation during childhood. *Head Neck Surg.* 1979; **1**:417–422.
90. Benninger, M. S., Lavertu, P., Linden, M. D. *et al.* Multiple parotid gland neoplasms after radiation therapy. *Otolaryngol. Head Neck Surg.* 1988; **98**:250–253.
91. Schneider, A. B., Favus, M. J., Stachura, M. E. *et al.* Salivary gland neoplasms as a late consequence of head and neck irradiation. *Ann. Intern. Med.* 1977; **87**:160–164.
92. Walker, M. J., Chaudhuri, P. K., Wood, D. C. *et al.* Radiation-induced parotid cancer. *Arch. Surg.* 1981; **116**:329–331.
93. Volpe, R. & Mazabraud, A. Primary sarcomas of the parotid gland. *Pathologica* 1981; **73**:541–546.
94. Auclair, P. L., Langloss, J. M., Weiss, S. W. *et al.* Sarcomas and sarcomatoid neoplasms of the major salivary gland regions. *Cancer* 1986; **58**:1305–1315.
95. Kauffman, S. L. & Stout, A. D. Tumors of the major salivary glands in children. *Cancer* 1963; **16**:1317–1331.
96. Luna, M. A., Tartoledo, E., Ordonez, N. G. *et al.* Primary sarcomas of the major salivary glands. *Arch. Otolaryngol. Head Neck Surg.* 1991; **117**:302–306.
97. Blasco, P. A. & Stansbury, J. C. Glycopyrrolate treatment of chronic drooling. *Arch. Pediatr. Adolesc. Med.* 1996; **150**:932–935.
98. Stern, L. M. Preliminary study of glycopyrrolate in the management of drooling. *J. Paediatr. Child Health* 1997; **33**: 52–54.
99. Reddihough, D., Johnson, H., Staples, M., Hudson, I., & Exarchos, H. Use of benzhexol hydrochloride to control drooling of children with cerebral palsy. *Dev. Med. Child Neurol.* 1990; **32**:985–989.
100. Arnrup, K. & Crossner, C. G. Caries prevalence after submandibular duct retroposition in drooling children with neurological disorders. *Pediatr. Dent.* 1990; **12**:98–101.
101. Burton, M. J., Leighton, S. E., & Lund, W. S. Long-term results of submandibular duct transposition for drooling. *J. Laryngol. Otol.* 1991; **105**:101–103.
102. Panarese, A., Ghosh, S., Hodgson, D., McEwan, J., & Bull, P. D. Outcomes of submandibular duct re-implantation for sialorrhoea. *Clin. Otolaryngol.* 2001; **26**:143–146.
103. Burton, M. J. The surgical management of drooling. *Dev. Med. Child Neurol.* 1991; **12**:1110–1116.
104. Blasco, P. A. & Allaire, J. H, Consortium on drooling. Drooling in the developmentally disabled: management practices and recommendations. *Dev. Med. Child Neurol.* 1992; **34**:849–862.
105. Jongerius, P. H., Rotteveel, J. J., van den Hoogen, F. *et al.* Botulinum toxin A: a new option for treatment of drooling in children with cerebral palsy. *Eur. J. Pediatr.* 2001; **160**:509–512.
106. Ellies, M., Rohrbach-Volland, S., Arglebe, C. *et al.* Successful management of drooling with botulinum toxin A in neurologically disabled children. *Neuropediatrics* 2002; **33**:327–330.
107. Wong, A. M., Chang, C. J., Chen, L. R., & Chen, M. M. Laser intraductal photocoagulation of bilateral parotid ducts for reducing drooling of cerebral palsied children. *J. Clin. Laser Med. Surg.* 1997; **15**:65–69.
108. Langdon, J. D. In Langdon, J. D., Patel, M. F., eds. *Operative Maxillofacial Surgery.* London: Chapman & Hall, 1998: 380–389.

10

Head and neck tumors

Robert Ord and Rui Fernandes

Department of Oral and Maxillo Facial Surgery, University of Maryland, Baltimore, MD, USA

Malignant tumors: an introduction

Childhood cancer is fortunately rare. In the USA, 129.5 cases per million of white children and 104.1 cases per million of black children under the age of 15 years develop a cancer,[1] only 5% of which occur in the head and neck.[2,3] Pediatric head and neck malignancies represent a spectrum of histological types, which are totally different from those found in adults. In adult patients, squamous cell carcinoma accounts for over 90% of head and neck cancers if facial skin cancers are excluded. In pediatric patients, the majority of malignancies consist of small, blue, round cell tumors (neuroblastoma, peripheral neuroendocrine tumor, Ewing's sarcoma, non-Hodgkin's lymphoma, and soft tissue sarcomas). If central nervous system and hematological malignancies are excluded, then retinoblastomas, rhabdomyosarcomas and neuroblastomas are the most common cancers. Below the age of 3 years, retinoblastomas are the most common, followed by rhabdomyosarcomas and neuroblastomas; from 3 to 11 years, rhabdomyosarcomas are the most common, followed by lymphomas, while from 12 to 21 years this order is reversed.

Recent advances in molecular biology have led to increased understanding of the role of chromosomal changes, suppressor genes, and oncogenes in the etiology of these neoplasms. In addition, electron microscopy, histochemical staining, identification of cell markers, immunofluorescence, etc., have enabled better tumor typing and classification. In the clinical arena, multimodal therapy incorporating surgery, radiation and chemotherapy has increased long-term survival. Recent advances with the use of positron emission tomography (PET) scanning have improved the surveillance and assessment of tumor response to various treatment modalities.

However, head and neck cancer therapy in childhood presents many unique challenges. In addition to the cosmetic, speech, and swallowing difficulties faced by all patients who undergo surgery or radiation to the head and neck, problems with growth and development of soft tissues, facial bones and dentition are manifested by the pediatric patient in the long term.[4,5] Mucosal and endocrine damage, learning disabilities, and psychosocial problems for the child and the family are all concerns in treating these tumors.

This section discusses the management and long term outcomes of rhabdomyosarcoma, osteosarcoma, and Ewing's sarcoma of the head and neck.

Rhabdomyosarcomas

Rhabdomyosarcomas (RMS) comprise 10–15% of all pediatric solid tumors and account for over 50% of all soft tissue sarcomas in children.[6,7] Two-thirds of all cases are diagnosed in children less than 6 years of age. In the USA there is an incidence of 4.5 per million in children below the age of 15 years, 35–40% of these arising in the head and neck.[8,9] Prognosis depends on the histological type, the site, and the stage at presentation.

Histology

Classification of the pediatric small, blue, round cell tumors is continually undergoing revision. RMS is conventionally

Pediatric Surgery and Urology: Long-term Outcomes, Mark Stringer, Keith Oldham, Pierre Mouriquand.
Published by Cambridge University Press.

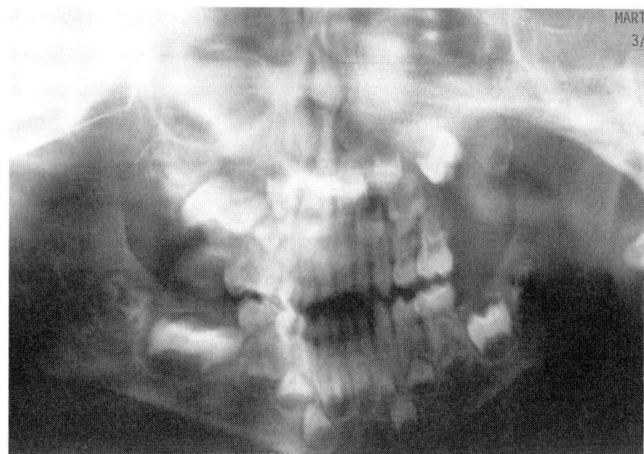

Fig. 10.1. Panoramic radiograph showing displacement of the left maxillary first molar by the tumor.

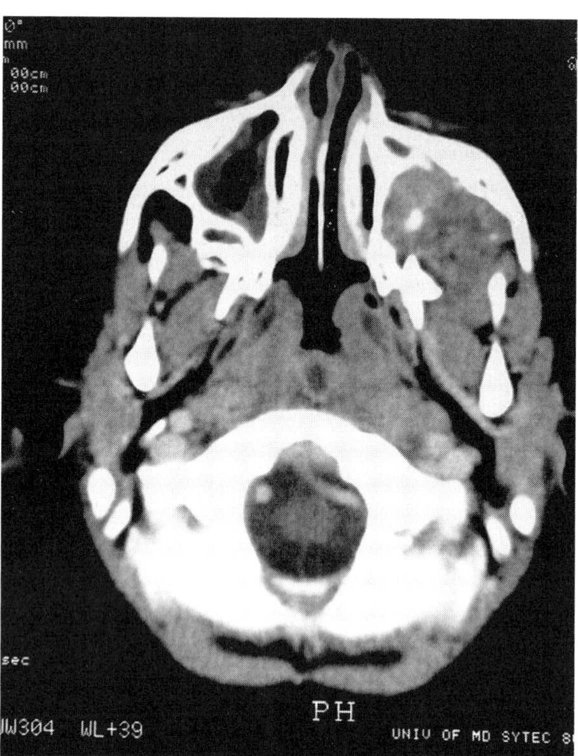

Fig. 10.2. CT scan of the patient in Fig. 10.1 shows extensive involvement of the maxillary sinus with destruction of the posterior bony wall; the tumor extended into the ethmoids.

divided into embryonal, botryoid, alveolar, and pleomorphic (adult) types. In the Intergroup Rhabdomyosarcoma studies, three other tumors that behave in an aggressive manner – extraosseous Ewing's sarcoma (EOE), sarcoma of undeterminate histology (SUH), and undifferentiated sarcoma (UD) – are included in the RMS group. The vast majority of head and neck RMS are embryonal or botryoid. The botryoid type has the most favorable prognosis, followed by the embryonal RMS; the alveolar type has a less favorable course; while EOE, SUH, and UD have the worst survival rates.

Site

In the head and neck, RMS is classified into three sites: 25% occur in the orbit, 50% in parameningeal sites, and 25% in other sites (non-parameningeal head and neck).

Orbital tumors are most commonly seen in younger patients, and usually arise behind the globe, although they may occur in the lids or conjunctiva. Extension posteriorly into the brain is rare, and these tumors are usually confined by the bony orbital walls from the nose and the paranasal sinuses. Lymph node metastases are extremely rare, and only 4% of orbital RMS show distant metastases.[10] Because of their localized nature, orbital RMS have the best prognosis for head and neck RMS with a 10-year event-free survival (EFS) and overall survival (OS) of 77% and 87%, respectively.[11]

Parameningeal sites include the nasopharynx, paranasal sinuses (Figs. 10.1 and 10.2), nasal cavity, middle ear, mastoid, parapharyngeal, and infratemporal regions. Rapid growth of RMS at these sites may lead to involvement of the skull base, the meninges, and in advanced cases the entire subarachnoid space. Patients may present at diagnosis with cranial nerve palsies, meningeal symptoms, or respiratory difficulties caused by brainstem infiltration.[12] RMS at these sites have the worst prognosis.

Tumors in other sites include RMS of the oral cavity (tongue), oropharynx, cheek, masseter, parotid, larynx, scalp, and neck. Rapid growth is common with these tumors, usually presenting as large masses.[13] Oral cavity RMS often occur in babies and infants, who may present with oral bleeding.[14] Eight percent of these patients will show lymph node metastases,[15] while 13% have distant metastases,[15] usually to the lung or bone marrow.

Staging

There are several staging systems for the soft tissue sarcomas. The UICC system incorporates the tumor grade (G) in addition to the standard TNM parameters.[16] The system most widely used in the USA is that of the Intergroup Rhabdomyosarcoma studies (IRS) I, II and III (Table 10.1).[17] Staging is assessed clinically, by special investigations, by imaging, and from pathological data after surgery. All RMS patients require a complete blood count, renal and liver panel, urinalysis, and bone marrow aspiration. In addition, the head and neck are evaluated with contrast computerized tomography (CT) and magnetic resonance imaging (MRI), while a chest CT and bone scan are undertaken as a metastatic screen. Recently, the use of fluorodeoxyglucose positron emission tomography (FDG-PET) is finding increasing use in diagnosing distinct metastasis both at presentation, as well as in assessment of chemotherapeutic response.[18] Patients with parameningeal RMS require a lumbar puncture and MRI of the brain with paramagnetic contrast medium.

Although it is not incorporated into the staging systems, the identification of gross bone erosion of the facial bones or skull base has been suggested to indicate a bad prognosis.[19]

Management

The prognosis for RMS has improved considerably with the implementation of multidisciplinary, multimodality, and multiagent chemotherapy protocols. All children with this diagnosis will receive chemotherapy with either surgery or radiation, or both, depending upon the stage, size and site of the tumor.

Surgery

When it is possible to resect the tumor widely with surrounding normal tissue, without sacrifice of essential structures causing severe functional or cosmetic problems, surgery plus chemotherapy gives the best overall survival. However, this is frequently impossible in parameningeal lesions, and extended biopsy for diagnosis, debulking and gene studies may be all that is feasible. Intraoral RMS, lesions of the scalp, and parotid lesions are frequently more amenable to surgery. In one recent review of 56 childhood RMS of the head and neck, complete resection with negative margins was possible in only three patients (5.4%), incomplete resection with microscopic residual disease in 13 (23.2%), while surgical margins were grossly positive in 40 patients (71.4%), the majority of which had incisional biopsy only.[20]

The surgical treatment for RMS has become progressively more conservative with each IRS study.[12] The extent of resection, however, varies by tumor site, although initial complete resection is recommended if feasible without loss of organ function. Initial surgical resection is not recommended in patients with tumors arising in the orbit

Table 10.1. Intergroup Rhabdomyosarcoma Study Group (IRSG) postsurgical grouping classification

Group	Description
I	Localized disease, completely excised, no microscopic residual
A	Confined to site of origin, completely resected
B	Infiltrating beyond site of origin, completely resected
II	Total gross resection
A	Gross resection with evidence of microscopic local residual
B	Regional disease with involved lymph nodes, completely resected with no microscopic residual
C	Microscopic local and/or nodal residual
III	Incomplete resection or biopsy with gross residual
IV	Distant metastases

because chemotherapy, with or without radiation therapy, or limited surgery performed after multiagent chemotherapy, offer an excellent chance of cure without a decrease in survival when compared with aggressive initial resection.[12]

In small, totally resectable lesions, chemotherapy is given postoperatively, while for larger lesions, induction chemotherapy, plus or minus radiation therapy, is used with surgery to remove residual disease only. However, radiation is associated with significant long-term complications in terms of subsequent growth and the induction of second malignancies.[21] Thus recent advances in craniofacial approaches, skull base surgery, microvascular reconstruction, and rigid fixation may allow more radical resection with decreased morbidity. This may be important as 50% of treatment failures are due to local recurrence.[20]

In the patient with an N0 neck, the low percentage of cervical metastases does not warrant elective neck dissection. Where clinically positive or suspicious nodes are present, neck dissection will give excellent control. Where there are multiple bulky nodes, radiation after neck dissection is indicated.

Radiation

Although radiation has proved very effective for RMS, dose schedules of at least 50 Gy in 28, 1.8 Gy daily fractions and wide fields (2 cm around the tumor) are necessary for local control. It is therefore difficult not to cause damage to the eye, parotid glands or growth regions such as the temporomandibular joint. The cure rate for orbital RMS with radiation is excellent, with overall survival at 87%, but with significant late sequela.[22] In parameningeal tumors, the skull base and 2 cm above are included in the field;

while in definite central nervous system involvement, the IRS II study included 30 Gy irradiation of the craniospinal axis.[23] The IRS evaluated the indications for radiotherapy and chemotherapy after complete resection in RMS looking at the data from the IRS studies I to III. The conclusions were that patients with group I embryonal RMS have an excellent prognosis when treated with adjuvant multiagent chemotherapy without radiotherapy. Patients with alveolar RMS or undifferentiated sarcoma fare worse; however, event-free survival and overall survival are improved substantially when RT is added to multiagent chemotherapy. The best outcome occurred in IRS-III when RT was used in conjunction with intensified chemotherapy.[24]

The IRS IV trial evaluated the use of conventionally fractionated radiotherapy (CFRT) vs. hyperfractionated radiotherapy (HFRT) in the treatment of group IV RMS. The study found no difference in the event-free survival and overall survival between the two RT methods when analyzed by age, gender, tumor size, tumor invasiveness, nodal status, histologic features, stage, or primary site. To date, the standard of care for group III RMS continues to be CFRT with chemotherapy.[25]

Chemotherapy

Prior to the 1960s, the use of wide surgical excision and radiation therapy yielded survival rates of only 5–9%.[26] Initial treatments with single and multiple chemotherapy agents showed good response rates. In 1974, a controlled clinical trial of chemotherapy in patients after surgery for Stage I disease clearly demonstrated improvement in survival.[29] This trial established the role of chemotherapy in RMS, and it has been considered unethical subsequently to carry out further trials with "no chemotherapy" arms for other stages or sites. All RMS patients are therefore given chemotherapy. In 1984, Flamant and Hill compared patients treated before 1972 without chemotherapy, or with chemotherapy not based on a systematic protocol related to stage, with patients treated after 1972 with systematic protocols incorporating chemotherapy; they reported 2-year and 5-year survival rates of 39% and 31% before 1972 and 63% and 52% after 1972.[30] Interestingly, head and neck patients had a greater increase in survival than for most other locations.

Standard regimens that have been used include vincristine, actinomycin D, and cyclophosphamide (VAC). The IRS study IV randomized patients to receive VAC, VAI (vincristine, dactinomycin, and ifosfomide), VIE (vincristine, ifosfomide, etoposide) with surgery (with or without RT) and found them to be equally effective for patients with local or regional RMS and more effective for the embryonal form. This study found the use of VAC + surgery + CFRT to be the gold standard therapy for most patients with non-metastatic embryonal rhabdomyosarcoma.[17]

Table 10.2. Five-year survival rates (%) in IRS studies I and II[30]

	Stage			
Disease site	I	II	III	IV
Orbit	100	91–95	88–90	0–50
Parameninges	100	70–92	45–66	11–29
Other	86–100	73–84	64–76	25–40

Long-term survival

Rhabdomyosarcoma has become increasingly more curable over the past quarter century, comparing a 25% survival probability in the 1970s to the 70% range in the 1990s.[17]

It is difficult to give overall figures for long-term survival as this will vary with site, stage and histology. Five-year survival data for IRS studies I and II[31] are given in Table 10.2. In IRS study II, because of the high rate of local recurrence in parameningeal RMS when there was CNS involvement, craniospinal axis radiation and intrathecal chemotherapy were added to the regimen. This improved survival from 33% to 57% at 3 years.[23] Although orbital RMS has an excellent prognosis (especially when localized), closely followed by other head and neck sites, parameningeal RMS still has a guarded prognosis. There are reports which indicate that RMS of the neck is also a site with lower survival rates.[32,33] The IRS studies have confirmed that completely resected tumors have the best prognosis, while patients with metastases at diagnosis have only a 29% chance of survival to 5 years.

The outlook for patients developing locoregional recurrence or distant metastases remains dismal, with 95% probability of death.[34] Most relapses are seen 2 years after the initiation of therapy, so that chemotherapy is usually continued for 1–2 years. However, relapse after 5–6 years has been reported,[35] and this may be more common in parameningeal RMS.[36]

The long-term complications of therapy are discussed at the end of the section on malignant tumors.

Osteosarcomas

Sarcomas of bone comprise 4.5% of all malignant pediatric tumors, and 2.6% of these are osteosarcomas.[37] Between

6% and 8% of osteosarcomas occur in the head or neck.[38,39] Prognosis will depend upon the stage and site of the tumor. Histology is less important than for rhabdomyosarcomas.

Histology

Although osteoblastic osteosarcoma is the most common histological type in long bones, in the jaws almost half of the osteosarcomas diagnosed are chondroblastic. In addition, fibroblastic and telangiectatic osteosarcomas are seen in the head and neck, although none of the patterns appears to have prognostic significance. In children, association with hereditary bilateral retinoblastoma (with or without prior radiation) or fibrous dysplasia are important etiological factors. A clear increase in the incidence of development of osteosarcoma in patients treated with radiation therapy for previous malignancies has also been shown. The median time between radiotherapy and the diagnosis of osteosarcoma was found to be 8 years with a range of 3.5 to 26 years.[40]

Site

The sites reported for osteosarcomas in the craniofacial region (CFOS) differ widely in the literature, and this is a disease mainly of adults (mean age 35 years). In one review of 329 cases of CFOS, 192 (58.3%) were mandibular, 106 (32%) were maxillary, and the remainder were found in the skull or other sites.[40] Figures from the Mayo Clinic show 36% mandibular osteosarcomas, 43% maxillary, and 21% skull tumors.[42] Smeele *et al.*[43] recently reported on 201 cases of CFOS, of which 35% were in the mandible, 34% in the maxilla, and 31% in the skull.

CFOS has a better prognosis than long bone osteosarcoma. This may be associated with its occurrence in older patients, its predominantly chondroblastic histology, and the lower incidence of distant metastases.[39] The mandible has the best overall survival as this is the easiest facial bone to resect with good margins and the easiest to reconstruct (Fig. 10.3). Juxtacortical osteosarcomas are variants of osteosarcoma, divided into parosteal (behaving as a low-grade malignancy) and periosteal (having an intermediate prognosis). Although these variants occur in the jaw, there are too few data to show whether they behave in a similar fashion to juxtacortical osteosarcomas of the long bones.[44]

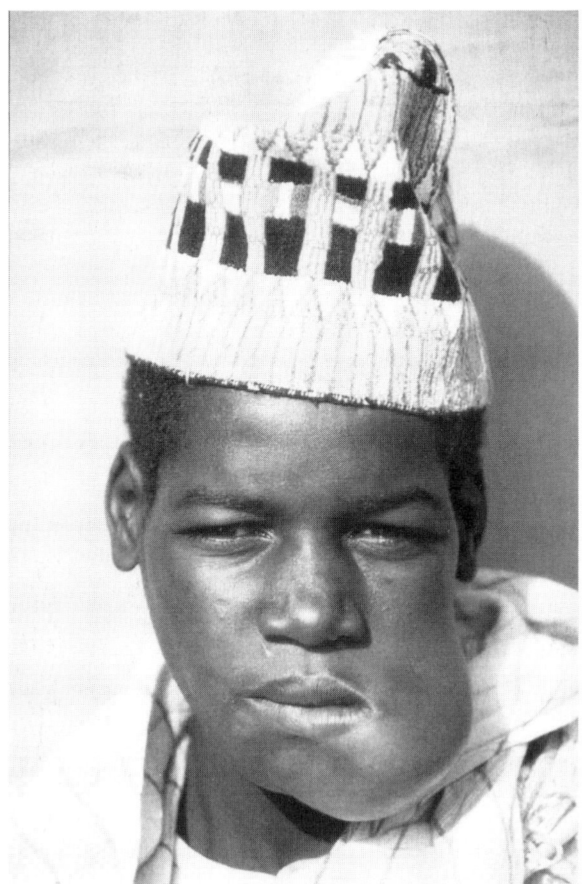

Fig. 10.3. Sixteen-year-old boy with a large osteosarcoma of the left mandible.

Staging

The system devised by Enneking and colleagues[45] divides malignant skeletal tumors into three stages: low-grade Stage I, high-grade Stage II, and distant metastasis Stage III. Stages I and II are subdivided into (A) and (B) on the basis of local invasion, either intramedullary (A) or extramedullary (B). The use of this system for osteosarcomas is controversial. An early radiological sign of osteosarcoma of the jaw is symmetric widening of the periodontal membrane, referred to as Garrington's sign[46,47] (Fig. 10.4). The true extent of the primary tumor is best seen on CT and MRI scan, which reveals marrow invasion (Fig. 10.5). An isotope scan both shows the extent of primary involvement and detects metastatic bone deposits. As the primary site for metastatic spread is the lung, a chest CT scan is essential. Staging should be completed prior to biopsy.

In the adult, a high serum alkaline phosphatase level is a useful prognostic marker and aids in follow-up in detecting recurrence and metastases. However, in the growing child, alkaline phosphatase is normally raised and is therefore

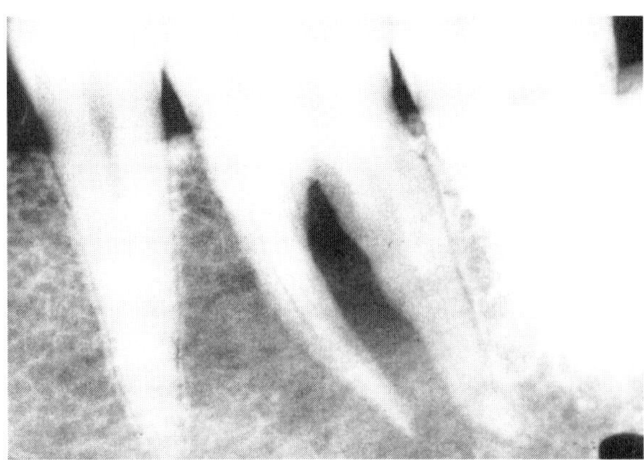

Fig. 10.4. Irregular bony destruction and a widened periodontal membrane on the first molar tooth is an early sign of osteosarcoma. Note the symmetric widening of the periodontal membrane – Garrington sign.

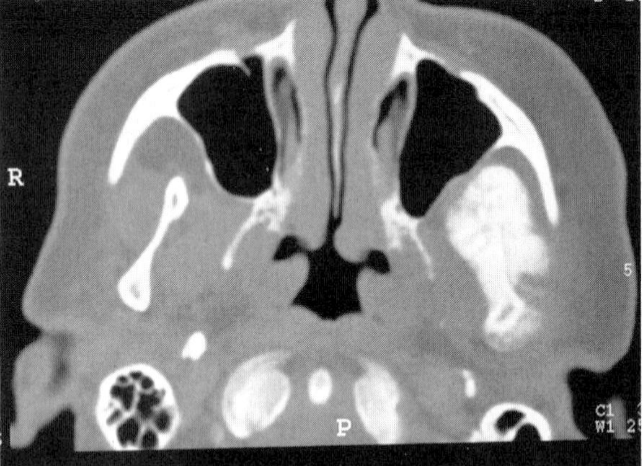

Fig. 10.5. CT scan reveals extensive tumor invasion of the mandibular ramus as well as the commonly seen sunray pattern.

less useful. Lymph node metastasis is rare and carries a poor prognosis.

Management

The most important modality of treatment is surgery. The role of radiation and chemotherapy in CFOS remains controversial. Due to the rarity of this disease in the head and neck, most of the treatment protocols are extrapolated from treatment trials of extremity osteosarcoma. The applicability of the proven therapies of osteosarcomas of the extremities remains controversial.

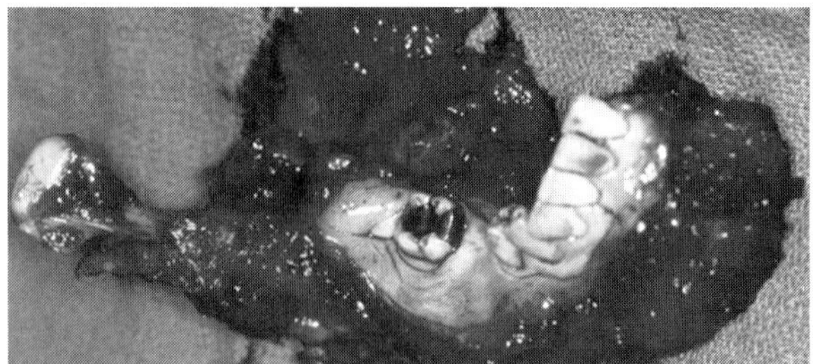

Fig. 10.6. Surgical specimen to show bony margins (osteosarcoma).

Surgery

Excision of the tumor with 3–5 cm of uninvolved bone, and removal of involved soft tissue with wide margins, will give the best chance of survival (Fig. 10.6). In CFOS, the overall incidence of distant metastases is 11–12% for a jaw primary and 36% for a skull primary.[41] Other authors have found metastatic rates of 7.1–40% for CFOS,[48] which is in contrast to the 80% of patients with long bone osteosarcoma who developed lung metastases prior to the use of chemotherapy.[49] Local control is therefore the most important factor in CFOS cure.

The mandible is the easiest of head and neck site to resect with good margins; maxillary lesions usually require maxillectomy with possible orbital exenteration. Resection of base-of-skull tumors, and of cervical vertebral osteosarcomas, may be impossible. It is hard to estimate clear margins owing to the bony nature of the tumor, and the inability to obtain frozen section analysis. When tumor remains at the primary site, survival rates are zero.[50] Despite the surgical necessity for tumor-free margins, most series illustrate that this is difficult to achieve in the head and neck, and the incidence of positive margins has varied, from 42.8% (6/14 patients)[48] to 55% (11/20 patients).[51] These figures are mirrored by a literature review examining sites of failure in CFOS which showed a local recurrence rate of 43% for the mandible, and 37%–55% for the maxilla.[41]

Surgery also has a large role to play in the management of pulmonary metastases from osteosarcomas, and aggressive surgical resection of chest lesions has improved survival and cure rates in children. In general, patients with late metastases more than 1 year after primary resection, and those who present with a solitary nodule, have the best prognosis and cure rate. Patients relapsing within 6 months of surgery with more than three nodules do badly.[52] It is important to monitor the patient with a chest CT scan every 3–4 months for the first 2 years to detect early metastatic disease.

Radiotherapy

Although high-dose radiation of 70 Gy for unresectable lesions has been advocated, and preoperative radiation has been claimed to increase local control,[53] it is generally felt that osteosarcoma is a radioresistant tumor. There appears to be little role for radiation in the management of the primary tumor if it is amenable to surgical resection.[52]

Chemotherapy

Chemotherapy has made a major impact on the survival of children with long bone osteosarcoma. The majority (80%) of these patients previously succumbed to metastatic disease, which was not evident on presentation. There are many protocols, most of which incorporate methotrexate, adriamycin, cisplatinum and ifosfamide. Bleomycin, cyclophosphamide and actinomycin D is another useful combination of chemotherapy. Presurgical chemotherapy has been recommended for patients with osteosarcoma because several trials that incorporated chemotherapy resulted in improved outcomes. The advantages of preoperative chemotherapy have been rationalized as: immediate treatment of micrometastatic disease; safer limb-resection procedure; postsurgical evaluation of tumor response to treatment.[54] The response of the tumor to preoperative chemotherapy is used to guide the choice of postoperative adjuvant chemotherapy. A recent prospective, randomized study by the Pediatric Oncology Group compared presurgical chemotherapy with immediate surgery and adjuvant chemotherapy for non-metastatic osteosarcoma. The study found that chemotherapy was effective in both treatment groups without demonstrable advantage in event free survival for patients given presurgical chemotherapy.[54] In craniofacial osteosarcomas, the use of chemotherapy is controversial and many authors have reported that chemotherapy has not been of benefit.[34,50,55] However, a recent retrospective study of 201 patients concludes that chemotherapy has improved survival,[43] and the report demonstrates improvement in survival for both completely and incompletely resected tumors. The choice between induction chemotherapy and postoperative chemotherapy remains unresolved. The authors advocate the use of preoperative chemotherapy, salvage surgery and postoperative chemotherapy based on an evaluation of necrosis. In view of the rarity of CFOS, prospective trials to confirm the value of chemotherapy are not available.

Long-term survival

It is generally accepted that CFOS has a much improved survival when compared with long bone osteosarcoma. The vast majority of local recurrences and distant metastases occur in the first 2 years and 68.8% at 5 years have been reported.[48] Actuarial 10-year survival of 206 cases in a literature review (1940–82) was approximately 50% for mandibular and maxillary alveolar ridge osteosarcomas, 20% for maxillary antrum, and 10% for those in the skull.[34] However, in one series in which over 50% of patients had tumors larger than 10 cm and in which 87% of tumors were histologically high grade, the 5-year survival for osteosarcoma of the jaw was only 10%.[56]

Ewing's sarcoma

Ewing's sarcoma occurs most commonly in the second decade of life and this cohort of patients represents about two-thirds of all cases. Only 27% of all cases present in the first decade of life and 9% in the third decade.[16] It is more common in males and rare in black patients. Using data from 1505 patients, 53% of tumors were found in the extremity and 47% in the central axis,[57] and only 9% of the central axis tumors were located in the head and neck.

Histology

Ewing's sarcoma of bone is one of the small, blue, round cell tumors of childhood, which is thought to arise from neural tissue. ES is considered to be part of the Ewing's family of tumors (EFT). The EFT is defined by the expression of *ews/ets* fusion genes. Recent experimental evidence suggests that the Ewing tumor cell is capable of neuroectodermal differentiation. The degree of neuroectodermal differentiation has been utilized for histological subclassification of the EFT into: classical Ewing sarcoma, atypical Ewing sarcoma, and malignant peripheral neuroectodermal tumor (PNET).[58] The PNET, which has more neural differentiation, may have the worst prognosis.

Site

The mandible is the most common head and neck site,[59] and 7% of all Ewing's sarcomas have been reported to occur here as either primary or secondary lesions.[60] In a collected series of 111 head and neck cases, 47.7% were mandibular, 20.7% arose in the skull, 15.5% were maxillary, 11.7% were found in the cervical spine, and 4.4% were located in the orbit and ethmoids.[41] Head and neck tumors appear to have a good overall prognosis.[61]

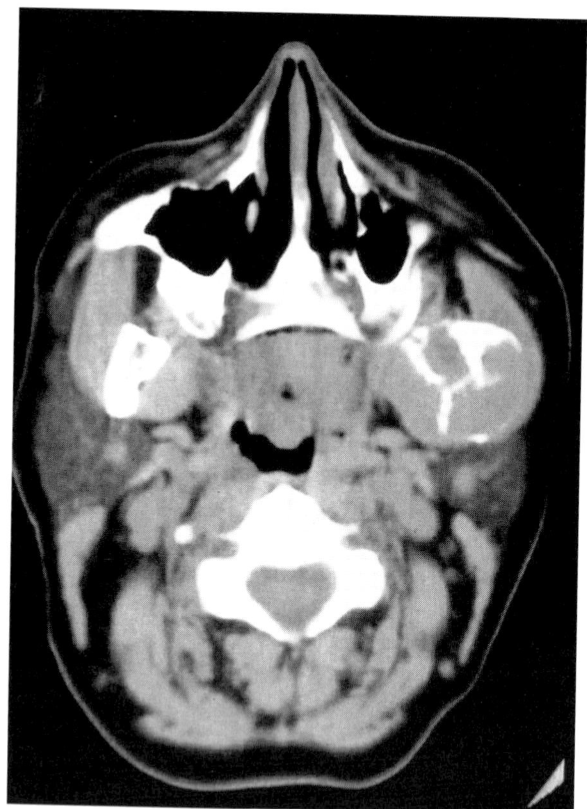

Fig. 10.7. PNET tumor of vertical ramus of mandible shows classical involvement of the masseter and pterygoid muscles.

Staging

There is no internationally accepted staging system for Ewing's sarcoma. The presence of metastases and the size of the primary tumor have great prognostic significance. Radiological evaluation of the jaw primary site does not usually show the typical onion skin appearance of Ewing's sarcoma of long bones. In the mandible, an osteolytic lesion is most common,[62,63] although "sunray"[64,65] and sclerotic lesions[66] have been reported. Because of associated fevers, increased local temperature, intermittent pain and swelling which may be stable for many months, dental infection is a common misdiagnosis, and definitive diagnosis is delayed.

Imaging of the primary tumor should include both MRI for bone marrow and soft tissue spread and CT scan for cortical bone invasion (Fig. 10.7). The most common sites of metastases are the lungs, bone and bone marrow. Chest X-ray, CT scan of the chest, bone scan and bone marrow aspiration are mandatory in tumor assessment. Serum LDH should be measured as raised serum levels are associated with a poor prognosis. Lymph nodes are involved in only 7% of cases.[67] Approximately 20% of cases will present with a clinically obvious metastasis, although it is estimated that 80%–90% of cases have micrometastases and Ewing's sarcoma should be regarded as a systemic disease.

Management

As the Ewing's sarcoma family of tumors are regarded as systemic diseases at diagnosis, all patients receive chemotherapy. Most authorities advocate the use of radiation therapy as the best treatment for the primary tumor, although this may not always be the case in the head and neck, where the long-term morbidity of radiation may be reduced by the use of aggressive "en bloc" surgical resection.[68] The outlook towards surgery in the management of ES has changed over the years from offering surgical treatment to selected cases to offering it generally to every patient as a form of local treatment.[69]

Radiation

There is no agreement on the optimum dose of radiation therapy,[64] but local control rates of 85%–90% for radiation when combined with multiagent chemotherapy have been reported.[70,71] Most radiation regimens use dosages in the range 50–55 Gy. A slightly higher total dose given with a twice-a-day hyperfractionation protocol has resulted in a 2-year local control rate of over 90%.[72]

Surgery

Although surgery has traditionally been used for salvage procedures following chemotherapy and radiation, the growth disturbances caused by radiation in the head and neck, and the induction of second cancers, have justified re-examination of its role in treatment. There are few good studies comparing radiation and surgery. A European study showed no differences in relapse-free survival between radiation alone, surgery alone or a combination of both.[73] An earlier report gave surgery a better relapse-free survival, but showed an increase in long-term local failure.[74] The mandible is particularly amenable to resection with immediate microvascular fibula flap reconstruction in children with Ewing's sarcoma.[63,68] Other indications for surgery are large tumors 8–10 cm in diameter, or tumors associated with pathological fracture of the bone. There is controversy about the extent of surgery for the tumor following induction chemotherapy. Surgeons have always followed the rule that resected margins should relate to the size of the tumor prior to chemotherapy. However, reports suggest that the tumor shrinks from the periphery without leaving marginal tumor islands.[75] If this is the case, then resection need only encompass the margins of the residual tumor, allowing a more conservative approach. Longer-term studies will allow analysis of this approach for Ewing's sarcoma.

Chemotherapy

The standard regimen for Ewing's sarcoma has been vincristine, actinomycin D, and cyclophosphamide (VAC) plus Adriamycin.[70] Other agents that are being investigated for use in Ewing's sarcoma are ifosfamide and etoposide.

Long-term survival

Prior to the use of multiagent chemotherapy, prognosis was extremely poor. The 5-year survival was 16%, mainly due to distant metastases, and a further 25% of survivors died after 5 years.[66] The 5-year survival rate in the early 1970s was regarded to be <10%. With current aggressive multimodality treatment, survival rates of 60 to 70% are expected; although in recent years the 5-year survival has reached a plateau.[77] Long-term overall survival at follow-up of 5, 10, 15, and 20 years have been reported to be 57.2, 49.3, 44.9, and 38.4%, respectively.[69] Patients with clinical metastatic disease have only a 30% 3-year progression-free survival;[76] while female patients have a statistically significant increased chance of becoming long-term survivors.[77] In the head and neck the prognosis is better, with a 72.8% long-term survival (24/29 patients).[61] The reason for this may be that most head/neck tumors are diagnosed when small, and lesions larger than 8 cm have a poor prognosis. The use of multimodality approach to the treatment of ES has had a positive impact on long-term survival. However, the long-term incidence of complications appears to increase steadily over time. This fact further emphasizes the need for continued long-term follow-up.

Morbidity and complications of malignant tumors

In discussing these three malignant tumors of the head and neck, rhabdomyosarcoma, osteosarcoma, and Ewing's sarcoma, many of the problems of multimodality therapy have been mentioned. Although combinations of surgery, radiation and chemotherapy have improved overall survival for these three tumors, and for other malignant head and neck tumors, long-term complications and morbidity have also increased.

Radiation doses of 20 Gy will cause bone damage and growth disturbances. These effects are most marked in children under 5 years of age when treated. Higher doses of radiation 40–60 Gy, and irradiation of the temporomandibular joint area are also associated with predictably problematic subsequent growth and development. The effects become increasingly obvious as the young child grows (Fig. 10.8) but are minimal if irradiation takes place after the age of 15 years when the majority of facial growth is complete. Soft tissue hypoplasia will also occur with high doses, and at doses of 60 Gy and above, radiation fibrosis will become more prominent. This may be associated with trismus if the masticatory muscles are involved.

The teeth can be affected with doses less than 20 Gy,[78] with malformation of crowns and roots, or failure of eruption all reported. Damage to the parotid gland begins at 30 Gy and xerostomia is often permanent for doses of 40–50 Gy. In addition, damage to the thyroid and pituitary glands may give rise to growth disturbances.

The eye may be damaged at doses of 45 Gy and above. Late effects of therapy in patients with localized RMS of the orbit was reported in the IRS III study.[22] The therapy consisted of chemotherapy using either VAC or VA regimen and CFRT ranging from 41.4 to 50.4 Gy. At a median follow-up of 7.6 years, 82% of patients developed cataracts, 66% underwent cataract surgery, and 70% had decreased visual acuity. The orbit was found to be hypoplastic in 59% of patients; however, the eye was preserved in 86% of patients.

Most of the chemotherapy agents have specific long-term complications. These include neuropathy (vincristine), hemorrhagic cystitis and infertility (cyclophosphamide), cardiac failure (doxorubicin), and renal damage (ifosfamide).

In addition, both radiation and chemotherapy have been implicated in the induction of second malignancies in children. The most common second primary cancers following radiation appear to be hard and soft tissue sarcomas, leukemias, lymphomas, thyroid cancer and skin cancers. The alkylating agents have been implicated in the induction of leukemia, lymphomas and bone sarcomas. The incidence of second cancers seems to be related to the total dose and volume treated by radiation, but appears to be lower for more modern radiation regimens. Newer surgical approaches with craniofacial access techniques, rigid fixation, calvarial grafting, microvascular reconstruction and dental implants have reduced surgical morbidity. Implants may be used to restore dentition in children older than 7 years.[79] Whether tumor shrinkage following induction chemotherapy will allow more conservative surgery in these tumors is unknown at present.

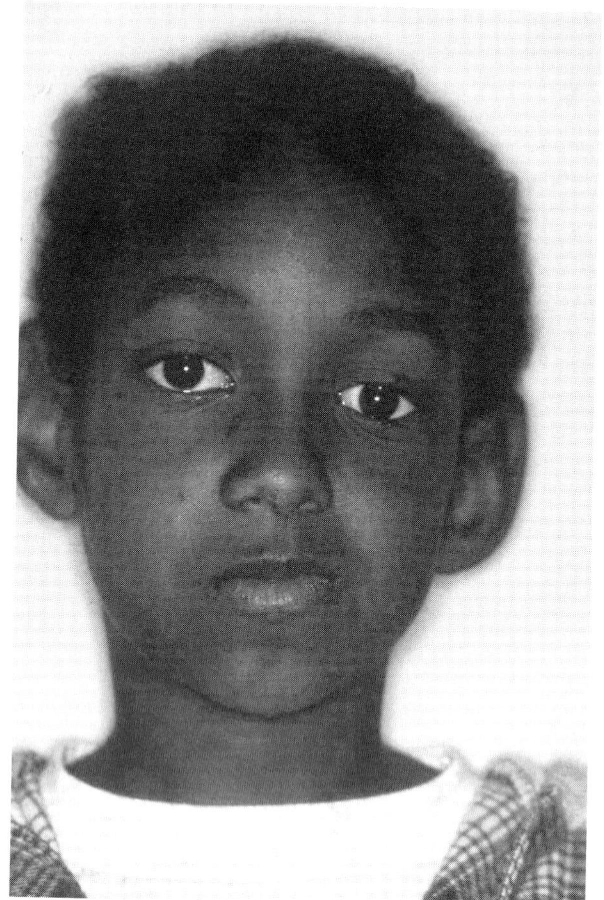

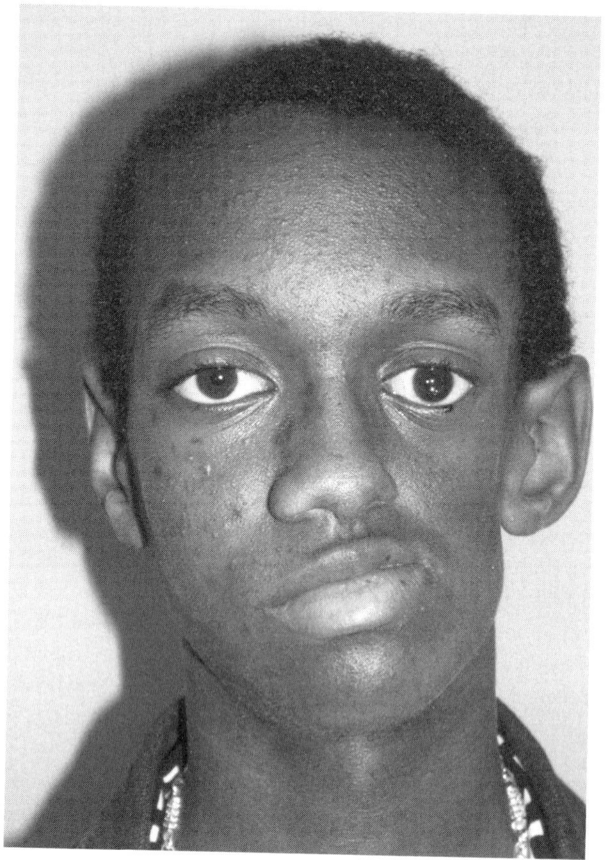

Fig. 10.8. Patient at 2 years (age 6 years) and 8 years (age 12 years) after irradiation and chemotherapy for a left maxillary sinus rhabdomyosarcoma, showing increasing hypoplasia of the left face.

Benign tumors

Although many benign tumors are common in the head and neck (e.g. vascular malformations) it is difficult to evaluate their long-term behaviors and outcomes owing to their diversity and the paucity of good, long-term follow-up reviews. The *ameloblastoma* in children has many unique features and will be discussed in this section.

The ameloblastoma is the most common odontogenic tumor. It is mostly seen in adults in the third and fourth decades of life. In the adult it is usually multicystic or solid and behaves aggressively like a non-metastasizing low-grade malignancy. Although regarded as rare in children,[80] some large series have been published. Individual cases of children as young as 4 and 6 years have been reported,[81,82] and in 1962 Young and Robinson reviewed 32 cases below the age of 17 years.[83] These authors emphasized the fact that ameloblastomas in children were most likely to arise as a unicystic dentigerous cyst. In a recent study carried out by the senior author, the figures from our institution as well as a review of the western and African literature, revealed a total of 173 cases of pediatric ameloblastomas. The mean age was found to be 14 years. A clear difference in occurrence of unicystic ameloblastoma was found between the Western and African groups, 76.5% and 19.5%, respectively. Analysis of recurrences after enucleation of unicystic ameloblastoma was found to be ~40% for cases followed up to 5 years[84] (Figs. 10.9–10.11).

The importance of this observation is that unicystic ameloblastoma is generally thought to have a much less aggressive behavior. Histologically, the whole cyst lining may show a flattened epithelium, which can be plexiform. The lining may also show mural thickening into the cyst wall, or projections into the cyst itself which may be free-floating. Islands of ameloblastoma, however, can also be seen in the fibrous capsule wall in some variants, and these

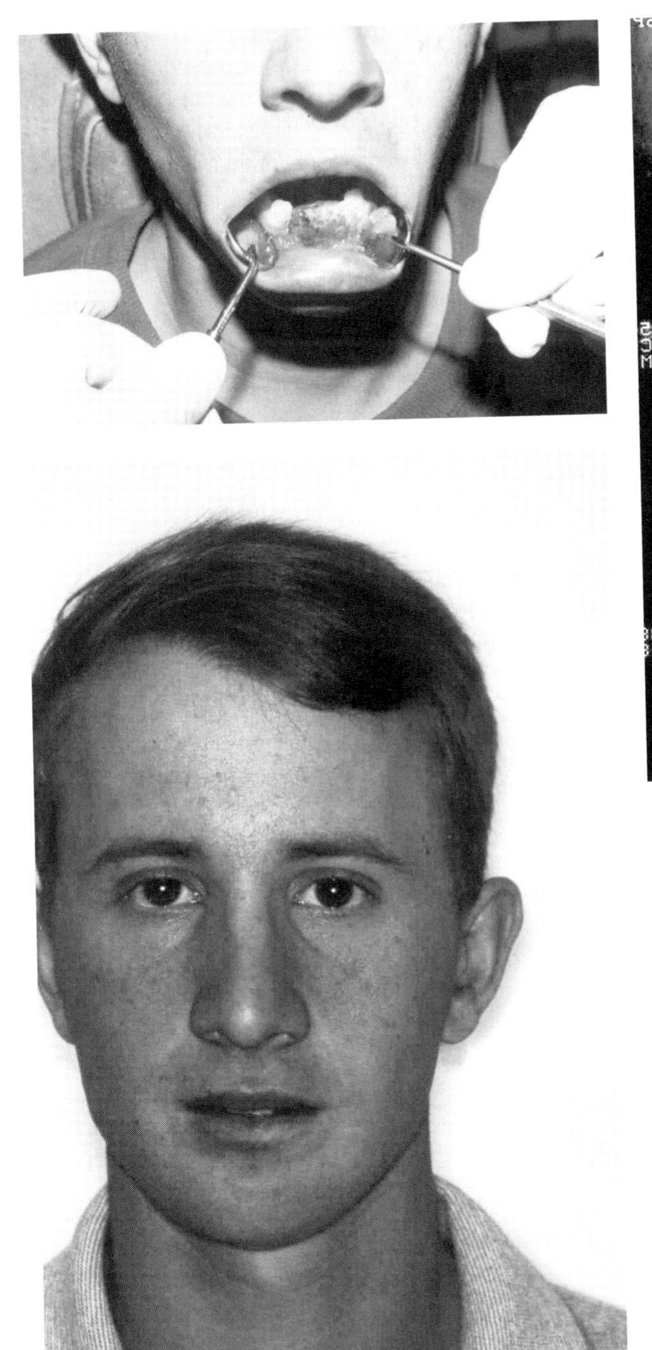

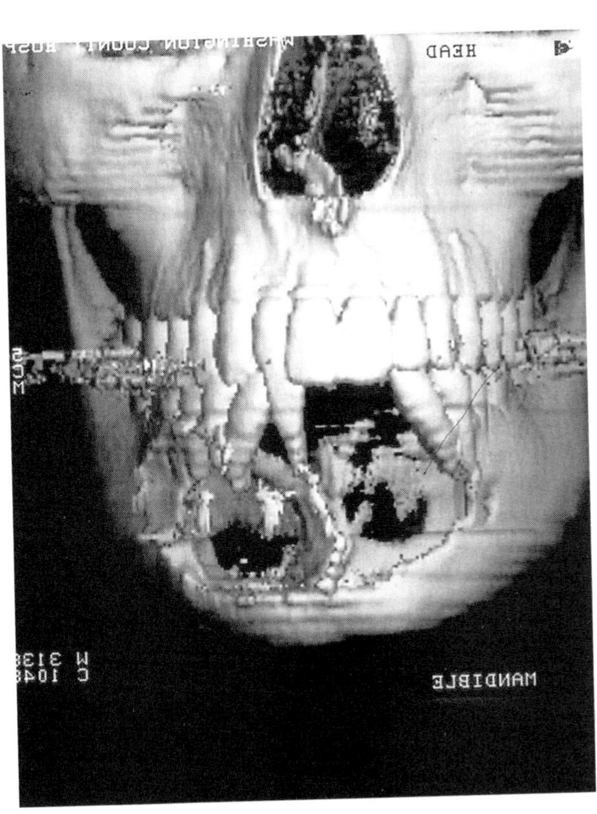

Fig. 10.9. A 16-year-old boy presented with tumor out of mandibular incisor sockets. The three-dimensional image reveals the extent of the ameloblastoma. The bottom picture was taken 2 years after resection and bone-grafting.

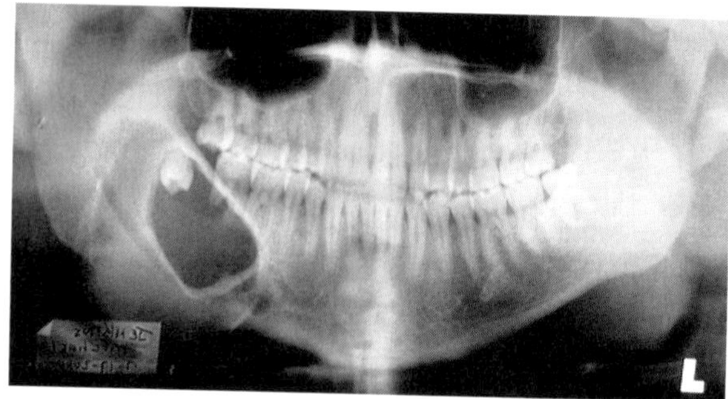

Fig. 10.10. Large right mandibular unicystic ameloblastoma.

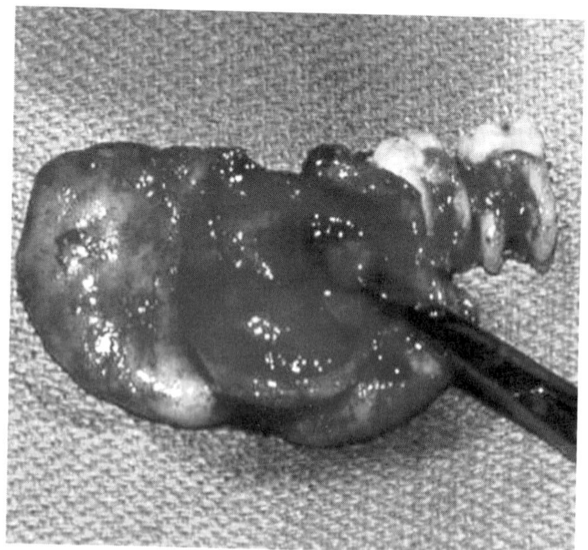

Fig. 10.11. This specimen shows only one nodule of ameloblastoma in the cyst wall, as indicated by the instrument.

may extend to the periphery. Simple enucleation should be curative for most of the cases, although where islands of tumor occur in the capsule – especially when the periphery is involved – the potential for recurrence exists. Long-term follow-up to assess recurrence is difficult as these tumors can recur 20 years after initial surgery.

When lesions are recurrent, or when initial diagnosis is of a solid or multicystic tumor, then more aggressive resection with 1–1.5 cm margins in medullary bone is required. If cortical bone is perforated, the overlying soft tissue should be resected to ensure complete tumor excision. The author's practice is to undertake enucleation only for unicystic ameloblastoma with intraluminal proliferation or ameloblastic changes of the epithelium. When epithelial proliferation or odontogenic islands occur in the connective tissue wall of the lesion, we believe that further bone removal, either keeping mandibular continuity or segmental resection is advisable. Unfortunately, the diagnosis of connective tissue wall invasion can be made reliably only on examination of the entire histological specimen. Frozen sections are subject to sampling error. This means that enucleation should be regarded as a diagnostic or possible staging procedure.[84]

Long-term outcome

When ameloblastoma is treated surgically by complete enucleation for unicystic lesions and by complete resection with a 1 cm margin for solid or multicystic lesions, recurrence should be minimal. However, if tumor extends to the periphery of unicystic ameloblastoma recurrence rates of 18%–40% are to be expected. In multicystic ameloblastoma, curettage or enucleation will give recurrences of 80%–90%, and resection is mandatory. Modern bone-grafting techniques with endosseous implant placement have improved reconstruction (see Fig. 10.9) and reduced morbidity. Long-term follow-up (20 years) is mandatory for late recurrence.

REFERENCES

1. Young, J. L., Ries, L. G., Silverberg, E. *et al.* Cancer incidence survival and mortality for children younger than age 15 years. *Cancer* 1986; **58**:598–602.
2. Cunningham, M. J., Myers, E. N., Bluestone, C. D. Malignant tumors of the head and neck in children: a twenty-year review. *Int J Pediat Otorhinolaryngol* 1987; **13**:279–292.
3. Robinson, L. D., Rightmire, J., Smith, R. J. M. Head and neck malignancies in children: an age-incidence study. *Laryngoscope* 1988; **98**:11–13.
4. Jaffe, N., Toth, B. B., Moar, R. E. *et al.* Dental and maxillofacial abnormalities in long term survivors of childhood cancer: effects of treatment with chemotherapy and radiation to the head and neck. *Pediatrics* 1984; **73**:816–823.
5. Paulino, A. C., Simon, J. H., Zhen, W., Wen, B. C. Long-term effects in children treated with radiotherapy for head and neck rhabdomyosarcomas. *Int. J. Radiat. Oncol. Biol. Phys.* 2000; **48**:1489–1495.
6. Sutow, W. W., Sullivan, M. P., Ried, H. G., *et al.* Prognosis in childhood rhabdomyosarcoma. *Cancer* 1970; **25**:1386–1390.
7. Maurer, H. M., Beltangady, M., Gehan, E. A., *et al.* The Intergroup Rhabdomyosarcoma Study-I: A final report. *Cancer* 1988; **61**:209–220.
8. Newton, W. A., Soule, E. H., Hamoudi, A. B., *et al.* Histopathology of childhood sarcomas: Intergroup Rhabdomyosarcoma studiesI andII: clinicopathologic correlation. *J. Clin. Oncol.* 1988; **6**:67–75.
9. Raney, R. B., Toffer, M., Hays, D. M., & Triche, T. J. Rhabdomyosarcoma and the undifferentiated sarcomas. In Pizzo,

P. A., & Poplack, D. G. (eds), *Principles and Practices of Pediatric Oncology*, 2nd edn. Philadelphia: J. B. Lippincott, 1993.

10. Sutow, W. W., Lindberg, R. D., Gehan, E. A. *et al.* Three-year relapse-free survival rates in childhood rhabdomyosarcoma of the head and neck: report from the Intergroup Rhabdomyosarcoma study. *Cancer* 1982; **49**:2217–2221.
11. Oberlin, O., Rey, A., Anderson, J. *et al.* Treatment of orbital rhabdomyosarcoma: survival and late effects of treatment – results of an international workshop. *J. Clin. Oncol.* 2001; **19**:197–204.
12. Andrassy, R. J. Advances in the surgical management of sarcomas in children. *Am. J. Surg.* 2002; **184**:484–491.
13. Wharman, M. D., Beltangady, M. S., Heyn, R. M. *et al.* Pediatric orofacial and laryngopharyngeal rhabdomyosarcomas: an Intergroup Rhabdomyosarcoma study report. *Arch. Otolaryngol. Head Neck Surg.* 1987; **113**:1225–1227.
14. Liebert, P. S. & Stool, S. E. Rhabdomyosarcoma of the tongue in an infant: results of combined radiation and chemotherapy. *Ann. Surg.* 1973; **178**:621–624.
15. Lawrence, W., Hays, D. M., Heyn, R. M. *et al.* Lymphatic metastases with childhood rhabdomyosarcoma: a report from the Intergroup Rhabdomyosarcoma study. *Cancer* 1987; **60**:910–915.
16. *UICC Manual of Clinical Oncology 7th edn*, 1999, Wiley-Liss.
17. Crist, W. M., Anderson, J. R., Meza, J. L. *et al.* Intergroup rhabdomyosarcoma study – IV: results for patients with nonmetastatic disease. *J. Clin. Oncol.* 2001; **19**:3091–3102.
18. Hawkins, D. S., Rajendran, J. G., Conrad, E. U., Bruckner, J. D., & Eary, J. F. Evaluation of chemotherapy response in pediatric bone sarcomas by [F-18]-fluorodeoxy-D-glucose positron emission tomography. *Cancer* 2002; **94**:3277–3284.
19. Mandell, L. R., Massey, V., & Ghaviri, F. The influence of extensive bone erosion on local control in non-orbital rhabdomyosarcoma of the head and neck. *Int. J. Radiat. Oncol. Biol. Phys.* 1989; **17**:649–653.
20. Lyos, A. T., Goepfert, H., Luna, M. A. *et al.* Soft tissue sarcoma of the head and neck in children and adolescents. *Cancer* 1996; **17**:193–200.
21. Ron, E., Modan, B., Boice, J. D. *et al.* Tumors of the brain and nervous system after radiotherapy in childhood. *N. Engl. J. Med.* 1988; **319**:1033–1039.
22. Raney, R. B., Anderson, J. R., Kollath, J. *et al.* Late effects of therapy in 94 patients with localized rhabdomyosarcoma of the orbit: report from the intergroup rhabdomyosarcoma study (IRS)-III, 1984–1991. *Med. Pediatr. Oncol.* 2000; **34**:413–420.
23. Raney, R. B., Tefft, M., Maurer, M. M. *et al.* Improved prognosis with intensive treatment of children with cranial soft tissue sarcomas arising in non-orbital parameningeal sites: a report from the Intergroup Rhabdomyosarcoma study. *Cancer* 1987; **59**:147–155.
24. Wolden, S. L., Anderson, J. R., Crist, W. M. *et al.* Indications for radiotherapy and chemotherapy after complete resection in rhabdomyosarcoma: a report from the intergroup rhabdomyosarcoma studies I toIII. *J. Clin. Oncol.* 1999; **17**:3468–3475.
25. Donaldson, S. S., Meza, J., Breneman, J. C. *et al.* Results from the ISR-IV randomized trial of hyperfractionated radiotherapy in children with rhabdomyosarcoma – a report from the IRSG. *Int. J. Radiat. Oncol. Biol. Phys.* 2001; **51**:718–728.
26. McGill, T. Rhabdomyosarcoma of the head and neck: an update. *Otolaryngol. Clin. N. Amer.* 1989; **22**:631–636.
27. Moore, O. & Grossi, C. Embryonal rhabdomyosarcoma of the head and neck. *Cancer* 1959; **12**:69–73.
28. Masson, J. K. & Soule, E. M. Embryonal rhabdomyosarcoma of the head and neck: report of 88 cases. *Am. J. Surg.* 1965; **110**:585–591.
29. Heyn, R. M., Holland, R., Newton, W. A. *et al.* The role of combined chemotherapy in the treatment of rhabdomyosarcoma in children. *Cancer* 1974; **34**:2128–2142.
30. Flamant, F. & Hill, C. The improvement in survival associated with combined chemotherapy in children rhabdomyosarcoma: a historical comparison of 345 patients in the same center. *Cancer* 1834; **53**:2417–2421.
31. Crist, W. M., Garnsey, L., Beltangady, M. S. *et al.* Prognosis in children with rhabdomyosarcoma: a report of the Intergroup Rhabdomyosarcoma studies I and II. *J. Clin. Oncol.* 1990; **8**:447–448.
32. Rao, B. N., Santana, V. M., Flemming, J. D. *et al.* Management and prognosis of head and neck sarcomas. *Am. J. Surg.* 1989; **158**:373–377.
33. Wharam, M. D., Foulkes, M. A., Lawrence, W. *et al.* Soft tissue sarcoma of the head and neck in children: non-orbital and nonparameningeal sites: a report of the Intergroup Rhabdomyosarcoma study IRS-I. *Cancer* **53**:1016–1019.
34. Raney, J. B., Crist, W. M., Maurer, H. M. *et al.* Prognosis of children with soft tissue sarcoma who relapse after achieving a complete response: a report from the Intergroup Rhabdomyosarcoma study I. *Cancer* 1983; **52**:444–450.
35. Sutow, W. W., Fugimoto, T., Wilbur, J. R. *et al.* Long-term evaluation of VAC-chemotherapy in childhood rhabdomyosarcoma. *Proc. AACR, ASCO* 1977; **18**:291 (abstract).
36. Sutton, W. W., Lindberg, R. D., Gehan, A. E. *et al.* Three-year relapse-free survival rates in childhood rhabdomyosarcoma of the head and neck: report from the Intergroup Rhabdomyosarcoma study. *Cancer* 1982; **49**:2217–2221.
37. Young, J. L. & Miller, R. W. Incidence of malignant tumors in US children. *J. Pediatr.* 1975; **86**:254–258.
38. Stark, A., Kreicberg, S. A., & Silfersward, C. The age of osteosarcoma patients is increasing: an epidemiological study of osteosarcomas in Sweden, 1971 to 1984. *J. Bone Joint Surg.* 1990; **72B**:89–93.
39. Clark, J. L., Unni, K. K., Dahlin, D. C. *et al.* Osteosarcoma of the jaw. *Cancer* 1983; **51**:2311–2316.
40. Tabone, M. D., Terrier, P., Pacquement, H. *et al.* Outcome of radiation-related osteosarcoma after treatment of childhood and adolescent cancer: a study of 23 cases. *J. Clin. Oncol.* 1999; **17**:2789–2795.
41. Marcus, R. B., Post, J. C., & Mancuso, A. A. Pediatric tumors of the head and neck. In Million, R. R. & Cassisi, N. J. (eds),

Management of Head and Neck Cancer: A Multidisciplinary Approach, 2nd edn. Philadelphia: J. P. Lippincott, 1994.

42. Dahlin, D. C. Osteosarcoma of bone and a consideration of prognostic variables. *Cancer Treat. Rep.* 1978; **62**:189–192.
43. Smeele, L. E., Kostense, P. J., van der Waal, I. *et al.* Effects of chemotherapy on survival of craniofacial osteosarcoma: a systematic review of 201 patients. *J. Clin. Oncol.* 1997; **15**:363–367.
44. Regizi, J. A. & Sciubba, J. W. Oral pathology. In Regizi, J. A., Sciubba, J. (eds), *Clinical–Pathological Correlations*, 2nd edn. Philadelphia: W. B. Saunders, 1993: 442.
45. Fechner, R. E. & Mills, S. E. (eds). Tumors of the bones and joints, In *Atlas of Tumor Pathology, 3rd series, fascicle 8.* Washington, DC: Armed Forces Institute of Pathology, 1993: 14–15.
46. Gardener, D. G. & Mills, D. M. The widened periodontal ligament of osteosarcoma of the jaws. *Oral. Surg.* 1976; **41**:652–656.
47. Garrington, G. E., Scofield, H. H., Cornyn, J., & Hooker, S. P. Osteosarcoma of the Jaws: analysis of 56 cases. *Cancer* 1967; **20**:377–391.
48. Smeele, L. E., Van der Wal, J. E., Van Diest P. J. *et al.* Radical surgical treatment in craniofacial osteosarcoma gives excellent survival: a retrospective cohort study of 14 patients. *Oral Oncol. Eur. J. Cancer.* 1994; **30B**:374–376.
49. Friedman, M. A. & Carter, S. K. The therapy of osteogenic sarcoma: current status and thoughts for the future. *J. Surg. Oncol.* 1972; **4**:482–510.
50. Goepfert, H., Raymond, A. K., Spires, J. R. *et al.* Osteosarcoma of the head and neck. *Cancer. Bull.* 1990; **42**:347–354.
51. Delgardo, R., Maafs, E., Alfeiran, A. *et al.* Osteosarcoma of the jaw. *Head Neck* 1994; **16**:246–252.
52. Link, M. P. & Eilber, F. Osteosarcoma. In Pizza, P. A. & Poplack, D. G. (eds), *Principles and Practice of Pediatric Oncology*, 2nd edn. Philadelphia: J. B. Lippincott, 1993.
53. Suit, D. G. Radiotherapy in osteosarcoma. *Clin. Orthop.* 1975; **111**:71–75.
54. Goorin, A. M., Schwartzentruber, D. J., Devidas, M. *et al.* Presurgical chemotherapy compared with immediate surgery and adjuvant chemotherapy for nonmetastatic osteosarcoma: pediatric oncology group study POG-8651. *J. Clin. Oncol.* 2003; **21**:1574–1580.
55. Veges, D. S., Borges, A. M., Aggrawal, K. *et al.* Osteosarcoma of the craniofacial bones: a clinico-pathological study. *J. Craniomaxillofac. Surg.* 1991; **19**:90–93.
56. Meyers, P. A., Hiller, G., Healey, J. *et al.* Chemotherapy for nonmetastatic osteogenic sarcoma: the Memorial Sloan–Kettering experience. *J. Clin. Oncol.* 1992; **10**:5–15.
57. Horowitz, M. E., Malower, M. M., Delaney, T. F., & Tsakos, M. G. Ewing's sarcoma family of tumors: Ewing's sarcoma of bone and soft tissue and the peripheral primitive neuroectodermal tumors. In Pizzo, P. A. & Poplack, D. G. (eds.), *Principles and Practice of Pediatric Oncology*, 2nd edn. Philadelphia: J. B. Lippincott, 1993.
58. Burdach, S. & Jurgens, H. High-dose chemotherapy (HDC) in the Ewing family of tumors (EFT). *Crit. Rev. Oncol. Hemat.* 2002; **41**:169–189.
59. Posnick, J. C., Louie, G., Zucker, R. M. *et al.* Ewing's sarcoma primary involvement of the zygoma undergoing resection and immediate reconstruction. *Plast. Reconst. Surg.* 1992; **89**:956–961.
60. Berstein, P. E., Bone, R. C., & Feldman, P. S. Ewing's sarcoma of the mandible. *Ann. Otol. Rhinol. Laryngeal.* 1979; **88**:105–108.
61. Siegal, G. P., Oliver, W. R., Reinus, W. R. *et al.* Primary Ewing's sarcoma involving the bones of the head and neck. *Cancer* 1987; **60**:2829–2840.
62. Crowe, W. W. & Harper, J. C. Ewing's sarcoma with primary lesion in the mandible: report of a case. *J. Oral. Surg.* 1965; **23**:156–161.
63. Berk, R., Heller, A., Heller, D. *et al.* Ewing's sarcoma of the mandible. *Oral Surg. Oral Med. Oral Pathol. Oral Radiol. Endod.* 1995; **79**:159–162.
64. Pottlar, G. G. Ewing's sarcoma of the jaws. *Oral Surg. Oral Med. Oral Pathol.* 1970; **29**:505–512.
65. Rapoport, A., Sobrinho, J., Carvalho, M. *et al.* Ewing's sarcoma of the mandible. *Oral Surg. Oral Med. Oral Pathol.* 1977; **44**:89–94.
66. Wood, R. E., Nortje, C. J., Messeling, P. *et al.* Ewing's tumor of the jaw. *Oral Surg.* 1990; **69**:120–127.
67. Miser, J. S., Kirsella, T. J., Triche, T. J. *et al.* Preliminary results of treatments of Ewing's sarcoma of bone in children and young adults: six months of intensive combined modality therapy without maintenance. *J. Clin. Oncol.* 1988; **6**:686–690.
68. Posnick, J. C. Pediatric craniomaxillofacial tumors in oral and maxillofacial surgery. In Kahan, L. B. (ed.), *Clinics of North America*, vol. 6:1. Philadelphia: W. B. Saunders, 1996.
69. Bacci, G., Forni, C., Longhi, A. *et al.* Lont-term outcome for patients with non-metastatic Ewing's sarcoma treated with adjuvant and neoadjuvant chemotherapies. 402 patients treated at Rizzoli between 1972 and 1992. *Eur. J. Cancer.* 2004; **40**:73–83.
70. Nesbit, M. E., Gehan, E. A., Burgert, E. O. *et al.* Multimodal therapy for the management of primary non-metastatic Ewing's sarcoma of bone: a long-term follow-up of the first intergroup study. *J. Clin. Oncol.* 1990; **8**:1664–1672.
71. Burgert, E. O., Nesbit, M. E., Garnsey, L. A. *et al.* Multimodal therapy for the management of non-pelvic, localized Ewing's sarcoma of bone: Intergroup study IESS-II. *J. Clin. Oncol.* 1990; **8**:1514–1521.
72. Marcus, R. B., Cantor, A., Heare, T. C. *et al.* Local control and function after twice-a-day radiotherapy for Ewing's sarcoma of bone. *Int. J. Radiat. Oncol. Biol. Phys.* 1988; **15**:53–59.
73. Duns, J., Sauer, R., Burgers, J. M. *et al.* Radiation therapy as local treatment in Ewing's sarcoma: results of the Cooperative Ewing's Sarcoma Studies CESS 81 and CESS 86. *Cancer* 1991; **67**:2828–2825.
74. Sailer, S. J., Harmon, D. C., Mankin, H. J. *et al.* Ewing's sarcoma: surgical resection as a prognostic factor. *Int. J. Radiat. Oncol. Biol. Phys.* 1988; **15**:43–48.

75. Hayes, F. A., Thompson, E. l., Meyer, W. H. *et al.* Therapy for localized Ewing's sarcoma of bone. *J. Clin. Oncol.* 1989; **7**:208–212.
76. Cangir, A., Vietti, T. J., Gehan, E. A., *et al.* Ewing's sarcoma metastatic at diagnosis. Results and comparisons of two intergroups: Ewing's sarcoma studies. *Cancer* 1990; **66**:887–893.
77. Fuchs, B., Valenzuela, R. G., Inwards, C., Sim, F. H., & Rock, M. G. Complications in longterm survivors of Ewing sarcoma. *Cancer* 2003; **98**:2687–2692.
78. Sonis, A. L., Tarbell, N., Valachovic, R. W. *et al.* Dentofacial development in longterm survivors of acute lymphoblastic leukemia: a comparison of three treatment modalities. *Cancer* 1990; **66**:2645–2652.
79. Perrott, D. H., Sharma, A. B. & Vargervik, K. Endosseous implants for pediatric patients: unknown factors, indications, contra-indications and special considerations. *Oral Maxillofac. Surg. Clin. N. Amer.* 1994; **6**:79–88.
80. Chuong, R. & Kaban, L. B. Diagnosis and treatment of jaw tumors in children. *J. Oral Maxillofac. Surg.* 1985; **43**:323–332.
81. Topazian, R. B. Ameloblastoma in a 4-year-old child. *Oral Surg.* 1964; **17**:581–583.
82. Dresser, W. J. & Segal, W. Ameloblastoma associated with a dentigerous cyst in a 6-year-old child. *Oral Surg.* 1967; **24**:388–391.
83. Young, D. R. & Robinson, M. Ameloblastomas in children. *Oral Surg.* 1962; **15**:1155–1159.
84. Ord, R. A., Blanchaert, R. H., Nikitakis, N. G., & Sauk, J. J. Ameloblastoma in children. *J. Oral Maxillofac. Surg.* 2002; **60**:762–770.

Part III

Thorax

11

Chest wall deformities

Donald Nuss

Children's Hospital of the King's Daughters, Norfolk, VA, USA

Chest wall deformities fall into two categories; those in which there is overgrowth of the ribs and cartilages causing either a depression (excavatum) or protrusion (carinatum) of the anterior chest wall, and those in which there is an absence (agenesis), deficiency (atresia), or failure of closure (dysplasia) of the various chest wall structures.

Pectus excavatum is by far the most common chest wall anomaly and occurs with a frequency of 1 in 1000[1] individuals (Fig. 11.1). Pectus carinatum is much less common, with about 10 pectus excavatum cases for each pectus carinatum in a large series, and usually presents during the pubertal growth spurt (Fig. 11.2).

The abnormalities in which there is partial agenesis or failure of fusion (ectopia cordis, Cantrell's pentalogy) are fortunately very rare because many of these conditions are incompatible with life (Fig. 11.3).

In Poland's syndrome, there is variable absence of breast tissue, pectoralis major muscle, pectoralis minor muscle, and ribs. Some patients lack only one structure and others lack all of them and have only skin covering the thoracic cavity (Fig. 11.4).

Pectus excavatum

Pathophysiology and symptoms

Anatomically, the depression of pectus excavatum may be mild, moderate, or severe, and it may be localized or diffuse, symmetric or asymmetric. Asymptomatic cases may be treated with an exercise and posture program, whereas anatomically severe cases may be symptomatic and require surgical correction. The deformity is often present at birth or may appear in early childhood or adolescence, progressing slowly as the child grows.[2,3] In many patients, it may require surgery before puberty, but in patients who are not surgical candidates before puberty, rapid progression of the deformity during the pubertal growth spurt causes them to present for repair. These families will sometimes present with a history that the patient's chest "suddenly caved in." Anatomically severe patients most frequently report shortness of breath with exercise and chest pain on exertion (Table 11.1). Other symptoms may include lack of endurance, frequent respiratory tract infections, and asthma. Puberty not only causes progression of the deformity but also increased rigidity of the chest wall, both of which contribute to the development of restrictive lung disease and worsening of symptoms.

A strong genetic predisposition to pectus excavatum was noted by Coulson in 1820.[4] Among the patients seen at Children's Hospital of the King's Daughters, 46% gave a family history of pectus excavatum (Table 11.2). There have been families where all the children of one family as well as the paternal cousins had a deformity severe enough to require surgery. The condition shows a male predisposition: more than 80% of patients are male. There is a 24.1% incidence of connective tissue disorder (Marfan's syndrome, Ehlers–Danlos syndrome) in our patients and a 29% incidence of scoliosis (see Table 11.2).

History of pectus excavatum repair

In 1931, Sauerbruch published the first description of the bilateral cartilage resection, with anterior sternal osteotomy technique.[5] In addition, he used external traction to splint the anterior chest wall for several weeks after repair. In 1948, Ravitch[6] extended the operation by

Pediatric Surgery and Urology: Long-term Outcomes, Mark Stringer, Keith Oldham, Pierre Mouriquand.
Published by Cambridge University Press.

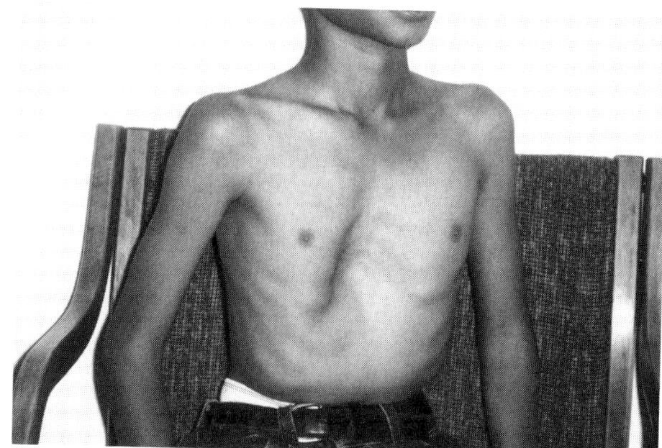

Fig. 11.1. Patient, age 9, with severe pectus excavatum.

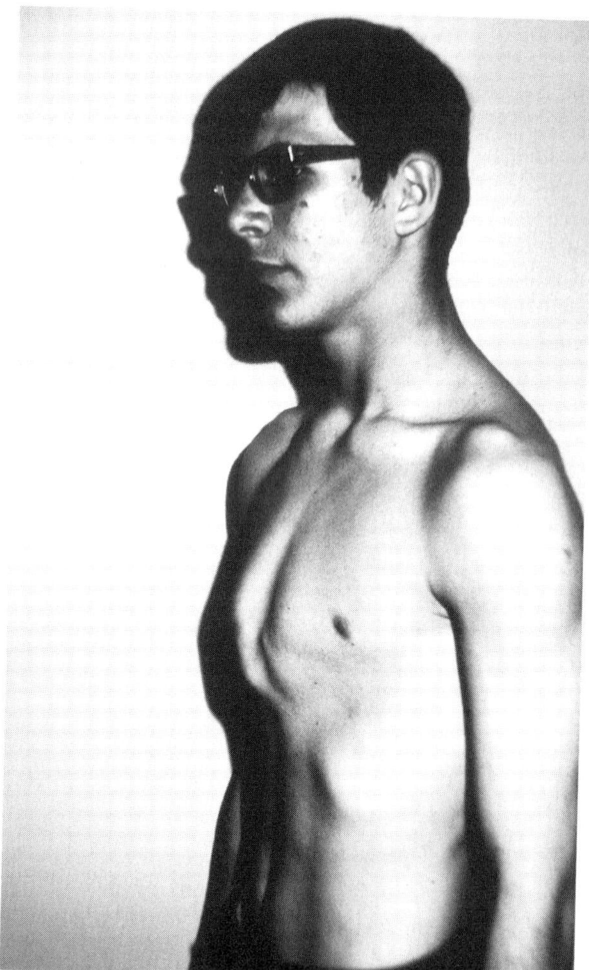

Fig. 11.2. Patient with severe pectus carinatum.

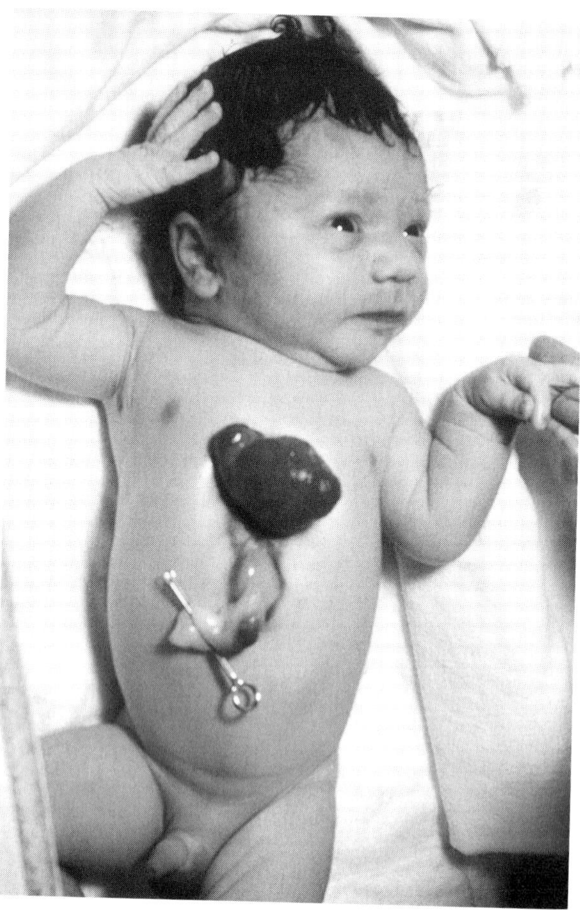

Fig. 11.3. Newborn with ectopia cordis.

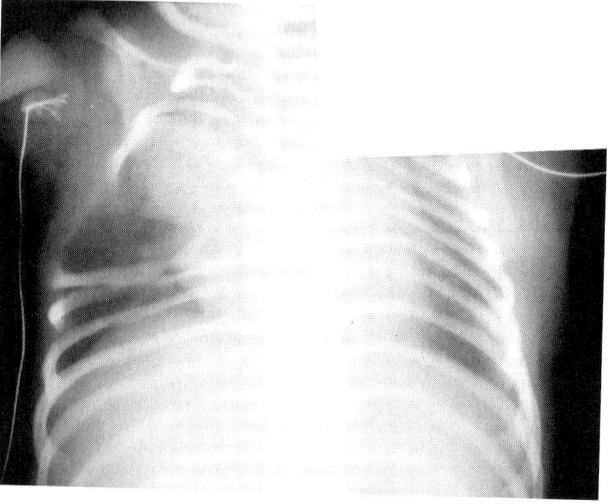

Fig. 11.4. Poland's syndrome: chest radiograph showing congenital absence of ribs on the right side.

Table 11.1. Presenting symptoms of 618 surgical patients with pectus excavatum

Shortness of breath, lack of endurance, exercise intolerance	571/618 (92.4%)
Chest pain, with or without exercise	433/618 (70.1%)
Asthma/asthma-like symptoms	208/618 (34.0%)
Frequent respiratory infections	198/618 (32.0%)
Cardiac indicators	
Cardiac compression (by CT, Echo)	523/618 (84.6%)
Cardiac displacement (by CT, Echo)	536/618 (86.7%)
Murmur on exam	169/618 (27.3%)
Mitral valve prolapse	89/618 (14.4%)
Other anomalies (BBB, aortic insufficiency, regurgitation, hypertrophy, malformations)	139/618 (22.5%)
Pulmonary indicators	
FVC below 80%	29.4%
FEV1% below 80%	36.3%
FEF_{25-75}% below 80%	50.2%

FVC: forced vital capacity.
FEV: forced expiratory volume.
FEF: forced expiratory flow.

Table 11.2. Incidence and etiology

	Number of patients	
Total evaluated	**1230**	
Total with pectus excavatum only	1077 (87.5%)	
Total with pectus carinatum only	83 (6.7%)	
Total with mixed pectus excavatum/pectus carinatum	70 (5.6%)	
Total with Poland's syndrome	9 (0.7%)	
Total with other deformities	8 (0.6%)	
Primary surgical patients	**618**	
Total with pectus excavatum only	610 (98.7%)	
Total with mixed pectus excavatum/pectus carinatum	7 (1.1%)	
Total with Poland's syndrome	3 (0.5%)	
Total with other deformities	1 (0.2%)	
Male to female ratio	510:109	4.6:1
Family history of pectus excavatum	285 (46.0%)	
Incidence of scoliosis	182 (29.4%)	
Incidence of Marfan's – diagnosed	21 (3.4%)	
Marfanoid (presumed Marfan's)	114 (18.4%)	
Patients with Ehlers–Danlos	14 (2.3%)	

performing not only the sternal osteotomy and cartilage resection but also completely isolated the sternum, which included transection of the intercostal and rectus muscular attachments of the sternum and excision of the xiphisternum. He thought that by cutting all the diaphragmatic ligaments and sternal attachments, he could do away with external traction.

In 1956, Wallgren and Sulamaa, concerned by the increased recurrence rate after abandoning external traction, were the first to advocate internal bracing by pushing a bar through the sternum and resting it on the rib ends on each side.[7] In 1961, Adkins and Blades placed the bar behind the sternum rather than through the sternum.[8] Concern about the extent of the resection advocated by Ravitch had already surfaced in 1958 when Welch[9] presented a less extensive approach. He removed the costal cartilages but did not cut through the muscular attachment to the sternum and did not isolate the sternum. He had very acceptable results in 75 patients. However, he and all authorities still advocated doing the procedure in very young patients at this time.

In 1990, Martinez, Juame, Stein, and Pena[10] drew attention to the danger of asphyxiating chondrodystrophy secondary to cartilage resection in young children and supported their hypothesis that cartilage resection contributed to the condition in an experimental study on baby rabbits. Subsequently, in 1996, Haller *et al.*, in a review entitled "Chest wall constriction after too extensive and too early operations for pectus excavatum,"[11] confirmed the association of extensive cartilage resections performed in young children with asphyxiating chondrodystrophy. After these two papers, many surgeons waited until patients had stopped growing before performing what was now called a "modified Ravitch" procedure in which only a limited amount of cartilage was resected without sternal isolation.

In 1998, Nuss *et al.*[12,13] published their 10-year experience of 42 patients with a minimally invasive procedure requiring no cartilage incision nor resection and no sternal osteotomy. Four years later the same group published an update of all the modifications that had occurred since the original publication, with special emphasis on the use of thoracoscopy, the use of stabilizers, modifications to the bar, and new instruments.[14]

Treatment

Selection of patients for surgery

Patients are evaluated clinically. Those who are asymptomatic and have a mild to moderate deformity are treated with a posture and exercise program and re-evaluated annually. If patients comply with our conservative treatment program, progression may be reversed.

If the patients are symptomatic and are judged to have a severe deformity with evidence of cardiopulmonary

Table 11.3. Evaluation and treatment pathway

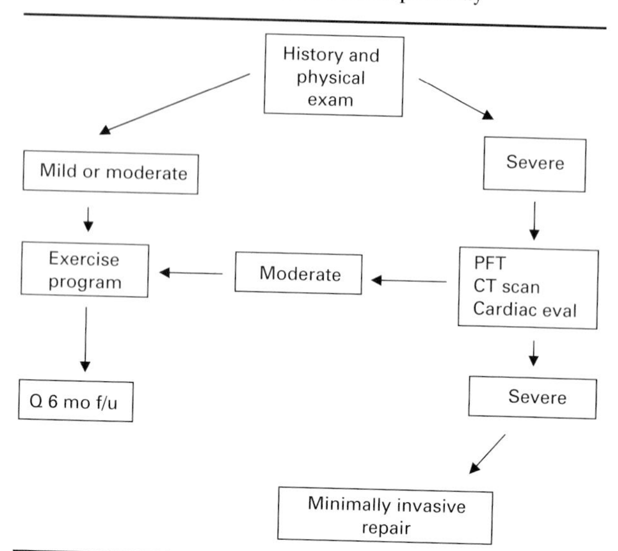

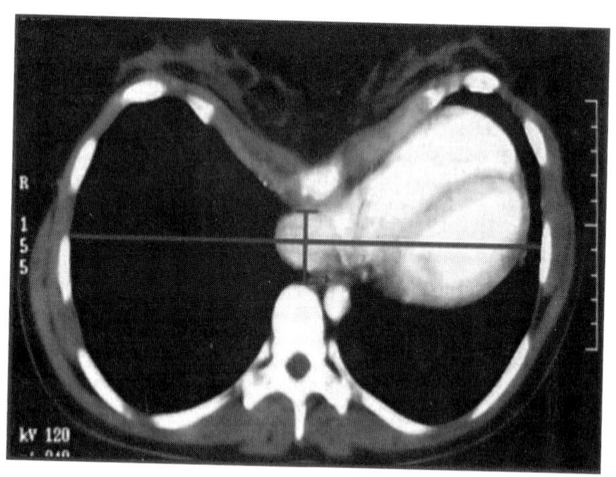

Fig. 11.5. Chest computer tomography (CT) scan with Haller index greater than 3.25.

compression or displacement, then they are evaluated by CT scan, pulmonary function studies, and cardiology evaluation including EKG and echocardiogram (Table 11.3). Patients are selected for surgical correction if they demonstrate two or more of the following criteria:

(a) symptomatic patients;
(b) history of progression of the deformity;
(c) paradoxical respiration with deep inspiration;
(d) a chest computer tomography (CT) scan with Haller index greater than 3.25, cardiac compression/displacement and/or pulmonary compression (Fig. 11.5);

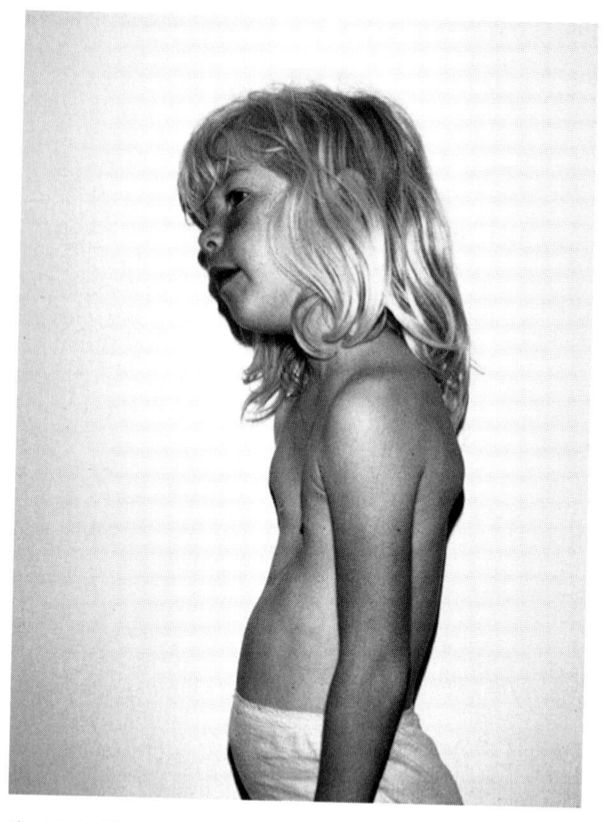

Fig. 11.6. Classic pectus posture.

(e) abnormal pulmonary function studies showing significant restrictive lung disease;
(f) mitral valve prolapse, bundle branch block, or other cardiac pathology secondary to compression of the heart;
(g) failed previous pectus repair(s).

Conservative treatment

All patients are started on an exercise and posture program when first seen in consultation and are encouraged to perform the following two exercises. (a) Every morning and evening, patients are to do five deep breathing exercises with 10 s. of breath holding, and (b) a posture exercise designed to strengthen their sacrospinalis muscles and to improve their posture. In addition, they are strongly encouraged to be involved in aerobic sports such as swimming, running, soccer, basketball, and so forth.

If patients have a classic pectus posture with kyphosis of the thoracic spine and forward sloping shoulders (Fig. 11.6), a figure-of-eight clavicular brace is also prescribed.

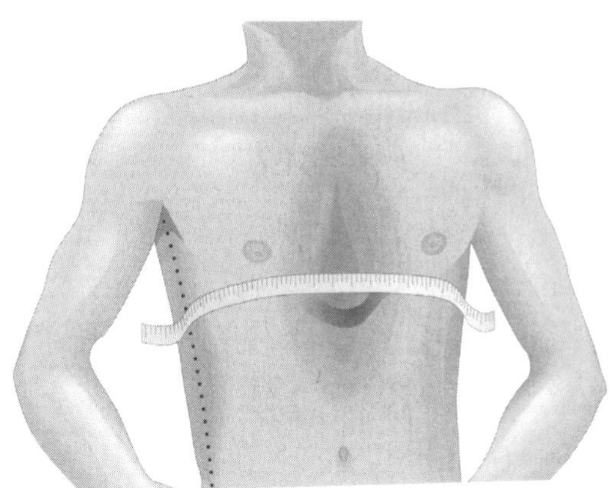

Fig. 11.7(a). Measurement of the chest.

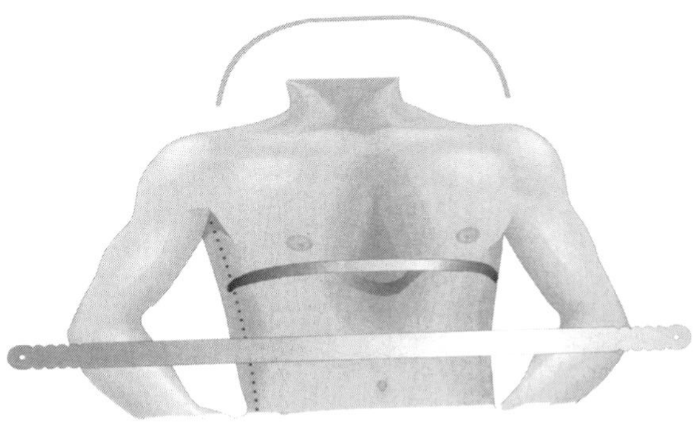

Fig. 11.7(b). Bending the bar. The bar should be bent to approximate a semicircle.

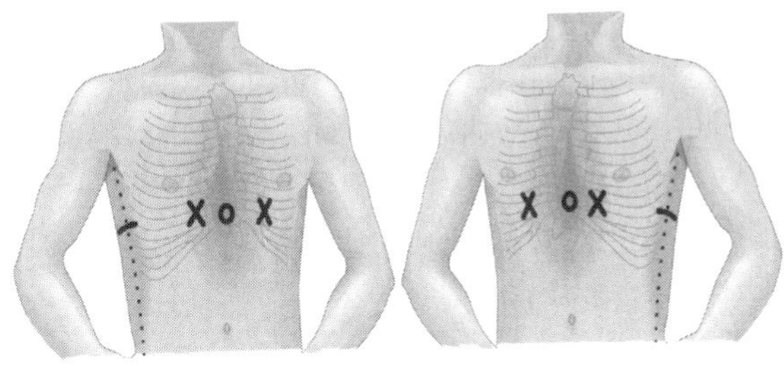

Fig. 11.7(c). Marking the site.

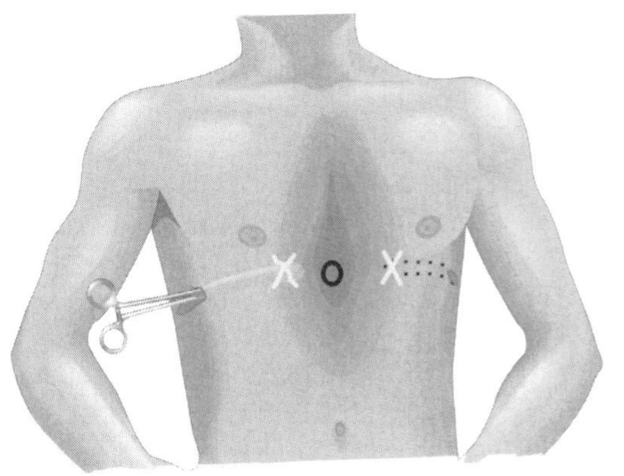

Fig. 11.7(d). Creating the tunnel.

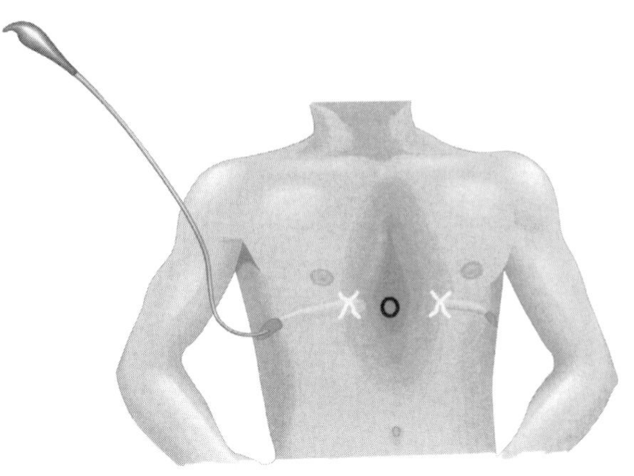

Fig. 11.7(e). Inserting the introducer.

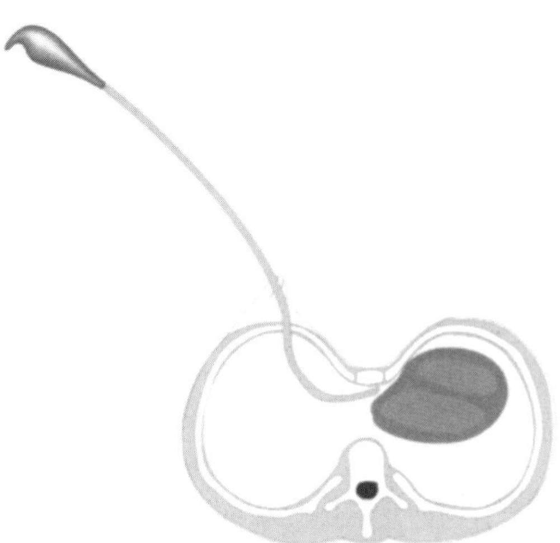

Fig. 11.7(f). Inserting the introducer.

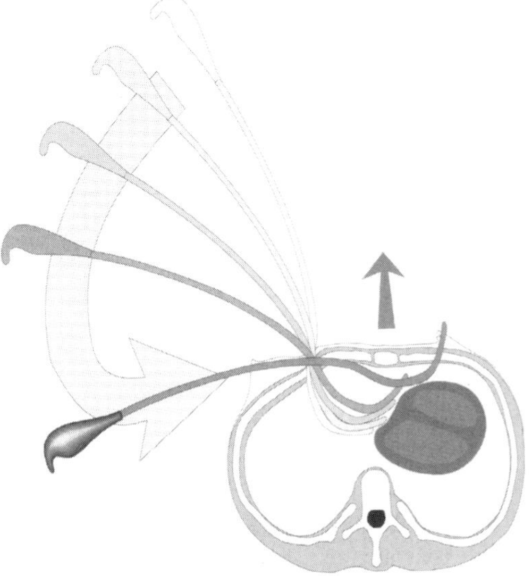

Fig. 11.7(g). Advancing the introducer.

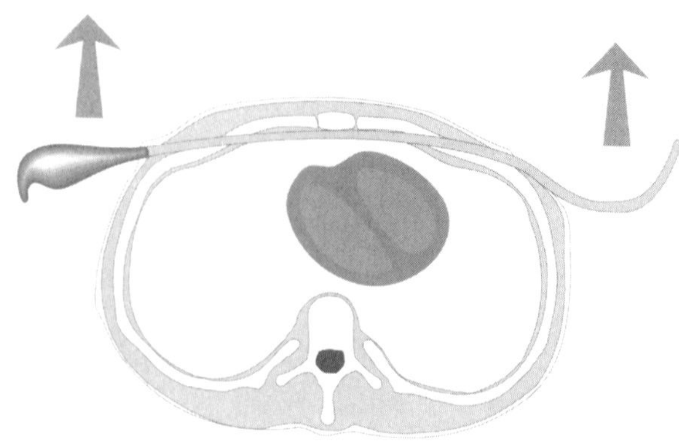

Fig. 11.7(h). Elevation of the sternum.

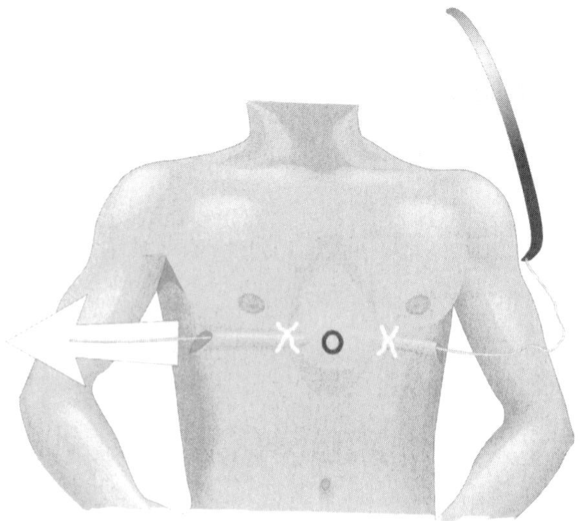

Fig. 11.7(i). Use of umbilical tape to guide the bar through the substernal tunnel.

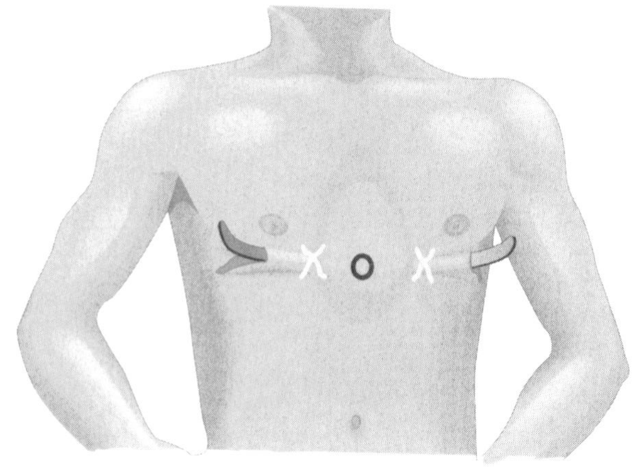

Fig. 11.7(j). Bar position, ready for rotation.

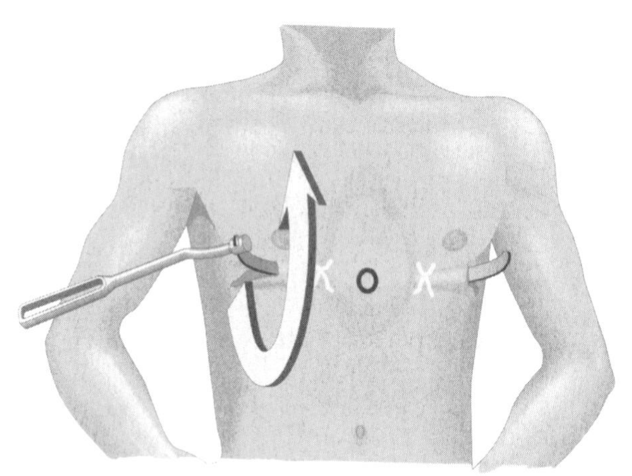

Fig. 11.7(k). Rotation of the bar.

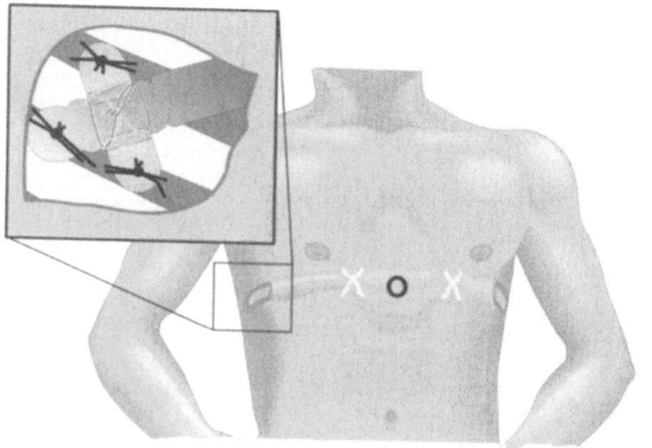

Fig. 11.7(l). Stabilization of the bar.

Surgical treatment

Minimally invasive procedure

Technique The minimally invasive procedure relies on the flexibility and malleability of the anterior chest wall and consists of insertion of a curved steel bar under the sternum. The patient is measured from mid-axillary line to mid-axillary line and 1 in (2 cm) is subtracted from the measurement to select the correct length substernal steel bar. The anesthesiologist inserts a thoracic epidural catheter prior to the start of the procedure to facilitate perioperative pain control. Under thoracoscopic guidance, a substernal tunnel is created with a specially designed introducer, which is inserted through small lateral thoracic incisions. The introducer is advanced subcutaneously to enter and exit the thoracic cavity just lateral to the sternum (Fig. 11.7(a)–11.7(l)). When the introducer has been

Table 11.4. Minimally invasive technique: materials and methods

1230 patients were evaluated for chest wall deformity
674 patients had minimally invasive pectus repair[a]
618 patients underwent primary operations
87 patients evaluated had prior pectus repairs.
51 have had redo operations:
28 failed Ravitch procedures
23 failed Nuss procedures[b]
2 failed Leonard procedures[c]

343 patients have had their bar(s) removed

Minimally invasive technique: operation and length of stay		
• Single pectus bar	80.4%	(497/618)
• Double pectus bar	19.5%	(121/618)
• No stabilizers	18.1%	(112/618)
• Stabilizers	81.9%	(506/618)
– wired	85.8%	(434/506)
– not wired	14.4%	(73/506)
– absorbable sutures	19.2%	(119/618)
• Median age	13.6 yrs	(22 mths–29 yrs)
• Median Haller CT index	4.7	(2.4–21)
• Epidural	3 days	(2–5)
• Length of stay	5 days	(3–10)

[a] there are five patients who have not yet been consented for inclusion in analysis
[b] 20 done elsewhere
[c] both patients had a prior Ravitch and are only counted once.

Table 11.5. Early complications

Deaths	0
Cardiac perforations	0
Pneumothorax	357 (57.8%)
Chest tube	17 (2.7%)
Aspiration	3 (0.5%)
Hemothorax	1 (0.2%)
Pleural effusion requiring drainage	4 (0.6%)
Pericarditis	6 (1.0%)
Wound infection	6 (1.0%)
Pneumonia	7 (1.1%)
Medication reactions	25 (4.0%)
Transient Horner's syndrome	161 (26.0%)

passed under the sternum and advanced out of the left lateral incision, it is used to elevate the sternum out of its depressed position. Before pulling the introducer out of the chest, an umbilical tape is attached to the end of the introducer. The introducer is slowly withdrawn from the chest cavity pulling the tape through the newly created substernal tunnel. The attached umbilical tape is cut loose from the introducer and used to guide the previously bent pectus support bar through the chest under thoracoscopic guidance. Once the bar is in position, it is rotated 180 degrees, thereby correcting the pectus excavatum. The bar is stabilized by wiring a rectangular steel stabilizer to the bar and by placing absorbable sutures around the bar and underlying ribs. Patients are kept on antibiotics for the duration of their hospitalization and are encouraged to do incentive spirometry to prevent pneumonia.

Demographics As of December 31, 2003, 1230 patients had been evaluated for chest wall deformity at our institution, of whom 674 patients underwent the minimally invasive procedure. Of these, 618 patients underwent primary operations and 51 underwent secondary operations (Table 11.4). Younger patients generally require only one bar whereas older patients and Marfan patients generally require two bars. Stabilizers were introduced in 1998 and are attached to the bar with #3 surgical steel sternal wire.

The median age of our patients was 13.6 years (see Table 11.4). The median CT Haller index was 4.7. Since 1994, all of our patients have received epidural analgesia for 3 to 5 days for postoperative pain management. The median length of hospital stay is 5 days.

Early complications (Table 11.5) Thoracoscopy is essential to prevent cardiac or pulmonary injury. In the 674 primary and secondary cases performed at our institution, there have been no cardiac or pulmonary injuries. However, prior to the use of thoracoscopy, one cardiac perforation occurred. The patient survived immediate sternotomy and repair of the cardiac injury. There are no reported cases of cardiac injury with the use of thoracoscopy.

A residual pneumothorax is almost always evident on X-ray after the use of thoracoscopy; however, only 2.7% of patients in this series required a chest tube. Recently a modification was introduced that has essentially eliminated the postoperative pneumothorax. This modification utilizes a "water seal" system combined with positive pressure respiration. At the end of the procedure, the CO_2 tubing is cut and the proximal end placed under water, while the anesthesiologist re-inflates the lungs until no more air bubbles escape from the end of the tubing.

Hemothorax from a bleeding intercostal vessel occurred in one patient. The patient did not require a transfusion. Thoracoscopy markedly reduces the risk of hemorrhage.

A small pleural effusion on routine post-op chest radiograph is frequently present and usually resolves spontaneously in 3 to 4 days. A significant pleural effusion

Table 11.6. Late complications

Bar displacement	67/618	(11.0%)
Requiring revision	48/618	(7.8%)
prior to stabilizer	15/112	(13.4%)
with stabilizer	33/506	(6.5%)
with wired stabilizer	21/434	(4.8%)
with absorbable sutures	2/119	(1.6%)
Hemothorax (post-traumatic)	2/618	(0.3%)
Bar infection	3/618	(0.5%)
Overcorrection	28/618	(4.5%)
Skin erosion	1/618	(0.2%)
Recurrences	9/343	(2.6%)

requiring chest tube drainage occurred in four (0.6%) of our patients.

Pericarditis occurred in 6 (1%) patients. It is thought to be due to pericardial injury and is a variant of the post-cardiomyotomy syndrome. Patients manifest with a fever, central chest pain, and a friction rub. An echocardiogram demonstrating fluid in the pericardial sac confirms the diagnosis. Patients respond well to indomethacin in most instances. Aspiration may be necessary if the pericardial effusion is large.[14]

Wound infection occurred in 6 (1%) patients. We emphasize prophylactic measures usually taken for patients undergoing implantation of foreign materials. Aseptic technique is stressed in the operating room. Adequate skin preparation with Duraprep® or Betadine® soap and solution is essential. During the procedure, the wounds are frequently bathed with antiseptic solution. All patients are given intravenous antibiotic (Cephalosporin – 2 ml generation) immediately after induction of anesthesia. The antibiotic is continued until the patient is discharged on day 4 or 5.

Vigorous incentive spirometry is encouraged to prevent pneumonia, which could result in a bar infection. Pneumonia occurred in 7 (1.1%) of the patients and responded well to antibiotics and incentive spirometry.

Transient Horner's syndrome secondary to the epidural analgesia was documented in 161 (26%) patients. It cleared in all cases when the epidural flow rate was reduced or when the catheter was removed.

Late complications Bar displacement has remained the biggest challenge with the minimally invasive approach (Table 11.6). A total of 67 patients (11%) had bar displacement, of whom 48 (7.8%) required repositioning. Prior to the use of stabilizers, the bar displacement rate was 15 out of 112 patients (13.4%). Since the use of wired stabilizers, the incidence of bar displacement has decreased to 4.8% and with the addition of absorbable sutures around the rib and bar, the incidence of bar displacement has dropped to 1.6%.

Allergy to one of the metallic components of the stainless steel bar occurred in three patients. It manifested as redness and pain in the area overlying the bar. All patients should be questioned as to their sensitivity to metallic jewelry and especially whether they have a nickel allergy. Bar allergy requires removal of the bar and replacement with a special titanium bar.

Overcorrection occurred in 28 patients, of whom four developed a true carinatum. These four patients had either been diagnosed with Marfan syndrome or exhibited symptoms consistent with Marfan syndrome; they also had a very severe or deep pectus excavatum preoperatively. They are presently still being treated conservatively to see if the protrusion will resolve once the bar is out.

Of 343 patients who have had their bars removed, nine have had a recurrence. We address the factors that we believe contributed to the recurrences in the next section.

Long-term results Our patients are asked to return for evaluation at 6 months, 24 months, and 36 months after repair. After bar removal, patients are asked to return at 1, 3, and 5 years, and every 2 years thereafter until they have completed puberty. Our median follow-up is 2 years from the time of repair, with a range of 5 days to 15 years postrepair.

As of December 31, 2003, we had removed bars in 343 patients after completion of treatment. Two hundred and sixty four patients have had their bar out for more than one year. Of these, 170 patients have returned for one or more visits (64.4% return rate), with a postbar removal follow-up of $12^1/_2$ years. The long-term results remain excellent in 76%, good in 14.7%, fair in 4.7%, and failed in 4.7% (of the nine recurrences, eight are more than 1 year postremoval; Fig. 11.8).

Eight of the 170 patients had a fair result. A result is considered to be fair if the chest shows some residual deformity. Five of these patients had had their repair and their bars removed before undergoing pubertal growth (Figs. 11.9, 11.10).

Of the nine patients who have had a recurrence, eight had undergone their initial repair and bar removal before undergoing pubertal growth. When the minimally invasive procedure was first developed, the most common age of the patients was 4 to 6 years and these patients therefore had many years of growth ahead of them. This taught us that age at initial surgery and bar removal are important factors in terms of long-term outcome. A recurrence or less

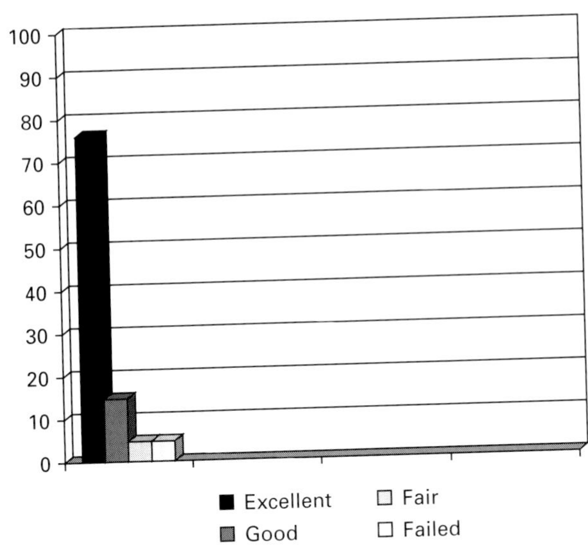

Fig. 11.8. Long-term results for patients who have had their bar out for >1 year.

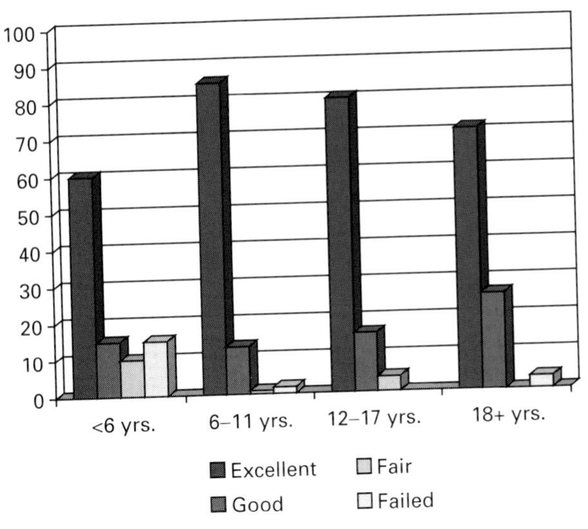

Fig. 11.10. Long-term results by age at time of surgery.

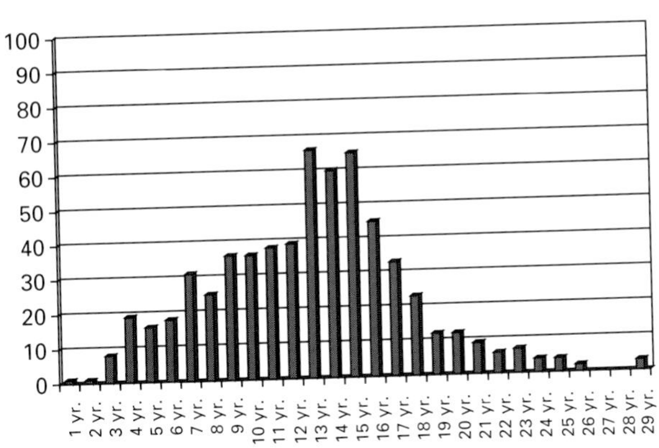

Fig. 11.9. Number of primary operations by age at time of surgery.

than ideal result is more likely in children with substantial somatic growth subsequent to bar removal.

It should be noted that, in addition to age, the recurrences also reflect both the early learning experience and technical factors that have subsequently been modified, such as when to remove the bar. Some patients with a recurrence had their bars removed prior to 1 year (Fig. 11.11). In addition, some of the patients who had recurrences underwent surgery while we were still refining the procedure, including bar material. Initially, the bar was too soft to maintain the correction, and when removed, some of these patients noticed a recurrence. Other modifications that have helped maintain the correction included the addition of stabilizers in 1998.

Our experience indicates that the bar should remain *in situ* for 2 to 4 years depending on growth patterns. Most patients now retain their bar for 3 years. Two additional factors that we have identified as important to ensuring an excellent long-term outcome include slight overcorrection at the time of the repair and also physical activity. Factors that appear to promote a poor outcome are poor posture and a sedentary lifestyle. We encourage all our patients to do the deep breathing and posture exercises every day and, in addition, we encourage them to participate in aerobic sporting activities.

Many investigators have shown that patients with pectus excavatum have "low normal" pulmonary function studies.[15,16] Since 1994, 541 patients have undergone routine preoperative pulmonary function testing and the results show that these patients do suffer from mild to severe restrictive lung disease. Only 20% of the patients have an FVC above average (100% predicted value), showing that the normal distribution has shifted markedly to the abnormal side in the pectus excavatum population (Table 11.7). After open surgical correction (Ravitch type) long-term studies have shown a reduced level of performance on PFTs, and this is thought to be due to scarring and rigidity of the anterior chest wall.[3,17–19] Following repair with the minimally invasive procedure, there is no significant improvement at 6 months, but after 12 months we have recently found significant improvement in pulmonary function (L. M. Lawson, unpublished data, 2004). This improvement is particularly significant in patients who are compliant with the exercise program.

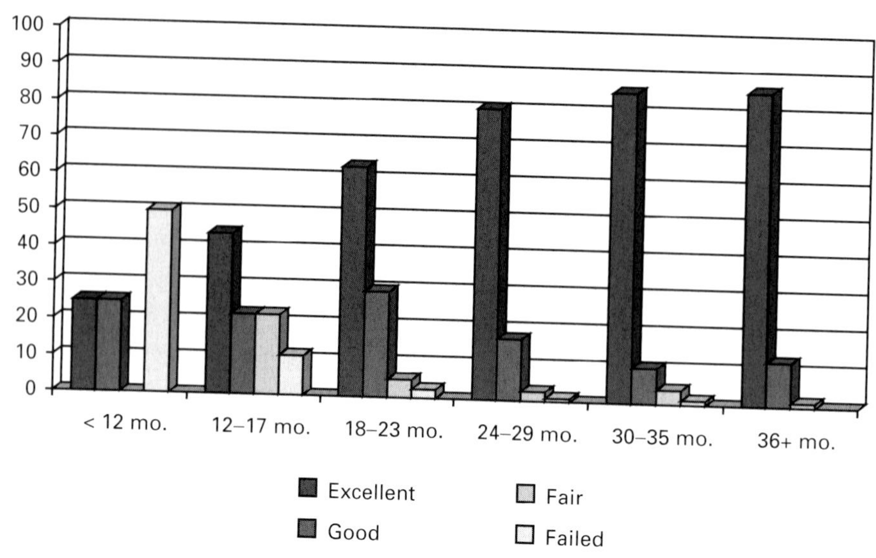

Fig. 11.11. Results after bar removal by time bar *in situ*.

Table 11.7. Preoperative pulmonary function study results for pectus excavatum surgical patients repaired primarily. $N = 541$

FVC%	FEV1%	FEF25–75%
100%+ = 20%	100%+ = 13.9%	100%+ = 22.9%
90–99% = 20.5%	90–99% = 22.5%	90–99% = 13.7%
80–89% = 30%	80–89% = 27.2%	80–89% = 13.1%
70–79% = 17.7%	70–79% = 18.3%	70–79% = 11.6%
60–69% = 4.8%	60–69% = 10.5%	60–69% = 14.6%
50–59% = 2.8%	50–59% = 3.1%	50–59% = 8.3%
40–49% = 1.5%	40–49% = 0.9%	40–49% = 3.7%
30–39% = 0%	30–39% = 0.4%	30–39% = 2.2%
<30% = 2.6%	<30% = 3.1%	<30% = 9.8%
29.4% with FVC% below 80%.	36.3% with FEV1% below 80%.	50.2% with FEF25%–75% below 80%.

Potential surgical candidates undergo a cardiac evaluation including EKG and Echo. These evaluations have confirmed the preoperative presence of mitral valve prolapse in 14.4%. Heart murmur or other cardiac symptoms are present in 22.5%. In all patients, there is significant improvement in cardiac compression and displacement noted on exam after surgery.

Many patients have significant body image concerns prior to surgery, causing them to withdraw from participation in sports and social activities, giving rise to depression that sometimes leads to suicidal thoughts. In addition, the preoperative symptoms of shortness of breath, exercise intolerance, lack of endurance, and chest pain hinder the activity of many of the patients. Preliminary results using the Pectus Excavatum Evaluation Questionnaire (PEEQ) indicate that surgical repair of pectus has a positive impact on the well-being of the patient.[20] In addition, of the 321 patients who have completed our postoperative evaluation questionnaire, 91.3% report being either happy or very happy with the results of their surgery, and 84% have noted an increase in exercise tolerance.

Conclusions The minimally invasive technique is simple in concept and requires neither rib resection nor sternal osteotomy. The blood loss is typically insignificant. However, the procedure requires meticulous attention to detail and there is a significant learning curve. Our experience indicates that timing of the repair and bar removal is critical to maintaining excellent long-term outcomes. The long-term outcome in a large series over 17 years shows good to excellent results in 90.7% of patients, fair results in 4.7%, and an overall recurrence rate of 2.6% (Fig. 11.12a, 11.12b).

Pectus carinatum

Pathophysiology and symptoms

Pectus carinatum is characterized by anterior protuberance and constitutes approximately 15% of chest wall deformities.[21] Pectus carinatum may involve the upper manubrium of the sternum,[22] which is called a chondromanubrial deformity. However, the most common

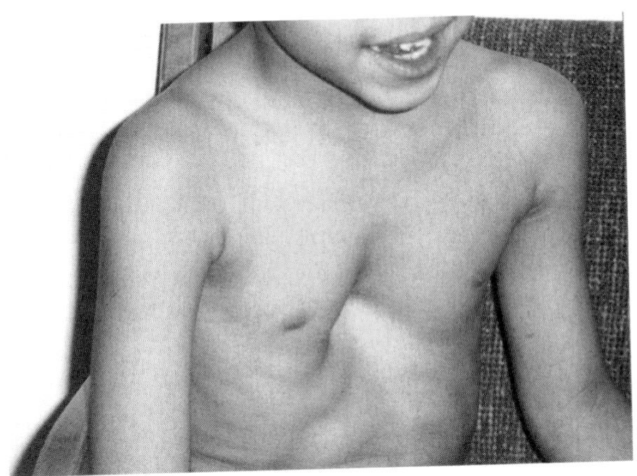

Fig. 11.12(a). Patient, age 5, with severe pectus excavatum before surgery.

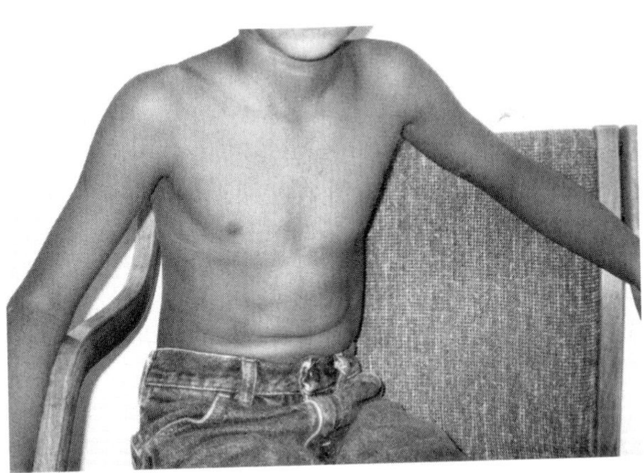

Fig. 11.12(b). Patient, age 7, 2 years after minimally invasive pectus repair.

protrusion occurs in the lower or body of the sternum (the gladiolus), and is called chondrogladiolar. The protrusion may be unilateral, bilateral, or mixed.[23] About 80% of patients are male. Although the etiology is unknown,[24] like pectus excavatum, there is a genetic component of causation as suggested by the one-fourth of patients who have a family history of chest wall defect.[21] In our patient population, 6.7% of our patients have noted a family history of this condition (see Table 11.1). Pectus carinatum has also been reported to occur following treatment of pectus excavatum.

The natural history of this condition differs from pectus excavatum. Unlike pectus excavatum, which is noted at birth, pectus carinatum is usually noted in childhood, especially around the time of a growth spurt. Symptoms are confined to tenderness at the site of the protrusion.[23,25] Associated mitral valve disease has been reported.[26] In patients without congenital heart disease, cardiopulmonary limitation due to the condition has not been reported. Other coexisting conditions include Marfan syndrome and scoliosis (in 15%).[21]

Treatment

Conservative treatment

There has been limited experience with orthotic bracing. Two reports have described correction or improvement in the deformity by means of a brace that exerts pressure in the anteroposterior direction, analogous to that used for treatment of scoliosis.[25,27] We have had limited success with bracing.

Surgical treatment

Open procedure Surgical treatment is usually by costochondral resection with sternotomy.[23,28,29] These studies emphasize the importance of performing a bilateral cartilage resection, even if there is unilateral deformity of the cartilages, to prevent recurrence.

The preoperative preparation and evaluation is the same as for the minimally invasive technique. However, because there is a risk of interference with growth plates in young children and of the development of asphyxiating chondrodystrophy,[10,11] the procedure should be reserved for patients who have completed their growth. The open procedure is better suited to the older patients, especially those who have asymmetric or eccentric deformities and patients with carinatum deformities.

Technique The open technique involves making an anterior thoracic incision and elevating skin and muscle flaps until all the costal cartilages from T3 to T6 are exposed. The perichondrium is incised longitudinally and the deformed cartilages are either partially or completely removed. A "V" shape sternal osteotomy is performed at the angle of Louis. The sternum is placed in a neutral position, and the osteotomy closed with non-absorbable sutures. A pectus bar is inserted under the sternum to bridge the gap between the ribs and the sternum and to prevent movement of the sternum. The perichondrial "sleeves" are re-sutured, drains are inserted, the muscle flaps sutured back into position, and the incisions are closed. Postoperative management is similar to the open excavation technique, except that patients are required to refrain from contact sports activities for at least 3 months.

Complications There have been very few postoperative problems associated with surgical correction of pectus carinatum, and recurrence has been reported to be 5 to 15% by centers with a large experience.[30]

Poland's syndrome

Pathophysiology

Poland's syndrome has an incidence of 1 in 30 000 live births and is sporadic in occurrence.[31] It is a constellation of anomalies including absence of the pectoralis major, pectoralis minor, serratus anterior, rectus abdominus, and latissimus dorsi muscles. In addition, there can be athelia or amastia, nipple deformities, and limb deformities such as syndactyly or brachydactyly, absent axillary hair, and limited subcutaneous fat.

In 1841, Alfred Poland, an English medical student, published a partial description of the deformity.[32] However, the syndrome was initially described in the French and German literature in 1826 and 1839 respectively.[33,34]

Poland's syndrome does not appear to be inherited, although there are rare family occurrences. The right side is more commonly affected. Seventy percent of patients are males.[35] One out of six patients with breast hypoplasia/aplasia has Poland's syndrome. The etiology is unclear, but some theories include abnormal migration of the embryonic tissues forming the pectoralis muscles, hypoplasia of the subclavian artery, or *in utero* injury.

There is no correlation between the extent of hand deformities and chest wall deformities. Varying degrees of either can occur with mild hypoplasia to total aplasia of muscles, ribs, and cartilage. The latter can lead to major depressions and paradoxical respiratory motion.

Treatment

Surgical repair is rarely required. Except in those patients with aplasia of the ribs or a major depression deformity,[36] chest wall reconstruction with correction of contralateral carinatum type protrusions can usually be performed at the same time. Autologous rib grafts, or a variety of bioprosthetic agents, can be used with or without a latissimus dorsi flap. The use of custom-made chest wall prostheses has been associated with significant problems such as migration, erosion of local tissues, and adverse cosmesis.[37] Chest wall reconstruction should take place prior to any breast reconstruction in a female with hypoplasia or aplasia of the breast.

Sternal defects

Pathophysiology and treatment

Sternal defects are midline defects of the upper torso that range from the relatively benign sternal cleft (sternal defect without displacement of the heart) to the rare and almost uniformally fatal thoracic ectopia cordis.

Cleft sternum (bifid sternum, partial ectopia cordis) is a rare malformation (15% of all chest wall malformations in some series) due to partial or total failure of sternal fusion at an early stage of embryonic development. Sternal clefts can be classified as either complete (the rarest form), superior, or inferior.[38] Superior clefts are either U-shaped (proximal to the fourth cartilage) or V-shaped (reaching the xiphoid process) and are most often isolated with only minor associated lesions such as vascular dysplasias and supra-umbilical-raphe.

The heart is in a normal position and cardiac anomalies are rare. Surgery, which is typically successful, is warranted once the diagnosis is made and can be done electively. Optimally, it is done in the neonate when the sternal bars can be approximated easily due to flexibility with minimal compression of mediastinal structures. After one year of age, primary repair is difficult and more extensive techniques may be needed such as use of autologous (costal cartilage, ribs) or prosthetic materials (Marlex® mesh, teflon).[39]

Thoracic ectopia cordis occurs when the heart has no overlying somatic structures. It is rare and there is usually some form of associated abdominal wall defect with the heart external to the chest and the apex pointed toward the chin. Intrinsic cardiac anomalies are frequent, especially tetralogy of Fallot, pulmonary artery stenosis, transposition of the great arteries, and ventricular septal defects.[40] Survival is reportable; only three survivors have been reported to date because the return of the heart to the thorax is poorly tolerated. Most affected patients die due to torsion of the great vessels and compression of the heart when attempting reduction. The goals of therapy are to cover the heart; preserve cardiac output by preventing kinking of the great vessels; repair the associated abdominal wall defect; and stabilize the thoracic cavity so that spontaneous ventilation can be effective.[41,42]

Thoracoabdominal ectopia cordis (Cantrell's pentalogy) refers to the situation where the heart is covered by an omphalocele-like membrane. Intrinsic cardiac anomalies are also common in these patients, with tetralogy of Fallot and ventricular septal defects being the most common.[40] Cantrell's pentalogy consists of inferior sternal cleft, ectopia cordis, midline abdominal wall defects or omphalocele, pericardial defects, and one or more cardiac defects. Repair is much more successful than in thoracic ectopia cordis. Initial surgical management addresses the lack of skin overlying the heart and abdominal cavity. After initial stabilization and cardiac echo, the goal of the initial operation is to provide coverage of the midline defects, to separate the abdominal and pericardial compartments, and to repair the diaphragm. Various techniques to gain closure include flap mobilization, skin closure only, and a variety of bioprosthetic agents. The congenital heart disease is repaired at a later date.

Thoracic insufficiency syndrome associated with diffuse skeletal disorders

Pathophysiology

Thoracic insufficiency syndrome may be defined as any disorder that produces the inability of the thorax to support normal respiration or lung growth.[43] It includes a spectrum of disorders including asphyxiating thoracic dystrophy (Jeune's syndrome), acquired asphyxiating thoracic dystrophy, for example following open techniques for pectus repair, spondylothoracic dysphasia (Jarcho–Levin syndrome), congenital scoliosis with multiple vertebral anomalies with fused or absent ribs (jumbled spine), and severe kyphoscoliosis.

These disorders have often been viewed and treated historically as separate entities with little coordinated effort between specialties. They are best addressed with a unified approach integrating pediatric general and orthopedic surgeons as well as the pulmonologist.

Jeune's syndrome[44] is an autosomal recessive inherited osteochondrodystrophy with variable expressions. In mild forms, the chest may support adequate respiration. In more severe cases, the thorax is narrowed both transversely and in height with short, wide horizontal ribs and irregular costochondral junctions. This chest wall configuration produces a rigid chest with very little intercostal excursion for normal respiration.[45] This leads to ventilatory dependence and death from respiratory failure.[46]

Pathologic examination has produced varied findings including pulmonary hypertension and normal bronchial development with variable alveolar density.[47] This suggests that the extrinsic chest wall plays a significant role in the underlying pulmonary hypoplasia.[48]

Other associated skeletal abnormalities in Jeune's syndrome include short stubby extremities, fixed elevated clavicles, hypoplastic iliac wings,[49–50] and a high incidence of C1 spinal stenosis.[51] These patients also have varying degrees of renal dysplasia.[52]

Spondylothoracic dysplasia (Jarcho–Levin) syndrome occurs in two forms with different inheritance patterns. Type I is an autosomal recessive deformity characterized by multiple vertebral hemivertebrae and posterior rib fusions.[53] This produces a marked shortening of the thoracic spine and a crab-like appearance of the chest on standard X-ray.[54] Associated malformations are noted in 30% and include cardiac and renal anomalies. The Type I form is often fatal by 15 months of age and there is a high incidence of this disorder reported in Puerto Rican families.[55] Type II spondylothoracic dysplasia has an autosomal dominant inheritance pattern and is associated with near normal longevity. It is mostly seen in Caucasian children.[55]

Thoracic insufficiency may also arise secondary from too early or too extensive pectus operations.[11] Complex spine anomalies producing the so-called "jumbled spine" unilateral thoracic hypoplasia seen with the VACTERL association, and kyphoscoliosis may also be a cause for thoracic insufficiency.[56–60]

Surgical treatment

Surgical techniques to correct the spectrum of these complex disorders have attempted to address the issue of thoracic volume by various approaches. In both congenital (Jeune's) and acquired (postpectus) thoracic dystrophy, one approach has been the use of an anterior longitudinal sternal split with widening of the sternum.

This has been done with methylmethacrylate, bone grafts or rib, and metal plates.[61–63] A staged approach with a methylmethacrylate plate followed by secondary removal of the plate and latissimus dorsi flaps to cover the created sternal cleft has also been described.[64] Sternal elevation has also been done in cases of acquired thoracic dystrophy by both open technique[11] and the minimally invasive technique used for standard pectus repair.[14] A lateral staged approach with staggered rib osteotomies, staggered division of the chest wall, intercostal muscles and pleura with transposition of alternating ribs using metal plate fixation has also been described.[65]

These approaches have had variable results due to the fact that they are not easily revised to allow for continued growth of the chest wall and permit lung expansion. The lateral thoracic expansion may also interfere with intercostal muscle function after division of multiple intercostal muscles and nerves.

With regard to patients with Jarcho–Levin syndrome, jumbled spine and kyphosis, pediatric general surgeons have done little to correct these problems, as they were either considered lethal or solely in the domain of the orthopedic surgeon.

A promising technique to address patients with the spectrum of causes for thoracic insufficiency syndrome rejoins the disciplines of pediatric general thoracic and orthopedic surgery. Expansion thoracoplasty and use of a vertical expandable prosthetic titanium rib (VEPTR) developed by Campbell and Smith addresses many problems in the spectrum of these disorders. This technique allows for serial expansion of the chest wall to allow for continued growth of the thorax and spine until skeletal maturity is achieved.[66]

Over 300 patients with various disorders have been treated with this technique. In Jeune's asphyxiating thoracic dystrophy, 14 patients have undergone staged bilateral expansions. Anterior rib osteotomies adjacent to the costochondral junction and posterior osteotomies adjacent to the transverse process of the spine in ribs 3–9 are performed, creating a mobilized segment of chest wall that is distracted posteriolaterally and anchored to a curved VEPTR that is attached to the second and tenth ribs. The segment is anchored to the VEPTR with 2 mm titanium rings stabilizing the segment and allowing re-ossification of the multiple osteotomies. The second stage is done 3 months later and then the devices are expanded every 6 months.

In patients with fused or absent ribs and scoliosis, a wedge thoracostomy through the fused segment of ribs not only allows expansion of the chest, but will correct the scoliosis and the rotational spinal deformity (producing a wind swept thorax).[60] It also stimulates increased spinal height in both congenital scoliosis and Jarcho–Levin syndrome where bilateral devices are placed.

REFERENCES

1. Williams, A. M. & Crabbe, D. C. G. Pectus deformities of the anterior chest wall. *Paediatr. Resp. Rev.* 2003; **4**(3):237–242.
2. Molik, K. A., Engum, S. A., Rescorla, F. J. *et al.* Pectus excavatum repair: Experience with standard and minimally invasive techniques. *J. Pediatr. Surg.* 2001; **36**(2):324–328.
3. Shamberger, R. C. Congenital chest wall deformities. In *Pediatric Surgery*. 5th edn. Philadelphia, PA: Elsevier, 1998: 787–817.
4. Coulson, W. Deformities of the chest. *Lond. Med. Gaz.* 1820; **4**:69–73.
5. Sauerbruch, F. Operative Beseitigung der Angeborenen Trichterbrust. *Deutsche Zeitschr. f. Chir.* 1931; **234**:760.
6. Ravitch, M. M. The operative treatment of pectus excavatum. *Ann. Surg.* 1949; **129**:429–444.
7. Wallgren, G. R. & Sulamaa, M. Surgical treatment of funnel chest. Exhib. VIII, *Int. Congr. Paediatr.* 1949: 32.
8. Adkins, P. C., & Blades, B. A. Stainless steel strut for correction of pectus excavatum. *Surg. Gynecol. Obstet.* 1961:111–113.
9. Welch, K. J. Satisfactory surgical correction of pectus excavatum deformity in childhood. *J. Thorac. Surg.* 1958; **36**:697–713.
10. Martinez, D., Juame, J., Stein, T., & Pena, A. The effect of costal cartilage resection on chest wall development. *Pediatr. Surg. Int.* 1990; **5**:170–173.
11. Haller, J. A., Colombani, P. M., Humphries, C. T. *et al.* Chest wall constriction after too extensive and too early operations for pectus excavatum. *Ann. Thorac. Surg.* 1996; **61**:1618–1625.
12. Nuss, D., Kelly, R. E., Jr., Croitoru, D. P., & Katz,, M. E. A 10-year review of a minimally invasive technique for the correction of pectus excavatum. *J. Pediatr. Surg.* 1998; **33**(4):545–552.
13. Nuss, D., Kelly, R. E., Jr., Croitoru, D. P., & Swoveland, B. Repair of pectus excavatum. *Pediatr. Endosurg. Innovat. Techn.* 1998; **2**:205–221.
14. Croitoru, D. P., Kelly, R. E., Jr., Goretsky, M. J. *et al.* Experience and modification update for the minimally invasive Nuss technique for pectus excavatum repair in 303 patients. *J. Pediatr. Surg.* 2002; **37**(3):437–445.
15. Malek, M. H., Fonkalsrud, E. W., & Cooper, C. B. Ventilatory and cardiovascular responses to exercise in patients with pectus excavatum. *Chest* 2003; **124**(3):870–882.
16. Malek, M. H. & Fonkalsrud, E. W. Cardiorespiratory outcome after corrective surgery for pectus excavatum: a case study. *Med. Sci. Sports Exerc.* 2004; **36**(2):183–190.
17. Borgeskov, S. & Raahave, D. Long-term result after operative repair of funnel chest. *Thorax* 1971; **26**:74–76.
18. Morshuis, W., Folgering, H., Barentsz, J. *et al.* Pulmonary function before surgery for pectus excavatum and at long-term follow-up. *Chest* 1994; **105**:1646–1652.
19. Quigley, P. M., Haller, J. A., Jelus, K. L. *et al.* Cardiorespiratory function before and after corrective surgery in pectus excavatum. *J. Pediatr.* 1996; **128**:638–643.
20. Lawson, M. L., Cash, T. F., Akers, R. *et al.* A pilot study of the impact of surgical repair on disease-specific quality of life among patients with pectus excavatum. *J. Pediatr. Surg.* 2003; **38**(6):916–918.
21. Shamberger, R. C. & Welch, K. J. Surgical correction of pectus carinatum. *J. Pediatr. Surg.* 1987; **22**:48–53.
22. Chin, E. F. Surgery of funnel chest and congenital sternal prominence. *Br. J. Surg.* 1957; **44**:360–376.
23. Robisek, F., Cook, J. W., Daugherty, H. K. *et al.* Pectus carinatum. *J. Thorac. Cardiovasc. Surg.* 1979; **78**:52–61.
24. Pena, A., Perez, L., Nurka, S., *et al.* Pectus carinatum and pectus excavatum: are they the same disease? *Am. Surg.* 1981; **47**:215–218.
25. Haje, S. A. & Bowen, J. R. Preliminary results of orthotic treatment of pectus deformities in children and adolescents. *J. Pediatr. Orthop.* 1992; **12**:795–800.
26. Currarino, G. & Silverman, F. N. Premature obliteration of the sternal sutures and pigeon-breast deformity. *Radiology* 1958; **70**:532–540.
27. Egan, J. C., DuBois, J. J., Morphy, M. *et al.* Compressive orthotics in the treatment of asymmetric pectus carinatum: a preliminary report with an objective radiographic marker. *J. Pediatr. Surg.* 2000; **8**:1183–1186.
28. Ravitch, M. M. The operative correction of pectus carinatum (pigeon breast). *Ann. Surg.* 1960; **151**:705–714.
29. Welch, K. J. & Vos, A. Surgical correction of pectus carinatum (pigeon breast). *J. Pediatr. Surg.* 1973; **8**:659–667.

30. Shamberger, R. C. Congenital chest wall deformities. *Curr. Probl. Surg.* 1996; **33**(6):469–542.
31. Freire-Maia, N., Chautard, E. A., & Opitz, J. M. The Poland Syndrome-clinical and genealogical data, dermatoglyphic analysis, and incidence. *Hum. Hered.* 1973; **23**:97–104.
32. Poland, A. Deficiency of the pectoralis muscles. *Guys. Hosp. Rep.* 1841; **6**:191–193.
33. Lallemand, L. M. Ephermerides Medicales de Montpellier 1826; **1**:144–147.
34. Froriep, R. Beobachtung eines Falles Von Mangel der Brustdrauuse 1839; **10**:9–14.
35. Golladay, E. S. Pectus carinatum and other deformities of the chest wall. In Zeigler, M. M., Azizkhan, R. G., & Weber, T. R., eds. *Operative Pediatric Surgery*. New York: McGraw-Hill,2003: 269–278.
36. Shamberger, R. C., Welch, K. J., & Upton, J., III. Surgical treatment of thoracic deformity in Poland's Syndrome. *J. Pediatr. Surg.* 1989; **24**:760–766.
37. Seyfer, A. E., Icochea, R., & Graber, G. M. Poland's anomaly: natural history and long-term results of chest wall reconstruction in 33 patients. *Ann. Surg.* 1988; **208**:776–782.
38. Samarrai, A. R., Charmockley, H. A., & Attr, A. A. Complete cleft sternum: classification and surgical repair. *Int. Surg.* 1985; **70**:71–73.
39. Knox, L., Tuggle, D., & Knott-Craig, C. J. Repair of congenital sternal clefts in adolescence and infancy. *J. Pediatr. Surg.* 1994; **29**:1513–1516.
40. Shamberger, R. C. & Welch, K. J. Sternal defects. *Pediatr. Surg. Int.* 1990; **5**:156–164.
41. Amato, J. J., Zelen, J., & Talwalker, N. G. Single-stage repair of thoracic ectopia cordis. *Ann. Thorac. Surg.* 1995; **59**:518–520.
42. Groner, J. I. Ectopia cordis and sternal defects. In Zeigler, M. M., Azizkhan, R. G., & Weber, T. R., eds. *Operative Pediatric Surgery*. New York: McGraw-Hill, 2003: 279–293.
43. Campbell, R. M. & Smith, M. Treatment of thoracic insufficiency syndrome associated with congenital scoliosis. *J. Bone. Joint. Surg.* 1997; **79B**(1):82.
44. Jeune, M., Carron, R., Beraud, C. *et al.* Polychondrodystrophie avec blocage thoracique d'evolution fatale. *Pediatrics* 1954:390–392.
45. Borland, L. M. Anesthesia for children with Jeune's Syndrome (asphyxiating thoracic dystrophy). *Anesthesiology* 1987; **66**:86–88.
46. Tahernia, A. C. & Stamps, P. Jeune's Syndrome (asphyxiating thoracic dystrophy). *Chin. Pediatr.* 1977; **16**:903–907.
47. Williams, A. J., Vawter, G., & Reid, L. M. Lung structure in asphyxiating thoracic dystrophy. *Arch. Pathol. Lab. Med.* 1984; **108**:658–661.
48. Finegold, J., Katzew, H., Genieser, N. B. *et al.* Lung structure in thoracic dystrophy. *Am. J. Dis. Child.* 1971; **122**:153–159.
49. Langer, L. O. Thoracic pelvic phalangeal dystrophy: asphyxiating thoracic dystrophy of the newborn, infantile thoracic dystrophy. *Radiology* 1968; **91**:447–456.
50. Oberklaid, F., Dnaks, D. M., Mayne, V. *et al.* Asphyxiating thoracic dysplasia. *Arch. Dis. Child.* 1977; **52**:758–765.
51. Campbell, R. M. The incidence of proximal cervical spine stenosis in Jeune's asphyxiating dystrophy, presented at The Scoliosis Research Society; 2001.
52. Herdman, R. C. & Langer, L. O. The thoracic asphyxiant dystrophy and renal disease. *Am. J. Dis. Child.* 1977; **52**:192–201.
53. Jarcho, S. & Levin, P. M. Hereditary malformations of the vertebral bodies. *Bull. Johns Hopkins Hosp.* 1938; **62**:216–226.
54. Roberts, A. P., Conner, A. N., Tolmie, J. L. *et al.* Spondylothoracic and spondylocostal dystosis: hereditary forms of spinal deformity. *J. Bone Joint Surg.* 1988; **70B**:123–126.
55. Heilbronner, D. M. & Renshaw, T. S. Spondylothoracic dysplasia. *J. Bone Joint Surg. Am.* 1984; **66**:302–303.
56. McMaster, M. J. Congenital scoliosis. In: Weinstein, S. L., ed. *The Pediatric Spine: Principles and Practice.* New York: Raven Press; 1994.
57. McMaster, M. J. Congenital scoliosis caused by unilateral failure of vertebral segmentation with contralateral hemivertibrae. *Spine* 1998; **23**:998–1005.
58. McMaster, M. J. & David, C. Hemivertebrae as a cause of scoliosis: a study of 104 patients. *J. Bone Joint Surg.* 1986; **68B**:588–595.
59. Campbell, R. M. Congenital scoliosis due to multiple vertebrae anomalies associated with thoracic insufficiency syndrome. *Spine: State Art Rev.* 2000; **14**:209–218.
60. Campbell, R. M., Smith, M. D., Mayes, T. *et al.* The characteristics of thoracic insufficiency syndrome associated with fused ribs and congenital scoliosis. *J. Bone Joint Surg.* 2003; **85**:399–408.
61. Todd, D. W., Tinguely, S. T., & Norberg, W. J. A thoracic expansion technique for Jeune's asphyxiating thoracic dystrophy. *J. Pediatr. Surg.* 1986; **21**:161–163.
62. Barnes, N. D., Hall, D., Milner, A. D. *et al.* Chest reconstruction in asphyxiating thoracic dystrophy. *Arch. Dis. Child.* 1971; **46**:833–837.
63. Weber, T. R. & Kurkchubasche, A. G. Operative management of asphyxiating thoracic dystrophy after pectus repair. *J. Pediatr. Surg.* 1998; **33**:262–265.
64. Sharoni, E., Erez, E., Chorer, G. *et al.* Chest reconstruction in asphyxiating thoracic dystrophy. *J. Pediatr. Surg.* 1998; **33**:1578–1581.
65. Davis, J. T., Heistein, J. B., Castile, R. G. *et al.* Lateral thoracic expansion for Jeune's syndrome: mid-term results. *Ann. Thorac. Surg.* 2001; **72**:872–878.
66. Campbell, R. M., Hell-Vocke, A. K. Growth of the thoracic spine in congenital scoliosis after expansion thoracoplasty. *J. Bone Joint Surg.* 2003; **85A**:409–419.

12

Congenital diaphragmatic hernia

Nikki Almendinger, Son Lee West and Jay Wilson

Department of Surgery, Children's Hospital and Harvard Medical School, Boston, MA, USA

Introduction

Despite recent advances in critical care, improved ventilatory support strategies, and ready access to extracorporeal life support (ECLS), the management of patients with congenital diaphragmatic hernia (CDH) continues to be a vexing problem for the clinician. Improvements in treatment strategies have been associated with an increase in overall survival probability for CDH patients in recent years; however, there has also been an unanticipated increase in morbidity in these survivors. The objective of this chapter is to briefly review the history and pathophysiology of CDH, as well as current management strategies, but most importantly to summarize current data related to the long-term outcome, morbidity, and recommended follow-up of these complex patients.

Etiology and embryology

The incidence of CDH is between 1 in 2000 and 5000 live births, yielding approximately 1000 affected infants per year in the USA.[1] It has been suggested that the in utero mortality rate is as high as 30%, although this is probably an overestimate.[1] Over 90% of the defects are posteriolateral and 85% of these are left sided.[2] The etiology of CDH is still not known. Exposure to teratogens such as insecticides, phenmetrazine, quinine, nitrofen and vitamin A deficiency has been implicated in the development of CDH. Although CDH has been reported to be associated with trisomies 18, 21 and 22, the genetic contribution to the lesion is likely to be quite complex. Consequently, sporadic occurrence is most common. It is believed that CDH results from failure of closure of the pleuroperitoneal canals, which occurs normally in the human fetus at 8–10 weeks' gestation. Consequently, the abdominal viscera herniate into the affected thorax, creating a shift of the mediastinum to the contralateral side and hypoplasia of both the ipsilateral and contralateral lung. Although the mass effect is thought to play a large role in creating pulmonary hypoplasia, there are contributing factors that are not yet well defined. Some believe that the timing and the degree of the intestinal herniation are related to the extent of lung hypoplasia. In addition to reduced bronchial branching and a lower number of alveoli in affected lungs, there is also a reduction in the total number of pulmonary arterial branches seen in both lungs in CDH patients. Among the preacinar and intraacinar arterioles, there is abnormal medial muscular hypertrophy. This hypertrophy, in combination with a decrease in the total number of pulmonary vessels, is thought to play a large role in the pathogenesis of high pulmonary vascular resistance and pulmonary hypertension in infants with CDH.[3,4]

Prenatal diagnosis and care

Comprehensive care of infants and children with CDH begins with the fetus. Proper identification of the defect and assessment of the likely severity and its impact on the neonate can improve perinatal management and avoid perinatal complications, which can have significant long-term consequences. Prenatal ultrasound readily identifies the fetus with CDH as early as 14 gestational weeks and follow-up fetal MRI can provide details about the severity of the defect. The finding of CDH in a fetus should also lead to a careful search for other anomalies as they have

Pediatric Surgery and Urology: Long-term Outcomes, Mark Stringer, Keith Oldham, Pierre Mouriquand.
Published by Cambridge University Press.

been reported to occur in up to 50% of cases.[5] The most common abnormalities associated with CDH are cardiac, genitourinary, gastrointestinal, central nervous system and chromosomal, in that order. Structural cardiac defects are the most prevalent associated anomaly, affecting approximately 25% of live born infants with CDH. For this reason, in addition to a level three ultrasound, a fetal echocardiogram should be performed for detailed cardiac evaluation in all CDH fetuses. An amniocentesis should also be performed to look for chromosomal abnormalities. Not surprisingly, the presence of associated anomalies is associated with a worse prognosis compared to isolated CDH.[6]

Despite vigorous attempts to identify consistent prenatal predictors of severity, none have been substantiated beyond single institutions. Polyhydramnios, intrathoracic liver and stomach, lung to head ratio (LHR) and the lung/transverse thorax ratio are values that have all been proposed as predictors but not yet validated. MRI has recently allowed for more accurate and detailed evaluation of the fetus and may allow better prediction of severity in the future.

Current management

Neonatal mechanical ventilation was not widely available until the 1960s and, prior to that time, most infants with respiratory distress at birth died before they could undergo repair. It wasn't until 1946 that Gross reported the first infant to survive CDH repair performed at less than 24 hours of age.[7] With improvements in neonatal intensive care in the 1970s and 1980s, sicker patients survived to receive surgery in tertiary centers. During this time, the mortality rate for infants with CDH was about 50%.[8,9] Because of this persistently high mortality, newer techniques for the management of neonatal respiratory failure including extracorporeal membrane oxygenation (ECMO), high frequency oscillatory ventilation (HFOV), exogenous surfactant, permissive hypercapnea, and inhaled nitric oxide were rapidly adopted. Although some authors disagree, survival to hospital discharge appears to have improved substantially during the past decade.[10–13] In fact, several authors have recently reported survival figures approaching or exceeding 90%.[14] While such high survival statistics are encouraging, the current nationwide survival is probably best estimated by the data contained in the CDH Study Group registry which calculates a 69% survival in 2676 live born infants reported from 50 tertiary centers (Lally, KP personal communication). The actual survival, were all affected infants to be counted, is probably lower than that.

Once a prenatal diagnosis of CDH has been made, delivery at a center that is prepared for advanced neonatal care should be arranged. Delivery should be planned at or near term to allow for maximal prenatal pulmonary development.

Following delivery, care is focused on respiratory and circulatory support. Most infants require intubation immediately after birth. Mask bagging should be avoided as it can result in distension of the intrathoracic intestines and a functional tension pneumothorax. Intravenous access is usually obtained via umbilical artery or vein. A naso/orogastric tube is placed to decompress the stomach and prevent intestinal distension within the chest. A chest radiograph is obtained to confirm the presence of CDH and to check endotracheal and nasogastric tube placement. An umbilical arterial line is placed to monitor blood gases and blood pressure. A head ultrasound is obtained to look for intraventricular hemorrhage (IVH). If present, IVH is a relative but not absolute contraindication to ECMO, as the necessary anticoagulation may worsen an existing bleed. An echocardiogram is also obtained to look for any occult structural cardiac abnormalities as well as to evaluate the degree of pulmonary hypertension and functional impact on the right ventricle. Some degree of pulmonary hypertension is present in virtually all infants with CDH.

Pulmonary hypoplasia and pulmonary hypertension are the most difficult aspects of CDH to manage. Because the hypoplastic lungs are quite vulnerable to barotrauma, appropriate manipulation of ventilatory support is probably the most crucial aspect of the care of the infant with CDH. The centers with the highest survival use "gentle ventilation," which involves permissive hypercapnea, spontaneous respiration and avoidance of hyperventilation and barotrauma.

Inhaled nitric oxide (iNO) acts as a pulmonary vasodilator and can be beneficial in the context of pulmonary hypertension but in a prospective randomized trial it was not shown to improve survival of infants with congenital diaphragmatic hernias.[15] In our experience, iNO can be an important adjunct in treating CDH if used with the guidance of echocardiography to evaluate its impact on pulmonary vascular resistance and right ventricular function when initiated. Frequently, when iNO is used there will be no clinical sign of decreasing pulmonary vascular resistance even though echocardiography demonstrates this to be so.

High frequency oscillatory ventilation (HFOV) is another mode of ventilation that can be effectively used in CDH infants to maintain preductal oxygenation while avoiding hyperventilation and barotraumas.[16] It is best used at low mean airway pressures and as a primary therapy. When used as a rescue therapy, the airway pressures required only add to the barotrauma. If iNO and HFOV fail, ECMO is the next consideration. Currently, we define "failure" as a pH < 7.25 in spite of optimal ventilatory management as defined by the following thresholds: peak inspiratory pressures < 30 cm H_2O, and preductal $S_aO_2 > 60\%$ with $F_iO_2 < 60\%$.

Extracorporeal membrane oxygenation (ECMO) has become a widely accepted mode of therapy for infants with CDH who fail maximal medical therapy. A prospective randomized trial from the UK in 1996 showed that there was a significant improvement in survival with the addition of ECMO.[17] Historically, veno-arterial ECMO has been more widely used than veno-venous ECMO in CDH patients, but in recent years, veno-venous ECMO has become more widely used.

Surfactant administration has not been shown to improve outcome in infants with CDH, despite a laboratory based hypothesis that it might be advantageous. In fact, a recent report from the CDH Study Group showed that children with CDH treated with surfactant actually fare worse.[18]

Operative management

Currently, the predominant practice for CDH affected infants worldwide is to defer repair until the child is hemodynamically stabilized. This often requires several days, but may necessitate up to several weeks in rare instances. In our practice, patients who are not on ECMO have an epidural catheter placed at the start of the operative repair in order to blunt the stress response and to aid in postoperative pain control and ventilator weaning. The repair is done via an open abdominal approach through a subcostal incision. The abdominal viscera are reduced into the abdomen, and primary repair is preferred if it can be done without significant tension. Frequently, repairs require a synthetic patch to close the defect because of its size. A 1 mm thick polytetrafluoroethylene patch is the most widely used material, but several other synthetic materials have been tried. All suffer from the inability to grow or expand as the patient grows. This leads to significant long-term morbidity including chest wall abnormalities and a very high recurrence rate. A chest tube is not always necessary and is generally placed only if the infant is on ECMO.

Long-term follow-up

Traditionally, the absence of coordinated multispecialty follow-up led to an underestimate of the many problems affecting survivors of neonatal CDH, repair. More recently, data from several long-term follow-up studies has identified several potential morbidities involving pulmonary, cardiac, neurologic, gastrointestinal, urogenital, and musculoskeletal systems. Because all are predictable, some are avoidable, and others are treatable, these infants are best cared for in a multidisciplinary follow-up clinic where coordinated care involving multiple specialties is possible. No individual clinician has all the skills necessary to provide optimum care for these complex patients.

Pulmonary morbidity

Pulmonary morbidity, including pulmonary hypoplasia, bronchopulmonary dysplasia (BPD), persistent pulmonary hypertension (PPHN), reactive airway disease, and limited postnatal alveolar growth, is the most significant problem in CDH survivors, especially in the first 1–2 years. While pulmonary hypoplasia has long been considered the principal determinant of survival and non-survival, recently observed improvements in survival associated with gentler ventilatory strategies suggest that ventilator inflicted barotrauma and consequent BPD actually play a much larger role than previously suspected in both mortality and morbidity.

In a retrospective analysis of CDH survivors followed in our multidisciplinary clinic, Muratore *et al.* found that the need for ECMO and a prosthetic patch repair were associated with significantly higher pulmonary morbidity. Jaillard *et al.* report similar findings in their 2-year follow-up of CDH survivors.[19,20] However, in both reports non-ECMO survivors were also noted to have frequent pulmonary problems in the first year of follow-up. Muratore *et al.* reported that 60% of all CDH survivors received bronchodilators and 40% received inhaled steroids at some point during the first year of life.[20]

ECMO survivors who required a patch repair were also likely to have a longer period of intubation and hospitalization, as well as an increased need for diuretics and supplemental oxygen at discharge. Obstructive airway disease is demonstrable in approximately 25% of CDH children at 5 years of age in our experience; a commonly reported morbidity in other series as well.[20–23] Consequently, all of the children in our clinic have pulmonary function tests performed at age 5 years. In the study by Muratore *et al.*, serial VQ scans corroborated the data from a smaller study by Falconer *et al.* showing progressive improvement in ventilation over time in the ipsilateral lung without a change in perfusion. This is similar to the findings in other smaller series.[20–25] Initially, this observation was thought to be clinically insignificant; however, more recent (unpublished) data from our institution suggest that some children with the most severe VQ mismatch develop significant limitations in exercise tolerance in their preteen and adolescent years. Because of this, we now perform an exercise stress evaluation in all children at about the age of 10 years.

Cardiac function in CDH patients has not been well studied at present. It is known that congenital cardiac heart disease (CHD) significantly increases the mortality compared to CDH alone.[5,36] The most common associated malformations are ventricular septal defect, aortic arch obstruction, hypoplastic left heart syndrome and tetralogy of Fallot.[5,36]. Evidence of right ventricular hypertrophy on electrocardiography at 1 and 2 years of age has been reported in up to 50% of CDH patients.[24] Schwartz *et al.* report that the incidence of pulmonary hypertension is 38% at long-term follow-up for CDH patients; however, we have not generally seen this beyond the neonatal period. We believe that persistent right ventricular pressures in excess of 50% of the corresponding systemic pressures are indicative of clinically significant pulmonary hypertension, and require pharmacologic intervention to prevent long term cardiac dysfunction. Potential therapies include nitric oxide (either inhaled or in the form of an NO donor pharmaceutical agent), supplemental oxygen, inotropes, and diuretics during hospitalization, and oxygen, diuretics, and in some cases nitric oxide after discharge. We tailor the interval between echocardiograms based on the findings at initial evaluation and on other clinical indicators, but recommend follow-up study at least once at 1 year of age, even if evaluation at time of discharge does not indicate residual pulmonary hypertension.

Nutritional morbidity and growth

Growth failure is common in CDH patients and the etiology appears to be multifactorial in cause. Chronic lung disease, pulmonary hypoplasia and the increased work of breathing, gastroesophageal reflux (GER), and oral aversion all play a role. In a retrospective analysis of 121 CDH survivors followed in our multidisciplinary clinic, over half of the patients were below the 25th percentile for height and weight in the first year of life. One-third of this population had problems severe enough to require gastrostomy tube placement to improve caloric intake. The requirement for ECMO and the need for O_2 at discharge were, in our clinic, predictive of growth failure in the first year of life.[26] Jaillard *et al.* and Van Meurs *et al.* reported similar trends in ECMO-treated CDH survivors, with over 40% of their patients weighing less than the fifth percentile for weight at 2 years of age.[24,27]

Oral aversion has been shown to play a significant role in the growth failure of CDH patients. Almost 25% of CDH patients followed in our clinic display behavior consistent with oral aversion.[12] These findings correspond to the results from a follow-up of 51 CDH survivors reported by Jaillard *et al.*[19,26] Although the etiology of this oral aversion is unknown, prolonged mechanical ventilation and O_2 requirement at discharge predicted the development of oral aversion in our patients.[26] This conclusion is supported by de Larminant *et al.* who found that prolonged intubation impaired the swallowing reflex in intubated adult patients.[28]

Since CDH survivors are at high risk for nutritional failure, they should all be monitored closely by a dietician or nutritionist. In our experience, it is often necessary to give these postoperative children with CDH approximately 20% more calories than is customary in order to counterbalance the increased respiratory work of breathing and achieve adequate growth. Typically, this is done using hyperosmolar formulas to limit fluid volume, as the respiratory status of these children can be fragile.

Gastroesophageal reflux (GER)

GER was rarely discussed in association with CDH prior to 1990. More recent literature, however, demonstrates that GER is now recognized as a common complication among survivors of CDH.[29,30] Despite its frequency, the pathogenesis of this GER is not clearly understood.[30,31] It is hypothesized that partial or complete obstruction of the distal esophagus secondary to extrinsic compression from the herniated intrathoracic viscera may result in GER. Malposition and abnormal anatomy of the GE junction, absence of the perihiatal diaphragm, recurrence of CDH, and increased intraabdominal pressure after closure of the defect are suggested as possible etiologies of GER in CDH patients.[32,33]

Stolar *et al.* has described in utero esophageal dilatation in association with poor gastric motility, apparently resulting from the extrinsic pressure created by the herniated viscera. GE reflux, confirmed by pH probe, was noted in 69% of his patients with an ectatic esophagus.[30] Keiffer *et al.* noted that GER occurred in 62% of patients whose stomach was in the chest pre-operatively.[7] Kamiyama reported that the preoperative position of the left liver lobe in the chest increased the risk of pathologic GER.[34] However, Koot *et al.* report an overall incidence of 55% for GER in CDH patients, but found no correlation between GER and preoperative position of the stomach, presence or absence of a sac, or size of the defect.[35]

In our population, diaphragmatic patch repair was significantly related to refractory GER and subsequent need for an antireflux procedure.[26] Jaillard *et al.* also found patch repair to correlate with severe GER and therefore proposed an antireflux procedure at the time of repair for large diaphragmatic defects or diaphragmatic agenesis, a recommendation we have not adopted.[19,26] Vanamo *et al.* reported that over half of adult CDH survivors demonstrated endoscopic or histologic evidence of esophagitis in routine investigations for the diagnosis of GER.[4]

Recurrent bronchitis, worsening bronchopulmonary dysplasia, and aspiration pneumonia are specific complications of GER in the CDH survivor population, in addition to the more general effects on nutrition and growth.[37,38] In this group of patients with already compromised pulmonary function, prompt diagnosis and treatment is paramount. We recommend H_2-blockers or proton pump inhibitors for all patients, and pursue further work-up if signs of pulmonary morbidity develop or if clear evidence of GER is seen during evaluation of the esophagus and upper GI tract. Anti-reflux surgery is reserved for pathologic GER that persists despite maximization of medical therapy. In our clinic, this is approximately 25% of all patients.[26]

Neurocognitive deficit

In addition to impaired growth, GER, and chronic pulmonary pathology in CDH survivors, developmental delay, and neurocognitive and behavioral disorders represent additional morbidities that have been documented in CDH survivors.[4,37,39–45] Nobuhara *et al.* reported mild or moderate developmental delay in more than one-third of CDH survivors followed in our multidisciplinary clinic.[35] The most common deficit was mildly decreased tone of the extremities. Of these patients with developmental delay, 72% had been treated with ECMO.[4] Similarly, McGahren *et al.* reported that the incidence of neurological delay was 67% of ECMO-treated infants, compared to 24% of CDH survivors not requiring ECMO.[43]

In a study of 23 survivors, Davenport *et al.* reported that only 9% of CDH infants had major disabilities, specifically hemiplegia and lower limb monoplegia. None of these patients had developmental delay, and none of the infants was treated with ECMO.[40] A retrospective review of 27 ECMO-treated survivors in the UK reported significant neurologic sequelae in 26% of patients.[1] Of survivors, 22% were reported to have developmental delay, with speech and language delay in all affected, and motor delay in half of the children. Jaillard *et al.* reported that neurologic examination at 2 years of age was normal in 88% of 51 CDH survivors. They reported that developmental delay was observed in 12% of CDH survivors in their series and was associated with growth failure and hyptonia.[19] D'Agostino *et al.* reported that patients with the largest diaphragmatic defects had the highest risk of cognitive and motor delay.[46] This finding is supported by McGahren *et al.* who reported a higher probability of diaphragmatic and abdominal patch repair in CDH survivors who required ECMO.[43] Taken together, these findings suggest that CDH disease severity plays a role in the development of neurologic sequelae.[43,46]

Some contributions to the neurologic deficits described in CDH survivors are likely from the underlying disease process and the critically ill nature of these infants; however, the contribution of ECMO and other treatments to neurologic morbidity in these infants is of particular concern.[4,44,45] The relationship between treatment decisions and neurological sequelae remains to be entirely elucidated. The reported incidence of neurologic abnormalities among ECMO survivors ranges from 10 to 50%.[27,47,48] These abnormalities include cerebral palsy, hearing loss, seizure disorders, cognitive delay, vision loss, and delayed motor skills.[4,39,40,42–45]

Bernbaum *et al.* reported in a 1-year follow-up of 82 ECMO CDH survivors that a subset of patients experienced significant delays in both motor and cognitive development when compared to infants requiring ECMO with other diagnoses. The CDH infants also had a lower overall survival rate and significant comorbidities.[49] Given the frequency of comorbidities in these infants, observed differences may be attributable to the severity of the primary disease. McGahren *et al.* also found a higher incidence of adverse neurologic sequelae in a retrospective review of 37 CDH infants comparing ECMO-treated infants to those who did not require ECMO treatment. Neither duration of ECMO nor incidence of complications during ECMO had any apparent affect on the neurologic outcome. However, the need for patch closure of either the diaphragm or the abdomen and the need for gastrostomy tube for nutrition were correlated with neurologic deficits.[43] Stolar *et al.* reported on 51 CDH survivors followed prospectively in a multidisciplinary clinic.[8] This report demonstrated an increased risk of cognitive disability in CDH survivors treated with ECMO when compared to ECMO survivors with other underlying diagnoses.[45] In particular, they found that the neurocognitive outcome was significantly worse for male patients and for those patients whose mother had a limited formal education.[45] Van Meurs *et al.* reported a 17% incidence of abnormal neurodevelopment among ECMO-treated CDH survivors, and abnormal neuroimaging was found in over 75% of those imaged.[24] However, they found no significant difference in the neurodevelopmental outcome among ECMO survivors when comparing CDH and non-CDH patients.[24] Jaillard *et al.* found no significant difference in neurologic outcome in CDH survivors treated with or without ECMO.[19] Of CDH survivors, 12% had an abnormal neurologic examination, and although there was a trend toward developmental delay in ECMO-treated children, this was not statistically significant.[19] Jaillard *et al.* suggested that neurodevelopmental outcome improves with age in CDH survivors, and other studies have shown that early delay in motor skills is not predictive of future disability.[19,24,42] These discrepancies in the current literature demonstrate that more comprehensive follow-up is needed to assess long-term outcomes in CDH survivors. Frequent monitoring in the outpatient setting coupled with specific therapy for developmental delay is necessary to determine the effectiveness of early intervention.[4,44] In addition, Van Meurs *et al.* recommend neuroimaging in all ECMO-treated survivors before discharge, given the high incidence of hemorrhagic and embolic intracranial abnormalities in ECMO survivors.[4,24]

Hearing loss

Walton *et al.* reported a 37% incidence of sensorineural hearing loss among 51 surviving neonates with persistent pulmonary hypertension. Only duration of hyperventilation was significantly different between children with hearing loss and those without. Five infants in this cohort developed progressive hearing loss.[50] Nobuhara *et al.* report a 28% incidence of significant hearing loss among CDH survivors.[35] Of these patients, 71% were treated with ECMO.[4] Of note, some patients have developed progressive hearing loss despite normal baseline brainstem auditory evoked responses (BAER), stressing the need for routine periodic evaluation to detect progressive delay.[4,52]

Recurrence

The reported incidence of recurrent diaphragmatic hernia after neonatal CDH repair, and the timing of these recurrences varies widely.[4,24,50] Van Meurs *et al.* reported a 22% incidence of recurrence for the diaphragmatic hernia. Of infants requiring patch repair, 40% had a recurrence before 1 year of age.[24] In a report by Moss *et al.* on the durability of patch repair over time, approximately half of all prosthetic patches showed evidence of reherniation and required revision within 3 years.[50] Nobuhara *et al.* report a 5% incidence of recurrence overall after CDH repair, and all affected patients had had patch repair initially.[4] Patients with recurrent hernia may present with gastrointestinal complaints, which may include evidence of bowel obstruction or progressively severe vomiting. Only a few such patients will present with pulmonary signs or symptoms. A significant number will have an asymptomatic recurrence demonstrated on a surveillance chest radiograph.[50] We recommend regular surveillance with chest radiographs in all CDH survivors, a follow-up strategy also employed by Van Meurs *et al.* who recommend chest films at 2, 6, and 12 months of age to monitor for hernia recurrence.[24] We recommend annual chest radiographs at least to the age of 5 years in CDH patients repaired with a prosthetic patch.

Orthopedic deformities

Chest asymmetry and pectus deformity are the most commonly described orthopedic problems in children with CDH.[4,42,51] CDH survivors are also prone to scoliosis.[4,50] Nobuhara *et al.* reported a 21% incidence of pectus deformities and a 10% incidence of mild to moderate scoliosis.[4] Vanamo *et al.* described asymmetry of the chest wall in 48% of CDH survivors and a 27% incidence of significant scoliosis. Chest asymmetry and pectus deformities were more common among patients with a large diaphragmatic defect. Scoliosis was reported more commonly in patients with ventilatory impairment and a large diaphragmatic defect.[50] Vanamo *et al.* found that the majority of chest deformities were mild and recommended surveillance of CDH survivors into adulthood.[51] Lund *et al.* suggest pectus deformities and scoliosis may be related to diaphragmatic tension when closing the defect.[42]

Summary

The treatment of CDH survivors has undergone many changes in recent years, resulting in survival of a greater number of these critically ill infants. A new cohort of CDH patients who now survive the neonatal period has been identified in recent years. However, significant long-term morbidities exist in some of these CDH survivors that are only now being recognized and described. Although many CDH survivors are healthy and lead normal lives, others are not so fortunate. These survivors are not "fine," but they do have predictable pulmonary, gastrointestinal, nutritional, developmental, and musculoskeletal problems, many of which respond well to careful follow-up and early intervention. Consequently, because these issues transcend any single subspecialty, this group of patients is best cared for in a multidisciplinary setting.

REFERENCES

1. Arensman, R. & Bambini, D. Congenital diaphragmatic hernia and eventration. In Ashcraft, K. W. & Holder, T. M. (eds.). *Pediatric Surgery*, 3rd edn. Philadelphia: W. B. Saunders, 1999: 300.
2. Torfs, C. P., Curry, C. J., Bateson, T. F. *et al.* A population-based study of congenital diaphragmatic hernia. *Teratology* 1992; **46**:555–565.
3. DiFiore, J. W., Fauza, D. O., Slavin, R. *et al.* Experimental fetal tracheal ligation and congenital diaphragmatic hernia: a pulmonary vascular morphometric analysis. *J. Pediatr. Surg.* 1995; **30**:917–923.
4. Nobuhara, K. K., Lund, D. P., Mitchell, J. *et al.* Long-term outlook for survivors of congenital diaphragmatic hernia. *Clin. Perinatol.* 1996; **23**:873–887.
5. Fauza, D. O. & Wilson, J. M. Congenital diaphragmatic hernia and associated anomalies: their incidence, identification, and impact on prognosis. *J. Pediatr. Surg.* 1994; **29**:1113–1117.
6. Wilson, J. M., Fauza, D. O., Lund, D. P. *et al.* Antenatal diagnosis of isolated congenital diaphragmatic hernia is not an indicator of outcome. *J. Pediatr. Surg.* 1994; **29**:815–819.
7. Gross, R. E. Congenital hernia of the diaphragm. *Am. J. Dis. Child.* **579**, 1946; **71**:579–592.
8. Mishalany, H. G., Nakada, K., & Woolley, M. M. Congenital diaphragmatic hernias: eleven years' experience. *Arch. Surg.* 1979; **114**:1118–1223.
9. Wilson, J. M., Lund, D. P., Lillehei, C. W. *et al.* Congenital diaphragmatic hernia–a tale of two cities: the Boston experience. *J. Pediatr. Surg.* 1997; **32**:401–405.
10. Boloker, J., Bateman, D. A., Wung, J. T. *et al.* Congenital diaphragmatic hernia in 120 infants treated consecutively with permissive hypercapnea/spontaneous respiration/elective repair. *J. Pediatr. Surg.* 2002; **37**:357–366.
11. Javid, P. J., Jaksic, T., Skarsgard, E. D. *et al.* Survival rate in congenital diaphragmatic hernia: the experience of the Canadian Neonatal Network. *J. Pediatr. Surg.* 2004; **39**:657–660.
12. Kays, D. W., Langham, M. R., Jr., Ledbetter, D. J. *et al.* Detrimental effects of standard medical therapy in congenital diaphragmatic hernia. *Ann. Surg.* 1999; **230**:340–348.
13. Stege, G., Fenton A., & Jaffray, B. Nihilism in the 1990s: the true mortality of congenital diaphragmatic hernia. *Pediatrics* 2003; **112**:532–535.
14. Downard, C. D., Jaksic, T., Garza, J. J. *et al.* Analysis of an improved survival rate for congenital diaphragmatic hernia. *J. Pediatr. Surg.* 2003; **38**:729–732.
15. The Neonatal Inhaled Nitric Oxide Study Group (NINOS). Inhaled nitric oxide and hypoxic respiratory failure in infants with congenital diaphragmatic hernia. *Pediatrics* 1997; **99**:838–845.
16. Azarow, K., Messineo, A., Pearl, R. *et al.* Congenital diaphragmatic hernia–a tale of two cities: the Toronto experience, *J. Pediatr. Surg.* 1997; **32**:395–400.
17. UK Collaborative ECMO Trial Group. UK collaborative randomised trial of neonatal extracorporeal membrane oxygenation. *Lancet* 1996; **348**:75–82.
18. Lally, K. P., Lally, P. A., Langham, M. R. *et al.* Surfactant does not improve survival rate in preterm infants with congenital diaphragmatic hernia. *J. Pediatr. Surg.* 2004; **39**:829–833.
19. Jaillard, S. M., Pierrat, V., Dubois, A. *et al.* Outcome at 2 years of infants with congenital diaphragmatic hernia: a population-based study. *Ann. Thorac. Surg.* 2003; **75**:250–256.
20. Muratore, C. S., Kharasch, V., Lund, D. P. *et al.* Pulmonary morbidity in 100 survivors of congenital diaphragmatic hernia monitored in a multidisciplinary clinic. *J. Pediatr. Surg.* 2001; **36**:133–140.
21. Falconer, A. R., Brown, R. A., Helms, P. *et al.* Pulmonary sequelae in survivors of congenital diaphragmatic hernia. *Thorax* 1990; **45**:126–129.
22. Ijsselstijn, H., Tibboel, D., Hop, W. J. *et al.* Long-term pulmonary sequelae in children with congenital diaphragmatic hernia. *Am. J. Respir. Crit. Care Med.* 1997; **155**:174–180.
23. Wischermann, A., Holschneider, A. M., & Hubner, U. Long-term follow-up of children with diaphragmatic hernia. *Eur. J. Pediatr. Surg.* 1995; **5**:13–18.
24. Van Meurs, K. P., Robbins, S. T., Reed, V. L. *et al.* Congenital diaphragmatic hernia: long-term outcome in neonates treated with extracorporeal membrane oxygenation. *J. Pediatr.* 1993; **122**:893–899.
25. Vanamo, K., Rintala, R., Sovijarvi, A. *et al.* Long-term pulmonary sequelae in survivors of congenital diaphragmatic defects. *J. Pediatr. Surg.* 1996; **31**:1096–1099.
26. Muratore, C. S., Utter, S., Jaksic, T. *et al.* Nutritional morbidity in survivors of congenital diaphragmatic hernia. *J. Pediatr. Surg.* 2001; **36**:1171–1176.
27. Glass, P., Wagner, A. E., Papero, P. H. *et al.* Neurodevelopmental status at age five years of neonates treated with extracorporeal membrane oxygenation. *J. Pediatr.* 1995; **127**:447–457.
28. de Larminat, V., Montravers, P., Dureuil, B. *et al.* Alteration in swallowing reflex after extubation in intensive care unit patients. *Crit. Care. Med.* 1995; **23**:486–490.
29. Muratore, C. S. & Wilson, J. M. Congenital diaphragmatic hernia: where are we and where do we go from here? *Semin. Perinatol.* 2000; **24**:418–428.
30. Stolar, C. J., Levy, J. P., Dillon, P. W. *et al.* Anatomic and functional abnormalities of the esophagus in infants surviving congenital diaphragmatic hernia. *Am. J. Surg.* 1990; **159**:204–207.
31. Fasching, G., Huber, A., Uray, E. *et al.* Gastroesophageal reflux and diaphragmatic motility after repair of congenital diaphragmatic hernia. *Eur. J. Pediatr. Surg.* 2000; **10**:360–364.
32. Kieffer, J., Sapin, E., Berg, A. *et al.* Gastroesophageal reflux after repair of congenital diaphragmatic hernia. *J. Pediatr. Surg.* 1995; **30**:1330–1333.

33. Sigalet, D. L., Nguyen, L. T., Adolph, V. *et al.* Gastroesophageal reflux associated with large diaphragmatic hernias. *J. Pediatr. Surg.* 1994; **29**:1262–1265.
34. Kamiyama, M., Kawahara, H., Okuyama, H. *et al.* Gastroesophageal reflux after repair of congenital diaphragmatic hernia. *J. Pediatr. Surg.* 2002; **37**:1681–1684.
35. Koot, V. C., Bergmeijer, J. H., Bos, A. P. *et al.* Incidence and management of gastroesophageal reflux after repair of congenital diaphragmatic hernia. *J. Pediatr. Surg.* 1993; **28**:48–52.
36. Cohen, M. S., Rychik, J., Bush, D. M. *et al.* Influence of congenital heart disease on survival in children with congenital diaphragmatic hernia. *J. Pediatr.* 2002; **141**:25–30.
37. Fonkalsrud E. W. & Ament, M. E. Gastroesophageal reflux in childhood. *Curr. Probl. Surg.* 1996; **33**:1–70.
38. St, Cyr., J. A., Ferrara, T. B., Thompson, T. *et al.* Treatment of pulmonary manifestations of gastroesophageal reflux in children two years of age or less. *Am. J. Surg.* 1989; **157**:400–403.
39. Bouman, N. H., Koot, H. M., Tibboel, D. *et al.* Children with congenital diaphragmatic hernia are at risk for lower levels of cognitive functioning and increased emotional and behavioral problems. *Eur. J. Pediatr. Surg.* 2000; **10**:3–7.
40. Davenport, M., Rivlin, E., D'Souza, S. W. *et al.* Delayed surgery for congenital diaphragmatic hernia: neurodevelopmental outcome in later childhood. *Arch. Dis. Child.* 1992; **67**:1353–1356.
41. Hunt, R. W., Kean, M. J., Stewart, M. J. *et al.* Patterns of cerebral injury in a series of infants with congenital diaphragmatic hernia utilizing magnetic resonance imaging. *J. Pediatr. Surg.* 2004; **39**:31–36.
42. Lund, D. P., Mitchell, J., Kharasch, V. *et al.* Congenital diaphragmatic hernia: the hidden morbidity. *J. Pediatr. Surg.* 1994; **29**:258–262.
43. McGahren, E. D., Mallik, K., & Rodgers, B. M. Neurological outcome is diminished in survivors of congenital diaphragmatic hernia requiring extracorporeal membrane oxygenation. *J. Pediatr. Surg.* 1997; **32**:1216–1220.
44. Rasheed, A., Tindall, S., Cueny, D. L. *et al.* Neurodevelopmental outcome after congenital diaphragmatic hernia: extracorporeal membrane oxygenation before and after surgery. *J. Pediatr. Surg.* 2001; **36**:539–544.
45. Stolar, C. J., Crisafi, M. A., & Driscoll, Y. T. Neurocognitive outcome for neonates treated with extracorporeal membrane oxygenation: are infants with congenital diaphragmatic hernia different? *J. Pediatr. Surg.* 1995; **30**:366–371.
46. D'Agostino, J. A., Bernbaum, J. C., Gerdes, M. *et al.* Outcome for infants with congenital diaphragmatic hernia requiring extracorporeal membrane oxygenation: the first year. *J. Pediatr. Surg.* 1995; **30**:10–15.
47. Bennett, C. C., Johnson, A., Field, D. J., *et al.* UK collaborative randomised trial of neonatal extracorporeal membrane oxygenation: follow-up to age 4 years. 2001; *Lancet* **357**:1094–1096.
48. Hofkosh, D., Thompson, A. E., Nozza, R. J. *et al.* Ten years of extracorporeal membrane oxygenation: neurodevelopmental outcome. *Pediatrics* 1991; **87**:549–555.
49. Bernbaum, J., Schwartz, I. P., Gerdes, M. *et al.* Survivors of extracorporeal membrane oxygenation at 1 year of age: the relationship of primary diagnosis with health and neurodevelopmental sequelae. *Pediatrics* 1995; **96**:907–913.
50. Moss, R. L., Chen, C. M., & Harrison, M. R. Prosthetic patch durability in congenital diaphragmatic hernia: a long-term follow-up study. *J. Pediatr. Surg.* 2001; **36**:152–154.
51. Vanamo, K., Peltonen, J., Rintala, R. *et al.* Chest wall and spinal deformities in adults with congenital diaphragmatic defects. *J. Pediatr. Surg.* 1996; **31**:851–854.
52. Cheung, P. Y., Haluschak, M. M., Finer, N. N. *et al.* Sensorineural hearing loss in survivors of neonatal extracorporeal membrane oxygenation. *Early Hum. Dev.* 1996; **44**:225–233.

13

Surgical management of airway obstruction

Dana Mara Thompson, Robin T. Cotton

Department of Pediatric Otolaryngology and the Aerodigestive and Sleep Center, Cincinnati Children's Hospital Medical Center and The University of Cincinnati College of Medicine, OH, USA

Surgical management of obstructive diseases of the pediatric airway is challenging and rewarding. These diseases may present with acute, life-threatening airway obstruction and warrant quick relief of obstruction often accomplished by endotracheal intubation or tracheotomy. The etiology of obstructive airway disease is often multifactorial, and includes anatomic, congenital, and inflammatory problems. Regardless of the cause and mode of presentation, diagnosis and successful surgical management requires a high index of suspicion and clinical experience to establish the correct diagnosis and formulate a surgical solution. To achieve good surgical outcomes, meticulous attention to detail, recognition and treatment of other medical comorbidities that affect healing, and complete dedication of the surgeon's time and resources are required. These resources include many other pediatric specialists and other allied health care individuals. The priority of intervention is to establish and maintain a safe and stable airway. One must also recognize that diseases causing airway obstruction and the surgical interventions to correct these problems may compromise voice, speech, and swallowing. The impact of these diseases and their surgical interventions may have tremendous socialization implications for children at a critical phase of growth and development. Because of the potential impact and devastating outcomes these diseases and interventions may have on medical and psychosocial development of children, we are obliged to examine our interventions to assume the best possible outcomes for airway, voice, swallowing, and socialization. The number of children who require surgical intervention for airway obstruction has increased. This is due in part to the development of long term intubation and ventilation techniques in the 1960s that increased the number of critically ill mature infants who survived. As a result of long-term intubation, these infants are now able to survive, however, with an entirely new spectrum of long-term health problems including those of the airway, particularly the larynx and trachea. Infants who develop laryngotracheal stenosis often require a tracheotomy. Tracheotomy allowed many such infants to be raised at home by their parents, but tracheotomy-associated morbidity and mortality become the next challenge in management of this patient population. These complications have been the catalyst for development of improved materials for endotracheal tubes and for better techniques of home tracheotomy management.

Beginning in the early 1970s, modern techniques for expansion of the narrowed subglottis were described. These airway expansion techniques allow for early decannulation of many such infants. With increased surgical experience and improved techniques, identification and management of comorbidities that affect outcomes, and improvement in postoperative care, the indications for airway expansion surgery have been extended to patients with laryngotracheal stenosis as the primary definitive operation, thus avoiding tracheotomy.[1–4] The next challenge in airway surgery is to develop innovative techniques that preserve and improve voice quality and communication ability, as these will have a positive impact on psychosocial development. This review will focus the discussion on evaluation, surgical management, and long-term outcomes of laryngotracheal airway obstruction. These airway problems are more commonly evaluated and managed at a tertiary care pediatric facility by a multidisciplinary

Pediatric Surgery and Urology: Long-term Outcomes, Mark Stringer, Keith Oldham, Pierre Mouriquand. Published by Cambridge University Press.

team. Descriptions of specific operative techniques for airway surgery will be brief. The reader is referred elsewhere for more details.[5]

Airway pathophysiology and diagnostic considerations

The larynx is the entry point for air into the tracheobronchial tree and respiratory system. Without a functioning larynx, the remainder of the respiratory system is compromised. The phylogenetic purposes of the larynx are respiration and protection of the lower airway from aspiration. Voice is an evolutionary and secondary function of the larynx. The pediatric airway differs from the adult airway in structure and function. The infant larynx is approximately one-third its adult size, measuring approximately 7 mm in the sagittal dimension and 4 mm in the coronal plane. The vocal cords are 6–8 mm long. The subglottic space is approximately 4.5 mm across and is bounded by the cricoid cartilage, the only complete ring of cartilage in the upper airway and the narrowest portion of the upper airway. Therefore, only 1 mm of mucosal edema in this portion of the infant airway can reduce the airway by 40%. As the airway dimensions increase with age, mucosal edema causes less compromise of the airway. The cartilaginous framework of the larynx and trachea is softer and more pliable in infancy. This can lead to a tendency to collapse under external compression or air pressure gradients which may lead to airway obstruction as seen in laryngomalacia and tracheomalacia. As the infant grows and the cartilage matures and becomes more rigid, symptoms of these conditions often spontaneously improve and resolve without intervention. In the infant, the larynx sits high in the neck at the level of vertebrae C2 and C3, directly behind the nose with approximation of the velum, tongue, and epiglottis, thereby functionally separating respiration from swallowing. Because neuromuscular function for airway protection is not fully developed at this stage, this intended anatomic relationship allows the infant to safely breathe and feed at the same time without aspirating. With this anatomic relationship, however, any obstruction of the nasal cavity can cause significant obstruction of the airway, which also causes feeding difficulty. In conjunction with neuromuscular maturation the position of the larynx descends in the neck. By the age of 2 years, the larynx descends to C4, thereby creating less of a functional separation between the acts of breathing and swallowing. By age 6, the larynx has descended to its adult location at C6. Airway and swallowing symptoms tend to be exaggerated if neuromuscular function is compromised or has not matured in conjunction with descent of the larynx.

A variety of clinical signs and symptoms are associated with airway obstruction and in the acute setting including stridor, respiratory distress, apnea, cyanosis, pallor, tachypnea, use of muscles accessory of respiration and retractions, and mental status changes. Chronically obstructed airways may present with similar signs and symptoms or patients may develop long-term complications of airway obstruction and hypoxia such as failure to thrive, poor weight gain, pulmonary hypertension, and pectus deformities. Regardless, if the airway is acutely or chronically obstructed, observation and characterization of the strider is the most useful non-invasive clinical examination for determining location of the obstruction in the airway. Stridor is caused by turbulent airflow through a narrowed lumen. It is present in virtually all children with airway obstruction, except those with little airflow who are on the verge of complete asphyxia. The phase of respiration in which the stridor is heard will help the astute examiner better determine the location of the lesion. Inspiratory stridor is typically heard in obstructive lesions above the glottis such as laryngomalacia and vocal cord paralysis. Biphasic stridor is heard in a fixed obstruction below the glottis in the subglottis or trachea. Expiratory stridor is typically heard in diseases of the intrathoracic airway such as tracheomalacia. Obstructive lesions of the airway may be mistakenly diagnosed as asthma on the basis of a respiratory "wheeze;" therefore, a high index of suspicion and correlation with other clinical examination findings are essential so as to not overlook a potentially critical or surgically correctable cause of airway obstruction.

Further evaluation begins with assessment of the degree of respiratory embarrassment. An extensive diagnostic evaluation is inappropriate for any child with severe airway obstruction, where attaining a safe airway is a critical priority. Common evaluations of airway obstruction include simple and sophisticated radiographs and aerodigestive track endoscopy. High kilovoltage airway films are useful to screen for airway pathology, but are not diagnostic and should be correlated with clinical examination and findings. These films can be useful to screen for supraglottic pathology, such as acute epiglottitis or tongue base cyst that may lead to retroflexed positioning of the epiglottis. Subglottic narrowing can be seen in inflammatory conditions of the subglottis such as croup, subglottic stenosis, and subglottic tumors such as a hemangioma. Narrowing or tapering of the tracheal airway may suggest tracheal stenosis or extrinsic compression of the trachea by lesions like a vascular ring. Dynamic airway fluoroscopy may help better determine the presence of tracheomalacia. Fluoroscopy of the airway may help detect dynamic tongue base problems that obstruct the supraglottic airway. Fluoroscopy is also helpful to screen for dynamic collapse of the trachea with respiration, which can be seen in tracheomalacia or extrinsic compression of the airway. Gastrointestinal contrast radiographic studies are not helpful to define obstructive lesions of the airway itself. However, this study may outline an indentation of the esophagus that may suggest a complete vascular ring compressing the airway in addition to the esophagus. Contrast esophagram is also a screening test for gastroesophageal reflux disease (GERD). GERD can cause inflammation of the airway. Reflux-related complications may cause acute or chronic airway obstruction. Aspiration of barium contrast into the airway may suggest the possibility of a laryngeal cleft, which is a surgically correctable cause of airway obstruction. Communication between the esophagus and trachea may suggest a tracheoesophageal fistula.

More sophisticated radiographic studies of the airway obstruction include MRI and CT scans. Cross-sectional imaging studies of the chest using either CT or MRI is useful for evaluating extrinsic compression from vascular structures or mediastinal tumors.[6] MRI of the head is indicated in a child with inspiratory stridor and on other lower cranial nerve symptoms such as dysphagia and aspiration or findings such as vocal cord paralysis. Studies have shown children with this combination of symptoms may have brainstem pathology such as a Chiari malformation or hydrocephalus that once identified and treated often results in complete reversal of the presenting airway symptom.[7,8]

Endoscopic evaluation of the airway has revolutionized the diagnosis and management of the obstructed airway. Endoscopic evaluations are separated into those done awake and those done under sedation or general anesthesia. Flexible fiberoptic nasopharyngoscopy and laryngoscopy is done with the child awake. This technique permits for safe, rapid examination of the nose, hypopharynx, supraglottis and glottis in virtually all children, despite age or the lack of cooperation. The awake state allows for evaluation of the dynamics of supraglottic tone, vocal fold mobility, and the impact of fixed obstructing lesions of the larynx. Examination under the influence of sedation or general anesthesia can alter the findings; therefore a significant cause of airway obstruction, particularly laryngomalacia and vocal cord paralysis could be overlooked. Application of this technique has even been expanded to evaluate swallowing function in relationship to airway obstruction, by feeding the child developmentally appropriate foods while observing laryngeal function.[9–11] Direct examination of the airway under general anesthesia or sedation remains the mainstay in diagnosis and confirmation of lesions that obstruct the airway, particularly those below the glottis that cannot be accurately evaluated by awake fiberoptic examination. Specifics in technique are not discussed here and the reader is referred elsewhere.[12,13] Airway endoscopy confirms the presence of suspected laryngotracheal pathology such as subglottic stenosis and tracheal stenosis. Endoscopic evaluation of the esophagus is warranted in selected cases. With increased understanding of the impact and role of gastroesophageal reflux disease in airway disease, endoscopic evaluation of the esophagus for GERD has become a more commonly performed evaluation in the child with airway obstruction.

The role of GERD in airway disease should not be underestimated.[14–16] Any obstruction of the airway promotes changes in intrathoracic pressure to facilitate breathing, and these in turn, promote GERD. Once acid reflux becomes extraesophageal and reaches the structures of the hypopharynx and larynx where it is aspirated into the subglottis and trachea, its impact can be quite deleterious. Extraesophageal reflux, more commonly known as laryngopharyngeal reflux (LPR) can cause local inflammation and mucosal edema that can lead to airway obstruction especially in the very small infantile larynx. Chronic acid exposure can lead to airway scarring and stenosis.[14,17–19] The most sensitive test for GERD in airway disease is 24-hour esophageal pH monitoring[20,21] with a dual probe, with the proximal probe in the upper esophageal sphincter region. Aggressive medical and sometimes surgical treatment of GERD is essential to achieve good outcomes of reconstructive airway surgery and to maintain airway patency after successful relief of airway obstruction.

Tracheotomy

Indications

Tracheotomy is the most commonly employed surgical means of management of an acute or critical airway obstruction by a non-airway surgeon. Because it is the definitive procedure to bypass an obstruction in the airway, indications, technique, complications, and functional and developmental implications of this procedure will be discussed first. There are three major indications for long-term tracheotomy in children: airway obstruction, need for ventilatory support, and pulmonary toilet. Most children with tracheotomy tubes in place for airway obstruction undergo the procedure as very young infants; either for acquired subglottic stenosis related to prolonged endotracheal intubation or for congenital lesions compromising the airway.

Patients requiring tracheotomy for ventilatory support are a more heterogeneous group. Respiratory failure may be associated with prematurity, central nervous system disease, or pulmonary infection. With medical advances in management of former premature infants with respiratory failure and more children developing respiratory compromise as a complication of other medical diseases that are being more aggressively treated, there has been a steady increase in this group of patients with tracheotomy. Most of these patients have the potential to get decannulated; however, they may develop trach tube related complications that may cause airway obstruction and require further surgical management to achieve decannulation. Children requiring tracheotomy for pulmonary toilet generally have some degree of aspiration. Most are neurologically impaired and aspirate because of a poorly coordinated swallowing mechanism, thereby requiring a way to remove the aspirated material. Critical airway obstruction is uncommon in this group of children, as they are rarely dependent on the tracheotomy tube for airway support. Even if they do acquire obstructive lesions of the airway, extensive surgical procedures to achieve decannulation are generally not recommended because of the potential compromise of the reconstructive effort by chronic aspiration.

Technique

The technique of pediatric tracheotomy that is preferred by the present authors is as follows. The patient is taken to the operating room and the airway is secured with an endotracheal tube. Because the typical landmarks for tracheotomy may be difficult to identify due to the small size of the larynx and cricoid, tracheotomy in the emergent setting is best done with an airway secured either by intubation or rigid bronchoscopy. A vertical incision is made over the midline of the neck, its superior extent at the cricoid cartilage. Subcutaneous fat is removed with electrocautery, and the fascia is divided in layers in the midline. The strap muscles are separated at the raphe, and the tyroid isthmus is divided with the electrocautery. Vertical 4–0 non-absorbable "stay sutures" are placed though the third and fourth tracheal cartilage rings on the right and left sides just off of the midline and tied loosely. Gentle tension is applied to these sutures to elevate the tracheal rings and then, the airway is entered with a blade in the midline between the third and fourth rings. As seen in Fig. 13.1 the stoma is created by placing 4–0 chromic gut sutures through the cut edge of the trachea and sewn to skin. Some authors note that the above technique fashions a more "permanent" stoma, and may result in a persistent tracheocutaneous fistula after decannulation. Since the major sources of mortality in pediatric tracheotomy are accidental decannulation or inability to replace an obstructed tube, the authors feel that the added margin of safety, particularly in the first few days, is justification for the approach outlined. In addition, pediatric tracheotomies are rarely short term, and even without the skin sutures, the tract tends to epithelialize over time.

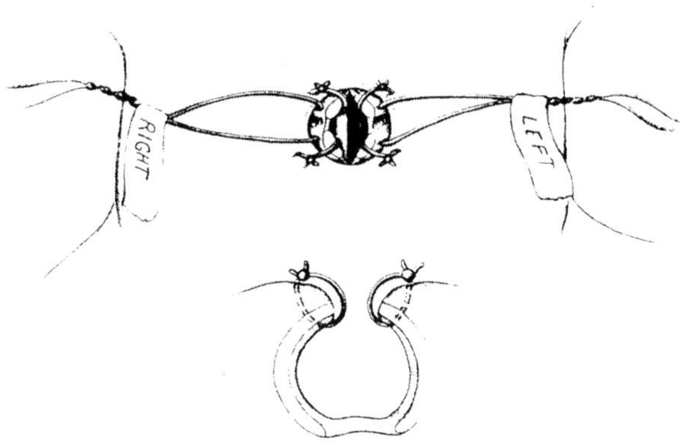

Fig. 13.1. Pediatric tracheotomy technique as preferred by the authors.[13]

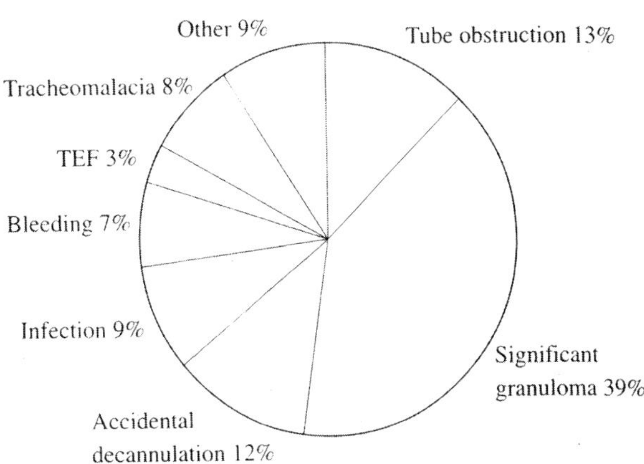

Fig. 13.2. Relative proportions of late complications derived from the literature review in Table 13.1. The data are derived from a total of 423 late complications in 1254 patients, excluding 42 patients with persistent tracheocutaneous fistula (since it was not uniformly considered in other series) and 15 patients with subglottic stenosis (since it cannot be determined that this was actually a complication of the tracheotomy itself).

The endotracheal tube (or bronchoscope) is withdrawn, an appropriate-sized tracheotomy tube is inserted, and ventilation is assured bilaterally. As seen in Fig. 13.2, the previously placed stay sutures labeled for both the right and left sides are then taped to the anterior chest wall to serve as emergency traction lines in the event of accidental decannulation. The tracheotomy tube is secured around the neck with cotton twill ties. A tracheotomy tube, particularly if it does not have an inner cannula, should never be

Table 13.1. Long-term follow-up in pediatric tracheotomy, with incidence of selected late complications

Author	Year	*n*	Airway obstruction	Age range (mo)	Patients with late complications	No. of late complications	Tube obstruction	Significant granuloma*	Accidental decannulation	Infection	Bleeding	Tracheo-esophageal fistula	Tracheo-malacia	Other	Trach related mortality
Gaudet *et al.*[a]	1978	123	63	0–144	30	36	1	5	1	1	0	0	1	27†	3
Wetmore *et al.*[b]	1982	420	164	0–252	n/a	222	23	54	40	18	22	0	12	53‡	8
Carter *et al.*[c]	1983	164	126	0–158	n/a	35	3	17	0	7	0	0	4	4	0
Kenna *et al.*[d]	1987	124	88	0–12	39	47	2	28	0	0	5	1	6	5	3
Crysdale *et al.*[e]	1988	319	222	0–240	74	101	18	50	5	9	1	10	7	1	3
Gianoli *et al.*[f]	1990	60	28	0–12	23	33	7	15	2	2	1	0	2	4	1
Zeitouni *et al.*[g]	1993	44	25	0–12	6	6	3	0	2	0	1	0	0	0	2
Totals		1254	716		n/a	480	57	169	50	37	30	11	32	94	20

* Some authors group suprastomal and distal granuloma together when reporting complications; †Includes 15 patients who developed subglottic stenosis, possibly related to underlying conditions or previous intubation; ‡Includes 42 patients with tracheocutaneous fistula, not considered as a complication in other series; n/a, not available.

[a] Gaudet, P. T. *et al. Laryngorcope* 1978; **88**:1633–1641.

[b] Wetmore, R. F. *et al. Ann. Otol. Rhinol. Laryngol.* 1982; **91**:628–632.

[c] Carter, P. *et al. Ann. Otol. Rhinol. Laryngol.* 1983; **92**:398–400.

[d] Kenna, M. A. *et al. Ann. Otol. Rhinol. Laryngol.* 1987; **96**:68–71.

[e] Crysdale, W. S. *et al. Ann. Otol. Rhinol. Laryngol.* 1988; **97**:439–443.

[f] Gianoli, G. J. *et al. Ann. Otol. Rhinol. Laryngol.* 1990; **99**:896–901.

[g] Zeitouni, A. *et al. J. Otolaryngol.* 1993; **22**: 431–443.

directly sewn to the skin of a child. In the scenario of a significant life-threatening mucous plug obstructing the trach tube, particularly in the immediate postoperative period as the tract has not fully mucosalized, having a tube secured to the skin presents a significant challenge for removal and replacement with a patent clean tube changed emergently. Postoperative deaths have occurred in this scenario. Ideally, the position of the tracheotomy tube is evaluated by passing a telescope through the glottis, along side of the tracheotomy tube. This allows the surgeon to assure that the tip of the tracheostomy tube is proximal to the carina. This technique also allows the surgeon to evaluate the fit of the trach tube within the lumen of the trachea. This relationship is ideally colinear and cocentric without any abrasion or encroachment on the anterior or posterior tracheal wall. If assessment by this method is not possible, a flexible bronchoscope can be passed through the tracheostomy tube to ensure that the tip is proximal to the carina. The tracheotomy tube is changed and the stay sutures are removed in about 5 days, once the tract has mucosalized. These patients should be managed in a monitored in-hospital setting at least until the tract has mucosalized and a successful change of the tracheotomy tube has occurred.

Rare complications of pneumothorax do occur, so a chest X-ray should be done at the end of the procedure. The most common and life-threatening immediate postoperative complications are mucus plugging and accidental decannulation.

Long-term complications

As seen in Table 13.1 several series report long-term follow-up of children with tracheotomy tubes detailing a variety of late complications. Early and perioperative complications were discussed above; however, it is important to note that risk of some complications is a reality throughout the entire time a child has a tracheotomy tube. The common complications that can occur at any time include mucous plugging leading to airway obstruction, accidental decannulation, granulation tissue formation, or occlusion of the trach tube due to inappropriate size tracheotomy tube. As seen in Fig. 13.3, tracheal granulomas and granulation tissue formation are the most common long-term complication and can cause significant airway obstruction. Accidental decannulation is probably the most common fatal late complication. Bleeding from a tracheo-innominate fistula is relatively uncommon but is the most lethal complication. Suprastomal collapse and suprastomal tracheomalacia are the late complications that are most likely to prevent decannulation, but sometimes can be corrected by a reconstructive procedure depending on the amount of malacia present.

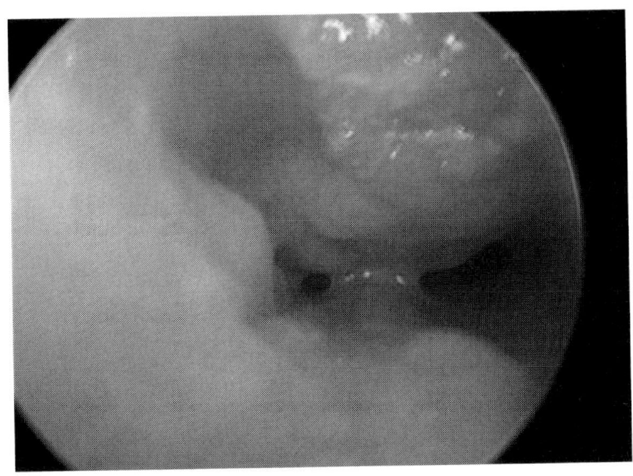

Fig. 13.3. Obstructing granulation tissue in distal trachea caused by aggressive suction trauma.

Because distal airway obstruction in the child with the tracheotomy is a potentially lethal complication, special care must be taken to prevent it. This risk is more pronounced in the very young child with a small margin for safety in the airway lumen. Granulation tissue is the most common culprit, related to either the irritating presence of the tracheotomy tube or to excessive suctioning (Fig. 13.3). For this reason, care should be taken when the tracheotomy tube is initially placed to ensure that the tip is well above the carina and the tube is colinear and cocentric within the lumen of the airway. Some tracheotomy tubes are supplied in various lengths for the same diameter, and a longer tube can be mistakenly placed during a routine change, leading to distal airway obstruction. It is of the utmost importance to ensure that whoever is changing the tube, understands the difference between neonatal and pediatric lengths and does not simply rely on the outer diameter in selecting a replacement.

Obstructing granulation tissue requires removal. Removal techniques vary based on the size of the airway, location, and extent. Removal of distal granulation has traditionally been done with electrocautery or laser. With the recent introduction of powered rotary instrumentation to laryngeal and tracheal surgery, a good option now exists for removal of the granulation without causing a thermal injury to the underlying trachea as with cautery or laser. Adjunctive therapy with the use of topical steroids may reduce granulation tissue and minimize the inflammatory response that encourages its formation. Recent studies suggest that the application of topical mitomycin C prevents reformation of granulation tissue, particularly in the setting of an acute inflammatory response. Final assessments of outcomes of this off label use of mitomycin C are not available.[22] Once the granulation tissue has been removed, caregivers should be cautioned against excessively vigorous suctioning.

Tracheal and bronchial stenosis below the tracheotomy site related to local trauma is rare but even more difficult than granulation tissue to manage successfully. It is usually caused by local trauma from overly aggressive suctioning. Since this results in mature scar, topical preparations are not helpful. Bronchial stenosis is difficult to repair by open techniques and may require ECMO or bypass support to allow sleeve resection with anastomosis. Bronchial stenosis can be successfully managed by endoscopic techniques. Open surgical and endoscopic techniques of surgery for tracheal stenosis described later in this chapter may be employed for management of the child who otherwise no longer requires a tracheotomy tube. If the tracheotomy tube is a necessity, the obstruction must be opened and then bypassed with a longer tracheotomy tube to prevent restenosis. If the stenosis extends beyond the trachea into the mainstem bronchus, a variety of stenting methods may be required to maintain patency and air exchange to the lungs.

Accidental decannulation remains a major concern, especially as a young child develops the manual dexterity to remove his or her own tracheotomy tube. This may be a fatal event in the child with near total obstruction of the airway above the tracheotomy tube. Although not universally adopted, many caregivers recommend home apnea monitors or pulse oximeters to assist caregivers in detecting such a situation. In many cases, the child will still be able to breathe comfortably through the stoma and care should be taken to replace the tube rapidly, but safely. Hastily performed insertion of the cannula may result in tracheal perforation and placement of the tube into a false tract, leading to airway compromise where none existed previously. Anecdotally, it is notable that patients have returned for a follow-up appointment months after an accidental decannulation, with a closed tracheotomy tract and no sign of respiratory distress.

Recent advances in engineering have made mechanical failure of the tracheotomy tube extremely rare. Metal tubes are rarely used in children because they are unable to conform to the airway and can cause significant anterior tracheal wall erosion. Metal tubes, by design, have an inner cannula that compromises the lumen diameter. A variety of tubes are available for the pediatric patient, but most utilize soft silicone (Argyle™, Bivona™), wire-reinforced silicone (Bivona™), or polyvinyl chloride (Shiley™, Portex™). These conform to the tract and do not promote the accumulation of inspissated secretions. Suctioning is made easier by their design and they avoid the need for an inner cannula, commonly found in adult and metal tubes, which compromises the lumen diameter. These materials avoid a stiff, brittle interface with the external neck plate. One-piece construction further reduces the risk of materials failure. Care must be taken with customized tubes, which may have weak points at fabrication joints.

Complications related to local infection of either the skin and soft tissue surrounding the stoma (cellulitis), the tracheal mucosa (tracheitis), or the tracheal cartilage (chondritis) are rare in the mature tracheotomy tract. By approximating the skin directly to the cut edge of the tracheal cartilage, epithelialization of the tract is accelerated and healing promoted. Nevertheless, some patients may develop local infections after the perioperative period. Typically, these individuals have some underlying predisposition to breakdown and bacterial invasion, such as drug-induced immunosuppression, primary immunodeficiency, or diabetes. Treatment is with local antimicrobial packing, frequent dressing and cannula changes, and systemic antibiotics. The choice of antibiotics is dictated by culture. *Staphylococcus* and *Pseudomonas* infections are frequently seen in the intensive care unit setting. Aggressive infections can lead to chondritis with breakdown of the wound, exposure of the great vessels, and extension of infection into the mediastinum.

Suprastomal granuloma formation is a nearly universal consequence of the presence of a chronic foreign body in the airway. Although some authors recommend routine removal of this tissue at regular intervals, this is not necessary in all patients. Overly aggressive removal of granulomas leads to more frequent recurrences, further arguing against routine excision.[23] Granulomas that completely obstruct the suprastomal airway require removal because of the potential for complete airway obstruction if the tube becomes blocked or displaced, as well as to preserve phonation. Parents are usually the first to note symptoms or findings that may suggest suprastomal granuloma formation. Most common are progressive loss of voice and difficulty changing the tracheotomy tube. Voice loss occurs because the granuloma prevents the necessary air passage around the trach tube that is required to vibrate the vocal cords for voice production. Perhaps the most dramatic and lethal of all late tracheotomy complications is that of innominate artery erosion. As seen in Fig. 13.4, this vessel arises from the aortic arch to cross in front of the trachea and give rise to the right common carotid and subclavian arteries. The

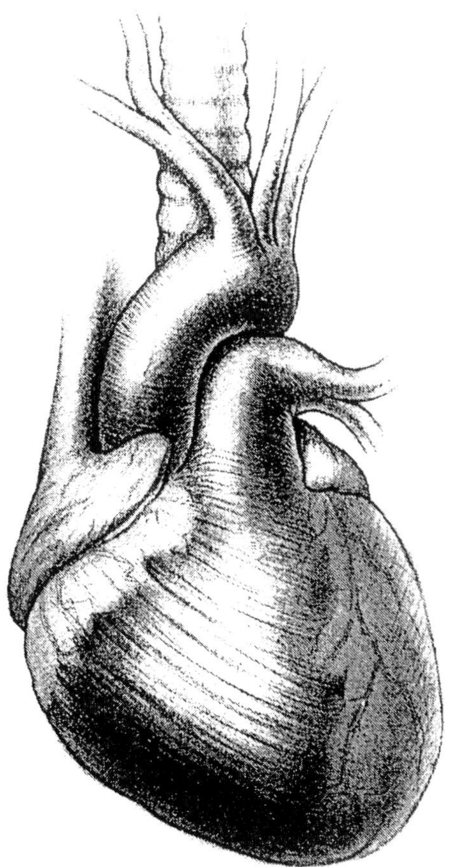

Fig. 13.4. The innominate artery crossing the trachea.[13]

tracheotomy cannula can generate pressure against the anterior tracheal wall causing granulation tissue formation, injury to the cartilage and eventual erosion if not identified. Rigid and inappropriately curved tubes are notorious for causing this, thus emphasizing the importance of appropriate tracheotomy tube size selection. If the anterior wall is eroded in the region of the innominate artery, the vessel will be exposed to the contaminated tracheal lumen. Similar to a carotid blowout following head and neck surgery, the vessel wall is progressively weakened by desiccation and local infection. Often, a sentinel bleed of bright red blood will alert the clinician to impending arterial rupture. For this reason, even small amounts of suctioned blood should be evaluated fully by a physician by removing the cannula and inspecting the tract with a flexible telescope to rule out major vessel exposure. If a tracheo-innominate fistula is suspected, further evaluation should be done in the operating room. Placing a small endotracheal tube in the tract to ensure ventilation and protect the airway best controls active bleeding. If the tract is large enough, a cuffed tube may be used to prevent aspiration of blood. Finger pressure should compress the vessel between the tracheal wall and the posterior surface of the manubrium. Definitive management requires sternotomy, with division or repair of the innominate artery. Although some authors describe the use of aortography as the initial step in the evaluation and management of patients with suspected tracheo-innominate fistula, we do not recommend this approach as delay in the diagnosis and management increases the risk of a fatality. If one's index of suspicion is this high, it is unwise to bring a potentially unstable patient to a radiology suite. Additionally, if bleeding from a fistula is intermittent, the study may be falsely negative. Any serious suspicion of an impending innominate artery rupture should undergo a mediastinal exploration with a thoracic surgeon available.

In the same manner that the anterior wall of the trachea can erode from the continued pressure of a tracheal cannula, the posterior wall can break down as well. This is fairly uncommon as a late complication, although the presence of an indwelling nasogastric tube worsens the situation by trapping the posterior wall between two rigid foreign bodies. The diagnosis is suspected in patients with unexplained recurrent pneumonia, pneumomediastinum, or if a ventilated patient has eructation with each inspiratory breath. This complication is traditionally managed by an open surgical procedure, with interposition of healthy muscle between the trachea and the esophagus.

Speech, and swallowing function with a tracheotomy

The concept of the "critical stage" has been applied to many areas of child development. A variety of studies suggests the importance of early stimulation of the sense organs in the acquisition of visual and communicative skills.[24] A tracheotomy alters the normal pathways for phonation, olfaction, and deglutition. Since many children with tracheotomies have been cannulated since early infancy, there is concern regarding the eventual long-term outcomes following decannulation.

Human oral communication is a complex process in which different anatomical structures work in synchrony to produce intelligible speech. Leaving aside problems with the cognitive control mechanism, the two types of speech dysfunction, which may be caused by tracheotomy, are dysphonia and dysarthria. The former refers to phonation or the production of pure tone by vibration of the vocal ligament mucosa in the transglottic airstream. Any injury to this delicate layer may result in interference with the sound-producing vibratory wave. Even in patients without glottic injury, obstruction to airflow past the tracheotomy tube can result in inadequate subglottic air pressure and ineffective phonation. This obstruction may be due to suprastomal tracheomalacia, granulation tissue, or a tracheotomy cannula that is large for airway lumen.

Dysarthria refers to problems with formation of speech elements by concerted muscular action on the entire vocal tract (including the mouth and tongue). Children with tracheotomies may develop adaptive patterns of speech while the tube is present. Once decannulated, they can have difficulties forming a variety of sounds.[25]

Long-term results in speech acquisition may be affected even after decannulation. A comparison of late outcomes in patients decannulated in both prelingual and linguistic stages of development have shown spoken language delays related to the time of removal of the tracheotomy tube. Children decannulated in the prelingual stage exhibited normal speech development, while those decannulated in the linguistic stage demonstrated an increased incidence of communication impairment. Speech and language therapy was successful in aiding 20 of 23 children with impairment to attain appropriate speech.[26] Other authors have similarly reported post decannulation acquisition of intelligible speech – appropriate for the patient's cognitive level – with appropriate instruction.[27]

Swallowing may also be affected by the presence of tracheal cannula. The majority of children who have a tracheotomy and swallowing problems have other medical co-morbidities that affect motor and sensory function in the head and neck region leading to dysphagia. However, even children without other medical problems can develop dysphagia and aspiration. This is multifactorial and likely due to diminution of the protective cough reflex by alterations in subglottic pressure because of the tube. Additionally, presence of the tracheotomy tube tethers the larynx to the skin therefore interfering with laryngeal elevation, a requirement for complete relaxation of the cricopharyngeus muscle. Fortunately, these difficulties tend to be transient and resolve as these patients accommodate to the presence of the tracheotomy tube. Videofluoroscopic evaluation of swallowing has been the gold standard to detect aspiration in children with tracheotomy tubes, but may not provide an accurate assessment of airway protection in the child who is unable to eat. Recent introduction of the flexible endoscopic evaluation of swallowing allows for a superior assessment of laryngeal function and airway protection in relationship to swallowing function without exposure to radiation. The additional advantage is that this examination technique can assess aspiration risk in those children who are unable to feed and swallow by visualizing the path of the patient's own secretions to see if they are aspirated into the trachea or spontaneously swallowed and cleared from access to the airway.[9,10,28]

Home care

Perhaps no development has contributed as much to the reduction in tracheotomy-related morbidity and mortality as has home care. Specialists in this area have developed both prophylactic strategies and methods to reduce problems related to plugging, accidental decannulation, local breakdown of the surgical site, mucosal suction trauma, and infection. Long-term outcomes in children needing tracheotomy for prolonged periods have markedly improved as a result of this work.

One of the most important jobs of the clinician coordinating home care of a child with a tracheotomy is to ensure that the parents or other caregivers are connected to an appropriate support network, which will be available at all times. The surgeon, pediatrician, nurses, speech and language pathologists, backup caregivers, and equipment providers should all be easily accessible to those primarily responsible for the child's welfare.

Education of the primary caregivers, particularly the parents, should be thorough and formalized and include teaching routine and emergent care. Even something as basic as suctioning can induce severe complications if done inexpertly. Optimal procedures for such things as tie securing, humidification, tracheotomy tube changes, and cardiopulmonary resuscitation are beyond the scope of this chapter, but are outlined elsewhere.[13]

Most experienced clinicians recommend home monitoring for the child with a tracheotomy. This may be achieved using a mechanical "apnea" type monitor, or transcutaneous pulse oximetry. A limitation of the use of an apnea monitor is that respiratory efforts may continue in the presence of a blocked or displaced tube for some time before the alarm is triggered, thereby a catastrophic event can be easily missed. Transcutaneous pulse oximetry is the monitoring device of choice for most experienced clinicians who manage children with tracheotomy tubes, because near fatal complications of accidental decannulation and mucous plugging are usually associated with hypoxia. Oximetry provides the most accurate non-invasive method of detecting hypoxia. The limitation and challenge of this monitoring system is that frequent false alarms are triggered by failure of the probe to find the pulse or accidental detachment of the measuring device. It must be understood that no alarm system is a substitute for adequate education and training of the caregivers to understand clinical problems and respond appropriately to respiratory distress. A danger is that this equipment may provide a false sense of security.

Decannulation

Suprastomal collapse is almost universally present in children with long-term tracheotomies. The superior edge of the tracheotomy tube tends to compress the tracheal cartilage of the anterior wall just above the stoma. In an older child or adult with fairly rigid tracheal rings and a large lumen, such limited tracheomalacia is unlikely to be problematic. In young children, however, suprastomal tracheomalacia is more likely to be problematic. Also, in young children, suprastomal tracheomalacia and granuloma formation may be limiting factors in decannulation of a patient whose primary airway pathology has improved through growth or surgical intervention.

Cervical tracheoplasty is the authors' preferred technique when a surgical procedure is required to achieve decannulation. This combines an excision of the epithelialized tract and granuloma with anterior reinforcement of the tracheal wall. Following bronchoscopic confirmation of the diagnosis of suprastomal tracheomalacia and/or granuloma, and exclusion of other significant obstructing pathology, the patient is nasotracheally intubated and the tracheotomy tube removed. The tract is excised with horizontal ellipse of skin and the airway skeletonized above the stoma. A small hemostat is placed in the airway, directed superiorly, and the malacic segment is divided vertically in the midline for a short distance (up to normal cartilage). Coexisting granuloma may be excised directly at this point. The two tracheal flaps are then pexed anteriorly to the strap muscles with long-acting absorbable sutures (such as Vicyl™). The wound is loosely closed with chromic gut sutures in two layers (skin and subcutaneous tissue), so as to avoid air trapping and possible pneumothorax or pneumomediastinum. The patient is brought into the intensive care unit and extubated in 24-hours, by which time the tract should be closed.

Significant suprastomal collapse may require laryngotracheoplasty with cartilage grafting to achieve decannulation. Techniques and applications of laryngotracheoplasty operations are presented later in the chapter.

Causes of airway obstruction and surgical management

Laryngomalacia

Laryngomalacia is the most common laryngeal anomaly and cause of stridor in infancy. The clinical presentation is that of inspiratory stridor that is worse with feeding, agitation, and supine position. The symptoms are usually present at birth or shortly thereafter. Symptoms peak at 6–8 months of age and usually resolve between 18 and 24 months of age.[29] Mild forms of the disease present with inspiratory stridor and usually no other constitutional symptoms. Those with moderate malacia usually have feeding problems, as it can be difficult for infants to coordinate the suck swallow breathe sequence in the setting of airway obstruction. Many of those infants have GERD and benefit from antireflux treatment, possibly including surgical therapy.[30,31] Why there is such a high incidence of GERD in this patient population is poorly understood. These children may have GERD because of more negative intrathoracic airway pressure as a consequence of the proximal airway obstruction. Another contributing factor could be immature reflexes that regulate esophageal motility, causing poor esophageal clearance. GERD in this patient population, like other infant populations with airway problems and apnea, may be related to frequent relaxation events of the lower esophageal sphincter.[32] Infants with severe laryngomalacia develop life-threatening complications of airway obstruction that can contribute to pectus abnormalities, failure to thrive, chronic hypoxia, pulmonary hypertension, and cor pulmonale. These patients require surgical intervention.[33–36] The diagnosis is suspected by auscultation of the stridor, but must be confirmed by flexible laryngoscopy. This examination must be done with the infant awake so as to demonstrate the cyclical collapse of the supraglottic tissues into the laryngeal inlet. The influence of general anesthesia can obscure these findings. Other typical findings include an omega shaped epiglottis and forward prolapsing arytenoid cartilages, which obstruct airflow and give an incomplete view of the vocal folds. This examination is also done to ensure that there is no other significant supraglottic pathology contributing to the stridor. The etiology of this condition remains elusive. Proposed theories include abnormal airway anatomy,[37,38] and immature cartilage formation. Because laryngomalacia is frequently seen in children with other neurologic diseases, some believe laryngomalacia has a neurologic etiology.

Laryngomalacia is usually a self-limiting disease that rarely requires surgical intervention. Surgical intervention is recommended in those who develop life-threatening episodes of airway obstruction or complications of hypoxia as described above. Tracheotomy was the treatment of choice for this condition until the mid 1980s when techniques of supraglottoplasty were introduced.[35,39,40] Tracheotomy bypasses the site of laryngeal obstruction until the condition resolves spontaneously, usually after 18–24 months of age. Tracheotomy can be avoided by performing a supraglottoplasty. This is accomplished by microsurgical removal of the redundant prolapsing tissue seen in the area of the arytenoid cartilages and release of the aryepiglottic folds which tether the epiglottis in position.[35] Long-term results with this approach have generally been excellent with symptom reversal in 80–100% of patients[33,35,36,41–44] although some authors report that as many as 50% of patients will require additional airway procedures, either revision supraglottoplasty or tracheotomy.[43,44] Supraglottic stenosis is the most severe complication of this operation and can occur after overzealous removal of tissue or failure to control for acid reflux which causes inflammatory injury and haphazard scarring. To minimize chances of scarring, some authors advocate staged operations with minimal tissue removal and from only one side at a time. These same authors found that a unilateral procedure is enough to alleviate symptoms and reserve bilateral operation for infants whose life-threatening symptoms persist.[45,46] Though supraglottoplasty is a superior alternative to tracheotomy, some children with multiple medical comorbidities, particularly those with severe neurologic impairment or syndromes that involve the airway, often fail supraglottoplasty and are better managed with a tracheotomy.[47]

Laryngeal atresia and webs

Laryngeal webs are congenital or acquired. Congenital laryngeal webs and atresias are rare and appear to result from the embryologic failure of recannulization of the larynx during prenatal development. An atresia or a web of sufficient size will present at birth as aphonia and rapid asphyxiation if not immediately addressed. A thin web with a small residual airway may be perforated by endotracheal intubation. Often this is the only treatment needed; however, these infants should be followed closely so appropriate intervention occurs if airway obstruction develops. Thick webs and atresias make emergent intubation by standard techniques difficult if not impossible. In this setting, survival of the infant may be dependent on securing the airway with a 2.5 rigid bronchoscope and if that is not possible, obtaining a surgical airway. Surgical management of thick webs and atresias requires a tracheostomy tube until the larynx is larger and amenable for surgical intervention.[48] Surgical correction usually requires a laryngofissure with open airway division of the atretic region and placement of costal cartilage in the anterior cricoid and cervical trachea, similar to a laryngotracheal reconstruction for subglottic stenosis discussed later in this chapter. Timing or reconstruction is dependent on many factors including age of the child and surgeon experience.

Thin and moderate anterior webs are not usually diagnosed or suspected at birth and may or may not create airway obstructive symptoms. The most common presenting symptom is hoarseness. The primary goals of management are to provide a patent airway and to achieve good voice quality. This is challenging because vocal cords have a tendency to fibrosis and granulation tissue formation after surgical interventions. Traditionally, the treatment of choice for thin and moderate laryngeal webs is laryngofissure and placement of a stent or keel when the surgeon feels the child has grown appropriately, usually greater than 12 months of age. Recent reports show that selected laryngeal webs can be managed with endoscopic lysis and off FDA label topical mitomycin-C application, even in infants under 1 year of age.[49] This technique may allow congenital webs to be successfully managed at a younger age. However, long-term outcomes of this technique are not available, and it is unknown if infants treated by this method eventually need laryngotracheal reconstruction to maintain a patent airway. Long-term results in the management of webs depend on the severity of the original lesion. Surgically treated thin webs often heal with minimal disruption of phonation, while thicker plates with associated subglottic stenosis have less satisfactory results.[50]

Acquired laryngeal webs are also uncommon. Etiology is usually from direct laryngeal trauma where the medial surfaces of both vocal cords are disrupted and they heal together forming a web. This is most commonly seen in the management and treatment of laryngeal papillomas, typically caused by overzealous treatment of papilloma disease at the anterior glottic commissure, particularly in the setting of laryngopharyngeal reflux.[51]

Vocal cord immobility: vocal cord paralysis and vocal cord fixation

Vocal cord movement requires intact neurologic function of the vagus nerve and free rotation of the cricoarytenoid joint. The action of abduction of the vocal cords from the midline opens the glottic inlet for airflow into the tracheobronchial tree. Airflow is restricted if vocal cord abduction does not occur. Vocal cord immobility is caused by failure of the vocal cords to abduct. There are two primary etiologies of vocal cord immobility, vocal cord paralysis and vocal cord fixation. Injury of the vagus nerve anywhere along its course from the skull-base to thoracic cavity causes neurogenic vocal cord paralysis. Paralysis can be congenital or acquired. Acquired immobility is usually caused by a stretch injury, pressure encroachment, inflammatory insult, and trauma or sectioning of the nerve itself. In this setting the cricoarytenoid joint is mobile, but the neuromuscular function is compromised. A traumatic or inflammatory process in the cricoarytenoid joint causes vocal cord fixation. In this setting, the function of the joint that is required for mobility is fixed, but the neuromuscular function is intact. Fixation and paralysis can coexist. Regardless of the etiology of immobility, failure for one or both of the vocal cords to abduct can lead to stridor and airway obstruction.

Unilateral vocal cord immobility rarely causes stridor or airway obstruction, except occasionally in very young infants particularly in the setting of mucosal edema where the cross-sectional diameter of the airway is already small. In the setting of bilateral vocal cord immobility, both cords lay near the midline thereby limiting airflow through the glottis. Bilateral vocal fold immobility may present with severe life-threatening symptoms and airway obstruction requiring an immediate artificial airway. Some infants and children have mild symptoms occurring only during periods of upper respiratory tract infection and may not require a tracheotomy. Most children with bilateral vocal cord immobility require tracheotomy early in the course of the disease, prior to definitive surgical therapy. Because it is bilateral immobility that most commonly leads to airway obstruction, the discussion of surgical treatment will be limited to management of bilateral immobility.

Management and treatment of airway symptoms of bilateral cord immobility is based on the etiology and site of involvement along the vagus nerve. In neonates and infants, bilateral vocal cord paralysis may have a central etiology, most commonly a Chiari malformation or hydrocephalus. Caudal displacement of the brainstem seen in a Chiari malformation causes pressure on the brainstem at the site of origin of the vagal nerve nuclei and nerves. Recognition and diagnosis of this is important to prevent other complications of a Chiari malformation. Vocal cord paralysis can be cured once the Chiari malformation is decompressed, if done in a timely fashion. Hydrocephalus leads to increased compression of the fourth ventricle. This can also cause compression of the vagal nerve nuclei and nerves. Decreasing the intracranial pressure by shunt placement is often curative.[8,52] Infants with a central etiology of bilateral vocal cord paralysis who fail central decompressive procedures will require a tracheotomy for airway safety. These patients also often go on to develop other lower cranial nerve problems and aspiration that keep them tracheotomy tube dependent and not good candidates for other surgical procedures to achieve decannulation. If the vagal nerve is intact, and the etiology of bilateral vocal cord paralysis is a localized insult to the vagal nerve such as a stretch injury from obstetrical trauma, infection, or extrinsic compression, an observational period is often warranted if there are no acute symptoms of airway obstruction. The paralysis is frequently transient in these patients who are otherwise healthy. If the etiology of vocal cord paralysis is traumatic with direct nerve injury where function is not expected to return, a tracheotomy is required until another procedure can be done to expand the glottic opening. This situation may be seen in "fixed wire" neck trauma,[53] with nerve injury as a complication of thyroid or other surgery.

Bilateral vocal fold immobility due to fixation occurs when the synovial joint surfaces of the cricoarytenoid joint become fixed, thereby not allowing vocal fold abduction or adduction. In this setting, the vagal nerve is usually fully functional and physically intact. The most common cause of fixation of the joint is some type of direct trauma to the joint area itself such as intubation or neck trauma dislocating the cricoarytenoid joint. Once the joint is injured, an inflammatory process occurs causing an arthritic-like process. Juvenile rheumatoid arthritis can also cause bilateral cricoarytenoid joint immobility.

Regardless of whether vocal fold immobility is paralysis or fixation, surgical approaches to treatment in children are similar. The fact that there is a wide variety of surgical approaches suggests that no one procedure is ideal. The goal is to open the posterior glottic airway enough to allow for adequate airflow without exposing the patient to increased risk of complications of aspiration. The procedures described are often done after the airway has been secured and is stable with a tracheotomy tube. More recently, many of these surgical techniques have been employed as the primary surgery with the goal of avoiding a tracheotomy. The decision to do definitive primary surgery depends on the acuity of airway obstruction, age of the child, and ability to protect the airway against aspiration.

Repositioning or removal of structures and tissue in the posterior glottis, namely the arytenoid cartilage and mucosa, are well-described techniques of opening the airway in the setting of bilateral vocal cord immobility. These include arytenoid lateralization, arytenoidopexy, partial arytenoidectomy, and cordotomy.[54–57] These procedures can be done alone or in combination with the goal of decannulation. The surgical approach can be external through a laryngofissure or endoscopic using a CO_2 laser or a combination of both. Endoscopic CO_2 laser removal of the vocal process of the arytenoid and a portion of the posterior vocal cord has been successfully employed in some series.[57] The management challenge of this technique is treatment of postoperative granulation tissue formation that may lead to airway obstruction.[58] Recent meta-analysis and retrospective studies evaluating outcomes of surgically managed bilateral vocal cord paralysis in children suggest that laryngofissure with partial arytenoidectomy combined with a vocal cord lateralization procedure results in the highest decannulation rates when compared to CO_2 arytenoidectomy and cordotomy procedures or arytenoidopexy procedures alone.[59] These same studies conclude that open external procedures appear to be more effective as a first-line treatment in pediatric vocal cord paralysis, with arytenoidopexy with or without partial arytenoidectomy offering an attractive first-line surgical option. They also conclude that CO_2 laser procedures, while having limited success as a primary procedure, are effective for revision. While these procedures have been effective in achieving decannulation and maintaining airway patency, long-term outcomes related to aspiration and voice are unknown.

Posterior graft laryngotracheoplasty is another effective technique to open the posterior glottis.[60,61] Through a laryngofissure with extension into the first two rings of the trachea, the posterior cricoid lamina is incised and distracted, thereby separating the arytenoid cartilages. Inserting a costal cartilage graft into the distracted posterior cricoid lamina stabilizes the position of the arytenoid cartilages. Although published series of this procedure are small, the decannulation rate after posterior approaches is near 100%.[62] Endoscopic posterior cricoid split and rib graft insertion has been successfully accomplished in a few children with posterior glottic and subglottic stenosis.[63]

Recurrent respiratory papillomatosis

Recurrent respiratory papillomatosis (RRP) is the expression of human papillomavirus (HPV) infection in the mucosa of the upper aerodigestive tract. Papillomas involving the larynx are the most common laryngeal tumor in children, and the larynx is the most common site of occurrence in the aerodigestive tract. Adult laryngeal papilloma disease is usually solitary whereas papillomas of childhood tend to occur in clusters and have a high propensity for recurrence. Clinical presentation of laryngeal papilloma is progressive airway obstruction, with dysphonia and progression to aphonia. RRP is most commonly associated with HPV-6 and HPV-11 subtypes. Subtypes 16 and 18 are rarely associated with RRP but, if present, have a higher risk of malignant transformation. These viral particles are present in adjacent and clinically normal sites of the respiratory tract but are expressed primarily in anatomical locations of juxtaposed epithelium, hence the high predilection for the vocal cord.[64] These sites include the lumen vestibule, the nasopharyngeal surface of the soft palate, the midline of the laryngeal surface of the epiglottis, the upper and lower margins of the ventricle, the undersurface of the true vocal folds, the carina, and the bronchial spurs. The other common location are sites of mucosal injury, such as a tracheotomy site.[64] Identification of the vector of transmission is a point of controversy. Pediatric RRP and vaginal condyloma accuminata are both caused by HPV subtypes 6 and 11, thus leading most researchers to believe that vertical transmission from mother to child occurs in most cases. Although unusual, vertical transmission to children born by cesarean section of mothers with vaginal warts has also been documented.[65]

The natural course of RRP is extremely variable, with no obvious patient-related risk factors to aid in prognosis. Many cases have been seen to regress spontaneously in adolescence, but others go on to extensive disease involving the trachea and pulmonary parenchyma with a high fatality rate from untreatable airway obstruction. Even more uncommonly, the papilloma may undergo malignant degeneration to squamous cell carcinoma. For this reason, interval histological examination of the obstruction tissue is important. The estimated mean number of procedures per child for their disease is 19.7, with an average 4.4 procedures per year. It was noted that children presenting at an age younger than 3 years were 3.6 times more likely to require more than four surgical procedures per year and 2.1 times more likely to have two or more anatomic sites involved than children diagnosed after their fourth birthday.[66] Other investigators have noted that a younger age of presentation correlates with more aggressive disease.[64]

Pediatric RRP continues to be an extremely difficult management problem. This disease process continues to be a significant burden on the health care system and is a significant cause of morbidity in affected patients and their families. The incidence of RRP is approximately 3.96 per 100 000 in the pediatric population. It has been noted recently that approximately 7 of every 1000 children born to mothers with vaginal condyloma develop pediatric RRP. The goal of surgical treatment is to maintain a patent airway while providing a usable voice and to prevent spread of disease into the distal airway.

Although the mainstay of surgical management has traditionally been the CO_2 laser, newer surgical techniques have demonstrated efficacy in the management of pediatric RRP patients, including powered instrumentation, the laryngeal shaver[67] and the pulse-dye laser.[68] A recent study has demonstrated that microdebrider resection of laryngeal papilloma in children allowed more rapid surgery with potentially reduced treatment costs. Other advantages of this technique include precise excision without thermal injury.[69]

Advocates of the pulsed dye laser believe that this technique enhances epithelial excision by improving hemostasis and by creating an optimal dissection plane between the basement membrane and the underlying superficial lamina propria. Long-term outcomes for this technique are unknown.[70,71]

Regardless of the surgical technique employed, scarring, stenosis, and web formation in the larynx result from overly aggressive or inexpertly performed endoscopic removal of the disease. Care must be taken to avoid injury to vital structures. Papillomas should be removed down to the level of the vocal ligaments, but the cords themselves should not be incised. When working in the anterior commissure, the far anterior glottis where the vocal cords meet, bilateral resection should not be done, so as to avoid web formation. Even in experienced hands, the incidence of minor scarring in the anterior glottis may be as high as 25%.[72] Aggressive resection beyond that necessary to maintain a safe airway will not improve the long-term prognosis for remission, but may contribute to morbidity.

The role of tracheotomy in the surgical management of laryngeal papilloma is controversial. It is believed that it is best to avoid tracheotomy if at all possible. The mucosal injury at the tracheotomy site encourages growth of papilloma outside of the larynx, thereby increasing the probability of distal spread of the disease. The rate of tracheal spread in patients requiring tracheotomy has been reported as high as 50%.[73] It is possible, given the variable natural history of RRP, that patients who have distal spread of disease represent a subset of the patient population with a predetermined propensity to disseminate beyond the larynx and would require a tracheotomy regardless. Patients who develop life-threatening airway obstruction from aggressive disease within or beyond the larynx that cannot be managed by endoscopic procedures, should have a tracheotomy placed until the disease can be controlled with further surgical intervention and adjunctive therapy. If a tracheotomy is placed, the clinician should make every attempt to decannulate as soon as possible, both to limit potential distal airway dissemination and to relieve the child of the burden of tracheotomy. The traditional adjuvant medical therapies used for pediatric RRP are interferon-[alpha]2a, retinoic acid, and indol-3-carbinol/diindolylmethane (I3C/DIM). The most recently introduced adjunctive therapy is Cidofovir™. Cidofovir is an acyclic nucleoside phosphonate derivative with antiviral activity used for the treatment of cytomegalovirus retinitis in patients with acquired immunodeficiency syndrome. Off-label use of Cidofovir™ injected directly into the region after removal of laryngeal papilloma has demonstrated efficacy in selected patients. In addition, promising research efforts are underway to develop vaccination therapy for pediatric RRP. Pediatric RRP continues to be a highly morbid disease; however, new surgical and medical therapies offer hope for better control. Recent advances offer the hope of immune modulation as a potential future treatment modality.

Table 13.2. Classification of congenital subglottic stenosis

Cartilaginous stenosis	Soft tissue stenosis
Cricoid cartilage deformity	Granulation tissue
Normal shape	Submucosal fibrosis
Small for infant's size	Submucosal gland hypoplasia
Abnormal shape	
Large anterior lamina	
Large posterior lamina	
Generalized thickening	
Elliptical shape	
Submucous cleft	
Other congenital cricoid stenoses	
Trapped first tracheal ring	

Laryngotracheal stenosis and subglottic stenosis

Laryngotracheal stenosis may be characterized by etiology and area involved. Areas of involvement include the supraglottis, glottis, subglottis, and upper trachea. A single area or multiple areas can be involved. Stenosis of the larynx is congenital or acquired. Congenital stenoses are believed to be the result of failure or incomplete recanalization of the laryngeal lumen that normally occurs by the tenth week of gestation in lumens. Congenital subglottic stenosis is histopathologically divided into a membranous stenosis and cartilaginous stenosis (Table 13.2).

Congenital stenosis exists when the lumen of the cricoid region of the airway measures less than 4 mm in a full-term infant or 3 mm in a premature infant with no prior history of intubation. As seen in Fig. 13.5, the typical appearance of a congenital cartilaginous stenosis is that of an elliptical shaped cricoid cartilage. The distinction between congenital and acquired stenosis can be somewhat arbitrary, because children with congential subglottic stenosis may develop secondary soft tissue stenosis and scarring from injury, thereby developing an acquired component. This most commonly occurs from prolonged intubation, so the true incidence of congenital subglottic stenosis is difficult to determine. Of the areas involved in stenosis, the subglottis is the most common. Most subglottic stenoses that require surgical management are acquired. An example of acquired stenosis is seen in Fig. 13.6. The principles of surgical management discussed are applicable to congenital and acquired disease.

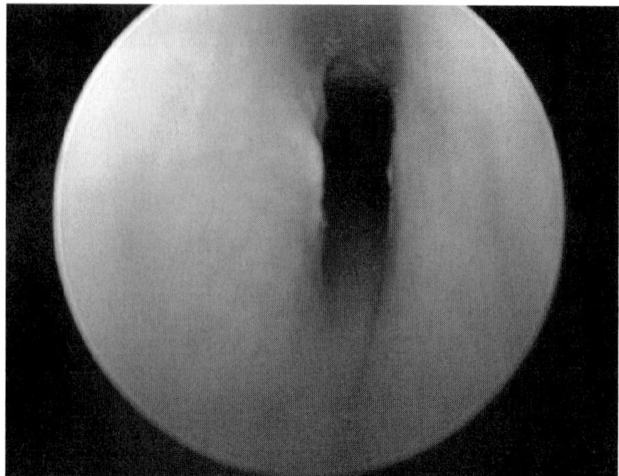

Fig. 13.5. Congenital cartilaginous stenosis. The elliptically shaped cricoid cartilage is demonstrated.

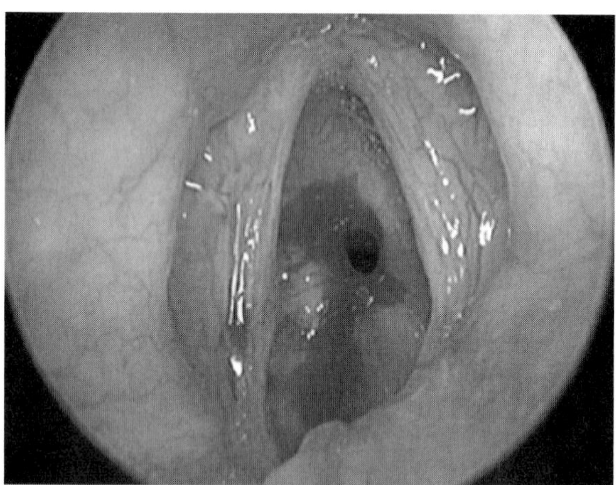

Fig. 13.6. Endoscopic photograph showing acquired subglottic stenosis.

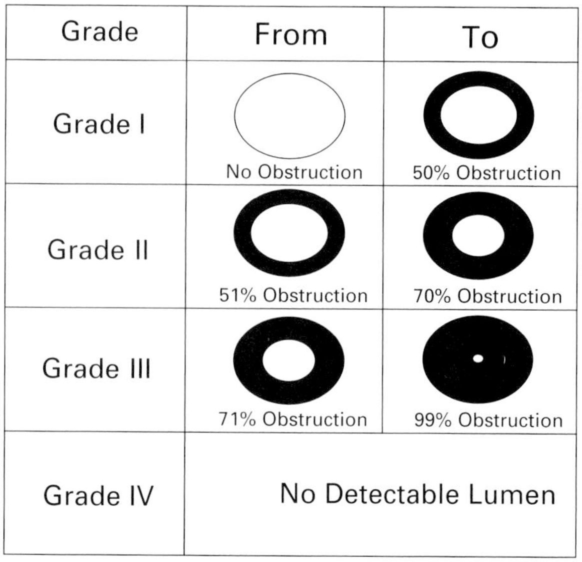

Grade	From	To
Grade I	No Obstruction	50% Obstruction
Grade II	51% Obstruction	70% Obstruction
Grade III	71% Obstruction	99% Obstruction
Grade IV	No Detectable Lumen	

Fig. 13.7. The Cotton–Myer grading system for subglottic stenosis.

Subglottic stenosis (SGS) essentially did not exist until after the mid 1960s as the prolonged endotracheal intubation and ventilation of neonates became feasible and then commonplace.[74] As very low birthweight infant survival increased, so did the number of patients with secondary laryngotracheal stenosis, with the incidence of SGS in surviving neonates as high as 97%.[75] Fortunately, advances in the techniques of endotracheal intubation and tube stabilization, along with the implementation of softer materials for endotracheal tubes, have decreased the incidence of tracheal laryngotracheal stenosis in surviving neonates to 0.9–8.3%.[76] With the proliferation of life saving advancements in medicine and surgery, we are seeing children survive disease processes who would not have done so previously. These children also develop other chronic diseases as a result of treatment, with subglottic stenosis being one of them. The number of toddlers, children, and adolescents who now develop stenosis of the larynx has increased, but the exact incidence is unknown. The nature of the stenosis can be soft or firm and a combination of both is common. Causes of soft tissue stenosis are submucosal mucous gland hyperplasia, ductal cysts, fibrous, granulation tissue, and laryngopharyngeal reflux of gastric acid causing mucosal edema. Firm stenoses are usually associated with an abnormally shaped or thickened cricoid cartilage or mature scar tissue. The Cotton–Myer grading system is most widely used for documentation of degree of obstruction (Fig. 13.7). Endotracheal tube sizing has become the most widely used means of grading and assessing degree of stenosis.[77]

Successful laryngotracheal reconstructive surgery requires a carefully formulated plan. This plan includes identification and management of significant medical comorbidities that have potential to contribute to poor outcomes. The plan also requires accurate identification of the type of stenosis and all areas of the larynx and upper trachea involved since the stenosis can be multilevel and require more than one type of intervention. The treatment plan is custom tailored to the specific patient, their medical comorbidities and the anatomic problem. This treatment plan is best developed by a multidisciplinary team approach including the pediatric otolaryngologist, pediatric surgeon, pulmonologist, gastroenterologist, anesthesiologist, intensivist, and appropriate allied health.

Any laryngeal stenosis can be effectively managed by placement of a tracheotomy. Morbidity and mortality associated with tracheotomy tube placement has encouraged advancements in laryngotracheal reconstructive procedures (LTR) to either avoid tracheotomy tube placement or to achieve decannulation.

Associated medical comorbidities, particularly cardiopulmonary disease, must be addressed, stabilized and managed prior to considering surgical intervention for laryngeal stenosis. Children who require significant ventilatory or medical support are not good candidates for laryngotracheal reconstruction. Evaluation of swallowing function is essential to help determine airway protection ability and aspiration risk so that preoperative and perioperative accommodations can be made to minimize the complications of aspiration. Patients with significant aspiration are usually not good candidates for LTR.

The influence of gastroesophageal reflux on laryngotracheal stenosis and wound cannot be overemphasized. GERD is an etiologic factor in acquired subglottic stenosis. Clinical and animal studies demonstrate that the presence of acid in the region of the larynx negatively affect healing.[14,15,17,78–81] Perioperative and postoperative aggressive medical and sometimes surgical antireflux therapy is recommended in the setting of LTR surgery. Prospective and retrospective studies correlating long-term outcomes and reflux control in LTR surgery are not available.

Surgical management of laryngotracheal stenosis is individualized to the patient and no one operative approach is exactly the same. Each individual patient presents with multiple variables that must be considered, including the location and extent of the stenotic area, medical comorbidities, airway protection plan, and swallowing function, age, and weight. Surgical options include endoscopic techniques, expansion surgery, and resection surgery. Methods employed are dependent on the degree and location of the stenosis. In general, grade I stenoses are usually managed by endoscopic techniques. Grade II stenoses may be approached with either endoscopic or open techniques depending on location and extent of the lesion. Grade III and IV lesions almost always require open surgical reconstruction (Table 13.3).

Multiple endoscopic techniques have been advocated in the past, including microcauterization,[82] cryosurgery,[83] and serial electrosurgical resection. The carbon dioxide (CO_2) and KTP lasers, because of their precision, have largely replaced these modalities. The laser is useful for treating early intubation injury with granulation tissue accumulation, subglottic cysts, thin circumferential webs, and crescent-shaped bands. Predisposing factors to failure of endoscopic laser treatment of SGS are previous failed endoscopic procedures, significant loss of the cartilaginous framework, thick, circumferential cicatricial scarring greater than 1 cm in vertical dimension, and posterior commissure involvement. A complication of laser treatment of SGS is exposure of perichondrium or cartilage causing perichondritis and chondritis that may lead to further scar formation. The limits of endoscopic management of laryngotracheal stenosis are being expanded. A recent report describes successful endoscopic expansion of the posterior glottic lumen through CO_2 division of the posterior cricoid lamina with a laser and inserting a rib cartilage graft through the laryngoscope.[63] Long-term outcomes for this approach are not known.

Table 13.3. Surgical options in laryngeal stenosis

Grades I and II
Endoscopic laser techniques
Anterior laryngotracheal decompression
Anterior laryngotracheal split with autologous cartilage grafting:
 costal cartilage
 auricular cartilage

Grades III and IV
Anterior and posterior laryngotracheal split:
 long-term stent alone
 anterior and/or posterior costal cartilage graft
Cricotracheal resection

Open surgical reconstruction is recommended when endoscopic methods to establish a patent airway are inappropriate or have failed. Anterior cricoid split is one of the open expansion surgical techniques. It is utilized predominantly in neonates with anterior subglottic narrowing who fail multiple attempts at extubation and have adequate pulmonary reserve. In this setting, the laryngotracheal problem is due to narrowing at the level of the cricoid cartilage. The airway lumen is expanded by dividing the anterior cricoid cartilage in the midline. An endotracheal tube is left in place for 5–10 days. Dexamethasone sodium phosphate is initiated 24 hours before extubation and continued for 5 days after extubation. This technique leads to successful extubation in 66–78% of patients.[84] As seen in Table 13.4, several clinical criteria must be met to maximize the probability of successful extubation following anterior cricoid split.

In the authors' hands, this technique has nearly been replaced by anterior cricoid split with the placement of a small auricular cartilage graft followed by endotracheal intubation for 7 days. Outcomes comparing decannulation

Table 13.4. Criteria for performing an anterior cricoid split in a neonate

Criteria
Extubation failure on at least two occasions secondary to subglottic laryngeal pathology
Weight greater than 1500 g
No ventilator support for at least 10 days before repair
Supplemental O_2 requirement less than 30%
No congestive heart failure for 1 month before repair
No acute respiratory tract infection
No antihypertensive medication for 10 days before repair

rates of cricoid split vs. cricoid split with placement of the auricular cap graft have not been formally reviewed.

Multiple open procedures have been described to expand the stenosed airway. These procedures and their applications have evolved over the past 30 years. Fearon and Cotton introduced laryngotracheal reconstruction (LTR) with cartilage interpositional grafting in 1972 with placement of a cartilage graft between a split anterior cricoid and upper trachea. This method has become one of the most common techniques of expanding stenotic airway segments. Anterior grafting alone is typically used in grade II and grade III stenoses that do not involve the posterior glottis or subglottis. If there is posterior glottic or subglottic involvement in addition to the anterior stenosis, the posterior cricoid plate lamina is split without the placement of an interpositional graft, depending on the degree of the stenosis. This problem is more commonly seen in grade III and grade IV stenosis. Partial cricotracheal resection (CTR) is another option for surgical management of selected grade III and IV stenosis.[85–90] In this operation the stenotic region of the anterior cricoid plate and any involved tracheal stenotic segment is resected, and the trachea is mobilized to allow for an end-to-end anastomosis. The posterior trachea and trachealis muscle is anastomosed with the posterior cricoid plate and its mucosa. The anterior mobilized trachea is then sewn into the removed segment of the cricoid and secured to the thyroid cartilage. The reader is referred elsewhere for surgical details of this operation.[85–87,90]

The traditional approach to LTR surgery involved staged reconstruction[91–94] where the expansion operation was done, and a stent (Silastic® sheeting or Teflon®) was placed to stabilize the reconstruction. The stent is left in place above a tracheotomy stoma and tube (suprastomal stent) for 4–6 weeks. With this strategy, after the stent is removed and once the surgical site has healed with a patent subglottis, the tracheotomy tube is downsized as the child tolerates and becomes able to breathe around a plugged trach tube. Once this is accomplished, the tracheotomy tube is removed. This process of reconstruction and decannulation can take weeks to several months. The morbidity and potential mortality of a tracheotomy tube is well recognized in children and discussed earlier in this chapter. With staged reconstruction and stent placement, the child is left with little or no airway above the tracheotomy tube, which is life threatening if the tube accidentally falls out or is occluded. Long-term stenting has additional morbidities of granulation tissue formation, infection, dislodgment of the stent, dysphagia, and aspiration. To address these risks and circumvent some of these problems, Single Stage LTR (SSLTR) evolved. In the authors' hands, staged procedures are still done in children with compromised pulmonary reserve or complex, multilevel stenosis that requires prolonged stenting.

Single stage LTR (SSLTR) involves surgical correction of the stenotic airway with a short period of endotracheal intubation, thus avoiding the need for prolonged laryngotracheal stenting and tracheotomy tube dependency. The airway must have adequate cartilaginous support to consider SSLTR as a surgical option. SSLTR requires a comprehensive understanding of the principles of airway reconstruction and extensive experience on the part of the surgeon, anesthesiologist, intensivist, and nursing staff. Postoperative care of these patients can be complicated. The reader is referred to other sources for details of postoperative management.[1,95,96] A recent study looking at outcomes of 200 SSLTR cases showed that after SSLTR, 29% of patients were reintubated and 15% required postoperative tracheostomy. The overall decannulation rate was 96%. This study also found that the use of anterior and posterior costal cartilage grafting, age less than 4 years, sedation for more than 48 hours, a leak pressure around the endotracheal tube at greater than 20 cm H_2O, and moderate/severe tracheomalacia significantly increased the rate of reintubation. The duration of stenting did not affect outcomes. Children with anterior and posterior grafts and those with moderate or severe tracheomalacia were more likely to need postoperative tracheostomy. This study shows that SSLTR is effective for the treatment of pediatric laryngotracheal stenosis and that diligent preoperative assessment of the patient comorbidities and the patient's airway and meticulous postoperative care are important to the success of this operation.

The ultimate goal of laryngotracheal reconstruction is either avoidance of tracheotomy or prompt tracheotomy decannulation if necessary. The rate of decannulation varies with the severity of stenosis and the method of reconstruction. Surgical management of pediatric subglottic stenosis is challenging. Multiple operations may be required to achieve eventual extubation or decannulation.

It is not possible to predict the outcome of pediatric airway reconstructive surgery with certainty; however, the results of a retrospective study of 1296 airway reconstruction procedures over a 12 year period provides the best data available. This study examined Myer–Cotton grade-specific SGS outcomes as determined by decannulation and extubation rates. Decannulation rates for two-stage laryngotracheal reconstruction for Myer–Cotton grades 2, 3, and 4 were 95%, 74%, and 86%, respectively. Decannulation rates for SSLTR for Myer–Cotton grades 2, 3, and 4 were 100%, 86%, and 100%. The conclusion of this study is that children with Myer–Cotton grade 3 or 4 disease represent a significant challenge, and refinements of techniques are needed to address this subset of children.

Surgical management of grade 4 stenosis represents the most difficult group to obtain good results. A recent study has shown that refinements in surgical technique and application of CTR as the primary operation for Grade 4 stenosis has improved the decannulation rates from 67% in the 1980s to 86% in 1990s.[97] This same study shows that patients who underwent CTR had a higher decannulation rate than patients who underwent laryngotracheal reconstruction (LTR) with anterior and posterior costal cartilage grafting (92% vs. 81%). CTR patients were less likely to need additional open procedures to achieve decannulation (18% vs. 46%).[97] Patients with Grade 4 stenosis and other areas of the larynx and trachea involved often require extended CTR with the application of cartilage grafting and arytenoid procedures.

Functional outcomes of LTR surgery are critical in determination of success. Studies evaluating post LTR exercise tolerance, speech, voice, and swallowing are limited. The ability to obtain accurate objective data of voice function is well established for adults but not children. However, adult-derived means of assessment are evolving in the evaluation of children. Interpretation of results is challenging, because no normative data are available in children. Early studies of voice function after LTR surgery were entirely subjective assessments.[98] Recent studies in children have included a combination of subjective findings with limited objective measures.[99–101,102] The available studies suggest that LTR surgery has a negative effect on vocal quality.[100,103,104] The adverse effect is dependent on the degree of stenosis. Seventy-five percent of children with grade I stenosis have an adequate voice, in contrast to 50% or fewer among children with stenosis grades 2–4.[104] Another study suggests that stenosis involving the posterior glottis has worse voice outcomes.[105] One of the future goals of LTR surgery is improving voice outcomes and developing a standard objective method of assessment of pre- and postoperative voice.

Transient dysphagia is common after laryngotracheal reconstruction.[11] A recent study demonstrated that patients with compromised feeding prior to LTR surgery tend to be those with tracheotomy tubes, children less than 2 years of age, and those with multiple medical comorbidities, neurological diagnoses being most common. Preoperative assessment of swallowing function can provide a method of identifying patients with poor airway protection that may compromise the patient after reconstruction. Specific findings on swallowing studies that predict poor airway protective mechanisms are pooling of secretions in the hypopharynx; poor oral motor skills, premature spillage of material into the hypopharynx where it penetrates the larynx; and residue that persists in the hypopharynx after multiple swallows.[11] Long-term effects of LTR surgery on swallowing function have not been studied.

Objective assessment of airway capacity and exercise tolerance following LTR surgery in children is also lacking. Subjective reports show that exercise tolerance is good in up to 96% of patients. The ideal objective assessment of airway capacity after LTR surgery would be the flow loop studies. The adult LTR literature suggests that flow volume loop studies are useful in evaluating pre- and postoperative outcomes.[106] A study that looked at airway capacity in children after LTR surgery suggests that objective assessment of functional capacity after laryngotracheal reconstruction in older children may serve as a basis for follow-up. They found that the assessment in younger children, was difficult to obtain and provided no significant value in the overall assessment of functional capacity of the airway.[107] No objective pre- and postoperative studies of airway capacity in children after LTR surgery have been done.

Hemangioma

Subglottic and tracheal hemangiomas are benign congenital vascular malformations that are derived from mesodermal rests. The lesions are relatively uncommon, accounting for 1.5% of all congenital laryngeal anomalies, with a 2:1 female predominance.[29] Patients are usually asymptomatic at birth but present with stridor within the first few months of life; 85% present in the first 6 months,[108] and 50% have cutaneous hemangiomas present at the time of diagnosis.[109] Asymmetric subglottic narrowing is the classic finding on soft tissue neck radiographs. Endoscopic diagnosis is usually made without biopsy because of the lesion's typical appearance of a compressible, asymmetric, submucosal mass with bluish or reddish discoloration, most often located in the posterolateral subglottis.

Subglottic and tracheal hemangiomas will have a rapid growth phase that slows by 12 months of age, followed by slow resolution over the subsequent months to years. Most will show complete resolution by five years. However, subglottic hemangiomas are associated with 30–70% mortality when left untreated. Therapeutic and surgical management of this problem is directed at maintaining the airway, while minimizing long-term sequelae of the treatment itself. Current management options include laser partial excision, open surgical resection, systemic or intralesional steroids, systemic interferon-[alpha] 2a, and tracheotomy.

Bypassing the obstructing lesion with a tracheotomy and waiting for the expected involution will provide for the optimal anatomical result and is considered by many to be the standard of care against which all other treatment options need to be measured. However, as previously discussed in this chapter, there are risks associated with a tracheotomy as well as delays in speech and language that are routinely encountered when children acquire tracheotomy at a young age. Methods of treatment that are no longer used because of the associated morbidity include external beam radiation, radium and gold implants and sclerosing agents.

Systemic corticosteroids for treatment of subglottic hemangiomas were introduced in 1969 by Cohen,[110] and are used both as primary and adjuvant therapy. Steroids decrease the size of the hemangioma and accelerate involution via an unknown mechanism. Steroids are thought to decrease hemangioma size by blocking estradiol-induced growth,[111] or by directly increasing capillary sensitivity to vasoconstrictors. Corticosteroid therapy with or without tracheotomy has been shown to be successful in 82–97% of cases. However, whether or not the period of tracheotomy cannulation is decreased with steroids is unknown.[112] Risks of long-term steroid use include growth retardation, Cushingoid face and increased susceptibility to infection.[113] Using an alternate-day dosing regimen in the smallest possible doses may minimize these effects. Recent reports suggest that systemic steroids, followed by short-term intubation after diagnostic bronchoscopy, can be used as a safe and effective alternative in the management of obstructive subglottic hemangiomas in pediatric patients.[114] Others[115] report successful avoidance of tracheotomy by endoscopic intralesional injection of corticosteroids, with or without short-term intubation.

Endoscopic surgical management with the CO_2 laser was first reported in 1980 by Healy and colleagues.[116] Since its introduction, the CO_2 laser alone or in combination with steroids or tracheotomy has become a standard therapy. Isolated unilateral subglottic hemangiomas are usually most favorable to CO_2 laser treatment. In carefully selected patients, partial resection of the hemangioma with CO_2 laser with or without systemic corticosteroids is successful.[117] Recent reports show that the KTP laser is a good tool for management of subglottic hemangiomas with a low incidence of complications.[118,119] The KTP generated light frequencies are preferentially absorbed by hemoglobin making this laser system well suited for the treatment of vascular tumors such as a hemangioma. Long-term outcomes of this technique are not available.

Interferon-[alpha] 2a has been used recently for obstructing hemangioma in children who were unresponsive to laser and/or corticosteroid therapy, achieving a 50% or greater regression of the lesion in 73% of patients.[120] Interferon-[alpha] 2a requires prolonged therapy because it does not promote involution, but rather inhibits proliferation by blocking various steps in angiogenesis. The potential side effects of interferon-[alpha] 2a therapy include neuromuscular impairment, skin slough, fever, and hepatocellular dysfunction,[120] and limit its use to larger, potentially fatal lesions.

Despite the more widespread use of steroids and other treatment modalities, the requirement for tracheostomy has remained unchanged over the last 20 years. The use of laser therapy does not appear to confer any additional therapeutic benefit over and above tracheostomy alone in bringing about resolution of subglottic hemangiomas. Systemic steroids may reduce the size of the hemangioma but are associated with multiple adverse effects. The decision to use the above techniques must, therefore, be made in the light of these observations.[121] To avoid the complications and provide a more definitive treatment, the possibility of open surgical excision has been revisited.[2–4,121–124] The surgical technique is similar to SSLTR. The airway is opened at the level of the cricoid cartilage, followed by a submucosal dissection with excision of the hemangioma. An anterior cartilage graft is usually placed and the patient is intubated for 5–7 days. A recent study concludes that surgical resection of severe subglottic hemangiomas is a reliable technique in selected patients and should be considered in corticosteroid resistant or dependent, circular or bilateral hemangiomas[2] and large life-threatening lesions.[3] The early experience with single-stage excision suggests that this technique represents an exciting and promising surgical alternative. Its more widespread adoption may be the only way of further improving the outcome of patients with subglottic hemangiomas.[121]

Laryngeal and laryngotracheoesophageal clefts

Congential laryngeal and laryngotracheoesophageal clefts are rare conditions that can be characterized by a posterior midline deficiency in the separation of the larynx and trachea from the hypopharynx and esophagus. The incidence is less than 0.1% and the majority of cases are sporadic. There is a strong association with other anomalies (56%), most commonly tracheoesophageal fistula in 20–27%.[125] Six percent of children with tracheoesophageal fistula have a coexisting laryngeal cleft. Of the children who present with tracheoesophageal fistula, the laryngeal cleft goes undetected in three-quarters until persistent aspiration, in spite of successful tracheoesophageal fistula repair prompts further investigation.[125] Laryngeal or laryngotracheoesophageal clefting is commonly associated with a syndrome. The most common associations include G syndrome, VATER, VACTERL and Pallister–Hall syndrome.[126]

The degree of clefting may be relatively minor, involving only a failure of interarytenoid muscle development or can extend to the carina and even into the mainstem bronchi. Multiple classification systems have been used to describe laryngeal clefts. Independent of the numbering system used, it is useful to differentiate to the length of the cleft as laryngeal (interarytenoid only, partial cricoid, or complete cricoid), and laryngotracheoesophageal clefts that extend into the cervical trachea, or the intrathoracic trachea.

Patients with laryngeal or laryngotracheoesophageal clefts present with congential inspiratory stridor, cyanotic attacks associated with feeding, aspiration, and recurrent pulmonary infections. As the length of the cleft increases, so does the severity of presenting symptoms, with aspiration present in 100% of laryngotracheoesophageal clefts. While radiographic contrast studies may suggest aspiration, the best single study for identifying a laryngeal cleft is careful endoscopic examination. The arytenoids need to be parted in order to obtain adequate visualization, as the larynx may be obscured by redundant esophageal mucosa prolapsing into the glottic and subglottic lumen. Smith and colleagues[127] developed an instrument for measuring interarytenoid notch height relative to the vocal folds when a minor laryngeal cleft is suspected.

Most clefts that are limited to the supraglottic larynx do not require surgical intervention. The anatomic depth of these small clefts is to the interarytenoid level and stops at the vocal processes. Treatment methods include evaluation and treatment of gastroesophageal reflux and swallowing therapy.[125] When surgical intervention is required for these small clefts, endoscopic repair is successful in over 80%, with open repair reserved for endoscopic failures.[125,128]

In contrast to the interarytenoid clefts, surgical repair is required in nearly all laryngeal clefts that extend below the vocal cords. A complete discussion of these surgical options is beyond the scope of this chapter. However, an anterior approach through a laryngofissure is most commonly used. The advantage of this approach is excellent exposure of the entire defect without risk to the laryngeal innervation. Complete laryngotracheoesophageal clefts that extend to the carina may require a posterolateral approach to allow for a two-layer closure without requiring intraoperative extracorporeal circulation. In most circumstances, a tracheotomy is present prior to or placed at the time of reconstructive surgery. However, single-stage repair utilizing endotracheal intubation as a short-term stent is being increasingly utilized.

The mortality of laryngeal clefts is usually from associated congenital anomalies, or related to delay in making the diagnosis. Overall, mortality has been reported to be between 11%[125] and 46%,[129] unlike the mortality associated with intrathoracic laryngotracheoesophageal clefts which has been reported as high as 93%.[129] The incidence of revision surgery also increases with the severity of the cleft,[125] with an overall incidence of 11%.[130] In addition to the length of the cleft, insufficiently treated gastroesophageal reflux correlates with a decreased success rate.

Congenital tracheal stenosis

Congential tracheal stenosis is a rare, potentially life-threatening anomaly that usually involves complete cartilaginous tracheal rings. Over the years this has proven to be difficult to treat. In 1964, Cantrell and Guild[131] classified congential tracheal stenosis into three categories: long-segment stenosis with generalized hypoplasia (22%), funnel-like stenosis (37%), and segmental stenosis (41%). Associated anomalies in children with congenital tracheal stenosis are common with 24% having coexistent vascular anomalies, most commonly pulmonary artery sling.[132]

Congenital tracheal stenosis usually presents with a history of biphasic stridor and possibly acute respiratory distress. A definitive diagnosis is best obtained with endoscopy; however, magnetic resonance imaging or contrast enhanced computed tomography, and echocardiography are frequently needed to identify associated cardiovascular abnormalities. In recent years, tremendous progress has been made in the treatment of congenital tracheal stenosis. Segmental resection with primary anastomosis has been shown to be the treatment of choice for stenosis involving up to 50% of the trachea. However, many difficult procedures have been advocated for long-segment stenosis because none has proven to be universally successful. In fact, Benjamin *et al.* in 1981[132a] recommended a non-surgical approach because the 57% survival in this group of patients was higher than in his operated group. A recent report reiterates that non-operative management of complete tracheal rings may be appropriate in selected patients. Through a retrospective study Rutter and colleagues[133] estimate that up to 10% of patients with complete tracheal rings will not require tracheoplasty. Selected patients must be asymptomatic or have minimal symptoms and demonstrate tracheal growth on serial examinations. The rate of growth, however, is yet to be determined. Anterior tracheoplasty using pericardium was first described by Idriss and colleagues in 1984.[134] Since then, reported results with this technique reveal survival rates of 47–76% in larger series.[135] Costal cartilage grafting for augmentation has yielded similar results[136] in a smaller number of patients. Other augmentation materials that have been tried include esophageal wall, rib, duramater, and periosteum. Slide tracheoplasty, as described by Tsang and colleagues[136a] involves a transverse division of the trachea in the middle of the stenosis with longitudinal incisions of the anterior portion on one end and the posterior portion on the other, sliding the two ends over each other halving the length and doubling the diameter. In its original description, slide tracheoplasty was used for funnel-shaped stenosis. This technique has evolved to become a preferred surgical approach for tracheal stenosis regardless of the length of narrowing.[137,138] Another alternative is the use of tracheal homograft for reconstruction in cases of severe long-segment and recurrent stenosis. An 83% success rate is reported with this technique.[139,140] Long-term outcomes after homograft reconstruction are not available at present.

Tracheobronchial vascular compression

Vascular compression of the tracheobronchial tree has been the subject of much discussion since 1945 when Gross first described the successful operation for a double aortic arch.[141] In 1963, Fearon and Shortreed[142] reviewed 104 cases and coined the term "reflex apnea" to describe the episodic apnea associated with airway vascular compression. In 1969, Mustard *et al.*[143] reviewed 285 cases and reported successful medical management in 86.3% of cases.

Suggested indications for surgical management were reflex apnea and recurrent bronchopulmonary infections. In 1971, MacDonald and Fearon[144] proposed absolute and relative operative criteria, adding failure of medical management, greater than 50% compression of tracheal lumen and associated airway and lung abnormalities to the existing indications. In 1975, Moes and colleagues[145] compared 60 children who were operated on for innominate artery compression of the trachea with 30 children who did not undergo surgery. They suggested that the need for surgical intervention was based not on the severity of compression judged at endoscopy or radiographically, but was best correlated with the severity of symptoms. In 1981, Strife and colleagues[146] concluded that the word "anomalous" should be omitted from discussion of innominate artery tracheal compression syndrome since the origin of the innominate artery partially or totally to the left of the trachea was a normal finding in 96% of children as seen on aortogram.

Clinically relevant compression of the tracheobronchial tree by a vascular structure has an overall incidence of 3%. The most common symptomatic true vascular ring is the double aortic arch. This results if the fourth branchial arches and the dorsal aortic root persist bilaterally. In 1 of 2500 persons, the left arch has an atretic segment, but the right arch persists. A right-sided arch with a descending right aorta does not cause airway compromise. However, if there is an associated left ductus or an aberrant left subclavian artery, a vascular ring is formed that generally results in less airway compromise than a true double aortic arch. The pulmonary artery sling is the most symptomatic of the non-circumferential vascular anomalies and occurs when the left sixth arch resorbs and the left pulmonary artery arises as a large collateral artery from the right pulmonary artery, passing between the esophagus and trachea to perfuse the left lung. This anomaly commonly results in significant compression of the right mainstem bronchus and yields symptomatic airway. In addition, 30% of patients with pulmonary artery slings have associated complete tracheal rings.[147] The aberrant right subclavian artery is the most common mediastinal vascular anomaly. However, because of its retroesophageal course, affected individuals may present with dysphagia but rarely with symptomatic airway compromise. Innominate artery compression of the trachea is not a true vascular anomaly. The innominate artery normally passes from its origin on the aortic arch left of midline, across the anterior trachea to the right side. It has been hypothesized that, in patients who are symptomatic, the innominate artery is more taut than normal and the tracheal cartilages are unusually compliant and more easily compressed, or that dilatation of other structures such as the heart, esophagus, or thymus cause mediastinal crowding.

Respiratory compromise from tracheobronchial vascular compression is potentially life threatening, but can present with subtle symptoms. Frequently, a high index of suspicion is required in order to make the diagnosis. Patients with significant vascular compression of the airway usually present early, with stridor, chronic cough, recurrent bronchitis or pneumonia, difficulty feeding, failure to thrive, and occasionally reflex apnea. Reflex apnea is described as a reflexive respiratory arrest of variable duration that is secondary to stimulation of vagal afferent nerve fibers during swallowing and other forms of transient intrathoracic pressure changes.

Chest radiographs may provide some evidence of tracheal compression and a barium esophagram can show characteristic filling defects that correspond to the various types of vascular compression. However, once vascular compression is suspected, the diagnostic modality of choice is magnetic resonance imaging. This will clearly demonstrate the mediastinal vascular anatomy as well as the size of the lower airway. Spiral computed tomography may be a useful adjunct or alternative to magnetic resonance.[6,148] In contemporary practice the diagnosis of vascular compression is usually known prior to undergoing endoscopy. However, bronchoscopy also has characteristic findings of compression depending on the type of vascular ring or sling. Bronchoscopy also provides an immediate visual assessment of the surgical results upon dividing a vascular ring and affords assessment of any residual tracheomalacia.

Non-surgical management may be effective for the majority of patients with innominate artery compression and vascular rings and slings that are mildly symptomatic. In contrast, moderately to severely symptomatic patients typically require surgical repair. Absolute indications for surgical treatment include reflex apnea, failure of medical management of severe respiratory distress after 48 hours, and prolonged intubation. Relative criteria include repeated episodes of lower respiratory tract infection, exercise intolerance, significant dysphagia with failure to thrive, or coexisting subglottic stenosis, asthma, cystic fibrosis, or previous tracheoesophageal repair.

Innominate artery compression is relieved by aortopexy or reimplantation, with success rates of 93–100% and no reports of operative mortality or long term morbidity.[149] Occasionally, aortopexy sutures can loosen and the procedure needs to be revised.

Results of surgical treatment of vascular rings are also encouraging, with 70–92% obtaining complete resolution of symptoms.[150] Double aortic arch requires surgical division of the smaller of the two arches. The ductus arteriosus or aberrant subclavian artery is divided in the case of right aortic arch with left ductus arteriosus or aberrant left subclavian artery. In cases of severe tracheobronchial compression, residual tracheomalacia may persist for a variable period of time, and occasionally a tracheotomy is required to stent the malacic segment.

The pulmonary artery sling is corrected by dividing the aberrant left pulmonary artery at its origin and reimplanting it anterior to the trachea. There is significant morbidity and mortality in these cases, usually due to the associated complete tracheal rings and/or malacia.

REFERENCES

1. Gustafson, L. M., Hartley B. E., Liu, J. H. *et al.* Single-stage laryngotracheal reconstruction in children: a review of 200 cases. *Otolaryngol. Head Neck Surg.* 2000; **123**(4):430–434.
2. Van Den Abbeele, T., Triglia J. M., Lescanne, E. *et al.* Surgical removal of subglottic hemangiomas in children. *Laryngoscope* 1999; **109**(8):1281–1286.
3. Froehlich, P., Seid, A. B., & Morgon, A. Contrasting strategic approaches to the management of subglottic hemangiomas. *Int. J. Pediatr. Otorhinolaryngol.* 1996; **36**(2):137–146.
4. Wiatrak, B. J., Reilly, J. S., Seid A. B. *et al.* Open surgical excision of subglottic hemangioma in children. *Int. J. Pediatr. Otorhinolaryngol.* 1996; **34**(1–2):191–206.
5. Postic, W. P., Cotton R. T., & Handler, S. *Surg. Pediatr. Otolaryngol.* 1997.
6. Gustafson, L. M., Lin, J. H., Link, D. T. *et al.* Spiral CT versus MRI in neonatal airway evaluation. *Int. J. Pediatr. Otorhinolaryngol.* 2000; **52**(2):197–201.
7. Bluestone, C. D., Delerme, A. N., & Samuelson, G. H. Airway obstruction due to vocal cord paralysis in infants with hydrocephalus and meningomyelocele. *Ann. Otol., Rhinol. Laryngol.* 1972; **81**(6):778–783.
8. Yamada, H., Tanaka, Y., & Nakamura, S. Laryngeal stridor associated with the Chiari II malformation. *Childs Nerv. Syst.* 1985; **1**(6):312–318.
9. Hartnick, C. J., Hartley, B. E., Miller, C. *et al.* Pediatric fiberoptic endoscopic evaluation of swallowing. *Ann. Otol., Rhinol. Laryngol.* 2000; **109**(11):996–999.
10. Link, D. T., Willging, J. P., Miller, C. K. *et al.* Pediatric laryngopharyngeal sensory testing during flexible endoscopic evaluation of swallowing (FEES): feasible and correlative. *Ann. Otol., Rhinol, Laryngol.* 2000; **109**(10):899–905.
11. Willging, J. P. Benefit of feeding assessment before pediatric airway reconstruction. *Laryngoscope.* 2000; **110**(5 Pt 1):825–834.
12. Holinger, L. D., Lusk, R. P., & Green, C. G. eds. *Pediatric Laryngology and Bronchoesophagology.* 1st edn. 1997, Philadelphia, New York: Lippincott-Raven: 402.
13. Myer C., Cotton R. T., & Shott S. R. *The Pediatric Airway: An Interdisciplinary Approach.* 1st edn, ed. C. Myer, R. T. Cotton, and S. R. Shott. 1995, Philadelphia: J.B. Lippincott Company: 372.
14. Yellon, R. F. & Goldberg, H. Update on gastroesophageal reflux disease in pediatric airway disorders. *Am. J. Med.* 2001; **111**(Suppl 8A):78S–84S.
15. Halstead, L. A. Gastroesophageal reflux: a critical factor in pediatric subglottic stenosis. *Otolaryngol. Head Neck Surg.* 1999; **120**(5):683–688.
16. Halstead, L. A. Role of gastroesophageal reflux in pediatric upper airway disorders. *Otolaryngol. Head Neck Surg.* 1999; **120**(2):208–214.
17. Little, F. B., Koufman, J. A., Kohut R. I. *et al.* Effect of gastric acid on the pathogenesis of subglottic stenosis. *Ann. Otol. Rhinol. Laryngol.* 1985; **94**:516–519.

18. Koufman, J. A. The otolaryngologic manifestations of gastroesophageal reflux disease (GERD): a clinical investigation of 225 patients using ambulatory 24-hour pH monitoring and an experimental investigation of the role of acid and pepsin in the development of laryngeal injury. *Laryngoscope* 1991; **101**(4 Pt 2 Suppl 53):1–78.
19. Koufman, J. A., Aviv, J. E., Casiano, R. R. *et al.* Laryngopharyngeal reflux: position statement of the committee on speech, voice, and swallowing disorders of the American Academy of Otolaryngology – Head and Neck Surgery. [Review] [60 refs]. *Otolaryngol. Head Neck Surg.* 2002; **127**(1):32–35.
20. Koufman, J. A. Laryngopharyngeal reflux is different from classic gastroesophageal reflux disease. *Ear, Nose, Throat J.* 2002; **81**(9 Suppl 2):7–9.
21. Koufman, J. A., Belafsky, P. C., Bach, K. K. *et al.* Prevalence of esophagitis in patients with pH-documented laryngopharyngeal reflux. *Laryngoscope* 2002; **112**(9):1606–1609.
22. Hartnick, C. J., Hartley, B. E., Lacy, P. D. *et al.* Topical mitomycin application after laryngotracheal reconstruction: a randomized, double-blind, placebo-controlled trial. *Arch. Otolaryngol. Head Neck Surg.* 2001; **127**(10):1260–1264.
23. Rosenfield, S. Should granulomas be excised in children with long term tracheotomy? *Arch Otolaryngol. Head Neck Surg.* 1992; **118**:1323–1327.
24. Fagiolini, M., Pizzoruss, T., Berardi, N. Functional postnatal development of the rat primary visual cortex and the role of visual experience: dark rearing and monocular deprivation. *Vision Resuscitate* 1994; **34**:709–720.
25. Karmen, W. Effects of long-term tracheostomy on spectral characteristics of vowel production. *J. Speech Hear Res.* 1991; **34**:1057–1065.
26. Simon, B. M., Fowler, S. M., & Handler, S. D. Communication development in young children with long-term tracheostomies: preliminary report. *Int. J. Pediatr. Otorhinolaryngol.* 1983; **6**:37–50.
27. Ross, E. R., Green, R., Auslander, M. O. *et al.* Cricopharyngeal myotomy: management of cervical dysphagia. *Otolaryngol. Head Neck Surg.* 1982; **90**(4):434–441.
28. Willging, J. P. Endoscopic evaluation of swallowing in children. *Int. J. Pediatr. Otorhinolaryngol.* 1995; **32** Suppl:S107–108.
29. Holinger, H. & P. Brown, W. Congenital webs, cyst, laryngoceles and other anomalies of the larynx. *Ann. Otol. Rhinol. Laryngol.* 1967; **76**:744–752.
30. Giannoni, C., Sulek, M., Friedman, E. M. *et al.* Gastroesophageal reflux association with laryngomalacia: a prospective study. *Int. J. Pediatr. Otorhinolaryngol.* 1998; **43**(1):11–20.
31. Remacle, M., Bodart, E., & Lawson, G. Use of the CO_2-laser micropoint micromanipulator for the treatment of laryngomalacia. *Europ. Arch. Otol. Rhinol. Laryngol.* 1996; **253**(7):401–404.
32. Rudolph, C. D., Mazur, I. L., Librak, G. S. *et al.* Guidelines for evaluation and treatment of gastroesophageal reflux in infants and children: recommendations of the North American Society for Pediatric Gastroenterology and Nutrition.[see comment]. *J. Pediatr. Gastroenterol. Nutrit.* 2001; **32**(2): PS1–S31.
33. Holinger, L. D. & Konior, R. J. Surgical management of severe laryngomalacia. *Laryngoscope* 1989; **99**(2):136–142.
34. Polonovski, J. M., Contencin, P., Francois, M. *et al.* Aryepiglottic fold excision for the treatment of severe laryngomalacia. *Ann. Otol., Rhinol. Laryngol.* 1990; **99**(8):625–627.
35. Zalzal, G. H., Anon, J. B. & Cotton, R. T. Epiglottoplasty for the treatment of laryngomalacia. *Ann. Otol., Rhinol. Laryngol.* 1987; **96**(1 Pt 1):72–76.
36. Roger, G., Denoyelle, F., Trigilia, J. M. *et al.* Severe laryngomalacia: surgical indications and results in 115 patients. *Laryngoscope* 1995; **105**(10):1111–1117.
37. Baxter, M. R. Congenital laryngomalacia. *Can. J. Anaesth.* 1994; **41**(4):332–339.
38. McSwiney, P. F., Cavanagh, N. P., & P. Languth, Outcome in congenital stridor (laryngomalacia). *Arch. Dis. Childh.* 1977; **52**(3):215–218.
39. Seid, A. B., Park, S. M., Kearns, M. J. *et al.* Laser division of the aryepiglottic folds for severe laryngomalacia. *Int. J. Pediatr. Otorhinolaryngol.* 1985; **10**(2):153–158.
40. Lane, R. W., Weider, D. J., Ochi, J. W. *et al.* Laryngomalacia. A review and case report of surgical treatment with resolution of pectus excavatum. *Arch. Otolaryngol.* 1984; **110**(8):546–551.
41. Jani, P., Koltai, P., Ochi, J. *et al.* Surgical treatment of laryngomalacia. *J. Laryngol. Otol.* 1991; **105**(12):1040–1045.
42. Marcus, C. L., Crockett, D. M., & Davidson, Ward, S. L. Evaluation of epiglottoplasty as a treatment for severe laryngomalacia. *J. Pediatr.* 1990; **117**(5):706–710.
43. McClurg, F. L. & Evans, D. A. Laser laryngoplasty for laryngomalacia. *Laryngoscope* 1994; **104**(3 Pt 1):247–252.
44. Toynton, S. C., Saunders, M. W., & Bailey, C. M. Aryepiglottoplasty for laryngomalacia: 100 consecutive cases. *J. Laryngol. Otolo.* 2001; **115**(1):35–38.
45. Reddy, D. K. & Matt, B. H. Unilateral vs. bilateral supraglottoplasty for severe laryngomalacia in children. *Arch. Otolaryngol. Head Neck Surg.* 2001; **127**(6):694–699.
46. Kelly, S. M. & Gray, S. D. Unilateral endoscopic supraglottoplasty for severe laryngomalacia.[see comment]. *Arch. Otolaryngol – Head & Neck Surg.* 1995; **121**(12):1351–1354.
47. Denoyelle, F., Mondain, M., Gresillon, N. *et al.* Failures and complications of supraglottoplasty in children. *Arch. Otolaryngolo. Head Neck Surg.* 2003; **129**(10):1077–1080; discussion 1080.
48. Milczuk, H. A., Smith, J. D., & Everts, E. C. Congenital laryngeal webs: surgical management and clinical embryology. *Int. J. Pediatr. Otorhinolaryngol.* 2000; **52**(1):1–9.
49. Unal, M. The successful management of congenital laryngeal web with endoscopic lysis and topical mitomycin-C. *Int. J. Pediatr. Otorhinolaryngol.* 2004; **68**(2):231–235.
50. Benjamin, C., Jackson, B. N. Congenital laryngeal webs. *Ann. Otol., Rhinol. Laryngol.* 1983; **92**:317–326.

51. Holland, B. W., Koufman, J. A., Postma, G. N. *et al.* Laryngopharyngeal reflux and laryngeal web formation in patients with pediatric recurrent respiratory papillomas. *Laryngoscope* 2002; **112**(11):1926–1929.
52. Pollack, I. F., Kinnunen, D., & Albright, A. L. The effect of early craniocervical decompression on functional outcome in neonates and young infants with myelodysplasia and symptomatic Chiari II malformations: results from a prospective series. *Neurosurgery* 1996; **38**(4):703–710; discussion 710.
53. Link, D. T. & Cotton, R. T. The laryngotracheal complex in pediatric head and neck trauma: securing the airway and management of external laryngeal injury. *Facial Plast. Surg. Clin. N. Am.* 1999; **7**(2):133–144.
54. Triglia, J. M., Belus, J. F., & Nicollas, R. Arytenoidopexy for bilateral vocal fold paralysis in young children. *J. Laryngol. Otolo.* 1996; **110**(11):1027–1030.
55. Bower, C. M., Choi, S. S., & Cotton, R. T. Arytenoidectomy in children. *Ann. Otol., Rhinol. Laryngol.* 1994; **103**(4 Pt 1):271–278.
56. Narcy, P., Contencin, P., & Viala, P. Surgical treatment for laryngeal paralysis in infants and children. *Ann. Otol., Rhinol. Laryngol.* 1990; **99**(2 Pt 1):124–128.
57. Friedman, E. M., de Jong, A. L., & Sulek, M. Pediatric bilateral vocal fold immobility: the role of carbon dioxide laser posterior transverse partial cordectomy. *Ann. Otol., Rhinol. Laryngol.* 2001; **110**(8):723–728.
58. Rimell, F. L. and Dohar, J. E., Endoscopic management of pediatric posterior glottic stenosis. *Ann. Otol., Rhinol. Laryngol.* 1998; **107**(4):285–290.
59. Brigger, M. T. & Hartnick, C. J. Surgery for pediatric vocal cord paralysis: a meta-analysis. *Otolaryngol. Head Neck Surg.* 2002;**126**(4):349–355.
60. Gray, S. D., Kelly, S. M., & Dove, H. Arytenoid separation for impaired pediatric vocal fold mobility. *Ann. Otol., Rhinol. Laryngol.* 1994; **103**(7):510–515.
61. Younis, R. T., Lazar, R. H., & Astor, F. Posterior cartilage graft in single-stage laryngotracheal reconstruction. *Otolaryngol. Head Neck Surg.* 2003; **129**(3):168–175.
62. Hartnick, C. J., Brigger, M. T., Willging, J. P. *et al.* Surgery for pediatric vocal cord paralysis: a retrospective review. *Ann. Otol., Rhinol. Laryngol.* 2003; **112**(1):1–6.
63. Inglis, A. F., Jr., Perkins, J. A., Manning, S. C. *et al.* Endoscopic posterior cricoid split and rib grafting in 10 children. *Laryngoscope* 2003; **113**(11):2004–2009.
64. Kashima, H., Mounts, P., Leventhal, B. *et al.* Sites of predilection in recurrent respiratory papillomatosis. *Ann. Otol., Rhinol. Laryngol.* 1993; **102**(8 Pt 1):580–583.
65. Shah, K., Kashima, H., Polk, B. F. *et al.* Rarity of cesarean delivery in cases of juvenile-onset respiratory papillomatosis. *Obst. Gynecol.* 1986; **68**(6):795–799.
66. Wiatrak, B. J. Overview of recurrent respiratory papillomatosis. *Curr. Opin. Otolaryngol. Head Neck Surg.* 2003; **11**(6):433–441.
67. Parsons, D. S. & Bothwell, M. R. Powered instrument papilloma excision: an alternative to laser therapy for recurrent respiratory papilloma. *Laryngoscope* 2001; **111**(8):1494–1496.
68. Derkay C. S., Darrow, D. H., Recurrent respiratory papillomatosis of the larynx: current diagnosis and treatment. *Otolaryngol. Clin. N. Am.* 2000; **33**:1127–1142.
69. Patel, N., Rowe, M., & Tunkel, D. Treatment of recurrent respiratory papillomatosis in children with the microdebrider. *Ann. Otol., Rhinol. Laryngol.* 2003; **112**(1):7–10.
70. Franco, R. A., Jr., Zeitels, S M., Farinellik, W. A. *et al.* 585-nm pulsed dye laser treatment of glottal papillomatosis. *Ann. Otol., Rhinol. Laryngol.* 2002; **111**(6):486–492.
71. Cohen, J. T., Koufman, J. A., & Postma, G. N. Pulsed-dye laser in the treatment of recurrent respiratory papillomatosis of the larynx. *Ear, Nose, Throat J.* 2003; **82**(8):558.
72. Wetmore, S. J. Key, J., & Suen, J. Y. Complications of laser surgery for laryngeal papillomatosis. *Laryngoscope* 1985; **95**:798–801.
73. Cole, R. R., Myer, C. M. 3rd, & Cotton, R. T. Tracheotomy in children with recurrent respiratory papillomatosis. *Head Neck* 1989; **11**(3):226–230.
74. McDonald I. H., Stock, J., Prolonged nasotracheal intubation. *Br. J. Anesth.* 1965; **37**:161–173.
75. Holinger, P. H., Kutnick, S. L., Schild, J. A. *et al.* Subglottic stenosis in infants and children. *Ann. Otol. Rhinol. Laryngol.* 1976; **85**:591–599.
76. Ratner, W. Acquired subglottic stenosis in the very-low-birth-weight infant. *Am. J. Dis. Child.* 1983; **137**:40–43.
77. Myer, C. M. 3rd, O'Connor, D. M., & Cotton, R. T. Proposed grading system for subglottic stenosis based on endotracheal tube sizes. *Ann. Otol., Rhinol. Laryngol.* 1994; **103**(4 Pt 1):319–323.
78. Gilger, M. A. Pediatric otolaryngologic manifestations of gastroesophageal reflux disease. *Curr. Gastroenterol. Rep.* 2003; **5**(3):247–252.
79. Maronian, N. C., Azaden, H., Waugh, P. *et al.* Association of laryngopharyngeal reflux disease and subglottic stenosis. *Ann. Otol., Rhinol. Laryngol.* 2001; **110**(7 Pt 1):606–612.
80. Suskind, D. L., Zeringue, G. P., Kluka, E. A. *et al.* Gastroesophageal reflux and pediatric otolaryngologic disease: the role of antireflux surgery. *Arch. Otolaryngol. Head Neck Surg.* 2001; **127**(5):511–514.
81. Walner, D. L., Stern, Y., Gerber, M. E. *et al.* Gastroesophageal reflux in patients with subglottic stenosis. *Arch. Otolaryngol. Head Neck Surg.* 1998; **124**(5):551–555.
82. Kirchner, F. R. & Toledo, P. S. Microcauterization in otolaryngology. *Arch. Otolaryngol.* 1974; **99**:198–202.
83. Rodgers, T. Clinical application of endotracheal cryotherapy. *J. Pediatr. Surg.* 1978; **13**:662–668.
84. Cotton, R. T., Myer, C. M., Bratcher, G. O. *et al.* Anterior cricoid split, 1977–1987. Evolution of a technique. *Arch. Otolaryngol. Head Neck Surg.* 1988; **114**(11):1300–1302.
85. Rutter, M. J., Hartley, B. E., & Cotton, R. T. Cricotracheal resection in children. *Arch. Otolaryngol. Head Neck Surg.* 2001; **127**(3):289–292.

86. Stern, Y., Gerber, M. E., Walner, D. L. *et al.* Partial cricotracheal resection with primary anastomosis in the pediatric age group. *Ann. Otol., Rhinol. Laryngol.* 1997; **106**(11):891–896.
87. Hartley, B. E., Rutter, M. J., & Cotton, R. T. Cricotracheal resection as a primary procedure for laryngotracheal stenosis in children. *Int. J. Pediatr. Otorhinolaryngol.* 2000; **54**(2–3):133–136.
88. Walner, D. L., Stern, Y., & Cotton, R. T. Margins of partial cricotracheal resection in children. *Laryngoscope* 1999; **109**(10):1607–1610.
89. Monnier, P., Lang, F., & Savary, M. Partial cricotracheal resection for pediatric subglottic stenosis: a single institution's experience in 60 cases. *Europ. Arch. Otol. Rhinol. Laryngol.* 2003; **260**(6):295–297.
90. Triglia, J. M., Nicollas, R., & S. Roman, Primary cricotracheal resection in children: indications, technique and outcome. *Int. J. Pediatr. Otorhinolaryngol.* 2001; **58**(1):17–25.
91. Cotton, R. T. Pediatric laryngotracheal stenosis. *J. Pediatr. Surg.* 1984; **19**(6):699–704.
92. Cotton, R. T. & Myer, C. M. 3rd Contemporary surgical management of laryngeal stenosis in children. *Am. J. Otolaryngol.* 1984; **5**(5):360–368.
93. Zalzal, G. H., Cotton, R. T., & McAdams, A. J. Cartilage grafts – present status. *Head Neck Surg.* 1986; **8**(5):363–374.
94. Cotton, R. T., Gray, S. D., & Miller, R. P. Update of the Cincinnati experience in pediatric laryngotracheal reconstruction. *Laryngoscope* 1989; **99**(11):1111–1116.
95. Jacobs, B. R., Salmon, B. A., Cotton, R. T. *et al.* Postoperative management of children after single-stage laryngotracheal reconstruction. *Crit. Care Med.* 2001; **29**(1):164–168.
96. Hartley, B. E., Gustafson, L. M., Liu, J. H. *et al.* Duration of stenting in single-stage laryngotracheal reconstruction with anterior costal cartilage grafts. *Ann. Otol., Rhinol. Laryngol.* 2001; **110**(5 Pt 1):413–416.
97. Gustafson, L. M., Hartley, B. E., & Cotton, R. T. Acquired total (grade 4) subglottic stenosis in children. *Ann. Otol., Rhinol. Laryngol.* 2001; **110**(1):16–19.
98. Cotton, R. T. The problem of pediatric laryngotracheal stenosis: a clinical and experimental study on the efficacy of autogenous cartilaginous grafts placed between the vertically divided halves of the posterior lamina of the cricoid cartilage. *Laryngoscope* 1991; **101**(12 Pt 2 Suppl 56):1–34.
99. Pech, C., Triglia, J. M., Bouanga, C. *et al.* [Phonetic results after surgery of laryngotracheal stenoses in children]. *Ann. Oto-Laryngolo. Chir. Cervico-Faciale* 1995; **112**(5):199–204.
100. MacArthur, C. J., Kearns, G. H., & Healy, G. B. Voice quality after laryngotracheal reconstruction. *Arch. Otolaryngol – Head Neck Surg.* 1994; **120**(6):641–647.
101. Smith, M. E., Marsh, J. H., Cotton, R. T., & Myer, C. M. Voice problems after pediatric laryngotracheal reconstruction: videolaryngostroboscopic, acoustic and perceptual assessment. *Int. J. Pediatr. Otorhinolaryngol.* 1993; **25**:173–181.
102. Zalzal, G. H., Loomis, S. R., & Fischer, M. Laryngeal reconstruction in children. Assessment of vocal quality. *Arch. Otolaryngol. Head Neck Surg.* 1993; **119**(5):504–507.
103. Smith, M. E., Clary, R. A., Dengilly, A. *et al.* Voice problems after pediatric laryngotracheal reconstruction: videolaryngostroboscopic, acoustic, and perceptual assessment. *Int. J. Pediatr. Otorhinolaryngol.* 1993; **25**(1–3):173–181.
104. Albert, D. M., Bailey, C. M., Clary, R. A. *et al.* Voice quality following laryngotracheal reconstruction. *Int. J. Pediatr. Otorhinolaryngol.* 1995; **32**(Suppl):S93–S95.
105. Thome, R. & Thome, D. C. Posterior cricoidotomy lumen augmentation for treatment of subglottic stenosis in children. *Arch. Otolaryngol. Head Neck Surg.* 1998; **124**(6):660–664.
106. Gregor, R. T., Plit, M., & Webster, T. The use of the flow-volume loop in assessing the results of laryngotracheal reconstruction. *S. Afri. J. Surg.* 1997; **35**(4):210–214.
107. Zalzal, G. H. Rib cartilage grafts for the treatment of posterior glottic and subglottic stenosis in children. *Ann. Otol., Rhinol. Laryngol.* 1988; **97**(5 Pt 1):506–511.
108. Choa, D. I., Smith, M. C., Evans, J. N., & Bailey, C. M. Subglottic hemangioma in children. *J. Laryngol. Otol.* 1986; **100**:447.
109. Leikensohn, B., Cotton, R. T. Subglottic hemangioma. *J. Otolaryngol.* 1976; **5**:487–492.
110. Cohen, S. R., Unusual lesions of the larynx, trachea, and bronchial tree. *Ann. Otol. Rhinol. Laryngol.* 1969; **78**:476–489.
111. Hawkins, D. B. Corticosteroid management of airway hemangiomas: long term follow-up. *Laryngoscope* 1984; **94**:633–637.
112. Shikhani, A. H., Infantile subglottic hemangiomas. *Ann. Otol. Rhinol. Laryngol.* 1986; **95**:336–347.
113. Aviles, R., Boyce, T. G., & Thompson, D. M. Pneumocystis carinii pneumonia in a 3-month-old infant receiving high-dose corticosteroid therapy for airway hemangiomas. *Mayo Clin. Proc.* 2004; **79**(2):243–245.
114. Al-Sebeih, K. & Manoukian, J. Systemic steroids for the management of obstructive subglottic hemangioma. *J. Otolaryngol.* 2000; **29**(6):361–366.
115. Meeuwis, J., Bos, C., Hoeve, L. *et al.* Subglottic hemangiomas in infants: treatment with intralesional corticosteroid injection and intubation. *Int. J. Pediatr. Otorhinolaryngol.* 1990; **19**:145–150.
116. Healy, G. B. Treatment of subglottic hemangioma with the carbon dioxide laser. *Laryngoscope* 1980; **90**:809–813.
117. Sie, M., McGill, T., & Healy, G. B. Subglottic hemangioma: ten year's experience with the carbon dioxide laser. *Ann. Otol. Rhinol. Laryngol.* 1994; **103**:167–172.
118. Kacker, A., April, M., & Ward, R. F. Use of potassium titanyl phosphate (KTP) laser in management of subglottic hemangiomas. *Int. J. Pediatr. Otorhinolaryngol.* 2001; **59**(1):15–21.
119. Madgy, D., Ahsan, S. F., Kest, D. *et al.* The application of the potassium-titanyl-phosphate (KTP) laser in the

management of subglottic hemangioma. *Arch. Otolaryngol. Head Neck Surg*. 2001; **127**(1):47–50.

120. Ohlms, L. A., Jones, D. T., McGill, J. J. Interferon Alfa-2A Therapy for airway hemangiomas. *Ann. Otol. Rhinol. Laryngol.* 1994; **103**:1–8.
121. Chatrath, P., Black, M., Jani, P. *et al.* A review of the current management of infantile subglottic haemangioma, including a comparison of CO_2 laser therapy versus tracheostomy. *Int. J. Pediatr. Otorhinolaryngol.* 2002; **64**(2):143–157.
122. Seid, A. B., Pransky, S. M., & Kearns, D. B. The open surgical approach to subglottic hemangioma.[comment]. *Int. J. Pediatr. Otorhinolaryngol.* 1993; **26**(1):95–96.
123. Seid, A. B., Pransky, S. M., & Kearns, D. B. The open surgical approach to subglottic hemangioma.[see comment]. *Int. J. Pediatr. Otorhinolaryngol.* 1991; **22**(1):85–90.
124. Naiman, A. N., Ayari, S., & Froehlich, P. Controlled risk of stenosis after surgical excision of laryngeal hemangioma. *Arch. Otolaryngol. Head Neck Surg*. 2003; **129**(12):1291–5.
125. Evans, K. L., Courteney-Harris, R., Bailey, C. M. *et al.* Management of posterior laryngeal and laryngotracheoesophageal clefts. *Arch. Otolaryngol.* 1995; **121**:1380–1385.
126. Eriksen, C. & Zwillenberg D., Robinson, N., Diagnosis and management of cleft larynx: literature review and case repoart. *Ann. Otol. Rhinol. Laryngol.* 1990; **103**(10):753–757.
127. Smith, R., Neville, M., & Bauman, N. Interarytenoid notch height relative ot the vocal folds. *Ann. Otol. Rhinol. Laryngol.* 1994; **103**:753–757.
128. Bent, J. P. Endoloscope repair of tpe IA laryngeal clefts. *Laryngoscope* 1997; **107**:282–286.
129. Roth, B. Laryngotracheoesophageal cleft, clinical features, diagnosis, and therapy. *Eur. J. Pediatr. Surg.* 1983; **140**:41–46.
130. Robie, D. K., Pearl, R. H., Gonsales, C. *et al.* Operative strategy for recurrent laryngeal cleft: a case report and review of the literature. *J. Pediatr. Surg.* 1991; **26**:973–974.
131. Cantrell, J. R. & Guild, H. G.Congenital stenosis of the trachea. *Am. J. Surg.* 1964; **108**:297–305.
132. Blumer, J. Distal tracheal stenosis in neonates and infants. *Otolaryngol. Head Neck Surg.* 1992; **107**:583–590.
132a. Benjamin, B., Pitkin, J., & Cohen, D. Congenital tracheal stenosis. *Ann. Otol. Rhinol. Laryngol.* 1981; **90**:364–371.
133. Rutter, M. J., Willging, J. P., & Cotton, R. T. Nonoperative management of complete tracheal rings. *Arch. Otolaryngol. Head Neck Surg*. 2004; **130**(4):450–452.
134. Indriss, F. Tracheoplasty with pericardial patch for extensive tracheal stenosis in infants and children. *J. Thorac. Cardiovasc. Surg.* 1984; **88**:527–536.
135. Dunham, M. Management of severe congenital tracheal stenosis. *Ann. Otol. Rhinol. Laryngol.* 1994; **103**:351–356.
136. Weber, T. Resection of congenital tracheal stenosis involving the carina. *J. Thorac. Cardiovasc. Surg.* 1982; **84**:200–203.
136a. Tsang, V., Murday, A., Gillbe, C., & Goldstraw, P. Slide tracheoplasty for congenital funnel-shaped tracheal stenosis. *Ann. Thorac. Surg.* 1989; **48**:632–635.
137. Rutter, M. J., Cotton, R. T., Manning, P. B. *et al.* Slide tracheoplasty for the management of complete tracheal rings. *J. Pediatr. Surg.* 2003; **38**(6):928–934.
138. Cunningham, M. J., Eavey, R. D., Vlahakes, G. J. *et al.* Slide tracheoplasty for long-segment tracheal stenosis. *Arch. Otolaryngol – Head Neck Surg*. 1998; **124**(1):98–103.
139. Jacobs, J. P. Pediatric tracheal homograft reconstruction: a novel approach to complex tracheal stenoses in children. *J. Thorac. Cardiovasc. Surg.* 1996; **112**:1546–1558.
140. Jacobs, J. P. Successful complete tracheal resection in a three-month-old infant. *Ann. Thorac. Surg.* 1996; **61**:1824–1826.
141. Gross, R. Surgical relief for tracheal obstruction from a vascular ring. *N. Engl. J. Med.* 1945; **233**:586–590.
142. Feron, B. & Shortreed R. Tracheobronchial compression by congenital cardiovasculare anomalies in children: syndrome of apnea. *Ann. Otol. Rhinol. Laryngol.* 1963; **72**:949–969.
143. Mustard, W., Bayliss C. E., Fearon B. *et al.* Tracheal compression by the innominate artery in children. *Ann. Thorac. Surg.* 1969; **8**:312–319.
144. MacDonald R. E. & Fearon B., Innominate artery compression syndrome in children. *Ann. Otol. Rhinol. Laryngol.* 1971; **80**:535–540.
145. Moes C. A. F., Trusler, G. A., & Izukawa T. Innominate artery compression of the trachea. *Arch. Otolaryngol.* 1975; **101**:733–738.
146. Strive J. L., Baumel A., & Dunbar, J. S. Tracheal compression by the innominate artery in infancy and childhood. *Radiology* 1981; **139**:73–75.
147. Backer, C. Vascular rings, slings, and tracheal rings. *Mayo Clin. Proc.* 1993; **68**:1131–1133.
148. Lee, K. H., Yoon, C. S., Choe, K. O. *et al.* Use of imaging for assessing anatomical relationships of tracheobronchial anomalies associated with left pulmonary artery sling. *Pediatr. Radiol.* 2001; **31**(4):269–278.
149. Adler, S. M., Isaacson, G., Balsara, R. K. Innominate artery compression of the trachea: diagnosis and treatment by anterior suspension: a 25-year experience. *Ann. Otol. Rhinol. Laryngol.* 1995; **107**:924–927.
150. Backer, C. Vascular anomalies causing tracheoesophageal compression. *J. Thorac. Cardiovasc. Surg.* 1989; **97**:725–731.

14

Pulmonary resection and thoracotomy

Frédérique Sauvat and Yann Revillon

Service de Chirurgie Pediatrique, Paris, France

Thoracic surgery in childhood has changed considerably in the last 50 years. In particular, surgical indications and techniques have altered dramatically. At the beginning of the twentieth century, the main indications for thoracic surgery were related to infectious diseases, especially bronchiectasis and tuberculosis, whereas congenital malformations now constitute the commonest reason for lung resection. Thoracic surgery has become more commonplace in younger patients, including neonates. Safe techniques have prompted the development of prophylactic surgery in asymptomatic patients and thoracoscopic techniques offer a minimally invasive approach.

The long-term consequences of pulmonary resection and thoracotomy are related to many different factors: the underlying disease process and its natural history; the effects of loss of parenchymal volume; and the physical sequelae of surgery on the chest wall. In addition, in younger patients there is the added dimension of the effects of somatic growth on future pulmonary function.

As in all branches of pediatric surgery, knowledge of long-term sequelae is limited because of the lack of studies following patients through to adulthood. The late consequences of thoracoscopic procedures and the relative merits of open surgery and thoracoscopic techniques are poorly understood. However, specific data are reported in two broad areas: the functional consequences of pulmonary resection and musculoskeletal abnormalities resulting from thoracotomy.

Lung development and compensatory lung growth

In order to understand the effects of lung resection during childhood, it is helpful to review the process of normal lung development.[1,2] The human lung is an organ which continues to mature after birth. Indeed, its principal function of gas exchange only exists after birth. In the embryo, the endodermal lung bud appears about 26 days after fertilization. The first phase of development, the pseudoglandular phase, begins from about the fifth week. Segmental bronchi are present from about the seventh week. The second phase of development, the canalicular phase, extends to 24 weeks of gestation and is characterized by flattening of the epithelium of the distal airways, thinning of the mesenchyme and growth of the capillary network that surrounds the terminal airways. Type II pneumocytes and surfactant appear during this period and are detectable in amniotic fluid. The last phase of development is the sac period, which refers to the appearance of a thin layer of respiratory epithelium apposed to a capillary network and capable of gas exchange. True alveolar formation begins shortly before birth and continues afterwards. At birth, 20 million saccules are present but by 8 years of age, there are about 300 million, which is close to the normal adult lung complement. Recently, a final process of microvascular maturation has been described, beginning at birth and progressing for 2 years; alveoli become fully functional when their capillary network is properly developed. After 3 years of age, no further major structural modifications occur and the child's lung is nearly the same as that of an adult, although smaller.

After lung resection, it is clearly established that compensatory growth occurs in both children and adults. The mechanism is not fully defined although it has been studied in animals and humans. Compensatory growth results from hyperplasia rather than hypertrophy. Pulmonary resection leads to an increase in the number and size of remaining alveoli. In children, compensatory growth is more

Pediatric Surgery and Urology: Long-term Outcomes, Mark Stringer, Keith Oldham, Pierre Mouriquand.
Published by Cambridge University Press.

prominent than emphysematous expansion. It has also been suggested that the complexity of the gas exchanging surface in the alveolus might be increased by mechanisms other than alveolar multiplication.[2] The cellular mechanisms inducing growth after pulmonary resection are still mysterious. The deformation of the cytoskeleton of certain cells probably initiates signal transduction pathways resulting in the release of substances (paracrine and autocrine) which promote cell multiplication and growth.

Traditionally, it has been stated that human newborns and young children have better compensatory growth than older patients. For example, Laros and Westermann showed that patients who had undergone a pneumonectomy before the age of five years had, 30 years later, similar pulmonary function to normal individuals.[3] The physiology of lung development and compensatory growth leads to the conclusion that lung resection at an early age optimizes eventual respiratory function. Progress in newborn surgery and anesthesia and the development of prenatal diagnosis now allow such procedures to be performed safely in very young patients.

Long-term respiratory function after pulmonary resection

The traditional view is that partial lung resection during childhood does not lead to significant respiratory impairment and has few physical consequences. However, few reports have precisely documented the volume of lung removed, the indication for surgery and the age at operation.

In our clinical experience of 75 patients operated for cystic adenomatoid malformation, 71% of whom were diagnosed prenatally, all were asymptomatic beyond 1 month postoperatively; mean follow-up was 16 months.[4] Surgery had consisted of a segmentectomy in 65% and a lobectomy in the remainder. Only one child subsequently developed asthma, which was unrelated to his previous segmental pulmonary resection. Chest radiographs taken two months or more postoperatively were considered normal. In a study of 47 children whose mean age was 90 days, Ayed and Owayed (2003) confirmed the safety of lung resection in infancy for congenital malformations.[5] A lobectomy was performed in 89% of cases. None of the patients had any physical limitations at a mean follow-up of four years. Verga *et al.* investigated pulmonary function in seven subjects three to 25 years after pulmonary lobectomy in childhood.[6] Resting and stress ECGs, chest radiographs, and arterial blood gases were normal. Spirometry and basal and stress pulmonary scintigraphy were more difficult to interpret but confirmed that the residual lung after lobectomy demonstrates a good functional recovery. In another study of 27 patients who underwent pulmonary lobectomy between birth and 14 years of age, Caussade *et al.* found normal spirometry values with a forced vital capacity ranging between 87% and 143% of normal, and a normal oxygen saturation during and after effort.[7] Radiographs suggested satisfactory lung growth and development.

Considering age at operation, one small series reported on 12 children who had undergone lobectomy before 10 years of age.[8] In those over 10 years old and more than 2 years out from surgery, a chest radiograph showed no evidence of compensatory lung regeneration or overdistension but vital capacity was increased, probably as a result of growth of the thorax and respiratory muscles. In contrast, children who had undergone surgery before 8 years of age had evidence of mild overdistension of the lung during the early postoperative period but this was no longer present two years later. The normality of pulmonary function tests after lobectomy has been confirmed by other authors.[9] Nakajima *et al.* found that vital capacity showed a transient decrease after surgery before recovering to within or above the normal range within 2 years. The ratio of residual volume to total lung capacity was also normal 2 years later. This study of 27 children suggested that overinflation of the residual lung compensates vital capacity early on after lobectomy and that alveolar multiplication occurs subsequently. These authors considered that the factors adversely affecting compensatory lung growth were surgery performed after 4 years of age, preoperative infection, and pre-existing thoracic deformity. The good prognosis for functional capacity after lobectomy during childhood seems to be confirmed in adults.[10] After empyema, most children show a restrictive pattern on pulmonary function testing within 3 months of hospital discharge but this decreases significantly over time and most patients have normal lung function after a year.[11]

These good functional outcomes are also found after a limited pulmonary resection such as a segmentectomy in adults[12] or children.[13] In one report of 14 children who had had a segmental lung resection at a mean age of 6.8 months, residual volume and functional residual capacity were larger than predicted-corrected values in most patients after a mean period of 11.6 years. However, decreased expiratory flows, regional ventilation abnormalities, and decreased perfusion localized to the region of resection suggested the presence of abnormal ventilation and perfusion at the resection site.

Pneumonectomy in children is relatively uncommon and most often required for complications of infection or bronchiectasis; rarely it is necessary for a tumor. Eren *et al.*

Table 14.1. Musculoskeletal sequelae of thoracotomy

Author	Side	Surgery performed	Cases (*n*)	Scoliosis	Synostosis	Chest deformity	Shoulder elevation
Seghaye *et al.*[29]	Left	PDA lign	27	3%	74%		
Chetcuti *et al.*[28]	Right	TEF	232	7.7%		20%	
Jaureguizar *et al.*[27]	Right	TEF	227	7.8%	10%	20%	23.8%
Durning *et al.*[25]	Right	TEF	18	50%			
Bal *et al.*[30]	Right	Cardiac	49	31%		14%	61%

PDA = patent ductus arteriosus, TEF = tracheoesophageal fistula, Cardiac = surgery for cardiac disease.

reported a series of 17 pediatric patients (mean age 9 years) after pneumonectomy for bronchiectasis or tuberculosis.[14] Two patients died but follow-up information was available for 13 patients between one and 12 years later. Quality of life had improved and growth and development were stated to be normal. In a larger series of 59 patients aged between six months and 14 years, Blyth *et al.* recorded no mortality and came to similar conclusions about longer term consequences.[15] Perioperative morbidity included pulmonary artery injury, intraoperative cardiac arrest and excessive bleeding, in one patient each. Postoperative complications, predominantly infective or a bronchopleural fistula, developed in 12% of cases.

The largest series of patients followed up after pneumonectomy was reported by Laros and Westermann.[16] They studied patients who had had a pneumonectomy at 2–40 years of age and were followed up for a mean of 33 years. From a group of 98 patients with a normal forced expiratory volume, the authors concluded that if a pneumonectomy had been performed before 5 years of age, the ventilatory capacity was only minimally smaller than that predicted for an individual with two lungs, suggesting that compensatory growth had occurred mainly as a result of hyperplasia. When surgery had been performed later in childhood, a significant difference in ventilatory function was still found compared to a group of patients operated on after 20 years of age. This difference indicates that compensatory growth, possibly as a result of simple hypertrophy, plays an important but gradually diminishing role with advancing age.

A striking finding from this study was the stability of the tidal volume/functional residual capacity ratio, which in the under 5-year group especially was very close to the predicted value for two lungs. The authors concluded that most individuals with one healthy remaining lung are able to lead a normal social life after pneumonectomy.

The long-term cardiac effects of childhood pneumonectomy were first reported in 1966 in a small series of eight patients.[17] Four had electrocardiogram abnormalities: three with an incomplete right bundle branch block, and one with right ventricular hypertrophy. Pulmonary artery pressures rose excessively during maximal exercise. Similar abnormal pulmonary artery pressures were reported by Sery *et al.*[18] but without clinical consequences.

One complication that does have physical consequences is the right pneumonectomy syndrome.[19] This syndrome is characterized by exertional dyspnea resulting from mediastinal shift into the empty hemi-thorax with rotation of the heart and great vessels.[20] Symptoms arise from compression of the left bronchus between the pulmonary artery, aorta, ductus arteriosus and spine. Similar symptoms have been described in some cases of unilateral pulmonary artery agenesis. Various surgical treatments have been used to correct this syndrome, including suspension of the great vessels, thoracoplasty, muscle flap transposition, or hemithorax prosthetic implants. The latter procedure seems to be effective in children.[21–23]

In conclusion, after lung resection during childhood, patients can expect to have normal physical development and vital capacity because of compensatory growth of the remaining lung. The increase in residual volume and decreased perfusion in the region of the resection are probably the result of simple expansion of the lung. Most studies indicate that few children are functionally impaired by lung resection.

Musculoskeletal morbidity after thoracotomy

Thoracotomy is usually very well tolerated in the short term in relation to musculoskeletal function. Recovery and return to normal physical and school activities after thoracotomy in children contrasts with the prolonged pain and disability described by many adults after surgery. However, this rapid recovery must be tempered by the possibility of long term growth abnormalities resulting from the thoracotomy (rather than the lung resection). Few reports have specifically investigated the musculoskeletal sequelae of thoracotomy for lung resection. Most publications refer to thoracotomy for cardiac surgery or esophageal atresia repair (Table 14.1). Several types of orthopedic deformity are recognized after thoracotomy: scoliosis (Figs. 14.1

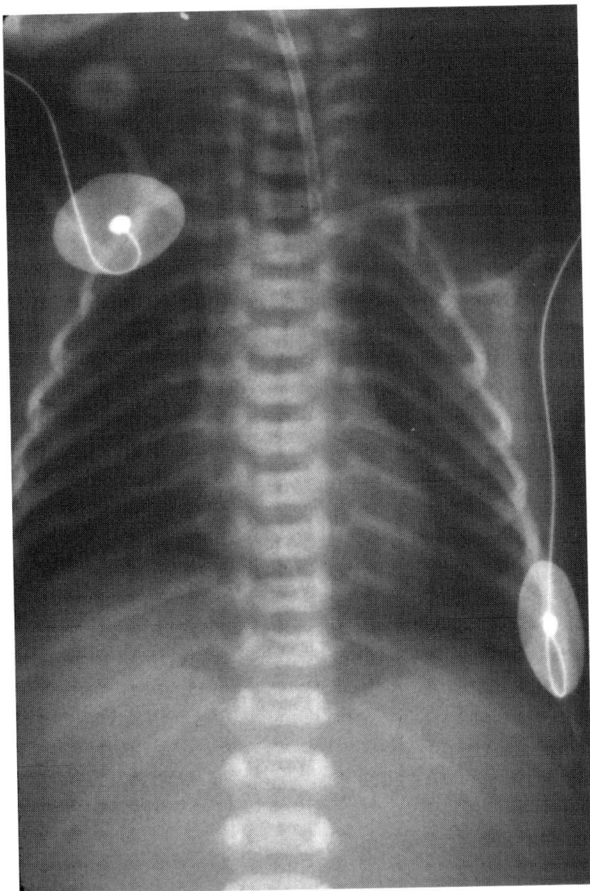

Fig. 14.1. Chest radiograph of a patient with esophageal atresia at birth.

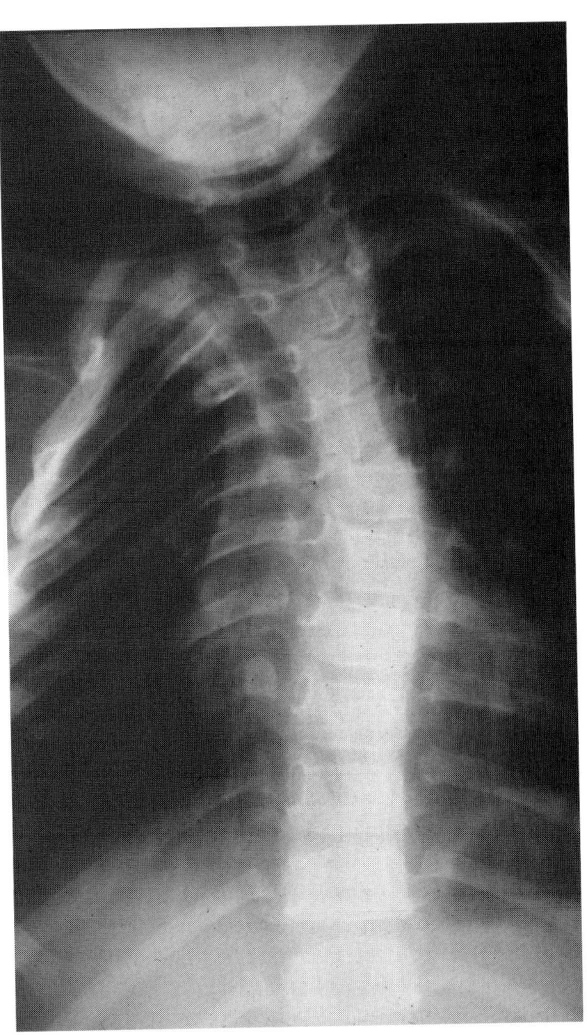

Fig. 14.2. The same patient as in Fig 14.1, at 10 years of age with scoliosis induced by thoracotomy.

and 14.2), rib deformities and synostosis, and shoulder deformities.

In 1969, Freeman and Walkden first reported right shoulder deformities after repair of esophageal atresia by right thoracotomy.[24] Orthopedic surgeons subsequently described severe scoliosis in 18 patients followed up for more than 10 years after repair of tracheoesophageal fistula.[25] A spinal curvature of more than 10 degrees had developed in nine patients and in eight of these cases the curves were convex away from the side of the incision. The scoliosis had appeared at any time from early childhood to skeletal maturity but was more likely to be progressive in those in whom it had developed before the adolescent growth spurt. Severe scoliosis was more likely in patients who had experienced postoperative infectious complications such as mediastinitis and empyema secondary to esophageal dehiscence; in these cases it was often accompanied by marked scarring and rib fusion.[26]

Two larger series of chest wall deformities after surgery for esophageal atresia or tracheoesophageal fistula have been reported (*see also Chapter on Esophageal Atresia*). Jaureguizar *et al.* reported a series of 89 patients operated on for esophageal atresia via a right dorso-lateral thoracotomy and followed up for 3 to 16 years.[27] Twenty-nine of the patients had significant musculoskeletal deformities: 21 (24%) had a "winged" scapula from partial paralysis of the latissimus dorsi muscle; 18 (20%) had marked asymmetry of the thoracic wall from atrophy of the serratus anterior muscle; 9 (10%) had rib fusion (with major respiratory dysfunction in one patient); and 7 (8%) had severe thoracic scoliosis. No patient required surgical correction but all needed physiotherapy. Chetcuti *et al.* reported a similar experience in a study of 232 patients with esophageal atresia but no congenital vertebral anomaly; in this series 77 (33%) patients developed chest wall deformities.[28] Anterior chest wall deformities were found in 47, scoliosis in 18 and a combination of both in 12 patients. Chest wall deformity appeared to be more common in patients after 25 years of age and scoliosis in patients who had had numerous thoracotomies. One patient required surgery for severe scoliosis.

Similar sequelae have been described after thoracotomy for congenital cardiac disease. Seghaye *et al.* prospectively followed 36 premature infants after left thoracotomy for patent ductus arteriosus.[29] One developed a thoracic scoliosis and 20 of 27 (74%) had minor radiologic skeletal abnormalities in the form of rib deformation or fusion; the latter carries a risk of long term scoliosis. No left shoulder elevation or left arm dysfunction was noticed. Bal *et al.* confirmed this high prevalence of musculoskeletal problems in a series of 49 children who had required posterolateral thoracotomy for cardiac surgery. After a mean follow-up period of 6 years, 94% had various deformities: 31% had a scoliosis, with a severe curve exceeding 25 degrees in two; 61% had shoulder elevation; 77% had a winged scapula; and 14% had asymmetry of the thoracic wall due to the atrophy of the serratus anterior muscle.[30]

From these studies, it is evident that children should be followed up for many years after thoracotomy because, even in the absence of vertebral anomalies, scoliosis and chest wall deformities may develop, especially if there is evidence of rib fusion on a postoperative chest radiograph. Most thoracotomies in children use a lateral or posterolateral skin incision and the latissimus dorsi muscle and a portion of the serratus anterior muscle are divided. The rhomboids, trapezius and paraspinal muscles are preserved intact. The intercostal muscles are divided to enter the chest. In order to decrease the rate of musculoskeletal deformities, greater attention must be paid to the thoracotomy procedure, particularly in relation to these muscles. Particular care must be taken when closing the intercostal space to avoid injury to nerves and to prevent synostosis (Fig. 14.3). A muscle sparing incision has been described using a true posterolateral approach with mobilization of latissimus dorsi and trapezius and is being used with increasing frequency in infants and children.[31,32]

Skeletal morbidity could be further reduced by the more widespread use of thoracoscopy for lung resection[33] and repair of esophageal atresia.[34,35] However, experience of thoracoscopy is still limited and long term studies will be required to demonstrate its potential advantages over open surgery.

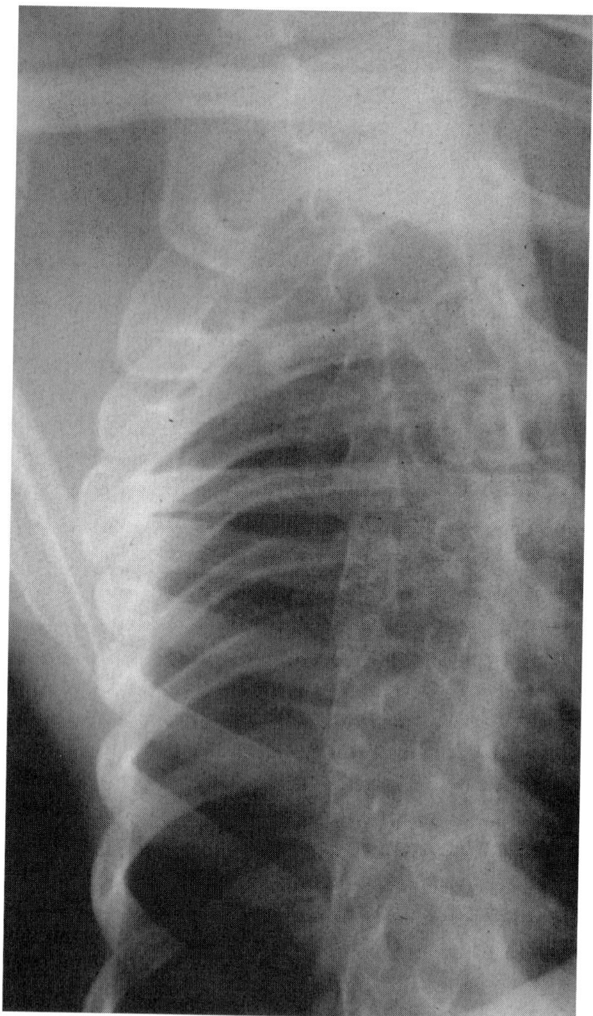

Fig. 14.3. Synostosis and scoliosis 8 years after thoracotomy.

Neurologic morbidity after thoracotomy

Thoracotomy may result in three main types of nerve injury: phrenic nerve injury causing diaphragmatic paralysis, recurrent laryngeal nerve injury, and damage to the sympathetic chain leading to Horner's syndrome.

Diaphragmatic paralysis has been described after cardiothoracic surgery in children, secondary to division, dissection or diathermy coagulation close to the phrenic nerve.

This complication is more commonly associated with cardiac surgery than with lung resection.[36] Tonz *et al.* reported a series of 1656 cardiac surgical procedures in children.[37] The rate of phrenic nerve injury, resulting in diaphragmatic paralysis was 1.5%. Plication of the diaphragm was performed in 11 (44%) of these patients, all of whom were under 2 years of age. The indications for surgery were inability to wean from mechanical ventilation and persistent or recurrent respiratory distress. De Leeuw *et al.* reported an almost identical rate of diaphragmatic paralysis (1.6%) in a series of 168 children.[38] Surgical treatment was necessary in 40% but the remainder recovered spontaneously within a few weeks. When diaphragmatic plication is necessary, it enables weaning from mechanical ventilation and stable respiratory function, even in adults.[39]

Recurrent laryngeal nerve injury after thoracic surgery is mainly described after right thoracotomy for esophageal atresia and left thoracotomy for ligation of a patent ductus arteriosus. It results in a paralysed vocal cord which may or may not be symptomatic. Bargy *et al.* reported a 20% incidence of recurrent nerve palsy in a series of 100 patients with esophageal atresia.[40] In a similar series of 65 patients, Robertson and Birck found a similar incidence: 10 (15%) of patients had laryngeal symptoms and half of these had vocal cord paresis confirmed by laryngoscopy (three of whom required surgical treatment).[41] Fan *et al.* investigated the prevalence of recurrent laryngeal nerve injury after thoracotomy for ligation of patent ductus arteriosus in 167 neonates; seven (4%) had evidence of vocal cord paralysis on laryngoscopy.[42]

Horner's syndrome has also been described in 1.3% of patients after thoracotomy[43] and in some patients after insertion of a thoracostomy tube.[44,45] The latter has mostly been reported in adults but children are occasionally affected.[46] In such cases, injury to the sympathetic chain is believed to be caused by the tip of the chest tube near the first thoracic intervertebral space.

Another neurologic injury has been described after thoracotomy but only in adults. Rarely, patients can develop involuntary twitching of the latissimus dorsi induced by contractions of adjacent muscles (serratus anterior or external intercostal) as a result of aberrant neural regeneration to the denervated latissimus dorsi from adjacent nerves.[47]

Esthetic morbidity after thoracotomy

Skin incisions for pediatric thoracotomy are usually short and devoid of major esthetic sequelae. Postoperative wound infection is uncommon after lung resection, thereby increasing the chance of a satisfactory scar. Posterolateral thoracotomy through an axillary skin incision has been described, allowing for access through the third or fourth intercostal space.[48]

Deformities caused by atrophy of chest wall muscles from nerve injuries during thoracotomy have been reported. Frola *et al.* reviewed a series of 58 adult CT scans in patients who had had a previous thoracotomy and compared muscle thickness on the side of surgery with that on the contralateral chest wall.[49] Muscle atrophy was found in 42 patients but in two cases this was confined to the serratus anterior muscle only. Signs of atrophy of the latissimus dorsi muscle and the inferior portion of the serratus anterior muscle were seen in all patients after posterolateral thoracotomy, whereas this pattern of atrophy was present in only two of 18 patients after anterolateral thoracotomy. No equivalent pediatric series has been published.

In order to preserve muscle, a muscle-sparing thoracotomy (see above) is an alternative and may be particularly important if rotational muscle flaps might be necessary.[50] Muscle-sparing thoracotomy has been reported in children.[51] The only specific morbidity described using this technique rather than the classical approach was the occurrence of seroma.[52]

A more serious esthetic complication of thoracotomy concerns breast development. Jaureguizar *et al.* reported scar disfiguration of the right breast in 3.3% of patients after right posterolateral thoracotomy for esophageal atresia; one patient had mammary maldevelopment.[27] Nipple asymmetry has been described in 63% of patients after thoracotomy for congenital cardiac disease.[30] After cardiac surgery via an anterolateral thoracotomy, Bleiziffer *et al.* reported a disturbance in breast development in 55% of women (left breast volume at least 20% greater than right breast), with an asymmetry of the lower part of the right breast in 61%.[53] These authors concluded that anterolateral thoracotomy can significantly interfere with ipsilateral breast development.

In conclusion, thoracotomy and lung resection during childhood remains a relatively safe procedure both in terms of subsequent respiratory function and chest wall growth and appearance. Nevertheless, the pediatric surgeon must maintain long-term follow-up of these patients to assess the true incidence of late sequelae such as musculoskeletal and cosmetic effects and any impact on breast development. In the future, the morbidity of thoracotomy must be compared with newer, less invasive thoracoscopic procedures.

REFERENCES

1. Burri, P. H. Structural aspects of prenatal and postnatal development and growth of the lung. In McDonald, J., ed. *Lung Growth and Development*. New York: M.Dekker, Inc., 1997: 1–35.
2. Addis, T. Compensatory hypertrophy of lung after unilateral pneumonectomy. *J. Exp. Med.* 1928; **47**:51–56.
3. Laros, C. D. & Westermann, C. J. J. Dilatation, compensatory growth, or both after pneumonectomy during childhood and adolescence. *J. Thorac. Cardiovasc. Surg.* 1987; **93**:570–576.

4. Sauvat, F., Michel, J. L., Benachi, A., Emond, S., & Revillon, Y. Management of asymptomatic cystic adenomatoid malformations. *J. Pediatr. Surg.* 2003; **38**:548–552.
5. Ayed, A. & Owayed, A. Pulmonary resection in infants for congenital pulmonary malformation. *Chest* 2003; **124**:98–101.
6. Verga, G., Minnitti, S., Donati, P., Spina, P., & Verga, L. Follow-up study of pulmonary function in individuals subjected to lobectomy in infancy and childhood. *Minerva Pediatr.* 1995; **47**:7–12.
7. Caussade, S., Zuniga, S., Garcia, C. *et al.* Pediatric lung resection. A case series and evaluation of postoperative lung function. *Arch. Bronchopneumol.* 2001; **37**:482–488.
8. Nonoyama, A., Tanaka, K., Osaka, T. *et al.* Pulmonary function after lobectomy in children under ten years of age. *Jpn J. Surg.* 1986; **16**:425–434.
9. Nakajima, C., Kijimoto, C., Yokoyama, Y. *et al.* Longitudinal follow up of pulmonary function after lobectomy in childhood – factors affecting lung growth. *Pediatr. Surg. Int.* 1998; **13**:341–345.
10. Bolliger, C. T., Jordan, P., Soler, M. *et al.* Pulmonary function and exercise capacity after lung resection. *Eur. Respir. J.* 1996; **9**:415–421.
11. Kohn, G. L., Walston, C., Feldstein, J., Warner, B. W., Succop, P., & Hardie, W. D. Persistent abnormal lung function after childhood empyema. *Am. J. Respir. Med.* 2002; **1**:441–445.
12. Takizawa, T., Haga, M., Yagi, N. *et al.* Pulmonary function after segmentectomy for small peripheral carcinoma of the lung. *J. Thorac. Cardiovasc. Surg.* 1999; **118**:536–541.
13. Werner, H. A., Pirie, G. E., Nadel, H. R., Fleisher, A. G., & LeBlanc, J. G. Lung volumes, mechanics, and perfusion after pulmonary resection in infancy. *J. Thorac. Cardiovasc. Surg.* 1993; **105**:737–742.
14. Eren, S., Eren, M. N., & Balci, A. E. Pneumonectomy in children for destroyed lung and the long-term consequences. *J. Thorac. Cardiovasc. Surg.* 2003; **126**:574–581.
15. Blyth, D., Buckels, N. J., Sewsunker, R., & Soni, M. A. Pneumonectomy in children. *Eur. J. Cardiothorac Surg.* 2002; **22**:587–594.
16. Laros, C. D. & Westermann, C. J. Dilatation, compensatory growth, or both after pneumonectomy during childhood and adolescence. A thirty-year follow-up study. *J. Thorac. Cardiovasc. Surg.* 1987; **93**:570–576.
17. Giammona, S. T., Mandelbaum, I., Battesby, J. S., & Daly, W. J. The late cardiopulmonary effects of childhood pneumonectomy. *Pediatrics* 1966; **37**:79–88.
18. Sery, Z. D., Ressl, J., & Vyhnaleck, J. Some late sequels of childhood pneumonectomy. *Surgery* 1969; **65**:343–351.
19. Morel, V. O., Jacobs, J. P., & Quintessenza, J. A. Right post-pneumonectomy syndrome and severe pectus excavatum in a child:surgical management. *J. Thorac. Cardiovasc. Surg.* 2002; **124**(1):203–204.
20. Stolar, C., Berdon, W., & Reyes, C. Right pneumonectomy syndrome:a lethal complication of lung resection in a newborn with cystic adenomatoid malformation. *J. Pediatr. Surg.* 1988; **23**:343–351.
21. Audry, G., Balquet, P., Vasquez, M. P. *et al.* Expandable prosthesis in right post-pneumonectomy syndrome in childhood and adolescence. *Ann. Thorac. Surg.* 1993; **56**:323–327.
22. Nichol, P. F., DeCock, D., Noon, J., & Gutenberg, J. E. Long term follow-up in a patient after pneumonectomy and SILASTIC prosthetic placement after unilateral pulmonary artery agenesis. *J. Pediatr. Surg.* 2004; **39**:1116–1118.
23. Morrow, S. E., Glynn, L., & Aschcraft, K. W. Ping-pong ball plombage for right post-pneumonectomy syndrome in children. *J. Pediatr. Surg.* 1998; **33**:1048–1051.
24. Freeman, N. V. & Walkden, J. Previously unreported shoulder deformity following right lateral thoracotomy for esophageal atresia. *J. Pediatr. Surg.* 1969; **4**:627–636.
25. Durning, R. P., Scoles, P. V., & Fox, O. D. Scoliosis after thoracotomy in tracheoesophageal fistula patients. A follow-up study. *J. Bone. Joint. Surg. Am.* 1980; **62**:1156–1159.
26. Gilsanz, V., Boechat, I. M., Birnberg, F. A., & King, J. D. Scoliosis after thoracotomy for esophageal atresia. *Am. J. Roentgenol.* 1983; **141**:457–460.
27. Jaureguizar, E., Vazquez, J., Murcia, J., & Diez Pardo, J. A. Morbid musculoskeletal sequelae of thoracotomy for tracheoesophageal fistula. *J. Pediatr. Surg.* 1985; **20**:511–514.
28. Chetcuti, P., Myers, N. A., Phelan, P. D., Beasley, S. W., & Dickens, D. R. Chest wall deformity in patients with repaired esophageal atresia. *J. Pediatr. Surg.* 1989; **24**:244–247.
29. Seghaye, M. C., Grabitz, R., Alzen, G. *et al.* Thoracic sequelae after surgical closure of the patent ductus arteriosus in premature infants. *Acta Paediatr.* 1997; **86**:213–216.
30. Bal, S., Elshershari, H., Celiker, R., & Celiker, A. Thoracic sequels after thoracotomies in children with congenital cardiac disease. *Cardiol. Young.* 2003; **13**:264–267.
31. Bianchi, A., Sowande, O., Alizai, N. K., Rampersad, B. Aesthetics and lateral thoracotomy in the neonate. *J. Pediat. Surg.* 1998; **33**:1798–1800.
32. Jawad, A. J. Experience with modified posterolateral muscle sparing thoracotomy in neonates, infants, and children. *Pediatr. Surg. Int.* 1997; **12**:337–339.
33. Rothenberg, S. S. Experience with thoracoscopic lobectomy in infants and children. *J. Pediatr. Surg.* 2003; **38**:102–104.
34. Bax, K. M. & Van Der Zee, D. C. Feasibility of thoracoscopic repair of esophageal atresia with distal fistula. *J. Pediatr. Surg.* 2002; **37**:192–196.
35. Bax, K. M., Van Der Zee, D. C. Feasibility of thoracoscopic repair of esophageal atresia with distal fistula. *J. Pediatr. Surg.* 2002; **37**:192–196.
36. Greene, W., L'Heureux, P., & Hunt, C. E. Paralysis of the diaphragm. *Am. J. Dis. Child.* 1975; **129**:1402–1405.
37. Tonz, M., Von Segesser, L. K., Mihaljevic, T. *et al.* Clinical implications of phrenic nerve injury after pediatric cardiac surgery. *J. Pediatr. Surg.* 1996; **31**:1265–1267.
38. De Leeuw, M., Williams, J. M., Freedom, R. M. *et al.* Impact of diaphragmatic paralysis after cardiothoracic surgery in children. *J. Thorac. Cardiovasc. Surg.* 1999; **118**:510–517.
39. Higgs, S. M., Hussain, A., Jackson, M., Donnelly, R. J., & Berrisford, R. G. Long term results of diaphragmatic plication for

unilateral diaphragm paralysis. *Eur. J. Cardiothorac. Surg.* 2002; **21**:294–297.

40. Bargy, F., Manach, Y., Helardot, P. G., & Bienaymé, J. Risk of recurrent laryngeal nerve palsy in surgery of esophageal atresia. *Chir. Pediatr*. 1983; **24**:130–132.
41. Roberstson, J. R. & Birck, H. G. Laryngeal problems following infant esophageal surgery. *Laryngoscope* 1976; **86**:965–970.
42. Fan, L. L., Campbell, D. N., Clarke, D. R. *et al.* Paralyzed left vocal cord associated with ligation of patent ductus arteriosus. *J. Thorac. Cardiovasc. Surg.* 1989; **98**:611–613.
43. Kaya, S. O., Liman, S. T., Bir, L. S. *et al.* Horner's syndrome as a complication in thoracic surgical practice. *Eur. J. Cardiothorac. Surg.* 2003; **24**:1025–1028.
44. Kahn, S. A. & Brandt, L. J. Iatrogenic Horner's syndrome:a complication of thoracostomy tube replacement. *N. Engl. J. Med.* 1985; **312**:245.
45. Campbell, P., Neil, T., & Wake, P N. Horner's syndrome caused by an intercostal chest drain. *Thorax* 1989; **44**:305–306.
46. Rossegger, H. & Fritsch, G. Horner's syndrome after treatment of tension pneumothorax with tube thoracosctomy in a newborn infant. *Eur. J. Pediatr.* 1980; **133**:67–68.
47. Kuwabara, S., Fukutake, T., Kasahata, N. *et al.* Associated movement as a sequel to thoracotomy: aberrant regeneration to the latissimus dorsi muscle. *Mov. Disord.* 1995: **10**:788–790.
48. Kalma, A. & Verebely, T. The use of axillary skin crease incision for thoracotomies of neonates and children. *Eur. J. Pediatr. Surg.* 2002; **12**:226–229.
49. Frola, C., Serrano, J., Cantoni, S. *et al.* CT findings of atrophy of chest wall muscle after thoracotomy:relationship between muscles involved and type of surgery. *Am. J. Roentgenol.* 1995; **164**:599–601.
50. Landreneau, R. J., Pigula, F., Luketich, J. D. *et al.* Acute and chronic morbidity differences between muscle-sparing and standard lateral thoracotomies. *J. Thorac. Cardiovasc. Surg.* 1996; **112**:1326–1350.
51. Rothenberg, S. S. & Pokorny, W. J. Experience with a total muscle-sparing approach for thoracotomies in neonates, infants and children. *J. Pediatr. Surg.* 1992; **27**:1157–1159.
52. Akcalli, Y., Demir, H., & Tezcan, B. The effect of standard posterolateral versus muscle-sparing thoracotomy on multiple parameters. *Ann. Thorac. Surg.* 2003; **76**:1050–1054.
53. Bleiziffer, S., Schreiber, C., Burgkart, R. *et al.* The influence of right anterolateral thoracotomy in prepubescent female patients on late breast development and on the incidence of scoliosis. *J. Thorac. Cardiovasc. Surg.* 2004; **127**:1474–1480.

15a

Esophageal atresia: Surgical aspects

Spencer W. Beasley

Department of Paediatric Surgery, Christchurch Hospital, New Zealand

Introduction and historical aspects

William Durston is credited with providing the earliest description of esophageal atresia (EA) when he observed its occurrence in one of conjoined twins in 1670.[1] In 1888, Charles Steele was the first to attempt surgical correction of EA. Although the child died, it gave an indication that the abnormality was potentially treatable. It was not until 1939 that Ladd and Leven independently obtained the first long-term survivors with EA. Two years later Cameron Haight successfully achieved a primary esophageal anastomosis.

Before 1939, esophageal atresia was considered a uniformly fatal condition. Nowadays, all patients with EA are expected to survive irrespective of their gestation, provided there are no major concomitant congenital abnormalities.[2] There has been a steady decline in the overall mortality from EA in most institutions, but there remains a significant group of patients who will die as a result of their associated abnormalities: the prognosis for many of these infants is considered so poor that no active treatment to correct the atresia is justified.

The eventual quality of life is good in the majority of survivors. Despite this, many have ongoing minor but troublesome symptoms, many of which relate to esophageal function (Table 15a.1). In particular, there are concerns about the ultimate risk of malignancy in the esophagus exposed to persisting gastroesophageal reflux. This chapters outlines how the early management of esophageal atresia influences long term outcome, and identifies some of the persistent difficulties that adults with repaired EA may suffer.

Operative repair techniques

Esophageal atresia with distal tracheoesophageal fistula

The initial approach to the operative management of esophageal atresia influences both the early postoperative complication rate and the long term outcome. Complete primary repair of the defect, without staged procedures and without having to resort to repeated thoracotomies, achieves the best results.

The infant is placed with the right side uppermost and a towel folded underneath the left chest to give lateral flexion. A transverse incision centered on the inferior angle of the scapula allows a fourth intercostal extrapleural approach. The serratus anterior is retracted anteriorly or its posterior fibers divided low at their origin to preserve its innervation – this helps to maintain a normal chest wall appearance. The extrapleural approach is favored over a transpleural approach because empyema is less likely to occur should there be an anastomotic leak.

The azygos vein is divided between ligatures to facilitate exposure of the fistulous connection of the lower esophageal segment to the trachea. The fistula is closed with transfixion sutures and divided. Ligation alone increases the chance of recurrent fistula. Care is taken to avoid damage to the vagus nerve and the blood supply to the distal esophageal segment.

The upper esophagus is mobilized enough to allow an end-to-end one-layer interrupted anastomosis between the upper and lower esophageal segments (Fig. 15a.1). The mucosal layer should be included in each suture. Where

Pediatric Surgery and Urology: Long-term Outcomes, Mark Stringer, Keith Oldham, Pierre Mouriquand. Published by Cambridge University Press.

Table 15a.1. Potential esophageal problems following repair of esophageal atresia

Early

Anastomotic leakage:

- Radiologic leak/persistent drainage of saliva in the chest drain
- Complete disruption of anastomosis
- Empyema/abscess, mediastinitis

Recurrent tracheoesophageal fistula

Esophageal stricture:

- From poorly constructed anastomosis
- From anastomotic leakage
- From gastroesophageal reflux

Late

Symptoms of dysphagia (various contributing causes)

Food impaction in the esophagus

Poor motility/delayed esophageal clearance

Esophagitis/gastroesophageal reflux

Risk of malignancy

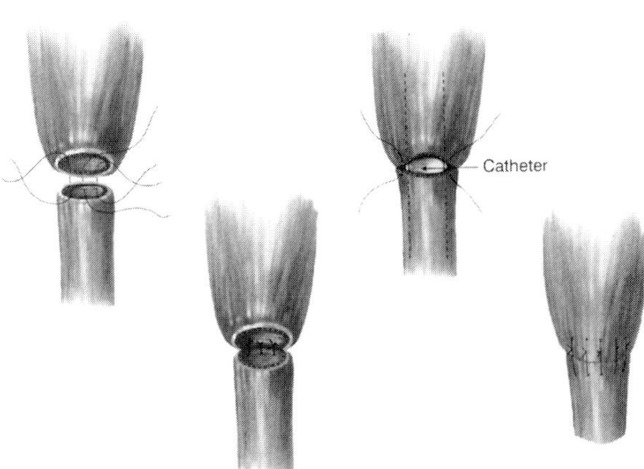

Fig. 15a.1. The technique of esophageal anastomosis in esophageal atresia. From left to right: sutures are first placed in the far wall of the esophagus (ensuring that mucosa is included with each suture) before the esophageal ends are gently apposed. Insertion of an orogastric tube facilitates completion of the front wall of the anastomosis. The tube can then be removed.

there is a significant gap between the esophageal ends, the upper esophageal segment is mobilized first. Sometimes the lower esophagus may require mobilization as well, to prevent undue tension on the anastomosis. A chest drain is not used routinely,[3] but may be placed at the discretion of the surgeon if there is concern about the integrity of the anastomosis. A trans-anastomotic tube is not required except in the very premature infant where it is used for gavage feeding. Oral feeds can be commenced on postoperative day 3 or 4, usually after a contrast study has confirmed that there is no leak from the esophagus.

There is increasing experience with a thoracoscopic approach to repair of esophageal atresia.[4,5]

Long-gap esophageal atresia

The surgeon's approach to the investigation and management of long-gap esophageal atresia is crucial if optimal long-term outcome is to be achieved. Failure to fully utilize the patient's own esophagus may lead to it being discarded unnecessarily, and introduces a number of long-term problems, some of which are difficult to manage. No air below the diaphragm on the initial plain X-ray of the torso suggests that there is no distal tracheoesophageal fistula, and this is the clue that the gap between the two esophageal ends is likely to be extensive.[6] In these infants an immediate primary esophageal anastomosis may not always be possible.

The absence of a distal tracheoesophageal fistula affects management and long term outcome in another respect as well: inability of the fetus to swallow amniotic fluid or for fluid to enter the stomach through a distal fistula means the stomach is smaller than normal. This may make it difficult to site the gastrostomy in a way that avoids compromising later gastric interposition or an anti-reflux operation,[6] should either be required.

Once an upper pouch fistula (proximal tracheo-esophageal fistula) has been excluded by endoscopy or by a contrast study under continuous fluoroscopic control, a gastrostomy is fashioned. Through this, the length of lower segment can be evaluated by introducing a metal bougie or sound into the lower esophagus at the same time as the anaesthetist introduces a radio-opaque catheter into the upper esophageal segment. This enables an assessment of how closely the esophageal ends can be approximated, and indicates whether it is safe to proceed to immediate primary end-to-end anastomosis.

The usual finding is that the gap between the ends is extensive so that thoracotomy is best delayed for 1–3 months, during which time it is conjectured there may be growth of both esophageal segments, particularly if there is gastroesophageal reflux and filling of the lower esophagus during bolus gastrostomy feeds.

The surgical approach to the esophagus is similar to that employed for the usual esophageal atresia with distal tracheoesophageal fistula. The upper esophageal segment is identified within the chest and mobilized as far into the neck as possible. A stay suture passed through the most dependent part of the upper esophageal segment facilitates this dissection and enables assessment of the amount of additional esophageal length necessary.

The fine white fibers of the vagus nerve course towards the lower esophageal segment and assist in its identification.[7] Usually the lower esophagus is found a few centimeters above the diaphragm in the lower thorax; a stay suture through its upper part may facilitate its gentle dissection. The dissection can be continued through the esophageal hiatus to allow the intra-abdominal esophagus to pass up into the thorax, with or without the proximal part of the stomach. Myotomy of the esophagus may provide additional length, but comes at a cost to both the vascular and nerve supplies to the esophagus, for which reason it is preferable to perform an extensive mobilization of the distal esophageal segment should additional length be requried.[8]

Where, despite these techniques, an esophageal anastomosis cannot be constructed, esophageal replacement is indicated.[6] This may be performed at the same operation or, alternatively, a cervical esophagostomy can be fashioned initially and the esophagus replaced when the infant is older. The stomach is currently favored for this purpose, usually as a gastric interposition using a greater curvature tube of the Heimlich–Gavriliu type brought into the neck either via the left pleural cavity or the anterior mediastinum (retrosternal route). This tube can be based upon the cardia[9] or the pylorus.[10] When the whole stomach is used the procedure is called "gastric transposition."[11]

Another method involves incomplete division of the fundus of the stomach from the lesser curve.[12] In earlier years esophagocoloplasty was a popular technique of esophageal replacement, and early results were encouraging, but with longer follow-up an increasing number of problems have been identified (Table 15a.2). Whether the long-term results of gastric tube replacement (which also has many potential problems) are any better is yet to be determined. This subject is covered in more detail in Chapter 17.

Table 15a.2. Complications of colonic replacement of esophagus

Early complications

Necrosis of colonic interposition (from ischemia)
Anastomotic leakage
Esophagocutaneous fistula
Strictures (usually proximal esophagocolonic anastomosis)
Transient malabsorption
Gastric outlet obstruction
Empyema

Late complications

Redundancy of upper esophagus, or esophageal pouch
Colonic dilatation
Halitosis
Acid reflux:
- Nocturnal coughing/wheezing
- Ulceration/erosion, heartburn, dysphagia

Graft-related complications:
- Colitis
- Iron-deficiency anemia
- Massive hemorrhage
- Inflammatory colonic polyps

Diaphragmatic hernia
?Risk of malignancy in esophageal remnant
Anterior chest wall deformity from multiple procedures

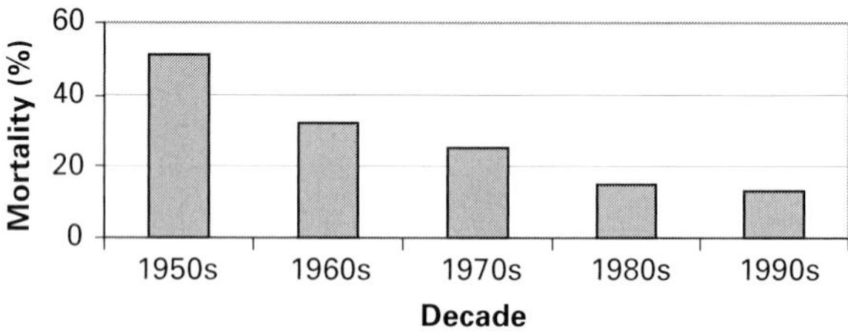

Fig. 15a.2. Decline in overall mortality in patients with esophageal atresia and distal tracheoesophageal fistula (includes patients in whom no active treatment was attempted).

Short-term outcomes

Mortality

There was a steady decline in the overall mortality from esophageal atresia until about 1985, since when it has changed little. Figure 15a.2 shows the reduction in overall mortality over time in patients with EA and distal tracheoesophageal fistula. If infants with major associated congenital abnormalities for whom the prognosis was considered so poor that they received no active treatment are excluded, the decline in mortality with each decade becomes even more impressive (Fig.15a.3).

Causes of early death

In the early years, most deaths were the result of respiratory failure and inadequate resuscitation, from soiling of the lungs, hyaline membrane disease, and other complications of prematurity.[2] The other major cause of mortality was from the complications of the esophageal surgery itself, particularly those related to dehiscence of the anastomosis and poor nutrition (Table 15a.3). Improvements in operative and anesthetic techniques, and sophisticated

Table 15a.3. Factors contributing to early deaths from esophageal atresia

Respiratory failure and inadequate resuscitation:
- Inadequate upper pouch suctioning
- Oral feeds prior to diagnosis
- Aspiration, repeated lung soiling
- Hyaline membrane disease
- Other complications of prematurity

Complications of surgery
- Anesthetic complications
- Anastomotic leak or dehiscence, empyema
- Recurrent tracheoesophageal fistula
- Sepsis
- Poor nutrition

Associated major congenital abnormalities
- Chromosomal aberrations (e.g. Trisomy 18)
- Congenital heart disease (e.g. hypoplastic left heart)
- Bilateral renal agenesis/multicystic dysplastic kidneys

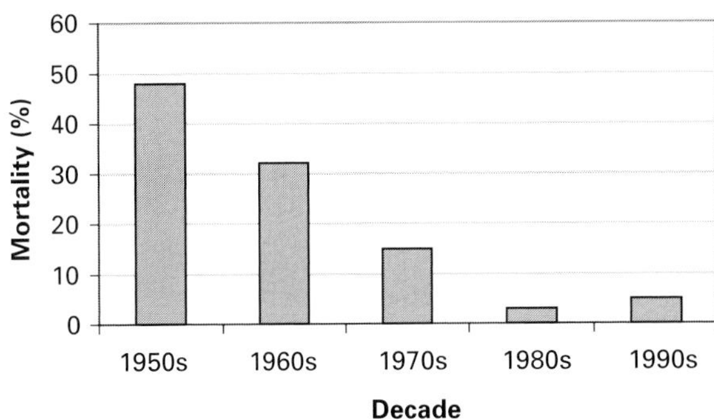

Fig. 15a.3. Decline in mortality in patients with esophageal atresia and distal tracheoesophageal fistula undergoing definitive treatment. Patients with major chromosomal or other congenital abnormalities which precluded active treatment have been excluded.

neonatology, have ensured that now the main cause of death is due to associated anomalies not amenable to treatment. As the treatment of congenital heart disease has improved, major chromosomal aberrations have assumed greater importance.[13] Table 15a.4 lists the coexisting abnormalities contributing to death in patients with esophageal atresia admitted to the Royal Children's Hospital, Melbourne, during a 15-year period, for whom definitive treatment to the esophagus was not offered.

As an indication of the effect of improvements in neonatology on survival, Figure 15a.4 shows the trend in mortality in Waterston Group C infants with EA and a distal tracheoesophageal fistula receiving treatment. This experience is consistent with that reported by others, and renders the Waterston classification no longer relevant in predicting outcome in esophageal atresia;[2,14,15,16] rather, it is the nature of any coexisting abnormalities that determines survival.

Table 15a.4. Coexisting abnormalities contributing to death in infants with esophageal atresia for whom no definitive treatment to the esophagus was undertaken (1974–1989)

Associated abnormality	Infants (*n*)
Trisomy 18	7
Trisomy 21	3
Congenital heart disease	9
CHARGE association	2
Other major (usually multiple) abnormalities	17
Severe hyaline membrane disease	1

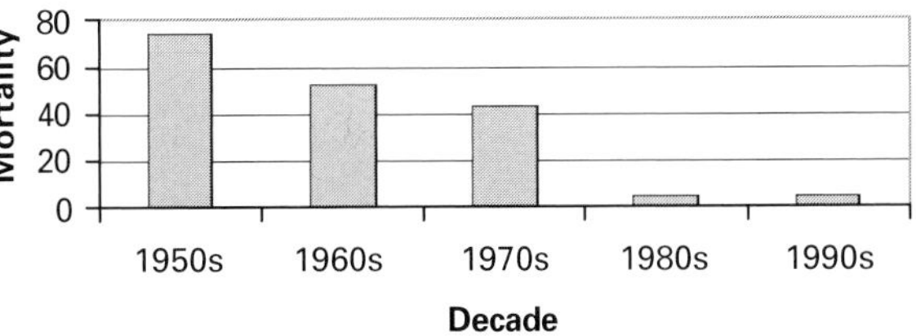

Fig. 15a.4. Trends in mortality in 118 infants with Waterston Group C esophageal atresia with distal tracheoesophageal fistula receiving treatment.[6]

Death during childhood

Death outside the neonatal period following repair of esophageal atresia is unusual. Most mortality occurs in the first year of life, the single most common cause being congenital heart disease. The next most common cause is respiratory failure, and recurrent pneumonia. A high incidence of so-called "cot deaths" has also been noted,[2] but in these patients the actual cause of death remains unknown. It is possible that in some of these babies death may be a complication of tracheomalacia or gastroesophageal reflux.

Early esophageal complications

As indicated in Table 15a.1, the three main surgical complications of repair of esophageal atresia are: (1) anastomotic leakage or dehiscence; (2) recurrent tracheoesophageal fistula; and (3) anastomotic stricture (Fig. 15a.5). The incidence of each of these is related to the adequacy of the blood supply to the esophageal ends, the degree of tension on the

Table 15a.5. Severity of leak after primary anastomosis in 200 consecutive patients with esophageal atresia and distal fistula

No leak	158	79.0%
Radiologic leak, infant asymptomatic	17	8.5%
Minor leak:		
Saliva in chest drain <1 week	14	7.0%
Saliva in chest drain >1 week	5	2.5%
Major leak:		
Empyema/mediastinitis	4	2.0%
Lung abscess	2	1.0%

From Beasley, Myers and Auldist (eds.), *Oesophageal Atresia*, Chapman & Hall 1991

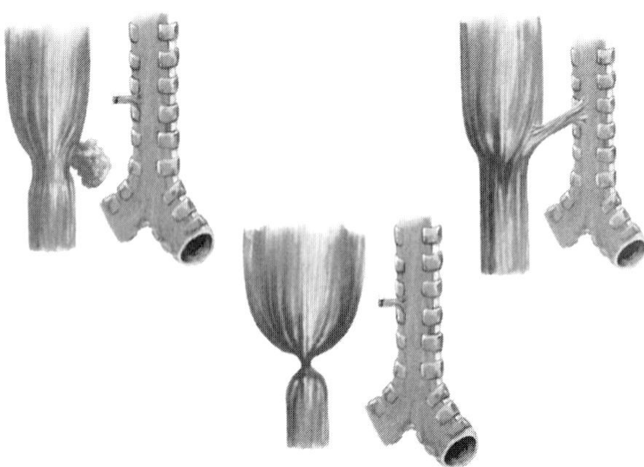

Fig. 15a.5. The three main esophageal complications of repair of esophageal atresia. From left to right: leakage at the anastomosis; esophageal stricture; recurrent tracheoesophageal fistula.

anastomosis, and the type of anastomosis performed. The blood supply to the anastomosis is affected by the extent of dissection required to mobilize the esophagus, trauma to the ends of the esophagus from handling, and by ongoing tension following completion of the anastomosis. The type of anastomosis influences the frequency and nature of subsequent anastomotic complications, as described below.

End-to-end anastomosis

An end-to-end anastomosis which includes the mucosa is the type of esophageal anastomosis which carries the lowest incidence of anastomotic leakage, recurrent fistula, and esophageal stricture at the level of the anastomosis.[17] In a series of 200 consecutive primary anastomoses for esophageal atresia with distal fistula reviewed at the Royal Children's Hospital, Melbourne, major anastomotic leakage occurred in 3% (Table 15a.5). Early leakage will occur

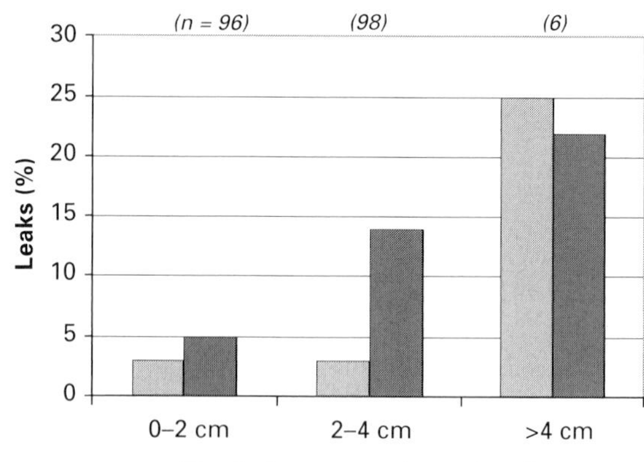

Fig. 15a.6. Relationship between length of gap between the esophageal ends and anastomotic leak in repaired esophageal atresia and distal tracheoesophageal fistula in 200 consecutive patients. Leakage is more likely to occur if the gap between the esophageal ends is more than 4 cm in length.[6]

if the anastomosis is poorly constructed and the sutures are not placed or tied correctly. The likelihood of anastomotic disruption increases if there is excessive tension on the esophageal ends or if they are ischemic. Not surprisingly, leakage is more likely to occur if the gap between the esophageal ends is more than 4 cm in length (Fig. 15a.6). Use of a circular myotomy significantly increases the likelihood of anastomotic leakage, esophageal stricture[18] and pseudodiverticulum formation, probably because the relative ischemia created by the myotomy impairs anastomotic healing.

The incidences of anastomotic leakage, recurrent fistula, and an anastomotic stricture requiring resection according to the type of anastomosis employed, are shown in Figs. 15a.7–15a.9, respectively.

End-to-side anastomosis

The end-to-side anastomosis is used infrequently nowadays, mainly because leakage of the anastomosis is more common (although often minor), as are recurrent tracheoesophageal fistulas and anastomotic strictures requiring resection (Figs. 15a.7–15a.9). The original Haight sleeve anastomosis had a high complication rate and is no longer used.

Anterior flap repair

This technique was devised primarily for use in overcoming a long gap in esophageal atresia. The anterior aspect

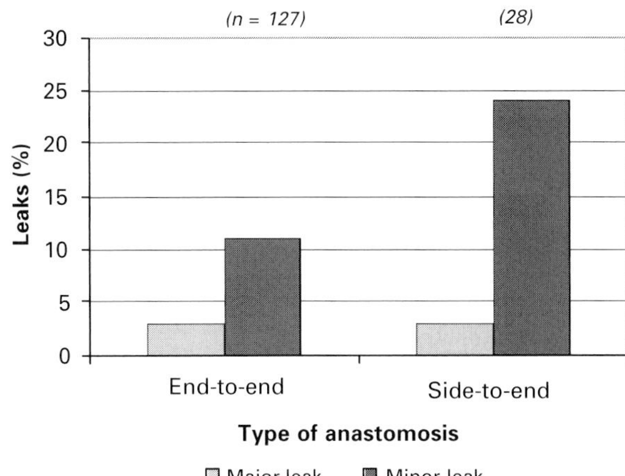

Fig. 15a.7. Incidence of leak according to type of anastomosis. Not included in this figure are five anastomoses in conjunction with circular myotomy (three of which leaked) and nine Haight anastomoses (one of which leaked). Modified from ref. 6

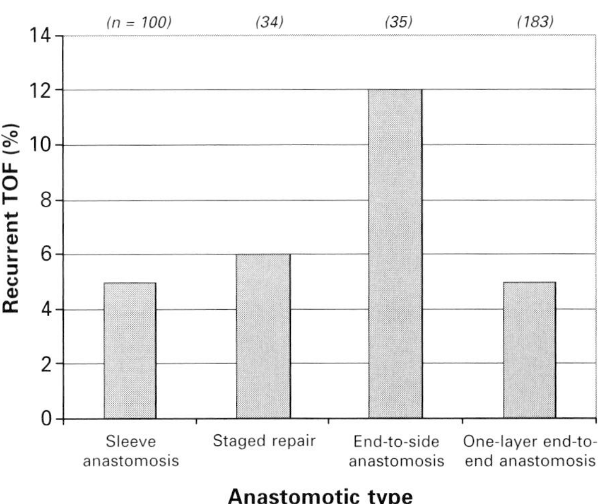

Fig. 15a.8. Relative incidence of recurrent tracheoesophageal fistula according to the type of anastomosis.[6]

of the upper pouch is rotated downwards to bridge the gap between the proximal and distal ends.[19,20] The technique has its advocates but is associated with a high rate of complications. Its main drawback is that it produces a long suture line, with convergence of three suture lines in an area of moderate tension and impoverished blood supply. Also, it creates an antiperistaltic segment of esophagus, another disadvantage of the technique. Anastomotic leaks can be expected in up to 30%, anastomotic stricture in 87%, and recurrent fistula in 8–14%. In the series reported by Davenport and Bianchi,[21] it was used routinely irrespective of gap

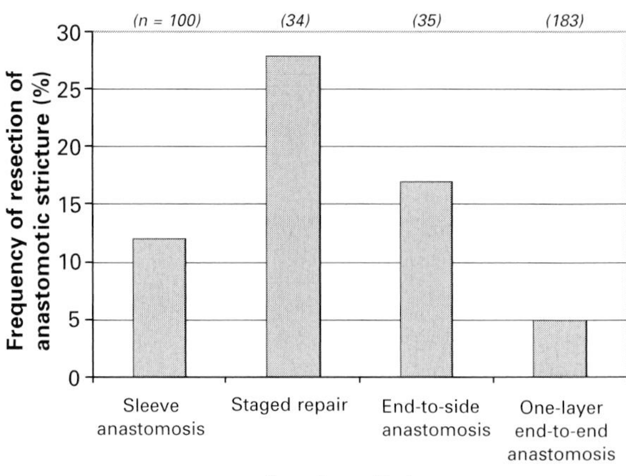

Fig. 15a.9. Frequency of resection of an anastomotic stricture according to the type of anastomosis. These data pertain to anastomoses performed over several decades: nowadays, the necessity for resection of an anastomotic stricture would be lower in all types of anastomoses because the current management of coexisting gastroesophageal reflux includes fundoplication.[6]

length, producing an unacceptably high complication rate for this type of patient. Brown *et al.*[20] reported esophageal incoordination in 7 of 15 patients (47%). Three children (20%) showed signs of failure to thrive, although the reasons for this were not described. Late deaths resulted from a recurrent fistula in two patients.

In summary, a well-performed all-layer end-to-end anastomosis would appear to be the method with the fewest complications and best long term results, even where extensive mobilization of the esophageal ends has been required. With all techniques, the complication rate increases if the gap between the esophageal ends is wide, or the anastomosis is under tension.

Implications of anastomotic complications

A major anastomotic disruption that becomes apparent very early in the post-operative period is best repaired surgically. However, the vast majority of anastomotic leaks are less severe and most close spontaneously and can be managed non-operatively. Total parenteral nutrition allows oral feeds to be stopped. Antibiotics should be administered until the leak has closed. Radical measures (e.g. cervical esophagostomy) are required rarely, being reserved for the patient in whom there is ongoing, poorly controlled sepsis or where supportive therapy has been unsuccessful. Occasionally, a longstanding leak may require gastrostomy to allow continuation of enteral feeds.

Spontaneous closure of a recurrent tracheoesophageal fistula is extremely unusual: therefore, a policy of indefinite waiting is not appropriate. The fistula is closed surgically, usually through the original thoracotomy incision, when the infant is in an optimal respiratory and general condition.

Anastomotic strictures may result from a poorly constructed anastomosis, or gastroesophageal reflux. Dilatation of a stricture is less likely to be successful in the long term unless any underlying reflux is corrected.[7,21,22] Radial balloon dilatation under fluoroscopic control is less traumatic to the esophagus than traditional bougienage.[23] Administration of Omeprazole 1.9–2.5 mg/kg/d reduces the need for esophageal dilatation.[24]

Recurrent tracheoesophageal fistula

A recurrent tracheoesophageal fistula is a potentially dangerous complication of repair of esophageal atresia. Most fistulas develop in the early postoperative period, but others may become apparent many months or years after the primary operation. The typical presentation is that of an infant who coughs and splutters with feeds. Other clinical features include gagging, choking, cyanosis, apnea, dying spells, wheezing and recurrent chest infections. Sometimes a recurrent fistula is diagnosed on a routine post-operative barium swallow. Second recurrence of tracheoesophageal fistula occurs occasionally.

Some recurrent fistulas probably result from anastomotic leakage and infection, particularly when the anastomosis is adjacent to the site of tracheal closure. Where there has been no clinical or radiologic evidence of a leak or stricture, the cause is less clear but occasionally may be due to a missed proximal tracheoesophageal fistula. The incidence after end-to-end anastomosis is about 4% but may be even lower with current techniques. The incidence of recurrent tracheoesophageal fistulas can be reduced by division (rather than ligation alone) of the original fistula, and by meticulous esophageal anastomosis. Interposition of mediastinal tissue is not normally needed with a primary repair.

The most reliable method of confirming a suspected recurrent tracheoesophageal fistula is to perform cineradiographic tube esophagography with the patient prone. A catheter in the esophagus is gradually withdrawn as contrast is introduced. The diagnosis can also be made on bronchoscopy. The recurrent fistula usually arises from the tracheal pouch of the original fistula and enters the esophagus at or just below the level of the anastomosis.

Management

Spontaneous closure of a recurrent fistula is unlikely to occur. Inflammation between the esophagus and trachea makes early operation difficult, and may increase the chance of causing damage to the original anastomosis. If the infant's condition allows, it is preferable to wait a month or so from the first operation, during which time the infant's respiratory and general condition can be improved: this may require intravenous nutrition. Nasogastric tube feeding is discouraged because reflux may lead to respiratory complications if gastric contents are aspirated through the fistula.

The fistula is repaired through the original fourth intercostal space incision. Prior to thoracotomy, some surgeons perform bronchoscopy to place a fine catheter through the fistula to facilitate its localization. The esophagus is mobilized no more than is necessary to identify the fistula which is divided and closed. Interposed mediastinal tissue (pleura, pericardium or intercostal muscle) may help separate the two ends of the fistula. Other techniques described include endoscopic obliteration using diathermy, tissue adhesives or sclerosing agents. These techniques may have special application in situations where repeat thoracotomy has an unacceptably high morbidity.

Long-term outcomes

Dysphagia and food impaction

Dysphagia is one of the most common gastrointestinal problems occurring after repair of esophageal atresia. It is probable that the motility of the esophagus is inherently abnormal to some degree in all patients with repaired esophageal atresia[25,27] and surgical dissection to repair the atresia may compromise it further. However, when a child or adult presents with ongoing or worsening dysphagia, an anastomotic stricture and reflux esophagitis must be excluded.

Dysphagia during childhood

Choking with feeds and pain on swallowing, as well as food impaction in the esophagus, are relatively common during childhood.[28,29] Most trapped foods (e.g. apple, bread, meat) can be removed by induction of vomiting, without medical help.[30] The frequency with which surgical intervention for swallowing problems is required declines as the child gets older, although the proportion of patients experiencing symptoms of dysphagia alters little (Fig. 15a.10).[28] Most swallowing problems first become evident when solids are introduced, although food impaction of the esophagus peaks in incidence around 2 years of age (Fig. 15a.11). As the child continues to grow, obstructive

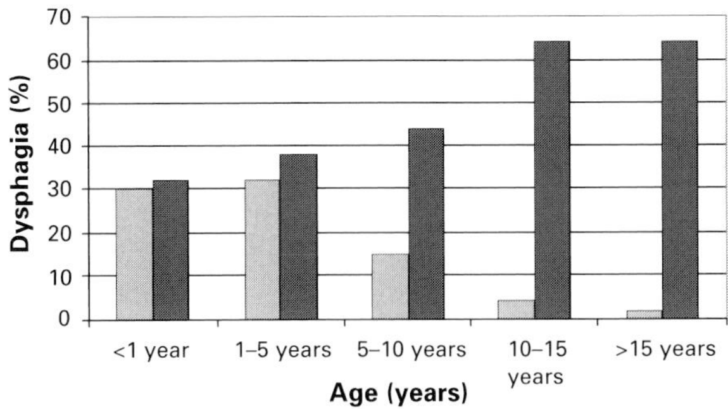

Fig. 15a.10. Incidence of dysphagia according to age. The overall prevalence of dysphagia changes little with age, whereas surgical intervention is rarely required outside childhood. Modified from ref. 6.

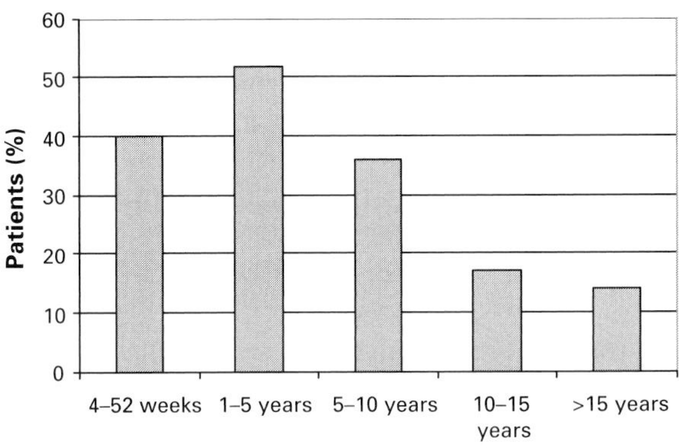

Fig. 15a.11. Incidence of food impaction in the esophagus according to age.[6]

episodes in the esophagus become progressively less common and less severe. Use of early "routine" upper GI studies have not been shown to be predictive of subsequent symptoms.[31]

Those who have persistent difficulties with swallowing are more likely to have had an esophageal stricture or severe gastroesophageal reflux during infancy.[29] In most instances, repeated esophageal dilatation alone for an esophageal stricture in the presence of persistent, untreated reflux is not effective in resolving the stricture;[22] these patients are better dealt with by treatment with a proton pump inhibitor[24] or, if medical treatment fails, by (laparoscopic) fundoplication to stop the reflux, after which the esophageal stricture will usually (but not always) resolve spontaneously.[7,32] In a few, further radial balloon dilatation of the esophagus under continuous fluoroscopic control may be necessary.

Table 15a.6. Persistent gastrointestinal symptoms in adult survivors with repaired esophageal atresia

Dysphagia:	
None	38%
< 1/week	38%
About 2/week	10%
Every day	7%
Every meal	7%
Symptoms of gastroesophageal reflux:	
None	45%
< 1/week	51%
About 2/week	2%
Daily symptoms	2%

Dysphagia during adulthood

Most adult survivors with repaired esophageal atresia have persistent gastrointestinal symptoms, but these are usually minor (Table 15a.6).[29,33] Difficulties with swallowing are frequent, and many patients find it useful to drink fluids with their meals. While the prevalence of feeding difficulties after repair of EA appears to vary only slightly with advancing age, the frequency with which surgical intervention is required decreases significantly.[20] A few adults will deliberately avoid certain foods because of discomfort during swallowing but, despite these difficulties, most enjoy normal diet and lifestyle, and seldom require medical attention. It is possible that the adult patient is better able to recognize and avoid those foods or situations which produce dysphagia.

Dysphagia is believed to be caused mainly by disordered esophageal peristalsis. Although dysphagia is more likely in patients who were hospitalized during childhood for an anastomotic or reflux stricture, not all patients who had these complications in childhood have dysphagia persisting into adulthood.[29] Moreover, absence of symptoms of dysphagia does not exclude significant esophageal dysmotility or aperistalsis.[34] The inter-relationship between esophageal dysmotility and gastroesophageal reflux is complex, and has many contributing factors (Table 15a.7). The symptomatology they produce is often a poor indicator of their underlying severity.

Foreign body impaction in adulthood

Obstructive episodes in the esophagus become progressively less common from the age of two years (Fig. 15a.11), but even beyond the age of 15 years, foreign body impaction has been recorded in 16% of patients.[28] Inadequately chewed meat, poultry and bread are the foods most likely to get stuck in the esophagus. An anastomotic stricture

Table 15a.7. Factors contributing to poor esophageal motility and gastroesophageal reflux after repair of esophageal atresia

Inherent esophageal dysmotility:
- Incomplete vagal innervation
- Abnormality of Auerbach's plexus

Injury to vagus nerve during surgery:
- Division during dissection
- Rough handling of tissues

Ischemic injury to esophagus:
- Tension on anastomosis
- Excessive mobilization of lower esophagus
- Myotomy

Surgical mobilization of lower esophagus
- Upwards displacement of lower esophagus
- Reduction in length of intra-abdominal esophagus
- Alteration of angle of His
- Traction on gastroesophageal junction. Reduced lower esophageal sphincter pressure

Use of gastrostomy
- Fixation of stomach exacerbates reflux

is an important cause of dysphagia or food-impaction in the early years after surgery, but is not so significant in subsequent years. There appears to be a relationship between gastroesophageal reflux, dysphagia, and foreign body impaction.

Food impaction of the esophagus in adulthood is not always associated with antecedent symptoms.[35] There is sudden onset of choking and gagging after swallowing solid food. In adults obstruction is often in the lower esophagus, perhaps reflecting the combination of the effects of gastroesophageal reflux and poor esophageal clearance. The food debris should be endoscopically removed from the esophagus at the time of esophagoscopy. Afterwards, esophageal manometry and pH monitoring should be undertaken to assess esophageal motility and to identify the presence of gastroesophageal reflux, unless this information is already known.

Relationship between gastroesophageal reflux, dysphagia, and esophageal dysmotility

While it is generally believed that persistent gastroesophageal reflux in patients with esophageal atresia contributes to dysphagia, there is surprisingly little objective evidence of this. In the general adult population, symptoms of gastroesophageal reflux are relatively common, with a prevalence of occasional symptoms in about one-third, and symptoms occurring more than once a week in 7%.[36] A review of adults with repaired esophageal atresia found that symptoms of gastroesophageal reflux were only slightly more frequent than in the normal population, and that this difference did not attain statistical significance.[29] Gastroesophageal reflux appears to be more common during childhood, and in most studies has been documented in nearly 50% of EA patients in the first 5 years after initial surgery.[29,37–39] This is a higher figure than their symptomatology would suggest. Symptomatic evidence of reflux occurs in a much smaller percentage (18%), which suggests that it may exist at a subclinical level in many children.[29]

In older patients, gastroesophageal reflux is symptomatic and recognized more often than in children. In part this may be due to an increased willingness of older patients to admit to symptoms,[20] and the inability of children to recognize the significance of retrosternal discomfort. In the majority of adults, symptoms tend to be mild and infrequent, and cause little interference with their daily activities.

Even if the actual incidence of gastroesophageal reflux in repaired EA is only a little higher than that of the general population, its effect on the lower esophagus may be more debilitating. Poor esophageal clearance means that when reflux occurs, the lower esophageal mucosa is exposed to acid for a longer period. If the development of Barrett's esophagus and the propensity for malignant degeneration later in life are related to acid exposure, the combination of poor esophageal clearance and gastroesophageal reflux assumes greater importance.

Late respiratory effects of gastroesophageal reflux

Children with gastroesophageal reflux are more likely to be admitted to hospital with respiratory complications than those without.[40] However, there is little evidence that gastroesophageal reflux causes progressive respiratory tract effects into adulthood. Lung function is similar to those with and without symptoms of gastroesophageal reflux, although there is a slight increase in airways obstruction and a reduction in lung volume in patients with radiologically proven reflux. It would be reasonable to assume that any lung function abnormalities are a reflection of damage received from recurrent inhalation during infancy and childhood, although the possibility on ongoing aspiration at a subclinical level cannot be excluded. Early diagnosis and management of gastroesophageal reflux may help to minimize subsequent lower airways disease and restrictive lung disease.[41]

Malignant risk after repair of esophageal atresia

Adults with repaired esophageal atresia might be at increased risk of developing esophageal malignancy. As the

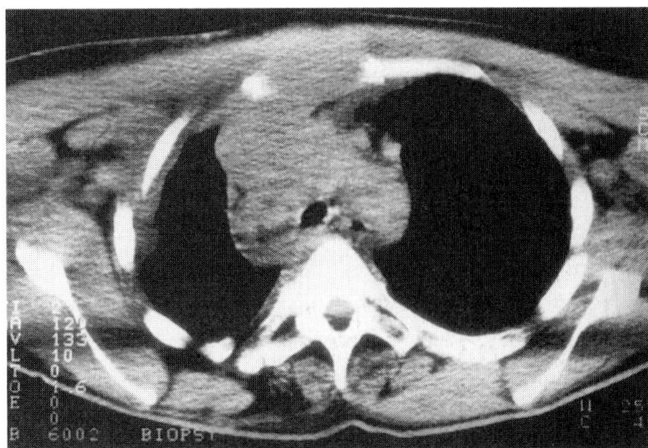

Fig. 15a.12. CT scan of aggressive lower thoracic malignancy, probably arising from the esophagus, in a 43-year-old man with repaired esophageal atresia.

oldest survivors of EA are in their 50s, it is too early to be certain whether this concern is justified but it is possible that, in some, the combination of persistent reflux from birth and poor esophageal clearance may predispose to esophageal malignancy.

Esophageal malignancy and gastroesophageal reflux

In 1989, Adzick *et al.*[42] reported the case of a woman who developed an esophageal adenocarcinoma 20 years after EA repair. In infancy, she had required esophageal dilatation several times for an esophageal stricture but, until presentation, had been largely asymptomatic with no overt evidence of gastroesophageal reflux. At 17 years of age she had a barium swallow which showed abnormal motility in the distal two-thirds of the esophagus. She presented at age 20 with dysphagia to solid foods, and weight loss. Endoscopy revealed an irregular exophytic adenocarcinoma near the cardia, with no evidence of Barrett's epithelium or esophagitis proximal to the tumor. She underwent esophagogastrectomy with colon interposition.

There are a number of other anecdotal reports of malignancy after repair of esophageal atresia. For example, a 43-year-old man with EA repaired at the Royal Children's Hospital, Melbourne, died of an aggressive lower thoracic malignancy. It was believed that this may have emanated from the lower esophagus, but it was too advanced at the time of diagnosis to be certain of its exact origin (Fig. 15a.12). In another report, a 38-year-old man was shown to have developed an esophageal squamous cell carcinoma near the anastomosis,[43] perhaps secondary to stasis caused by impaired esophageal motility.

It is well recognized that, in adults, the columnar epithelium-lined Barrett's esophagus is associated with an increased risk of the development of adenocarcinoma.[44] Barrett's esophagus is considered to be an acquired phenomenon due to chronic mucosal injury secondary to gastroesophageal reflux. In the case reported by Adzick,[42] Barrett's esophagus was not seen, but it is probable that the adenocarcinoma arose in an area of columnar epithelium-lined esophagus which was then obliterated by tumour.

Esophageal dysmotility, poor esophageal peristalsis and clearance, often in conjunction with a reduced lower esophageal sphincter pressure, and gastroesophageal reflux may occur at a subclinical level in many patients with EA.[45] The esophageal dysfunction persists for many years, if not forever. Now that there are many adults with repaired EA entering middle age, it would seem sensible that they have regular surveillance of the esophagus to detect chronic inflammation and dysplasia. Follow-up should be vigilant and lifelong[42] until we know exactly what is the risk of malignant degeneration in these adults with repaired esophageal atresia.

To date, it has been assumed that the relationship between EA and esophageal cancer is related to gastroesophageal reflux. Whether early surgical correction of the reflux prevents these changes from occurring is yet to be established.

Malignancy in the esophageal remnant after replacement

There is a second situation where malignancy may occur in EA patients. The distal esophageal remnant is often left in-situ after esophageal replacement using a colonic segment. Esophagitis may develop in this remnant, the mucosa may ulcerate and stricture, and gastric mucosa may replace the squamous epithelium to produce a Barrett's esophagus.[46] The presence of chronic inflammation and metaplastic squamous epithelium in the residual esophagus raises concern about the possible long term complication of malignant degeneration. For this reason it may be best to completely excise the esophageal remnant at the time of esophageal replacement if feasible, or later if symptoms occur or barium studies show esophagitis or ulceration.[46]

Carcinoma of skin-tube conduits

Early descriptions of repair of esophageal atresia included a multi-stage approach, involving a feeding gastrostomy, ligation of the tracheoesophageal fistula, and a cervical esophagostomy.[47] These procedures enabled survival, but required eventual re-establishment of gastrointestinal continuity. One of the former procedures advocated to achieve this was an antethoracic tubularized bipedicled skin flap.[48] Although this is rarely employed these days, there are a number of adult survivors of the procedure. LaQuaglia *et al.*[49] reported a 45-year-old woman with EA who had an antethoracic skin-tube connecting a cervical esophagostomy to a Roux-en-Y loop of jejunum. She presented with dysphagia, investigation of which showed severe inflammation of the lining of the neo-esophagus. Because of continued symptoms and ongoing severe inflammation the skin tube was resected. Histologic examination of the tube showed extensive pseudo-epitheliomatous hyperplasia with areas of well-differentiated squamous cell carcinoma. The authors identified 12 previously reported cases of malignant degeneration in such conduits, 11 of which occurred in skin-tubes created to treat benign esophageal strictures. Nine patients had developed squamous cell carcinoma, and in all patients, resection of the conduit with interposition of jejunum or colon was required. The interval between creation of the skin-tube and the development of carcinoma was about three decades. Surgeons should be aware of this complication of skin-tube interposition, and ensure that these patients receive careful long term follow up. The presence of severe inflammatory change and pseudo-epitheliomatous hyperplasia might be considered as precursors to subsequent malignant degeneration. Endoscopic biopsy cannot be relied on to rule out carcinoma,[49] necessitating removal of the conduit where there is gross inflammatory change, polyp formation, or unexplained induration or thickening. Incidentally, LaQuaglia also warned of the possibility of malignant degeneration of heterotopic skin used in other types of reconstruction, such as urethroplasty.

Effect of type of definitive repair for long-gap atresia on long term outcome

Primary anastomosis in long-gap atresia

It is the impression of many pediatric surgeons that the long term results of primary esophageal anastomosis are better than those of esophageal replacement, irrespective of the type of replacement chosen. For example, the Melbourne review found that patients in whom esophageal anastomosis had been achieved had less morbidity and fewer continuing problems than those with esophageal replacement, but acknowledged that the former group involved most of the more recent patients.[6,50] Likewise, Delahunt *et al.*[51] found, in a review of 14 patients with long-gap esophageal atresia treated by delayed primary anastomosis and followed up from two to 17 years, that all children were established on full oral feeds. Boyle *et al.*[40] reviewed eight infants who had a primary single layer repair without myotomy for long-gap esophageal atresia where the gap ranged from 3.5 cm to 6 cm: they recorded no anastomotic leaks or disruptions, recurrent fistulas or deaths. All had marked anastomotic tension, and five required a Nissen fundoplication for gastroesophageal reflux. At between one and 11 years' follow-up, all children were eating a normal diet for age.

However, there has been no controlled study directly comparing outcome after primary anastomosis with that of esophageal replacement, and most reviews have an inherent historical bias. In many institutions the initial intention has been to obtain gastrointestinal continuity with a primary esophageal anastomosis, but if this fails, as it does occasionally, an alternative conduit is sought; this adds a further bias to any comparison, as those patients undergoing esophageal replacement are predominantly those who failed primary anastomosis.

Esophageal dysfunction is evident early after delayed primary repair of long-gap atresia, but swallowing improves during childhood. These children have a high incidence of gastroesophageal reflux, possibly contributed to by the extensive mobilization of the lower esophageal segment required to achieve esophageal continuity (Table 15a.7). This mobilization and the upwards traction on the lower esophagus may interfere with the neurovascular supply of the lower esophagus,[53] exacerbating esophageal dysmotility and worsening esophageal clearance. These factors exaggerate the adverse effects of reflux on the anastomosis and lower esophagus, and a significant proportion will develop a stricture and require prolonged treatment with a proton pump inhibitor such as Omeprazole. A few will require an antireflux procedure.[7] The dilemma is that the fundoplication itself may make the esophageal dysmotility more apparent[54] and delay clearance from the lower esophagus. Many of these patients have difficulty swallowing for many months even after a loose fundoplication in infancy. For this reason some surgeons perform a Toupet fundoplication rather than a Nissen fundoplication. Ongoing gastrostomy supplementation of enteral feeding may be necessary in these children for many months, or even a year or more.

In acknowledging these frustrating but transient disadvantages of fundoplication, the implications of not controlling the reflux are worse. For example, a review from Dublin[55] highlighted the effects of inadequate treatment of gastroesophageal reflux in long-gap EA treated by delayed primary anastomosis. Anastomotic stricture developed in eight of the 11 patients reviewed, of whom seven required between one and five esophageal dilatations and one underwent resection of an esophageal stricture. There were three patients with swallowing difficulties who had esophageal strictures and gross gastroesophageal reflux. The purpose of the report was to suggest that the patients may have benefited from a more aggressive approach to the management of their gastroesophageal reflux. The use of proton pump inhibitors in children with repaired esophageal atresia and symptomatic gastroesophageal reflux appears to have reduced the number who need fundoplication.

Swallowing improves in the longer term, as reflected in several reports.[6,51,52] There would seem to be consensus that the eventual function of an intact native esophagus is virtually always better than that following esophageal replacement[52] and should be the preferred alternative if possible. In summary, primary repair of long-gap esophageal atresia may cause short term problems of esophageal stricture and gastroesophageal reflux but as the years progress, the function of the native esophagus continues to improve, making it the conduit of choice where technically feasible.

Esophageal replacement

The wide variety of techniques for esophageal replacement is an indication that none is entirely satisfactory. Each has its proponents, but as with the results of primary esophageal anastomosis, there are no prospective or controlled studies of outcome.

In a retrospective review of 39 such children with esophageal atresia aged between three and 19 years of age[56] who had either colonic or gastric tube interposition, most children needed to chew food well. The gastric tube has a reputation of being more frequently associated with reflux than transposed colon, but this was not confirmed in this study. Nocturnal coughing or wheezing was reported in 41% of children, helped by sleeping on two pillows. The problem tended to become less prevalent in later years. Diet can be unrestricted for the most part, and problems of reflux appear to be manageable and to diminish over time. Redundancy of the upper esophageal pouch and colon may be severe enough to require surgical revision because of the severe dysphagia and space-occupying effect it produces (Table 15a.2). Children can develop ulcers in either transposed colon or gastric tube. This complication is considered a potentially lifelong threat and careful follow-up is required to detect the development of mucosal erosion from acid reflux. Bleeding or erosion of adjacent structures from ulceration of the esophageal substitute can be disastrous. This subject is covered in more detail in Chapter 17.

Chest wall deformity

Until the Melbourne review of chest wall deformity after repair of esophageal atresia, there had been only sporadic reports documenting the final appearance of the chest wall and back after surgery for EA. Scoliosis is a recognized complication of thoracotomy with rib resection in children,[57] and breast maldevelopment has been observed following thoracotomy in the newborn period.[58]

Table 15a.8. Surgical factors which will minimize chest wall deformity

Use the intercostal approach, avoiding rib resection
Limit thoracotomy numbers:
- avoid staged procedures
- focus on good surgical techniques to reduce incidence of anastomotic complications

An extrapleural approach to the esophagus reduces the likelihood of empyema if anastomotic disruption occurs
Keep the serratus anterior innervated – retract the muscle anteriorly or divide it low at its origin on the chest wall

Anterior chest wall asymmetry

Anterior chest wall asymmetry was evident in 59 of 232 patients with repaired esophageal atresia who had no coexisting congenital vertebral anomalies,[28] although in the majority it was minor. Partial denervation of the serratus anterior during thoracotomy may contribute to anterior chest wall asymmetry,[59] which would account for the higher incidence and greater severity seen in patients older than 25 years, as it was these patients who had the serratus anterior divided in the line of the incision. Factors which minimize the risk of chest wall deformity are summarized in Table 15a.8 and discussed further in Chapter 14 (*Pulmonary resection and thoracotomy*).

The approach employed for any thoracotomy in a neonate is dictated by the need for good exposure and the effect that incision will have on subsequent growth and function of the chest wall. An intercostal approach offers little morbidity and satisfactory exposure. Rib resection is not necessary, and the posterior fibers of serratus anterior should be either retracted anteriorly or divided low at their origin on the chest wall to preserve their innervation.[7] Where there are no coexisting vertebral abnormalities and an intercostal approach has been used, anterior chest wall deformity is non-existent or minor.[7] The thoracoscopic approach may have even less effect on chest wall development.

Many years ago, multiple thoracotomies with rib resection were performed deliberately as part of staged repairs and in the management of major esophageal complications such as anastomotic dehiscence, empyema or recurrent fistula (Fig. 15a.13).[28] It is now evident that both multiple thoracotomies and rib resection are associated with an increase in the likelihood and severity of subsequent anterior chest wall deformity and scoliosis even in the absence

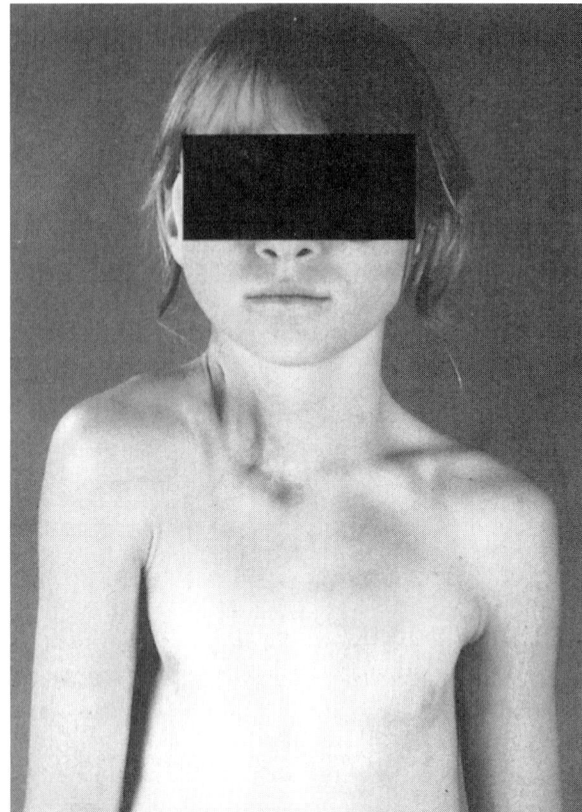

Fig. 15a.13. Example of anterior chest wall deformity caused by staged procedures, multiple thoracotomies, rib resection and intrathoracic complications of surgery.

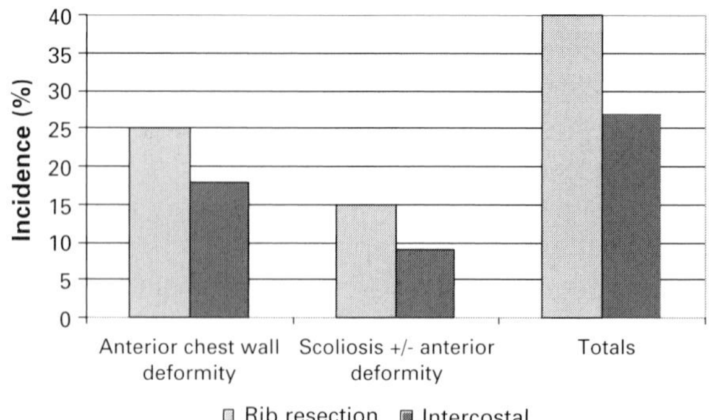

Fig. 15a.14. Effect of rib resection on anterior chest wall deformity and scoliosis in the absence of a congenital vertebral abnormality in repaired esophageal atresia.[6]

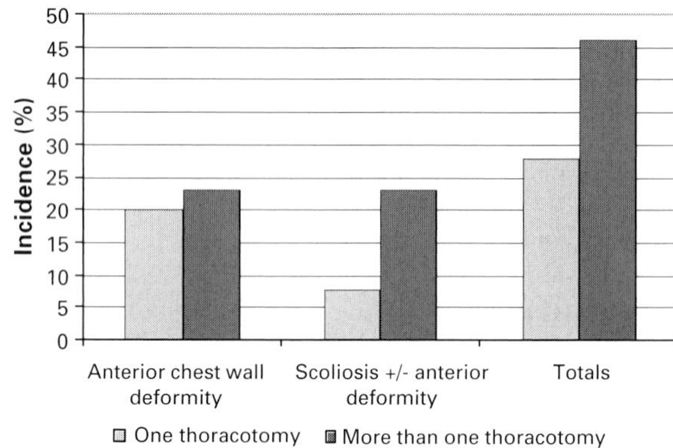

Fig. 15a.15. Effect of thoracotomy number on scoliosis and/or anterior chest wall deformity in the absence of a congenital vertebral abnormality in repaired esophageal atresia.[6]

of hemivertebrae (Fig. 15a.14). Moreover, total lung capacity and vital capacity are decreased, in part perhaps as a consequence of the reasons for which the multiple thoracotomies were performed, such as anastomotic dehiscence and empyema.[7] Improvements in neonatal care and surgical technique have meant that staged thoracic procedures for repair of esophageal atresia are now performed rarely, and are used only for specific situations, such as in the extremely premature infant with gastric perforation where the infant's clinical condition sometimes precludes esophageal anastomosis at the time of division of the fistula.[60]

Scoliosis

In the absence of a congenital veretebral anomaly, scoliosis tends to be minor and does not progress. Scoliosis is more common in patients who have had multiple thoracotomies (Fig. 15a.15). Where there are coexisting vertebral anomalies (e.g., hemivertebrae), scoliosis is often progressive and may become severe. In about 15% it becomes sufficiently severe to require spinal fusion.[61] Scoliosis associated with mixed vertebral anomalies in the lower thoracic spine have the worst prognosis.[62] Early detection of vertebral abnormalities is crucial, and these patients need careful follow-up throughout childhood and into adult life.

Parent support groups[63–66]

Throughout the world a number of esophageal atresia support groups have been set up. The primary role of these groups has been to provide information and support for the parents of children with esophageal atresia, but many of these organizations have also contributed to fundraising for research into the causes of esophageal atresia and its long term outcomes. Some are extremely active, with regular newsletters (e.g., CHEW[63]) and meetings which help to alleviate parental feelings of isolation,[30,67] and have been instrumental in setting up sophisticated follow-up studies of esophageal atresia patients who have survived into adulthood (e.g., OARA).[64]

Conclusions

Survival in esophageal atresia is largely determined by the presence of concomitant major congenital abnormalities, but long-term morbidity is influenced more by the way the atresia is managed surgically in the neonatal period and during infancy. At present we cannot influence the nature and severity of associated anomalies, but it is important to recognize early those infants for which the prognosis is so poor that no active treatment of the atresia is justified. On the other hand, there is much we can do about the way we manage the atresia itself, and this will affect the ultimate quality of life of the survivors.

It is widely acknowledged that the esophagus is inherently abnormal in EA, and no matter how carefully the surgical procedure is performed there will be some degree of ongoing esophageal dysmotility. Yet it is equally recognized that the surgical procedure itself may influence eventual esophageal function. The fibers of the vagi are vulnerable as they course through the mediastinum and along the esophagus – excessive or rough handling of the esophagus may damage them. Surgery can affect outcome in other ways as well: transfixion and division of the tracheo-esophageal fistula, rather than ligation alone, reduces the likelihood of a recurrent fistula; and minimal handling of the esophageal ends with well-placed interrupted sutures which include the mucosa produces a secure anastomosis and minimizes the incidence of anastomotic dehiscence and stricture. Avoidance of staged procedures, use of the intercostal approach (rather than rib resection), and preservation of the innervation to serratus anterior, ensure that the child will not develop significant chest wall deformity or scoliosis, in the absence of hemivertebrae. An extrapleural approach to the esophagus probably limits the magnitude of sepsis following anastomotic leakage. In addition, treatment with proton pump inhibitors and the surgical correction of gastroesophageal reflux controls reflux esophagitis and allows an anastomotic stricture to resolve. Finally, a successful primary esophageal anastomosis in long-gap EA obviates the need for esophageal replacement, with its many long-term drawbacks and complications.

There are other areas where we can be less certain about the long-term implications of management. Prime amongst these is concern regarding the possible deleterious effects of ongoing gastroesophageal reflux on an esophagus that is already relatively dysfunctional and empties poorly. Until the risk of malignancy is better defined, it would seem prudent that adults with repaired EA should have lifelong surveillance of their esophagus.

Despite these concerns, and the recognition that children with EA have more learning, emotional and behavioral problems than children in the general population[68], it is evident that most adults with repaired esophageal atresia lead a fairly normal lifestyle.

REFERENCES

1. Myers, N. A. The history of oesophageal atresia and tracheo-oesophageal fistula – 1670–1984. *Progr. Pediatr. Surg.* 1986; **20**:106–157.
2. Beasley, S. W. & Myers, N. A. Trends in mortality in oesophageal atresia. *Pediatr. Surg. Int.* 1992; **7**:86–89.
3. Patel, S. B., Ade-Ajayi, N., & Kiely, E. M. Oesophageal atresia: a simplified approach to early management. *Pediatr. Surg. Int.* 2002; **18**:87–89.
4. Bax, K. M. & Van Der Zee, D. C. Feasibility of thoracoscopic repair of oesophageal atresia with distal fistula. *J. Pediatr. Surg.* 2002; **37**:192–196.
5. Rothenberg, S. S. Thorascopic repair of tracheoesophageal fistula in newborns. *J. Pediatr. Surg.* 2002; **37**:869–872.
6. Beasley, S. W. Oesophageal atresia without fistula. In Beasley, S. W., Myers, N. A., & Auldist, A. W., eds. *Oesophageal Atresia.* London: Chapman & Hall Medical, 1991:137–159.
7. Beasley, S W. Influence of anatomy and physiology on the management of oesophageal atresia. *Progr. Pediatr. Surg.* 1991; **27**:53–61.
8. Farkash, U., Lazar, L., Erez, I., Gutermacher, M., & Freud, E. The distal pouch in esophageal atresia – to dissect or not dissect, that is the question. *Eur J. Pediatr. Surg.* 2002; **12**:19–23.
9. Anderson, K. D. Oesophageal substitution. *Aust. NZ. J. Surg.* 1984; **54**:447–449.
10. Cohen, D. G., Middleton, A. W., & Fletcher, J. Gastric tube esophagoplasty. *J. Pediatr. Surg.* 1974; **9**:451–460.
11. Spitz, L. Gastric transposition via the mediastinal route in infants with long gap esophageal atresia. *J. Pediatr. Surg.* 1984; **19**:149–154.
12. Scharli, A. F. Esophageal reconstruction in very long atresia by elongation of the lesser curvature. *Pediatr. Surg. Int.* 1992; **7**:101–105.
13. Beasley, S. W., Allen, M., & Myers, N. A. The effect of Down syndrome and other chromosomal abnormalities on survival and management in oesophageal atresia. *Pediatr. Surg. Int.* 1997; **12**:550–551.
14. Luzzatto, C. C., Ronconi, M. E. Tuvr, S. O. Guglielmi, M. E., & Zanardo, V. Longterm follow-up results after surgical repair of esophageal atresia. *Pediatr. Radiol.* 1990; **25**:313–320.

15. Ensure, S. A., Grosfeld, J. L., West, R. W., Rescorla, F. J., & Scherer, L. R. Analysis of morbidity and mortality in 227 cases of esophageal atresia and/or tracheo-esophageal fistula over 2 decades. *Arch. Surg.* 1995; **130**:502–508.
16. Konkin, D. E., O'Hali, W. A., Webber, E. M., & Blair, G. K. Outcomes in esophageal atresia and tracheoesophageal fistula. *J. Pediatr. Surg.* 2003; **38**:1726–1729.
17. Auldist A. W. & Beasley, S. W. Oesophageal complications. In Beasley, S. W., Myers, N. A., & Auldist, A. W., eds., *Oesophageal Atresia*. London: Chapman & Hall Medical, 1991; 305–330.
18. Janik, J., Filler, R. M., Ein, S. R., & Simpson, J. S. Longterm follow up of circular myotomy for esophageal atresia. *J. Pediatr. Surg.* 1980; **15**:835–841.
19. Gough, M. H., Esophageal atresia: use of an anterior flap in the difficult anastomosis. *J. Pediatr. Surg.* 1980; **15**:310–311.
20. Brown, A. K., Gough, M. H., Nicholls, G., & Tam, P. K H. Anterior flap repair of esophageal atresia: a 16-year evaluation. *Pediatr. Surg. Int.* 1995; **10**:525–528.
21. Davenport, M. & Bianchi, A. Early experience with esophageal flap esophagoplasty for repair of esophageal atresia. *Pediatr. Surg. Int.* 1990; **5**:332–335.
22. Said, M., Meeki, M., Golli, M. *et al.* Balloon dilatation of anastomotic strictures secondary to surgical repair of oesophageal atresia. *Br. J. Radiol.* 2003; **26**:26–31
23. Lang, T., Hummer, J. P., & Behrens, R. Balloon dilatation is preferable to bougienage in children with esophageal atresia. *Endoscopy* 2001; **33**:329–335.
24. Van Biervliet, S., Van Winkel, M., Robberecht, E., & Kerremans, I. High-dose Omeprazole in esophagitis with stenosis after surgical management of esophageal atresia. *J. Pediatr. Surg.* 2001; **36**; 1416–1418.
25. Stokes K. B. Pathophysiology of oesophageal atresia. In Beasley, S. W., Myers, N. A., & Auldist, A. W., eds. *Oesophageal Atresia*. London: Chapman & Hall Medical, 1991: 59–73.
26. Nakazato, Y., Landing, B. H., & Wells, T. R. Abnormal Auerbach plexus in the esophagus and stomach of patients with esophageal atresia and tracheoesophageal fistula. *J. Pediatr. Surg.* 1986; **21**:831–837.
27. Romeo, G., Zuccarello, B., & Proetto, F. Disorders of the esophageal motor activity in atresia of the esophagus. *J. Pediatr. Surg.* 1987; **22**:120–124.
28. Beasley, S. W., Phelan, P. D., & Chetcuti, P. Late results following repair of oesophageal atresia. In Beasley, S. W., Myers, N. A., Auldist, A. W., eds. *Oesophageal Atresia*. London: Chapman & Hall Medical, 1991: 369–394.
29. Chetcuti, P. & Phelan, P. D. Gastrointestinal morbidity following repair of esophageal atresia and tracheoesophageal fistula. *Arch. Dis. Child.* 1993; **68**:163–166.
30. Schier, F., Korn, S., & Michel, E. Experiences of a parent support group with the long-term consequences of esophageal atresia. *J. Pediatr. Surg.* 2001; **36**:605–610.
31. Yanchar, N. L., Gordon, R., Cooper, M., Dunlap, H., & Soucy, P. Significance of the clinical course and early upper gastrointestinal studies in predicting complications associated with repair of esophageal atresia. *J. Paediatr. Surg.* 2001; **36**:815–822.
32. Veit, F., Schwagten, K., Auldist, A. W., Beasley, S. W. Trends in the use of fundoplication in children with gastro-oesophageal reflux. *J. Paediat. Child Health* 1995; **31**:121–126.
33. Chetcuti, P., Myers, N. A., Phelan, P. D., & Beasley, S. W. Adults who survived repair of congenital esophageal atresia and tracheo-esophageal fistula. *Br. Med. J.* 1988; **297**:344–346.
34. Montgomery, M., Frenckner, B., Freyschuss, U., & Mortensson, W. Esophageal atresia: long term follow-up of respiratory function, maximal working capacity, and esophageal function. *Pediatr. Surg. Int.* 1995; **10**:519–522.
35. Harries, P. G. & Frost, R. A. Foreign body impaction arising in adulthood: a result of neonatal repair of tracheo-oesophageal fistula and oesophageal atresia. *Ann. R. Coll. Surg. Eng.* 1996; **78**:217–220.
36. Nebel, O., Fornes, M., & Castell, D. Symptomatic gastroesophageal reflux: incidence and precipitating factors. *Dig. Dis.* 1976; **21**:953–956.
37. Leendertse-Verloop, K., Tibboel, D., Hazebroek, F., & Molenaar, J. Post-operative morbidity in patients with oesophageal atresia. *Pediatr. Surg. Int.* 1987; **2**:2–5.
38. McKinnon, L. & Kosloske, A. Prediction and prevention of anastomotic complications of esophageal atresia and tracheoesophageal fistula. *J. Pediatr. Surg.* 1990; **25**:778–781.
39. Jolley, S. G., Johnson, D., Roberts, C., & Herbst, L. Patterns of gastroesophageal reflux in children following repair of esophageal atresia and tracheoesophageal fistula. *J. Pediatr. Surg.* 1980; **15**:857–862.
40. Chetcuti, P. & Phelan, P. D. Respiratory morbidity after repair of oesophageal atresia and tracheo-oesophageal fistula. *Arch. Dis. Child.* 1993; **68**:167–170.
41. Chetcuti, P., Phelan, P. D., & Greenwood, R. Lung function abnormalities in repaired esophageal atresia and tracheo-esophageal fistula. *Thorax* 1992; **47**:1030–1034.
42. Adzick, N. S., Fisher, J. H., Winter, H. S., Sandler, R. H., & Hendren, W. H. Esophageal adenocarcinoma years after esophageal atresia repair. *J. Pediatr. Surg.* 1989; **24**:741–744.
43. Deurloo, J. A., van Lanschot, J. J., Drillenburg, P., & Aronson, D. C. Esophageal squamous cell carcinoma 38 years after primary repair of esophageal atresia. *J. Pediatr. Surg.* 2001; **26**:629–630.
44. Haggett, R. C., Tryzelaar, J., Ellis, F. H. *et al.* Adenocarcinoma complicating columnar epithelium lined (Barrett's) esophagus. *Am. J. Clin. Pathol.* 1978; **70**:1–5.
45. Orringer, M., Kirsh, M., & Sloan, H. Longterm esophageal function following repair of esophageal atresia. *Ann. Surg.* 1977, **186**:436–443.
46. Shamberger, R. C., Eraklis, J., Kozakewrch, H. P., & Hendren, W. H. Fate of the distal esophageal remnant following esophageal replacement. *J. Pediatr. Surg.* 1988; **23**:1210–1214.
47. Ladd, W. E. The surgical treatment of esophageal atresia and tracheoesophageal fistula. *Engl. J. Med.* 1944; **230**:625–637.
48. Sauerbruch, F., Osophago-dermato-jejuno-gastrostomie. In *Chirurgerie der Brustorgane*. Berlin: Springer, 1925: 568–570.

49. LaQuaglia, M. P., Gray, M., & Schuster, S. R. Esophageal atresia and ante-thoracic skin tube esophageal conduits: squamous cell carcinoma in the conduit 44 years following surgery. *J. Pediatr. Surg.* 1987; **22**:44–47.
50. Myers, N. A., Beasley, S. W., Auldist, A. W. *et al.* Oesophageal atresia without fistula: anastomosis or replacement.? *Pediatr. Surg. Int.* 1987; **2**:216–222.
51. Delahunt, M. N., Sleet, M. S., & Wagget, J. Delayed primary anastomosis for wide defect esophageal atresia: a 17 year experience. *Pediatr. Surg. Int.* 1994; **9**:21–23.
52. Boyle, E. M., Irwin, E. D., & Foker, J. E. Primary repair of ultra long-gap esophageal atresia: results without a lengthening procedure. *Ann. Thorac. Surg.* 1994; **57**:576–579.
53. Holder, T. M. & Ashcraft, K. W. Developments in the care of patients with esophageal atresia and tracheoesophageal fistula. *Surg. Clin. North. Am.* 1981; **61**:1051–1061.
54. Carci, M. R. & Dibbins, A. W. Problems associated with a Nissen fundoplication following tracheoesophageal fistula and esophageal atresia repair. *Arch. Surg.* 1988; **123**:618–620.
55. Puri, P., Ninan, G. K., Blake, N. S. *et al.* Delayed primary anastomosis for esophageal atresia: 18 months to 11 years follow-up. *J. Pediatr. Surg.* 1992; **27**:1127–1130.
56. Anderson, K. D., Noblett, H., Belsey, R., & Randolph, J. G. Longterm follow-up of children with colon and gastric tube interposition for esophageal atresia. *Surgery* 1992; **111**:131–136.
57. De Rosa, G. P., Progressive scoliosis following chest wall resection in children. *Spine* 1985; **20**:618–622.
58. Cherup, L. L., Siewers, R. D., & Futrell, J. W. Breast and pectoral muscle maldevelopment after anterolateral and posterolateral thoracotomies in children. *Ann. Thorac. Surg.* 1986; **41**:492–497.
59. Freeman, N. V. & Walken, J. Previously unreported shoulder deformity following right lateral thoracotomy for esophageal atresia. *J. Pediatr. Surg.* 1969; **4**:627–636.
60. Maoate, K., Myers, N. A., & Beasley, S. W. Gastric perforation in infants with esophageal atresia and distal tracheo-oesophageal fistula. *Pediatr. Surg. Int.* 1999; **15**:24–27.
61. Chetcuti, P., Myers, N. A., Phelan, P. D., Beasley, S. W., & Dickens, D. R V. Chest wall deformity in patients with repaired esophageal atresia. *J. Pediatr. Surg.* 1989; **23**:244–247.
62. Chetcuti, P., Dickens, D. R. V., & Phelan, P. D. Spinal deformity in patients born with esophageal atresia and tracheoesophageal fistula. *Arch. Dis. Child.* 1989; 1427–1430.
63. www.tofs.org.uk.
64. Oesophageal Atresia Research Auxiliary (OARA), Victoria, Australia. www.rch.unimelb.edu.au/oara/.
65. www.keks.org.
66. www.voks.nz.
67. Little, D. C., Rescorla, F. J., Grosfeld, J. L., West, K. W., Scherer, L. R., & Engum, S. A. Long-term analysis of children with esophageal atresia and tracheo-esophageal fistula. *J. Pediatr. Surg.* 2003; **38**:852–856.
68. Bouman, N. H., Koot, H. M., & Hazebroek, F. W. Long-term physical, psychological and social functioning of children with esophageal atresia. *J. Pediatr. Surg.* 1999; **34**:399–404

15b

Esophageal atresia: nutrition, growth, and respiratory function

Philip A. J. Chetcuti and John W. L. Puntis

Clarendon Wing, Leeds General Infirmary, UK

There was an old man of Tobago
Who lived on rice, gruel and sago;
Til, much to his bliss
His physician said this –
To a diet of lamb you may go
The Oxford Book of Nursery Rhymes

A late progression from soft to lumpy food is characteristic of esophageal dysfunction following surgical correction of esophageal atresia (EA). Maintenance of an adequate nutritional intake is crucial for normal growth and development, and survival without food impossible. Prior to the first successful repair in 1943 EA was universally fatal. Despite the availability of effective surgical intervention for over 60 years, there has until recently been a paucity of data regarding long-term outcomes. Overall, survival following surgery is now greater than 90% and a high proportion of adults appear to enjoy an excellent quality of life. [1] Preoperative prognostic classification systems are important when it comes to prediction of outcome.[2] Feeding difficulties[3] and respiratory disorders[4,5] in childhood place a considerable burden of care on families.[6] It is uncertain how much these problems affect growth and pulmonary function and at what stage, and to what extent they resolve.

Many infants with EA exhibit poor intrauterine growth. For example, in one study of 294 cases, 36% were found to have a birthweight below the fifth centile, while only 15% were above the 50th centile.[7] The explanation for this observation is unclear, but it is unlikely to be fully explained by coexisting congenital anomalies (found in up to two-thirds of cases)[7–9] and the effect of premature birth. Detailed anthropometric data are needed to more accurately define growth and nutritional status at birth. This has some relevance to long-term outcome since epidemiologic evidence points to a link between poor fetal growth and later cardiovascular[10] and respiratory disease.[11] In addition, the particular patterns of intrauterine growth failure with respect to effects on body proportions appear to have specific health implications in adult life.[10]

Feeding difficulties

Underlying mechanisms

Vomiting and choking are the presenting features in around one-sixth of infants with EA.[8] Following surgery, feeding problems are both common and a source of considerable parental anxiety. Esophageal dysmotility is one of the principal reasons for difficulty at feed times,[12] and leads to dysphagia, aspiration and choking episodes. Motor abnormalities can be demonstrated in adult survivors, even those who regard themselves as being well.[13] Videofluoroscopy shows that while the oral phase of deglutition is normal, pharyngeal function is often disturbed and associated with aspiration.[14] Gastroesophageal reflux (GER) makes an additional important contribution in some children, as does anastomotic stricture. Congenital abnormalities in innervation of the esophagus, gastroesophageal junction and stomach increase the likelihood of dysmotility and GER.[15] Repeated episodes of distress during feeding may quickly lead to learned food aversions and reluctance to feed. This is well recognized in children with primary GER[16] and is probably the basis for eating difficulties in a wide range of children.[17] It is important to note that following esophagostomy, sham feeding is essential if normal taste sensations, sucking and swallowing are to be

Pediatric Surgery and Urology: Long-term Outcomes, Mark Stringer, Keith Oldham, Pierre Mouriquand.
Published by Cambridge University Press.

Table 15b.1. Some details of the TOFS group feeding questionnaire[18]

These questions were asked in relation to both milk feeds and introduction of solid foods:
- Did your child take a long time to finish a feed?
- Did your child refuse to feed at times?
- Did your child experience coughing or choking during feeds?
- Did your child vomit during or after feeds?

Parents were asked to indicate for each question whether symptoms occurred with:
- all feeds
- most feeds
- half of feeds
- 1–2 feeds/day
- 1–2 feeds/week
- occasionally
- never

developed and oral hypersensitivity and subsequent food refusal avoided. A combination of mechanical and behavioral factors underlie feeding problems, and the early involvement of a speech therapist and dietitian should be encouraged.

Feeding difficulties in infancy

An attempt to define the frequency and severity of feeding difficulties in children with EA was made with the help of a patient group in the UK.[18] All 230 families who were members of the Tracheo-Oesophageal Fistula Support (TOFS) group were sent a questionnaire regarding growth, surgery, complications, feeding history and experiences at feed/mealtimes; 124 questionnaires were completed, and the "feeding" part of the questionnaire was also administered to parents of 50 healthy controls for comparison (Table 15b.1).

Almost half of the 124 mothers had been able to breastfeed their infant, whether following a primary anastomosis or esophagostomy. However, 15% of women reported that they were actively discouraged from breastfeeding. Although there are many different factors influencing the rate of breastfeeding on the neonatal unit,[19] sympathetic support from nursing staff is crucial. Help may be needed with expressing milk during the infant's early postoperative period when suckling is precluded; mechanical breastpumps should be available.

Ninety-two children in this study had undergone a primary anastomosis. During at least two feeds each day almost two-thirds were considered to be slow feeders and one-third experienced coughing and choking. These symptoms were significantly more common than in the controls. Solid and lumpy food was introduced later in the EA children, and slowness, feed refusal, choking and vomiting were all reported more frequently. Of the 88 children who had reached 1 year of age, only 20% were completely free of symptoms at mealtimes.

Thirty-two children had an esophagostomy with a later esophageal substitution procedure. The frequency with which specific feed-related symptoms occurred in children after closure of esophagostomy was similar to that seen in the primary anastomosis group, although they were less likely to be perceived as slow milk-feeders. For solids, 50% were considered to be slow by parents, 31% vomited, 28% choked and 19% refused feeds at least twice a day. Compared with controls, only slowness to feed and vomiting appeared more common. At 1 year of age, no child was completely free of feed-related symptoms.

Feeding difficulties in childhood

Among both the primary anastomosis group and those who had a delayed repair, almost two-thirds of children who had reached 7 years of age (19/33) were symptom-free at mealtimes.[18] This indicates a tendency for resolution of feeding difficulties with increasing age, one of the findings also highlighted in another large cohort.[20] In this study, 67% of patients had required admission to hospital (one-fifth of these for more than 20 days) with esophageal complications in the years after initial surgery. The prevalence of feeding difficulties (dysphagia, food impaction, prolonged mealtimes) according to age group, and surgical intervention, are shown in Fig. 15b.1. The prevalence of feeding difficulties in the 12 months prior to the study, including the numbers with daily symptoms, are shown in Fig. 15b.2 for various age groups.

Various centers have reported experience with EA, including some long-term outcome data. End-to-side anastomosis is an operative approach which has been claimed to reduce the risk of esophageal dysmotility. Touloukian[21] provided follow-up data on 68 infants who were operated on in this way. Mild dysphagia and occasional respiratory symptoms were common during the first year of life. All patients were eating table foods after 12 months of age, although 15% had required removal of impacted food. Whether or not this represents a significantly better functional result than end-to-end anastomosis is uncertain.

In 10 survivors of delayed primary anastomosis followed up for 18 months to 11 years,[22] three had swallowing difficulties. All three were found to have strictures, and two

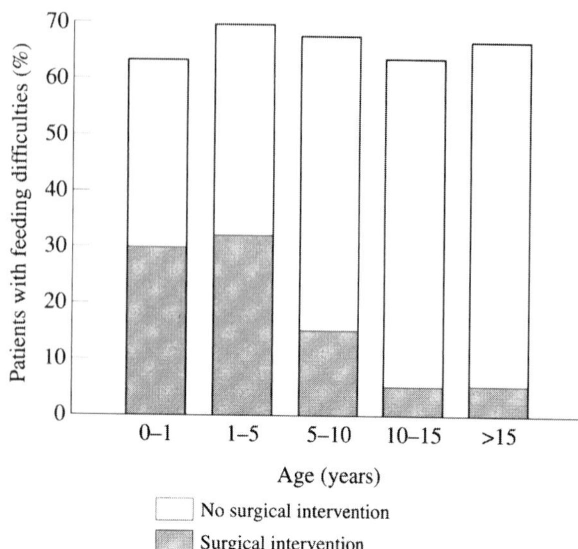

Fig. 15b.1. Prevalence of feeding difficulties.[20]

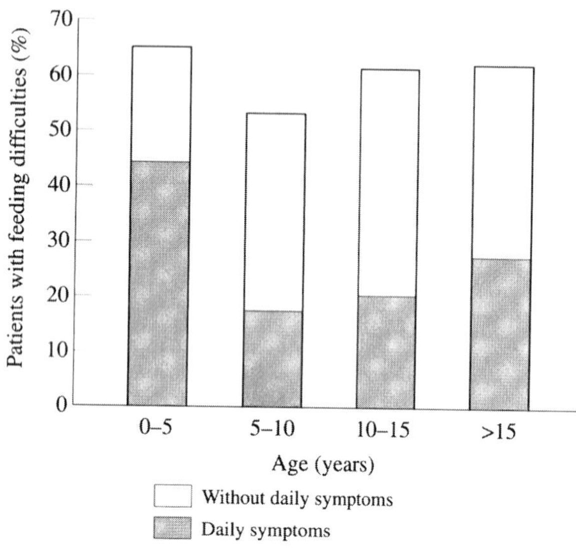

Fig. 15b.2. Age of the patient and prevalence of feeding difficulties in the 12 months prior to review.[20]

also had gross GER. One was a child with Down syndrome who was nasogastrically fed; the other two were described as having only occasional dysphagia and vomiting.

An investigation of 59 patients with a colon interposition for either EA or caustic stricture documented mild dysphagia in 17, after follow-up periods ranging from 18 months to 37 years.[23] Forty of the 57 survivors reported normal eating and swallowing habits; four had dysphagia with specific foods, and 13 had experience of food suddenly sticking. Anderson *et al.*[24] compared outcomes in 24 patients from the UK with esophageal atresia who had undergone a colon interposition with 15 patients from the USA who had a reversed gastric tube as their esophageal substitute. Age range at follow-up was from 3 to 19 years. Although normal diets were tolerated by most children, three avoided specific foods, three were troubled by food sticking, and 12 (10 colon, 2 gastric) ate slowly when compared with the rest of the family; over 90% were regarded as having minor dysphagia. This suggests a higher rate of problems in patients who have had colon grafts, perhaps not surprising given the less "physiologic" nature of this operation.

Feeding difficulties in adulthood

Approximately 70% of 145 patients operated on in one center[1] were interviewed regarding gastro-intestinal symptoms when they were over 18 years of age. Just over half complained of occasional dysphagia, while 16% had dysphagia on a daily basis. Heartburn was only a little more frequent than in the normal population, with almost half experiencing occasional discomfort and 11% admitting to more than one episode per week. Difficulty with swallowing was, therefore, a common complaint, and many patients drank fluids with meals to assist deglutition. However, only two deliberately avoided certain foods because they associated them with swallowing problems. Even though many older patients continued to have frequent symptoms, the majority did not consider them to be problematic.

Tovar *et al.*[13] investigated 22 patients aged 9–26 years who had been operated on for EA and in whom GER was undetected or untreated. All considered themselves to be healthy and were studying or working normally. Despite this, questioning revealed frequent symptoms of esophageal dysfunction. Two-thirds had dysphagia or heartburn, one-third vomiting, and almost half had experienced foreign body impaction. Manometry revealed uniformly disorganized propulsive activity with failure to clear acid from the esophagus.

In 26 patients investigated at a mean of 15.8 years after surgery, Tomaselli *et al.*[25] found without exception that esophageal peristaltic activity was disorganized, and that the amplitude of contractions was also reduced in 58%. Although such abnormalities on manometric investigation may cause little functional disturbance and have no long-term nutritional significance, poor acid clearing in combination with GER leads to chronic inflammation in up to 50% of patients.[26] In addition, 6% of 60 long-term survivors were found to have Barrett's esophagus,[26] a group requiring regular endoscopic follow up.[27]

Growth

Growth during childhood

Assessment of growth is an important indicator of nutritional status in children. On the basis of weight and height as reported by parents of 100 children in the TOFS group study, 32 showed evidence of growth failure.[18] The primary repair group was significantly smaller than the normal reference population with *z*-scores (standard deviation scores) for height-for-age and weight-for-height being −0.5 (SD 1.8) and −0.4 (SD 1.6), respectively. They were, however, better grown than those children who had an esophagostomy. The prevalence of growth retardation did not appear to decrease with increasing age, although few subjects had reached adulthood. Chetcuti *et al.*[20] studied over 300 children and adults born with EA and found that 11% were stunted (height <third percentile), and 13% were wasted (weight-for-height >2 standard deviations below the mean). Of those who were wasted, 20 were under 5 years of age, ten were between 5 and 10 years, seven were 10–15 years of age, and only one was over the age of 15. Patients identified by anthropometry as nutritionally compromised in this way were more likely to have experienced severe esophageal complications than those who were normally grown.

Other, smaller, studies have suggested an even higher prevalence of growth failure in childhood after EA repair. For example, of ten children undergoing a delayed primary anastomosis reported by Puri *et al.*,[22] three showed evidence of growth failure. In another study, 44% of 25 children who had a colon interposition for EA were found to be below the fifth centile for height and weight, whilst those operated on for caustic burns of the esophagus were better grown.[23] In a comparison between children with a gastric tube or colon graft esophageal substitution,[24] weight data were reported for 17 out of 39. The weight graph is striking and shows that all 17 fell close to or below the fifth centile; three were markedly underweight in late teenage years. The height data as published do not correspond exactly in age with the weight data, but most points were above the fifth centile, with five falling below (i.e., almost one-third of those measured were stunted). No details of birthweight or gestational age were given, but the authors also noted that children with EA tend to have a low birthweight; they suggested (unconvincingly) that the poor growth observed in their patients reflected prematurity. In another study, the mean birthweight of 227 infants with EA was 2557 g (range 1110–4460 g) but no details of subsequent growth were provided.[8]

Growth by adulthood

In the only large follow-up study of adult survivors of EA, 74% of 145 patients had height and weight measurements performed.[1] Both height and weight appeared normally distributed, and there was only one patient who was growth retarded. The above data can be interpreted as indicating that, for the most part, growth faltering in childhood is a temporary phenomenon associated with feeding difficulties and early esophageal complications, with catch-up growth likely to occur as feeding and respiratory symptoms (see below) improve throughout early life.

Respiratory problems

Mechanisms underlying respiratory problems

A number of different factors combine to produce respiratory illness in the years following initial surgical repair of EA. GER may result in the inhalation of gastric contents and cause an increase in bronchial hyper-reactivity, recurrent lower airways infection, and pneumonia, together with longer term bronchiolar and lung parenchymal damage. Reflux sometimes initiates vagally mediated laryngospasm or bronchospasm in the absence of inhalation.[28,29] Abnormal esophageal peristalsis and impaction of food above an anastomotic stricture also predisposes to inhalation. Impacted food may lead to external compression of the trachea, causing narrowing.

Tracheomalacia is often widespread, involving both the intrathoracic and extrathoracic trachea,[30] and may be exacerbated by congenital denervation abnormalities of the trachea.[31] Whilst all these factors contribute to variable narrowing of the trachea, the nature and severity of symptoms depend upon the location and degree of tracheomalacia as well as the age of the patient. The mildest form is associated with the presence of the characteristic harsh brassy cough alone (the "TOF cough"). Next is the presence of stridor (extrathoracic obstruction) or wheeze (intrathoracic obstruction) associated with intercurrent respiratory infection. At its most severe, stridor and/or wheeze are present continuously with exacerbations of severe obstruction associated with cyanosis. This is rarely present over the age of 2 years as the trachea becomes more stable with age. Severe intrathoracic tracheomalacia may exacerbate GER, compounding the airway problems, and GER may increase the severity of airway obstruction. Tracheomalacia is associated both with a relatively ineffective cough and with squamous metaplasia of the tracheal mucosa with loss of ciliary activity.[32] The result is retention of secretions with the risk of secondary bacterial infection. Finally, although uncommon, recurrence of the tracheoesophageal fistula should always be considered in a child experiencing an excess of symptoms, particularly if associated with abnormalities on the chest X-ray.

Other factors sometimes contribute to lower respiratory tract problems, including low birthweight and prematurity, both of which are independently associated with an excess of illness in the early years of life. Airway and lung damage is usually present in infants who have required prolonged ventilation.

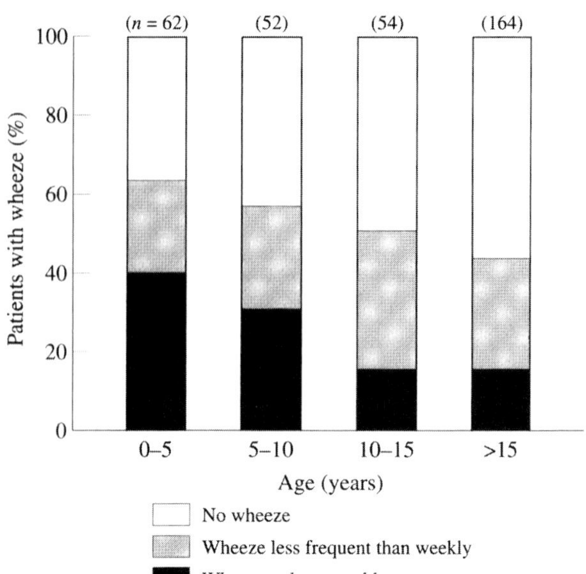

Fig. 15b.3. Age of the patient and prevalence of wheeze in the 12 months prior to review.[33]

Respiratory problems in infants

Infancy is the most hazardous period for respiratory disorders. Complications in the upper gastrointestinal tract are usually at their peak, with a high proportion of infants experiencing difficulties in swallowing, vomiting and choking with feeds. Tracheomalacia is also at its worst and the combination of all these problems leads to an increased likelihood of hospitalization,[20,33] the occurrence of "near death" episodes,[34] and even sudden unexpected death. A minority of children will experience persistent respiratory distress making feeding more difficult. Together with increased energy requirements resulting from the work of breathing, this inevitably poses a threat to nutritional status. Frequent intercurrent infections exacerbate all of these difficulties.

Few studies have examined the prevalence of respiratory disorders in this group of patients during infancy. In a very large follow-up study, 8% of parents recalled cyanotic episodes in early childhood.[33] In the same group late deaths in infancy were extremely uncommon, occurring in only one of over 300 patients. In a smaller study, 11 of 16 infants developed respiratory symptoms and/or GER.[35] Two children died, and five were operated upon (two requiring Nissen fundoplication, and three tracheopexy).

Respiratory problems in childhood

Respiratory morbidity following surgery for EA was first highlighted in 1966 with a description of aspiration pneumonia in 14 patients.[36] Several other reports have also drawn attention to respiratory problems.[4,37] A long-term follow-up study of over 300 children and adults by Chetcuti *et al.*[33] included details of the prevalence of respiratory symptoms and illnesses; 44% were hospitalized with respiratory illnesses and 10% were admitted on more than five occasions. Admissions occurred mainly in the first 5 years of life and were unusual over the age of 10 years. Individuals with a low birthweight and those known to have GER were more likely to require hospital admission. Alternative risk factors such as a history of atopy or parental smoking were no more common in patients hospitalized than those not.

In this study, pneumonia had been confirmed radiologically in 31% of children under 5 years of age, with more than two-thirds experiencing two or more episodes. This complication decreased in frequency with increasing age, occurring in only 3% of patients over 10 years of age. Fortunately, bronchiectasis was rare, being present in less than 1%. The prevalence and frequency of episodes of wheezing and bronchitis in the 12 months prior to the study for different age groups are shown in Figs. 15b.3 and 15b.4. The prevalence of wheeze was more than twice the prevalence of asthma in Australia at the time of the study. Whilst wheezing was still common in older children, the frequency was reduced compared with younger children. The prevalence and frequency of bouts of bronchitis decreased significantly with increasing age. Two-thirds of subjects of all ages reported a normal exercise tolerance, with only a small number describing considerable limitation.

Lung function studies on small numbers of patients have confirmed the presence of mild restrictive lung disease and

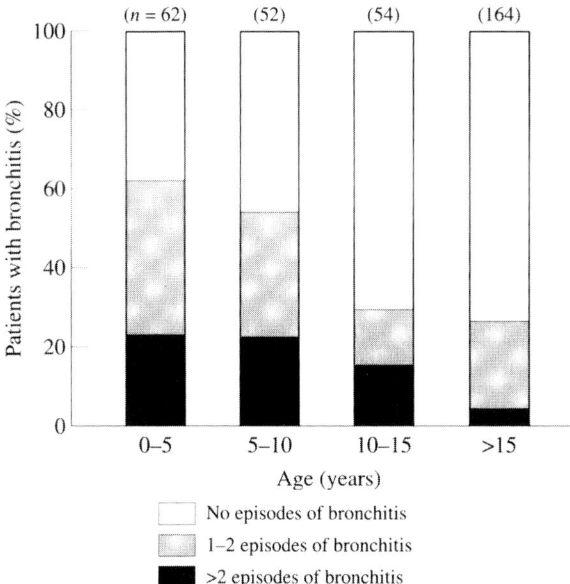

Fig. 15b.4. Age of the patient and prevalence of bronchitis in the 12 months prior to review.[33]

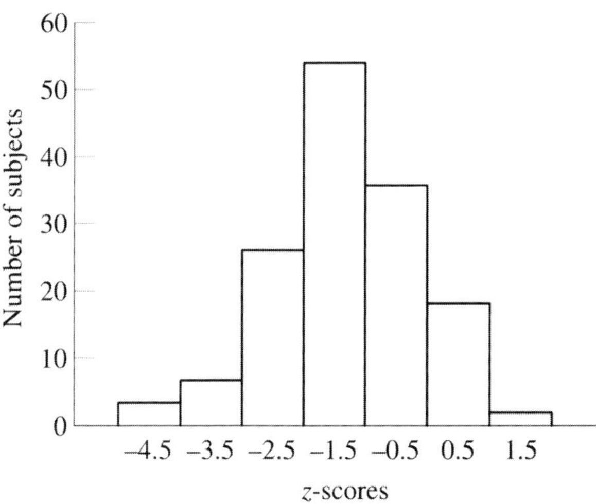

Fig. 15b.5. Distribution of FEV_1 expressed as standardized scores (z-scores), in children over 6 years of age, following EA repair. Mean z score = –1.32 (SD 1.11).

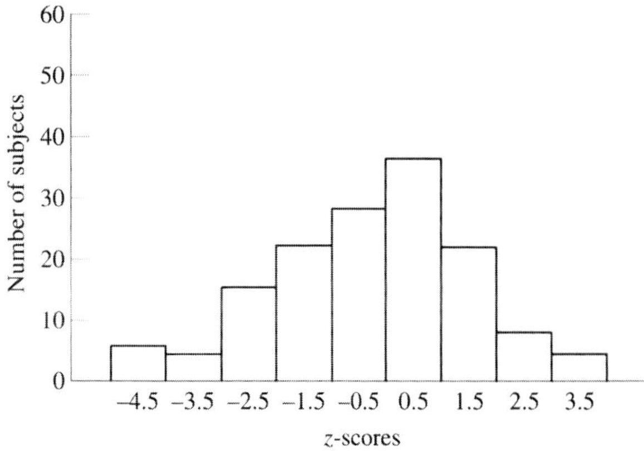

Fig. 15b.6. Distribution of TLC after EA repair expressed as standardized scores (z-scores), for the children in Fig.15b.5. Mean z score = –0.38 (SD 1.95).

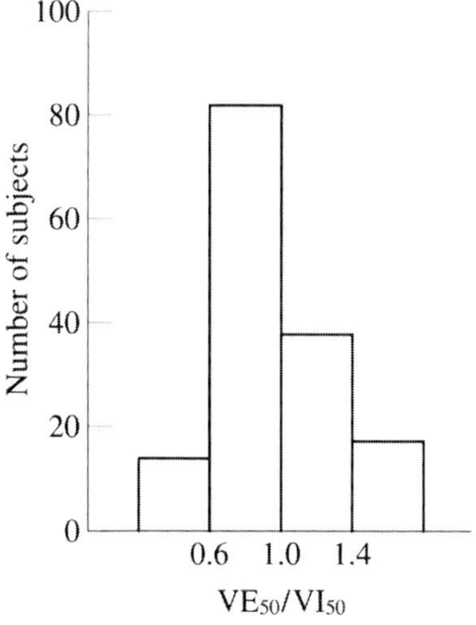

Fig. 15b.7. Distribution of VE_{50}/VI_{50} for the children in Fig.15b.5. Mean ratio = 1.0 (SD 0.3).

extrathoracic and intrathoracic airways obstruction.[38–42] In a much larger study,[43] lung function tests were performed on over 150 children and adults. Subjects with scoliosis were excluded from this analysis because of the known association with reduced lung volumes. Children under the age of 6 years were also excluded as they were unable to cooperate with the lung function measurements. Total lung capacity (TLC) and forced expiratory volume in one second (FEV_1) were measured as an index of lung volume and lower airways function, respectively. The data were expressed as standard deviation scores (z-scores) to permit comparisons between subjects of different age, sex and height, and were based on normal data (95% of the normal population would be expected to have a score between –2 and +2). Mid-expiratory to mid-inspiratory flows (VE_{50}/VI_{50}) were calculated to give an index of upper airway narrowing, the normal range being 0.6–1. Less than 0.6 suggests that lower airways narrowing is more significant than upper airways narrowing; a ratio of >1 suggests the reverse. Figures 15b.5 – 15b.7 illustrate the results.

The group showed evidence of significant airways narrowing, with a mean z-score for FEV_1 of -1.32 (25% had z-scores below −2). The mean z-score for TLC was −0.38, suggesting overall that subjects had slightly smaller lung volumes (18% had values for TLC below 2). Upper airway narrowing was more significant than lower airway narrowing in 38%, and lower airway narrowing was the most significant in 10% of patients.

FEV_1 was significantly reduced in subjects still experiencing respiratory symptoms, in those with previous hospital admissions for respiratory disease, and in those with documented GER. Total lung capacity was significantly reduced in subjects with documented GER in the past. Lung volumes were also reduced in those who had more than one thoracotomy.

Respiratory problems in adults

The Melbourne study reviewed 125 adults born with EA.[1] One in four had attended a general practitioner for respiratory symptoms in the preceding 12 months; 5% had experienced an episode of radiologically confirmed pneumonia during adult life. Only two considered themselves to have a significant reduction in exercise tolerance, one with severe scoliosis and one with bronchiectasis. Two had required hospital admission for respiratory illness since the age of 18 years, and 5 had more than 10 days off work in the preceding 12 months as a result of respiratory problems. An appreciable daily cough affected 9% of patients, and 6% reported having a daily productive cough for longer than one month. Occasional wheezing was present in 26%, and occurred at least once a week in 14%. Two or more episodes of bronchitis in the 12 months prior to review were experienced by 10%.

Symptomatic adults were compared with the asymptomatic group. The symptomatic group were much more likely to have experienced lower respiratory tract illnesses in early childhood. This implies that the symptoms are secondary to permanent damage to the airways and lung sustained from the repeated problems in childhood, including the effects of recurrent episodes of inhalation of esophageal and gastric contents. Adults with persisting respiratory symptoms were no more likely to have current symptoms of GER than those with no respiratory symptoms, further supporting the view that the current symptoms dated from damage originating in early childhood.

Adults with respiratory symptoms were more likely to have hayfever and eczema or a family history of allergic illnesses, suggesting that a number had asthma. The prevalence of smoking in this cohort was slightly higher than the national average at the time of the study. Whilst the symptomatic group were not more likely to be cigarette smokers than the asymptomatic group, there are concerns about the potential long-term adverse effects of smoking in these patients.

Seventy-four patients who had lung function tests showed evidence of mild airways obstruction with a mean z-score for FEV_1 of −1.28. Their lung volume measurements, however, were within the normal range. A significant reduction in FEV_1 was present in those who had experienced respiratory symptoms in the previous 12 months, and those admitted with respiratory illnesses in childhood.

Conclusions

With few exceptions, most children born with EA with or without tracheal fistula should survive. Feeding difficulties in infancy relate to both esophageal dysmotility and GER, together with learned aversive behavior. Some children fail to thrive, possibly as a result of their feeding difficulties, but many learn to avoid the foods and textures which cause them distress. Feeding problems show a tendency to spontaneous resolution during childhood, persistence suggesting mechanical complications such as anastomotic stricture or GER. Despite the fact that abnormalities of esophageal function are universal in adult survivors, only a small minority seem to regard themselves as having anything other than mild swallowing problems. This may in part be explained by them having developed mealtime strategies which minimize the risk of dysphagia and choking, such as a liberal fluid intake.

In a number of studies concerned with long-term outcome, growth is either not mentioned or dealt with superficially. Improved growth surveillance of children during follow-up and a greater willingness to consider nutritional support[44] might prevent or reverse growth failure which occurs in as many as a third of children. In those cases where primary repair of the esophagus is not possible, the superiority of one type of esophageal substitution over another with regard to effects on feeding and growth is not established. In one large follow-up study of adults which included detailed anthropometric assessment, there was no increased risk of poor nutritional status as indicated by growth. It appears overall that the long-term prognosis for normal eating and fulfillment of growth potential in children with EA is excellent.

Major respiratory morbidity is seen particularly during early childhood. These symptoms improve with increasing age and the majority enjoy a normal lifestyle. Significant lower respiratory tract illnesses in early life are an important contributing factor to persistent respiratory symptoms in adulthood, so all efforts should be directed towards early diagnosis and treatment. This might involve detailed assessments for the early detection of esophageal, gastroesophageal and tracheal complications when indicated. Medical treatment for GER, anti-reflux procedures, and tracheal stabilization surgery can all be required. The role of routine chest physiotherapy in these children is uncertain, but together with early identification and treatment of respiratory pathogens it may play a role in preventing chronic problems. Whether adults are at risk of deteriorating lung function in later life remains to be determined.

Postscript

The Tracheo-Oesophageal Fistula Support group in the UK have produced an excellent book for families: *The TOF Child*, V Martin (ed). Published by TOFS, St George's Centre, 91 Victoria Road, Netherfield, Nottingham NG4 2NN. Tel 0115 961 3092; fax 0115 961 3097; e-mail: info@tofs.org.uk Website: www.tofs.org.uk.

REFERENCES

1. Chetcuti, P., Myers, N. S., Phelan, P. D., & Beasley, S. W. Adults who survived repair of congenital oesophageal atresia and tracheo-oesophageal fistula. *Br. Med. J.* 1988; **297**:344–346.
2. Konkin, D. E., O'Hali, W. A., Webber, E. M., & Blair, G. K. Outcomes in esophageal atresia and tracheoesophageal fistula. *J. Pediatr. Surg.* 2003; **38**:1726–1729.
3. Smith, I. J. & Beck, J. Mechanical feeding difficulties after primary repair of oesophageal atresia. *Acta Paediatr. Scand.* 1985; **74**:237–239.
4. Shermeta, D. W., Whitington, P. F., Seto, D. S., & Haller, J. A. Lower esophageal sphincter dysfunction in esophageal atresia: nocturnal regurgitation and aspiration pneumonia. *J. Pediatr. Surg.* 1977; **12**:871–876.
5. Dudley, N. E. & Phelan, P. D. Respiratory complications in long term survivors of oesophageal atresia. *Arch. Dis. Child.* 1976; **51**:279–282.
6. Koop, C. E., Schnaufer, L., Thompson, G., Haecker, T., & Dalrymple, D. The social, psychological and economic problems of the patient's family after successful repair of esophageal atresia. *Z. Kinderchir.* 1975; **17**:125–131.
7. David, T. J. & O'Callaghan, S. E. Oesophageal atresia in the South West of England. *J. Med. Gen.* 1975; **12**:1–11.
8. Engum, A. S., Grosfeld, J. A., West, K. M. *et al.* Analysis of morbidity and mortality in 227 cases of esophageal atresia and/or tracheoesophageal fistula over two decades. *Arch. Surg.* 1995; **130**:502–508.
9. van Heurn, L. W., Cheng, W., de Vries, B. *et al.* Anomalies associated with oesophageal atresia in Asians and Europeans. *Pediatr. Surg. Int.* 2002; **18**:241–243.
10. Barker, D. J. P., Gluckman, P. D., Godfrey, K. M. *et al.* Fetal nutrition and cardiovascular disease in adult life. *Lancet* 1993; **341**:938–941.
11. Barker, D. J. P., Godfrey, K. M., Fall, C. *et al.* Relation of birth weight and childhood respiratory infection to adult lung function and death from chronic obstructive airways disease. In Barker, D. J. P., ed. *Fetal and infant origins of adult disease.* Br. Med. J., 1992: 150–161.
12. Orringer, M. B., Kirsh, M. M., & Sloan, H. Long-term esophageal function following repair of esophageal atresia. *Ann. Surg.* 1977; **186**:436–433.
13. Tovar, J. A., Diez Pardo, J. A., Murcia, J. *et al.* Ambulatory 24-hour manometric and pH metric evidence of permanent impairment of clearence capacity in patients with esophageal atresia. *J. Pediatr. Surg.* 1995; **30**:1224–1231.
14. Hormann, M., Pokieser, P., Scharitzer, M. *et al.* Videofluoroscopy of deglutition in children after repair of esophageal atresia. *Acta. Radiol.* 2002; **43**:507–510.
15. Nakazato, Y., Landing, B., & Wells, T. Abnormal Auerbach plexus in the esophagus and stomach of patients with esophageal atresia and tracheo-esophageal fistula. *J. Pediatr. Surg.* 1986; **21**:831–837.
16. Dellert, S. F., Hyams, J. S., Treem, W. R., & Geertsma, M. A. Feeding resistance and gastroesophageal reflux in infancy. *J. Pediatr. Gastroenterol. Nutr.* 1993; **17**:66–71.
17. Douglas, J. E. & Bryon, M. Interview data on severe behavioural eating difficulties in young children. *Arch. Dis. Child.* 1996; **75**:304–308.
18. Puntis, J. W. L., Ritson, D. G., Holden, C. E., & Buick, R. G. Growth and feeding problems after repair of oesophageal atresia. *Arch. Dis. Child.* 1990; **65**:84–88.
19. Lucas, A., Cole, T. J., Morley, R. *et al.* Factors asociated with maternal choice to provide breast milk for low birthweight infants. *Arch. Dis. Child.* 1988; **63**:48–52.
20. Chetcuti, P., Beasley, S., & Myers, W. Gastrointestinal morbidity and growth after repair of oesophageal atresia and tracheo-oesophageal fistula. *Arch. Dis. Child.* 1993; **69**:163–166.
21. Touloukian, R. J. Reassessment of the end-to-side operation for esophageal atresia with distal tracheo-esophageal fistula: 22 years experience with 68 cases. *J. Pediatr. Surg.* 1992; **27**:562–567.
22. Puri, P., Ninan, G. K., Blake, N. S. *et al.* Delayed primary anastomosis for esophageal atresia: 18 months to 11 years follow-up. *J. Pediatr. Surg.* 1992; **27**:1127–1130.
23. Raffensperger, J. G., Luck, S. R., Reynolds, M., & Schwarz, D. Intestinal bypass of the esophagus. *J. Pediatr. Surg.* 1996; **31**:38–47.
24. Anderson, K. D., Noblett, H., Belsey, R., & Randolph, J. G. Long-term follow-up of children with colon and gastric tube interposition for esophageal atresia. *Surgery* 1992; **111**:131–136.
25. Tomaselli, V., Volpi, M. L., Dell'Agnola, C. A., Bini, M., Rossi, A., & Indriolo, A. Long-term evaluation of esophageal function inpatients treated at birth for esophageal atresia. *Pediatr. Surg. Int.* 2003; **19**:40–43.

26. Somppi, E., Tammela, O., Ruuska, T. *et al.* Outcome of patients operated on for esophageal atresia: 30 years' experience. *J. Pediatr. Surg.* 1998; **33**:1341–1346.
27. Little, D. C., Rescorla, F. J., Grosfeld, F. J., West, K. W., Scherer, L. R., & Engum, S. A. Long-term analysis of children with esophageal atresia and tracheoesophageal fistula. *J. Pediatr. Surg.* 2003; **38**:852–856.
28. Danus, O., Lasou, C., Lauvom, A., & Pope, C. Esophageal reflux: an unrecognised cause of recurrent obstructive bronchitis in children. *J. Pediatr.* 1976; **89**:220–224.
29. Mansfield, L. & Stein, M. Gastro-esophageal reflux and asthma: a possible reflux mechanism. *Ann. Allergy* 1978; **41**:224–226.
30. Wailoo, M. & Emery, J. The trachea in children with tracheo-esophageal fistula. *Histopathology* 1979; **3**:329–338.
31. Nakazoto, Y., Wells, T., & Landing, B. Abnormal tracheal innervation in patients with esophageal atresia and tracheo-esophageal fistula: study of the intrinsic tracheal nerve plexuses by a microdissection technique. *J. Pediatr. Surg.* 1986; **21**:838–844.
32. Emery, J. & Haddadin, A. Squamous epithelium in the respiratory tract of children with tracheo-oesophageal fistula. *Arch. Dis. Child.* 1971; **41**:236–242.
33. Chetcuti, P. & Phelan, P. Respiratory morbidity after repair of oesophageal atresia and traceho-oesophageal fistula. *Arch. Dis. Child.* 1993; **68**:167–170.
34. Blair, G., Cohen, R., & Filler, K. M. Treatment of tracheomalacia: eight years experience. *J. Pediatr. Surg.* 1986; **21**:781–785.
35. Beardsmore, C., Macfadyen, U., Johnstowe, M., Williams, A., & Simpson, H. Clinical findings and respiratory function in infants following repair of oesophageal atresia and tracheo-oesophageal fistula. *Eur. Respir. J.* 1994; **7**:1039–1047.
36. Crispin, A., Friedland, G., & Waterston, D. Aspiration pneumonia and dysphagia after technically successful repair of oesophageal atresia. *Thorax* 1966; **81**:104–110.
37. Laks, H., Wilkinson, R., & Schuster, S. Long term results following correction of esophageal atresia with tracheo-esophageal fistula: a clinical and cine-fluorographic study. *J. Pediatr. Surg.* 1972; **7**:591–597.
38. Milligan, D. & Levinson, H. Lung function in children following repair of tracheo-oesophageal fistula. *J. Pediatr.* 1979; **95**:24–27.
39. Couriel, J., Hibbert, M., Olinsky, A., & Phelan, P. Long term pulmonary consequences of oesophageal atresia with tracheo-oesophageal fistula. *Acta. Paediatr. Scand.* 1982; **71**:973–978.
40. Le Souef, P., Myers, N., & Landon, L. Etiological factors in long-term respiratory function abnormalities following esophageal atresia repair. *J. Pediatr. Surg.* 1987; **22**:918–922.
41. Biller, J., Allen, A., Schuster, S. Treves, S., & Winter, H. Long term evaluation of esophageal and pulmonary function in patients with repaired esophageal atresia and tracheo-esophageal fistula. *Dig. Dis. Sci.* 1987; **32**:985–990.
42. Robertson, D., Mobaireek, K., Davis, G., & Coates, A. Late pulmonary function following repair of tracheo-esophageal fistula or esophageal atresia. *Pediatr. Pulmon.* 1995; **20**:21–26.
43. Chetcuti, P., Phelan, P., & Greenwood, R. Lung function abnormalities in repaired oesophageal atresia and tracheo-oesophageal fistula. *Thorax* 1992; **47**:1030–1034.
44. Booth, I. W. Enteral nutrition in childhood. *Br. J. Hosp. Med.* 1991; **46**:111–113.

16

Antireflux procedures

Adam Goldin

Department of Surgery, University of Washington, Seattle, WA, USA

Historically, operative management for gastroesophageal reflux disease (GERD) has been directed towards restoration of anatomical and functional norms. Many publications describe excellent short-term outcomes following medical and surgical therapy. Unfortunately, few studies have addressed the long-term outcomes in children who suffer from GERD. As our understanding of GERD has grown more sophisticated, and as we begin to focus on long-term outcomes, we have begun to re-evaluate the indications for our operative management. Fortunately, our ability to evaluate outcomes has also grown more sophisticated, and as we are beginning to find that not all children benefit equally from anti-reflux procedures (ARP), long-term evaluation is helping to delineate various subpopulations of children with GERD that may benefit to a greater degree than others. Hopefully such studies will modify the algorithms by which we choose which children are likely to benefit, and by which interventions.

A proper understanding of the published work on long-term outcomes for antireflux procedures thus requires a thorough discussion and understanding of the underlying disease, the indications for operative intervention, the various technical options available to perform an anatomic repair, and our goals in doing so. All of these need also to be considered within the context of the history of the understanding of the diagnosis of GERD, as well as the advances in the technology available for repair.

Gastroesophageal reflux disease (GERD) is the abnormal reflux of gastric content proximally into the esophagus. While a degree of reflux is normal, there is a spectrum of abnormal physiology that leads to discomfort and other problems within our patients. In general terms, GERD has three types of clinical manifestations – reflux that is sufficient to cause emesis, reflux that does not lead to emesis, but is high enough to spill over into the tracheobronchial tree, and reflux that simply irritates the esophagus alone. Each of these three general categories has several clinical manifestations that suggest the diagnosis of GERD. Generally, these lead to a medical treatment of the disorder, and, if that fails, often to a surgical treatment. The goals of medical therapy are to decrease acid production, to improve peristalsis and motility, to decrease the volume of secretions, and to minimize reflux via changes in positioning, or changes in the consistency of the feedings. The aim of surgical therapy, as stated previously, is to correct abnormal anatomy. The anatomical elements responsible for a competent lower esophageal sphincter (LES) are (i) normal antegrade peristalsis/ neuromuscular function, (ii) an adequate length of intra-abdominal esophagus, (iii) a normal (acute) angle of HIS, (iv) normal approximation of the diaphragmatic crura, and (v) no downstream obstruction, e.g., gastroparesis/gastric outlet obstruction. An abnormality of any one of these components can lead to GERD. Surgical therapies attempt to correct all but the first.

The problem then becomes not only making the correct diagnosis of GERD, but also understanding the underlying cause of GERD in each patient, as this will lead the clinician to the correct therapeutic intervention. Diagnostic tools available include (i) complete history and physical examination, (ii) upper gastrointestinal (UGI) contrast study (including oral-pharyngeal swallowing studies), (iii) 24 hour pH probe analysis, (iv) esophageal manometry, (v) esophagoscopy with or without biopsies, and (vi) gastric emptying scan with scintigraphy. Each of these tools highlights a different aspect of the possible etiology of the disease. As a single patient can have multiple causes of

Pediatric Surgery and Urology: Long-term Outcomes, Mark Stringer, Keith Oldham, Pierre Mouriquand.
Published by Cambridge University Press.

GERD, and since we can not identify the physiologic or anatomic abnormality by clinical examination, arguably each patient should undergo the full spectrum of diagnostic tests in order to correctly treat the disease. For example, several authors suggest that early surgical failures can be related to poor gastric emptying causing gastric contents to reflux despite an appropriate fundoplication.[1–10] The conclusion offered was that patients undergoing an antireflux procedure should therefore also undergo prospective gastric emptying scan, and if abnormal, have a gastric emptying procedure performed at the time of the antireflux operation. Similarly, many have argued that there is a higher rate of wrap failure among children with developmental delay because their problem is related to poor esophageal and gastric motility rather than simply an incompetent LES.[11–14]

As stated, an operation can only correct the anatomic abnormality. This is accomplished via one, or perhaps several of the following steps in performing an ARP: (i) reduction of the hiatal hernia, if present, (ii) re-approximation of the diaphragmatic crura thereby preventing further herniation, (iii) lengthening of the intra-abdominal component of the esophagus, (iv) re-creation of an acute angle of HIS, (v) buttressing of the LES with the fundus of the stomach, and (vi) performing a gastric emptying procedure if delayed gastric emptying is present. If the patient suffers from a primary motility disorder, none of the above maneuvers will restore completely normal function to the LES. In this latter circumstance, if the patient suffers from excessive salivation and aspiration, an ARP may even exacerbate the patient's risk.

The natural history

Unfortunately, relatively little is known about the natural history of untreated childhood GERD. Most citations regarding this topic refer to an article published in 1959 in which Carre described a number of children with a partial thoracic stomach (PTS).[15] Because this paper has served as the foundation of much of our understanding and many of the assumptions regarding the natural history of GERD, it compels a more detailed discussion. His study was a retrospective review in which he divided 235 children into three groups – group I were children with PTS, group II were children with PTS complicated by an esophageal stricture, and group III were children with PTS who died. As Carre's intention with this paper was to outline the clinical progress of children with PTS, he chose not to include any children who received either postural or surgical therapy, both of which were available to this population starting in 1951. He therefore included only children who had been evaluated prior to 1951. In addition to children with documented PTS, Carre increased his study population by identifying children who had been evaluated between 1930 and 1950 for either emesis of unknown etiology or an esophageal abnormality. He reassessed them clinically and radiographically, and then included them if the findings confirmed the diagnosis of PTS. Carre then examined each patient personally, and interviewed one or both parents. For this part of the study, he only included children who were at least 4 years old at the time of their most recent visit. His conclusions for this retrospective aspect of his paper were that 73% of children who successfully weaned to solid food showed improvement in clinical symptoms without intervention, whereas only 7% of children who did not wean successfully showed improvement. Furthermore, among the children who did not wean successfully, 94% still had symptoms at age 2 years, 78% at age 4, and 47% at age 7.

Carre also attempted a "prospective" study of 9 patients diagnosed with PTS within the first 3 months of life who had not been treated with postural or surgical therapy. One child died at 11 weeks of age, five had minimal symptoms by 12 months, and three children continued to have symptoms up to and beyond 4 years of age.

Despite the problems with Carre's paper in terms of its design and conclusions, it remains a landmark achievement and deserves its respected place within the history of our medical literature. Most importantly, it has served as a resource for many others who followed.

In 1997, for example, Nelson *et al.* performed a cross-sectional study of eight clinic-based practices, gathering information on the prevalence of reflux symptoms in infants.[16] She then performed a follow-up of these patients 1 year later. They found that 50% of children between 0 and 3 months of age had at least one episode of regurgitation per day, decreasing to 5% at 10–12 months of age. The prevalence of regurgitation peaked at 4 months of age at 67%, and there was not a statistically significant difference in eating behavior between children with and without regurgitation. The subpopulation of children that regurgitated at least four times per day demonstrated a similar pattern. Twenty-three percent of children 4–6 months of age regurgitated at least four times per day, whereas only 7% of children 7–9 months of age regurgitated this often. The two most important factors contributing to parental reporting of regurgitation as a problem were the frequency and the volume of regurgitation (see Table 16.1 and Fig 16.1).

Miyazawa and colleagues[17] interviewed the mothers of 921 Japanese infants at 1, 4, 7, and 12 month well-baby check-up visits. They found that 47% of infants regurgitate at least once per day at 1 month of age. The prevalence of regurgitation in their population decreased rapidly to 29% at 4 months, and 6% at 7 months. They also found that there

Table 16.1. Factors contributing to multiple logistic regression model for reporting regurgitation as a problem*

Factor	Adjusted odds ratio	95% CI
Frequency of regurgitation (>1 time/day)	21.02	9.92–44.53
Volume of regurgitation (>30 mL/day)	7.26	2.68–19.70
Increased crying/fussiness	2.77	1.39–5.55
Discomfort with spitting up	2.5	1.15–5.46
Frequent back arching	2.37	1.44–3.91

* Odds ratio obtained from multiple logistic regression; $P < 0.001$
From Nelson SP, Chen EH, Syniar GM, Christoffel KK. Prevalence of symptoms of gastroesophageal reflux during infancy. A pediatric practice-based survey. Pediatric Practice Research Group. *Arch Pediatr Adolesc Med* 1997; **151**(6):569–572.

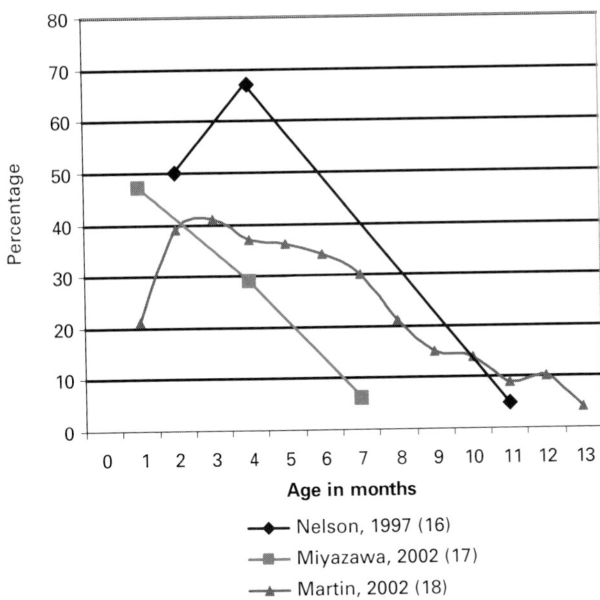

Fig. 16.1. Percentage of children with regurgitation.

was not a correlation of reflux patterns between children who were breast-fed versus formula fed, who were upright or supine after feeds, or between the body-weight-gain at 3 months.

In 2002, Martin *et al.* performed the only population-based longitudinal study designed to examine the prevalence and natural history of infant emesis.[18] They prospectively followed a cohort of 836 children from birth to two years of age, and subsequently followed up with 693 at a mean of 9.7 years of age. They found that 41% of children between 3 and 4 months of age were regurgitating or vomiting about half of their feedings daily. By 13–14 months of age, <5% had symptoms, and this became negligible by 19 months. The children who were classified as having frequent "spilling" (i.e., regurgitation/vomiting) during the first two years of life were more likely to have symptoms at 9 years of age. Specifically, when compared to children who did not have symptoms during the first two years of life, the frequent "spilling" group was 2.3 times more likely to have at least one symptom of reflux at 9 years of age, 4.6 times more likely to have heartburn, 2.7 times more likely to have vomiting, and 4.7 times more likely to have acid regurgitation.[18]

Considered together, these studies suggest that about half of all infants will regurgitate or have emesis in the first 1–4 months of life, after which the prevalence decreases to around 5% at 1 year of age (see Fig. 16.1). It is important to note, however, that these studies that illuminate the natural history of infant GERD do not include objective measures of reflux.

Outcome measures

If we were to define a reflux "event" as the abnormal and non-induced reflux of gastric content proximal to the LES, the ideal study of the natural history of reflux, as well as the efficacy of medical and surgical intervention, would measure the number of reflux events that occur over time. Specifically in regard to ARPs, one would want to compare the rate of reflux events before an operation, with the rate of similar events after an operation. This would be ideal because it would allow one to measure that which the operation is designed to do – reduction in the frequency of these "events". Knowing when an event occurs, however, is nearly impossible. True reflux "events" are demonstrable only over a defined period of time, such as during an esophageal pH study that measures these events over a 24-hour period.

Studies have therefore used other "events" as proxies for esophageal reflux. Common proxies are the signs and symptoms that clinicians have come to ascribe to GERD, such as emesis, hematemesis, chest pain/burning, Sandifer's posturing, and gagging/retching. Others have gone further to use the sequelae of GERD as a proxy by evaluating the rate or frequency of apnea, failure to thrive, feeding intolerance, and aspiration pneumonia. To make these proxies plausible, we must first confirm the association between GERD and its signs and symptoms, and then establish a link to the sequelae. Examples of this are readily found in the literature, such as the study by Euler demonstrating an association between reflux disease and recurrent pulmonary disease.[19]

Comparisons between the many published articles regarding outcomes after antireflux surgery are therefore extremely difficult given the non-uniform definitions of symptoms, as well as the range in outcomes measured. Additionally, several different populations are available for comparison, in each of which the underlying etiology of reflux may be different, and thus not amenable for a rigorous comparison.

Most published reviews have assessed the effectiveness of antireflux procedures based on the relief of symptoms. Generally, these symptoms are delineated by clinical and/or parental observation, and are not objectively measured by any of the diagnostic procedures listed above. One interesting study by Lochegnies *et al.* illuminates the difficulty in comparing subjective reports of symptoms evaluated in 31 adult patients using a quality of life index.[20] This study found that patients who suffered from GERD had a quality of life index score much lower than controls, and this remained significantly lower even after an ARP. Interestingly, although there was postoperative improvement among these patients in terms of reflux symptoms, the preoperative symptoms were replaced by different complaints such as flatulence and gas-bloating postoperatively. Yet it is the symptoms, above and beyond any objective measure of the presence of reflux, that compel surgeons to perform ARPs.

Few papers compare objective measurements of reflux before and after an antireflux procedure, and fewer still make this comparison more than a year from surgery. From the beginning of the use of antireflux operations in the treatment of GERD, surgeons recognized that the indications varied with age and underlying medical condition. In order to properly understand the outcomes of antireflux operations, one must therefore first understand the indications, and the variation in indication for specific groups within the 0–18-year-old population.

Overall outcomes

A few studies stand out that compare objective measurements of the sequelae of GERD. In an attempt to clarify the understanding of the natural history of GERD by more objective measures, Treem *et al.*[21] addressed some of the findings of Carre. They studied the progression of symptoms of reflux in older children (3.5–16 years of age, mean 9.8) without neurological abnormalities. Their report was based on a retrospective chart review of 32 patients followed and treated medically for an average of 3.5 years from the time of diagnosis (range 1–8 years). Medical treatment included the use of prokinetic agents such as metoclopramide, as well as H2-receptor antagonists. These patients then had a follow-up for this study including an UGI contrast study, 18–22 hour pH probe testing, and EGD with biopsy. Of these 32 older patients, 13 had complete or sufficient enough resolution of symptoms to discontinue medical therapy. Another 13 described moderate resolution of symptoms, but continued to require medication for symptom control. Four children were found to have no improvement in symptoms, and two others continued to have severe symptoms and refractory esophagitis requiring an anti-reflux operation. GERD was present in 12/32 (38%), and an esophageal stricture in 1/32 (3%) by UGI. Esophagitis was documented in 16/32 (50%) by mucosal biopsy after EGD, and was equally present in patients with and without symptoms of abdominal pain, heartburn, dysphagia, chest pain, or wheezing. Similarly, abnormal pH tests were not correlated with the finding of biopsy proven esophagitis. Ultimately, they found that greater than 50% of an older population required continuous medication or fundoplication to control symptoms.

In another review of the effectiveness of medical therapy, Andze *et al.*[22] reviewed 1153 children between the ages of 1 month and 20 years who underwent 20-hour pH monitoring for evaluation of GER. These patients were referred for either digestive symptoms, failure to thrive, or respiratory symptoms. They limited their review to the 500 children with respiratory symptoms. All of these children underwent 8 weeks of non-operative therapy, with resolution of symptoms in 81%. This escalating therapy began with changes in positioning and thickening of feeds, followed by administration of medications such as metoclopramide, cisapride, and domperidone. The remaining patients continued to be symptomatic and had persistent reflux by repeat pH monitoring, and went on to ARP.

Among the published reviews describing long-term outcomes of infants and children that have undergone ARP, the study by Turnage *et al.* is noteworthy.[23] These authors evaluated 46 patients who had undergone ARP and evaluated the 35 survivors a mean of 6.7 years later. This evaluation included an interview with the parents, physical examination, UGI, and 24-hour pH study. Seventy-four percent of these survivors had no symptoms, 14% had mild symptoms requiring little or no treatment, and 11% had symptoms requiring repeat ARP, with a 75% success rate after the second ARP as defined by resolution of symptoms.

Another study in the surgical literature compared the rates of hospitalization with a diagnosis of a symptom or sequelae of GERD before and after ARP.[24] This study was a population-based evaluation of 590 patients (mean

3.99 +/–5.6 years of age) over 15 years in the state of Washington. These authors found that overall, patients who have had an ARP were hospitalized an average of 4.8 times for every 1000 days of life before their operation with a diagnosis of pneumonia, aspiration pneumonia, or mechanical ventilation, and 1.7 times every 1000 days after ARP for these same diagnoses. When the population was divided into two groups – those who were hospitalized less frequently after ARP (65%), and those who were hospitalized as or more frequently after ARP (35%), the change in hospitalization rates are predictably more dramatic. For the population that benefited, the rate of hospitalizations with a diagnosis of aspiration pneumonia, or mechanical ventilation dropped from 7.1 to 0.6 per 1000 days of life. The group that did not benefit, however, experienced an increase in the number of hospitalizations with these diagnoses from 0.7 to 3.8 for every 1000 days of life. This difference is noteworthy given our understanding of these data within the context of the natural history of GERD as described above. Since infants and children have been shown to have a decrease in symptoms over time, we would expect the rate of complications, and therefore the rate of hospitalizations, also to decline with time even among those that might not benefit from surgical intervention. The finding that 35% of a state-wide population is being hospitalized at a significantly higher rate after ARP compels a more thorough evaluation of the indications for these procedures.

Comparing neurologically impaired vs. neurologically normal

There is a general consensus among pediatric surgeons and pediatricians that the neurologically impaired (NI) population of infants and children have a higher incidence of GERD, and more importantly, are less likely to have a successful long-term outcome after ARP. Several theories have been postulated to explain these observations. Among these, the diagnosis of NI may be associated with: (i) decreased lower esophageal sphincter pressure, (ii) esophageal dysmotility, (iii) increased abdominal pressure from either scoliosis, abdominal wall muscle spasticity, seizure disorder, chronic pulmonary disease, or chronic constipation, (iv) delayed gastric emptying, (v) increased duration of supine posture.[25,26] Many papers have been written to compare the outcome of antireflux operations in NI and neurologically normal (NN) children. The majority of these papers are single physician or single institution retrospective case-series reviews.

Martinez *et al.* performed a retrospective review of 198 NI children and reported that 141 (71%) of their population had a return of pre-operative symptoms at a mean of 11 months after surgery.[27] Additionally, the prevalence of symptoms of choking–gagging–retching increased from 13% to 29% following ARP. Objective tests (UGI, pH study, or gastric emptying scan) were performed in 86 of the 141 patients with post-operative symptoms (61%). No follow-up tests were performed in the 57 asymptomatic patients. Almost half (43%) of the tested symptomatic patients did not have reflux by the same diagnostic tests used to diagnose them preoperatively. This finding leads us to question what percentage of the asymptomatic population would have a positive test – information that would clarify either our use of tests or our use of symptoms as the defining indication for an antireflux operation in this population.

Pearl *et al.* reviewed 234 children who underwent ARP over a 5-year period, comparing NI ($n = 153$) and neurologically normal (NN) ($n = 81$) children.[28] They reported that children in their NI population more frequently underwent gastrostomy tube placement (86% vs. 30%), had late postoperative complications (26% vs. 12%), required re-operation (19% vs. 5%), and had death attributable to aspiration (9% vs. 1%).

Two studies have compared the number of hospitalizations after ARP, and have specifically commented on the impact of neurological impairment on this. Rice *et al.*[25] retrospectively reviewed 77 children treated in their institution over 18 years. When comparing the 6 months before ARP to the 6 months after, both the mean number of hospitalizations and the mean number of days hospitalized after ARP was lower for both NN and NI children, although the difference was statistically significant only in NI children. This study also compared the growth rates in the subset of children that were diagnosed preoperatively with failure to thrive (FTT). These authors found that a significant increase in the rate of postoperative growth compared to the preoperative rate was seen only in NI children, and only within 6 months of their procedures. No difference was seen at one and two years of follow-up. The second study, discussed above, was a population-based study that showed no difference between NI and NN children with regard to rates of hospitalization for aspiration pneumonia, pneumonia, or respiratory failure requiring mechanical ventilation before and after ARP.[24]

Esophageal atresia

Despite the known association between esophageal atresia (EA) and gastroesophageal reflux, little has been written about the long-term outcomes of patients who have undergone ARP after EA repair. Schier *et al.* sent a questionnaire to 128 former EA patients 10–34 years of age (median 14 years).[29] They found that 46% of patients had GERD, and 7% had Barrett's esophagus. Sixteen percent had undergone an ARP, though only 25% of these were considered to have been successful. The authors concluded that the most successful means of reflux prevention was abstinence from eating late in the evening.

Deurloo *et al.* performed a similar questionnaire obtaining long-term follow-up data on a group of 38 former EA patients greater than 28 years after repair.[30] Whereas 25% of patients had no complaints, 75% described dysphagia, heartburn, or retrosternal chest pain. None of the patients, however, was using an antireflux medication. Sixty-one percent of those surveyed ($n = 23$) agreed to undergo esophagogastroscopy revealing Barrett's in one patient, and squamous cell carcinoma in another.

Wheatley *et al.* reviewed the records of 80 patients treated for EA over a 15-year period at C. S. Mott Children's Hospital in Michigan.[31] Only 62 patients in this cohort, however, were used for their analysis (eight were not treated or died shortly after repair secondary to underlying medical conditions, five had isolated EA and underwent gastric transposition or colon interposition, and five were lost to follow-up shortly after surgery). Of the 62 patients available for analysis, 34 (55%) were diagnosed with GERD. Medical therapy was attempted in all children, was successful in seven, and failed in 27. Twenty-two of these 27 patients underwent an ARP, and 1 died intra-operatively. After a mean follow-up period of 62 months, primary ARP successfully eliminated symptoms of reflux in 14 of the surviving 21 patients (67%). Seven of the 21 (33%) were found to have recurrent reflux symptoms, and wrap disruption. Of these seven patients, four underwent a second ARP with elimination of reflux symptoms, and the remaining three patients either died of sepsis or postoperative complications (two patients), or continued to have symptoms despite three attempts at an ARP (one patient). Therefore, of the 21 patients who underwent surgical management, reflux symptom control was achieved in 18 of 21 (86%) after initial or repeat ARP. Overall, 88% (30/34) achieved control of reflux symptoms with either medical or surgical management. Wheatley considered recurrence of reflux after the primary ARP a failure, and therefore concluded that in comparison to the 10% failure rate after ARP described in 220 patients at this same institution, the observed 33% failure rate in patients with EA suggests that operative intervention for reflux may not be appropriate in this population.

Similarly, Kubiak *et al.*[32] found poor results in their population that underwent ARP after EA repair in terms of relief of symptoms. They reported 19 patients under 4 months of age, and only 58% of the infants improved symptomatically after ARP.

Congenital diaphragmatic hernia

Like EA, patients with congenital diaphragmatic hernia (CDH) are known to have a higher incidence of GERD than the normal population. Rather than a defect of the lower esophageal sphincter mechanism, patients with EA and CDH are thought to have a complete field defect resulting in foregut dysmotility from the mouth to the ligament of Treitz. In 1990, Stolar *et al.* described 22 of 30 survivors after CDH repair.[35] Sixty-nine percent of the patients were demonstrated to have severe GERD by 24 hour pH monitoring, each of whom was managed medically. None of the patients underwent ARP, and long-term follow-up after these procedures was therefore not reported. Though follow-up after a mean of 32 months showed weight gain to be slower in children with GERD, all but one child was asymptomatic. This group has since accrued approximately 400 patients, nearly all of whom are considered to have severe reflux by objective measures (pH testing and UGI studies). It has therefore become standard within this institution to place every child with CDH on proton pump inhibitors, H_2-receptor blockers, and metoclopramide. Antireflux procedures are still avoided at all costs, with only 5 out of *c.* 400 patients (1%) progressing on to surgery. The foregut dysmotility and reflux symptoms are overcome in most patients by a slow progression from continuous drip gastric feeds to an appropriate goal rate that is subsequently condensed to bolus feeds. On rare occasions, children who fail gastric feeds are converted to jejunal feeds, and transitioned to gastric feeds in time. If children ultimately require an operation, the procedure of choice in this group includes a partial fundoplication in conjunction with a pyloroplasty and gastrostomy tube. Long-term, two patients from this institution have developed Barrett's esophagus (at ages 14 and 16), and therefore underwent photoablation and partial fundoplication, and a third patient developed severe esophagitis compelling ARP (Stolar, personal communication).

Fasching *et al.* reviewed 54 patients who underwent repair of CDH at a single institution over a 12 year period.[33] Twenty-five of the 35 survivors were seen in follow-up an average of 9.4 years after repair. Sixteen of these 25 patients (64%) were found to have GERD by 24-hour pH monitoring or upper GI series, and seven (28%) went on to have an ARP performed. Unfortunately, long-term follow-up of the ARP was not reported.

Similarly, Nagaya *et al.* described 86 survivors of CDH repair at their institution, 10 (11.6%) of whom were shown to have GERD postoperatively.[34] Three of these patients (3.5%) responded to medical therapy, and (8%) went on to an ARP. Again, no long-term follow-up for these patients was reported.

Cystic fibrosis and chronic pulmonary disease

An association between cystic fibrosis (CF) and GERD has been described. Little is known about the relationship between these two diseases and the long-term outcomes for this subset of children. Vinocur *et al.*[36] were among the first to describe this association. In their population of 40 children diagnosed with CF, eight (20%) were found to have significant GERD with symptoms of vomiting, recurrent pneumonia, and/or failure to thrive. Three children in their series responded to medical therapy, and five went on to require ARP, all with complete postoperative resolution of symptoms. Based on findings of a 25% frequency of GERD in patients with CF older than 5 years, Malfroot *et al.*[37] evaluated 23 patients with CF at their institution younger than 5 years of age. GERD as defined by abnormal pH testing was present in 21 (81%). Symptoms in this population improved with medical management without ARP.

Olsen *et al.* described their institutional experience and found that many fewer children with CF required ARP.[38] A 15-year review found 578 operations performed on 210 children with CF. Only five of these operations were ARPs. Outcomes after the procedures were not discussed.

Taylor *et al.*[39] retrospectively reviewed their institution's experience with ARP between 1985 and 1992. All patients with relevant GERD symptoms at a mean post-ARP follow-up of 3 years (range 1–7.5) were re-evaluated by UGI. Those patients with a normal UGI study but with clinically suspected recurrence were worked-up further by 24-hour pH studies. Of the 239 patients who underwent ARP, 39 patients had documented recurrent GERD. Of these 39 children with recurrent GERD, 64% had chronic pulmonary disease (CPD). When comparing recurrence rates in patients with and without CPD, patients with CPD had a statistically significant higher frequency of GERD (32% vs. 7%, $p < 0.001$).

Technical surgical factors in ARP outcomes

Bliss *et al.*[40] described 28 patients who underwent an anterior gastric fundoplication at their institution over a 2-year period. This study used historical controls who had undergone circumferential fundoplication at the same institution reported in a prior publication.[23] Though no significant differences were found between the two groups, they reported a trend towards improved efficacy, decreased re-operative rate, and less severe complications.

The study by Fonkalsrud *et al.*[41] reviewing 7467 children operated on at seven large centers around the United States found no difference in results or complications between patients who received partial and complete wraps. The patients underwent Nissen fundoplication in 64% of cases, and partial wraps (Thal in 34%, and Toupet in 2%) in the remainder.

Perhaps the most rigorous study was a prospective randomized trial of 200 adult patients in Germany.[42] These authors postulated that post-operative dysphasia is more common in patients with esophageal dysmotility, and these patients would therefore be better served by a partial 270 degree Toupet wrap. All patients underwent endoscopy, 24 pH studies, and manometry preoperatively and postoperatively. 100 patients underwent Nissen, and 100 Toupet. Half of the patients in each of these two groups were diagnosed with motility disorders. Dysphagia was not associated with a preoperative diagnosis of dysmotility, though it was slightly more common after a Nissen than after a Toupet partial fundoplication. Both operations were equal in terms of control of reflux symptoms.

Watson *et al.*[43] randomized 102 adult patients to anterior or posterior crural repair during laparoscopic Nissen ARP. They found no difference in terms of postoperative dysphagia, relief of heartburn, or overall patient satisfaction 6 months after surgery.

Laparoscopic vs. open operations

The application of laparoscopy to ARP in infants and children has blossomed since the first published report of the successful laparoscopic treatment of GERD in 1991.[44] As the effectiveness of open ARP had already been accepted, early reports focused on comparing the laparoscopic approach to the open approach, i.e., the historical "gold standard".[45–47] These reports conclude generally that the short-term outcomes of the laparoscopic approach are similar in terms of rates of complications, postoperative time to goal nutritional regimens, and are better in terms of recovery time and length of hospital stay. Subsequent reports have gone on to show the safety of the laparoscopic approach in subpopulations such as infants under 8 kg,[48] and children under 2 yrs of age.[49] Both of these latter publications are case reports, without a control population.

At present, there are no published data that specifically address the difference in long-term outcomes between laparoscopic and open ARP in infants and children.

One of the more notable aspects of the laparoscopic approach is the learning curve associated with a safely performed operation. Champault[50] divided his adult patients into three groups based on ordered chronology, and found that the duration of surgery, the rate of conversion to an open procedure, morbidity, and proportion of relapses in symptoms was significantly reduced with each consecutive group. Flum performed a population-level study evaluating over 86 000 adult patients and found that adverse operative events were significantly more likely to occur during the first 15 procedures done by a single surgeon.[51] Adverse events were defined as splenectomy, esophageal laceration repair, and in-hospital death. A surgeon was 2.7 times more likely to perform a splenectomy, 2.3 times more likely to repair an esophageal laceration, and 5.6 times more likely to have a patient die in the hospital during the first 15 laparoscopic procedures, compared to after the 15th procedure. With each subsequent case performed, the risk of these adverse events was shown to decrease by 1.6%–1.7%. Allal *et al.*[46] described his first 142 pediatric cases and found a similar improvement with surgeon experience with a decrease in mean operative time from 125 minutes for his first 60 cases to 93 minutes for the second 79. He reported only one intraoperative complication, and three postoperative complications.

Summary

Before drawing conclusions from the studies summarized above, we must ask ourselves what is the true goal of an antireflux procedure (ARP)? Is it to increase the LES pressure and thereby decrease the events of GERD, or is it to decrease the sequelae of GERD, or is it even more removed, to decrease the rate of hospitalizations or missed days of work due to either the symptoms or the sequelae? For example, is it important how often a child refluxes if he has minimal discomfort and has never been hospitalized for aspiration pneumonia? Would we call an ARP a success if a child is referred for an ARP, and is hospitalized after the procedure with equal or greater frequency for aspiration pneumonia, even though the symptoms of gagging and emesis for which he was originally referred are resolved? Is it significant that 43% of patients who have recurrent symptoms after an ARP do not have reflux by any objective measures? Is it significant that we have not asked ourselves how many of the asymptomatic patients continue to have reflux by these same objective measures after an ARP? Herein lies a primary difficulty in assessing the long-term outcomes of ARP in the pediatric population.

In general, antireflux procedures (ARP) successfully alleviate the symptoms and sequelae of GERD. A critical evaluation of the efficacy of ARPs, however, requires an understanding of both the population that is being considered, as well as the indications for undergoing a procedure. Moreover, when evaluating the literature, it is important to note if the ultimate outcome is the subjective or objective measure of symptoms and/or sequelae. This review of the literature illuminates much of what has been described, but more importantly, it attempts to refocus and question some of our conclusions, and therefore our decision-making algorithms.

Choosing the correct approach for treating patients with gastroesophageal reflux must take the reason for evaluation and treatment into consideration. Whereas many patients are referred for clinical symptoms thought to be due to GERD, others are referred either to prevent, or more often to attenuate the secondary complications of GERD. Assessing the outcome of these operations must therefore also take these details into consideration. For example, if a procedure is done for a patient noted to have Barrett's esophagus, as an outcome we are more interested in the resolution of the metaplasia rather than the resolution of symptoms.

As our understanding of GERD has grown more sophisticated in recent years, and as our understanding of the underlying diseases that contribute to reflux has matured, so now must our approach to treating the disease.

REFERENCES

1. Dunn, J. C., Lai, E. C., Webber, M. M., Ament, M. E., & Fonkalsrud, E. W. Long-term quantitative results following fundoplication and antroplasty for gastroesophageal reflux and delayed gastric emptying in children. *Am. J. Surg.* 1998; **175**(1):27–29.
2. Byrne, W. J., Kangarloo, H., Ament, M. E. *et al.* "Antral dysmotility." An unrecognized cause of chronic vomiting during infancy. *Ann. Surg.* 1981; **193**(4):521–524.
3. Alexander, F., Wyllie, R., Jirousek, K., Secic, M., & Porvasnik, S. Delayed gastric emptying affects outcome of Nissen fundoplication in neurologically impaired children. *Surgery* 1997; **122**(4):690–697; discussion 697–698.
4. Fonkalsrud, E. W., Foglia, R. P., Ament, M. E., Berquist, W., & Vargas, J. Operative treatment for the gastroesophageal reflux syndrome in children. *J. Pediatr. Surg.* 1989; **24**(6):525–529.
5. Fonkalsrud, E. W., Berquist, W., Vargas, J., Ament, M. E., & Foglia, R. P. Surgical treatment of the gastroesophageal reflux syndrome in infants and children. *Am. J. Surg.* 1987; **154**(1):11–18.

6. Fonkalsrud, E. W., Ament, M. E., & Vargas, J. Gastric antroplasty for the treatment of delayed gastric emptying and gastroesophageal reflux in children. *Am. J. Surg.* 1992; **164**(4):327–31.
7. Fonkalsrud, E. W., Ament, M. E., & Berquist, W. Surgical management of the gastroesophageal reflux syndrome in childhood. *Surgery* 1985; **97**(1):42–8.
8. Fonkalsrud, E. W., & Ament, M. E. Gastroesophageal reflux in childhood. *Curr. Probl. Surg.* 1996; **33**(1):1–70.
9. Fonkalsrud, E. W. Surgical treatment of the gastroesophageal reflux syndrome in childhood. *Z. Kinderchir.* 1987; **42**(1):7–11.
10. Fonkalsrud, E. W. Nissen fundoplication for gastroesophageal reflux disease in infants and children. *Semin. Pediatr. Surg.* 1998; **7**(2):110–114.
11. Richards, C. A., Andrews, P. L., Spitz, L., & Milla, P. J. Nissen fundoplication may induce gastric myoelectrical disturbance in children. *J. Pediatr. Surg.* 1998; **33**(12):1801–1805.
12. Richards, C. A., Carr, D., Spitz, L., Milla, P. J., & Andrews, P. L. Nissen-type fundoplication and its effects on the emetic reflex and gastric motility in the ferret. *Neurogastroenterol. Motil.* 2000; **12**(1):65–74.
13. Richards, C. A., Milla, P. J., Andrews, P. L., & Spitz, L. Retching and vomiting in neurologically impaired children after fundoplication: predictive preoperative factors. *J. Pediatr. Surg.* 2001; **36**(9):1401–1404.
14. Kawahara, H., Nakajima, K., Yagi, M., Okuyama, H., Kubota, A., & Okada, A. Mechanisms responsible for recurrent gastroesophageal reflux in neurologically impaired children who underwent laparoscopic Nissen fundoplication. *Surg. Endosc.* 2002; **16**(5):767–771.
15. Carre, I. J. The natural history of the partial thoracic stomach (Hiatus hernia) in children. *Arch. Dis. Child.* 1959; **34**:344–353.
16. Nelson, S. P., Chen, E. H., Syniar, G. M., & Christoffel, K. K. Prevalence of symptoms of gastroesophageal reflux during infancy. A pediatric practice-based survey. Pediatric Practice Research Group. *Arch. Pediatr. Adolesc. Med.* 1997; **151**(6):569–572.
17. Miyazawa, R., Tomomasa, T., Kaneko, H., Tachibana, A., Ogawa, T., & Morikawa, A. Prevalence of gastro-esophageal reflux-related symptoms in Japanese infants. *Pediatr. Int.* 2002; **44**(5):513–516.
18. Martin, A. J., Pratt, N., Kennedy, J. D. *et al.* Natural history and familial relationships of infant spilling to 9 years of age. *Pediatrics* 2002; **109**(6):1061–1067.
19. Euler, A. R., Byrne, W. J., Ament, M. E. *et al.* Recurrent pulmonary disease in children: a complication of gastroesophageal reflux. *Pediatrics* 1979; **63**(1):47–51.
20. Lochegnies, A., Hauters, P., Janssen, P., Nakad, A., Farchack, E., & Defrennes, M. Quality of life assessment after Nissen fundoplication. *Acta. Chir. Belg.* 2001; **101**(1):20–24.
21. Treem, W. R., Davis, P. M., & Hyams, J. S. Gastroesophageal reflux in the older child: presentation, response to treatment and long-term follow-up. *Clin. Pediatr. (Phila).* 1991; **30**(7):435–440.
22. Andze, G. O., Brandt, M. L., St Vil, D., Bensoussan, A. L., & Blanchard, H. Diagnosis and treatment of gastroesophageal reflux in 500 children with respiratory symptoms: the value of pH monitoring. *J. Pediatr. Surg.* 1991; **26**(3):295–299; discussion 299–300.
23. Turnage, R. H., Oldham, K. T., Coran, A. G., & Blane, C. E. Late results of fundoplication for gastroesophageal reflux in infants and children. *Surgery* 1989; **105**(4):457–464.
24. Goldin, A. B, Sawin, R., & Flum, D. Do antireflux operations decrease the rate of reflux-related hospitalizations in children? submitted.
25. Rice, H., Seashore, J. H., & Touloukian, R. J. Evaluation of Nissen fundoplication in neurologically impaired children. *J. Pediatr. Surg.* 1991; **26**(6):697–701.
26. Smith, C. D., Othersen, H. B., Jr., Gogan, N. J., & Walker, J. D. Nissen fundoplication in children with profound neurologic disability. High risks and unmet goals. *Ann. Surg.* 1992; **215**(6):654–658; discussion 658–659.
27. Martinez, D. A., Ginn-Pease, M. E., & Caniano, D. A. Sequelae of antireflux surgery in profoundly disabled children. *J. Pediatr. Surg.* 1992; **27**(2):267–271; discussion 271–273.
28. Pearl, R. H., Robie, D. K., Ein, S. H. *et al.* Complications of gastroesophageal antireflux surgery in neurologically impaired versus neurologically normal children. *J. Pediatr. Surg.* 1990; **25**(11):1169–1173.
29. Schier, F., Korn, S., & Michel, E. Experiences of a parent support group with the long-term consequences of esophageal atresia. *J. Pediatr. Surg.* 2001; **36**(4):605–610.
30. Deurloo, J. A., Ekkelkamp, S., Bartelsman, J. F. *et al.* Gastroesophageal reflux: prevalence in adults older than 28 years after correction of esophageal atresia. *Ann. Surg.* 2003; **238**(5):686–689.
31. Wheatley, M. J., Coran, A. G., & Wesley, J. R. Efficacy of the Nissen fundoplication in the management of gastroesophageal reflux following esophageal atresia repair. *J. Pediatr. Surg.* 1993; **28**(1):53–55.
32. Kubiak, R., Spitz, L., Kiely, E. M., Drake, D., & Pierro, A. Effectiveness of fundoplication in early infancy. *J. Pediatr. Surg.* 1999; **34**(2):295–299.
33. Fasching, G., Huber, A., Uray, E., Sorantin, E., Lindbichler, F., & Mayr, J. Gastroesophageal reflux and diaphragmatic motility after repair of congenital diaphragmatic hernia. *Eur. J. Pediatr. Surg.* 2000; **10**(6):360–364.
34. Nagaya, M., Akatsuka, H., & Kato, J. Gastroesophageal reflux occurring after repair of congenital diaphragmatic hernia. *J. Pediatr. Surg.* 1994; **29**(11):1447–1451.
35. Stolar, C. J., Levy, J. P., Dillon, P. W., Reyes, C., Belamarich, P., & Berdon, W. E. Anatomic and functional abnormalities of the esophagus in infants surviving congenital diaphragmatic hernia. *Am. J. Surg.* 1990; **159**(2):204–207.
36. Vinocur, C. D., Marmon, L., Schidlow, D. V., & Weintraub, W. H. Gastroesophageal reflux in the infant with cystic fibrosis. *Am. J. Surg.* 1985; **149**(1):182–186.
37. Malfroot, A. & Dab, I. New insights on gastro-oesophageal reflux in cystic fibrosis by longitudinal follow up. *Arch. Dis. Child.* 1991; **66**(11):1339–1345.

38. Olsen, M. M., Gauderer, M. W., Girz, M. K., & Izant, R. J., Jr. Surgery in patients with cystic fibrosis. *J. Pediatr. Surg.* 1987; **22**(7):613–618.
39. Taylor, L. A., Weiner, T., Lacey, S. R., Azizkhan, R. G. Chronic lung disease is the leading risk factor correlating with the failure (wrap disruption) of antireflux procedures in children. *J. Pediatr. Surg.* 1994; **29**(2):161–164; discussion 164–166.
40. Bliss, D., Hirschl, R., Oldham, K. *et al.* Efficacy of anterior gastric fundoplication in the treatment of gastroesophageal reflux in infants and children. *J. Pediatr. Surg.* 1994; **29**(8):1071–1074; discussion 1074–1075.
41. Fonkalsrud, E. W., Ashcraft, K. W., Coran, A. G. *et al.* Surgical treatment of gastroesophageal reflux in children: a combined hospital study of 7467 patients. *Pediatrics* 1998; **101**(3 Pt 1):419–422.
42. Zornig, C., Strate, U., Fibbe, C., Emmermann, A., & Layer, P. Nissen vs Toupet laparoscopic fundoplication. *Surg. Endosc.* 2002; **16**(5):758–766.
43. Watson, D. I., Jamieson, G. G., Devitt, P. G. *et al.* A prospective randomized trial of laparoscopic Nissen fundoplication with anterior vs posterior hiatal repair. *Arch. Surg.* 2001; **136**(7):745–751.
44. Dallemagne, B., Weerts, J. M., Jehaes, C., Markiewicz, S., & Lombard, R. Laparoscopic Nissen fundoplication: preliminary report. *Surg. Laparosc. Endosc.* 1991; **1**(3):138–143.
45. Meehan, J. J. & Georgeson, K. E. Laparoscopic fundoplication in infants and children. *Surg. Endosc.* 1996; **10**(12):1154–1157.
46. Allal, H., Captier, G., Lopez, M., Forgues, D., & Galifer, R. B. Evaluation of 142 consecutive laparoscopic fundoplications in children: effects of the learning curve and technical choice. *J. Pediatr. Surg.* 2001; **36**(6):921–926.
47. Somme, S., Rodriguez, J. A., Kirsch, D. G., & Liu, D. C. Laparoscopic versus open fundoplication in infants. *Surg. Endosc.* 2002; **16**(1):54–56.
48. Thompson, W. R., Hicks, B. A., & Guzzetta, P. C., Jr. Laparoscopic Nissen fundoplication in the infant. *J. Laparoendosc. Surg.* 1996; **6** Suppl 1:S5–57.
49. Zamir, O., Udassin, R., Seror, D., Vromen, A., & Freund, H. R. Laparoscopic Nissen fundoplication in children under 2 years of age. *Surg. Endosc.* 1997; **11**(12):1202–1205.
50. Champault, G. G., Barrat, C., Rozon, R. C., Rizk, N., & Catheline, J. M. The effect of the learning curve on the outcome of laparoscopic treatment for gastroesophageal reflux. *Surg. Laparosc. Endosc. Percutan. Tech.* 1999; **9**(6):375–381.
51. Flum, D. R., Koepsell, T., Heagerty, P., & Pellegrini, C. A. The nationwide frequency of major adverse outcomes in antireflux surgery and the role of surgeon experience, 1992–1997. *J. Am. Coll. Surg.* 2002; **195**(5):611–618.

17

Esophageal replacement

Steven W. Bruch and Arnold G. Coran

University of Michigan Medical School C.S. Mott Children's Hospital, USA

Esophageal replacement

Esophageal replacement is an infrequent procedure required after great effort has been put forth to save the native esophagus. The most frequent indications for esophageal replacement include long-gap esophageal atresia with or without tracheoesophageal fistula, and esophageal strictures most often due to caustic ingestion or secondary to gastroesophageal reflux disease. Although children with esophageal atresia, gastroesophageal reflux disease, and to a lesser degree, caustic ingestion, are commonly encountered in pediatric surgery, they rarely require esophageal replacement. Our ability to anastomose the two ends of the esophagus in infants with esophageal atresia has improved over the years with techniques such as circular myotomies,[1] upper pouch flaps,[2] and dilation or stretching of the upper pouch and distal esophagus prior to anastomosis.[3,4] Caustic ingestions have become more infrequent with the changes in packaging of hazardous materials in the home. Peptic strictures due to acid reflux are on the decline due to our heightened awareness of the long-term damage caused by gastroesophageal reflux disease, and our improved medical armamentarium available to control acid reflux. In addition, novel procedures to save the strictured esophagus have been reported. These include stricturoplasty with placement of a vascularized colonic patch,[8] and stenting of caustic esophageal strictures combined with steroid and acid reducing therapy.[5] Despite these improvements, and our understanding that even a somewhat compromised native esophagus may be desirable when compared to the alternatives, there is a distinct subset of infants and children who will require an esophageal replacement.

Over the years, several different conduits, including skin, jejunum, colon (ascending, transverse, and descending), a tube fashioned from the stomach, and the entire stomach, have been placed in multiple positions, including subcutaneously on the chest wall, immediately behind the sternum, in the right or left posterior chest, or in the bed of the native esophagus in the posterior mediastinum, to replace the inadequate native esophagus. None of these combinations is clearly better than all of the others. Ideally, one would like to compare the various methods in a randomized prospective fashion, but that is not practical in this instance due to the rarity of the problem. So, we would like to briefly go over the procedures now commonly in use to replace the esophagus, and then compare their early and late complications as well as their long-term outcomes based on an accumulation of cases from a collection of recent series published in the literature.[6–18] This includes 214 cases of colonic interposition grafts, 64 cases of gastric tube interpositions, and 124 cases of gastric transpositions.

The three main procedures now utilized for esophageal replacement are, as noted above, colon interposition grafts, gastric tube interpositions, and gastric transpositions. The colon interposition utilizes either the right colon based on the middle colic vessels, or the transverse and descending colon based on the left colic vessels as depicted in Fig. 17.1. Each surgeon goes into the operation with his or her preference, but must remain adaptable depending on the adequacy of the arcades feeding the desired length of colon. The colon graft is then placed retrosternally, in the left posterior chest, or in the posterior mediastinum in the bed of the native esophagus. The final position depends on the anatomy, prior procedures, and the preference of

Pediatric Surgery and Urology: Long-term Outcomes, Mark Stringer, Keith Oldham, Pierre Mouriquand.
Published by Cambridge University Press.

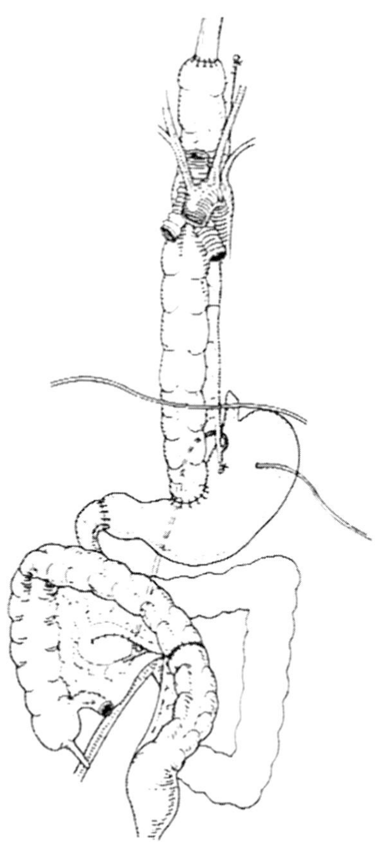

Fig. 17.1. Depiction of colon interposition graft using transverse and descending colon based on the left colic vessels.

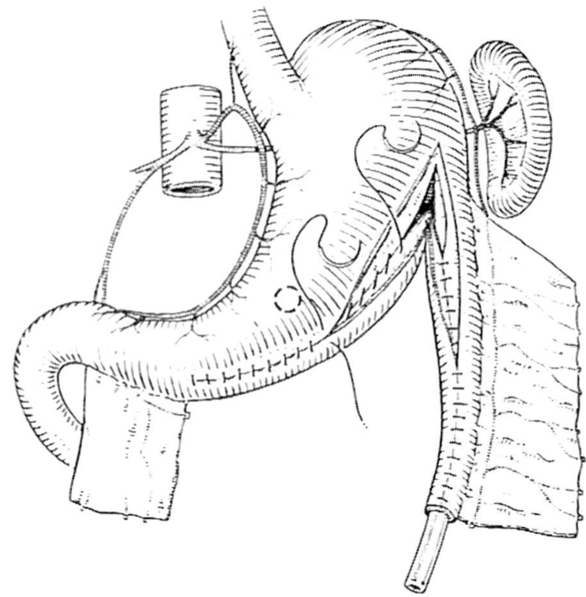

Fig. 17.2. Creation of a antiperistaltic gastric tube based on the left gastroepiploic vessels. This tube easily reaches the neck for an anastomosis to the cervical esophagus.

the surgeon. The proximal anastomosis occurs above the thoracic inlet in the neck. The distal anastomosis is performed to either the native esophagus above the diaphragm (less commonly), or in the abdomen to the stomach on the lesser curve. The proximal anastomosis may or may not be staged depending on the appearance of the graft at the end of the case.[19]

The gastric tube interposition is created by tubularizing a portion of the greater curvature of the stomach based on the gastroepiploic vessels as shown in Fig. 17.2. The tube may be based on the proximal stomach making it antiperistaltic and fed by the left gastroepiploic vessel, or alternatively on the distal stomach resulting in an isoperistaltic tube and fed by the right gastroepiploic vessel. The gastric tube is fashioned over a chest tube of appropriate size and divided using a stapling device. The gastric tube is then brought through the diaphragm, and placed either directly behind the sternum (usually for the isoperistaltic tube), or in the posterior mediastinum (more commonly), and anastomosed to the proximal esophagus in the neck.[20]

The gastric transposition, as depicted in Fig. 17.3, begins with mobilization of the stomach by dividing the greater omentum at a distance from the stomach wall to avoid injury to the right and left gastroepiploic vessels. The short gastric vessels are then divided, followed by division of the lesser omentum including the left gastric vessels at their origins. The duodenum is then widely mobilized, a pyloroplasty or pyloromyotomy is completed, and the distal esophagus is divided. A tunnel is then made in the posterior mediastinum using blunt dissection from both above and below. The native esophagus is removed, and the stomach is brought up through the native esophageal bed. The uppermost portion of the fundus is anastomosed to the cervical esophagus. If there is extensive scarring in the esophageal bed, the stomach may be placed in the left chest behind the hilum of the lung, or in the retrosternal position. This is rarely required.[21]

The three procedures have similar overall mortality rates of 5–8%, and procedure-related mortality rates of 3–4%. This mortality speaks to the extensive nature of the procedures, and to the underlying disease states in this patient population. Many of the babies with esophageal atresia were born prematurely resulting in associated pathology including chronic lung disease and cardiac defects that limit the reserve in these infants and children.

Overall, graft necrosis occurs infrequently. One would expect the colon interpositions to be at higher risk of

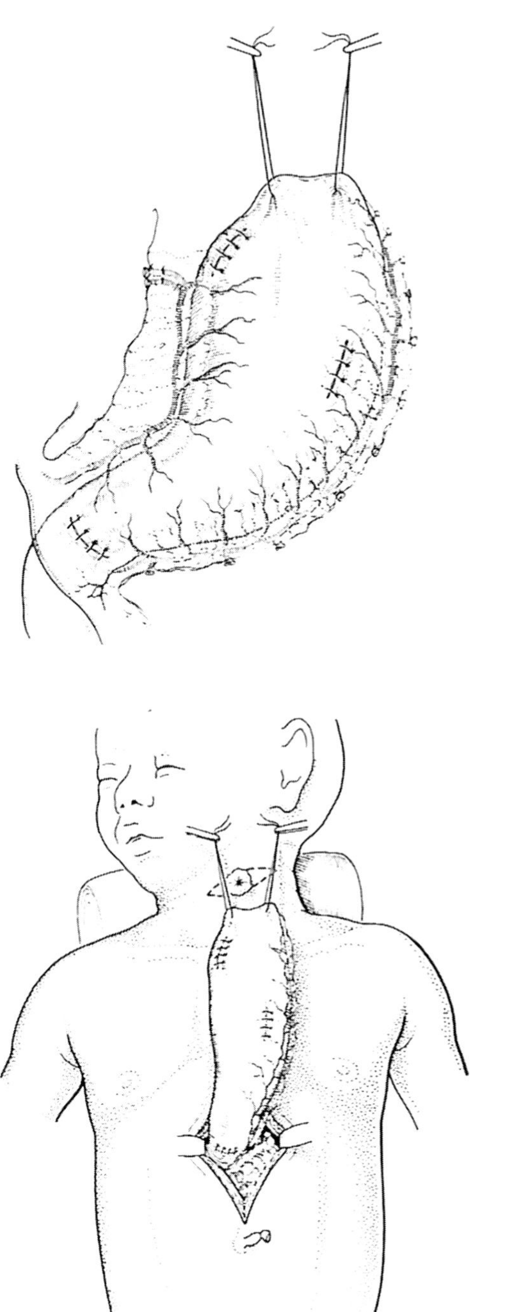

Fig. 17.3. Depiction of a gastric transposition based on the right gastric vessels. The stomach is brought up to the neck in the posterior mediastinum and placed in the bed of the native esophagus.

necrosis due to the more tenuous blood supply of the graft originating from the mesenteric vessels. The gastric tube relies on a blood supply from the gastroepiploic arcades, and the rich submucosal plexus of the stomach. This combination generally provides an excellent blood supply. The gastric transposition relies on the right gastric vessels and the same submucosal plexus of the stomach which also provides excellent blood supply. The colonic interposition has a low but definite risk of graft necrosis of 4%, compared to a 2% rate in gastric tubes, and no graft necrosis in the gastric transpositions.

Early complications occurred frequently in all three groups. By far the most common problem seen in the early period is an anastomotic leak occurring primarily at the cervical anastomosis. The majority of these leaks in all three groups were well-controlled leaks through the cervical incisions. These leaks are anticipated and a drain is routinely left in place in the cervical incision at the completion of all three procedures. The leak rate is highest in the gastric tubes, 56%, followed by the colon interpositions, 27%, and the gastric transpositions, 20%. It has been theorized that swelling in the gastric tube leads to a partial obstruction that then predisposes to the increased leak rate. However, the leak rates are no different when the cervical anastomosis is staged, or performed at the time of the original procedure. Two factors play a part in the anastomotic leaks in the colon graft: ischemia and positioning of the graft. The distal end of the colon graft used for the cervical anastomosis is farthest from the origin of blood supply in the abdomen. The route the graft takes, retrosternal vs. transthoracic, appears to affect the propensity of the coloesophageal anastomosis to leak. When the colon graft is placed retrosternally, there is a more acute forward angle from the esophagus to the conduit that is not present when the colon graft is brought up through the posterior chest. The retrosternally placed colonic grafts leaked 35% of the time compared to a leak rate of 19% when the graft is in the posterior thorax. The seriousness of a leak from the colon interposition appears to be greater than the seriousness of a gastric tube or a gastric transposition leak. In the colon interposition group, 21% of the cervical anastomotic leaks required surgical revision for control, compared to 5% in the gastric tube group, and none in the gastric transposition group where all leaks healed spontaneously. This again may be due to the varying quality of the blood supply in the three conduits. The gastric tube interpositions leaked into the chest along the staple line in 5% of the cases. Of these, one-third required treatment with operative intervention and two-thirds healed spontaneously. There was a 2% incidence of leak from the abdominal portion of the gastric staple line. The colon interpositions had a 1% incidence of cologastric anastomotic leak.

Postoperative pneumonias and pulmonary complications occurred more frequently in colon interpositions,

10%, compared to gastric transpositions, 3%, and gastric tube interpositions, 2%. Wound infection rates were similar occurring in up to 6% of the cases after each procedure. Nerve injuries also occurred at similar rates in all three procedures ranging from 2 to 4% overall. The recurrent laryngeal nerve was the most frequently injured. This injury usually occurs during the mediastinal dissection around the arch of the aorta and the subclavian vessels. Other nerves injured included the phrenic nerve, and the sympathetic chain resulting in a Horner's syndrome. The colon interposition procedure also had rare occurrences of gastric outlet obstruction, gastrointestinal bleeding, pancreatitis, and pericarditis that occurred in the immediate postoperative period.

Late complications were again dominated by anastomotic problems. Cervical anastomotic strictures were the most frequent late postoperative complication. Strictures developed in 41% of gastric tube interpositions, 24% of gastric transpositions, and 21% of colon interpositions. Again the sequelae of these strictures tended to be more serious in the colon interposition procedures with 64% of those developing strictures requiring operative intervention. Strictures that developed after gastric tubes required operative intervention in 23% of the cases, while no stricture occurring after a gastric transposition required a subsequent operative procedure. There was a 3% incidence of distal anastomotic stricture in the colon interposition group with 70% of these requiring a subsequent operation to treat the stricture. Of note, dilation of the gastric tubes should be done with care as 2 of the children with gastric tubes suffered a tube perforation during dilation of a postoperative stricture. One perforation was not recognized initially, and eventually led to the death of that child. Graft redundancy is frequently mentioned as an eventual outcome of the colon interposition. This occurred in only 6% of the children after a colon interposition. Graft redundancy did not occur in either of the gastric procedures. Redundancy of the colon grafts required operative treatment in 70% of the cases. Fistula formation was an infrequent occurrence, but required operative treatment. Fistulas to the trachea occurred in 2% of the gastric tube interpositions, and 1% of the colon interpositions. The gastric transpositions do not have a suture line in the chest and no one in this group developed a fistula to the trachea. Fistulas from the stomach or the bowel to the skin formed in 2% of the colon interposition grafts. There were no entero- or gastrocutaneous fistulas in the gastric tube interposition group, or the gastric transposition group. Bowel obstructions occurred in 12% of the colon interpositions, and 2% of the gastric transpositions. There were no reports of bowel obstructions following a gastric tube interposition. The gastric transposition group developed paraesophageal hernias in 1%, required prolonged ventilation and eventual tracheostomy in 2%, and required long-term feeding by enteral tube in 6%. These problems were not reported in the colon interposition or gastric tube interposition groups.

Both reflux and gastrointestinal bleeding occurred more often in the colon interposition grafts, 13% and 8% respectively, compared to gastric tubes, 3% and 5%, and gastric transposition, 0% and 1%. Recurrent aspiration was a problem after a colon interposition, occurring in 12%, and gastric tube interposition, with an 8% incidence, but did not occur in the gastric transposition group. However, the gastric transposition group complained of frequent unexplained episodes of breathlessness and tiredness. Delayed gastric emptying and early satiety was an issue in the gastric transposition group, occurring in 7%, and in the gastric tube interpositions, occurring in 5%, but not in the colonic interpositions, occurring in only 1%. Dumping and/or, diarrhea occurred in 10% of the colonic interposition grafts and was a frequent occurrence early on in the gastric transposition group. The dumping and diarrhea turned out to be a long-term problem in only 1% of the gastric transposition group, and did not occur in the gastric tube interpositions.

Reoperations were required in all three groups, but at varying rates. A subsequent operation for a complication was required most frequently in the colonic interposition group, 36%, followed by gastric tube interpositions with 20%, and gastric transposition with only 5% requiring a subsequent operation. In the colonic interposition group, 57% of the reoperations were related to the anastomosis. A revision of the cervical anastomosis for an initial leak made up 15% of the reoperations, a revision of the cervical anastomosis for a stricture made up 36% of the reoperations, and a revision of the gastric anastomosis for stricture made up 6% of the reoperations. The remaining causes of reoperation include: redundancy 12%, bowel obstruction 10%, antireflux operations 6%, procedures for poor gastric emptying 6%, and repair of colotracheal fistula 3%. Graft failure requiring removal of the initial colon interposition occurred in 5% of the entire group of colon interpositions. The causes included necrosis, stricture, ulcer, and perforation. Again, in the gastric tube interposition group, the main reason for reoperation is centered around anastomotic issues. Revisions for anastomotic leaks were required in 23% of the reoperations, while revisions for anastomotic strictures were required in 46% of the reoperations. The remaining operations were a revision for necrosis of the gastric tube, repair of a gastric tube–right lower lobe bronchial fistula, resection of the omohyoid muscle to relieve dysphagia, and repair of a gastric tube perforation after dilation. The reoperations in the gastric transposition group did not center around anastomotic issues. Of the 5% that required reoperation, two-thirds required revision for poor gastric drainage with either a pyloroplasty, or a Roux-en-Y gastrojejunostomy, and the other one-third required lysis of adhesions for a bowel obstruction.

The long-term outcome in these children with esophageal replacement appears to be similar; however, it is difficult to determine this because it was not uniformly presented in the different series. Based on growth, requirement for tube feedings, and dysphagia, children were placed into one of three outcomes: excellent, good, and fair. The breakdown for the three groups was as follows: colonic interpositions – excellent 63%, good 31%, and fair 7%, gastric tube interpositions – excellent 73%, good 19%, and fair 8%, and gastric transposition – excellent 64%, good 24%, and fair 4%.

Esophageal replacement remains a rare procedure used only after considerable effort has been exerted in attempts to salvage the native esophagus. The usual indications for esophageal replacement are long-gap esophageal atresia, and strictures due to gastroesophageal reflux disease and caustic ingestion. Presently, three conduits are commonly used to span the defect left by the absent or damaged esophagus. Each of these conduits has its own advantages and drawbacks. The majority of the complications both in the short term and long term involve the cervical anastomosis. Despite a small but defined risk of graft failure and mortality owing to the extensiveness of the procedure and the underlying disease in these infants and children, the long-term outcomes of a well-constructed esophageal replacement using any of the three conduits results in a good to excellent quality of life.

REFERENCES

1. Livaditis A., Radburg L., & Odensjo G. Esophageal end-to-end anastomosis, reduction of anastomotic tension by circular myotomy. *Scand. J. Thorac. Cardiovasc. Surg.* 1972; **6**:206–214.
2. Gough M. H. Esophageal atresia – use of an anterior flap in the difficult anastomosis. *J. Pediatr. Surg.* 1980; **15**:310–311.
3. Mahour G. H., Woolley M. M., & Gwinn J. L. Elongation of the upper pouch and delayed anastomotic reconstruction in esophageal atresia. *J. Pediatr. Surg.* 1974; **9**:373–383.
4. Othersen H. B. Jr, Parker E. F., Chandler J. *et al.* Save the child's esophagus, part II: Colic patch repair. *J. Pediatr. Surg.* 1997; **32**:328–333.
5. DePeppo F., Zaccara A., Dall'Oglio L. *et al.* Stenting for caustic strictures: esophageal replacement replaced. *J. Pediatr. Surg.* 1998; **33**:54–57.
6. Hendren W. H. & Hendren W. G. Colon interposition for esophagus in children. *J. Pediatr. Surg.* 1985; **20**:829–839.
7. Stone M. M., Mahour G. H., Weitzman J. J. *et al.* Esophageal replacement with colon interposition in children. *Ann. Surg.* 1987; **203**:346–351.
8. Mitchell I. M., Goh D. W., Roberts K. D. *et al.* Colon interposition in children. *Br. J. Surg.* 1989; **76**:681–686.
9. Ahmed S. A., Sylvester K. G., Herba A. *et al.* Esophageal replacement using the colon: is it a good choice? *J. Pediatr. Surg.* 1996; **31**:1026–1031.
10. Khan A. R., Stiff G., Mohammed A. R. *et al.* Esophageal replacement with colon in children. *Pediatr. Surg. Int.* 1998; **13**:79–83.
11. Anderson K. D., Randolph J. G. Gastric tube interposition: a satisfactory alternative to the colon for esophageal replacement in children. *Ann. Thorac. Surg.* 1978; **25**:521–525.
12. Ein S. H., Shandling B., Simpson J. S. *et al.* Fourteen years of gastric tubes. *J. Pediatr. Surg.* 1978; **13**:638–642.
13. Anderson K. D., Noblett H., Belsey R. *et al.* Long-term follow-up of children with colon and gastric tube interposition for esophageal atresia. *Surgery* 1992; **111**:131–136.
14. Ein S. E. Gastric tubes in children with caustic esophageal injury: a 32-year review. *J. Pediatr. Surg.* 1998; **33**:1363–1365.
15. Schettini S. T. & Pinus J. Gastric-tube esophagoplasty in children. *Pediatr. Surg. Int.* 1998; **14**:144–150.
16. Spitz L. Gastric transposition for esophageal substitution in children. *J. Pediatr. Surg.* 1992; **27**:252–259.
17. Spitz L. Gastric transposition for oesophageal replacement. *Pediatr. Surg. Int.* 1996; **11**:218–220.
18. Hirschl R. B., Yardeni D., Oldham K. *et al.* Gastric transposition for esophageal replacement in children, experience with 41 consecutive cases with special emphasis on esophageal atresia. *Ann. Surg.* 2002; **236**:531–541.
19. Othersen H. B. Jr, Smith C. D., Tagge E. P. Esophageal replacement with colon. In Spitz, L. & Coran, A. G., ed. *Rob and Smith's Operative Surgery, Pediatric Surgery*, 5th edn. London: Chapman & Hall, 1995.
20. Ein S. E. Gastric tube. In Spitz, L. & Coran, A. G., ed. *Rob & Smith's Operative Surgery, Pediatric Surgery*, 5th edn. London: Chapman & Hall, 1995.
21. Spitz L. Gastric replacement of the esophagus. In Spitz, L. & Coran, A. G., ed. *Rob & Smith's Operative Surgery, Pediatric Surgery*, 5th edn. London: Chapman & Hall, 1995.

18

Esophageal achalasia

Thomas T. Sato

Children's Hospital of Wisconsin, Milwaukee, WI, USA

Introduction

Esophageal achalasia is an uncommon pediatric surgical condition characterized by abnormality of, specifically failure of, the distal esophagus to relax with swallowing, associated with abnormal esophageal motility. The initial case description of achalasia was reported in 1674 by Sir Thomas Willis[1] who treated the patient with esophageal bougienage using a whalebone dilator. The incidence of achalasia in children under 15 years of age has been reported at between 0.02 and 0.31 per 100 000 in Ireland and Britain.[2] Approximately one-fifth of children with achalasia will present during infancy with symptoms of regurgitation, cough, aspiration, or failure to thrive; however, definitive diagnosis and subsequent treatment is rarely accomplished in infancy as these symptoms may be confused with feeding difficulty or gastroesophageal reflux.[3] Older children and adolescents with achalasia typically present with dysphagia, substernal chest pain, regurgitation and weight loss.

Treatment of esophageal achalasia is aimed at resolving the clinical symptoms of dysphagia, odynophagia, and regurgitation. This is accomplished by reducing the resting lower esophageal sphincter (LES) pressure by either medical or surgical means. There is no currently available treatment that directly reverses the pathophysiologic mechanism responsible for achalasia in children. As such, all treatment modalities are aimed at symptom control by reducing the effective LES resting pressure. Rendering the LES incompetent allows the esophagus to empty more readily via gravity and residual esophageal motility. Improved esophageal emptying should alleviate or greatly reduce symptoms related to distal esophageal obstruction.

Whether early, definitive intervention in achalasia leads to at least some recovery of esophageal motility in children remains to be fully determined; generally, the intrinsic esophageal motility disorder should be considered a persistent, lifelong disease with surgical treatment aimed at symptom resolution.

Three major invasive therapies have been used in the surgical treatment of achalasia in infants and children: (1) intrasphincteric injection of botulinum toxin; (2) esophageal dilatation with either bougienage or pneumatic dilators; and (3) esophagomyotomy. Endoscopic injection of botulinum toxin into the distal esophageal musculature is a potentially effective treatment in selected patients with achalasia but generally requires sequential injections for durable relief of symptoms. Esophageal dilatation was the first treatment for achalasia and has enjoyed increased interest in the pediatric surgical community with the development of smaller, low-compliance pneumatic balloon dilators. Division of the distal esophageal musculature by esophagomyotomy is considered in the surgical literature to offer the highest probability of definitive symptom control; however, esophagomyotomy is often reserved for patients not responding to botulinum toxin injection, dilatation, or both. Recent advances in minimally invasive techniques may substantially reduce the perioperative morbidity previously associated with esophagomyotomy. The role of performing a concomitant antireflux procedure with esophagomyotomy remains controversial.

Diagnosis and medical management

The most common finding reported with histological examination of the distal esophagus in patients with

Pediatric Surgery and Urology: Long-term Outcomes, Mark Stringer, Keith Oldham, Pierre Mouriquand.
Published by Cambridge University Press.

achalasia is a decrease or loss of myenteric ganglion cells; however, this is not a consistent finding. Infection with *Tryptanosoma cruzi* can lead to the development of Chaga's disease in some areas of Central and South America and may be associated with the development of a distal esophageal motility disorder with progressive esophageal dilatation that mimics achalasia. Although the etiology of esophageal achalasia remains largely unknown, there are sporadic familial cases[4,5] and an intriguing, occasional relationship of achalasia with adrenocortical insufficiency, alacrima, and other disorders of the autonomic and peripheral nervous system.[6] Investigation of myectomy specimens from the distal esophagus in children with autosomal recessive Allgrove's syndrome (a triad of achalasia, Addisonianism, and alacrima) demonstrate esophageal intermuscular fibrosis and either absent or decreased neuronal nitric oxide synthase.[7] These data are consistent with an intrinsic, pathophysiologic relationship between esophageal innervation and musculature causing ineffective, uncoordinated distal esophageal relaxation in response to swallowing in this subgroup of patients with hereditary disease.

Because of the complex nature of pediatric feeding and swallowing problems, objective diagnostic assessment of oral, pharyngeal, and esophageal phases of swallowing is essential to establish the diagnosis of achalasia. Three contemporary diagnostic tests should be considered in any infant or child suspected of having achalasia:

(1) videofluoroscopic swallowing study; (2) esophageal manometry; and (3) esophagogastroduodenoscopy. The accepted diagnostic standard in the work-up of pediatric dysphagia is currently videofluoroscopic swallowing analysis.[8] Scout films of the chest may reveal evidence of aspiration pneumonia or chronic lung disease from recurrent pulmonary infection. Normal oropharyngeal swallowing with a dilated, contrast-filled esophagus and a distal, "bird's beak" tapering near the gastroesophageal junction is characteristic of achalasia. Retained food debris may be observed in the esophagus. Esophageal manometry will demonstrate absent peristalsis of the distal esophagus with either normal or increased lower esophageal sphincter (LES) resting pressure and a lack of coordinated LES relaxation during swallowing. Incomplete LES relaxation during swallowing is characteristic of achalasia and gives rise to the functional distal esophageal obstruction in response to swallowing. More proximal esophageal peristaltic waves may be pronounced or may be nearly absent, depending upon the degree of esophageal dilatation. Esophagogastroscopy typically demonstrates a dilated thoracic esophagus without mechanical obstruction to the stomach. Importantly, this finding excludes fixed anatomic causes of dysphagia in infants and children such as cartilaginous esophageal rings, webs, leiomyoma, or reflux-associated strictures. There may be substantial food debris and secretions in the proximal esophagus and mild to moderate stasis esophagitis. Biopsies are recommended to exclude other treatable causes of dysphagia such as eosinophilic esophagitis.

Current medical management includes use of long-acting nitrates such as isosorbide dinitrate, and calcium channel blockers (i.e., nifedipine) as smooth muscle relaxing agents. Both of these drugs achieve reductions in LES pressure in patients with achalasia that are approximately one-half the magnitudes achieved by dilatation or myotomy. In a randomized, double-blind, placebo-controlled, crossover study evaluating the role of nifedipine in achalasia, ten patients demonstrated a statistically significant decrease in dysphagia frequency and had an associated decrease in resting LES pressure. However, symptoms of dysphagia, regurgitation, and nocturnal cough persisted despite the reduction in LES pressure, leading the investigators to conclude that nifedipine cannot be recommended as a standard alternative to other treatment options that may provide more durable and complete relief of symptoms.[9] From the pediatric standpoint, the chronic use of pharmacologic therapy in achalasia has been disappointing due to lack of durable response, substantial side effects, and compliance issues.

Outcome issues

A review of the reported outcomes of the most widely used interventions for achalasia in children is the focus for the remainder of this chapter. This analysis is limited statistically by the relative absence of well-controlled, randomized clinical trials comparing one surgical approach with another in the treatment of achalasia in children. Therefore, the vast majority of studies reporting the surgical treatment and outcome of pediatric achalasia in the literature reflect category IV evidence, composed of retrospective reviews and case series. The nature of these studies reflects in part the uncommon occurrence of pediatric achalasia.

The ability to measure and meaningfully compare the effectiveness of different treatments for achalasia is dependent on several factors, including: (1) use of the same diagnostic criteria for achalasia; (2) accurate definition of symptom control; (3) uniformity in pre- and postoperative assessment techniques; and (4) critical, long-term follow-up in carefully designed, randomized clinical trials. To date, there are no studies of pediatric achalasia treatment that meet these criteria. The uniform adoption of a relatively simple, descriptive symptom classification

Table 18.1. Symptom scale for achalasia

Score	Description	Symptoms
1	Excellent	Asymptomatic
2	Good	Symptoms less than once a week
3	Moderate	Symptoms more than once a week
4	Poor	Daily symptoms

(adapted from Ref. 10)

similar to that proposed[10] and listed in Table 18.1 may allow for more meaningful comparative analysis. This is particularly important when reliance upon parental reporting of symptoms for an infant or young child is required. Future studies may also benefit from the use of a standard, objective, preoperative work-up for achalasia that is ideally repeated in long-term, postoperative follow-up. These studies should generally include a history, physical examination, weight, videofluoroscopic swallowing study, manometry, and endoscopy. Repeating these studies postoperatively would create data for longitudinal comparison between and within investigational sites. Finally, there have been no controlled trials comparing the two most widely used procedures to treat achalasia, namely pneumatic dilatation and esophagomyotomy, in the pediatric population. Therefore, extrapolation of data from the singular adult controlled trial and several published uncontrolled case series is often accepted as the basis for best current pediatric management of achalasia.

Botulinum toxin

The use of botulinum toxin for the treatment of achalasia relies on the ability of the toxin to inhibit the release of acetylcholine from presynaptic nerve terminals. The toxin binds to the presynaptic nerve terminals and produces neuromuscular blockade as well as smooth muscle relaxation.[11,12] The concept is to induce neuromuscular blockade of the esophageal LES musculature, allowing for decreased LES resting tone and improvement of esophageal emptying. From a physiologic standpoint, neuromuscular blockade from a singular botulinum toxin injection is expected to be transient, and on the order of several weeks to months in effectiveness. Delivery of intrasphincteric botulinum toxin in children requires general anesthesia and endoscopic visualization of the gastroesophageal junction. Aliquots of botulinum toxin are injected radially in four quadrants at the LES using 25-gauge, 3- to 5-mm sclerotherapy needles deployed through the endoscopic instrument channel. The dose is generally a total of 80 to 100 units of toxin; some investigators also prefer to deliver injections inferior to the LES with the endoscope retroflexed for visualization.

Experience in adult patients with achalasia demonstrates that intrasphincteric injection of 80 to 100 units of botulinum toxin produces short- and medium-term relief of dysphagia in over 50% of patients, although durability is quite variable. Annese[13] *et al.* treated 57 achalasia patients with an age range of 10 to 91 years with intrasphincteric injection of 100 units botulinum toxin and demonstrated a statistically significant decrease in dysphagia symptoms and mean LES pressure. Relapse of symptoms led to repeat injection. With a mean follow-up of 24 months, 30 patients required greater than or equal to two repeat injections. On average, repeat injection was required at 10-month intervals to remain symptom-free. A multicenter, randomized dose study of intrasphincteric botulinum toxin injection in 118 adult patients with achalasia using 50 units, 100 units, or 200 units of botulinum toxin demonstrated an overall clinical response rate of 82%, without a demonstrable dose–effect relationship.[14] With a mean follow-up of 12 months, symptom relapse was much less common in patients receiving two injections of 100 units botulinum toxin 30 days apart compared to singular injections, suggesting that a substantial limitation of botulinum toxin injection is the lack of durable, long-term symptom relief.

The use of intrasphincteric botulinum toxin injection in the treatment of pediatric achalasia was initially reported in 1997.[15,16] These two studies report on the treatment of four pediatric patients with achalasia. Botulinum toxin injection produced effective symptom control at 6 to 8 months of follow-up. A retrospective survey review of 23 infants and children with achalasia treated with botulinum toxin injection between June 1995 and November 1998 demonstrated an 83% initial clinical response rate, as measured by symptom resolution or reduction, and post-injection weight gain.[17] Mean duration of response after a single injection was 4.2 months. Four patients did not respond, and twelve patients underwent more than one injection procedure. Eleven patients ultimately underwent esophagomyotomy during the study period. No patients were asymptomatic at the conclusion of the study without having undergone an additional procedure. The authors recommended that botulinum toxin injection be used only in children with achalasia who are considered poor candidates for dilatation or surgery. Importantly, this includes the patients in whom transient control of symptoms using botulinum toxin injection may decrease the risk of future dilatation or esophagomyotomy, i.e., recovery from aspiration pneumonia or establishment of adequate preoperative nutritional status.

Other studies have verified the initial effectiveness of botulinum toxin injection in the control of symptoms in pediatric achalasia. Ip *et al.* (2000)[18] treated seven children aged 2 to 15 years with 100 units intrasphincteric botulinum toxin. Three of the seven (43%) children had sustained improvement of symptoms for greater than 6 months. Response appeared to be independent of whether associated conditions such as Allgrove's syndrome were present. There was an inverse correlation between the pretreatment LES pressure and the duration of response to botulinum toxin.

In summary, intrasphincteric injection of botulinum toxin in the infant or child with achalasia may produce an initial favorable response, but the majority of patients will have relatively prompt recurrence of their presenting symptoms. There may be selected patients in whom transient improvement in swallowing induced by botulinum toxin may help improve preoperative management and risk reduction for future pneumatic dilatation or esophagomyotomy. Without repeat botulinum toxin injection within 1 to 6 months, the majority of children with achalasia will not have long-term symptom control with this modality alone. No major complications or deaths related to the esophageal botulinum toxin injection have been reported in the pediatric population.

Esophageal dilatation

The aim of esophageal dilatation in the treatment of achalasia is to forcefully distend the dysfunctional LES and render it incompetent, allowing for a reduction in LES resting pressure and consequent improvement in esophageal emptying. Successful treatment of achalasia from forced esophageal dilatation is commonly believed to cause disruption of the LES musculature. However, investigation using high-resolution endoscopic ultrasonographic examination of the esophageal wall following pneumatic dilatation for achalasia failed to demonstrate evidence of muscular tearing or disruption.[19] Historical review of esophageal dilatation reveals that a wide variety of devices have been used, ranging from the whalebone bougie used by Willis in 1674 to fixed-size blunt and taper-tipped dilators, and more recently, to contemporary pneumatic dilators. Pneumatic balloon dilators are capable of being deployed over an intraesophageal guidewire with fluoroscopic or endoscopic visualization. Given the current variety and size of available balloon catheters, radial esophageal dilatation is attractive in the pediatric population because graduated dilatation can be performed over the same guidewire in even the smallest infants and children. With real time fluoroscopy, the progress of dilatation can be directly controlled and visualized. In addition, mucosal traction injury from pulsion-type dilators is avoided.

Pneumatic dilatation for achalasia can generally be performed on an outpatient basis with little reported morbidity or mortality. Immediate technical complications include esophageal bleeding or perforation, with late complications of gastroesophageal reflux. Speiss and Kahrilas[20] reviewed the published English literature from 1966 to 1997 and selected 18 uncontrolled studies examining treatment of pneumatic dilatation for achalasia in adults based upon a reported good to excellent response. Individual studies were weighted proportional to their sample size. The pooled estimate of response rate of pneumatic dilatation to achalasia for 1276 patients was 72% ± 26%. Approximately 21% of achalasia patients undergoing pneumatic dilatation required repeat treatment. The incidence of esophageal perforation with pneumatic dilatation was 3%.

Pneumatic dilatation in adult achalasia has been demonstrated via randomized clinical trial to have a more durable response when compared to intrasphincteric botulinum toxin injection.[21] At 12 months follow-up, 70% of patients treated with pneumatic dilatation were in remission with regard to symptoms, compared to 32% of the patients treated with intrasphincteric botulinum toxin. Objectively, dilatation was associated with significant improvement of esophageal emptying at 12 months, as assessed by esophagram, when compared to the group treated by botulinum toxin.

Experience with pneumatic esophageal dilatation as primary therapy for childhood achalasia was reported from the Children's Hospital of Philadelphia using a Brown-McHardy dilator placed under fluoroscopic guidance.[22] Ten pediatric patients were treated over a 10-year period, with follow-up ranging from 9 months to 10 years. Four patients reported an excellent response and were either asymptomatic or having only occasional dysphagia or pain; two patients required multiple dilatations to maintain an excellent response. Two patients reported good response with persistent dysphagia to certain foods or environmental stimuli, and two patients underwent Heller myotomy for persistent symptoms. Three patients had either postprocedure substernal chest pain or fever without demonstrable esophageal leak. The authors recommended pneumatic dilatation as primary therapy in late-onset childhood achalasia, reserving surgery for younger children or children with a poor clinical response to two dilatations. Similar results using pneumatic dilatation for achalasia in children have been reported and are listed in Table 18.2, with an overall success rate of 60% to 83%. Overall, these pediatric data are quite similar to the adult experience, despite the

Table 18.2. Selected outcomes for primary pneumatic dilatation in childhood achalasia

Author	*N*	Multiple dilatations	Excellent	Good/ moderate	Fair/poor	Complication	Surgery
Boyle *et al.* (1981)[22] (Follow-up range 9 mo to 10 yr)	10	2	6 (60%)	2	2	0	2
Nakayama *et al.* (1987)[24] (Follow-up range 1 to 5 yr)	15[a]	8	11 (73%)	0	0	0	4
Perisic *et al.* (1996)[44] (Follow-up range 2 to 8 yr)	12	3	10 (83%)	0	2	1[b]	2
Hamza *et al.* (1999)[45] (Follow-up range 2 to 7 yr)	11	11	8 (72%)	2	1	0	1
Upadhyaya *et al.* (2002)[46] (Follow-up range 3 mo to 8 yr)	12	2	10 (83%)	2	0	0	0

[a] excludes two patients undergoing primary esophagomyotomy and two patients treated with bougienage and subsequent myotomy.
[b] one patient developed reflux esophagitis with ulceration.

differences in clinical presentation for infants and younger children.

In contrast, results with esophageal dilatation in 20 children with achalasia treated at the Children's Hospital of Boston were less encouraging.[23] Pneumatic dilatation was used in children older than 5 years of age or greater than 20 kg weight; pulsion dilatation with filiform and followers was used in smaller infants and children. Five children, all over 9 years of age, had symptomatic relief with 2 dilatations; 15 children responded poorly to esophageal dilatation and 12 children ultimately required operative management. The authors concluded that initial dilatation is appropriate therapy but that it should be reserved for older children with achalasia; primary operative therapy was recommended for younger infants and children. This study highlights the potential age-related differences in response to dilatation, and in particular, the observation that patients unresponsive to initial dilatation or who experience rapid recurrence of symptoms are unlikely to respond to repeat dilatation.[24]

Pneumatic dilatation has also been described anecdotally as a useful secondary treatment in the setting of the symptomatic child following unsuccessful esophagomyotomy.[25,26] The reported esophageal perforation rate during pneumatic dilatation in children over the past 25 years remains minimal and is likely equivalent to adult series. Recognizing the substantial anatomic differences between esophageal stricture and achalasia, a recent, large series of infants and children undergoing pneumatic dilatation for either esophageal stricture or achalasia reported an esophageal perforation rate of 1.5% for 260 procedures.[27] Long-term follow-up regarding gastroesophageal reflux disease following dilatation suggests a relatively low incidence, but these data are notable for the lack of objective assessment in most pediatric trials.

In summary, pneumatic esophageal dilatation for childhood achalasia remains an acceptable treatment given its overall initial success rate and reported low morbidity. The efficacy and long-term outcome of pneumatic dilatation compared to esophagomyotomy as a primary treatment for pediatric achalasia has not been effectively studied. Most children require general anesthesia for esophageal dilatation and the procedure may be performed on an outpatient basis. Results are generally more durable that botulinum toxin injection. While pediatric data available for review are scant, approximately 60% to 83% of selected patients have a favorable response, as characterized by symptom relief, and this may be lower than response rates in adults. Approximately 20% will require repeat treatment for recurrent symptoms. The esophageal perforation rate appears to be less than 3%. There appear to be age-specific issues, and patients with initial dilatation failure or rapid symptom recurrence following dilatation appear less likely to have an acceptable response to repeat dilatation. There are currently no identifiable, consistent characteristics to determine which children will either not respond to dilatation or have prompt relapse of symptoms following initial dilatation.

Esophagomyotomy

Ernest Heller reported the successful surgical management of esophageal achalasia in 1913 by creating two longitudinal extramucosal esophagomyotomies that did not

Table 18.3. Reported outcome of selected series using esophagomyotomy for childhood achalasia

Author	*N*	Excellent	Good/ moderate	Fair/poor	Complications	Follow-up
Tachovsky (1968)[31]	15	12	1	1	3	mean 6.9 yr
Azizkhan (1980)[23]	12	11	1[a]	0	3	mean 4 yr
Buick and Spitz (1985)[32]	15	9	3	3	1	mean 2.1 yr
Vane *et al.* (1988)[33]	21	18	3[b]	0	9[c]	mean 6.3 yr
Nihoul-Fekete *et al.* (1989)[38]	35	32	2[d]	1	5	range 1 to 25 yr
Emblem *et al.* (1993)[39]	12	9	2	1[e]	4	mean 3.9 yr
Morris-Stiff *et al.* (1997)[40]	10	8	2	0	3	median 8 yr
Lelli (1997)[47]	19	17	2[f]	0	0	mean 9 yr
Karnak *et al.* (2001)[48]	19	14	3	2[g]	0	range 2 mo to 16 yr
Hussain (2002)[49]	29	15	4	2	0	mean 4.7 yr

[a] one patient required re-operation 4 months after initial operation.
[b] one patient required postop dilatation; two patients required second esophagomyotomy.
[c] fever and atelectasis; three patients developed significant gastroesophageal reflux.
[d] two patients required postop Nissen fundoplication; an antireflux procedure was performed in 33 patients.
[e] two patients required postop dilatation for pain; one patient required postop gastric transposition for pain.
[f] 17 patients had resolution of presenting symptoms. Patients subjectively rated their overall result as either excellent (68%) or good (32%).
[g] two patients developed esophageal stenosis requiring esophagocardioplasty.

extend onto the gastric wall.[28] The modification to a single, anterior esophagomyotomy by De Brune Groenveldt[29] is the operation most commonly performed today for achalasia. The esophagomyotomy may be performed either through the left chest, transabdominally, and more recently, via thoracoscopic or laparoscopic approaches.

Because of the perceived morbidity of operative esophagomyotomy via thoracotomy or laparotomy, pneumatic dilatation has been recommended historically by many authors as the initial treatment of choice for achalasia. There are currently no data available to definitively conclude that pneumatic dilatation is superior or inferior to esophagomyotomy as primary therapy for pediatric achalasia. The efficacy of esophagomyotomy in the treatment of achalasia in children and adults has been demonstrated predominantly by retrospective case series. Collectively, these studies offer strong argument that esophagomyotomy is predictable, definitive treatment for the vast majority of patients with achalasia. There is a single, prospective, randomized adult clinical trial comparing pneumatic esophageal dilatation to esophagomyotomy in 81 adults.[30] At approximately 5-year follow-up (range 24 to 156 months), symptom resolution was noted in 65% of the dilatation group compared to 95% in the esophagomyotomy group. Including this singular controlled trial, selective review of 30 additional uncontrolled trials of esophagomyotomy was performed by Speiss and Kahrilas.[20] Individual studies were weighted proportional to their sample size. The pooled estimated response rates of esophagomyotomy to correct symptoms of dysphagia for a total of 2124 patients with achalasia was 84% ± 20% for Heller myotomy via thoracotomy, 85 ± 18% for laparotomy, and 92 ± 18% for laparoscopic myotomy. These pooled data appear to support the contention that esophagomyotomy is a highly effective treatment for symptoms of dysphagia secondary to achalasia. Notably, a few children and adults with achalasia will continue to have specific problems with dysphagia, regurgitation, and proximal esophageal distension, despite aggressive treatment, including repeated dilatation, esophagectomy, or both. While surgical revision remains possible, the experience is quite limited and unpredictable. Anecdotal use of esophagectomy with either colonic interposition graft or gastric transposition procedures has been reported.

Several case series of esophagomyotomy are reported in the pediatric surgical literature. Larger, selected studies with recorded longitudinal follow-up data are summarized in Table 18.3. Given the differences in perioperative measurements of symptoms, operative approach (thoracotomy vs. laparotomy), and treatment outcome, comparative outcome analysis is limited to tabulation of the reported efficacy of esophagomyotomy to control symptoms of dysphagia. Despite current limitations in comparative analysis, historical review of surgical treatment options in pediatric achalasia demonstrates a consistent transition from thoracotomy or laparotomy to minimally invasive approaches. Additionally, there appears to be growing acceptance or consensus over time to support the routine performance of a concomitant antireflux procedure, most commonly a partial fundoplication, following esophagomyotomy.

There are no compelling data to suggest that symptomatic relief from dysphagia is different based upon the use of a thoracotomy vs. laparotomy in the treatment of pediatric achalasia. An adequate esophagomyotomy that traverses the distal esophagus for a length of 6 to 8 cm and typically extends for 1 to 2 cm onto the gastric fundus can be performed through either approach. Tachovsky, Lynn, and Ellis[31] described the Mayo Clinic experience between 1950 and 1967 with 15 pediatric patients with achalasia using thoracotomy. Mean length of postoperative hospitalization was less than 7.5 days, with one reported complication secondary to empyema. Excluding this patient, the mean hospitalization was 6.4 days. Fourteen of the patients were followed for a mean period of 6.9 years, with 12 patients reporting excellent relief of symptoms. Some centers adopted a transabdominal approach in the following two decades. Reports included either thoracic or transabdominal approaches to correct pediatric achalasia.[23,32,33] There are no discernable differences in outcome between thoracotomy vs. laparotomy in these uncontrolled studies with the exception that more children treated via laparotomy underwent either selective or routine concomitant fundoplication. Given the concern of either immediate or delayed gastroesophageal reflux following esophagomyotomy, some surgeons advocate the transabdominal approach as more favorable for fundoplication. Ballantine, Fitzgerald, and Grosfeld[34] reported the use of a transabdominal approach in nine children with achalasia; three children had concomitant fundoplication and two children required subsequent fundoplication within the first postoperative 13 months to control gastroesophageal reflux symptoms.

There is a compelling anatomic argument that an operation designed to render the LES incompetent should be expected to increase the incidence of gastroesophageal reflux. Furthermore, there are no preoperative factors, in the absence of hiatal hernia, that allow identification of achalasia patients at higher risk for the development of postoperative gastroesophageal reflux. Therefore studies reporting selective application of fundoplication with esophagomyotomy are generally ancecdotal. Studies describing the incidence of postoperative gastroesophageal reflux following esophagomyotomy have significant range. This is due, in part, to substantial variation in the subjective and objective measurements used to define gastroesophageal reflux perioperatively. Reported rates of gastroesophageal reflux following esophagomyotomy with or without fundoplication in several adult series range from 0% to 52% with an estimated mean incidence rate of 10% to 12%.[35] Limiting the length of myotomy to several millimeters onto the stomach has been proposed as a means of reducing postoperative gastroesophageal reflux and eliminating the need for fundoplication. This approach has not been demonstrated to completely eliminate gastroesophageal reflux when measured with postoperative pH probe monitoring.[36] In addition, recent experience with a 3 cm extension of the gastric myotomy was reported to reduce the frequency and severity of postoperative dysphagia when compared historically to a 1.5 cm gastric myotomy in adults.[37]

Performance of fundoplication with esophagomyotomy generally reflects individual or institutional preference. Experience in France using esophagomyotomy without fundoplication in four children led to severe postoperative gastroesophageal reflux in two, causing the investigators to use esophagomyotomy with fundoplication in the remaining 31 children reported in their series.[38] Experience from London[39] and Cardiff[40] in children with achalasia treated by esophagomyotomy with Nissen fundoplication has demonstrated good to excellent results in symptom relief as well as control of postoperative gastroesophageal reflux disease, without apparent increase in postoperative dysphagia from the fundoplication. In a large, adult case series of thoracoscopic esophagomyotomy without fundoplication versus laparoscopic esophagomyotomy with partial fundoplication for achalasia, both groups experienced good to excellent symptomatic relief from dysphagia; however, in the subset of patients having postoperative 24-hour pH probe monitoring, 60% of patients treated with thoracoscopic myotomy alone had gastroesophageal reflux compared to 17% of patients treated by laparoscopic myotomy with partial fundoplication.[41] These data suggest that: (1) an effective esophagomyotomy designed to reduce resting LES pressure appears to increase the postoperative incidence of gastroesophageal reflux disease; (2) esophagomyotomy extended 1 to 3 cm distal to the gastroesophageal junction reduces the probability of "incomplete" myotomy and symptomatic postoperative dysphagia; and (3) use of concomitant fundoplication with esophagomyotomy is becoming more common.

In 1996, the successful treatment of two children with achalasia using laparoscopic esophagomyotomy was reported.[42] Minimally invasive approaches to this disease led rapidly to recognition that these approaches are associated with reductions in postoperative morbidity, and particularly by less pain and shorter hospital length of stay. Selected pediatric studies reporting experience with

Table 18.4. Selected series of laparoscopic/thoracoscopic esophagomyotomy for pediatric achalasia

Author	*N*	TS	Fundo	Postoperative function excellent/good	Complications	Follow-up
Holcomb (1996)[42]	2	0	0	2 (100%)	0	mean 17.5 mo
Esposito *et al.* (2000)[50]	10	0	10	9 (90%)	3	6 mo to 6 yr
Rothenberg *et al.* (2001)[53]	9	4	5	7 (78%)	2	
Mehra *et al.* (2001)[51]	22	4	18	18 (82%)	2	mean 17 mo
Mattioli *et al.* (2003)[52]	20	0	20	20 (100%)	2	45 mo

TS = thoracoscopic.
Fundo = fundoplication.

laparoscopic and/or thoracoscopic esophagomyotomy are listed in Table 18.4. These studies have generally demonstrated good to excellent functional results with substantial reduction in dysphagia, along with earlier institution of oral feeding and marked reduction in hospital stay. As with open esophagomyotomy, esophageal mucosal perforation is a reported complication of laparoscopic or thoracoscopic myotomy. The incidence of esophageal mucosal perforation may be initially higher in the minimally invasive series due to a learning curve effect. As in contemporary adult laparoscopic series, there is a tendency for performance of a concomitant partial fundoplication, either anterior (Dor) or posterior (Toupet) with laparoscopic esophagomyotomy in children. Early results with laparoscopic esophagomyotomy and fundoplication for children with achalasia are encouraging, but will need continued evaluation of efficacy in long-term follow-up. If the long-term outcome is similar to the adult experience, the laparoscopic approach may become accepted as standard, primary therapy for childhood achalasia.

Summary

The treatment of childhood achalasia remains a challenging surgical problem. Effective treatment of pediatric achalasia relies on the reduction of resting LES tone by either medical or surgical intervention, allowing for improved esophageal emptying. The esophageal motility disorder associated with achalasia is a lifelong issue. Essential to making rational treatment decisions in this setting is consideration of the efficacy, durability, and associated morbidity of therapeutic interventions. Accurate assessment of subjective and objective symptom control of dysphagia and gastroesophageal reflux during the postoperative period is essential for meaningful conclusions regarding the long-term outcome. Pneumatic dilatation has been recognized as an effective therapy for childhood achalasia, but the efficacy and durability of dilatation appears less predictable than Heller myotomy. Esophagomyotomy is an efficacious and durable treatment for achalasia, and with contemporary laparoscopic technique, the associated morbidity appears low.

Limiting the length of myotomy to several millimeters onto the stomach has been proposed as a means of reducing postoperative gastroesophageal reflux and eliminating the need for fundoplication. This approach has not been demonstrated to completely eliminate gastroesophageal reflux when measured with postoperative pH probe monitoring.[36] In addition, recent experience with a 3 cm extension of the gastric myotomy was reported to reduce the frequency and severity of postoperative dysphagia when compared historically to a 1.5 cm gastric myotomy in adults.[37] Experience from London[39] and Cardiff[40] in children with achalasia treated by esophagomyotomy with Nissen fundoplication has demonstrated good to excellent results in symptom relief and control of postoperative gastroesophageal reflux disease without apparent increase in postoperative dysphagia from the fundoplication. These data suggest that (1) esophagomyotomy extended 1 to 3 cm distal to the gastroesophageal junction will reduce the probability of "incomplete" myotomy and symptomatic dysphagia; (2) an effective esophagomyotomy to reduce resting LES pressure will consequently increase the probability of gastroesophageal reflux; and (3) a concomitant antireflux procedure performed at the time of an esophagomyotomy reduces the incidence of postoperative gastroesophageal reflux.

Lemmer *et al.*[43] performed transthoracic esophagomyotomy in 6 children and at a mean follow-up of nearly two years, none of the children had symptomatic gastroesophageal reflux.

REFERENCES

1. Willis, T. *Pharmaceutical Rationalis. Sive Diatriba de Medicamentorum Operationibus in Humano Corpore. Editio tertia.* Oxford, E Theatro Sheldoniano, Prostant apud Ric. Davis, 1679.
2. Mayberry, J. F. & Mayell, M. J. Epidemiological study of achalasia in children. *Gut*. 1988; **29**(1):90–93.
3. Myers, N. A., Jolley, S. G., & Taylor R. Achalasia of the cardia in children: a worldwide survey. *J. Pediatr. Surg*. 1994; **29**(10):1375–1379.
4. Monning, P. J. Familial achalasia in children. *Ann. Thorac. Surg*. 1990; **49**(6):1019–1022.
5. Galanakis, E., Gardikis, S., Vlachakis, J. *et al.* A local cluster of achalasia in a province of Crete. *Acta Paediatr*. 2000; **89**:246–247.
6. Gazarian, M., Cowell, C. T., Bonney, M. *et al.* The "4A" syndrome: adrenocortical insufficiency associated with achalasia, alacrima, autonomic and other neurological abnormalities. *Eur. J. Pediatr*. 1995; **154**:18–23.
7. Khelif, K., De Laet, M. H., Chaouachi, B. *et al.* Achalasia of the cardia in Allgrove's (triple A) syndrome: histopathologic study of 10 cases. *Am. J. Surg. Pathol*. 2003; **27**(5):667–672.
8. Miller, C. K. & Willging, J. P. Advances in the evaluation and management of pediatric dysphagia. *Curr. Opin. Otolaryngol. Head Neck Surg*. 2003; **11**:442–446.
9. Traube, M., Dubovik, S., Lange, R. C. *et al.* The role of nifedipine therapy in achalasia: results of a randomized, double-blind, placebo-controlled study. *Am. J. Gastroenterol*. 1989; **84**:1259–1262.
10. Vantrappen, G. & Hellemans, J. Treatment of achalasia and related motor disorders. *Gastroenterology*. 1980; **79**:144–154.
11. Pasricha, P. J., Rai, R., Ravich, W. J. *et al.* Botulinum toxin for achalasia: long-term outcome and predictors of response. *Gastroenterology*. 1996; **110**:1410–1415.
12. Pasricha, P. J., Ravich, W. J., & Kalloo, A. N. Effects of intrasphincteric botulinum toxin on lower esophageal sphincter in piglets. *Gastroenterology*. 1993; **105**:1045–1049.
13. Annese, V., Basciani, M., and Borrelli, O. *et al.* Intrasphincteric injection of botulinum toxin is effective in long-term treatment of esophageal achalasia. *Muscle Nerve*. 1998; **21**:1540–1542.
14. Annese, V., Bassotti, G., and Coccia, G. *et al.* A multicenter randomized study of intrasphincteric botulinum toxin in patients with oesophageal achalasia. *Gut*. 2000; **46**:597–600.
15. Khoshoo, V., LaGarde, D. C., & Udall, J. N. Intrasphincteric injection of botulinum toxin for treating achalasia in children. *J. Pediatr. Gastroenterol. Nutrit*. 1997; **24**:439–444.
16. Walton, J. M. & Tougas, G. Botulinum toxin use in pediatric esophageal achalasia: a case report. *J. Pediatr. Surg*. 1997; **32**:916–917.
17. Hurwitz, M., Bahar, R. J., & Ament, M. E. *et al.* Evaluation of the use of botulinum toxin in children with achalasia. *J. Pediatr. Gastroenterol. Nutrit*. 2000; **30**:509–514.
18. Ip, K. S., Cameron, D. J. S., Catto-Smith, A. G. *et al.* Botulinum toxin for achalasia in children. *J. Gastroenterol. Hepatol*. 2000; **15**(10):1100–1104.
19. Schiano, T. D., Fisher, R. S., Parkman, H. P. *et al.* Use of high-resolution endoscopic ultrasonography to assess esophageal wall damage after pneumatic dilation and botulinum toxin to treat achalasia. *Gastrointest. Endosc*. 1996; **44**:151–57.
20. Speiss, A. E. & Kahrilas, P. J. Treating achalasia. *J. Am. Med. Assoc*. 1998; **280**:638–642.
21. Vaezi, M. F., Richter, J. E., & Wilcox, C. M. *et al.* Botulinum toxin versus pneumatic dilatation in the treatment of achalasia: a randomized trial. *Gut*. 1999; **44**:231–239.
22. Boyle, J. T., Cohen, S., & Watkins, J. B. Successful treatment of achalasia in childhood by pneumatic dilatation. *J. Pediatr*. 1981; **99**:35–40.
23. Azizkhan, R. G., Tapper, D., and Eraklis, A. Achalasia in childhood: a 20-year experience. *J. Pediatr. Surg*. 1980; **15**:452–456.
24. Nakayama, D. K., Shorter, N. A., Boyle, J. T., Watkins, J. B., & O'Neill, J. A. Jr. Pneumatic dilatation and operative treatment of achalasia in children. *J. Pediatr. Surg.* 1987; **22**:619–622.
25. Gelfand, M. D. & Christie, D. L. Pneumatic dilation under general anesthesia after unsuccessful cardiomyotomy for achalasia. *J. Clin. Gastroenterol*. 1979; **1**:317–319.
26. Babu, R., Grier, D., & Cusick, E. *et al.* Pneumatic dilatation for childhood achalasia. *Pediatr. Surg. Int*. 2001; **17**:505–507.
27. Lan, L. C. L., Wong, K. K. Y., & Lin, S. C. L. *et al.* Endoscopic balloon dilatation of esophageal strictures in infants and children: Experience and literature review. *J. Pediatr. Surg*. 2003; **38**:1712–1715.
28. Heller, E. Extramukose cardiaplastik beim chonischen cardiospasmus mit dilatation des oesophagus. *Mitteilungen Grenzgebieten Med Chir*. 1913; **27**:141–149.
29. De Brune Groenveldt, J. R. Over cardiospasmus. *Nederlands Tijdschrift voor Geneeskunde*. 1918; **54**:1281–1282.
30. Csendes, A., Braghetto, I., and Henriquez, A. *et al.* Late results of a prospective randomised study comparing forceful dilatation and oesophagomyotomy in patients with achalasia. *Gut*. 1989; **30**:299–304.
31. Tachovsky, T. J., Lynn, H. B., & Ellis, F. H. Jr. The surgical approach to esophageal achalasia in children. *J. Pediatr. Surg*. 1968; **3**:226–231.
32. Buick, R. G. & Spitz, L. Achalasia of the cardia in children. *Br. J. Surg*. 1985; **72**:341–343.
33. Vane, D. W., Cosby, K., & West, K. *et al.* Late results following esophagomyotomy in children with achalasia. *J. Pediatr. Surg*. 1988; **23**:515–519.
34. Ballantine, T. V. N., Fitzgerald, J. F., & Grosfeld, J. L. Transabdominal esophagomyotomy for achalasia in children. *J. Pediatr. Surg*. 1980; **15**:457–461.

35. Abir, F., Modlin, I., and Kidd, M. *et al.* Surgical treatment of achalasia: Current status and controversies. *Dig. Surg.* 2004; **21**:165–176.
36. Patti, M. G., Molena, D., Fisichella, P. M. *et al.* Laparoscopic Heller myotomy and Dor fundoplication for achalasia: analysis of successes and failures. *Arch. Surg.* 2001; **136**:870–877.
37. Oelschlager, B. K., Chang, L., & Pellegrini, C. A. Improved outcome after extended gastric myotomy for achalasia. *Arch. Surg.* 2003; **138**:490–497.
38. Nihoul-Fekete, C., Bawab, F., Lortat-Jacob, S. *et al.* Achalasia of the esophagus in childhood: surgical treatment in 35 cases with special reference to familial cases and glucocorticoid deficiency association. *J. Pediatr. Surg.* 1989; **24**:1060–1063.
39. Emblem, R., Stringer, M. D., & Hall, C. M. *et al.* Current results of surgery for achalasia of the cardia. *Arch. Dis. Child.* 1993; **68**:749–751.
40. Morris-Stiff, G., Khan, R., & Foster, M. E. *et al.* Long-term results of surgery for childhood achalasia. *Ann. Roy. Colle. Surg. Engl.* 1997; **79**:432–434.
41. Patti, M. G., Pellegrini, C. A., & Horgan, S. *et al.* Minimally invasive urgery for achalasia. An 8-year experience with 168 patients. *Ann. Surg.* 1999; **230**:587–594.
42. Holcomb, G. W. 3rd., Richards, W. O., & Riedel, B. D. Laparoscopic esophagomyotomy for achalasia in children. *J. Pediatr. Surg.* 1996; **31**:716–718.
43. Lemmer, J. H., Coran, A. G., Wesley, J. R., Polley, T. Z., Jr., & Byrne W. J. Achalasia in children: treatment by anterior esophageal myotomy (modified Heller operation). *J. Pediatr. Surg.* 1985; **20**:333–338.
44. Perisic, V. N., Scepanovic, D., & Radlovic, N. Nonoperative treatment of achalasia. *J. Pediatr. Gastroenterol. Nutr.* 1996; **22**:45–47.
45. Hamza, A. F., Awad, H. A., & Hussein, O. Cardiac achalasia in children. Dilatation or surgery? *Eur. J. Pediatr. Surg.* 1999; **9**:299–302.
46. Upadhyay, M., Fataar, S., & Sajwany, M. J. Achalasia of the cardia: experience with hydrostatic balloon dilatation in children. *Pediatr. Radiol.* 2002; **32**:409–412.
47. Lelli, J. L., Jr, Drongowski, R. A., & Coran, A. G. Efficacy of the transthoracic modified Heller myotomy in children with achalasia – a 21-year experience. *J. Pediatr. Surg.* 1997; **32**:338–341.
48. Karnak, I., Senocak, M. E., Tanyel, F. C., & Buyukpamukcu, N. Achalasia in childhood: surgical treatment and outcome. *Eur. J. Pediatr. Surg.* 2001; **11**:223–229.
49. Hussain, S. Z., Thomas, R., & Tolia, V. A review of achalasia in 33 children. *Dig. Dis. Sci.* 2002; **47**:2538–2543.
50. Esposito, C., Mendoza-Sagaon, M., Roblot-Maigret, B. *et al.* Complications of laparoscopic treatment of esophageal achalasia in children. *J. Pediatr. Surg.* 2000; **35**:680–683.
51. Mehra, M., Bahar, R. J., Ament, M. E. *et al.* Laparoscopic and thoracoscopic esophagomyotomy for children with achalasia. *J. Pediatr. Gastroenterol. Nutr.* 2001; **33**:466–471.
52. Mattioli, G., Esposito, C., Pini Prato, A. *et al.* Results of the laparoscopic Heller-Dor procedure for pediatric esophageal achalasia. *Surg. Endosc.* 2003; **17**:1650–1652.

19

Congenital malformations of the breast

Younghoon R. Cho and Arun K. Gosain

Department of Plastic Surgery, Medical College of Wisconsin, Milwaukee, WI, USA

Introduction

The mammary glands begin their development early in organogenesis and progress through several developmental stages, both in the uterus and in subsequent life. From a biologic standpoint, the mammary glands serve as a source of nourishment and provide passive immunity to our offspring. From a social perspective, mammary glands serve as a means of nurturing these bonds between mother and infant. In addition, they play an important role in defining femininity and our perceptions of beauty and attraction.

The importance of normal breast development can be demonstrated further by the psychosocial impact that results when normal development is interrupted. Congenital breast malformations may become manifest at different stages of breast development. These can be characterized in terms of symmetry, shape variations, over- or underdevelopment, multiple sites of development, unilateral development, or absence of development. Abnormal breast development may affect either sex. In this chapter, we will discuss normal breast development in more detail as well as some of the more common congenital breast disorders encountered in the pediatric population.

Breast development

The development of the mammary glands is initially identical for both sexes, and is a result of complex interplay of growth factors including TGF-α, TGF-β1, tenascin-C and extracellular matrix proteins such as collagen IV during organogenesis.[1] This interplay begins in the fourth week of gestation, when the human embryo measures between 4.5 and 6 mm. Paired ectodermal thickenings develop on the ventral surface of the embryo from the axillae to the inguinal crease to form the milk line or mammary ridges. This line eventually disappears and only a small remnant remains at the level of the fourth intercostal space in the pectoral region, where it matures to form the primary mammary bud by the fifth gestational week. The persistence of this ridge or milk line results in supernumerary breast or nipples.

During the seventh week the primary breast bud begins a downward descent towards the underlying dermis and by the tenth week begins to branch and form secondary buds that will develop into lactiferous ducts. By the twelfth week the breast buds mature into the mammary lobules. The surrounding adipose tissue in the underlying mesoderm is an important source of hormones and growth factors that eventually promote and regulate further development of the mammary gland. By the twentieth week of gestation placental hormones induce the formation of lactiferous ducts within the mammary buds. The mesoderm in this area forms the nipple-areola complex and the ectoderm forms the surrounding breast. By term, approximately 15–20 lobes of glandular tissues containing lactiferous ducts have formed in each breast. The lactiferous ducts drain into retroareolar ampullae, which coalesce into a mammary pit.

At birth, both sexes have measurable amounts of breast tissue that persists for weeks to months. It is not entirely clear whether this presence is attributable to the exposure of maternal hormones in utero, breast-feeding, or the presence of endogenous estradiol in the growing infant. A recent study by Schmidt *et al.*[2] demonstrated the presence of breast tissue in 85% of girls and 73% of boys at 3 months of age, with girls having a higher median serum

Pediatric Surgery and Urology: Long-term Outcomes, Mark Stringer, Keith Oldham, Pierre Mouriquand.
Published by Cambridge University Press.

estradiol level than boys. Median testosterone levels were significantly higher in boys than girls. Only estradiol levels in girls correlated with breast tissue size.

In girls, the onset of puberty marks another stage of breast development and glandular maturation in response to circulating hormones including estrogens, growth hormone and prolactin. During this period, there is a marked growth, elongation and branching of the ductal systems to form terminal end buds and enlargement of the lobules and an increase of the stromal component. The terminal end buds further differentiate to form alveolar buds, which are lined by epithelial cells that contain the cytoplasmic organelles necessary for lactation in the postpartum period. The alveolar buds cluster around a terminal duct to form lobules, which become evident within 1 to 2 years after the menarche. Full maturation of the mammary gland takes years and only reaches the final stage of maturation with the onset of pregnancy.

After menopause, in response to an absence of ovarian estradiol and progesterone secretion, the glandular tissue of the breast begins to atrophy with a decrease in the number of lobules and fibrous connective tissue of the stroma. There is gradual replacement of the glandular tissues with connective tissue and fat.

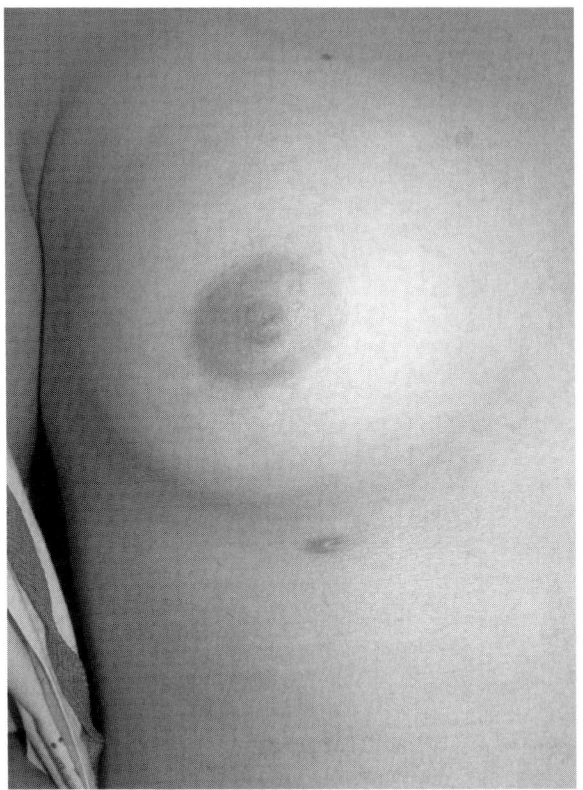

Fig. 19.1. 14-year-old girl with a supernumerary nipple below her right breast.

Congenital breast malformation

Malformations of the nipple

Congenital malformations of the nipple include athelia, polythelia, microthelia, macrothelia and the inverted nipple. Athelia is the congenital absence of the nipple and is among the rarest of the breast malformations.[3] It can present unilaterally or bilaterally and may occur in the setting of normal breast tissue. It is thought to be caused by a failure of the development of the lower cervical and upper thoracic somites.

Polythelia is the congenital presence of multiple nipples or supernumerary nipples and is far more common than athelia. The prevalence of supernumerary nipples vary in different populations; 0.22% in a Hungarian population,[4] 1.62% in African American neonates,[5] 2.5% in Israeli neonates,[6] 4.7% in Israeli Arabic children,[7] 5.6% in German children[8] and 11–16% in a Native American population in Chile.[9] Clinically, these supernumerary nipples appear most commonly along the embryonic milk line that extends bilaterally from a point slightly beyond the axillae on the arms to the proximal inner sides of the thigh (Fig. 19.1).[6,7,10] They appear as a small pigmented or pearl-colored mark or as a concave or umbilicated spot. In most cases, their diameter is less than a third of the normal nipple and can often be mistaken for other small cutaneous lesions. Most appear as a single lesion and are located below the normal nipple with a preponderance on the right side;[11] however, 13% appear above the nipple along the milk line.[6] Approximately 5% can be found outside the embryonic milk line in places including the limbs, shoulder, back, neck, face and vulva.[12,13] With the exception of cosmetic issues, the supernumerary nipple rarely is a cause of concern. However, some pathologic changes may occur as with the development of a regular nipple or breast. These include inflammation, mastitis, abscess formation, cysts, fibroadenoma, and Paget's disease. Occasionally, these lesions may be familial or syndromic. Three modes of familial inheritance have been described: autosomal dominant with variable penetration,[8] X-linked dominant,[10] and autosomal rescessive.[14] Syndromic polythelia include Turner's syndrome, trisomy 8, partial chromosome 3p trisomy, Fanconi's anemia, Kaufman-McKusick syndrome, and Char syndrome. There are also associated lesions such as ectodermal dysplasia, aplasia cutis with syndactyly, scalp defect, and microcephaly, or developmental delay.[9]

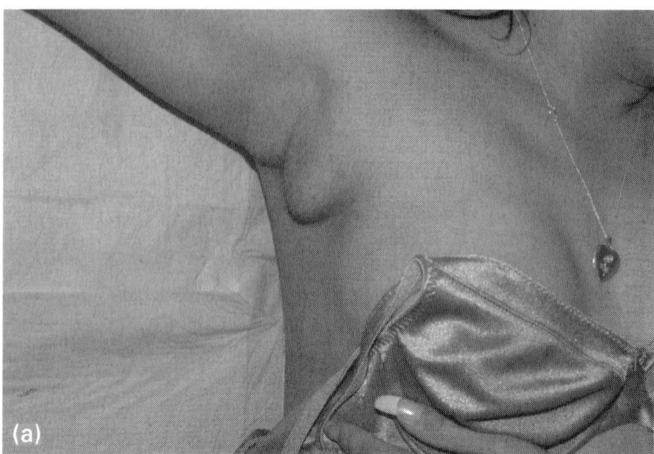

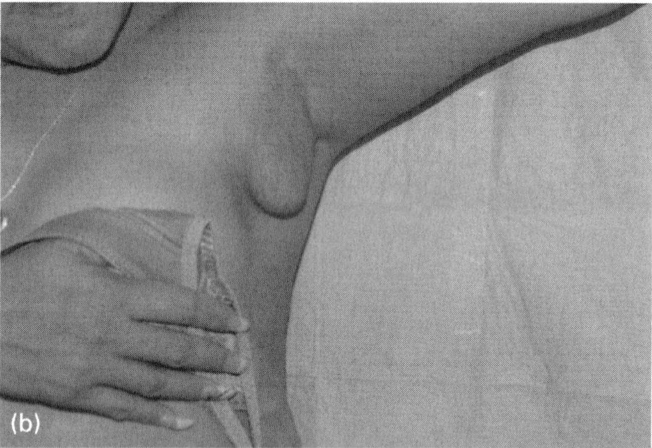

Fig. 19.2. (a), (b) 36-year-old woman with bilateral axillary polymastia.

The supernumerary nipple need only be removed surgically if the lesion causes embarrassment or cosmetic concern. Simple excision is performed along Langer's lines.

Although much more rare, intra-areolar polythelia involves a supernumerary nipple within the areola.[15] There are also reports of supernumerary areolae.[16] Microthelia and macrothelia refer to abnormally small or large nipples, respectively. The average nipple diameter measures 7 mm or more in full-term infants and 6 mm or less in preterm infants. Microthelia tends to present symmetrically with poorly pigmented nipples with a small or absent areolar zone and breast tissue. Microthelia is a rare presentation of a hypertrophic, bulbous, and flabby nipple.[3]

The nipple commonly presents as an inverted nipple at birth and everts within the first few days to weeks. Inverted nipples that persist into adulthood have been found in 1.8–3.3% of unmarried women aged 19–26 years,[17,18] with 87% of patients having bilateral presentation. Inverted nipples are generally sporadic but there are reports of familial autosomal dominant transmission and of several syndromes including Robinow syndrome and congenital disorders of glycosylation.[19] Inverted nipples arise as a result of failure of the underlying mesenchyme to proliferate, hindering nipple eversion.

Inverted nipples merit surgical correction. The Namba surgical technique involves three simple half-Z-plasties to elongate the nipple in conjunction with a tightening of the nipple base to evert the nipple. This technique spares the duct system and does not add any additional bulk to the nipple.[20] A less invasive technique, which has even been used in women in their third trimester of pregnancy, involves the use of nipple piercing devices.[21]

Malformations of the breast

Amastia

Amastia is defined as complete absence of the breast and may present unilaterally or bilaterally. This is a very rare condition with a five-fold female predominance. Trier[22] reported only 43 cases over a 126-year period. At birth, it presents with complete absence of the breast and nipple–areola complex. At puberty, there is no breast development on the affected side, though other secondary sexual characteristics are not affected. Familial amastia has been observed in patterns of both autosomal dominant and recessive inheritance.[9,23] Cases of unilateral amastia are often associated with Poland syndrome.

Polymastia

Polymastia is defined by the presence of more than two breasts. Two patterns have been described: supernumerary breast and aberrant mammary tissue.[24] Of the supernumerary breasts, the incidence of a complete breast including a well-formed nipple–areola complex is less than one percent.[12] Polymastia may occur along the embryonic milk line or present as an ectopic breast.[25] Aberrant mammary tissue may contain ducts and lobules that are less organized than in normal breasts and do not have a nipple or areola (Fig. 19.2). It becomes clinically apparent only when there is associated pathology at the affected site.[24] Some problems associated with polymastia include discomfort, secretions, and psychological embarrassment.[9] Surgical correction is directed at excision of the aberrant tissue.

Gynecomastia

Gynecomastia is the growth of glandular breast tissue in males. The term stems from the Greek words *gyne* (female) and *mastos* (breast) which translates roughly into female-like breasts. This is a benign condition and accounts for 60% of all disorders of the male breast and 85% of male breast masses. It can present at any age, but 40% of patients present in adolescent boys aged 14–15.5 years. Approximately 40% of healthy men and 70% of hospitalized men have palpable breast tissue. By the seventh decade of life, approximately 60% of men have palpable breast tissue. Autopsy of military personnel have shown an incidence of gynecomastia in 30–55% of men.[26,27]

The main sex hormone in males, testosterone, is secreted by the testes, while the main sex hormone in females, estrogen, is secreted by the ovaries. However, both sex hormones are produced in the gonads of each sex. Estradiol stimulates breast tissue development while testosterone antagonizes this development. Gynecomastia is felt to arise when there is an imbalance of the androgen/estrogen ratio, although it is likely that multiple hormones play a role. Physiologic gynecomastia occurs commonly in both neonates secondary to transplacental estrogen effect, and, subsequently during puberty. In neonates, gynecomastia will revolve spontaneously in several weeks. In pubertal boys, most cases will resolve within 16–18 months. Prepubertal gynecomastia is much more rare and merits additional evaluation, including a search for chromosomal abnormalities, medications that induce gynecomastia, and endogenous endocrine abnormalities. In a small series of prepubertal boys with gynecomastia, the authors found that, in five of six boys affected, the breast contained neurofibromatosis, and in the remaining boy the affected breast had lymphangioma circumscriptum. Of the neurofibromatosis-associated gynecomastia, four (80%) boys were black, suggesting a racial predilection, and three (60%) had a unilateral presentation.

Gynecomastia may occur secondary to numerous concurrent conditions. These include primary testicular failure as found in Klinefelter's syndrome, and secondary testicular failure due to orchitis and mumps.[28] Endocrine diseases such as hypo- and hyperthyroidism and hypercortisemia can cause gynecomastia. Drugs associated with gynecomastia include anabolic steroids, cimetidene, haldol, opiates, marijuana, phenothiazines, spironolactone, tricyclic antidepressants, and exogenous estrogens. Liver disease including alcohol-induced cirrhosis is also associated with gynecomastia.

Evaluation for patients with gynecomastia should include blood, chromosomal and urine studies. Blood studies should include liver function tests, follicle-stimulating hormone, luteinizing hormone, human chorionic gonodatropin, thyroid-stimulating hormone, thyroxine, estrogen, estradiol, and testosterone. Chromosomal studies should include karyotype to screen for Klinefelter's and testicular feminization, while urine studies should screen for elevated estrogen and 17-ketosteroid levels which may indicate the presence of an adrenal tumor. Imaging studies such as ultrasound can also aid in assessing the testes and breasts. For the most part, gynecomastia is a benign condition without an increased incidence of breast cancer. In Klinefelter's syndrome, however, the incidence of cancer is at least 20 times greater than in the general male population.[29]

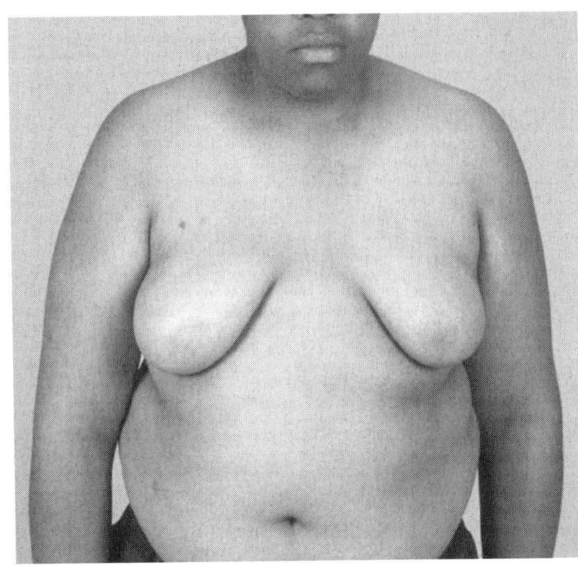

Fig. 19.3. 12-year-old boy with bilateral group 3 gynecomastia.

Several classification systems are used to describe gynecomastia. Webster[30] defines gynecomastia based on the presence of glandular breast tissue and/or adipose tissue. Type I gynecomastia is glandular alone; type II is both fatty and glandular; type III is fatty tissue alone. Simon *et al.*[31] used size as a means for classification. Group 1 patients have minimal yet visible breast enlargement. Group 2A has moderate breast enlargement without skin redundancy, whereas Group 2B has mild skin redundancy. Group 3 patients have gross breast enlargement with skin redundancy (Fig. 19.3). Histologically there are three recognized patterns in gynecomastia: florid, fibrous, and intermediate. The florid type has increased number and length of ducts, proliferation of ductal epithelium, periductal edema, a highly cellular fibroblastic stroma and hypervascularity, and formation of pseudolobules. The fibrous pattern differs from the florid type in that it has dilated ducts with minimal epithelial proliferation, an absence of periductal edema, and adipose tissue with an acellular fibrous stroma. The intermediate pattern is a combination of the florid and fibrous patterns. The florid pattern is more common for early onset of gynecomastia, of age less than 4 months; whereas the fibrous pattern is more common between age 4 and 12 months.

Treatment of gynecomastia depends on the severity of the condition and degree of psychosocial impact or embarrassment conferred upon the patient. In mild to moderate cases, observation is indicated for up to one year, since many undergo spontaneous regression. Additionally, medical management by withdrawal of an offending agent or by administering testosterone has been shown to help those with testicular failure. Other drugs such as tamoxifen, clomiphen, testolactone, and danazol have been tried with varying degrees of success.

Early reports by Paulas Aegineta [32] of reduction mammoplasty for treatment of gynecomastia date back to the seventh century; contemporary surgical treatment focuses on removal of the breast tissue and preservation of the normal breast contour while minimizing the scar. Though there are several surgical techniques to treat gynecomastia, they essentially entail a mastectomy with or without the aid of liposuction. For minimal to moderate gynecomastia, a periareolar incision can be used to access and excise the excess breast tissue. Through this incision, circumferential skin flaps are developed over the breast tissue down to the pectoral fascia and dissected free. It is important to preserve adequate soft tissue below the nipple–areola complex to avoid nipple retraction. In cases where there is significant adipose tissue, preliminary suction assisted lipectomy can be a useful means to smooth out the resection margin.[33] More contemporary techniques involve the use of liposuction alone[34,35] or ultrasound-assisted liposuction[36] to correct the breast deformity.

In more severe gynecomastia, both the excess breast tissue and skin require resection necessitating repositioning of the nipple–areola complex. Several techniques have been described including excising excess skin in a superior crescent excision, an elliptical excision described by Letterman and Schurter[37] with a resultant transverse or oblique chest wall scar; and the vertical reduction mastopexy described by LeJour.[38] In Letterman's technique, the nipple–areola complex is rotated superiorly and medially based on a pedicle consisting of dermis and breast parenchyma. LeJour's technique involves basing the nipple–areola complex on a superiorly-based pedicle. *En bloc* breast tissue and skin excision with free-nipple

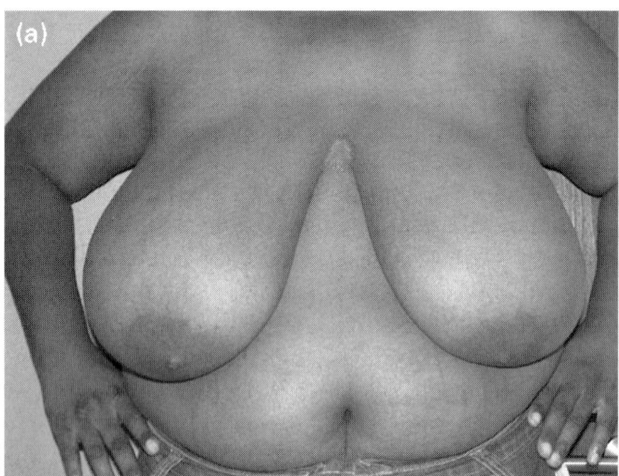

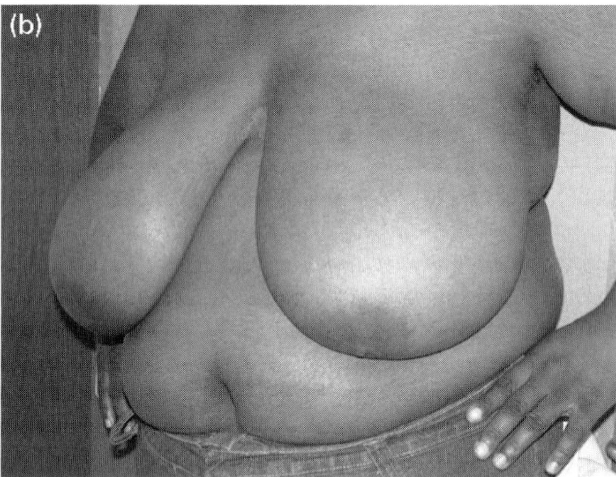

Fig. 19.4. (a), (b) 17-year-old girl with bilateral macromastia.

grafting may be necessary for massive gynecomastia. The latter techniques described for severe gynecomastia are essentially the same as those used in female breast reduction. Criticisms of these techniques when applied to male gynecomastia are that scars are placed on the chest, which are more difficult to hide in a male chest, and that the pedicle required to maintain the repositioned nipple–areola complex gives the appearance of a retained breast mound. Regardless of technique, postoperative compression garments will minimize hematoma formation. Activity restrictions should remain in place for several weeks, though normal activities of daily living can be resumed within days.

Macromastia

Whereas gynecomastia involves excess breast development in males, macromastia involves excess breast development in females, disproportional to other parts of the body (Fig. 19.4). More frequently, macromastia is seen and treated in the adult population, but can develop during puberty. Symptoms associated with macromastia include upper body pain, back pain, poor posture, and headache.[39] Like other breast disorders, there is also a strong psychological burden on body image. This can interfere with simple habits like buying clothes or participating in sports. Macromastia may present with unilateral or bilateral development. Unlike gynecomastia, spontaneous remission rarely occurs. The etiology is unclear, but may be caused by end-organ hypersensitivity during a period of intense endocrine regulatory stress and may also have an inherited component.[40] Obesity may accentuate both gynecomastia and macromastia. O'Hare and Frieden[41] report two cases of macromastia involving a 14-year-old with alpha (or) 1-antitrypsin deficiency and a 12-year-old with hyperthyroidism.

In adults, the recommended treatment is reduction mammoplasty. This treatment often results in significant symptomatic relief.[39,42] In adolescent girls, it is prudent to wait until the breast is mature before undergoing surgical treatment. If surgery is done too early in puberty, subsequent breast development may necessitate additional surgical correction. As described for the correction of severe gynecomastia, techniques for reduction mammoplasty involve repositioning of the nipple–areola complex based on an underlying pedicle consisting of breast parenchyma with or without an overlying strip of dermis, and excision of excess skin and breast tissue. These techniques usually result in a circumareolar scar, a vertical scar from the areola to the inframammary fold, and a scar along the inframammary fold. Whereas the circumareolar scar is well hidden, the remaining scars can be noticeable. Variations in technique have been proposed to avoid one or both of the latter scars. Depending on the amount of breast parenchyma retained beneath the nipple–areola complex, breast feeding may still be an option in these patients. In cases of very severe macromastia in which nipple perfusion may be difficult to preserve due to the length of pedicle that would be required, *en bloc* breast tissue and skin excision with free-nipple grafting remains an option. If the latter technique is chosen, patients should be informed that nipple sensation will be impaired, the nipple–areola complex may darken in color and that they will not be able to breastfeed after pregnancy.

Poland syndrome

Sir Alfred Poland,[43] as a medical student, described in Guy's Hospital Gazette a chest wall anomaly based on a cadaver dissection. He found an absence of the sternocostal portion of the pectoralis major muscle with an intact clavicular origin, an absent pectoralis minor, and hypoplastic serratus anterior and external oblique muscles. Poland syndrome is the most frequent etiology of congenital breast aplasia or hypoplasia (Fig. 19.5). Today, the classical features of Poland syndrome are defined by a spectrum of anomalies with varying degrees of severity. Muscular anomalies include absence of the sternal head of the pectoralis major and hypoplasia or aplasia of the pectoralis minor, serratus anterior external oblique, latissimus dorsi, infraspinatus, and/or supraspinatus muscles. Soft tissue anomalies include hypoplasia or aplasia of the breast or nipple and deficiency of subcutaneous fat and axillary hair. Bony abnormalities include the absence of

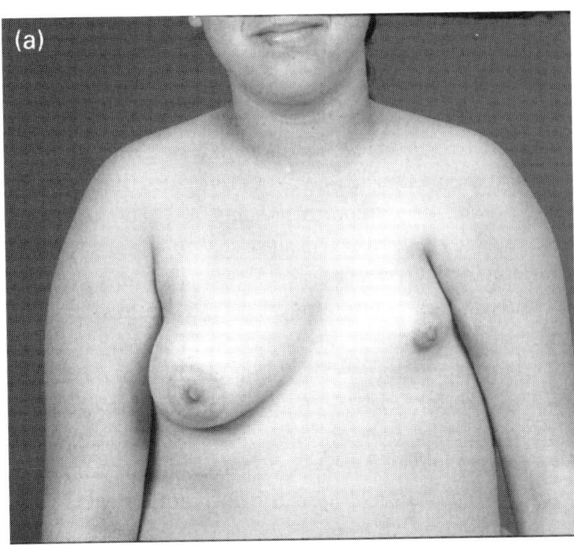

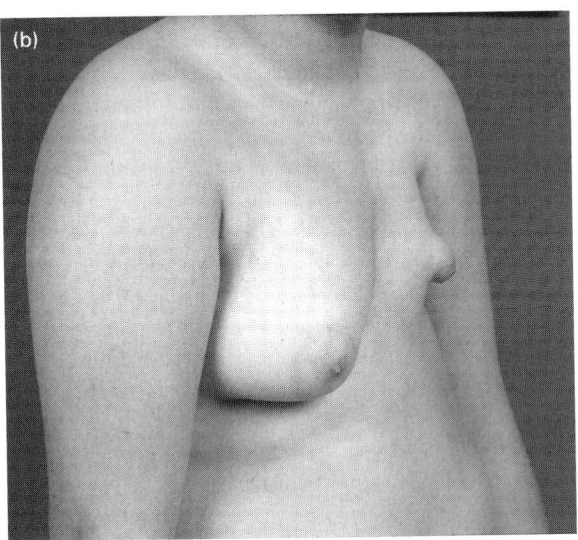

Fig. 19.5. (a), (b) 14-year-old girl with Poland syndrome.

the anterior chest wall with possible herniation of lung, and anomalies of the vertebral column or shoulder blade. Associated hand anomalies can include syndactyly, symbrachydactyly, and hypoplasia of the ipsilateral upper arm, forearm or fingers. Poland's original description did not mention breast hypoplasia or aplasia.[43] The incidence of Poland syndrome is approximately 1 in 30 000 live births with the right side affected more than the left. It is more common in males by a 3:1 ratio.[44] Although most cases are sporadic, there are some familial cases in which autosomal dominant transmission is reported.

It has been hypothesized that a vascular event during the sixth week of gestation, with hypoplasia of the subclavian artery, may be the etiology of Poland syndrome. This event, known as subclavian artery supply disruption sequence, coincides with the medial and forward growth of the ribs forcing the subclavian vessel into a U-shaped configuration. Interruption of the subclavian artery proximal to the origin of the internal mammary and distal to the origin of the vertebral artery leads to Poland's anomaly.[45] Several mechanisms may lead to the disruption of the subclavian artery including edema, hemorrhage, cervical rib, aberrant musculature, amniotic band, intrauterine compression or tumor.[46] Similar subclavian artery disruptions may also cause other syndromes including Mobius and Klippel–Feil syndromes.[46,47] The higher incidence of right-sided anomalies and relatively high associations of dextrocardia and left-sided anomalies also support a vascular etiology of Poland syndrome, since the embryologic development of the aortic arch and subclavian arteries are asymmetric.[45,48]

Spear *et al.*[49] recently described another clinical entity with similar features as Poland syndrome in which there is unilateral posterior depression of the third through seventh anterior ribs and hypoplasia of the breast. However, these authors reported the pectoralis muscles to be completely normal. At surgery, the presence of the sternal head of the pectoralis major muscle was confirmed. This clinical disorder was called anterior thoracic hypoplasia; and like Poland syndrome, the authors also found a higher preponderance of right-sided involvement.[49]

Although there is a threefold increased incidence of Poland syndrome in males, males with less severe anomalies often do not seek treatment. Some boys may find the absence of the pectoralis muscles particularly distressing, and there are reports of using the ipsilateral latissimus dorsi muscle to repair this defect.[50–52] In girls, the reconstruction is more challenging, especially in the setting of the growing breast. Definitive reconstruction is usually reserved until the age of 18 or 19 years when the breast has fully matured. During the pubertal years, a tissue expander may be used to provide some semblance of symmetry during breast development. The latissimus dorsi muscle can be used in conjunction with a tissue expander if there is inadequate subcutaneous tissue coverage, or to reconstruct the anterior axillary fold in the absence of the pectoralis muscle. The tissue expander is later exchanged for a permanent breast implant when the contralateral breast is fully mature. If the latissimus dorsi muscle is hypoplastic, then the use of rectus abdominis muscle flaps has been described.[53] A free autologous tissue transfer using the gluteus maximus muscle has also been described, obviating the need for a prosthetic device.[54] Other microvascular free flaps which have been used in Poland syndrome include the rectus abdominis, superior gluteal, inferior gluteal and the contralateral latissimus dorsi flap.[48] It may be warranted to avoid the rectus abdominis flap in patients who intend to become pregnant. The specific free flap choice depends largely on the body habitus, degree of chest deformity, and breast asymmetry. To achieve symmetry, the contralateral breast may require reduction mammoplasty, mastopexy, or augmentation.

Tuberous breast

The tuberous breast was first described in 1976 by Rees and Aston,[55] and in the same year Vecchione[56] described this as a "domed nipple." The tuberous breast results from a deformity involving the nipple–areola complex. A constricting ring around the base of the breast causes narrowing of the mammary base and herniation of the hypoplastic breast tissue into the areola, resulting in hypertrophy of the nipple–areola complex.[57] The tuberous breast is first recognized during puberty and can affect one or both breasts (Fig. 19.6). The exact incidence has not been properly investigated, although it is believed to be rare.[58,59]

During breast development, the breast tissue is contained within a fascial envelope, which is continuous with Camper's fascia and consists of a deep and superficial layer of the superficial fascia. The deep layer forms the posterior boundary of the breast parenchyma, and lies superficial to the pectoralis and serratus anterior fascia. The superficial layer covers the breast parenchyma. In the tuberous breast, the superficial layer of the superficial fascia is absent in the region under the nipple–areola complex and hence allows herniation of the mammary bud in the mesenchyme. Clinically, this correlates with a constricting ring of dense fibrous tissue around the periphery of the areola. This prevents the normal breast from expanding inferiorly and peripherally during puberty and causes the breast tissue to herniate superficially and expand the nipple–areola complex.[57,60,61]

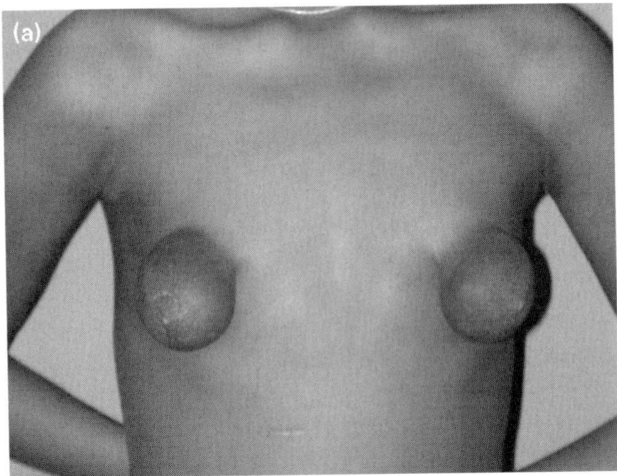

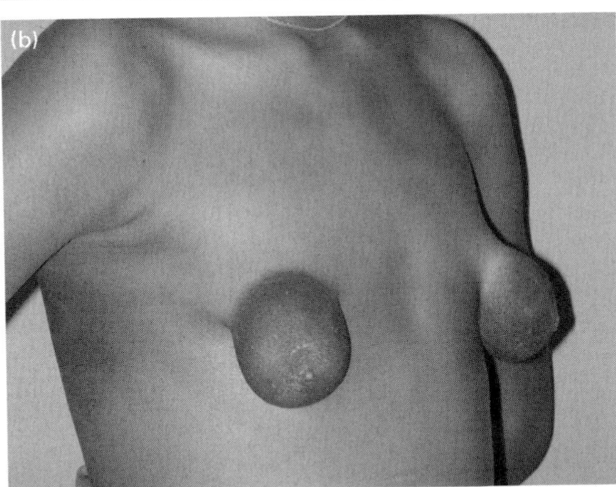

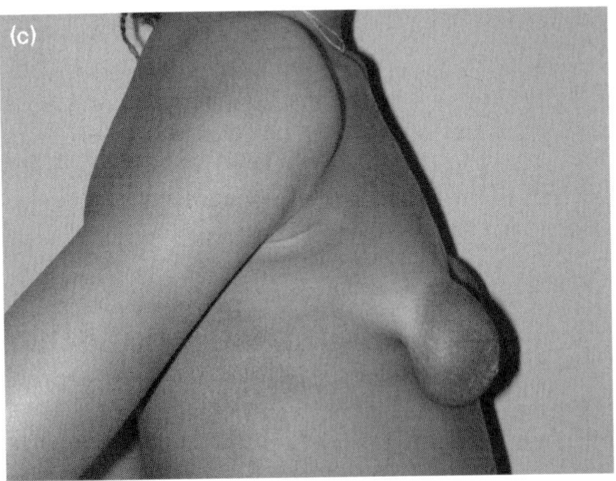

Fig. 19.6. (a) (b)–(c) 13-year-old girl with bilateral tuberous breasts.

Grolleau *et al.*[61] have developed a classification system in which a deficiency of breast parenchyma in lower medial quadrant is defined as type I. Deficiency of both medial and lateral lower quadrants with the areola pointing downwards is classified as type II. Involvement of all four quadrants with both vertical and horizontal constriction is classified as type III.

Surgical correction of the tuberous breast depends on whether there is unilateral or bilateral involvement, whether the affected breast is type I, II or III, the breast volume present, the degree of asymmetry between the two breasts, and size of the nipple–areola complex. Surgical goals include re-sizing of the areola, repositioning of the inframammary fold, and achieving comparable volume and breast symmetry. In patients who are more concerned with surgical scar than with breast size, Rebiero *et al.*[60] have described a one-stage operation without the use of a prosthetic device. They use a periareolar incision and develop an inferiorly based flap, using the medial and lateral extensions to disrupt the constricting ring that caused the initial herniation. The inferior flap is then folded on itself to allow for greater breast projection.[60] Mandrekas *et al.*[57] described a similar technique in which the constricting ring at the base of the breast is disrupted at the six o'clock position, creating two pillars at the inferior portion of the breast. The two pillars are then loosely approximated or folded over one another to achieve breast projection at the inferior portion of the breast. In some cases implants are utilized when additional breast volume is desired. Symmetry may be achieved with the adjunct of a reduction mammoplasty or prosthetic augmentation of the contralateral breast.[57,61,62]

Conclusions

This chapter has described several congenital malformations of the breast. Although these are all benign malformations, they cause significant social embarrassment to the patient, especially during puberty. Early diagnosis and proper surgical reconstruction can provide a valuable service to these patients. Whereas the simplest of these malformations can be treated with simple excision, such as in polythelia, more complex deformities, such as the tuberous breast, warrant referral to a surgeon with experience in breast reconstruction.

REFERENCES

1. Osin, P. P., Anbazhagan, R., Bartkova, J., Nathan, B., & Gusterson, B. A. Breast development gives insights into breast disease. *Histopathology* 1998; **33**:275–283.
2. Schmidt, I. M., Chellakooty, M., Haavisto, A.-M. *et al.* Gender difference in breast tissue size in infancy: correlation with serum estradiol. *Pediatr. Res.* 2002; **52**:682–686.

3. Huffman, J. W., Dewhurst, C. J., & Caprano, V. J. (eds.) *The Gynecology of Childhood and Adolescence.* 2nd edn. Philadelphia: W. B. Saunders Co., 1981.
4. Mehes, K. Association of supernumerary nipples with other anomalies. *J. Pediatr. Surg.* 1979; **95**:274–275.
5. Rahbar, F. Clinical significance of supernumerary nipples in black neonates. *Clin. Pediatr.* 1982; **21**:46–47.
6. Mimouni, F., Merlob, P., & Reisner, S. H. Occurence of supernumerary nipples in newborns. *Am. J. Dis. Child.* 1983; **137**:952–953.
7. Jaber, L. & Merlob, P. The prevalence of supernumerary nipples in Arab infants and children. *Eur. J. Pediatr.* 1988; **147**:443.
8. Schmidt, H. Supernumerary nipples: prevalence, size, sex and side predilection – a prospective clinical study. *Eur. J. Pediatr.* 1998; **157**:821–823.
9. Merlob, P. Congenital malformation and developmental changes of the breast: a neonatological view. *J. Pediatr. Endocrinol. Metab.* 2003; **16**:471–485.
10. Leung, A. K. & Robson, W. L. Polythelia. *Int. J. Dermatol.* 1989; **28**:429–433.
11. Armoni, M., Filk, D., Schlesinger, M., Pollak, S., & Metzker, A. Accessory nipples: any relationship to urinary tract malformation? *Pediatr. Dermatol.* 1992; **9**:239–240.
12. Hanson, E. & Segovia, J. Dorsal supernumerary breast. Case report. *Plast. Reconstr. Surg.* 1978; **61**:441–445.
13. Schewach-Millet, M. & Fisher, B. K. Supernumerary nipple on the shoulder. *Cutis* 1976; **17**:384–385.
14. Toumbis-Joannou, E. & Cohen, P. R. Familial polythelia. *J. Am. Acad. Dermatol.* 1994; **30**:667–668.
15. Urbani, C. E. & Betti, R. Sporadic unilateral intra-areolar polythelia. *Acta. Dermatol. Venerol.* 1996; **76**:156.
16. Shewnake, S. W. & Izuno, G. T. *Supernumerary areolae. Arch. Dermatol.* 1977; **113**:823–825.
17. Schwager, R. C., Smith, J. W., Gray, G. F., & Goulian, D. J. Inversion of the human female nipple, with a simple method of treatment. *Plast. Reconstr. Surg.* 1984; **54**:164–168.
18. Park, H. S., Yoon, C. H., & Kim, H. J. The prevalence of congenital inverted nipples. *Aesth. Plast. Surg.* 1999; **23**:144–146.
19. Shafir, R., Bonne-Tamir, B., Ashbel, S., Tsur, H., & Goodman, R. M. Genetic studies in a family with inverted nipples (mammillae invertita). *Clin. Genet.* 1979; **15**:346–350.
20. Lee, K. Y. & Cho, B. C. Surgical correction of inverted nipples using the modified Namba or Teimourian technique. *Plast. Reconstr. Surg.* 2004; **113**:328–336.
21. Scholten, E. A contemporary correction of inverted nipples. *Plast. Reconstr. Surg.* 2001; **107**:551–513.
22. Trier, W. C. Complete breast absence: case report and report of literature. *Plast. Reconstr. Surg.* 1965; **36**:431–439.
23. Tawil, H. M. & Najjar, S. S. Congenital absence of the breasts. *J. Pedriatr.* 1968; **73**:751–753.
24. Rosen, P. P. *Rosen's Breast Pathology.* 2nd edn. Philadelphia: Lippincott Williams & Wilkins, 2001.
25. Leung, W., Heaton, J. P. W., & Morales, A. An uncommon urologic presentation of a supernumerary breast. *Urology* 1997; **50**:122–124.
26. Carlson, H. E. Gynecomastia. *N. Engl. J. Med.* 1980; **303**:795–759.
27. Anderson, J. A. & Gram, J. B. Male breast at autopsy. *Acta. Pathol. Microbiol. Immunol. Scand.* 1982; **90**:191–197.
28. McGrath, M. H. *Gynecomastia.* St. Louis: CV Mosby, 1990.
29. Scheike, O., Visfeldt, J., & Petersen, B. Male breast cancer. 3. Breast carcinoma in association with the Klinefelter syndrome. *Acta Pathol. Microbiol. Immunol. Scand.* 1973; **81**:352–358.
30. Webster, G. V. Gynecomastia in the Navy. *Milit. Surg.* 1944; **95**:375–379.
31. Simon, B. E., Hoffman, S., & Kahn, S. Classification and surgical correction of gynecomastia. *Plast. Reconstr. Surg.* 1973; **51**:48–52.
32. Gurunluoglu, R. & Gurunluoglu, A. Paulus Aegineta, a seventh century encyclopedist and surgeon: his role in the history of plastic surgery. *Plast. Reconstr. Surg.* 2001; **108**:2072–2079.
33. Teimourian, B. & Pearlman, R. Surgery for gynecomastia. *Aesth. Plast. Surg.* 1983; **7**:155–157.
34. Courtiss, E. H. Gynecomastia: analysis of 159 patients and current recommendations for treatment. *Plast. Reconstr. Surg.* 1987; **79**:740–753.
35. Rosenberg, G. J. Gynecomastia: suction lipectomy as a contemporary solution. *Plast. Reconstr. Surg.* 1987; **80**:379–386.
36. Rohrich, R. J., Ha, R. Y., Kenkel, J. M., & Adams, W. P. Jr. Classification and management of gynecomastia: defining the role of ultrasound-assisted liposuction. *Plast. Reconstr. Surg.* 2003; **111**:909–923.
37. Letterman, G. & Schurter, M. *Gynecomastia.* St Louis: CV Mosby, 1982.
38. LeJour, M. Vertical mammaplasty and liposuction of the breast. *Plast. Reconstr. Surg.* 1994; **94**:100–114.
39. Blomqvist, L., Eriksson, A., & Brandberg, Y. Reduction mammaplasty provides long-term improvement in health status and quality of life. *Plast. Reconstr. Surg.* 2000; **106**:991–997.
40. Corriveau, S. & Jacobs, J. S. Macromastia in adolescence. *Clin. Plast. Surg.* 1990; **17**:151–160.
41. O'Hare, P. M. & Frieden, I. J. Virginal breast hypertrophy. *Pediatr. Dermatol.* 2000; **17**:277–281.
42. Collins, E. D., Carolyn, L. K., Kim, M. *et al.* The effectiveness of surgical and nonsurgical interventions in relieving the symptoms of macromastia. *Plast. Reconstr. Surg.* 2002; **109**:1556–1566.
43. Poland, A. Deficiency of the pectoral muscles. *Guys Hosp. Rep.* 1841; **6**:191.
44. DerKaloustia, V. M., Hoyme, H. E., Hogg, H., Entin, M. A. & Guttmacher, A. E. Possible common pathogenetic mechanisms for Poland sequence and Adams-Oliver syndrome. *Am. J. Med. Gen.* 1991; **38**:69–73.
45. Bouvert, J-P, Leveque, D., Bernetieres, F., & Gros, J. J. Vascular origin of Poland syndrome? A comparative rheographic study of the vascularization of the arms in eight patients. *Eur. J. Pediatr.* 1978; **128**:17–26.
46. Bavinck, J. N. B. & Weaver, D. D. Subclavian artery supply disruption sequence: hypothesis of a vascular etiology for Poland,

Klippel–Feil, and Mobius anomalies. *Am. J. Med. Genet.* 1986; **23**:903.

47. Issaivanan, M., Virdi, V. S., & Parmar, V. R. Subclavian artery supply disruption sequence–Klippel–Feil and Mobius anomalies. *Ind. J. Pediatr.* 2002; **65**:441–442.
48. Longaker, M. T., Glat, P. M., Colen, L. B., & Siebert, J. W. Reconstruction of breast asymmetry in Poland's chest-wall deformity using microvascular free flaps. *Plast. Reconstr. Surg.* 1997; **99**:429–436.
49. Spear, S. L., Pelletiere, C. V., Lee, E. S., & Grotting, J. C. Anterior thoracic hypoplasia: a separate entity from Poland syndrome. *Plast. Reconstr. Surg.* 2004; **113**:69–77.
50. Hester, T. R. J. & Bostwick, J.3rd. Poland's syndrome: correction with latissimus muscle transposition. *Plast. Reconstr. Surg.* 1982; **69**:226–233.
51. Ohmori, K. & Takada, H. Correction of Poland's pectoralis major muscle anomaly with latissimus dorsi musculocutaneous flaps. *Plast. Reconstr. Surg.* 1980; **65**:400–404.
52. Corso, P. F. Plastic surgery for the unilateral hypoplastic breast. A report of eight cases. *Plast. Reconstr. Surg.* 1972; **50**:134–141.
53. Mestak, J., Zadorozna, M., & Cakrtova, M. Breast reconstruction in women with Poland's syndrome. *Acta Chir. Plast.* 1991; **33**:137–144.
54. Fujino, T., Harashina, T., & Aoyagi, F. Reconstruction for aplasia of the breast and pectoral region by microvascular transfer of a free flap from the buttock. *Plast. Reconstr. Surg.* 1975; **56**:178–181.
55. Rees, T. D. & Aston, S. The tuberous breast. *Clin. Plast. Surg.* 1976; **3**:339–347.
56. Vecchione, T. R. A method for recontouring the domed nipple. *Plast. Reconstr. Surg.* 1976; **57**:30–32.
57. Mandrekas, A. D., Zambacos, G. J., Anastasopoulos, A., Hapsas, D., Lambrinaki, N., & Ioannidou-Mouzaka, L. Aesthetic reconstruction of the tuberous breast deformity. *Plast. Reconstr. Surg.* 2003; **112**:1099–1108.
58. Toranto, I. R. Two-stage correction of tuberous breast. *Plast. Reconstr. Surg.* 1981; **67**:642–646.
59. Atiyeh, B. S., Hashim, H. A., El-Douaihy, Y., & Kayle, D. I. Perinipple round-block technique for correction of tuberous/tubular breast deformity. *Aesth. Plast. Surg.* 1998; **22**:284–288.
60. Ribeiro, L., Canzi, W., Buss, A. Jr., & Accorsi, A. Jr. Tuberous breast: a new approach. *Plast. Reconstr. Surg.* 1998; **101**:42–50.
61. Grolleau, J. L., Lanfrey, E., Lavigne, B., Chavoin, J. P., & Costagliola, M. Breast base anomalies: treatment strategy for tuberous breasts, minor deformities, and asymmetry. *Plast. Reconstr. Surg.* 1999; **104**:2040–2048.
62. Puckett, C. L. & Concannon, M. J. Augmenting the narrow-based breast: the unfurling technique to prevent the double-bubble deformity. *Aesth. Plast. Surg.* 1990; **14**:15–19.

Part IV

Abdomen

20

Abdominal surgery: general aspects

Mark D. Stringer

Children's Liver and GI Unit, St James's University Hospital, Leeds, UK

Introduction

The morbidity and mortality of abdominal surgery in infants and children continues to decline. This is partly due to overall socioeconomic progress and general improvements in health. Medical advances such as more effective antimicrobial therapy, better imaging techniques, progress in surgery and anesthesia, and improved nutritional care have also contributed. Other less obvious factors which may have contributed to improved long-term outcomes in children undergoing abdominal surgery include the development of specialist training programs and accreditation systems, and the regulation of operative procedures, equipment, and standards of care. However, medical advances have also generated new challenges: managing the problems of children with congenital and acquired conditions who would previously have died; greater societal expectations and demands; and iatrogenic complications.

This chapter has two main aims: first, to stress the importance of studying long-term outcomes in pediatric surgery and, second, to consider some of the general long-term issues of abdominal surgery in children.

Long-term outcomes

Mortality and postoperative morbidity are traditional and essential outcome measures in pediatric surgery but long-term results and quality of life issues – physical, psychological and social – are becoming increasingly important to parents, surgeons, and health economists.

Why are long-term outcomes important in pediatric surgery?

(i) To inform parents (and patients) about future health expectations.

(ii) To anticipate potential long-term complications that might be avoidable by monitoring and timely intervention, e.g., renal impairment secondary to neurogenic bladder in spinal dysraphism.

(iii) To guide current surgical practice, e.g., the long-term life-threatening consequences of choledochocystojejunostomy for congenital choledochal dilatation have caused it to be replaced by radical excision of the extrahepatic bile ducts and hepaticoenterostomy.

(iv) To provide information on when to operate, e.g., the optimum time to perform an orchidopexy or repair an anorectal malformation. Neonatal repair of anorectal anomalies may facilitate earlier development of neural pathways between the anorectum and the developing brain, thereby improving subsequent bowel control;[1]

(v) . . . . and when not to operate, e.g., the natural history of conditions such as gastroesophageal reflux, vesicoureteric reflux, and some antenatally diagnosed structural abnormalities can only be defined by careful longitudinal follow-up studies. Only when the natural history is clear, can we be confident about who needs surgical intervention.

Why are there so few long-term outcome studies in pediatric surgery?

The definition of long-term outcome is variable. Strictly, it means outcome at maturity, i.e., during adulthood. In

Pediatric Surgery and Urology: Long-term Outcomes, Mark Stringer, Keith Oldham, Pierre Mouriquand.
Published by Cambridge University Press.

Table 20.1. Factors influencing functional long-term outcomes after repair of an anorectal malformation[3]

- Type of malformation (this demands a practical, clinical classification)
- Sex
- Age at diagnosis
- Sacral/spinal defects
- Other associated anomalies
- Type and timing of surgery
- Internal sphincter preservation
- Surgical complications
- Evaluation: methods, age of patient, independence of assessor
- Psychosocial and cognitive factors

practice, the paucity of available data encourages the use of relatively short-term results as surrogate measures of long-term outcomes. In many instances we currently have to depend on follow-up studies that extend over several years only.

Information on long-term outcomes is difficult to obtain. Studies require meticulous data collection over many years and the cooperation of patients who may already feel over exposed to medical facilities. Studies are hampered by poor continuity of patient care (which, in turn, is encouraged by overstretched health care systems), and a mobile patient population. There is often no clearly defined pathway for pediatric surgical patients once they become adults and they may become lost to follow-up. Their care may become fragmented and taken over by specialists who are unfamiliar with the congenital malformation and its treatment. Ideally, there should be arrangements for providing seamless care through adolescence and beyond for children with complex surgical problems. In some countries, children with conditions such as congenital heart disease and cystic fibrosis are managed in this way.[2] This approach would encourage the study of long-term outcomes.

Various methodologic problems hamper the study of long-term outcomes.

- It can be difficult to evaluate the long-term impact of a single intervention in pediatric surgery because (a) surgical outcomes are the result of multiple interdependent factors, not simply those related to the operation, and (b) many changes in practice occur over time.
- Comparing outcomes between centers may be hindered by different methods of classification and assessment. The number of variables affecting the long-term outcome of a condition can be large; long-term studies must include sufficient information about these descriptors in order to interpret the data. Table 20.1 illustrates some of the many variables that influence the long-term outcome of infants with an anorectal malformation (*see chapter on Anorectal Malformations*).
- Normative data from control subjects is frequently difficult to obtain, especially when investigating continence, sexuality and fertility.
- Ascertainment bias is a significant hazard when selecting individuals for investigation; willingness to participate in follow-up studies may reflect a hidden bias.
- Relatively few clinical interventions and treatments in pediatric surgery are supported by adequately powered, randomized controlled trials (category I evidence).[4,5] If the evidence-base for a particular surgical technique is weak,[6] this will undermine any subsequent analysis of its long-term outcome.
- Quality of life assessments and economic studies require specialist techniques not readily available to most pediatric surgeons.

Are there common themes in the evaluation of long-term outcomes in pediatric surgery?

Common themes repeatedly emerge in the assessment of long-term outcomes. As well as disease/operation specific consequences (and in newborns, gestation/birthweight-specific consequences), long-term issues that typically arise include: growth and nutrition; psychosocial and cognitive development; risk of malignancy; effects on sexuality and fertility; genetic aspects; quality of life concerns; and medicolegal considerations.

Categorization of long-term outcomes in pediatric surgery

Long-term outcomes may relate to the condition itself, to its surgical treatment, or both. Four broad categories exist. First, there are a few conditions with almost no long-term sequelae. For example, small cutaneous hemangiomas on the trunk and small, simple parenchymal cysts in the spleen or liver appear to have no practical long-term effects. Second, there are conditions with variable sequelae; these constitute the largest group and include most major congenital malformations. Third, there are pediatric surgical conditions that may present for the first time in adult life. Intestinal malrotation[7] and Hirschsprung's disease[8] are examples. Finally, there are pediatric surgical conditions or interventions which currently have unknown long-term consequences. For example, developmental delay is relatively common after extracorporeal membrane oxygenation for diaphragmatic hernia[9] but the implications of this for adult life are unknown. The potential problems during pregnancy and childbirth after neonatal repair of an anorectal malformation or excision of a sacrococcygeal teratoma are poorly understood. The prion mediated neurodegenerative brain disease, variant Creutzfeldt–Jakob disease, is now known to be transmissible by blood transfusion or surgical instruments but the magnitude of this risk in pediatric surgery is unknown.[10]

Pediatric abdominal surgery

Surgical techniques

In adults, mass closure of the abdomen is associated with fewer wound complications (category Ia evidence).[11] In infants and children, abdominal wounds can be safely closed with absorbable sutures using either a layered or mass closure technique.[12] Non-absorbable sutures may occasionally be necessary, such as in the malnourished adolescent on steroids undergoing surgery for inflammatory bowel disease. Wound dehiscence is rare and usually due to poor surgical technique. The wound infection rate in clean pediatric surgical operations is about 3% but significantly higher after contaminated procedures.[13]

The use of interrupted, single layer, extramucosal sutures for intestinal anastomosis is highly effective in both small and large bowel surgery, resulting in few anastomotic leaks or strictures.[14] Improved suture materials, particularly monofilament sutures such as non-absorbable prolene and absorbable polydioxanone, have largely replaced traditional materials such as silk and catgut. In the surgery of esophageal atresia, the use of polyglycolic acid or prolene sutures in preference to silk results in fewer anastomotic complications.[15]

The development and application of surgical stapling devices has had a major impact on pediatric gastrointestinal surgery. The prototypes of these instruments originated in Russia in the 1950s and included both linear and circular anastomotic staplers. American manufacturers subsequently created lighter, disposable instruments with preloaded, sterilized cartridges.[16] The Duhamel operation for Hirschsprung's disease and ileo-anal pouch construction are just two procedures that have been revolutionized by the application of stapling instruments.

In addition to improved suture materials and surgical instruments, surgical techniques have advanced as a result of the introduction of magnification loupes which permit greater accuracy, particularly in neonatal surgery. Technologic progress has encouraged the development of definitive operations in the newborn such as primary pull-through procedures for Hirschsprung's disease, which may ultimately lead to better long-term outcomes.

The most recent technical revolution in pediatric abdominal surgery has been the development of therapeutic laparoscopy. Although previously established as a diagnostic tool in children, only in the last 15 years have appropriate instruments and techniques been devised to permit safe and reliable laparoscopic operations in children. Almost all abdominal operations can now be performed using minimal access surgery, including many neonatal procedures. There are clear short-term gains in terms of speed of recovery, postoperative pain, and cosmesis but the impact of these techniques on long-term functional outcomes have, with few exceptions, yet to be evaluated.

Scars

Provided safe operative access is assured, cosmesis is a key consideration when planning the site, extent, and method of closure of a surgical incision. If possible, incisions should be sited in skin creases and closed without tension using fine absorbable monofilament subcuticular sutures or subcutaneous sutures and adhesive tapes/glue. Scarpa's fascia should be sutured to avoid the skin becoming tethered to the underlying rectus sheath or muscle layers in patients with little subcutaneous fat. Scar migration may occur with future growth, e.g., scars located just below the costal margin in infants tend to migrate upwards.

Skin scarring can have physical, esthetic, psychologic and social consequences.[17] The psychosocial sequelae of surgical and traumatic scars are not simply related to the severity, size, or location of scarring.[18] Distress from a scar cannot be accurately predicted by the surgeon but depends on how self-conscious the patient feels. Little is known about children's perception of their surgical scars, particularly as they reach maturity. In one long-term analysis of 23 gastroschisis survivors with a median age of 16 years, the abdominal scar *per se* had caused few problems (in contrast to the absence of an umbilicus which was a source of considerable distress).[19] Cosmetic concerns are likely to become more important in the future. This will encourage wider adoption of minimal access surgery and more cosmetic incisions, e.g., circumumbilical pyloromyotomy.[20]

Abnormal scars occasionally mar the long-term result of otherwise successful abdominal surgery in children. These scars may be stretched, hypertrophic (remaining confined to the area of the initial wound and increasing in size by pushing out the margins of the scar), or keloid (a raised scar spreading beyond the margins of the original wound and progressively invading surrounding normal skin). Risk factors include: race, particularly African descent; age, the risk being greatest in adolescents and young adults; site, particularly the sternal and deltoid areas, the back, ears and neck; and type of incision, the risk being greater across lines of election. Many scars take 2 years to pale and fully mature and invasive treatments should be avoided in most cases for a year. Stretched scars may be improved by revisional surgery. Hypertrophic scars tend to slowly regress but this process may be facilitated by the use of pressure garments or the application of silicone gel sheeting. Keloids remain elevated and unsightly, and almost invariably recur after simple excision, unless this is combined with intralesional corticosteroids[17] or postoperative, single-fraction radiotherapy.[21] Other therapies have insufficient evidence to recommend them at present.[22]

Significant advances in our understanding of wound healing and scar formation have come from studies of fetal wound healing, where scarless skin healing is known to occur *(see chapter on Fetal Surgery)*.[23] Transforming growth factor β plays a central role in wound healing. Various manipulations of this cytokine are under evaluation in clinical trials in an effort to reduce skin scarring in response to surgery or trauma.

Incisional hernia

An incisional hernia in the abdominal wall occurs in 5–7% of adults after major laparotomy.[24] Recognized risk factors include obesity, long incisions, abdominal distension, respiratory complications and wound sepsis.[25] Left untreated, these hernias often progressively increase in size. There is limited information on the incidence and outcome of incisional hernias in infants and children. Peritoneal dialysis is known to be a potent cause.[26] Kiely and Spitz (1985) found only four cases of incisional hernia after 507 laparotomies in children and all four healed spontaneously within 4 months.[12] In an animal model, Tsui and Ellis (1991) found evidence of spontaneous healing of incisional hernias in infant rats but not in adult animals, but late recurrence developed in some.[24] A conservative approach to asymptomatic incisional hernias in infants appears reasonable but may not be justified in the older child. Ventral hernias following repair of abdominal wall defects are considered elsewhere *(see chapter on Abdominal Wall Defects)*.

Incisional hernia is also a rare complication of laparoscopic surgery. They generally occur through trocar sites of 10 mm or more in size but have been described at 5 mm port sites in infants.[27] They can be prevented by closing the incisions at fascial level.

Postoperative intra-abdominal adhesions

Mechanism of formation

The parietal and visceral peritoneum consists of a single continuous layer of mesothelial cells supported by a basement membrane overlying loose connective tissue; it possesses excellent regenerative properties. After injury, healing takes place by migration of phagocytes, principally macrophages, which are then "replaced" by new mesothelium within 3–7 days (Fig. 20.1). Unlike skin repair, the peritoneal defect becomes epithelialized throughout and not just from its margins. The inflammatory response to peritoneal injury leads to the release of a fibrin-rich serous exudate, which causes the formation of fibrinous adhesions within hours. Plasminogen activator released from mesothelial cells results in the conversion of plasminogen to plasmin, which in turn causes fibrinolysis and the removal of this fibrin matrix. Peritoneal trauma and infection not only reduce the release of plasminogen activator from mesothelial cells but also prompt the release of plasminogen activator inhibitors.[28] The net balance is the deposition of a fibrin matrix, which is gradually replaced by vascular granulation tissue containing fibroblasts which lay down collagen.

The most potent stimulus for the development of adhesions is peritoneal trauma, particularly from ischemia, inflammation or foreign bodies (e.g., surgical glove powder, lint from gauze swabs, or suture material). Genetic or constitutional factors may play a role in determining the severity of adhesions.[29] Adhesions are to some extent beneficial since they encourage neovascularization after injury but they are also a major source of surgical morbidity.

Incidence

Between one- and two-thirds of all intestinal obstructions in *adults* are due to peritoneal adhesions.[28,30] A study of all patients who underwent open abdominal or pelvic surgery in Scotland in 1986 revealed that 5.7% were readmitted with complications from adhesions during a 10-year follow-up period, and 3.8% required surgery.[30] Twenty two percent of these readmissions occurred within a year of the initial surgery, but the remainder were distributed throughout the 10-year period.

The vast majority of adhesions are a result of preceding operations rather than inflammatory or congenital in origin. Symptomatic adhesions are a distressing problem for the patient, family and surgeon, even more so because their occurrence is unpredictable and difficult to prevent. Not only is there significant mortality and morbidity from adhesive bowel obstruction but the problem is also a major economic burden. A United States study of 1988 data calculated that $1.2 billion of expenditure resulted from hospitalizations during which adhesiolysis was performed.[31]

The incidence of adhesive intestinal obstruction in children has been underestimated in many reports for two main reasons. First, only patients requiring reoperation

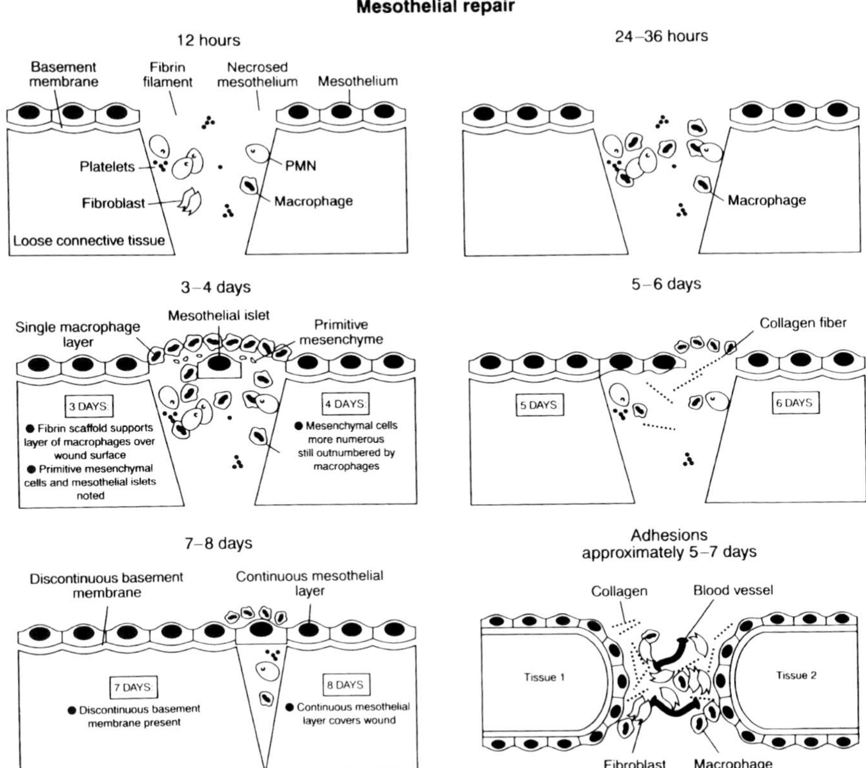

Fig. 20.1. Proposed sequence of events involved in mesothelial repair of the peritoneum. Reproduced by kind permission of Genzyme BV and Gardiner-Caldwell Communications Ltd, Cheshire, UK.

have been included in most studies, but many episodes of adhesive obstruction settle spontaneously. In one series from Toronto, 131 infants and children had adhesive small bowel obstruction proven at laparotomy or autopsy but during the same 12-year period there were another 207 patients who had clinical and/or radiologic signs of obstruction which resolved with conservative measures.[32] Second, studies of adhesive bowel obstruction in childhood have been limited to relatively short follow-up periods and yet we know that postsurgical adhesions may cause obstruction 30 or more years after abdominal surgery.[28]

In a study of 1476 abdominal operations in children spanning an 11-year period, adhesive small bowel obstruction requiring reoperation complicated 2.1% of all laparotomies; 80% of episodes developed within three months of surgery.[33] In another series with a similar follow-up period, two-thirds of obstructions occurred within 6 months of the original laparotomy.[32] In a recent analysis of children under 16 years who underwent abdominal surgery in Scotland in the year 1996–97, 1.1% of 1581 cases required readmission within four years because of adhesions.[34] The incidence of reoperation for adhesions was highest in the first year after surgery but remained significant during the subsequent 3 years. Risk factors for adhesive obstruction include multiple operations, peritonitis, and prolonged postoperative ileus.[33,35,36] In Festen's study, a single band adhesion was responsible for more than two-thirds of cases.[33] No recurrent episode of adhesive small bowel obstruction requiring surgery was documented in the latter study but in other series this occurs in 5–15% of cases.[32,37–39]

Of 649 neonates undergoing laparotomy in a 10-year period at the Hospital for Sick Children, London, 54 (8.3%) developed adhesive intestinal obstruction requiring surgery.[35] Seventy five percent of obstructions occurred within six months and 90% of obstructions developed within one year of surgery. Recurrent adhesive small bowel obstruction affected 5 (9%) patients. In a smaller study of 304 neonates from the Netherlands, adhesive intestinal obstruction was recorded in 3.3% of cases during a similar period.[33] A recent retrospective study of 414 neonates from Oxford, UK, followed up for a median of 39 months showed that 23 (5.6%) required reoperation for adhesive intestinal obstruction; recurrent adhesive obstruction occurred

Table 20.2. Incidence of postoperative adhesive small bowel obstruction after various open abdominal operations in children

Operation (reference)	Incidence	Comment
Appendectomy[32,34,41]	0.3–1%	Risk doubled after perforated appendicitis
Nissen fundoplication[42,43]	2–10%	Risk increased with concomitant surgical procedures
Total colectomy[32,44,45]	15–20%	Similar risk for straight ileo-anal pull-through, ileo-anal pouch and subtotal colectomy alone
Gastroschisis repair[19,32,35]	5–15%	Adhesive small bowel obstruction may occur many years later
Diaphragmatic hernia repair[32,35,36,46]	4–9%	Late incidence of adhesive obstruction indicates the long-term figure may be >10% if adult survivors included
Ladd's procedure[32,35]	8–15%	
Wilms' nephrectomy[38]	5%	Not increased by postoperative radiation therapy
Intussusception[47]	3–6%	In those undergoing operative intervention

Figures refer to episodes of obstruction requiring operative intervention during variable follow-up periods.

in four patients.[40] Seventy-four percent of obstructions developed within 6 months of the primary operation and 87% within one year.

Type of operation

The incidence of adhesive small bowel obstruction complicating various intra-abdominal operations is detailed in Table 20.2. Several procedures merit further comment.

Open appendectomy

Adhesive small bowel obstruction is uncommon after appendectomy. Janik *et al.* (1981) reported an incidence of less than 1% during a 12-year period.[32] However, because appendectomy is such a frequent operation, numerically it is an important cause of adhesive obstruction.[39] Perforated appendicitis is associated with a doubling of the risk of adhesion-related small bowel obstruction.[32,41] It has been suggested that adhesive small bowel obstruction after appendectomy in adults is usually due to a band adhesion and rarely settles with conservative management.[48]

Open transabdominal Nissen fundoplication

Wilkins and Spitz identified a 10.3% incidence of adhesive small bowel obstruction occurring after a mean interval of 10 months in 156 children undergoing Nissen fundoplication.[42] Additional procedures performed concomitantly with the fundoplication substantially increased the risk of developing obstruction; the risk was 21% for patients who had a Ladd's procedure and 12% for those who had an incidental appendectomy. The incidence in those patients who underwent no additional procedure other than the fundoplication was 1.8%. Inability to vomit in most of the children led to delay in diagnosing intestinal obstruction and this proved fatal in two cases. Other series have reported adhesive small bowel obstruction rates of 2%–10% after Nissen fundoplication.[43]

In a personal series of 80 infants and children undergoing Nissen fundoplication in Leeds (two-thirds of whom had a Stamm gastrostomy) there was not a single case of adhesive bowel obstruction during a median follow-up of more than 2 years. Restricting the operative field to the left upper quadrant of the abdomen and deliberately avoiding handling of the small bowel, which is retained within the infracolic compartment, appear to be important factors in preventing this complication.

Nephrectomy for Wilms' tumor

In a report from the Third National Wilms' Tumor Study, 104 (5.4%) of 1910 children developed adhesive small bowel obstruction after transperitoneal nephrectomy for Wilms' tumor.[38] Important risk factors were higher local tumor stage, extrarenal vascular involvement, and en bloc resection of other organs at the time of nephrectomy. The incidence of adhesive bowel obstruction was not increased in children who received postoperative radiation therapy.

In neonates, meconium ileus, necrotizing enterocolitis and intestinal malrotation are more likely to be complicated by adhesive obstruction than other pathologies.[40]

Morbidity and mortality

Postoperative adhesive small bowel obstruction is associated with a mortality of between 2 and 6%[32,33,42,49] and a much greater morbidity from intestinal resection, intra-abdominal sepsis, and wound complications. In addition, there are potential but controversial long-term risks from pelvic adhesions such as infertility and chronic abdominal/pelvic pain *(see chapter on Appendix)*.[50] The morbidity associated with surgical treatment has encouraged some authors to challenge the traditional surgical approach to adhesive bowel obstruction in children and advocate a more conservative policy in selected cases.[39,49] However, in the absence of reliable clinical signs of intestinal strangulation, this approach must be adopted with caution. For those that require surgery, laparoscopic adhesiolysis is possible in selected cases.[51]

Prevention

Attempts to prevent the development of adhesions have focused on (i) minimizing peritoneal injury during surgery,

(ii) separating adhesiogenic surfaces and, (iii) promoting fibrinolysis.

Minimizing peritoneal trauma

This requires meticulous surgical technique with gentle handling and careful hemostasis. The use of powder-free surgical gloves, wet gauze swabs and fine absorbable sutures may help to reduce the risk of postoperative adhesions. Avoiding tissue desiccation and covering raw surfaces with omentum may also be beneficial. Although omental adhesions are the most common, they are at low risk of producing intestinal obstruction.[28]

Laparoscopic techniques result in fewer adhesive complications than open procedures but the risk of adhesions is not eliminated. Several large studies of children undergoing laparoscopic appendectomy have been reported but there are no long-term data on the risk of subsequent adhesion obstruction. In one French multicenter study of 1379 pediatric laparoscopic appendectomies followed up for only 15 days, two cases required adhesiolysis and gut resection.[52] Moore *et al.* (1995) reviewed 41 pediatric patients who had undergone second-look procedures after laparoscopic urologic interventions.[53] Adhesions were noted in 4 (10%) patients either at the operative site or at trocar sites; the risk of adhesions was related to the extent of dissection. These authors considered that the incidence of adhesions was lower than that which would be expected with open surgery. A reduction in foreign body contamination of the peritoneum may be one factor contributing to the lower incidence of adhesions after laparoscopic surgery.[54]

Separating adhesiogenic surfaces

Two approaches have been used to separate adhesiogenic surfaces after abdominal surgery: (a) the use of liquid or mechanical barriers and (b) the administration of prokinetic agents. Peritoneal lavage with normal saline or macromolecular dextran solution has no major role in preventing adhesions.[55] Hyaluronan, a polysaccharide found throughout the body, facilitates cell migration and increases mesothelial cell proliferation.[56] A hyaluronic acid–carboxymethylcellulose membrane (Seprafilm) has been shown to reduce intra-abdominal adhesion formation in adults undergoing colectomy without increasing the risk of intra-abdominal sepsis.[57] A recent randomized controlled study of 122 children in Japan showed that the incidence and severity of intra-abdominal adhesions under the abdominal incision site was significantly reduced by the use of Seprafilm® but the frequency of clinical adhesive small bowel obstruction was not affected.[57a] Seprafilm® did not cause an increase in surgical complications. Wrapping a bowel anastomosis or staple line with this bioresorbable membrane should be avoided since this may increase the risk of leakage.[58] This material is approved in the United States and Europe for use in adults undergoing laparotomy for benign, non-infectious conditions but it is not currently licensed for use in children. In Europe, intraperitoneal 4% icodextrin solution (Adept®) is also licensed for use in adults to reduce adhesions after abdominal surgery. At present, it is uncertain whether these agents will result in fewer episodes of adhesive bowel obstruction. Recently, fibrin-sealant plication of the small bowel has been proposed as a method of preventing the formation of obstructing adhesions in children but evidence for this technique is from retrospective, uncontrolled data only.[59]

In experimental animals, early introduction of enteral feeding and the use of Cisapride, a prokinetic agent, have been shown to reduce the duration of postoperative ileus and adhesion formation but the clinical validity of these findings is uncertain.[60] In comparison with intravenous opiates, epidural analgesia is associated with earlier recovery of gut function after major abdominal surgery and this may be beneficial in reducing postoperative adhesion formation.[61]

Promoting fibrinolysis

The rationale for the primary prevention of adhesions with fibrinolytic agents is based on the recognition that damaged peritoneum is unable to generate plasmin from plasminogen, and consequently fibrinolytic activity is impaired. Studies of recombinant tissue plasminogen activator have shown promise in experimental animals but there are no reports as yet of randomized controlled clinical trials.[28] Attempts to minimize the inflammatory response using corticosteroids, thereby enhancing intrinsic fibrinolytic activity, have not been successful.

There are a few reports on the secondary prevention of adhesive intestinal obstruction in children using intraluminal tube-stent plication of the small bowel.[62] Short follow-up periods and uncontrolled data limit conclusions on the efficacy of this technique but it may have a place as an adjunct to adhesiolysis in patients requiring repeated operations for the relief of obstruction due to extensive, dense adhesions.

Intestinal resections

The physiology and long-term complications of short bowel syndrome are discussed elsewhere (see Chapter 28). However, extensive gut resection may have significant long-term consequences in children without overt intestinal failure. The length of resected ileum and the presence of an ileocecal valve or colon are important factors affecting outcome.[63] There is less potential for adaptation in the jejunum than in the ileum. Potential long-term sequelae of intestinal resection in infants include the following.

Vitamin deficiencies

Ileal resection leads to the loss of some or all of the capacity for receptor-mediated absorption of intrinsic factor–cobalamin complex. Vitamin B_{12} deficiency is usually associated with a low serum concentration and an abnormal Schilling test result. Valman and Roberts found impaired vitamin B_{12} absorption in seven of ten infants who had more than 45 cm of ileum resected but they documented normal vitamin B_{12} absorption in two children in whom only 15 cm of terminal ileum was preserved.[64] In their patients with impaired absorption, the serum level of vitamin B_{12} did not fall below the normal range for several years, puberty being a particularly vulnerable time. Parashar *et al.* (1990) found only one child with vitamin B_{12} deficiency in a series of 27 children who had undergone ileocolic resection for various etiologies followed up for a mean of 6 years.[65] Impaired absorption of vitamin B_{12} may recover after several years, probably because of intestinal adaptation.[66] Vitamin B_{12} status should be checked periodically in children who have undergone ileal resection.

Disturbance of the normal enterohepatic circulation of bile salts after ileal resection predisposes to fat-soluble vitamin deficiencies. This may be exacerbated by cholestyramine used to control bile salt diarrhea. Vitamin D deficiency and rickets can occur in children who achieve full enteral feeding with a short gut[67] but does not appear to be a particular hazard after extensive ileal resection alone.[68] Vitamin E malabsorption may manifest many years after apparently successful surgery for jejunal atresia.[69] Deficiency of vitamin E may lead to mitochondrial degeneration and the deposition of brown lipofuscin pigment within intestinal smooth muscle which exacerbates intestinal dysmotility. A combination of intestinal tapering and vitamin E supplementation appears to be an effective treatment.

Gallstones

Cholelithiasis is a well-recognized late complication of ileal resection, disease or bypass in adults and, to a lesser extent, in children. Pathogenesis is multifactorial and may be related to perioperative gallbladder stasis and starvation, the disturbance of the normal enterohepatic circulation of bile salts, and increased absorption of bilirubin from the gut.

Hyperoxaluria and renal stones

Fat malabsorption secondary to ileal resection encourages the formation of insoluble calcium soaps in the lumen of the gut. One consequence of this is increased absorption of dietary oxalate which, under normal circumstances, would form insoluble calcium oxalate in the bowel lumen; bile salts in the colon may also increase oxalate absorption. Hyperoxaluria and renal oxalate stones may develop in patients with a retained functioning colon after extensive small bowel resection. A quarter of adults with less than 200 cm jejunum anastomosed to colon develop symptomatic renal stones.[70] The risk in children is uncertain but in one small series approximately half the patients had evidence of hyperoxaluria.[71] Bohane *et al.* (1979) found hyperoxaluria in four out of ten children who had undergone ileal resection but could not correlate this with the length of resected ileum or the interval since surgery.[72]

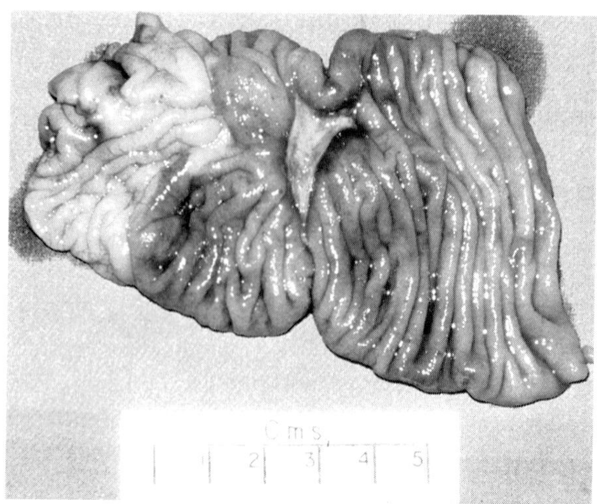

Fig. 20.2. Resected ileocolic anastomosis from a boy with bleeding from an ileocolic anastomotic ulcer 5 years after neonatal surgery. Reproduced by kind permission of Dr John WL Puntis, Leeds General Infirmary, UK.

Perianastomotic ulceration

Perianastomotic ulceration is a rare long-term complication of ileocolic or jejunocolic anastomosis in infancy (Fig. 20.2).[75] All reported cases have presented between 3 and 13 years after their original surgery with severe iron deficiency anemia from overt or occult lower gastrointestinal bleeding, with or without abdominal pain and diarrhea (Table 20.3). Colonoscopy is the most useful investigation. The etiology of this complication is unknown but the pathology of the ulceration suggests a process of chronic inflammation and repair. Treatment is problematic: antibiotics, H_2-blockers and sulphasalazine are not curative and resection and reanastomosis may be complicated by recurrence.[78]

Other potential late sequelae

Anastomotic strictures and other mechanical problems are rarely encountered as late complications of intestinal

Table 20.3. Reported cases of peri-anastomotic ileo/jejuno-colic ulceration[78]

Author	Sex	Age at operation	Primary condition	Anastomosis	Suture material	Age (y) at presentation	Type & site of ulcer	Treatment	Outcome
Parashar[73]	M	1 m	Volvulus	Jejuno-colic	Silk	4	Multiple, small, ileal & colic	Resection	Well 18 m
	M	4 m	Intussusception	Ileo-colic	–	13	Multiple, small, ileal & colic	Sulphasalazine & iron	"Symptoms relieved"
	M	2d	Colonic atresia	Ileo-colic	Dexon	12	Single, large, anastomotic	Resection	Well 18 m
	F	6w	NEC	Jejuno-colic	Dexon	11	Multiple, small, ileal & colic	–	–
	M	4 m	Gastroschisis	Ileo-colic	–	3	–	–	–
Couper[74]			Gastroschisis	Ileo-colic	–	8	Single, anastomotic	Resection	Recurrence 4 m
	M > F	Infancy	Ileal atresia	Jejuno-colic	–	10	Two small bowel	Resection	Well 7 m
			Gastroschisis	Ileo-colic	–	5	Single, large, ileal	–	–
Hamilton[75]	M	9 w	NEC	Ileo-colic	Silk	7	Single, large, ileal	Resection	Recurrence 3 m
	M	2 d	Gastroschisis	Ileo-colic	Silk	5	Single, large, ileal	Resection	Recurrence 8 y
Paterson[76]	M	3 y	Volvulus	Ileo-colic	CCG & silk	10	Single, large, ileal	Resection	Well 7 m
	F	2 d	NEC	Ileo-colic	CCG & silk	8	Single, anastomotic	Lactose-free diet Cholestyramine & iron	Well 3 y
Arnbjornsson[77]	M	9 m	Gastroschisis	Ileo-colic	–	8	Multiple perianastomotic	Resection Ranitidine	Recurrence 4 m Asymptomatic 2 y

resection but should be excluded in a child with chronic diarrhea, malabsorption or failure to thrive. Infants undergoing extensive ileal resection survive with few developmental scars,[79] although some authors have suggested a more guarded prognosis.[80] These children may be shorter and lighter than their siblings.[80] Assessment of these patients is complicated by differences in maternal and intrauterine environments, prematurity, variability of neonatal nutrition, and complications other than those related to the gut.

Until recently, only extensive small bowel resection in infants was considered to be associated with significant long-term sequelae. Davies *et al.* (1999) studied the long-term nutritional and metabolic effects of limited ileal resection (<50 cm) after neonatal necrotizing enterocolitis (NEC).[81] Seventeen children with a median age of 7 (5.5 to 13.7) years were compared with seven control subjects of similar age who had developed neonatal NEC but had been managed non-operatively. Five of the 17 surgical cases had undergone an isolated ileal resection; 12 had also had variable lengths of colon removed. The median length of resected ileum was 10 (3–44) cm. Median height, weight and body mass index after ileal resection were between the 25th and 50th centiles; no child was stunted or wasted. Hematologic and biochemical parameters were normal. No renal calculi were detected and bone mineral density measurements were normal in all except one child. However, limited ileal resection was associated with asymptomatic vitamin B_{12} deficiency in one child and cholelithiasis in four (two after isolated ileal resection and two after ileocolic resection). At a median age of 7.0 years, the prevalence of cholelithiasis after limited ileal resection for NEC was 24%. Potential etiologic factors for gallstones in these children include prematurity, parenteral nutrition/prolonged fasting, ileal resection, phototherapy, and frusemide therapy. However, the absence of cholelithiasis in the small group of medically treated NEC controls suggests that limited ileal resection and/or neonatal surgery is a major predisposing factor.

Intestinal stomas

Most intestinal stomas are required only temporarily in the management of anorectal malformations, NEC, and Hirschsprung's disease. Short-term complications are well documented[82] but there are almost no long-term data on children with long-standing or permanent stomas. Permanent intestinal stomas are rare but may be necessary in a few children with a high anorectal malformation, cloacal anomaly, intestinal dysmotility, Crohn's disease, or because of failed pelvic pouch surgery or intractable fecal incontinence not manageable by alternative techniques such as the antegrade colonic enema (*see chapter on The Malone ACE Procedure*).[83] Long-term stomas should be end-colostomies or ileostomies sited through the rectus abdominis muscle away from scars, skin creases, and bony prominences. Careful initial siting and construction will help to prevent complications: avoiding ischemia, tension, diseased bowel, and loop stomas, and properly spouting an ileostomy. Early involvement of a stoma therapist is advisable.

Table 20.4. Potential long-term complications of intestinal stomas

Peristomal dermatitis
Poor stoma location
Retraction
Stenosis
Prolapse
Parastomal hernia
Dehydration/electrolyte disturbances (sodium deficit and poor growth in infants)[84]
Small bowel obstruction (adhesions, parastomal hernia, lateral space herniation, volvulus)
Stomal disease, e.g., Crohn's, varices
Psychosocial morbidity

Mechanical complications can occur many years later in patients with ileostomies or colostomies (Table 20.4). In adults, stoma complications are more likely within the first five years, but there is a small continuing risk of problems thereafter.[85] Parastomal hernias are more common with colostomies whilst peristomal dermatitis is a more frequent complication of ileostomies. Peristomal skin irritation may be due to leakage of effluent, mechanical irritation from the stoma appliance, allergy, infection, or skin disease. A skilled stoma therapist is usually able to cure these problems. In a study of adults with permanent ileostomies for inflammatory bowel disease, the cumulative rate of surgical revision after 8 years was 44% for those with ulcerative colitis and 75% for those with Crohn's disease.[86] Ileostomy stenosis and recession were the two most common indications for reconstruction. Surgical revision could often be carried out as a local procedure without the need for laparotomy. Local stapling techniques may be useful in the prevention and treatment of these problems.[87] In adults with left iliac fossa sigmoid colostomies the complication rate is as high as 51% after 13 years, paracolostomy hernia being the commonest.[88] A more detailed account of the management of stoma complications in adults is provided by Shellito (1998).[85] Stoma associations, inflammatory bowel disease societies and self-help groups are useful resources for older patients.

In children, a permanent colostomy or ileostomy is compatible with good long-term growth. Fluid balance and nutritional problems are a short-term hazard with an ileostomy,[89] and cholelithiasis and urolithiasis are potential long-term risks.[90] Whilst the results of the continent Kock ileostomy have steadily improved in the hands of enthusiasts, up to two-thirds of patients require revisional surgery in the longer term[91] and experience in children is limited.[92] Quality of life issues and effects on schooling have been neglected in children with long-term stomas and little is known about their psychosocial adjustment. In one small study of young people with inflammatory bowel disease, 12 patients aged between 9 and 29 years with a stoma established 2–15 years earlier were compared with two matched groups – patients who had had an ileorectal anastomosis, and others managed medically.[93] No differences in psychological adjustment, self-esteem, or quality of life were found between the groups. Anxieties about leakage, noise, odour and what to tell others were common, as were concerns about social acceptability, employment and sexual desirability. The services of a stoma nurse with pediatric experience can be invaluable for these patients.[94]

Neoplasia

Malignant change is a rare complication of several conditions in pediatric abdominal surgery. Although this complication can occur in children, more typically it affects adults and underlines the importance of good links between pediatric and adult specialists. In conditions associated with well-recognized risks, appropriate surveillance programs may allow timely intervention and prevention of this serious long-term complication. Several examples of this hazard are highlighted.

Alimentary tract duplications are rare congenital malformations that may be found anywhere from mouth to anus. They are usually single, variable in size, and more often spherical than tubular. Typically, they are lined by alimentary tract mucosa and share a common smooth muscle wall and blood supply with the adjacent bowel, with which they may communicate. Whilst some duplications never cause symptoms, most present in infancy or early childhood with obstruction, hemorrhage or inflammation.[95] Hazards of incomplete excision include meningitis, gastrointestinal bleeding, and perforation. Malignant change is reported to occur in duplication cysts after a latent interval of many years. Duplications arising from the rectum or stomach may be particularly hazardous.[96–99] At least nine cases of adenocarcinoma arising in a rectal duplication cyst have been reported in adults aged between 30 and 60 years.[100] This complication may be unavoidable if the duplication cyst is clinically silent, but when dealing with a manifest rectal duplication it is important, whenever possible, to attempt complete excision rather than marsupialisation.

Malignant change is a well-described complication of congenital choledochal dilatation (choledochal cysts), mostly affecting adults. However, teenagers are at risk.[101,102] The age-related cancer risk has been estimated to be 0.7% in the first decade, 7% in the second decade, and 14% after 20 years of age.[103] Iwai *et al.* (1990) reported a 12-year-old girl with a type IV choledochal cyst and extensive carcinomatous change in the extrahepatic biliary tree.[104] Pancreatobiliary ductal malunion predisposes to choledochal cyst and gallbladder malignancy. Early radical excision of the choledochal cyst minimizes the risk of malignancy and other complications. However, even after cyst excision, malignancy may affect incompletely excised extrahepatic ducts or dilated intrahepatic ducts, indicating the need for lifelong surveillance (*see chapter on Choledochal Cysts*).

Early onset inflammatory bowel disease is a major risk factor for the subsequent development of colorectal cancer; panproctocolitis and more than 10 years of disease are others. In some cases, cancer can be predicted by the finding of dysplasia in colorectal mucosal biopsies. This has prompted the development of regular endoscopic review of at risk patients *(see chapter on Inflammatory Bowel Disease)*.[105] Endoscopic surveillance programs are also critical for patients with familial adenomatous polyposis since they are prone to develop large bowel cancer. Colonoscopy can help determine the timing of prophylactic colectomy.

Other pediatric abdominal surgical conditions with a long-term risk of malignancy include: the occurrence of perianastomotic adenocarcinoma 20 years after ureterosigmoidostomy urinary diversion;[106] mid-esophageal squamous cell carcinoma 20 to 40 years after caustic ingestion *(see chapter on Esophageal Replacement)*;[107] malignant degeneration of the intra-abdominal testis (*see chapter on Undescended Testis*); and the small risk of malignancy in mesenteric cysts.[108] Other conditions are associated with less well defined risks of malignancy, e.g., adenocarcinoma complicating childhood Barrett's esophagus.[109] The risk for some conditions has yet to be defined, e.g., the potential for esophageal cancer in patients with repaired esophageal atresia,[110,110a] and the long-term risk of gastric cancer in children with *Helicobacter pylori* gastritis.[111]

Benign neoplasia is a very rare long-term sequel of abdominal surgical conditions in children. The development of inflammatory pseudotumors has been linked to previous inflammation or surgery.[112] Potentially fatal desmoid tumours are known to develop in about 10% of patients with familial adenomatous polyposis, mostly in association with previous surgery.[113] Desmoids arise most commonly within the small bowel mesentery or the abdominal wall and are benign, poorly demarcated, fibrous lesions; they can cause death from local invasion. They pose a major threat to polyposis patients and now represent one of the leading causes of death after prophylactic colectomy.

Medicolegal and economic aspects

Pediatric surgical patients may first present with a long-term complication to an adult specialist. It is imperative therefore that detailed, accurate records are kept and not destroyed. Parents and children should be given adequate information about their condition and its treatment together with an understanding of long-term hazards.

The medicolegal aspects of long-term consequences of surgical interventions continue to attract increasing attention. For example, in the UK claims relating to intra-abdominal adhesions have increased. The basis of these have included failure to warn of risk and failure to take precautions to prevent adhesion formation.[114] In view of the potential long-term hazards of blood transfusion, we have a legal and clinical duty to minimize the requirements for blood product transfusion and to keep up to date with contemporary guidelines.[114a] Detailed informed consent is essential and independent consent in older children is advisable. Economic pressures have led to a greater emphasis on day-case surgery which requires careful patient selection and skilled community nursing if complications and their sequelae are to be avoided. In future years, surgical interventions are likely to become increasingly driven by cost-effectiveness. Such analyses must include long-term outcomes and not simply rely on duration of hospital stay and other measures of short-term recovery. Economic analyses, such as that carried out for diaphragmatic hernia,[115] are likely to have a greater influence in shaping treatment strategies.

Conclusions

Pediatric surgeons, perhaps more than any other surgical specialists, must be aware of the long-term consequences of congenital and acquired surgical conditions and operative interventions. In abdominal surgery, the paucity of long-term data and lack of information about the quality of our patients' lives is disconcerting. As new technologies and basic scientific research in molecular biology and genetics capture our attention, we must not lose sight of the importance of long-term outcomes in pediatric surgery.

REFERENCES

1. Freeman, N. V. & Bulut, M. "High" anorectal anomalies treated by early "neonatal" operation. *J Pediatr Surg* 1986; **21**:218–220.
2. Viner, R. Barriers and good practice in transition from paediatric to adult care. *J. Roy. Soc. Med.* 2001; **94** (Suppl.40):2–4.
3. Stringer, M. D. Long-term outcomes in newborn surgery. In Puri, P., ed. *Newborn Surgery*. 2nd edn., Arnold: London, 2003: 915–924.
4. Moss, R. L., Henry, M. C. W., Dimmitt, R. A. *et al.* The role of prospective randomized clinical trials in pediatric surgery: state of the art? *J. Pediatr. Surg.* 2001; **36**:1182–1186.
5. Curry, J. I., Reeves, B., & Stringer, M. D. Randomized controlled trials in pediatric surgery: could we do better? *J. Pediatr. Surg.* 2003; **38**:556–559.
6. Baraldini, V., Spitz, L., & Pierro, A. Evidence-based operations in paediatric surgery. *Pediatr. Surg. Int.* 1998; **13**:331–335.
7. Gilbert, H. W., Thompson, M. H., & Armstrong, C. P. The presentation of malrotation of the intestine in adults. *Ann. Roy. Coll. Surg. Engl.* 1990; **72**:239–242.
8. Hawley, P. R. & Ritchie, J. K. Hirschsprung's disease in adults. In Kamm, M. A. & Lennard-Jones, J. E., eds. *Constipation*. Petersfield: Wrightson Biomedical Publishing Ltd, 1994: 199–203.
9. Van Meurs, K. P., Robbins, S. T., Reed, V. L. *et al.* Congenital diaphrafgmatic hernia: long-term outcome in neonates treated with extracorporeal membrane oxygenation. *J. Pediatr.* 1993; **122**:893–899.
10. Lumley, J. S. P. Creutzfeldt–Jakob Disease (CJD) in surgical practice. *Ann. R. Coll. Surg. Engl. (Suppl.)* 2004; **86**:86–88.
11. Weiland, D. E., Bay, R. C., & Del Sordi, S. Choosing the best abdominal closure by meta-analysis. *Am. J. Surg.* 1998; **176**:666–670.
12. Kiely, E. M. & Spitz, L. Layered versus mass closure of abdominal wounds in infants and children. *Br. J. Surg.* 1985; **72**:739–740.
13. Horwitz, J. R., Chwals, W. J., Doski, J. J. *et al.* Pediatric wound infections. A prospective multicenter study. *Ann. Surg.* 1998; **227**:553–558.
14. Brain, A. J. L. & Kiely, E. M. Use of a single layer extramucosal suture for intestinal anastomosis in children. *Br. J. Surg.* 1985; **72**:483–484.
15. Spitz, L., Kiely, E., & Brereton, R. J. Esophageal atresia: five year experience with 148 cases. *J. Pediatr. Surg.* 1987; **22**:103–108.
16. Steichen, F. M. & Ravitch, M. M. Staplers in gastrointestinal surgery. In Schwartz, S. I. & Ellis, H., *Maingot's Abdominal*

Operations, 8th edn. Connecticut: Appleton-Century Crofts, 1985: 1537–1575.

17. Bayat, A., McGrouther, D. A., & Ferguson, M. W. J. Skin scarring. *Br. Med. J.* 2003; **326**:88–92.
18. Partridge, J. & Rumsey, N. Skin scarring: new insights may make adjustment easier. *Br. Med. J.* 2003; **326**:765 (letter).
19. Davies, B. W. & Stringer, M. D. Where are they now? The survivors of gastroschisis. *Arch. Dis. Child.* 1997; **77**:158–160.
20. Tan, K. C. & Bianchi, A. Circumumbilical incision for pyloromyotomy. *Br. J. Surg.* 1986; **73**:399.
21. Ragoowansi, R., Cornes, P. G., Moss, A. L., & Glees, J. P. Treatment of keloids by surgical excision and immediate postoperative single-fraction radiotherapy. *Plast. Reconstr. Surg.* 2003; **111**:1853–1859.
22. Mustoe, T. A., Cooter, R. D., Gold, M. H. *et al.* International clinical recommendations on scar management. *Plast. Reconstr. Surg.* 2002; **110**:560–571.
23. Adzick, N. S. & Lorenz, H. P. Cells, matrix, growth factors, and the surgeon. The biology of scarless fetal wound repair. *Ann. Surg.* 1994; **220**:10–18.
24. Tsui, S. & Ellis, H. Healing of abdominal incisional hernia in infant rats. *Br. J. Surg.* 1991; **78**:927–929.
25. Ellis, H., Bucknall, T. E., & Cox, P. J. Abdominal incisions and their closure. *Curr. Probl. Surg.* 1985; **22**:28–30.
26. von Lilien, T., Salusky, I. B., Yap, H. K., Fonkalsrud, E. W., & Fine, R. N. Hernias: a frequent complication in children treated with continuous peritoneal dialysis. *Am. J. Kidney. Dis.* 1987; **10**:356–360.
27. Waldhaussen, J. H. Incisional hernia in a 5-mm trocar site following pediatric laparoscopy. *J. Laparoendosc. Surg.* 1996; **6** Suppl 1:S89–S90.
28. Menzies, D. Postoperative adhesions: their treatment and relevance in clinical practice. *Ann. Roy. Coll. Surg. Eng.* 1993; **75**:147–153.
29. Erdogan, E., Celayir, S., Eroglu, E., & Yilmaz, E. The relation between human leukocyte antigen (HLA) distribution and intestinal obstruction and adhesions in childhood: preliminary report. *Pediatr. Surg. Int.* 2000; **16**:374–376.
30. Ellis, H., Morgan, B. J., Thompson, J. N. *et al.* Adhesion related hospital readmissions after abdominal and pelvic surgery: a retrospective cohort study. *Lancet* 1999; **353**:1476–1480.
31. Ray, N. F., Larsen, J. W., Stillman, R. J., & Jacobs, R. J. Economic impact of hospitalizations for lower abdominal adhesiolysis in the United States in 1988. *Surg. Gynecol. Obstet.* 1993; **176**:271–276.
32. Janik, J. S., Ein, S. H., Filler, R. M., Shandling, B., Simpson, J. S., Stephens, C. A. An assessment of the surgical treatment of adhesive small bowel obstruction in infants and children. *J. Pediatr. Surg.* 1981; **16**:225–235.
33. Festen, C. T. Postoperative small bowel obstruction in infants and children. *Ann. Surg.* 1982; **196**:580–583.
34. Grant, H. W., Parker, M. C., Wilson, M. S. *et al.* Population-based analysis of the risk of adhesions following abdominal surgery in children. Presented at British Association of Surgeons 51st Annual International Congress, Oxford, UK, July 2004.
35. Wilkins, B. M. & Spitz, L. Incidence of postoperative adhesion obstruction following neonatal laparotomy. *Br. J. Surg.* 1986; **73**:762–764.
36. Vanamo, K., Rintala, R. J., Lindahl, H., & Louhimo, I. Long-term gastrointestinal morbidity in patients with congenital diaphragmatic defects. *J. Pediatr. Surg.* 1996; **31**:551–554.
37. Devens, K. Recurrent intestinal obstruction in the neonatal period. *Arch Dis. Child.* 1963; **38**:118–119.
38. Ritchey, M. L., Kelalis, P. P., Eltzioni, R., Breslow, N., Shochat, S., & Haase, G. M. Small bowel obstruction after nephrectomy for Wilms' tumor. *Ann. Surg.* 1993; **218**:654–659.
39. Akgur, F. M., Tanyel, F. C., Buyukpamukcu, N., & Hicsonmez, A. Adhesive small bowel obstruction in children: the place and predictors of success for conservative treatment. *J. Pediatr. Surg.* 1991; **26**:37–41.
40. Choudhry, M. S., Kader, M., & Grant, H. W. Retrospective study of incidence of adhesions following neonatal laparotomy. Presented at British Association of Surgeons 51st Annual International Congress, Oxford, UK, July 2004.
41. Andersson, R. E. B. Small bowel obstruction after appendicectomy. *Br. J. Surg.* 2001; **88**:1387–1391.
42. Wilkins, B. M. & Spitz, L. Adhesion obstruction following Nissen fundoplication in children. *Br. J. Surg.* 1987; **74**:777–779.
43. Mira-Navarro, J., Bayle-Bastos, F., Frieyro-Segui, M., Garramone, N., & Gambarini, A. Long-term follow-up of Nissen fundoplication. *Eur. J. Pediatr. Surg.* 1994; **4**:7–10.
44. Morgan, R. A., Manning, P., & Coran, A. G. Experience with the straight endorectal pullthrough for the management of ulcerative colitis and familial polyposis in children and adults. *Ann. Surg.* 1987; **206**:595–599.
45. Telander, R. L., Spencer, M., Perrault, J., Telander, D., & Zinsmeister, A. R. Long-term follow-up of the ileoanal anastomosis in children and young adults. *Surgery* 1990; **108**:717–725.
46. Lund, D. P., Mitchell, J., Kharasch, V., Quigley, S., Kuehn, M., & Wilson, J. M. Congenital diaphragmatic hernia: the hidden morbidity. *J. Pediatr. Surg.* 1994; **29**:258–264.
47. Stringer, M. D., Pablot, S. M., & Brereton, R. J. Paediatric intussusception. *Br. J. Surg.* 1992; **79**:867–876.
48. Meagher, A. P., Moller, C., & Hoffmann, D. C. Non-operative treatment of small bowel obstruction following appendicectomy or operation on the ovary or tube. *Br. J. Surg.* 1993; **80**:1310–1311.
49. Shieh, C.-S., Chuang, J.-H., & Huang, S.-C. Adhesive small-bowel obstruction in children. *Pediatr. Surg. Int.* 1995; **10**:339–341.
50. Monk, B. J., Berman, M. L., & Montz, F. J. Adhesions after extensive gynecologic surgery: clinical significance, etiology, and prevention. *Am. J. Obstet. Gynecol.* 1994; **170**:1396–1403.
51. van der Zee, D. C. & Bax, N. M. Management of adhesive bowel obstruction in children is changed by laparoscopy. *Surg. Endosc.* 1999; **13**:925–927.

52. El Ghoneimi, A., Valla, J. S., Limonne, B. *et al.* Laparoscopic appendectomy in children: report of 1,379 cases. *J. Pediatr. Surg.* 1994; **29**:786–789.
53. Moore, R. G., Kavoussi, L. R., Bloom, D. A. *et al.* Postoperative adhesion formation after urological laparoscopy in the pediatric population. *J. Urol.* 1995; **153**:792–795.
54. Torre, M., Favre, A., Pini Prato, A., Brizzolara, A., & Martucciello, G. Histologic study of peritoneal adhesions in children and in a rat model. *Pediatr. Surg. Int.* 2002; **18**:673–676.
55. Watson, A., Vandekerckhove, P., & Lilford, R. Liquid and fluid agents for preventing adhesions after surgery for subfertility. *Cochrane Database Syst. Rev.* 2000;(3):CD001298.
56. Reijnen, M. M., Bleichrodt, R. P., & van Goor, H. Pathophysiology of intra-abdominal adhesion and abscess formation, and the effect of hyaluronan. *Br. J. Surg.* 2003; **90**:533–541.
57. Becker, J. M., Dayton, M. T., Fazio, V. W. *et al.* Prevention of postoperative abdominal adhesions by a sodium hyaluronate-based bioresorbable membrane: a prospective, randomized, double-blind multicenter study. *J. Am. Coll. Surg.* 1996; **183**:297–306.
57a. Inoue, M., Uchida, K., Miki, C., & Kusunoki, M. Efficacy of Seprafilm® for reducing reoperative risk in pediatic surgical patients undergoing abdominal surgery. *J. Pediatr. Surg.* 2005; **40**:1301–1306.
58. Beck, D. E., Cohen, Z., Fleshman, J. W. *et al.* A prospective, randomized, multicenter, controlled study of the safety of Seprafilm adhesion barrier in abdominopelvic surgery of the intestine. *Dis. Colon. Rectum.* 2003; **46**:1310–1319.
59. Holland-Cunz, S., Boelter, A. V., & Waag, K. L. Protective fibrin-sealed plication of the small bowel in recurrent laparotomy. *Pediatr. Surg. Int.* 2003; **19**:540–543.
60. Springall, R. G. & Spitz, L. The prevention of post-operative adhesions using a gastrointestinal prokinetic agent. *J. Pediatr. Surg.* 1989; **24**:530–533.
61. Steinbrook, R. A. An opioid antagonist for postoperative ileus. *N. Engl. J. Med.* 2001; **345**:988–989.
62. Grosfeld, J. L., Cooney, D. R., & Csicsko, J. F. Gastrointestinal tube stent plication in infants and children. *Arch. surg.* 1975; **110**:594–599.
63. Stringer, M. D. & Puntis, J. W. L. Short bowel syndrome. *Arch. Dis. Child.* 1995; **73**:170–173.
64. Valman, H. B. & Roberts, P. D. Vitamin B_{12} absorption after resection of ileum in childhood. *Arch. Dis. Child.* 1974; **49**:932–935.
65. Parashar, K., Booth, I. W., Corkery, J. J., Gornall, P., & Buick, R. G. The long-term sequelae of ileocolic anastomosis in childhood: a retrospective survey. *Br. J. Surg.* 1990; **77**:645–646.
66. Ooi, B. C., Barnes, G. L., & Tauro, G. P. Normalization of vitamin B_{12} absorption after ileal resection in children. *J. Pediatr. Child Health* 1992; **28**:168–171.
67. Touloukian, R. J. & Gertner, J. M. Vitamin D deficiency rickets as a late complication of the short gut syndrome during infancy. *J. Pediatr. Surg.* 1981; **16**:230–236.
68. Preece, M. A. & Valman, H. B. Vitamin D status after resection of ileum in childhood. *Arch. Dis. Child.* 1975; **50**:283–285.
69. Ward, H. C., Leake, J., Milla, P. J., & Spitz, L. Brown bowel syndrome: a late complication of intestinal atresia. *J. Pediatr. Surg.* 1992; **27**:1593–1595.
70. Nightingale, J. M. D., Lennard-Jones, J. E., Gertner, D. J., Wood, S. R., & Bartram, C. I. Colonic preservation reduces need for parenteral therapy, increases incidence of renal stones but does not change high prevalence of gall stones in patients with short bowel. *Gut* 1992; **33**:1493–1497.
71. Valman, H. B., Oberholzer, V. G., & Palmer, T. Hyperoxaluria after resection of ileum in childhood. *Arch. Dis. Child.* 1974; **49**:171–173.
72. Bohane, T. D., Haka-Ikse, K., Biggar, W. D., Hamilton, J. R., & Gall, D. G. A clinical study of young infants after small intestinal resection. *J. Pediatr.* 1979; **94**:552–558.
73. Parashar, K., Kyawhla, S., Booth, I. W., Buick, R. G., & Corkery, J. J. Ileocolic ulceration: a long-term complication following ileocolic anastomosis. *J. Pediatr. Surg.* 1988; **23**:226–228.
74. Couper, R. T., Durie, P. R., Stafford, S. E. *et al.* Late gastrointestinal bleeding and protein loss after distal small-bowel resection in infancy. *J. Pediatr. Gastroenterol. Nutr.* 1989; **9**:454–460.
75. Hamilton, A. H., Beck, J. M., Wilson, G. M., Heggarty, H. J., & Puntis, J. W. L. Severe anaemia and ilecolic anastomotic ulceration. *Arch. Dis. Child.* 1992; **67**:1385–1386.
76. Paterson, C. A., Langer, J. C., Cameron, G. S., Issenman, R. M., & Marcaccio, M. J. Late anastomotic ulceration after ileocolic resection in childhood. *Can. J. Surg.* 1993; **36**:162–164.
77. Arnbjornsson, E. & Larsson, L. T. Ulceration in an ileocolic anastomosis treated with ranitidin. *J. Pediatr. Surg.* 1999; **34**:1532–1533.
78. Ceylan, H., Puntis, J. W. L., Abbott, C., & Stringer, M. D. Recurrent peri-anastomotic ileo/jejuno-colic ulceration. *J. Pediatr. Gastroenterol. Nutr.* 2000; **30**:450–452.
79. Valman, H. B. Intelligence after malnutrition caused by neonatal resection of ileum. *Lancet* 1974; **1**:425–427.
80. Tejani, A., Dobias, B., Nangia, B. S., & Mahadevan, R. Growth, health, and development after neonatal gut surgery: a long-term follow-up. *Pediatrics* 1978; **61**:685–693.
81. Davies, B. W., Abel, G., Puntis, J. W. L. *et al.* Limited ileal resection in infancy; the long-term consequences. *J. Pediatr. Surg.* 1999; **34**:583–587.
82. Nour, S., Beck, J. M., & Stringer, M. D. Colostomy complications in infants and children. *Ann. R. Coll. Surg. Engl.* 1996; **78**:526–530.
83. Malone, P. S., Ransley, P. G., & Kiely, E. M. Preliminary report: the antegrade continence enema. *Lancet* 1990; **336**:1217–1218.
84. Bower, T. B., Pringle, K. C., & Soper, R. T. Sodium deficit causing decreased weight gain and metabolic acidosis in infants with ileostomy. *J. Pediatr. Surg.* 1988; **23**:567–572.
85. Shellito, P. C. Complications of abdominal stoma surgery. *Dis. Colon. Rectum.* 1998; **41**:1562–1572.
86. Carlstedt, A., Fasth, S., Hulten, L., Nordgren, S., & Palselius, I. Long-term ileostomy complications in patients with

ulcerative colitis and Crohn's disease. *Int. J. Colorectal Dis.* 1987; **2**:22–25.

87. Ecker, K. W., Schmid, T., Xu, H. S., & Feifel, G. Improved stabilization of conventional (Brooke) ileostomies with the stapler technique. *World J. Surg.* 1992; **16**:525–529.
88. Londono-Schimmer, E. E., Leong, A. P., & Phillips, R. K. Life table analysis of stomal complications following colostomy. *Dis. Colon Rectum* 1994; **37**:916–920.
89. Husmann, D. A., McLorie, G. A., Churchill, B. M., & Ein, S. H. Management of the hindgut in cloacal exstrophy: terminal ileostomy versus colostomy. *J. Pediatr. Surg.* 1988; **23**:1107–1113.
90. Giunchi, F., Balbi, B., Giulianini, G., & Cacciaguerra, G. Cholelithiasis and urolithiasis in ileostomy patients. *Ital. J. Surg. Sci.* 1989; **19**:37–40.
91. Sivula, A. Long-term results of continent ileostomy. *Int. J. Colorectal Dis.* 1986; **1**:40–43.
92. Ein, S. H. A ten-year experience with the pediatric Kock pouch. *J. Pediatr. Surg.* 1987; **22**:764–766.
93. Lask, B., Jenkins, J., Nabarro, L., & Booth, I. Psychosocial sequelae of stoma surgery for inflammatory bowel disease in childhood. *Gut*. 1987; **28**:1257–1260.
94. O'Brien, B. K. Coming of age with an ostomy. *Am. J. Nursing* 1999; **99**:71–74.
95. Stringer, M. D., Spitz, L., Abel, R. *et al.* Management of alimentary tract duplication in children. *Br. J. Surg.* 1995; **82**:74–78.
96. Orr, M. M. & Edwards, A. J. Neoplastic change in duplications of the alimentary tract. *Br. J. Surg.* 1975; **62**:269–274.
97. Coit, D. G. & Mies, C. Adenocarcinoma arising within a gastric duplication cyst. *J. Surg. Oncol.* 1992; **50**:274–277.
98. Gibson, T. C., Edwards, J. M., & Shafiq, S. Carcinoma arising in a rectal duplication cyst. *Br. J. Surg.* 1986; **73**:377.
99. LaQuaglia, M. P., Feins, N., Eraklis, A., & Hendren, W. H. Rectal duplications. *J. Pediatr. Surg.* 1990; **25**:980–984.
100. Stringer, M. D. Adenocarcinoma within a rectal duplication. *Ann. Roy. Coll. Surg. Engl.* 1999; **81**:436.
101. Yamaguchi, M. Congenital choledochal cyst. Analysis of 1,433 patients in the Japanese literature. *Am. J. Surg.* 1980; **140**:653–657.
102. Bismuth, H. & Krissat, J. Choledochal cystic malignancies. *Ann. Oncol.* 1999; **10** Suppl. 4:S94–S98.
103. Voyles, C. R., Smadja, C., Shands, W. C., & Blumgart, L. H. Carcinoma in choledochal cysts: age related incidence. *Arch. Surg.* 1983; **118**:986–988.
104. Iwai, N., Deguchi, E., Yanagihara, J. *et al.* Cancer arising in a choledochal cyst in a 12-year-old girl. *J. Pediatr. Surg.* 1990; **12**:1261–1263.
105. Axon, A. T. R. Cancer surveillance in ulcerative colitis – a time for reappraisal. *Gut* 1994; **35**:587–589.
106. Woodhouse, C. R. J. Urinary diversion. In Woodhouse, C. R. J., ed. *Long-term Paediatric Urology*. Blackwell Scientific Publications, Oxford, 1991: 80–96.
107. Appelqvist, P. & Salmo, M. Lye corrosion carcinoma of the esophagus. *Cancer* 1980; **45**:2655–2658.
108. Kurtz, R. J., Heimann, T. M., Beck, A. R., & Holt, J. Mesenteric and retroperitoneal cysts. *Ann. Surg.* 1986; **203**:109–112.
109. Hassall, E., Dimmick, J. E., & Magee, J. F. Adenocarcinoma in childhood Barrett's esophagus: case documentation and the need for surveillance in children. *Am. J. Gastroenterol.* 1993; **88**:282–288.
110. Adzick, N. S., Fisher, J. H., Winter, H. S., Sandler, R. H., & Hendren, W. H. Esophageal adenocarcinoma 20 years after esophageal atresia repair. *J. Pediatr. Surg.* 1989; **24**:741–744.

110a. Pultrum, B. B., Bijleveld, C. M., de Langen, Z. J., & Plukker, J. T. Development of an adenocarcinoma of the esophagus 22 years after primary repair of a congenital atresia. *J. Pediatr. Surg.* 2005; **40**:E1–E4.

111. Parsonnet, J., Harris, R. A., Hack, H. M., & Owens, D. K. Modelling cost-effectiveness of Helicobacter pylori screening to prevent gastric cancer: a mandate for clinical trials. *Lancet* 1996; **348**:150–154.
112. Stringer, M. D., Ramani, P., Yeung, C. K., Capps, S. N. J., Kiely, E. M., & Spitz, L. Abdominal inflammatory myofibroblastic tumours (inflammatory pseudotumours) in children. *Br. J. Surg.* 1992; **79**:1357–1360.
113. Clark, S. K., Neale, K. F., Landgrebe, J. C., & Phillips, R. K. Desmoid tumours complicating familial adenomatous polyposis. *Br. J. Surg.* 1999; **86**:1185–1189.
114. Ellis, H. Medicolegal consequences of postoperative intra-abdominal adhesions. *J. Roy. Soc. Med.* 2001; **94**:331–332.

114a. McClelland, B. & Contreras, M. Appropriateness and safety of blood transfusion. *Br. Med. J.* 2005; **330**:104–105.

115. Metkus, A. P., Esserman, L., Sola, A., Harrison, M. R., & Adzick, N. S. Cost per anomaly: what does a diaphragmatic hernia cost? *J. Pediatr. Surg.* 1995; **30**:226–230.

21

Abdominal wall defects

David K. Magnuson

Rainbow Babies and Children's Hospital, Cleveland, OH, USA

Although abdominal wall defects have been recognized and described since ancient times, virtually all significant anomalies of abdominal wall development were fatal until the last century. The first substantial advancement in the care of infants with large abdominal wall defects was the development by Gross of a staged technique for the closure of omphaloceles with skin flaps. The resulting ventral hernia defect and lateral displacement of abdominal wall musculature often caused considerable morbidity, but this was acceptable in light of the alternative. The second development that had a major impact on survival was the introduction of temporary coverage by prosthetic materials, allowing gradual reduction of the eviscerated structures and delayed fascial closure. Both of these techniques were applicable to omphaloceles with functional intestinal tracts protected by intact amniotic membranes. Improvements in survival for gastroschisis awaited the advent of techniques for parenteral nutrition to provide metabolic and nutritional support and allow time for the injured intestinal tract to become functional. Currently, survival with an acceptable quality of life is expected for most infants with isolated abdominal wall defects, and mortality is primarily related to associated anomalies.

Embryology and pathogenesis

Formation of the normal ventral abdominal wall requires the successful orchestration of many complex events that occur primarily from the fourth to the twelfth week of fetal development. These events include the folding, fusion, growth, and differentiation of embryonic tissues destined to become abdominal wall musculature, umbilicus, and the intestinal tract. Failure of the normal sequence of events can result in a wide variety of congenital malformations that include not only gastroschisis and omphalocele, but also umbilical hernia, Meckel's diverticulum, exstrophy of the bladder and cloaca, and "prune belly" syndrome.

By the end of the third week of gestation, a trilaminar germ disc comprising ectoderm, mesoderm, and entoderm is suspended within the chorionic cavity, attached to the trophoblastic shell by a connecting stalk that contains the developing umbilical vessels. At this stage the embryo appears nearly spherical. The amniotic cavity forms one hemisphere in association with the ectodermal aspect of the germ disc, and the secondary yolk sac forms the other hemisphere in association with the entodermal surface. The interposed mesodermal layer divides axially into two parasagittal sheets separated by the neural tube as it invaginates from the ectoderm. To each side of the neural tube, the mesoderm condenses into a medial segmented mass of somites and a contiguous lateral sheet that divides into somatic and splanchnic components.

During the fourth week, a complicated process of folding begins. Craniocaudal folding occurs as a result of differential growth between ectoderm and entoderm, while lateral folding is related to somite growth patterns. The result of both processes is to internalize the splanchnic mesoderm, entoderm, and part of the yolk sac (destined to become the intestinal wall, epithelium, and lumen, respectively). The internalized portion of the chorionic cavity becomes intraembryonic coelom, and later, the peritoneal cavity. The ectoderm and associated amnion thereby become the outer layer of the folded embryo.

By the fifth week, the leading edges of the folding embryo converge around the center of the ventral surface. The

Pediatric Surgery and Urology: Long-term Outcomes, Mark Stringer, Keith Oldham, Pierre Mouriquand.
Published by Cambridge University Press. © Cambridge University Press, 2006.

circular edge of the converging ectoderm and amnion is referred to as the primitive umbilical ring, and during the fifth week both the connecting stalk and yolk sac pass through it into the interior of the folded embryo. The internalized yolk sac/entoderm (gut) rapidly retreats away from the remainder of the yolk sac, which remains in the shrinking chorionic cavity. The residual connection between gut and yolk sac narrows into the vitelline (or omphalomesenteric) duct. During the fifth week, progressive constriction at the primitive umbilical ring promotes fusion of the vitelline duct and connecting stalk. The vitelline duct then regresses by the beginning of the sixth week. When this common stalk is then covered by the reflecting edge of amnion, the primitive umbilical cord is formed.

During the sixth week of gestation, two processes begin that have important roles in the pathological development of clinically significant abdominal wall defects. First, the mesodermal somites differentiate and give rise to a new layer, the myotome, that migrates laterally, invades the somatopleure (ectoderm plus somatic mesoderm) of the primitive body wall, and differentiates into the various muscular layers of the thorax and abdomen. The rectus muscles differentiate early during migration, the oblique layers forming later. The rectus muscles remain widely separated until growth of the embryo produces a relative reduction in the size of the primitive umbilical cord. Midline fusion of the recti proceeds from both cranial and caudal ends, converging on the umbilical ring at about 12 weeks' gestational age. Formation of the lower body wall between the umbilical ring and genitalia is somewhat more complex, and involves an initial migration and deposition of mesoderm from the region of the cloaca. Failure of this process may contribute to the unique features of bladder and cloacal exstrophy.

The second event with relevance to abdominal wall defects is the physiologic herniation of the developing midgut into the extra embryonic coelom of the umbilical cord. Rapid cellular proliferation during the fourth and fifth weeks causes marked elongation of the midgut, which herniates into the umbilical cord as abdominal wall growth cannot keep pace. This process eventually reverses, with retraction of the midgut into the expanded abdominal cavity by 12 weeks' gestational age. There is considerable controversy regarding the nature of the forces responsible for the return of the intestine to the abdomen, but they may include contributions from the growth of the abdominal wall, the regression of the mesonephros, the relative shrinkage of the liver, and the retraction of the mesentery.

The exact pathogenesis of both omphalocele and gastroschisis is conjectural. In omphalocele, the abdominal muscles are essentially intact but displaced. The umbilical ring is dilated, and abdominal contents herniate into a sac composed of amnion, with an intact umbilical cord inserting into the top of the sac (Fig. 21.1). The sac invariably contains small intestine (midgut), which is variably accompanied by liver, stomach, spleen, colon, and gonads. The abdominal cavity is correspondingly small, and in the case of a giant defect the thoracic cavity may also be abnormally shaped and reduced in size (Fig. 21.2). Rarely, the omphalocele is part of a more complex ventral wall defect including ectopia cordis or bladder/cloacal exstrophy. Whether the cause of omphalocele is failure of abdominal wall folding and fusion, umbilical ring closure, abdominal cavity growth, or mesenteric retraction is speculative. Prevailing opinion favors the failure of whatever forces are responsible for the retraction of the normally herniated intestine into the abdominal cavity around the twelfth week of gestation.

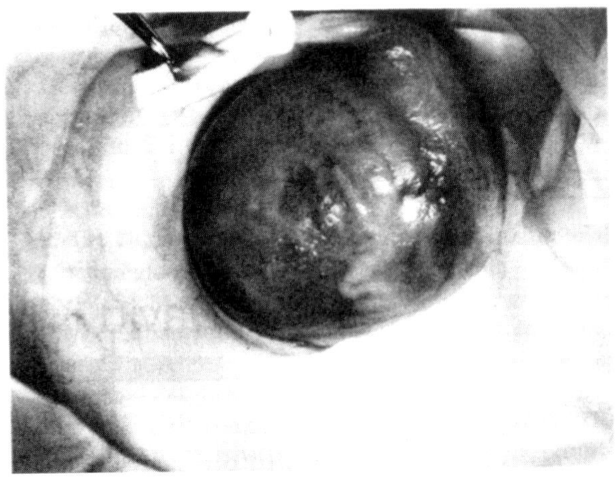

Fig. 21.1. The typical appearance of an omphalocele containing liver and intestine within intact amnion.

Gastroschisis is characterized by a circular defect in the abdominal wall immediately lateral to the umbilical cord, which is usually intact. Approximately 90% of these defects occur on the right side. Although a skin bridge commonly separates the defect from the base of the cord, the underlying rectus muscle is intact and displaced laterally. The defect is usually significantly smaller than that found in omphalocele. No trace of an amnion remains. The evisceration is usually limited to small intestine, though stomach and gonads are occasionally observed. The intestine itself is characterized by a variable degree of injury (Fig. 21.3). The spectrum of intestinal wall morphology extends from complete normalcy to complete atresia and resorption of the midgut (Fig. 21.4). The usual case is associated with an inflammatory "peel" on the surface of the entire eviscerated mass. The peel is occasionally thick enough to

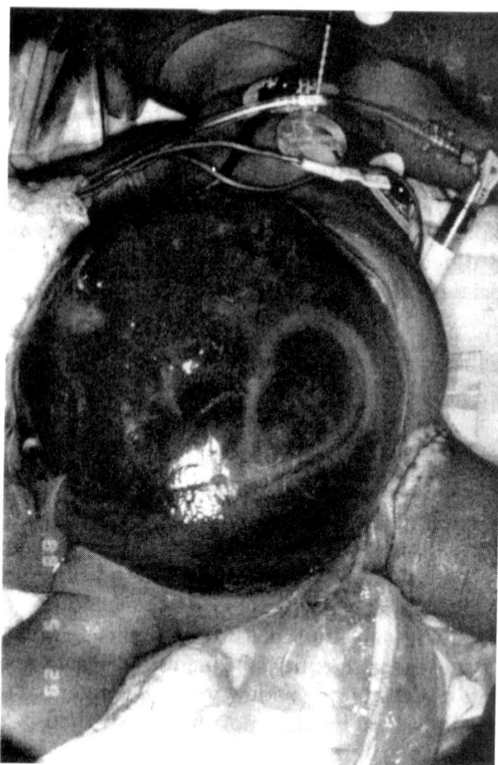

Fig. 21.2. A giant omphalocele with narrow thorax. The infant died from lethal pulmonary hypoplasia.

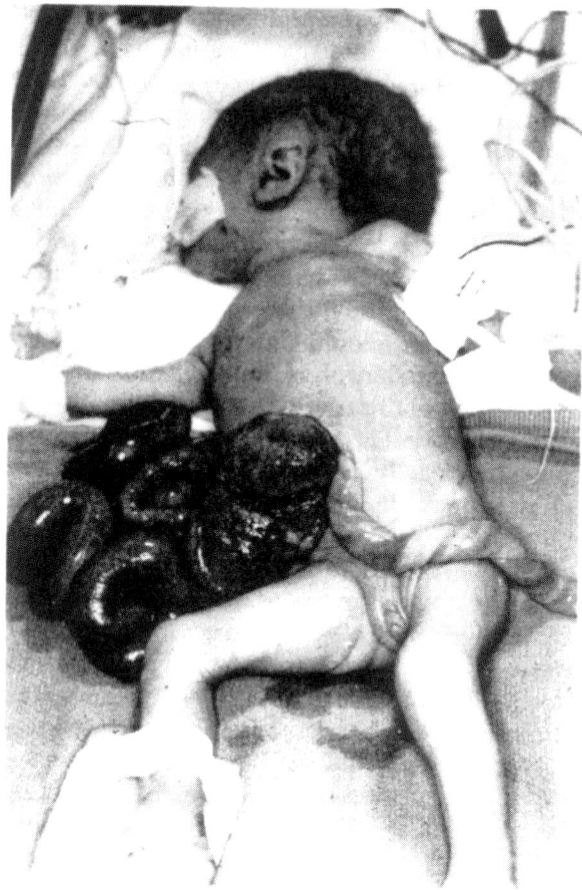

Fig. 21.3. The typical appearance of a gastrostroschisis with the defect to the right of an intact umbilical cord. The intestine is slightly edematous and thickened, exhibiting a mild degree of peel.

obscure completely the individual underlying bowel loops, producing the appearance of a phlegmonous mass. One or more intestinal atresias may be present within the mass. As is the case with omphaloceles, the abdominal cavity is small.

The pathogenesis of gastroschisis is also obscure. Hypotheses invoking a failure of mesodermal migration into the embryonic somatopleure or an ischemic injury to the developing abdominal wall resulting from thromboembolic occlusion of a vitelline or umbilical artery are not supported by the presence of a normally developed but displaced rectus muscle column lateral to the defect. A more satisfactory explanation may be the evisceration of physiologically herniated midgut from the extraembryonic coelom of the umbilical stalk through a tear in the amnion, followed by closure and healing of the amnion defect.

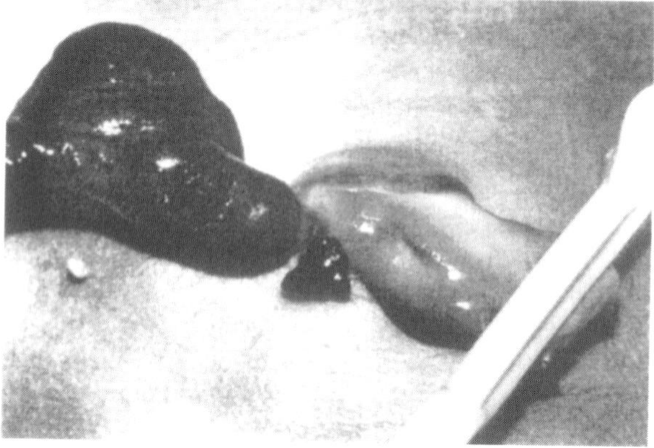

Fig. 21.4. A gastroschisis defect that spontaneously closed *in utero*, causing infarction and resorption of the entire midgut.

Pathophysiology

Perhaps the most striking distinction between omphalocele and gastroschisis is the severe intestinal injury frequently associated with the eviscerated bowel in gastroschisis, often referred to as the "peel." While intestinal structure and function are largely preserved in omphalocele, injury to the externalized bowel accounts for most of the morbidity and mortality associated with gastroschisis. The nature of the intestinal injury causing peel formation, absorption abnormalities, and dysmotility in gastroschisis is the subject of much speculation.

Morphologically, the eviscerated bowel appears matted, edematous, and foreshortened. In a variety of fetal models, observed changes include villous blunting and atrophy, submucosal thickening due to increased collagen deposition, venous and lymphatic dilatation, smooth muscle hyperplasia and hypertrophy, and a thickened serosal layer containing inflammatory cells, fibrin, collagen, and squamous epithelial cells.[1,2] When the effects of exposure to amniotic fluid are distinguished from those due to constriction of the mesentery, the formation of a serosal peel was found to be caused by amniotic fluid exposure, while all other changes were secondary to mechanical compression. The relative effects of luminal obstruction and venous/lymphatic outflow impedance due to constriction have not been precisely defined. A causal relationship between amniotic fluid exposure and peel formation is supported by the finding that peel formation is prevented by amniotic fluid exchange in experimental gastroschisis.[3]

The observation that many infants born with gastroschisis do not exhibit a significant peel has prompted many to question why amniotic fluid exposure does not consistently produce intestinal injury. Recent clinical studies have documented a close linkage between peel formation and meconium staining of the amniotic fluid, suggesting some fetal gastrointestinal constituent (e.g., activated digestive enzymes) is responsible for inducing an inflammatory process in the exposed bowel.[4] Anal ligation in a fetal rat model of gastroschisis has demonstrated that intestinal shortening and wall thickening are related to the degree of meconium contamination of the amniotic fluid.[5] The inflammatory nature of the underlying injury is suggested by the fact that peel formation can be prevented in experimental gastroschisis by either maternal or amniotic dexamethasone administration.[6,7] The thickening and edema of the intestinal wall may also be related to reduced oncotic pressure due to protein loss from the evisceration.[8]

How these structural and histological changes produce the functional correlates of malabsorption and dysmotility is unclear. Mucosal absorption is abnormal in both pre- and postnatal periods in experimental gastroschisis, and may be related both to abnormal villous architecture and impaired expression of enterocyte genes coding for digestive enzymes.[9,10] The delayed development of peristaltic activity in patients with gastroschisis is another major cause of postnatal morbidity. Prenatal intestinal dysmotility has also been documented in fetuses with gastroschisis.[11] Recent findings have strongly suggested that delayed maturation of neuromuscular components of the intestinal wall occurs in gastroschisis. These studies document delayed differentiation of interstitial cells of Cajal (intestinal pacemaker cells) and smooth muscle cells, delayed formation of neurofilaments, delayed synaptic vesicle activity, and delayed maturation of ganglion cells and myenteric neural organization.[12,13] Derangements in nitric oxide activity have also been implicated in the prolonged motility disorder that accompanies gastroschisis.[14]

Epidemiology and risk factors

Abdominal wall defects are uncommon malformations, though the incidence of gastroschisis has increased over the last three decades. Most recent studies report an omphalocele incidence rate of approximately 1.5–2.5 per 10 000 live births, and this rate is stable or declining slowly. From the 1960s to the 1990s, gastroschisis rates increased slowly from approximately 0.5 per 10 000 to 1.0–1.5 per 10 000.[15] The incidence of gastroschisis has increased sharply, however, from approximately 1990 to the present, with current studies reporting incidence rates of up to 5 per 10 000.[16–19] The incidence of gastroschisis in Japan, which has historically been reported to be about one-fourth to one-half the incidence observed in the United States and Europe, has also tripled over roughly the same period.[20]

Studies have reached different conclusions with respect to risk factors for abdominal wall defects. Isolated defects have generally been considered sporadic in nature, while those (particularly omphaloceles) associated with multiple anomalies are thought to have a genetic etiology. Recent reports, however, have supported a non-genetic etiology in some cases of multiple defects and a genetic etiology in cases of sporadic omphalocele and gastroschisis.[21] Clearly, a strong genetic component prevails in cases of syndromic omphalocele, as is discussed below.

Because of its largely sporadic nature, gastroschisis has been exhaustively studied with respect to environmental risk factors, again with conflicting results. Most studies agree on a correlation between gastroschisis and young maternal age. The majority of excess cases of gastroschisis accounting for the dramatic increase in incidence over the last decade are related to infants born to young mothers. Other factors include a disadvantaged socioeconomic background, use of vasoconstrictive decongestants, use of some cyclooxygenase inhibitors (aspirin and ibuprofen), and prenatal substance abuse (alcohol and cocaine).[22,23] Tobacco exposure has also been implicated in gastroschisis. Typical gastroschisis defects can be produced in fetal mice by maternal exposure to carbon monoxide and malnutrition.[24] A separate study noted a seasonal correlation between gastroschisis and conception in the late spring and summer, suggesting a possible association with exposure to teratogenic chemicals in pesticides and herbicides.[25]

Associated anomalies

Another point of divergence between omphalocele and gastroschisis is the coexistence of other major structural and/or chromosomal anomalies. Abnormal intestinal rotation is obligate in both. Numerous studies document an association between omphalocele and other major abnormalities that range from 50 to 75%.[15,26–28] Approximately one-third of patients with omphalocele and normal chromosomes will have an associated structural anomaly.[29] Structural malformations commonly associated with omphalocele include cardiac, gastrointestinal, genitourinary, and central nervous system defects. The associated malformations, not the abdominal wall defect, are the most significant determinants of prognosis.

Syndromic associations have been found with the VACTERL association (vertebral, anorectal, cardiac, tracheoesophageal, renal, limb defects), Beckwith–Wiedemann syndrome (macrosomia, macroglossia, visceromegaly, hemihypertrophy, hypoglycemia), EEC syndrome (ectodermal dysplasia, ectodactyly, cleft palate), and OEIS complex (omphalocele, exstrophy, imperforate anus, spinal defects). Uncommon comalformations include inferior vena caval anomalies and "prune belly" syndrome. A clinically important association between giant omphalocele, thoracic dystrophy, and pulmonary hypoplasia is well recognized.[30] A long-suspected association between abdominal wall defects and undescended testes remains unclear. A specific association between omphalocele, cryptorchidism, and brain malformations is well documented.[31] Some retrospective studies have found a generally increased incidence of cryptorchidism in both omphalocele and gastroschisis, though the increased incidence in gastroschisis may be partially accounted for by prematurity.[32] Other studies have failed to find correlation between abdominal wall defects and undescended testes.[33]

Chromosomal abnormalities are also frequently associated with omphalocele. Studies of fetuses with an omphalocele diagnosed by prenatal ultrasound document a coexistence of chromosomal abnormalities in 20–54%, and suggest that small defect size, the absence of liver in the sac, and the presence of other malformations strongly predict an abnormal karyotype.[34,35] In one recent study, the overall incidence of chromosomal abnormalities in infants with omphalocele was approximately 30%; two-thirds of those with associated structural anomalies displayed abnormal karyotypes, while no infant with an isolated omphalocele had a chromosomal abnormality.[36] The most common chromosomal abnormalities are trisomy 13, 18, and 21.

In contrast, the association between gastroschisis and other malformations was historically reported to be 5%–10%, although incidences as high as 20%–30% have been cited.[15] Most of the reported abnormalities with gastroschisis are intestinal atresias, felt to be caused by vascular compromise of the externalized bowel. Neither chromosomal abnormalities nor cryptorchidism are relatively increased in infants with gastroschisis.

Prenatal diagnosis and management

The ultrasonographic features of both gastroschisis and omphalocele are well-documented, allowing an accurate prenatal diagnosis in the majority of cases. In instances where ambiguity exists, elevated amniotic fluid levels of alpha-fetoprotein and acetylcholinesterase can help distinguish gastroschisis from an intact omphalocele.[37] When an omphalocele is detected on screening ultrasonography, a more extensive sonographic examination is essential to identify associated defects. Karyotyping may be helpful in planning postnatal management or considering elective termination. In gastroschisis, oligohydramnios, bowel dilatation, intrauterine growth retardation, and prematurity are common and may require a change in perinatal management.

Few issues related to the management of abdominal wall defects engender as much debate as do the obstetrical decisions regarding route and timing of delivery of fetuses with gastroschisis. The suggestion that elective cesarean delivery is preferable to spontaneous vaginal delivery owing to the avoidance of the mechanical effects of labor and membrane rupture has been refuted.[38] Although some continue to advocate elective cesarean delivery, the weight of evidence confirming the equivalency of cesarean and vaginal delivery with respect to outcome (primary closure, time to enteral feeds, length of stay, mortality) is well documented in a recent meta-analysis and independent reports.[39–44]

The logical assumption that bowel injury in gastroschisis should be mitigated by early delivery and repair has prompted some enthusiasm for planned early delivery at 34–38 weeks' gestation, after documentation of lung maturity.[45,46] Others have advocated a more selective approach involving serial ultrasonographic assessments of bowel dilatation, thickness, and echogenicity.[47,48] Early delivery (cesarean or vaginal) may then be recommended if these parameters suggest intestinal compromise. To date, however, retrospective studies have not confirmed a reduction in morbidity or mortality in infants delivered preterm.[49,50] On the contrary, the outcome for fetal gastroschisis in these studies was negatively affected by prematurity but not intrauterine growth retardation, suggesting that early delivery may have an adverse effect on gut function and survival.[42,43] Since a potential problem with retrospective methodology is the lack of adequate controls, a strategy of early, selective preterm delivery in fetuses with gastroschisis cannot be fairly evaluated by comparison with the outcomes of infants who are born early due to fetal distress and/or *in utero* compromise. A more recent uncontrolled prospective trial of selective preterm delivery for infants with gastroschisis documented reductions in peel formation, time to enteral feedings, and length of hospitalization.[51] Although the rationale for this approach remains appealing, proof of its efficacy awaits an adequately controlled, prospective randomized trial.

The rationale for selective preterm delivery in gastroschisis is predicated on the ability to assess accurately the *in utero* condition of the eviscerated bowel. Although several trials have utilized sonographic findings such as bowel dilation, wall thickness, and "matting" as a basis for advocating early delivery,[47,48,51] the reliability of the prenatal ultrasound appearance of the bowel in predicting the postnatal clinical course or prognosis has been questioned by others.[52,53] Additional fetal ultrasound findings that may predict peel formation and increased postnatal morbidity include a dilated fetal stomach and the presence of polyhydramnios.[53,54] Increased amniotic fluid beta-endorphin levels, possibly a sign of fetal stress, have also been found to correlate with increase postnatal morbidity.[55] As the progressive nature of intestinal injury and fetal compromise in gastroschisis becomes better understood, the use of frequent sonography, cardiotocography, and fetal home monitoring has been recommended by some to detect fetal distress sooner and direct the use of preterm delivery.[56,57]

As bowel injury in gastroschisis is convincingly linked to prolonged exposure to amniotic fluid components (digestive enzymes, meconium, fetal urine), another potentially useful intervention may be amniotic fluid exchange. Several reports of this technique in gastroschisis combined with severe oligohydramnios confirm its feasibility.[58] Encouraging results in these limited studies has led to a more routine application of amnioexchange for fetal gastroschisis in some institutions, and has generally been associated with improved outcomes.[59] The identification of clinical indicators that allow for the selective application of amnioexchange may promote a more widespread adoption of this technique.

Surgical treatment

The goal of surgical management for all abdominal wall defects is to provide complete fascial and skin closure without causing further injury due to excessive intra-abdominal pressure or abdominal wall tension. Ideally, this goal is realized at the time of the first operation, but can be accomplished in a staged fashion if necessary. Despite sharing this common goal, the operative management of gastroschisis and omphalocele differ substantially.

Gastroschisis

The clinical debate over the preferred strategy for abdominal wall closure – primary vs. staged – rivals that over early delivery in terms of the enthusiastic engagement of its participants. Early studies demonstrating improved outcomes following primary closure were interpreted by many to indicate that prolonged evisceration, no matter how treated, resulted in delayed gut function, and that aggressive attempts to close the defect primarily were justified. Over the last decade, however, a significant trend towards gentle, staged closure has gained widespread acceptance with the realization that most of the mortality, and much of the morbidity, in gastroschisis is related to the complications associated with increased intra-abdominal pressure and decreased visceral perfusion.[60] Careful selection of individual patients with respect to closure strategy provides optimal outcome.

Preoperative evaluation

The objectives of preoperative care in gastroschisis are resuscitation, protection of the eviscerated bowel from injury, and expeditious closure of the defect or coverage of the bowel. Approximately 50%–70% of fetuses with gastroschisis are born prior to 37 weeks' gestation, and greater than 50% are in the lowest quartile for gestational age-adjusted birthweight.[43] As a large number of newborns with gastroschisis are both premature and small for gestational age, the usual postnatal issues related to these problems must be rapidly addressed.

Intravenous access must be established immediately for administration of fluids, glucose, and albumin. The loss of fluid and heat by evaporation and convection from the exposed bowel and peritoneal cavity add significantly to the pre-existing need for fluid resuscitation and external warming. A nasogastric tube is necessary to prevent gaseous distention of the bowel due to crying and mask ventilation, and to reduce the risk of aspiration of gastric contents.

The presence of meconium-stained fluid in the oropharynx or trachea of newborns with gastroschisis is a common finding at delivery, but true meconium aspiration syndrome is unusual. Other significant pulmonary disease, including infant respiratory distress syndrome, may be present, especially in premature infants. Intubation and surfactant administration may be warranted in affected newborns who are significantly premature.

The care of the eviscerated bowel itself is critical. Ideally, it should be aseptically covered while still allowing for visualization to prevent unrecognized torsion and vascular compromise during the transport phase. The authors favor placing the entire baby below the axillae into a sterile, transparent bag with a drawstring closure, such as is used to contain the small intestine during abdominal surgery, and closing the drawstring at the chest level. This covers the bowel, prevents evaporative and convective losses, and allows observation of intestinal viability. A lateral position may be better tolerated than a supine one. In the event of vascular compromise due to a tightly constricting defect, opening the skin and fascia for a short distance superiorly may prevent intestinal loss.

Primary closure

Primary fascial closure in gastroschisis is technically feasible in the majority of cases. In many of these, however, primary closure is accomplished with significant difficulty and under substantial pressure. The factors that interfere with primary closure are abdominovisceral disproportion, the degree of fibrin peel, prematurity, and the presence of severe pulmonary disease. Excessive surgical delay reduces the chance of satisfactory primary closure owing to progressive swelling of the viscera. For this reason, repair of the defect in the delivery room immediately after birth has been advocated by some.[61] Others have noted that, within reason, the time to surgical closure is not associated with outcome, and stress the importance of appropriate resuscitation prior to operative intervention.[62]

A bladder catheter should be placed prior to surgery in addition to the nasogastric tube. Reduction of the gut back into the abdomen may be facilitated by preoperative evacuation of meconium by anal dilation and warm saline rectal irrigation. Manually stretching the abdominal wall from within the abdomen may increase the space available for the externalized viscera. The fascial defect may be extended either vertically or horizontally to facilitate reduction of the abdominal contents. Anesthetic management should include complete neuromuscular blockade with non-depolarizing agents.

After reducing the viscera into the abdomen, primary closure of the gastroschisis defect is usually performed by first dividing the umbilical cord structures deep to the fascia. The edges of the fascial defect must be defined by separating the skin and subcutaneous tissue from the fascia. Whether one chooses to leave the umbilical skin in place depends on the preferred method of creating a neoumbilicus at the end of the procedure. Fascial closure is then attempted while monitoring abdominal, ventilatory, and systemic blood pressures. Gastric or bladder pressure may be transduced to detect increases in intra-abdominal pressure that might compromise intestinal and renal perfusion, venous return from the inferior vena cava, and ventilation.[63]

Staged closure

If preoperative risk factors, intraoperative pressure measurements, or cardiopulmonary deterioration suggest that primary closure is not well-tolerated, the creation of a silo from prosthetic material is a safe alternative. This allows the bowel to be covered in an aseptic manner and to be gradually reduced over an extended period. The fascial defect is usually extended vertically prior to suturing the prosthetic material to the fascia. Cautious skin flap mobilization is performed. The base of the silo should be slightly larger than the top.

A variety of materials may be used for the silo. Reinforced silicone (Silastic) is commonly used because the smooth, non-porous surface prevents fluid and heat loss, as well as intestinal adherence that might result in the formation of an enterocutaneous fistula. A composite material, such as polypropylene mesh lined with silicone has the advantage of promoting tissue ingrowth at the edges, which prevents premature separation of the silo from the fascia and allows for a more gradual reduction of viscera. Various methods of reduction have been described, including twisting of the silo and tying umbilical tape after each successive reduction, suturing or stapling the silo at progressively lower levels. Once the abdominal fascia is approximated, the silo can be removed and a delayed primary repair can be accomplished. A small patch of a permanent prosthetic material such as expanded polytetrafluoroethylene (PTFE, Gore-Tex®) may be necessary to complete closure. At either the first operation or at the time of delayed primary closure, central venous access is advisable to facilitate total parenteral nutrition.

The recent development of preformed Silastic silos with spring-loaded bases of various diameters has

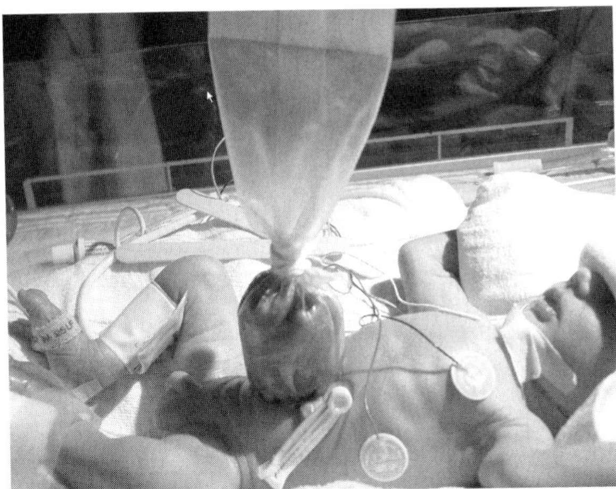

Fig. 21.5. Wringer clamp used to gradually reduce eviscerated bowel contained in the silo.

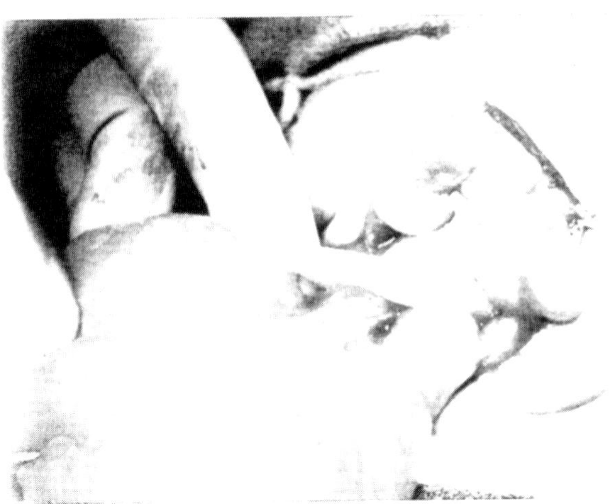

Fig. 21.6. Appearance of gastroschisis complicated by jejunal atresia.

revolutionized both primary and staged closure techniques. Because the spring-loaded base fits underneath the fascial rim without enlarging the defect and holds its position against tension without suturing to the fascia, these silos may be placed in the delivery room or neonatal intensive care unit instead of the operating room (Fig. 21.5). They can be used for protective coverage while transporting the patient to the operating room for primary closure, or can be used for staged closure by standard techniques. Routine use of a preformed silo at the time of delivery and elective closure of the defect after gentle reduction has been reported to result in improved outcomes, including reduced need for ventilatory support, time to enteral feeds, and hospital discharge.[64,65] In addition, the complications of excessive abdominal pressure and decreased visceral perfusion are effectively avoided.

Intestinal atresia

Intestinal atresia occurs in 5%–20% of infants with gastroschisis and presents a challenging problem for which several options exist (Fig. 21.6). Resection and primary anastomosis or proximal enterostomy may be combined with either primary or delayed closure. Resection and anastomosis combined with a tight primary closure is ill advised. Primary or staged closure alone, temporarily deferring management of the atresia, is an increasingly popular approach. After 2–4 weeks, the peel resolves and allows better definition of the anatomy and safer anastomosis. This approach is most appropriate for proximal atresias that can be effectively decompressed for a prolonged time by continuous nasogastric suction. Distal ileal and colonic atresias cannot be effectively managed by nasogastric decompression and are more commonly associated with perforation or segmental necrosis, necessitating surgical management at the outset. Creation of an enterostomy is most conservative, but the coexistence of a stoma and a prosthetic silo theoretically increases the risk of potentially life-threatening sepsis.

Postoperative care

The physiologic consequences of increased abdominal pressure associated with closure of gastroschisis or omphalocele are potentially life-threatening. Central venous and arterial pressure monitoring are therefore desirable in cases with a difficult reduction. A bladder catheter is recommended to monitor urine output. Frequent arterial blood gas measurements in the early postoperative period may reveal metabolic acidosis caused by intestinal ischemia due to impaired perfusion. Oliguria may indicate hypovolemia or increased renal vein pressures. Albumin is an excellent volume expander in these children since most have marked hypoalbuminemia.

Advances in ventilator management have had a significant impact on short term survival. Elevated intra-abdominal pressures impair diaphragmatic excursion and result in reduced extrinsic compliance and functional residual capacity. Mechanical ventilation with positive end-expiratory pressure (PEEP) is frequently required to overcome this problem; high-frequency oscillatory ventilation may be helpful in selected cases. As the abdomen stretches over the first several days after closure, compliance usually improves and inspiratory pressures and inspired oxygen can be reduced. Every effort is made to reduce barotrauma and oxygen toxicity during mechanical ventilation. Continued neuromuscular paralysis may be necessary to permit adequate ventilation, especially when the intra-abdominal pressures are high. While infants who were closed primarily required a shorter period of ventilation in most studies, the presence of a silo does not preclude extubation during the reduction phase unless high intra-abdominal pressures are necessary to achieve closure before dehiscence of the silo occurs.

Parenteral nutrition is administered until regular intestinal function is documented. This may occur within a few days of surgery, but more typically begins 1–2 weeks after closure, and normal peristalsis may not be achieved for 3–6 weeks. If stooling does not occur within 2 weeks, a retrograde water-soluble contrast study is advisable to determine whether an unrecognized intestinal atresia is present. The combination of gastroschisis and Hirschsprung's disease has been reported and may be mistaken for routine dysmotility.[66] Since the ability to tolerate enteral feedings may be quite delayed, the avoidance of TPN-associated cholestatic liver disease should be attempted. Cyclical administration of TPN, addition of taurine, avoidance of sepsis, and reduction of copper and manganese are all factors which have been purported to reduce the risk of cholestasis. Early initiation of partial enteral feedings is perhaps the most important factor in avoiding this serious complication.

Omphalocele

Preoperative evaluation

The presence of associated anomalies such as aneuploidy, pulmonary hypoplasia, Beckwith–Wiedemann syndrome, cardiac, or renal lesions takes precedence over the abdominal wall defect in dictating initial postnatal management. The presence of an intact amnion obviates the need for urgent primary repair in the first few hours of life. Instead, a detailed sonographic and radiologic evaluation should be performed to rule out concurrent malformations. In patients with a lethal anomaly or a physiologic deficit that might interfere with a complete recovery from surgery, a non-operative treatment strategy is favored. The rare coexistence of omphalocele with Beckwith–Wiedemann syndrome may necessitate aggressive diagnosis and treatment of hypoglycemia to prevent neurologic injury. Pulmonary hypoplasia, which may be indicated by a narrow thorax on a chest radiograph, is often associated with a giant defect. If the omphalocele is ruptured, the same issues of resuscitation and intestinal coverage pertain as for gastroschisis, and urgent operative intervention is usually indicated. Occasionally, a small tear in an otherwise intact amnion may be suture repaired at the bedside.

Primary and delayed closure

The operative approach for omphalocele closure is similar to that for gastroschisis, with several exceptions. The amnion can be removed entirely or left to cover the intestine and liver. Leaving the amnion in place is particularly beneficial in large defects or when prosthetic material is used to close the defect. The fascial edges are then approximated using interrupted sutures in a similar fashion to gastroschisis. If fascial approximation results in excessive intra-abdominal pressure, a patch of prosthetic material may be used. A smooth, non-adhering material such as Gore-Tex® is best, but mesh materials such as Marlex can be used, provided the amnion is left in place to protect against the formation of an enterocutaneous fistula. Primary closure of the skin is usually possible regardless of the size of the defect. Construction of a neoumbilicus is also desirable. The use of tissue expanders to promote the growth and enlargement of the muscular abdominal wall as an adjunct to staged closure has been reported.[67]

Skin closure alone, as described by Gross, is an alternative to primary fascial repair. Skin flaps can be raised and mobilized sufficiently to bring the skin edges together, covering even large defects. This approach was developed in response to ventilatory dysfunction in children with large omphaloceles, as well as the infections which resulted when prosthetic materials were used. These children had large ventral hernias which eventually required fascial repair. Unfortunately, the amnion was usually removed and the skin became densely adherent to underlying bowel and liver. Subsequent repair was uniformly difficult, bloody, and complicated. More recent advocates of skin closure without fascial repair have stressed the importance of leaving the amnion in place, which makes later fascial closure substantially safer. As the skin flaps are more elastic than the fascia, the defect and overlying skin tend to enlarge with time at the expense of abdominal cavity growth. Ultimate fascial closure should, therefore, be delayed no longer than necessary.

Initial non-operative management

The non-operative approach to omphalocele is based on the ability of the amnion to support epithelial proliferation and migration from the skin edges. Topical antimicrobial agents such as silver sulfadiazine cream that promote the development of an aseptic eschar are used (Fig. 21.7). Other topical agents have been used, but many have toxic side effects. The use of acellular dermal matrix to accommodate

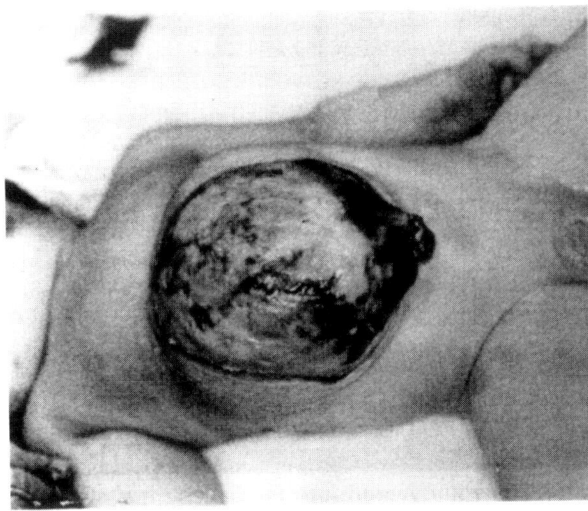

Fig. 21.7. Eschar formation after application of silver sulfadiazine cream to intact amnion in a baby with a large omphalocele and multiple associated anomalies.

early epithelial grafting has been reported.[68] The fascial defect does not enlarge with age, so that its relative size decreases. Circumferential binding with elastic bandages helps to gently force the abdominal organs back into the abdomen, gradually increasing the size of the abdominal cavity. The residual ventral hernia can be closed at a later age when reduction of the abdominal organs beneath the level of the fascia is better tolerated. This approach has proven particularly beneficial for infants with pulmonary hypoplasia who experience significant parenchymal lung growth in the period before fascial closure. In severe cases, in which children have required tracheostomy and long term ventilation, definitive repair has been deferred for up to 2 years, at which time it is better tolerated (Fig. 21.8).

Postoperative care

The postoperative concerns about increased intra-abdominal pressure are equally important for omphalocele patients as for those with gastroschisis. The central venous pressure and volume issues discussed above are often more problematic in omphalocele patients since the inferior vena cava (IVC) may be anatomically abnormal. As the liver is replaced in the abdomen, the IVC may easily become distorted, compromising venous return to the heart and obstructing renal vein flow. The ventilatory issues are also important, especially since some of these children have pulmonary hypoplasia. Fortunately, intestinal function for omphalocele patients is usually well preserved and most can be fed in the early postoperative period.

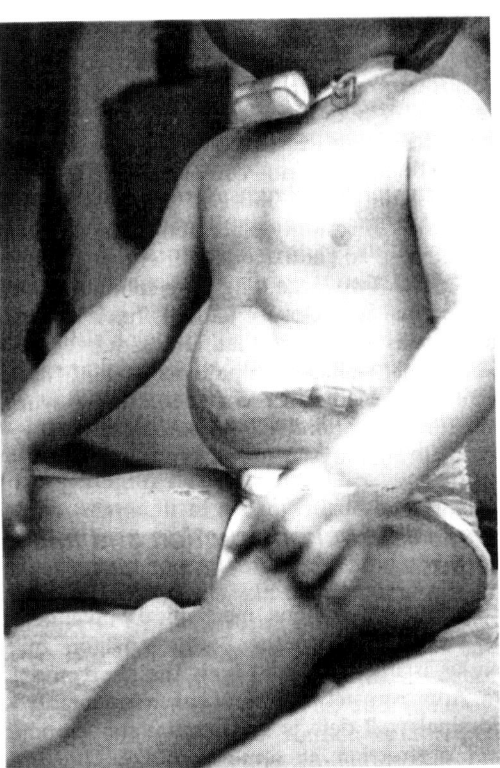

Fig. 21.8. Epithelialized amnion and residual ventral hernia after non-operative treatment of a large omphalocele in an infant with concurrent pulmonary hypoplasia.

Results, complications, and long-term outcome

It is difficult to extrapolate current survival rates for abdominal wall defects from retrospective data because of historical and regional differences in perinatal and perioperative management, and evolving trends in elective termination of pregnancy based on prenatal diagnosis. In general, survival for infants with gastroschisis is much higher than that for infants with omphalocele, and this difference is explained in large part by the frequent coexistence of lethal chromosomal abnormalities and congenital malformations in the latter. Current mortality rates cited for gastroschisis are 5%–10%,[69,70] while those cited for omphalocele range from 20%–70%.[15,26,29] Both gastroschisis and omphalocele can be segregated into low and high risk groups. For gastroschisis, the 20%–30% of patients with intestinal atresia, stenosis, or perforation constitute a higher-risk group with a mortality rate of approximately 30%.[71] Patients without these complicating features have a nearly 100% survival. Patients with omphalocele and normal chromosomes have a mortality rate of approximately

20%, considerably lower than the overall rate.[29] When infants with both chromosomal abnormalities and major anatomic anomalies are excluded, the mortality rate for isolated omphalocele approaches that of gastroschisis. Causes of perioperative mortality related to the closure of the abdominal wall defect itself include the development of necrotizing enterocolitis, sepsis from silo-related abdominal wall infections, and the acute effects of increased intra-abdominal pressure on visceral perfusion, venous return and pulmonary function.

Gastrointestinal function

Morbidity due to alterations in gastrointestinal function is more common in gastroschisis than omphalocele, in which the intestinal tract is protected by amnion.[72] The observed delay in full enteral feeding may be related to temporary deficiencies in mucosal absorption, motility, and intestinal length, and is recognized even in infants with minimal or no apparent peel. Although these deficiencies are widely recognized in clinical practice, little objective data exist to explain them. Measurements of intestinal length in gastroschisis infants are artificially low because the peel tethers the mesentery and foreshortens the bowel. The disappearance of the peel and the enteroendocrine response to enteral substrate causes elongation of the bowel. A significant increase in intestinal length is commonly observed in infants who are re-explored after closure of gastroschisis. Intestinal motility and myoelectric activity have also been observed to normalize over time.[73] Since developmental immaturity of the intestinal wall has been well described in experimental gastroschisis, it is possible that the delayed onset of intestinal motility observed clinically may be related to an obligate period of postnatal neuromuscular maturation.

It is unlikely that gastrointestinal function is improved by primary closure compared with delayed closure, and patients have not been randomly assigned to these two strategies in any published series. Several reports suggest a more rapid initiation of enteral feedings, shorter hospital stays, and fewer complications in patients who were closed primarily. Retrospective studies, however, have not consistently documented a correlation between primary closure and reduced time to full enteral feedings or the need for parenteral nutrition.[74,75] Postnatal gastrointestinal function, as measured by time to full enteral feedings, has been shown to correlate with gestational age and not with intrauterine growth retardation or type of abdominal wall closure.[76] It is evident that infants in whom primary closure is feasible and safe exhibit less intestinal injury than infants who require delayed fascial closure. Newborns with massive abdomino-visceral disproportion, respiratory insufficiency, or intestinal atresia are preferentially treated by the more conservative method of staged repair. The apparent advantages of primary closure may therefore reflect patient selection bias.

Eventually, the vast majority of infants with gastroschisis not complicated by atresia or resection can be weaned from intravenous nutritional support. In a few infants with sustained gastrointestinal dysfunction, however, prolonged TPN dependence and the concomitant development of cholestatic liver disease characterize a subset of patients with a much poorer prognosis. Short bowel syndrome, which prolongs TPN dependence and increases both morbidity and mortality, has been studied in patients with abdominal wall defects, and is usually due to the ischemic complications of excessively tight primary closure.[77] Interestingly, fetuses with abdominal wall defects and intrauterine growth retardation do as well as appropriate size fetuses with respect to primary closure, postoperative complications, and duration of hospitalization.[78]

Intestinal atresia

The coexistence of intestinal atresia with gastroschisis is not uncommon, occurring in 5%–25%. Atresias may occur anywhere from the duodenum to the distal colon, and are frequently multiple. As the pathophysiological consequences of intestinal atresia are nearly identical to those of gastroschisis, deleterious effects on gastrointestinal function and nutrition are additive. Bowel length is short and intestinal dysmotility severe and prolonged in those with combined lesions; all reported series have noted substantial delays in enteral feeding and discharge from hospital. A large number of infants continue to require prolonged parenteral nutrition following discharge. Recurrent operations for adhesive obstruction, anastomotic dysfunction, and persistent bowel dysmotility and dilatation are common in survivors. Dilated bowel loops are often akinetic, and some of these children respond favorably to plication of the dilated bowel which improves peristaltic efficiency and reduces stasis.

Numerous reports identify the presence of intestinal atresia as the most important parameter determining a poor prognosis in gastroschisis.[79–81] Morbidity and mortality in these series were mostly related to the hepatic complications of long-term parenteral nutrition in those infants with short-bowel syndrome or persistent malabsorption and dysmotility. Catheter-related sepsis is another common cause of morbidity and mortality in this particular group.

Necrotizing enterocolitis

A less well-recognized but important contributor to postoperative morbidity in gastroschisis is the development of necrotizing enterocolitis (NEC).[82] When defined as gastrointestinal dysfunction with radiographic evidence of pneumatosis intestinalis, NEC may occur in up to 15%–20% of infants following gastroschisis repair; the typical clinical features of NEC without pneumatosis may occur in another 20%.[83] Surprisingly, increased intra-abdominal pressure does not correlate with the development of NEC, as the incidence of the condition following primary closure is no different than that following delayed closure. The only variables that correlated with NEC in one study were the delayed onset of enteral feeds and the development of TPN-related liver disease.[83] The incidence of NEC may be less in patients with gastroschisis fed with maternal breast milk than in those fed with commercial formulas.[84] Episodes of NEC are often characterized by late presentation, a benign clinical course, successful non-operative management, and no negative impact on overall survival. These factors, coupled with the observation that mortality was weakly correlated with TPN-related liver disease, have led some authors to adopt the somewhat aggressive posture of advancing enteral feedings in the face of active pneumatosis. The efficacy of this approach has not been validated.

Gastroesophageal reflux

Gastroesophageal reflux is a relatively common problem in infants with abdominal wall defects.[85] Whether this is related to an increased abdominothoracic pressure gradient or to altered anatomy at the gastroesophageal junction is unclear, though the transient effects of the former have been documented in an animal model.[86] In the early postoperative period, when these changes might be expected to be most acute, reflux may compound the problems of dysmotility already present. For this reason, administration of prokinetic and acid antisecretory agents may be beneficial in infants with abdominal wall defects and delayed enteral function.

It is uncommon for gastroesophageal reflux to remain a clinically significant problem during later childhood. One study documented a high incidence of gastroesophageal reflux by esophageal pH measurements in both symptomatic and asymptomatic infants following closure of an abdominal wall defect.[87] Reflux was not common after the age of 2 years. Additionally, most of these patients had undergone gastrostomy placement, which is known to predispose to reflux independent of abdominal wall closure. Two large long-term follow-up studies of patients with abdominal wall defects have not identified reflux as a significant late problem.[88,89]

Adhesive bowel obstruction and midgut volvulus

Contrary to expectations, mechanical bowel obstruction secondary either to adhesions or midgut volvulus is uncommon in both the short and long term. Approximately 5%–10% of surviving infants with an abdominal wall defect will require reoperation for bowel obstruction at some point.[88,89] The risk of late bowel obstruction may be highest in patients with gastroschisis complicated by intestinal atresia, although late adhesive intestinal obstruction may occur many years after uncomplicated primary gastroschisis repair. The presence of extensive adhesions has been documented in two patients undergoing gynecological surgery as adults after repair of gastroschisis and ruptured omphalocele as infants.[90]

Midgut volvulus is an uncommon consequence of the intestinal malrotation that necessarily accompanies abdominal wall defects. The long-term studies by Tunell *et al.*[88] and Larsson and Kullendorff[89] mention no patients with this complication. In an extensive retrospective study, only 1% of patients who underwent repair of a congenital abdominal wall defect without a concurrent Ladd's procedure subsequently developed an acute midgut volvulus, though the duration of follow-up was variable.[91] Both instances occurred in infants who had had an omphalocele with an intact sac, and both were fatal. Whether or not a Ladd's procedure or appendectomy should be done at the time of abdominal closure or ventral herniorrhaphy depends on the presence of inflammatory changes, the ease of abdominal closure, and the surgeon's clinical judgment. At a minimum, the parents of a child with a repaired abdominal wall defect must be made aware of the rotational abnormality and the potential for intestinal volvulus.

Abdominal wall hernias

Residual or recurrent abdominal wall hernias are another long-term complication of congenital abdominal wall defects, though morbidity is small and mortality negligible. Ventral hernias are either intentional, as a result of initial skin-flap coverage or preservation of the amnion, or unintentional after fascial or silo dehiscence. The reported incidence of ventral hernias has historically ranged from 10% to 30%, depending on the number of infants initially treated by Gross's method. While initial non-operative management of omphaloceles or skin-flap coverage alone always resulted in a ventral hernia, several patients with skin-flap coverage of a gastroschisis defect exhibited spontaneous closure of their ventral hernia.[89] Although skin-flap coverage alone is rarely used at present, current interest in initial non-operative management of giant omphaloceles may result in a larger number of children who ultimately require delayed ventral herniorrhaphy.

When treatment of a congenital abdominal wall defect results in a ventral hernia, whether intentional or not, the defect can be closed in one stage in the majority of patients.[92] In the remainder, sequential, staged closure with progressively smaller patches is usually successful. Morbidity has largely been limited to intestinal injury during dissection of the densely adherent skin layer, and can be prevented by preserving the amnion or interposing prosthetic material between skin and bowel during initial surgical treatment. Given the risk of enterocutaneous fistula formation with prosthetic mesh, non-porous Gore-Tex® or Silastic should be used alone or as a composite prosthesis when intentionally creating a ventral defect.

Pulmonary complications

Impaired pulmonary function is an important cause of postoperative complications in both gastroschisis and omphalocele. Increased intra-abdominal pressure following primary fascial closure in both conditions results in decreased compliance and increased positive pressure requirements in the early postoperative period, but the effect is transient.[93] Interestingly, measured compliance is also reduced preoperatively. This may be due in part to the fact that prematurity and hyaline membrane disease may also be present, particularly in gastroschisis. The role of exogenous surfactant administration in reducing the need for assisted ventilation has not been determined.

Another study confirmed a significant reduction in lung volumes, flow rates, and compliance following primary repair of both gastroschisis and omphalocele.[94] Although the reductions in volumes and flow rates were transient, compliance remained decreased over the 4-week study period. Bronchodilators were moderately effective in improving lung volumes and flow rates in the short term, and may improve pulmonary function in some ventilator-dependent infants following primary repair.

Overly aggressive attempts at primary closure in order to avoid a silo can result in extreme reductions in pulmonary compliance which may require ventilation with pressures sufficiently high to cause short- and long-term complications of barotrauma: maldistribution of pulmonary blood flow resulting in inefficient gas exchange, pneumothorax, and parenchymal changes consistent with interstitial emphysema and bronchopulmonary dysplasia. Impairment of venous return also reduces cardiac output and pulmonary blood flow, compounding respiratory insufficiency. Pulmonary hypertension resulting in persistent fetal circulation and right-to-left shunting has been reported as a complication of increased intra-abdominal pressure after primary closure.[95]

Apart from acquired abnormalities in pulmonary function caused by increased intra-abdominal pressure, there exists a well-documented association between giant omphalocele and pulmonary hypoplasia. Babies with a giant omphalocele containing liver and a narrow thoracic cage on a chest radiograph are at high risk of respiratory distress from pulmonary hypoplasia.[30] Reduced bronchial branchings, acinar complexity, and acinar maturation have been documented in these patients. Infants with pulmonary hypoplasia complicating giant omphalocele tend to require longer periods of ventilatory support and supplemental oxygen administration, and have higher mortality rates.[96,97]

Growth and development

The long-term outcome of gastroschisis and omphalocele with respect to growth and development is generally good, and tends to improve with time. An early report of impaired physical growth after abdominal wall repair documented that the majority of children were more than two standard deviations below the norms in length and weight for their ages despite normal liver function studies, normal intestinal absorption, and a virtual absence of infants with atresias in the sample.[98] Little "catch-up" growth occurred over time. Whether or not poor growth was simply related to prematurity and intrauterine growth retardation was not determined.

More recent surveys have found abdominal wall defect survivors to be normal in weight, height, and other anthropometric parameters.[99] Whether this difference is attributable to improvements in nutritional care or to the older age of the sample group in the latter studies is unclear. The vast majority of children who underwent abdominal wall repair as neonates report good or excellent health. Some gastroschisis patients, however, express subjective complaints regarding minor gastrointestinal symptoms, social maladjustment, and the cosmetic appearance of an absent umbilicus. In spite of normal measured lung volumes and function, children with large abdominal wall defects appear to develop reduced exercise tolerance, possibly due to a more sedentary lifestyle.[100] Intellectual development in these patients is average, but learning disabilities and behavioral problems may occur with increased frequency. The pediatric surgeon's role, therefore, does not end when abdominal wall integrity is restored, but should extend to making parents and pediatricians aware of potential problems that may occur in later childhood. When all of these issues are adequately addressed, the eventual quality of life for most infants with isolated abdominal wall defects should be little different from that of other healthy children. Improvements in the long-term outcome for infants with complicated abdominal wall defects await more objective appraisals of controversial techniques, such as planned early delivery and amniotic fluid exchange, which may alter the pathophysiology of intestinal injury in these challenging patients.

REFERENCES

1. Langer, J. C., Longaker, M. T., Crombleholme, T. M. *et al.* Etiology of intestinal damage in gastroschisis. I: Effects of amniotic fluid exposure and bowel constriction in a fetal lamb model. *J. Pediatr. Surg.* 1989; **24**:992–997.
2. Srinathan, S. K., Langer, J. C., Blennerhassett, M. G. *et al.* Etiology of intestinal damage in gastroschisis. III: Morphometric analysis of the smooth muscle and submucosa. *J. Pediatr. Surg.* 1995; **30**:379–383.
3. Aktug, T., Erdag, G., Kargi, A. *et al.* Amnio-allantoic fluid exchange for the prevention of intestinal damage in gastroschisis: an experimental study on chick embryos. *J. Pediatr. Surg.* 1995; **30**:384–387.
4. Nichol, P. F., Hayman, A., Pryde, P. G. *et al.* Meconium staining of amniotic fluid correlates with intestinal peel formation in gastroschisis. *Pediatr. Surg. Int.* 2004; **20**:211–214.
5. Correia-Pinto, J., Tavares, M. L., Baptista, M. J. *et al.* Meconium dependence of bowel damage in gastroschisis. *J. Pediatr. Surg.* 2002; **37**:31–35.
6. Yu, J., Gonzales-Reyes, S., Diez-Pardo, J. A., & Tovar, J. A. Effects of prenatal dexamethazone on the intestine of rats with gastroschisis. *J. Pediatr. Surg.* 2003; **38**:1032–1035.
7. Yu, J., Gonzales-Reyes, S., Diez-Pardo, J. A., & Tovar, J A. Local dexamethazone improves the intestinal lesions of gastroschisis in chick embryos. *Pediatr. Surg. Int.* 2004; **19**:780–784.
8. Carroll, S. G., Kuo, P. Y., Kyle, P. M., & Soothill, P. W. Fetal protein loss in gastroschisis as an explanation of associated morbidity. *Am. J. Obstet. Gynecol.* 2001; **184**:1297–1301.
9. Shaw, K., Buchmiller, T. L., Curr, M. *et al.* Impairment of nutrient uptake in a rabbit model of gastroschisis. *J. Pediatr. Surg.* 1994; **29**:376–378.
10. Srinathan, S. K., Langer, J. C., Wang, J. L., & Rubin, D. C. Enterocytic gene expression is altered in experimental gastroschisis. *J. Surg. Res.* 1997; **68**:1–6.
11. Oyachi, N., Lakshmanan, J., Ross, M. G., & Atkinson, J. B. Fetal gastrointestinal motility in a rabbit model of gastroschisis. *J. Pediatr. Surg.* 2004; **39**:366–370.
12. Midrio, P., Faussone-Pellegrini, M. S., Vannucchi, M. G., & Flake, A. W. Gastroschisis in the rat model is associated with a delayed maturation of intestinal pacemaker cells and smooth muscle cells. *J. Pediatr. Surg.* 2004; **39**:1541–1547.
13. Vannucchi, M. G., Midrio, P., Flake, A. W., & Faussone-Pellegrini, M. S. Neuronal differentiation and myenteric plexus organization are delayed in gastroschisis: an immunochemical study in a rat model. *Neurosci. Lett.* 2003; **339**:77–81.
14. Bealer, J. F., Graf, J., Bruch, S. W. *et al.* Gastroschisis increases small bowel nitric oxide synthase activity. *J. Pediatr. Surg.* 1996; **31**:1043–1045.
15. Calzolari, E., Bianchi, F., Dolk, H., & Milan, M. Omphalocele and gastroschisis in Europe: a survey of 3 million births 1980–1990. EUROCAT Working Group. *Am. J. Med. Genet.* 1995; **58**:187–194.
16. Kazaura, M. R., Lie, R. T., Irgens, L. M. *et al.* Increasing incidence of gastroschisis in Norway: an age-period-cohort analysis. *Am. J. Epidemiol.* 2004; **159**:358–363.
17. Salihu, H. M., Pierre-Louis, B. J., Druschel, C. M., & Kirby, R. S. Omphalocele and gastroschisis in the State of New York, 1992–1999. *Birth Defects Res. A Clin. Mol. Teratol.* 2003; **67**:630–636.
18. Reid, K. P., Dickinson, J. E., & Doherty, D. A. The epidemiologic incidence of congenital gastroschisis in Western Australia. *A. M. J. Obstet. Gynecol.* 2003; **189**:764–768.
19. Laughon, M., Meyer, R., Bose, C., *et al.* Rising birth prevalence of gastroschisis. *J. Perinatol.* 2003; **23**:291–293.
20. Suita, S., Okamatsu, T., Yamamoto, T. *et al.* Changing profile of abdominal wall defects in Japan: results of a national survey. *J. Pediatr. Surg.* 2000; **35**:66–71.
21. Reece, A., Thornton, J., & Stringer, M. D. Genetic factors in the aetiology of gastroschisis: a case report. *Eur. J. Obstet. Gynecol. Reprod. Biol.* 1997; **73**:127–128.
22. Torfs, C. P., Katz, E. A., Bateson, T. F. *et al.* Maternal medications and environmental exposures as risk factors for gastroschisis. *Teratology* 1996; **54**:84–92.
23. Werler, M. M., Sheehan, J. E., & Mitchell, A A. Association of vasoconstrictive exposures with risks of gastroschisis and small intestinal atresia. *Epidemiology* 2003; **14**:349–354.
24. Singh, J. Gastroschisis is caused by the combination of carbon monoxide and protein–zinc deficiencies in mice. *Birth Defects Res. B Dev. Reprod. Toxicol.* 2003; **68**:355–362.
25. Goldblum, G., Darling, J., & Milham, S. Risk factors for gastroschisis. *Teratology* 1990; **42**:397–403.
26. Hwang, P. J. & Kousseff, B. G. Omphalocele and gastroshisis: an 18-year review study. *Genet. Med.* 2004; **6**:232–236.
27. Blazer, S., Zimmer, E. Z., Gover, A., & Bronshtein, M. Fetal omphalocele detected early in pregnancy: associated anomalies and outcomes. *Radiology* 2004; **232**:191–195.
28. Stoll, C., Alembik, Y., Dott, B., & Roth, M. P. Risk factors in congenital abdominal wall defects (omphalocele and gastroschisis): a study in a series of 265,858 consecutive births. *Ann. Genet.* 2001; **44**:201–208.
29. Heider, A. L., Strauss, R. A., & Kuller, J. A. Omphalocele: clinical outcomes in cases with normal karyotypes. *Am. J. Obstet. Gynecol.* 2004; **190**:135–141.
30. Argyle, J. C. Pulmonary hypoplasia in infants with giant abdominal wall defects. *Pediatr. Pathol.* 1989; **9**:43–55.
31. Hadziselimovic, F., Duckett, J. W., Snyder, H. M. *et al.* Omphalocele, cryptorchidism, and brain malformations. *J. Pediatr. Surg.* 1987; **22**:854–856.

32. Koivusalo, A., Taskinen, S., & Rintala, R. J. Cryptorchidism in boys with congenital abdominal wall defects. *Pediatr. Surg. Int.* 1998; **13**:143–145.
33. Aliotta, P. J., Piedmont, M., Karp, M., & Greenfield, S. P. Cryptorchidism in newborns with gastroschisis and omphalocele. *Urology* 1992; **40**:84–86.
34. Nicolaides, K. H., Snijders, R. J., Cheng, H. H., & Gosden, C. Fetal gastrointestinal and abdominal wall defects: associated malformations and chromosomal abnormalities. *Fetal Diag. Ther*. 1992; **7**:107–115.
35. Nyberg, D. A., Fitzsimmons, J., Mack, L. A. *et al.* Chromosomal abnormalities in fetuses with omphalocele: significance of omphalocele contents. *J. Ultrasound Med.* 1989; **8**:299–308.
36. DeVeciana, M., Major, C. A., & Porto, M. Prediction of an abnormal karyotype in fetuses with omphalocele. *Prenat. Diag*. 1994; **14**:487–492.
37. Tucker, J. M., Brumfield, C. G., Davis, R. O. *et al.* Prenatal differentiation of ventral abdominal wall defects: are amniotic fluid markers useful adjuncts? *J. Reprod. Med.* 1992; **37**:445–448.
38. Strauss, R. A., Balu, R., Kuller, J. A., & McMahon, M. J. Gastroschisis: the effect of labor and ruptured membranes on neonatal outcome. *Am. J. Obstet. Gynecol.* 2003; **189**:1672–1678.
39. Dunn, J. C., Fonkalsrud, E. W., & Atkinson, J. B. The influence of gestational age and mode of delivery on infants with gastroschisis. *J. Pediatr. Surg.* 1999; **34**:1393–1395.
40. Moore, T. C., Collins, D. L., Catanzarite, V., & Hatch, E. I. Jr. Pre-term and particularly pre-labor cesarean section to avoid complications of gastroschisis. *Pediatr. Surg. Int.* 1999; **15**:97–104.
41. Segal, S. Y., Marder, S. J., Parry, S., & Macones, G. A. Fetal abdominal wall defects and mode of delivery: a systematic review. *Obstet. Gynecol.* 2001; **98**:867–873.
42. Salihu, H. M., Emusu, D., Aliyu, Z. Y. *et al.* Mode of delivery and neonatal survival in infants with isolated gastroschisis. *Obstet. Gynecol.* 2004; **104**:678–683.
43. Puligandla, P. S., Janvier, A., Flageole, H. *et al.* Routine cesarean delivery does not improve the outcome of infants with gastroschisis. *J. Pediatrr. Surg.* 2004; **39**:742–745.
44. Adra, A. M., Landy, H. J., Nahmias, J., & Gomez-Marin, O. The fetus with gastroschisis; impact of route of delivery and prenatal ultrasonography. *Am. J. Obst. Gyn.* 1996; **174**:540–546.
45. Fitzsimmons, J., Nyberg, D. A., & Hatch, E. Perinatal management of gastroschisis. *Obstet. Gynecol.* 1988; **71**:910–913.
46. Swift, R. I., Singh, M. P., Ziderman, D. A. *et al.* A new regime in the management of gastroschisis. *J. Pediatr. Surg.* 1992; **27**:61–63.
47. Bond, S. J., Harrison, M. R., & Filly, R. A. Severity of intestinal damage in gastroschisis: correlation with prenatal sonographic findings. *J. Pediatr. Surg.* 1988; **23**:520–525.
48. Pryde, P. G., Bardicef, M., Treadwell, M. C. *et al.* Gastroschisis: can antenatal ultrasound predict infant outcomes? *Obstet. Gynecol.* 1994; **84**:505–510.
49. Simmons, M. & Georgeson, K. E. The effect of gestational age at birth on morbidity in patients with gastroschisis. *J. Pediatr. Surg.* 1996; **31**:1060–1062.
50. Huang, J., Kurkchubasche, A. G., Carr, S. R. *et al.* Benefits of term delivery in infants with antenatally diagnosed gastroschisis. *Obstet. Gynecol.* 2002; **100**:695–699.
51. Moir, C. R., Ramsey, P. S., Ogburn, P. L. *et al.* A prospective trial of preterm delivery for fetal gastroschisis. *Am. J. Perinatol.* 2004; **21**:289–294.
52. Alsulyman, O. M., Monteiro, H., Ouzounian, J. G. *et al.* Clinical significance of prenatal ultrasonographic intestinal dilatation in fetuses with gastroschisis. *Am. J. Obstet. Gynecol.* 1996; **175**:982–984.
53. Japaraj, R. P., Hockey, R., & Chan, F. Y. Gastroschisis: can prenatal sonography predict neonatal outcome? *Ultrasound Obstet. Gynecol.* 2003; **21**:329–333.
54. Aina-Mumuney, A. J., Fisher, A. C., Blakemore, K. J. *et al.* A dilated fetal stomach predicts a complicated postnatal course in cases of prenatally diagnosed gastroschisis. *Am. J. Obstet. Gynecol.* 2004; **190**:1326–1330.
55. Mahieu-Caputo, D., Muller, F., Jouvet, P. *et al.* Amniotic fluid beta-endorphin: a prognostic marker for gastroschisis? *J. Pediatrr. Surg.* 2002; **37**:1602–1606.
56. Salomon, L. J., Mahieu-Caputo, D., Jouvet, P. *et al.* Fetal home monitoring for the prenatal management of gastroschisis. *Acta. Obstet. Gynecol. Scand.* 2004; **83**:1061–1064.
57. Brantberg, A., Blass, H. G., Salvesen, K. A. *et al.* Surveillance and outcome of fetuses with gastroschisis. *Ultrasound Obstet. Gynecol.* 2004; **23**:4–13.
58. Sapin, E., Mahieu, D., Borgnon, J. *et al.* Transabdominal amnioinfusion to avoid fetal demise and intestinal damage in fetuses with gastroschisis and severe oligohydramnios. *J. Pediatrr. Surg.* 2000; **35**:598–600.
59. Luton, D., Guibourdenche, J., Vuillard, E. *et al.* Prenatal management of gastroschisis: the place of the amnioexchange procedure. *Clin. Perinatol.* 2003; **30**:551–572.
60. Kidd, J. N. Jr, Jackson, R. J., Smith, S. D., & Wagner, C. W. Evolution of stage versus primary closure of gastroschisis. *Ann. Surg*. 2003; **237**:759–764.
61. Coughlin, J. P., Drucker, D. E., Jewell, M. R. *et al.* Delivery room repair of gastroschisis. *Surgery* 1993; **114**:822–826.
62. Driver, C. P., Bowen, J., Doig, C. M. *et al.* The influence of delay in closure of the abdominal wall on outcome in gastroschisis. *Pediatr. Surg. Int.* 2001; **17**:32–34.
63. Lacey, S. R., Carris, L. A., Beyer, A. J., III, & Azizkhan, R. G. Bladder pressure monitoring significantly enhances care of infants with abdominal wall defects: a prospective clinical study. *J. Pediatr. Surg.* 1993; **28**:1370–1374.
64. Minkes, R. K., Langer, J. C., Mazziotti, M. V. *et al.* Routine insertion of a silastic spring-loaded silo for infants with gastroschisis. *J. Pediatr. Surg.* 2000; **35**:843–846.
65. Schlatter, M., Norris, K., Uitvlugt, N. *et al.* Improved outcomes in the treatment of gastroschisis using a preformed silo and delayed repair approach *J. Pediatr. Surg.* 2003; **38**:459–464.

66. Hipolito, R., Haight, M., Dubois, J. *et al.* Gastroschisis and Hirschprung's disease: a rare combination. *J. Pediatr. Surg.* 2003; **36**:638–640.
67. De Ugarte, D. A., Asch, M. J., Hedrick, M. H., & Atkinson, J. B. The use of tissue expanders in the closure of a giant omphalocele. *J. Pediatr. Surg.* 2004; **39**:613–615.
68. Ladd, A. P., Rescorla, F. J., & Eppley, B. L. Novel use of acellular dermal matrix in the formation of a bioprosthetic silo for giant omphalocele coverage. *J. Pediatr. Surg.* 2004; **39**:1291–1293.
69. Snyder, C. L. Outcome analysis for gastroschisis. *J. Pediatr. Surg.* 1999; **34**:1253–1256.
70. Driver, C. P., Bruce, J., Bianchi, A. *et al.* The contemporary outcome of gastroschisis. *J. Pediatr. Surg.* 2000; **35**:1719–1723.
71. Molik, K. A., Gingalewski, C. A., West, K. W. *et al.* Gastroschisis: a plea for risk categorization. *J. Pediatr. Surg.* 2001; **36**:51–55.
72. Dimitriou, G., Greenough, A., Mantagos, J. S. *et al.* Morbidity in infants with antenatally-diagnosed anterior abdominal wall defects. *Pediatr. Surg. Int.* 2000; **16**:404–740.
73. Cheng, G., Langham, M. R. Jr, Sninsky, C. A. *et al.* Gastrointestinal myoelectric activity in a child with gastroschisis and ileal atresia. *J. Pediatr. Surg.* 1997; **32**:923–927.
74. Bryant, M. S., Tepas, J. J., III, Mollitt, D. L. *et al.* The effect of initial operative repair on the recovery of intestinal function in gastroschisis. *Am. Surg.* 1989; **55**:209–211.
75. Sauter, E. R., Falterman, K. W., & Arensman, R. M. Is primary repair of gastroschisis and omphalocele always the best treatment? *Am. Surg.* 1991; **57**:142–144.
76. Puligandla, P. S., Janvier, A., Flageole, H. *et al.* The significance of intrauterine growth restriction is different from prematurity for the outcome of infants with gastroschisis. *J. Pediatr. Surg.* 2004; **39**:1200–1204.
77. Thakur, A., Chiu, C., Quiros-Tejeir, R. E. *et al.* Morbidity and mortality of short-bowel syndrome in infants with abdominal wall defects. *Am. Surg.* 2002; **68**:75–79.
78. Fries, M. H., Filly, R. A., Callen, P. W. *et al.* Growth retardation in prenatally diagnosed cases of gastroschisis. *J. Ultrasound. Med.* 1993; **12**:583–588.
79. Cusick, E., Spicer, R. D., & Beck, J. M. Small-bowel continuity: a crucial factor in determining survival in gastroschisis. *Pediatr. Surg. Int.* 1997; **12**:34–37.
80. Hoehner, J. C., Ein, S. H., & Kim, P. C. Management of gastroschisis with concomitant jejuno-ileal atresia. *J. Pediatr. Surg.* 1998; **33**:885–888.
81. Snyder, C. L., Miller, K. A., Sharp, R. J. *et al.* Management of intestinal atresias in patients with gastroschisis. *J. Pediatr. Surg.* 2001; **36**:1542–1545.
82. Amoury, R. A. Necrotizing enterocolitis following repair of gastroschisis. *J. Pediatr. Surg.* 1989; **24**:513–514.
83. Oldham, K. T., Coran, A. G., Drongowsky, R. A. *et al.* The development of necrotizing enterocolitis following repair of gastroschisis: a surprisingly high incidence. *J. Pediatr. Surg.* 1988; **23**:945–949.
84. Jayanthi, S., Seymour, P., Puntis, J. W., & Stringer, M. D. Necrotizing enterocolitis after gastroschisis repair: a preventable complication? *J. Pediatr. Surg.* 1998; **33**:705–707.
85. Beaudoin, S., Kieffer, G., Sapin, E. *et al.* Gastroesophageal reflux in neonates with congenital abdominal wall defects. *Eur. J. Pediatr. Surg.* 1995; **5**:323–326.
86. Qi, B., Diez Pardo, J. A., Soto, C., & Tovar, J. A. Transdiaphragmatic pressure gradients and the lower esophageal sphincter after tight abdominal wall closure in the rat. *J. Pediatr. Surg.* 1985; **31**:1666–1669.
87. Jolley, S. G., Tunell, W. P., Thomas, S. *et al.* The significance of gastric emptying in children with intestinal malrotation. *J. Pediatr. Surg.* 1985; **20**:627–631.
88. Tunell, W. P., Puffinbarger, N. K., Tuggle, D. W., *et al.* Abdominal wall defects in infants: survival and implications for adult life. *Ann. Surg.* 1995; **221**:525–530.
89. Larsson, L. T. & Kullendorff, C. M. Late surgical problems in children born with abdominal wall defects. *Ann. Chir. Gynecol.* 1990; **79**:23–25.
90. Chandler, P., Coddington, C. C., Hansen, K., & Tollison, S. Gynecologic surgery after repair of gastroschisis or omphalocele. *J. Reprod. Med.* 1991; **36**:679–682.
91. Rescorla, F. J., Shedd, F. J., Grosfeld, J. L. *et al.* Anomalies of intestinal rotation in childhood: analysis of 447 cases. *Surgery* 1990; **108**:710–715.
92. Swartz, K. R., Harrison, M. W., Campbell, J. R., & Campbell, T. J. Ventral hernia in the treatment of omphalocele and gastroschisis. *Ann. Surg.* 1985; **201**:347–350.
93. Dimitriou, G., Greenough, A., Giffin, F. *et al.* Temporary impairment of lung function in infants with anterior abdominal wall defects who have undergone surgery. *J. Pediatr. Surg.* 1996; **31**:670–672.
94. Nakayama, D. K., Mutich, R., Motoyama, E. K. Pulmonary dysfunction after primary closure of an abdominal wall defect and its improvement with bronchodilators. *Pediatr. Pulmonol.* 1992; **12**:174–218.
95. Janik, J. S., Adamkin, D. H., Nagaraj, H. S., & Groff, D. B. Pulmonary hypertension after primary closure of a gastroschisis. *South. Med. J.* 1982; **75**:77–78.
96. Hershenson, M. B., Brouillette, R. T., Klemka, L. *et al.* Respiratory insufficiency in newborns with abdominal wall defects. *J. Pediatr. Surg.* 1985; **20**:348–353.
97. Tsakayannis, D. E., Zurakowski, D., & Lillehei, C W. Respiratory insufficiency at birth: a predictor of mortality for infants with omphalocele. *J. Pediatr. Surg.* 1996; **31**:1088–1090.
98. Berseth, C. L., Malachowski, N., Cohn, R. B., & Sunshine, P. Longitudinal growth and late morbidity of survivors of gastroschisis and omphalocele. *J. Pediatrr. Gastroenterol. Nutr.* 1982; **1**:375–379.
99. Davies, B. W. & Stringer, M. D. The survivors of gastroschisis. *Arch. Dis. Child.* 1997; **77**:158–160.
100. Zaccara, A., Iacobelli, B. D., Calzolari, A. *et al.* Cardiopulmonary performances in young children and adolescents born with large abdominal wall defects. *J. Pediatr. Surg.* 2003; **38**:478–481.

22

Inguinal and umbilical hernias

Emma J. Parkinson and Agostino Pierro

Department of Paediatric Surgery, Institute of Child Health, London, UK

Inguinal hernia

The patent processus vaginalis is the common element in the pathogenesis of both congenital indirect inguinal hernia and congenital hydrocele. A wide patent processus creates a hernia by permitting the passage of intra-abdominal organs into the hernia sac, a hydrocele has a narrower processus permitting the passage of intraperitoneal fluid only.[1] An inguinal hernia commonly presents as a reducible groin mass emerging from the external inguinal ring, lateral to the pubic tubercle, and may extend into the scrotum.

Congenital indirect inguinal hernias are one of the most common surgical conditions in infancy with a peak incidence in the first three months of life, occurring in approximately 3.5 to 5% of full-term neonates.[2,3] In premature infants the incidence increases further, up to approximately 30%.[4]

Boys have an increased incidence (male to female ratio between 8:1 and 12:1).[5,6] In both sexes the incidence of right-sided inguinal hernia is higher than left (right 64%, left 29%, bilateral 7%). Consequently, patients presenting initially with a left-sided hernia have a higher probability of developing a metachronous hernia.[7]

Specific abnormalities predispose to the development of inguinal hernia early in life. Prematurity is the most important risk factor (Table 22.1).[2] These conditions represent part of a whole spectrum of incomplete obliteration of the processus vaginalis which leads to the potential development of both hydroceles and inguinal hernias.

Historical aspects

There is evidence from 1552 BC that the Egyptians described inguinal hernias controlled by external pressure. Susrata first described surgical treatment in the fifth century.[1] In the nineteenth and twentieth centuries, significant advances were made in the management of inguinal hernia. Czerny, in 1877, recommended ligation of the hernia sac at the external ring and in 1884 Banks described splitting the external ring to allow full dissection of the sac within the inguinal canal. In children, McLennan recognized in 1922 that herniotomy was sufficient treatment. It was also demonstrated at this time that children could be treated safely on a daycare basis. The gold standard of operative management was set by Gross in 1953 when he reported a recurrence rate of 0.15% in a review of 3874 children.[8] The challenge in the twenty-first century is achieving minimal complications of inguinal hernia in the expanding population of very low birthweight preterm infants.

This chapter reviews the outcome of both the untreated inguinal hernia and herniotomy in infants and older children. It highlights current areas of debate including the management of the incarcerated hernia, the exploration of the asymptomatic contralateral side and the particular difficulties of inguinal hernia in the preterm infant.

Surgical technique

Although inguinal herniotomy is the most commonly performed operation by pediatric surgeons, several surveys of senior surgeons have demonstrated a remarkable lack of consensus on many basic aspects of surgical management.[9]

Open inguinal herniotomy

A skin crease incision is made above and lateral to the pubic tubercle and the external inguinal ring identified. Some

Pediatric Surgery and Urology: Long-term Outcomes, Mark Stringer, Keith Oldham, Pierre Mouriquand. Published by Cambridge University Press.

Table 22.1. Risk factors for development of congenital inguinal hernia

Prematurity	
Urogenital	
	– Androgen insensitivity syndrome
	– Cryptorchidism
Increased abdominal pressure	
	– Ventriculoperitoneal shunts
	– Ascites
	– Peritoneal dialysis
	– Exomphalos/gastroschisis repair
	– Meconium peritonitis
Connective tissue disorders	
	– Congenital dislocation of the hip
	– Ehlers–Danlos syndrome
	– Marfan syndrome
	– Mucopolysaccharidoses
Chronic respiratory disease	
	– Cystic fibrosis
Abdominal wall defects	
	– Bladder exstrophy
	– Prune belly syndrome

surgeons approach the spermatic cord through an incision in the external oblique whilst others expose the hernial sac outside the external ring. The spermatic cord is mobilized with or without exteriorizing the testis in boys. The hernial sac is dissected free from the vas deferens and testicular vessels in boys and the round ligament in girls. The proximal part of the hernial sac is dissected free and any contents inspected and reduced. The sac is then transected, leaving the distal part open. The proximal sac is then twisted and ligated at the level of the internal inguinal ring, and any redundant tissue excised. Before closing the wound in boys the testis is correctly positioned in the scrotum.

Laparoscopic inguinal hernia repair

A Hasson cannula is inserted above the umbilicus under direct vision using an open technique. A pneumoperitoneum is created (10 mmHg) and a 3 mm 0° telescope is introduced. A 3 mm needle driver and 3 mm Kelly forceps are inserted in the right and left flanks with no ports. The open internal ring of the inguinal hernia is closed with a purse-string or Z-type suture of non-absorbable monofilament material. The Kelly elevates the peritoneum so that the stitch is applied without injuring the vas deferens and testicular vessels. The contralateral internal ring is also inspected; it may be considered patent if there is an obvious opening or if bubbles are seen on external manipulation of the scrotum and/or groin.

Current controversies

Laparoscopic approach

A recent large multicenter series indicated that laparoscopic hernia repair in children was safe and reproducible, with a recurrence rate of 3%.[10] Although this is slightly higher than the overall recurrence rate in children of 1%,[1] it is lower than the reported recurrence rates in infants of up to 9%.[11] The advantages of this technique compared to a conventional open repair are: (i) clear visualization of the vas deferens and testicular vessels and reduced risk of injury to these structures; (ii) easier to perform after incarcerated or strangulated inguinal hernia, facilitating inspection of reduced structures and obviating the difficult dissection of edematous tissues; (iii) permits assessment of the contralateral side and closure of a patent processus vaginalis; (iv) allows inspection of the adnexae in girls. The disadvantages include the need for endotracheal intubation and the potential risks of injury to intra-abdominal organs from trocar or instruments (which are greatly reduced if the operation is performed by an experienced surgeon).

Contralateral exploration

The issue of how to manage the contralateral groin in a child with a unilateral hernia has been debated for over 50 years and remains controversial. The advantage of contralateral exploration is that complications from a contralateral inguinal hernia and subsequent surgery can be avoided. The disadvantage is the perhaps unnecessary risk of injury to the vas deferens and testicular vessels.

In 1996, a survey of the Section of Surgery of the American Academy of Pediatrics[9] indicated that most surgeons performed open exploration in selected cases, but criteria varied widely. Various methods have been used to detect a patent processus vaginalis including herniography, transperitoneal probing, pneumoperitoneum (Goldstein test), and ultrasonography. Many studies have concluded that given the low incidence of metachronous hernia following unilateral repair, the invasiveness of open contralateral exploration and the possibility of damage to vas and vessels, contralateral exploration cannot be recommended.[12, 13] However, during the last 12 years, diagnostic laparoscopy has been used to evaluate the internal ring for the presence of an indirect hernia or patent processus vaginalis. A systematic review of laparoscopic exploration indicated that 40% of children with unilateral inguinal hernia have a contralateral patent processus vaginalis.[14] Although not every patent processus will go on to become a clinically relevant hernia, closure (either open or laparoscopic) ensures that this will not occur.[15]

Table 22.2. Incidence of metachronous inguinal hernia (adapted from Miltenberg *et al*[15])

Author	Year	Number of cases	Metachronous hernia	Percentage	Duration of follow-up (years)
Sparkman[19]	1962	259	31	12	15
DeBoer and Potts[20]	1963	100	9	9	10–14
Rowe *et al.*[21]	1969	2484	83	3.3	5
Simpson *et al.*[22]	1969	300	15	5	7
Harvey *et al.*[23]	1985	365	17	5	2–7
Given and Rubin[6]	1989	904	57	6.3	2
Surana and Puri[24]	1993	116	12	10.3	12
Hrabovsky and Pintér[25]	1995	2554	138	5	9

It is known that the incidence of a metachronous hernia is higher in infants compared to older children. A meta-analysis of the risk of a metachronous hernia in infants and children found 35 studies published between 1941 and 1996.[14] The incidence of a metachronous hernia varied widely from 1 to 31% (Table 22.2). Some of these studies were retrospective and many of the patients were lost to follow-up. Notably, some studies from this meta-analysis excluded premature infants and patients with left-sided hernias from their analyses because of the high risk of developing a metachronous hernia. The cumulative risk of developing a metachronous hernia appears to be 10% among children younger than 2 years of age.[15] However, the meta-analysis did not provide an assessment of the risk in infants. In this group, the incidence of a metachronous hernia can be as high as 68%.[16] Some surgeons have recommended routine contralateral exploration in girls presenting with a unilateral hernia because of a perceived increased risk in this group.[17] However, a recently published series by Chertin *et al.* reported an 8% incidence of metachronous hernia among a series of 300 unilateral herniotomies in girls, and the authors concluded that contralateral exploration in girls is unnecessary.[18]

Prematurity and low birth weight infants

Inguinal herniotomy in premature infants is technically challenging for both the surgeon and anesthetist. It is the most commonly performed operation in this high-risk group. The timing of surgery is controversial.

The incidence of inguinal hernia varies according to gestational age and birth weight. Kumar *et al.* described an incidence of 11% in very low birth weight infants (<1500 g) and 17% in extremely low birthweight infants (<1000 g).[26] Testicular descent and obliteration of the patent processus is less likely to be complete if gestation is shortened or if growth and development are impaired.[26] Prematurity is recognized as the single most important predisposing factor for the development of inguinal hernia.[2]

Due to the technical challenges in these very small infants there is a high recurrence rate, 8.6% reported by Phelps,[11] and a high risk of damaging the vas and testicular vessels.[27] It has therefore been common practice to delay surgery until the time of discharge from the neonatal unit, after the infant has grown and his/her respiratory status has improved. However, with this approach there remains a potential risk of incarceration before elective surgery.[28] Coren *et al.* reported two very low birth weight infants who suffered major morbidity when their hernias became incarcerated and bowel perforation ensued.[29] The incidence of incarceration in premature infants is reportedly uncommon at about 13%[28], and the risk of strangulated or perforated gut as a consequence of an incarcerated inguinal hernia in this age group is very small.[30]

Earlier surgery is recommended in premature infants who have developed an incarcerated hernia, in those with a very large hernia where discomfort may occur and prolong the need for supplementary oxygen[31], or where it is difficult to be sure that all the sac contents are fully reducible.[30]

Genetic testing in girls

Female infants with an inguinal hernia present another area of controversy requiring careful decision making. In 21% of female infants with an inguinal hernia the fallopian tube, ovary and rarely the uterus lie within the hernial sac.[1] Careful surgical technique is needed to prevent damage to these structures.

An additional consideration is that approximately 1.6% of girls with inguinal hernia have the complete form of androgen insensitivity syndrome (CAIS).[30] These are phenotypically normal females who have an XY genotype and intra-abdominal testes which produce testosterone that fails to masculinize the genitalia. It has been shown that female infants with bilateral inguinal hernias are no more likely to have CAIS than those with unilateral hernias and that approximately 75% of patients with CAIS initially present with an inguinal hernia.[33]

A survey of 32 United Kingdom pediatric surgeons showed that the commonest method of detecting CAIS was by assessment of the ovary or fallopian tube at the time of surgery, either via the groin incision or laparoscopy. If this was inconclusive, further investigation by karyotyping was advocated by 43% of surgeons, whilst others used rectal examination or vaginoscopy to identify the cervix, or ultrasound to identify the uterus.[34] However, whether it is necessary to exclude CAIS in all females presenting with inguinal hernia remains controversial. Laparoscopic inguinal hernia repair is advantageous in this respect since it facilitates intra-abdominal inspection of the uterus and ovaries. Failure to identify CAIS at the time of inguinal hernia repair may result in delayed presentation at puberty with primary amenorrhea, sexual dysfunction and the associated psychologic consequences of a late diagnosis. In addition, there is a potential risk of gonadal malignancy; a comprehensive review in 1987 stated that the risk was 2%–5% in CAIS patients over 25 years of age.[35] The timing of gonadectomy in CAIS patients is also controversial.

Complications

Preoperative

Most commonly inguinal hernias present as an asymptomatic intermittent groin bulge which is easily reducible in a child who is otherwise well. Symptoms of poor feeding and irritability, occasionally described in infants with reducible hernias, often persist after herniotomy. Older children may complain of groin pain particularly after exercise. Elective herniotomy should follow as promptly as possible after detection because of the risk of incarceration. With the exception of premature infants this may be performed safely as a day-case procedure, and the results are excellent.

An incarcerated hernia may present with an irreducible lump, irritability, pain and symptoms of intestinal obstruction. Strangulation of a hernia occurs when the blood supply to its contents is impaired. Testicular infarction and ultimately atrophy may also develop secondary to compression of the testicular vessels by the incarcerated hernia.[1] Strangulation of an intestinal loop may be suspected if the overlying skin is red and edematous, the pain is severe, bilious or fecalant vomiting develops, or if blood is visible in the stools. Intestinal strangulation may also progress and present with the signs of perforation and peritonitis. In girls, the incidence of incarceration is higher (and more likely to involve the ovary than intestine) but the incidence of strangulation is lower as the blood supply to the ovary is not usually compromised[36]. In an older child the hernial sac may contain omentum.

The incidence of incarceration in an inguinal hernia was reported by Rowe and Clatworthy as 12% among 2764 patients[7] and by Stephens as 17% among 228 patients.[37] The greatest risk is in infants under the age of 3 months. In full term infants the incidence of incarceration is 6%–18%[38,39] whilst in premature infants it ranges between 18% and 31%.[40,41] The incidence of testicular atrophy after an incarcerated inguinal hernia varies from 0% to 11.7%, and the testis is often described as cyanotic at surgery in approximately 2.2% to 5% of cases.[39,42,43] The reported incidence of intestinal infarction requiring resection after incarceration is 1.4%.[39]

Reduction by manipulation (taxis), with effective sedation, is successful in up to 96% of incarcerated inguinal hernias (incarcerated ovaries may be more difficult to reduce than intestine).[43,44] If there are no obvious signs of strangulation gentle persistent taxis should therefore succeed in eliminating the need for emergency surgery in the majority of cases. In those cases where taxis fails or if strangulation is suspected then resuscitation should be followed promptly by an emergency operation. Where taxis is successful the patient should be operated on after 24–48 hours once the edema has settled; close observation is needed in the interim.[45]

Incarcerated inguinal hernia is associated with a significant morbidity and mortality both before and after surgery. The overall death rate associated with incarcerated inguinal hernia is 0.3% to 3%.[46] A national audit in the United Kingdom carried out between 1980 and 1984 revealed 8 preoperative deaths from complications of inguinal hernia among a population of approximately 9000 elective pediatric inguinal herniotomies.[47] The authors commented on the delay in diagnosis and treatment in all cases. Two children were noted to have an inguinal hernia at a previous hospital examination. The authors emphasized the importance of gastrointestinal symptoms in children with a previously diagnosed inguinal hernia.

Postoperative

Early complications

The early complications of inguinal herniotomy may be relatively minor such as local edema, hematoma, and wound infection. A large hernial space may become filled with interstitial fluid creating an alarming appearance, which may be mistaken for a recurrent hernia. The reported rate of infection following routine inguinal herniotomy is low. Kvist *et al.* found no wound infections among 497 children[48] and Koulack *et al.* reported one stitch abscess in 145 children after elective repair.[49] The risk of all of these complications increases after emergency surgery for incarceration. Stylianos *et al.* reported 4 (5%) infections in 85 such patients.[50]

Injury to neighboring viscera is uncommon in elective inguinal hernia repair. However, intestine, bladder, ovary and rarely uterus may be present in the hernial sac and may potentially be damaged. To avoid these complications careful inspection of the contents of the hernial sac is recommended. Redman *et al.* described two infants in whom almost all of the bladder was excised following excessive

Table 22.3. Incidence of ipsilateral inguinal hernia recurrence

Author	Year	Number of cases	Recurrence	Percentage	Duration of follow-up (years)
Gross[8]	1953	3874	6	0.15	11
Lynn and Johnson[58]	1961	1000	6	0.3	5
Simpson *et al.*[22]	1969	992	1	0.1	7
Bronsther *et al.*[59]	1972	1000	3	0.3	5
Harvey *et al.*[23]	1985	436	11	2.52	2–7
Wright[60]	1994	1600	13	0.8	16
Grosfeld *et al.*[54]	1991	3577	23	0.6	12
Kviest *et al.*[48]	1989	398	15	3.7	7

mobilization of the inguinal sac.[51] Injuries to the vas deferens and testicular vessels are described in the following section.

Late complications

The late complications of inguinal herniotomy include: ipsilateral recurrence, testicular ascent, testicular atrophy, damage to the vas deferens resulting in infertility, damage to neighboring nerves, postoperative hydrocele and stitch granuloma.

Ipsilateral recurrence Recurrence of inguinal hernia after herniotomy is due to technical failure: the hernial sac is not completely closed. This may be due to incomplete dissection, a tear in the hernial sac, a displaced ligature or as a consequence of infection.

Recurrent hernia after uncomplicated inguinal herniotomy in children is uncommon, typically less than 1%[52] (Table 22.3). In neonates the incidence of recurrence is higher. In term infants less than 2 months of age recurrence rates of 1–2% are reported.[40] In premature infants, it is significantly greater at 11–15%.[53,54] A recurrence rate of 21.9% has been reported after surgery for incarcerated inguinal hernia.[53] Most of these data are derived from retrospective studies and vary in their inclusion criteria and follow-up periods. Davies *et al.* reported a recurrence rate of 4% in a prospective follow-up study of male infants weighing less than 3 kg at the time of inguinal herniotomy.[55]

Steinau *et al.* highlighted the importance of an extended follow-up with 34% of recurrent hernias presenting within 6 months of repair, 38% between 6 months and 2 years later, and 28% in the period of 2 to 9 years later.[53] Grosfeld *et al.* reported that 50% of all recurrent hernias appeared within 6 months and 76% within 2 years.[54]

Table 22.4. Risk factors for ipsilateral inguinal hernia recurrence

Patient factors	
Age	(less than 1 year)
Prematurity	(less than 31 weeks' gestation)
Clinical factors	
Incarcerated hernia	
Ventriculoperitoneal shunt	
Surgical factors	
Postoperative complications	(hemorrhage or wound infection)
Technical skill	(not seniority of surgeon)

The majority of ipsilateral recurrent hernias will be indirect but direct hernias have been reported in children after inguinal herniotomy. Fonkalsrud *et al.* found that 4 of 14 children undergoing direct hernia repair had previously had surgery for an indirect hernia.[56] A direct hernia occurring after repair of an indirect hernia may be due to concomitant pathology not previously noted or secondary to iatrogenic damage to the posterior wall of the inguinal canal.[57] Several factors contribute to the development of ipsilateral recurrence (Table 22.4).

Testicular ascent Secondary testicular ascent is a known complication of inguinal herniotomy. The small mobile prepubertal testis is either dislocated from its normal scrotal position and/or tethering by scar tissue prevents its scrotal position being maintained with growth, resulting in an iatrogenic undescended testis.[61] The incidence of iatrogenic undescended testis is 0.8% to 2.8% in boys after inguinal herniotomy.[28, 62] However, some of these "iatrogenic" undescended testes may represent a low form of congenital cryptorchidism which may be difficult to detect in the presence of a large or complicated hernia in early infancy. The position of each testis should therefore be documented before, during, and after inguinal herniotomy. Descent of the iatrogenic undescended testis does not occur with time and orchidopexy is therefore indicated.[61]

Imthurn *et al.* examined testicular biopsies obtained at orchidopexy for testicular ascent secondary to inguinal hernia repair in 15 boys. They demonstrated that germ cell loss occurs more slowly in secondary as opposed to primary undescended testes. The changes were related to the duration of displacement – after 5 years there was evidence of significant dysfunction.[63]

Testicular atrophy and ovarian trauma Testicular atrophy is a recognized complication of inguinal herniotomy but occurs rarely after elective repair. In contrast, the incidence of this complication after emergency herniotomy varies from 1% to 20%.[27,43,50] Morecroft *et al.* identified only one case (0.2%) in a retrospective series of emergency and elective herniotomies in 556 boys.[52]

Few reports document testicular volume after inguinal herniotomy. Clinical assessment may underestimate the frequency of testicular atrophy.[55] Ultrasound has been advocated as a more accurate measure of testicular volume as opposed to the Prader orchidometer. Using ultrasound to determine testicular volume in 173 boys, Leung *et al.* reported 0.6% of cases where testicular volume decreased to 50% of the contralateral testis and 6% where there was a 25%–50% reduction. In this study testicular atrophy was not significantly greater in infants or after emergency operations.[64]

Walc *et al.* stated that neither the operative findings nor early postoperative testicular assessment correlated with ultimate testicular development. Testicular pathology may become more evident after puberty, when the real incidence of atrophy may increase.[27]

Damage to the vas deferens The vas deferens is vulnerable to handling, crushing by forceps and accidental transection and ligation during division of the hernial sac. A 1.7% incidence of injury to the vas deferens has been reported on the basis of pathologic examination of excised hernial sacs.[65] Partrick *et al.* described an incidence of only 0.13% in a population operated on by pediatric surgeons but these injuries were only those recognized at the time of the initial surgery.[66] This may therefore be an underestimate of the true incidence of vas deferens injury.

Obstruction of the vas deferens caused by inguinal herniotomy in childhood is one of the most common causes of seminal tract obstruction in adults. Matsuda *et al.* found evidence of unilateral obstruction of the vas deferens after childhood inguinal herniotomy in 10 of 724 subfertile men.[67] Jequier described five patients who had previously undergone unilateral inguinal hernia repair out of a total 102 with obstructive azoospermia.[68] The success of vasal reanastomosis is poor in post-inguinal herniotomy patients as compared to vasectomy reversal patients.[69] This is because of the increased technical difficulty of performing microsurgical anastomosis in the inguinal region with a retracted proximal vas and also because long term obstruction can cause secondary epididymal obstruction or spermatogenic failure.

Damage to neighboring nerves Nerve damage during inguinal herniotomy is well recognized but pediatric data are limited[70]. The incidence of neural damage after laparoscopic repair in children is unknown.

The ilioinguinal, iliohypogastric, genitofemoral and lateral femoral cutaneous nerves are all potentially at risk. The anatomical course of these nerves is highly variable and they may be difficult to identify in small infants.[71] In addition, the consequences of damage to these nerves, sensory disturbances and/or neuralgic pain, may not be identified for many years in the pediatric population.

Postoperative hydrocele Davies *et al.* performed a prospective follow-up study on 38 male infants less than 3 kg undergoing inguinal herniotomy with a minimum follow-up period of 1 year.[55] They reported that 14% of infants developed an ipsilateral hydrocele within 12 months after inguinal herniotomy. Two of these boys underwent a negative inguinal exploration and the authors commented that repeat surgery should be reserved for those cases where hernia recurrence is suspected. Postoperative hydrocele is likely to be due to fluid accumulating in the distal hernial sac and the majority of these cases will resolve spontaneously. Applebaum *et al.* considered that post operative hydroceles may be more common after direct closure of the internal ring from within the sac using laparoscopic techniques rather than after conventional herniotomy.[72]

Stitch granuloma Using modern suture materials, stitch granuloma after inguinal herniotomy is very rare. Nagar found a 0.6% incidence of stitch granuloma in 2447 children undergoing inguinal herniotomy during a 10-year period.[73] The source in these cases was thought to be 3/0 silk and the problem became apparent at an average of 2.5 years after operation.

Specialist vs. generalist repair

There continues to be a debate as to who should perform common elective pediatric surgical procedures such as inguinal and umbilical herniotomy and where they should be performed. Central to this debate is the safety of the child. There is indirect evidence that mortality associated with complicated inguinal hernias is reduced in children treated in specialist centres.[47,74] The repair of the neonatal inguinal hernia requires expert skills in terms of anesthesia, intensive care, and surgery. Specialist units have recently reported excellent outcomes in these complex cases.[28] There is no evidence to suggest that repair of the uncomplicated inguinal hernia in otherwise healthy older children is detrimental when performed by general surgeons experienced in pediatric surgery.

Postoperative mortality

The overall death rate in children with an incarcerated inguinal hernia varies between 0.3% and 3.0% in the literature.[46] Mortality has decreased over time. In 1938, Thorndike and Ferguson reported a mortality of 2.8% in children with an incarcerated inguinal hernia.[75] In 1954, Clatworthy and Thompson reported one death (0.9%) in 135 patients treated for an incarcerated hernia.[76] From the same institution in 1970 no deaths were reported among a consecutive series of 351 children.[39]

In 1989, the National Confidential Enquiry into Perioperative Deaths in the United Kingdom reported five deaths in infants with a strangulated inguinal hernia. The risk factors identified were age less than 6 months and lack of pediatric experience of both the surgeon and the anesthetist.[76] In 1999, this same confidential enquiry documented two postoperative deaths associated with inguinal hernia repair in children. The details of these cases are not provided but the report states that the great majority of the children who died postoperatively were severely ill with associated respiratory and cardiovascular disease in addition to their primary diagnosis.[77] The mortality rate of elective inguinal herniotomy is extremely low, quoted as 0.1% by Jona who believes that major complications and death are avoidable if a strategy of early repair of all inguinal hernias is implemented.[46]

Umbilical hernia

Umbilical hernias in childhood occur with equal frequency in both sexes.[78] The incidence in Caucasian newborns is approximately 5–10%; a greater incidence of 26.6% has been recorded in African infants.[79]

The earliest reference to the surgical management of umbilical hernias is Celsus who described simple ligature of the hernia. Prior to the end of the nineteenth century the treatment was most commonly a truss. In 1890, Nota first performed an operative repair in a newborn by tightening a purse-string suture around the umbilical ring as the abdominal contents were reduced. Nota operated on 244 children and had only one recurrence. The modern surgical approach is attributed to Mayo who in 1901 described an overlapping transverse fascial closure.[80,81]

The umbilical ring is open throughout gestation but becomes progressively relatively smaller as gestation progresses. At birth the umbilicus is surrounded by a dense fascial ring, consisting of a defect in the linea alba. The umbilical opening is reinforced by remnants of the umbilical vessels and urachus and a layer of fascia overlying the peritoneum. An umbilical hernia develops if the supporting fascia of the umbilical defect is weak or absent. Most umbilical hernias are noted in the first few weeks of life after cord separation, almost all by 6 months of age. Most undergo spontaneous closure during the first 3 years of life as the umbilical ring continues to close over time.[82] There are reports of umbilical hernias closing spontaneously between 5 and 11 years of age.[78] Umbilical hernias with a small ring diameter (<1.0 cm) are more likely to close spontaneously and sooner than those with large diameter (>1.5 cm).[82]

There is a close association between umbilical hernias and low birthweight. Vohr *et al.* reported that 75% of infants with a birthweight of less than 1500 g presented with an umbilical hernia by 3 months of age. Gradual spontaneous resolution of these hernias occurred during the subsequent 12 months.[83] Umbilical hernias are also associated with Down syndrome, trisomy 18, trisomy 13, mucopolysaccharidoses, congenital hypothyroidism, Beckwith–Wiedemann syndrome and the presence of ascites.[82]

Complications

Reducible umbilical hernias are rarely painful. Incarceration of an umbilical hernia is rare. Lassaletta *et al.* reported 28 cases of incarceration in 377 umbilical hernias, an incidence of 7.4%.[84] Strangulation of hernial contents, intestine or omentum, is extremely rare and was found in only one case (0.26%) in this same series.

The relationship between childhood umbilical defects and symptomatic umbilical hernias in adults is unknown. It is of note that umbilical hernias in late adolescence are extremely uncommon and it has been suggested that in adults factors such as obesity and multiple childbirth are of greater etiologic significance than the pre-existence of an infantile umbilical hernia.[84]

Surgical management

Incarceration requiring reduction or resulting in intestinal strangulation or perforation are absolute indications for operative repair. An incarcerated umbilical hernia can usually be reduced by gentle manipulation with analgesia and operation performed the next day. If reduction fails emergency surgery is required. Persistence and the appearance of an umbilical hernia are relative indications for surgical repair. Most pediatric surgeons avoid operating on an asymptomatic umbilical hernia unless it persists as a large defect (>1.5 cm diameter) beyond 4 years of age.[81]

Umbilical hernia repair is usually performed as a day-case procedure under general anesthesia via an infraumbilical skin crease incision. The umbilical hernial sac is dissected free and opened, any contents reduced, and the fascia is closed transversely. Inversion of the umbilicus is maintained by using an absorbable suture from the underside of the umbilical skin to the middle of the fascial closure. Repair of huge umbilical hernias that occur particularly in African children can present a surgical challenge; management of the large amounts of redundant skin and the potential for keloid formation may impair the cosmetic result.[85]

Postoperative complications

Postoperative complications after umbilical hernia repair are uncommon but include wound infection (0.8%) and hematoma (1.3%). Recurrence of the umbilical hernia is rare, occurring in one out of 377 repairs in the series from Lassaletta *et al.*[84] Data regarding mortality and the complications of umbilical hernia repair are relatively scarce. Lassaletta *et al.* reported no perioperative deaths.[84]

REFERENCES

1. Lloyd, D. A. & Rintala R. J. *Inguinal hernia and hydrocele.* In O'Niell, J. A. Jr., Rowe, M. L., & Grosfield, J. L., eds. *Pediatric Surgery.* St Louis, MO: Mosby-Year Book Inc, 1998; 1071–1086.
2. Grosfeld, J. L. Current concepts in inguinal hernia in infants and children. *World J. Surg.* 1989; **13**:506–515
3. Cox, J. A. Inguinal hernia of childhood. *Surg. Clin. North Am.* 1985; **65**:1331–1342.
4. Harper, R. G., Garcia, A., & Sia, C. Inguinal hernia: a common problem of premature infants weighing 1,000 grams or less at birth. *Pediatrics* 1975; **56**:112–115.
5. Knox, G. The incidence of inguinal hernia in Newcastle children. *Arch. Dis. Child.* 1959; **34**:482–486.
6. Given, J. P. & Rubin, S. Z. Occurrence of contralateral inguinal hernia following unilateral repair in a pediatric hospital. *J. Pediatr. Surg.* 1989; **24**:963–965.
7. Rowe, M. I. & Clatworthy, H. W., Jr. The other side of the pediatric inguinal hernia. *Surg. Clin. North Am.* 1971; **51**:1371–1376.
8. Gross, R. E. Inguinal Hernia. *The Surgery of Infancy and Childhood.* Philadelphia: W.B. Saunders, 1953; 449–462.
9. Wiener, E. S. Touloukian, R. J., Rodgers, B. M. *et al.* Hernia survey of the Section on Surgery of the American Academy of Pediatrics. *J. Pediatr. Surg.* 1996; **31**:1166–1169.
10. Schier, F. Montupet, P., & Esposito, C. Laparoscopic inguinal herniorrhaphy in children: a three-center experience with 933 repairs. *J. Pediatr. Surg.* 2002; **37**:395–397.
11. Phelps, S. & Agrawal, M. Morbidity after neonatal inguinal herniotomy. *J. Pediatr. Surg.* 1997; **32**:445–447.
12. Ballantyne, A., Jawaheer, G., & Munro, F. D. Contralateral groin exploration is not justified in infants with a unilateral inguinal hernia. *Br. J. Surg.* 2001; **88**:720–723.
13. Nassiri, S. J. Contralateral exploration is not mandatory in unilateral inguinal hernia in children: a prospective 6-year study. *Pediatr. Surg. Int.* 2002; **18**:470–471.
14. Miltenburg, D. M., Nuchtern, J. G., Jaksic, T. *et al.* Laparoscopic evaluation of the pediatric inguinal hernia – a meta-analysis. *J. Pediatr. Surg.* 1998; **33**:874–879.
15. Miltenburg, D. M., Nuchtern, J. G., Jaksic, T. *et al.* Meta-analysis of the risk of metachronous hernia in infants and children. *Am. J. Surg.* 1997; **174**:741–744.
16. Jona, J. Z. The incidence of positive contralateral inguinal exploration among preschool children: a retrospective and prospective study. *J. Pediatr. Surg.* 1996; **31**:656–660.
17. Weber, T. R. & Tracy, T. F. *Groin hernias and hydroceles.* In Ashcraft, K. W., Murphy, J. P. & Sharp, R. J., eds. *Pediatric Surgery.* Philadelphia: Saunders WB, 2000; 654–662.
18. Chertin, B., De Caluwe, D., Gajaharan, M. *et al.* Is contralateral exploration necessary in girls with unilateral inguinal hernia? *J. Pediatr. Surg.* 2003; **38**:756–757.
19. Sparkman, R. S. Bilateral exploration in inguinal hernia in juvenile patients. Review and appraisal. *Surgery* 1962; **51**:393–406.
20. DeBoer, A. & Potts, W. J. Inguinal hernias in children. *Arch. Surg.* 1963; **86**:1072–1074.
21. Rowe, M. I., Copelson, L. W., & Clatworthy, H. W. The patent processus vaginalis and the inguinal hernia. *J. Pediatr. Surg.* 1969; **4**:102–107.
22. Simpson, T. E., Gunnlaugsson, G. H., Dawson, B. *et al.* Further experience with bilateral operations for inguinal hernia in infants and children. *Ann. Surg.* 1969; **169**:450–454.
23. Harvey, M. H., Johnstone, M. J., & Fossard, D. P. Inguinal herniotomy in children: a five year survey. *Br. J. Surg.* 1985; **72**:485–487.
24. Surana, R. & Puri, P. Is contralateral exploration necessary in infants with unilateral inguinal hernia? *J. Pediatr. Surg.* 1993; **28**:1026–1027.
25. Hrabovsky, Z. & Pinter, A. B. Routine bilateral exploration for inguinal hernia in infancy and childhood. *Europ. J. Pediatr. Surg.* 1995; 152–155.
26. Kumar, V. H., Clive, J., Rosenkrantz, T. S. *et al.* Inguinal hernia in preterm infants (≤ 32-week gestation). *Pediatr. Surg. Int.* 2002; **18**:147–152.
27. Walc, L., Bass, J., Rubin, S. *et al.* Testicular fate after incarcerated hernia repair and/or orchiopexy performed in patients under 6 months of age. *J. Pediatr. Surg.* 1995; **30**:1195–1197.
28. Misra, D., Hewitt, G., Potts, S. R. *et al.* Inguinal herniotomy in young infants, with emphasis on premature neonates. *J. Pediatr. Surg.* 1994; **29**:1496–1498.
29. Coren, M. E., Madden, N. P., Haddad, M. *et al.* Incarcerated inguinal hernia in premature babies – a report of two cases. *Acta Paediatr.* 2001; **90**:453–454.

30. Misra, D. Inguinal hernias in premature babies: wait or operate? *Acta. Paediatr.* 2001; **90**:370–371.
31. Emberton, M., Patel, L., Zideman, D. A. *et al.* Early repair of inguinal hernia in preterm infants with oxygen-dependent bronchopulmonary dysplasia. *Acta Paediatr.* 1996; **85**:96–99.
32. Kaplan, S. A. Testicular feminization syndrome. *Am. J. Dis. Child.* 1969; **118**:531.
33. Jagiello, G. & Atwell, J. D. Prevalance of testicular feminisation. *Lancet* 1962; **1**:329.
34. Burge, D. M. & Sugarman, I. S. Exclusion of androgen insensitivity syndrome in girls with inguinal hernias: current surgical practice. *Pediatr. Surg. Int.* 2002; **18**:701–703.
35. Verp, M. S. & Simpson, J. L. Abnormal sexual differentiation and neoplasia. *Cancer. Genet. Cytogenet.* 1987; **25**:191–218.
36. Kapur, P., Caty, M. G., & Glick, P. L. Pediatric hernias and hydroceles. *Pediatr. Clin. North Am.* 1998; **45**:773–789.
37. Stephens, B. J., Rice, W. T., Koucky, C. J. *et al.* Optimal timing of elective indirect inguinal hernia repair in healthy children: clinical considerations for improved outcome. *World J. Surg.* 1992; **16**:952–956.
38. Farrow, G. A. & Thomson, S. Incarcerated inguinal hernia in infants and children: a five-year review at the hospital for sick children, Toronto, 1955 to 1959 inclusive. *Can. J. Surg.* 1963; **6**:63–67.
39. Rowe, M. I. & Clatworthy, H. W. Incarcerated and strangulated hernias in children. A statistical study of high-risk factors. *Arch. Surg.* 1970; **101**:136–139.
40. Rescorla, F. J. & Grosfeld, J. L. Inguinal hernia repair in the perinatal period and early infancy: clinical considerations. *J. Pediatr. Surg.* 1984; **19**:832–837.
41. Rajput, A., Gauderer, M. W., & Hack, M. Inguinal hernias in very low birth weight infants: incidence and timing of repair. *J. Pediatr. Surg.* 1992; **27**:1322–1324.
42. Palmer, B. V. Incarcerated inguinal hernia in children. *Ann. R. Coll. Surg. Engl.* 1978; **60**:121–124.
43. Murdoch, R. W. Testicular strangulation from incarcerated inguinal hernia in infants. *J. R. Coll. Surg. Edin.* 1979; **24**:97–101.
44. Puri, P., Guiney, E. J., & O'Donnell, B. Inguinal hernia in infants: the fate of the testis following incarceration. *J. Pediatr. Surg.* 1984; **19**:44–46.
45. Stringer, M. D., Higgins, M., Capps, S. N. *et al.* Irreducible inguinal hernia. *Br. J. Surg.* 1991; **78**:504–505.
46. Jona, J. Z. Letter: The neglected inguinal hernia. *Pediatrics* 1976; **58**:294–295.
47. Harper, S. J. & Bush, G. H. Deaths in children with inguinal hernia. *Br. Med. J. (Clin. Res. Ed.)* 1988; **296**:210.
48. Kvist, E., Gyrtrup, J. H., Mejdahl, S. *et al.* Outpatient orchiopexy and herniotomy in children. *Acta. Paediatr. Scand.* 1989; **78**:754–758.
49. Koulack, J., Fitzgerald, P., Gillis, D. A. *et al.* Routine inguinal hernia repair in the pediatric population: is office follow-up necessary? *J. Pediatr. Surg.* 1993; **28**:1185–1187.
50. Stylianos, S., Jacir, N. N., & Harris, B. H. Incarceration of inguinal hernia in infants prior to elective repair. *J. Pediatr. Surg.* 1993; **28**:582–583.
51. Redman, J. F., Jacks, D. W., & O'Donnell, P. D. Cystectomy: a catastrophic complication of herniorrhaphy. *J. Urol.* 1985; **133**:97–98.
52. Morecroft, J. A., Stringer, M. D., Higgins, M. *et al.* Follow-up after inguinal herniotomy or surgery for hydrocele in boys. *Br. J. Surg.* 1993; **80**:1613–1614.
53. Steinau, G., Treutner, K. H., Feeken, G. *et al.* Recurrent inguinal hernias in infants and children. *World J. Surg.* 1995; **19**:303–306.
54. Grosfeld, J. L., Minnick, K., Shedd, F. *et al.* Inguinal hernia in children: factors affecting recurrence in 62 cases. *J. Pediatr. Surg.* 1991; **26**:283–287.
55. Davies, B. W., Fraser, N., Najmaldin, A. S. *et al.* A prospective study of neonatal inguinal herniotomy: the problem of the postoperative hydrocele. *Pediatr. Surg. Int.* 2003; **19**:68–70.
56. Fonkalsrud, E. W., Delorimier, A. A., & Clatworthy, H. W., Jr. Femoral and direct inguinal hernias in infants and children. *J. Am. Mid. Assoc.* 1965; **192**:597–599.
57. Wright, J. E. & Gill, A. W. Direct inguinal hernias in the newborn. *Aust. N Z J. Surg.* 1991; **61**:78–81.
58. Lynn, H. B. & Johnson, W. W. Inguinal herniorrhaphy in children. A critical analysis of 1,000 cases. *Arch. Surg.* 1961; **83**:573–579.
59. Bronsther, B., Abrams, M. W., & Elboim, C. Inguinal hernias in children – a study of 1,000 cases and a review of the literature. *J. Am. Med. Womens Assoc.* 1972; **27**:522–525.
60. Wright, J. E. Recurrent inguinal hernia in infancy and childhood. *Pediatr. Surg. Int.* 1994; **9**:164–166.
61. Fenig, D. M., Snyder, H. M., III, Wu, H. Y. *et al.* The histopathology of iatrogenic cryptorchid testis: an insight into etiology. *J. Urol.* 2001; **165**:1258–1261.
62. Surana, R. & Puri, P. Iatrogenic ascent of the testis: an under-recognized complication of inguinal hernia operation in children. *Br. J. Urol.* 1994; **73**:580–581.
63. Imthurn, T., Hadziselimovic, F., & Herzog, B. Impaired germ cells in secondary cryptorchid testis after herniotomy. *J. Urol.* 1995; **153**:780–781.
64. Leung, W. Y., Poon, M., Fan, T. W. *et al.* Testicular volume of boys after inguinal herniotomy: combined clinical and radiological follow-up. *Pediatr. Surg. Int.* 1999; **15**:40–41.
65. Steigman, C. K., Sotelo-Avila, C., & Weber, T. R. The incidence of spermatic cord structures in inguinal hernia sacs from male children. *Am. J. Surg. Pathol.* 1999; **23**:880–885.
66. Partrick, D. A., Bensard, D. D., Karrer, F. M. *et al.* Is routine pathological evaluation of pediatric hernia sacs justified? *J. Pediatr. Surg.* 1998; **33**:1090–1092.
67. Matsuda, T., Horii, Y., & Yoshida, O. Unilateral obstruction of the vas deferens caused by childhood inguinal herniorrhaphy in male infertility patients. *Fertil. Steril.* 1992; **58**:609–613.
68. Jequier, A. M. Obstructive azoospermia: a study of 102 patients. *Clin. Reprod. Fertil.* 1985; **3**:21–36.
69. Matsuda, T., Muguruma, K., Hiura, Y. *et al.* Seminal tract obstruction caused by childhood inguinal herniorrhaphy:

results of microsurgical reanastomosis. *J. Urol.* 1998; **159**:837–840.

70. Van Hoff, J., Shaywitz, B. A., Seashore, J. H. *et al.* Femoral nerve injury following inguinal hernia repair. *Pediatr. Neurol.* 1985; **1**:195–196.
71. Al-dabbagh, A. K. Anatomical variations of the inguinal nerves and risks of injury in 110 hernia repairs. *Surg. Radiol. Anat.* 2002; **24**:102–107.
72. Applebaum, H., Bautista, N., & Cymerman, J. Alternative method for repair of the difficult infant hernia. *J. Pediatr. Surg.* 2000; **35**:331–333.
73. Nagar, H. Stitch granulomas following inguinal herniotomy: a 10-year review. *J. Pediatr. Surg.* 1993; **28**:1505–1507.
74. Campling, E. A., Devlin, H. B., & Lunn, J. N. The 1989 report of the national confidential enquiry into perioperative deaths. p 58, 1990, The King's Fund.
75. Thorndike, A. & Ferguson, C. F. Incarcerated inguinal hernia in infancy and childhood. *Am. J. Surg.* 1938; **39**:429.
76. Clatworthy, H. W. & Thompson, A. G. Incarcerated and strangulated inguinal hernia in infants: a preventable risk. *J. Am. Med. Assoc.* 1954; **154**:123.
77. Callum, K. G., Gray, A. J. G., Hoile, R. W. *et al.* Extremes of age: The 1999 report of the national confidential enquiry into perioperative deaths. 1999.
78. Hall, D. E., Roberts, K. B., & Charney, E. Umbilical hernia: what happens after age 5 years? *J. Pediatr.* 1981; **98**:415–417.
79. Crump, E. P. Umbilical hernia. I. Occurrence of the infantile type in Negro infants and children. *J. Pediatr.* 1952; **40**:214–223.
80. Mayo, W. J. An operation for the radical cure of umbilical hernia. *Ann. Surg.* 1901; **34**:276–280.
81. Skinner, M. A. & Grosfeld, J. L. Inguinal and umbilical hernia repair in infants and children. *Surg. Clin. North Am.* 1993; **73**:439–449.
82. Cilley, R. E. & Krummel, T. M. Disorders of the umbilicus. In O'Niell, J. A.Jr., Rowe, M. I., Grosfeld, J. L., Fonkalsrud, E. W., & Coran, A. G., eds. *Pediatric Surgery.* Mosby, 1998; 1029–1043.
83. Vohr, B. R., Rosenfield, A. G., & Oh, W. Umbilical hernia in the low-birth-weight infant (less than 1,500 gm). *J. Pediatr.* 1977; **90**:807–808.
84. Lassaletta, L., Fonkalsrud, E. W., Tovar, J. A. *et al.* The management of umbilicial hernias in infancy and childhood. *J. Pediatr. Surg.* 1975; **10**:405–409.
85. Blanchard, H., St Vil., D. Carceller, A. *et al.* Repair of the huge umbilical hernia in black children. *J. Pediatr. Surg.* 2000; **35**:696–698.

23

Infantile hypertrophic pyloric stenosis

David C. G. Crabbe

The General Infirmary at Leeds, UK

Introduction

Although there were undoubtedly earlier descriptions, Hirschsprung gave the first accurate account of pyloric stenosis in 1887.[1] The first reports of successful surgical treatment of pyloric stenosis appeared in the late nineteenth century. Various surgical techniques were described including gastroenterostomy and forcible dilatation of the pylorus (Loreta's operation). In 1902 Dent treated a baby with pyloric stenosis by performing a Heineke–Mickulicz pyloroplasty. Over the following decade various extramucosal pyloroplasties were reported until, in 1912, Ramstedt described the pyloromyotomy that has become the standard treatment today.[2]

In the early years perioperative mortality was unacceptably high and medical therapy for pyloric stenosis was favored in many centers. This involved assiduous attention to feeding, anticholinergic drugs (of which atropine methylnitrate was most favored) and often long periods of time in hospital. Surgical treatment for pyloric stenosis became increasingly popular in North America and Britain after the Second World War, although a few pediatricians continued to report successful use of atropine into the 1950s. Medical treatment remained commonplace in Europe into the early 1970s before being superseded by surgery.

Ramstedt's procedure is now firmly established as the treatment of choice for pyloric stenosis. With appropriate preoperative rehydration and skilled anesthesia the perioperative mortality is negligible. Recent study has centered on the use of ultrasound for early diagnosis and the choice of incisions (transverse, circumumbilical or laparoscopic) for exposure of the pylorus.

Treatment

It is a testimonial to the success of Ramstedt's operation that it remains the procedure of choice for pyloric stenosis. Interest briefly centered on balloon dilatation of the pylorus. Tam and Carty[3] reported unsatisfactory results, with eight of their twelve cases subsequently requiring open pyloromyotomy and the procedure was abandoned.

Although the success of the extramucosal pyloromyotomy is undisputed the choice of incision remains a subject of debate. Many incisions have been recommended over the years. Robertson[4] popularized a right subcostal incision with a grid-iron approach through the abdominal wall muscles. In 1986 Tan and Bianchi[5] described the circumumbilical incision for pyloromyotomy.

The first laparoscopic pyloromyotomy was reported by Alain in 1991.[6] Since then several series of laparoscopic pyloromyotomies have been published.[7–11] The technique is clearly feasible, safe and growing in popularity. In experienced hands, laparoscopic pyloromyotomy takes no longer than open pyloromyotomy. Purported advantages of laparoscopic pyloromyotomy include shorter postoperative stay and minimal cosmetic deformity. The former contention has yet to be supported by scientific evidence showing less disturbance of gastric peristalsis than open pyloromyotomy and the latter contention is dubious when three incisions for laparoscope and instruments are compared to the circumumbilical incision.

Short-term outcomes

There have been many series published reporting the short-term results of surgery for pyloric stenosis. Complication

Pediatric Surgery and Urology: Long-term Outcomes, Mark Stringer, Keith Oldham, Pierre Mouriquand.
Published by Cambridge University Press.

Table 23.1. Short term complications of pyloromyotomy

Authors	Period	Number of patients	Technique	Deaths (%)	Wound infection (%)	Wound dehiscence (%)	Incisional hernia (%)	Perforation (%)	Bleeding (%)	Incomplete myotomy (%)	Negative laparotomy (%)
Paediatric surgeons											
Fitzgerald[12]	1984–88	50	conv	0	2	0	0	2	0		
Leinwand[13]	1993–98	254	conv	0	1.2	0	0	1.6	0	0	0
Huddart[14]	1984–91	182	conv	0.5	5.5	–	2.7	–	–	–	–
Nour[15]	1987–92	150	conv	0	5.3	0	0	2.0	–	–	–
Poli-Merol[16]	1990–93	40	conv	0	2.5	0	0	0	–	–	–
Hulka[17]	1969–94	901	conv	0	0.89	–	–	4.3	–	0	0.11
Ford[8]	1993–95	51	conv	–	0	0	–	5.9	–	2	–
Sitsen[9]	1993–96	36	conv	0	–	–	–	5.6	–	0	–
Campbell[11]	1997–00	52	conv	–	0	–	0	4.0	–	–	–
TOTAL		**1716**		**0.06**	**2.2**	**0**	**0.3**	**3.2**	**0**	**0.1**	**0.06**
Fitzgerald[12]	1984–88	50	umbil	0	4	0	0	4.0	0		
Leinwand[13]	1993–98	90	umbil	0	6.7	1.1	4.4	8.9	0	0	0
Huddart[14]	1984–91	138	umbil	0	16	–	0.7	–	–	–	–
Poli-Merol[16]	1990–93	40	umbil	0	0	2.5	0	2.5	–	–	–
Fujimoto[10]	1994–97	30	umbil	–	7.0	–	–	3.5	–	–	–
TOTAL		**348**		**0**	**9.2**	**0.6**	**1.4**	**3.4**	**0**	**0**	**0**
Najmaldin[7]	1991–93	37	lap	0	0	0	0	0	0	0	0
Alain[6]	1991–96	70	lap	0	0	0	0	2.9	–	0	–
Ford[8]	1993–95	33	lap	–	0	6.1	–	9.1	–	3.0	–
Sitsen[9]	1990–96	36	lap	0	–	–	–	8.3	–	5.6	–
Fujimoto[10]	1994–97	30	lap	–	0	–	–	3.5	–	–	–
Campbell[11]	1997–00	65	lap	–	4.6	–	3.1	8.0	–	1.5	–
TOTAL		**271**		**0**	**1.1**	**0.7**	**0.7**	**5.2**	**0**	**1.4**	**0**
BAPS 1996[18]	1994–95	309	various	0	2.6	0.65	0.3	1.0	–	1.0	0
General surgeons											
Eriksen[19]	1984–89	46	conv	0	15.0	4.4	2.2	24.0	0	–	–
Harvey[20]	1978–87	170	conv	–	15.5	6.7	–	12.8	0	–	–
Mason[21]	1976–89	54	conv	0	15.0	3.0	0	35.0	0	–	–
O'Donoghue[22]	1979–91	120	conv	0	9.2	0	0	6.6	–	1.6	0.8
Curley[23]	1980–90	79	conv	0	8.9	2.5	2.5	5.1	1.3	3.8	–
Maxwell-Armstrong[24]	1995–98	64	conv	–	3.1	–	1.6	3.1	–	3.1	–
Whyte[25]	1979–95	160	conv	–	4.4	1.9	–	19	–	0.6	–
TOTAL		**693**		**0**	**9.8**	**2.7**	**0.6**	**15**	**0.1**	**1.2**	**0.1**

Conv, conventional incisions; lap, laparoscopic pyloromyotomy; umbil, circumumbilical incisions.
Footnote: This table includes series of ≥ 30 patients published since 1990 with sufficient details on complications for analysis. Series are listed in chronological order of year of publication.

rates from larger representative series of infants treated by pediatric and general surgeons published since 1990 are shown in Table 23.1. It is distressing that many authors have simply accepted relatively high rates of complications without acknowledging that, in most cases, this reflects errors of surgical judgement and operative technique. Complication rates following laparoscopic pyloromyotomy are higher than average rates following open surgery but this is almost certainly due to the learning curve and an enthusiasm to report early clinical results. The wound infection rate is significantly higher with the circumumbilical incision and this probably reflects the degree of manipulation which is often necessary to deliver the pylorus.

The perioperative mortality rate following pyloromyotomy is close to zero. From a total of 2644 babies treated in specialist pediatric surgical centers since 1990, there has been only one reported death. This infant died preoperatively during resuscitation from severe dehydration and alkalosis.[14]

Perioperative complications include negative laparotomy, perforation of the duodenal mucosa and bleeding from the pyloromyotomy. Negative laparotomy is an infrequent event. Palpation of a typical pyloric tumor is a highly specific method for diagnosing pyloric stenosis. False-positives are very rare but aberrant pancreatic tissue,[26] duplication cysts[27] and the upper pole of the kidney[28] have all been mistaken for a pyloric tumor. Mucosal perforation during pyloromyotomy is an avoidable complication which occurs because of penetration of the duodenal fornix in an attempt to ensure complete myotomy. The average incidence of duodenal perforation was 3.2% in 1716 cases operated on by pediatric surgeons through conventional incisions versus 15% in 693 cases reported by general surgeons (Table 23.1). Pranikoff *et al.*[29] recently confirmed this difference in a study of infants treated by pediatric and general surgeons in North Carolina with mucosal perforation rates of 0.55% vs. 2.9%, respectively. In a recent study of 11 003 babies Safford *et al.*[29a] showed a clear correlation between case volume and outcome. Babies undergoing surgery in hospitals receiving less than five cases of pyloric stenosis per year were 1.6 times more likely to suffer a complication than babies treated in hospitals receving five or more cases. These discrepancies almost certainly reflect expertise gained by familiarity with the operation. However, provided the complication is recognized and treated at the time of pyloromyotomy, no long-term sequelae ensue, although the risk of wound infection is probably higher.

Postoperative wound complications figure prominently in most reported series and account for most of the short-term morbidity from pyloromyotomy. Wound infection rates vary from zero to 16%, the commonest organism being *Staphylococcus aureus*. Retrospective studies are a notoriously unreliable method of documenting wound infection rates so the true incidence is probably higher. Several factors may influence wound infection rates including gentle handling of the infant's tissues, bacterial colonization of the umbilicus and immune function in the neonate.[30] The use of prophylactic antibiotics to prevent wound infection is common practice. In a recent retrospective analysis Ladd *et al.*[30a] compared wound infection rates in three groups of babies undergoing pyloromyotomy: group I pyloromyotomy through a right upper quadrant incision, no prophylactic antibiotics ($N = 258$), group II pyloromyotomy through a circum-umbilical incision, no prophylactic antibiotic ($N = 85$) and group III pyloromyotomy through a circum-umbilical incision, given prophylactic antibiotics ($N = 42$). The recorded wound infection rates were 2.3%, 7.0% and 2.3%, respectively. Nour *et al.*[15] however, found no significant difference in wound infection rates in infants receiving prophylactic antibiotics in a prospective randomized study. These authors also demonstrated that in most infants with pyloric stenosis the umbilicus is colonized with gut and skin flora and not Staph, aureus, refuting the popular belief that the umbilicus is the source of wound infection. There is no evidence to demonstrate a reduction in infection rates following use of prophylactic antibiotics but this remains common practice. In a recent prospective randomized study Nour *et al.*[15] found no significant difference in wound infection rates in those infants receiving prophylactic antibiotics. Furthermore, these authors demonstrated that in most infants with pyloric stenosis the umbilicus is colonized with gut and skin flora and not *Staphylococcus aureus*, refuting the popular belief that the umbilicus is the source of wound infection.

Table 23.2. Reported late sequelae of pyloromyotomy

Persisting radiological deformity of pyloric canal
Altered gastric emptying
Elevated basal and peak gastric acid output
Minor reduction in final adult height
Impairments of short-term memory and attention
Increased incidence of enuresis
Impaired glucose tolerance
Increased incidence of peptic ulcer disease
Prolonged retention of swallowed foreign bodies
Recurrence in future generations

Wound dehiscence and incisional hernia are problems mainly associated with the circumumbilical incision, although there can be no doubt this reflects poor surgical technique. Adherence to the standard principles and techniques of wound closure should prevent this complication.

Postoperative vomiting is a frequent occurrence after pyloromyotomy but almost invariably self-limiting. Gastric peristalsis is reduced for 16–24 hours after pyloromyotomy and consequently it is common practice to withhold oral feeds for 24 hours after surgery.[31] Many different postoperative feeding regimens have been advised after pyloromyotomy and it has been shown that post operative vomiting is not influenced by the pattern in which feeds are re-established.[32] Spitz[33] studied vomiting after pyloromyotomy and concluded that the only significant risk factors were the presence of esophagitis at endoscopy and a history of preoperative hematemesis. Persistent vomiting after pyloromyotomy delays discharge from hospital. Earlier tolerance of oral feeding is reported after laparoscopic pyloromyotomy.

Incomplete pyloromyotomy is uncommon. Radiological studies are unhelpful for diagnosis because the postoperative appearance of the pylorus does not differ from the preoperative appearance for several weeks following successful myotomy.[34] Providing the baby is otherwise well, it is sensible to wait 10–14 days, attempting to control vomiting by medical means, before considering an inadequate myotomy and re-exploring the pylorus.

Long-term outcomes

Ramstedt's procedure is widely regarded as a satisfactory operation with few long-term sequelae (Table 23.2). In broad terms this appears to be true but there have been relatively few studies examining long-term outcome following pyloromyotomy. There are serious flaws in the methodology of many of these reports. Studies that have sought to identify late symptoms after pyloromyotomy all suffer from an ascertainment bias and most have not included normal control populations. However, it must be acknowledged that there are considerable difficulties in trying to attribute symptoms in adult life to the effects of an operation carried out in infancy.

Anatomy

Healing of the pylorus after pyloromyotomy appears to be rapid and complete. In an autopsy study from the 1920s Wollstein reported findings in 23 infants who died between 24 hours and 2 years after pyloromyotomy.[35] The pyloromyotomy heals by granulation. Wound contraction occurs, bringing the edges of the myotomy together to leave only a narrow furrow to mark the site of the incision. Within 2 weeks of operation, the pylorus softens and by 25 days the pylorus appears normal. It is interesting to note, although of historical importance only, that the pylorus is reported to remain permanently hypertrophied and obstructed after gastroenterostomy is performed for infantile pyloric stenosis.

The radiological appearance of the pylorus after pyloromyotomy has been studied by ultrasonography and conventional radiology. Steinicke and Roelsgaard[36] organized a radiological follow-up of 253 children treated for pyloric stenosis in Denmark between 1935 and 1951. This included a group of 80 children treated surgically, examined at 2–10 years after pyloromyotomy, and 173 patients treated with antispasmodics, examined at 5–22 years of age. They reported characteristic changes in the appearance of the gastric outlet after pyloric stenosis – an abrupt transition from antrum to pylorus, persistent pyloric narrowing and reduced peristalsis in the region of the pylorus. These appearances were found less frequently in children studied after pyloromyotomy than children treated medically. The changes became less prominent with age although 13% of the adults had persistent abnormalities.

Several ultrasonographic studies have documented changes in dimensions of the hypertrophied pylorus after myotomy. Okorie *et al.*[37] followed 25 infants after pyloromyotomy and concluded that the hypertrophy regresses at a variable rate but normal measurements were consistently reached within 12 weeks. Ludtke *et al.*[38] carried out a study of 48 adults treated for pyloric stenosis between 17 and 27 years previously; the study included 12 cases treated medically and 36 cases treated surgically. Muscle thickness and pyloric diameter were normal in both groups. Tander *et al.*[39] performed ultrasound scans on 22 babies with pyloric stenosis preoperatively and then postoperatively at intervals for 6 months. They found that pyloric muscle thickness began to decrease by the end of the first postoperative week and had returned to normal in most cases by 12 weeks. Pyloric length and diameter measurements, however, were still above normal by 12 weeks.

Gastric emptying

The effect of pyloromyotomy on gastric emptying has been studied in a number of ways. The earliest reports followed the passage of barium from the stomach. Delayed gastric emptying was noted in 9/40 patients studied by Herrmann and Schickedang,[40] 21/129 patients studied by Léderer *et al.*,[41] 2/14 patients studied by Wanscher and Jensen,[42] and in 1/31 by Solowiejczyk *et al.*[43] Unfortunately, this is widely regarded as an unsatisfactory method of assessing gastric emptying because barium emulsions tend to adhere to the gastric mucosa and separate in the stomach, following neither the kinetics of liquid nor solid phase emptying. Presumably this explains the widely differing results.

Tam *et al.*[44] studied gastric emptying in seven children between 5 and 11 years after pyloromyotomy. They compared results with data from 16 normal children who acted as controls. Liquid gastric emptying was measured by a double sampling technique. Four children who had undergone pyloromyotomy were found to have accelerated gastric emptying. Rasmussen *et al.*[45] used scintigraphy to study gastric emptying for both liquids and solids in 25 adults and concluded that previous pyloromyotomy had no effect on subsequent gastric emptying. Ludtke *et al.*[46] used similar methods and again found normal gastric emptying in 38 adults who had undergone pyloromyotomy in infancy.

Asai *et al.*[47] evaluated gastric emptying of liquids using a two-step serial ultrasound technique to follow changes in gastric volume. They studied 30 patients between 1 and

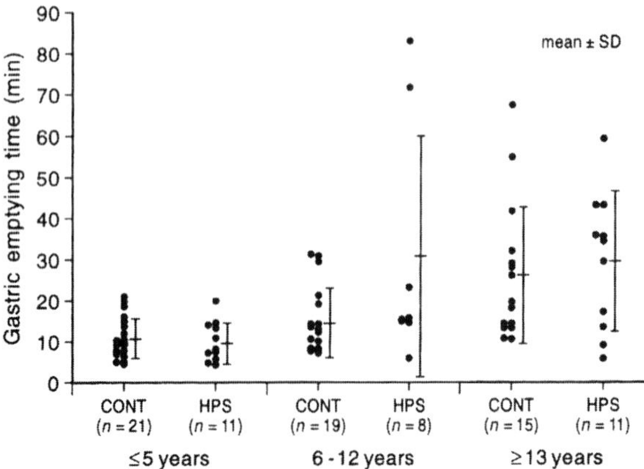

Fig. 23.1. Gastric emptying half-time in normal control children and in patients who had undergone pyloromyotomy for hypertrophic pyloric stenosis (HPS). From Asai *et al.*[47]

19 years after pyloromyotomy and 41 controls of similar age. Overall, they found normal rates of gastric emptying in both subjects and controls (Fig. 23.1). However, two children in the pyloromyotomy group had significant delay in gastric emptying but no symptoms. Barium studies were performed that confirmed slow gastric emptying, although there was no evidence of pyloric deformity in either child.

Sun *et al.*[48] studied gastric emptying and pyloric motility in six adults 24–26 years after pyloromyotomy and compared the results with six normal controls. Gastric emptying of liquids was measured by scintigraphy and pyloric motility by manometry. The authors found normal gastric emptying rates in both subjects and controls. Abnormal patterns of pyloric motility were found in the subjects. Resting pyloric tone was higher than controls and the amplitude and frequency of phasic pyloric pressure waves were both reduced. They concluded that, despite the reduction in phasic pyloric motor activity in adults who had undergone pyloromyotomy for hypertrophic pyloric stenosis in infancy, the stomach is able to compensate to maintain normal gastric emptying. In dogs pyloroplasty causes a reduction in amplitude but not frequency of phasic pyloric activity and this may partly explain the changes seen in the subjects. However, the cause of the elevated basal pyloric tone is less clear and the authors speculate that this may be a long-term consequence of the neonatal pyloric hypertrophy.

Gastric acid output

The late effects of pyloromyotomy on gastric acid output have been reported in two studies. Wanscher and Jensen[42] examined 12 adults aged 21–27 years. Although there was no control group in this study, they reported higher basal acid secretion rates, basal acid outputs and poststimulation acid secretion rates when compared to previously published data from normal adults. The peak acid output was not significantly raised. Tam *et al.*[44] reported normal basal and maximal acid output and secretion rates in seven children studied after pyloromyotomy when compared to a control group of healthy children.

Peptic ulceration

The most contentious aspect of the literature published on the late consequences of pyloric stenosis is the incidence of peptic ulcer disease. Several studies have sought to ascertain the incidence of upper gastrointestinal symptoms and they are summarized in Table 23.3. In retrospective studies based on postal questionnaire and interview an ascertainment bias is inevitable. Definitions of dyspepsia vary, with some authors distinguishing "ulcer dyspepsia" as symptoms relieved by food or antacids from "dyspepsia," which may include epigastric pains, fullness, eructation and pyrosis. Few studies have included a control population and certainly none has attempted to control for the effects of lifestyle and smoking, which are known to predispose to peptic ulcer disease in adult life. In these studies the diagnosis of peptic ulcer disease is based almost exclusively on barium meal examination. The true incidence of peptic ulcer disease documented by endoscopy is unknown.

Two reports included normal control populations. Steinicke Nielson and Roelsgaard[50] sought dyspeptic symptoms in 45 adults who had been treated with antispasmodics for pyloric stenosis in infancy and a control group of 45 adults attending hospital for non-gastrointestinal reasons. Dyspeptic symptoms were more common in the adults previously treated for pyloric stenosis (19/45) than in the control group (6/45) but the difference was not significant. Barium meals were performed in each case. Peptic ulcers were found in three control patients (all symptomatic) and in 14 index cases (nine symptomatic, five asymptomatic). In a more recent study Lüdtke *et al.*[46] inquired about gastrointestinal symptoms in 18 adults who received medical treatment for pyloric stenosis in infancy and 38 adults who underwent pyloromyotomy in infancy. A matched number of healthy controls were given the same questionnaire. There was no significant difference in the incidence of dyspeptic symptoms between the groups.

Growth and development

The effects of pyloric stenosis on subsequent growth and development appear to be related to starvation in infancy.

Table 23.3. Dyspeptic symptoms and peptic ulcer disease after pyloric stenosis

Authors	Number of patients	Age at follow-up	Treatment	Dyspeptic symptoms	Barium studies	Radiological findings
Bendix & Necheles 1947[49]	17	18–28 y	P	3 (18%)	3*	2 DU
Steinicke Nielsen & Roelsgaard 1956[50]	45	25–50 y	M	19 (42%)	45	1 GU. 5 pyloric ulcers, 8 DU
Wansher & Jensen 1971[42]	14	21–27 y	P	10 (71%)	14	No ulcers found
Berglund & Rabo 1973[51]	176	Mean 35.5 y	M	36 (20%)	–	–
Léderer *et al.* 1975[41]	128	1–17 y	P	–	25	1 DU
Solowiejczyk *et al.* 1980[43]	41	15–30 y	P	24 (59%)	31	1 GU, 4 DU
Vilmann *et al.* 1986[52]	72	24–46 y	P	44 (61%)	34	2 duodenal deformity
Rasmussen *et al.* 1988[53]	80	19–35 y	M	11 (14%)	5*	1 "duodenitis"
Rasmussen *et al.* 1988[53]	204	19–35 y	P	19 (9%)	5*	1 "duodenitis"
Lüdtke *et al.* 1994[46]	18	16–26 y	M	5 (28%)	–	–
Lüdtke *et al.* 1994[46]	38	16–26 y	P	8 (21%)	–	–
Dietl *et al.* 2000[54]	31	19–66 y	P	8 (26%)		2 GU, 1 DU, 1 "benign stenosis of the gastric outlet"

* Only symptomatic patients studied. DU, duodenal ulcer; GU, gastric ulcer; M, medical treatment; P, pyloromyotomy.

Surgical treatment of pyloric stenosis would seem advantageous to minimize the period of starvation. Dodge[55] studied 246 children in Belfast who had undergone pyloromyotomy in infancy and reported that height and weight were within normal limits at follow-up later in childhood. Berglund and Rabo[51] examined the military medical records of 180 conscripts who had received medical treatment for pyloric stenosis in Gothenburg. The authors found minor, but statistically significant, reductions in mean adult height proportional to the degree of malnutrition in infancy. There was no significant reduction in mental development which they assessed using a standard military intelligence test. In a separate paper these authors noted an excess of deaths from violent causes in the same cohort of patients although they were unable to offer an explanation.[56]

Klein *et al.*[57] reported the results of detailed cognitive assessments of 50 children at 5–14 years of age who underwent pyloromyotomy in infancy and compared them to carefully matched control groups. They concluded that severe malnutrition, with loss of more than 10% body weight, was associated with significant impairments of short term memory and attention at the time of follow-up. Brooks and Sims reported[58] a higher than expected incidence of enuresis in children treated for pyloric stenosis.

One study has suggested that the incidence of diabetes mellitus may be increased after pyloromyotomy. Chimènes *et al.*[59] noted an increased incidence of diabetes in military conscripts and arranged oral glucose tolerance tests on 49 subjects with a previous history of pyloric stenosis. Glucose tolerance was normal in 35 cases but impaired in 14 (Fig. 23.2). The glucose tolerance curves did not follow patterns

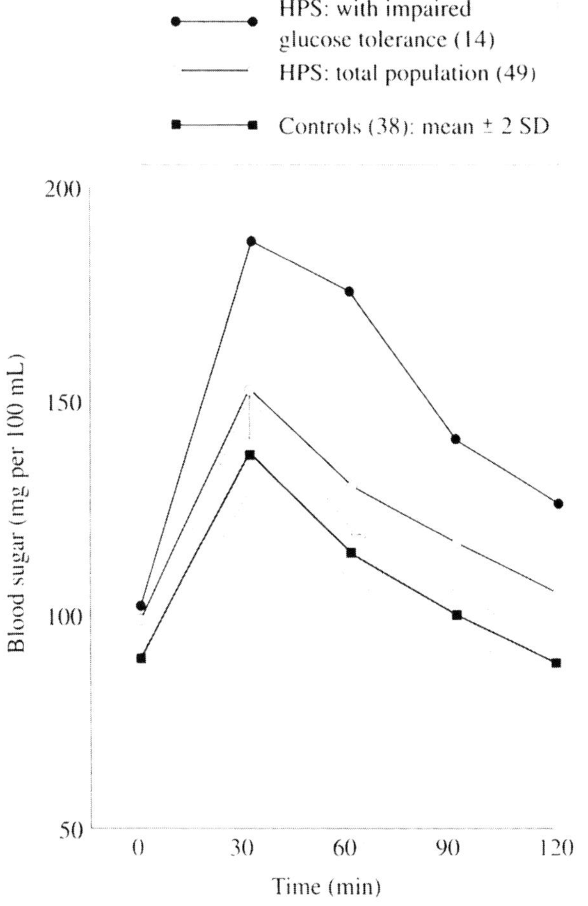

Fig. 23.2. Blood glucose concentrations during oral glucose tolerance tests in 49 adult males with previous hypertrophic pyloric stenosis (HPS) (mean±SEM), and 38 control subjects (mean±2SD, in tinted area). From Chimènes *et al.*[59]

typical of dumping so the results cannot be explained on the basis of altered gastric emptying. None of the cases required treatment but the authors recommended surveillance of children after pyloromyotomy.

Other late sequelae

Late surgical consequences of pyloromyotomy appear remarkably rare. Adhesive intestinal obstruction is vanishingly rare, with a single case reported in the Pittsburgh series of over 1200 patients[28] and a further case reported by Hulka *et al.*[17] There have been a number of reports of prolonged gastric retention of swallowed foreign bodies in children.[60] Endoscopic removal is probably advisable after a suitable period of observation. The cosmetic consequences of pyloromyotomy are the subject of much debate among surgeons advocating alternative approaches but objective information is wanting.

The etiology of pyloric stenosis is unknown. There is undoubtedly a genetic component to the condition but so far no candidate genes have been clearly identified. One study has suggested that the neuronal nitric oxide synthase gene (NOS1) might be a susceptibility locus for the condition.[61] Of the various theories that have been proposed, the most popular is the multifactorial threshold inheritance model. This model assumes the liability to pyloric stenosis is determined by the additive effects of numerous genetic and environmental factors, with the trait expressed when an individual's liability exceeds a threshold. The prevalence is consistently two to five times greater in males than females. Carter and Evans[62] concluded that the risk to offspring of patients inheriting the disease was 20% of sons and 7% of daughters born of a female proband and 5% of sons and 2.5% of daughters born of a male proband.

Conclusions

Ramstedt's operation is simple, safe, effective, and the treatment of choice for pyloric stenosis. Alternative methods to treat pyloric stenosis have not shown satisfactory results and the basic technique of pyloromyotomy remains unmodified since the original description in 1912. The short-term morbidity from pyloromyotomy is almost entirely due to wound complications. The ideal incision and the place of laparoscopic pyloromyotomy have yet to be defined. Apart from the risk of inheritance of pyloric stenosis in future generations, long-term sequelae are infrequent or unproven.

REFERENCES

1. Ravitch, M. M. The story of pyloric stenosis. *Surgery* 1960; **48**:1117–1143.
2. Ramstedt, C. Zur operation der angeborenen pylorusstenose. *Med. Klin.* 1912; **8**:1702.
3. Tam, P. K. H., Carty, H. Endoscopy-guided balloon dilatation for infantile hypertrophic pyloric stenosis. *Pediatr. Surg. Int.* 1991; **6**:306–308.
4. Robertson, D. E. Congenital pyloric stenosis. *Ann. Surg.* 1940; **112**:687–699.
5. Tan, K. C. & Bianchi, A. Circumumbilical incision for pyloromyotomy. *Br. J. Surg.* 1986; **73**:399.
6. Alain, J. L., Grousseau, D., Longis, B., Ugazzi, M., & Terrier, G. Extramucosal pyloromyotomy by laparoscopy. *Euro. J. Pediatr. Surg.* 1996; **6**:10–12.
7. Najmaldin, A. & Tan, H. L. Early experience with laparoscopic pyloromyotomy for infantile hypertrophic pyloric stenosis. *J. Pediatr. Surg.* 1995; **30**:37–38.
8. Ford, W. D., Crameri, J. A., & Holland, A. J. The learning curve for laparoscopic pyloromyotomy. *J. Pediatr. Surg.* 1997; **32**:552–554.
9. Sitsen, E., Bax, N. M. A., & van der Zee, D. C. Is laparoscopic pyloromyotomy superior to open surgery? *Surg. Endosc.* 1998; **12**:813–815.
10. Fujimoto, T., Lane, G. J., Segawa, O., Esaki, S., & Miyano, T. Laparoscopic extramucosal pyloromyotomy versus open pyloromyotomy for infantile hypertrophic pyloric stenosis: which is better? *J. Pediatr. Surg.* 1999; **34**:370–372.
11. Campbell, B. T., McLean, K., Barnhart, D. C., Drongowski, R. A., & Hirschl, R. B. A comparison of laparoscopic and open pyloromyotomy at a teaching hospital. *J. Pediatr. Surg.* 2002; **37**:1068–1071.
12. Fitzgerald, P. G., Lau, G. Y. P., Langer, J. C., & Cameron, G. S. Umbilical fold incision for pyloromyotomy. *J. Pediatr. Surg.* 1990; **25**:1117–1118.
13. Leinwand, M. J., Shaul, D. B., & Anderson, K. D. The umbilical fold approach to pyloromyotomy: is it a safe alternative to the right upper-quadrant approach? *J. Am. Coll. Surg.* 1999; **189**:362–367.
14. Huddart, S. N., Bianchi, A., Kumar, V., & Gough, D. C. S. Ramstedt's pyloromyotomy: circumumbilical versus transverse approach. *Pediatr. Surg. Int.* 1993; **8**:395–396.
15. Nour, S., MacKinnon, A. E., Dickson, J. A. S., & Walker, J. Antibiotic prophylaxis for infantile pyloromyotomy. *J. Roy. Coll. Surg. Ed.* 1996; **41**:178–180.
16. Poli-Merol, M. L., Francois, S., Lefebvre, F., Bouche Pillon-Persyn, M. A., Lefort, G., & Daoud, S. Interest of umbilical fold incision for pyloromyotomy. *Europ. J. Pediatr. Surg.* 1996; **6**:13–14.
17. Hulka, F., Harrison, M. W., Campbell, T. J., & Campbell, J. R. Complications of pyloromyotomy for infantile hypertrophic pyloric stenosis. *Am. J. Surg.* 1997; **173**:450–452.

18. British Association of Paediatric Surgeons. Comparative Audit Service – Paediatric Surgery. Surgical Epidemiology Unit, Royal College of Surgeons of England, London, UK, 1996.
19. Eriksen, C. A. & Anders, C. J. Audit of results of operations for infantile pyloric stenosis in a district general hospital. *Arch. Dis. Child.* 1991; **66**:130–133.
20. Harvey, M. H., Humphrey, G., Fieldman, N., George, J. D., & Ralphs, D. N. L. Abdominal wall dehiscence following Ramstedt's operation: a review of 170 cases of infantile hypertrophic pyloric stenosis. *Br. J. Surg.* 1991; **78**:81–82.
21. Mason, P. F. Increasing infantile hypertrophic pyloric stenosis? Experience in an overseas military hospital. *J. Roy. Coll. Surg. Ed.* 1991; **36**:293–294.
22. O'Donoghue, J. M., O'Hanlon, D. M., Gallagher, M. M., Connolly, K. D., Doyle, J., & Flynn, J. R. Ramstedt's pyloromyotomy: a specialist procedure? *Br. J. Clin. Pract.* 1993; **47**:192–194.
23. Curley, P. J., McGregor, B., Ingoldby, C. J. H., & MacFaul, R. The management of pyloric stenosis in a district hospital. *J. Roy. Coll. Surg. Ed.* 1997; **42**:265–268.
24. Maxwell-Armstrong, C. A., Cheng, M., Reynolds, J. R., & Holliday, H. W. Surgical management of infantile hypertrophic pyloric stenosis – can it be performed by general surgeons? *Ann. Roy. Coll. Surg. Engl.* 2000; **82**:341–343.
25. White, J. S., Clements, W. D. B., Heggarty, P., Sidhu, S., Mackle, E., & Stirling, I. Treatment of infantile hypertrophic pyloric stenosis in a district general hospital: a review of 160 cases. *J. Pediatr. Surg.* 2003; **38**:1333–1336.
26. Scharli, A., Sieber, W. K., & Kiesewetter, W. B. Hypertrophic pyloric stenosis at the Children's Hospital of Pittsburgh from 1912 to 1967. *J. Pediatr. Surg.* 1969; **4**:108–114.
27. Ramsay, G. S. Enterogenous cyst of the stomach stimulating pyloric stenosis. *Br. J. Surg.* 1957; **44**:632–633.
28. Benson, C. D. & Lloyd, J. R. Infantile pyloric stenosis. A review of 1120 cases. *Am. J. Surg.* 1964; **107**:429–433.
29. Pranikoff, T., Campbell, B. T., Travis, J., & Hirschl, R. B. Differences in outcome with subspecialty care: pyloromyotomy in North Carolina. *J. Pediatr. Surg.* 2002; **37**:352–356.
29a. Safford, S. D., Pietrobon, R., Safford, K. M., Martins, H., Skinner, M. A., & Rice, H. E. A study of 11,003 patients with hypertrophic pyloric stenosis and the associations between surgeon and hospital volume and outcomes. *J. Pediatr. Surg.* 2005; **40**:967–973.
30. Rao, N. & Youngson, G. G. Wound sepsis following Ramstedt pyloromyotomy. *Br. J. Surg.* 1989; **76**:1144–1146.
30a. Ladd, A. P., Nemeth, S. A., Kirincich, A. N. *et al.* Suprumbilical pyloromyotomy: a unique indication for antimicrobial prophylaxis. *J. Prediatr. Surg.* 2005; **40**:947–977.
31. Scharli, A. F. & Leditschke, J. F. Gastric motility after pyloromyotomy in infants: a reappraisal of postoperative feeding. *Surgery* 1968; **64**:1133–1137.
32. Wheeler, R. A., Najmaldin, A., Stoodley, N., Griffiths, D. M., Burge, D. M. & Atwell, J. D. Feeding regimens after pyloromyotomy. *Br. J. Surg.* 1990; **77**:1018–1019.
33. Spitz, L. Vomiting after pyloromyotomy for infantile hypertrophic pyloric stenosis. *Arch. Dise. Childh.* 1979; **54**:886–889.
34. Bishop, H. C. & Hope, J. W. Pyloric stenosis: postoperative roentgen studies and their significance. *J. Pediatr.* 1962; **60**:62–68.
35. Wollstein, M. Healing of hypertrophic pyloric stenosis after the Fredet–Rammstedt operation. *Am. J. Dis. Child.* 1922; **23**:511–517.
36. Steinicke, O., Roelsgaard, M. Radiographic follow-up in hypertrophic pyloric stenosis. *Acta. Paediatrica.* 1960; **49**:4–16.
37. Okorie, N. M., Dickson, J. A. S., Carver, R. A., & Steiner, G. M. What happens to the pylorus after pyloromyotomy? *Arch. of Dis. in Childh.* 1988; **63**:1339–1340.
38. Lüdtke, F. E., Bertus, M., Michalski, S., Dapper, F. D., & Lepsien, G. Long-term analysis of ultrasonic features of the antropyloric region 17–27 years after treatment of infantile hypertrophic pyloric stenosis. *J. Clin. Ultrasound* 1994; **22**:229–305.
39. Tander, B., Akalin, A., Abbasoğlu, L., & Bulut, M. Ultrasonographic follow-up of infantile hypertrophic pyloric stenosis after pyloromyotomy: a controlled prospective study. *Europ. J. Pediatr. Surg.* 2002; **12**:379–382.
40. Herrmann, K. & Schickedang, H. Radiological findings of the stomach in late follow-up studies of children who have undergone pyloromyotomy. *Z. Kinderchir.* 1968; **6**:34–38.
41. Léderer, L., Négyesi, M., & Felházy, L. Congenital hypertrophic pyloric stenosis: a follow up study. *Gyermekgyógyászat* 1975; **26**:309–313.
42. Wanscher, B. & Jensen, H. Late follow-up studies after operation for congenital pyloric stenosis. *Scand. J. Gastroenterol.* 1971; **6**:597–599.
43. Solowiejczyk, M., Holtzman, M., & Michowitz, M. Congenital hypertrophic pyloric stenosis: a long-term follow up of 41 cases. *Am. Surg.* 1980; **10**:567–571.
44. Tam, P. K. H., Saing, H., Koo, J., & Ong, G. B. Pyloric function five to eleven years after Ramstedt's pyloromyotomy. *J. Pediatr. Surg.* 1985; **20**:236–239.
45. Rasmussen, L., Öster-Jörgensen, E., Hansen, L. P., Qvist, N., & Pederson, S. A. Gastric emptying in adults treated for infantile hypertrophic pyloric stenosis. *Acta. Chir. Scand.* 1989; **155**:471–473.
46. Lüdtke, F. E., Bertus, M., Voth, E., Michalski, S., & Lepsin, G. Gastric emptying 16 to 26 years after treatment of infantile hypertrophic pyloric stenosis. *J. Pediatr. Surg.* 1994; **29**:523–526.
47. Asai, A., Takehara, H., Harada, M., & Tashiro, S. Ultrasonographic evaluation of gastric emptying in normal children and children after pyloromyotomy. *Pediatr. Surg. Int.* 1997; **12**:344–347.
48. Sun, W. M., Doran, S. M., Jones, K. L., Davidson, G., Dent, J., & Horowitz, M. Long-term effects of pyloromyotomy on pyloric motility and gastric emptying in humans. *Am. J. Gastroenterol.* 2000; **95**:92–100.

49. Bendix, R. M. & Necheles, H. Hypertrophic pyloric stenosis. *J. the Am. Med. Assoc.* 1947; **135**:331–333.
50. Steinicke Nielson, O. & Roelsgaard, M. Roentgenologically demonstrable gastric abnormalities in cases of previous congenital pyloric stenosis. *Acta. Radiol.* 1956; **45**:273–282.
51. Berglund, G. & Rabo, E. A long-term follow-up investigation of patients with hypertrophic pyloric stenosis – with special reference to heredity and later morbidity. *Acta. Paediat. Scand.* 1973; **62**:130–132.
52. Vilmann, P., Hjortrup, A., Altmann, P., Anderson, F. H., & Sorenson, C. A long term gastrointestinal follow up in patients operated on for congenital hypertrophic pyloric stenosis. *Acta. Paediatr. Scand.* 1986; **75**:156–158.
53. Rasmussen, L., Hansen, L. P., Qvist, N., & Pedersen, S. A. Infantile hypertrophic pyloric stenosis and subsequent ulcer dyspepsia. *Acta. Chir. Scand.* 1988; **154**:657–658.
54. Dietl, K. H., Borowski, U., Menzel, J., Wissing, C., Senninger, N., & Brockmann, J. Long-term investigations after pyloromyotomy for infantile pyloric stenosis. *Europ. J. Pediatr. Surg.* 2000; **10**:365–367.
55. Dodge, J. A. Infantile hypertrophic pyloric stenosis in Belfast, 1957–1969. *Arch. Dis. Childh.* 1975; **50**:171–178.
56. Berglund, G. & Rabo, E. A long-term follow-up investigation of patients with hypertrophic pyloric stenosis – with special reference to the physical and mental development. *Acta. Paediatr. Scand.* 1973; **62**:125–129.
57. Klein, P. S., Forbes, G., & Nader, P. R. Effects of starvation in infancy (pyloric stenosis) on subsequent learning abilities. *J. Paediatr.* 1975; **87**:8–15.
58. Brooks, J. H., Sims & A.C.P. Nocturnal enuresis and congenital pyloric stenosis. *Developm. Med. and Child Neurol.* 1969; **11**:262–263.
59. Chimènes, H., Gautier, D., Bon, R., & Fromantin, M. Abnormalities of glucose tolerance as a late consequence of hypertrophic pyloric stenosis surgically treated in the neonate. *Diabetologia* 1980; **18**:513–514.
60. Stringer, M. D., Kiely, E., & Drake, D. P. Gastric retention of swallowed coins after pyloromyotomy. *Br. J. Clin. Pract.* 1991; **45**:66–67.
61. Chung, E., Curtis, D., Chen, G. *et al.* Genetic evidence for the neuronal nitric oxide synthase gene (NOS1) as a susceptibility locus for infantile pyloric stenosis. *Am. J. Hum. Genet.* 1996; **58**:363–370
62. Carter, C. O. & Evans, K. A. Inheritance of congenital pyloric stenosis. *J. Med. Genet.* 1969; **6**:233–254.

24

Small bowel disorders

Julie R. Fuchs[1] and Jacob C. Langer[2]

[1]Department of Pediatric Surgery, J. W. Riley Hospital for Children, Indianapolis, IN, USA,
[2]Department of Surgery, University of Toronto and Department of Pediatric General Surgery, Hospital for Sick Children, Toronto, Ontario, Canada

There is a wide variety of conditions which affect the small bowel in children, from the newborn period to adolescence. Many of these, including abdominal wall defects, meconium ileus, Crohn's disease, and the general topic of short bowel syndrome, are discussed elsewhere in this text. This chapter will review the long-term outcomes associated with congenital duodenal obstruction (i.e., atresia and webs), jejunoileal atresia and webs, Meckel's diverticulum, intussusception, malrotation, and intestinal duplication. Most children recover from these problems and go on to live a normal healthy life. For this reason, relatively few studies exist documenting long-term outcomes. In this chapter the authors have used a combination of the existing literature, and their own institutional experience, to document outcome in an objective way.

Long-term problems associated with small bowel disorders can be classified into several categories:

- those specific to the disorder itself (e.g., motility disturbances associated with atresia or malrotation);
- those that are a result of surgical intervention (e.g., short bowel syndrome following massive resection, or peritoneal adhesions following laparotomy);[1]
- those related to underlying disease processes or associated anomalies.

Complications and survival can also be divided into early and late time periods. Since both may influence long-term outcomes, some disease processes require a discussion of both early and late morbidity and mortality.

Congenital duodenal obstruction

Although infants with complete duodenal atresia present in the neonatal period, duodenal web or stenosis may present later during the first years of life. The obstruction is postampullary in approximately 80% of patients and preampullary in 20%. Type I is the most common, although types II and III as well as mucosal atresias are also seen. Because polyhydramnios is common, approximately 45% of these infants are born before term.[2] Additional structural or chromosomal anomalies are seen in 52% of patients. Trisomy 21 is present in approximately 30% of children with duodenal atresia and duodenal atresia occurs in approximately 5% of children with Trisomy 21.[3] Annular pancreas, malrotation, and anterior portal vein are frequently associated with duodenal atresia, but they may also cause duodenal obstruction without an intrinsic defect of the duodenum. Other associated anomalies include congenital heart disease, esophageal atresia, anorectal malformations, renal anomalies, biliary atresia, jejunal duplication, vertebral anomalies, and the situs inversus/polysplenia complex.[4,5]

The surgical procedures most commonly performed for duodenal atresia include duodenoduodenostomy, duodenojejunostomy, and much less commonly gastrojejunostomy.[6] For cases of duodenal web, it is appropriate to do a web excision, web incision with duodenoplasty,[7] or one of the previously mentioned bypass procedures. Some surgeons add an antimesenteric tapering duodenoplasty or plication in an effort to improve motility in the dilated proximal duodenum.[8,9]

Recently Rothenberg and Gluer *et al.* have reported successful laparoscopic duodenoduodenostomy for duodenal obstruction in both newborns and young children.[10,11] The authors suggest that this approach may be accompanied by a decrease in the time to feeding due to the minimal amount of bowel manipulation.

Pediatric Surgery and Urology: Long-term Outcomes, Mark Stringer, Keith Oldham, Pierre Mouriquand.

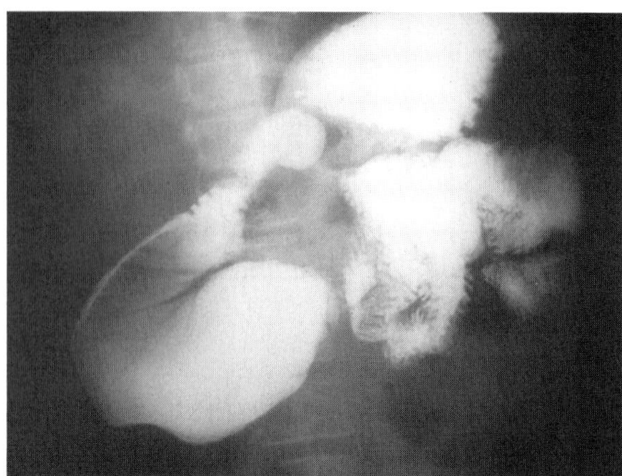

Fig. 24.1. Barium swallow in a 15-year-old child with a neonatal history of duodenal atresia treated by duodenoduodenostomy, who presented with bilious vomiting. Note the dilated proximal duodenum without evidence of anastomotic obstruction. The child's symptoms improved after duodenal tapering, although he continued to present with intermittent episodes of "ileus," probably due to a panintestinal motility disorder.

Early postoperative survival after repair of duodenal atresia has steadily improved over the past 4 decades from approximately 60% to over 90% in contemporary practice, owing to improved neonatal and anesthetic management, total parenteral nutrition (TPN), and more aggressive treatment of associated anomalies.[1,12–14]

Long-term outcomes

Long-term outcomes for most patients with congenital duodenal obstruction are excellent, with the majority of patients reported to be asymptomatic with normal growth.[1,15–17] Problems generally occur for two reasons: abnormalities of gastrointestinal function, and difficulties due to associated structural or chromosomal anomalies.

Late gastrointestinal complications include megaduodenum, duodenogastric reflux, gastritis, blind loop syndrome, peptic ulcer, and gastroesophageal reflux. Megaduodenum is a particularly troublesome problem, which may result either from anastomotic obstruction or from an inherent motility disorder of the proximal duodenum[18] (Fig. 24.1). Symptoms are poor weight gain, frequent vomiting, and less commonly abdominal pain or blind-loop syndrome. Frequency varies considerably (0%–30%) depending on the diagnostic technique employed, the use of tapering or plication at the initial procedure, and the type of operation done. Kimura *et al.*[19] reported no instances of megaduodenum in a series of patients undergoing diamond-shaped anastomosis, although Weber *et al.*[20] did not demonstrate any difference in complications with this compared with two other techniques. The present authors have had several children develop megaduodenum after using the Kimura-type of anastomosis. Spigland and Yazbeck[18] reported an unusually high rate of megaduodenum in children initially treated by duodenojejunostomy. Megaduodenum is usually managed effectively by revision of the anastomosis (if stenotic) and/or duodenal tapering[21] or plication.[22] Alexander and colleagues have recently reported a new method of tapered duodenoduodenostomy, triangular tapered duodenoplasty, as an alternative to diamond-shaped duodenoplasty that has been reported to provide superior results in terms of time to feeding, gastric emptying, and gastroesophageal reflux compared with standard side-to-side duodenoplasty.[23] A prospective trial examining this question has not been done.

Other late gastrointestinal complications have been reported after repair of congenital duodenal obstruction, which may or may not require surgical intervention. Adhesive intestinal obstruction has been reported in some of these children, a complication which may decrease with more frequent use of a minimal access approach.[10] Duodenogastric reflux has been noted with particular frequency by Kokkonen *et al.*,[17] who performed routine endoscopy as part of their follow-up routine. However, the majority of the patients with this finding were asymptomatic. Blind-loop syndrome has been described by a number of authors. Kokkonen *et al.*[17] cultured *Escherichia coli* or bacteroides species in the duodenal fluid in 6/41 such patients. This problem appears to be more common in children treated by duodenojejunostomy, and may be improved by conversion to a duodenoduodenostomy.[24] Gastric and duodenal ulcers have been reported in several series, and gastroesophageal reflux is also commonly seen on late follow-up. In some cases, these problems may be related to anastomotic obstruction or megaduodenum, but in others they are present without anatomic or functional duodenal obstruction. Most such patients can be treated medically, but surgical intervention may be necessary in a few.

Long-term problems may also occur because of other structural or chromosomal anomalies, the most common of which is Trisomy 21. In older series, children with duodenal obstruction associated with Trisomy 21 had a significantly higher rate of reoperation, as well as a relatively high mortality rate, when compared to those without Trisomy 21.[4,16] This was largely due to the significant incidence of congenital heart disease in these children, although other complications such as pneumonia, empyema, and Hirschsprung's enterocolitis have been reported. In more recent times, medical care for children with Trisomy 21 has improved, and the mortality rate has decreased.[2,25] Other congenital anomalies may also occur in the absence of Trisomy 21, and have been shown to have a strong impact on both short- and long-term survival. However, as with the Trisomy 21 population, overall survival of infants with duodenal atresia and cardiac defects, esophageal atresia, biliary atresia, anorectal malformations, and other anomalies has improved dramatically over the past few decades. For this reason, the mortality for duodenal atresia has decreased from 36% in 1969,[4] to 25% in 1977,[16] to 10% in 1993.[2]

Jejunoileal atresia and web

Jejunoileal atresia is usually classified into five major types: type I (a completely occluding web), type II (proximal and distal segments separated by a cord), type IIIa (complete separation with a mesenteric defect), type IIIb (proximal jejunal atresia with complete absence of the mesentery to the distal small bowel, the so-called "Christmas tree" or "apple peel" atresia), and type IV (multiple atresias).[26] In type IIIb the distal bowel survives on the marginal branches from the ileocolic vessels, and is prone to volvulus and necrosis. Unlike congenital duodenal obstruction, associated anomalies are uncommon with jejunoileal atresia and they tend to involve the gastrointestinal system when they do occur.[12,27] Most of these, such as cystic fibrosis, abdominal wall defects, and malrotation, may actually be involved in the genesis of the atresia. A recent study by Sweeney and colleagues found that there was a significantly higher incidence of associated congenital extraintestinal malformations in jejunal atresia compared with ileal atresia (42 vs 2%), suggesting that some cases of jejunal atresia may arise from a different, malformative process.[28]

Surgical repair of jejunoileal atresia involves performing an anastomosis between the two affected segments of bowel. For type I cases, simple web excision or incision is done,[7] and for stenosis, an enteroplasty can be performed. In many cases, particularly with proximal jejunal atresia, the proximal end is massively dilated and a concomitant resection or tapering procedure is recommended[29] (Fig. 24.2). In children with a Christmas tree deformity, great care must be taken to avoid torsion of the distal bowel. For type IV atresia, short intervening segments may be resected, and as few anastomoses as possible are done as long as adequate small bowel length is maintained.[30] Recent reports have described the successful use of intraluminal stents in multiple intestinal atresia to preserve maximum small bowel length either with[31] or without[32,33] sutureless anastomoses.

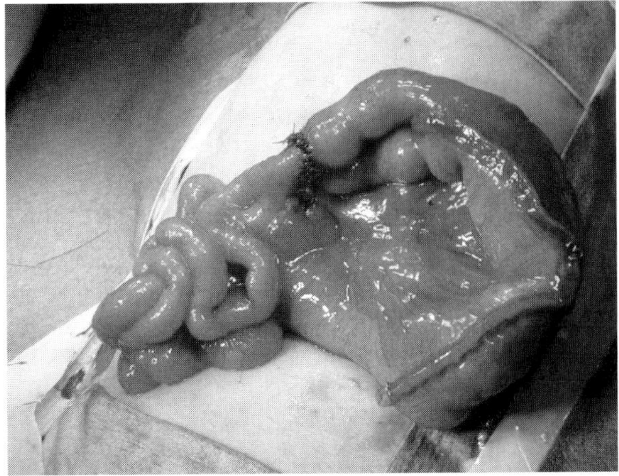

Fig. 24.2. Repaired jejunal atresia with a massively dilated proximal jejunum. The proximal bowel has been tapered using a stapling device.

Long-term outcomes

Few studies have been done reporting long-term outcomes in children with jejunoileal atresia. Overall, survival has increased from 10% in 1950 to 90% in the 1990s,[34] largely owing to improvements in neonatal care and nutritional support. Kumaran *et al.* reported a significant reduction in mortality from the condition when comparing their patients from 1976 to 82 (19%), vs. 1983 to 90 (10%), vs. 1991 to 1998 (0%), similarly attributed primarily to advances in perioperative management, TPN, and improved surgical techniques to preserve bowel length in cases of foreshortened gut.[35] Dalla Vecchia reported a long-term survival rate of 84% with an experience of 128 small bowel atresia patients over 25 years,[36] with the majority of late deaths due to ultrashort bowel syndrome with associated TPN-induced cholestasis and liver failure. Recent reports have described antenatal diagnosis of jejunoileal atresias in approximately 28%–32% of affected patients.[35,37] Potential benefits of antenatal diagnosis include earlier recognition and parental counseling, prompt intervention and the reduction of associated metabolic disturbances.[35]

Most long-term problems in these patients are related to abnormal intestinal function, both absorptive and propulsive. Some infants suffer from short bowel syndrome due to resection (most commonly with type IV defects) or to necrosis (most commonly with type IIIb anomalies). Improved survival in this group is due to the use of total parenteral nutrition,[38] although these children continue to have morbidity and mortality due to sepsis, liver failure and metabolic disturbances (see Chapter 28).

The "apple peel" type of atresia has had an improved long-term outcome in two recent reports. Festen and colleagues reviewed 15 such cases in the Netherlands with a follow-up of 7.8 years.[39] They reported an 80% survival rate with low rates of late morbidity and concluded that, if the patients survive the operative and early postoperative period, and they survive the morbidity associated with malnutrition and use of TPN, they have an excellent long-term probability of normal bowel function with normal growth, without dietary restrictions.[39] Similarly, Waldhausen and Sawin reviewed 12 of these patients with a mean follow-up of 5.1 years. They found that TPN was essential for initial nutritional management, that use of an enterostomy led to an increased incidence of complications, that gastrostomy tubes were necessary for initial management, and that early morbidity was common, although excellent long-term outcome and normal growth and development were seen in 8 of 11 available patients.[40]

Motility problems occur in a small percentage of children with jejunoileal atresia. These may occur many years after surgical repair,[41] are more common with proximal than with distal atresia, and appear to be most common in type IIIb lesions.[42] As with duodenal atresia, these patients usually present with persistent dilatation of the proximal intestine. Experimental work has suggested that both the proximal and distal intestine may be involved, although the mechanisms are unclear.[43–45] In a few cases, there may be evidence of stenosis at the anastomosis, although the modern use of end-to-end rather than side-to-side techniques has made this a relatively rare occurrence.[34] In most children with abnormal motility, there is significant dilatation of the proximal bowel without anastomotic narrowing.[46] Surgical management involves revision of the anastomosis, if necessary, and either plication[47] or tapering[48] of the proximal bowel. Normalizing the caliber of the proximal bowel may improve the mechanical properties of peristalsis, or may prevent kinking of the anastomosis. Late reoperation may also be required for adhesive obstruction in these patients, with a reported incidence of 7% in one study by Wilkins and Spitz.[1] In a report by Sato and colleagues of a 27-year experience with 88 patients, 4 underwent reoperation for anastomotic leakage, 2 for stricture, and 2 for adhesive obstruction. None required long-term treatment for malnutrition secondary to short bowel syndrome.[49]

The present authors followed 26 patients at St. Louis Children's Hospital with jejunoileal atresia for 3–18 years (mean 10 years). Of these, 3 children had associated gastroschisis, 5 had atresia complicating meconium ileus due to cystic fibrosis, and one had malrotation and atresia. Of the remaining 17, 4 (24%) had type I, 9 (53%) had type II, 2 (12%) had type IIIb, and 2 (12%) had type IV jejunoileal atresia. All 26 patients underwent surgery within the first 48 hours of life. Eighteen (69%) underwent primary resection and anastomosis, 2 (8%) underwent web excision, and 6 (23%) underwent stoma formation with delayed anastomosis. Nine patients (35%) underwent tapering of the proximal bowel during the initial procedure. Early postoperative complications included two wound infections, three anastomotic strictures requiring surgical revision, and two adhesive small bowel obstructions. Late complications included three anastomotic strictures requiring surgical revision, one child with chronic constipation, and one child with chronic diarrhea in the absence of short bowel syndrome. One patient with an apple peel jejunal atresia and severe short gut syndrome died at 1 year of age from progressive TPN-induced liver failure. Of the patients without cystic fibrosis, 85% were completely asymptomatic long term. Four of the five patients with cystic fibrosis reported chronic, crampy abdominal pain and diarrhea after meals, and one reported multiple episodes of distal intestinal obstruction syndrome which were relieved by enemas. On long-term follow-up, quality of life and functional status were unaffected by jejunoileal atresia. All patients were functioning normally with the exception of the five cystic fibrosis patients (who had pulmonary disease), one patient with a left hemiparesis, and one with attention deficit disorder.

Meckel's diverticulum

Meckel's diverticulum is a congenital anomaly which is caused by failure of the omphalomesenteric duct to completely regress, leaving an antimesenteric diverticulum of ileum proximal to the ileocecal junction. In a small number of cases the diverticulum may contain heterotopic gastric mucosa, and in some cases there may be an associated congenital band attached to the anterior abdominal wall or to the mesentery. Although most people with a Meckel's diverticulum remain asymptomatic, some patients present with intestinal bleeding due to ulceration from ectopic gastric mucosa, inflammation due to obstruction of the outlet from the diverticulum (usually due to ulceration as above), intussusception with an inverted diverticulum as a lead point, or intestinal obstruction from volvulus around a Meckel's band. Treatment of all these symptomatic conditions is resection of the diverticulum, with or without segmental ileal resection. Resection of an incidentally identified Meckel's diverticulum is controversial.[50,51]

Recent reports have described successful laparoscopic Meckel's diverticulectomy.[52,53] Some authors advocate resection using an endoscopic linear stapler if the diverticulum is asymptomatic with a narrow base, while recommending exteriorization to resect a pathologic Meckel's diverticulum, as heterotopia is more frequent in these cases.[52] Additionally, Hirschl and colleagues suggest that laparoscopy may be a viable alternative to the Meckel's scan in children who present with gastrointestinal bleeding and a high suspicion for a Meckel's diverticulum, as ^{99m}Tc pertechnetate scintigraphy has a low negative predictive value in this group.[54]

Long-term outcomes

Many authors have documented an extremely low rate of complications or death after excision of Meckel's diverticulum.[55,56] No long-term problems have been identified in any of these studies. In one study of patients operated on for complications of Meckel's diverticulum, the incidence of early postoperative complications was 12%, including wound infection (3%), ileus (3%), and anastomotic leak (2%).[57,58] The mortality rate was 1.5%, and the cumulative incidence of late postoperative complications was 7%. The overall rate of morbidity after incidental removal of a Meckel's diverticulum was 2%, with a postoperative mortality rate of 1%. The risk of developing long-term complications at 20 years after an incidental Meckel's diverticulectomy was 2%.[57,58]

The present authors contacted 31 patients for long-term follow-up 5–25 years (mean 13.5) after resection of a Meckel's diverticulum. Nine patients (29%) were asymptomatic preoperatively, and the diverticulum was an incidental finding at laparotomy, while 22 (71%) were symptomatic (7 with closed-loop obstruction from a Meckel's band, 5 with intussusception, 4 with rectal bleeding, 4 with Meckel's diverticulitis, and 2 with patent omphalomesenteric duct). Ectopic gastric mucosa was present in 11 (50%) of the symptomatic cases and in none of the asymptomatic cases. Twenty-two patients underwent Meckel's diverticulectomy alone, and 9 underwent ileal resection. Early postoperative complications were limited to one anastomotic leak (suture line dehiscence), and one death from multiple trauma which was unrelated to the incidental Meckel's diverticulectomy.

There was no long-term mortality, and the majority of patients had no gastrointestinal complaints. One patient had a small bowel obstruction 11 years postoperatively requiring adhesiolysis. Three patients complained of chronic diarrhea after the surgery; two of these had extensive ileal resection. Quality of life and functional status were normal in all patients, except for two patients with severe pre-existing neurological disability.

Intestinal duplication

Duplications can occur anywhere along the gastrointestinal tract from the esophagus to the rectum. Small bowel duplications may be cystic or tubular, are usually situated between the leaves of the mesentery. Patients may present with an asymptomatic abdominal mass, intestinal obstruction or bleeding due to ectopic gastric mucosa with an acid-ulcer diathesis.[59] In the majority of cases, the duplication involves a relatively short segment of intestine, which can be resected easily with a low rate of complications. Less commonly, the duplication may involve a long segment of intestine, and in these cases more extensive resection may be necessary. Other options include creating a common channel between the duplication and the normal intestine, draining the duplication into the stomach, or stripping the mucosal lining of the duplication if there is ectopic gastric mucosa.[59] An important point stressed by many groups is to carefully protect the common blood supply shared by the duplication and the native bowel.[60,61]

Recently, numerous groups have reported the prenatal diagnosis of abdominal enteric duplications by ultrasound.[60,62,63] This ability has provided an opportunity to treat these lesions before they produce symptoms or cause complications.[63] Foley *et al.* reviewed 12 patients with antenally diagnosed gastrointestinal duplications.[60] In four patients, the duplications were resected early due to symptoms of small bowel obstruction. The remaining patients were resected electively between 6 weeks and 14 months. The authors noted the presence of gastric mucosa in approximately half of asymptomatic patients, concluding that they should not be left indefinitely. However, the present authors have managed some patients with prenatally diagnosed duplications with observation alone, and have not experienced any known adverse outcomes during this period of follow-up, suggesting that the natural history of asymptomatic prenatally diagnosed duplications is uncertain.

A number of groups have reported safe and effective laparoscopically assisted resection of ileocecal and colonic duplications.[60,64]

Long-term outcomes

Mortality following resection of an intestinal duplication is extremely low. Although there are no reports in the literature which include long-term outcome, the present authors have followed seven patients with intestinal duplication from 3 to 17.5 years (mean 9). The age of presentation ranged from the neonatal period to 4 years, and the diagnosis was made prenatally in three of the neonates. All seven cases underwent surgical excision of the duplication; in four the mass was excised alone, and in three a segmental bowel resection was performed. There were no deaths in this series. No gastrointestinal symptoms were reported, and there were no long-term surgical complications. Quality of life and functional status were unaffected and all patients were functioning at a normal level at follow-up. Complex tubular duplications of the esophagus or primitive hindgut present a more complex problem and require individualized reconstruction; however, these are rare and there are no published data on long-term outcome.

Malrotation

The normal process of intestinal rotation begins between the sixth and tenth weeks after conception while the intestine has migrated into the umbilical cord, and this is usually completed by the end of the twelfth gestational week. During this process, the cecum moves counterclockwise from the left side of the abdomen, anterior to the superior mesenteric vessels, to reside in the right lower quadrant. At the same time the duodenum also moves counterclockwise, posterior to the superior mesenteric vessels, forming its characteristic "C-loop." Finally, fixation of the cecum and duodenal jejunal junction to the posterior body wall occurs in the right lower and left upper quadrants, respectively. Malrotation occurs when this process is incomplete or otherwise altered. Malrotation may present in a number of ways:

- duodenal obstruction from Ladd's bands (peritoneal bands derived from the dorsal mesogastrium extend from the cecum to the right abdominal wall, potentially coursing over the duodenum and compressing it);
- volvulus of the midgut around the superior mesenteric vessels, resulting in ischemia or necrosis;
- chronic symptoms such as abdominal pain or constipation with rare reports of mesenteric venous thrombosis secondary to chronic midgut volvulus;[65]
- incidental discovery in an asymptomatic patient.

Although the majority of children present during infancy, the diagnosis may be made later in childhood or adulthood.[66] Once the diagnosis has been made, most patients undergo a Ladd's procedure, which consists of untwisting of the bowel (if volvulus exists), division of the Ladd's bands, placement of the bowel into non-rotation (thereby separating the ligament of Treitz and the ileocecal junction and, importantly, broadening the base of the small bowel mesentery), and appendectomy. Recently, several groups have reported success in performing the Ladd's procedure laparoscopically in infants[67–68] and children[69–71] with malrotation without volvulus. Some authors report earlier feeding and decreased hospital stays,[67] absence of complications,[70] usefulness in verifying the diagnosis in patients without classic radiographic findings, often with vague abdominal pain,[68 69] and usefulness in assessing the width of the mesenteric base to prevent midgut volvulus without the associated morbidity of a laparotomy.[69,72]

Malrotation has been associated with other anomalies in 30%–62% of cases.[73] These include defects which directly contribute to the genesis of malrotation by interfering with the normal process of rotation (omphalocele, gastroschisis, diaphragmatic hernia), gastrointestinal abnormalities which are probably not etiologically important (biliary atresia, Hirschsprung's disease, congenital chloride diarrhea, or esophageal, duodenal, intestinal, and anal atresia), and anomalies involving other organ systems. The most common example of the latter is the association of intestinal malrotation with congenital heart disease, midline liver, and asplenia or polysplenia (the Ivemark or heterotaxia syndrome).

Long-term outcomes

Mortality in children with malrotation has diminished from approximately 25% to 3% over the past 50 years, owing to earlier recognition and aggressive surgical management of children with volvulus, as well as better supportive measures such as modern critical care and total parenteral nutrition.[74] Long-term follow-up or outcome studies have not been reported, although several problems are known to occur. The most important of these is massive intestinal necrosis which results in short bowel syndrome. Approximately 2% of children with malrotation survive with inadequate intestinal length, and malrotation accounts for approximately 18% of all children with short bowel syndrome.[74] These children continue to suffer ongoing morbidity and mortality due to sepsis, liver failure, and metabolic disturbances (see Chapter 28). In a study by Prasil and colleagues, patients operated on for malrotation younger than 2 years of age were compared with those older than 2 years of age.[75] There was a trend toward more postoperative complications in the younger group in comparison to the older group. Additionally, they found that five of the older patients presented with midgut volvulus, and therefore recommended that older children require surgical attention (with laparoscopy where appropriate) even if asymptomatic, as they have a significant risk of volvulus which is difficult to anticipate radiologically.[75]

Intestinal obstruction can occur following a Ladd procedure, owing to adhesions or to recurrent volvulus. Fortunately, both of these occur infrequently.[76] Persistent gastrointestinal symptoms can also occur following

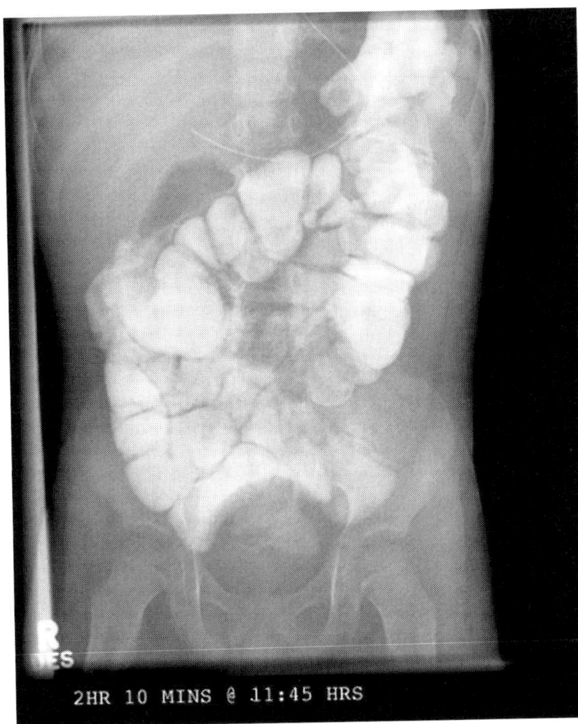

Fig. 24.3. Gastrointestinal contrast study in a 5-year-old child who had been operated on for malrotation without volvulus at 6 months of age. This 24-hour film demonstrates retention of the barium, indicating that the child has chronic intestinal pseudo-obstruction.

correction of malrotation. These include obstructive symptoms, diarrhea, or abdominal pain. In some cases no obvious cause of these postoperative symptoms is found, and it can be assumed that they are unrelated to the malrotation. In other patients, postoperative symptoms are due to an inherent abnormality of intestinal motility (pseudo-obstruction)[77,78] (Fig. 24.3). Whether there is an etiological association between these two conditions remains unknown.

Mehall *et al.* reviewed 176 consecutive operations for malrotation over five years with available radiologic studies. "Typical" malrotation (assessed radiographically) was present in 75 patients, while "atypical" malrotation (a low or high ligament of Treitz) was present in 101 patients.[79] They found that atypical malrotation patients were at a significantly lower risk of volvulus and internal hernia compared with typical malrotation patients. Additionally, they found that postoperative complications occurred in 13% of typical versus 22% of low (atypical) and 21% of high (atypical) patients which included obstruction, intussusception, and wound infection.[79] Atypical malrotation patients had a significantly higher incidence of persistent symptoms postoperatively when compared with typical malrotation, calling into question the efficacy of this operation in resolving all types of symptoms in a disparate population.

Long-term outcome can also be influenced by other associated anomalies particularly those which are associated with morbidity or mortality. Examples may include diaphragmatic hernia, biliary tract anomalies,[80] and complex cardiac anomalies.

Intussusception

Intussusception is characterized by invagination of a segment of intestine into the distal adjacent bowel. It can occur at any age, although 90% of patients present between 3 months and 3 years of age. In some cases there is a lead point (usually a polyp, benign or malignant tumor, or inverted Meckel's diverticulum). However, in most patients a lead point is not identifiable and the etiology is therefore idiopathic. In many of these, the intussusception may be caused by a hypertrophied Peyer's patch. The incidence of an identifiable anatomical lead point increases with the patient's age, and is present in over 95% of adult intussusceptions.[81]

Diagnosis is usually made by contrast enema, and in over half of the cases the intussusception can be reduced by the radiologist using barium or air. Recently, air enema has been reported to be highly effective with a success rate of 84% in 181 cases. Mean fluoroscopy time was only 2.8 minutes in successful procedures and 4.9 minutes in unsuccessful procedures.[82] The use of carbon dioxide insufflation is associated with similar success and has the advantage of more rapid absorption after the procedure.[83] Ultrasound-guided pneumatic reduction has been added recently to the armentarium, with a reported success rate of 92% and the additional radiation-sparing benefit.[84] The presence of an anatomical lead point is associated with a much lower rate of successful reduction. Irreducible cases require laparotomy, at which time the intussusception can be either manually reduced or resected, depending on the surgeon's assessment of bowel viability. Occasionally, the attempted hydrostatic or pneumatic reduction will be complicated by perforation (incidence 1% or less), in which case emergency laparotomy is required. A dreaded complication, life threatening tension pneumoperitoneum, can occur in this situation, and is emergently treated with immediate needle decompression of the abdominal compartment.[85] A recent study by Bratton and colleagues showed that children who received care for intusscusception in a large children's hospital (>10 000 annual admissions), had a lower probability of operative care, shorter length of stay, and lower hospital charges compared with children who received care in hospitals with smaller pediatric caseloads (<10 000 admissions).[86]

Controversy exists regarding the role of laparoscopy in the management of childhood intussusception.[87] van der Laan *et al.* concluded that patients 3 years of age or older often need resection and will not benefit from the laparoscopic approach. Additionally, they suggest that there is little role in those under 3 years of age if there is an experienced pediatric radiology staff, because intussusceptions that are easily reduced laparoscopically are most likely to be those that could have been reduced by non-surgical methods.[87] They conclude that there is a place for the laparoscopic approach in cases of recurrent intussusception or questionable but probable reduction.[87]

Long-term outcomes

Mortality from intussusception is approximately 1%. Most deaths are due to late recognition and inadequate resuscitation, leading to sepsis and multisystem organ failure.[88] Intussusception may recur in up to 10% of cases, as much as several years after initial reduction.[89] Recurrence is less likely after surgical management, but it still occurs in 1%–4% of cases. The principles of management for recurrent intussusception should be the same as for the initial episode, i.e., attempted hydrostatic or pneumatic reduction. Some authors recommend surgical management of recurrence in children who are at high risk for an anatomical lead point.[90] Intussusception in premature neonates is an exceedingly rare entity (occurring even less than the 1.3% of all cases reported in term neonates). Intussusception in preterm infants has a higher reported mortality (20%) due to misdiagnosis as NEC which often delays operative intervention, and yields a higher probability of necrotic bowel.[91]

The vast majority of children with intussusception have an excellent long-term outlook. This is true even for those with recurrent episodes. In the small group of children who have a tumor or systemic disease involved in the etiology of the intussusception, the prognosis is dictated by the underlying disease. Examples include Burkitt's lymphoma, Peutz–Jeghers syndrome, cystic fibrosis, and Henoch–Schönlein purpura.

REFERENCES

1. Wilkins, B. M. & Spitz, L. Incidence of postoperative adhesion obstruction following neonatal laparotomy. *Br. J. Surg.* 1986; **73**:762–764.
2. Grosfeld, J. L. & Rescorla, F. J. Duodenal atresia and stenosis: reassessment of treatment and outcome based on antenatal diagnosis, pathologic variance, and long-term follow-up. *World J. Surg.* 1993; **17**:301–309.
3. Chhabra, R., Suresh, B. R., Weinberg, G., Marion, R., & Brion, L. P. Duodenal atresia presenting as hemate-mesis in a premature infant with Down syndrome. *J. Perinatol.* 1992; **12**:25–27.
4. Fonkalsrud, E. W., DeLorimier, A. A., & Hays, D. M. Congenital atresia and stenosis of the duodenum: a Review compiled from the members of the surgical section of the American Academy of Pediatrics. *Pediatrics* 1969; **43**:79–83.
5. Atwell, J. D. & Klidjian, A. M. Vertebral anomalies and duodenal atresia. *J. Pediatr. Surg.* 1982; **17**:237–240.
6. Puri, P. & Sweed, Y. Duodenal obstructions. In Puri, P. (ed.), *Newborn Surgery*. Oxford, UK: Butterworth-Heinemann, 1996: 290–297.
7. Langer, J. C. & Winthrop, A. L. A simplified surgical technique for the management of gastrointestinal Webs. *Pediatr. Surg. Int.* 1993; **8**:180–181.
8. Aubrespy, P., Derlon, S., & Seriat-Gautier, B. Congenital duodenal obstruction: a review of 82 cases. *Prog. Pediatr. Surg.* 1978; **11**:109–124.
9. Weisgerber, G. & Boureau, M. Immediate and secondary results of duodeno-duodenostomies with tapering in the treatment of total congenital duodenal obstructions in newborn infants. *Chir. Pediatr.* 1982; **23**:369–372.
10. Rothenberg, S. S. Laparoscopic duodenoduodenostomy for duodenal obstruction in infants and children. *J. Pediat. Surg.* 2002; **37**:1088–1089.
11. Gluer, S., Petersen, C., & Ure, B. M. Simultaneous correction of duodenal atresia due to annular pancreas and malrotation by laparoscopy. *Eur. J. Pediatr. Surg.* 2002; **12**:423–425.
12. Nixon, H. H. & Tawes, R. Etiology and treatment of small intestinal atresia: analysis of a series of 127 jejunoileal atresias and comparison with 62 duodenal atresias. *Surgery* 1970; **69**:41–51.
13. Wesley, J. R. & Mahour, G. H. Congenital intrinsic duodenal obstruction: a twenty-five year review. *Surgery* 1977; **82**:716–720.
14. Mooney, D., Lewis, J. E., Connors, R. H., & Weber, T. R. Newborn duodenal atresia: an improving outlook. *Am. J. Surg.* 1987; **153**:347–349.
15. Feggetter, S. A review of the long-term results of operations for duodenal atresia. *Br. J. Surg.* 1969; **56**:68–72.
16. Stauffer, U. G. & Irving, I. Duodenal atresia and stenosis: long-term results. *Prog. Pediatr. Surg.* 1977; **10**:49–60.
17. Kokkonen, M. L., Kalima, T., Jaaskelainen, J., & Louhimo, I. Duodenal atresia: late follow-up. *J. Pediatr. Surg.* 1988; **23**:216–220.
18. Spigland, N. & Yazbeck, S. Complications associated with surgical treatment of congenital intrinsic duodenal obstruction. *J. Pediatr. Surg.* 1990; **25**:1127–1130.
19. Kimura, K., Mukohara, N., Nishijima, E. *et al.* Diamond-shaped anastomosis for duodenal atresia: an experience with 44 patients over 15 years. *J. Pediatr. Surg.* 1990; **25**:977–979.

20. Weber, T. R., Lewis, J. E., Mooney, D., & Connors, R. Duodenal atresia: a comparison of techniques of repair. *J. Pediatr. Surg.* 1986; **21**:1133–1136.
21. Adzick, N. S., Harrison, M. R., & deLorimier, A. A. Tapering duodenoplasty for megaduodenum associated with duodenal atresia. *J. Pediatr. Surg.* 1986; **21**:311–312.
22. Ein, S. H. & Shandling, B. The late nonfunctioning duodenal atresia repair. *J. Pediatr. Surg.* 1986; **21**:798–801.
23. Alexander, F., DiFiore, J., & Stallion, A. Triangular tapered duodenoplasty for the treatment of congenital duodenal obstruction. *J. Pediat. Surg.* 2002; **37**:862–864.
24. Rescorla, F. J. & Grosfeld, J. L. Duodenal atresia in infancy and childhood: improved survival and long-term follow-up. *Contemp. Surg.* 1988; **33**:22–27.
25. Puri, P. & O'Donnell, B. Outlook after surgery for congenital intrinsic duodenal obstruction in Down's syndrome (letter). *Lancet* 1982; **10**:802.
26. Grosfeld J. L. Jejunoileal atresia and stenosis. In Welch, K. J., Randoph, J. G., Ravitch, M. M., O'Neill, J. A., & Rowe, M. I. (eds.), *Pediatric Surgery*. Chicago: YearBook Medical, 1986: 838–848.
27. de Lorimier, A. A., Fonkalsrud E. W., & Hays, D. M. Congenital atresia and stenosis of the jejunum and ileum. *Surgery* 1969; **65**:819–827.
28. Sweeney, B., Surana, R., & Puri, P. Jejunoileal atresia and associated malformations: correlation with the timing of in utero insult. *J. Pediatr. Surg.* 2001; **36**:774–776.
29. Cywes, S., Rode, H., & Millar, A. J. W. Jejuno-ileal atresia and stenosis. In Puri, P. (ed.), *Newborn Surgery*. Oxford, UK: Butterworth-Heinemann, 1996: 307–317.
30. El Shafie, M. & Rickham, P. P. Multiple intestinal atresias. *J. Pediat. Surg.* 1970; **5**:655–659.
31. Alexander, F., Babak, D., & Goske, M. Use of intraluminal stents in multiple intestinal atresia. *J. Pediatr. Surg.* 2002; **37**:E34.
32. Dinsmore, J. E., Jackson, R. J., & Wagner, C. W. Management of multiple intestinal atresias and perforations with intraluminal stenting. *Pediatr. Surg. Int.* 1998; **13**: 226–228.
33. Federici, S., Domenichelli, V., Antonellini, C. *et al.* Multiple intestinal atresia with apple peel syndrome: successful treatment by five end-to-end anastomoses, jejunostomy, and transanastomotic silicone stent. *J. Pediatr. Surg.* 2003; **38**:1250–1252.
34. Touloukian, R. J. Diagnosis and treatment of jejunoileal atresia. *World J. Surg.* 1993; **17**:310–317.
35. Kumaran, N., Shankar, K. R., Lloyd, D. A. *et al.* Trends in the management of jejuno-ileal atresia. *Eur. J. Pediatr. Surg.* 2002; **12**:163–167.
36. Dalla Vecchia, L. K., Grosfeld, J. L., West, K. W. *et al.* Intestinal atresia and stenosis: a 25-year experience with 277 cases. *Arch. Surg.* 1998; **133**:490–497.
37. Tam, P. K. H. & Nicholls, G. Implications of antenatal diagnosis of small-intestinal atresia in the 1990s. *Pediatr. Surg. Int.* 1999; **15**:486–487.
38. Smith, G. H. H. & Glasson, M. Intestinal atresia: factors affecting survival. *Aust. NZ J. Surg.* 1989; **59**:151–156.
39. Festen, S., Brevoord, J. C. D., Goldhoorn, G. A. *et al.* Excellent long-term outcome for survivors of apple peel atresia. *J. Pediatr. Surg.* 2002; **37**:61–65.
40. Waldhausen, J. H. T. & Sawin, R. S. Improved long-term outcome for patients with jejunoileal apple peel atresia. *J. Pediatr. Surg.* 1997; **32**:1307–1309.
41. Ward, H. C., Leake, J., Milla, P. J., & Spitz, L. Brown bowel syndrome: a late complication of intestinal atresia. *J. Pediatr. Surg.* 1992; **27**:1593–1595.
42. Ahlgren, L. S. Apple peel jejunal atresia. *J. Pediatr. Surg.* 1987; **22**:451–453.
43. Nixon, H. H. An experimental study of propulsion in isolated small intestine and applications to surgery in the newborn. *Ann. Roy. Coll. Surg. Engl.* 1960; **27**:105–124.
44. Cloutier, R. Intestinal smooth muscle response to chronic obstruction: possible applications in jejunoileal atresia. *J. Pediatr. Surg.* 1975; **10**:3–8.
45. Doolin, E. J., Ormsbee, H. S., & Hill, J. L. Motility abnormality in intestinal atresia. *J. Pediatr. Surg.* 1987; **22**:320–324.
46. Carmon, M., Krauss, M., Aufses, A. H., & Katz, L. B. Jejunal obstruction as a late result of neonatal jejunal atresia. *J. Pediatr. Surg.* 1994; **29**:1613–1615.
47. De, Lorimier, A. A. & Harrison, M. R. Intestinal plication in the management of atresia. *J. Pediatr. Surg.* 1983; **18**:734–737.
48. Weber, T. R., Vane, D. W., & Grosfeld, J. L. Tapering enteroplasty in infants with bowel atresia and short gut. *Arch. Surg.* 1982; **117**:684.
49. Sato, S., Nishijima, E., Muraji, T. *et al.* Jejunoileal atresia: a 27-year experience. *J. Pediatr. Surg.* 1998; **33**:1633–1635.
50. Cullen, J. J., Kelly, K. A., Moir, C. R., Hodge, D. O., Zinsmeister, A. R., & Melton, J. Surgical management of Meckel's diverticulum: an epidemiologic, population-based study. *Ann. Surg.* 1994; **220**:564–569.
51. Bemelman, W. A., Hugenholtz, E., Heij, H. A., Wiersma, P. H., & Obertop, H. Meckel's diverticulum in Amsterdam: experience in 136 patients. *World J. Surg.* 1995; **19**:734–737.
52. Valla, J. S., Steyaert, H., Leculee, R. *et al.* Meckel's diverticulum and laparoscopy of children. What's new? *Eur. J. Pediatr. Surg.* 1998; **8**:26–28.
53. Schmid, S. W., Schafer, M., Krahenbuhl, L. *et al.* The role of laparoscopy in symptomatic Meckel's diverticulum. *Surg. Endosc.* 1999; **13**:1047–1049.
54. Swaniker, F., Soldes, O., & Hirschl, R. B. The utility of technetium 99m pertechnetate scintigraphy in the evaluation of patients with Meckel's diverticulum. *J. Pediatr. Surg.* 1999; **34**:760–765.
55. Vane, D. W., West, K. W., & Grosfeld, J. L. Vitelline duct anomalies: experience with 217 childhood cases. *Arch. Surg.* 1987; **122**:542–547.
56. St-Vil, D., Brandt, M. L., Panic, S., Bensoussan, A. L., & Blanchard, H. Meckel's diverticulum in children: a 20-year review. *J. Pediat. Surg.* 1991; **26**:1289–1292.
57. Yahchouchy, E. K., Marano, A. F., Etienne, J. F. *et al.* Meckel's diverticulum. *J. Am. Coll. Surg.* 2001; **192**:658–662.

58. Cullen, J. J., Kelly, K. A., Moir, C. R. *et al.* Surgical management of Meckel's diverticulum. An epidemiologic, population-based study. *Ann. Surg.* 1994: **220**:564–569.
59. Heiss, K. Intestinal duplications. In Oldham, K. T., Colombani, P. M., & Foglia, R. P. (eds.), *Surgery of Infants and Children.* Philadelphia: Lippincott-Raven, 1997: 1265–1274.
60. Foley, P. T., Sithasanan, N., McEwing, R. *et al.* Enteric duplications presenting as antenatally detected abdominal cysts: is delayed resection appropriate? *J. Pediatr. Surg.* 2003; **38**:1810–1813.
61. Iyer, C. P. & Mahour, G. H. Duplications of the alimentary tract in infants and children. *J. Pediatr. Surg.* 1995; **30**:1267–1270.
62. Correia-Pinto, J., Tavares, M. L., Monteiro, J. *et al.* Prenatal diagnosis of abdominal enteric duplications. *Prenat. Diagn.* 2000; **20**:163–167.
63. Puligandla, P. S., Nguyen, L. T., St-Vil, D. *et al.* Gastrointestinal duplications. *J. Pediatr. Surg.* 2003; **38**:740–744.
64. Diamond, I. R., Teckman, J., & Langer, J. C. Laparoscopy in the management of colonic duplication. *Pediatr. Endosurg. Innov. Tech.* 2003; **7**:439–44.
65. Walsh, D. S. & Crombleholme, T. M. Superior mesenteric venous thrombosis in malrotation with chronic volvulus. *J. Pediatr. Surg.* 2000; **35**:753–755.
66. Maxson, R. T., Franklin, P. A., & Wagner, C. W. Malrotation in the older child: surgical management, treatment, and outcome. *Am. Surg.* 1995; **61**:135–138.
67. Bass, K. D., Rothenberg, S. S., & Chang, J. H. T. Laparoscopic Ladd's procedure in infants with malrotation. *J. Pediatr. Surg.* 1998; **33**:279–281.
68. Gross, E., Chen, M. K., & Lobe, T. E. Laparoscopic evaluation and treatment of intestinal malrotation in infants. *Surg. Endosc.* 1996; **10**:936–937.
69. Mazziotti, M. V., Strasberg, S. M., & Langer, J. C. Intestinal rotation abnormalities without volvulus: the role of laparoscopy. *J. Am. Coll. Surg.* 1997; **185**:183–187.
70. Bax, N. M. A. & van der Zee, D. C. Laparoscopic treatment of intestinal malrotation in children. *Surg. Endosc.* 1998; **12**:1314–1316.
71. Tsumura, H., Ichikawa, T., Kagawa, T. *et al.* Successful laparoscopic Ladd's procedure and appendectomy for intestinal malrotation with appendicitis. *Surg. Endosc.* 2003; **17**:657–658.
72. Chen, L. E., Minkes, R. M., & Langer, J. C. Laparoscopic vs open surgery for malrotation without volvulus. *Pediat. Endosurg. Innov. Tech.* 2003; **7**:433–438.
73. Warner, B. W. Malrotation. In Oldham, K. T., Colombani, P. M., & Foglia, R. P. (eds.), *Surgery of Infants and Children.* Philadelphia: Lippincott-Raven, 1997: 1229–1240.
74. Ford, E. G., Senac, M. O., Srikanth, M. S., & Weitzman, J. J. Malrotation of the intestine in children. *Ann. Surg.* 1992; **215**:172–178.
75. Prasil, P., Flageole, H., Shaw, K. S. *et al.* Should malrotation in children be treated differently according to age? *J. Pediatr. Surg.* 2000; **35**:756–758.
76. Torres, A. M. & Ziegler, M. M. Malrotation of the intestine. *World J. Surg.* 1993; **17**:326–331.
77. Devane, S. P., Coombes, R., Smith, V. V. *et al.* Persistent gastrointestinal symptoms after correction of malrotation. *Arch. Dis. Child.* 1992; **67**:218–221.
78. Singh, G., Hershman, M. J., Loft, D. E. *et al.* Partial malrotation associated with pseudo obstruction of the small bowel. *Br. J. Clin. Pract.* 1993; **47**:274–275.
79. Mehall, J. R., Chandler, J. C., Mehall, R. L. *et al.* Management of typical and atypical intestinal malrotation. *J. Pediatr. Surg.* 2002; **37**:1169–1172.
80. Campbell, K. A., Sitzmann, J. V., & Cameron, J. L. Biliary tract anomalies associated with intestinal malrotation in the adult. *Surgery* 1993; **113**:312–317.
81. Lang, L.-C. Intussusception revisited: Clinicopathologic analysis of 261 cases, with emphasis on pathogenesis. *South. Med. J.* 1989; **82**:215–228.
82. Lui, K., Wong, H., Cheung, Y. *et al.* Air enema for diagnosis and reduction of intussusception in children: clinical experience and fluoroscopy time correlation. *J. Pediatr. Surg.* 2001; **36**:479–481.
83. Paterson, C. A., Langer, J. C., Somers, S. *et al.* Pneumatic reduction of intussusception using carbon dioxide. *Pediatr. Radiol.* 1994; **24**:296–297.
84. Yoon, C. H., Kim, H. J., & Goo, H. W. Intussusception in children: US-guided pneumatic reduction – initial experience. *Radiology* 2001; **218**:85–88.
85. Ng, E., Kim, H. B., Lillehei, C. W. *et al.* Life threatening tension pneumoperitoneum from intestinal perforation during air reduction of intussusception. *Paediatr. Anaesth.* 2002; **12**:798–800.
86. Bratton, S. L., Haberkern, C. M., Waldhausen, J. H. T. *et al.* Intussusception: hospital size and risk of surgery. *Pediatrics* 2001; **107**:299–303.
87. van der Lann, M., Bax, N. M. A., van der Zee D. C. *et al.* The role of laparoscopy in the management of childhood intussusception. *Surg. Endosc.* 2001; **15**:373–376.
88. Stringer, M. D., Pledger, G., & Drake, D. P. Childhood deaths from intussusception in England and Wales, 1984–9. *Br. Med. J.* 1992; **304**:737–739.
89. Ein, S. H. Recurrent intussusception in children. *J. Pediatr. Surg.* 1975; **10**:751–755.
90. Beasley, S. W., Auldist, A. W., & Stokes, K. B. Recurrent intussusception: barium or surgery? *Aust. NZ J. Surg.* 1987; **57**:11–14.
91. Avansino, J. R., Bjerke, S., Hendrickson, M. *et al.* Clinical features and treatment outcome of intussusception in premature neonates. *J. Pediatr. Surg.* 2003; **38**:1818–1821.

25

Cystic fibrosis

Mark Davenport and Hilary Wyatt

King's College Hospital, London, UK

"Das Kind stirbt bald wieder, dessen Stirne beim Küssen salzig ist"
(The child will die soon, whose forehead tastes salty when kissed)
German children's song

Introduction

Cystic fibrosis (CF) is the most common lethal inherited condition in Caucasians. In the 1960s patients rarely survived their first decade, succumbing to the effects of malnutrition and lung disease.[1–3] At the end of the 1980s there were approximately 5000 patients with CF within the UK with an estimated 6000 by the year 2000.[3] In practice, in 2002, almost 7000 patients had been registered on the UK Cystic Fibrosis database (personal communication). Similar changes have been observed in North America.[4] Improvements to treatment over the last 40 years have led to a dramatic increase in life expectancy such that the median survival is now around 32 years.[5] Further improvements in survival are expected for babies born in the past decade. The treatment of CF is, however, complex, time-consuming and intrusive to the sufferer's daily life. With advancing age, more complications of CF develop and a number of these require surgical intervention. Discovery of the abnormal gene responsible for CF in 1989[6] has resulted in a much greater understanding of this multisystem disease, as well as hope of a cure for the major cause of morbidity and mortality, lung disease.

Pathophysiology

CF is an autosomal recessive condition with an incidence of about 1 in 2500 live births in the UK and Canada and 1 in 3400 live births in the USA white population. The carrier frequency is therefore about 1 in 25 in the UK. It is much less common in non-white populations with frequencies of about 1 in 14 000 in Afro-Caribbeans and 1 in 25 000 in Asian populations. The CF gene spans 250 000 base pairs on the long arm of chromosome 7, and codes for a 1480 amino acid protein called the cystic fibrosis transmembrane conductance regulator (CFTR). In health, CFTR acts primarily as a cyclic AMP-activated chloride channel, although it is recognized as having a number of other functions. CFTR is located in many tissues, but is associated particularly with disease of the lungs, pancreas, biliary tract, and vas deferens. The presence of two abnormal CF genes in an individual leads to impaired secretion of chloride from the cell and enhanced absorption of sodium into the cell. The net inward flux of ions is accompanied by water, causing dehydration of secretions on the epithelial cell surface. Abnormalities of secreted glycoproteins also contribute to an increase in viscosity of these secretions and consequent obstruction of small lumina. It is also proposed that abnormal CFTR in the lung is associated with cell surface receptors for organisms, in particular *Pseudomonas aeruginosa*.

More than 1300 disease-causing CFTR gene mutations have been reported. These are divided into five classes depending on the site within the cell at which abnormal, or absent, production of the CFTR protein occurs.[7] The most frequent gene mutation, found in about 75% of patients in the UK and USA, is the ΔF_{508} mutation.[8] The level of functioning CFTR at the apical membrane of epithelial cells is thought to be one of the determinants of disease expression. Other functions of CFTR and modifier genes are also thought to contribute to the phenotype. In general, there is no clear genotype–phenotype relationship,

Pediatric Surgery and Urology: Long-term Outcomes, Mark Stringer, Keith Oldham, Pierre Mouriquand.
Published by Cambridge University Press.

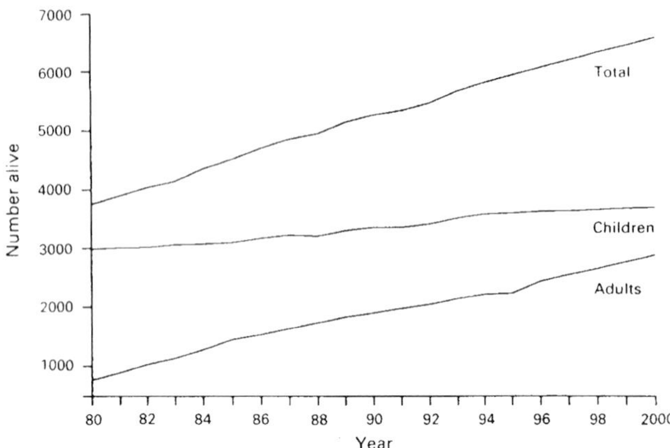

Fig. 25.1. Estimated numbers of patients with cystic fibrosis in England and Wales by year from 1980 to 2000. (Reproduced with permission from ref. 3.)

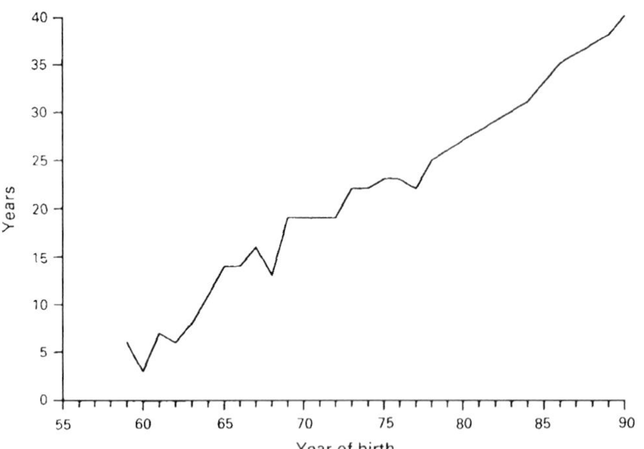

Fig. 25.2. Median survival by year of birth from 1959 to 1990 (England and Wales). (Reproduced with permission from ref. 3.)

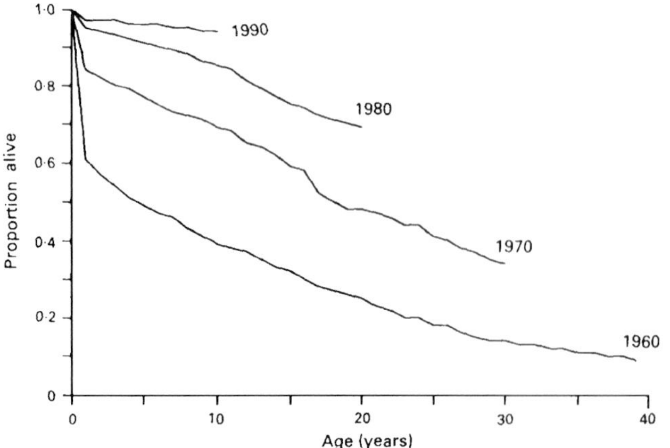

Fig. 25.3. Survival curves for cohorts born in England and Wales at the beginning of each decade, extrapolated to the year 2000. (Reproduced with permission from ref. 3.)

and only in relation to pancreatic exocrine function is there some correlation.[9] CFTR gene mutations have been classified as "mild" or "severe" according to whether they produce pancreatic sufficiency (PS) or insufficiency (PI), where the presence of one "mild" allele confers pancreatic sufficiency. People with CF who are PS tend to have lower sweat chloride levels and less lung disease. "Severe" mutations include ΔF508 and G551D; whereas R117H is considered "mild." A relationship between genotype and meconium ileus has not been shown.[9,10]

Overview of cystic fibrosis

Worldwide there are about 70 000 people affected with CF, with about half of them living in the USA. In terms of the age spectrum, at least half are adolescents and adults (Figs. 25.1, 25.2, 25.3). Neonatal screening for CF has been performed in a few areas in the UK and throughout the world for many years.[11] In these areas, research has indicated some health benefit from the early diagnosis of CF. There remains, however, controversy about the long-term outcomes, and similarly the financial benefits. Despite this, neonatal screening has been planned to commence across the UK once funding and practical issues have been resolved. Antenatal screening, other than for family members of known carriers, is impractical and the actual incidence of new cases of CF seems unlikely to change.

Most children in unscreened populations with CF present in the first 18 months of life with recurrent chest infections (40%–50%), malabsorption (20%–25%) and failure to thrive (40%–50%). About 10%–20% of infants born with CF will present with meconium ileus.

In a child with an affected first-degree relative, positive neonatal screening test, or typical clinical features, the diagnosis is confirmed by an abnormal sweat test or the presence of two known disease-forming CF gene mutations. Sweat chloride is considered more discriminatory than sodium and must be obtained through pilocarpine iontophoresis with a minimum sweat weight of 1 g/m^{2}per min. The sweat test can be less reliable in the first few months of life, but only because of difficulties collecting a sufficient volume of sweat. A revised upper limit of normal for infants of 40 mmol/l has been suggested.[11] Other techniques can be useful in borderline cases. These include measurement of nasal transepithelial potential difference, which is raised in CF, and, in neonates, measurement of serum immunoreactive trypsin (IRT) or identification of the common CF genes. IRT levels are higher than normals in first 6 weeks of life, perhaps because of back-leakage of enzymes from obstructed pancreatic acini.

Identification of the common alleles for CF, accounting for about 85% of all potential abnormal genes, is now also a practical method of diagnosis whatever the age of the infant. Using similar techniques it is possible to make an antenatal diagnosis in the affected fetus either by chorionic villus or percutaneous umbilical cord blood sampling. There is a risk of fetal loss of between 1% and 2% with such invasive tests. A possibility for the future comes from the demonstration of trophoblasts and fetal cells in the maternal circulation; such cells can be separated and identified and can provide a source of fetal DNA which would enable genetic diagnosis.

Long-term survival statistics

There has been a remarkable improvement in the survival expectation of children born with CF over the last 40 years. The current median survival for the CF population in the UK and USA is about 32 years.[5] In the USA, the median survival in 1969 was only 14 years, which had doubled to 28 years by 1990.[4] Similarly, a study from Denmark estimated that a newborn child with CF now has an 80% probability of survival to the 45th birthday.[12] This improvement is a result of aggressive treatment to delay lung disease, optimization of nutrition, and management by specialist multidisciplinary teams. This care should now be available to all newborns with CF.

There is a consistent gender difference in expected survival with affected males living longer than females.[5] This has been shown in British,[1, 13] American[4, 5] and European studies.[14] However, there is also some demographic evidence to suggest that survival among females is improving faster than males and may even be better beyond 20 years of age.[1] The anticipation of long-term survival of children born with this disease has modified attitudes to management in recent decades (Fig. 25.3) from relative nihilism to optimism.

Management of cystic fibrosis

Correction of the CFTR ion transport defect by gene therapy was first demonstrated in mice by a group from Oxford in 1993.[15] Since then much work in experimental models and human studies has been published using viral (e.g., adenovirus, lentivirus, retroviruses) and non-viral (plasmids, cationic liposomes[16]) vectors; and direct insertion of compacted naked DNA (e.g., PLASmin, *Copernicus Therapeutics Inc.*). Without doubt, such techniques currently provide the best chance of actually curing CF.[17] Nevertheless, most human trials have actually been largely unsuccessful in terms of fundamentally altering the disease process and we are some way off achieving real practical benefits.

Respiratory failure remains by far the most common cause of mortality in CF, accounting for more than 90% of deaths. The dramatic improvement in survival has been achieved largely through aggressive treatment of respiratory tract infection directed by multidisciplinary teams from specialist CF centers. The development of improved formulations of pancreatic enzyme replacement therapy has also made it possible to correct malabsorption and potentially achieve normal nutritional status. Current management strategies are therefore aimed at the complications of established disease; of prime importance to the surgeon are those of the lungs, the gastrointestinal tract and the hepatobiliary system.

Respiratory complications

Progressive bronchopulmonary sepsis remains the primary cause of morbidity and mortality in CF. The underlying failure of the mucociliary clearance mechanism causes abnormal bacterial colonization and an increased frequency of respiratory infections. *Staphylococcus aureus* and *Pseudomonas aeruginosa* are the most common pathogens, increasing in prevalence with advancing age. *Burkholderia cepacia* is an organism that can cause an accelerated, or even fatal, deterioration in CF patients. Transmission of *B. cepacia* between patients was recognized from an early stage, but more recently the identification of cross-infection of *P. aeruginosa* has required the segregation of most CF patients from each other.[18] Methicillin resistant *Staphylococcus aureus* (MRSA) does not appear to be more virulent than its methicillin-sensitive counterpart, but requires further isolation of affected patients in clinic and ward environments. Survival varies greatly according to the presence of bacterial infection. It has recently been shown that, if respiratory cultures remained negative (suggesting the absence of bacterial infection) the average survival was 39 years but survival was reduced to 28 years if chronically infected with *P. aeruginosa* and only 16 years if infected by *B. cepacia*.[19] Other infectious agents may also cause respiratory problems in CF and, although viral infections may be no more common, this does seem to precipitate deterioration in lung function. Mycobacterial infections are also found in up to 10% of the CF population if screened for acid-fast bacilli but these are usually due to atypical, non-tuberculous organisms. Infection with, and hypersensitivy to, *Aspergillus fumigatus* is another increasing problem, particularly for those patients being considered for organ transplantation. No defect of cellular or humoral immunity has been demonstrated in CF despite the fact that one of the hallmarks of the disease is the failure of the respiratory tract to eliminate pathogens. Infection is contained within the airways by an intense inflammatory response, but failure to eradicate the inciting organisms leads to a continuing neutrophil influx. Such leuokocytes release large amounts of enzymes and other chemicals and their toxic effects can cause as much, or more, local tissue damage as the pathogens.

The consequences of progressive lung infection include increased mucus production, airway obstruction, atelectasis and bronchiectasis. The mainstays of respiratory therapy are aggressive, regular airway clearance and antibiotics. The frequency and route of the latter depend on the condition of the patient and the organisms present.

Although pulmonary pathology is typically multifocal, surgical resection of involved parenchymal tissue may be indicated if the disease is localized and has been resistant to intensive medical therapy. Marmon *et al.* described 11 pulmonary resections, typically for segmental bronchiectasis, with marked clinical improvement in all.[20] Similarly, Lucas *et al.* described six children, ranging in age from 20 months to 12 years, who underwent limited pulmonary resection with clinical benefit but suggested that such surgery is only needed in less than 2% of the children seen in typical CF centers in the UK.[21] The criterion for considering resectional surgery is persistent lobar changes (typically right upper lobe disease) on serial imaging not responding to aggressive physiotherapy and antibiotic regimens. Only minimal lung disease, as evidenced by high resolution CT scanning, should be present in other lobes. *Pseudomonas* colonization is not, in itself, a contraindication.

General anesthesia, for any reason, can lead to an acute deterioration in respiratory status in CF. This may be caused by the use of antimuscarinic drugs and periods of restricted fluid intake leading to dehydration of respiratory tract secretions and by postoperative pain, which may inhibit coughing and impair airway clearance. A fall in lung function following even upper gastrointestinal endoscopy has been shown.[22] Parenteral antibiotics, intensive physiotherapy and fluid support should therefore be commenced prior to surgery and continued with effective analgesia after the procedure. If the patient is intubated, pulmonary toilet by experienced physiotherapists can be of great benefit, and provides an opportunity to obtain lower respiratory tract secretions for culture.

Intravenous antibiotics are required for the treatment of exacerbations of pulmonary infection by *Pseudomonas aeruginosa*, or other infections that fail to respond to oral antibiotics. The need for repeated courses of intravenous antibiotics often leads to increasing difficulty with venous access. Needle phobia can rapidly develop in children who have had previous traumatic attempts at peripheral cannulation. Insertion of a totally implanted permanent venous access device (e.g., *Port-A-Cath (Deltec), PAS-PORT (Deltec))* should be considered when the administration of intravenous antibiotics becomes compromised by lack of reliable vascular access (see Chapter 71). Children with needle phobia can be reassured by the ease of accessing the device. The undoubted benefits of these devices need to be balanced against the rare, but real, risks of general anesthesia, line infection, thrombosis, or catheter fracture and migration into the right heart or pulmonary artery. The latter most commonly occurs as a result of the "pinch-off" effect, where the catheter is compressed between the intersection of the clavicle and first rib. Placing the catheter in the subclavian vein, via the percutaneous route makes the pinch off syndrome more likely. Attention should also be given to the site of the Port, in order to achieve a satisfactory cosmetic result, as well as ease of access, and avoidance of interference with chest physiotherapy. The site will depend to some extent on the age of the patient and the activities in which they participate.

Hemoptysis is a known complication of bronchiectasis, and is usually due to rupture of dilated bronchial arteries. Minor episodes are not uncommon in older children and adults and are often associated with exacerbations of infection. About 60% of patients in one study had this particular symptom.[23] A clotting profile should obviously be checked, particularly in children with coexisting liver disease. Most episodes of bleeding settle with conservative treatment but more troublesome cases may respond to tranexamic acid. Rarely, hemoptysis can be life-threatening when bronchoscopy may reveal an isolated bleeding point. Bronchial artery embolization may need to be considered, although it carries the reported risk of spinal artery occlusion.

Pneumothorax is not uncommon in older patients, although unusual in children. Around 16%–20% of adults with CF will suffer a pneumothorax,[24] usually caused by spontaneous rupture of a subpleural or apical bleb or bulla. Much less commonly, it may arise following trauma such as barotrauma from mechanical ventilation or lung puncture during central line insertion. As well as causing classical signs and symptoms of sudden onset chest pain, respiratory distress and general deterioration, a pneumothorax may be completely asymptomatic and detected on a chest radiograph taken for other reasons. The risk of spontaneous pneumothorax and its clinical effects increase

Table 25.1. Lung and heart–lung transplantation for cystic fibrosis

Series	Centre	Period	Surgery	N	Actuarial survival	
					1 year	3 year
Madden *et al.* [25]	Harefield, UK	1984–1991	Heart–lung	79	69%	50%
Egan *et al.* [26]	North Carolina, USA	1990–1994	BSLT*	44	85%	67%
Balfour-Lynn *et al.* [28]	London, UK	1988–1995	Heart–lung	13 (< 10 yrs)	76%	41%
				24 (10–18 yrs)	63%	46%
Starnes *et al.* [27]	Los Angeles, USA	1993–1996	LDLLT**	32	68%	–
Huddleston *et al.* [30]	St Louis, USA	1990–2000	Isolated LT	89	77	62
Wiebe *et al.* [31]	Hanover, Germany	1988–1997	BSLT	35	91	83
Egan *et al.* [29]	North Carolina, USA	1993–2001	BSLT	114	81%	59% (5 year)
			LDLLT	9		
De Perrot *et al.* [32]	Toronto, Canada	1983–2003	BSLT	124	–	55% (5 year)

* BSLT – bilateral sequential lung transplantion (cadaveric)
** LDLLT – living donor lobar lung transplantation

with worsening lung disease. In patients with extensive parenchymal lung changes a CT scan may be needed to reach a diagnosis, and can also be useful in determining the optimal site of placement of a drainage tube. Management of a pneumothorax depends largely on the size of the air leak, although an apparently small pneumothorax in a patient with advanced lung disease can cause severe respiratory compromise. In such cases, pre-existing pleural adhesions and poor elastic recoil of lung parenchyma prevent the lung from collapsing, despite the development of increasing positive pressure within the pleural space.

A small, asymptomatic pneumothorax can be observed for spontaneous resolution, with the initial 24 hours in hospital in case of deterioration. Insertion of a chest drain, with or without suction, will be required if the air leak is larger or symptomatic. The suction pressure should not exceed 20 cm of water. A large pneumothorax should usually be drained initially without suction to minimize patient discomfort and edema of the affected lung if suddenly reinflated. A pneumothorax that does not resolve with relatively conservative treatment is best treated by limited surgical abrasion pleurodesis, and/or apical stapling of the pleura via thoracoscopy. To minimize an exacerbation of pulmonary infection, intravenous antibiotics and gentle physiotherapy should be continued, ensuring adequate analgesia if the patient has a chest drain. A recurrent pneumothorax also indicates the need for surgery in view of the high risk of further episodes. Pleurodesis is no longer an absolute contraindication to lung transplantation if a limited surgical procedure has been performed. Pleurodesis achieved through chemical irritation (e.g., talc or bleomycin) is occasionally used in very sick patients but the extensive pleural adhesions produced make subsequent lung transplantation extremely hazardous due to difficulty in dissecting the pleura and consequent bleeding.

Lung transplantation, either bilateral sequential or in combination with heart transplantation, has become an increasingly used option for end-stage, incapacitating lung disease in both children and adults with CF (see also Chapter 67 on *Heart and Lung Transplantation*). Table 25.1 illustrates recently published experience from the UK, USA and European centers.[25–32] Although 1-year survival rates have been acceptable (55%–90%) the key statistic should include those who are accepted onto a transplant waiting list but who die before a donor is found. For instance, Ryan *et al.*[33] reported the lung transplant experience of a West Midlands CF center in the UK between 1987 and 1994. Of the 49 patients who were referred for consideration of transplant, 47 were accepted onto the program and 14 (30%) of these died before being transplanted.

Problems of the upper airway may not cause dramatic effects but can contribute significantly to morbidity. Sinus disease is almost universal in CF with most being infected with the same pathogens as in the patient's lower respiratory tract. Nasal polyps are also very common in children and adults with CF,[23] and their presence in a child not known to have CF should prompt investigation for this condition. The etiology of polyps is obscure, they can be difficult to remove fully and are therefore prone to recurrence. Surgical treatment of upper airway disease tends to be reserved for particularly symptomatic cases.[34]

Table 25.2. Surgical alternatives for meconium ileus

1. Enterotomy (proximal ileal/ appendiceal[45] and luminal lavage)
2. Ileal resection and primary anastomosis
3. Enterostomies:
   (a) *Complete diversion*
   Ileostomy and mucous fistula
   (b) *Incomplete diversion*
   Bishop–Koop ileostomy[38]
   Santulli ileostomy[41]
   T-tube enterostomy[43,44]

Table 25.3. Results of treatment of meconium ileus

Series	Period	n	(i) Uncomplicated (ii) Complicated	% Survival @ 1 year (i) Uncomplicated (ii) Complicated
Del Pin *et al.*[49]	1959–1989	59	(i) 11 (19%)	(i) 100%
Philadelphia, USA			(ii) 48 (81%)	(ii) 77%
Caniano *et al.*[48]	1969–1984	42	(i) 24 (57%)	97%
Colombus, USA			(ii) 18 (43%)	
Gross *et al.*[36]	1972–1983	36	(i) 15 (42%)	(i) 87%
Indiana, USA			(ii) 21 (58%)	(ii) 86%
Rescorla *et al.*[50]	1972–1991	60	(i) 25 (42%)	(i) 92%
Indiana,[a] USA			(ii) 35 (58%)	(ii) 89%
Docherty *et al.*[54]	1972–1990	53	(i) 44 (83%)	(i) 81%
Glasgow, UK			(ii) 9 (17%)	(ii) 75%

[a] Reference[50] is an update of the preceding series (reference[36]).

Meconium ileus in the neonate

The gastrointestinal manifestations of CF were historically the first to be recognized when Landsteiner reported the association between meconium ileus and pancreatic abnormalities in 1905.[35]

Meconium ileus (MI) is the classical surgical presentation of infants with CF occurring in about 1 in 10 000–20 000 live births (i.e., about 6%–20% of patients with CF).[4] The small bowel obstruction is due to viscid, inspissated meconium that has impacted within the terminal ileum. Such meconium has an increased albumin and decreased water content, which is a result of abnormal intestinal mucus secretion rather than a deficiency in prenatal pancreatic exocrine secretion. The obstruction, beginning in intrauterine life, is simple and uncomplicated in up to half of affected neonates. However, complications may occur, such as intestinal volvulus, atresia or stenosis; intestinal perforation and meconium peritonitis; or giant meconium pseudocyst formation.[36]

As the obstruction develops during gestation, it may be diagnosed using ultrasonography. The postnatal diagnosis of MI is suggested by plain radiography which will show a "soap bubble" pattern in the right lower quadrant (Neuhauser's sign) but should be confirmed by contrast enema. This shows a small, unused microcolon and progressive ileal distension due to impacted meconium.

The management of MI has changed considerably over the past 40 years. Early reports[37–40] of survivors were achieved by surgical means alone and a range of operative techniques were developed (Table 25.2) to clear the ileum of meconium and achieve intestinal continuity either in stages.[38,41] or *ab initio*.[37,42–45] A simpler non-surgical approach was developed in the late 1960s and 1970s by Helen Noblett and became used increasingly for uncomplicated MI.[46] This technique uses a hyperosmolar contrast solution (e.g., meglumine diatrizoate – *Gastrografin, Schering Ltd*), which is introduced in a retrograde fashion as an enema. Liquefaction and disruption of the meconium is achieved in 40%–90% of uncomplicated cases and hence avoids the need for operation.[46–50]

Currently, most surgeons use a hyperosmolar contrast enema following diagnosis but, if this treatment is unsuccessful or there is prior evidence of complications (e.g., meconium cyst, perforation, etc.), a laparotomy is performed. The aim of surgical treatment is to clear the gastrointestinal tract of obstruction and restore continuity. This may be achieved by various techniques including the use of temporary stomas (Table 25.2). However, the most recent trend (which is, in fact, a reapplication of the original surgical treatment[37]) has been either to perform a simple enterotomy and meconium clearance or resection of bowel and primary anastomosis.[42,51] This shift away from the use of stomas has occurred largely because of complications related to the stoma (e.g., dehydration, sodium deficit and skin excoriation) rather than to the underlying disease.

Earlier surgical series[52,53] emphasized the significant mortality of infants with meconium ileus, although most series published in the 1980s and 1990s have shown 1-year survivals of over 80% (Table 25.3).[36,37,48–50,54] As an example, Rescorla *et al.*[50] described the outcome of 60 infants with MI treated between 1972 and 1992. The obstruction was uncomplicated in 25 (42%) and complicated in 35 (58%). Ten (17%) uncomplicated cases were treated successfully with conservative measures alone and the remainder came to surgery. One-year survival was 92% for uncomplicated and 89% for complicated MI. Long-term survival statistics for neonates with MI are generally not available separately as these infants tend to be subsumed into the general population of CF patients. However, Harry Shwachman reported a personal series of ten patients, originally

Table 25.4. Gastrointestinal problems in children and adults with cystic fibrosis

Common
1. constipation
2. rectal prolapse
3. distal intestinal obstruction syndrome (meconium ileus equivalent)

Uncommon
4. intussusception
5. appendiceal pathology: mucus distension, acute appendicitis, appendix mass / abscess
6. fibrosing colonopathy
7. ? celiac disease
8. Crohn's disease
9. intestinal malignancy

treated at the Boston Children's Hospital for MI.[55] All had reached 28 years of age with the oldest at the time of the report (1983) being 36 years old. All had suffered a variety of subsequent problems and complications.

Gastrointestinal tract disorders in older children and adults

Nutrition

The gastrointestinal tract remains abnormal throughout childhood and into adulthood and may be a continuing source of acute or chronic problems (Table 25.4). It is important that such problems are minimized as malnutrition and failure to thrive may have profound effects on the general health of the patient with CF. Children with CF have an increased energy requirement some 25%–50% higher, and adults about 20% higher, than normal.[56] This is due largely to the increased work of breathing and the catabolism associated with an increased frequency of acute lung infections.[56] Chronic pancreatic exocrine insufficiency requires enzyme supplementation to avoid steatorrhea and about 80%–90% of patients take such enzymes regularly. Modern enteric coated microsphere preparations (e.g., *Creon, Solvay*) introduced in the mid 1980s, allow an unrestricted fat diet and have contributed greatly to the long-term diminution in morbidity. Many children with CF have a poor appetite, particularly with chest infections, and fail to meet even their basic calorie requirements. Unremitting pressure to achieve a good, daily nutritional intake can easily lead to eating disorders particularly in toddlers and adolescents.

Invasive techniques that provide overnight enteral feeding by nasogastric tube or gastrostomy have become used increasingly where diet and oral nutritional supplements have failed to maintain adequate nutrition. The ability to ensure a reliable, high calorie intake can give immense relief to parent and child from the unremitting pressure to eat. Percutaneous endoscopic gastrostomy is the usual first procedure, but subsequent conversion to a low-profile device (e.g., Mic-Key Button, *Kimberley-Clark Inc.*) is popular, particularly with adolescents and adults.[4,56]

Gastroesophageal reflux

Gastroesophageal reflux is frequent in CF, particularly in infants and young children. Calorie intake may be impaired due to vomiting or a reduced appetite consequent on esophagitis. Reflux of gastric contents into the lungs will cause irritation, chemical pneumonitis, and progressive lung damage. A chronic cough may be a consequence of the problem and the increase in intra-abdominal pressure that this provokes will exacerbate reflux. Twenty-four-hour pH monitoring with an intraesophageal probe is considered by many the most effective method of diagnosing acid reflux. Barium swallow and detection of esophagitis by endoscopy can give valuable additional information. Initial treatment is with acid reduction therapy; a proton pump inhibitor is used most routinely except in infants where an H2 antagonist is probably more acceptable. Resolution of inflammation helps to restore the effectiveness of the physiological esophageal sphincter. Many pediatricians would also use a drug with prokinetic properties, such as domperidone or erythromycin. Failure of conservative treatment and progressive lung disease are indications for surgery, the most popular operation being a fundoplication. The ability to perform this laparoscopically has the potential to reduce respiratory morbidity associated with the operation.[57]

Constipation and distal intestinal obstruction syndrome

Constipation is the commonest gastrointestinal problem among older children and adults, and about one-third of patients will have chronic symptoms requiring long term laxative therapy.[23] Distal intestinal obstruction syndrome (DIOS), previously termed meconium ileus equivalent, can cause very similar symptoms but generally responds to conservative treatment, avoiding the need for general anesthesia and surgery.[58] Inspissated intestinal contents in the distal ileum and proximal colon cause complete or partial obstruction. There is often, but not invariably, a preceding history of worsening malabsorption over days or weeks, usually due to inadequate pancreatic enzyme therapy, and obstruction may be precipitated by an episode of mild dehydration. Malabsorptive stools give way to increasing constipation and worsening colicky abdominal pain. Sixteen percent of the Brompton Hospital series of adolescents and adults[23] with CF had at least one episode of DIOS. It is an uncommon complication before 5 years of age, and there appears to be a male predominance. A number of factors have been suggested as causal including a reduced pancreatic bicarbonate and water load, faulty lysosomal digestion of mucoproteins in the ileum, and a reduced bile acid pool.[59,60]

Most patients with DIOS can be treated effectively by conservative methods although surgery remains an option for resistant cases. Intravenous hydration is often required. For relatively mild episodes, oral *N*-acetyl-cysteine (e.g., *Parvolex, Celltech*) and lactulose can be sufficient, although may need to be continued for several weeks. More severe episodes will often respond to one or more doses of oral *Gastrografin* with additional oral fluid. *Gastrografin* and *N*-acetyl-cysteine can also be used as enemas. More resistant cases may need to be treated with large volumes of a balanced electrolyte intestinal lavage solution such as *Klean Prep* (polyethylene glycol), although a nasogastric tube is usually required to administer the required volume.

The prokinetic agent, cisapride (*Prepulsid – Janssen-Cilga Ltd*) was reported to be useful in reducing the frequency of obstructive episodes,[60,61] but has since been withdrawn because of side effects. There has been some interest in the use of a surgically implanted access device in the cecum or appendix stump to enable easy application of intraluminal lavage fluids in older children with recurrent obstructive symptoms. This is analogous to the antegrade continent enema (ACE) technique and regimen used in resistant cases of chronic constipation (see Chapter 33 *the Malone antegrade continence enema*).

Rectal prolapse

Intermittent rectal prolapse is not unusual in children and adults with CF (4% in the Brompton Hospital series).[23] In an early series, Shwachman and Kulczycki[62] found that 85 (22%) of 386 CF patients had suffered rectal prolapse and in 16 (4%) it was the presenting feature of the disease. The mean age at onset of symptoms was 31 months in one study.[36] Rectal prolapse occurs for a number of reasons such as frequent bowel movements, high intra-abdominal pressure, poor nutrition and poor anal muscle tone. Medical management which includes correction of constipation and straining is beneficial although some patients may require injection sclerotherapy to the prolapsing rectal mucosa. With the advent of early diagnosis of CF and good nutrition, this complication has become much less common.

Fibrosing colonopathy

Ten years ago, a new gastrointestinal complication of CF was described. Fibrosing colonopathy is manifest by colonic strictures, particularly affecting the ascending colon.[63,64] Initially, a temporal association with the introduction of high-strength pancreatic enzymes (e.g., *Creon 25 000, Solvay; Pancrease HL, Cilag Ltd; Nutrizym 22, Merck Pharmaceuticals*) was identified, and these agents were withdrawn. Further case-controlled studies suggested that the complication only occurred with certain preparations, in particular those that contained *Eudragit* in the coating of the microspheres. A high total daily intake of lipase was also implicated, and was more easily achieved with the "high-strength" formulations. A few cases were reported where high-strength preparations had not been used, and even one case in a pancreatic-sufficient patient not receiving enzymes.

Fibrosing colonopathy appears more often to affect the ascending colon. Histologic features include a relatively uninflamed epithelium and submucosal thickening caused by deposition of connective tissue.[64] In some patients there are also features suggestive of a neuropathy (e.g., ganglion cell hyperplasia) or a vasculopathy (e.g., venous intimal hyperplasia). It presents with symptoms and signs of intestinal obstruction, colitis or occasionally ascites and the diagnosis may be established by contrast enema or ultrasound of the colonic wall. Surgical resection is indicated for established strictures.

Creon 25 000 has now been relicensed and a preparation with 40 000 units of lipase per capsule has recently been launched by the same manufacturer. A maximum intake of 10 000 IU of lipase per kg per day, however, is strongly recommended. The actual incidence of fibrosing colonopathy appears to have declined and recently there have been few reports of this complication.

Appendiceal pathology

Appendiceal pathology is probably commoner in children and adults with CF than normal, although it may be that acute appendicitis itself is less common.[65] The incidence of acute appendicitis in a study of 1220 patients with CF was 1.8%, which is lower than in the non-CF population (variously quoted as about 5%–7%).[66,67] The appendix in CF may certainly become swollen, tense and distended by retained mucus and this in itself may become symptomatic either as abdominal pain or as a mass in the right iliac fossa.[66–68] Acute appendicitis in CF is often complicated by perforation or an appendix mass probably because of diagnostic delay rather than any difference in the appendiceal flora.[65,69] For instance, McCarthy *et al.*[65] described six children and adolescents with CF and appendicitis and, of these, three had had symptoms for more than 5 days before the correct diagnosis was made. All had perforated and formed a periappendiceal abscess.

Intussusception

Intussusception, usually ileo-colic, is a recognized complication of CF that occurs in a much older age group than intussusception in the normal population. Once again there is often diagnostic difficulty and most are confirmed only at laparotomy.[36,59,70] Bowel ischemia is uncommon despite the delayed presentation and most cases can be treated without intestinal resection.

Other gut disorders

Celiac disease has been reported in association with CF and may be commoner than in the normal population although no large studies have been performed.[71]

Both Crohn's disease and an increased risk of intestinal malignancy have been associated with CF in epidemiologic studies of adults. In a prospective study of over 11 000 CF patients, Lloyd-Still *et al.*[72] found 28 patients with coexisting inflammatory bowel disease, 25 of whom had Crohn's disease. This was about 17 times the incidence of Crohn's disease in age-matched controls. The origin of this association is obscure but may be related to known changes in bile acid metabolism, increased intestinal permeability and impaired protein digestion. From the literature, such cases usually have a neonatal history of MI and an onset of Crohn's disease in early adolescence. Most have required resectional surgery for fistulas and stricture.

There also appears to be an increased long-term risk of developing pancreatic or intestinal malignancy in CF, which has been uncovered by the increased survival. Although early small-scale studies were contradictory[73] a large study from Neglia *et al.*[74] confirmed the relationship. They reported an analysis of over 28 000 patients with CF from Europe and North America which showed an odds ratio of 6.6 for the observed to expected incidence of digestive tract (including pancreatic) cancers. They also noted an absence of any association with lung cancer, lymphoma or leukemia.

Liver and pancreatic disease in cystic fibrosis

Hepatobiliary disorders

Cystic fibrosis may cause conjugated hyperbilirubinemia in infants and early series reported an incidence of up to 20% in infants with meconium ileus.[40] The cholestasis in such cases usually has a good prognosis, although jaundice may be prolonged.[75] An unusual and specific cause of jaundice in the infant with CF is inspissated bile syndrome; surgical intervention and clearance of the biliary tree have been required in some patients. *N*-acetyl cysteine and intravenous cholecystokinin may be useful in selected cases.[76]

Approximately 1%–4% of patients with CF will develop significant liver disease in later life. Symptoms are usually apparent by adolescence.[77,78] Boys appear to be more susceptible[77,79] but the reason for this is unclear. Liver injury is due to the abnormal CFTR present in intrahepatic bile ducts and to a lesser extent in gallbladder epithelial cells. This causes portal tract fibrosis with relative preservation of hepatic architecture. A history of meconium ileus seems to increase the risk of liver disease fourfold although there is no defined predilection for a particular genotype.[79] The accumulation of abnormal ductular secretions causes cholestasis and hepatic fibrosis, which leads to severe portal hypertension. The gallbladder in CF is usually small, shrunken and often contains "white" bile. The term "microgallbladder" has been used to describe this appearance.[59] Gallstones and their complications are therefore relatively uncommon,[77] although this has been disputed by some authors.[78] There are also anomalies in bile acid metabolism with an increase in bile acid turnover due to an increase in fecal bile acid loss. The clinical consequences of this are still not clear.[59]

Hepatosplenomegaly, and occasionally ascites, are the first clinical manifestations of liver disease. Gastrointestinal bleeding due to esophageal (less commonly gastric or anorectal) varices may also occur although usually in patients with known liver disease. These features are unusual before 10 years of age and clinically important liver disease in CF is usually a problem of adolescents and young adults.[77] The median age at first variceal bleed in one study was 11 years.[80] Jaundice may occur, and is either indicative of severe hepatocyte loss and end-stage liver disease or acute bile duct obstruction secondary to gallstones or inspissated bile. Ultrasound, radio-nuclide hepatobiliary imaging and ERCP help to delineate such complications. Most cases of variceal bleeding in CF can be treated successfully with a course of either injection sclerotherapy[81] or endoscopic variceal banding. Portosystemic shunting (either open or more latterly via a transjugular intrahepatic approach[82]) is another option for CF patients with varices[34] although nowadays this has been superseded by liver transplantation.[83]

Liver transplantation, either alone or as part of a multi-organ procedure, has been used in children and adults with end-stage liver disease due to CF.[78,83,84] Although immunosuppression is a concern in patients with chronic colonization with microbial pathogens (e.g., *Pseudomonas* spp. and *Staphylococcus* spp.), this has not been a significant cause of morbidity and short-term survival rates are similar to those in non-CF liver transplantation.[83] Indeed, isolated liver transplantation in CF is often associated with an improvement in lung disease. Various factors such as suppression of the potent pulmonary inflammatory process by anti-rejection therapy and improved diaphragmatic function have even been considered beneficial to lung disease. Immunosuppression, however, is hazardous in patients with atypical mycobacteria or *Aspergillus fumigatus* in view of their resistance to antimicrobial agents.

Pancreatic disorders

Damage to the pancreas in CF occurs prenatally and impaired secretion of pancreatic enzymes in utero probably causes impaired digestion of intra-luminal intestinal contents which contributes to the development of MI. Breast-fed infants with CF may have little evidence of malabsorption at first due to the presence of a lipase in breast milk. Pancreatic insufficient infants produce frequent loose, offensive and fatty stools and failure to thrive is usual, although some are able to maintain their weight gain through a greatly increased oral intake.

The histologic appearances of the pancreas are characterized by an extensive loss of acini, scattered groups of dilated ducts with inspissated calcium material and a relative increase in islet cells. There is also a gradual replacement of pancreatic tissue with adipocytes beginning in the body and tail. Continuing pancreatic destruction may lead to the formation of macrocysts and this condition has been termed pancreatic cystosis.[85] Uncommonly, calcium deposition visible on a radiograph may occur as a later phenomenon. This finding has been associated clinically with the development of diabetes mellitus in adults.[86] There are, therefore, three clinically important long-term manifestations of pancreatic damage: loss of pancreatic function, both exocrine and endocrine, and a susceptibility to pancreatitis.

Exocrine pancreatic insufficiency can be expected in up 85% of patients[87] and in these there is total dependence on pancreatic enzyme supplementation. A small minority do not require supplements.[23] There is a suggestion that, in the long term, the need for supplementation declines, perhaps as a result of adaptation of gut regulatory peptides and activation of lingual lipase, and that adults have a milder degree of malabsorption than children.[23,56]

Endocrine pancreatic failure and diabetes mellitus occurs with a prevalence of over 10% in adults and about 2% in children with CF.[23,56] However, about one-third of adults will have an abnormal glucose tolerance test.[59] Penketh *et al.*[23] described 36 adults with diabetes and CF where the onset was mostly in adolescence. Only one-third of these required insulin and the remainder were managed with diet and oral hypoglycemic agents.

CF patients with diabetes are now living long enough to develop microvascular complications. In the UK, an annual oral glucose tolerance test is recommended in all children over the age of 12 years in order to detect diabetes at an early stage and thereby reduce its impact on future health. Insulin is the mainstay of treatment particularly as the high calorie CF diet needs to be maintained. Inevitably, the addition of another major medical disease and the implications of treatment often result in significant psychological problems for young patients.

Acute and chronic pancreatitis occur with an increased frequency although usually in adolescents and adults. Shwachman *et al.* reported ten patients from a series of over 2000 who suffered clinical episodes of acute pancreatitis.[87] The pulmonary features of CF in most of these patients were relatively mild. The age at onset of pancreatitis ranged from 7 to 25 years. Pancreatic function was relatively well preserved and pancreatic calcification was not a feature on the abdominal radiograph. In two patients (one child and one adult) the first episode of pancreatitis was the presenting feature of their CF. A similar presentation has also been described in two young adults aged 20 and 22 years who showed typical clinical and radiographic features of chronic pancreatitis and were later shown to have CF.[88] Although initial reports suggested that symptomatic pancreatic pathology only occurred in patients with preserved pancreatic function, this has subsequently been disputed.[4,87]

Chronic pancreatitis in CF can cause complications including obstructive jaundice due to compression of the intrapancreatic common bile duct. Lambert *et al.*[89] described a 29-year-old man with CF who had a 4-year history of recurrent episodes of jaundice due to mechanical compression of the duct demonstrated by ERCP.

Pancreatic cystosis may be symptomatic. Ade-Ajayi *et al.*[85] described an 11-year-old boy with disabling episodic epigastric pain and total pancreatic failure (both exocrine and endocrine). He was rendered pain free and fully rehabilitated by the radical surgical option of total pancreatectomy.

An increased frequency of CF gene mutations has been noted in patients with chronic, idiopathic pancreatitis.[90] A few of these patients have been found to have two CF gene mutations, abnormal sweat chloride levels and other features of CF such as mild bronchiectasis or absence of the vas deferens. The spectrum of CF disease has led to the term "CFTR-disease" to describe patients with biochemical or genetic features of CF but only isolated clinical manifestations.

Finally, in view of the hepatobiliary abnormalities described above there may be a long-term risk of malignancy. There has been a single case report of a carcinoma of the extrahepatic biliary tree in a patient with CF.[91]

Reproduction

The characteristic genital tract abnormality in males is absence or aplasia of the vas deferens leading to obstructive azoospermia.[23] Therefore, in most men with CF, conventional fertility is not possible but biologic fatherhood has been reported using microsurgical epididymal sperm aspiration and in vitro fertilization by intracytoplasmic sperm injection. In addition, Stern *et al.*[92] have reported a particular genetic mutation which is associated with mild pulmonary disease and some preservation of sperm production.

Fertility in women with CF was previously considered to be impaired due to abnormally thick cervical and tubal mucus. The menarche in girls with CF was reported to be delayed with an average age of 15 years in the Brompton Hospital series.[23] However, improved nutrition and general health in girls with CF has been associated with normal progression of puberty and conception in women with CF is now considered to be similar to unaffected females. Pregnancies have been relatively frequent since the first report of a successful outcome in 1960.[23,93] Although there are risks from pregnancy, these are few if lung function tests are greater than 60% of predicted and a good nutritional status is maintained.[92] The offspring from such pregnancies will inherit one of their mother's CF mutations and screening of partners for their CF gene carrier status is recommended prior to conception so that the risk of an affected baby can be determined.

Conclusions

Cystic fibrosis is a very serious disease with major morbidity and a high potential for mortality. However, over the past 20 years the outlook for a child with CF has changed radically. Median survival in 1969 was estimated at only 14 years but by 2000 this had more than doubled to about 32 years.[5] A child with CF born today will therefore have a probable life expectancy of 40 years or more (Fig. 25.3).

The long-term survivor is no longer exceptional and surgeons treating the newborn infant with meconium ileus should be no more pessimistic about the child reaching adulthood than other cases of neonatal intestinal obstruction. However, there must be a realistic acceptance of the profound changes in lifestyle and family involvement that are vital to achieve a good long-term outcome. Early diagnosis and expert management of potential long-term complications is essential (Table 25.5). The pediatric surgeon has an important role in the multidisciplinary care of CF patients throughout childhood whether it is by placement of vascular access devices, insertion of gastrostomies, endoscopy, and thoracic or intestinal surgery.

Table 25.5. Approximate long-term incidence of complications in cystic fibrosis

Complication	Long-term incidence	References
Respiratory infection	99–100%	23
Pseudomonas colonisation	60–80%	4,10,14,23
Pancreatic insufficiency	85–90%	4,23,79
Rectal prolapse	4–20%	23,36
Distal intestinal obstruction syndrome	4–30%	4,23,60
Diabetes	10–11%	4,23
Liver disease	4–18%	10,23,79
Appendicitis	2–4%	34,36,66
Intussusception	1–4%	23,36
Pancreatitis	0.1–2%	4,87
Malignancy	< 0.1%	73,74
Crohn's disease	< 0.1%	72

REFERENCES

1. BPA working party on cystic fibrosis. Cystic fibrosis in the United Kingdom 1977–85: an improving picture. *Br. Med. J.* 1988; **297**:1599–1602.
2. Conway, S. Cystic fibrosis in teenagers and young adults. *Arch. Dis. Child.* 1996; **75**:99–101.
3. Elborn, J. S., Shale, D. J., & Britton, J. R. Cystic fibrosis: current survival and population estimates to the year 2000. *Thorax* 1991; **46**:881–885.
4. FitzSimmons, S. C. The changing epidemiology of cystic fibrosis. *J. Pediatr.* 1993; **122**:1–9.

5. Fogarty, A., Hubbard, R., & Britton, J.. International comparison of median age at death from cystic fibrosis. *Chest* 2000; **117**:1656–1660.
6. Rommens, J. M., Iannuzzi, M. C., Kerem, B.-S. *et al.* Identification of the cystic fibrosis gene: chromosome walking and jumping. *Science* 1989; **245**:1059–1065.
7. http://www.genet.sickkids.on.ca/cgi-bin/WebObjects/MUTATION)
8. Schwarz, M. J., Malone, G. M., Haworth, A. *et al.* Cystic fibrosis mutation analysis: report from 22 UK regional genetics laboratories. *Hum. Mutation.* 1995; **6**:326–333.
9. Cystic Fibrosis Genotype–Phenotype Consortium. Correlation between genotype and phenotype in patients with cystic fibrosis. *N. Engl. J. Med.* 1993; **329**:1308–1313.
10. Johansen, H. K., Nir, M., Hoiby, N. *et al.* Severity of cystic fibrosis in patients homozygous and heterozygous for ΔF508 mutation. *Lancet* 1991; **337**:631–634.
11. Farrell, M. H. & Farrell, P. M. Newborn screening for cystic fibrosis. *J. Pediatr.* 2003; **143**:707–712.
12. Frederickson, B., Lanng, S., Koch, C., & Hoiby, N.. Improved survival in the Danish center-treated cystic fibrosis patients: results of aggressive treatment. *Pediatr. Pulmon.* 1996; **21**:153–158.
13. Britton, J. R. Effects of social class, sex and region of residence on age at death from cystic fibrosis. *Br. Med. J.* 1989; **298**:483–487.
14. Nir, M., Lanng, S., Johansen, H. K., & Koch, C. Long term survival and nutritional data in patients with cystic fibrosis treated in a Danish centre. *Thorax* 1996; **51**:1023–1027.
15. Hyde, S. C., Gill, D. R., Higgins, C. F. *et al.* Correction of the ion transport defect in cystic fibrosis transgenic mice by gene therapy. *Nature* 1993; **362**:250–255.
16. Gill, D. R., Southern, K. W., Moffard, K. A. *et al.* A placebo-controlled trial of liposome-mediated gene transfer to the nasal epithelium of patients with cystic fibrosis. *Gene. Ther.* 1997; **4**:199–209.
17. Colledge, W. H. & Evans, M. J. Cystic fibrosis gene therapy. *Br. Med. Bull.* 1995; **51**:82–90.
18. McDowell, A., Mahenthiralingam, E., Dunbar, K. E. *et al.* Epidemiology of Burkholderia cepacia complex species recovered from cystic fibrosis patients: issues related to patient segregation. *J. Med. Microbiol.* 2004; **53**:663–668.
19. Cystic Fibrosis Foundation, Patient Registry 1996 Annual Report. Bethesda, Maryland August 1997.
20. Marmon, L., Schidlow, D., Palmer, J. *et al.* Pulmonary resection for complications of cystic fibrosis. *J. Pediatr. Surg.* 1983; **18**:811–815.
21. Lucas, J., Connett, G. J., Lea, R. *et al.* Lung resection in cystic fibrosis patients with localised pulmonary disease. *Arch. Dis. Child.* 1996; **74**:449–451.
22. Richardson, V. F., Robertson, C. F., Mowat, A. P., Howard, E. R., & Price, J. F. Deterioration in lung function after general anaesthesia in patients with cystic fibrosis. *Acta. Paediatr. Scand.* 1984; **73**:75–79.
23. Penketh, A. R. L., Wise, A., Mearns, M. B. *et al.* Cystic fibrosis in adolescents and adults. *Thorax* 1987; **42**:526–532.
24. Schidlow, D. W., Taussig, L. M., & Knowles, M. R. Cystic Fibrosis Foundation consensus conference report on pulmonary complications of cystic fibrosis. *Pediatr. Pulmonol.* 1993; **15**:187–198.
25. Madden, B. P., Hodson, M. E., Tsang, V. *et al.* Intermediate term results of heart-lung transplantation for cystic fibrosis. *Lancet* 1992; **339**:1583–1587.
26. Egan, T. M., Detterbeck, F. C., Mill, M. R. *et al.* Improved results of lung transplantation for patients with cystic fibrosis. *J. Thorac. Cardiovasc. Surg.* 1995; **109**:224–234.
27. Starnes, V. A., Barr, M. L., Cohen, R. G. *et al.* Living-donor lobar lung transplantation experience: intermediate results. *J. Thorac. Cardiovasc. Surg.* 1996; **112**:1284–1291.
28. Balfour-Lynn, I. M., Martin, I., Whitehead, B. F. *et al.* Heart–lung transplantation for patients under 10 with cystic fibrosis. *Arch. Dis. Child.* 1997; **76**:38–40.
29. Egan, T. M., Detterbeck, F. C., Mill, M. R. *et al.* Long-term results of lung transplantation for cystic fibrosis. *Eur. J. Cardiovasc. Surg.* 2002; **22**:602–609.
30. Huddleston, C. B., Bloch, J. B., Sweet, S. C. *et al.* Lung transplantation in children. *Ann. Surg.* 2002; **236**:270–276.
31. Wiebe, K., Wahlers, T., Harringer, W. *et al.* Lung transplantation for cystic fibrosis – a single center experience. *Eur. J. Cardiothorac. Surg.* 1998; **14**:191–196.
32. De Perrot, M., Chaparro, C., McRae, K. *et al.* Twenty-year experience of lung transplantation at a single center: influence of recipient diagnosis on long-term survival. *J. Thorac. Cardiovasc. Surg.* 2004; **127**:1493–1501.
33. Ryan, P. J. & Stableforth, D. E. Referral for lung transplantation: experience of the Birmingham Adult Cystic Fibrosis centre between 1987 and 1994. *Thorax* 1996; **51**:302–305.
34. Olsen, M. M., Gauderer, M. W., Girz, M. K., & Izant, R. J. Jr. Surgery in patients with cystic fibrosis. *J. Pediatr. Surg.* 1987; **22**:613–618.
35. Landsteiner, K. Darmverschluss durch Eingedicktes Meconium: pankreatitis. *Zentralbl. Allg. Pathol.* 1905; **16**:903.
36. Gross, K., Desanto, A., Grosfeld, J. L. *et al.* Intrabdominal complications of cystic fibrosis. *J. Pediatr. Surg.* 1985; **20**:431–435.
37. Hiatt, R. B. & Wilson, P. E. Celiac syndrome. Therapy of meconium ileus: report of eight cases with a review of the literature. *Surg. Gynecol. Obstet.* 1948; **87**:317–327.
38. Bishop, H. C. & Koop, C. E. Management of meconium ileus: resection, Roux-en-Y anastomosis and ileostomy irrigation with pancreatic enzymes. *Ann. Surg.* 1957; **145**:410–414.
39. Holsclaw, D. S., Eckstein, H. B., & Nixon, H. H. Meconium ileus. *Am. J. Dis. Child.* 1965; **109**:101–113.
40. Donnison, A. B., Shwachman, H., & Gross, R. E. A review of 164 children with meconium ileus seen at the Children's Hospital Medical Centre of Boston. *Pediatrics* 1966; **37**:833–850.
41. Santulli, T. V. & Blanc, W. A. Congenital atresia of the intestine: pathogenesis and treatment. *Ann. Surg.* 1961; **154**:939–948.

42. Nuygen, L. T., Youssef, S., Guttman, F. M., Laberge, J. M., *et al.* Meconium ileus: is a stoma necessary? *J. Pediatr. Surg.* 1986; **21**:766–768.
43. Millar, A. J. W., Rode, H., & Cywes, S. Management of uncomplicated meconium ileus with T tube ileostomy. *Arch. Dis. Child.* 1988; **63**:309–310.
44. Mak, G. Z., Harberg, F. J., Hiatt, P. *et al.* T-tube ileostomy for meconium ileus: four decades of experience. *J. Pediatr. Surg.* 2000; **35**:349–352.
45. Fitzgerald, R. & Conlon, K.. Use of the appendix stump in the treatment of meconium ileus. *J. Pediatr. Surg.* 1989; **24**:899–900.
46. Noblett, H. Treatment of uncomplicated meconium ileus by Gastrografin enema: a preliminary report. *J. Pediatr. Surg.* 1969; **4**:190–197.
47. Waggett, J., Bishop, H. C., & Koop, C. E. Experience with Gastrografin enema in the treatment of meconium ileus. *J. Pediatr. Surg.* 1970; **5**:649–654.
48. Caniano, D. A. & Beaver, B. L. Meconium ileus: a fifteen-year experience with forty two neonates. *Surgery* 1987; **102**:699–703.
49. Del Pin, C. A., Czyrko, C., Ziegler, M. M., Scanlin, T. F., & Bishop, H. C. Management and survival of meconium ileus. A 30 year review. *Ann. Surg.* 1992; **215**:179–185.
50. Rescorla, F. J. & Grosfeld, J. L. Contemporary management of meconium ileus. *World. J. Surg.* 1993; **17**:318–325.
51. Venugopal, S. & Shandling, B. Meconium ileus: laparotomy without resection, anastomosis or enterostomy? *J. Pediatr. Surg.* 1979; **14**:715–719.
52. O'Neil, J. A., Grosfeld, J. L., Boles, E. T. *et al.* Surgical treatment of meconium ileus. *Am. J. Surg.* 1970; **119**:99–105.
53. Kalayoglu, M., Sieber, W. K., Rodnan, J. B., & Kiesewetter, W. B. Meconium ileus: a critical review of treatment and eventual prognosis. *J. Pediatr. Surg.* 1971; **6**:290–300.
54. Docherty, J. G., Zaki, A., Coutts, J. A. *et al.* Meconium ileus: a review 1972–1990. *Br. J. Surg.* 1992; **79**:571–573.
55. Shwachman, H. Meconium ileus: ten patients over 28 years of age. *J. Pediatr. Surg.* 1983; **18**:570–575.
56. Elborn, J. S. & Bell, S. C. Nutrition and survival in cystic fibrosis. *Thorax* 1996; **51**:971–972.
57. Powers, C. J., Levitt, M. A., Tantoco, J. *et al.* The respiratory advantage of laparoscopic Nissen fundoplication. *J. Pediatr. Surg.* 2003; **38**:886–891.
58. Levy, E. A case of fibrocystic disease of the pancreas with intestinal obstruction. *Arch. Dis. Child.* 1951; **26**:335–339.
59. Park, R. W. & Grand, R. J. Gastrointestinal manifestations of cystic fibrosis: a review. *Gastroenterology* 1981; **81**:1143–1161.
60. Khoshoo, V. & Udall, J. N. Meconium ileus equivalent in children and adults. *Am. J. Gastroenterol.* 1994; **89**:153–157.
61. Koletzko, S., Corey, M., Ellis, L., & Durie, P. R. Effect of cisapride in patients with cystic fibrosis and distal intestinal obstruction. *J. Pediatr.* 1990; **117**:815–822.
62. Shwachman, H. & Kulczycki, L. L. Long term study of 105 patients with cystic fibrosis. *Am. J. Dis. Child.* 1958; **96**:6–15.
63. Smyth, R. L., van Velzen, D., Smyth, A. R., Lloyd, D. A. *et al.* Strictures of ascending colon in cystic fibrosis and high-strength pancreatic enzymes. *Lancet* 1994 **343**:85–86.
64. Smyth, R. L. Fibrosing colonopathy in cystic fibrosis. *Arch. Dis. Child.* 1996; **74**:464–468.
65. McCarthy, V. P., Mischler, E. H., Hubbard, V. S., Chernick, M. S., di Sant'Agnese, P. A. Appendiceal abscess in cystic fibrosis. *Gastroenterology* 1984; **86**:564–568.
66. Coughlin, J. P., Gauderer, M. W. L., Stern, R. C. *et al.* The spectrum of appendiceal diseae in cystic fibrosis. *J. Pediatr. Surg.* 1990; **25**:835–839.
67. Martens, M., De Boeck, K., Van der Steen, K. *et al.* A right lower quadrant mass in cystic fibrosis: a diagnostic challenge. *Eur. J. Pediatr.* 1992; **151**:329–331.
68. Rimmer, J. A. P., Gilbert, J. M., & Allen-Mersh, T. G. Appendicitis complicating meconium ileus equivalent. *Br. J. Surg.* 1989; **76**:168.
69. Holshaw, D. S. & Habboushe, C. Occult appendiceal abscess complicating cystic fibrosis. *J. Pediatr. Surg.* 1976; **11**:217–220.
70. Holmes, M., Murphy, V., Taylor, M., & Denham, B. Intussusception in cystic fibrosis. *Arch. Dis. Child.* 1991; **66**:726–727.
71. Littlewood, J. M. Gastrointesinal complications. *Br. Med. Bull.* 1992; **48**:847–859.
72. Lloyd-Still, J. D. Crohn's disease and cystic fibrosis. *Dig. Dis. Sci.* 1994; **39**:880–885.
73. Sheldon, C. D., Hodson, M. E., Carpenter, L. M., & Swerdlow, A. J. A cohort study of cystic fibrosis and malignancy. *Br. J. Cancer.* 1993; **68**:1025–1028.
74. Neglia, J. P., FitzSimmons, S. C., Maisonneuve, P. *et al.* The risk of cancer among patients with cystic fibrosis. *N. Eng. J. Med.* 1995; **332**:494–499.
75. Nagel, R. A., Javaid, A., Meire, H. B. *et al.* Liver disease and bile duct abnormalities in adults with cystic fibrosis. *Lancet* 1989; **ii**:1422–1425.
76. Evans, J. S., George, D. E., & Mollit, D. Biliary infusion therapy in the inspissated bile syndrome. *J. Pediatr. Gastroenterol. Nutr.* 1991; **12**:131–135.
77. Scott-Jupp, R., Lama, M., & Tanner, M. S. Prevalence of liver disease in cystic fibrosis. *Arch. Dis. Child.* 1991; **66**:698–701.
78. Sharp, H. L. Cystic fibrosis liver disease and transplantation. *J. Pediatr.* 1995; **127**:944–946.
79. Colombo, C., Apostolo, M. G., Ferrari, M. *et al.* Analysis of risk factors for the development of liver disease associated with cystic fibrosis. *J. Pediatr.* 1994; **124**:393–399.
80. Stringer, M. D. Pathogenesis and management of esophageal and gastric varices. In *Surgery of the Liver, Bile Ducts and Pancreas in Children*, ed E. R. Howard, M. D. Stringer, P. M. Colombani. London: Arnold 2002: 287–314.
81. Stringer, M. D., Price, J. F., Mowat, A. P., & Howard, E. R. Liver cirrhosis in cystic fibrosis. *Arch. Dis. Child.* 1993; **69**:407.
82. Pozler, O., Krajina, A., Vanicek, H. *et al.* Transjugular intrahepatic portosystemic shunt in five children with cystic fibrosis:

long-term results. *Hepatogastroenterology* 2003; **50**:1111–1114.

83. Noble-Jamieson, G., Valente, J., Barnes, N. D. *et al.* Liver transplantation for hepatic cirrhosis in cystic fibrosis. *Arch. Dis. Child.* 1994; **71**:349–352.
84. Fridell, J. A., Bond, G. J., Mazariegos, G. V. *et al.* Liver transplantation in children with cystic fibrosis: a long-term longitudinal review of a single center's experience. *J. Pediatr. Surg.* 2003; **38**:1152–1156.
85. Ade-Ajayi, N., Law, C., Burge, D. M. *et al.* Surgery for pancreatic cystosis with pancreatitis in cystic fibrosis. *Br. J. Surg.* 1997; **84**:312.
86. diSant'Agnese, P. A. & Lepore, M. J. Involvement of abdominal organs in cystic fibrosis of the pancreas. *Gastroenterology* 1961; **40**:64–68.
87. Shwachman, H., Lebenthal, E., & Khaw, K. T. Recurrent acute pancreatitis in patients with cystic fibrosis with normal pancreatic enzymes. *Pediatrics* 1975; **55**:86–95.
88. Masaryk, T. J. & Achkar, E.. Pancreatitis as initial presentation of cystic fibrosis in young adults: a report of 2 cases. *Dig. Dis. Sci.* 1983; **28**:874–878.
89. Lambert, J. R., Cole, M., Crozier, D. N., Connon, J. J. Intrapancreatic common bile duct compression causing jaundice in an adult with cystic fibrosis. *Gastroenterology* 1981; **80**:169–172.
90. Cohn, J. A., Freidman, K. J., Noone P. G. *et al.* Relation between mutations of the cystic fibrosis gene and idiopathic pancreatitis. *N. Eng. J. Med.* 1998; **339**:653–658.
91. Abdul-Karim, F. W., King, T. A., Dahms, B. B. *et al.* Carcinoma of extrahepatic biliary system in an adult with cystic fibrosis. *Gastroenterology* 1982; **82**:758–762.
92. Stern, R. C., Doershuk, C. F., & Drumm, M. L. 3849+10 kb CT mutation and disease severity in cystic fibrosis. *Lancet* 1995; **346**:274–276.
93. Edenborough, F. P., Stableforth, D. E., Webb, A. K. *et al.* The outcome of pregnancy in cystic fibrosis. *Thorax* 1995; **50**:170–174.

26

Necrotizing enterocolitis

Marion C. W. Henry and R. Lawrence Moss

Department of Pediatric Surgery, Yale University School of Medicine, New Haven, CT, USA

Introduction

For more than 30 years, necrotizing enterocolitis (NEC) has been the most common surgical emergency in the neonatal intensive care unit (NICU). Despite decades of clinical advances and research, the management of NEC continues to pose a significant challenge to the pediatric surgeon. Currently, NEC is the major cause of death for all neonates undergoing surgery with a surgical mortality rate of 20–60%.[1–14] The mortality from this disease is greater than that from all of the congenital anomalies of the gastrointestinal tract combined. Infants who do survive may be plagued by the chronic condition of short-bowel syndrome, with its associated complications of total parenteral nutrition and the possible need for liver and/or intestinal transplantation. Additionally, infants surviving necrotizing enterocolitis may have significant long-term gastrointestinal, growth and neurodevelopmental sequelae.

Epidemiology

Necrotizing enterocolitis affects 1–3 in 1000 live births and up to 8% of NICU admissions.[8,15–18] In 2001, NEC was the tenth leading cause of neonatal deaths.[19] As advances in neonatology and the modern intensive care unit have led to the increased survival of smaller and younger infants, the number of babies at risk for NEC and, therefore, the incidence has increased.[20–22]

During the last 20 years, the infant mortality rate attributable to NEC increased from an average of 11.5 per 100 000 live births in the early 1980s to an average of 12.3 deaths per 100 000 live births during 1990–1992.[23] The most recent data suggests improvement in the last five years as the mortality rate from NEC was 9.4 per 100 000 live births in 2001 and 8.7 per 100 000 live births in 2002 (Table 26.1).[19] Although the data from 2002 is still preliminary, there does appear to be a trend downward in the mortality rate from NEC. Continued examination of these rates will reveal whether this is a true decline in the infant mortality rate or whether the decrease is due to incomplete coding of infant death certificates.

More than 90% of babies with NEC are premature infants weighing less than 2000 grams.[17,24] Most commonly, NEC affects infants between 30 and 32 weeks' gestational age.[16,25,26] Prematurity is the only risk factor for necrotizing enterocolitis that is consistently identified in case control studies of infants in neonatal intensive care units.[16,21,27] NEC is rare in countries where prematurity is uncommon, such as Sweden and Japan.[15,28,29] The rare case of NEC in a term infant tends to be accompanied by a predisposing condition, such as congenital heart disease.[24,30] When a term infant develops NEC, the disease tends to present earlier, perhaps due to an earlier initiation and more rapid progression of feeds.[24,31–33]

Necrotizing enterocolitis has significant financial costs. The incremental cost per case for acute hospital care compared to age-matched controls is estimated to be $74 000 to $186 000, not including the costs of long-term care for infants with lifelong morbidity.[14]

Clinical diagnosis

The diagnosis of necrotizing enterocolitis is primarily based on clinical presentation and characteristic

Pediatric Surgery and Urology: Long-term Outcomes, Mark Stringer, Keith Oldham, Pierre Mouriquand. Published by Cambridge University Press. © Cambridge University Press, 2006.

Table 26.1. Mortality rates for neonates with NEC, 1981–2003

Series	Year	Patients (surgical NEC)	Surgical mortality (%)
Stevenson *et al.*[2]	1981	71	30
Schullinger *et al.*[1]	1981	40	63
Gregory *et al.*[4]	1981	42	38
Kleigman *et al.*[16]	1981	123	46
Cikrit *et al.*[5]	1984	101	50
Dykes *et al.*[6]	1985	80	31
Kanto *et al.*[7]	1985	148	51
Pokorny *et al.*[8]	1986	74	35
Jackman *et al.*[9]	1990	74	23
Ricketts *et al.*[10]	1990	100	30
Kurscheid *et al.*[11]	1993	73	26
Horwitz *et al.*[12]	1995	252	28
Ladd *et al.*[25]	1998	249	45
Patel *et al.*[13]	1998	69	39
Bisquera *et al.*[14]	2002	37	41
Guthrie *et al.*[129]	2003	145	23

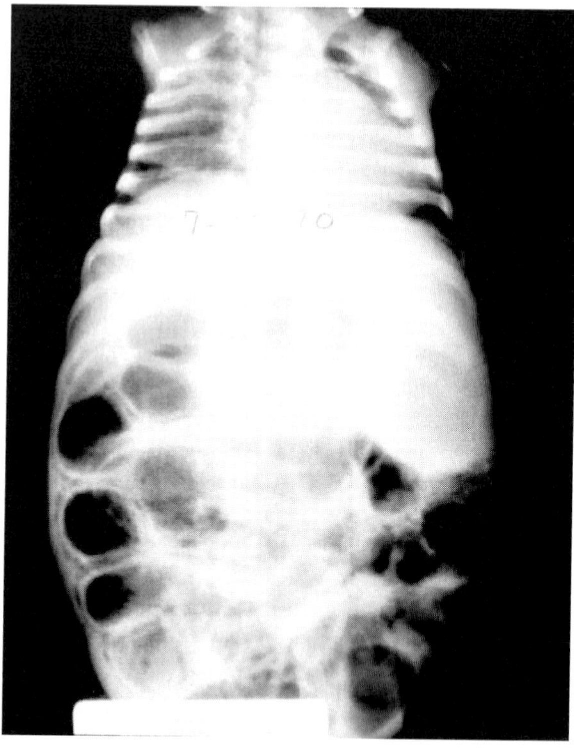

Fig. 26.1. Radiograph showing pneumatosis intestinalis.

radiographic findings. Initially, non-specific gastrointestinal findings suggest the disease, including feeding intolerance with large or bilious gastric aspirates, abdominal distension, and occasionally, bilious vomiting. Systemic signs include apnea, temperature instability, bradycardia, and lethargy. Occult or gross blood may occur in the stools 25–60% of the time.[34]

Laboratory tests include indicators of an inflammatory process and sepsis such as thrombocytopenia, elevated white blood cell count with a bandemia, or neutropenia. A rapid fall in the platelet count has been found to be a poor prognostic factor.[35] Metabolic acidosis is common.

Standard anteroposterior and cross-table lateral or left lateral decubitus radiographs are the cornerstone of diagnosing necrotizing enterocolitis. The most specific radiographic finding in NEC is pneumatosis intestinalis, either cystic or linear (Fig. 26.1). Other characteristic radiographic findings include ileus, portal venous gas (PVG), persistently dilated loops of bowel, ascites, and pneumoperitoneum. These findings can be used to stage NEC, but do not reliably predict prognosis. Early non-specific radiographic findings are gas-filled loops of bowel and air fluid levels consistent with ileus. While pneumatosis intestinalis is reasonably specific to NEC, it has been noted in infants with Hirschsprung's enterocolitis, pyloric stenosis, severe diarrhea, and carbohydrate intolerance.

Portal venous gas (Fig. 26.2) may be a transient radiographic finding, which may explain the low reported incidence of up to 20%. This finding has generally been considered a poor prognostic sign and a strong indication for surgery.[36] In the experience of one large institution, PVG had an incidence rate of 19%. Of the patients with PVG, 52% had NEC involving more than 75% of the intestine, and 90% of these patients died. Overall, the mortality of patients with PVG was 52%.[36] In a comparison study of premature infants and micro-premature infants, portal venous gas indicated pan-intestinal involvement in 40% of the premature infants and in 71% of the micro-premature infants. Thus, PVG may be a predictor of higher mortality when seen in micro-premature infants.[37] The findings of these studies have led some surgeons to advocate surgery as soon as PVG is noted. PVG, however, is not considered an absolute indication for operation, and many babies with NEC and PVG recover without operative intervention.

The criteria specified by Bell remain the accepted standard for diagnosis and staging of necrotizing enterocolitis.[38] Stage I NEC is characterized by abdominal distension, vomiting, feeding intolerance, and findings of ileus on plain abdominal radiographs. Stage II NEC includes all the stage I findings plus gastrointestinal bleeding and either intestinal pneumatosis or portal venous air on X-ray. Stage III, or advanced NEC, is characterized by pneumoperitoneum on radiographs with a concomitant clinical deterioration into septic shock. Other radiographic studies such as ultrasound and MRI have not been found to be more advantageous than plain radiographs.[39,40]

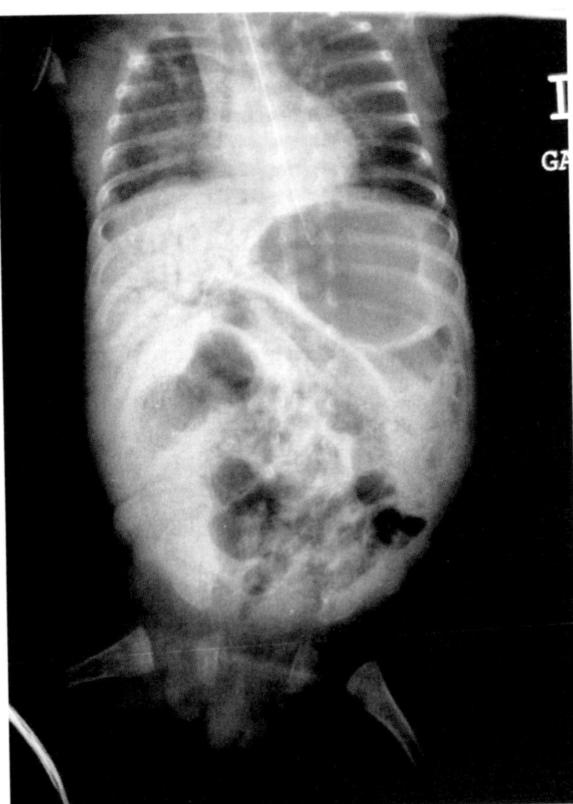

Fig. 26.2. Portal venous gas and pneumatosis evident on abdominal radiograph.

Medical management

Most cases of necrotizing enterocolitis can be effectively treated with medical management.[41] The hallmarks of medical management include bowel rest, intestinal decompression, intravenous fluid administration, and antibiotic therapy. Blood products should be transfused as necessary. A crucial part of medical management is close observation with serial abdominal examination to monitor for any deterioration in status and abdominal radiographs to monitor for perforation.

Clinical deterioration or worsening abdominal radiographs may indicate the need for surgical management. In the event of clinical deterioration without radiographic evidence of perforation, abdominal paracentesis may be performed at the bedside to assist with a diagnosis of perforation. However, no standards exist for the use of this modality. Paracentesis has a reported specificity of 100%. Thus, evidence of stool, bile or a gram stain positive for organisms is an absolute indication for surgery. A negative tap, however, does not rule out perforation and should not be considered absolute evidence against surgical exploration.[10]

Surgical management

Absolute indications for surgical management include evidence of intestinal perforation, confirmed either by abdominal radiograph or positive paracentesis. Relative indications include deterioration in clinical condition, oliguria, hypotension, metabolic acidosis, thrombocytopenia, leukopenia, leukocytosis, ventilatory failure, portal venous gas on radiograph, persistently dilated loops of bowel, fixed abdominal masses, or erythema of the abdominal wall. Pneumatosis alone confirms the diagnosis of NEC but is not an indication for operation. While portal venous gas in the presence of extensive pneumatosis is an ominous sign, its presence is not an absolute indication for operation. There has been disagreement about the prognosis associated with the presence of portal venous gas on radiographs,[42] but Rowe found that panintestinal involvement was significantly more common in the presence of PVG in the very low birthweight infants.[37] Cikrit also found that presence of PVG was associated with a significant increase in mortality rate.[5,43] As previously discussed, these findings of increased mortality in the presence of PVG, has led some surgeons to consider PVG to be an indication for operative intervention.[36] A fixed loop of bowel seen on abdominal radiographs, and abdominal wall erythema are suggestive of intestinal ischemia, but these signs are not absolute indications for surgical intervention.

In the face of these many relative indications, a wide disparity in surgical management between centers has emerged. There is no definitive evidence identifying the optimal time for surgical intervention and when absolute indications are absent this decision remains based on subjective clinical judgment. Approximately 25–60% of patients with NEC will deteriorate and receive surgical intervention.[3,44]

The principles of surgical management of necrotizing enterocolitis have traditionally been resection of the areas of clearly gangrenous bowel, exteriorization of any marginally viable intestinal ends with preservation of as much intestinal length as possible. More recently, some surgeons have turned to peritoneal drainage as a first-line treatment of NEC. Initially described in 1977 by Ein as a treatment for perforation in infants thought to be too ill to tolerate laparotomy,[45] it has subsequently been described as a temporizing procedure in the sickest and smallest patients and, more recently, as a definitive treatment strategy.[46–54] Though many studies have reported on outcomes with this technique, these reports contain significant bias influencing the patient selection and it is not possible, even through meta-analysis, to determine whether peritoneal drainage or laparotomy is the better technique for any size infant.[32,46–53,55–59] Currently, there are randomized trials under way in both the USA and the UK to determine whether peritoneal drainage or laparotomy is a better treatment for perforated necrotizing enterocolitis.

The actual surgical intervention used should be determined by the clinical condition of the patient and the possible extent of affected bowel. Many studies have shown that the most important factor influencing mortality rate is the extent of bowel involvement.[5,37,60,61]

Impact of surgical strategy on gastrointestinal function

Any segment of the intestinal tract can be involved in necrotizing enterocolitis, but the ileocecal region is most commonly affected. Approximately half of patients present with an isolated area of necrosis and perforation and half with multi-segmental disease.[22,41,62] "NEC totalis," or massive necrosis of nearly all of the intestines, presents in 5–20% of cases, and is almost uniformly fatal.[22,32,37] Recently, a separate entity of focal intestinal perforation has been reported in the literature. It is not clear whether this represents a separate entity or simply NEC with limited intestinal involvement. Patients presenting with "focal" disease have been shown to have a better prognosis than those with wider involvement.[55,63–72]

The management of infants who present with multisegmental NEC or pan-involvement is challenging for the pediatric surgeon. These patients are more likely to develop short bowel syndrome postoperatively and have a greater dependence on total parenteral nutrition. The principle of surgical management in this situation is to minimize the amount of bowel resected and several strategies have been proposed to accomplish this goal. Limited resection followed by second-look laparotomy is one method used to limit the lengths of intestinal resection.[73] A similar technique has been termed the "clip and drop-back" technique. In this case, all non-viable bowel is resected at the initial operation with neither stomas nor anastomoses being created. Blind-ending segments are then returned to the abdomen and re-exploration occurs in 48–72 hours with bowel continuity restored at that time.[74] A strategy of very proximal diversion without any resection has also been attempted in cases of pan-involvement with anecdotal reports of recovery of significant amounts of bowel at the time of ostomy closure.[75]

Preservation of as much bowel as possible is critical to patients with necrotizing enterocolitis in order to prevent short-bowel syndrome. However, NEC is a global intestinal disease that can cause severe injury to portions of non-gangrenous bowel. It is, therefore, not always possible to predict the ultimate gastrointestinal (GI) outcome based solely on the length and segment of bowel resected. Sometimes patients with massive resections do better than expected while patients with limited resections have poor outcomes.

Additionally, the portion of intestine that is resected plays a role in later GI function. In a series of patients reported on by Fasching, mortality rate was higher when the ileum was involved, whereas none of the patients with only colonic disease died.[76] Horwitz also showed that patients with colonic disease had a better survival rate than those with either only small bowel disease or combined small and large bowel disease.[12] Beasley has also shown that whenever the jejunum was involved in the disease process, the prognosis was worse.[77] In another series of patients, de Souza also showed results suggesting that small bowel involvement may be an important predictor of mortality, though the numbers were relatively small in this study.[78]

Preservation of the ileocecal valve during intestinal resection has been considered crucial to the patient's outcome.[36] Several studies have suggested that the duration of parenteral nutrition requirement is shorter when the ileocecal valve can be preserved.[79–83] However, in a small series of patients, Fasoli showed no difference in duration of TPN, length of hospital stay, or survival between those infants who had their ileocecal valve resected and those who did not. Furthermore, they showed that the incidence of post-NEC strictures was less in those neonates who had their ileocecal valve resected than those who did not.[84] These findings were consistent with those of Ladd, who also found, in a small series, that retention of the ileocecal valve did not significantly shorten the length of time on parenteral nutrition or in the hospital.[25] Andorsky also did not find a relationship between having an ileocecal valve and the duration of parenteral nutrition.[85] Other studies have also questioned the importance of retaining the ileocecal valve.[86–88] These findings need to be investigated more fully and in a greater number of patients before it will be clear whether preservation of the ileocecal valve is truly crucial.

The difficulties of determining how much intestine to resect can raise ethical dilemmas for the pediatric surgeon. The clinical uncertainty caused by the variability in outcomes for patients following bowel resection for NEC compounds the difficult decisions a surgeon faces. With this uncertainty, surgeons are faced with "tough calls" when it comes to advising parents on the projected outcomes for their children. It is difficult to tell which child may do well with the amount of bowel they have left and which may have viable, but poorly functioning, bowel. This uncertainty makes promoting the patient's best interest more difficult as the prognosis remains an unknown. Furthermore, as advances are made in the fields of intestinal adaptation and transplantation, some treatment options may become more widely available and more reasonable options for greater numbers of affected infants.

Postoperative management

The hallmarks of postoperative management in NEC are hemodynamic support, antibiotic therapy, intestinal decompression, and bowel rest until the ileus resolves and there is evidence of a functioning stoma.

Recurrent necrotizing enterocolitis occurs approximately 5% of the time, an average of five weeks after the initial occurrence.[3,89] There is no apparent correlation between the initial site of disease and the area of reoccurrence.[89] Neither operative technique nor time of initiation of feeding appears to influence the reoccurrence rate.[89] Recurrent disease can be managed non-operatively the majority of the time.[10,89–94]

Stomal complications

In the surgical management of necrotizing enterocolitis, creation of a properly constructed stoma can be life-saving. However, enterostomies are associated with a high rate of both early and late complications. In the case of necrotizing enterocolitis, stomas are used for decompression and diversion. There are different types of stoma that may be used for these purposes, and several ways to bring the proximal stoma through the abdominal wall and mature it (see Table 26.2).

The optimal method for enterostomy formation in this situation remains controversial. Several different methods have been suggested including bringing out the functional stoma and the mucous fistula through opposite ends of the surgical incision, bringing out two separate stomas together at one end of the surgical incision, bringing the proximal stoma through a separate right lower quadrant incision, and doing a double-barreled Mikulicz stoma brought out either through the surgical incision or a separate incision.[95,96] Most surgeons caution against maturing a stoma primarily in small neonates as it will interfere with the already tenuous blood supply.[95]

Some surgeons advocate bringing the end stoma out through a separate incision, citing an increased incidence of wound complications when the stoma is brought out through the main incision. Another consideration in this matter is that if the stoma remains for a long period of time, the fold created by the celiotomy incision may lead to the inability to properly fit a stoma appliance.[95]

Table 26.2. Options for enterostoma formation

Type of stoma
End stoma, single opening
Double-barrel (Mikulicz) stoma
End stoma with anastomosis below abdominal wall
Loop stoma over a small catheter or skin bridge
Exit of stoma and mucous fistula
Through celiotomy incision
Through separate opening
Proximal and distal limbs together
Proximal and distal limbs separated
Multiple stomas

In a comparison study of two methods of stoma creation, a double-barrel Mikulicz enterostomy brought out through a counter incision versus a proximal stoma with distal mucous fistula brought out through the surgical incision, Musemeche found no difference in the incidence of stoma complications, including retractions, prolapse, hernia, or wound infections or dehiscence.[96]

The use of a loop enterostomy has been suggested as a safe and effective alternative to an end stoma, when it is difficult to adequately mobilize an end ostomy due to shortening of the diseased mesentery. Furthermore, the diseased mesentery may have poor blood flow leading to tenuous bowel. In this situation, a loop enterostomy provides a more effective method of forming a viable stoma. In a small series of patients treated by this method, there was a 20% complication rate that consisted of two incidences of wound dehiscence and one prolapsed stoma.[97] Another benefit to this method may also be easier closure at the time of the stoma takedown.

Problems and complications related to stomas of either the small or large intestine in neonates can lead to significant morbidity (see Table 26.3). Review of series of infants treated for NEC using enterostomies reveals complication rates up to and exceeding 50%.[12,98–101] The more common and serious complications are prolapse, stricture and retraction. These complications may require surgical revision or early closure of the stoma.

Very proximal jejunostomies can cause significant fluid and electrolyte losses leading to difficulty with fluid homeostasis and inadequate weight gain.[36,102] Jejunostomies can cause significant peristomal skin complications. Aggressive skin care and replacement of the fluid and

Table 26.3. Enterostomal complications

Prolapse
Stricture
Retraction
Wound separation or dehiscence
Wound infection
Parastomal hernia
Intestinal obstruction
Intestinal torsion
Fistula formation
Skin excoriation, moniliasis, dermatitis
Mucosal excoriation and bleeding
Electrolyte imbalance
Dehydration

electrolyte losses, however, can make proximal jejunostomy a viable approach to managing severe NEC.[36,103]

The optimal timing for enterostomy closure remains undetermined. Some surgeons advocate waiting up to 2 months in order to observe for stricture formation.[104] Some have suggested waiting up to 4 months and a weight of 6 to 10 lb.[105–107] Most recommendations are for closure between 3 and 8 weeks after surgery, and a weight of 2000 g, as long as the infant is tolerating feeds and growing.[36,102,104,108] However, particularly with a very proximal stoma, there may be difficulty establishing feeds, or serious fluid and electrolyte derangements that call for earlier closure.[36,102,109]

A very proximal stoma that causes serious fluid and electrolyte derangements should be closed sooner, usually after 4 to 6 weeks. Many individual factors, including ileostomy diarrhea, failure to thrive and coexisting medical problems must also be considered in determining optimal time to closure. The timing of stoma closure is not standardized. Earlier reanastomosis may lead to better absorption of enteral feeds enabling further weaning from parenteral nutrition. Additionally, some studies show that reestablishment of the continuity of the intestines can ameliorate TPN-associated cholestasis.[85]

Intestinal strictures

Intestinal strictures occur in many patients after necrotizing enterocolitis, whether treated medically or surgically. It is believed that strictures are a result of fibrosis and cicatricial healing of ischemic areas of intestine. The incidence of stricture formation in patients managed medically for NEC has been reported to be from 12 to 35%.[1,99,110–115] The incidence following surgical management for NEC varies according to the type of surgical management. In one series of patients treated for severe NEC by a proximal diverting enterostomy, the incidence of stricture formation was 55%.[111] Despite this high rate of stricture formation, these patients with severe NEC had a much higher survival rate than most reported series, suggesting this may be an effective strategy to treat severe NEC. Most studies report a stricture formation incidence of 10%–35% after intestinal resection with either primary anastomosis or enterostomy formation.[1,10–12,84,98,99,106,107,111–121]

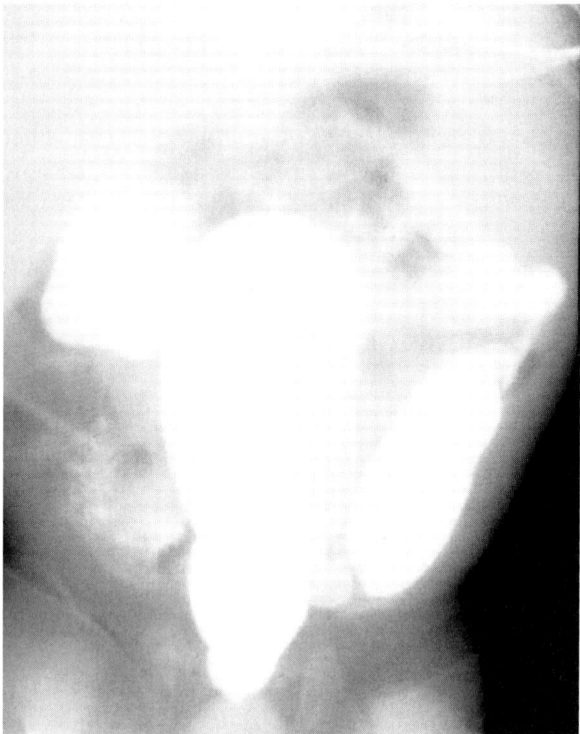

Fig. 26.3. Barium enema showing post-NEC stricture in the descending colon.

Some studies suggest that strictures occur more frequently in those patients who have undergone peritoneal drainage vs. resection.[12,120] It is possible that this occurs because the damaged areas which are prone to stricture formation upon healing would have been resected at the time of laparotomy. These infants present with symptoms of feeding intolerance including abdominal distension and vomiting, and evidence of a partial bowel obstruction on X-ray. The majority of post-NEC strictures, regardless of management, occur in the colon, most commonly the left colon (Fig. 26.3).[22,106,113,120,122]

While medically managed infants with strictures usually exhibit the symptoms described above, there have been some reported series of infants presenting in distress with perforations due to strictures.[113] Incidences such as those cases have led some surgeons to advocate for routine contrast studies prior to feeding in medically treated NEC patients.[110,112,113,115] Others, however, cite the incidence of strictures of 14–25%, the potential for false-negatives, and a reluctance to submit asymptomatic infants to a relatively invasive procedure as reasons not to do routine imaging of these patients.[122,123] The timing of such imaging studies also is controversial. In one prospective study of medically treated patients, an upper GI series was performed two weeks post-NEC, with suspicious examinations being followed by a lower GI examination.[112] In this study of 50 infants, 28% (14 patients) had a suspicious upper GI and proceeded to lower GI. The lower GI confirmed a stricture in 9 patients, for an overall stricture incidence of 18%. None of the remaining 41 patients had a delayed presentation of stricture.[112] In another study, there was a stricture incidence of 36% (10 pts out of 28) found on contrast enemas 3 to 4 weeks after the acute phase of NEC.[110] Six of these ten patients were asymptomatic at the time of the study and were followed closely. Three later presented with symptoms and underwent resection, while the other three remained asymptomatic.

Resection of strictures is standard management, though spontaneous resolution has been reported.[110,118,124] Furthermore, depending on how and when they are identified, not all lesions have been symptomatic.[110,125] Some resected segments of bowel have also appeared on pathology to have minimal or no scarring. Thus, other approaches to the management of strictures have developed. Schwartz and colleagues advocate close follow-up of patients with radiographically identified strictures who remain asymptomatic.[110] Ball and colleagues have used a balloon catheter dilatation technique for strictures that were focal and non-obstructing.[125] This technique, however, was only used on a small number of patients and needs further study before being widely adopted.

Patients who were managed surgically, with an enterostomy, for their NEC must undergo routine imaging of the intestine distal to the enterostomy to determine whether they have a stricture. As this part of their intestine is defunctionalized, strictures can occur without any symptoms; thus, imaging is required prior to closure of their stoma and return of their bowel continuity.[114]

When enterostomy takedown occurs after 6–8 weeks, most strictures can be identified prior to this operation and resected at the time of ostomy closure. Some surgeons may choose to address the problems in two separate operations, however. Earlier ostomy closure could lead to later stricture formation requiring a second operation for resection. Some surgeons have suggested that early restoration of intestinal continuity may actually decrease the incidence of stricture formation through the earlier passage of fecal material through the healing areas and the subsequent endogenous healing this provides.[96] However, in a study by Fasoli, 20.5% (9 of 44) of their patients who underwent intestinal resection and primary anastomosis at their initial operation for NEC had to undergo another operation for resection of a stricture.[84]

Despite the high incidence of stricture formation, there is little evidence about the impact of strictures on the long-term outcomes of patients with NEC. For patients in whom stricture development requires a new operation, this development will delay their time to full enteral feeding and prolong their hospital stay. However, many infants have these strictures resected at the time of their stoma takedown, and such a delay may not be seen. Resection of strictures may also impact the ultimate GI outcome of patients, as these patients are already at risk of short-bowel syndrome and resection of more intestine increases that risk.

Length of hospital stay

Neonates who suffer from necrotizing enterocolitis have tended to have longer hospitalizations than neonates of the same gestational age that did not get NEC. Additionally, the patients requiring surgical intervention tend to have even longer and more expensive hospital stays. This longer stay corresponds with a requirement for parenteral nutrition and longer delay to full enteral feeds.

The average length of stay after primary surgery in the Ladd cohort was 74.0 ± 75.4 days, with a range from 4 to 460 days. The few term infants who underwent surgical intervention for NEC had the shortest length of stay.[25] In the series reported by Bisquera, the patients treated medically had an average length of stay of 95 days ± 42 days, while those treated surgically had an average stay of 142 days ± 65 days.[14] The patients in the Limpert series had a similar length of stay of 104 days ± 66 days for the surgical patients vs. 74 days ± 29 days for the non-surgical patients.[126]

Parenteral nutrition was required on average 42 ± 87 days in Ladd's patients. Enteral nutrition was generally started around day 10 postoperatively. All but 5% of infants achieved full enteral feedings prior to discharge from the hospital.[25]

Corresponding to their longer hospitalizations, patients in the series reported by Bisquera who were treated surgically also had a higher average cost at $448 000 ± $210 000 compared to the average cost for the medically treated patients of $304 000 ± $137 000.[14]

Mortality

While the incidence of necrotizing enterocolitis has been rising in the postsurfactant era, survival from this disease has not seen a concurrent rise. Estimates and reports of mortality from NEC remain steady over the last two decades at 20%–50%.[12–14,25,123,127] The overall mortality from NEC has been cited as 10%–50% of all NEC cases.[28] Surgical mortality initially decreased from the 70% rate cited in the 1960s[128] to more recent rates of 20%–50% (see Table 26.1).[1,2,4–14]

In a study of 400 patients using a national database, Guthrie *et al.* found a mortality rate of 24% for medically managed NEC and 37% for surgically treated NEC.[129] The highest mortality occurs in those infants with the lowest gestational age and the smallest birthweight. Specifically, micropremature infants (those born at or before 28 weeks' gestational age) have significantly lower survival than premature infants, with some reported mortality rates as high as 84%.[5,10,12,32,37,62,78,120,130] Infants suffering from intrauterine growth retardation also have been shown to have an increased risk of mortality.[78]

Survival rate also tends to be adversely affected by increasing extent of disease. In most studies, this factor was the strongest independent predictor of mortality.[78] In the series reported by Cikrit, infants with localized disease had a mortality rate of 30% compared to >95% mortality in those with extensive disease.[5]

In a 15-year cohort reported by Ladd *et al.* approximately one-third of the mortality was due to NEC totalis. Another third died from sepsis and consequential cardiovascular collapse and 10% from multisystem organ failure. Roughly half of the deaths in their series occurred more than 1 month postoperatively.[25] In a series by Camberos, 26% of their patients died within the first week postoperatively. The average time of postoperative deaths was 46.9 ± 91.5 days.[131]

The greatest predictor of survival and eventual growth is the period of intestinal adaptation. Those patients, who survive the insults of surgery, the risks of parenteral nutrition and undernourishment during intestinal adaptation, can be expected to have some degree of normal growth. Patients that could be discharged from their primary hospitalization have a greater than 80%–95% chance of long-term survival.[25]

Short-bowel syndrome

Short-bowel syndrome develops after necrotizing enterocolitis when an infant has inadequate intestine to absorb enteral nutrients that are required for growth. NEC is the leading cause of short-bowel syndrome in children, accounting for half of all pediatric short-bowel syndrome cases. Short-bowel syndrome occurs in up to one-quarter of all patients who suffer from necrotizing enterocolitis.[61]

In a 1970s review, Wilmore showed that in infants without an ileocecal valve and with less than 40 cm of residual small intestine, there were no survivors. If the ileocecal valve was retained, infants with small intestine between 20 and 40 cm could survive, and most infants who had more than 40 cm of small intestine and an ileocecal valve survived.[132] Following this report, other investigators have used age-adjusted lengths of small intestine in order to define short-bowel syndrome. For infants between 27 and 35 weeks' gestational age, this length was defined as less than 50 cm, and for neonates over 35 weeks' gestation, less than 72 cm.[133] These age distinctions have been suggested since the length of the intestine grows by a factor of two during the last trimester of pregnancy.[134,135] Therefore, patients under 35 weeks' gestation should have a significant postoperative increase in the length of their small intestine.[136]

Despite these definitions, experience has shown that this syndrome should be defined by functional outcome more than by length. The gastrointestinal dysfunction in these patients occurs at varying lengths and is also influenced by factors such as the region of the intestine remaining, the presence of an ileocecal valve, the presence of the colon, the patient's age at time of resection and the time allowed for adaptation.[137]

The loss of small bowel length leads to a series of physiologic events resulting in the short-bowel syndrome. There is a loss of absorptive surface area. Additionally, there is an increase in the volume of gastric and small bowel secretions to which the remaining bowel is exposed. Depending on the section of bowel resected, there are specific absorptive losses that are unique to individual bowel segments such as the loss of the absorption of B12, bile salts and fat soluble vitamins when the terminal ileum has been resected.

In response to intestinal resection, there is an up-regulation of nutrient absorption by the remaining segments of intestine. This adaptation includes an increase in crypt cell production rate, which leads to an increased villus height and an increase in the functional surface area. This process invariably leads to an increase in the diameter of the bowel and occasionally an increase in the length of the intestine. During adaptation, the ileum responds most prominently showing the greatest changes. For this reason, children who undergo jejunal resection and retain their ileum adapt better than those who undergo ileal resection.[137] The ability of the small intestine to undergo adaptation is great enough that some patients are able to achieve normal gastrointestinal functioning even after losing 70%–80% of their intestinal mass.[137]

The colon has also shown ability to take on increased absorptive function by prolonging transit time and by deriving energy from short chain fatty acids. Functionally, the colon has the absorptive capacity of an additional foot of small intestine .[138]

Residual small bowel length after surgery has been associated with duration of dependence on parenteral nutrition. Generally, the longer the residual small bowel, the greater chance of successful weaning and the earlier the weaning tends to be.[81–83,85,133,135,139] Residual length has also been associated with survival and the need for small bowel transplantation.[81,132,140] In one study, Georgeson found a trend toward a negative correlation between bowel length and the time spent on parenteral nutrition.[82] Although it has been suggested that younger infants may do better with shorter lengths of intestine due to their greater likelihood for intestinal growth,[136] Georgeson did not find this to hold true in his series of patients.[82]

The presence of an ileocecal valve has been found by some to decrease the duration of TPN dependency,[79–83,85] but this finding has not always been upheld.[88,135,141] In a series of 26 patients with short-bowel syndrome, Georgeson and colleagues found that the absence of an ileocecal valve resulted in a threefold longer duration of parenteral nutrition, but did not preclude their ability to wean from parenteral nutrition, or affect their overall survival.[82] However, Andorsky did not find a relationship between the presence of an ileocecal valve and shorter duration of parenteral nutrition.[85]

Both the route and the content of feeding may correlate with an ability to wean a child from parenteral nutrition. Early enteral feeding has been found to be correlated with earlier weaning from TPN.[135] Enteral feeding with breast milk or an amino acid-based formula have also been associated with shorter duration of parenteral nutrition.[85] Amino acid-based formulas may also improve outcomes in infants with short-bowel syndrome, though further testing of this hypothesis is still required.[142]

Some patients cannot be weaned off of TPN despite maximal medical therapy and may benefit from surgical attempts at ameliorating their short-bowel syndrome. These techniques include procedures to reduce the diameter of dilated, non-functioning bowel and procedures to increase the absorptive surface area, prolong intestinal transit, reduce stasis and improve intestinal motility. Procedures to improve the functioning of the intestinal remnant lead to at least transient improvement some of the time.[138] The Bianchi procedure, originally described in 1980, has been used in children with short-bowel syndrome to increase intestinal length.[143] The procedure involves longitudinal division of the dilated section of bowel while carefully preserving the mesenteric blood supply to the two divided segments. The two divided segments are then anastomosed end-to-end to provide a length of bowel that is twice as long but half the diameter of the original bowel. This procedure has met variable success in increasing the amount of enteral nutrition children are able to tolerate.[144] However, this is believed to be due to an increase in transit time and motor disruption in the intestine and not due to improved absorption.[79,138]

In 2003, a new technique was described for intestinal lengthening. The serial transverse enteroplasty, or STEP, technique takes advantage of the natural tendency of the bowel to dilate in the course of adaptation. In fact, with this technique, the more dilated the bowel, the more the lengthening that can be done. This procedure involves serial transverse application of a linear stapler from opposite directions, thus dividing the bowel from the mesenteric and antimesenteric sides. While this technique has been shown to be feasible and safe, it is still in the process of being studied for its physiologic impact and long-term outcomes.[145,146]

Intestinal lengthening is the most frequently performed non-transplant procedure for short-bowel syndrome.[138] In the short term, 90% of patients demonstrate improvements in nutritional status, but long-term results suggest that less than half of the patients will have sustained benefit up to 20 years.[138]

TPN-related liver disease

Cholestatic liver disease occurs frequently in children who are TPN dependent. Along with sepsis, this complication is a leading cause of death in these children.[147] Of children requiring long-term parenteral nutrition 40%–60% will have hepatic dysfunction.[148] Since it was first described, many investigators have tried to determine its cause, and efforts have focused in two main areas. Some believe that TPN itself is toxic and leads to liver disease, while others have argued that it is a lack of enteral stimulation that leads to cholestasis. Without enteral stimulation, gut hormone production is decreased which may contribute to the development of liver disease. Additionally, bacterial overgrowth may result from intestinal stasis. This bacterial overgrowth can lead to translocation and the leakage of endotoxins, contributing to cholestatic liver disease. These theories led to the conclusion that partial enteral feeds may protect the liver against cholestasis. However, studies by Moss and Hode both showed progression of cholestasis despite enteral feeds.[149,150] Several factors likely contribute to the development of cholestasis including altered gut hormone production, intestinal permeability with bacterial overgrowth, translocation, and leakage of endotoxins, and secondary responses of the liver, particularly to other problems such as sepsis.[82,135,151,152]

Without a clear-cut etiology for TPN associated cholestasis, it has been difficult to identify successful treatments for the disease. An early study of cholecystokinin (CCK) suggested that it could prevent biliary sludge formation in adults on TPN. Unfortunately, CCK has not proved to be as successful in further animal studies [153,154] or human studies.[155,156] A prospective, non-randomized trial examining CCK as a prophylactic agent for TPN-AC showed no significant difference in the incidence of TPN-AC.[156] A subsequent randomized trial reported a similar lack of efficacy (D. H. Teitelbaum, personal communication).

Ursodeoxycholic acid has also been studied for treatment of TPN-AC. In animal studies it has been shown to have protective effects against liver dysfunction and it has been shown to be beneficial in adult liver disease. However, studies focusing on its use as treatment in children with TPN cholestasis have not been able to demonstrate a therapeutic effect.[148]

Balanced amino acid solutions in TPN have been suggested to decrease the incidence of cholestatic jaundice.[157] Treatment of intestinal bacterial translocation with oral antibiotics such as neomycin also has sporadically improved cholestatic jaundice.[82] However, the only known effective treatment of TPN-AC is to discontinue TPN use and advance children as rapidly as possible to enteral feedings. Other measures that may be useful in slowing the rate of progression of cholestasis and avoiding fulminant liver failure include preventing line sepsis, reducing small bowel bacterial overgrowth, promoting intestinal motility, cycling TPN and avoiding excess glucose and protein in the TPN.[147,158]

Central venous catheter sepsis

Sepsis related to the presence of a central venous catheter is a common and potentially life-threatening complication in children with short-bowel syndrome who are TPN dependent. Sepsis is implicated as the cause of death in 3%–14% of children with short-bowel syndrome.[81,82,133,159] Contamination of the central venous catheter is the most common cause of septic complications.[134,160–164] Cohort studies of pediatric inpatients on parenteral nutrition for gastrointestinal problems have revealed a range of 0.81–7.59 cases of sepsis per 1000 days on parenteral nutrition, for an average overall rate of 1.66 cases of sepsis per 1000 days of PN.[165] A study by Klein of newborn surgical patients showed an even higher rate of sepsis due to central venous catheters at 9.9 episodes per 1000 catheter days.[163] Strict aseptic technique in managing these catheters is important to minimize line sepsis, but catheter sepsis often occurs even in the absence of apparent breaches in sterile technique.

Investigators have suggested that TPN itself may increase the risk of sepsis by compromising immune function.[166,167] Okada found that, in normal infants, the whole-blood killing of coagulase-negative staphylococci correlated with neutrophil counts but that this is not true in infants on TPN. In infants on TPN, neutrophil phagocytosis was decreased. Thus, TPN appears to cause an underlying neutrophil dysfunction that may also contribute to an increased risk of infection.[166]

Sepsis in children with short-bowel syndrome may also be related to bacterial overgrowth in the intestines.[134,161,162,167,168] Pierro found that there was an association between microorganisms found in the digestive tract and those found in the bloodstream of infants with sepsis on parenteral nutrition.[168] Moreover, carriage in the digestive tract always preceded the episode of infection. Additionally, microbial overgrowth was observed in at least two-thirds of the septic patients.[168] Terra observed that in comparing children with more than 50 cm of remaining bowel after surgery with those who had less than 50 cm remaining, there were significantly more episodes of infection in those with the shorter amount of bowel remaining.[161] Sigalet also found that patients with the shortest amount of remaining bowel had the greatest number of episodes of sepsis suggesting that these infections may result from increased intestinal permeability and bacterial translocation.[134] Klein found that the presence of an enterostomy was highly related to having septic episodes.[163] However, it is unclear whether these episodes are due to contamination from the stoma or whether the stoma is simply associated with gastrointestinal disease which could be contributing to the sepsis.

Sepsis may also contribute to the development of cholestasis in children who are receiving total parenteral nutrition. Sondheimer reported that in their series of patients, liver cholestasis followed the first infection in 89%, on average 13.5 ± 3.4 days. In the three patients in whom cholestasis did not follow an infection, two had acute obstruction of the superior vena cava that led to their development of cholestasis.[169] Other researchers have also seen a greater incidence of cholestasis in patients who have had infections than in those who have not.[170]

Transplantation

The survival rate for short-bowel syndrome is reported as 80% to 94%.[171,172] However, for patients who are parenteral nutrition dependent, the mortality rate is reported to be as high as 25% per year.[173,174] Overall, 40 to 60% of these parenteral nutrition dependent patients develop liver failure in the long term.[175] These results have led to an increased interest and development of transplantation as an option for these children.

Isolated intestinal transplantation for children with intestinal failure, and combined intestinal and liver transplantation for those children who have also developed TPN-associated liver failure have become part of the armamentarium against short-bowel syndrome. Since the natural history of TPN-associated liver disease is progressive liver failure and death within 6 to 12 months after the onset of cholestasis,[172] there is some rationale for offering isolated intestinal transplantation before patients develop irreversible liver disease, particularly if they have intestinal anatomy that is unlikely to adapt and allow for weaning off of TPN.[172] Researchers in Japan have also shown that isolated intestinal transplantation can reverse cholestasis and steatosis in the liver, though fibrosis remains unchanged.[176]

The waiting time for intestinal transplantation can be quite lengthy, and mortality rates for children on the intestinal transplant list are high. In children who have TPN-associated liver disease that is getting progressively worse, there may be some compelling argument for an isolated liver transplantation first.[172,177] Liver transplantation alone can lead to return to normal liver function and resolution of portal hypertension such that the intestine can either have a longer period of time for adaptation or the child can survive while awaiting an appropriate intestinal donor.[177]

Currently, small bowel transplantation is indicated for children with moderate liver dysfunction or compromised vascular access who are dependent on total parenteral nutrition. The recommendations for referral to a transplant center for assessment, as determined by the Sixth International Small Bowel Transplant Symposium, are when a child has lost more than two central intravenous sites, if they have had recurrent septic episodes, or if they have cholestasis, before they show signs of end-stage liver disease.[172,178,179]

Early referral is essential, as there is a high mortality rate for patients while on the waiting list. Researchers in Toronto reported a 53% mortality rate for patients on the waiting list for intestinal transplantation. These patients died within 6 months, and did not have a chance for transplantation as the average waiting time for surgery was 212 days.[178] Pittsburgh researchers noted that the mean wait for an intestinal transplant in their center was 10.1 ± 1.3 months.[179] 47% of referred patients died while on the waiting list at their institution.[180]

Rejection occurs at a rate of 70%–95% in intestinal transplantation, though there has been some improvement in these rates with better immunosuppressive regimens usually involving triple agents: tacrolimus, steroids and either cyclophosphamide, mycophenolate mofetil, or rapamycin.[181] Rejection of an isolated intestinal graft is higher than in a composite intestinal/liver graft or in a multivisceral graft. Despite this fact, the isolated intestinal transplant carries less perioperative risk and complication rate, leading to an overall superior survival with isolated intestinal transplants than with composite grafts.[181] While survival rates for isolated intestinal transplantation are roughly 70%–90% at 1 year, the rates for combined liver and intestine are only half of that at one year.[182–184] Therefore, it is better to transplant children early, before they develop liver failure. Unfortunately, this is often not possible as approximately 70% of infants receiving an intestinal transplant also require a simultaneous liver transplant due to end-stage liver disease.[180]

Overall, the most recently reported rates of patient and graft survival from the major pediatric transplant centers range from 72 to 86% patient survival at 1 year decreasing to 50%–55% at 2 and 3 years.[179,180,185]

Age at the time of intestinal transplantation is an important prognostic factor.[172,185] Intestinal transplantation in infants has the worst prognosis, particularly if they also have liver failure.[172] At one center, 32% of pediatric intestinal transplant recipients underwent transplant before the age of 1, and 75% of these children had concomitant liver failure.[172] Necrotizing enterocolitis was the disease with the worst prognosis in the Pittsburgh experience. Survival rates were 28.7% and 14.4% at 1 and 2 years.[180] Researchers in Miami also saw decreased survival in their patients who had short gut syndrome due to NEC vs. other patients.[186]

Among survivors of intestinal transplantation, greater than 90% achieve freedom from parenteral nutrition.[171,181,187,188] Despite this fact, growth and development of children undergoing intestinal transplantation remains a difficult issue. Researchers in both Nebraska and

Miami report that only a small percentage of these patients show positive trends in their catch-up and maintenance growth.[172,187,188]

As survival rates are increasing after intestinal transplantation, there has been increased focus on quality of life following transplantation. In the Pittsburgh experience with 84 transplanted children, there was a high incidence of affective disorders in the early post-operative period. However, ultimately over 80% of their school-age patients who are 3 years post-transplant are attending school full-time at the appropriate level.[181] These researchers do describe, though, that for the first 6–12 months children may be taking 7–15 daily medications, have tube feedings, stomas, and venous access, all requiring daily care and very frequent endoscopic examinations to monitor for rejection. While these routines decrease over time, at 3 years post-transplant a mean of seven daily or twice daily medications are still required and 17% of patients still require enteral feeding due to oral aversion.[181]

As intestinal transplantation becomes more frequent and outcomes improve, it will become more of an option for children with short-bowel syndrome. This may change the management algorithms of pediatric surgeons as they approach children with NEC. Survival rates in intestinal transplantation are now similar to those of lung transplantation.[178,189] Alternative strategies such as isolated liver transplantation as a bridge to intestinal adaptation or early intestinal transplantation are under consideration. Improvements in immunosuppression are constantly made. With transplantation becoming a more viable management option, children with more extensive disease may have a better prognosis due to the addition of transplant as an option. Unfortunately, organ availability will likely remain a problem, and mortality rates will remain high while children wait on the transplant list. Pediatric surgeons must consider the current survival rates and the challenges of organ transplantation as they present this potential therapy to parents.

Growth

Children with short-bowel syndrome consistently fall behind their peers in growth. In a cohort of patients followed by Ladd for 4.2 ± 3.8 years, with a median follow-up of 2.9 years, the median percentile weight was less than the 25th percentile at each follow-up timepoint.[25] Stanford found that all children in their series of patients treated medically and surgically for NEC were below the 50th percentile for height and weight at a mean follow-up age of 7.5 ± 2.5 years. The mean percentile for height was 33.5% ± 10 inches. The mean percentile for weight was 22% ± 10 kg. All children in this follow-up study were able to receive their daily caloric requirements orally.[190] Orellana found that, in a comparison of extremely low birthweight infants with and without NEC, the children who had NEC had significantly lower height and weight measurements at 6 or 8 year visits, despite the lack of differences in gastrointestinal or neurodevelopmental outcomes.[191] Whiteman has also reported height and weight retardation at 4 years of age in patients with NEC.[192]

In contrast to those studies, Sonntag found no difference in weight gain in a group of 20 children with NEC and a control group at 20 months follow-up. However, less than half of their patients had surgery, and none of their patients had short-bowel syndrome.[193] Walsh and colleagues found that while infants who had suffered from stage II NEC had demonstrated "catch up" growth by 8 months of age, those who suffered from stage III NEC continued to be significantly smaller in height and weight even out to twenty months of age.[194]

Though all of these studies are relatively small observational studies, it appears that NEC may have long-term consequences in growth patterns. Children who had more severe NEC (stage III) seem to be affected to a greater degree than those with more moderate disease. Children who develop short-bowel syndrome as a result of intestinal resections and their disease appear to be the most severely affected. However, even those children who have normal gastrointestinal function afterward still may have delayed or decreased growth. Larger long-term follow-up evaluations are needed, though, to examine the impact of birthweight, NEC severity, length of resected intestine, and other illnesses on the growth outcomes of these children.

Neurodevelopmental outcomes

As advances in neonatology have led to the survival of greater numbers of premature infants, examination of the long-term outcomes in these patients has become more crucial. In 1980, Stevenson and colleagues raised concerns that quality of survival for patients with NEC was as important as the concern for the prevention of death, citing that fewer than 50% of their patients were completely normal on follow-up of three years. Furthermore, 81% of the morbidity they found was not gastrointestinal in nature. Stevenson did not attribute the non-gastrointestinal injury that these children suffered to their NEC, since a control group of patients without NEC had comparable morbidity.[2] However, the findings from this study sparked further studies of neurodevelopmental outcomes in patients treated for necrotizing enterocolitis.

Several observational studies of NEC survivors have found these children to suffer from developmental delays on long-term follow-up. In a study of 48 children followed at a mean of 2.7 years (range 4 months to 10 years), Cikrit found that 33.3% had developmental delays and 31.5% had intellectual delays.[195] The study did not specify, though, how either developmental delay or intellectual delay was defined.

In a 4-year follow-up of 28 NEC survivors, Patel found, from interviewing parents, that 10 patients (35.7%) had some neurodevelopmental problem, including two children with "moderate-to-severe developmental delay with speech and motor impairment," one with cerebral palsy, one with a moderate speech and hearing deficit, four children requiring speech therapy, three children with reading problems, and two children having repeated 1 grade.[13]

In a long-term follow-up of forty-three children, with a mean follow-up time of 7.5 years, Stanford found that 83% of children aged 5–10 were enrolled in school full-time. However, 14% of the children had developmental delay, with 28% requiring special education classes.[190] Though they state that they did not find any specific factors that predicted the likelihood of requiring special education classes, they did not identify which factors were examined.

These observational series of survivors of NEC raise some concerns about the neurodevelopmental outcomes of these children. However, the retrospective nature of these studies means that a large portion of patients were not available for follow-up. Additionally, there was no formal developmental testing done, and in some of the studies, the definition of developmental delay was not given. Finally, there were no control groups for the studies, so it is not possible to determine whether these rates of neurodevelopmental problems are due to NEC or simply the result of prematurity. There was also no differentiation between surgically treated patients or medically treated patients, which may also influence their outcome.

In his initial study on long-term outcomes, Stevenson found that six of 40 children (15% of survivors) followed for three years had moderate to severe neurological impairment.[2] These impairments included three children with spasticity, one with diffuse encephalopathy, one with hydrocephalus, and one with seizures. However, the morbidity in these children was similar to a control group of children, matched for degree of prematurity and level of perinatal stress; thus he found that their neurodevelopmental outcomes could not be attributed to their necrotizing enterocolitis.

Abbasi compared 22 NEC survivors with 18 control patients, matched for birthweight and gestational age and found 3 NEC survivors and 2 controls with neurodevelopmental delays at 1 year of age.[196] They did not describe the details of these delays, however. It is important to note, though, that 18 of the NEC survivors were treated medically and 4 were treated surgically, which may give some indication to their degree of illness.

Orellana found no neurodevelopmental differences at 6- or 8-year follow-up visits when comparing 25 prior extremely low birthweight (ELBW) infants with NEC to 50 ELBW children without NEC. The group of NEC patients followed in this study, as in the Abbasi study, were mostly treated medically (84% medical treatment).[191] The fact that these patients were mainly those who were treated medically speaks to the severity of their disease and is important to consider in evaluating their outcomes.

In a follow-up of 36 patients with NEC who were evaluated at 20 months of age, Walsh and colleagues found that the Bayley developmental scores of survivors of NEC did not differ significantly from those infants who did not have NEC. However, they did find that the percentage of infants with lower scores was greater in those with more severe disease (stage III versus stage II NEC), suggesting that these infants need to be closely followed and evaluated for neurodevelopmental sequelae.[194] Additionally, of twelve patients with either abnormal neurosensory status or a score of less than 80 on the Bayley scale of infant development, ten had stage III NEC.

Sonntag found significant neurodevelopmental impairment in NEC survivors in their case control study of 22 very low birthweight (VLBW) infants with NEC compared to 40 VLBW infants.[193] This study found that the NEC patients scored lower on tests of locomotor skills and general scales at 12-month follow-up, and on all subscales as well as the general scale at 20-month follow-up. Of infants who suffered from NEC 55% were severely retarded compared to 22.5% of their control group. In this group of patients, the delays at 12 months were on scales assessing "locomotor" and "general" function. At 20 months, however, these locomotor delays had resolved and the delays at this time were in the areas of "hearing and speech," "intellectual performance" and "personal and social" on the Griffiths developmental scale.[193]

In the Sonntag study, less than half of the NEC patients had had surgery, and the developmental delays were consistent in those who had been treated both surgically and

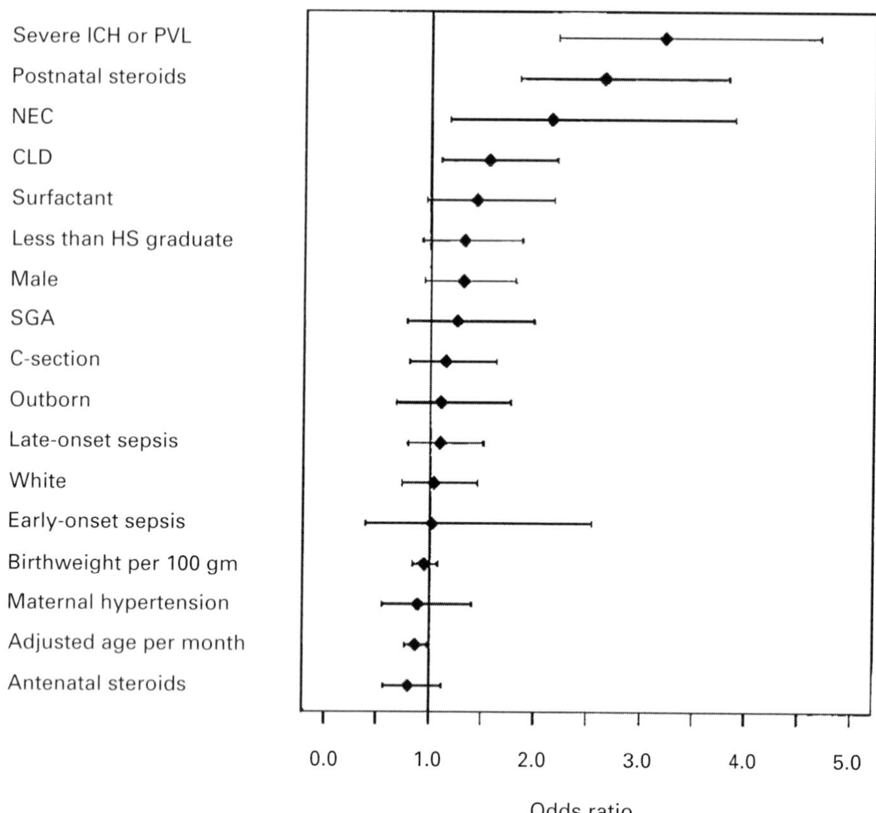

Fig. 26.4. Adjusted risk factors for Psychomotor Development Index <70 (Odds Ratios and 95% Confidence Intervals [CI]): NICHD Neonatal Research Network. Antenatal steroids indicates beta-methasone (2 doses, 12 or 24 hours apart) or dexamethasone (4 doses, 6 hours apart); surfactant, any surfactant preparation given at location (delivery room, neonatal intensive care unit, or referring hospital); early-onset sepsis, positive blood culture result within the first 72 hours; late-onset sepsis, positive blood culture result >72 hours obtained in the presence of clinical signs of septicemia; postnatal steroids, any doses or courses of steroids for CLD.[203]

medically. Therefore, they postulated that these delays resulted from having NEC itself, not from the effects of surgery.[193]

Comparing ten children who had laparotomy for necrotizing enterocolitis and 20 controls matched for gestational age, birthweight and year of birth, Chacko found that a greater percentage of those undergoing laparotomy had mild or severe neurologic impairment. Comparing infants with NEC managed surgically versus medically, an even greater difference was found in the incidence of neurologic impairment.[197] However, these surgically managed patients also had a significant difference in their incidence of hypotension and inotrope requirement during their acute illness. Thus, this hypotension and the resulting acidosis of these patients may have contributed to their different neurological outcome, as both of these factors have been correlated with neurologic impairment in other studies.[198–201]

A prospective study in London investigated developmental outcomes in neonates undergoing emergency surgery for any cause with examinations at 6 and 12 months of age. This study found that the surgical group scored significantly lower in 5 of 7 areas on the Griffiths Mental Development Scales. The factor that was most strongly correlated with impaired development, though, was length of hospital admission.[202]

Finally, the NIHCD carried out a large multicenter cohort study to look at neurodevelopmental outcomes in over 1100 extremely low birthweight survivors. In this study, necrotizing enterocolitis was an independent risk factor for an abnormal neurologic examination and a low score on one of four developmental tests administered. Logistic regression analysis found that necrotizing enterocolitis was a risk factor for an abnormal neurologic examination, particularly on the psychomotor development index (Fig. 26.4). NEC was not a

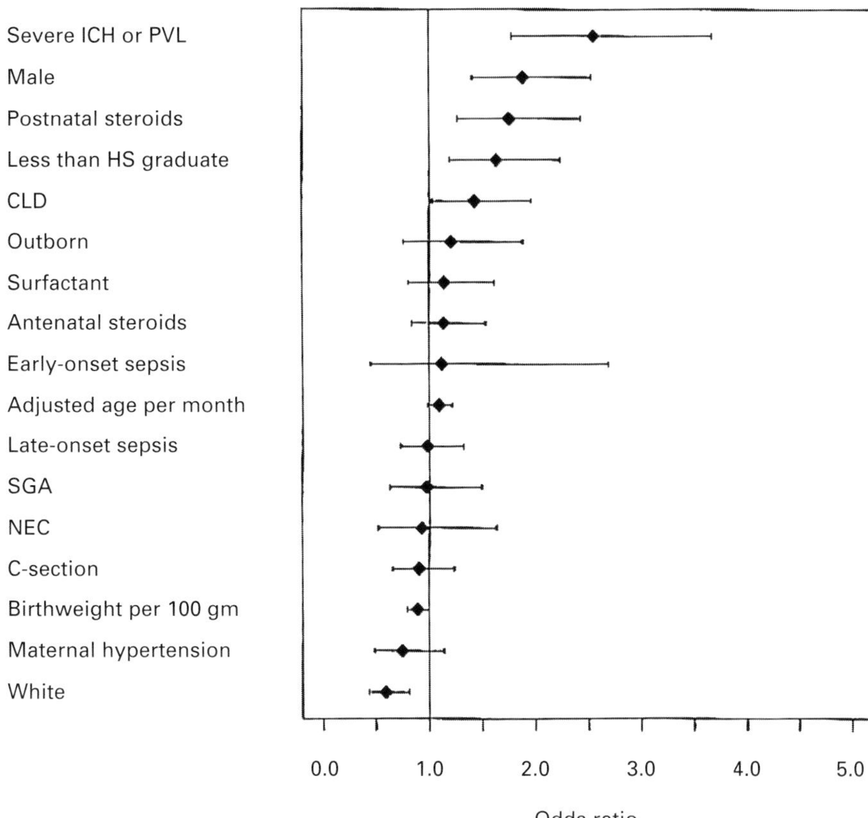

Fig. 26.5. Adjusted risk factors for Mental Developmental Index <70 (ORs and 95% CIs): NICHD Neonatal Research Network.[203]

significant risk factor on the mental development index (Fig. 26.5).[203]

There are several difficulties in assessing long-term neurodevelopmental outcomes in children who had necrotizing enterocolitis. Several factors that must be considered include the associated disease processes that these ELBW, VLBW and premature infants suffer. Multiple factors including hypoperfusion, acidosis, shock, hypoxemia, a systemic inflammatory response, malnutrition, parenteral nutrition and prolonged hospitalization could all play an etiologic role in the developmental outcome of these children. Another challenge comes from the changing nature of neurodevelopmental outcomes such that those children who may appear normal at 12 months of age have a disability detected when they reach school age. In the Sonntag study, the nature of neurodevelopmental delays changed completely between the 12 month check-up and the 20 month check-up.[193] Additional large prospective studies are needed to determine the true relation between necrotizing enterocolitis and poor neurodevelopmental outcomes.

While the neurodevelopmental delays identified in these studies may not be solely attributable to NEC, they are likely multifactorial, with prematurity, intraventricular damage from hemorrhage, hypoxia, acidosis, a systemic inflammatory response, and the effects of surgery and prolonged hospitalization all possibly contributing. Long-term studies comparing to those with premature infants who suffer from NEC vs. other diseases of prematurity could help to further elucidate which factors are most highly related. Large multicenter cohort studies such as that by the NIHCD will yield the most helpful evidence in this problem. As advances continue to be made, further investigation of this nature should be carried out. In the interim, parents should be counseled that children with NEC are at risk for neurodevelopmental disabilities and appropriate follow-up for evaluation and treatment should be advised.

Conclusions

Necrotizing enterocolitis remains a challenge for neonatologists and pediatric surgeons. As advances in neonatal care are improving survival rates of premature infants, these patients face the long-term challenges of their disease.

However, many of these long-term challenges and outcomes are still only described by small, single-institution, descriptive studies. As new therapies and technologies evolve, such as the STEP procedure, peritoneal drainage, and intestinal transplantation, hopefully more patients will survive with fewer debilitating consequences. With the increase in survival, though, it is crucial to have evidence regarding outcomes in the areas of growth, development, and quality of life. Parents are faced with challenging decisions when such a severe disease occurs in their children. As the professionals caring for their children, we are obligated to provide the best available information to them so that they can make informed and ethical decisions. Further, large-scale, investigations into the long-term consequences of this disease are critical to providing this information to parents and practitioners.

REFERENCES

1. Schullinger, J. N., Mollitt, D. L., Vinocur, C. D., Santulli, T. V., & Driscoll, J. M., Jr. Neonatal necrotizing enterocolitis. Survival, management, and complications: a 25-year study. *Am. J. Dis. Childr.* 1981; **135**(7):612–614.
2. Stevenson, D. K., Kerner, J. A., Malachowski, N., & Sunshine, P. Late morbidity among survivors of necrotizing enterocolitis. *Pediatrics* 1980; **66**(6):925–927.
3. Lee, J. S. & Polin, R. A. Treatment and prevention of necrotizing enterocolitis. *Semin. Neonatol.* 2003; **8**(6):449–459.
4. Gregory, J. R., Campbell, J. R., Harrison, M. W., & Campbell, T. J. Neonatal necrotizing enterocolitis. A 10 year experience. *Ame. J. Surg.* 1981; **141**(5):562–567.
5. Cikrit, D., Mastandrea, J., West, K. W., Schreiner, R. L., & Grosfeld, J. L. Necrotizing enterocolitis: factors affecting mortality in 101 surgical cases. *Surgery* 1984; **96**(4):648–655.
6. Dykes, E. H., Gilmour, W. H., & Azmy, A. F. Prediction of outcome following necrotizing enterocolitis in a neonatal surgical unit. *J. Pediatr. Surg.* 1985; **20**(1):3–5.
7. Kanto, W. P., Jr., Wilson, R., & Ricketts, R. R. Management and outcome of necrotizing enterocolitis. *Clin. Pediatr.* 1985; **24**(2):79–82.
8. Pokorny, W. J., Garcia-Prats, J. A., & Barry, Y. N. Necrotizing enterocolitis: incidence, operative care, and outcome. *J. Pediatr. Surg.* 1986; **21**(12):1149–1154.
9. Jackman, S., Brereton, R. J., & Wright, V. M. Results of surgical treatment of neonatal necrotizing enterocolitis. *Br. J. Surg.* 1990; **77**(2):146–148.
10. Ricketts, R. R. & Jerles, M. L. Neonatal necrotizing enterocolitis: experience with 100 consecutive surgical patients. *World J. Surg.* 1990; **14**(5):600–605.
11. Kurscheid, T. & Holschneider, A. M. Necrotizing enterocolitis (NEC) – mortality and long-term results. *Eur. J. Pediatr. Surg.* 1993; **3**(3):139–143.
12. Horwitz, J. R., Lally, K. P., Cheu, H. W., Vazquez, W. D., Grosfeld, J. L., & Ziegler, M. M. Complications after surgical intervention for necrotizing enterocolitis: a multicenter review. *J. Pediatr. Surg.* 1995; **30**(7):994–998; discussion 998–999.
13. Patel, J. C., Tepas, J. J., 3rd, Huffman, S. D., Evans, J. S. Neonatal necrotizing enterocolitis: the long-term perspective. *Am. Surg.* 1998; **64**(6):575–579; discussion 579–580.
14. Bisquera, J. A., Cooper, T. R., & Berseth, C. L. Impact of necrotizing enterocolitis on length of stay and hospital charges in very low birth weight infants. *Pediatrics* 2002; **109**(3):423–428.
15. Kosloske, A. M. Epidemiology of necrotizing enterocolitis. *Acta. Paediatr. Suppl.* 1994; **396**:2–7.
16. Kliegman, R. M. & Fanaroff, A. A. Neonatal necrotizing enterocolitis: a nine-year experience. *Am. J. Dis. Child.* 1981; **135**(7):603–607.
17. Ryder, R. W., Shelton, J. D., & Guinan, M. E. Necrotizing enterocolitis: a prospective multicenter investigation. *Am. J. Epidemiol.* 1980; **112**(1):113–123.
18. Sweet, D. G., Craig, B., Halliday, H. L., & Mulholland, C. Gastrointestinal complications following neonatal cardiac catheterisation. *J. Perinat. Med.* 1998; **26**(3):196–200.
19. Arias, E., Anderson, R. N., Hsiang-Ching, K., Murphy, S. L., & Kochanek, K.D. Final death data for 2001. *National Vital Statistics Reports.* Vol. 52, No. 3. Hyattsville, Maryland: National Center for Health Statistics, 2003.
20. Nadler, E. P., Upperman, J. S., & Ford, H. R. Controversies in the management of necrotizing enterocolitis. *Surg. Infect.* 2001; 2(2):113–119; discussion 119–120.
21. Holman, R. C., Stoll, B. J., Clarke, M. J., & Glass, R. I. The epidemiology of necrotizing enterocolitis infant mortality in the United States. *Am. J. Public Hlth.* 1997; **87**(12):2026–2031.
22. Albanese, C. T. & Rowe, M. I. Necrotizing enterocolitis. *Semin. Pediatr. Surg.* 1995; **4**(4):200–206.
23. Holman, R. C., Stehr-Green, J. K., & Zelasky, M. T. Necrotizing enterocolitis mortality in the United States, 1979–85. *Am. J. Public Hlth.* 1989; **79**(8):987–989.
24. Ostlie, D. J., Spilde, T. L., St, Peter, S. D. *et al.* Necrotizing enterocolitis in full-term infants. *J. Pediatr. Surg.* 2003; **38**(7):1039–1042.
25. Ladd, A. P., Rescorla, F. J., West, K. W., Scherer, L. R., 3rd, Engum, S. A., & Grosfeld, J. L. Long-term follow-up after bowel resection for necrotizing enterocolitis: factors affecting outcome. *J. Pediatr. Surg.* 1998; **33**(7):967–972.
26. Kliegman, R. M., Pittard, W. B., & Fanaroff, A. A. Necrotizing enterocolitis in neonates fed human milk. *J. Pediatr.* 1979; **95**(3):450–453.
27. Stoll, B. J., Kanto, W. P., Jr., Glass, R. I., Nahmias, A. J., & Brann, A. W., Jr. Epidemiology of necrotizing enterocolitis: a case control study. *J. Pediatr.* 1980; **96**(3 Pt 1):447–451.
28. Caplan, M. S. & Jilling, T. New concepts in necrotizing enterocolitis. *Curr. Opin. Pediatr.* 2001; **13**(2):111–115.
29. Shimura, K. Necrotizing enterocolitis: a Japanese survey. *NICU* 1990; **3**:5–7.
30. Bolisetty, S., Lui, K., Oei, J., & Wojtulewicz, J. A regional study of underlying congenital diseases in term neonates with

necrotizing enterocolitis. *Acta. Paediatr.* 2000; **89**(10):1226–1230.

31. Wilson, R., Kanto, W. P., Jr., McCarthy, B. J., Burton, A., Lewin, P., & Feldman, R. A. Age at onset of necrotizing enterocolitis: an epidemiologic analysis. *Pediatr Res.* 1982; **16**(1):82–85.
32. Snyder, C. L., Gittes, G. K., Murphy, J. P., Sharp, R. J., Ashcraft, K. W., & Amoury, R. A. Survival after necrotizing enterocolitis in infants weighing less than 1,000 g: 25 years' experience at a single institution. *J. Pediatr. Surg.* 1997; **32**(3):434–437.
33. Ruangtrakool, R., Laohapensang, M., Sathornkich, C., & Talalak, P. Necrotizing enterocolitis: a comparison between full-term and pre-term neonates. *J. Med. Assoc. Thailand* 2001; **84**(3):323–331.
34. Kafetzis, D. A., Skevaki, C., & Costalos, C. Neonatal necrotizing enterocolitis: an overview. *Curr. Opin. Infect. Dis.* 2003; **16**(4):349–355.
35. Ververidis, M., Kiely, E. M., Spitz, L., Drake, D. P., Eaton, S., & Pierro, A. The clinical significance of thrombocytopenia in neonates with necrotizing enterocolitis. *J. Pediatr. Surg.* 2001; **36**(5):799–803.
36. Albanese C. T. & Rowe, M. I. Necrotizing enterocolitis. In O'Neill, J. A., Jr., Rowe, M. I., Grosfeld, J., Fonkalsrud, E. W., & Coran, A. G., eds. *Pediatric Surgery*. 5th edn. St. Louis: Mosby, 1998; 1297–1320.
37. Rowe, M. I., Reblock, K. K., Kurkchubasche, A. G., & Healey, P. J. Necrotizing enterocolitis in the extremely low birth weight infant. *J. Pediatr. Surg.* 1994; **29**(8):987–990; discussion 990–991.
38. Bell, M. J., Ternberg, J. L., Feigin, R. D. *et al.* Neonatal necrotizing enterocolitis. Therapeutic decisions based upon clinical staging. *Ann. Surg.* 1978; **187**(1):1–7.
39. Moss, R. L. The role of magnetic resonance imaging in necrotizing enterocolitis. *Pediatrics* 2000; **106**(5):1170.
40. Maalouf, E. F., Fagbemi, A., Duggan, P. J. *et al.* Magnetic resonance imaging of intestinal necrosis in preterm infants. *Pediatrics* 2000; **105**(3 Pt 1):510–514.
41. Ballance, W. A., Dahms, B. B., Shenker, N., & Kliegman, R. M. Pathology of neonatal necrotizing enterocolitis: a ten-year experience. *J. Pediatr.* 1990; **117**(1 Pt 2):S6–S13.
42. Chandler, J. C. & Hebra, A. Necrotizing enterocolitis in infants with very low birth weight. *Semin. Pediatr. Surg.* 2000; **9**(2):63–72.
43. Cikrit, D., Mastandrea, J., Grosfeld, J. L., West, K. W., & Schreiner, R. L. Significance of portal vein air in necrotizing entercolitis: analysis of 53 cases. *J. Pediat. Surg.* 1985; **20**(4):425–430.
44. Kosloske, A. M. Necrotizing enterocolitis in the neonate. *Surg., Gynecol. Obstet.* 1979; **148**(2):259–269.
45. Ein, S. H., Marshall, D. G., & Girvan, D. Peritoneal drainage under local anesthesia for perforations from necrotizing enterocolitis. *J. Pediatr. Surg.* 1977; **12**(6):963–967.
46. Morgan, L. J., Shochat, S. J., & Hartman, G. E. Peritoneal drainage as primary management of perforated NEC in the very low birth weight infant. *J. Pediatr. Surg.* 1994; **29**(2):310–314; discussion 314–315.
47. Takamatsu, H., Akiyama, H., Ibara, S., Seki, S., Kuraya, K., & Ikenoue, T. Treatment for necrotizing enterocolitis perforation in the extremely premature infant (weighing less than 1,000 g). *J. Pediatr. Surg.* 1992; **27**(6):741–743.
48. Janik, J. S. & Ein, S. H. Peritoneal drainage under local anesthesia for necrotizing enterocolitis (NEC) perforation: a second look. *J. Pediatr. Surg.* 1980; **15**(4):565–566.
49. Ein, S. H., Shandling, B., Wesson, D., & Filler, R. M. A 13-year experience with peritoneal drainage under local anesthesia for necrotizing enterocolitis perforation. *J. Pediatr. Surg.* 1990; **25**(10):1034–1036; discussion 1036–1037.
50. Cheu, H. W., Sukarochana, K., & Lloyd, D. A. Peritoneal drainage for necrotizing enterocolitis. *J. Pediatr. Surg.* 1988; **23**(6):557–561.
51. Azarow, K. S., Ein, S. H., Shandling, B., Wesson, D., Superina, R., & Filler, R. M. Laparotomy or drain for perforated necrotizing enterocolitis: who gets what and why? *Pediatr. Surg. Int.* 1997; **12**(2–3):137–139.
52. Demestre, X., Ginovart, G., Figueras-Aloy, J. *et al.* Peritoneal drainage as primary management in necrotizing enterocolitis: a prospective study. *J. Pediatr. Surg.* 2002; **37**(11):1534–1539.
53. Lessin, M. S., Luks, F. I., & Wesselhoeft, C. W. Peritoneal drainage as definitive treatment for intestinal perforation in infants with extremely low birth weight (<750 gms). *J. Pediatr. Surg.* 1998; **33**:370–372.
54. Sharma, R., Tepas, J. J., 3rd, Mollitt, D. L., Pieper, P., & Wludyka, P. Surgical management of bowel perforations and outcome in very low-birth-weight infants (< or =1,200 g). *J. Pediatr. Surg.* 2004; **39**(2):190–194.
55. Rovin, J. D., Rodgers, B. M., Burns, R. C., & McGahren, E. D. The role of peritoneal drainage for intestinal perforation in infants with and without necrotizing enterocolitis. *J. Pediatr. Surg.* 1999; **34**(1):143–147.
56. Moss, R. L., Dimmitt, R. A., Henry, M. C., Geraghty, N., & Efron, B. A meta-analysis of peritoneal drainage versus laparotomy for perforated necrotizing enterocolitis. *J. Pediatr. Surg.* 2001; **36**(8):1210–1213.
57. Downard, C. & Campbell, T. *Peritoneal drainage for neonatal intestinal perforation*. Las Vegas, NV: 33rd Annual Meeting of Pacific Association of Pediatric Surgeons, 2000.
58. Dimmitt, R. A., Meier, A. H., Skarsgard, E. D., Halamek, L. P., Smith, B. M., & Moss, R. L. Salvage laparotomy for failure of peritoneal drainage in necrotizing enterocolitis in infants with extremely low birth weight. *J. Pediatr. Surg.* 2000; **35**(6):856–859.
59. Ahmed, T., Ein, S. & Moore, A. The role of peritoneal drains in treatment of perforated necrotizing enterocolitis: recommendations from recent experience. *J. Pediatr. Surg.* 1998; **33**(10):1468–1470.
60. Kabeer, A., Gunnlaugsson, S., & Coren, C. Neonatal necrotizing enterocolitis. A 12-year review at a county hospital. *Dise. Colon Rectum* 1995; **38**(8):866–872.
61. Ricketts, R. R. Surgical treatment of necrotizing enterocolitis and the short bowel syndrome. *Clin. Perinatol.* 1994; **21**(2):365–387.

62. Grosfeld, J. L., Cheu, H., Schlatter, M., West, K. W., & Rescorla, F. J. Changing trends in necrotizing enterocolitis. Experience with 302 cases in two decades. *Ann. Surg.* 1991; **214**(3):300–6; discussion 306–7.
63. Buchheit, J. Q. & Stewart, D. L. Clinical comparison of localized intestinal perforation and necrotizing enterocolitis in neonates [see comment]. *Pediatrics* 1994; **93**(1):32–36.
64. Aschner, J. L., Deluga, K. S., Metlay, L. A., Emmens, R. W., & Hendricks-Munoz, K. D. Spontaneous focal gastrointestinal perforation in very low birth weight infants. *J. Pediatr.* 1988; **113**(2):364–367.
65. Meyer, C. L., Payne, N. R., & Roback, S. A. Spontaneous, isolated intestinal perforations in neonates with birth weight less than 1,000 g not associated with necrotizing enterocolitis. *J. Pediatr. Surg.* 1991; **26**(6):714–717.
66. Mintz, A. C. & Applebaum, H. Focal gastrointestinal perforations not associated with necrotizing enterocolitis in very low birth weight neonates. *J. Pediatr. Surg.* 1993; **28**(6):857–860.
67. Novack, C. M., Waffarn, F., Sills, J. H., Pousti, T. J., Warden, M. J., & Cunningham, M. D. Focal intestinal perforation in the extremely-low-birth-weight infant. *J. Perinatol.* 1994; **14**(6):450–453.
68. Raghuveer, T. S., McGuire, E. M., Martin, S. M. *et al.* Lactoferrin in the preterm infants' diet attenuates iron-induced oxidation products. *Pediatr. Res.* 2002; **52**(6):964–972.
69. Uceda, J. E., Laos, C. A., Kolni, H. W., & Klein, A. M. Intestinal perforations in infants with a very low birth weight: a disease of increasing survival?[see comment]. *J. Pediatr. Surg.* 1995; **30**(9):1314–1316.
70. Hwang, H., Murphy, J. J., Gow, K. W., Magee, J. F., Bekhit, E., & Jamieson, D. Are localized intestinal perforations distinct from necrotizing enterocolitis? *J. Pediatr. Surg.* 2003; **38**(5):763–767.
71. Cass, D. L., Brandt, M. L., Patel, D. L., Nuchtern, J. G., Minifee, P. K., & Wesson, D. E. Peritoneal drainage as definitive treatment for neonates with isolated intestinal perforation. *J. Pediatr. Surg.* 2000; **35**(11):1531–1536.
72. Pumberger, W., Mayr, M., Kohlhauser, C., & Weninger, M. Spontaneous localized intestinal perforation in very-low-birth-weight infants: a distinct clinical entity different from necrotizing enterocolitis. *J. Am. Coll. Surg.* 2002; **195**(6):796–803.
73. Weber, T. R. & Lewis, J. E. The role of second-look laparotomy in necrotizing enterocolitis. *J. Pediatr. Surg.* 1986; **21**(4):323–325.
74. Vaughan, W. G., Grosfeld, J. L., West, K., Scherer, L. R., 3rd, Villamizar, E., & Rescorla, F. J. Avoidance of stomas and delayed anastomosis for bowel necrosis: the 'clip and drop-back' technique. *J. Pediatr. Surg.* 1996; **31**(4):542–545.
75. Luzzatto, C., Previtera, C., Boscolo, R., Katende, M., Orzali, A., & Guglielmi, M. Necrotizing enterocolitis: late surgical results after enterostomy without resection. *Eur. J. Pediatr. Surg.* 1996; **6**(2):92–94.
76. Fasching, G., Hollwarth, M. E., Schmidt, B., & Mayr, J. Surgical strategies in very-low-birthweight neonates with necrotizing enterocolitis. *Acta. Paediatr. Suppl.* 1994; **396**:62–64.
77. Beasley, S. W., Auldist, A. W., & Ramanjuan, T. M. The surgical management of neonatal necrotizing enterocolitis: 1975–1984. *Pediatr. Surg. Int.* 1994; **1**:210–217.
78. de Souza, J. C., da Motta, U. I., & Ketzer, C. R. Prognostic factors of mortality in newborns with necrotizing enterocolitis submitted to exploratory laparotomy. *J. Pediatr. Surg.* 2001; **36**(3):482–486.
79. Thompson, J. S., Quigley, E. M. M., & Adrian, T. E. Effect of intestinal tapering and lengthening on intestinal structure and function. *Am. J. Surg.* 1995; **169**:111–119.
80. Mayr, J., Fasching, G., & Hollwarth, M. E. Psychosocial and psychomotoric development of very low birthweight infants with necrotizing enterocolitis. *Acta Paediatr. Suppl.* 1994; **396**:96–100.
81. Goulet, O. J., Revillon, Y., Jan, D. *et al.* Neonatal short bowel syndrome. *J. Pediatr.* 1991; **119**(1 (Pt 1)):18–23.
82. Georgeson, K. E. & Breaux, C. W., Jr. Outcome and intestinal adaptation in neonatal short-bowel syndrome. *J. Pediatr. Surg.* 1992; **27**(3):344–348; discussion 348–350.
83. Chaet, M. S., Farrell, M. K., Ziegler, M. M., & Warner, B. W. Intensive nutritional support and remedial surgical intervention for extreme short bowel syndrome. *J. Pediatr. Gastroenterol. Nutrit.* 1994; **19**(3):295–298.
84. Fasoli, L., Turi, R. A., Spitz, L., Kiely, E. M., Drake, D., & Pierro, A. Necrotizing enterocolitis: extent of disease and surgical treatment. *J. Pediatr. Surg.* 1999; **34**(7):1096–1099.
85. Andorsky, D. J., Lund, D. P., Lillehei, C. W. *et al.* Nutritional and other postoperative management of neonates with short bowel syndrome correlates with clinical outcomes.[see comment]. *J. Pediatr.* 2001; **139**(1):27–33.
86. Cooper, A., Floyd, T. F., Ross, A. J., 3rd, Bishop, H. C., Templeton, J. M., Jr., & Ziegler, M. M. Morbidity and mortality of short-bowel syndrome acquired in infancy: an update. *J. Pediatr. Surg.* 1984; **19**(6):711–718.
87. Sondheimer, J. M., Sokol, R. J., Narkewicz, M. R., & Tyson, R. W. Anastomotic ulceration: a late complication of ileocolonic anastomosis. *J. Pediatr.* 1995; **127**(2):225–230.
88. Weber, T. R., Tracy, T., Jr., & Connors, R. H. Short-bowel syndrome in children. Quality of life in an era of improved survival. *Arch. Surg.* 1991; **126**(7):841–846.
89. Stringer, M. D., Brereton, R. J., Drake, D. P., Kiely, E. M., Capps, S. N., & Spitz, L. Recurrent necrotizing enterocolitis. *J. Pediatr. Surg.* 1993; **28**(8):979–981.
90. Frantz, I. D., 3rd, L'Heureux, P., Engel, R. R., & Hunt, C. E. Necrotizing enterocolitis. *J. Pediatr.* 1975; **86**(2):259–263.
91. Vollman, J. H., Smith, W. L., & Tsang, R. C. Necrotizing enterocolitis with recurrent hepatic portal venous gas. *J. Pediatr.* 1976; **88**(3):486–487.
92. Mollitt, D. L. & Golladay, E. S. Postoperative neonatal necrotizing enterocolitis. *J. Pediatr. Surg.* 1982; **17**(6):757–763.
93. Oldham, K. T., Coran, A. G., Drongowski, R. A., Baker, P. J., Wesley, J. R., & Polley, T. Z., Jr. The development of necrotizing enterocolitis following repair of gastroschisis: a surprisingly high incidence. *J. Pediatr. Surg.* 1988; **23**(10):945–949.

94. Shanbhogue, L. K., Tam, P. K., & Lloyd, D. A. Necrotizing enterocolitis following operation in the neonatal period. *Br. J. Surg.* 1991; **78**(9):1045–1047.
95. Gauderer, M.W. Stomas of the small and large intestine. In O'Neill, J. A., Jr., Rowe, M. I., Grosfeld, J., Fonkalsrud, E. W., & Coran, A. G., eds. *Pediatric Surgery*. 5th edn. St. Louis: Mosby, 1998: 1349–1359.
96. Musemeche, C. A., Kosloske, A. M., & Ricketts, R. R. Enterostomy in necrotizing enterocolitis: an analysis of techniques and timing of closure. *J. Pediatr. Surg.* 1987; **22**(6):479–483.
97. Alaish, S. M., Krummel, T. M., Bagwell, C. E., Michna, B. A., Drucker, D. E., & Salzberg, A. M. Loop enterostomy in newborns with necrotizing enterocolitis. *J. Am. Coll. Surg.* 1996; **182**(5):457–458.
98. O'Connor, A. & Sawin, R. S. High morbidity of enterostomy and its closure in premature infants with necrotizing enterocolitis. *Arch. Surg.* 1998; **133**(8):875–880.
99. Lemelle, J. L., Schmitt, M., de Miscault, G., Vert, P., & Hascoet, J. M. Neonatal necrotizing enterocolitis: a retrospective and multicentric review of 331 cases. *Acta. Paediatr. Suppl.* 1994; **396**:70–73.
100. Haberlik, A., Hollwarth, M. E., Windhager, U., & Schober, P. H. Problems of ileostomy in necrotizing enterocolitis. *Acta. Paediatr. Suppl.* 1994; 396:74–76.
101. Cogbill, T. H. & Millikan, J. S. Reconstitution of intestinal continuity after resection for neonatal necrotizing enterocolitis. *Surg., Gynecol. Obstetr.* 1985; **160**(4):330–334.
102. Gertler, J. P., Seashore, J. H., & Touloukian, R. J. Early ileostomy closure in necrotizing enterocolitis. *J. Pediatr. Surg.* 1987; **22**(2):140–143.
103. Sugarman, I. D. & Kiely, E. M. Is there a role for high jejunostomy in the management of severe necrotising enterocolitis? *Pediatr. Surg. Int.* 2001; **17**(2–3):122–124.
104. O'Neill, J. A., Jr., & Holcomb, G. W., Jr. Surgical experience with neonatal necrotizing enterocolitis (NNE). *Ann. Surg.* 1979; **189**(5):612–619.
105. Rowe, M. I. Necrotizing enterocolitis. In Welch, K. J., Randolph, J. G., & Ravitch, M. M., eds. *Pediatric Surgery*. 4th edn. Chicago: Year Book Medical, 1986: 944–958.
106. Ricketts, R. R. Surgical therapy for necrotizing enterocolitis. *Ann. Surg.* 1984; **200**(5):653–657.
107. Gobet, R., Sacher, P., & Schwobel, M. G. Surgical procedures in colonic strictures after necrotizing enterocolitis. *Acta. Paediatr. Suppl.* 1994; **396**:77–79.
108. Philippart, A. Necrotizing enterocolitis. In Ravitch, M. M., Welch, K. J., & Benson, C. D., eds. *Pediatric Surgery*. 3rd edn. Chicago: Year Book Medical, 1979: 970–976.
109. Rothstein, F. C., Halpin, T. C., Jr., Kliegman, R. J., & Izant, R. J., Jr. Importance of early ileostomy closure to prevent chronic salt and water losses after necrotizing enterocolitis. *Pediatrics* 1982; **70**(2):249–253.
110. Schwartz, M. Z., Hayden, C. K., Richardson, C. J., Tyson, K. R., & Lobe, T. E. A prospective evaluation of intestinal stenosis following necrotizing enterocolitis. *J. Pediatr. Surg.* 1982; **17**(6):764–770.
111. Schimpl, G., Hollwarth, M. E., Fotter, R., & Becker, H. Late intestinal strictures following successful treatment of necrotizing enterocolitis. *Acta. Paediatr. Suppl.* 1994; **396**:80–83.
112. Radhakrishnan, J., Blechman, G., Shrader, C., Patel, M. K., Mangurten, H. H., & McFadden, J. C. Colonic strictures following successful medical management of necrotizing enterocolitis: a prospective study evaluating early gastrointestinal contrast studies. *J. Pediatr. Surg.* 1991; **26**(9):1043–1046.
113. Hartman, G. E., Drugas, G. T., & Shochat, S. J. Post-necrotizing enterocolitis strictures presenting with sepsis or perforation: risk of clinical observation. *J. Pediatr. Surg.* 1988; **23**(6):562–566.
114. Butter, A., Flageole, H., & Laberge, J. M. The changing face of surgical indications for necrotizing enterocolitis. *J. Pediatr. Surg.* 2002; **37**(3):496–499.
115. Kosloske, A. M., Burstein, J., & Bartow, S. A. Intestinal obstruction due to colonic stricture following neonatal necrotizing enterocolitis. *Ann. Surg.* 1980; **192**(2):202–207.
116. Weber, T. R., Tracy, T. F., Jr., Silen, M. L., & Powell, M. A. Enterostomy and its closure in newborns. *Arch. Surg.* 1995; **130**(5):534–537.
117. Bell, M. J., Ternberg, J. L., Askin, F. B., McAlister, W., & Shackelford, G. Intestinal stricture in necrotizing enterocolitis. *J. Pediatr. Surg.* 1976; **11**(3):319–327.
118. Schwartz, M. Z., Richardson, C. J., Hayden, C. K., Swischuk, L. E., & Tyson, K. R. Intestinal stenosis following successful medical management of necrotizing enterocolitis. *J. Pediatr. Surg.* 1980; **15**(6):890–899.
119. Kosloske, A. M. Surgery of necrotizing enterocolitis. *World J. Surg.* 1985; **9**(2):277–284.
120. Janik, J. S., Ein, S. H., & Mancer, K. Intestinal stricture after necrotizing enterocolitis. *J. Pediatr. Surg.* 1981; **16**(4):438–443.
121. Robertson, J. F., Azmy, A. F., & Young, D. G. Surgery for necrotizing enterocolitis. *Br. J. Surg.* 1987; **74**(5):387–389.
122. Born, M., Holgersen, L. O., Shahrivar, F., Stanley-Brown, E., & Hilfer, C. Routine contrast enemas for diagnosing and managing strictures following nonoperative treatment of necrotizing enterocolitis. *J. Pediatr. Surg.* 1985; **20**(4):461–463.
123. Kliegman, R. M. & Fanaroff, A. A. Necrotizing enterocolitis. *N. Engl. J. Med.* 1984; **310**(17):1093–1103.
124. Tonkin, I. L., Bjelland, J. C., Hunter, T. B., Capp, M. P., Firor, H., & Ermocilla, R. Spontaneous resolution of colonic strictures caused by necrotizing enterocolitis: therapeutic implications. AJR. *Am. J. Roentgenol.* 1978; **130**(6):1077–1081.
125. Ball, W. S., Jr., Kosloske, A. M., Jewell, P. F., Seigel, R. S., & Bartow, S. A. Balloon catheter dilatation of focal intestinal strictures following necrotizing enterocolitis. *J. Pediatr. Surg.* 1985; **20**(6):637–639.
126. Limpert, J. N., Limpert, P. A., Weber, T. R. *et al.* The impact of surgery on infants born at extremely low birth weight. *J. Pediatr. Surg.* 2003; **38**(6):924–927.
127. Santulli, T. V., Schullinger, J. N., Heird, W. C. *et al.* Acute necrotizing enterocolitis in infancy: a review of 64 cases. *Pediatrics* 1975; **55**(3):376–387.

128. Touloukian, R. J. Neonatal necrotizing enterocolitis: an update on etiology, diagnosis, and treatment. *Surg. Clin. North Am.* 1976; **56**(2):281–298.
129. Guthrie, S. O., Gordon, P. V., Thomas, V., Thorp, J. A., Peabody, J., & Clark, R. H. Necrotizing enterocolitis among neonates in the United States. *J. Perinatol.* 2003; **23**(4):278–285.
130. Kosloske, A. M. Operative techniques for the treatment of neonatal necrotizing enterocolitis. *Surg., Gynecol. Obstet.* 1979; **149**(5):740–744.
131. Camberos, A., Patel, K., & Applebaum, H. Laparotomy in very small premature infants with necrotizing enterocolitis or focal intestinal perforation: postoperative outcome. *J. Pediatr. Surg.* 2002; **37**(12):1692–1695.
132. Wilmore, D. W. Factors correlating with a successful outcome following extreme intestinal resection in newborn infants. *J. Pediatr.* 1972; **80**:88–95.
133. Galea, M., Holliday, H., & Carachi, L. Short-bowel syndrome: a collective review. *J. Pediatr. Surg.* 1992; **27**:592–596.
134. Sigalet, D. L. Short bowel syndrome in infants and children: an overview. *Semin. Pediatr. Surg.* 2001; **10**(2):49–55.
135. Sondheimer, J. M., Cadnapaphornchai, M., Sontag, M., & Zerbe, G. O. Predicting the duration of dependence on enteral nutrition after neonatal intestinal resection. *J. Pediatr.* 1998; **132**:80–84.
136. Touloukian, R. J. & Smith, G. J. Normal intestinal length in preterm infants. *J. Pediatr. Surg.* 1983; **18**(6):720–723.
137. Georgeson, K.E. Short-bowel syndrome. In O'Neill, J. A., Jr., Rowe, M. I., Grosfeld, J., Fonkalsrud, E. W., & Coran, A. G., eds. *Pediatric Surgery*. 5th edn. Mosby, 1998; 1223–1232.
138. Thompson, J. S. Surgical rehabilitation of intestine in short bowel syndrome. *Surgery* 2004; **135**:465–470.
139. Kaufman, S. S., Loseke, C. A., & Lupo, J. V. Influence of bacterial overgrowth and intestinal inflammation on duration of parenteral nutrition in children with short bowel syndrome. *J. Pediatr.* 1997; **131**:356–361.
140. Kurkchubasche, A. G., Rowe, M., & Smith, S. Adaptation in short-bowel syndrome: reassessing old limits. *J. Pediatr. Surg.* 1993; **28**:1069–1071.
141. Cooper, A., Ross, A. J., 3rd, O'Neill, J. A., Jr., & Schnaufer, L. Resection with primary anastomosis for necrotizing enterocolitis: a contrasting view. *J. Pediatr. Surg.* 1988; **23**(1 Pt 2):64–68.
142. Bines, J., Francis, D., & Hill, D. Reducing parenteral requirement in children with short-bowel syndrome: impact of an amino acid-based complete infant formula. *J. Pediatr. Gastroenterol. Nutrit.* 1998; **26**:123–128.
143. Bianchi, A. Intestinal loop lengthening – a technique for increasing small intestinal length. *J. Pediatr. Surg.* 1980; **15**:145–151.
144. Figueroa-Colon, R., Harris, P. R., Birdsong, E., Franklin, F. A., & Georgeson, K. E. Impact of intestinal lengthening on the nutritional outcome for children with short bowel syndrome. *J. Pediatr. Surg.* 1996; **31**(7):912–916.
145. Kim, H. B., Lee, P. W., & Garza, J. Serial transverse enteroplasty for short bowel syndrome: a case report. *J. Pediatr. Surg.* 2003; **38**:881–885.
146. Kim, H. B., Fauza, D., & Garza, J. Serial transverse enteroplasty (STEP): a novel bowel lengthening procedure. *J. Pediatr. Surg.* 2003; **38**:425–529.
147. Hwang, S. T. & Shulman, R. J. Update on management and treatment of short gut. *Clin. Perinatol.* 2002; **29**:181–194.
148. Moss, R. L. & Amii, L. A. New approaches to understanding the etiology and treatment of total parenteral nutrition-associated cholestasis. *Semin. Pediatr Surg.* 1999; **8**:140–147.
149. Hodes, J. E., Grosfeld, J. L., & Weber, T. R. Hepatic failure in infants on total parenteral nutrition: clinical and histopathological observations. *J. Pediatr. Surg.* 1982; **17**:463–468.
150. Moss, R. L., Das, J. B., & Raffensperger, J. G. Total parenteral nutrition-associated cholestasis: clinical and histopathologic correlation. *J. Pediatr. Surg.* 1993; **28**(10):1270–1274; discussion 1274–1275.
151. Kubota, A., Yonekura, T., Hoki, M. *et al.* Total parenteral nutrition-associated intrahepatic cholestasis in infants: 25 years' experience. *J. Pediatr. Surg.* 2000; **35**:1049–1051.
152. Amii, L. A. & Moss, R. L. Nutritional support of the pediatric surgical patient. *Curr. Opin. Pediatr.* 1999; **11**:237–240.
153. Curran, T. J., Uzoaru, I., & Das, J. B. The effect of cholecystokinin-octapeptide on the hepatobiliary dysfunction caused by total parenteral nutrition. *J. Pediatr. Surg.* 1995; **30**:242–247.
154. Dawes, L. G., Muldoon, J. P., & Greiner, M. A. Cholecystokinin increases bile acid synthesis with total parenteral nutrition but does not prevent stone formation. *J. Surg. Res.* 1997; **67**:84–89.
155. Teitelbaum, D. H., Han-Markey, T., & Schumacher, R. Treatment of parenteral nutrition-associated cholestasis with cholecystokinin-octapeptide. *J. Pediatr. Surg.* 1995; **30**:1082–1085.
156. Teitelbaum, D. H., Han-Markey, T., & Drowngowski, R. A. Use of cholecystokinin to prevent the development of parenteral nutrition-associated cholestasis. *J. Parenteral Enteral Nutrit.* 1997; **21**:100–103.
157. Beck, R. Use of a pediatric parenteral amino acid mixture in a population of extremely low birth weight neonates: frequency and spectrum of direct bilirubinemia. *Am. J. Perinatol.* 1990; **7**:84–86.
158. Vanderhoof, J. A. & Langnas, A. N. Short bowel syndrome in children and adults. *Gastroenterology* 1997; **113**:1767–1778.
159. Meehan, J. J. & Georgeson, K. Prevention of liver failure in parenteral nutrition-dependent children with short bowel syndrome. *J. Pediatric. Surg.* 1997; **32**:473–475.
160. Vanderhoof, J. A., Young, R. J., & Thompson, J. S. New and emerging therapies for short bowel syndrome in children. *Pediatr. Drugs* 2003; **5**:525–531.
161. Terra, R. M., Plopper, C., Waitzberg, D. L. *et al.* Remaining small bowel length: association with catheter sepsis in patients receiving home total parenteral nutrition: evidence of bacterial translocation. *World J. Surg.* 2000; **24**:1537–1541.

162. Lloyd, D. A. Central venous catheters for parenteral nutrition: a double-edged sword. *J. Pediatr. Surg.* 1997; **32**:943–948.
163. Klein, M. D., Rood, K., & Graham, P. Central venous catheter sepsis in surgical newborns. *Pediatr. Surg. Int.* 2003; **19**:529–532.
164. Attar, A. & Messing, B. Evidence-based prevention of catheter infection during parenteral nutrition. *Curr. Opin. Clini. Nutrit. Metab. Care* 2001; **4**:211–218.
165. Moukarzel, A. A., Haddad, I., Ament, M. E. *et al.* 230 patient years of experience with home long-term parenteral nutrition in childhood: natural history and life of central venous catheters. *J. Pediatr. Surg.* 1994; **29**:1323–1327.
166. Okada, Y., Klein, N. J., & Pierro, A. Neutrophil dysfunction: the cellular mechanism of impaired immunity during total parenteral nutrition in infancy. *J. Pediatr. Surg.* 1999; **34**:242–245.
167. Pierro, A., van Saene, H. K., Jones, M. O., Brown, D. R., Nunn, A. J., & Lloyd, D. A. Clinical impact of abnormal gut flora in infants receiving parenteral nutrition. *Ann. Surg.* 1998; **227**:547–552.
168. Pierro, A., van Saene, H. K., Donnell, S. C. *et al.* Microbial translocation in neonates and infants receiving long-term parenteral nutrition. *Arch. Surg.* 1996; **131**:176–179.
169. Sondheimer, J. M., Asturias, E., & Cadnapaphornchai, M. Infection and cholestasis in neonates with intestinal resection and long-term parenteral nutrition. *J. Pediatr. Gastroenterol. Nutrit.* 1998; **27**:131–137.
170. Wolf, A. & Pohlandt, F. Bacterial infection: the main cause of acute cholestasis in newborn infants receiving short term parenteral nutrition. *J Pediatr. Gastroenterol. Nutrit.* 1989; **8**:297–303.
171. Sokal, E. M., Cleghorn, G., Goulet, O. J., Silveira, T. R., McDiarmid, S., & Whitington, P. F. Liver and intestinal transplantation in children: Working group report of the first world congress of pediatric gatroenterology, hepatology, and nutrition. *J. Pediatr. Gastroenterol. Nutrit.* 2002; **35**:S159–S172.
172. Mittal, N., Tzakis, A., Kato, T., & Thompson, J. F. Current status of small bowel transplantation in children: an update. *Pediatr. Clin. N. Am.* 2003; 50.
173. Howard, L. & Hassan, N. Home parenteral nutrition – 25 years later. *Gastroenterol. Clini. N. Am.* 1998; **27**:481–512.
174. Howard, L., Ament, M. E., Fleming, C.Rea. Current use and clinical outcome of home parenteral and enteral nutrition therapies in the United States. *Gastroenterology* 1995; **109**:355–365.
175. Iyer, K. R., Srinath, C., Horslen, S. *et al.* Late graft loss and long-term outcome after isolated intestinal transplantation in children. *J. Pediatr. Surg.* 2002; **37**:151–154.
176. Hasegawa, T., Sasaki, T., Kimura, T. *et al.* Effects of isolated small bowel transplantation on liver dysfunction caused by intestinal failure and long-term total parenteral nutrition. *Pediatr. Transpl.* 2002; **6**:235–239.
177. Muiesan, P., Dhawan, A., Novelli, M., Mieli-Vergani, G., Rela, M., & Heaton, N. Isolated liver transplantation and sequential small bowel transplantation for intestinal failure and related liver disease in children. *Transplantation* 2000; **69**:2323–2326.
178. Fecteau, A., Atkinson, P., & Grant, D. Early referral is essential for successful pediatric small bowel transplantation: the Canadian experience. *J. Pediatr. Surg.* 2001; **36**:681–684.
179. Reyes, J., Bueno, J., Kocoshis, S. *et al.* Current status of intestinal transplantation in children. *J. Pediatr. Surg.* 1998; **33**(2):243–254.
180. Bueno, J., Ohwada, S., Kocoshis, S. *et al.* Factors impacting the survival of children with intestinal failure referred for intestinal transplantation. *J. Pediatr. Surg.* 1999; **34**(1):27–32; discussion 32–33.
181. Reyes, J., Mazariegos, G., Bond, G. M. *et al.* Pediatric intestinal transplantation: historical notes, principles, and controversies. *Pediatr. Transpl.* 2002; **6**:193–207.
182. Fishbein, T. M., Schiano, T., & LeLeiko, N. S. An integrated approach to intestinal failure: results of a new program with total parenteral nutrition, bowel rehabilitation and transplantation. *J. Gastrointestinal Surg.* 2002; **6**:554–562.
183. Fishbein, T. M., Kaufman, S. S., Florman, S. S. *et al.* Isolated intestinal transplantation: proof of clinical efficacy. *Transplantation* 2003; **76**:636–640.
184. Nishida, S., Levi, D., Kato, T. *et al.* Ninety-five cases of intestinal transplantation at the University of Miami. *J. Gastrointestinal Surg.* 2002; **6**(2):233–239.
185. Kato, T., Mittal, N., Nishida, S. *et al.* The role of intestinal transplantation in the management of babies with extensive gut resections. *J. Pediatr. Surg.* 2003; **38**(2):145–149.
186. Vennarecci, G., Kato, T., Misiakos, E. P. *et al.* Intestinal transplantation for short gut syndrome attributable to necrotizing enterocolitis. *Pediatrics* 2000; **105**(2):E25.
187. Nucci, A. M., Barksdale, E. M., Beserock, N. *et al.* Long-term nutritional outcome after pediatric intestinal transplantation. *J. Pediatr. Surgery.* 2002; **37**:460–463.
188. Iyer, K. R., Horslen, S., Iverson, A. *et al.* Nutritional outcome and growth of children after intestinal transplantation. *J. Pediatr. Surg.* 2002; **37**:464–466.
189. Grant, D. Intestinal transplantation: 1997 report of the international registry. *Transplantation* 1999; **67**:1061–1064.
190. Stanford, A., Upperman, J. S., Boyle, P., Schall, L., Ojimba, J. I., & Ford, H. R. Long-term follow-up of patients with necrotizing enterocolitis. *J. Pediatr. Surg.* 2002; **37**(7):1048–1050; discussion 1048–1050.
191. Orellana, C. B., Orellana, F. A., & Friesen, C. Long-term follow-up: neurodevelopmental outcome and gastrointestinal function in infants <801 grams diagnosed with necrotizing enterocolitis. *Pediatr. Res.* 2003; **54**:773–782.
192. Whiteman, L., Wuethrich, M., & Egan, E. Infants who survive necrotizing enterocolitis. *Maternal–Child Nurs. J.* 1985; **14**(2):123–133.
193. Sonntag, J., Grimmer, I., Scholz, T., Metze, B., Wit, J., & Obladen, M. Growth and neurodevelopmental outcome of very low birthweight infants with necrotizing enterocolitis. *Acta. Paediatr.* 2000; **89**(5):528–532.

194. Walsh, M. C., Kliegman, R. M., & Hack, M. Severity of necrotizing enterocolitis: influence on outcome at 2 years of age. *Pediatrics* 1989; **84**(5):808–814.

195. Cikrit, D., West, K. W., Schreiner, R., & Grosfeld, J. L. Long-term follow-up after surgical management of necrotizing enterocolitis: sixty-three cases. *J. Pediatr. Surg.* 1986; **21**(6):533–535.

196. Abbasi, S., Pereira, G. R., Johnson, L., Stahl, G. E., Duara, S., & Watkins, J. B. Long-term assessment of growth, nutritional status, and gastrointestinal function in survivors of necrotizing enterocolitis. *J. Pediatr.* 1984; **104**(4):550–554.

197. Chacko, J., Ford, W. D., & Haslam, R. Growth and neurodevelopmental outcome in extremely-low-birth-weight infants after laparotomy. *Pediatr. Surg. Int.* 1999; **15**(7):496–499.

198. Kitchen, W., Ford, G., & Orgill, A. Outcome in infants with birth weight 500 to 999 gm: a regional study of 1979 births. *J. Pediatr.* 1984; **104**:921–927.

199. Group VICS. Surgery and the tiny baby: sensorineural outcome at 5 years of age. *J. Paediatr. Child Hlth.* 1996; **32**:167–172.

200. Doyle, L. W. for the Victorian Infant Collaborative Study Group. Outcome to five years of age of children at 24–16 weeks' gestational age in Victoria. *Med. J. Aust.* 1995; **163**:11–14.

201. Goldstein, R. F., Thompson, R. J., & Oehler, J. M. Influence on acidosis, hypoxemia, and hypotension on neurodevelopmental outcome in very low birth weight infants. *Pediatrics* 1995; **95**:238–243.

202. Ludman, L., Spitz, L., & Lansdown, R. Developmental progress of newborns undergoing neonatal surgery. *J. Pediatr. Surg.* 1990; **25**:469–471.

203. Vohr, B. R., Wright, L. L., Dusick, A. M. *et al.* Neurodevelopmental and functional outcomes of extremely low birth weight infants in the National Institute of Child Health and Human Development Neonatal Research Network, 1993–1994. *Pediatrics* 2000; **105**(6):1216–1226.

Inflammatory bowel disease in children

Frederick Alexander

Department of Pediatric Surgery, Cleveland Clinic, OH, USA

Introduction

Inflammatory bowel disease is a chronic intestinal disease of unknown etiology that takes several different forms including Crohn's disease and ulcerative colitis. Typically the inflammation in Crohn's disease is panenteric and full-thickness while in ulcerative colitis it is usually limited to colorectal mucosa. These archetypal diseases may sometimes be difficult to distinguish because they may have similar presenting features, especially when there is colonic involvement and both are associated with similar extra-intestinal manifestations. Histologically, Crohn's disease is characterized by apthous ulceration and cobblestoning with rectal sparing while ulcerative colitis is manifested by crypt abscesses and depletion of goblet cells with continuous inflammation always involving the rectum. However, in as many as 10% or more of patients, the histology may be indeterminate. The surgical treatment for Crohn's disease and ulcerative colitis and the outcomes vary considerably, and these are the subjects of this chapter.

Crohn's disease

Epidemiology

Crohn's disease is more common than ulcerative colitis, occurring in 11 cases per 100 000 population per year, versus 2.3 cases of ulcerative colitis per 100 000 population per year in the pediatric age group.[1] The incidence of Crohn's disease is age specific, occurring in 2.5 cases per 100 000 population per year in persons less than 15 years of age compared to 16 cases per 100 000 population per year in persons 15–19 years of age.[2] Males and females are equally affected and Crohn's disease occurs more commonly in the Caucasian and Jewish populations compared to other ethnic groups. Finally, the incidence of juvenile Crohn's disease appears to be rising in Western cultures as evidenced by a threefold rise in Scotland between 1968 and 1983.[3]

Etiology of Crohn's disease

The etiology of Crohn's disease is unknown; however, there are a number of risk factors that appear to be relevant. For example, there appears to be a genetic predisposition such that patients with Crohn's disease have a 5%–25% chance of having a first degree relative risk with inflammatory bowel disease.[4] The likelihood of a sibling developing Crohn's disease is 7%, while that of offspring is 9%. In addition, there is a high concordance between monozygotic twins. Moreover, certain infectious agents such as mycobacterium paratuberculosis and measles virus, have been implicated, both of which may cause granulomatous inflammation, sepsis, and fistulas. Tissue destruction in patients with Crohn's disease occurs in areas heavily infiltrated by lymphocytes that appear to lose the usual self-limited response to antigenic stimulation. The hypothesis has been offered that poorly controlled release of cytokines, arachidonic acid metabolites, and reactive oxygen intermediates leads to the local histological perturbations characteristic of the disease. Recent studies[5] have shown that cytokines such as IL1, IL4, IL8, IL12, TNF, and gamma IFN recruit inflammatory cells, promote collagen production, and induce local eosinophil degranulation, stimulating chloride secretion and causing diarrhea. The sequence of steps involved in the progression from immune activation to tissue injury are not well understood but likely involve abnormal T-helper

Pediatric Surgery and Urology: Long-term Outcomes, Mark Stringer, Keith Oldham, Pierre Mouriquand.
Published by Cambridge University Press.

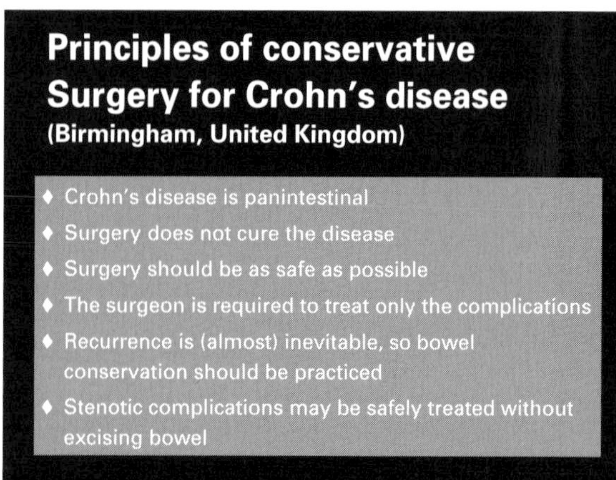

Fig. 27.1. Conservative therapy for Crohn's disease.

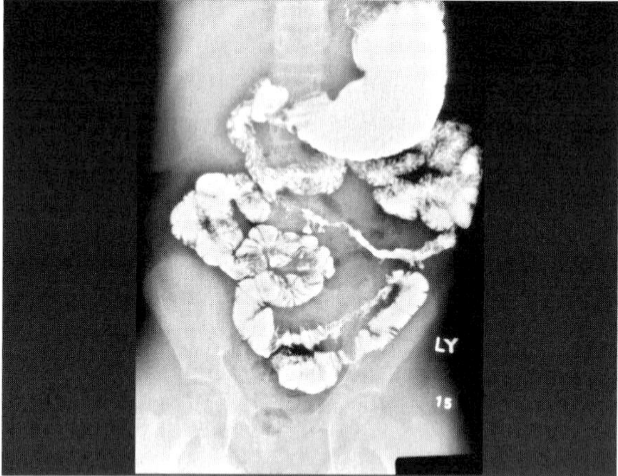

Fig. 27.2. Panenteric Crohn's disease.

cell responses and/or release of oxygen metabolites that are potent cytotoxins.[6] Finally, although there is no direct evidence that Crohn's disease is stimulated by dietary allergens, it is known that serum antibodies to cow's milk protein are elevated in many patients with Crohn's disease.

Pathology

In a series of 361 patients treated for Crohn's disease at The Cleveland Clinic Foundation, the disease involved the terminal ileum and colon in 60% of patients, the small bowel only in 30% of patients, and the large bowel only in 10% of patients.[7] The involved bowel and mesentery is thickened from collagen deposition and edema along with fat migration over serosal surfaces (fat wrapping). Histologically, there is extensive apthous ulceration of mucosa that grossly has a cobblestone appearance due to adjacent areas of mucosal ulceration and regeneration. This is sometimes referred to as a "bear claw" deformity. Often, the inflammation is interspersed with normal appearing mucosa giving the appearance of skip areas. The inflammation is usually transmural and tends to erode into adjacent structures, resulting in fistulas from bowel to other structures including the bowel, bladder, abdominal wall, vagina, or perineum. Fistulas may also end blindly to form localized areas of inflammation or phlegmon. Histologic evidence of granulomas is found in 40% of affected small bowel specimens, 60%–80% of endoscopic biopsies taken from the stomach, and 25% of endoscopic biopsies taken from the colon.[8]

Clinical presentation

Crohn's disease occurs with increasing frequency in older age groups within a pediatric population. Four percent of new cases occur at 6–10 years of age, 31% between 11 and 15 years, and 65% in the 15–20 year age group.[2] Most young people have been symptomatic for 2 years when the diagnosis of Crohn's disease is made. The diagnosis is suggested by a history of chronic, intermittent, crampy abdominal pain associated with diarrhea, weight loss, rectal bleeding, and a family history of inflammatory bowel disease. Clinical findings include abdominal tenderness or a mass with perianal disease, clubbing, stomatitis, or rash. Serial measurements of height and weight may demonstrate weight loss or growth failure. Growth failure appears to result from anorexia, malnutrition and diarrhea as well as corticosteroid inhibition of IGF-1 and collagen metabolism. Approximately 10% of children develop arthralgias and arthritis that may present several years prior to the bowel disease. Skin manifestations such as erythema nodosum and pyoderma gangrenosum occur in 1%–4% of patients and eye manifestations such as iritis and uveitis occur in less than 10% of patients.[9] Renal stones composed of calcium oxylate and uric acid occur in up to 5% of patients with Crohn's disease and gallstones are also seen in 2%–5% of patients.[9]

Diagnosis

Laboratory studies for patients with Crohn's disease are non-specific but often contributory. Seventy percent of patients are anemic, 60% have thrombocytosis, and 80% have an elevated erythrocyte sedimentation rate. Nutritional markers such as albumin and pre-albumin are abnormally low in more than one half of all patients with Crohn's disease. Stool guaiac is positive in one-third of patients and all stools should be thoroughly evaluated for enteric pathogens such as *Clostridium difficile*, Rotavirus, and *Campylobacter*.

Radiographic studies are useful screening tools in patients with Crohn's disease. More than 80% of patients with Crohn's disease have small bowel involvement and thus upper gastrointestinal contrast series and small bowel follow-through should be performed in most cases. Positive findings include terminal ileal nodularity and narrowing, with thickening and separation of bowel loops. CT scan with IV/GI contrast may show thickened bowel loops and is helpful in identifying phlegmon or abscess formation.

Finally, upper and lower endoscopy allows direct mucosal observation and histologic sampling. The finding of rectal sparing by colonoscopy effectively eliminates the possibility of ulcerative colitis and documentation of ileal involvement or granulomas is functionally adequate to establish the diagnosis of Crohn's disease. A small number of patients lack sufficiently distinctive clinical and pathological features to differentiate between Crohn's disease and ulcerative colitis, thus resulting in a diagnosis of indeterminate colitis.

Operative indications and treatment

Surgery does not cure Crohn's disease and should be reserved only for complications of the disease (Fig 27.1). Further, since recurrence of Crohn's disease is inevitable, a conservative surgical strategy is generally warranted. The specific surgical procedure indicated in each case depends upon the site of involvement and the type of complications. The most common complications of Crohn's disease include bowel obstruction, perforation, intra-abdominal and perirectal abscess, fistula, and megacolon. In many cases, these complications present with fulminant signs and symptoms that resolve completely with surgical treatment.

Of children and adolescents with Crohn's disease, 50%–60% present with right lower quadrant pain due to localized disease in the terminal ileum and caecum. Disease in this region of the intestine is frequently complicated by mechanical bowel obstruction, abscess, phlegmon, and/or fistulae formation. Many patients with these complications and associated symptoms may be successfully treated with intravenous antibiotics and steroids. If the symptoms do not completely resolve with medical therapy and/or become associated with growth failure, then surgery becomes necessary. The recommended procedure in this situation is ileocecectomy and primary anastomosis with resection of phlegmon and/or fistulae. The resection margin of the involved small intestine should encompass gross

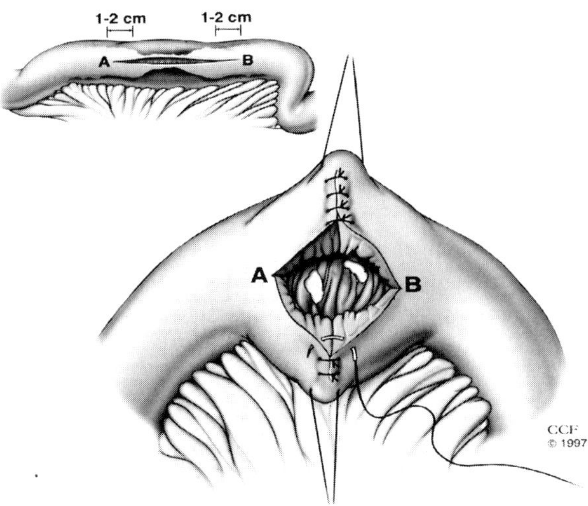

Fig. 27.3. Heineke–Mikulicz strictureplasty.

disease only, since resection of microscopic disease offers no protection against recurrence.[10] Fistulae may be safely resected without the need for wide resection of the wall of the end organ whether it be small intestine, large intestine, bladder, or vagina. In these patients, the fistulae may be transected flush with the end organ and the defect simply closed.

Approximately 20%–30% of children and adolescents with Crohn's disease present with acute and/or chronic small bowel obstruction due to multiple small bowel strictures (Fig. 27.2). Once again, these patients may respond initially to anti-inflammatory agents and immunotherapy. However, most patients will develop chronic bowel obstruction with intermittent but prolonged abdominal pain and growth failure. In the past, surgical treatment was limited to small bowel resection of each stricture, sometimes resulting in short gut syndrome as the result of multiple bowel resections. Currently, small bowel resection is indicated only in patients with small bowel perforation, fistulae formation, or extreme bowel wall thickening that precludes strictureplasty. In virtually all other situations, strictureplasty is the surgical treatment of choice. Short strictures up to 7–10 cm in length may be treated by Heineke–Mikulitz strictureplasty (Fig. 27.3). This procedure is performed by making a longitudinal incision across the stricture and 1–2 cm into "normal" bowel on either side of the stricture. The bowel is then closed transversely using a single layer of closely spaced interrupted full-thickness dissolvable sutures. Longer strictures up to 25–30 cm may be treated by Finney side-to-side anastomosis performed with a back wall of seromuscular sutures and then full thickness dissolvable sutures on the back and front wall of the bowel. Strictureplasty is recommended for all strictures with a linear diameter of 2 cm or less measured by a Foley catheter balloon. However, because of the progressive nature of the disease, it may be advisable to treat all strictures except where the caliber is not compromised. Strictureplasty provides relief of obstructive symptoms and allows discontinuation of corticosteroids in 85% of patients while preserving small intestinal length.[11] Complications of strictureplasty include anastomotic leak and hemorrhage, with an incidence of about 5%–10% which is comparable to bowel resection. The overall frequency of recurrent disease at the site of previous strictureplasty does not differ from that following resection. Further, anecdotal reports have described complete healing of bowel that had undergone previous strictureplasty. Thus, preservation of the diseased bowel does not appear to predispose to early recurrence of disease at the strictureplasty site.

In 10%–20% of children with Crohn's disease, inflammation is limited to the colon and rectum. Crohn's colitis may be patchy or diffuse and is often associated with rectal sparing that does not occur in patients with ulcerative colitis. Crohn's colitis may be associated with perianal disease; however, perianal disease does not necessarily signal the presence of Crohn's colitis. Complications such as perforation, abscess, and fistulae formation are rare with this form of disease, although strictures may occasionally develop in the descending and sigmoid colon. Most patients with Crohn's colitis require surgery for intractable abdominal pain and diarrhea. When Crohn's colitis is unresponsive to medical therapy, surgical options include partial colectomy, total colectomy with ileostomy or ileal rectal anastomosis, and total proctocolectomy with end ileostomy. Partial colectomy should be avoided since it is associated with a high recurrence rate, approaching 60% in 5 years.[12] Total colectomy is an excellent alternative procedure that preserves the possibility of reconstituting the normal fecal stream. When the rectum is severely diseased or there is severe perianal Crohn's disease, total colectomy should be performed with end-ileostomy and Hartmann's pouch as a first stage procedure. When the rectum is spared as judged by normal sphincter and rectal distensibility with insufflation, then primary ileo-rectal anastomosis may be safely performed. Ileo-rectal anastomosis may also be performed as a second stage procedure after the resolution of the rectal disease. Total proctocolectomy and permanent ileostomy is the treatment of choice for patients with severe unrelenting rectal or perianal disease, failed ileo-rectal anastomosis due to recurrent Crohn's disease, or biopsy proven carcinoma *in situ*. It is important when performing this procedure to preserve all tissue extrinsic to the muscular wall of the rectum including the sphincter muscles, in order to avoid the problem of postoperative perineal sinus tracts. Although the ileal pouch–anal anastomosis (IPAA) has become the procedure of choice for ulcerative colitis, this procedure is not appropriate for patients with Crohn's colitis in whom high risk of recurrent disease within the pouch may require excision of the pouch and loss of precious small bowel. Indeterminate colitis does not appear to be a contraindication for IPAA.[13] However, if Crohn's disease is suspected because of rectal sparing or perianal disease, then total colectomy with end ileostomy and Hartmann's pouch is indicated. Subsequently, the decision to perform an ileo-rectal anastomosis with an ileal pouch–anal anastomosis can be made based on the specimen pathology.

Severe perianal disease occurs in 5%–10% of patients with adolescent Crohn's disease, often in association with ileal or distal colonic disease. Similar to intra-abdominal Crohn's disease, perianal Crohn's disease typically responds to medical therapy and surgery is reserved for complications. The most common indication for surgery is perianal abscess requiring incision, drainage and debridement. Small abscesses may be loosely packed with gauze that is removed in 24–48 hours. Larger abscesses involving the ischiorectal space should be intubated with drains depending upon the extent of involvement. In order to accomplish this, water-soluble contrast studies are performed in the operating room using fluoroscopy in order to identify horseshoe abscesses that may require secondary drains. Drains should be left in place for 4–8 weeks in order to create a controlled fistula. Patients are then treated with either metronidazole or ciprofloxacin and frequent daily baths until the abscess cavity completely resolves as documented by follow-up contrast studies. At this point, the drains may be removed and drain tract(s) treated with silver nitrate and injection of Fibrin glue.[14] Fistulae in ano are another complication of perianal Crohn's disease that may respond to antibiotics (Flagyl®) or ciprofloxacin) and immunosuppressive therapy (corticosteroids and Inflixiniab). Infrasphincteric fistulae in ano respond quite well to fistulotomy/fistulectomy as long as the intestinal component of the disease is well controlled medically. Suprasphincter fistulae in ano are more difficult to treat and carry the risk of fecal incontinence when fistulotomy/fistulectomy is performed. These are best treated by placement of a seton stitch or by debridement and installation of silver nitrate and Fibrin glue.[14] Proximal diversion (i.e., end colostomy) is indicated for patients who fail to respond to the medical or surgical therapy described above. This may be done in conjunction with limited bowel resection or partial versus subtotal colectomy depending upon the site and extent of disease. In many cases, fistulae will resolve within 6–12 months after diversion, at which time patients may be considered for intestinal reconstruction using colocolostomy or ileo-rectal anastomosis. Fissures in patients with Crohn's disease are best treated with medical therapy. Fissurectomy is not recommended in patients with Crohn's disease since poor wound healing and recurrence is extremely common. Severe fissures may be treated with similar efficacy by dietary restriction and total parenteral nutrition or by proximal diversion depending upon the circumstances of the case.

Surgical outcomes

The cumulative risk of recurrence requiring re-operation following resection for Crohn's disease approaches 20% at 5 years, 35% at 10 years, and nearly 45% by 15 years.[7] Moreover, it appears that this progressive risk of recurrence is not diminished after a second operative procedure for Crohn's disease.[15] Several studies including one at The Cleveland Clinic Foundation have shown that the risk of recurrence after surgery is not dependent upon the clinical features of the case.[10] For example, recurrence is not affected by sex, age at onset, time from symptoms to resection, or indications for surgery including obstruction, mass, fistulae or intractability. Further, it appears that the risk of recurrence following intestinal resection is equivalent between patients with combined terminal ileal and large bowel disease, small bowel, and large bowel disease.[7] Finally, histologic studies have shown that the margin of resection does not affect recurrence and thus a resection margin of greater than 3–5 cm in length is not necessary to prevent recurrence. The only surgical procedure that appears to decrease recurrence is creation of a permanent stoma. This procedure is eventually required to salvage nearly 25% of patients with juvenile onset Crohn's disease by ten years following the onset of disease.[15]

Given its panintestinal nature and high risk of recurrence, Crohn's disease confers a significant risk of short bowel syndrome. In several large adult series reviewed by Dr. Douglas Wilmore,[16] patients with Crohn's disease comprised 24% of those with less than 200 cm of jejunum ileum and 90% of patients with less than 50 cm of jejunum ileum with colon in continuity. In order to reduce the risk of short gut syndrome in patients with Crohn's disease, a consensus group at the University of Birmingham recommended routine use of strictureplasty for the treatment of small intestinal stenoses without excision of bowel.[17] Strictureplasty is safe and effective and is complicated by hemorrhage or recurrent stenosis of the strictureplasty site in less than 5% of patients, with fistulae/leak/abscess occurring in less than 10% of patients.[18] Strictureplasty successfully relieves obstruction in nearly 100% of patients and has been shown to increase growth and weight gain in nearly

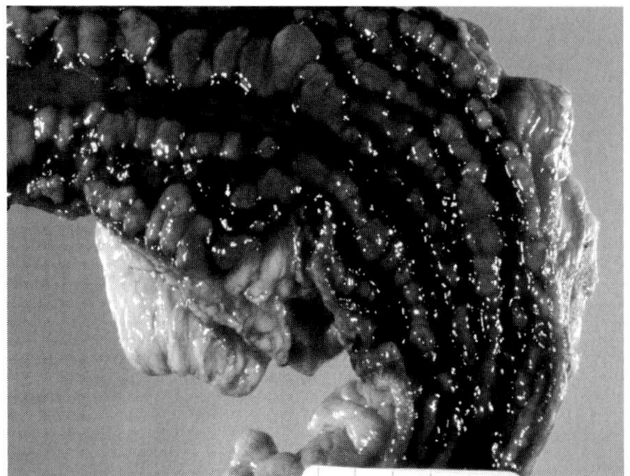

Fig. 27.4. Bear claw deformity in Crohn's colitis.

75% of young patients with Crohn's disease.[11] Postoperative recurrence of Crohn's disease following strictureplasty follows the same pattern as it does after intestinal resection, approaching a 50% incidence at 10 years.[18] However, in many cases the strictureplasty site was found to be free of active disease at the time of re-exploration.

Crohn's colitis differs from small bowel disease in that the major indications for surgery in adolescents are intractable disease and poor response to therapy, rather than intestinal obstruction. Surgical strategies may include partial colectomy, total colectomy with ileo-rectal anastomosis (Fig. 27.5) or ileostomy and Hartmann's pouch and total proctocolectomy with ileostomy. Most clinical studies have shown that proctocolectomy is attended by the lowest recurrence rate approximating 15% at 5 years and 20% at 10 years.[19] Recurrence after total colectomy approximates 30% at 5 years and 50% at 10 years. Finally, partial colectomy is attended by the highest recurrence rates approximating 50% at 5 years and 65% at 10 years.[18]

Total colectomy and ileo-rectal anastomosis are currently the most commonly performed procedures in one or two stages with an overall complication rate of 15%, including an incidence of 3% for anastomotic leak, 4% sepsis, 2% bowel obstruction, and 6% others.[20] Ileo-rectal anastomosis functions at least as well as an ileal pouch with complete daytime and night-time continence and approximately four bowel movements per day. In a report of 131 patients who underwent ileo-rectal anastomosis, 72 had functioning and 36 had non-functioning anastomoses at a mean follow-up of 7.5 years.[20] Indications for proctectomy or fecal diversion in this series included poor function, excessive steroid requirement, and bleeding. In these patients, perineal proctectomy provides excellent salvage therapy.

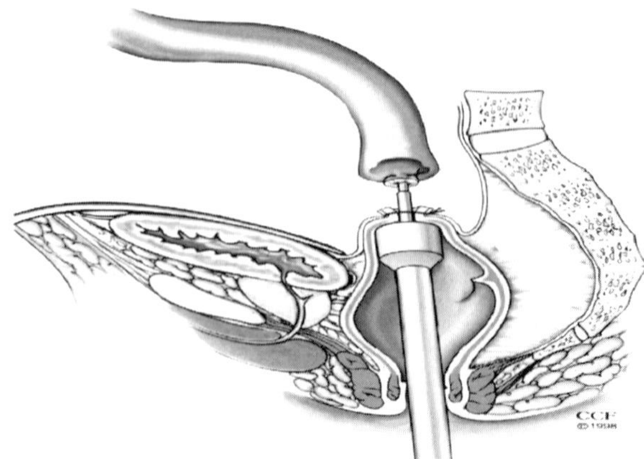

Fig. 27.5. Ileo-rectal anastomosis.

Severe perianal Crohn's disease is exceedingly difficult to treat. Approximately 20–30% of patients will resolve their perianal disease when treated either by resection of proximal small or large bowel or intestinal diversion.[21] If these surgical procedures fail to palliate perianal disease, then proctectomy or proctocolectomy may be used for salvage, with a 10% risk of further surgery at five years and a 30% risk at 10 years.[14]

Ulcerative colitis

Introduction

Unlike Crohn's disease, ulcerative colitis is potentially curable by surgery. The inflammation in ulcerative colitis is limited to colonic and rectal mucosa that may be completely excised without affecting normal growth and development. Historically, total proctocolectomy with permanent ileostomy has restored good health to many adolescent children, but has been largely abandoned in favor of ileal pouch–anal anastomosis (IPAA) in order to preserve bowel continuity and avoid permanent ileostomy. At the same time, earlier diagnosis and more effective medical management has reduced the number of patients with ulcerative colitis who require an emergent colectomy and staged procedures for life-threatening toxic megacolon, hemorrhage, or colonic perforation.

Epidemiology

Ulcerative colitis occurs in 2.3 cases per 100 000 population/year in children 10–19 years of age.[22] It is relatively uncommon in children 5–10 years of age, as this group account for only 12% of new diagnoses. Only 1% of newly diagnosed patients with ulcerative colitis are less than 5 years of age. The overall prevalence of the disease in the USA is 50–75 cases per 100 000 population.[14] Males and females are equally affected and the disease has a predilection for Jews and Caucasians.

Pathology

Ulcerative colitis is characterized by proctitis that invariably extends into the left colon in 25% of patients and into the entire colon in 60% of patients.[2] Of children who present with proctosigmoiditis 73% develop extension of the inflammation into the proximal colon within 5 years.[23] In ulcerative colitis, the inflammation is virtually always limited to the colon with continuous involvement of the rectum. Rectal sparing may occur but is extremely unusual. The mucosa is granular in appearance due to edema and erythema, with areas of superficial sloughing and ulceration. Microscopically, there is inflammation in the crypts with depletion of goblet cells. Pseudopolyps often occur due to isolated islands of mucosal preservation with surrounding areas of ulceration. Similar to Crohn's disease, the etiology of ulcerative colitis is unknown. There are no known specific infectious, allergic, or psychologic causes although there is an increased prevalence of ulcerative colitis in third-degree relatives. Recent investigations have demonstrated the presence of antineutrophil antibodies in the serum of many patients with ulcerative colitis.[24,25] This finding has led to the development of an immunologic test that is 60% sensitive and 90% specific for ulcerative colitis.

Clinical presentation

Abdominal pain, diarrhea, and rectal bleeding are the most common presenting clinical features of ulcerative colitis, occurring in 90% of patients. Weight loss and growth failure do not occur as frequently in patients with ulcerative colitis as compared to those with Crohn's disease. Arthralgia and arthritis may present several years prior to the bowel disease in patients with ulcerative colitis, and are twice as common as in patients with Crohn's disease (9% vs. 4%).[26] Other extraintestinal manifestations such as skin, ocular and hepatic involvement, and biliary stone disease occur with equal frequency in patients both with ulcerative colitis and Crohn's disease.

Skin manifestations of ulcerative colitis including erythema nodosum and pyoderma gangrenosum occur in 1%–4% of patients. Ocular complications occur in less than 10% of patients and include iritis, episcleritis, uveitis and orbital pseudotumors. Sclerosing cholangitis is rare, occurring in only 1%–2% of patients with ulcerative colitis. Gallstones do occur, but less commonly in patients with ulcerative colitis (occurring in only 4% versus 14% in patients with Crohn's disease). Similarly, calcium oxalate and uric acid renal stones are less common in patients with ulcerative colitis compared to Crohn's disease and may present at any time during the patient's course.

Surgical indications

Intractable crampy abdominal pain and bloody diarrhea are not only the most common presenting features of ulcerative colitis, but also the most common indications for surgery. In the past, many children with ulcerative colitis required emergent surgery for life-threatening hemorrhage or toxic megacolon. Improved medical therapy has virtually eliminated these complications and has shifted the primary indication for surgery to intractable disease and failure of medical management.

The timing of surgery is highly individualized depending upon the patient's response to medical therapy and the family's desires and expectations. In this regard, it is important for the surgeon to have a frank discussion with the family regarding the realistic expectations of surgery including the functional results and all possible postoperative complications. There are no data to indicate what optimal timing of surgery should be once the diagnosis of ulcerative colitis is made. Certainly, patients who require multiple blood transfusions, chronic hospitalization, and/or prolonged total parenteral nutrition should be considered strong candidates for surgery. Further, complications related to medical therapy such as soft tissue or central venous catheter infections, spinal compression fractures, glaucoma, or hepatitis are indications for discontinuation of immuno-suppressive agents and surgery in children. However, it would be preferable to embark upon surgery before these complications occur. Thus it becomes paramount for surgeons, gastroenterologists, and pathologists to work together as a team in order to make the best decisions for each individual patient.

Surgical treatment

Total colectomy and ileal pouch–anal anastomosis (IPAA) with sphincter preservation has replaced total proctocolectomy and end-ileostomy as the treatment of choice for ulcerative colitis. IPAA may be performed using several operative approaches including mucosal proctectomy or extra-rectal proctectomy. Mucosal proctectomy for ulcerative colitis was first developed by Ravitch and Sabiston[27] and subsequently refined by Martin who described the critical level of IPAA required to preserve continence and prevent recurrent proctitis.[28]

In this procedure, a total colectomy is performed by dividing and ligating the colonic mesentery from the ileocecal valve to the rectosigmoid junction. The colon is transected at the ileocecal valve and rectosigmoid junction and sent to pathology. The terminal ileum is then mobilized by dividing branches of the ileocecal artery and preserving the marginal vessels. An ileal pouch is then constructed in an S- or J-configuration depending upon the surgeon's preference (Figs. 27.6 and 27.7). A J-pouch is usually constructed using two 10–15 cm ileal limbs depending upon the patient's size, and these are anastomosed in side-to-side fashion using a stapling device. An S-pouch is constructed using three hand sewn 8–10 cm ileal limbs with a short anal spout less than 2 cm in length to facilitate emptying and prevent pouchitis due to stasis. The J-pouch is quicker and easier to construct, whereas the S-pouch provides a longer ileal pedicle that may reduce anastomotic tension in patients with a deep pelvis or mesenteric foreshortening due to prolonged inflammation or steroid therapy. At this point, a sphincter saving proctectomy is performed. This can be done using an extramuscular dissection from the rectosigmoid junction to within 2.5–3.0 cm of the dentate line where an end-to-end anastomosis between the pouch and the anal cuff is constructed using an EEA Stapler®. Again, this is relatively quick and easy to perform, but leaves a cuff of native rectal mucosa that may be prone to dysplasia. It is currently recommended that all patients who undergo extramuscular proctectomy and EEA anastomosis require surveillance on a yearly or every other year basis.

To avoid this issue, a mucosal proctectomy is often done. In this circumstance, the extramuscular dissection is shifted to the submucosal plane at the mid-sacral level and carried down to the anal canal. The mucosal proctectomy is completed from below beginning from the top of the columns of Morgagni, thus preserving the anal transition zone. Once the upper plane of dissection is reached, the rectal specimen is everted out of the rectum and discarded. The pouch is pulled through and anastomosed to the anal transition zone using dissolvable sutures and hand-sewn technique. The great advantage of the mucosal proctectomy and hand sewn anastomosis is that all native rectal mucosa is removed sparing the anal transition zone and eliminating the need for routine surveillance. In either case, an end or loop ileostomy is generally constructed at a comfortable distance above the pouch (usually 20–25 cm) and is closed 2–3 months later.

Recently, pediatric surgeons have pioneered laparoscopic assisted total colectomy and IPAA. In this procedure,

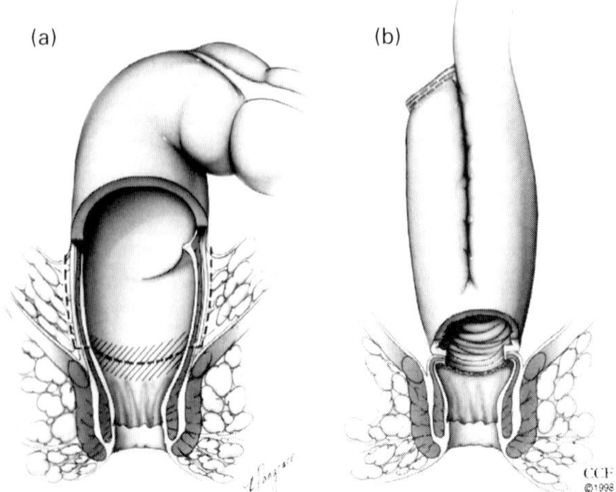

Fig. 27.6. Extramuscular proctectomy with stapled J-pouch IPAA.

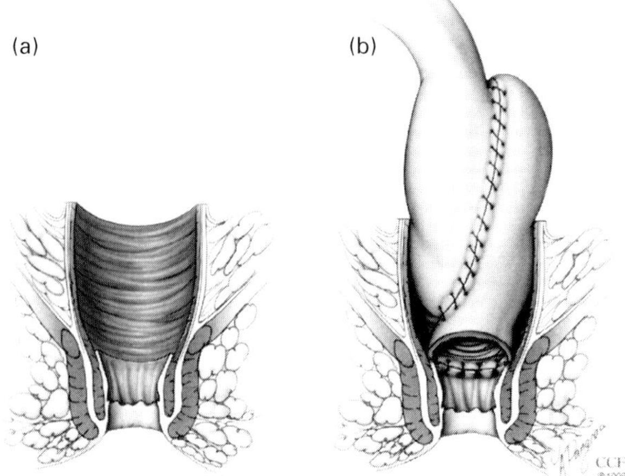

Fig. 27.7. Mucosal proctectomy with hand-sewn S-pouch IPAA.

the patient is placed in the modified lithotomy position using Allen stirrups and after appropriate preparation, trocars are placed in the supra-umbilical, left upper and lower, and right upper and lower quadrants. The colon is completely mobilized laparoscopically and the terminal ileum is divided using a roticulating GIA Stapler®. The colonic mesentery is divided and ligated from the ileocolic vessels on the right to the superior hemorrhoidals on the left. The dissection is extended circumferentially as far distal on the rectum as may be safely done. A transanal mucosectomy is performed from below and the muscular wall of the rectum is circumferentially incised above the puborectalis muscle whereupon the dissection is carried proximally up in the extra-muscular layer to the distal margin of the laparoscopic dissection. The colon is then removed through the anal canal. The ileal pedicle is lengthened by dividing the ileal cecal artery and the terminal ileum is configured into a J-pouch with a holding suture. The terminal ileum is pulled into the rectal cuff and a J-pouch is created by firing a GIA Stapler® through the anus. A hand-sewn anastomosis is performed and, finally, a loop ileostomy is created through the left or right lower abdominal trocar site.

Clinical outcome

The overall functional results of total colectomy IPAA for ulcerative colitis are excellent, regardless of the type of pouch used (S or J) or the type of proctectomy used (mucosal or extra-muscular) as long as the transition zone is preserved. Daytime continence approaches 100% within 1 year following both types of procedures.[29] Night-time continence approaches 80% at one year after mucosal proctectomy and 95% after extramuscular proctectomy.[30] Continence does improve over time after both procedures and may return more slowly after mucosal proctectomy compared to extra-muscular proctectomy due to the more limited dissection required. At the same time, mucosal proctectomy may reduce the risk of dysplasia since it leaves behind no retained rectal mucosa in the anal canal. Low grade dysplasia has been found in 8 of 254 patients who have undergone extramuscular proctectomy with ileo-anal pouch over 15 years at The Cleveland Clinic Foundation.[30] For this reason, periodic proctoscopy is recommended for patients who undergo this type of procedure. The average number of bowel movements is four per day at one year following both mucosal and extramuscular proctectomy.[29] The number of bowel movements is related to the mechanical compliance of the ileal pouch as well as dietary factors. Mechanical compliance is difficult to measure given the limitations of current manometric techniques, but is presumed similar for both S- and J-pouches. Patients are advised to maintain a high fiber diet and to limit their intake of chocolate, tomatoes, and cathartic fruits in order to decrease the number of daily bowel movements. Fiber substitutes and antidiarrheal agents such as Lomotil® and Imodium® may be used in patients who have difficulty complying with the prescribed diet. Similar long-term results have been reported in patients with a straight pull through, that is neither a J- nor S-ileal pouch, but a large majority of surgeons in contemporary practice construct a pouch.

Pouchitis occurs in approximately 10%–40% of all patients after IPAA for ulcerative colitis. The etiology of pouchitis is unknown, but interestingly, it is rarely observed in patients following IPAA for familial polyposis.[31] Also,

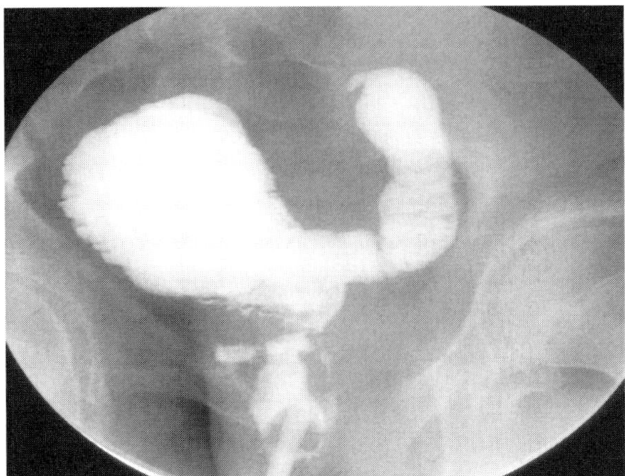

Fig. 27.8. Gastrografin pouch study demonstrating pouch fistulae.

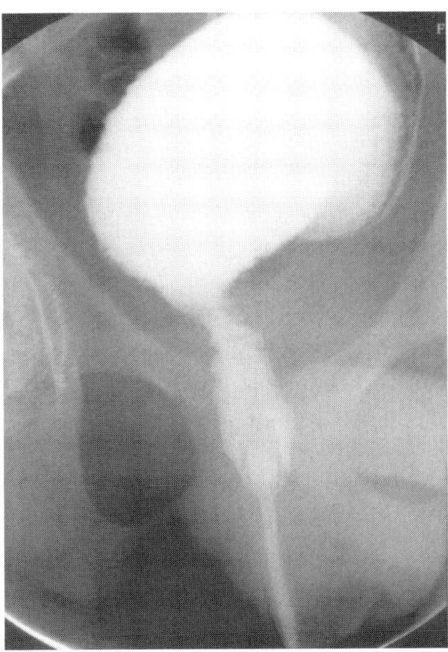

Fig. 27.9. Gastrografin pouch study demonstrating stricture in an abnormally long efferent spout.

the occurrence of pouchitis is independent of the type of pouch performed.[13] Pouchitis usually presents with crampy lower abdominal pain, increased stool frequency, and intermittent bright red blood per rectum. In many cases, it is episodic occurring within the first post-operative year, and is successfully managed with 2–8 weeks of oral antibiotic therapy including either metronidazole and or ciprofloxacin. Chronic or intractable pouchitis is a much more difficult problem to treat and may be associated with incomplete evacuation and fecal stasis or previously unrecognized Crohn's disease. In fact, a significant number of

Clinical and endoscopic features which suggest Crohn's disease

Clinical	Perianal disease (fissures / fistulas / abscesses / tags)
	Previous anal surgery
	Abdominal mass
	Oral ulcer
	Extra-intestinal symptoms
X-ray	Small bowel disease
Endoscopic	Rectal sparing
	Cobblestoning of mucosa
	Serpiginous ulcers
	Colonic strictures
	Skip lesions

Fig. 27.10. Features of Crohn's disease.

patients with chronic pouchitis may develop pouch fistulae (Fig. 27.8). If chronic pouchitis responds to intermittent intubation and/or the anal spout appears to be elongated on a pouch study (Fig. 27.9), then revision of the pouch should be considered.[32,33,34] In some cases, intermittent anal dilatation in conjunction with topical steroids may be successful in eliminating symptoms of pouchitis. Unremitting, chronic pouchitis should be periodically investigated by proctoscopy and biopsy since histologic evaluation will sometimes demonstrate findings indicative of Crohn's disease (Fig. 27.10). These patients may benefit from systemic medication and/or excision of the pouch and permanent ileostomy.

Pouch failure may be caused by technical problems such as anastomotic tension and/or ischemia, pelvic sepsis, multiple complications such as leaks or fistulae and Crohn's disease. On the other hand, pouch failure does not appear related to the type of procedure used whether S- vs. J-pouch, the anastomotic technique whether hand-sewn vs. stapled, or the occurrence of pouchitis.[13] Clinical studies have shown that the incidence of anastomotic leaks and pouch failure decreases as the surgeon's experience increases.[35] Complications are not infrequent following IPAA; however, most complications do not lead to pouch failure. For example, anal stricture is the most common complication, occurring in 15% of patients following IPAA and usually responds to dilatation or ileal pouch advancement flap.[36] The most common complications leading to re-diversion for pouch failure are pouch fistulae and pelvic sepsis. Overall, re-diversion is required in 3%–5% of patients following IPAA.[33] Some of these patients may heal spontaneously and others may be salvaged by ileal pouch advancement flap. Most patients who are salvaged and undergo un-diversion for such complications as pouch

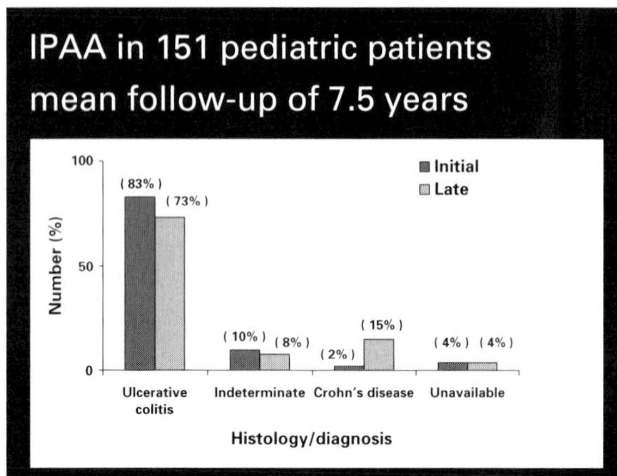

Fig. 27.11. Diagnostic progression in a large series of pediatric patients who underwent IPAA.

IPAA in 151 pediatric patients
Effect of Crohn's disease and indeterminant colitis on outcome

	Crohn's disease $n = 151$	P	Indeterminant colitis $n = 151$	P
No pouchitis	2/54		5/54	
Mild acute pouchitis	1/73		4/73	
Chronic pouchitis	10/11		2/11	
Ileostomy +/- pouch excision	10/13	<0.001	1/13	NS

Fig. 27.12. Crohn's disease, not indeterminate, colitis is an independent risk factor for chronic pouchitis and pouch failure.

fistulae and anastomotic stricture or anastomotic separation can expect no functional disadvantage, as opposed to those with pelvic sepsis and multiple complications who usually exhibit an increased number of bowel movements per 24 hours and increased leakage or seepage as compared to controls who did not require revisional surgery.[36] Patients with unsalvageable pouch failure are usually found to have Crohn's disease and ultimately require pouch excision (Figs. 27.11 and 27.12). It is important to recognize that indeterminate colitis does not carry the same risk of pouch failure as does Crohn's disease. Clinical studies have shown that the risk of complications and pouch failure is not significantly higher in patients with indeterminate colitis compared to those with ulcerative colitis following IPAA.[13]

Cancer

The most important factor in assessing the risk of cancer in patients with Crohn's disease or ulcerative colitis is duration of disease. It is estimated that the risk of cancer in patients with ulcerative colitis increases at a rate of 1% per year after the first ten years of disease.[37] Patients with total colonic disease are at highest risk, but those with partial colonic disease have a higher risk of cancer compared to the normal population.[38,39] Additionally, patients with Crohn's disease also have a higher risk of cancer compared to the normal population.[40] In a 20-year retrospective study conducted at The Cleveland Clinic Foundation, 10 of 454 adolescents with ulcerative colitis and 2 of 834 adolescents with Crohn's disease developed colorectal cancer.[41] Thus, yearly surveillance should be performed in all patients with ulcerative colitis beginning 8–10 years after diagnosis whether or not they are symptomatic.[42] Further, patients with severe perianal or rectal Crohn's disease should be periodically examined and any suspicious anorectal mass should be promptly biopsied.

REFERENCES

1. Grand, R. J., Ramakrishna, J., Calenda, K. A. Inflammatory bowel disease in the pediatric patient. *Gastoenterol. Clin. N. Am.* 1995; **24**(3):613–632.
2. Michner, W. M., Caulfield, M., Wyllie, R., & Farmer, R. G. Management of inflammatory bowel disease: 30 years of observation. *Clevel. Clin. J. Med.* 1990; **57**:685–691.
3. Gilat, T. Incidence of inflammatory bowel disease: going up or down? *Gastroenterology* 1983; **85**(1):196–197.
4. Michener, W. M., Caufield, M., Farmer, R. G., Wyllie, R., Cotman, K., & Hertzer, J. Genetic counseling and family history in IBD: 30 years experience at The Cleveland Clinic. *Can. J. Gastroenterol.* 1990; **4**:350–354.
5. Fiocchi, C. From immune activation to gut tissue injury: the pieces of the puzzle are coming together. *Gastroenterology* 1999; **117**:1238–1241.
6. Levin, K. E., Pemberton, J. H., Phillips, S. F., Zinmeister, A. R., & Pezim, M. E. Role of oxygen free radicals in the etiology of pouchitis. *Dis. Colon Rectum* 1992; **35**(5):452–456.
7. Lock, M. R., Farmer, R. G., Fazio, V. W., Jagelman, D. G., Lavery I. C., & Weakley, F. L. Recurrence and reoperation for Crohn's Disease: the role of disease location in prognosis. *N. Engl. J. Med.* 1981; **304**(26):1586–1588.
8. Michener, W. M. & Wyllie, R. Management of children and adolescents with inflammatory bowel disease. *Med. Clin. N. Am.* 1990; **74**:103–117.
9. Hyams, J. S. Extaintestinal manifestations of inflammatory bowel disese. *J. Pediatr. Gastroenterol. Nutr.* 1994; **19**:7–21.

10. Kotanagi, H., Kramer, K., Fazio, V. W., & Petras, R. E. Do microscopic abnormalities at resecton margins correlate with increased anastomotic recurrence in Crohn's Disease? *Dis. Colon Rectum* 1991; **34**(10):909–916.
11. Oliva, R. T., Wyllie, R., Alexander, F. *et al.* The results of strictureplasty in pediatric patients with multifocal Crohn Disease. *J. Pediatr. Gastroenterol. Nutrit.* 1994; **18**:307–311.
12. Tiandra, J. J., Fazio, V. W. *et al.* Surgery for Crohns colitis. *Int. Surg.* 1992; **77**:9–14.
13. Alexander, F., Sarigol, S., DiFiore, J. *et al.* Fate of the pouch in 151 pediatric patients after ileal pouch anal anastomosis. *J. Pediatr. Surg.* 2003; **38**(1):78–82.
14. Cintron, J. R., Park, J. J., Orsay, C. P. *et al.* Repair of fistulas–in-ano using fibrin adhesive. *Dis. Colon Rectum* 2000; **43**(7):944–950.
15. Sedgwick, D. M., Barton, J. R., Hamer-Hodges, D. W. *et al.* Population-based study of surgery in juvenile onset Crohn's Disease. *Br. J. Surg.* 1991; **78**(2):171–175.
16. Wilmore, D. Short bowel syndrome. *World J. Surg.* 2000; **24**:1487–1493.
17. Fazio V. W. Galandiuk, S. *et al.* Strictureplasty in Crohn's disease. *Ann. Surg.* 1989; **210**:621–625.
18. Alexander-Williams, J. & Haynes, I. G. Conservative operations for Crohn's disease of the small bowel. *World. J. Surg.* 1985; **9**:945–951.
19. Dietz, D. W., Lauret, S., Strong, S. A. *et al.* Safety and long term efficacy of strictureplasty in 314 patients with obstructing small bowel Crohn's disease. *J. Am. Coll. Surg.* 2001; **192**:333–337.
20. Longo, W. E., Oakley, J. R., Lavery, I. C., Church, J. M., & Fazio, V. W. Outcome of ileorectal anastomosis for Crohns Colitis. *Dis. Colon Rectum* 1992; **35**(11):1066–1070.
21. Orkin, B. A. & Telander, R. L. The effect of intra-abdominal resection or fecal diversion on perianal disease in pediatric Crohn's disease. *J. Pediatr. Surg.* 1985; **20**(4):343–347.
22. Canfield, M. E. & Michener, W. Ulcerative colitis. In Wyllie, R. & Hyams, J. S., eds. *Pediatric Gastrointestinal Disease: Pathophysiology, Diagnosis and Management.* Philadelphia: W.B. Saunders, 1993: 765–787.
23. Mir-Madjlessi, S. H., Michener, W. M., & Farmer, R. G. Course and prognosis of idiopathic ulcerative proctosigmoiditis in young patients. *J. Pediatr. Gastroenterol. Nutr.* 1986; **5**:570–575.
24. Provjansky, R., Fawcett, P. T., Gibney, K. M., Treem, W. R., & Hyams, J. S. Examination of anti-neutrophil cytoplasmic antibodies in childhood inflammatory bowel disease. *J. Pediatr. Gastroenterol. Nutr.* 1993; **17**:193–197.
25. Broekroelofs, J., Mulder, A. H., Nelis, G. F., Westerveld, B. D., Tervaert, J. W., & Kallenberg, C. G. Anti-neutrophil cytoplasmic antibiodies (ANCA) in sera from patients with inflammatory bowel disease (IBD). Relation to disease pattern and disease activity. *Dig. Dis. Sci.* 1994; **39**:545–549.
26. Michener, W. M., Whelan, G., Greenstreet, R. L., & Farmer, R. G. Comparison of the clinical features of Crohn's Disease and Ulcerative Colitis with onset in childhood or adolescence. *Clevel. Clin. J. Med.* 1982; **49**:13–16.
27. Ravitch, M. M. & Sabiston, D. C. Anal ileostomy with preservation of the sphincter. *Surg. Gynecol. Obstet.* 1947; **84**:1095–1099.
28. Martin, L. W., Torres, A. M., Fischer, J. E., Alexander, F. The critical level for preservation of continence in the ileo anal anastomosis. *J. Pediatr. Surg.* 1985; **20**:664–667.
29. Davis, C., Alexander, F., Lavery, I. C., & Fazio, V. W. Results of mucosal proctectomy versus extra rectal dissection for ulcerative colitis and familial polyposis in children and young adults. *J. Pediatr. Surg.* 1994; **29**(2):305–309.
30. Ziv, Y., Fazio, V. W., Sirimarco, M. T., Lavery, I. C., Goldblum, J. R., & Petras, R. E. Incidence risk factors, and treatment of dysplasia in the anal transition zone after ileal pouch anal anastomosis. *Dis. Colon Rectum* 1994; **37**(12):1281–1285.
31. Dozois, R. R., Kelly, K. A., Welling, D. R. *et al.* Ileal pouch-anal anastomosis: comparison of results in familial adenomastous polyposis and chronic ulcerative colitis. *Ann. Surg.* 1989; **210**(3):268–271.
32. Ozuner, G., Hull, T., Lee, P., & Fazio, V. W. What happens to a pelvic pouch when a fistula develops? *Dis. Colon Rectum* 1997; **40**(5):543–547.
33. Foley, E. F., Schoetz, D. J., Roberts, P. L. *et al.* Rediversion after ileal pouch–anal anastomosis. Causes of failures and predictors of subsequent pouch salvages. *Dis. Colon Rectum* 1995; **28**(8):793–798.
34. Fazio, V. W. & Tjandra, J. J. Pouch advancement and neoileal-anal anastomosis for anastomosed stricture and anovaginal fistula complicating restorative proctocolectomy. *Br. J. Surg.* 1992; **79**:694–696.
35. Macrae, H. M., McLeod, R. S., Cohen, Z., O'Connor, B. I., & Cheong, E. N. Risk factors for pelvic pouch failure. *Dis. Colon Rectum* 1997; **40**(3):257–262.
36. Breen, E. M., Schoetz, D. J., Marcello, P. W. *et al.* Functional results after perineal complications of ileal pouch anal anastomosis. *Dis. Colon Rectum.* 1998; **41**(6):691–695.
37. Devroede, G. J., Taylor, W. T., Sauer, W. G., Jackman, R. J., & Stickler, G. B. Cancer risk and life expectancy of children with ulcerative colitis. *N. Engl. J. Med.* 1971; **285**(1):17–21.
38. Collins, R. H., Feldman, M., & Fordtran, J. S. Colon cancer, dysplasia, and surveillance in patients with ulcerative colitis. A critical review. *N. Engl. J. Med.* 1987; **316**(26):1654–1658.
39. Bansai, P. & Sonnenberg, A. Risk factors of colorectal cancer in inflammatory bowel disease. *Am. J. Gastroenterol.* 1996; **91**(1):44–48.
40. Greenstern, A. J., Sachar, D. B., Smith, H., Janowitz, H. D., & Aufses, A. H. Jr. A comparison of cancer risk in Crohn's disease and ulcerative colitis. *Cancer* 1981; (**12**):2742–2745.
41. Michener, W. M., Farmer, R. G., & Mortimer, E. A. Long-term prognosis of ulcerative colitis with onset in childhood or adolescence. *J. Clin. Gastroenterol.* 1979; **1**:301–305.
42. Jonsson, B., Ahsgren, L., Anderson, L. O., Stenberg, R., & Rutegard, J. Colorectal cancer surveillance in patients with ulcerative colitis. *Br. J. Surg.* 1994; **81**:689–691.

28

Intestinal failure

Jacqueline Saito

Division of Pediatric Surgery, University of Alabama, Birmingham, AL, USA

Introduction

The outcome of intestinal failure due to short bowel syndrome has changed dramatically over the past half century. Following massive intestinal resection, survival of infants and children was rare[1] and led Potts to conclude in 1955, ". . . an infant cannot part with more than about 15 in (38 cm) and live".[2] The development of total parenteral nutrition (TPN) introduced a new era in the management of children with short bowel syndrome. In 1968, Wilmore reported a pediatric case of parenteral nutritional support,[3] and followed this with a series of 18 patients that were successfully treated with TPN for as long as 400 days.[4] With new therapy came new complications, such as transient glycosuria and catheter-associated infections. The development of intestinal transplantation added yet another therapeutic option for children with intestinal failure. Goulet reported one of the first pediatric survivors of a cadaveric intestinal transplant in 1989.[5] Advances in immunosuppression have improved both patient and graft survival over the past 15 years.

The outcome of short bowel syndrome is difficult to determine in infants and children. First, the definition of short bowel syndrome is variable, sometimes based on absolute bowel length, percentage of bowel resected, or necessity for support with parenteral nutrition, a more functional parameter. Absolute length and even percentage of bowel remaining are imprecise parameters, as a range of "normal" bowel length exists. In the neonate, small bowel length is influenced by gestational age and increases from an average of 114.8± 21 cm in neonates born between 19 and 27 weeks' gestation, to 248 cm ± 40 cm at greater than 35 weeks' gestation.[6] A simple measurement of intestinal function has not been well established. The etiology of short bowel syndrome may influence outcome through impact on intestinal function, motility, and comorbidities. Finally, most reports consist of case series originating from a single institution, with outcomes that may be influenced by local practice patterns.

The problems encountered with short bowel syndrome fall into two broad categories. First, there are consequences of the loss of intestinal length itself, often due to malabsorption, such as dehydration, electrolyte disorders, vitamin deficiencies, growth retardation, bacterial overgrowth, osteopenia, and oxalate renal stones. Second, there are complications from support with parenteral nutrition, such as catheter-associated sepsis, venous thrombosis, gallstone or biliary sludge formation, and cholestatic liver disease.

Etiology

Few reports of the incidence of pediatric short bowel syndrome have been published. In Ontario, Canada, neonatal short bowel syndrome is estimated to occur in 15–29 per 1000 nursery admissions, or 24.5 per 100 000 live births.[7] When comparing preterm (<37 weeks' gestation) and term infants, the frequency of short bowel syndrome is 43.6 vs. 3.1 per 1000 admissions. The most common underlying causes of pediatric short bowel syndrome are necrotizing enterocolitis (NEC), intestinal atresia, gastroschisis, malrotation and volvulus, and long-segment Hirschsprung's disease. Table 28.1 summarizes data from North America,[7–10] Europe,[11–13] and the International Intestinal Transplant Registry.[14] The variable frequency of etiologies may reflect

Pediatric Surgery and Urology: Long-term Outcomes, Mark Stringer, Keith Oldham, Pierre Mouriquand.
Published by Cambridge University Press.

Table 28.1. Etiology of short bowel syndrome

Causes	USA Andorsky[8]	USA Kaufman[9]	USA Georgeson[10]	Canada Wales[7]	Italy Gambara[11]	Greece Anagn.[12]	Austria Mayr[13]	Transplant Registry[14]
n	30	49	52	40	41	59	17	
NEC	47%	41%	50%	35%	15%	41%	23%	12%
Atresia	30%	25%	12%	10%	60%	22%	23%	8%
Gastroschisis	17%	18%	22%	12.5%	5%	8%	29%	21%
Malrotation/volvulus	10%	15%	8%	10%	10%	10%	18%	17%
Hirschsprung's disease			6%	2.5%		12%		7%

regional differences in practice patterns, especially with regard to NEC and support of the very sick preterm infant. In children who had NEC, the remaining intestine may have abnormal absorption or motility due to scarring in the healed intestine. Intestinal atresias can be extensive, as with "apple-peel" or "Christmas tree" variant (type IIIb), and multiple atresias (type IV). Intestinal atresias as well as motility disturbances can occur with gastroschisis and lead to shortened bowel length and abnormal function. Infrequent causes of pediatric short bowel syndrome include Crohn's disease,[15] traumatic injury to the bowel or its mesentery,[16] extensive tumors, and mesenteric vessel thrombosis.[17]

Early management

Immediately after intestinal resection, the short bowel state leads to several potential problems. Depending on the length and region of intestine remaining, severe diarrhea may occur with subsequent dehydration and electrolyte abnormalities. Proximal ostomies typically produce a voluminous watery output. The jejunum has a porous epithelium, allowing fluid loss that is exacerbated by hypertonic and hyperosmolar nutrients.[18] Loss of fluid, bicarbonate, and potassium from diarrhea can cause dehydration, metabolic acidosis, and hypokalemia. Initial management is directed at maintaining normovolemia and normal electrolytes. Peripherally inserted central catheters (PICC) and surgically placed cuffed silastic central venous catheters are short- and long-term venous access options appropriate for administration of parenteral nutrition. Gastric acid hypersecretion, stimulated by increased gastrin following massive intestinal resection, may be diminished by administration of H2-blockers.[19]

When enteral nutrition is started, short bowel patients may initially have better tolerance of elemental rather than standard infant formulas.[18] Malabsorption due to decreased absorptive surface area may be diminished by predigested nutrients within elemental formulas. Medium chain triglycerides are directly absorbed from the intestinal lumen. Formulas with hydrolyzed protein are more hypoallergenic. However, the theoretical benefits of elemental formulas are not always clinically realized. When studied in a small randomized trial, formulas with hydrolyzed vs. intact protein did not result in better nitrogen absorption or intestinal permeability.[20] Experimentally, more complex nutrients, such as long-chain triglycerides and high fat diets, stimulate intestinal adaptation.[21] Continuous administration of formula allows for saturation of mucosal transport proteins, thereby maximizing absorption. Alternatively, oral or intermittent feedings may minimize oral aversion and stimulate release of gastrointestinal hormones such as cholecystokinin.[22]

The management of a high-output ostomy can prove a challenge. A well-fitted ostomy appliance facilitates output monitoring and skin protection. Accurate measurement of stool production aids in the management of fluid, electrolytes, and enteral feeds. However, optimal ostomy positioning can be restricted by small patient size.

Surgical closure of ostomies within months of an initial procedure helps maximize enteral feeding tolerance. The benefits of stoma closure extend beyond simple addition of intestinal length. The terminal ileum slows motility and increases intestinal transit time through release of factors such as peptide YY, the so-called "ileal brake," and possibly glucagon-like peptide 2 (GLP-2).[23] Closure of ostomies may decrease stasis and bacterial overgrowth in diverted segments of intestine. Once thought a passive conduit for fluids, the colon is now recognized as a potential contributor to nutrient absorption. Colonic bacteria metabolize indigestible fiber through fermentation into short chain fatty acids (SCFA). SCFA, such as acetate, propionate, and butyrate, are important energy sources for colonocytes. SCFA facilitate colonic sodium and water absorption and may enhance intestinal adaptation.[24]

Intestinal adaptation

Intestinal adaptation encompasses a spectrum of changes that occur following intestinal resection. These processes start 24 to 48 hours following intestinal resection[18] and may continue in children for several years. Clinically, bowel adaptation becomes evident from decreasing stool output and increased tolerance of enteral feedings. Grossly, the small bowel and colon dilate, lengthen and thicken. Histologically, small intestinal mucosa develops increased villus length and surface area.[22,24] Enterocytes change functionally with increased carrier capacity of individual transport proteins.[24] The jejunum is more adaptive than ileum in terms of nutrient absorption. The ileum is more resistant to fluid loss and produces factors that slow intestinal transit. Epithelial hyperplasia starts soon after intestinal resection and is promoted by enteral nutrition, gastrin, enteroglucagon, GLP-2, epidermal growth factor (EGF), insulin-like growth factor 1 (IGF-1), prostaglandins, and polyamines.[18,19] Prostaglandin inhibitors and corticosteroids may inhibit epithelial hyperplasia.[18]

Factors that may impact intestinal adaptation include region of intestine present,[25] presence of the colon[25] and preservation of the ileocecal valve.[26] The importance of the ileocecal valve is attributed to its ability to prevent reflux of colonic bacteria into the ileum. However, several series[8,10,27] have not shown the ileocecal valve to significantly impact ability to achieve independence from parenteral nutrition. An easily obtained, functional parameter to assess bowel adaptation is still lacking. Serum measurements of 3-methylglucose uptake,[28] citrulline,[29] and GLP-2[30] correlate with intestinal length. In children, tolerance of enteral feeds correlates with GLP-2 level well[30] and with 3-methylglucose uptake weakly.[28] Citrulline negatively correlates with percentage of calories from parenteral nutrition in adult short bowel patients.[29]

Longer-term management: medical treatment

The long-term management of short bowel syndrome focuses on achieving normal growth. Additional goals include attaining independence from parenteral nutrition and prevention of complications. Careful monitoring of weight gain and height increase is essential to guide the adjustment of parenteral and enteral caloric intake. Energy requirements may be altered by age, illness and other stresses.[31] On the other hand, overfeeding should be avoided, since this may exacerbate bacterial translocation from the bowel.[32]

Gradual increases in enteral feedings are tolerated as intestinal adaptation occurs, though several strategies can enhance enteral tolerance. As mentioned previously, use of elemental formulas may minimize malabsorption, though these are generally less conducive to intestinal adaptation. Furthermore, breast milk, though highly complex in nutrient composition, contains growth factors and hormones that may promote adaptation.[19] Breast milk was associated with shorter time on TPN in Andorsky's series.[8] Stool output and reducing substances are useful parameters to guide adjustment of enteral intake. Tracking stool output helps avoid dehydration from malabsorption and diarrhea. Assessment of stool reducing substances detects the presence of non-digested carbohydrate before malabsorption leads to massive diarrhea. Agents that slow intestinal motility, such as loperamide and diphenoxylate/atropine, may decrease fluid losses by increasing intestinal transit time. Bile salt diarrhea, a result of disrupted enterohepatic circulation following ileal resection, can be controlled with cholestyramine; its administration should be spaced from other medications, especially those that are fat soluble, to prevent competitive binding.

Depending on the deficient region of intestine, patients are at risk for development of certain vitamin and mineral deficiencies. Iron and folate are absorbed in the duodenum, calcium in the proximal small bowel, and vitamin B_{12} in the terminal ileum. Bile salt depletion can lead to deficiencies of the fat-soluble vitamins (A, D, E, and K). Finally zinc, magnesium and selenium deficiencies may occur as a consequence of gastrointestinal losses.[18] Periodic assessment of vitamin and micronutrient levels, combined with supplementation, can prevent development of these deficiencies.

Use of supplements to promote intestinal adaptation, such as glutamine, growth hormone (GH), growth hormone releasing factor (GRF) and GLP-2, has been the subject of substantial research. Glutamine is an important substrate for developing intestine and is mitogenic to enterocytes; however, glutamine has not reproducibly increased nutrient absorption in adults with short-bowel syndrome.[33] GH is an anabolic hormone that may indirectly promote intestinal adaptation by increasing IGF-1.[34,35] GH, alone and in combination with glutamine, has increased intestinal lengthening[36] and enhanced intestinal adaptation[34] in experimental animals. In adult short bowel syndrome, GH improved absorption of energy, nitrogen, carbohydrate, and D-xylose and increased lean body mass.[35] However, GH and glutamine administered together did not improve intestinal absorption in a small, randomized trial with adult short bowel patients.[37] In children, Nucci *et al.* reported enhanced linear growth with GH or GRF, though without increasing independence from TPN.[38] GLP-2, a proglucagon derived peptide, increases mucosal epithelial proliferation and inhibits gastrointestinal motility and secretion.[23] In adults with short bowel syndrome and no colon in continuity, GLP-2 increased intestinal energy absorption, improved nutritional status, but had no effect on intestinal transit time.[23] More information regarding the efficacy of these supplements in pediatric short bowel patients and optimal dosing is needed.

Education of caretakers of children with short bowel syndrome is a priority. Initial training includes central venous catheter and gastrostomy care, administration of parenteral nutrition, and use of infusion pumps. Monitoring of serum and urine glucose, and patient temperature is necessary. Frequent outpatient follow-up, often with a multidisciplinary team, aids in optimizing overall nutritional and developmental status. Many infants develop oral aversion due to lack of oral feedings in the neonatal period. Instituting small oral feedings or oral stimulation exercises, with the guidance of an occupational therapist, can facilitate the transition to oral diet.

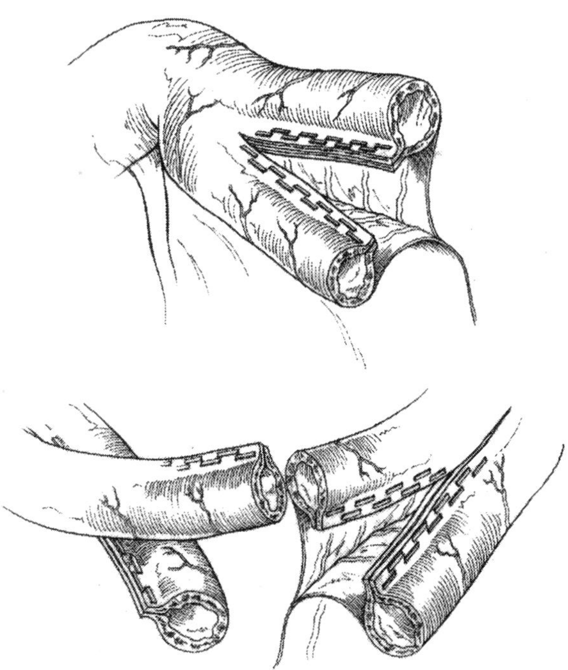

Fig. 28.1. Longitudinal intestinal lengthening and tailoring (Bianchi procedure).[39] (Reprinted with permission from Elsevier.)

Longer-term management: surgical treatment

Surgical interventions for short bowel syndrome consist of autologous bowel procedures and intestinal transplantation, a form of bowel replacement. Non-transplantation options include bowel tapering, longitudinal intestinal lengthening and tailoring (LILT), and serial transverse enteroplasty (STEP).

Autologous bowel procedures may improve enteral feeding tolerance in several ways. Bowel length, transit time of nutrients, and surface area to volume ratio can be increased. By decreasing stasis of intestinal contents, bacterial overgrowth may be diminished. Tapering and plication does not increase length but may improve tolerance through improved motility.[39] In 1980, Bianchi first described LILT in a pig model.[40] The operation, commonly referred to as the Bianchi procedure, requires use of dilated bowel, a typical feature in short bowel syndrome due to intestinal adaptation.[41] The dilated bowel, usually >5 cm in diameter, is divided longitudinally by separating the two leaves of the bowel mesentery and creating two lumens (Fig. 28.1). An isoperistaltic anastomosis is constructed to reestablish bowel continuity. The STEP procedure, recently reported by Kim *et al.*,[42] utilizes bowel dilation to similarly increase bowel length, though with a different geometry (Fig. 28.2). Other bowel lengthening procedures include initial use of a surgically created partial intestinal obstruction to induce bowel dilation, followed by LILT or the Kimura procedure, in which bowel develops a parasitic blood supply from the abdominal wall or liver.[39]

Intestinal transplantation is an intervention that continues to evolve (see Chapter 66). In 1995, approximately 35 intestinal transplants were performed in children worldwide.[14] Within 7 years, this annual number has more than doubled. Indications for intestinal transplant include impending or overt hepatic failure, thrombosis of major central venous channels, recurring catheter-associated sepsis, extreme short bowel syndrome, congenital intractable epithelial (mucosal) disorders, and frequent, severe dehydration.[43] Clinical signs of liver failure include dilated abdominal wall veins, splenomegaly in infants and toddlers, and varices in older children. Liver biopsies typically reveal fibrosis. Ascites and synthetic dysfunction, such as hypoalbuminemia and coagulopathy, are late signs of hepatic failure in children. Many indications such as extreme short bowel, recurring catheter-associated sepsis, and frequent severe diarrhea are defined qualitatively rather than by specific numerical criteria.

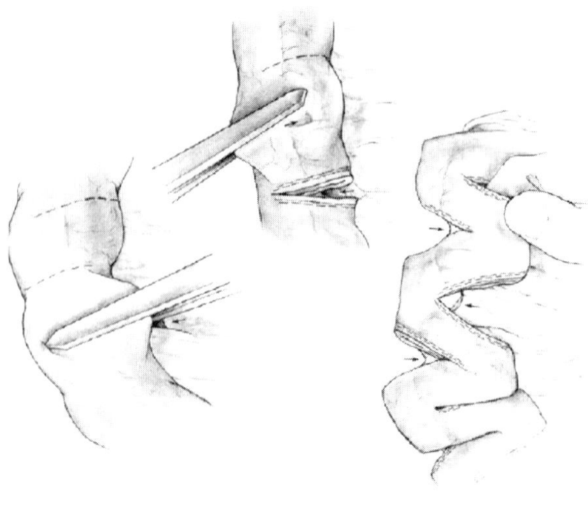

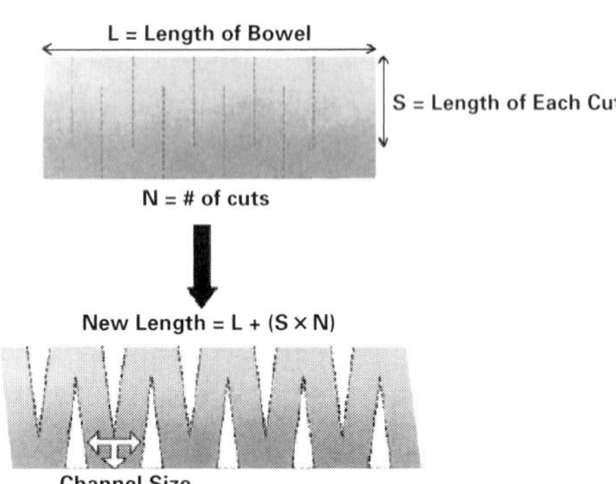

Fig. 28.2. Serial transverse enteroplasty increases bowel length and decreases luminal diameter through application of GIA stapling device.[42] (Reprinted with permission from Elsevier.)

Contraindications to intestinal transplant include profound neurologic disabilities, comorbidities that are life threatening or non-correctable and unrelated to the gastrointestinal system, severe congenital or acquired immunologic deficiencies, non-resectable malignancies, and insufficient vascular patency to maintain central venous access for 6 months.

Complications

The complications encountered in short bowel syndrome are varied in complexity. The major complications can be loosely grouped into those related to shortened bowel length itself, treatment with TPN, and central venous catheters.

Because of shortened bowel length, patients are susceptible to diarrhea with subsequent dehydration and electrolyte abnormalities. This may occur even after substantial intestinal adaptation; Mayr reported a 35% incidence of recurrent diarrhea in a series of 17 patients.[13] Viral gastroenteritis, from infections such as rotavirus, is often more severe and persistent in the short bowel patient.[12] Depending on the degree of TPN-dependence and severity of diarrhea, patients are at risk of electrolyte abnormalities.

The types and amount of bacteria within the intestine are often altered in patients with short bowel syndrome.[9] Increased strict and facultative anaerobes within the intestine can lead to bowel distension, cramping and malabsorption.[22] The ^{13}C xylose breath test has a high sensitivity and moderate specificity in diagnosing bacterial overgrowth.[44] Bacterial overgrowth is treated with a variety of antibiotics, including metronidazole, trimethoprim-sulfamethoxazole, oral aminoglycosides, extended penicillins, and cephalosporins.[45] Probiotics such as lactobacillus GG and lactobacillus plantarum 299V may alter bacterial populations and decrease bacterial adherence to mucosa.[46] Anti-inflammatory agents, such as sulfasalazine and steroids, can be used to decrease mucosal inflammation. When stasis of luminal contents and poor intestinal motility are significant, cathartics such as magnesium citrate, diversion with an ostomy, or surgical bowel tapering or lengthening may diminish bacterial overgrowth.[45] D-lactic acidosis is an unusual phenomenon that may occur in short bowel syndrome patients. Symptoms include altered mental status, confusion, weakness, ataxia, and slurred speech. Metabolic acidosis and dehydration are clinical features. D-lactic acid is produced by fermentation of malabsorbed carbohydrate by colonic bacteria such as lactobacilli and streptococci. Absorbed D-lactic acid is poorly cleared due to a lack of degradation enzymes and slow renal clearance. Treatment includes bowel rest, fluid resuscitation, and luminal antibiotics. A low carbohydrate diet and chronic luminal antibiotics may be useful in preventing D-lactic acidosis.[47]

Short bowel patients are at risk for osteopenia from deficiencies of vitamin D, calcium and magnesium. With vitamin D toxicity, parathyroid hormone (PTH) and 1,25-OH vitamin D levels are decreased. Magnesium deficiency reduces PTH secretion and function, thereby reducing renal conservation of calcium and production of 1,25-OH vitamin D.[48]

Urinary oxalate stone formation may occur in patients who lack ileum. Renal oxalate stones form from precipitation of calcium and oxalate in urine. Following ileal resection, increased colonic absorption of dietary oxalate is multifactorial. Normally, intraluminal calcium binds oxalate; when dietary fat is increased, unabsorbed free fatty acids bind calcium in the colon and leave unbound oxalate. Other factors include increased colonic permeability from unabsorbed bile acids, reduced bacterial breakdown of oxalate, deficiencies of thiamine and pyridoxine, hypocalciuria, and dehydration. Citrate excretion and urine pH are reduced by systemic acidosis and hypomagnesemia; citrate prevents nucleation, an initial step in urinary stone formation. Dehydration promotes stone formation through decreased production and increased concentration of urine. Preventative measures include avoiding dehydration, increasing dietary calcium, ingestion of a low oxalate diet, and use of cholestyramine.[48]

The hepatobiliary consequences of prolonged TPN administration include liver and gall stone disease. TPN-associated liver disease is exacerbated by the short bowel state[49] and has an increased incidence in young patients.[18] TPN-associated liver disease ranges in severity from cholestasis, fatty change, portal fibrosis and bile duct proliferation, to cirrhosis.[50] Histologic changes include acute and chronic inflammation.[46] Patients develop jaundice, splenomegaly, and other manifestations of portal hypertension, such as dilated abdominal wall veins and esophageal varices.[43] The mechanism leading to TPN-associated liver disease has not been established. Potential candidate factors include disrupted enterohepatic circulation of bile acids, sepsis, bacterial overgrowth/dysmotility, deficiencies in TPN such as taurine, and toxic components in TPN such as lipid phytosterols, manganese, and copper.[46]

The impact of TPN-associated liver disease is substantial, though the reported incidence varies widely. Sondheimer *et al.* reported a series of 42 patients who required TPN for at least 3 months following neonatal bowel resection.[51] Thirty patients (71%) had resection or atresia of greater than 50% estimated bowel length. Cholestasis, as reflected by conjugated bilirubin >2 mg/dl, occurred in 28 patients (67%). Seven patients (17%) developed liver failure, of whom five had a very short bowel length (9–51 cm). Four patients died, and three were listed for combined liver/intestine transplant. Fortunately, 21 patients had resolution of cholestasis despite continuation of TPN. Patients who did not develop cholestasis tended to develop infections at an older age. Gestational age, birth weight, presence of the ileocecal valve, and mean length of residual intestine were not correlated with the development of cholestasis. Duration of TPN was shorter in the population of patients with cholestasis. Knafelz *et al.* reported data from a series of 58 pediatric home TPN patients, 21 of whom had short bowel syndrome.[52] Only 11 of 58 patients (19%) developed liver disease ranging from biochemical abnormality to cirrhosis. Decreased bile flow may contribute to the development of gallstones and biliary sludge in short bowel patients.[48] The reported incidence of gall stones and biliary sludge ranges from 1.7%[52] to 54%.[50] Roslyn *et al.* prospectively evaluated 21 long-term pediatric TPN patients for gallstones; 11 had short bowel syndrome.[53] Nine patients (43%) developed gallstones. Risk factors for gallstones were increased length of time on TPN, fasting or aberrant eating patterns, and prior ileal resection.

Proven therapies for preventing or treating TPN liver disease are limited. Ursodeoxycholic acid, a choleretic, decreased conjugated bilirubin and hepatic transaminases in a small series of children with TPN-associated liver disease.[54] Cholecystokinin may provide some benefit in the absence of end-stage liver disease.[55] Preventative measures include control of bacterial overgrowth and cyclic administration of TPN.[46] Cessation of TPN through successful transition to enteral nutrition can be effective in diminishing liver disease. In cases where liver disease is progressive, combined liver/intestine transplant is often necessary.

The necessity for a central venous catheter to administer TPN introduces another set of complications. Catheter-associated problems may be mechanical, infectious or thrombotic. Moukarzel *et al.* reported catheter complications in a series of 27 pediatric home TPN patients.[56] Mean life-span of a central venous catheter was 22.4 ± 14.7 months with a range of 1.5 to 178 months. Of 123 catheters, 96 were removed. Mechanical complications, such as catheter displacement or breakage, accounted for 13 catheter removals (14%). Twenty-three catheters (24%) were clotted and not able to be cleared with urokinase or hydrochloric acid. Infectious causes of catheter removal were exit-site/tunnel infection (17%) or catheter-associated sepsis (45%). The average rate of infection was 0.41 infections/year or 1 infection per 884 catheter days. All fungal and mycobacterial infections resulted in catheter removal. With pediatric home TPN, Knafelz *et al.* reported a complication rate of 0.79 per patient, with a high proportion due to mechanical (52%) and infectious catheter problems.[52] Short bowel patients, in particular, are at risk of catheter sepsis. Two series have reported an increased rate of catheter-associated infections in short bowel syndrome patients compared to controls (3.1 vs. 1.3 catheter infections per patient,[57] and 7.8 vs. 1.3 infections per 1000 catheter–days).[58] Possibly a reflection of altered bowel flora, short bowel patients are at particular risk of fungal and gram-negative bacterial infections. Kurkchubasche *et al.* found that enteric organisms were causative in 62% of the infections in short bowel patients, compared to 12% in non-short bowel patients.[58] Catheter infections with *Candida* and coagulase-negative *Staphylococcus* had a lower rate of catheter salvage.[58] Vessel thrombosis, if recurrent or extensive, can pose a major problem for TPN-dependent

Table 28.2. Mortality associated with short bowel syndrome

Causes	USA Andorsky[8]	USA Kaufman[9]	USA Georgeson[10]	Canada Wales[11]	Greece Anagn.[12]	Austria Mayr[13]
Overall	30%	6%	17%	37.5%	20%	24%
Liver failure	20%	4.1%	3.8%	23%	8%	24%
Sepsis	6.7%	2%	3.8%	20%	10%	
Cardiac arrest	3.3%					
Transplant	3.3%					

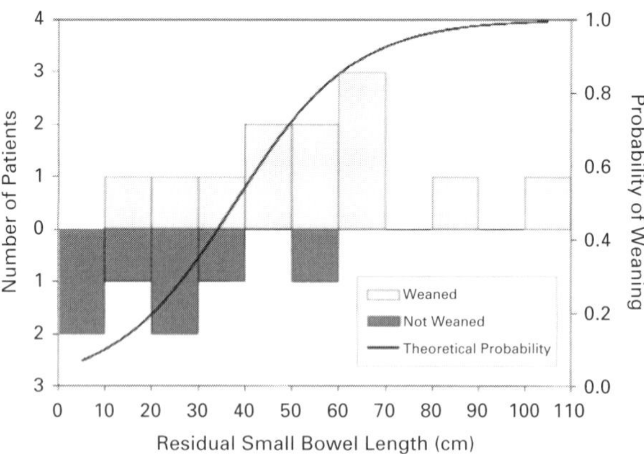

Fig. 28.3. Probability of weaning from TPN versus residual small bowel length.[8] (Reprinted with permission from Elsevier.)

patients. Swaniker and Fonkalsrud reviewed a series of 756 catheters in 510 infants under the age of 1 year. Significant caval thrombosis was identified in 35 patients (6 superior vena cava [SVC], 23 inferior vena cava [IVC], and 6 both SVC and IVC).[59] Thrombosis rates were 1 per 565 catheter–days for SVC, and 1 per 1550 catheter–days for IVC. Highlighting the severity of this complication, combined thrombosis of the SVC and IVC was uniformly fatal within 6 months.[59]

Variable success has been reported following bowel lengthening procedures. Early complications include anastomotic leak and stricture; redilation of bowel with poor motility and bacterial overgrowth may occur as a late complication.[60] In a series of 20 patients with short bowel syndrome from atresia and gastroschisis, Bianchi reported anastomotic stenosis in two patients and air/bile leak in one patient after LILT.[41] In a series of 9 patients who underwent LILT alone or following a partially obstructing ileal valve to induce bowel dilation, postoperative complications included bowel obstruction, duodenal stenosis, bowel perforation, and ileal nipple prolapse.[61]

Common complications following intestinal transplantation are acute and chronic rejection, post-transplant lymphoproliferative disease (PTLD), infections, and graft vs. host disease (see Chapter 66). The incidence of PTLD varies with type of transplant and ranges from 13.5 to 20.8%.[14] Cytomegalovirus (CMV) and Epstein–Barr virus are frequent opportunistic infections with an incidence of 22% and 31%, respectively.[5] Graft versus host disease has been reported in 8% of pediatric patients following intestinal transplant.[5]

Outcome and survival

Survival rates reported for short bowel syndrome are influenced by the variable severity of the condition, underlying disorders, and comorbidities. In 1972, Wilmore published observations regarding factors associated with survival of short bowel patients. In 50 patients with short bowel syndrome, no patient survived with less than 15 cm of small bowel and an intact ileocecal valve, or less than 40 cm without an ileocecal valve.[26] Features associated with survival included higher birthweight, lack of postoperative complications, and lack of associated anomalies. Later studies have refuted the absolute length associated with poor outcome.[8,12,15,27,50] Reported survival in multiple series varies widely (Table 28.2). The most common causes of death were liver failure and sepsis, highlighting the severity of these complications. Less frequent causes of death were acute abdomen, vena cava injury, respiratory failure,[10] cardiac failure,[11] and multisystem organ failure.[7] Another relevant outcome measure is acquisition of TPN independence. Again, success in weaning from TPN varies in reports from different institutions (Table 28.3). Andorsky *et al.* summarized the probability of weaning from TPN as a function of small bowel length (Fig. 28.3); remarkably, even patients with very short bowel length have some chance, albeit low, of weaning from TPN.[8]

In autologous bowel procedures, death is often related to hepatic dysfunction or sepsis. Bianchi reported overall survival of 45% in 20 patients with a mean follow-up of 6.8 years. Features that were associated with survival included >40 cm residual jejunum, longer colonic length, older age at time of operation, and presence of minimal hepatic dysfunction. Out of 11 deaths, 10 were attributed to hepatic dysfunction, and a single patient died of sepsis. Seven patients (77% of survivors, or 35% of total group) were weaned off TPN.[41] Figueroa-Colon *et al.* reported nine patients who underwent LILT, some in combination with a partially obstructing ileal valve; two patients died due to respiratory arrest and an unknown cause, respectively.[62] In Waag *et al.*'s series from Germany, 18 of 25 patients survived

Table 28.3. Weaning from TPN

	Weaned (%)	Mean bowel length (all cases)	Bowel length (weaned)	Bowel length (not weaned)	Comment
Andorsky[8]	20/30 (67%)	83 ± 67 cm			
Kaufman[9]	42/47 (86%)		81±65 cm	31 ± 30 cm	
Georgeson[10]	39/52 (75%)	48 ± 20.6 cm			
Gambara[11]	14/41 (34%)				Weaned after <6 months TPN
Mayr[13]	11/17 (64%)				

Table 28.4a. Pediatric intestinal transplant survival – University of Pittsburgh[5]

	Overall patient survival $n = 84$	Patient survival 1990–1994 $n = 34$	Patient survival 1995–2000 $n = 50$	Graft survival $n = 89$
1 year	74%	66%	77%	67%
5 year	56%	47%	64%	47%

Table 28.4b. Pediatric intestinal transplant patient survival – University of Miami[65]

Era	1994–1997 $n = 19$	1997–2000 $n = 28$	2001– $n = 23$
6 month	55%	58%	86%
1 year	50%	50%	86%
2 year	38%	46%	N/A

(72%).[63] Causes of death were liver failure (3 patients), central venous catheter-associated sepsis (1), pneumonia with sepsis (1), aspiration (1), and heart failure with multiple venous thromboses (1). Autologous bowel procedures appear to improve enteral feeding tolerance. In Figueroa-Colon's series, the percentage of total calories via enteral nutrition increased from an average of 9% to 50% by 9 months after the bowel lengthening procedure.[62] Waag *et al.* weaned the majority of survivors, 17 of 18 patients, off TPN.[63] Weber had success in weaning 14 of 16 patients off TPN; this was paralleled by an increase in D-xylose absorption from 5.4 mg/dl to 25.5 mg/dl by 12 months following the procedure.[64]

Outcome measures after intestinal transplant include graft and patient survival. The most common reasons for graft removal are rejection, vessel thrombosis, organ ischemia, and bleeding. Causes of death include sepsis, rejection, technical problems, lymphoma, respiratory failure, and multi-system organ failure. The type and era of transplant impact graft and patient survival. With approximately 40% graft survival at 5 years, combined transplantation of the intestine and liver has a better outcome than intestine only or multivisceral grafts. In contrast, patient survival is best with isolated intestine (approximately 50% at 5 years) versus combined intestine/liver or multivisceral grafts. Both graft and patient survival have been highest in the most recent era of transplantation.[14] Reported pediatric patient and graft survival from the University of Pittsburgh[5] and University of Miami[65] are summarized in Table 28.4a and 4b. A hidden mortality exists with intestinal transplants, as patients may die whilst awaiting donor organs. In the Miami series, 19 patients referred for transplant died, with 8 on the waiting list for donor organs.[65] A series from Spain recorded 4 deaths from 18 patients prior to transplant.[66] All deaths were in patients under the age of 1 year, highlighting the difficulty in obtaining appropriate organs for infants. Following intestinal transplant, the majority of patients are eventually supported with enteral nutrition alone; Nucci *et al.* reported 87% (20/23) weaned off TPN.[67]

Growth/development

Achievement of normal somatic growth is a challenge in the short bowel patient. Colomb *et al.* examined growth patterns in 16 prepubertal patients supported with TPN, of whom 8 had short bowel syndrome or Hirschsprung's disease. Seventy-five percent of patients had periods of alternating regular and slow growth.[68] Ralston *et al.* observed 9 patients on home TPN for 36 months; 6 patients had short bowel syndrome.[69] Time to achieve normal rate of growth varied from <1 to 40 weeks, and two-thirds of patients had normal growth by 8 weeks of age. At 6 months, 44% of patients had marginal height, though the mean height improved with increasing age to the 50th centile by

36 months.[69] In a series of 16 patients with short bowel syndrome, height and weight were over the 50th centile in 11 patients 2–10 years after bowel resection.[27] After discontinuing TPN, prepubertal patients with short bowel syndrome had a shorter stature and lower body weight compared to normal controls; however, bone mineral content was not significantly different when adjusted for height and weight.[70] Increased caloric needs associated with growth spurts, for example during puberty, may necessitate added TPN support to maintain growth velocity.[31] Following intestinal transplant, ongoing difficulty with maintaining linear growth has been observed.[67]

The impact of multiple hospitalizations and complications, such as infection, in short bowel patients is not known. Intellectual and developmental delay has been detected in some patients with short bowel syndrome and may reflect underlying comorbidities. In Mayr *et al.*'s series, 6 of 11 short bowel patients weaned off TPN had intellectual or motor retardation.[13] In contrast, Dorney *et al.* found that 4 of 5 short bowel patients weaned off TPN were able to attend a normal school.[50] Weber's report of 16 short bowel patients included 7 that attended regular school, and 2 who were deaf, one of whom also had mild developmental delay.[27] Ralston *et al.* assessed home TPN patients with the Gesell development schedules and found high variability in 6 month scores.[69] At 24 months, 2 of 9 children had a declining trend with scores <85; at 36 months, 4 patients had scores <85. One child had a persistently small head circumference that was associated with slow behavioral development.[69]

Economic issues

Care of the short bowel patient can entail substantial expense. Charges for supplies, including disposable sterile equipment, parenteral nutrition, enteral formulas, time and labor associated with training, hospitalization and diagnostic testing all contribute to costs. Because charges can vary widely based on location, accurate estimates of the true economic impact of short bowel syndrome are lacking. In 1992, the annual direct cost per home parenteral nutrition (HPN) patient averaged \$100 000.[71] Costs of nursing care, physician services, laboratory tests and hospitalization were not included. In Austria, hospital-based TPN cost was reported as \$205 000 annually compared to \$90 000 for HPN.[72] In Mexico in 1998, the mean annual cost for care of the pediatric short bowel patient ranged from \$12 000 to \$165 000, with a mean of \$50 000, a huge expense in the context of the annual minimum wage of \$1616. Shorter intestinal length was associated with higher costs.[73] Estimates of transplant cost were \$132 285 for isolated intestine and \$214 746 for composite grafts in the United States[31] and up to \$45 000 with a 30 day hospitalization in Austria.[72] It is unclear whether these figures accounted for the added expense from complications.

Quality of life

For the pediatric short bowel patient, complex medical needs and potential complications have an obvious impact on quality of life. The development of HPN programs has provided greater independence from the hospital for patients, though with increased responsibility for parents and caretakers. For patients who gain independence from TPN, there is often reliance on elemental or special diets. Few rigorous assessments of the psychosocial impact of this chronic illness have been made. In 1991, Weber detailed several parameters that impact quality of life, such as duration of initial hospitalization (range 62–395 days), number of rehospitalizations (range 2–14 for 13 of 16 patients), and the need for operations (range 2–14).[27] However, no direct assessment of the psychological, financial or social impact of short bowel syndrome was obtained. More information regarding quality of life in adult HPN patients has been collected using SF-36 and other instruments. Scores for social function, emotional function, and systemic symptoms were lower in patients on HPN, i.e. a poorer quality of life, compared to those with short bowel syndrome not on HPN.[74] In adults with short bowel syndrome, HPN patients had lower SF-36 scores for perceived quality of life, general health, and health concern for bowel disease compared to non-HPN patients.[75] Expressed concerns included being a burden to others, having surgery and energy level. Short bowel syndrome patients compared to matched controls had lower assessments of seven of eight health dimensions, including body pain, general health, vitality, social function, and emotional health. Among adult HPN patients, age may play a role in determining quality of life, as younger patients (<45 years) had SF-36 scores that approached those for the normal population.[76]

Quality of life has also been evaluated after intestinal transplant. Using the Child Health questionnaire, Sudan *et al.* obtained quality of life information from 29 "successful" pediatric intestinal transplant patients.[77] Inclusion criteria included an intact graft and more than a 1 year follow-up. Pediatric self-assessment by intestinal transplant patients was comparable to norms in physical function, role/social limitation due to physical function, general health, bodily pain, role/limitations due to emotions, self-esteem, mental health, and behavior. However, the assessment of the parental proxy was generally lower than the child's in general health perception and role limitations resulting from physical problems. The parental proxy had significantly lower scores than parents of normal children in physical function, role limitations owing to physical problems, general health perception, negative impact in terms of emotion and time, and negative impact on family activities. Bodily pain, general behavior, mental health, self-esteem, and family cohesion were comparable between parents of transplanted children and norms. A direct comparison of intestinal transplant and short bowel patient quality of life has not yet been reported.

Ethics

As the efficacy of treatment for short bowel syndrome has improved, new ethical issues have evolved. Previously held notions regarding absolute bowel length necessary for long-term survival[26] have been challenged in more recent reports.[8] As detailed in this chapter, the available treatments for short bowel syndrome each have potential morbidity. Ethical discussions in the 1980s regarding whether or not to support an infant or child with short bowel syndrome occurred in the context of intestinal transplant as an "experimental" therapy.[78] However, even at the present time, the application of intestinal transplantation is hampered by donor shortage with resultant long waiting-times on transplant lists, as well as the challenges of transplant rejection and post-transplant lymphoproliferative disorders. The number of centers offering pediatric intestinal transplant is limited. As recently as 2003, withholding total parenteral nutrition from a child with short-bowel syndrome was advocated;[79] in this case, intestinal transplant was not available within the patient's country. An important consideration while making ethical decisions is that quality of life may vary with social circumstances and underlying diagnosis.[80] From a public health standpoint, high costs may impact future decisions regarding the allocation of medical resources in general.

Summary

The management of infants and children with short bowel syndrome requires meticulous attention to optimize patient growth and development, work towards independence from parenteral nutrition, and minimize or prevent complications. The ongoing and ever-changing needs of patients and their families can be managed through a multidisciplinary approach engaging medical and surgical physicians, nurse clinicians, nutritionists, occupational and physical therapists, and pharmacists. As intestinal transplant outcomes continue to improve, prompt referral for specific indications may help to avoid clinical deterioration to the point that transplant is precluded, especially in the light of waiting times for cadaveric organs. Further development of living donation may facilitate prompt transplantation.

Future directions in medical management include the development and identification of agents that enhance intestinal adaptation, and methods to prevent liver disease and catheter-associated sepsis. For surgical therapy in short bowel syndrome, more information regarding the long-term effects of the STEP procedure will clarify its impact on motility and nutrient absorption, and whether redilation of bowel occurs. Improvements in immunosuppression and treatment of post-transplant lymphoproliferative disorder will continue to improve outcome after intestinal transplantation. Finally, advances in tissue engineering may make regrowth of autologous, functional tissue a reality.[81]

REFERENCES

1. Pilling, G. P. & Cresson, S.L. Massive resection of the small intestine in the neonatal period. *Pediatrics* 1957; **19**:940–948.
2. Potts, W. J. Pediatric surgery. *J. Am. Med. Assoc.* 1955; **157**:627–630.
3. Wilmore, D.W. & Dudrick, S. J. Growth and development of an infant receiving all nutrients exclusively by vein. *J. Am. Med. Assoc.* 1968; **203**:140–144.
4. Wilmore, D.W., Groff, D. B., Bishop, H. C., & Dudrick, S. J. Total parenteral nutrition in infants with catastrophic gastrointestinal anomalies. *J Pediatr. Surg.* 1969; **4**:181–189.
5. Reyes, J., Mazariegos, G.V., Bond, G. M. *et al.* Pediatric intestinal transplantation: historical notes, principles and controversies. *Pediatr. Transpl.* 2002; **6**:193–207.
6. Touloukian, R. J. & Smith, G. J. Normal intestinal length in preterm infants. *J. Pediatr. Surg.* 1983; **18**:720–723.
7. Wales, P. W., de Silva, N., Kim, J. *et al.* Neonatal short bowel syndrome: population-based estimates of incidence and mortality rates. *J. Pediatr. Surg.* 2004; **39**:690–695.
8. Andorsky, D. J., Lund, D. P., Lillehei, C. W. *et al.* Nutritional and other postoperative management of neonates with short bowel syndrome correlates with clinical outcomes. *J. Pediatr.* 2001; **139**:27–33.
9. Kaufman, S. S., Loseke, C. A., Lupo, J. V. *et al.* Influence of bacterial overgrowth and intestinal inflammation on duration of parenteral nutrition in children with short bowel syndrome. *J. Pediatr.* 1997; **131**:356–361.
10. Georgeson, K. E. & Breaux, C.W. Outcome and intestinal adaptation in neonatal short-bowel syndrome. *J. Pediatr. Surg.* 1992; **27**:344–350.
11. Gambara, M., Diamanti, A., Castro, M. *et al.* Clinical outcome and etiology of chronic non-malignant intestinal failure: a pediatric series. *Transpl. Proc.* 2002; **34**: 3363–3365.

12. Anagnostopoulos, D., Valioulis, J., Sfougaris, D. *et al.* Morbidity and mortality of short bowel syndrome in infancy and childhood. *Eur. J. Pediatr. Surg.* 1991; **1**:273–276.
13. Mayr, J. M., Schober, P. H., Weibensteiner, U., & Hollwarth, M. E. Morbidity and mortality of the short-bowel syndrome. *Eur. J. Pediatr. Surg.* 1999; **9**:231–235.
14. Intestinal Transplant Registry. Results presented at the 8th International Small Bowel Transplant Symposium, September 10–13, 2003. www.intestinaltransplant.org.
15. de Agustin, J. C., Vazquez, J. J., Rodriguez-Arnao, D. *et al.* Severe short-bowel syndrome in children: clinical experience. *Eur. J. Pediatr. Surg.* 1999; **9**:236–241.
16. Pomberger, G., Hallwirth, U., Pumberger, W., & Horcher, E. Short-bowel syndrome associated with subtotal necrosis of small intestine after rectal trauma. *Eur. J. Pediatr. Surg.* 1999; **9**:251–252.
17. Oguzkurt, P., Senocak, M. E., Ciftci, A. O. *et al.* Mesenteric vascular occlusion resulting in intestinal necrosis in children. *J. Pediatr. Surg.* 2000; **35**:1161–1164.
18. Vanderhoof, J. A. & Langnas, A. N. Short-bowel syndrome in children and adults. *Gastroenterology* 1997; **113**:1767–1778.
19. Lentze, M. J. Intestinal adaptation in short-bowel syndrome. *Eur. J. Pediatr.* 1989; **148**:294–299.
20. Ksiazyk, J., Piena, M., Kierkus, J., & Lyszkowska, M. Hydrolyzed versus nonhydrolyzed protein diet in short bowel syndrome in children. *J. Pediatr. Gastroenterol. Nutr.* 2002; **35**:615–618.
21. Sukhotnik, I., Mor-Vaknin, N., Drongowski, R. A. *et al.* Effect of dietary fat on early morphological intestinal adaptation in a rat with short bowel syndrome. *Pediatr. Surg. Int.* 2004; **20**: 419–424.
22. Goulet, O., Ruemmele, F., Lacaille, F., & Colomb, V. Irreversible intestinal failure. *J. Pediatr. Gastroenterol. Nutr.* 2004; **38**:250–269.
23. Jeppesen, P. B., Hartmann, B., Thulesen, J. *et al.* Glucagon-like peptide 2 improves nutrient absorption and nutritional status in short-bowel patients with no colon. *Gastroenterology*, 2001; **120**:806–815.
24. Robinson, M. K., Ziegler, T. R., & Wilmore, D. W. Overview of intestinal adaptation and its stimulation. *Eur. J. Pediatr. Surg.* 1999; **9**:200–206.
25. Cosnes, J., Gendre, J. P., & Le Quintrec, Y. Role of the ileocecal valve and site of intestinal resection in malabsorption after extensive small bowel resection. *Digestion* 1978; **18**:329–336.
26. Wilmore, D. W. Factors correlating with a successful outcome following extensive intestinal resection in newborn infants. *J. Pediatr.* 1972; **80**:88–95.
27. Weber, T. R., Tracy, T., Connors, R. H. Short-bowel syndrome in children: quality of life in an era of improved survival. *Arch. Surg.* 1991; **126**:841–846.
28. Sigalet, D. L., Martin, G. R., Meddings, J. B. 3-0 Methylglucose uptake as a marker of nutrient absorption and bowel length in pediatric patients. *JPEN* 2004; **28**:158–162.
29. Crenn, P., Coudray-Lucas, C., Thuillier, F. *et al.* Postabsorptive plasma citrulline concentration is a marker of absorptive enterocyte mass and intestinal failure in humans. *Gastroenterology* 2000; **119**:1496–1505.
30. Sigalet, D. L., Martin, G., Meddings, J. *et al.* GLP-2 levels in infants with intestinal dysfunction. *Pediatr. Res.* 2004; **56**:1–6.
31. Warner, B. W., Vanderhoof, J. A., & Reyes, J. D. What's new in the management of short gut syndrome in children. *J. Am. Coll. Surg.* 2000; **190**:725–736.
32. Yamanouchi, T., Suita, S., & Masumoto, K. Non-protein energy overloading induces bacterial translocation during total parenteral nutrition in newborn rabbits. *Nutrition* 1998; **14**:443–447.
33. Scolapio, J. S., McGreevy, K., Tennyson, G. S., & Burnett, O. L. Effect of glutamine in short-bowel syndrome. *Clin. Nutr.* 2001; **20**:319–323.
34. Gu, Y., Wu, H., Xie, J. X. *et al.* Effects of growth hormone (rhGH) and glutamine supplemented parenteral nutrition on intestinal adaptation in short bowel rats. *Clin. Nutr.* 2001; **20**:159–166.
35. Seguy, D., Vahedi, K., Kapel, N. *et al.* Low-dose growth hormone in adult parenteral nutrition-dependent short bowel syndrome patients: a positive study. *Gastroenterology* 2003; **124**:293–302.
36. Benhamou, P. H., Canarelli, J. P., Richard, S. *et al.* Human recombinant growth hormone increases small bowel lengthening after massive small bowel resection in piglets. *J. Pediatr. Surg.* 1997; **32**:1332–1336.
37. Szudlarek, J., Jeppesen, P. B., & Mortensen, P. B. Effect of high dose growth hormone with glutamine and no change in diet on intestinal absorption in short bowel patients: a randomised, double blind, crossover, placebo controlled study. *Gut* 2000; **47**:199–205.
38. Nucci, A. M., Finegold, D. N., Yaworski, J. A. *et al.* Results of growth trophic therapy in children with short bowel syndrome. *J. Pediatr. Surg.* 2004; **39**:335–339.
39. Vernon, A. H. & Georgeson, K. E. Surgical options for short bowel syndrome. *Semin. Pediatr. Surg.* 2001; **10**:91–98.
40. Bianchi, A. Intestinal loop lengthening – a technique for increasing small intestinal length. *J. Pediatr. Surg.* 1980; **15**:145–151.
41. Bianchi, A. Experience with longitudinal intestinal lengthening and tailoring. *Eur. J. Pediatr. Surg.* 1999; **9**:256–259.
42. Kim, H., Fauza, D., Garza, J. *et al.* Serial transverse enteroplasty (STEP): a novel bowel lengthening procedure. *J. Pediatr. Surg.* 2003; **38**:425–429.
43. Kaufman, S. S., Atkinson, J. B., Bianchi, A. *et al.* Indications for pediatric intestinal transplantation: a position paper of the American Society of Transplantation. *Pediatr. Transpl.* 2001; **5**:80–87.
44. Dellert, S. F., Nowicki, M. J., Farrell, M. K. *et al.* The ^{13}C-xylose breath test for the diagnosis of small bowel bacterial overgrowth in children. *J. Pediatr. Gastroenterol. Nutr.* 1997; **25**:153–158.
45. Vanderhoof, J. A., Young, R. J., Murray, N., & Kaufman, S. S. Treatment strategies for small bowel bacterial overgrowth in short bowel syndrome. *J. Pediatr. Gastroenterol. Nutr.* 1998; **27**:155–160.
46. Kaufman, S. S. Prevention of parenteral nutrition-associated liver disease in children. *Pediatr. Transpl.* 2002; **6**:37–42.

47. Zhang, D. L., Jiang, Z. W., Jiang, J. *et al.* D-lactic acidosis secondary to short bowel syndrome. *Postgrad. Med. J.* 2003; **79**:110–112.
48. Nightingale, J. M. D. Hepatobiliary, renal and bone complications of intestinal failure. *Best. Pract. Res. Clin. Gastroenterol.* 2003; **17**:907–929.
49. Stanko, R., Nathan, G., Mendelow, H., & Adibi, S. A. Development of hepatic cholestasis and fibrosis in patients with massive loss of intestine supported by prolonged parenteral nutrition. *Gastroenterology* 1987; **92**:197–202.
50. Dorney, S. F., Ament, M. E., Berquist, W. E. *et al.* Improved survival in very short small bowel of infancy with use of long-term parenteral nutrition. *J. Pediatr.* 1985; **107**:521–525.
51. Sondheimer, J. M., Asturias, E., & Cadnapaphornchai, M. Infection and cholestasis in neonates with intestinal resection and long-term parenteral nutrition. *J. Pediatr. Gastroenterol. Nutr.* 1998; **27**:131–137.
52. Knafelz, D., Gambarara, M., Diamanti, A. *et al.* Complications of home parenteral nutrition in a large pediatric series. *Transpl. Proc.* 2003; **35**:3050–3051.
53. Roslyn, J. J., Berquist, W. E., Pitt, H. A. *et al.* Increased risk of gallstones in children receiving total parenteral nutrition. *Pediatrics* 1983; **71**:784–789.
54. Spagnuolo, M. I., Iorio, R., Vegnente, A., & Guarino, A. Ursodeoxycholic acid for treatment of cholestasis in children on long-term total parenteral nutrition: a pilot study. *Gastroenterol* 1996; **111**:716–719.
55. Teitelbaum, D. H., Han-Markey, T., & Schumacher, R. E. Treatment of parenteral nutrition-associated cholestasis with cholecystokinin-octapeptide. *J. Pediatr. Surg.* 1995; **30**:1082–1085.
56. Moukarzel, A. A., Haddad, I., Ament, M. E. *et al.* 230 patient years of experience with home long-term parenteral nutrition in childhood: natural history and life of central venous catheters. *J. Pediatr. Surg.* 1994; **29**:1323–1327.
57. Piedra, P. A., Dryja, D. M., & LaScolea, L. J. Incidence of catheter-associated gram-negative bacteremia in children with short bowel syndrome. *J. Clin. Microbiol.* 1989; **27**:1317–1319.
58. Kurkchubasche, A. G., Smith, S. D., & Rowe, M. I. Catheter sepsis in short-bowel syndrome. *Arch. Surg.* 1992; **127**:21–25.
59. Swaniker, F. & Fonkalsrud, E.W. Superior and inferior vena caval occlusion in infants receiving total parenteral nutrition. *Am. Surg.* 1995; **61**:877–881.
60. Huskisson, L. J., Brereton, R. J., Kiely, E. M., & Spitz, L. Problems with intestinal lengthening. *J. Pediatr. Surg.* 1993; **28**:720–722.
61. Georgeson, K., Halpin, D., Figueroa, R. *et al.* Sequential intestinal lengthening procedures for refractory short bowel syndrome. *J. Pediatr. Surg.* 1994; **29**:316–321.
62. Figueroa-Colon, R., Harris, P. R., Birdsong, E. *et al.* Impact of intestinal lengthening on the nutritional outcome for children with short bowel syndrome. *J. Pediatr. Surg.* 1996; **31**:912–916.
63. Waag, K. L., Hosie, S., Wessell, L. What do children look like after longitudinal intestinal lengthening? *Eur. J. Pediatr. Surg.* 1999; **9**:260–262.
64. Weber, T. R. Isoperistaltic bowel lengthening for short bowel syndrome in children. *Am. J. Surg.* 1999; **178**:600–604.
65. Kato, T., Mittal, N., Nishida, S. *et al.* The role of intestinal transplantation in the management of babies with extensive gut resections. *J. Pediatr. Surg.* 2003; **38**:145–149.
66. Lopez-Santamaria, M., Gamez, M., Murcia, M. *et al.* Pediatric intestinal transplantation. *Transpl. Proc.* 2003; **35**:1927–1928.
67. Nucci, A. M., Barksdale, E. M., Beserock, N. *et al.* Long-term nutritional outcome after pediatric intestinal transplantation. *J. Pediatr. Surg.* 2002; **37**:460–463.
68. Colomb, V., Dabbas, M., Goulet, O. *et al.* Prepubertal growth in children with long-term parenteral nutrition. *Horm. Res.* 2002; **58**:2–6.
69. Ralston, C. W., O'Connor, M. J., Ament, M. *et al.* Somatic growth and developmental functioning in children receiving prolonged home total parenteral nutrition. *J. Pediatr.* 1984; **105**:842–846.
70. Dellert, S. F., Farrell, M. K., Specker, B. L., & Heubi, J. E. Bone mineral content in children with short bowel syndrome after discontinuation of parenteral nutrition. *J. Pediatr.* 1998; **132**:516–519.
71. Howard, L. & Malone, M. Current status of home parenteral nutrition in the United States. *Transpl. Proc.* 1996; **28**:2691–2695.
72. Schalamon, J., Mayr, J. M., & Hollwarth, M. E. Mortality and economics in short bowel syndrome. *Best Pract. Res. Clin. Gastroenterol.* 2003; **17**:931–942.
73. Varela-Fascinetto, G., Greenawalt, S. R., & Villegas-Alvarez, F. Short bowel syndrome in patients studied at the National Institute of Pediatrics in Mexico: care, cost and perspectives. *Arch. Med. Res.* 1998; **29**:337–340.
74. Jeppesen, P. B., Langholz, E., & Mortensen, P. B. Quality of life in patients receiving home parenteral nutrition. *Gut* 1999; **44**:844–852.
75. Carlsson, E., Bosaeus, I., & Nordgren, S. Quality of life and concerns in patients with short bowel syndrome. *Clin. Nutr.* 2003; **22**:445–452.
76. Richards, D. M. & Irving, M. H. Assessing the quality of life of patients with intestinal failure on home parenteral nutrition. *Gut* 1997; **40**:218–222.
77. Sudan, D., Horslen, S., Botha, J. *et al.* Quality of life after pediatric intestinal transplantation: the perception of pediatric recipients and their parents. *Am. J. Transpl.* 2004; **4**:407–413.
78. Caniano, D. A. & Kanoti, G. A. Newborns with massive intestinal loss: difficult choices. *N. Engl. J. Med.* 1988; **318**:703–707.
79. Severijnen, R., Hulstijn-Dirkmaat, I., Gordijn, B. *et al.* Acute loss of the small bowel in a school-age boy. Difficult choices: to sustain life or to stop treatment? *Eur. J. Pediatr. Surg.* 2003; **162**:794–798.
80. Irving, M. Ethical problems associated with the treatment of intestinal failure. *Aust. NZ. J. Surg.* 1986; **56**:425–427.
81. Grikscheit, T. C., Siddique, A., Ochoa, E. R. *et al.* Tissue-engineered small intestine improves recovery after massive small bowel resection. *Ann. Surg.* 2004; **240**:748–754.

29

Appendicitis

Prem Puri and Alan Mortell

Children's Research Centre, Our Lady's Hospital for Sick Children, Dublin, Ireland

Acute appendicitis is the most common surgical emergency in childhood. Appendicitis may present at any age, although it is uncommon in preschool children. Approximately one-third of children with acute appendicitis have perforation by the time of operation. Despite improved fluid resuscitation and better antibiotics, appendicitis in children, especially in preschool children, is still associated with significant morbidity.

Historical aspects

Early reports of appendicitis were usually based on autopsy findings. In 1736, Amyand reported an operation on a boy with a perforated appendix in a scrotal hernia.[1] Several important contributions toward the diagnosis and treatment of appendicitis were made during the 1880s. The term appendicitis was first used in 1886 by the Harvard pathologist Reginald Fitz,[2] who provided an extraordinary description of the signs and symptoms of both acute and perforated appendicitis and, in addition, appreciated the role of luminal obstruction in the pathogenesis of appendicitis. He stressed the importance of early diagnosis and treatment by laparotomy. Although drainage of an appendiceal abscess had been performed earlier, Mortin,[3] in 1887, did the first successful appendectomy for perforated appendicitis. In 1889, McBurney[4] published his classical description of the typical tenderness in the right lower quadrant and recommended early operation. Although modern antibiotics and intravenous administration of fluids have improved the outcome for children with appendicitis, the basic principles of early diagnosis and appendectomy remain the same as described by McBurney over 100 years ago.

Epidemiology

The incidence of acute appendicitis has been reported to vary substantially by country, geographic region, race, sex and season, but the reasons for these variations are unknown. An epidemiologic study of acute appendicitis in California revealed that the incidence of appendicitis in blacks and Asians was less than half that in whites.[5] Epidemiologic studies of acute appendicitis and perforation rates in California and New York have shown higher incidence rates of appendicitis among Hispanics than African Americans and Whites with Hispanics, Asians and African Americans having a higher risk of perforation than Whites.[6,7] The incidence of acute appendicitis may also vary with time. For example, since the 1950s the incidence of acute appendicitis in the United Kingdom has decreased by about 60%.[8]

Etiology

The exact etiology and pathogenesis of appendicitis are poorly understood. While invasion of the appendiceal wall by micro-organisms is the ultimate pathologic event, the primary initiating condition is not known. Obstruction of the appendix lumen, from whatever cause, with resulting distension and disturbance of blood flow, is still considered the major factor in the pathogenesis of acute appendicitis. Other factors include low dietary fiber intake[9,10]

Pediatric Surgery and Urology: Long-term Outcomes, Mark Stringer, Keith Oldham, Pierre Mouriquand.
Published by Cambridge University Press.

and bacterial[11,12] and viral[13] infections. Andersson et al[14] found that appendicitis occurs in space-time clusters and outbreaks (characteristics of infectious diseases), thus supporting an infectious etiology. Recently, Gauderer *et al.*[15] investigated the relationship between heredity and appendicitis and found that children with appendicitis are at least twice as likely to have a positive family history of appendicitis as compared with children with right lower quadrant pain without appendicitis or controls without abdominal pain. Tsuji *et al.*[16] reported significant perturbation of the local inflammatory response in acute appendicitis. Whilst this was not a surprising observation in the context of an acutely inflamed organ, it was particularly interesting that abnormal immunocyte infiltration was seen throughout the entire organ in focal appendicitis. Focal appendicitis refers to those appendices that appear normal microscopically and are classified as normal histologically, if only a few sections are examined but when extensive sectioning is performed, a small focus of inflammation is seen. The finding of selective lymphocyte infiltration of the lamina propria throughout the entire appendix in focal appendicitis suggests that focal appendicitis probably represents the earliest recognizable pathologic manifestation of acute appendicitis. Wang *et al.*[17] provided new insights into the immunopathologic events occurring in appendicitis. They investigated cytokine expression by *in situ* hybridization in normal appendices and appendiceal specimens removed from patients with a clinical diagnosis of appendicitis. They demonstrated TNF-α and IL-2 messenger RNA expression in the germinal centers, submucosa and lamina propria in 7 of 31 histologically normal appendices from patients with clinical features of acute appendicitis. The abnormal cytokine expression in these patients was similar to that seen in typical acute appendicitis specimens. These results suggest that antigenic stimulation from luminal sources could be a major factor in the pathogenesis of appendicitis. Nemeth *et al.*[18] demonstrated increased expression of inflammatory markers (COX 1 and 2, PGE_2, iNOS and MHC Class II antigens) in appendices which were removed for suspected appendicitis but histologically classified as normal. Their findings support the concept that there is a sub-group of so-called histologically normal appendices in which there is evidence of an inflammatory pathologic condition at a molecular level. Other recent studies have reported a significant increase in mast cell numbers with associated neuronal hypertrophy of the myenteric plexus in a high proportion of acutely inflamed and some histologically normal appendices (removed because of suspected appendicitis).[19,20] These findings were unlikely to have developed during a single acute inflammatory episode, suggesting the presence of an underlying abnormality as a secondary response to chronic luminal obstruction or repeated inflammation.

Diagnosis

The diagnosis of acute appendicitis in childhood can sometimes be difficult. Definite diagnosis is made in only 43–72% of patients at the time of initial assessment.[21] The rate of negative appendectomy in children is in the range of 4–50% in various reports.[22–26] The patient's history and clinical examination are the most important tools for the diagnosis of appendicitis. Periumbilical pain is often the first symptom, followed by vomiting and fever. When the inflammation progresses, the pain localizes to the right lower quadrant where tenderness develops. Laboratory investigations and plain radiographs are neither sensitive nor specific in the diagnosis of appendicitis.[27] Barium enema is an unreliable test because of its high false-positive and false-negative rates.[28] In recent years, graded compression ultrasonography of the right lower quadrant has been shown to be a useful tool in the evaluation of patients with clinical findings that are suggestive but not diagnostic of appendicitis, with a sensitivity of 80–100%, a specificity of 78–98%, and an overall accuracy of 91%.[29] Ultrasound is portable, fast, free of irradiation, of modest incremental cost, and useful in detecting gynecologic disease. However, it is of limited use in obese adolescents and highly user dependent. The only sonographic sign that is specific for appendicitis is an enlarged, non-compressible appendix measuring greater than 6 mm in maximal diameter.[30] The appendix may not be visible following perforation. Recently, computed tomography (CT) has been used as an adjunct to the diagnosis of appendicitis, reducing negative appendectomy rates to 4.1% and perforation rates to 14.7%.[31] The principal advantages of CT are its operator independency and enhanced delineation of disease extent in perforated appendicitis. Sensitivity, specificity and accuracy for unenhanced limited CT have approached 97%, 100% and 99%, respectively. However, with this improved diagnostic accuracy came a reduction in the degree of significance put on the initial clinical evaluation by the responsible surgical team. Also, CT exposes the child to a significant dose of ionizing radiation. Garcia Pena *et al.* suggested that diagnostic CT should be used according to a patient risk-stratification protocol.[32] Other recent studies have suggested that CT has not increased the accuracy of diagnosing appendicitis when compared to a careful history and physical examination performed by an experienced surgeon.[33,34]

In patients with an uncertain cause of acute abdominal pain, a policy of active observation in hospital is usually practiced.[22] A repeated structured clinical examination is simple and non-invasive. However, the argument against this policy is that it may lead to a delay in specific management of these patients and may result in a higher incidence of perforation. Using active observation alone, Bachoo *et al.*[35] achieved a positive predictive value of 97.9% and a normal appendectomy rate of 2.6% and showed no correlation between postoperative morbidity and timing of surgery with this protocol. We have shown that delay in appendectomy in children observed in a hospital setting does not increase the incidence of complicated appendicitis.[36]

Operative techniques

Children with appendicitis are assessed for degree of sepsis and dehydration. Intravenous fluids are indicated preoperatively because most patients have vomited and taken little fluid in the preceding 24 hours. Broad-spectrum antibiotics should be administered pre- and postoperatively in order to prevent infectious complications.

Open appendectomy

A transverse right lower quadrant skin crease incision is recommended. The muscular layers are split in the direction of their fibers. The peritoneum is opened and fluid sent for culture; recent studies have questioned the value of routine peritoneal fluid culture.[37] The mesoappendix is divided and the appendiceal base clamped and ligated. Stump inversion is optional. Engstrom and Fenyo found no difference in rates of wound infection and postoperative fever between one group in which the appendix was ligated and doubly invaginated and another group in which it was simply ligated.[38] If pus is present, the abdomen should be irrigated with saline. The abdominal wall is closed in layers. The skin is usually closed by subcuticular absorbable sutures even in the case of perforation. Primary wound closure after perforated appendicitis is safe, economical and advantageous in pediatric practice.[39,40]

Laparoscopic appendectomy

An infraumbilical port is inserted using an open rather than percutaneous technique. Two 5 mm infraumbilical incisions are placed on either side of the midline. A third right lower quadrant incision is optional. After mobilization of the appendix, the mesoappendix is divided, the appendiceal stump is ligated with endoloops or an endoscopic stapler, and the appendix is removed.

In recent years, laparoscopic appendectomy has emerged as a safe alternative in the pediatric age group.[41–43] Although the rate at which laparoscopy is utilized in the treatment of appendicitis varies dramatically from center to center (range 0%–95%),[44] it is undoubtedly a reasonable surgical alternative to open appendectomy for the treatment of acute appendicitis in children. Recent studies have demonstrated that laparoscopic appendectomy is at least as safe and effective as open appendectomy.[45,46] Despite the fact that laparoscopic appendectomy takes longer to perform (57minutes vs. 34 minutes) at a marginally increased cost (1023 Euro vs. 970 Euro) compared to open appendectomy, it has multiple advantages.[47,48] A large database study of adults and children in the United States showed laparoscopic appendectomy to be associated with a shorter median hospital stay and lower rates of wound infection, gastrointestinal complications and overall complications.[49] The increased operative expense of laparoscopic appendectomy appeared to be offset by an earlier return to normal daily activities.

Appendicitis in preschool children

Acute appendicitis in the preschool child accounts for a small fraction of all pediatric admissions with this diagnosis. Children under 2 years of age account for 1% of all cases of appendicitis in childhood.[50] In a large series from Dublin, Puri *et al.* found that only 4.3% of their patients with appendicitis presented during the first three years of life.[51] A recent 28-year review of appendicitis in children less than 3 years of age showed that all had perforated appendicitis at presentation.[52] This resulted in very high morbidity (wound infection/abscess/dehiscence, pneumonia, small bowel obstruction, incisional hernia and enterocutaneous fistula) affecting 59% of these patients. Although appendicitis is uncommon in this age group, it should be considered in the differential diagnosis in a preschool child presenting with abdominal pain, tenderness, and vomiting.

The diagnosis of appendicitis in preschool children can be difficult, resulting in delay and more severe disease. The young child's inability to communicate adequately with its parents, atypical disease presentation, and associated illnesses may delay the diagnosis. Surana *et al.* reviewed 132 children under 5 years of age treated for acute appendicitis in two Dublin children's hospitals between 1987 and 1991 in order to identify factors contributing to more serious disease in this age group.[53] Sixty three (48%) of these children had perforated appendicitis, 29 (22%) had an appendix mass, 36 (27%) had uncomplicated appendicitis,

Table 29.1. Presenting symptoms in 132 preschool children with appendicitis[53]

Symptoms	Patients
Abdominal pain	117 (89%)
Nausea/vomiting	115 (87%)
Fever	25 (19%)
Diarrhea	35 (27%)
Anorexia	38 (29%)
Dysuria	4 (3%)
Cough/sore throat	15 (11%)
Earache	2 (1.5%)
Headache	2 (1.5%)
Rash	1 (0.8%)
Irritability	20 (15%)
Lethargy/drowsiness	9 (7%)

and 4 (3%) had a normal appendix. All the classic symptoms were present in the majority of patients. However, atypical symptoms were found in many children including diarrhea, cough/sore throat, dysuria, headache and earache (Table 29.1). A diagnosis other than appendicitis was suspected in 53 (40%) patients, leading to a delay in management. Mean duration of symptoms before admission was as follows: acute appendicitis 39 hours, perforated appendicitis 53 hours, and appendix mass 82 hours. Postoperatively, an intra-abdominal abscess occurred in 5% of patients with perforated appendicitis and none with uncomplicated appendicitis; these patients were treated using antimicrobial agents, with complete resolution clinically and on ultrasound in all cases. One patient required a laparotomy for adhesive intestinal obstruction. There were no deaths.

In view of the frequency of atypical presentation and the increased incidence of advanced appendicitis, a high index of suspicion is necessary in preschool children presenting with acute abdominal pain. Early diagnosis is the key to reducing morbidity from appendicitis in this age group.

Perforated appendicitis

The reported incidence of perforated appendicitis in children is 18–40%.[23,39,54] Two recent large series of appendicitis in children have reported an 18%[39] and 20%[23] incidence, respectively. The incidence is much higher in preschool children (see above).[53,55]

Nowadays, mortality is very rare.[56] Several controversies have arisen over the years regarding the best approach to reduce the morbidity from appendicitis, especially infectious complications such as intra-abdominal abscess and wound infection. Many of these controversies relating to perforated appendicitis have now been resolved. Several studies have confirmed the efficacy of antibiotics in reducing morbidity. Probably, the first preoperative dose of antibiotics is the most important. There is still some disagreement about the duration of antibiotic therapy and which agents to use. Routine wound drainage is no longer regarded as beneficial, and is associated with an increased risk of infection. Current opinion overwhelmingly favors confining the use of drains to those cases in which there is a clearly localized abscess cavity.[57] Insertion of a peritoneal drain does not improve the outcome after perforated appendicitis, and is not associated with a reduction in the duration of nasogastric drainage or period of hospitalization. Intraoperative irrigation of the peritoneal cavity is beneficial in perforated appendicitis. The majority of pediatric surgeons currently favor irrigation, with or without antibiotics, until a clear effluent is returned. Subcuticular skin closure is safe after perforated appendicitis; wound infection rates are low and thus there is no compelling reason to opt for delayed closure of the appendectomy incision.[39,58]

In Dublin, our protocol for the management of perforated appendicitis consists of preoperative administration of antibiotics that are continued for 5 days postoperatively. Intraoperative irrigation of the peritoneal cavity is carried out and the appendectomy wound is closed using subcuticular absorbable sutures. During a 5-year period (1987–91), a total of 870 patients underwent emergency appendectomy for appendicitis at Our Lady's Hospital for Sick Children.[39] One hundred and fifty-eight (18%) of the patients (98 boys) were found to have a perforated appendix. Their ages ranged from 18 months to 15 years (mean 7.8 y). Thirteen (8%) developed postoperative complications: 9 (5.6%) had a wound infection, which was managed by local drainage and antibiotics and 5 (3.2%), including one with a wound infection, developed an intra-abdominal abscess, which was confirmed by ultrasonography and resolved with antibiotic therapy. Nine of the 13 patients with postoperative infective complications were readmitted to hospital; their mean hospital stay was 9.4 days (range 3–18). The mean duration of hospital stay in the 158 patients with perforated appendicitis, including those who were readmitted, was 6.8 days (range 3–47). There were no deaths.

An analysis of three recent studies of perforated appendicitis which used a protocol of preoperative antibiotics, intraoperative irrigation of the peritoneal cavity, primary subcuticular skin closure and a short course of postoperative antibiotics showed an intra-abdominal abscess rate of 1.3–3.2%, a wound infection rate of 1.3–5.7%, no deaths, and a mean hospital stay of 6.8–11.4 days.[29,39,54] These results set new standards in wound management, infectious complications and length of hospital stay in perforated appendicitis.

Appendix mass

An appendix mass results from appendicitis that is localized by edematous, adherent omentum and loops of small bowel.[51] In contrast, appendiceal abscess is a localized suppurative process that may occur at any time in the course of appendicitis, or may complicate an appendiceal mass. Clinically, it is not possible in most cases to distinguish with certainty between the two conditions. An appendiceal mass is discovered at presentation in about 10% of children with appendicitis.[59,60] The incidence is higher during the first three years of life, when one-third of the patients with appendicitis may present with an appendiceal mass.[51]

The management of an appendiceal mass in children is controversial. Many authors recommend non-operative management, with antibiotics followed by delayed appendectomy. Others favor immediate appendectomy in every case of appendicitis. Controversy around the conservative management of appendiceal mass has arisen mainly from the belief that children, and particularly infants, have a poor ability to localize intraperitoneal inflammatory processes, and so those with an appendiceal mass should be managed operatively. The senior author has previously shown that a child's ability to localize appendiceal inflammation is well developed, even in infancy, and that half of the patients developing appendicitis during the first two years of life,[50] and one-third of those developing appendicitis during the first three years of life,[51] have an appendiceal mass at presentation.

Initial conservative management of an appendix mass, followed by interval appendectomy, has been practiced at the authors' institution for over 30 years.[50] Gillick *et al.* recently reviewed these results.[61] During the period 1982–2000, 427 children presented to one of Dublin's three pediatric hospitals with a diagnosis of appendix mass. There were 222 boys and 205 girls ranging in age from 2 months to 18 years (mean 7.3 years). Duration of symptoms ranged from a few hours to 21 days, with 266 (62%) having had symptoms for longer than 3 days. The diagnosis was made clinically in 136 (32%) children, by ultrasonography in 61 (14%), by examination under anesthesia in 229 (54%), and by computed tomography in one child. All were initially managed conservatively with intravenous antibiotics, nasogastric suction as required and intravenous fluids until oral fluids and diet were tolerated. In 346 (84%) of 411 patients the mass resolved completely. The mean duration of hospital stay in this group was 6 days. Three hundred and thirty-one children had an elective appendectomy as planned, 4–6 weeks after discharge; 15 (4.5%) of these elective appendectomies were performed laparoscopically. The complication rate following elective appendectomy was 2.3% (five wound infections, two intra-abdominal abscesses and one hematoma). Histological assessment of the appendices removed electively demonstrated acute or subacute inflammation in 51% of the specimens. Two specimens had a carcinoid tumor. Sixty-five (16%) children with an appendix mass failed to respond to initial non-operative management: 17 required early appendectomy for ongoing symptoms and 27 developed an appendix abscess that required drainage and subsequent appendectomy. These data, as well as other studies, support the contention that initial non-operative management of an appendiceal mass, followed by an appendectomy, is a safe and effective policy.

We recommend interval appendectomy following resolution of the appendiceal mass. Some investigators have questioned the need for appendectomy after conservative management, on the assertion that the incidence of recurrent appendicitis is low and the complication rate after interval appendectomy is high. However, complications after interval appendectomy in children in our series were uncommon. Moreover, histologic evidence of inflammation was present in 51% of these appendices. It is possible that the inflammation in some cases might have resolved spontaneously, but some patients develop recurrent appendicitis (see later). Therefore, we recommend initial non-operative management of appendiceal masses with antibiotics, followed by appendectomy 6–8 weeks later.

Mortality

In the United Kingdom, the number of deaths from acute appendicitis in children has decreased dramatically since the 1930s, largely as a result of the decline in incidence of appendicitis but also because of a marked reduction in the hospital case-fatality rate during the last 30 years.[8] Three national audits between 1963 and 1997 covering all children dying of appendicitis in England and Wales showed an 85% decrease in the hospital case-fatality rate (Table 29.2).[56] This almost certainly reflects improvements in clinical care which have occurred in parallel with the expansion of specialist pediatric surgery and anesthesia. Delay in referral to hospital and/or diagnosis of acute

Table 29.2. Hospital death rates in England and Wales per 1,000 discharges with acute appendicitis (actual number of deaths in parentheses)[56]

	Age (yr)			
Period	0–4	5–9	10–14	All
1963–67	6.5 (71)	0.96 (56)	0.53 (54)	1.06 (181)
1980–1984	3.13 (8)	0.35 (8)	0.15 (9)	0.30 (25)
1993–1997	0.44 (1)	0.12 (2)	0.15 (6)	0.16 (9)
Fall in death rate 1963–1997	−93%	−87%	−72%	−85%

appendicitis are the dominant factors responsible for the residual small number of avoidable deaths.[8]

Long-term outcomes

The long-term outcome of the vast majority of patients who undergo appendectomy for childhood appendicitis is excellent. A small number of patients develop late adhesive intestinal obstruction. The belief that perforated appendicitis in girls is associated with reduced fertility in later life has been based on few reports that do not stand up to critical analysis.

Intestinal obstruction

Intestinal obstruction requiring surgery has been reported in 0.68% of patients after open appendectomy[62] and 1.6%–2% of patients with perforated appendicitis.[23,63] Adhesive intestinal obstruction requiring surgery has also been reported after removing a normal appendix. Most cases of intestinal obstruction occur relatively soon after appendectomy. Lund and Murphy reported 6 patients out of 373 children (1.6%) with perforated appendicitis who developed small bowel obstruction that required operative intervention.[63] This occurred 1–11 months postoperatively. In a historical cohort study of 245,400 patients who underwent open appendectomy, Andersson found that the risk of postoperative small bowel obstruction needing surgical treatment was lower than previously thought.[64] The cumulative risk of surgically treated small bowel obstruction after appendectomy was 0.41% after 4 weeks, 0.63% after 1 year and 1.3% after 30 years. This compared with 0.003% at 1 year and 0.21% after 30 years in non-operated population-based matched controls. The risk was low after non-perforated appendicitis and higher after perforated appendicitis, and after appendectomy performed at operations for other diagnoses, including non-specific abdominal pain and mesenteric lymphadenitis. The cause of increased adhesions after perforated appendicitis is evident as peritonitis induces adhesions. When a macroscopically normal appendix is found at laparotomy, a wider exploration of the abdomen may be undertaken to determine the cause of the symptoms. It has been suggested that this exploration may predispose to more widespread adhesions due to damage to the peritoneum. Band adhesions were more often the cause of small bowel obstruction after appendectomy than in controls; this type of adhesive bowel obstruction is less likely to settle with non-operative management. Previously, it had been suggested that adhesion formation was considerably less after laparoscopic appendectomy.[65] A recent retrospective review of intestinal obstruction after laparoscopic surgery demonstrated a prevalence of early postoperative obstruction of 0.16% after appendectomy.[66] Appendectomy was in third place after cholecystectomy and transperitoneal hernia repair as one of the most likely laparoscopic procedures to be followed by intestinal obstruction. Obstruction was most commonly due to adhesions or fibrotic bands and mostly affected the umbilical trocar site. The small intestine was most frequently involved.

Perforated appendicitis and subsequent fertility in girls

It is often stated that perforated appendicitis in girls is associated with an increased risk of tubal infertility, although there is little evidence base in the literature. Most early studies that examined the frequency of infertility in women who had undergone appendectomy for perforated appendix in adult life were based on a small number of cases and lacked detailed investigations of infertility. For example, in a study of 158 women with primary infertility, Mueller *et al.* reported that those who had had an operation for a perforated appendix were five times more likely to be infertile, relative to women who had never had appendicitis.[67] Critical analysis of their study showed that 20% of their patients with primary infertility had a history of pelvic inflammatory disease compared with only 3% of controls. Since pelvic inflammatory disease is a well-known cause of infertility, a higher incidence of infertility due to tubal disease in this group of patients is to be expected.

Owing to the proximity of the appendix to the right fallopian tube, one might expect an appendectomy to be associated with unilateral tubal disease, rather than bilateral disease. Consistent with this was a WHO study that found that 11% of 7570 women attending for fertility investigations had undergone appendectomy, 18% of which were classified as complicated.[68] In this study bilateral tubal occlusion was found significantly less often in those who had had an appendectomy compared to those who had not. Furthermore, the incidence of pelvic adhesions was not significantly different between those who had had a complicated appendectomy and those in whom the procedure had been uncomplicated.

There are only a few reports in the literature that have specifically examined the risk of infertility in women who have undergone appendectomy in childhood. Puri *et al.*[69] and Geerdson and Hanson[70] reported that perforated appendicitis in girls was not associated with an increased incidence of subsequent infertility. However, an earlier study by Thompson and Lynn found that 6 out of 37 women who had undergone appendectomy for perforated appendicitis in childhood were infertile.[71] Close scrutiny of this report shows that two of the six patients had evidence of salpingitis, and in the other four women, infertility investigations were inadequate.

Puri *et al.* reviewed 389 girls operated on for perforated appendicitis between 1957 and 1975.[72] Their ages at the time of appendectomy ranged from 10 months to 13 years. Of these, 276 were between 20 and 43 years old when the study was undertaken and it proved possible to contact 181 of them. One hundred and two were married and 79 were unmarried. Eighty-four (82%) of the married women had one or more children. Eighteen married women who had no children were studied in detail (Table 29.3): five were using contraceptives; two desired pregnancy but had not conceived; one woman was separated from her husband; two patients had conceived and aborted; and two were married to infertile men. The remaining six patients had been investigated for infertility: no demonstrable cause was found in three, one showed evidence of bilateral tubal occlusion secondary to pelvic inflammatory disease, one had had a right ectopic pregnancy followed by two abortions, and one was found to have a pituitary adenoma.

Recently, Andersson *et al.* investigated fertility patterns in three cohorts of women ($n = 9840$) who had undergone appendectomy when aged less than 15 years between 1964 and 1983.[73] For each patient, five age-matched controls were randomly selected from the Swedish Fertility Registry ($n = 47\,590$). The patients were divided into three groups, based on their discharge diagnosis of non-perforated, perforated or normal appendix. Women with a history of perforated appendicitis had a similar rate of first births as the control women and a similar distribution of parity at the end of follow-up (mean age 31.6 years). Women who had had a normal appendix removed had an increased rate of first births and on average had their first child at an earlier age and reached a higher parity than control women. This study concluded that a history of perforated appendicitis in childhood does not seem to have long-term negative consequences on female fertility and supports our own findings.

Although the fallopian tubes may be affected by inflammation as a result of perforated appendicitis in childhood, the inflammatory process usually resolves completely after appendectomy and adequate antibiotic treatment, and does not have the same implications as salpingitis or endometriosis in adults. After the introduction of antibiotics directed against anaerobes, particularly Bacteroides species, the incidence of intra-abdominal abscess complicating perforated appendicitis fell significantly. This is likely to have contributed further to minimizing any risk of tubal damage arising from a perforated appendix.

It is possible that women who have borne children may nevertheless have sustained damage to their right fallopian tube from appendicitis. However, the left tube in such cases should function normally, a situation analogous to ectopic pregnancy in which a salpingectomy has previously been performed but the remaining tube retains its normal physiologic function. In summary, these data indicate that perforated appendicitis before puberty has little if any role in the etiology of tubal infertility.

Appendectomy and subsequent development of right inguinal hernia

Some investigators have suggested an increased incidence of right inguinal hernia after appendectomy. The cause of the right-sided inguinal hernia is thought to be damage to the nerve supply of the inguinal muscles during appendectomy. Malazgirt *et al.* investigated the effect of appendectomy on the subsequent development of right inguinal hernia in 583 patients.[74] They found that the incidence of right inguinal hernia was no greater in those who had previously undergone appendectomy compared with those who had not.

Nerve entrapment after appendectomy

A rarely reported complication of appendectomy is entrapment of the ilioinguinal nerve.[75] These patients have the classic triad of the entrapment syndrome: pain accurately localized near the incision; objective sensory impairment in the appropriate area of the skin; and temporary relief by injection of local anesthetic agents. The symptoms may arise immediately after operation or several years later, implying that the nerve may be involved either directly by a suture, or indirectly by pressure from mature scar tissue.

Table 29.3. Clinical data in 18 childless married women after childhood appendectomy for perforated appendicitis[72]

Patient no	Age at appendectomy (y)	Age at follow-up (y)	Duration of marriage (y)	Postoperative abscess	Comment
1	5	24	1	–	FP-pill
2	8	26	1	Pelvic	FP-pill
3	11	29	$1^1/_2$	–	FP-pill
4	4	29	1	Pelvic	FP-pill
5	7	27	$1^1/_2$	–	FP-none
6	$2^1/_2$	26	2	–	FP-none
7	10	25	$2^1/_2$	–	FP-pill 2 years
8	8	29	Separated	–	–
9	$12^1/_2$	35	$7^1/_2$	–	3 miscarriages
10	3	31	4	–	1 miscarriage
11	$7^1/_2$	35	6	Pelvic	REP, 2 miscarriages, (L) salpingolysis, bilateral ovariolysis HSG-NAD
12	$9^1/_2$	39	15	Intra-abdominal	Male sterility
13	11	37	13	–	Male sterility
14	3	28	7	–	PID, (L) ovarian cystectomy, bilateral tubal occlusion, microsurgery, endometriosis
15	12	26	6	Pelvic	(L) ovarian cystectomy, HSG-bilateral tubal spill, pituitary adenoma, IVF
16	8	28	4	Subphrenic	No demonstrable cause
17	4	29	$4^1/_2$	–	No demonstrable cause
18	6	28	4	–	No demonstrable cause

FP, family planning; HSG, hysterosalpingography: IVF, *in vitro* fertilization; PID, pelvic inflammatory disease; REP, right ectopic pregnancy.

Recurrent appendicitis

It is important to avoid leaving a significant remnant of the appendix at operation since recurrent appendicitis in the stump has been reported after both open appendectomy[76–78] and laparoscopic appendectomy.[79–81] This complication has been described after an interval of up to 21 years and may be a particular hazard in pediatric surgery because of the growth potential in children. Other pathology of the appendix stump has also been rarely described, including intussusception[82] and malignancy.[83]

Inflammatory bowel disease

The etiology and pathogenesis of ulcerative colitis (UC) and Crohn's disease (CD) are poorly understood. Recent studies have suggested a link between appendectomy and the subsequent risk of developing inflammatory bowel disease.[84–86] In a large cohort study of 212 963 patients who underwent appendectomy before the age of 50 years, Andersson *et al.* found that those who had had an appendectomy for an inflammatory condition (appendicitis or lymphadenitis) had a lower risk of subsequent UC.[84] This inverse relation was limited to patients who had surgery before the age of 20 years. These findings are supported by case-control studies, which have shown that appendectomy under the age of 20 years was associated with a significantly reduced risk of subsequent UC.[85] In contrast to this, an increased risk of CD was found in patients who had undergone appendectomy at the age of 20 years or more.[86] Crohn's disease patients with a history of perforated appendicitis generally had a worse prognosis. Further studies of the potential association between inflammatory bowel disease and appendicitis are warranted, not least because they may give clues to the etiology and pathogenesis of both inflammatory bowel disease and appendicitis.[87]

Medicolegal aspects

Missed appendicitis

Missed appendicitis remains a high-risk area in professional liability. Failure to diagnose appendicitis is routinely listed among the important reasons for a malpractice suit to be brought against the accident and emergency physician.[88] In the United Kingdom, delay in diagnosis is the most common reason for complications of appendicitis resulting in litigation.[89] Diagnosing appendicitis accurately and early is therefore very important.

Although classic symptoms are present in the majority of patients with appendicitis, atypical symptoms are not uncommon, especially in preschool children (see above). For example, approximately 15% of all children and 25% of preschool children with appendicitis have diarrhea on presentation. In a recent report on appendicitis in preschool children, a diagnosis other than appendicitis was suspected by attending medical practitioners in 40% of the patients, leading to a delay in management.[53] The various diagnoses in these patients included gastroenteritis, upper respiratory tract infection, urinary tract infection, gastritis, intussusception, meningitis and pneumonia. In view of the atypical presentation and increased incidence of complicated appendicitis and associated morbidity, a high index of suspicion is necessary in preschool children presenting with acute abdominal pain.[90]

REFERENCES

1. Amyand, C. Cited by Moir, C. R. Appendicectomy: open and laparoscopic techniques. In Spitz, L. & Coran, A. G. *Operative Pediatric Surgery*. London: Chapman & Hall, 1995; 402–410.
2. Fitz, R. H. Perforating inflammation of the vermiform appendix: with special reference to its early diagnosis and treatment. *Am. J. Med. Sci.* 1886; **1**:321–346.
3. Mortin, T. Cited by Cloud, D. T. Appendicitis. In Ashcraft, K. W. & Holder, T. M. *Pediatric Surgery*, Philadelphia: W. B. Saunders, 1993; 470–477.
4. McBurney, C. Disease of the vermiform appendix. *NY Med. J.* 1889; **50**:676–684.
5. Luckmann, R. & Davis, P. The epidemiology of acute appendicitis in California: racial, gender and seasonal variation. *Epidemiology* 1994; **2**:323–330.
6. Gerst, P. H., Mukherjee, A., Kumar, A., & Albu, E. Acute appendicitis in minority communities: an epidemiologic study. *J. Natl. Med. Assoc.* 1997; **89**:168–172.
7. Guagliardo, M. F., Teach, S. J., Huang, Z. J., Chamberlain J. M., & Joseph, J. G.. Racial and ethnic disparities in pediatric appendicitis rupture rate. *Acad. Emerg. Med.* 2003; **10**:1218–1227.
8. Stringer, M. D. & Pledger, G. Childhood appendicitis in the United Kingdom: fifty years of progress. *J. Pediatr. Surg.* 2003; **38** (Suppl. 1):65–69.
9. Burkitt, D. P. The aetiology of appendicitis. *Br. J. Surg.* 1971; **58**: 695–699.
10. Adamidis, D., Roma-Giannikou, E., Karamolegou, K., Tselalidou, E., & Constantopoulos, A. Fiber intake and childhood appendicitis. *Int. J. Food Sci. Nutr.* 2000; **51**:153–157
11. Attwood, S. E., Mealy, K., Cafferkey, M. T. *et al. Yersinia* infection and acute abdominal pain. *Lancet* 1987; **1**:529–533.
12. Lamps, L. W., Madhusudhan, K. T., Greenson, J. K. *et al.* The role of *Yersinia enterocolitica* and *Yersinia pseudotuberculosis* in granulomatous appendicitis: a histologic and molecular study. *Am. J. Surg. Pathol.* 2001; **25**:508–515.
13. Jackson, R. H., Gardner, P. S., Kennedy, J., & McQuillan, J. Viruses in the aetiology of acute appendicitis. *Lancet* 1996; **ii**:711–715.
14. Andersson, R., Hugander, A., Thulin, A., Nystrom, P. O., & Olaison, G. Clusters of acute appendicitis: further evidence for an infectious aetiology. *Int. J. Epidemiol.* 1995; **24**:829–833.
15. Gauderer, M. W. L., Crane, M. M., Green, J. A., DeCou, J. M., & Abrams, R. S. Acute appendicitis in children: the importance of family history. *J. Pediatr. Surg.* 2001; **36**:1214–1217.
16. Tsuji, M., Puri, P., & Reen, D. J. Characterisation of the local inflammatory response in appendicitis. *J. Pediatr. Gastroenterol. Nutr.* 1993; **16**:43–48.
17. Wang, Y., Reen, D. J., & Puri, P. Is a histologically normal appendix following emergency appendicectomy always normal? *Lancet* 1996; **347**:1076–1079.
18. Nemeth, L., Reen, D. J., O'Brian, S., McDermott, M., & Puri, P. Evidence of an inflammatory pathologic condition in "normal" appendices following emergency appendectomy. *Arch. Pathol. Lab. Med.* 2001; **125**:759–764.
19. Nemeth, L., Rolle, U., Reen, D. J., & Puri, P. Nitrergic hyperinnervation in appendices histologically classified as normal. *Arch. Pathol. Lab. Med.* 2003; **127**:573–578.
20. Xiong, S., Puri, P., Nemeth, L., O'Briain, D. S., & Reen, D. J. Neuronal hypertrophy in acute appendicitis. *Arch. Pathol. Lab. Med.* 2000; **124**:1429–1433.
21. Rothrock, S. G. & Pagane, J. Acute appendicitis in children: emergency department diagnosis and management. *Ann. Emerg. Med.* 2000; **36**:39–51.
22. Surana, R., O'Donnell, B., & Puri, P. Appendicitis diagnosed following active observation does not increase morbidity in children. *Pediatr. Surg. Int.* 1995; **10**:76–78.
23. Pearl, R. H., Hale, D. A., Molloy, M., Schutt, D. C., & Jacques, D. P. Pediatric appendectomy. *J. Pediatr. Surg.* 1995; **30**:173–181.
24. Paajanen, H. & Somppi, E. Early childhood appendicitis is still a difficult diagnosis. *Acta Pediatr.* 1996; **85**:459–462.
25. Kosloske, A. M., Love, C. L., Rohrer, J. E., Goldthorn, J. F., & Lacey, S. R. The diagnosis of appendicitis in children: outcomes of a

strategy based on pediatric surgical evaluation. *Pediatrics* 2004; **113**:29–34.
26. Bendeck, S. E., Nino-Murcia, M., Berry, G. J., & Jeffrey, R. B. Jr. Imaging for suspected appendicitis: negative appendectomy and perforation rates. *Radiology* 2002; **225**:131–136.
27. Oncel, M., Degirmenci, B., Demirhan, N., Hakyemez, B., Altuntas, Y., & Aydinli, M. Is the use of plain abdominal radiographs (PAR) a necessity for all patients suspected acute appendicitis in emergency services? *Curr. Surg.* 2003; **60**:296–300.
28. Okamoto, T., Utsunomiya, T., Inutsuka, S. *et al.* The appearance of a normal appendix on barium enema examination does not rule out a diagnosis of chronic appendicitis: report of a case and review of the literature. *Surg. Today* 1997; **27**: 550–553.
29. Lowe, L. H., Penney, M. W., Stein, S. M. *et al.* Unenhanced limited CT of the abdomen in the diagnosis of appendicitis in children: comparison with sonography. *Am. J. Roentgenol.* 2001; **176**:31–35.
30. Sivit, C. J. & Applegate, K. E. Imaging of acute appendicitis in children. *Semin. Ultrasound CT MR* 2003; **24**:74–82.
31. Garcia-Pena, B. M., Mandl, K. D., Kraus, S. J. *et al.* Ultrasonography and limited computed tomography in the diagnosis and management of appendicitis in children. *J. Am. Med. Assoc.* 1999; **282**:1041–1046.
32. Garcia-Pena, B. M., Cook, E. F., & Mandl, K. D. Selective imaging strategies for the diagnosis of appendicitis in children. *Pediatrics* 2004; **113**:24–28.
33. Partrick, D. A., Janik, J. E., Janik, J. S., Bensard, D. D., & Karrer, F. M. Increased CT scan utilization does not improve the diagnostic accuracy of appendicitis in children. *J. Pediatr. Surg.* 2003; **38**:659–662.
34. Stephen, A. E., Segev, D. L., Ryan, D. P. *et al.* The diagnosis of acute appendicitis in a pediatric population: to CT or not to CT. *J. Pediatr. Surg.* 2003; **38**:367–371.
35. Bachoo, P., Mahomed, A. A., Ninan, G. K., & Youngson, G. G. Acute appendicitis: the continuing role for active observation. *Pediatr. Surg. Int.* 2001; **17**:125–128.
36. Surana, R., Quinn, F., & Puri, P. Is it necessary to perform appendicectomy in the middle of the night in children? *Br. Med. J.* 1993; **306**:1168.
37. Celik, A., Ergun, O., Ozcan, C., Aldemir, H., & Balik, E. Is it justified to obtain routine peritoneal fluid cultures during appendectomy in children? *Pediatr. Surg. Int.* 2003; **19**:632–634.
38. Engstrom, L. & Fenyo, G. Appendicectomy. Assessment of stump invagination versus simple ligation: a prospective, randomized trial. *Br. J. Surg.* 1985; **72**:971–972.
39. Surana, R. & Puri, P. Primary wound closure after perforated appendicitis in children. *Br. J. Surg.* 1994; **81**:440.
40. Rucinski, J., Fabian, T., Panagopoulos, G., Schein, M., & Wise, L. Gangrenous and perforated appendicitis: a meta-analytic study of 2532 patients indicates that the incision should be closed primarily. *Surgery* 2000; **127**:136–141.
41. Moir, C. R. Appendicectomy: open and laparoscopic approaches. In Spitz, L. & Coran A. G. *Rob & Smith's Operative Surgery*, 5th edn. London: Chapman & Hall, 1995; 402–410.
42. Gilchrist, B. F., Lobe, T. E., Schropp, K. P. *et al.* Is there a role for laparoscopic appendicectomy in pediatric surgery? *J. Pediat. Surg.* 1992; **27**:209–216.
43. Humphrey, G. M. E. & Najmaldin, A. Laparoscopic appendicectomy in childhood. *Pediat. Surg. Int.* 1995; **10**:86–89.
44. Newman, K., Ponsky, T., Kittle, K. *et al.* Appendicitis 2000: variability in practice, outcomes, and resource utilization at thirty pediatric hospitals. *J. Pediatr. Surg.* 2003; **38**:372–379.
45. Canty, T. G. Sr, Collins, D., Losasso, B., Lynch, F., & Brown, C. Laparoscopic appendectomy for simple and perforated appendicitis in children: the procedure of choice? *J. Pediatr. Surg.* 2000; **35**:1582–1585.
46. Lintula, H., Kokki, H., Vanamo, K., Antila, P., & Eskelinen, M. Laparoscopy in children with complicated appendicitis. *J. Pediatr. Surg.* 2002; **37**:1317–13120.
47. Lintula, H., Kokki, H., Vanamo, K., Valtonen, H., Mattila, M., & Eskelinen, M. The costs and effects of laparoscopic appendectomy in children. *Arch. Pediatr. Adolesc. Med.* 2004; **158**: 34–37.
48. Vegunta, R. K., Ali, A., Wallace, L. J., Switzer, D. M., & Pearl, R. H. Laparoscopic appendectomy in children: technically feasible and safe in all stages of acute appendicitis. *Am. Surg.* 2004; **70**:198–201.
49. Guller, U., Hervey, S., Purves, H. *et al.* Laparoscopic versus open appendectomy: outcomes comparison based on a large administrative database. *Ann. Surg.* 2004; **239**:43–52.
50. Puri, P. & O'Donnell, B. Appendicitis in infancy. *J. Pediat. Surg.* 1978; **13**:173–174.
51. Puri, P., Boyd, E., Guiney, E. J., & O'Donnell, B. Appendix mass in the very young child. *J. Pediatr. Surg.* 1981; **16**:55–57.
52. Alloo, J., Gerstle, T., Shilyansky, J., & Ein, S. H. Appendicitis in children less than 3 years of age: a 28-year review. *Pediatr. Surg. Int.* 2004; **19**:777–779.
53. Surana, R., Quinn, F., & Puri, P. Appendicitis in preschool children. *Pediatr. Surg. Int.* 1995; **10**:68–70.
54. Neilson, I. R., Laberge, J. M., Nguyen, L. T. *et al.* Appendicitis in children: current therapeutic recommendations. *J. Pediatr. Surg.* 1990; **25**:1113–1116.
55. Williams, N. & Kapila, L. Acute appendicitis in the under-5 year old. *J. Roy. Coll. Surg. Edin.* 1994; **39**:168–170.
56. Pledger, G. & Stringer, M. D. Childhood deaths from acute appendicitis in England and Wales 1963–1997: observational population based study. *Br. Med. J.* 2001; **323**:430–431.
57. Tander, B., Pektas, O., & Bulut, M. The utility of peritoneal drains in children with uncomplicated perforated appendicitis. *Pediatr. Surg. Int.* 2003; **19**:548–550.
58. Meier, D. E., Guzzetta, P. C., Barber, R. G., Hynan, L. S., & Seetharamaiah, R. Perforated appendicitis in children: is there a best treatment? *J. Pediatr. Surg.* 2003; **38**:1520–1524.
59. Puri, P. & O'Donnell, B. Management of appendiceal mass in children. *Pediatr. Surg. Int.* 1989; **4**:306–308.
60. Surana, R. & Puri, P. Appendiceal mass in children. *Pediat. Surg. Int.* 1995; **10**:79–81.
61. Gillick, J., Velayudham, M., & Puri, P. Conservative management of appendix mass in children. *Br. J. Surg.* 2001; **88**:1539–1542.

62. Tingstedt, B., Johansson, J., Nehez, L., & Andersson, R. Late abdominal complaints after appendectomy – readmissions during long-term follow-up. *Dig. Surg.* 2004; **21**:23–27.
63. Lund, D. P. & Murphy, E. U. Management of perforated appendicitis in children: a decade of aggressive treatment. *J. Pediatr. Surg.* 1994; **29**:1130–1134.
64. Andersson, R. E. Small bowel obstruction after appendicectomy. *Br. J. Surg.* 2001; **88**:1387–1391.
65. De Wilde, R. L. Goodbye to the late bowel obstruction after appendicectomy. *Lancet* 1991; **338**:1012.
66. Duron, J. J., Hay, J. M., Msika, S. *et al.* Prevalence and mechanisms of small intestinal obstruction following laparoscopic abdominal surgery: a retrospective multicenter study. French Association for Surgical Research. *Arch. Surg.* 2000; **135**:208–212.
67. Mueller, B. A., Daling, J. R., Moore, D. E. *et al.* Appendicectomy and the risk of tubal infertility. *N. Engl. J. Med.* 1986; **315**:1506–1508.
68. Cooke, I. D. Investigation of the subfertile couple: results from the female partner. WHO Task Force on the diagnosis and treatment of fertility. In Shan Ratnam, S., Teoh, E. S., & Anandakumar, C., eds. *Infertility.* New Jersey: Parthenon, 1987; 143–150.
69. Puri, P., Guiney, E. J., O'Donnell, B., & McGuinness, E. P. J. Effects of perforated appendicitis in girls on subsequent fertility. *Br. Med. J.* 1984; **288**:25–26.
70. Geerdson, J. & Hanson, J. B. Incidence of sterility in women operated on in childhood for perforated appendicitis. *Acta. Obstet. Gynecol. Scand.* 1977; **56**:523–524.
71. Thompson, W. M. & Lynn, H. B. The possible relationship of appendicitis with perforation in childhood to infertility in women. *J. Pediatr. Surg.* 1971; **6**:458–461.
72. Puri, P., McGuinness, E. P. J., & Guiney, E. J. Fertility following perforated appendicitis in girls. *J. Pediatr. Surg.* 1989; **24**:547–549.
73. Andersson, R., Lambe, M., & Bergstrom, R. Fertility patterns after appendicectomy: historical cohort study. *Br. Med. J.* 1999; **318**:963–967.
74. Malazgirt, Z., Ozen, N., & Ozkan, K. Effects of appendicectomy on development of right inguinal hernia. *Eur. J. Surg.* 1992; **158**:43–44.
75. Stulz, P. & Pfeiffer, K. M. Peripheral nerve injuries resulting from common surgical procedures in the lower portion of abdomen. *Arch. Surg.* 1982; **17**:324–327.
76. Feigin, E., Carmon, M., Szold, A., & Seror, D. Acute stump appendicitis. *Lancet* 1993; **341**:757.
77. Durgun, A. V., Baca, B., Ersoy, Y., & Kapan, M. Stump appendicitis and generalized peritonitis due to incomplete appendectomy. *Tech. Coloproctol.* 2003; **7**:102–104.
78. Gupta, R., Gernshiemer, J., Golden, J., Narra, N., & Haydock, T. Abdominal pain secondary to stump appendicitis in a child. *J. Emerg. Med.* 2000; **18**:431–433.
79. Devereaux, D. A., McDermott, J. P., & Caushaj, P. F. Recurrent appendicitis following laparoscopic appendicectomy: report of a case. *Dis. Col. Rectum.* 1994; **37**:719–720.
80. Greenberg, J. J. & Esparito, T. J. Appendicitis after laparoscopic appendectomy: a warning. *J. Laparoendosc. Surg.* 1996; **6**:185–187.
81. Mangi, A. A. & Berger, D. L. Stump appendicitis. *Am. Surg.* 2000; **66**:739–741.
82. Forshall, I. Intussusception of the vermiform appendix with a report of seven cases in children. *Br. J. Surg.* 1953; **40**:305–312.
83. Thomas, S. E., Denning, D. A., & Cummings, M. H. Delayed pathology of the appendiceal stump: a case report of stump appendicitis and review. *Am. Surg.* 1994; **60**:842–844.
84. Andersson, R. E., Olaison, G., Tysk, C., & Ekbom, A. Appendectomy and protection against ulcerative colitis. *N. Engl. J. Med.* 2001; **344**:808–814.
85. Kurina, L. M., Goldacre, M. J., Yeates, D., & Seagroatt, V. Appendicectomy, tonsillectomy, and inflammatory bowel disease: a case-control record linkage study. *J. Epidemiol. Commun. Health* 2002; **56**:551–554.
86. Andersson, R. E., Olaison, G., Tysk, C., & Ekbom, A. Appendectomy is followed by increased risk of Crohn's disease. *Gastroenterology* 2003; **124**:40–46.
87. Frisch, M. Inverse association between appendicectomy and ulcerative colitis. *Br. Med. J.* 2006; **332**, 561–562.
88. Reynolds, S. L. Missed appendicitis in a pediatric emergency department. *Pediatr. Emerg. Care* 1993; **9**:1–3.
89. Keddie, N. A vestigial organ which causes a lot of claims. *J. Medi. Defence Union*, 1990; Winter:52–54.
90. Puri, P. Appendicitis: editorial comments. *Pediatr. Surg. Int.* 1995; **10**:61.

30

Hirschsprung's disease

Risto J. Rintala and Mikko Pakarinen

Children's Hospital, University of Helsinki, Finland

Introduction and historical aspects

Hirschsprung's disease (HD) is characterized by an absence of ganglion cells in the nerve plexuses of the distal large bowel. The lack of ganglion cells produces a functional obstruction and leads to dilatation of the bowel that is proximal to the aganglionic zone. The commonly quoted incidence of HD is 1:5000.[1] The classic description of HD was first presented in detail by a Danish pediatrician, Harald Hirschsprung in 1886.[2] The absence of ganglion cells in the distal large bowel was first reported by Tittel,[3] but the crucial role of this finding as the primary pathology was not appreciated until the late 1940s. In 1948 the first successful operation for HD was performed by Swenson and Bill.[4] This was a rectosigmoidectomy and later became known as the Swenson operation.

The functional obstruction caused by a lack of enteric ganglion cells in the distal bowel results in severe constipation and failure to thrive and may be fatal because of enterocolitis. The exact embryologic mechanism of the development of HD is controversial but the most favored theory is defective neuronal migration. Several genes (RET, GDNF, EDN3, ETRB) have been shown to cause HD both in humans and animal models. However, single gene defects explain only a minority of HD cases; in the majority, the cause of HD is probably multifactorial and multigenic.

In its classic form HD is restricted to the rectosigmoid region. Classic HD comprises 75–80% of all patients. Long segment HD and total colonic HD (in which a variable length of ileum is also involved) both occur in 10–15% of patients. More extensive proximal aganglionosis is exceedingly rare.

The severity of the clinical picture of HD is variable and not necessarily related to the length of the aganglionic segment. Almost all patients have symptoms immediately after birth but, in some, symptoms are initially alleviated and the patients present later in infancy or childhood. The variation in clinical presentation of HD is poorly understood.

Operative techniques

There are four major types of operative procedure in common use for the repair of HD. Each procedure has unique features in terms of the need for intrapelvic dissection and preservation of anal canal length. Each technique can be used as a primary operation or in multistage surgery and each technique is also suitable for laparoscopic-assisted repair of HD.

Swenson's rectosigmoidectomy

Swenson's operation was the first consistently successful operation for treating HD.[4] The original concept of elimination of the functional obstruction by bringing ganglionic bowel down to or near the anus is the basis of all later surgical modifications for the management of HD. The sigmoid colon and rectum are mobilized and resected trans-abdominally down to the anal canal. The anal canal is temporarily everted and the anastomosis between pulled-through ganglionic colon and the anal canal is performed outside the anus. The level of the anastomosis is 1–2 cm above the dentate line.

Duhamel's retrorectal pull-through

The Duhamel procedure was described by Bernard Duhamel in 1956.[5] The operation was later modified by

Pediatric Surgery and Urology: Long-term Outcomes, Mark Stringer, Keith Oldham, Pierre Mouriquand.
Published by Cambridge University Press.

Grob[6] and Martin.[7] The Duhamel operation requires much less pelvic dissection than Swenson's procedure. The dissection is retrorectal and preserves the extrinsic innervation of the pelvic organs. The ganglionic bowel is brought down to the level of the anal canal behind the aganglionic rectum and anastomosed side-to-side to the aganglionic bowel. The lower level of the anastomosis is about 1 cm above the dentate line.

Soave's endorectal pull-through

The Soave endorectal pull-through operation was described in 1964.[8] The procedure was modified by Boley[9] and Denda.[10] The principle of the Soave procedure is to protect the pelvic innervation and organs by keeping the rectal dissection in the submucosal plane within the bowel wall. The submucosal dissection is extended down to the anal canal. The ganglionic bowel is pulled-through the rectal muscle sleeve and anastomosed to the mucosa of the anal canal about 1 cm above the dentate line. In the original Soave procedure a 5–10 cm length of bowel was left hanging outside the anus and the anastomosis was performed by secondary trimming of the bowel. Later modifications advocated primary anastomosis, with or without splitting of the aganglionic muscular cuff. More recently, the Soave operation has been modified by undertaking the entire endorectal dissection transanally, leaving either a short or long muscular cuff.[11,12] Other recent developments include laparoscopic-assisted transanal endorectal pull-through[13] and a totally transanal endorectal pull-through.[14]

Rehbein's anterior resection

The Rehbein anterior resection for HD was first described by Fritz Rehbein in 1959.[15] The operation comprises a low anterior rectosigmoid resection and end-to-end anastomosis between the residual rectum and the proximal ganglionic bowel 5–7 cm above the dentate line. There is no dissection in the lower pelvis which leaves the extrinsic innervation intact. The remaining aganglionic rectum is potentially obstructive and repeated anorectal dilatations are therefore required in the long term in many patients who have undergone Rehbein's operation for HD.

The role of primary pull-through procedures

Primary pull-through procedures without preliminary diversion or protective diversion during the definitive repair of confirmed HD have gained popularity in recent decades. In many centers, primary pull-through is the preferred method of repair.[16–19] The safety of this approach is well established.[16,19,20] All standard methods of repair are suitable for primary pull-through.

There has been a clear trend to timing the primary pull-through as early as possible. The results of neonatal pull-through operations have been shown to be comparable to those of multistage repair or primary pull-through later in infancy in terms of the frequency of complications and short- or medium-term bowel function.[16–20] A higher incidence of enterocolitis following primary neonatal pull-through has been reported[16,21] but this finding has not been confirmed in other series.[22] The potential advantages of primary neonatal pull-through are evident: multistage procedures with frequent colostomy complications are avoided; the potential hazards and stress from multiple anesthetics and operations for the patient are decreased; and the cumulative length of hospital stay and costs are reduced. It has also been suggested that the development of critical brain-anus neural circuitry with cortical synaptic connections is optimized if HD repair is performed soon after birth.

The most recent trend in the repair of HD is mini-invasive primary surgery. The first stage of this development was laparoscopic-assisted repair.[13] Primary laparoscopic pull-through gives excellent cosmesis and is possibly associated with less pain, faster return to normal activities and feeding, and a shorter postoperative hospital stay although these conclusions have not been challenged in randomized controlled trials. All standard operations for HD can be performed as laparoscopic-assisted procedures. In 1998, de la Torre-Mondragon and Ortega-Salgado published a novel approach for the repair of classic rectosigmoid HD, namely totally transanal endorectal pull-through.[14] Since then an increasing number of reports of this technique have appeared in the literature.[23–25] Early experience suggests that there is less blood loss and pain, faster return to normal feeding, and a significantly shorter hospital stay than after open or possibly also laparoscopic-assisted surgery. The totally transanal operation does not leave a scar. In addition to endorectal transanal repair, transanal Swenson operations have also been reported.[26]

Short-term outcomes

Mortality

The major causes of death in HD patients include pre- and postoperative enterocolitis and associated malformations and diseases that occur especially in syndromic HD patients. Down syndrome patients have an increased

Table 30.1. Early complications

1st author	Year	Surgical technique	Patients	Study period	Wound infection (%)	Wound dehiscence (%)	Perineal excoriation (%)	Rectal prolapse (%)	Anastomotic leakage (%)	Stoma revisions (%)	Preoperative enterocolitis (%)
Sherman[34]	1989	Swenson	880	1947–85	7	2			9		
Tariq[33]	1991	ERPT	60	1978–88	7		49	11	7		
Rescorla[46]	1992	Multiple	260	1972–91	1					2	6
Marty[35]	1995	Multiple	135	1971–93	1				3		13
Reding[37]	1997	Multiple	59	1972–92					4		15
Baillie[41]	1999	Duhamel	91	1980–91						13	
Yanchar[32]	1999	Multiple	107	1974–97			43	8	2	3	9
Shankar[17]	2000	ERPT	136	1988–98	7						
Teitelbaum[16]	2000	ERPT	181	1989–99	4	1	42	1	8		15
Total/mean			**1909**		**4**	**<1**	**45**	**7**	**5**	**6**	**11**

Complications are percentages. ERPT = endorectal pull-through.

risk of Hirschsprung's disease; a typical cardiac abnormality in these patients is an atrioventricular septal defect that requires open heart surgical repair. Down syndrome patients also have an attenuated immune defence system that makes them vulnerable to infectious complications following repair of HD and more susceptible to enterocolitis than otherwise healthy patients.[27,28] Cartilage-hair hypoplasia is a cartilage-bone dysplasia that is associated with HD; a defective immune system is the cause of an exceptionally high mortality in this specific group of patients.[29] Most but not all reported series of HD patients indicate that enterocolitis and its associated morbidity and mortality are more common in patients with total colonic aganglionosis (TCA).[30,31] Operative mortality was reported in earlier series but with improved overall management and better anesthesia and antibiotics operative deaths are now very rare. Recent large series of patients with HD show a very low mortality in patients who are otherwise healthy or suffer from classic HD.[16,23]

Complications

Most series of patients with HD report a significant incidence of early postoperative enterocolitis.[16,32–36] It has been suggested that postoperative enterocolitis is more common in patients who have had preoperative attacks of enterocolitis, but this is not supported by the literature. Other serious postoperative complications include anastomotic leak, anastomotic stricture and pelvic sepsis. The incidence of early complications depends on how carefully minor complications such as wound infections or postoperative perianal excoriation are reported. The frequency of preoperative enterocolitis and early postoperative complications in recent large series is summarized in Table 30.1.

All surgical techniques have inherent complications. Anastomotic leaks tend to be more common after Swenson's operation. Enterocolitis and protracted postoperative diarrhea tend to be more frequent following classic endorectal pull-through. Patients who have undergone Duhamel's operation have more constipation and may develop recurrence of the rectocolonic spur. Patients who have been treated by Rehbein's anterior resection often require long-term anorectal dilatations to treat the constipation associated with the retained aganglionic distal rectum.

Bowel function

Early bowel function following a pull-through procedure for HD is extremely unpredictable. In most cases, early bowel function is characterized by frequent bowel movements. This reflects the absence of a rectal reservoir. A bowel frequency of 5–15 times a day is normal during the early postoperative phase after an endorectal pull-through or Swenson operation. Patients who have had a Duhamel operation may have fewer bowel movements since they have a side-to-side anastomosis between ganglionic pulled-through bowel and aganglionic rectum.

A typical early problem that is related to frequent bowel movements and occurs especially after neonatal or infant one-stage operations is perineal excoriation. Early postoperative excoriation occurs in almost all newborns and small infants but usually subsides within weeks if there is no residual anastomotic stenosis.[16,24,25,32,33] Typical signs of an early anastomotic stenosis requiring anal dilatations are explosive loose stools and perineal excoriation unresponsive to standard skin care measures.

Frequent bowel movements should gradually subside within 6–12 months. Two to three years after the pull-through procedure 80% of patients should have less than three or four bowel movements per day.[16,17] Persistent frequent bowel movements are associated with (i) sphincter insufficiency that is usually caused by a failure in the surgical technique or anastomotic complications, (ii) recurrent or chronic enterocolitis, or (iii) bacterial overgrowth in the retained colon. Recurrent or chronic enterocolitis is typical in syndromic HD patients, especially in those with Down syndrome.[27–29]

Long-term outcomes

Basic concepts

Fecal continence

Fecal continence is a complex physiologic function that is dependent on sphincteric function, sensation, spinal reflexes, and control from higher cerebral centers. Cultural and psychological factors also play a role in the timing of independent fecal continence. The complexity of the continence mechanism makes it vulnerable to dysfunction that may cause variable degrees of incontinence.

In a normal child the development of fecal continence is a maturation process. Independent fecal control requires toilet training that may be possible at any time between 1 and 4–5 years. Usually, it is not possible to consider a child younger than 3 or 4 years of age as having full control of bowel function. If a child has undergone a pull-through procedure for HD, it is evident that many physiologic factors involved in fecal continence are disturbed and/or damaged. All operations for HD either remove or by-pass the rectal reservoir and very likely significantly affect its sensory input pathways. In the Duhamel and Swenson operations, the proximal part of the internal sphincter is damaged. The endorectal pull-through creates a double-walled distal bowel outlet that alters the compliance of the neorectum. Keeping these major physiologic alterations in mind, it is not surprising that many children with repaired HD suffer from defective bowel control especially during early childhood.

It is important when assessing fecal continence in patients with HD to consider the social and practical impact of potentially defective bowel control on the patient's life. Minor degrees of soiling or staining without major fecal accidents are relatively well tolerated in preschool children. When the social circumstances of a child change to include more contacts with peers outside the home, fecal continence becomes a major issue. The older the child, the more important is the absence of fecal soiling. Teenage culture and social relationships during adolescence do not tolerate any kind of fecal soiling. Soiling at this age usually leads to social discrimination and may isolate the patient from his or her peers. Very often, these patients carry the social consequences of defective fecal control into adult life.

Constipation

Although the objective of the operative management of HD is to overcome the functional obstruction that causes recalcitrant constipation, recurrent constipation is not uncommon. This problem occurs following each type of procedure for HD but appears to be more frequent in patients after Duhamel and Rehbein operations. As with the definition of fecal continence, the definition of constipation is difficult. Moreover, constipation is very common in otherwise healthy children in the Western World.[36] A reasonably well-accepted definition of constipation is that of Loening-Baucke:[36] two or less bowel movements per week and the presence of other symptoms that are related to constipation. In terms of HD, significant or recurrent constipation exists when the patient requires regular management in excess of dietary manipulation. The disability related to constipation varies significantly. If the postoperative constipation can be controlled by oral laxatives and there is no associated fecal incontinence, the psychosocial impact of symptoms is insignificant in most instances. On the other hand, if the patient requires regular bowel washouts or has had a continent appendicostomy for the administration of antegrade enemas, there are significant lifestyle restrictions. However, constipation is in the great majority of cases more easily manageable than significant fecal soiling and causes less psychosocial disturbance.

Length of follow-up

The length of follow-up is an important issue when considering long-term outcomes after pull-through operations for HD. The development of more or less normal bowel function compatible with normal social life requires a significant period, in many cases several years, of adaptation. The earliest possible time that functional outcome can be reliably assessed is when the patient is toilet trained and weaned from nappies. In patients with HD this assessment is usually possible at the age of 3–5 years. Although it is important to evaluate early or medium-term outcome following surgery for HD, the results may not reflect outcome beyond childhood. There are several reasons for this. Reliable assessment of bowel function is difficult in a child who is not able to fully understand the social consequences of an abnormal bowel function. In early childhood, information concerning bowel function comes from the parents who may not be able to give a realistic picture of the magnitude of any bowel dysfunction. Moreover, the bowel function of HD patients tends to improve significantly with age. Early and medium-term results only provide an approximate estimate of the proportion of patients with HD who will require specific bowel management during childhood. This information is nevertheless important for caregivers and medical personnel because both groups need a realistic picture of the likelihood of significant bowel dysfunction during childhood.

The follow-up of HD patients needs to be extended into adolescence or adulthood if the true end point of management of the condition is to be assessed. Adolescents and adults are able to assess the physical and psychosocial impact of their bowel function as independent individuals. The social and quality of life consequences of possible bowel dysfunction are best and most reliably evaluated in adults.

Methods of evaluating bowel function

In the literature there is great variation in the functional results after the treatment of HD. There is no generally agreed method for assessing the bowel function of patients with HD and the main problem in comparing different series is the highly variable criteria used in the evaluation of bowel function. Evaluation of bowel function during childhood may be biased because the information is mainly derived from the parents; they may not want to report unfavorable results to a surgeon who has been responsible for the treatment of their child. The parents may also ignore mild to moderate incontinence in a child whose bowel function has been abnormal from birth or, in the case of younger children, may consider defective bowel control as part of the normal maturation of defecation.

There are several ways to overcome these difficulties. The evaluation should be performed by an independent person, who is not a member of the team responsible for the care of the child. A questionnaire with detailed questions concerning bowel function may give more reliable information than a visit to a busy hospital outpatient clinic. If a questionnaire is used, it should be validated by applying it to a control group of healthy children of similar age and sex distribution as the patients.

Most long-term studies of patients with HD are either institutional or single surgeon reviews. Methods of evaluating long-term outcomes typically include chart reviews, questionnaires and interviews of the patients either personally or by telephone. Criteria used to assess the functional outcome vary tremendously. Some authors have designed their own scoring systems,[37,38] whilst others use scoring systems that were originally designed to assess fecal continence in patients with an anorectal malformation.[39–41] Simple stratification of patients into those with normal bowel function, i.e., clean, and those with variable degrees of soiling or constipation is commonly performed.[16,17,19,34,35,42] Long-term follow-up studies that assess the outcome of HD patients in comparison to age-matched controls are still few.[37,38,41,42,43]

Late complications

Intestinal obstruction

Intestinal obstruction is not uncommon following repair of HD. Reports in the literature show considerable variation in the incidence of this complication and do not always denote if surgery was required to relieve the obstruction. The incidence of late postoperative intestinal obstruction requiring hospital management ranges between 4% and 21%.[16,32,33,34,35,37,40] The mean incidence of intestinal obstruction in HD patients is 10%. There is no obvious difference between the types of repair. The incidence of bowel obstruction following repair of HD appears to be somewhat higher than the overall incidence following laparotomy during childhood. In a large series of 1476 pediatric surgical patients the overall incidence of bowel obstruction was 2.1%.[44] After neonatal laparotomy adhesive bowel obstruction affects between 3.3 and 8.3% of patients.[44,45]

Outlet obstruction

Beyond the immediate postoperative period outlet obstruction is one of the most frequent complications after repair of HD, whatever surgical method has been used. The symptoms of outlet obstruction include recurrent constipation, abdominal distension, diarrhea and postoperative enterocolitis. Outlet obstruction may be due to one or more specific causes related to the operative procedure. After Swenson's operation, mechanical outlet obstruction is usually caused by anastomotic stenosis. The incidence of late stenosis following Swenson's operation varies between 7.6% and 13%.[34,40] After Duhamel's retrorectal pull-through, outlet obstruction may be caused by regrowth of the rectocolonic spur; the incidence of symptomatic rectal spur formation requiring surgery varies between 9% and 35%.[32,41,43,46] Another cause of outlet obstruction after Duhamel's operation is anorectal achalasia which is probably related to poor motility in the side-to-side anastomosis between the aganglionic rectal stump and the pulled-through colon. A typical feature of outlet obstruction in these patients is the development of a fecaloma within the anterior rectal pouch. Organic

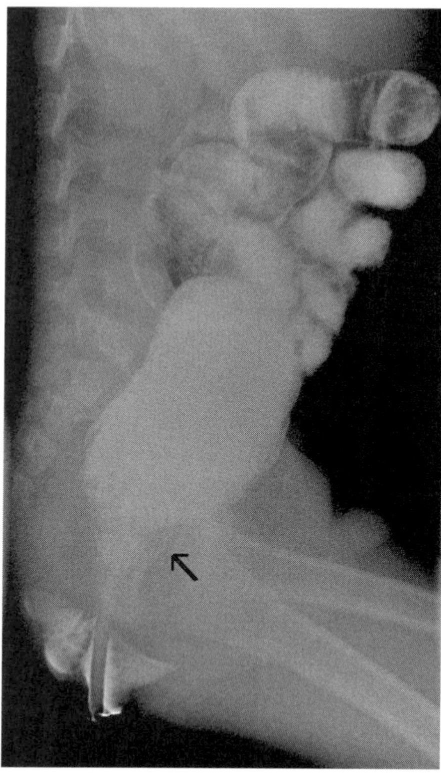

Fig. 30.1. Stenosis of the aganglionic cuff (arrow) following pull-through of the hepatic flexure for long-segment aganglionosis.

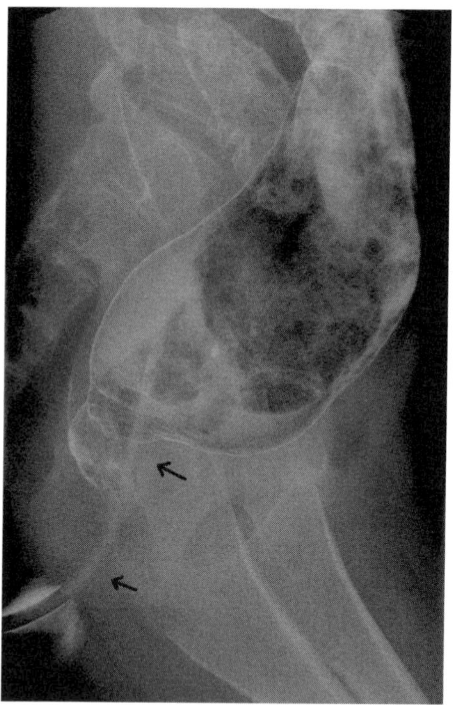

Fig. 30.2. Retained aganglionic segment (between arrows) following a Swenson procedure for classic HD.

outlet obstruction after endorectal pull-through may be caused by anastomotic stenosis or stricture, stenosis of the aganglionic rectal cuff (Fig. 30.1), colonic retraction, and dysfunction of the aganglionic muscle cuff, especially if it is long. The incidence of organic outlet obstruction after endorectal pull-through ranges between 6% and 22%.[16,17,32,33,47] After Rehbein's operation, organic outlet obstruction is almost invariably caused by the relatively long aganglionic bowel segment retained between the anastomosis and the anus. Functional outlet obstruction without any identifiable mechanical cause (e.g., stenosis, rectal spur, etc.) may occur after treatment of HD by any surgical technique. The pathophysiology of functional outlet obstruction is obscure. Although generally attributed to internal sphincter hypertonicity and non-relaxation, no manometrically detectable differences between obstructed and non-obstructed HD patients have been found.[48]

The diagnosis of outlet obstruction is mainly based on clinical symptoms and findings. Radiologic assessments include barium enema and transit time studies. Barium enema typically shows rectosigmoid dilatation. Transit time studies are useful in assessing colonic motility but are relatively cumbersome to perform. Moreover, there are no well-standardized methods that have sufficient healthy pediatric control data. A few controlled studies have been performed but have not shown any correlation between functional outcome and total or segmental colonic motility.[41] As stated previously, anorectal manometry has not been found to be a good method of diagnosing functional outlet obstruction.[48]

Outlet obstruction has been attributed to abnormalities in the innervation of the pulled-through colon in a significant proportion of cases. Abnormalities of innervation include acquired/retained aganglionosis (Fig. 30.2), hypoganglionosis, and intestinal neuronal dysplasia.[48–50] Hypoganglionosis and aganglionosis are common findings if the transitional zone has been anastomosed to the anal canal; transitional zone pull-throughs are associated with a poor outcome.[51] However, there is no general agreement about the significance of residual neuronal abnormalities on the functional outcome of HD. There is also no evidence that any clear pattern of dysmotility is directly related to neuronal dysplasia.[52] Some surgeons suggest that biopsy mapping of the colon prior to the pull-through procedure is essential if good functional results are to be expected.[53,54] These surgeons suggest that if the ganglionic colon shows features of neuronal dysplasia, then this segment should be resected along with the aganglionic bowel. This approach has not been tested in any controlled trial. There are several problems in diagnosing neuronal dysplasia. The main criteria for identifying neuronal dysplasia are the presence of hyperganglionosis, i.e., an excess number of ganglion cells in one ganglion and giant ganglia in the submucous plexus. However, the number of ganglion cells per ganglion is an age-dependent phenomenon; the older the patient, the fewer the ganglion cells in the ganglia.[55] This makes the interpretation of biopsies difficult. Moreover, it has been shown that there is significant interobserver variability in the diagnosis of neuronal dysplasia despite the published criteria.[56]

The overall incidence of symptomatic outlet obstruction varies between 6% and 42%.[16,17,32–35,40,46] The incidence tends to be lower in reports that include historical patient series.[34,35] This probably reflects underreporting of this problem. The incidence of symptomatic late outlet obstruction following repair of HD according to major reports in the literature is summarized in Table 30.2. The break-up of the results is performed according to the surgical method. The table shows that, overall, there is very little difference in the incidence of late outlet obstruction between different surgical methods. The incidence of functional outlet obstruction following Rehbein's anterior resection is excluded from the table. There are only a few reports concerning late outcome of the Rehbein operation. In these series up to 40% of the patients have developed recurrent rectoanal achalasia that has required repeated anal dilatations under general anesthesia.[57,58]

Table 30.2. Outlet obstruction and local anastomotic reoperations in relation to the primary surgical procedure

Operation	Study	Patients	Follow-up (years)	Outlet obstruction (%)[a]	Anastomotic reoperative procedure (%)[b]
Duhamel	Mishalany[65]	14	1–30		21
	Moore[40]	21	1–36	5	
	Fortuna[47]	27	1–20	22	33
	Yanchar[32]	28	1–15	46	43
	Minford[21]	34	1–15	18	18
	Total/mean	**124**		**23**	**29**
ERPT	Mishalany[65]	33	1–30		24
	Moore[40]	75	1–36	21	
	Fortunal[47]	55	1–20	22	20
	Yanchar[32]	40	1–15	33	35
	Minford[21]	37	1–15	19	19
	Total/mean	**240**		**24**	**25**
Swenson	Mishalany[65]	15	1–30		47
	Moore[40]	13	1–36	62	
	Yanchar[32]	8	1–15	0	0
	Total/mean	**36**		**31**	**24**

ERPT = endorectal pull-through.
[a]Includes anastomotic stenosis and stricture, rectal spur and postoperative achalasia.
[b]Includes dilatation, myotomy, myectomy and division of rectal spur.

Management of outlet obstruction

The primary treatment of symptomatic late outlet obstruction in HD patients is conservative. Simple constipation related to outlet obstruction may respond to stool softeners and laxatives. Outlet obstruction may also be associated with diarrhea. Loose stools, diarrhea and flatulence without any general symptoms suggestive of enterocolitis may be caused by colonic bacterial overgrowth and usually respond to oral antibiotics such as metronidazole. Dietary measures are often helpful in reducing bacterial overgrowth. A low residue diet and avoidance of lactose and artificial sweeteners such as sorbitol and xylitol reduces bacterial substrates.

An anastomotic stenosis or stricture may respond to anal dilatations. More recalcitrant stenoses and long strictures may require repeat pull-through surgery.[59,60] Duhamel patients with symptomatic regrowth of the rectal spur generally require operative division of the spur,[32,41,43,46] which can usually be accomplished with a linear stapler. However, the spur may recur after successful stapling. Patients with retained or acquired aganglionic segments may respond to anorectal myectomy, but in cases where there is a long segment of aganglionosis a repeat pull-through is usually required.

The management of resistant functional outlet obstruction is more problematic. Functional obstruction does not usually respond to dilatations except in patients who have had Rehbein's anterior resection. Many surgeons using Rehbein's procedure routinely perform anal dilatations under general anesthesia after the pull-through and also later on if the patient develops recurrent constipation. Anal stretch has been advocated for functional outlet obstruction but there is little evidence to support its use. Many surgeons recommend aggressive management especially if the patient has recurrent enterocolitis. A typical approach is anorectal myotomy or myectomy. However, in the long term, only about two-thirds of such patients are cured by myectomy or myotomy. Results appear to be better in patients with recurrent enterocolitis than in those who present with severe constipation with or without a retained aganglionic segment.[61] Recently, intrasphincteric injections of botulinum toxin have been advocated for the management of functional outlet obstruction in HD patients.[62] Preliminary results are promising and a significant proportion of patients improve, at least temporarily, with no side effects. One disadvantage of this treatment modality is the need for repeated injections. The overall incidence of local redo-procedures for problems related to outlet obstruction is summarized in Table 30.2.

Repeat pull-through operations have been used as a rescue therapy for failed primary pull-through. Typical indications for redo pull-through include retained or acquired aganglionosis unresponsive to local measures, and recalcitrant strictures. The most commonly used repeat pull-through method is Duhamel's operation. Although the incidence of postoperative complications is higher than following primary surgery, late functional outcomes appear to be favorable in at least two-thirds of patients.[59,60] Restorative proctocolectomy with ileoanal J-pouch anastomosis has been reported to be an effective salvage procedure in HD patients who have severe colonic dysfunction following surgery for long-segment colonic disease or who have lost significant length of bowel due to technical or vascular problems. Functional outcome appears to be at least as good as following restorative proctocolectomy for ulcerative colitis.[63]

Enterocolitis

Enterocolitis is a complication unique to HD. Together with congenital malformations, enterocolitis is still a major source of morbidity and mortality. The etiology is poorly understood but the clinical picture resembles the fulminant colitis associated with inflammatory bowel disease. Several bacteria have been implicated in the pathogenesis of enterocolitis but cultures taken in the acute phase usually do not reveal any specific causative organism. Enterocolitis is not precisely defined and the reported incidence of postoperative enterocolitis therefore varies significantly. Enterocolitis is an inflammation of the bowel mucosa, but few surgeons perform routine endoscopies in patients who have acute symptoms suggestive of the condition. Milder clinical symptoms such as temporary loose stools or diarrheal episodes without systemic upset may be caused by colonic bacterial overgrowth; this is supported by a good response to a short course of oral metronidazole in many cases.

Patients with a defective immune response, such as those with Down syndrome and some other groups with syndromic HD, are particularly susceptible to late enterocolitis. In immunodeficient patients enterocolitis may become a chronic problem. Continuing loose stools and flatulence may damage the functional outcome in these patients whose reduced mental capacity interferes with the acquisition of normal bowel function. Patients with TCA appear to have an increased risk of postoperative enterocolitis. Recent large series of patients with TCA report incidences of postoperative enterocolitis as high as 54%–70%.[30,64]

The overall incidence of postoperative enterocolitis is about 15%. There is a clear trend towards a diminishing frequency of attacks with time. On the other hand, the recent trend toward performing repair of HD during the neonatal period as a one-stage operation appears to be associated with an increased risk of enterocolitis.[16,21] Enterocolitis also appears to be more frequent in patients who have undergone an endorectal pull-through or Swenson operation than in those who have had a Duhamel operation.[32,47,65] The reason for this is unclear since bowel outlet obstruction which is commonly invoked as one of the main pathophysiologic factors causing enterocolitis is not less frequent in patients who have had a Duhamel operation. Furthermore, Duhamel patients require secondary local anorectal procedures as often as Swenson and endorectal pull-through patients. The incidence of enterocolitis in relation to the primary surgical procedure is shown in Table 30.3.

Table 30.3. Postoperative enterocolitis in relation to the primary surgical procedure

Operation	Study	Patients	Follow-up (years)	Enterocolitis (%)
Duhamel	Mishalany[65]	14	1–30	21
	Fortuna[47]	27	1–20	19
	Yanchar[32]	28	1–15	7
	Minford[21]	34	1–15	3
	Total/mean	**103**		**13**
ERPT	Mishalany[65]	33	1–30	33
	Fortunal[47]	55	1–20	27
	Yanchar[32]	40	1–15	8
	Minford[21]	37	1–15	35
	Total/mean	**165**		**26**
Swenson	Mishalany[65]	15	1–30	47
	Yanchar[32]	8	1–15	50
	Total/mean	**23**		**49**

ERPT = endorectal pull-through.

Management of enterocolitis

The treatment of clinically severe attack of enterocolitis includes bowel decompression, parenteral antibiotics and bowel rest. For patients with recurrent attacks of enterocolitis many pediatric surgeons advocate repeat anorectal surgery: anal dilatations and internal sphincter myotomy or myectomy. The general view has been that these procedures are successful in preventing further episodes of enterocolitis. A recent long-term follow-up study of patients who had undergone internal sphincter myotomy or myectomy for recalcitrant constipation or recurrent enterocolitis showed moderate success: two-thirds of patients gained symptomatic relief.[61] However, the policy of treating recurrent episodes of enterocolitis by further anorectal procedures is not supported by controlled studies. Moreover, sphincter myectomy may cause fecal incontinence. The senior author has employed a conservative approach to recurrent enterocolitis for over 20 years. Patients with symptoms suggestive of enterocolitis have generally been treated as outpatients with short courses of oral metronidazole. Only patients with significant systemic upset have been hospitalized and treated with parenteral antibiotics. In non-syndromic HD patients recurrence of enterocolitis has been extremely uncommon after two to three years of age. Between 1981 and 2003 only two of our 168 patients with HD have undergone internal sphincter myectomy for recurrent enterocolitis. The procedure was moderately successful in one but failed in the other who subsequently required a restorative proctocolectomy.

Patients with recurrent or chronic enterocolitis may benefit from immunosuppressive therapy. The locally acting mast-cell stabilizing agent, sodium cromoglycate, has been used with success to treat chronic enterocolitis in patients with syndromic HD.[66] More recalcitrant cases may require local or systemic corticosteroids for the control of symptoms.

Long-term bowel function

Constipation

Recurrence of constipation in patients with repaired HD is a frustrating problem. The incidence of late constipation appears to be related to the type of reconstruction. It is particularly common after Duhamel and Rehbein operations. In the mid term, the incidence of constipation requiring treatment in patients with a Duhamel repair ranges between 20% and 57%.[32,40,65] After Rehbein's operation, 40%–50% of patients require sphincter dilatations under general anesthesia during the early postoperative period and 16%–23% of patients suffer from constipation in the medium term.[57,58] Some series report a high incidence of constipation after Swenson's operation,[40,65] but in most reports the number of patients who have had this operation is so small that definitive conclusions cannot be made. On the other hand, the large multinational series of Sherman *et al.*[34] reports no late constipation at all. Least affected by long-standing constipation are patients who have undergone an endorectal pull-through; recurrent constipation has been reported in 2%–15% of these patients.[32,33,40]

Most series agree that constipation in most patients with HD improves or resolves completely with time. Reports of outcomes in adolescence or adulthood show a low incidence of constipation.[32,34,42,43] However, these reports indicate that during childhood a significant proportion of patients suffered from constipation.[32,43] The reason for the disappearance of constipation is unclear. This feature is similar to that which occurs in patients suffering from functional constipation: the symptoms usually disappear before or at the onset of puberty.[67] On a speculative level, this consistent clinical progress in these patients suggests that the maturation of bowel function might in part be related to hormonal changes at puberty. Alternatively, improvement could be due to enhanced social motivation when the patients are approaching adolescence. However, it is difficult to understand how mental and social maturation affect constipation.

The management of constipation is usually conservative. Stool softeners, laxatives and sometimes enemas, can usually control recurrent constipation following repair of HD. Bowel washouts through a continent appendicostomy (ACE procedure) have been used to control intractable constipation in selected cases (see Chapter 33).[68] Prokinetic medication has been suggested for cases where constipation is associated with intestinal neuronal dysplasia.[48] Local anorectal procedures such as anal dilatations, rectal spur division, and sphincter myotomy or myectomy have been used to treat cases resistant to medical management. If an anastomotic stricture or regrowth of the rectal spur is the cause of the constipation the results of redo procedures appear to be good. On the other hand, further local surgery for unremitting constipation without any identifiable cause is not rewarding.[61] This also applies to cases where constipation is associated with a retained or acquired aganglionic segment – a redo pull-through operation may be a better alternative in such patients.[59,60]

Frequent bowel actions

Frequent bowel movements due to loose stools and chronic diarrhea are typical in the early postoperative period after repair of HD. In some patients this stooling pattern persists leading to fecal urgency and perianal skin problems, especially if the child still wears diapers. Frequent bowel movements are typical during the first few years after endorectal pull-through.[16] This is possibly due to decreased compliance of the neorectum which basically has two muscle layers, at least in the lower rectum and

Table 30.4. Long-term functional outcome of Hirschsprung's disease in uncontrolled retrospective studies

Study	Year	Surgical technique	Patients	Follow-up period/age (y)	Data collection method	Fecal incontinence (%)	Constipation (%)	Normal bowel control (%)	Comment
Sherman[34]	1989	Swenson	477	6–40	Interview Chart review	2–8	3–6	90–94	Improved outcome with increasing age
Tariq[33]	1991	ERPT	30	5–10	Not defined	17	0	68	–
Rescorla[46]	1992	Duhamel	55	5–20	Interview	0–9	–	91–100	Improved outcome with increasing age
Catto-Smith[69]	1995	Multiple	60	10 (5–26)	Questionnaire Diary	53	20	–	No improvement with increasing age
Moore[40]	1996	Multiple	115	> 4 years	Chart review	6–19	35	75	Improved outcome with increasing age
Yanchar[32]	1999	Multiple	45	> 5 years of age	Chart review Questionnaire	8–58	8–22	–	Improved outcome with increasing age
Van der Zee[19]	2000	Duhamel	29	6 (5–7)	Chart review Questionnaire	27	21	52	–
Shankar[17]	2000	ERPT	51	> 4 years of age	Chart review	24	0	76	Improved outcome with increasing age

If results show range, the higher figure implies outcome during childhood and the lower outcome beyond childhood.

anal canal. Stool frequency persists in only a minority and more than 80% of patients have three or fewer bowel movements per 24 hours three years later. Persistent bowel frequency occurs much more commonly in patients with long-segment aganglionosis or TCA. Chronic enterocolitis is another cause of long-term bowel frequency.

The management of persistent bowel frequency is aimed at slowing down colonic motility. Antipropulsive medication, such as loperamide, is usually helpful and well tolerated even in the long term. Enterocolitis as a cause of diarrhea has to be ruled out if loperamide is used because slowing colonic motility may increase bacterial overgrowth and aggravate the symptoms of enterocolitis. Instituting low-residue diet slows down colonic motility and decreases the risk of bacterial overgrowth. Avoidance of non-absorbable short-chain carbohydrates, sorbitol and xylitol, that are commonly used as artificial sweeteners, may also be helpful in controlling stool consistency.

Overall bowel function and fecal incontinence

There are conflicting reports regarding the outcome of surgery for HD. Older studies of patients who have undergone repair of HD indicate that the great majority gain more or less normal bowel function in the long term.[34,40,46,47] The average follow-up time in these reports ranges between 5 and 10 years and the percentage of patients with "good" or "normal" bowel function varies between 65% and 100%. The widely held view that long-term outcome is generally favorable has been strongly challenged by several recent reports with a similar length of follow-up.[32,37,38,41,69,70] There are no simple explanations to account for the observed differences. Data concerning the patients' bowel function in some of the older studies were retrieved from retrospective case note reviews. Hospital notes may significantly underestimate problems with bowel function.[69] Telephone and letter inquiries without a structured questionnaire may not give a reliable picture of the patient's problems. Many of the older reports grade the functional outcome as good, fair or poor without providing the criteria used in the evaluation. More recent critical reports have used structured questionnaire based scoring systems for the evaluation of functional outcomes. Weekly diaries have been used to verify the data retrieved from questionnaires. Some studies have also included healthy control subjects who have completed a similar questionnaire as the patients.[37,38,41,43] These recent critical or controlled studies have shown that only between 27% and 50% of patients have normal bowel control during early childhood and school years (5–10 years of age) (Table 30.4).[32,37,38,41,69,70] The common finding in all studies that have used scoring systems and healthy controls has been that the scores of HD patients are significantly lower than those of the controls (Table 30.5).[37,38,41,43]

It is a commonly accepted view that the bowel function of patients with HD improves with age. This is an almost uniform finding in long-term follow-up studies. Only one study has not reported a clear improvement in bowel function with increasing age.[69] The critical age when the

Table 30.5. Summary of long-term functional outcome in follow-up studies of patients with Hirschsprung's disease and age-matched controls

Author	Year	Surgical technique	Patients	Controls	Follow-up period/age (y)	Outcome	Follow up (%)	Comment
Heikkinen[43]	1995	Multiple	100	81	31 (15–39)	Significantly decreased continence score vs. healthy controls	87%	Positive correlation between age and outcome
Reding[37]	1997	Multiple	37	39	8.7 (1.2–22)	Significantly decreased continence score vs. healthy controls	70%	Positive correlation between age and outcome
Diseth[42]	1997	Duhamel	19	14	16 (10–20)	Significantly increased incidence of incontinence vs. healthy controls	59%	–
Baillie[41]	1999	Duhamel	80	22	8.4 (4.8–16)	Significantly decreased continence score vs. healthy controls	100%	Positive correlation between age and outcome
Bai[38]	2002	Swenson	45	44	9.1 (4–16)	Significantly decreased continence score vs. healthy controls	not defined	–

final improvement takes place is puberty.[43] Most reports describing outcome in adult or adolescent patients show few limitations with regard to occupation, social contacts or physical activities.[42,43] In contrast, controlled manometric studies performed in adult and adolescent patients have clearly demonstrated impaired performance of the anal sphincters.[71] Both resting anal canal and maximum squeeze pressures have been significantly lower than in healthy controls. The low resting pressure reflects mainly internal sphincter dysfunction; this is not unexpected, as a principal aim in the surgical repair of HD is to overcome the functional obstruction caused by achalasia of the internal sphincter. This is accomplished by resecting or bypassing the proximal part of the internal sphincter. It is obvious that this dysfunction is permanent. Overall fecal continence is probably salvaged by voluntary sphincters that remain undisturbed in uncomplicated surgery for HD and can thus compensate for the low resting pressure caused by internal sphincter dysfunction.

Fecal incontinence is psychosocially the most disturbing sequel of any type of anorectal surgery in childhood. Fecal soiling is incompatible with normal social life and has a profound effect on family dynamics. In early childhood, when the patient wears diapers, the problem is less overt but the patient may require considerably more care than a healthy child. This may include frequent nappy changes and skin care to avoid excoriation. In pre-school aged children minor defects in fecal continence such as occasional soiling or staining rarely cause any problems. On the other hand, in school-aged children even relatively minor soiling may be very embarrassing. According to the author's experience, minor soiling and staining do not cause social problems if the child does not need a change of underwear or protective pads to stay clean during school days. Any soiling in excess of this requires special treatment modalities.

The occurrence of fecal soiling in patients who have undergone repair of HD is not unexpected. Complete or partial loss of a rectal reservoir is an inevitable sequel of all pull-through procedures for HD. Internal sphincter function is disturbed by partial resection or bypass. Older studies report a relatively low incidence of fecal incontinence.[34,40,46,47] More recent critical or controlled reports show a significant incidence of fecal incontinence during childhood. When fecal soiling has been critically and independently assessed, the proportion of patients with fecal incontinence exceeds 50% during childhood.[21,32,37,38,41,69,70] These figures include patients with all grades of incontinence, i.e., not only those with frank incontinence and fecal accidents but also patients with occasional soiling or staining. Less severe fecal soiling may still be associated with social problems during childhood.[32] In the long term there are no significant differences in the incidence of incontinence between the main operative techniques. The problems with fecal incontinence appear to diminish significantly after puberty. Socially disturbing fecal soiling is much less common in adults and appears to have much less impact on psychosocial functioning.[42,43] In terms of psychological and social problems, adolescent and adult patients with HD appear to fare significantly better than those with an anorectal malformation. Unlike the latter, mental or psychosocial problems are not over-represented in adolescents and adults with HD in comparison to the normal population.[42]

The management of fecal soiling in patients with HD is usually conservative. The amount of soiling is not usually very extensive as the voluntary sphincter system is more or less undamaged. If soiling is associated with loose or liquid stools, a low residue diet and antipropulsive medication is helpful. Overflow soiling is typical in patients who have had a Duhamel operation. Fecal material may accumulate in the anterior rectal segment, especially in the presence of a retained or reconstituted rectal spur. In such cases, the rectal spur should be divided. Patients with significant outlet obstruction may also develop fecal collections and overflow soiling, especially if there is a stricture. Surgical treatment of the outlet obstruction by anorectal myectomy and elimination of the stricture may decrease the severity of soiling. Repeat pull-through may be indicated in selected cases that are unresponsive to more conservative approaches.[59,60] Recalcitrant fecal soiling may be related to surgical complications. Functional sphincter damage may occur after an anastomotic leak or retraction of the pulled-through bowel, and following local surgical procedures. Non-compliance of the rectum may be caused by an anastomotic leak and postoperative pelvic sepsis. If anorectal function is very poor, the best option for the patient may be permanent diversion or a bowel management program, preferably using antegrade washouts through a continent appendicostomy or Monti–Yang tube. Every major series of patients with HD includes some patients who have required permanent fecal diversion or a washout program.

Long-term functional outcomes in uncontrolled studies are shown in Table 30.4. Table 30.5 summarizes comparative results in studies where age-matched controls have been included in the evaluation of long-term functional outcomes.

Special groups

Total colonic aganglionosis

Total colonic aganglionosis (TCA) accounts for 8%–12% of all patients with HD. The male to female ratio of 1.5:1 is different from classic HD where 80% of the patients are males. In TCA the aganglionosis usually extends into the ileum; in 30%–50% of cases the aganglionosis extends for more than 30 cm up the ileum. The overall mortality in TCA is much higher than in classic HD. During the last two decades the reported mortality rate in TCA has ranged from 6% to 40%.[30,31,64] The survival rate continues to improve but surgical management remains challenging and long-term outcomes in terms of growth and bowel function are not well documented. Many ingenious methods have been devised for the surgical management of TCA; some have included a long longitudinal anastomosis between the aganglionic bowel and the proximal, ganglionic, pull-through segment. The high frequency of complications associated with these long aganglionic patches outweigh the potential benefit of increased fluid absorption. Most surgeons currently use standard methods of HD repair for TCA.[30,64] The senior author has used an endorectal pull-through with J-pouch ileoanal anastomosis during the last 8 years in nine consecutive patients with TCA.[72] Short- to medium-term functional outcome is favorable: the frequency of bowel movements is 2–5 per 24 hours, five patients are clean and four suffer from occasional, mainly night-time soiling. Only three patients have had episodes of enterocolitis.

Long-term outcome following operations for TCA is clearly inferior to that after surgery for classic HD. Many TCA patients require multiple operations and prolonged periods of hospitalization, which may include temporary total parenteral nutrition because of surgical and metabolic complications.[30,31,64] Fecal incontinence during childhood is very common in TCA patients and the majority require special dietary measures and antipropulsive medication to decrease fecal soiling. At adolescence, approximately one-third of patients still suffer from fecal soiling.[30,64] Functional outcome appears to be better in patients without an extensive common channel between ganglionic and aganglionic bowel.[64] One-fifth of patients with TCA end up with a permanent ileostomy.[30,64] Metabolic complications are common. Growth retardation manifesting largely as poor weight gain may be apparent. The incidence of problematic anemia ranges between 12% and 55%; this is possibly due to poor iron absorption and in some cases vitamin B_{12} deficiency.

Syndromic Hirschsprung's disease

Down syndrome (trisomy 21) is the syndrome most commonly associated with HD. The incidence of Down syndrome in patients with HD ranges from 2 to 15% and appears to be much higher in recent series. It is unlikely that this represents a true increase in the incidence of HD in Down syndrome and it is more likely that HD was previously underdiagnosed in Down syndrome patients or they died before a definitive diagnosis of HD was made. In the authors' series of 168 patients over the last 22 years the incidence of Down syndrome is 12%.

The mortality of Down syndrome patients with HD is higher than in other HD patients. This reflects the comorbidity in these patients, such as the presence of cardiac defects, especially atrioventricular septal defect. Many of the fatalities in Down syndrome patients with HD are attributed to cardiac problems.[26,27] Another significant problem in Down syndrome patients is an impaired immune defence system, rendering them more susceptible to enterocolitis. Enterocolitis is more likely to be fatal or become chronic in Down syndrome patients compared to otherwise healthy children with HD.[66] Chronic enterocolitis may lead to the development of inflammatory bowel disease; two of the authors' adolescent Down syndrome patients with HD and chronic enterocolitis have clear histologic findings of Crohn's disease. An increased incidence of inflammatory bowel disease in this group of patients has also been reported by Sherman *et al.*[34]

It is commonly accepted that the prognosis for bowel function in patients with both HD and Down syndrome is significantly inferior to those with isolated HD.[26,27] Opposing views have been reported – one study found that the bowel function in Down syndrome was not worse than in patients with a normal karyotype, at least in the short term.[73] The senior author's experience is that Down syndrome patients acquire bowel control at a much slower rate than other HD patients. Many of them, and especially those with chronic enterocolitis, suffer from fecal incontinence as adolescents or adults.

HD is also associated with other less common syndromes. Shah–Waardenburg syndrome is an audiopigmentary syndrome associated with HD and caused by mutations in the genes for endothelin-3 or its receptors. Mowat–Wilson syndrome patients have typical dysmorphic features in association with severe intellectual impairment; nearly all have microcephaly and seizures and many have HD. Mowat–Wilson syndrome is a result of deletions or mutations in the SIP 1 gene on chromosome 2q22. The authors' series includes five patients with Mowat–Wilson syndrome; clinically, the pattern of HD in these patients is similar to that seen in Down syndrome. Affected patients have frequent bouts of enterocolitis and develop bowel control very slowly. Cartilage-hair hypoplasia is a metaphyseal chondrodysplasia with growth failure, impaired immunity and a high incidence of HD. It is caused by a mutation in the RMRP gene. Affected patients with HD have a worse prognosis than patients with isolated HD.[29] They have an extremely high incidence of pre- and postoperative enterocolitis that may lead to fatal septic infections.

Urinary continence and sexual function

Although day- or night-time enuresis and urodynamic abnormalities have been reported in children with HD,[33,69,74] urinary incontinence and sexual dysfunction occur in only a small minority of adult and adolescent patients with HD. Some series report no older patients with these complications.[34,35,43] In their detailed analysis, Moore *et al.* found that a small percentage of patients suffered from disturbances of micturition and sexual dysfunction.[40] Sexual dysfunction, mainly in the form of dyspareunia, appeared to be more common in females. Sexual and urinary dysfunction were more common in patients after Swenson or Duhamel operations than in those who had undergone an endorectal pull-through.

Inheritance of Hirschsprung's disease

The overall recurrence risk of HD in siblings of the proband is about 4%. In isolated HD, the risk of recurrent disease in siblings depends on the sex and length of the aganglionic segment in the proband and the gender of the sibling. The highest recurrence risk is for a male sibling of a female proband with a long segment HD (33%). With typical isolated HD in a male proband with short segment involvement, the risk of HD in a male sibling is 5% and in a female sibling 1%.[75]

Both familial medullary thyroid cancer and MEN 2A syndrome can be associated with HD in some kindreds.[76] These families have a germline RET mutation on chromosome 10 in the same region as the mutation found in 50% of patients with familial HD and in 15%–20% of those with sporadic disease. Medullary thyroid cancer in adults has been reported in these families and also in adults with HD without any family history of MEN 2A syndrome.[76] This raises the question of whether all subjects with HD, regardless of family history, should be screened for the typical RET mutations to rule out cancer predisposition. Another question is whether all adult HD patients should be screened for medullary thyroid cancer and pheochromocytoma that occur in 70%–100% and 50% of patients with MEN 2A syndrome, respectively.

Conclusions

The surgical management of HD is still an evolving process. Since the 1980s, multistage operations have been replaced by primary pull-through procedures, often undertaken in the neonatal period. Long-segment and total colonic aganglionosis can now also be successfully managed by neonatal repair. The surgery for HD has also become less invasive. In the early 1990s laparoscopic-assisted pull-through procedures were introduced and gradually became popular in institutions with laparoscopic expertise. In the late 1990s, a totally transanal pull-through procedure for classic HD was developed; this operation has rapidly gained popularity as it is evidently associated with less postoperative discomfort, a shorter hospital stay, and lower costs than the previous procedures for HD. The long-term outcome following mini-invasive surgery for HD is still unclear but it appears that the functional results will be very similar to those following the classic operations.

Despite significant advances in the management of HD, the long-term functional outcome remains far from perfect. No individual surgical procedure is associated with superior long-term results. The main difference between the major operative procedures for HD is the profile of postoperative complications. Earlier reports described the long-term functional outcome as excellent in the great majority of patients who have been followed-up for more than 4–7 years. Recently, more critical prospective studies and studies with healthy controls have given a different picture of the late bowel function in patients with HD. Both constipation and fecal soiling are common late consequences. HD patients of all ages have uniformly lower bowel function scores than healthy controls. Urinary and sexual dysfunction occur in a small percentage of patients. Fortunately, the great majority of adults with HD appear to be able to function as normal members of society in terms of psychosocial, occupational and recreational activities. Nevertheless, the high incidence of functional problems throughout childhood demands careful follow-up of all patients with HD.

REFERENCES

1. Spouge, D. & Baird, P. A. Hirschsprung's disease in a large birth cohort. *Teratology* 1985; **32**:171–177.
2. Hirschsprung, H. Stuhltragheit Neugeborener in Folge von Dilatation und Hypertrophie des Colons. *Jahrb. Kinderh.* 1887; **27**:1–3.
3. Tittel, K. Uber eine eingeborene Missbildung des Dickdarmes. Wien *Klin. Wochenschr.* 1901; **14**:903–907.
4. Swenson, O. & Bill, A. H. Resection of rectum and rectosigmoid with preservation of the sphincter for benign spastic lesions producing megacolons: an experimental study. *Surgery* 1948; **24**:212–220.
5. Duhamel, B. New operation for congenital megacolon: retrorectal and transanal lowering of the colon, and its possible application to the treatment of various other malformations. *Presse Med.* 1956; **64**:2249–2250.
6. Grob, M., Genton, N., & Vontobel, V. Experiences with surgery of congenital megacolon and suggestion of a new surgical technique (modification of Duhamel's procedure). *Zentralbl. Chir.* 1959; **84**:1781–1789.
7. Martin, L. W. & Caudill, D. R. A method for elimination of the blind rectal pouch in the Duhamel operation for Hirschsprung's disease. *Surgery* **62**:951–953.
8. Soave, F. A new surgical technique for treatment of Hirschsprung's disease. *Surgery* 1964; **56**:1007–1014.
9. Boley, S. J. New modification of the surgical treatment of Hirschsprung's disease. *Surgery* 1964; **56**:1015–1017.
10. Denda, T. Surgical treatment of Hirschsprung's disease: a modification of Soave procedure. *Geka Shinryo* 1966; **8**:295–301.
11. Saltzman, D. A, Telander, M. J., Brennom, W. S., & Telander, R. L. Transanal mucosectomy: a modification of the Soave procedure for Hirschsprung's disease. *J. Pediatr. Surg.* 1996; **31**:1272–1275.
12. Rintala, R. & Lindahl, H. Transanal endorectal coloanal anastomosis for Hirschsprung's disease. *Pediatr. Surg. Int.* 1993; **8**:128–131.
13. Georgeson, K. E., Fuenfer, M. M., & Hardin, W. D. Primary laparoscopic pull-through for Hirschsprung's disease in infants and children. *J. Pediatr. Surg.* 1995; **30**:1017–1021.
14. De la Torre-Mondragon, L. & Ortega-Salgado, J. A. Transanal endorectal pull-through for Hirschsprung's disease. *J. Pediatr. Surg.* 1998; **33**:1283–1286.
15. Rehbein, F. & von Zimmermann, V. H. Ergebnisse der intraabdominellen Resektion bei der Hirschsprungschen Krankheit. *Zentralblatt Chir.* 1959; **84**:1744–1752.
16. Teitelbaum, D. H., Cilley, R. E., Sherman, N. J. *et al.* A decade of experience with the primary pull-through for Hirschsprung disease in the newborn period: a multicenter analysis of outcomes. *Ann. Surg.* 2000; **232**:372–380.
17. Shankar, K. R., Losty, P. D., Lamont, G. L. *et al.* Transanal endorectal coloanal surgery for Hirschsprung's disease: experience in two centers. *J. Pediatr. Surg.* 2000; **35**:1209–1213.
18. Santos, M. C., Giacomantonio, J. M., & Lau, H. Y. Primary Swenson pull-through compared with multiple-stage pull-through in the neonate. *J. Pediatr. Surg.* 1999; **34**:1079–1081.
19. van der Zee, D. C. & Bax, K. N. One-stage Duhamel–Martin procedure for Hirschsprung's disease: a 5-year follow-up study. *J. Pediatr. Surg.* 2000; **35**:1434–1436.
20. Pierro, A., Fasoli, L., Kiely, E. M., Drake, D., & Spitz, L. Staged pull-through for rectosigmoid Hirschsprung's disease is not safer than primary pull-through. *J. Pediatr. Surg.* 1997; **32**:505–509.
21. Minford, J. L., Ram, A., Turnock, R. R. *et al.* Comparison of functional outcomes of Duhamel and transanal endorectal coloanal anastomosis for Hirschsprung's disease. *J. Pediatr. Surg.* 2004; **39**:161–165.
22. Wulkan, M. L. & Georgeson, K. E. Primary laparoscopic endorectal pull-through for Hirschsprung's disease in infants and children. *Semin. Laparosc. Surg.* 1998; **5**:9–13.

23. Langer, J. C., Durrant, A. C., de la Torre, L. *et al.* One-stage transanal Soave pullthrough for Hirschsprung disease: a multicenter experience with 141 children. *Ann. Surg.* 2003; **238**:569–583.
24. Hadidi, A. Transanal endorectal pull-through for Hirschsprung's disease: experience with 68 patients. *J. Pediatr. Surg.* 2003; **38**:1337–1340.
25. Wester, T. & Rintala, R. J. Early outcome of transanal endorectal pull-through with a short muscle cuff during the neonatal period. *J. Pediatr. Surg.* 2004; **39**:157–160.
26. Weidner, B. C. & Waldhausen, J. H. Swenson revisited: a one-stage, transanal pull-through procedure for Hirschsprung's disease. *J. Pediatr. Surg.* 2003; **38**:1208–1211.
27. Quinn, F. M, Surana, R., & Puri, P. The influence of trisomy 21 on outcome in children with Hirschsprung's disease. *J. Pediatr. Surg.* 1994; **29**:781–783.
28. Caniano, D. A., Teitelbaum, D. H., & Qualman, S. J. Management of Hirschsprung's disease in children with trisomy 21. *Am. J. Surg.* 1990; **159**:402–404.
29. Makitie, O., Heikkinen, M., Kaitila, I., & Rintala, R. Hirschsprung's disease in cartilage-hair hypoplasia has poor prognosis. *J. Pediatr. Surg.* 2002; **37**:1585–1588.
30. Tsuji, H., Spitz, L., Kiely, E. M., Drake, D. P., & Pierro, A. Management and long-term follow-up of infants with total colonic aganglionosis. *J. Pediatr. Surg.* 1999; **34**:158–161.
31. Suita, S., Taguchi, T., Kamimura, T., & Yanai, K. Total colonic aganglionosis with or without small bowel involvement: a changing profile. *J. Pediatr. Surg.* 1997; **32**:1537–1541.
32. Yanchar, N. L. & Soucy, P. Long-term outcome after Hirschsprung's disease: patients' perspectives. *J. Pediatr. Surg.* 1999; **34**:1152–1560.
33. Tariq, G. M., Brereton, R. J., & Wright, V. M. Complications of endorectal pull-through for Hirschsprung's disease. *J. Pediatr. Surg.* 1991; **26**:1202–1206.
34. Sherman, J. O., Snyder, M. E., Weitzman, J. J. *et al.* A 40-year multinational retrospective study of 880 Swenson procedures. *J. Pediatr. Surg.* 1989; **24**:833–838.
35. Marty, T. L., Seo, T., Matlak, M. E., Sullivan, J. J., Black, R. E., & Johnson, D. G. Gastrointestinal function after surgical correction of Hirschsprung's disease: long-term follow-up in 135 patients. *J. Pediatr. Surg.* 1995; **30**:655–658.
36. Loening-Baucke, V. Functional constipation. *Semin. Pediatr. Surg.* 1995; **4**:26–34.
37. Reding, R., de Ville de Goyet, J., Gosseye, S. *et al.* Hirschsprung's disease: a 20-year experience. *J. Pediatr. Surg.* 1997; **32**:1221–1225.
38. Bai, Y., Chen, H., Hao, J., Huang, Y., & Wang, W. Long-term outcome and quality of life after the Swenson procedure for Hirschsprung's disease. *J. Pediatr. Surg.* 2002; **37**:639–642.
39. Rintala, R. J., & Lindahl, H. Is normal bowel function possible after repair of intermediate and high anorectal malformations. *J. Pediatr. Surg.* 1995; **30**:491–494.
40. Moore, S. W., Albertyn, R., & Cywes, S. Clinical outcome and long-term quality of life after surgical correction of Hirschsprung's disease. *J. Pediatr. Surg.* 1996; **31**:1496–1502.
41. Baillie, C. T., Kenny, S. E., Rintala, R. J., Booth, J. M., & Lloyd, D. A. Long-term outcome and colonic motility after the Duhamel procedure for Hirschsprung's disease. *J. Pediatr. Surg.* 1999; **34**:325–329.
42. Diseth, T. H., Bjornland, K., Novik, T. S., & Emblem, R. Bowel function, mental health, and psychosocial function in adolescents with Hirschsprung's disease. *Arch. Dis. Child.* 1997; **76**:100–106.
43. Heikkinen, M., Rintala, R. J., & Louhimo, I. Bowel function and quality of life in adult patients with operated Hirschsprung's disease. *Pediatr. Surg. Int.* 1995; **10**:342–344.
44. Festen, C. Postoperative small bowel obstruction in infants and children. *Ann. Surg.* 1982; **196**:580–583.
45. Wilkins, B. M., & Spitz, L. Incidence of postoperative adhesion obstruction following neonatal laparotomy. *Br. J. Surg.* 1986; **73**:762–764.
46. Rescorla, F. J., Morrison, A. M., Engles, D., West, K. W., & Grosfeld, J. L. Hirschsprung's disease. Evaluation of mortality and long-term function in 260 cases. *Arch. Surg.* 1992; **127**:934–941.
47. Fortuna, R. S., Weber, T. R., Tracy, T. F. Jr, Silen, M. L., & Cradock, T. V. Critical analysis of the operative treatment of Hirschsprung's disease. *Arch. Surg.* 1996; **131**:520–524.
48. Moore, S. W., Millar, A. J., & Cywes, S. Long-term clinical, manometric, and histological evaluation of obstructive symptoms in the postoperative Hirschsprung's patient. *J. Pediatr. Surg.* 1994; **29**:106–111.
49. Schmittenbecher, P. P., Sacher, P., Cholewa, D. *et al.* Hirschsprung's disease and intestinal neuronal dysplasia – a frequent association with implications for the postoperative course. *Pediatr. Surg. Int.* 1999; **15**:553–558.
50. Schulten, D., Holschneider, A. M., & Meier-Ruge, W. Proximal segment histology of resected bowel in Hirschsprung's disease predicts postoperative bowel function. *Eur. J. Pediatr. Surg.* 2000; **10**:378–381.
51. Ghose, S. I., Squire, B. R., Stringer, M. D., Batcup, G., & Crabbe, D. C. Hirschsprung's disease: problems with transition-zone pull-through. *J. Pediatr. Surg.* 2000; **35**(12):1805–1809.
52. Cord-Udy, C. L., Smith, V. V., Ahmed, S., Risdon, R. A., & Milla, P. J. An evaluation of the role of suction rectal biopsy in the diagnosis of intestinal neuronal dysplasia. *J. Pediatr. Gastroenterol. Nutr.* 1997; **24**:1–6.
53. Martucciello, G., Favre, A., Torre, M., Pini Prato, A., & Jasonni, V. A new rapid acetylcholinesterase histochemical method for the intraoperative diagnosis of Hirschsprung's disease and intestinal neuronal dysplasia. *Eur. J. Pediatr. Surg.* 2001; **11**:300–304.
54. Carvalho, J. L., Campos, M., Soares-Oliveira, M., & Estevao-Costa, J. Laparoscopic colonic mapping of dysganglionosis. *Pediatr. Surg. Int.* 2001; **17**:493–495.
55. Wester, T., O'Briain, D. S., & Puri, P. Notable postnatal alterations in the myenteric plexus of normal human bowel. *Gut* 1999; **44**:666–674.
56. Koletzko, S., Jesch, I., Faus-Kebetaler, T. *et al.* Rectal biopsy for diagnosis of intestinal neuronal dysplasia in children: a prospective multicentre study on interobserver variation and clinical outcome. *Gut* 1999; **44**:853–861.

57. Rassouli, R., Holschneider, A. M., Bolkenius, M. *et al.* Long-term results of Rehbein's procedure: a retrospective study in German-speaking countries. *Eur. J. Pediatr. Surg.* 2003; **13**:187–194.
58. Fuchs, O. & Booss, D. Rehbein's procedure for Hirschsprung's disease. *An appraisal of 45 years. Eur. J. Pediatr. Surg.* 1999; **9**:389–391.
59. Langer, J. C. Repeat pull-through surgery for complicated Hirschsprung's disease: indications, techniques, and results. *J. Pediatr. Surg.* 1999; **34**:1136–1141.
60. Wilcox, D. T. & Kiely, E. M. Repeat pull-through for Hirschsprung's disease. *J. Pediatr. Surg.* 1998; **33**:1507–1509.
61. Wildhaber, B. E., Pakarinen, M., Rintala, R. J., Coran, A. G., & Teitelbaum, D. H. Posterior myotomy/myectomy for persistent stooling problems in Hirschsprung's disease. *J. Pediatr. Surg.* 2004; **39**:920–926.
62. Minkes, R. K. & Langer, J. C. A prospective study of botulinum toxin for internal anal sphincter hypertonicity in children with Hirschsprung's disease. *J. Pediatr. Surg.* 2000; **35**:1733–1736.
63. Fonkalsrud, E. W., Thakur, A., & Beanes, S. Ileoanal pouch procedures in children. *J. Pediatr. Surg.* 2001; **36**:1689–1692.
64. Hoehner, J. C., Ein, S. H., Shandling, B., & Kim, P. C. Long-term morbidity in total colonic aganglionosis. *J. Pediatr. Surg.* 1998; **33**:961–965.
65. Mishalany, H. G. & Woolley, M. M. Postoperative functional and manometric evaluation of patients with Hirschsprung's disease. *J. Pediatr. Surg.* 1987; **22**:443–446.
66. Rintala, R. J. & Lindahl, H. Sodium cromoglycate in the management of chronic or recurrent enterocolitis in patients with Hirschsprung's disease. *J. Pediatr. Surg.* 2001; **36**:1032–1035.
67. Abrahamian, F. P. & Lloyd-Still, J. D. Chronic constipation in childhood: a longitudinal study of 186 patients. *J. Pediatr. Gastroenterol. Nutr.* 1984; **3**:460–467.
68. Dey, R., Ferguson, C., Kenny, S. E. *et al.* After the honeymoon – medium-term outcome of antegrade continence enema procedure. *J. Pediatr. Surg.* 2003; **38**:65–68.
69. Catto-Smith, A. G., Coffey, C. M., Nolan, T. M., & Hutson, J. M. Fecal incontinence after the surgical treatment of Hirschsprung disease. *J. Pediatr.* 1995; **127**:954–957.
70. Heij, H. A., de Vries, X., Bremer, I., Ekkelkamp, S., & Vos, A. Long-term anorectal function after Duhamel operation for Hirschsprung's disease. *J. Pediatr. Surg.* 1995; **30**:430–432.
71. Heikkinen, M., Rintala, R., & Luukkonen, P. Long-term anal sphincter performance after surgery for Hirschsprung's disease. *J. Pediatr. Surg.* 1997; **32**:1443–1446.
72. Rintala, R. J., & Lindahl, H. G. Proctocolectomy and J-pouch ileo-anal anastomosis in children. *J. Pediatr. Surg.* 2002; **37**:66–70.
73. Hackam, D. J., Reblock, K., Barksdale, E. M., Redlinger, R., Lynch, J., & Gaines, B. A. The influence of Down's syndrome on the management and outcome of children with Hirschsprung's disease. *J. Pediatr. Surg.* 2003; **38**:946–949.
74. Boemers, T. M., Bax, N. M., & van Gool, J. D. The effect of rectosigmoidectomy and Duhamel-type pull-through procedure on lower urinary tract function in children with Hirschsprung's disease. *J. Pediatr. Surg.* 2001; **36**:453–456.
75. Badner, J. A., Sieber, W. K., Garver, K. L., & Chakravarti, A. A genetic study of Hirschsprung's disease. *Am. J. Hum. Genet.* 1990; **46**:568–580.
76. Amiel, J. & Lyonnet, S. Hirschsprung's disease, associated syndromes and genetics: a review. *J. Med. Genet.* 2001; **38**:729–739.

31

Anorectal malformations: experience with the posterior sagittal approach

Alberto Peña and Marc A. Levitt

Cincinnati Children's Hospital Medical Center, Cincinnati, OH, USA

The management of anorectal malformations has, for many years, been a challenge for pediatric surgeons The most common and feared sequela is fecal incontinence. Urinary incontinence, sexual inadequacy, and fertility problems may also affect patients born with these defects.

Long-term outcomes in all congenital defects have been neglected by the pediatric surgical community, mostly because of the difficulty of follow-up. Also, once the patients reach a certain age they are no longer considered "pediatric" surgical patients, and they see adult specialists who continue their care. This seems true for all congenital defects, but with anorectal and genital malformations, long-term follow-up seems to be even more difficult to achieve, perhaps because the patients protect their privacy and do not like to disclose what could be considered embarrassing. Once patients reach puberty and/or adolescence they tend to hide their problems because the functional sequelae of an anorectal malformation are considered shameful. As a consequence, publications related to the long-term outcome of these patients have been rather scarce.[1–8]

Learning about the long-term functional sequelae suffered by these patients is mandatory for all pediatric surgeons in order to plan strategies for their management. The prevention and treatment of these functional sequelae is much more challenging, demanding, and expensive than the anatomical reconstruction upon which we have previously placed such emphasis. The challenge for the new generation of pediatric surgeons rests in understanding the intrinsic mechanisms of functional disorders that can be determined only through basic science research. Long-term follow-up of children after operations to repair congenital defects should be a fundamental part of our responsibility.

Historical introduction

Anorectal malformations have been known for many centuries; they are very obvious. There are multiple historical documents in the literature indicating that surgery to repair these defects has been attempted for many centuries.[9,10] In the past, surgeons tried to create an orifice in the place where they thought the rectum should be located. Many patients died from such operations, but a few survived. In retrospect, those who survived with good results most probably represented the group that we now call "low," meaning that the rectum was located very close to the skin. The patients who died or had poor functional results were probably those who had a rectum located far away from the perineum.

During the first 50 years of the twentieth century, surgeons tried to save a patient's life when faced with a "high" defect by opening a colostomy at birth. Later, usually when the child was 1 year old, an attempt was made to repair the malformation with an abdominoperineal pull-through, and subsequently the colostomy was closed. Functional results were rather poor. In so-called "low" defects surgeons tried to create an anus directly through the perineum without opening a protective colostomy.

In 1953, Douglas Stephens published his concept of the anatomy of "high" anorectal malformations.[11] He suggested that preservation of the puborectalis sling should be the main goal in the repair of high defects in order to achieve bowel control. It took several years for the pediatric surgical

Pediatric Surgery and Urology: Long-term Outcomes, Mark Stringer, Keith Oldham, Pierre Mouriquand.
Published by Cambridge University Press. © Cambridge University Press, 2006.

Table 31.1. Classification of anorectal malformations used in this chapter

Condition	Colostomy required?
Males	
Perineal (cutaneous) fistula	No
Rectourethral fistula (bulbar or prostatic)	Yes
Rectovesical fistula	Yes
Imperforate anus without fistula	Yes
Rectal atresia	Yes
Females	
Perineal (cutaneous) fistula	No
Vestibular fistula	Sometimes
Persistent cloaca	Yes
Imperforate anus without fistula	Yes
Rectal atresia	Yes

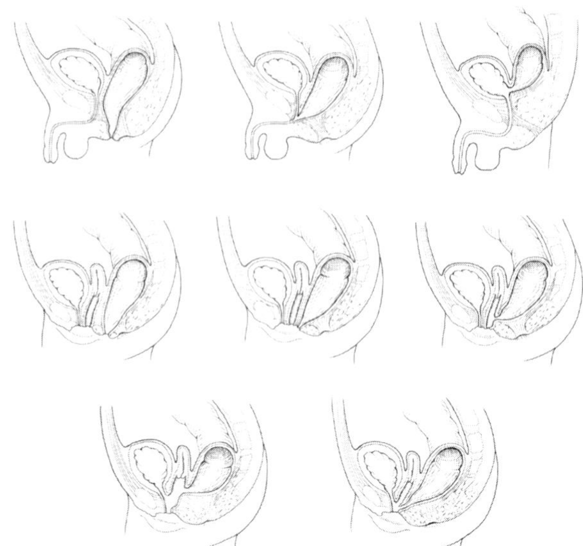

Fig. 31.1. Examples of anorectal malformations: boys (top row left to right): perineal fistula, rectourethral (bulbar) fistula, and rectobladder neck fistula; girls (middle row left to right): perineal fistula, rectovestibular fistula, rectovaginal fistula (very rare); cloacal malformations in girls (bottom row): a long common channel (left) and a short common channel (right). [Adapted from Pena 1990.[27]]

community worldwide to become aware of Dr. Stephens' ideas, but by the 1960s most pediatric surgeons were performing operations with his concept in mind. Functional results from these operations varied.[7,12–21]

In 1982, the posterior sagittal approach for the treatment of these malformations was developed, based on attempts to learn more about the basic anatomy of these defects and to improve the functional results.[22,23] The posterior sagittal approach allows direct visualization of the anatomy of these patients and precisely defines the relationship between rectum and genitourinary tract. Once the anatomy was widely exposed, the optimal way to repair each defect became obvious. In addition, many misconceptions about the anatomy of these defects were eradicated.

The assumption has been that a better and more precise anatomical reconstruction should lead to improved functional results.[24,25] Some authors believe, however, that this new approach has not changed the prognosis of children with anorectal malformations.[26] The first repair of an anorectal malformation via a posterior sagittal approach was performed in August 1980.

Terminology and classification issues

Comparing the results of reported series has always been a problem with anorectal malformations because different surgeons use different terminology when referring to types of imperforate anus. This problem is exacerbated by the use of various criteria and methods of evaluation. The most clear fact is that there is a spectrum of defects, so every attempt to classify them is arbitrary and somewhat inaccurate. Consequently, the traditional classification of "high," "intermediate" and "low" defects renders the results dubious. The classification presented in this chapter attempts to group together defects that have common diagnostic, therapeutic, and prognostic features (Table 31.1) (Fig. 31.1).

The posterior approach and direct visualization of the anatomy have allowed us to learn about important features. For instance, rectovaginal fistulas are almost nonexistent; in retrospect it seems that most of the previously reported "vaginal fistula" cases were misdiagnosed cloacas, or misdiagnosed vestibular fistulas. This assertion is supported by the senior author's experience of cloaca reoperations, where it has been found that most patients who were originally operated on by a surgeon who classified the defect as a "rectovaginal fistula" had only had the rectal component of the cloaca repaired and had been left with a persistent urogenital sinus.[27a] Such patients had become categorized as instances of "rectovaginal fistula" and the true diagnosis of cloaca had become evident only many years later. In addition, many patients had undergone an abdominoperineal pull-through at another institution to repair a "rectovaginal fistula," and years later had been referred because of fecal incontinence. When these girls were examined, the little pouch of what used to be the rectum was found opening in the vestibule, indicating that these patients had been born with a rectovestibular fistula.

Unfortunately, the abdominoperineal approach wrongly used for such patients had rendered them fecally incontinent. The cloaca itself represents a spectrum and certainly defies the classification of "high," "intermediate" and "low."

Also included in the "high" category in male patients were those with completely different defects requiring different treatments and carrying a different prognosis (e.g., rectourethral fistula and rectobladder neck fistula). A rectourethral fistula can be treated without a laparotomy, but a rectobladder neck fistula always requires the abdomen to be opened either with laparoscopy or laparetomy. The results of treatment are dramatically different, and so we cannot group these two defects into a single category.

The posterior sagittal approach has also allowed us to determine the precise incidence of cases without a fistula. The high incidence of such cases in previous reports is possibly related to misdiagnosis because of the inability of the surgeon to exactly define the type of malformation through lack of adequate exposure.[28] We now know that only 5% of all patients are born without a fistula.[24,25]

Surgical treatments

Perineal fistulas

Perineal fistulas in both males and females have traditionally been called "low" defects. In these cases the rectum opens in a small orifice, usually stenotic and located anterior to the center of the sphincter. Most of these patients have excellent sphincter mechanisms and a normal sacrum. A simple anoplasty enlarges the stenotic orifice and relocates the rectal orifice posteriorly within the limits of the sphincter complex. The operation is called a "minimal posterior sagittal anoplasty." It is performed with the patient positioned prone with the pelvis elevated; multiple fine silk sutures are placed at the mucocutaneous junction of the bowel orifice for traction. A short (1–2 cm) midsagittal incision is made posterior to the fistula site, dividing the entire external sphincter complex. The fistula and lower part of the rectum are carefully dissected to permit mobilization of the rectum for backward placement within the limits of the sphincter complex. The perineal body, that area where the fistula was located, is repaired with a few long-term absorbable sutures.[27]

Imperforate anus with a rectourethral fistula (prostatic or bulbar)

This is by far the most frequent defect seen in male patients. In these cases the rectum opens into the posterior urethra. Above the fistula, there is a common wall between rectum and urethra about 5–8 mm long. Sometimes the rectum opens into the lowest part of the posterior urethra, and this is termed a rectourethral bulbar fistula. Sometimes the rectum opens into the upper part of the posterior urethra, arbitrarily called a rectoprostatic fistula. Patients with a bulbar fistula have a better prognosis since patients with a prostatic fistula have a higher incidence of sacral dysplasia and abnormal sphincters.[24,25] In both cases, however, a colostomy is done soon after birth. One month later, provided the patient is growing and developing well, the posterior sagittal operation is performed. The patient is positioned prone with a Foley catheter in the bladder. A midline incision divides the entire sphincter complex. The use of an electric muscle stimulator helps to confirm that the muscles are bisected in the midline. The rectum is meticulously separated from the urethra and mobilized to reach the perineum. The urethra is repaired, and the rectum is placed within the limits of the sphincter complex, which may require tailoring of the rectum. An anoplasty is performed. Approximately 2 months after this operation, the colostomy is closed.

In cases of rectourethral bulbar fistula, the mobilization required to bring the rectum down is usually a relatively easy task. In cases of rectoprostatic fistula the mobilization requires a significant degree of circumferential dissection. The reader is referred to an earlier publication for detailed information about this surgical technique.[27]

Rectobladder-neck fistulas

Boys with a rectobladder-neck fistula represent approximately 10% of all male patients with an anorectal malformation. These children are frequently born with a poor sacrum and a poor sphincter mechanism. The incidence of associated defects, especially urological, is extremely high (about 90%).[29]

These patients require a laparoscopy or laparotomy in addition to the posterior sagittal approach in order for the rectum to reach the perineum, because it is located very high in the pelvis. The operation begins with a posterior sagittal approach. The entire sphincter complex is divided in the midline until the urethra is visualized. No attempt is made to find the rectum since this could expose the patient to injury of the vas deferens, prostate, seminal vesicles, and ectopic ureters. The presacral space behind the urethra is defined which is the path that the rectum should follow within the limits of the sphincter complex, and this incision is meticulously closed. The abdomen is then entered and the rectum is separated from the bladder-neck, which is an easy task because the rectum connects to the bladder-neck in a "T" fashion and has no common wall with the urinary tract. In addition, the end of the rectum is located approximately only 1 cm below the peritoneal reflection. The rectum is then mobilized and pulled down in position immediately behind the urethra along the track previously defined. An anoplasty is performed with 16 circumferential stitches.[28] The colostomy is closed about 2 months after surgery.

All patients are subjected to anal dilations starting 2 weeks after surgery and performed twice daily. The size of the dilator is increased every week to a level appropriate for the size of the patient.

Imperforate anus without fistula

This is a unique defect, accounting for 5% of all anorectal malformations.[24,25] The rectum in these patients is usually located 1–2 cm away from the perineal skin. The sacrum is uniformly good and so is the sphincter mechanism. These patients have a prognosis similar to those born with a rectourethral bulbar fistula. Of patients with Down syndrome and an anorectal malformation 95% have this specific type of defect. Operative repair is very similar to that described above for patients with a rectourethral fistula, except that there is no communication between the rectum and the urinary tract. Separation of the rectum from the urethra is nevertheless very demanding because both structures share a common wall. The prognosis for this type of defect is good.

Rectal atresia or rectal stenosis

Patients suffering from rectal atresia or rectal stenosis are a unique group of children who are born with an anorectal malformation and with an anal canal. They have a completely normal sphincter mechanism and normal sacrum. They have all the necessary anatomical and functional elements to be totally continent. Operative repair is performed via the posterior sagittal approach. The entire sphincter complex is divided and an end-to-end anastomosis is performed between the dilated proximal rectum and the narrow anal canal.

Rectovestibular fistula

Rectovestibular fistula is by far the most common defect seen in females. The rectum opens in the area called the vestibule, located between the hymen and the skin of the perineum, inside the genitalia. The rectum and vagina share a common wall for their distal 1–2 cm. The sacrum is usually normal and the sphincter mechanism is good. The prognosis in these patients is excellent.[24,25]

Depending on the surgeon's experience, management is either with a colostomy at or soon after birth, and the definitive repair is performed within a month, or with a primary repair. In the prone position, and with the pelvis elevated, multiple fine silk sutures are placed at the edge of the rectal opening in order to exert uniform traction, which facilitates dissection of the rectum. The entire sphincter mechanism is divided in the midline posterior to the rectum which is then dissected carefully, particularly the common wall between the rectum and the vagina. The rectum is completely separated from the vagina and then mobilized enough to be placed within the limits of the sphincter complex. Tapering of the rectum has not been required in the authors' experience. The perineal body is reconstructed. Anal dilations are started two weeks postoperatively and the colostomy is closed as with other malformations.

Cloacal malformations

The repair of cloacal malformations represents the most formidable technical challenge in dealing with these defects. A cloaca is defined as a defect in which rectum, vagina, and urethra are fused into a single common channel, which opens at the site of the normal female urethra. There is a broad spectrum of malformations in this category. The main concerns in dealing with patients with a cloaca are bowel function, urinary function, menstrual flow sexual function, and child-bearing capacity.

Retrospective analysis has shown that the length of the common channel measured from the external opening to the point where it bifurcates or trifurcates has a definite influence on the final prognosis of these patients; the turning point seems to be 3 cm. When the common channel is shorter than 3 cm, the patients have a better prognosis for bowel and urinary function, whereas when the patients have a common channel longer than 3 cm the prognosis is not as good.[24,25]

In cases of a short common channel, the operation has a level of difficulty similar to that of rectovestibular fistula repair. The defect is approached via a posterior sagittal incision. The rectum is separated from the vagina, and when the common channel is only 1 cm long there is no need to separate the vagina from the urinary tract. It is better to mobilize only the posterior and lateral walls of the vagina to create a large introitus. When the common channel is longer than larger, the rectum is mobilized as previously described, and then the vagina and urethra are mobilized as a unit (total urogenital mobilization) and placed below the clitoris.

This "total urogenital mobilization," was introduced to repair this malformation several years ago.[27b] This consists of the dissection of both urethra and vagina together. This maneuver has proved very useful, and the operation time has been considerably reduced. There have been no instances of urethrovaginal fistula, which used to occur in about 10% of cases in the past.[24,25] The blood supply of the vagina and urethra is also very well preserved with this technique. However, total urogenital mobilization gains only 2–3 cm of length. Therefore, when the common channel is longer than 3 cm, it is frequently necessary to use extra maneuvers to reconstruct the urethra and the vagina.

The vagina is sometimes located so high in the pelvis (in cases of a very long common channel) that the patient requires a laparotomy to reach it. A laparotomy is also sometimes necessary to reach a very high rectum. About 50% of patients with a cloaca suffer from hydrocolpos, which is a dilated vagina filled with fluid. This structure sometimes compresses the ureters at the point where they enter the bladder, producing megaureter(s). In addition, more than 50% of these patients suffer from various degrees of septation of the genitalia (hemivaginas and hemiuterus). Patients with a double hydrocolpos located very high in the pelvis may benefit from a maneuver called "vaginal switch." In this, one hemiuterus is resected along with the vaginal septum, both dilated hemivaginas are horizontally tubularized, and what used to be the dome of a hemivagina is switched down to the perineum.

In patients in whom the vagina is small and located very high in the pelvis, some form of vaginal replacement is needed. This can be performed by using small bowel or preferably sigmoid colon. Occasionally, the vagina can be replaced by the rectum, but this is feasible only in patients who have a very dilated rectum that can be longitudinally divided into a neovagina and rectum.

Sacral abnormalities

Sacral features appear to have a direct influence on the final functional outcome. Patients without a sacrum have no possibility of developing bowel and urinary control. Patients with a normal sacrum, on the other hand, are not guaranteed normal bowel control but certainly have a much better prognosis. Traditionally, it has been thought that the number of sacral vertebrae correlates well with the final functional outcome in these children. However, it is often difficult to count accurately the number of sacral vertebrae, particularly in patients with a very dysmorphic sacrum with fused vertebrae or hemivertebrae. A sacral ratio has therefore been devised in an attempt to provide an objective sacral measurement. Sacral measurements are compared with fixed bony parameters from the same patient's pelvis.

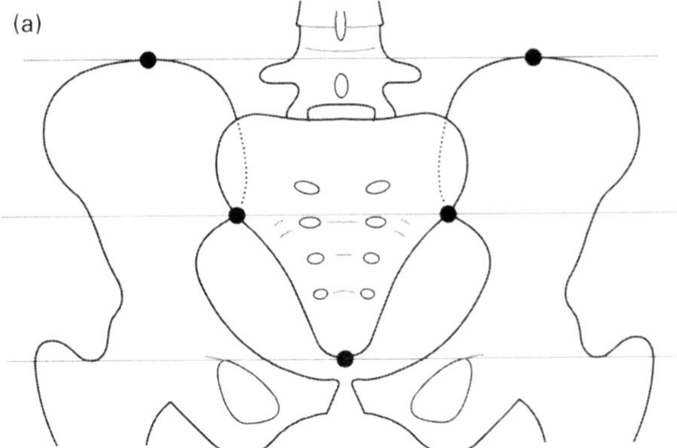

Fig. 31.2(a). The sacral ratio in the anteroposterior view.

The sacral ratio of a normal pelvis in anteroposterior view (AP film) is shown in Fig. 31.2(a). A line is traced from the uppermost portion of one iliac crest to the other. A second line is drawn across between the lowest point of each sacroiliac joint (posterior and inferior iliac spine). A third line runs parallel to the other two and touches the lowermost radiologically visible point of the sacrum. A ratio is obtained by dividing the distance between the two lower lines by the distance between the two upper lines. In 100 normal children at the authors' institution, the average ratio was 0.74; children with anorectal malformations show a spectrum of values. Lower ratios represent different degrees of sacral hypodevelopment and are associated with defects that have a poor functional outcome. The same sacral ratio in a normal child in the lateral position is shown in Fig. 31.2(b). This lateral ratio is a more reliable value because, in the AP position, the pelvis may be tilted in the anteroposterior direction to give a distorted ratio. The normal ratio in this lateral view is 0.77. Sacral hemivertebrae and hemisacra are also associated with a worse functional prognosis.

Evaluation of function

Bowel function should be evaluated independently of any medical treatment, such as suppositories, laxatives, or enemas. The parameters used for this evaluation include the following:

Voluntary bowel movements are defined as the act of "feeling" the urge to use the toilet for a bowel movement and the capacity to verbalize it and to hold it until the patient

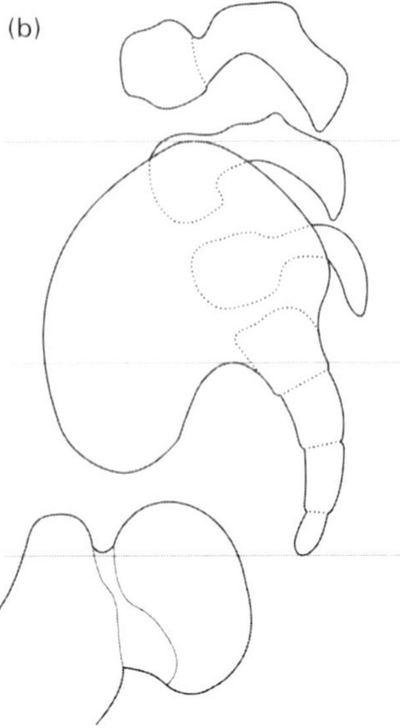

Fig. 31.2(b). The sacral ratio in the lateral view.

reaches the bathroom. This is considered the most valuable sign of fecal control.

Soiling is defined as the involuntary leakage of small amounts of stool, which produces smearing of the underwear.

Constipation is the incapacity to empty the rectum spontaneously (without help) every day.

Urinary incontinence is the incapacity to hold urine in the bladder and is considered Grade I when the patient has mild dribbling and wetness of the underwear day and night. Grade II is when the patient is completely incontinent.

For patients who have reached the age of sexual maturity, males should be asked about erections, ejaculation, sexual performance, and fertility. Females are asked about menstruation and associated symptoms, sexual activity, and fertility.

Long-term outcomes

Following patients long term is one of the most satisfying and rewarding aspects of a physician's professional life. Pediatric surgeons have reached a high degree of sophistication in the technical aspects of the repair of all anorectal malformations. There is no question that almost all anatomic malformations can be repaired. Yet the challenge of restoration to normal function remains. The long-term follow-up of our patients has taught us that functional sequelae are more complicated than first realized. The real imperative for the future consists in successfully treating these functional sequelae.

The first posterior sagittal anorectoplasty for the repair of an anorectal malformation was performed in Mexico City on August 10, 1980. We have been doing our best to follow all of the patients operated on by the senior author since this time. At the time of writing this chapter, our files include information relating to 1730 patients. From these, we have been in regular contact with 835. As the reader can imagine, these patients represent a spectrum in ages and complexity.

Patients operated on early in this series are now adults or teenagers; some of them are even older because we operated on them when they were already school age or later. This has been a unique opportunity to learn about the entire spectrum of anorectal malformations and the variety of problems encountered as these patients mature. We have learned to avoid words such as "never" and "always." New types of malformation are still seen and the spectrum of anomalies continues to expand.

This experience has been very satisfactory. It has been very rewarding to receive letters from women who have gotten married and had children or hear from others who have graduated from medical school or achieved some other professional milestone, expressing their gratitude for and satisfaction with the operation performed when they were infants. In contrast, we have been learning more and more about unpredicted sequelae; for example, sexual disorders in male and female adult patients. Adult urologists and gynecologists know little about these issues, and we are not adult urologists or gynecologists. We need sensitive, dynamic, ambitious gynecologists and urologists to help take care of this fascinating group of patients. The psychological impact of an anorectal malformation and the required social adaptation have also impressed us enormously. Since most sequelae are functional, we have been obligated to learn a great deal about the physiology of the anorectum and genitourinary system. We believe that it is imperative for surgeons to follow all such patients after anorectal reconstruction. Patients with anorectal malformations are patients for life.

Fecal continence

It is common knowledge that one of the most serious functional consequences of an anorectal malformation is fecal incontinence. The follow up of our patients has always centered on the evaluation of bowel control. There have been many meetings and roundtables to try to define bowel control and to create unified criteria to quantify and evaluate bowel control.

Table 31.2. Voluntary bowel movement and type of defect

Defect	Patients with voluntary bowel movement		
	Cases	n	(%)
Atresia or stenosis	8	8	(100.0)
Perineal fistula	41	41	(100.0)
Vestibular fistula	98	90	(91.8)
Imperforate anus without fistula	35	30	(85.7)
Bulbar fistula	83	68	(81.9)
Vaginal fistula	4	3	(75.0)
Prostatic fistula	72	53	(73.6)
Cloaca common channel < 3 cm	73	53	(72.6)
Cloaca common channel > 3 cm	41	17	(41.5)
Bladder-neck fistula	29	9	(31.0)
Totals	484	372	(77.0)

Table 31.3. Soiling and type of defect

Defect	Soiling		
	Cases	n	(%)
Perineal fistula	45	4	(8.9)
Atresia or stenosis	8	2	(25.0)
Vestibular fistula	101	37	(36.6)
Imperforate anus without fistula	37	18	(48.6)
Bulbar fistula	89	48	(53.9)
Cloaca common channel < 3 cm	77	47	(61.0)
Prostatic fistula	88	68	(77.3)
Vaginal fistula	5	4	(80.0)
Cloaca common channel > 3 cm	40	35	(87.5)
Bladder-neck fistula	41	36	(87.8)
Totals	531	299	(56.0)

We decided to evaluate two parameters related to bowel control. The first is the capacity for voluntary bowel movements. If a patient can verbalize the desire to pass stool, goes to the toilet, and has a voluntary bowel movement, he/she has a significant advantage. However, that does not mean that the patient is completely normal. We have encountered a significant number of patients who never have voluntary bowel movements after the repair of an anorectal malformation (Table 31.2). We consider these patients totally incontinent and they represent a specific category. However, different degrees of soiling (as defined above) may occur in patients with voluntary bowel movements. We have categorized them into grade 1 soiling, when the caregiver tells us that sometimes (once or twice a week) There is a spot or smear of stool on the underwear that happened because the child did not clean himself/herself well or is a manifestation of fecal incontinence. We have also found that these episodes of soiling are often related to constipation (see below). A patient who soils every day is considered to have grade 2 soiling (Table 31.3).

Many pediatric surgeons may disagree with the way we evaluate bowel control, believing that the presence of soiling alone defines fecal incontinence. However, we strongly disagree. There is a significant functional difference between a patient who never has a voluntary bowel movement and passes all stools in the underwear, and a patient who has voluntary bowel movements with occasional soiling. We therefore use the categorization outlined in this chapter.

We do not use any specific score to quantify bowel control because we do not believe that any of the available scores are clinically useful. Most of these scores include parameters that are not well correlated with bowel control such as manometric parameters. Furthermore, the presence or absence of constipation and diarrhea may affect bowel control but are not adequately addressed by conventional scoring systems. Therefore, we try not to quantify bowel control numerically, but rather in a more simplistic way.

- Does the patient have voluntary bowel movements?
- Does the patient soil and if so, how often?
- If the patient never soils and has voluntary bowel movements, he/she is for all practical purposes, a normal child from the perspective of bowel function and we regard this child as totally continent (Table 31.4).

In our series, about 75% of all anorectal patients have voluntary bowel movements. However, about half of these soil their underwear occasionally. This means that at least 25% of patients are incontinent after anorectal reconstruction. Only about 40% of our patients are totally continent (voluntary bowel movements and no soiling) (Table 31.4). Each specific type of defect has a different prognosis.

We do not use terms such as "high" and "low" because we consider that they represent an oversimplification of a much more complex spectrum of defects. This spectrum includes patients with severe, complex, very high malformations, who have a very poor functional prognosis. At the other extreme are patients with simple defects who have an excellent functional prognosis (traditionally known as "low malformations"). Between these two extremes, there are a variety of defects each with a different prognosis.

One of the great benefits of long-term follow-up in our patients is the ability to tell parents, in a fairly accurate way, what the future holds in terms of bowel function. By doing so, we believe one can avoid what we call the saga of

Table 31.4. Continence[a] and type of defect

	Totally continent		
Defect	Cases	n	(%)
Perineal fistula	41	36	(87.8)
Atresia or stenosis	8	6	(75.0)
Vestibular fistula	98	63	(64.3)
Imperforate anus without fistula	35	18	(51.4)
Bulbar fistula	83	34	(41.0)
Cloaca common channel < 3 cm	73	28	(38.4)
Vaginal fistula	4	1	(25.0)
Prostatic fistula	72	16	(22.2)
Cloaca common channel > 3 cm	41	4	(9.8)
Bladder-neck fistula	29	2	(6.9)
Totals	484	208	(43.0)

[a] Voluntary bowel movement and no soiling.

children with anorectal malformations. This refers to the scenario in which a patient is born with an anorectal defect and the surgeon tells the parents that the patient is going to be operated on and the operation is going to be "successful." The surgeon performs the operation, the patient recovers, is sent home, and then by the age of 3 years, the parents notice that the child has no bowel control. They go back to the surgeon, who inserts his finger in the child's rectum, feels some squeeze, and says that the child has an intact "puborectalis sling" (a structure that we have never seen). Yet the patient has fecal incontinence. The surgeon states that, from the anatomic point of view, everything is okay and advises referral to a gastroenterologist. The gastroenterologist performs rectal manometry, which may or may not indicate how "good or bad" the sphincter is. The gastroenterologist then suggests biofeedback, trying to improve the bowel function of the patient and yet the patient continues to be incontinent. At that point, the gastroenterologist alters the child's diet, and orders suppositories, enemas, and/or medications. This is both expensive and creates unrealistic expectations. At this point, the gastroenterologist may decide that the problem is psychological and the child is then referred to a psychologist or a psychiatrist. The latter find that the patient has psychological disturbances for which psychotherapy and behavior modification are advised. It is not unusual for us to see such patients coming to our clinic when they are 10 years old, still in diapers. The patients (and parents) are frustrated, often shy, and isolated at school. They do not talk to other people because their problem is considered shameful. Because of this, we believe that the pediatric surgeon must make an early, accurate diagnosis, which determines the specific prognosis for each type of defect. This makes it easier for the parents to adjust their expectations and to plan future care.

We maintain that all children born with an anorectal malformation should be completely clean of stool and dry of urine in the underwear after three years of age. This functional goal can be achieved either because they were born with a malformation that is considered to have a good functional prognosis and successfully potty train or because we keep them clean and dry with the implementation of what we call the Bowel and Urinary Management Program.[29]

We decided that 3 years of age should be the time to evaluate bowel control in our patients. Patients with mental retardation are not included in this analysis. As expected, the proportion of patients with voluntary bowel movements is higher in those nearer the good side of the anatomic spectrum. This is important to recognize because, if a patient is born with a "good defect" parents can expect bowel control by the age of three. In this kind of patient, we expend considerable effort in the toilet training process because we know that that there is a high likelihood of success. Also, in dealing with patients predicted to have a good prognosis on the basis of their anatomical defect, the surgeon should know that a major operative complication such as infection or dehiscence is unacceptable because it may change the functional prognosis. A similar complication in a patient with a bad prognosis type of defect does not have such a serious impact on the functional prognosis. If a baby is born with a "bad" type of malformation, less investment is made in time, money, and toilet training, and the bowel management program is started as soon as the patient reaches the age of three years. We believe that we should try to avoid the negative psychological experience of an incontinent child having embarrassing "accidents" in front of his toilet trained classmates. This can be a dramatic, deleterious, psychological event in the life of the child.

Some patients have an anatomic lesion associated with an uncertain functional outcome. For example, those who are born with a rectoprostatic fistula have about a 70% chance of having voluntary bowel movements by the age of three years (Table 31.2). We believe that these patients deserve the opportunity to become toilet trained. We try hard to encourage toilet training between the ages of $2^1/_2$ and 3 years. When the parents decide to send the child to school, if he/she is still not toilet trained, we offer the child our bowel management program so that the child can go to school wearing normal underwear. Because the patient has a 70% chance of achieving bowel control, we stop the bowel management program during the next summer vacation and try to toilet train again.

If a child has a poor prognosis based on the type of malformation, such as a rectobladder neck fistula in a male patient (associated with only a 30% chance of having voluntary bowel movements), we do not encourage the false expectations by trying to toilet train the patient, because it is unlikely to be successful. In such cases, we encourage the family to continue with the bowel management. Table 31.3 shows the incidence of soiling in our patients, distributed according to the type of anorectal malformation. Table 31.4 shows the incidence of totally continent patients according to type of defect.

The classification that we have used was selected because of its important therapeutic and prognostic implications. In other words, patients suffering from anatomically similar types of defect require the same operation and have very similar results. We have repeatedly tried to convince the pediatric surgical community to avoid the over simplifications inherent in the traditional classification that divides these malformations into "high," "intermediate," and "low." The so-called "high" group, for instance, includes malformations that must be treated differently and carry very different functional prognoses.

The Bowel Management Program has been in place at our institution for the last 20 years.[29] We use it in the 25% of our own patients who have no bowel control. In those that we have been able to follow, nearly all have found it successful. However, the majority of our patients come from other institutions and other countries. It has been extremely satisfying to observe how we can change the quality of life of a patient by the implementation of this bowel management program. The program consists principally of teaching the parents how to evacuate the child's colon once a day, and to try to decrease the motility of the colon by the use of a constipating diet and medications when necessary.

Most patients who come for the implementation of our program suffer from fecal incontinence and constipation. Because most patients have a hypomotile colon, once we have taught the family to empty the child's colon with an enema every day, the child will most likely stay completely clean for 24 hours or more. A few patients have colonic hypermotility with a tendency to diarrhea. This may be the consequence of some sort of inflammatory process or because they have lost a significant part of the colon during the original reconstruction. Fortunately, more and more pediatric surgeons try to preserve as much colon as possible in these patients. This is a key recommendation on our part. In the past, however, many surgeons sacrificed part of the rectosigmoid colon in reconstructive operations. This produced many fecally incontinent patients with a tendency to diarrhea.

A very important lesson we have learned is that in dealing with patients with an anorectal malformation, families and patients must accept that even in the best of circumstances, no patient can be considered completely normal. Many of our patients who are considered fecally continent may experience frequent "accidents" in their underwear during a bout of diarrhea. A few of our patients manage to control this diarrhea without any accidents, but this is extremely unusual. We have seen occasional patients who enjoy good bowel control until they become teenagers when they develop symptoms consistent with irritable bowel syndrome; some of these patients then become incontinent.

We have also treated 21 patients who were referred to us when they were 50 or 60 years old. These patients were born with a favorable anorectal malformation and underwent repair of the defect by a general surgeon. They indicate that they have been "continent" throughout their life but present to us because they have lost bowel control during the last 2 or 3 years. When we questioned these patients in detail, we found that the only thing that had really changed was the pattern of bowel movements and the consistency of the stool. We know that there is a tendency to suffer from an irritable colon and to become intolerant to certain foods with advancing age. These observations indicate that, even though these patients behaved as if they had normal bowels, they were not completely normal.

Patients with an anorectal malformation have two major functional threats: diarrhea and constipation. Both can produce fecal incontinence. The explanation seems to be the loss of one or more of the three key elements for fecal continence – normal anal sensation, intact sphincters, and normal bowel motility. All patients with an anorectal malformation have deficiencies in these three areas to a variable degree.

Constipation

Constipation is the commonest functional sequela in patients with an anorectal malformation treated by an operation in which the entire colon was preserved. Table 31.5 shows the incidence of constipation in our patients. Constipation is largely underestimated as a source of problems in patients with an anorectal malformation. Constipation is intimately linked with bowel control, a fact that is overlooked by many physicians. If constipation is treated inadequately it results in overflow pseudoincontinence. Thus, "normal" children who suffer from severe, idiopathic constipation and fecal impaction can have chronic soiling. They behave, for all practical purposes, like fecally

Table 31.5. Constipation and type of defect

Defect	Cases	n	(%)
Vestibular fistula	101	64	(63.4)
Bulbar fistula	91	53	(58.2)
Perineal fistula	53	30	(56.6)
Imperforate anus without fistula	40	22	(55.0)
Atresia or stenosis	8	4	(50.0)
Prostatic fistula	94	42	(44.7)
Cloaca common channel < 3 cm	87	33	(37.9)
Cloaca common channel > 3 cm	45	17	(37.8)
Bladder-neck fistula	45	7	(15.6)
Vaginal fistula	4	0	0
Totals	568	269	(47.9)

incontinent patients even though they have a normal sphincter and normal sensation.

Rectosigmoid motility is perhaps the most important factor in bowel control in children with an anorectal malformation. Patients born with a poor prognosis type of defect, with an almost undetectable anal sphincter and certainly absent sensation, can behave with a bowel management regimen almost like normal children, mainly because they have one or two bowel movements every day at a predictable time. The patients and/or the families learn that by taking meals consisting of the same types of food at the same time each day, they are able to have predictable bowel movements. By doing so, they behave for practical purposes like normal individuals. If they develop diarrhea, however, they will manifest incontinence.

At the other end of the spectrum are patients with a rectoperineal fistula who have undergone a technically good operation and should have an excellent functional prognosis but who are referred with "incontinence." Assessment of these patients shows that they actually have severe chronic fecal impaction and overflow pseudoincontinence. Once they are disimpacted and established on the right amount of laxatives to empty the colon every day, they become continent. It is very impressive to see patients who have been suffering chronically from overflow pseudoincontinence rendered continent by appropriate doses of laxatives. Some of these patients have even been subjected previously to operations such as gracilis muscle neosphincter formation, with or without electrical stimulation, placement of an artificial anal sphincter or "levatorplasty" in misguided attempts to improve bowel control. These operations, we have found, make the patient's condition worse.

It was noted previously that approximately 75% of all of our patients have voluntary bowel movements and about half occasionally soil their underwear (Table 31.3). Soiling is frequently a consequence of poorly treated constipation. Constipation and its secondary consequences are potentially so serious that we proactively overemphasize our concerns about constipation to the parents of our patients. When the colostomy is closed, we stress that it is extremely important to be sure that the baby empties his/her colon every day. The presence of bowel movements does not rule out the existence of constipation. In fact, some babies have two or three bowel movements every day and, as time goes by, this number increases. However, their degree of constipation and fecal impaction also increase. The patient is actually having tiny bowel movements that reflect fecal impaction and overflow. Parents are encouraged to distinguish between old stool retained in the rectum (usually dark and smelly) from fresh normal stool. Parents are also taught to do rectal examinations. We stress the importance of being sure that the baby empties the rectum, even if this requires the administration of laxatives every day.

We have tried to find an explanation for why some patients are more constipated than others and why some have no constipation. A retrospective analysis of our patients yielded the following conclusions:

- Patients who were left for many months with a transverse colostomy before undergoing definitive anorectal reconstruction develop a characteristic microcolon distal to the colostomy followed more distally by a mega rectosigmoid. A transverse colostomy makes the irrigation and cleaning of the distal colon very difficult. Meconium remains in the distal part of the bowel and the mucus produced in the colon generates the equivalent of fecal impaction in the distal colon, leading to a mega rectosigmoid. The preoperative degree of mega rectosigmoid correlates directly with the degree of constipation postoperatively. Therefore, we consider it imperative to keep the distal rectosigmoid completely decompressed from the first day of life. Constipation produces dilatation of the rectosigmoid which, in turn, produces more constipation, creating a vicious cycle.
- A loop colostomy usually allows the passage of some stool from the proximal to distal bowel. This results in more fecal impaction distally causing more rectosigmoid dilatation and eventually more constipation.
- Patients born with no fistula represent only 5% of all anorectal anomalies. Most of these children have Down syndrome. They suffer from more constipation than might otherwise have been expected.
- As can be seen in Table 31.5 we have found to our surprise that constipation is more severe with lower malformations. Initially, we thought that perhaps the dissection of the most distal rectum produces a degree of denervation which causes constipation. However, if this were so, patients with higher defects requiring more dissection

should experience more constipation. Clinical observations suggest exactly the opposite, i.e. patients with lower defects have more constipation than those with higher defects. A possible explanation is that patients with lower defects have a more dilated bowel from the moment they are born.

- Patients with a favorable type of anorectal anomaly have voluntary bowel movements, but the parents must be vigilant to detect and treat constipation in order to avoid undesirable consequences. Parents learn very early that the moment a child starts soiling, it is most likely to be due to constipation. If they increase the dose of laxatives, the soiling disappears. On the other hand, if too much laxative is given and the patient suffers from diarrhea, then the patient will become temporarily incontinent. These patients used laxatives rather than stool softener to effect the hypomotility.

Importance of colonic motility

We have learned to recognize the relevance of colonic motility to functional bowel control. Three examples demonstrate this point. One, already mentioned, is the pseudoincontinent patient with fecal overflow related to constipation. The second is the individual who has bowel control for a few years and then suddenly becomes incontinent due to development of an irritable colon. We know now that patients with an anorectal malformation have a great deal of difficulty controlling liquid stool. The third example is the child who remains clean despite the fact that he/she has no sphincter. This is because he/she has formed stool and has one or two bowel movements every day at a predictable time because of an appropriate diet and bowel management regimen. Although this patient has no normal bowel control, he/she behaves like a continent person.

Urinary function

For the purpose of evaluating urinary control, we have divided our patients into two groups: those with a cloaca and patients with other malformations. The reason for this is that we found very early on in our practice that patients with a cloaca may suffer from a unique type of urinary dysfunction.

Cloacal malformations

The overwhelming majority of babies with a cloaca have a large smooth bladder with a variable degree of emptying dysfunction. Table 31.6 summarizes urinary function in our patients with a cloaca. These girls do not have the hypertonic, trabeculated, "christmas tree" type of bladder seen in patients with a myelomeningocele. Fortunately, most infants with a cloaca have a good bladder neck. The combination of a large, floppy bladder and a good bladder neck allows these patients to hold a large amount of residual urine. When the bladder becomes full, the patient is prone to overflow and dribbling of urine. Passage of a urethral catheter and complete emptying of the bladder keeps the baby completely dry for several hours, until the bladder is full again. These two elements (a good bladder neck and a large, hypotonic bladder) make these patients ideal candidates for clean intermittent catheterization. Not all girls with a cloaca require intermittent catheterization (Table 31.6). Those with a common channel shorter than 3 cm have a much better functional prognosis in terms of urinary function.[30]

Table 31.6. Urinary continence in cloacal anomalies

Common channel →	< 3 cm		> 3 cm		Total	
Normal	59	72%	11	20%	70	51.5%
Dry with intermittent catheterization	16	20%	20	37%	36	26.5%
Dry with continent diversion	7	8%	23	43%	30	22.0%
Totals	82		54		136	

Two specific groups of patients with a cloaca do not have a good bladder neck. Firstly, there are those with separated pubic bones. All patients with this particular type of defect have no bladder neck. They can be described as having an essentially "covered exstrophy." These patients require either bladder neck reconstruction or permanent closure of the bladder neck with vesicostomy followed, at the age of social continence, by bladder augmentation and creation of a continent catheterizable conduit (Mitrofanoff). We favor the latter approach. Table 31.6 shows the number of patients who required this kind of reconstruction in our series.

The other type of cloacal defect that does not do well with intermittent catheterization is the patient with an extremely long common channel. In these cases, the vagina(s) and rectum are both connected to the urinary tract at the level of the bladder neck. Separation of these structures leaves the patient with no functional bladder neck. Therefore, management options are similar to those outlined for patients with separated pubic bones.

Patients with other anorectal malformations

The vast majority of patients with an anorectal malformation other than a cloacal anomaly have clinically normal urinary function. Table 31.7 summarizes urinary function in our patients. The few who suffer from urinary incontinence in our series are those who have either an absent sacrum or severe associated defects such as ectopic

Table 31.7. Urinary incontinence and type of defect (excluding cloacas)

Defect	Cases	*n*	(%)
Atresia or stenosis	8	0	(0.0)
Perineal fistula	38	0	(0.0)
Bulbar fistula	85	2	(2.4)
Imperforate anus without fistula	37	1	(2.7)
Vestibular fistula	94	4	(4.3)
Prostatic fistula	85	7	(8.2)
Bladder-neck fistula	38	7	(18.4)
Vaginal fistula	5	1	(20.0)
Totals	390	22	(5.6)

Table 31.8. Sexual function in male patients with an anorectal malformation: 41 patients older than 15 yrs

	Primary operations				
	Bulbar urethral fistual	Prostatic fistula	Bladder-neck fistula	Redo operations	Total
Normal sex[a]	5	8	1	21	35
No ejaculation	1	0	0	3	4
Retrograde ejaculation	0	0	1	2	1
Total	6	8	2	26	40

[a] Have erection, orgasm, ejaculation and satisfactory intercourse.

ureters opening in the bladder neck or a ureterocele affecting the bladder neck. There is a clear explanation for urinary incontinence in these patients. In contrast, we have reviewed a series of male patients who were referred to our hospital after having an operation for an anorectal malformation at another institution and we found that a significant proportion had urinary incontinence. Serious errors in the management of these patients accounted for their problems.[31] In male patients, the principal associations with urinary tract dysfunction were anorectal reconstruction with a blind technique or a posterior sagittal approach without an accurate distal colostogram.[32] In the latter circumstance, posterior sagittal exploration failed to identify the rectum; and the urethra, seminal vesicles, vas deferens, prostate, and nerves that innervate the bladder were encountered instead, presumably causing injury. Some of these patients suffered from urinary incontinence because of injury to the posterior urethra or bladder. In some cases, the urethra had been completely divided, and the bladder or a megaureter was pulled down instead of the rectum. A less frequent technical error was incomplete removal of the distal rectum, leaving a posterior urethral diverticulum causing persistent urinary dribbling.[31]

All of these intraoperative complications are preventable. A technically correct, high pressure, distal colostogram will allow the surgeon to precisely define rectal anatomy and thus minimize the risk of such injuries. When patients with an anorectal malformation other than a cloaca are well managed, urinary control is expected.

Sexual function

Males

The long-term follow-up of patients with an anorectal malformation has highlighted several important outcomes with respect to sexual function.

In addition to the follow-up of 424 male patients in our own series, we have significant experience of the follow-up of another group of approximately 400 male patients operated on at other institutions who were subsequently referred to our center. It is clear to us that patients operated on with previous blind techniques (sacroabdominoperineal type of operations) frequently suffered damage to the genitourinary tract.[31]

Table 31.8 documents the problems that we have encountered in a small group of our own patients who have reached adolescence. In general, we expect most male patients to have satisfactory sexual function. Among patients operated on at other institutions we have encountered multiple problems including impotence, lack of ejaculation or retrograde ejaculation. Upon evaluation, we have found that the latter group of men had suffered various injuries in the region of the junction of the rectum with the posterior urethra.[31] We believe that operative injury to the prostate, seminal vesicles, vas deferens, bladder nerves, and/or the penis is the most likely explanation. Some parents reported that their child no longer had erections after anorectal surgery. We maintain that the majority of sexual problems in these patients are avoidable.

We discovered that the first two patients we operated upon for a bladder neck fistula (the highest defect in our series) had no apparent ejaculation when they reached adolescence (Table 31.8). They had erection and orgasm, but no ejaculation. Investigation showed that they had a verumontanum located either at the bladder neck or in the trigone, at the site where the rectum originally joined the bladder. Ejaculation was occurring, but inside the bladder. Ten percent of all our male patients have a rectobladder neck fistula and a growing cohort are reaching maturity. This particular problem can be diagnosed endoscopically and, with modern techniques, sperm can be recovered from the bladder for artificial insemination, perhaps allowing

Table 31.9. Menstruation in girls with an anorectal malformation: 79 patients

	Normal	Abnormal
Cloaca	26	15[a]
Vestibular	28	–
Complex malformation	3	–
Rectal atresia	2	–
Vaginal fistula	2	–
Cloaca exstrophy	2	–
Unknown	1	–

[a] Retained menstrual blood due to atresias of Mullerian structures or amenorrhea. Six required an operation.

these men to father children. At present, this problem has not been surgically repaired.

Many of our own adult male patients have normal sexual function (Table 31.8) and a number of them now have children. In the coming years, at least another 600 of our patients will reach adult life and we will endeavor to assess their sexual function and fertility.

Epidydimitis is a frequent problem seen in males with an anorectal malformation. We have seen 21 patients with this problem. It occurs in patients with urinary tract infections, obstructive uropathy and/or an ectopic vas deferens communicating with the bladder or ureter.

Females

Since we are dealing with an anatomic spectrum of defects, we expected to find a spectrum of outcomes in terms of sexual function. Among 803 female patients operated by us, 87 are older than 11 years of age. From these, we have been able to obtain information about menstruation in 79. The results are summarized in Table 31.9.

Patients with a perineal or vestibular fistula have successful and satisfying sexual intercourse. A number of them have become pregnant and delivered vaginally without problems (Table 31.10). The vast majority of female patients with an anorectal malformation have normal ovaries and have progressed through puberty normally.

We have also followed up patients operated on at other institutions. Many of the girls with a cloaca born before 1980 were misdiagnosed as having a rectovaginal fistula.[33] These patients had the rectal component of the malformation repaired but were left with a persistent urogenital sinus. The patients grew up to find, when they became teenagers, that they had no vaginal opening. They have subsequently required reoperation to mobilize a normal vagina that was inside the pelvis, but connected to the urethra. The results have been very rewarding and many such patients have since become sexually active.

Table 31.10. Pregnancy and delivery in patients with an anorectal malformation, 11 patients

		Primary operations	
	Redo operations	Vestibular	Cloaca
Pregnancy[a]	1	3	2
Cesarean section	3	–	1
Vaginal delivery	1	–	–

[a] No outcome reported.

Some girls treated at other institutions for a vestibular fistula had had an inadequate repair. A limited procedure had been performed to enlarge the size of the rectal opening in order to facilitate the passage of stools; the rectum was left anteriorly mislocated and intimately attached to the vagina. Many of these patients suffer from a degree of fecal incontinence. Some have experienced serious rectal injuries and disruption of the perineal body during vaginal delivery. We have operated on 26 of these patients as adolescents or adults and they have been extremely happy with the anatomical results of reconstruction. Surgical reconstruction has improved their self-esteem and increased their satisfaction with sexual intercourse; many have also gained a significant improvement in bowel control.

Among the first 22 female patients with a cloaca to reach puberty, nine required an operation to drain trapped menstrual blood and/or resect a hemiuterus with an atretic cervix or vagina.[34] Six patients in this group had amenorrhea (Table 31.9).

Among 370 of our patients with a cloaca, approximately 20 have had a bladder augmentation, 125 have had a vaginal replacement (they menstruate through a neovagina constructed from bowel), and 22 have had a Malone procedure (see Chapter 33). These patients may present difficult management problems as they mature and become pregnant, perhaps requiring cesarean section for delivery. This is an area requiring collaboration between pediatric surgeons and gynecologists.

Orthopedic sequelae

About 30% of our patients with an anorectal anomaly suffer from spinal and sacral malformations. Eighty-two of our patients have spinal abnormalities including hemivertebra with scoliosis. These patients require advice from orthopedic surgeons. Nine of them have undergone spinal surgery with variable success.

Psychological sequelae and adaptation

It has been an extraordinary but also concerning experience to follow our patients with an anorectal malformation over many years and see what degrees of adaptation have been achieved and the different types of psychological problems they have experienced. We have seen patients who are completely maladapted to their environment, considering themselves segregated from society, and living relatively isolated lives. Even if they are clean and dry because of our bowel management program and/or intermittent catheterization, the burden of their condition can still make them very unhappy.

The quality of life for all of these patients with severe malformations is clearly abnormal. On the other hand, many patients have confronted and adapted to their adversity. Many have not only coped with their physical and functional limitations, but also been optimistic, using their experience to help others. Some have become leaders in self-help organizations for parents of patients with an anorectal malformation. They are uniquely qualified because they have a moral authority on the subject and they can help others cope with the problems engendered by an anorectal malformation.

REFERENCES

1. Iwai, N., Yanagihara, J., Tokiwa, K., Deguchi, E., & Takahashi, T. Results of surgical correction of anorectal malformations: a 10–30 year follow up. *Ann. Surg.* 1988; **207**:219–222.
2. Rintala, R., Lindahl, H., & Louhimo, I. Anorectal malformations: results of treatment and long-term follow up in 208 patients. *Pediatr. Surg. Int.* 1991; **6**:36–41.
3. Elly, A., Hassink, M. S., Rieu, P. N. *et al.* Are adults content or continent after repair for high anal atresia? A long-term follow-up study in patients 18 years of age and older. *Ann. Surg.* 1993; **218**:196–200.
4. Rinlala, R., Mildh, L., & Lindahl, H. Fecal continence and quality of life in adult patients with an operated low anorectal malformation. *J. Pediatr. Surg.* 1992; **27**:902–905.
5. Varma, K. K. Long-term continence after surgery for anorectal malformations. *Pediatr. Surg. Int.* 1991; **6**:32–35.
6. Diseth, T. H., Emblem, R., Solbraa, I. B., & Vandvik, I. H. A psychosocial follow-up of ten adolescents with low anorectal malformations. *Acta. Paediatr.* 1994; **83**:216–221.
7. Nixon, H. H. & Puri, P. P. The results of treatment of anorectal anomalies: a thirteen to twenty-year follow-up. *J. Pediatr. Surg.* 1977; **12**:27–37.
8. Karkowski, J., Pollock, W. F., & Landon, C. W. Imperforate anus: eighteen to thirty year follow-up study. *Am. J. Surg.* 1973; **126**:141–147.
9. Aegineta, P. On the imperforate anus. In Admas, F. (trans), *The Seven Books*. Book VI, Section LXXXI London: The Sydenham Society, 1844; 405.
10. Amussat, J. Z. Gustiure d'une operation d'anus artificial practique avec succes par un nouveau procede. *Gaz. Med. Paris* 1835; **3**:735.
11. Stephens, F. D. Imperforate rectum: a new surgical technique. *Med. J. Austral.* 1953; **1**:202–206.
12. Kiesewetter, W. B. & Turner, C. R. Continence after surgery for imperforate anus: a critical analysis and preliminary experience with sacroperineal pull-through. *Ann. Surg.* 1963; **158**:498–512.
13. Santulli, T. V., Schullinger, J. N., Kiesewetter, W. B., & Bill, A. H. Imperforate anus: a survey from the members of the Surgical Section of the American Academy of Pediatrics. *J. Pediatr. Surg.* 1971; **6**:484–487.
14. Templeton, J. M. & Ditesheim, J. A. High imperforate anus: quantitative results of long-term fecal continence. *J. Pediatr. Surg.* 1985; **20**:645–652.
15. Nai-Theow, O. & Beasley, S. Long-term continence in patients with high and intermediate anorectal anomalies treated by sacroperineal (Stephens) rectoplasty. *J. Pediatr. Surg.* 1991; **26**:44–48.
16. Iwai, N., Yanagihara, J., Tokiwa, K., Deguchi, E., & Takahashi, T. Voluntary anal continence after surgery for anorectal malformations. *J. Pediatr. Surg.* 1988; **23**:393–397.
17. Smith, E. I., Tunell, W. P., & Williams, G. R. A clinical evaluation of the surgical treatment of anorectal malformations (imperforate anus). *Ann. Surg.* 1978; **187**:583–591.
18. Ackroyd, R. & Nour, S. Long-term faecal continence in infants born with anorectal malformations. *J. Roy. Soc. Med.* 1994; **87**:695–696.
19. Cywes, S., Cremin, B. J., & Louw, J. H. Assessment of continence after treatment for anorectal agenesis: a clinical and radiological correlation. *J. Pediatr. Surg.* 1971; **6**:132–137.
20. Taylor, I., Duthie, H. L., & Zachary, R. B. Anal continence following surgery for imperforate anus. *J. Pediatr. Surg.* 1973; **8**:497–503.
21. Mollard, P., Meunier, P., Mouriquand, P., & Bonnet, J. P. High and intermediate imperforate anus: functional results and postoperative manometric assessment. *Eur. J. Pediatr. Surg.* 1991; **1**:282–286.
22. deVries, P. A. & Pena, A. Posterior sagittal anorectoplasty. *J. Pediatr. Surg.* 1982; **5**:638–643.
23. Pena, A. & deVries, P. Posterior sagittal anorectoplasty: important technical considerations and new applications. *J. Pediatr. Surg.* 1982; **17**:796–811.
24. Pena, A. Results in the management of 322 cases of anorectal malformations. *Pediatr. Surg. Int.* 1988; **3**:105–109.
25. Pena, A. Anorectal malformations. *Semin. Pediatr. Surg.* 1995; **4**:35–47.
26. Langemeijer, R. A. & Molenaar, J. C. Continence after posterior sagittal anorectoplasty. *J. Pediatr. Surg.* 1991; **26**:587–590.
27. Pena, A. *Atlas of Surgical Management of Anorectal Malformations.* New York: Springer Verlag, 1990.

27a. Levitt, M. A. & Peña, A. Pitfalls in the management of newborn cloacas. *Pediatr. Surg. Int.* 2005; **21**:264–269.

27b. Peña, A. Total urogenital mobilization: an easier way to repair cloacas. *J. Pediatr Surg.* 1997; **32**(2):263–268.

28. Stephens, F. D. & Smith, E. D. *Anorectal Malformations in Children: Incidence, Frequency of Types, Etiology.* Chicago: Year Book Medical, 1971; 160–171.

29. Peña, A., Guardino, K., Tovilla, J. M., Levitt, M. A., Rodriquez, G., & Torres, R. Bowel management for fecal incontinence in patients with anorectal malformations. *J. Pediatr. Surg.* 1998; **33**:133–137.

30. Peña, A., Levitt, M. A., Hong, A. R., & Midulla, P. Surgical management of cloacal malformations: a review of 339 patients. *J. Pediatr. Surg.* 2004; **39**:470–479.

31. Hong, A. R., Rosen, N., Acuña, M. F., Peña, A., Chaves, L., & Rodriquez, G. Urological injuries associated with the repair of anorectal malformations in male patients. *J. Pediatr. Surg.* 2002; **37**:339–344.

32. Gross, G. W., Wolfson, P. J., & Peña, A. Augmented-pressure colostogram in imperforate anus with fistula. *Radiology* 1991; **21**:560–562.

33. Rosen, N. G., Hong, A. R., Soffer, S. Z., Rodriquez, G., & Peña, A. Recto-vaginal fistula: a common diagnostic error with significant consequences in female patients with anorectal malformations. *J. Pediatr. Surg.* 2002; **37**:961–965.

34. Levitt, M. A., Stein, D. M., & Peña, A. Gynecologic concerns in the treatment of teenagers with cloaca. *J. Pediatr. Surg.* 1998; **33**:188–193.

32

Gastrointestinal motility disorders

Manu R. Sood[1] and Paul E. Hyman[2]

[1]Children's Hospital of Wisconsin, Milwaukee, WI, USA
[2]Department of Pediatrics, University of Kansas Hospital, Kansas City, KS, USA

During the past decade there have been advances in the understanding of gastrointestinal (GI) motility and sensory disorders in children. Newly validated diagnostic techniques can accurately diagnose previously misunderstood patients, and progress is being made in the treatment of enteric neuromuscular disorders. In this chapter pediatric GI motility disorders are discussed according to the anatomy of the GI tract.

Esophageal disorders

The esophagus includes three functional regions: the upper esophageal sphincter (UES), the esophageal body, and the lower esophageal sphincter (LES). The UES consists of striated muscle, which relaxes in response to swallowing. The esophageal body is lined by striated muscle in the proximal third, mixed striated and smooth muscle in the middle third, and smooth muscle in the lower third. Esophageal peristalsis is initiated by swallowing and is independent of intrinsic myoelectrical activity. The coordinated motor pattern of the esophagus is called primary peristalsis. Secondary peristalsis is usually induced by luminal distention or incomplete clearance of luminal contents by primary peristalsis. This is an important mechanism for the clearance of gastric contents during gastroesophageal reflux. The lower esophageal sphincter (LES), a band of smooth muscle located at the junction of the distal esophagus and gastric cardia, is tonically contracted except during swallowing when it relaxes momentarily to allow the food bolus to pass into the stomach. Inappropriate LES relaxation independent of swallowing is the mechanism responsible for the majority of gastroesophageal reflux episodes both in adults and children.[1,2]

Cricopharyngeal dysfunction

The most common disorder of the UES is failure to open completely or in synchrony with pharyngeal contractions, resulting in choking, repeated cough and aspiration. Upper esophageal sphincter achalasia or failure to relax is usually seen in patients with cerebral palsy and other neuromuscular disorders. Chiari malformation[3] can be associated with cricopharyngeal dysfunction.

Videofluoroscopy and nasopharyngeal endoscopy are helpful investigations. Findings include delayed passage of contrast through the UES, pharyngoesophageal incoordination and a "horizontal bar" caused by a non-relaxing sphincter.

Spontaneous improvement may occur, thickened feeds are usually better tolerated and safer to prevent aspiration. In older symptomatic children surgical and laser treatment have been used successfully.

Achalasia and other esophageal motility disorders

Achalasia,[4] diffuse esophageal spasm,[5] nutcracker esophagus[6] (Fig. 32.1), and non-specific esophageal motor disorders[7] all occur in pediatric patients. Esophageal motility disorders may be associated with dysphagia, chest pain, vomiting, and decreased oral intake. These conditions may cause food refusal in infants and in preschool children too young to provide an accurate pain history.[8] The management of achalasia is covered in Chapter 18.

Rumination syndrome in healthy children and adolescents

Rumination in otherwise healthy schoolchildren and adolescents is a diagnosis based on symptoms, and has become

Pediatric Surgery and Urology: Long-term Outcomes, Mark Stringer, Keith Oldham, Pierre Mouriquand.
Published by Cambridge University Press.

Very high amplitude distal esophageal contractions in nutcracker esophagus

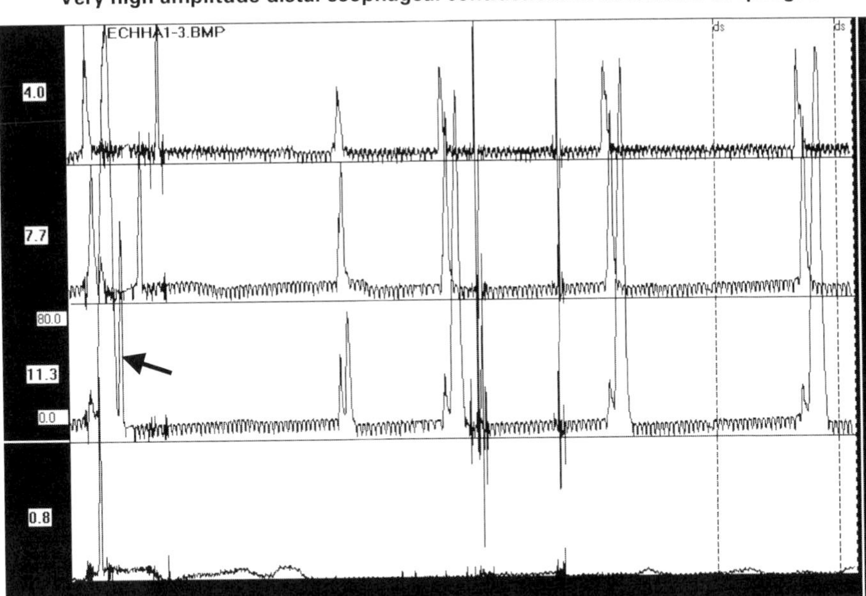

Fig. 32.1. (Channels from top to bottom): 1–3 esophageal body, 4 – stomach. Four propagating contractions and one non-propagating esophageal body contraction. Note that the amplitude of the first contraction in the lower third of the esophagus is 240 mm Hg (arrow). The next three contractions at the same level are above 200 mm Hg.

more widely recognized in recent years. Rumination syndrome is characterized by the effortless regurgitation into the mouth of recently ingested food, followed by its rechewing and reswallowing or expulsion. There are three variants of rumination syndrome. Infant rumination, with onset between 3 and 8 months, is self-stimulatory, secretive behavior caused by chronic neglect.[9] Infant rumination is life threatening but responds to a relationship with a loving caretaker. It was the first rumination syndrome to be described but is rare. Second, rumination syndrome occurs as a self-stimulatory behavior in neurologically devastated or retarded children. It is difficult to treat, but usually pleasurable for the child and not dangerous. Third, rumination syndrome in healthy schoolchildren and adolescents is often confused with motility disorders including gastroesophageal reflux disease, gastroparesis, and chronic intestinal pseudo-obstruction.[10] However, the history is characterized by regurgitation during and immediately after meals, and never during sleep. Rumination is caused by relaxation of the lower esophageal sphincter, together with tonic contraction of the crural diaphragm and increasing intra-abdominal pressure to initiate retrograde movement of gastric contents.

Extensive medical testing is unnecessary because the diagnosis is based on symptoms. In contrast to gastroparesis, in which the vomiting is delayed until long after eating, rumination emesis occurs during or immediately after eating. In contrast to gastroesophageal reflux disease there is no heartburn or esophagitis. Antroduodenal manometry is often diagnostic. The motility patterns are normal except that during or after eating there are brief, low amplitude, simultaneous increases in pressure called r-waves that occur coincidentally with rumination events (Fig. 32.2).

Recovery is achieved in most patients who wish to eliminate the behavior. Treatment involves teaching diaphragmatic breathing and relaxation, because rumination cannot take place if the patient is attending to their breathing in a deep slow rhythm. Fundoplication eliminates rumination, but worsens dyspepsia and distress in most cases.[11]

Gastric disorders

The stomach can be divided functionally into two regions: (i) the proximal portion containing the fundus and upper third of the body and (ii) the distal portion comprising of the rest of the body, antrum and pylorus. The proximal stomach relaxes to accommodate a meal. It then slowly, tonically contracts and moves its contents to the distal portion, which liquefies the solid food with phasic, powerful and coordinated contractions before emptying it into the duodenum, a process called trituration.

R-WAVES CORRELATING WITH SYMPTOMS

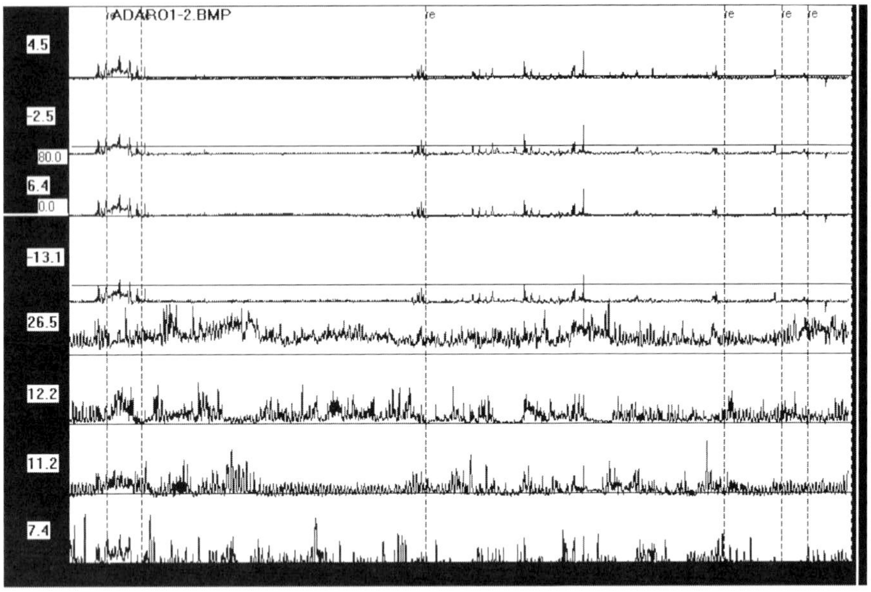

Fig. 32.2. Postprandial antroduodenal manometry. Recording sites: 1 and 2 – corpus, 3 – antrum, 4 – close to pylorus, 5 through 8 – duodenum and jejunum. Note the low-amplitude pressure waves in the stomach correlating with the occurrence of nausea and regurgitation marked with dotted line as soon as the patient signaled the symptoms.

Gastroparesis

Gastroparesis is a syndrome resulting from impaired gastric emptying, in the absence of a mechanical obstruction. It is a condition seldom found in children except in the preterm neonate.[12–16] In older children, it may be found in association with diabetes mellitus, hypothyroidism, during or following a viral enteritis,[17] eosinophilic gastroenteropathy, and muscular dystrophy or after surgery and vagotomy. Symptoms of gastroparesis include postprandial fullness, anorexia, early satiety, bloating, emesis several hours after meals, halitosis, and epigastric pain. Signs include failure-to-thrive and weight loss.

The most accurate and sensitive measure of gastric emptying in adults and cooperative children is the gastric emptying scan. A solid meal, usually containing Tc^{99m} labeled eggs, is used in cooperative children Formula is used in infants. Scintigraphic studies in pediatrics are fraught with shortcomings. Infants and uncooperative toddlers may not be able to lie motionless under the gamma camera for the required time periods. Standard test meals cannot be given to infants with dietary protein allergies or to children who refuse to eat. There are no normal values for gastric emptying in healthy children. The initial delay in solid meal emptying, known as the lag phase, is the time it takes the stomach to liquefy the solid meal. The lag time varies from person to person, and day to day, from a few minutes to 2 hours. Therefore, a solid gastric emptying test must be carried out for 4 hours.[18] Extrapolation of data curves from tests of shorter duration yield uninterpretable results.

Antroduodenal manometry may reveal hypomotility in the antrum or duodenum or hypermotility such as tonic duodenal contractions and unremitting, constant bands of phasic duodenal contractions causing a high-pressure zone. Either too much or too little motility inhibits gastric emptying.[19,20]

Sonography in experienced hands can be used to evaluate gastric emptying in young infants.[21] ^{13}C-octanoic acid breath test is a newer, safe, non-radiologic test that can be used to measure gastric emptying using a liquid or solid meal.[22]

Postviral gastroparesis usually takes weeks or months to resolve. Some children with prolonged, severe symptoms may require nutritional support by feeding tube. Prokinetic drugs such as domperidone, metoclopramide, cisapride and erythromycin improve gastric emptying. However, few controlled trials have documented their efficacy in gastroparesis. Surgical intervention is rarely effective, because changing the anatomy does not alter the physiology responsible for gastroparesis.[23] Gastric electrical stimulation relieves symptoms, but does not alter motility.[24]

Dumping syndrome

Rapid gastric emptying associated with dumping syndrome is uncommon in children. The most common cause of dumping syndrome in children is the accidental migration of a gastrostomy tube through the pylorus in a child who receives bolus tube feeds. The rapid digestion of starches to simple sugars in the small intestine results in osmotic forces that induce intraluminal fluid accumulation and symptoms of abdominal fullness, pain and nausea. The late symptoms result from insulin-induced secondary hypoglycemia causing tachycardia, diaphoresis, lethargy, or even syncope. Dumping syndrome may be due either to decreased gastric compliance and accommodation, most commonly caused by vagal denervation, or to loss of trituration caused by pyloroplasty or pyloromyotomy for gastroparesis. Dumping syndrome has been reported as a complication following fundoplication.[24,25] An oral glucose tolerance test documents postprandial hypoglycemia. Gastric emptying scans demonstrate rapid transit.

Dietary changes are usually successful in providing symptom relief.[24] Uncooked cornstarch can be beneficial in children fed exclusively by gastrostomy, by minimizing symptoms, enhancing weight gain and controlling glucose shifts.[26] Octreotide, a long acting somatostatin analogue, has been found effective in some children with dumping.[27]

Dumping syndrome following fundoplication is under recognized and the diagnosis is usually delayed. In one large retrospective multicenter study of surgically treated gastroesophageal reflux in children, transient dumping was reported in only 0.9% (range 0%–5%) of cases. However, in a follow-up study of 50 children which looked specifically for symptoms of dumping after Nissen fundoplication, Samuk *et al.* also performed a glucose tolerance test and gastric emptying scan in symptomatic children.[28] Twenty eight percent of children were symptomatic and had an abnormal glucose tolerance test following fundoplication. After 3 months of dietary treatment, 50% of the patients had complete resolution of their symptoms, 43% showed significant improvement and only 7% had persistent symptoms.

Small intestinal disorders

Fasting motility patterns in healthy infants, children and adults are characterized by the cyclical, repetitive, strong phasic contractions and quiescence, called the migrating motor complex (MMC).[29,30] The MMC consists of three phases. Phase 1 is a period of motor quiescence. Phase 2 is a period of random, irregular contractions, varying in amplitude, frequency and propagation. Phase 3 is a distinctive pattern of clustered contractions repeating at a maximal rate for several minutes, propagating from proximal to distal bowel (Fig. 32.3). Each phase propagates in sequence from proximal to distal. The postprandial pattern is an active but variable amplitude sequence of random contractions. Premature infants with a postconceptional age of less than 32 weeks do not have the MMC and exhibit nearly continuous activity.[31,32] The dominant motility pattern in fasted and fed infants is a short duration, non-migrating cluster. Readiness to feed appears to be correlated with an increase in inhibitory tone and the appearance of the MMC.

Antroduodenal manometry requires fluoroscopy and/or endoscopy facilitated catheter placement into the antrum and duodenum. Propofol is the anesthetic of choice, because narcotics disorganize motility, and inhalants suppress inhibitory tone, resulting in continuous clusters of non-propagating duodenal contractions for several hours following anesthesia. When using fluoroscopy, erythromycin 1 mg/kg intravenously over 30 minutes aids catheter passage.[33]

Four hours are sufficient in most children with normal motility to observe at least one MMC.[24] However, arousal due to anxiety or anger will suppress phase 3. The meal is individualized based on age and the patient's clinical condition, with an attempt being made to administer a meal with at least 10 kcal/kg or 400 kcal, ≥30% kcal from fat. Drugs, such as intravenous erythromycin and/or subcutaneous octreotide, are often administered during a motility study to test their potential as therapeutic agents. Antroduodenal manometry includes an evaluation of fasting and postprandial motility. During fasting the examiner observes for phase 3 of the MMC, its site of origin, direction of propagation, duration and frequency of contractions, and for discrete abnormalities such as continuous, non-migrating clusters or a persistent tonic contraction in one recording site. After the meal, conversion to a "fed" state is determined by the absence of MMCs and the presence of an increase in number and strength of antral and duodenal contractions. A trained observer watches and queries about symptoms associated with manometric patterns throughout the test session. For example, normal amplitude gastric antral contractions are associated with pain in some children with dyspepsia. Emesis may be associated with giant retrograde contractions (in a centrally-mediated vomiting reflex), r waves (in rumination syndrome), or no manometric event (in gastroesophageal reflux). Computer analysis quantitates motility and generates a "motility index," a value that takes account of the frequency and amplitude of contractions. Caution should be exercised in interpreting manometry studies performed in dilated bowel because the ability to increase intraluminal pressure is inversely

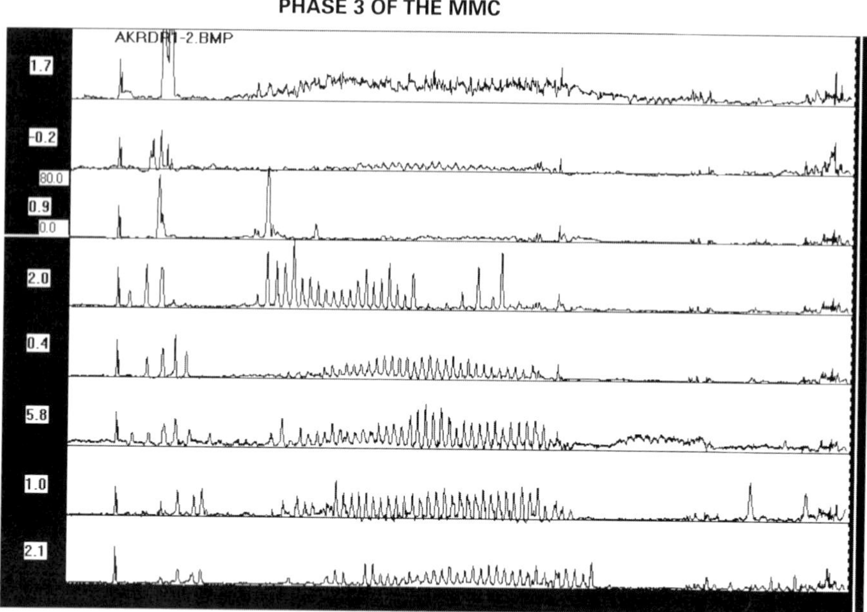

Fig. 32.3. Phase 3 of the migrating motor complex. 10 min of recording time. Recording sites: 1 and 2 – antrum, 3 – close to pylorus, 4 through 8 – duodenum. Note the organized uniform contractions of frequency 12 per min consistent with phase 3, followed by motility quiescence, phase 1.

proportional to the diameter (Laplace's law). Studies from dilated bowel are frequently uninterpretable.

Chronic intestinal pseudo-obstruction

Chronic intestinal pseudo-obstruction (CIP) refers to a heterogeneous group of gastrointestinal nerve and muscle disorders with similar phenotypic presentation of obstructive intestinal symptoms.[34] Based on a strict definition of the syndrome, CIP should be diagnosed only when a mechanical obstruction has been ruled out.[35] It is marked by repetitive episodes or continuous signs of bowel obstruction, often including radiographic evidence of dilated bowel with air–fluid levels, in the absence of a fixed lumen-occluding lesion.[34]

Over 50% of pediatric patients develop symptoms as neonates and about 40% of these have associated intestinal malrotation. Those less severely affected present months to years later with constipation or diarrhea, vomiting, and failure to thrive. The most common presenting symptom is abdominal distention and vomiting in almost 75% of patients; 60% describe constipation, intermittent abdominal pain, and poor weight gain; and one third complain of diarrhea. Twenty percent of pediatric patients with neuropathic and 80% of those with myopathic pseudo-obstruction have urinary tract and bladder involvement. In most children with congenital disease, the clinical course has an illness plateau with intermittent increases in acuity. Triggers for acute decompensation include intercurrent infections, general anesthesia, psychological stress, and poor nutrition. Non-specific radiographic signs include air-fluid levels, and dilated stomach, small intestine, and colon. Stasis of the contrast material may be prolonged.

In most children with congenital pseudo-obstruction there is no family history, suggesting that these cases are due to a new mutation. Rarely, autosomal recessive and dominant patterns of inheritance occur in myopathic and neuropathic pseudo-obstruction.[34] In utero exposure to toxins such as alcohol has been associated with neonatal pesudo-obstruction.[36] Children with chromosomal abnormalities may suffer from pseudo-obstruction or neuropathic constipation. Cytomegalovirus, herpes zoster and Epstein–Barr virus infection have been linked to acquired causes of pseudo-obstruction.[34] Patients with mitochondrial neurogastrointestinal encephalopathy (MNGIE) may have intestinal pseudo-obstruction as part of the syndrome.[37] Acquired aganglionosis may be caused by a T-cell mediated inflammatory response against enteric neurons, leading to enteric ganglionitis and subsequent loss of colonic and intestinal neurons.[38]

Diagnosis

Intestinal pseudo-obstruction is a clinical diagnosis based on symptoms of bowel obstruction in the absence of an

Table 32.1. Indications for motility testing in children as proposed by a Working Group of the American Motility Society[38]

Esophageal manometry
1. To diagnose achalasia and other primary motility disorders.
2. To evaluate dysphagia and chest pain of non-cardiac origin in children and adolescents.
3. To place pH electrodes for esophageal pH-metry when there are anatomical malformations (i.e. hiatal hernia) or to place it without x-rays.
4. To aid in the diagnosis of diseases that may have esophageal dysmotility, e.g., connective tissue diseases, Down syndrome, or chronic intestinal pseudo-obstruction.
Antroduodenal manometry
1. To confirm the pathophysiology underlying intestinal failure in children with chronic intestinal pseudo-obstruction.
2. To assess upper gastrointestinal motility when colectomy is being considered for intractable constipation.
3. To help distinguish between rumination and vomiting.
4. In patients with unexplained symptoms, which might be related to dysmotility.
Colonic manometry
1. To evaluate persistent constipation unresponsive to conventional treatment and of uncertain cause.
2. To characterize the physiology responsible for symptoms of chronic intestinal pseudo-obstruction and to assess the presence or absence of colonic involvement.
3. To determine the physiology associated with persistent symptoms following successful surgery for Hirschsprung's disease.
4. Prior to intestinal transplantation, to decide whether to retain the colon at the time of transplantation.
Anorectal manometry
1. To diagnose a non-relaxing internal anal sphincter
2. To evaluate postoperative patients with Hirschsprung's disease who have obstructive symptoms or fecal incontinence
3. To evaluate postoperative patients after repair of anorectal malformations
4. To decide if the patient is a candidate for biofeedback therapy

anatomic lesion. Manometric studies should be used to evaluate strength and coordination of contractions and relaxation in the esophagus, gastric antrum, small intestine, and colon (Table 32.1).[38,39] Abnormalities on manometry of the small bowel and colon usually correlate with the clinical severity of the disease, and help in treatment planning. Normal manometry of the small bowel and colon does not occur in pseudo-obstruction,[40] and behavioral observations of the child and family during testing will often suggest an alternative diagnosis such as pediatric condition falsification (formerly known as Munchausen's syndrome by proxy)[41] or pain-associated disability syndrome.[42] In subjects with neuropathy, there are normal amplitude, uncoordinated contractions. Often MMCs are absent and are replaced by prolonged clusters of non-propagating contractions. In children with myopathy, manometry reveals hypomotility, with persistent, low amplitude contractions. Antroduodenal manometry may also provide prognostic information, determine the areas of the gastrointestinal tract involved in the disease, and assess the potential for a drug to provide therapeutic benefit.[43,44]

Full thickness intestinal biopsies for routine histology, enzyme histochemistry and immunohistochemistry by light microscopy and ultrastructural studies by electron microscopy may show evidence of neuropathy or enteric muscle disease.[45] Visceral myopathies refer to degenerative disorders of visceral smooth muscle accompanied by thinning of the bowel wall. As myocytes drop out, the matrix substance collapses and the tissue appears fibrotic. Visceral neuropathies encompass both congenital maturational defects and degenerative disorders of the enteric plexi, and are characterized by absence, immaturity, or degeneration and loss of neurons.

Treatment and outcome

Nutrition must be adequate to optimize gut neuromuscular function. One-third of patients require parenteral nutrition (PN) and one-third require tube feeding. Continuous feeding by a gastrostomy or jejunostomy should be attempted if bolus feeding fails. A gastrostomy decompresses the bowel during acute episodes and provides access for enteral feeding during plateaus in disease. Ileostomy or colostomy is often necessary to decompress distal bowel and for the success of enteral feeding.[34,45] Attempts to improve motility with drugs have, in general, been disappointing. Mineral oil, polyethylene glycol, suppositories, and/or enemas are used to treat constipation. Cisapride increases intestinal contractions and improves symptoms in a minority of patients. Erythromycin and octreotide may improve bowel motility.[46] Bacterial overgrowth may be treated with antibiotics[46,34] or probiotics.

Pain management is an area requiring improvement in survivors of chronic intestinal pseudo-obstruction.[46] Bowel decompression is effective for acute abdominal pain. Chronic visceral pain responds to low-dose tricyclic antidepressants and gabapentin. Narcotics disrupt motility and are not useful for chronic neuropathic pain.

Surgery for chronic intestinal pseudo-obstruction usually begins in infancy, when the neonate presents with bowel obstruction. Between one and three exploratory laparotomies are commonly performed before pseudo-obstruction is considered. In older children, it may appear that segmental resections of dilated areas may provide some relief. However, chronic intestinal pseudo-obstruction is a condition which affects the entire gastrointestinal tract, so segmental small bowel resections are not advisable. A short time after a segmental resection, the disease again mainfests in nearby segments. Gallstones are common by age three in children totally dependent on PN, and elective cholecystectomy is advisable before an acute and life-threatening episode of cholecystitis occurs. Elective surgery for gastrostomy, feeding jejunostomy, ileostomy, or colostomy may provide an opportunity to resect tissue for histological analysis. With irreversible intestinal failure and recurrent sepsis secondary to bacterial translocation, total enterectomy may be necessary.

The mortality associated with chronic intestinal pseudo-obstruction occurs almost exclusively in PN-dependent children, so there is a compelling reason to maximize enteral feeding and attempt to avoid the parenteral route. In a large study from the USA which included 85 children with chronic intestinal pseudo-obstruction investigated at three different centers, 22 deaths were reported. Thirteen (59%) deaths were from liver failure or central venous catheter-related sepsis in patients receiving total PN.[47] Three other patients on partial PN also died of sepsis whilst five patients died after small bowel transplantation. There was no significant difference in mortality between the neuropathic and myopathic pseudo-obstruction groups. Absent phase 3 of the MMC was reported as a poor prognostic sign. Heneyke *et al.* reported on 44 children from the UK:[45] 20 had a good outcome defined as being alive and enterally fed; 10 had poor outcome defined as recurrent symptoms and being dependent on parenteral nutrition; and 14 patients had died. The cause of death was not reported. The presence of midgut malrotation, short small intestine, involvement of the urinary system, onset under 1 year of age, and the presence of myopathy on histology were associated with a poor prognosis. For life-threatening intestinal pseudo-obstruction, intestinal transplantation is a high-risk procedure with potential for cure.[48] Post small bowel transplant complications and survival in children with intestinal pseudo-obstruction appear to be similar to those in children transplanted for other causes of intestinal failure.

The quality of life for children with chronic intestinal pseudo-obstruction and their parents has not been as good as for other chronic diseases[51] but may be improved by appropriate treatment of chronic pain, and attention to relieving the family's burden of chronic illness and emotional distress.[49] Several investigational treatments hold promise. Electrically pacing the small bowel has been of interest for several decades, and clinical trials for children with pseudo-obstruction are planned. More remote, but just as exciting, are stem cell transplants of myocytes for myopathies and neurons for neuropathies which may one day be used to cure pseudo-obstruction.

Colonic disorders

Colon motility and gut transit time change with age. Features of normal colon motor activity include: (i) low amplitude tonic and phasic segmental contractions, mixing luminal contents; (ii) high amplitude propagated contractions, propelling stools from the right side of the colon to the distal sigmoid colon; they stop short of the rectum which is the storage area (Fig. 32.4); and (iii) increase in colonic motility after ingestion of a meal, the "gastrocolonic response."[52,53]

Functional constipation and functional fecal retention

Constipation is a very common problem in children, but rarely caused by a colonic motility disorder. Instead, it is due to a maladaptive behavior triggered by painful or otherwise unpleasant defecation. After experiencing an uncomfortable evacuation, some infants, toddlers, and children are unable or unwilling to relax their pelvic floors, but instead respond to each defecatory urge with retentive posturing, tightening the gluteal muscles to avoid defecation. As a consequence of the fear of defecation and retentive posturing, children with this condition pass large stools at infrequent intervals, less than twice a week. Children with this functional disorder, called functional fecal retention by the Rome pediatric working team,[9] have normal colon motility. A child who meets symptom-based criteria for functional fecal retention needs no testing.

A thorough history and physical examination is generally sufficient to establish whether the child requires further evaluation.[52] Abdominal examination may reveal a rectal fecal mass in children with functional fecal retention. Anorectal examination, although not required in every

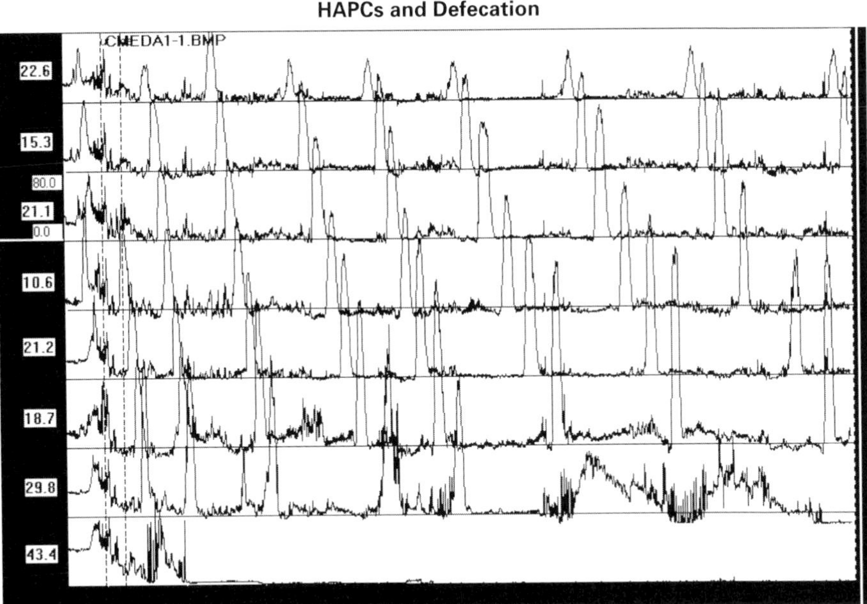

Fig. 32.4. Eight high amplitude propagating contractions stimulated by bisacodyl during colon manometry. HAPCs are the marker for colon neuromuscular health. In a 20 min panel (from top to bottom) 1, 2 – ascending colon; 3, 4 – transverse colon, 5, 6 – descending colon; 7 – sigmoid colon; 8 – rectum. Note that the recording site 8 and consecutively 7 were expelled out of the body by the HAPC.

patient, assesses perianal sensation, anal tone, size of the rectum and the presence of the anal wink.[54] Rectal examination may be postponed in a fearful child who meets diagnostic criteria for functional fecal retention. In many toddlers, successful treatment is linked to their ability to trust the examiner, and to rid themselves of the fear of defecation. Rectal examination may delay both. If the child does not improve after education and assuring painless defecation for a few weeks, rectal examination may be performed. Detection of a physical abnormality might lead to the identification of an organic disorder.

The approach to a child with functional fecal retention includes the following steps: (i) provide education to the parent and child, (ii) treat the impaction, melting it away with oral polyethylene glycol solution, (iii) initiate maintenance treatment to assure painless defecation (Table 32.2) and (iv) use behavioral modification that includes frequent follow up.[52] The education of the parents and the demystification of constipation (e.g., the colon never bursts, toxins do not leak back into the body, it does not cause cancer), including an explanation of the pathogenesis of functional fecal retention, should be the first steps in treatment. It is especially important for the parents to understand that soiling and overflow incontinence is neither a willful and defiant maneuver, nor a sign of laziness. Soiling is a consequence of attempts to pass gas around a fecal impaction. Rectal disimpaction may be quicker than the oral route but it is invasive and traumatic for a child who already has fear of defecation and withholding behavior. Moreover, it takes control away from the child, medicalizing a developmental problem in toilet learning, and creating learned helplessness.

There are no controlled studies demonstrating the efficacy of dietary manipulations, increased fiber, or increased fluids in otherwise healthy children with functional fecal retention.[52] After all, the problem is not the stool, but a pelvic floor contracted because of fear of painful defecation. An important component of treatment includes behavior modification and regular toileting. Behavior modification in addition to laxative therapy may achieve better results in children with soiling.[53] Unhurried time on the toilet after meals helps. It is helpful to have children or their caregivers keep diaries of stool frequency. This can be combined with a reward system for the child.

Several studies have reported the outcome of children with constipation and soiling managed by different treatment strategies. In a study of 110 children with soiling, Levine and Bakow reported a 77% success rate after one year of treatment with high dose mineral oil.[54] Sondheimer *et al.* randomized 37 children with chronic constipation, with and without soiling, to receive mineral oil or senna.[55] After 6 months, 89% of patients in the mineral oil group were having daily bowel movements compared to 50% in the senna group. Soiling was reported by 6% of the patients in the mineral oil group compared to 44% in the senna group. Our preferred treatment for children with functional

Table 32.2. Medicines used for treatment of constipation

Medication	Category	Presentation	Smell	Taste	Tips for use
Lactulose	Osmotic	Syrup. Thick clear liquid	No smell	Very sweet	Plenty of fluids. May cause dental decay. Advise dental hygiene & sugar free chewing gum. May cause gaseous distension
Movicol ® (Europe)	Osmotic	Granules in sachets	Lemon or no smell	Salty lemon flavour or flavour free	Mix with water, fruit juice or colas
Polyethylene glycol North America	Osmotic	Granules	None	None	Mix with water, fruit juice or colas
Mineral oil (Liquid Paraffin, Kondremul plain®)	Softener	Colorless liquid	None	Cooking oil	Avoid in patients with risk of aspiration.
Klean Prep ®	Bowel cleansing solution	Powder to be mixed with water	None	Salty	Administered through a nasogastric tube
Senna	Stimulant	Liquid syrup or brown tablets	Smells like cough medicine	Taste like coffee very sweet	Tolerance may develop. Griping pain. Tablets better for older children.
Bisacodyl (Dulcolax®)	Stimulant	Small yellow tablet	No smell	No taste if swallowed whole	Tolerance
Sodium Picosulphate	Stimulant and softener	Orange liquid	Fruity	Sweet orange squash	

fecal retention is to use stool softeners to ensure the regular passage of soft stools. Senna in children with fecal retention may cause abdominal pain, which may defeat the primary goal of ensuring painless defecation. Abrahamian and Lloyd-Still reported only 47% success in symptom resolution in 185 patients seen over a 7-year period treated with senna and dioctyl sodium sulfosuccinate.[56] Presence of soiling at the time of initial presentation was the only predictor of poor outcome. Staiano *et al.* used lactulose after initial disimpaction to treat chronic constipation in 62 children: 52% had persistent symptoms 5 years later.[57] Pashankar *et al.* used polyethylene glycol 3350, a tasteless, odorless, osmotic laxative, to treat 43 children with constipation and 31 with constipation and soiling.[58] Treatment was successful in 93% overall – 52% of children with constipation and soiling reported resolution of soiling and 84% had improvement in the frequency of soiling and bowel movements. Excellent compliance rates were achieved with this medication. Recently, Ginkel *et al.* reported the results of a large follow-up study of 418 children, aged 5 years and over with constipation.[59] The median duration of follow-up was 5 years. After an initial bowel clear out using enemas and/or laxatives, patients were treated with oral laxatives. Symptoms resolved within a year in 60% of patients and in 80% at 8 years. Treatment was more likely to be successful in children without soiling and in whom symptoms started after 4 years of age. Studies are required to determine what proportion of children with chronic constipation go on to become constipated adults.

Colonic neuromuscular disease

In children with colonic neuromuscular disease constipation is most often present from birth, the child has no retentive posturing, and there is little or no improvement after laxatives. Stools are typically soft, and the fecal impaction typical of functional fecal retention is absent. There may be extrarectal fecal masses (Table 32.3). Specific diagnosis requires histopathology or colon manometry.

Rectal biopsies are helpful only for Hirschsprung's disease, the most common neuropathy. Rectal biopsies showing intestinal neuronal dysplasia are potentially misleading, and do not correlate with symptoms or outcome.[60] The pathologic diagnosis of other neuromuscular colonic diseases is challenging due to the lack of age and location-matched control specimens.[61]

There are no validated age-specific normal values for total and segmental colonic transit studies using radio-opaque markers or scintigraphy techniques in children. It is difficult to standardize diet in children. A stool-filled rectosigmoid causes markers to accumulate in the proximal colon, so the colon must be empty at the time of testing. In functional fecal retention, the pelvic floor is the cause of the obstruction, so markers accumulate in the rectum.

In colonic neuromuscular disease markers are scattered throughout the colon and transit is prolonged.

Colon manometry differentiates causes of intractable constipation[50,51] and helps to select patients who will benefit from colon surgery[64] (Table 32.1). For isolated colonic neuromuscular disease, subtotal colectomy with ileoproctostomy is often curative. It is important to assess antroduodenal motility prior to colon resection to ensure that there is no evidence of latent small bowel neuromuscular disease. Evidence of small bowel disease may alter the plan for colectomy in some cases.

The Malone appendicostomy for antegrade colonic enemas (ACE) may be used to manage children with intractable constipation[63,64] (see Chapter 33). In the Malone procedure, the appendix is used as a catheterizable conduit between the abdominal wall and the cecum; enemas can be administered directly into the colon while the patient sits on the toilet. Using the ACE, the large bowel can be cleaned at regular intervals with irrigation solutions, such as polyethylene glycol, glycerin and saline, or phosphate enemas. Most patients evacuate stools within a few minutes to an hour after the irrigation solution is administered, depending on the type of solution used and the presence of normal colonic motility. Complete cleansing of the entire colon is a reliable method to avoid unpredictable "accidents." More recently, laparoscopic techniques and percutaneous endoscopic cecostomy devices have been used to achieve access to the cecum for ACE administration. Regular colonic lavage allows children to have regular bowel habits. Stoma complications include stenosis, mucus leak, fecal leak and catheter related pain in a minority of patients.

Defecation problems following surgery for Hirschsprung's disease

After surgery, 60% to 70% of children have continuing difficulties with constipation, soiling, and/or abdominal pain. These problems appear to be independent of the operation, age at operation, or sex of the child. About 10% of children continue to suffer from constipation due to a neuropathy proximal to the aganglionic segment.[65] Ganglion cells are present, but colonic contractions are low amplitude, and simultaneous. There are no high amplitude propagating contractions, the marker for colonic neuromuscular health. These patients may be more prone to enterocolitis, because colon transit is delayed. They are unresponsive to both prokinetic drugs and laxatives. They grow to hate rectal irrigations. It may be necessary to resect the remaining colon to provide a satisfactory quality of life for these patients. Another 10% have constipation due to functional fecal retention.[65,66] Toddlers with Hirschsprung's disease

Table 32.3. Differentiating functional constipation from colonic neuromuscular disease

Signs and symptoms	Functional fecal retention	Colonic neuromuscular disease
Soiling	Common	Rare
Obstructive symptoms	Rare	Common
Large caliber stool	Common	Rare
Stool withholding behavior	Common	Rare
Enterocolitis	Never	Possible
Symptoms from birth	Rare	Common
Localization of stool	Rectum	Rectal and extrarectal
Radio-opaque transit study	Markers in rectum	Throughout the colon
Colon manometry	Normal	Abnormal

are more likely to get functional fecal retention than healthy children because: (i) most miss normal toilet learning during infancy, (ii) postsurgery interventions such as dilations, irrigations, episodes of enterocolitis, etc. may cause painful defecation and fear of defecation.

As many as 50% of Hirschsprung's disease patients have difficulties with fecal soiling lasting into adult life.[65] The most common reason for soiling is that high amplitude propagating contractions, which normally end in the sigmoid and dump stool into the rectosigmoid reservoir can no longer work in this way after the rectosigmoid segment has been resected. Instead, high amplitude (averaging 150 mm Hg) propagating contractions continue through the neorectum to the anus, which has a resting pressure about 60 mm Hg with a maximal squeeze pressure of 120 mm Hg. The child must choose whether to give up and allow soiling, or to hold tight and bear the cramping pain. In general, toddlers' soil and toilet training is slow; school-age children hold tight and get chronic abdominal pains rather than soil themselves at school. These children often soil during sleep, because after losing the rectosigmoid, the normal protective rectal motor complex is gone.[65,66] In patients with fecal soiling due to high amplitude propagating contractions through the neorectum, drugs such as amitriptyline firm up the stools and reduce soiling episodes as well as reduce the crampy pain associated with attempts to avoid soiling. Amitriptyline is started at 10 mg at bedtime and increased by 10 mg each week until the pain and soiling stop or the dose reaches 1 mg/kg.[64] Loperamide works transiently, but tolerance develops rapidly, limiting its usefulness.

Another reason for fecal soiling is functional fecal retention. For the reasons given above functional fecal retention is common after successful surgery for Hirschsprung's disease. It is important to discriminate between the two causes of fecal soiling after Hirschsprung's disease because the treatments are different. If the history is inconclusive, colon manometry will reliably discriminate between functional fecal retention and high amplitude propagating contractions through the neorectum.

Hirschsprung patients also continue to have an incomplete rectosphincteric inhibitory reflex, a hallmark of the disease, after surgery. Because the inner sphincter provides only a fraction of the pressure, and the total anal sphincter pressure is far less than the pressure of a high amplitude propagating contraction, the sphincter rarely contributes to constipation following Hirschsprung's disease surgery. Rarely, the anal sphincter may have pressures exceeding 100 mm Hg, when it will contribute to constipation.[65] In these cases, sphincterotomy is still the procedure of choice. *Botulinum* toxin reduces sphincter pressure for weeks or months, and may provide a temporary window of time that helps a minority of children to learn appropriate toilet habits.

Internal anal sphincter achalasia/ultrashort segment Hirschsprung's disease

Absence of the recto-anal inhibitory reflex in children with a normal rectal biopsy and chronic constipation not responding to conventional medical therapy has been termed internal anal sphincter achalasia or ultra short segment Hirschsprung's disease. *Clostridium botulinum* toxin injection and sphincterotomy have been used to relieve symptoms.[68,69]

Conclusions

Motility disorders are common in children and may affect any area of the gastrointestinal tract. More sophisticated testing techniques have helped to differentiate normal from abnormal motility and further our understanding of pediatric motility disorders. Manometry studies can be used to clarify the pathophysiologic defect underlying dysphagia, rumination, gastroparesis, chronic intestinal pseudo-obstruction and colonic neuromuscular disorders. Motility testing may also be useful in evaluating patients with persistent symptoms after surgery for gastroesophageal reflux and Hirschsprung's disease.

Gastroparesis is a relatively rare disorder in children and the majority of affected patients improve with time. In experienced centers, almost two-thirds of the patients with intestinal pseudo-obstruction survive, but quality of life may be poor. The majority of these patients will require enteral and/or parenteral feeding support and currently available prokinetics are generally not helpful in the long term. Since mortality and morbidity are associated with parenteral feeding, every attempt should be made to feed these patients enterally. Functional constipation and fecal retention is a very common problem in children but, with appropriate management, a successful outcome can be anticipated in most. The primary goal in such patients should be to ensure the painless passage of soft stools by using stool softeners. A small proportion may have persistent symptoms and motility testing may then be helpful to differentiate functional disorders from colonic neuromuscular disease and when planning surgical interventions. It is not clear what proportion of children with constipation become constipated adults. Most patients with Hirschsprung's disease have continuing problems with defecation after surgery. Persistent constipation may be due to residual neuropathic bowel. Some patients develop functional constipation after surgery. Loss of the rectosigmoid reservoir after surgery may result in persistent soiling until the child is old enough to voluntarily reinforce the anal sphincter by contracting the gluteal muscles during high amplitude colonic contractions. More than half of the patients with Hirschsprung's disease have problems with soiling in adult life.

REFERENCES

1. Kawahara, H., Dent J., Davidson, G. Mechanisms responsible for gastroesophageal reflux in children. *Gastroenterology* 1997; **113**:399–408.
2. Mittal, R. K., McCallum, R. W. Characteristics and frequency of transient relaxations of the lower esophageal sphincter in patients with reflux esophagitis. *Gastroenterology* 1988; **95**:593–599.
3. Putnam, P. E., Orenstein, S. R., Pang, D., Pollack, I. F., Proujansky, R., & Kocoshis, S. A. Cricopharyngeal dysfunction associated with Chiari malformations. *Pediatrics* 1992; **89**:871–876
4. Boyle, J. T., Cohen, S., & Watkins, J. B. Successful treatment of achalasia in childhood by pneumatic dilation. *J. Pediatr.* 1981; **99**:35–40.
5. Glassman, M. S., Medow, M. S., Berezin, S., & Newman, L. J. Spectrum of esophageal disorders in children with chest pain. *Dig. Dis. Sci.* 1992; **37**:663–666.
6. Solzi, G. F. & Di Lorenzo, C. Nutcracker esophagus in a child with insulin-dependent diabetes mellitus. *J. Pediatr. Gastroenterol. Nutr.* 1999; **29**:482–484.
7. Rosario, J. A., Medow, M. S., Halata, M. S. *et al.* Nonspecific esophageal motility disorders in children without gastroesophageal reflux. *J. Pediatr. Gastroenterol. Nutr.* 1999; **28**:480–485.
8. Zangen, T., Ciarla, C., & Zangen, S. Motility and sensory disorders may cause food refusal in medically fragile toddlers *J. Pediatr. Gastroenterol. Nutr.* 2003; **37**:287–293.

9. Rasquin-Weber, A., Hyman, P. E., Cucchiara, S. *et al.* Childhood functional gastrointestinal disorders. *Gut* 1999; **45** (suppl II): II60-II68.
10. Chial, H. J., Camilleri, M., Williams, D. E. *et al.* Rumination syndrome in children and adolescents: diagnosis, treatment, and prognosis. *Pediatrics* 2003; **111**:158–162.
11. Oelschlager, B. K., Chan, M. M., Eubanks, T. R. *et al.* Effective treatment of rumination with Nissen fundoplication. *J. Gastrointest. Surg.* 2002; **6**:638–644.
12. Ittmann, P. I., Amarnath, R., & Berseth, C. L. Maturation of antroduodenal motor activity in preterm and term infants. *Dig. Dis. Sci.* 1992; **37**:14–19.
13. Berseth, C. L., & Nordyke, C. K. Enteral nutrients promote postnatal maturation of intestinal motor activity in preterm infants. *Am. J. Physiol.* 1993; **264**:G1046–G1051.
14. Koenig, W. J., Amarnath, R. P., Hench, V., & Berseth, C. L. Manometrics for preterm and term infants: a new tool for old questions. *Pediatrics* 1995; **95**:207–209.
15. Berseth, C. L. & Nordylee, C. K. Manometry can predict feeding readiness in preterm infants. *Gastroenterology* 1992; **103**:1523–1528.
16. Baker, J. & Berseth, C. L. Postnatal change in inhibitory regulation of intestinal motor activity in human and canine neonates. *Pediatr. Res.* 1995; **38**:133–139.
17. Sigurdsson, L., Flores, A., Putnam, P. E. *et al.* Postviral gastroparesis: presentation, treatment, and outcome. *J. Pediatr.* 1997; **131**:751–755.
18. Tougas, G., Eaker, E. Y., Abell, T. L. *et al.* Assessment of gastric emptying using a low fat meal: establishment of international control values. *Am. J. Gastroenterol.* 2000; **95**:1456–1462.
19. Di Lorenzo, C., Hyman, P. E., Flores, A. F. *et al.* Antroduodenal manometry in children and adults with severe non-ulcer dyspepsia. *Scand. J. Gastroenterol.* 1994; **29**:799–806.
20. Cucchiara, S., Bortolotti, M., Colombo, C. *et al.* Abnormalities of gastrointestinal motility in children with nonulcer dyspepsia and in children with gastroesophageal reflux disease. *Dig. Dis. Sci.* 1991; **36**:1066–1073.
21. Cucchiara, S. Ultrasound. In Hyman, P. E., & DiLorenzo, C. eds: *Pediatric Gastrointestinal Motility Disorders.* New York: Academy of Professional Information Services, 1994: 313–318.
22. Veereman-Wauters, G., Ghoos, Y., van der Schoor, S. *et al.* The ^{13}C-octanoic acid breath test: a noninvasive technique to assess gastric emptying in preterm infants. *J. Pediatr. Gastroenterol. Nutr.* 1996; **23**:111–117.
23. Jones, M. P. & Maganti, K. A. systematic review of surgical therapy for gastroparesis. *Am. J. Gastroenterol.* 2003; **98**:2122–2129.
24. Lin, Z., Forester, J., Sarosiek, I., & McCallum, R. W. Treatment of gastroparesis with electrical stimulation. *Dig. Dis. Sci.* 2003; **48**: 837–848.
25. Samuk, I., Afriat, R., Horne, T. *et al.* Dumping syndrome following Nissen fundoplication, diagnosis, and treatment. *J. Pediatr. Gastroenterol. Nutr.* 1996; **23**:235–240.
26. Borovoy, J., Furuta, L., & Nurko, S. Benefit of uncooked cornstarch in the management of children with dumping syndrome fed exclusively by gastrostomy. *Am. J. Gastroenterol.* 1998; **93**:814–818.
27. Lamers, C. B., Bijlstra, A. M., & Harris, A. G. Octreotide, a long-acting somatostatin analog, in the management of postoperative dumping syndrome. An update. *Dig. Dis. Sci.* 1993; **38**:359–364.
28. Fonkalsrud, E. W., Ashcraft, K. W., Coran, A. G. *et al.* Surgical treatment of gastroesophageal reflux in children: a combined hospital study of 7467 patients. *Pediatrics* 1998; **101**:419–422.
29. Uc, A., Hoon, A., Di Lorenzo, C., & Hyman, P. E. Antroduodenal manometry in children with no upper gastrointestinal symptoms. *Scand. J. Gastroenterol.* 1997; **32**:681–685.
30. Tomomasa, T., Di Lorenzo, C., Morikawa, A. *et al.* Analysis of fasting antroduodenal manometry in children. *Dig. Dis. Sci.* 1996; **41**:2195–2203.
31. Ittmann, P. I., Amarnath, R., & Berseth, C. L. Maturation of antroduodenal motor activity in preterm and term infants. *Dig. Dis. Sci.* 1992; **37**:14–19.
32. Berseth, C. L. & Nordyke, C. K. Enteral nutrients promote postnatal maturation of intestinal motor activity in preterm infants. *Am. J. Physiol.* 1993; **264**:G1046–G1051.
33. Di Lorenzo, C., Lachman, R., & Hyman, P. E. Intravenous erythromycin for postpyloric intubation. *J. Pediatr. Gastroenterol. Nutr.* 1990; **11**:45–47.
34. Di Lorenzo, C. Pseudo-obstruction: current approaches. *Gastroenterology* 1999; **116**:980–987.
35. Rudolph, C. D., Hyman, P. E., Altschuler, S. M. *et al.* Diagnosis and treatment of chronic intestinal pseudo-obstruction in children: report of consensus workshop. *J. Pediatr. Gastroenterol. Nutr.* 1997; **24**:102–112.
36. Uc, A., Vasiliauskas, E., Piccoli, D. A. *et al.* Chronic intestinal pseudoobstruction associated with fetal alcohol syndrome. *Dig. Dis. Sci.* 1997; **42**:1163–1167.
37. Verma, A., Piccoli, D. A., Bonilla, E., Berry, G. T., DiMauro, S., & Moraes, C. T. A novel mitochondrial G8313A mutation associated with prominent initial gastrointestinal symptoms and progressive encephaloneuropathy. *Pediatr. Res.* 1997; **42**:448–454.
38. Smith, V. V., Gregson, N., Foggensteiner, L., Neale, G., & Milla, P. J. Acquired intestinal aganglionosis and circulating autoantibodies without neoplasia or other neural involvement. *Gastroenterology* 1997; **112**:1366–1371.
39. Di Lorenzo, C., Hillemeier, C., Hyman, P. E. *et al.* Manometry studies in children: minimum standards for procedures. *J. Neurogastroenterol. Motil.* 2002; **14**:411–420.
40. Cucchiara, S., Borrelli, O., Salvia, G. *et al.* A normal gastrointestinal motility excludes chronic intestinal pseudoobstruction in children. *Dig. Dis. Sci.* 2000; **45**:258–264.
41. Hyman, P. E., Bursch, B., Beck, D. *et al.* Discriminating pediatric condition falsification from chronic intestinal pseudo-obstruction in toddlers. *Child Maltreatment* 2002; **7**:132–137.
42. Hyman, P. E., Bursch, B., Sood, M. *et al.* Visceral pain-associated disability syndrome: a descriptive analysis. *J. Pediatr. Gastroenterol. Nutr.* 2002; **35**:663–668.

43. Hyman, P. E., Di Lorenzo, C., McAdams, L., Flores, A. F., Tomomasa, T., & Garvey, T. Q. 3rd. Predicting the clinical response to cisapride in children with chronic intestinal pseudo-obstruction. *Am. J. Gastroenterol.* 1993; **88**:832–836.
44. Fell, J. M., Smith, V. V., & Milla, P. Infantile chronic idiopathic pseudo-obstruction: the role of small intestinal manometry as a diagnostic tool and prognostic indicator. *Gut* 1996; **39**:306–311.
45. Heneyke, S., Smith, V. V., Spitz, L., & Milla, P. J. Chronic intestinal pseudo-obstruction: treatment and long term follow up of 44 patients. *Arch. Dis. Child.* 1999; **81**:21–27.
46. Di Lorenzo, C., Lucanto, C., Flores, A. F. *et al.* Effect of octreotide on gastrointestinal motility in children with functional gastrointestinal symptoms. *J. Pediatr. Gastroenterol. Nutr.* 1998; **27**:508–512.
47. Mousa, H., Hyman, P. E., Cocjin, J., Flores, A. F., & Di Lorenzo, C. Long-term outcome of congenital intestinal pseudoobstruction. *Dig. Dis. Sci.* 2002; **47**:2298–2305.
48. Sigurdsson, L., Reyes, J., Kocoshis, S. A. *et al.* Intestinal transplantation in children with chronic intestinal pseudo-obstruction. *Gut* 1999; **45**:570–574.
49. Schwankovsky, L., Mousa, H., Rowhani, A., Di Lorenzo, C., & Hyman, P. E. Quality of life outcomes in congenital chronic intestinal pseudo-obstruction. *Dig. Dis. Sci.* 2002; **47**:19645–19648.
50. Di Lorenzo, C., Flores, A. F., Reddy, S. N., & Hyman, P. E. Use of colonic manometry to differentiate causes of intractable constipation in children. *J. Pediatr.* 1992; **120**:690–695.
51. Hamid, S. A., Di Lorenzo, C., Reddy, S. N., Flores, A. F., & Hyman, P. E. Bisacodyl and high-amplitude-propagating colonic contractions in children. *J. Pediatr. Gastroenterol. Nutr.* 1998; **27**:398–402.
52. Baker, S., Liptak, G. S., Colletti, R. B. *et al.* Constipation in infants and children: evaluation and treatment. *J. Pediatr. Gastroenterol. Nutr.* 1999; **29**:612–626.
53. Brazzelli, M. & Griffiths, P. Behavioural and cognitive intervention with or without other treatments for defecation disorders in children. In *The Cochrane Library*, Issue 2, 2002.
54. Levine, M. D. & Bakow, H. Children with encopresis: a study of treatment outcome. *Pediatrics* 1976; **58**(6):845–852.
55. Sondheimer, J. M. & Gervaise, E. P. Lubricant versus laxative in the treatment of chronic functional constipation of children: a comparative study. *J. Pediatr. Gastroenterol. Nutr.* 1982; **1**:223–226.
56. Abrahamian, F. P. & Lloyd-Still, J. D. Chronic constipation in childhood: a longitudinal study of 186 patients. *J. Pediatr. Gastroenterol. Nutr.* 1984; **3**:460–467.
57. Staiano, A., Andreotti, M. R., Greco, L., Basile, P., & Auricchio, S. Long-term follow-up of children with chronic idiopathic constipation. *Dig. Dis. Sci.* 1994; **39**:561–564.
58. Pashankar, D. S., Bishop, W. P., & Loening-Baucke, V. Long-term efficacy of polyethylene glycol 3350 for the treatment of chronic constipation in children with and without encopresis. *Clin. Pediatr.* 2003; **42**:815–819.
59. van Ginkel, R., Reitsma, J. B., Buller, H. A. *et al.* Childhood constipation: longitudinal follow-up beyond puberty. *Gastroenterology* 2003; **125**:357–363.
60. Cord-Udy, C. L., Smith, V. V., Ahmed, S. *et al.* An evaluation of the role of suction rectal biopsy in the diagnosis of intestinal neuronal dysplasia. *J. Pediatr. Gastroenterol. Nutr.* 1997; **24**:1–8.
61. Koletzko, S., Ballauff, A., Hadziselimovic, F., & Enck, P. Is histological diagnosis of neuronal intestinal dysplasia related to clinical and manometric findings in constipated children? *J. Pediatr. Gastroenterol. Nutr.* 1993; **17**:59.
62. Villarreal, J., Sood, M., Zangen, T. *et al.* Colonic diversion for intractable constipation in children: colonic manometry helps guide clinical decisions. *J. Pediatr. Gastroenterol. Nutr.* 2001; **33**:588–591.
63. Malone, P. S., Ransley, P. G., & Kiely, E. M. Preliminary report: the antegrade continence enema. *Lancet* 1990; **336**:1217–1218.
64. Squire, R., Kiely, E. M., Carr, B. *et al.* The clinical application of the Malone antegrade colonic enema. *J. Pediatr. Surg.* 1993; **28**:1012–1015.
65. Di Lorenzo, C., Solzi, G. F., Flores, A. F., Schwankovsky, L., & Hyman, P. E. Colonic motility after surgery for Hirschsprung's disease. *Am. J. Gastroenterol.* 2000; **95**:1759–1764.
66. Catto-Smith, A. G., Coffey, C. M., Nolan, T. M., & Hutson, J. M. Fecal incontinence after the surgical treatment of Hirschsprung disease. *J. Pediatr.* 1995; **127**:954–957.
67. Di Lorenzo, C. & Benninga, M. A. Pathophysiology of pediatric fecal incontinence. *Gastroenterology* 2004; **126**:S33–S40.
68. Ciamarra, P., Nurko, S., Barksdale, E., Fishman, S., & Di Lorenzo, C. Internal anal sphincter achalasia in children: clinical characteristics and treatment with *Clostridium botulinum* toxin. *J. Pediatr. Gastroenterol. Nutr.* 2003; **37**:315–319.
69. De Caluwe, D., Yoneda, A., Akl, U., & Puri, P. Internal anal sphincter achalasia: outcome after internal sphincter myectomy. *J. Pediatr. Surg.* 2001; **36**:736–738.

33

The Malone antegrade continence enema (MACE) procedure

Ashok Rajimwale and Padraig S. J. Malone

Southampton University Hospitals, UK

Intractable constipation and fecal incontinence are socially embarrassing and are commonly associated with spinal cord anomalies, anorectal malformations, Hirschsprung's disease and sacral agenesis. Initial conservative management of chronic constipation and fecal incontinence involves daily enemas, diet modification, stool softeners, suppositories, laxatives, and biofeedback. However, these programs are more unpleasant and difficult to manage as children get older. In the pre-MACE era when conservative management failed, children either faced the future wearing pads for fecal soiling or were doomed to permanent diverting colostomy as a last resort. The MACE procedure has allowed patients to become continent and independent with improved self-esteem.

Approximately 50% of patients with a neuropathic bladder secondary to myelomeningocele, who require bladder reconstructive surgery to establish continence or create a safe bladder, will also suffer from a neuropathic bowel with resultant chronic constipation and/or fecal incontinence, that does not respond to conservative measures.[1,2] Conversely, up to 50% of patients born with an anorectal malformation will have long-term fecal incontinence, and as many as 50% of these will also have a neuropathic bladder, many of whom will require bladder reconstructive surgery.[3,4] It is logical that these coexisting lower urinary tract and bowel problems should be managed simultaneously and not in isolation; in the majority of cases definitive bowel management usually rests with the reconstructive urologist.[5] It is within this setting of holistic care that the MACE procedure was conceived and developed.[6]

Principles of the MACE procedure

The MACE procedure simply combines three well-established surgical principles:

(a) the Mitrofanoff principle of a continent catheterizable abdominal stoma and conduit[7]

(b) the knowledge that complete colonic emptying can produce fecal continence[8]

(c) complete colonic emptying can be achieved by antegrade colonic irrigation.[9]

In general terms, after the MACE procedure patients had continent intermittent catheter access to their proximal colon (usually the cecum) through which they administered antegrade washouts, achieved colonic emptying and thus fecal continence.

Following the initial description, a large number of reports which included results from well over a thousand children appeared in the literature, and success rates of about 80% were reported.[10–17] The MACE was subsequently used successfully in the management of chronic constipation and fecal incontinence in adults.[18–20]

The results of simultaneous combined bladder reconstruction and MACE procedure have been reported in a number of series which have achieved double continence rates of up to 80%.[21–24] There is no doubt that the MACE is effective in producing fecal continence and that it can be combined with bladder reconstruction, including the Mitrofanoff procedure. Numerous publications have objectively demonstrated significant improvements in quality of life following the MACE.[25–27] Current evidence indicates that it should always be considered when

Pediatric Surgery and Urology: Long-term Outcomes, Mark Stringer, Keith Oldham, Pierre Mouriquand.
Published by Cambridge University Press.

a patient with fecal incontinence is undergoing bladder reconstruction.

Surgical techniques

The original description of the MACE involved detaching the appendix from the cecum, reversing it and reimplanting it back into a submucosal tunnel in the cecum.[6,28] The procedure has since been significantly modified in various ways both to simplify the technique and reduce the high complication rates initially reported.[10]

If the appendix is being used at the level of the cecum it is no longer necessary to disconnect it: it can simply be folded onto the cecum and a cecal wrap performed around its base to create a valve mechanism – the *in situ* appendix.[29] This is the recommended approach when a Mitrofanoff procedure is also required,[23] with the Mitrofanoff being constructed from either a split appendix[24] or a Yang–Monti conduit.[30,31] Alternatively, Sheldon *et al.* described a technique for constructing a MACE in cases where there is insufficient appendiceal length or when a concomitant appendiceal Mitrofanoff stoma is required. This technique involves tubularization of the cecum in continuity with the orthotopic appendix at its base using a stapling device. Initial results of this technique are encouraging as all six patients became continent after this procedure during a follow-up period of 16 months.[32] If the appendix is unsuitable for splitting, or if it is absent, alternative techniques such as the tubularized cecal or colonic flap are not recommended because of associated unacceptably high complication rates.[10]

There remains controversy as to whether any continence manouver is required at all. Some authors now advocate that the tip of the appendix is simply excised and brought out to the abdominal wall. Conduit incontinence rates appear to be slightly higher using this approach but if a minimally invasive laparoscopic technique is used the benefits of this approach may offset the slightly increased risk of stoma leakage. Therefore, if only a MACE procedure is needed, a laparoscopic ACE (LACE) offers a simple and effective method.[33]

One of the problems encountered by some patients with the MACE, particularly those with constipation, is the time it takes for the washout to work.[34] In an attempt to overcome this problem some surgeons have fashioned a Monti-MACE conduit in the left colon to reduce the length of bowel that has to be irrigated, and thus the duration of the washout. Preliminary results with this approach are very encouraging and, in the authors' experience, this has salvaged the procedure in five patients in whom an original cecal MACE failed.[35,36] A left-sided MACE should always be considered in patients with intractable constipation since this may be due to very slow transit through the sigmoid colon. It has been suggested that colonic transit studies should be performed before deciding on the site of the MACE.[36] The distal MACE stoma is not without its problems; Lemelle *et al.* and Perez *et al.* reported late accumulation of liquid mainly in the cecum and sigmoid colon causing long lasting leakage after enema administration via a transverse colon ACE.[37,38]

The commonest problem encountered in all catheterizable conduits is stomal stenosis, which occurs in up to 30% of patients.[39] In an attempt to overcome stomal stenosis, and in patients in whom the appendix was absent, a minimally invasive technique for placing a cecostomy tube under radiologic control was developed.[40] Once the tract has matured, the tube can then be replaced with a cecostomy button. Although the results are not perfect the technique offers a satisfactory alternative to a catheterizable conduit.[41] For patients with recurrent stomal stenosis it is also possible to leave a button in the conduit following dilation and this works well.

Recently, a new development embracing the principles of minimally invasive surgery and the left-sided MACE has been described. Following bowel preparation, a colonoscopy is performed and with the scope in the distal descending colon a colostomy tube is inserted, as one would insert a percutaneous endoscopic gastrostomy. Bowel washouts through this percutaneous endoscopic colostomy (PEC) tube can commence the next day. Once the tract has matured and the ACE irrigations shown to be effective, the patient has a choice of either keeping the tube, exchanging it for a button or having a formal conduit created.

There are therefore various different approaches to the ACE today. If the patient requires a synchronous bladder reconstruction, a formal conduit is constructed using the *in situ* appendix or a left-sided Monti-MACE if constipation is a severe problem. If only an ACE is required, a LACE would be the procedure of choice for cecal placement or a PEC if the patient is constipated and a left-sided site is needed.

Regional differences

Koyle *et al.* introduced the technique of simply wrapping the cecal wall around the folded appendix using non-absorbable sutures in North America in 1991.[11] Malone *et al.* had previously described making a submucosal tunnel along one of the tenia, laying the appendix into this, and closing the seromuscular layer over it.[6] In 1996, Shandling and colleagues from Canada described the technique of percutaneous placement of a cecostomy tube and button[40,41] – this has met with variable success on both sides of the Atlantic.[42] In a UK survey of 300 ACE procedures, cecal buttons were used in 19 cases and were reported to work well in most.[17] However, concern has been raised about skin erosion from the cecostomy button as the abdominal wall girth increases with age.[42]

Colonic irrigation fluids have been used alone or in combination and include sodium phosphate solutions, saline, tap water, and polyethylene glycol-electrolyte solution. In the UK, phosphate enema solutions are used most often for colonic irrigation whilst in North America either saline or tap water is popular.

Complications

Minor complications are not uncommon and range from 0% to 81%. The majority of complications involve the stoma, most commonly stomal stenosis (30%).[43] Van Savage *et al.* suggested that stomal location may play a role in the development of stomal stenosis, with an incidence of 13% at the umbilicus and 4% at a lower quadrant location.[44] They speculated that this was possibly due to the poorer blood supply of the umbilical skin flaps resulting in excessive scarring. However, further studies with follow-up periods of approximately 3 years have shown no significant differences between umbilical and abdominal stomas.[39] Regardless of whether daily enemas are administered, daily catheterization has been recommended to prevent stomal stenosis.[30] It has also been observed that stomal stenosis is more common in obese patients probably due to greater tension at the level of the skin anastomosis.[45]

Other reported complications include: stoma leak (6.6%), difficulty in catheterizing the conduit (3.7%), pain with enema administration (3%), adhesive bowel obstruction (1.5%), appendiceal necrosis (0.7%), cecal volvulus (0.7%), hyperphosphatemia (0.7%),[43] and necrosis of a Monti tube causing peritonitis.[36]

Results

As the first MACE was reported in 1990 and the procedure has evolved considerably since the original description, long-term results are not available for many of the techniques in current practice. However, some intermediate term results are available. These are best considered under two headings: (i) objective improvement in patient satisfaction and quality of life scores and (ii) continued use of the MACE and its ability to sustain fecal continence.

Quality of life

Three publications have assessed this issue objectively.[25,27,46] In the first study, the results of 40 patients who underwent a MACE procedure were assessed using a quality of life improvement (QOLI) score.[25] The mean score for all the patients was 3.5 where a score of 5 denoted a perfect result. The score was significantly lower in wheelchair-dependent patients with spinal cord pathologies (2.5) when compared to all other mobile patients. This paper does not indicate the time interval after the MACE procedure when the QOLIs were assessed. In another publication from the same unit, where the mean follow-up period was 5.4 years (3.25–8.25 years), 82% of 62 patients continued to use their MACE with a mean satisfaction score of 9, complete satisfaction being denoted by a score of 10.[46] In a further study, Aksnes *et al.* assessed the results of 20 patients 6 months after a MACE procedure.[27] They used several validated questionnaires including the Youth Self Report, Child Behaviour Check List, and Self Perception Profile for Adolescents. They concluded that following a MACE procedure there were important improvements in self-esteem and psychosocial functioning. Similarly Mitrofanoff's unit also published results of their survey to assess the level of satisfaction in patients who underwent a MACE procedure.[47] Twenty four of 28 patients returned the questionnaire and all considered themselves to have benefited from the operation, mainly in respect of personal, family and social well-being. All except three patients had acquired fecal continence (83%) on follow-up at 3.7 years. A review of the literature failed to identify any studies with longer follow-up that have objectively addressed these quality of life issues.

Achieving and sustaining fecal continence

The results of the MACE can be classified as: full success, partial success and failure. Full success denotes being totally clean or experiencing only minor leakage on the night of the washout. Partial success indicates being clean but having significant rectal leakage, occasional major leak, and/or still wearing protection, but perceived by the parent or child to be significantly improved from before the procedure. Based on these criteria, in 1998 Curry *et al.* reported a 39% failure rate in 31 patients with a mean

Table 33.1. Medium-term success of the MACE procedure in different series

Study	No. of patients (age in years)	Follow-up period	Conduits	Continence
Dick *et al.*[12]	13 (6–14)	3 years	ACE	86%
Ellsworth *et al.*[13]	18 (5–31)	2 years	ACE & Mitrofanoff	100% (93%)
Gerharz *et al.*[19]	16 (14–54)	6.6 years	ACE	50%
Wedderburn *et al.*[23]	46 (4–30)	4.3 years	ACE and Mitrofanoff	76% (both)
Kajbafzadeh *et al.*[24]	40 (4–22)	2 years	ACE and Mitrofanoff	95% (both)
Bau *et al.*[26]	19 (5–40)	6mo – 3 years	ACE and Mitrofanoff	88% (not known)
Curry *et al.*[48]	31 (1.3–18.3)	3.25 years	ACE	61%
Driver *et al.*[50]	29 (5–16)	6 years	ACE	79%
Levitt *et al.*[51]	20 (3–16)	Not known	ACE	95%
Tackett *et al.*[52]	45 (3.8–25.8)	2.4 years	ACE	87%

follow-up of more than 3 years. The majority of the failed patients had been treated either for chronic idiopathic constipation or Hirschsprung's disease.[48] A survey of MACEs performed by UK members of the British Association of Paediatric Surgeons found that the success of the procedure is dependent on the original diagnosis.[17] When patients with a neuropathic bowel or anorectal malformation were analyzed separately, partial and full success rates were 75% and 70%, respectively.[48] The overall success rate for this large national series was 79%.[17] Reviewing the literature on MACE with or without a Mitrofanoff conduit, the continence rate was found to be in the range of 61%–95% during follow-up periods of between 2 and 6 years (Table 33.1).

Conclusions

It is clear that long-term results are not currently available for the MACE procedure, particularly the newer modifications. It is important that these long-term results are collected to optimize our current indications and techniques. With the advent of further technical developments, it is important to remember the original principles that contribute to a successful MACE.[48,49] Patients who are over 5 years of age with a neuropathic bowel or an anorectal malformation, and who are motivated to be continent, do best. In depth preoperative counseling and continued postoperative support, usually provided by nurse specialists, are essential. The washout regimen used is individualized for each patient. If these guidelines are followed, the simultaneous use of the Mitrofanoff and MACE procedures can achieve double continence in the majority of patients.

REFERENCES

1. Stellman, G. R., Gilmore, M., & Bannister, C. M. A survey of the problems of bowel management experienced by families of spina bifida children. *Zeitschrift fur Kinderchir*. 1983; **38** (Suppl 2):96–97.
2. Malone, P. S., Wheeler, R. A., & Williams, J. E. Continence in patients with spina bifida: longterm results. *Arch. Dis. Child.* 1994; **70**:107–110.
3. Rintala, R. J. Fecal incontinence in anorectal malformations, neuropathy, and miscellaneous conditions. *Semin. Pediatr. Surg.* 2002; **11**:75–82.
4. Boemers, T. M. Urinary incontinence and vesicourethral dysfunction in pediatric surgical conditions. *Semin. Pediatr. Surg.* 2002; **11**:91–99.
5. Malone, P. S. J. The management of bowel problems in children with urological disease. *Br. J. Urol.* 1995; **76**:220–225.
6. Malone, P. S., Ransley, P. G., & Kiely, E. M. Preliminary report: the antegrade continence enema. *Lancet* 1990; **336**:1217–1218.
7. Mitrofanoff, P. Cystostomie continente trans-appendiculare dans le traitement des vessies neurologiques. *Chir. Pediatr.* 1980; **21**:297–305.
8. Shandling, B. & Gilmour, R. F. The enema continence catheter in spina bifida: successful bowel management. *J. Pediatr. Surg.* 1987; **22**:271–273.
9. Radcliffe, A. G. & Dudley, H. A. F. Intraoperative antegrade irrigation of the large intestine. *Surg. Gynecol. Obstet.* 1983; **156**:721–723.
10. Squire, R., Kiely, E. M., Carr, B., Ransley, P. G., & Duffy, P. G. The clinical application of the Malone antegrade continence enema. *J. Pediatr. Surg.* 1993; **28**:1012–1015.
11. Koyle, M. A., Kaji, D. M., Duque, M., Wild, J., & Galansky, S. H. The Malone antegrade continence enema for neurogenic and structural fecal incontinence and constipation. *J. Urol.* 1995; **154**:759–761.
12. Dick, A. C., McCallion, W. A., Brown, S., & Boston, V. E. Antegrade Colonic Enemas. *Br. J. Surg.* 1996; **83**:642–643.

13. Ellsworth, P. I., Webb, H. W., Crump, J. M. *et al.* The Malone antegrade colonic enema enhances the quality of life in children undergoing urological incontinence procedures. *J. Urol.* 1996; **155**:1416–1418.
14. Schell, S. R., Toogood, G. J., & Dudley, N. E. Control of fecal incontinence: continued success with the Malone Procedure. *Surgery* 1997; **122**:626–631.
15. Goepel, M., Sperling, H., Stoher, M. *et al.* Management of neurogenic fecal incontinence in myelodysplastic children by a modified continent appendiceal stoma and antegrade colonic enema. *Urology* 1997; **49**:758–761.
16. Sheldon, C. A., Minevich, E., Wackson, J., & Lewis, A. G. Role of the antegrade continence enema in the management of the most debilitating childhood recto-urogenital anomalies. *J. Urol.* 1997; **158**:1277–1279.
17. Curry, J. L., Osborne, A., & Malone, P. S. J. The MACE Procedure: experience in the United Kingdom. *J. Pediatr. Surg.* 1999; **34**:338–340.
18. Williams, N. S., Hughes, S. F., & Stuchfield, B. Continent colonic conduit for rectal evacuation in severe constipation. *Lancet* 1994; **343**:1321–1324.
19. Gerharz, E. W., Vik, V., Webb, G. *et al.* The value of the MACE (Malone antegrade colonic enema) procedure in adult patients. *J. Am. Coll. Surg.* 1997; **185**:544–547.
20. Krogh, K. & Laurberg, S. Malone antegrade continence enema for faecal incontinence and constipation in adults. *Br. J. Surg.* 1998; **85**:974–977.
21. Roberts, J. P., Moon, S., & Malone, P. S. Treatment of neuropathic urinary and faecal incontinence with synchronous bladder reconstruction and the antegrade continence enema procedure. *Br. J. Urol.* 1995; **75**:386–389.
22. Mor, Y., Quinn, F. M. J., Carr, B. *et al.* Combined Mitrofanoff and antegrade continence enema procedures for urinary and fecal incontinence. *J. Urol.* 1997; **158**:192–195.
23. Wedderburn, A., Lee, R. S., Denny, A. *et al.* Synchronous bladder reconstruction and antegrade continence enema. *J. Urol.* 2001; **165**:2392–2393.
24. Kajbafzadeh, A. M. & Chubak, N. Simultaneous Malone antegrade continent enema and Mitrofanoff principle using the divided appendix: report of a new technique for prevention of stoma complications. *J. Urol.* 2001; 165: 2404–2409.
25. Shankar, K. R., Losty, P. D., Kenny, S. E. *et al.* Functional results following the antegrade continence enema procedure. *Br. J. Surg.* 1998; **85**:980–982.
26. Bau, M. O., Younes, S., Aupy, A. *et al.* The Malone antegrade colonic enema isolated or associated with urological incontinence procedures: Evaluation from patient point of view. *J. Urol.* 2001; **165**:2399–2403.
27. Aksnes, G., Diseth, T. H., Helseth, A. *et al.* Appendicostomy for antegrade enema – effects on somatic and functioning in children with myelomeningocele. *Pediatrics* 2002; **109**:484–489.
28. Malone, P. S. The Malone procedure for antegrade continence enema. In Spitz, L. & Coran, A. *Rob & Smith's Operative Surgery, Pediatric Surgery*. London: Chapman & Hall, 1994.
29. Gerharz, E. W., Vik, V., Webb, G., & Woodhouse, C. R. J. The *in situ* appendix in the Malone antegrade continence enema procedure for faecal incontinence. *Br. J. Urol.* 1997; **79**:985–986.
30. Yang, W. H. Yang needle tunnelling technique in creating antireflux and continent mechanisms. *J. Urol.* 1993; **150**:830–834.
31. Monti, P. R., Lara, R. C., Dutra, M. A. *et al.* New techniques for construction of efferent conduits based on the Mitrofanoff principle. *Urology* 1997; **49**:112–115.
32. Sheldon, C. A., Minevich, E., & Wacksman, J. Modified technique of antegrade continence enema using a stapling device. *J. Urol.* 2000; **163**:589–591.
33. Webb, H. W., Barraza, M. A., & Crump, J. M. Laparoscopic appendicostomy for management of fecal incontinence. *J. Pediatr. Surg.* 1997; **32**:457–458.
34. Griffiths, D. M. & Malone, P. S. The Malone antegrade continence enema. *J. Pediatr. Surg.* 1995; **30**:68–71.
35. Mouriquand, P., Mure, P. Y., Feyaerts, A. *et al.* The left Monti-Malone. *BJU Int.* 2000; **85**(suppl):65.
36. Liloku, R. B., Mure, P. Y., Braga, L. *et al.* The left Monti-Malone procedure: Preliminary results in seven cases. *J. Pediatr. Surg.* 2002; **37**:228–231.
37. Lemelle, J. L., Olivier, P., David, N. *et al.* Analyse scintigraphique du lavement colique antegrade apres intervention de Malone. Presented at the Annual Meeting of the French Society of Paediatric Surgeons, Paris, Sept 1998.
38. Perez, M., Lemelle, J. L., Barhteleme, H. *et al.* Bowel management with anterograde colonic enema using a Malone or a Monti conduit. Clinical results. *Eur J. Pediatr. Surg.* 2001; **11**:315–318.
39. McAndrew, H. F. & Malone, P. S. J. Continent catheterisable conduits: which stoma, which conduit and which reservoir. *BJU Int.* 2002; **89**:86–89.
40. Chait, P. G., Shandling, B., Richards, H. M., & Connolly, B. E. Fecal incontinence in children: treatment with percutaneous cecostomy tube placement – a prospective study. *Radiology* 1997; **203**:621–624.
41. Chait, P. G., Shandling, B., & Richards, H. M. The cecostomy button. *J. Pediatr. Surg.* 1997; **32**:849–851.
42. Koyle, M. A. & Malone, P. S. J. The Malone antegrade continence enema. In Belman, A. B., King, L., & Kramer, S. A., eds. *Clinical Pediatric Urology*. 4th edn. Martin Dunitz Ltd, 2002: 529.
43. Graf, J. L., Strear, C., Bratton, B. *et al.* The antegrade continence enema procedure: a review of literature. *J. Pediatr. Surg.* 1998; **33**:1294–1296.
44. Van Savage, J. G., Khoury, A. E., Mc, Lorie, G. A. *et al.* Outcome analysis of Mitrofanoff principle applications using appendix and ureter to umbilicus and lower quadrant stomal sites. *J. Urol.* 1996; **156**(5):1794–1797.

45. Clark, T., Pope, J. C., Adams, M. C. *et al.* Factors that influence outcomes of the Mitrofanoff and Malone antegrade continence enema reconstructive procedures in children. *J. Urol.* 2002; **168**:1537–1540.
46. Dey, R., Kenny, S. E., Shankar, K. R. *et al.* After the honeymoon-medium-term outcome of antegrade continence enema procedure. *J. Pediatr. Surg.* 2003; **38**:65–68.
47. Liard, A., Bocquet, I., Bachy, B., & Mitrofanoff, P. Survey on satisfaction of patients with Malone continent cecostomy. *Prog. Urol.* 2002; **12**:1256–1260.
48. Curry, J. L., Osborne, A., & Malone, P. S. How to achieve a successful Malone antegrade continence enema. *J. Pediatr. Surg.* 1998; **33**:138–141.
49. Malone, P. S. J., Curry, J. L., & Osborne, A. The antegrade continence enema procedure; why, when and how. *World J. Urol.* 1998; **16**:274–278.
50. Driver, C. P., Barrow, C., Fishwick, J., *et al.* The Malone antegrade colonic enema procedure: outcome and lessons of 6 years' experience. *Pediatr. Surg. Int.* 1998; **13**:370–372.
51. Levitt, M. A., Soffer, S. Z., & Pena, A. Continent appendicostomy in the bowel management of fecal incontinent children. *J. Pediatr. Surg.* 1997; **32**:1630–1633.
52. Tackett, L. D., Minevich, E., Benedict, J. F., Wacksman, J., & Sheldon, C. A. Appendiceal versus ileal segment antegrade continence enema. *J. Urol.* 2002; **167**:683–686.

34

Splenectomy

Jennifer H. Aldrint and Henry E. Rice

Department of Surgery, Duke University Medical Center, Durham, NC, USA

Introduction

The first attempt to define the role of the spleen was made by Hippocrates around 400BC, who taught that the spleen "drew the watery part of food from the stomach."[1] Aristotle believed that the spleen had no function, and the ancient Greeks felt that the weight of the spleen hindered a man's athletic abilities and therefore applied hot irons to reduce its size.[1] Although many believed the spleen played a role in "cleansing the blood and spirit from unclear and obscuring matter," the belief that the spleen was a non-essential organ that could be removed without adverse affects persisted until the early 1900s.[1]

Morris and Bullock in 1919 were the first to recognize the spleen's role in infection based upon animal studies stating, "It is an observation of great antiquity that the operation of splenectomy is not followed by death . . . but this does not settle the problem as to whether or not a splenectomized person can weather a critical illness."[2] Following the landmark report by King and Shumaker in 1952 of five cases of sepsis in splenectomized infants, the association between fulminate bacterial sepsis following splenectomy has been firmly established.[3]

Embryology and anatomy

The primordial spleen appears as a mesodermal proliferation arising from the dorsal mesogastrium during the fifth and sixth weeks of embryologic development.[4] As the stomach rotates and the dorsal mesogastrium lengthens, the spleen is carried to the left upper quadrant of the abdomen where it fuses with the peritoneum of the posterior abdominal wall. The splenic artery and vein, and short gastric vessels, course through the lienorenal ligament and the gastrolienal ligament, the visceral attachments of the spleen.

The splenic artery arises from the celiac axis, and follows a course along the cephalad pancreas before entering the spleen at the hilum. The parenchyma of the spleen is divided into segments by fibrous bands along which course the trabecular arteries, the first order branches of the splenic artery. These trabecular arteries further divide into the central arteries of the spleen. The parenchyma of the spleen consists of lymphoid tissue adjacent to the central arterioles known as the white pulp, a marginal zone and a region of red pulp. The white pulp is composed largely of aggregates of T lymphocytes with interspersed antigen presenting dendritic cells. These lymphoid aggregates function as an immune barrier which detects and processes foreign antigen and antigen–antibody complexes. The marginal zone is rich in B-cells at varying stages of development. The large red pulp area, comprising 75% of the splenic parenchyma, is made up of splenic or Billroth cords with interspersed splenic sinuses.[5] These splenic cords are composed of fibroblasts and macrophages, while the sinuses contain large numbers of erythrocytes that are filtered and removed if defective or damaged.

Function

The major functions of the spleen can be broadly classified as either hematologic or immunologic, and are outlined in Table 34.1.

These hematologic and immune functions of the spleen are closely linked to its unique anatomy. The reticular

Pediatric Surgery and Urology: Long-term Outcomes, Mark Stringer, Keith Oldham, Pierre Mouriquand.
Published by Cambridge University Press.

Table 34.1. Functions of the spleen

Hematologic
Hematopoieses during fetal life
Removal of senescent or diseased RBCs
Removal of abnormal inclusion bodies from RBCs
Maturation of reticulocytes
Reservoir for platelets and granulocytes
Iron metabolism
Immunologic
Filtration and processing of antigen
Lymphocyte stimulation and activation
Production of antibodies
Production of opsonins (tuftsin and properdin)

Table 34.2. Indications for splenectomy

Disease treatment	Treatment of hypersplenism
Idiopathic thrombocytopenic purpura	Lymphoproliferative disorders
Thrombotic thrombocytopenic purpura	Felty syndrome
Hereditary spherocytosis	Sickle cell disease
Autoimmune hemolytic anemia	Gaucher disease
Hereditary spherocytosis	Thalassemia major
Trauma, splenic bleeding or rupture	Sarcoidosis
Splenic tumors	Splenic vein thrombosis
Splenic cysts	Chronic myeloid leukemia
Infection/abscess	Chronic lymphocytic leukemia

meshwork of red pulp serves as an excellent filter, enabling the removal of red cells and microorganisms that come into contact with the macrophages lining the Billroth cords. Similarly, antigens that are captured and processed in the red pulp are concentrated in the white pulp where T- and B-cell interactions stimulate an immune response.[6,7] The ability of the spleen to synthesize antibodies against polysaccharide antigens plays an important role in the host defense against encapsulated bacteria, including *Streptococcus pneumoniae, Haemophilus influenzae*, and *Neisseria meningitidis*. Opsonization of bacteria with specific antibody and complement enhances phagocytosis by splenic macrophages. Asplenic subjects are deficient in specific antibody to these organisms and have defective activation of complement, leaving them susceptible to infection with encapsulated pathogens.[6]

Indications for splenectomy

As knowledge regarding the critical immune functions of the spleen has increased, the indications for splenectomy have gradually evolved, yielding an approach which favors splenic preservation whenever possible. The indications for splenectomy can be divided into two broad categories: (1) treatment of disease, and (2) treatment of associated hypersplenism (Table 34.2). Overall, hypersplenism accounts for between 5 and 50% of all splenectomies, trauma 10%–30%, malignancy 19%–34%, and incidental to other surgery 20%–36%.[1]

Operative technique

The operative approach to splenectomy has become increasingly varied in recent years. The surgical repertoire includes total or partial splenectomy, resection via an open technique or a laparoscopic approach, splenic embolization, splenorraphy, or in many cases of blunt trauma, close observation alone without removal of the spleen.[8–11]

Open splenectomy

The traditional open total splenectomy is performed via either a midline or a left subcostal incision. The components of open splenectomy include complete mobilization of the spleen by division of the avascular posterior and lateral attachments, ligation of the short gastric arteries, and ligation of the splenic hilar vessels.

In certain immune mediated diseases such as immune thrombocytopenic purpura (ITP), it is critical to remove any accessory spleens, as any remaining splenic tissue can be responsible for relapse of disease following splenectomy. Accessory spleens are present in approximately 20% of individuals, and are often found in the splenic hilum, lesser sac, or omentum.

Laparoscopic splenectomy

Laparoscopic splenectomy was first introduced to the adult population in 1991, and has become the preferred approach for most patients requiring total splenectomy,[12–15] including the pediatric population.[16,17] Results of a large meta-analysis comparing outcomes of laparoscopic splenectomy vs. open splenectomy demonstrated a complication rate of 26.6% for the open group vs. 15.5% for the laparoscopic group ($P < 0.0001$), with equivalent mortality rates.[15] Numerous non-randomized prospective studies that have compared open splenectomy with laparoscopic splenectomy have reported decreased postoperative pain and a shorter recovery time with a laparoscopic approach.[15–20] Two series evaluating this approach in children have demonstrated a decrease in the postoperative stays and use of less pain medication for laparoscopic procedures.[16,17] Disadvantages of the laparoscopic approach include slightly longer operating times and higher total hospital charges.[15,16,19] Identification of accessory spleens during laparoscopic splenectomy is comparable to open splenectomy.[15–20]

Partial splenectomy

Partial splenectomy has been proposed as an alternative to total splenectomy in certain children with congenital hemolytic anemias, with the goal of removing enough spleen to gain a desired hematological effect while preserving splenic function.[21–23] However, the widespread application of partial splenectomy remains limited because of technical difficulties and concerns of splenic regrowth.[22,24,25] For most disease states, the objective of partial splenectomy is to remove 80%–90% of the splenic volume.[26]

At our institution, 23 children with various diseases have undergone partial splenectomy.[26] To date, only one child in our experience has required later conversion to a total splenectomy, similar to the rate of other series.[23] With the use of serial ultrasonography, we have found a variable rate of regrowth of the splenic remnant; in a small number of patients the splenic remnant has regrown up to almost the original splenic size.[26] However, importantly, in almost all children with congenital hemolytic anemias, this splenic regrowth does not appear to be associated with recurrent hemolysis, possibly due to parenchymal remodeling or altered blood flow following partial resection.[22,23,26] For children with hereditary spherocytosis, the mean hemoglobin concentrations in our series increased by more than 2 g/dl, and persisted for 5 years of follow-up.[26] Likewise, serum bilirubin levels and reticulocyte counts decreased, and there was a reduction in signs and symptoms of hypersplenism.[26] It is increasingly evident that a partial splenectomy is safe, and can provide long-term desired hematological effects in carefully selected patients.[23,26]

Splenic embolization

As immunologic complications of total splenectomy have become increasingly recognized, efforts to salvage the spleen have become more frequently employed. Splenic embolization has emerged as an alternative to surgery for both traumatic splenic injuries as well as select non-traumatic diseases, such as portal hypertension with hypersplenism.[27–30]

Non-operative management is preferred for traumatic splenic injuries in hemodynamically stable children whenever possible, with the goal of splenic preservation.[31] In the case of traumatic splenic bleeding, options include surgical total or partial splenectomy, splenorraphy, or angiographic embolization. The use of angiography to characterize the extent of splenic injury and predict the success of non-operative management has been shown to improve the splenic salvage rate in several series.[31–33] The absence of contrast extravasation on arteriography is a reliable predictor of successful conservative management of splenic injuries.[32,33] If contrast extravasation is seen, splenic artery embolization can control splenic hemorrhage. The non-operative management of hemodynamically stable patients with CT-diagnosed splenic injury in one study demonstrated that 56 of the 60 patients treated by splenic artery occlusion and bed rest had a successful outcome, with an overall splenic salvage rate of 88%.[33]

Partial splenic embolization procedures have also been used for children with portal hypertension and hypersplenism. Brandt *et al.* have shown that the use of partial splenic embolization for children with hypersplenism associated with portal hypertension resulted in the normalization of hematologic parameters throughout a follow-up of 2 years, and a decrease in the episodes of variceal hemorrhage per year from 2.4 to 0.5.[27] Similarly, Nio *et al.* reported that partial splenic embolization for children with hypersplenism secondary to portal hypertension resulted in initial improved hematologic indices in all 36 patients. However, recurrence of thrombocytopenia occurred in 30.6% of patients, thought to be related to proliferative potential of the remaining spleen; and in select cases this was amenable to repeat embolization. No patient died of complications related to splenic embolization, and long-term efficacy was demonstrated in 70% of the surviving patients.[30]

Splenorrhaphy

The option of splenic repair for traumatic injury has been increasingly encouraged because of concerns of postsplenctomy infection. In cases of traumatic injury to the spleen, operative salvage techniques include the use of partial splenectomy, splenorrhaphy, and topical hemostatic agents. The most important aspect of performing a splenic repair is the necessity for complete mobilization of the spleen from its attachments.[7] Once the spleen has been mobilized, the surgeon is able to adequately assess and control the injury. Surgical approaches include repair with sutures alone or in combination with omentum inserted into the parenchyma, enveloping the spleen in an absorbable mesh wrap that exerts its effect by tamponading the injury, or performing a hemisplenectomy with the use of stapler or other parenchyma ligation techniques.

Long-term outcomes following splenectomy for specific disorders

Hereditary spherocytosis

Hereditary spherocytosis (HS) is an autosomal dominant disorder in which there is an abnormality in the red blood cell membrane affecting the spectrin, ankyrin, or protein 3 component, which results in diminished capacity for deformation of the red blood cells and trapping within the spleen.[34–36] The clinical features of severe HS include anemia, jaundice, and splenomegaly. Less severe symptoms and signs include fatigue, increased rate of viral infection, and poor growth.

Classic indications for splenectomy in HS include severe anemic crises and recurrent transfusion requirements. In the past, it has been recommended that in the absence of life-threatening symptoms, total splenectomy be deferred at least until age 4 or 5 years in order to preserve immunologic function in young children who are at highest risk for overwhelming postsplenectomy sepsis.[34] However, the option of partial splenectomy in selected young children with HS has led to a recent reevaluation of indicators for surgical therapy. Following either total or partial splenectomy for HS, resolution of hemolysis and the associated symptoms is nearly 100%.[34,36]

Thalassemia major

Beta-thalassemia major, an inherited disorder that results in decreased or absent production of beta-globin and increased accumulation of alpha-globin chains, ineffective erythropoiesis, and reduced red blood cell survival is one of the most prevalent hemoglobinopathies throughout the world.[37,38] Traditional therapy for β-thalassemia major consists of red blood cell transfusions to maintain an adequate hemoglobin level, parenteral iron chelation therapy with deferoxamine, and splenectomy if growth and development are delayed or if symptoms of hypersplenism develop.[39] Death usually occurs between the second and fourth decades of life from cardiac arrhythmias caused by excessive iron accumulation in myocardial tissue.

Removal of the spleen for children with beta-thalassemia major has been shown to reduce transfusion requirements and consequent iron deposition. Partial splenectomy has been proposed as an alternative to total splenectomy in patients with thalassemia and its variant forms, especially in children less than 5 years of age.[40–42] Partial splenectomy improves hematological parameters in patients with thalassemia major, with an increase in mean hemoglobin value from 5.5 g/dl to 7.7 g/dl, and reduction in average transfusion requirements from 317 ml/kg per yr to 230 ml/kg per yr in one report.[40] Partial splenic embolization has also been explored as an alternative to total or partial splenectomy with advantages of preservation of a splenic remnant.[43,44] However, disadvantages of both surgical partial splenectomy and partial splenic embolization include regrowth of the splenic remnant with recurrence of anemias and symptoms of hypersplenism, often resulting in the need for subsequent total splenectomy. For these reasons, routine partial splenectomy is generally not performed in patients with thalassemia major, with the exception of children under 5 years of age, whose risk of overwhelming postsplenectomy infection is greatest.[42]

Although splenectomy is beneficial in terms of improvement of transfusion requirements and symptoms of hypersplenism, it does not alter the cardiac pathology which is the typical cause of death in these patients.[5] Bone marrow transplantation is the only curative therapy for β-thalassemia major, and is best performed prior to the onset of a pathologic condition from the disease or complications related to transfusion therapy, most notably hemosiderosis and alloimmunization.

Sickle cell anemia

Classic sickle cell anemia is a hereditary hemolytic anemia in which a genetic mutation results in a single amino acid substitution (glutamine to valine) in the beta chain of the hemoglobin molecule. In homozygous Hgb SS individuals, red blood cells are prone to sickling under hypoxic or acidic conditions. Sickle cell disease is characterized by chronic hemolysis and anemia, often highlighted by acute "crises" related to events of vascular occlusion. The sickled red blood cells become sequestered within the spleen, leading to acute splenic sequestration, the most common indication for splenectomy in this population.[25] Severe anemia, thrombocytopenia, and hypersplenism develop during acute splenic sequestration, resulting in significant morbidity and mortality. Other indications for splenectomy in these children include hypersplenism, splenic abscess, and massive splenic infarction.[45]

Genetic variants of the homozygous form of sickle cell disease exist, including hemoglobin SC disease in which hemoglobin C is produced and combined with Hgb S- β-thalassemia. Both of these variants result in less severe symptoms compared to the homozygous Hgb SS disease, with fewer pain crises, milder anemia, and longer life expectancy. The syndrome of acute splenic sequestration also occurs less frequently in children with Hgb SC disease than in their homozygous counterparts, with incidence rates reported between 3% and 6%.[46] making the role of splenectomy for these children less clear.

Several studies evaluating the outcome of total splenectomy in all types of sickle cell disease have demonstrated that in carefully selected individuals, the use of total splenectomy results in a reduction in transfusion requirements, elimination of hypersplenism, and avoidance of recurrent splenic sequestration crises.[45,47] In a series of 32 patients who underwent total splenectomy for sickle cell disease, Kar reported an increase in the hemoglobin value by 2 g/dl in 81% of patients, an increase in height in 90%, and an increase in weight in 61%.[48] In addition, the frequency of pain, anemia, and the need for blood transfusions improved in 79% of patients.

In contrast to the use of total splenectomy, the use of partial splenectomy has been proposed to control symptoms of hypersplenism and reduce splenic sequestration complications in selected children with sickle cell disease.[26] Svarch *et al.* reported a series of 50 patients with Hgb SS or Hgb S-beta thalassemia who underwent partial splenectomy.[49] In this series, there were no postoperative episodes of acute splenic sequestration, a significant reduction in the number of blood transfusions, and a significant reduction in hospitalizations with a mean follow-up of 8.3 years. Mean hemoglobin concentration and platelet counts were also significantly increased following partial splenectomy. There was one case of non-fatal overwhelming post-splenectomy sepsis in this series.

Despite the positive results of this study, the high long-term rate of splenic autoinfarction in homozygous Hgb SS disease has limited the use of partial splenectomy for this disease.[26] In our program, we generally do not use partial splenectomy for Hgb SS children, and limit the use of this procedure to children with Hgb SC or combined Hgb S-beta thalassemia. Others, however, argue that the use of partial splenectomy is a reasonable option for children with Hgb SS disease, because some element of reticuloendothelial activity is retained, and preservation of part of the spleen for several years prior to autoinfarction of the splenic remnant may provide temporary protection against serious infections.[49]

Immune thrombocytopenic purpura

Immune thrombocytopenic purpura (ITP) is one of the most common acquired bleeding disorders of childhood, resulting from the accelerated destruction of platelets.[19] Children with ITP have monoclonal and polyclonal antibodies directed mainly against the GPIIb/IIIa and GPIb/IX complexes of the platelet membrane.[19] These antibodies coat the surfaces of platelets, which upon entry into the spleen are sequestered from the circulation by macrophages. Clinical manifestations include easy bruising, purpura, ecchymoses, bleeding gums, hematuria, and gastrointestinal bleeding.

The majority of children with ITP (80%) will have an acute, self-limited course with normalization of the platelet count and the absence of severe bleeding with drug therapy or observation alone.[36] Initial therapy consists of corticosteroids, intravenous gamma globulin, anti-D immunoglobulin, or plasmapheresis.[50] Splenectomy is generally not required for the treatment of acute ITP. Approximately 20% of children with ITP develop thrombocytopenia that persists beyond six months and are defined as having chronic ITP.[50] Children with chronic ITP are managed according to the severity of the thrombocytopenia. Those who display no evidence of clinical bleeding and are capable of maintaining platelet counts above 50 000/ml may be closely followed. In symptomatic or severely thrombocytopenic patients, total splenectomy has resulted in normalization of the platelet count in greater than 75% of cases.[50,51] During the procedure a careful search for any accessory spleens is mandatory to ensure success. Partial splenectomy is not an option for patients with ITP, because any remaining splenic tissue will continue to function as an immune source for antibody production and platelet trapping and result in recurrence or persistence of disease.

For the 20%–25% of patients with chronic ITP who do not respond to splenectomy and remain thrombocytopenic, other alternative therapies are available. Azathioprine has been demonstrated to achieve long-term remissions in adults with chronic ITP with minimal associated toxicity, but similar efficacy in children has not yet been proven.[50]

Malignancies

Hodgkin's disease

Historically, staging laparotomy with splenectomy to evaluate the extent of abdominal disease for Hodgkin's disease was required to provide information necessary to stage patients and to select appropriate therapy. With advances in alternative imaging techniques including CT scan, magnetic resonance imaging (MRI), and fluorodeoxyglucose positron emission tomography (PET) imaging, the use of staging laparotomy for Hodgkin's disease has been virtually eliminated. A prospective, randomized study for the treatment of early stage Hodgkin's disease demonstrated no relapse or survival benefit with laparotomy and splenectomy compared to non-operative methods of staging.

Long-term consequences of staging laparotomy with splenectomy in patients with Hodgkin's disease include the risk of overwhelming postsplenectomy sepsis and an increased risk of secondary cancers, most commonly acute non-lymphocytic leukemias (ANLL) or solid tumors.[52,53] One study of 503 patients comparing the incidence of secondary ANLL reported a frequency of 5.86% in splenectomized patients and a frequency of 0.69% in non-splenectomized patients.[52]

Non-Hodgkin's lymphoma

Children with non-Hodgkin's lymphoma (NHL) may present with isolated splenic disease, and NHL is the most common primary splenic neoplasm. In addition, NHL may develop as a secondary malignancy following therapy for a variety of primary cancers. Children with diffuse NHL can develop splenomegaly and associated symptoms of abdominal pain and early satiety, and splenectomy is indicated for symptoms of hypersplenism in these children. Splenectomy has been shown to be effective in the management of patients who develop anemia, thrombocytopenia, and neutropenia in association with hypersplenism secondary to lymphatic infiltration.[54]

The long-term outcomes of splenectomy for NHL are similar to other hematological diseases for which splenectomy is performed. One series evaluated 59 patients with NHL with predominant splenic involvement, 40 of whom underwent splenectomy.[55] Of the patients in this series who underwent splenectomy 82% had a correction in their cytopenias, a finding that was associated with a significantly prolonged survival. This is similar to other reports citing a decrease in transfusion requirements in up to 80% of patients, with relief of gastric compression and pain associated with splenomegaly.[54] Similarly, a study of 26 patients with mantle cell NHL who underwent splenectomy reported a correction of anemia in 69.2% and a correction of thrombocytopenia in 90%.[56] Furthermore, 15% of these patients did not require any additional chemotherapy following splenectomy, and an additional 30% remained free of disease for >13 months following splenectomy, suggesting that splenectomy may provide durable remission in selected patients with refractory cytopenias or symptoms related to splenomegaly, and that some patients may experience a prolonged disease stabilization after splenectomy.[56] It should be noted, however, that correction of pancytopenias is somewhat dependent on the reserve of the bone marrow, which may have been heavily treated with chemotherapy or radiation therapy. This is difficult to predict prior to splenectomy, however, and the only means of assessing adequate reserve is a favorable response following splenectomy.

Gaucher's disease

Gaucher's disease is a familial disorder in which there is a deficiency of the enzyme β-glucosidase, leading to an abnormal storage or retention of glycolipid cerebrosides within reticuloendothelial cells, thereby resulting in significant splenomegaly. Splenectomy had historically been the procedure of choice for these patients, but the concern for postsplenectomy sepsis led many to advocate partial splenectomy for this condition.[57–59] However, partial splenectomy has been less successful for this condition compared to more common congenital anemias, and some have hypothesized that the splenic remnant tends to enlarge with Gaucher's disease due to tissue regeneration and/or continued deposition of the glucocerebrosides in the reticuloendothelial system.[57,59] Some suggest that by leaving a splenic remnant for continued deposition of lipid, the bone marrow is spared from deposition and therefore protected, offering an additional benefit to partial splenectomy in these patients.[5] With alglucerase enzyme therapy now widely instituted, rates of splenomegaly have decreased ameliorating much of the need for splenectomy in this disease.[60,61]

Overwhelming postsplenectomy sepsis

Overwhelming postsplenectomy infection (OPSI) is a fulminate, life-threatening complication occurring after anatomic splenectomy or functional asplenia. King and Shumaker first reported the association between splenectomy and fulminate, lethal sepsis in their 1952 report of five splenectomized infants who dramatically succumbed to infection.[3] Since that report, awareness of the association between splenectomy and risk of infection has led to improved prophylactic measures, better education of patients and families, and aggressive treatment. Surgical removal of the spleen clearly results in reduced clearance of extracellular and intracellular antigens, diminished response to new polysaccharide antigens, and impaired phagocytosis of unopsonized and opsonized bacteria.[62] The most common organism is *Streptococcus pneumonia*, accounting for 50%–90% of cases and 60% of the mortality associated with OPSI, but other encapsulated organisms such as *Haemophilus influenzae* and *Neisseria meningitidis* are also significant pathogens.[1,62–67] Less common infectious agents causing OPSI include *Escherichia coli*, *Pseudomonas aeruginosa*, *capnocytophaga canimorsus* (formerly called DF-2), group B streptococci, *Enterococcus* spp., *Bacteroides* spp., *Bartonella*, and others.[67]

Despite the widespread concern for OPSI, the true overall incidence of serious infections following splenectomy is somewhat difficult to ascertain, although the risk of fulminate OPSI has been reported to be between 0.1% and 8.5%.[1] A large meta-analysis of postsplenectomy sepsis series that included 19 680 cases reported a serious infection rate of 3.2% and an overall mortality of 1.4%.[67] The incidence of infection among children and adults was found to be similar, although the incidence of deaths was significantly higher among children (1.7%) than adults (1.3%) ($P < 0.001$). Other studies have supported these numbers, reporting overall risks of OPSI of 0.13% to 8.1% in children and 0.28% to 1.9% in adults.[1,63–66]

The majority of OPSI presents within the initial 2 years following splenectomy, with 50%–70% of cases occurring during that time period.[1] However, splenectomized patients are at lifelong risk, as postsplenectomy sepsis has been reported more than 40 years after surgery.[1] Overall lifetime risk of OPSI has been estimated to be 5%,[62] with a mean time interval between splenectomy and infection of 22.6 months.[67]

The incidence of OPSI is dependent on the underlying disease process, and several studies have stratified the risk of OPSI by the disease state for which splenectomy was performed.[1,67] Infection risk is highest among patients with thalassemia major (8.2%) and sickle cell anemia (7.3%) who exhibit alterations in complement activation, abnormal levels of immunoglobulin, and impaired phagocytic function placing them at increased risk for severe infection and death following splenectomy.[1,67] The lowest infection rates are observed among patients with ITP (2.1%) and trauma (2.3%).[67]

The clinical manifestations of OPSI begin with a prodrome of fever and mild, non-specific symptoms including chills, malaise, myalgias, headache, nausea, vomiting, diarrhea, and abdominal pain, rapidly evolving into overwhelming septic shock. Although the onset may be insidious and non-specific, rapid deterioration remains the hallmark of OPSI with hypotension, respiratory distress, disseminated intravascular coagulation, coma, and death occurring within hours of presentation. A high index of suspicion with any febrile illness leading to rapid diagnosis and aggressive treatment is critical in preventing decompensation and death in splenectomized patients. Diagnostic work-up should not delay the initiation of empiric antibiotic therapy. Initial diagnostic work-up should include a peripheral blood smear evaluation for the presence of bacteria. Visualization of organisms on Gram stain of the buffy coat suggests a quantitative bacteremia of $>10^6$ organisms/ml. Blood cultures should always be collected and are generally positive within 24 hours, aiding in the identification of the pathogen and guiding subsequent antibiotic therapy. Additional studies should be obtained as appropriate, in efforts to identify all possible sources of infection.

The critical point in management of these patients is early recognition followed by aggressive intervention. All asplenic patients with fever of unidentifiable source should be treated as medical emergencies. Initial empiric therapy should always include a broad-spectrum antibiotic with activity against *S. pneumonia*, *H. influenzae*, and *N. meningitidis*. Intravenous penicillin has been the cornerstone of antibiotic therapy due to its excellent activity against pneumococci and meningococci, but local resistance patterns must be taken into account, and inclusion of an antibiotic active against penicillin-resistant pneumococci and beta-lactamase-resistant organisms, such as ceftriaxone, should be considered.[1,68] In areas with concern for highly resistant pneumococci, vancomycin and rifampicin should be considered as empiric therapy.[1,68]

Prevention of OPSI

In general, risk reduction for OPSI in asplenic patients is multifaceted, including immunization, the use of prophylactic antibiotic regimens, education of the patient and family, and prompt recognition of early signs and symptoms of illness with institution of aggressive treatment. Although general clinical guidelines for the use of these risk reduction strategies exist, complete agreement on all aspects of risk reduction has not been reached. No prophylactic regimen will completely eliminate the risk of sepsis in asplenic patients, but with the institution of adequate vaccinations, the use of prophylactic antibiotics when appropriate, and the education of patients and families the morbidity and mortality of severe infection may be significantly reduced.

Immunoprophylaxis

The major approach to the prevention of severe infections in the asplenic host is vaccination against the most frequent causative agents. Highly immunogenic capsular vaccines are available for the three major organisms responsible for the morbidity and mortality of OPSI: *S. pneumoniae* (23 most common serotypes accounting for 85% of infections),

H. influenzae (type B), and *N. meningiditis* (groups A, C, Y, and W135). In children less than two years of age, a pneumococcal 7-valent conjugate vaccine should be used.[68] All pathologic strains are not included in the vaccines, however, so infection may occur despite immunization. Whenever possible, it is recommended for vaccinations to be given two weeks prior to elective splenectomy, in order to optimize antibody response.[69,70] In cases of emergent splenectomy, patients should be vaccinated prior to discharge from the hospital to ensure that they receive the vaccine, as many of these patients become lost to follow-up.[36] Reimmunization with pneumococcal and meningococcal vaccines is recommended at 5–10 year intervals, and after 2 years, respectively.[68] The need for reimmunization with the *H. influenzae* vaccine is not clear. The influenza vaccine is recommended annually for immunocompromised patients and may be valuable to asplenic patients by reducing the risk of secondary bacterial infection.[68]

Vaccination does not always result in protective levels of antibodies. Konradsen *et al.* evaluated pneumococcal and *Haemophilus influenzae* type B antibody levels following vaccination in splenectomized patients, and reported that only 52% of patients who had been properly vaccinated had protective levels of pneumococcal antibodies, and that only 60% of patients had Hib antibody levels high enough to confer long-term protection.[71] Pneumococcal vaccination without antibiotic prophylaxis does not provide full protection against late sepsis, as up to 20–40% of the septicemias may be caused by bacteria other than pneumococci, emphasizing the need for additional prophylactic measures in splenectomized patients.[72]

Chemoprophylaxis

Because vaccinations do not completely protect against infection, many authorities have recommended antibiotic prophylaxis for asplenic patients, especially for the first two years following splenectomy.[1,68–70] Although the value of prophylactic antibiotics has been demonstrated in a clinical trial setting only for sickle cell disease, most investigators advocate their use in all children who have undergone splenectomy regardless of the indication until 5 years of age, and many propose continuation of antibiotic chemoprophylaxis until adulthood.[68,70–73] Current guidelines for chemoprophylaxis include 125 mg twice-daily oral penicillin VK until age 3, and 250 mg twice daily thereafter.[66] Problems with the use of orally administered penicillin in children have included poor compliance, the risk of selecting antibiotic-resistant strains, and providing the patient with a false sense of security should a febrile illness develop.[70]

Education

Patient education in the prevention and early management of serious infection has a great potential to decrease the morbidity and mortality in OPSI. Studies have documented that from 11% to 50% of postsplenectomy patients remain unaware of the increased risk for serious infection, and the necessity for preventative strategies.[74–79] Deodhar *et al.* found that in their series of asplenic patients, less than half had received pneumococcal immunization, were currently on antibiotic prophylaxis, or had received education and instructions regarding their increased risk for serious infection.[69] Patients and families must be clearly informed about the risk of rapidly progressing, life-threatening infections, that the risk of infection is higher in the first 2 years after splenectomy but is still present life long, and about the need to inform doctors of splenectomizied status.[70]

It must be emphasized that despite the use of antibiotic prophylaxis and vaccination against *S. pneumoniae*, *H. influenzae* type B, and *N. meningiditis*, splenectomy still places the patient at life long risk for serious infection. Despite all of these measures, the true benefits of these risk reduction strategies remain poorly defined. The vaccines for *S. pneumoniae* and *N. meningiditis* are not effective against all bacterial strains, antimicrobial resistance develops, and the use of prophylactic antibiotics may generate a false sense of security in patients, families, and physicians. Therefore, careful and thorough education of patients and families, a rigorous vaccination policy, knowledge of regional antibiotic resistance patterns from which to tailor prophylactic coverage, and early recognition and aggressive initiation of therapy with the onset of any febrile illness are each vitally important in reducing the incidence and mortality of overwhelming postsplenectomy sepsis in asplenic patients.

Conclusions

Splenectomy remains a critical procedure for several hematologic and non-hematologic diseases, although an emphasis is now placed on splenic preservation whenever possible. The current surgical repertoire includes total and partial splenectomy, open and laparoscopic techniques, splenorraphy, and splenic embolization. When making decisions regarding which approach to use, it is imperative that patients and families are aware of the risks and benefits of each procedure, as well as the long-term consequences of splenectomy. The major long-term complication following splenectomy is overwhelming sepsis, but through awareness, education, and proper use of immunoprophylaxis and chemoprophylaxis, the risk of this devastating outcome may be minimized.

REFERENCES

1. Lynch, A. M. & Kapila, R. Overwhelming postsplenectomy infection. *Infect. Dis. Clin. N. Am.* 1996; **10**:693–707.
2. Morris, D. H. & Bullock, F. D. The importance of the spleen in resistance to infection. *Ann. Surg.* 1919; **50**:513.
3. King, H. & Shumacker, H. B. Splenic studies. I. Susceptibility to infection after splenectomy performed in infancy. *Ann. Surg.* 1952; **136**:239.
4. Sadler, T. W. *Langman's Medical Embryology*, 7th edn. Baltimore: Williams and Wilkins, 1995: 245–250.
5. Fraker, D. L. Spleen. In Greenfield, L. J. ed. *Surgery Scientific Principles and Practice*, ed. 3rd edn. Philadelphia, PA: Lippincott, Williams and Wilkins, 2001; 1236–1257.
6. Cullis, J. O. & Mufti, G. J. Splenectomy. In Stringer, M. D. Oldham, K. T. Mouriquand, P. D. E. Howard, E. R. eds. *Pediatric Surgery and Urology: Long Term Outcomes*, London: W. B. Saunders, 1998; 394–401.
7. Schwartz, S. I. The Spleen. In Cameron, J. L. *Current Surgical Therapy*, 1998; 545–556. St. Louis: Mosby, Inc.
8. Carroll, A. & Thomas, P. Decision-making in surgery: Splenectomy. *Br. J. Hosp. Med.* 1995; **54**:147.
9. Uranus, S., Pfeifer, J., Schauer, C. *et al.* Laparoscopic partial splenic resection. *Surg. Laparosc. Endosc.* 1995; **5**:133.
10. Farhi, D. C. & Ashfaq, R. Splenic pathology after traumatic injury. *Am. J. Clin. Pathol.* 1996; **105**:474.
11. Petroianu, A. Subtotal splenectomy for treatment of patients with myelofibrosis and myeloid metaplasia. *Int. Surg.* 1996; **81**:177.
12. Beanes, S., Emil, S., Kosi, M. *et al.* A comparison of laparoscopic versus open splenectomy in children. *Am. Surg.* 1995; **61**:908–910.
13. Berman, R. S., Yahanda, A. M., Mansfield, P. F. *et al.* Laparoscopic splenectomy in patients with hematologic malignancies. *Am. J. Surg.* 1999; **178**:530–536.
14. Cogliandolo, A., Berland-Dai, B., Pidoto, R. R. *et al.* Results of laparoscopic and open splenectomy for nontraumatic diseases. *Surg. Laparosc. Endosc. Percutan. Tech.* 2001; **11**:256–261.
15. Winslow, E. R. & Brunt, L. M. Perioperative outcomes of laparoscopic versus open splenectomy: a meta-analysis with an emphasis on complications. *Surgery* 2003; **134**:647–653.
16. Yoshida, K., Yamazaki, Y., Mizuno, R. *et al.* Laparoscopic splenectomy in children. Preliminary results and comparison with the open technique. *Surg. Endosc.* 1995; **9**:1279–1282.
17. Curran, T. J., Foley, M. I., Seanstrom, L. L., & Campbell, T. J. Laparoscopy improves outcomes for pediatric splenectomy. *J. Pediatr. Surg.* 1998; **33**:1498–1500.
18. Watson, D. I., Coventry, B. J., Chin, B. J. *et al.* Laparoscopic versus open splenectomy for immune thrombocytopenic purpura. *Surgery* 1997; **121**:18–22.
19. Lozano-Salazar, R. R., Herrera, M. F., Vargas-Vorackova, F., & Lopez-Karpovitch, X. Laparoscopic versus open splenectomy for immune thrombocytopenic purpura. *Am. J. Surg.* 1998; **176**:366–369.
20. Knauer, E. M., Ailawadi, G., Yahanda, A. *et al.* 101 laparoscopic splenectomies for the treatment of benign and malignant hematologic disorders. *Am. J. Surg.* 2003; **186**:500–504.
21. Tchernia, G., Gauthier, F., Mielot, F. *et al.* Initial assessment of the beneficial effect of partial splenectomy in hereditary spherocytosis. *Blood* 1993; **81**:2014–2020.
22. Tchernia, G., Bader-Meunier, B., Berterottiere, P. *et al.* Effectiveness of partial splenectomy in hereditary spherocytosis. *Curr. Opin. Hematol.* 1997; **4**:136–141.
23. Bader-Meunier, B., Gauthier, F., Archambaud, F. *et al.* Long-term evaluation of the beneficial effect of subtotal splenectomy for the management of hereditary spherocytosis. *Blood* 2001; **97**:399–403.
24. Guzzetta, P. C., Ruley, E. J., Merrick, H. F. W. *et al.* Elective subtotal splenectomy – indications and results in 33 patients. *Ann. Surg.* 1990; **211**:34–42.
25. Svarch, E., Vilorio, P., Nordet, I. *et al.* Partial splenectomy in children with sickle cell disease and repeated episodes of splenic sequestration. *Hemoglobin* 1996; **20**:393–400.
26. Rice, H. E., Oldham, K. T., Hillery, C. A. *et al.* Clinical and hematologic benefits of partial splenectomy for congenital hemolytic anemias in children. *Ann. Surg.* 2003; **237**:281–288.
27. Brandt, C. T., Rothbarth, L. J., Kumpe, D., Karrer, F. M., & Lilly, J. R. Splenic embolization in children: long-term efficacy. *J. Pediatr. Surg.* 1989; **24**:642–644.
28. Petersons, A., Volrats, O., & Bernsteins, A. The first experience with non-operative treatment of hypersplenism in children with portal hypertension. *Eur. J. Pediatr. Surg.* 2002; **12**:299–303.
29. Tajiri, T. Long-term hematological and biochemical effects of partial splenic embolization in hepatic cirrhosis. *Hepatogastroenterology* 2002; **49**:1445–1448.
30. Nio, M., Hayashi, Y., Sano, N., Ishii, T., Sasaki, H., & Ohi R. Long-term efficacy of partial splenic embolization in children. *J. Pediatr. Surg.* 2003; **38**:1760–1762.
31. Shanmuganathan, K., Mirvis, S. E., Boyd-Kranis, R., Takada, T., & Scales, T. M. Nonsurgical management of blunt splenic injury: use of CT criteria to select patients for splenic arteriography and potential endovascular therapy. *Radiology* 2000; **217**:75–82.
32. Sclafani, S. J., Weisberg, A., & Scalea, T. M. Blunt splenic injuries: nonsurgical treatment with CT, arteriography, and transcatheter arterial embolization of the splenic artery. *Radiology* 1991; **181**:189.
33. Sclafani, S. J., Shaftan, G. W., Scalea, T. M. *et al.* Nonoperative salvage of computed tomography – diagnosed splenic injuries: utilization of angiography for triage and embolization for hemostasis. *J. Trauma* 1995; **39**:818–827.
34. Delaunay, J. Genetic disorders of the red cell membrane. *Crit. Rev. Oncol. Hematol.* 1995; **19**:79–110.
35. Sackey, K. Hemolytic anemia: part I. *Pediatr. Rev.* 1999; **20**:152–158.

36. Rice, H. E. Pediatric spleen surgery. In Oldham, K. T., Colombani, P. M., Foglia, R. P., Skinner, M. A., eds. *Surgery of Infants and Children*, Philadelphia: Lippincott Williams & Wilkins, 2005; 1511–1522.
37. Dover, G. & Valle, D. Therapy for β-thalassemia – a paradigm for the treatment of genetic disorders. *N. Engl. J. Med.* 1994; **331**:609–610.
38. Gaziev J. & Lucarelli G. Stem cell transplantation for hemoglobinopathies. *Curr. Opin. Pediatr.* 2003; **15**:42–31.
39. Forget B. G. Thalassemia syndromes. In *Hematology: Basic Principles and Practice*, ed. R. Hoffman, 3rd edn. pp.488–499. Oxford: Churchill Livingstone, 2000.
40. Hoe, T. S., Lammi, A., & Webster, B. Homozygous beta-thalassemia: a review of patients who had splenectomy at the Royal Alexandra Hospital for Children, Sydney. *Singapore Med. J.* 1994; **35**:59–61.
41. Idowu, O. & Jordan-Hayes, A. Partial splenectomy in children under 4 years of age with hemoglobinopathy. *J. Pediatr. Surg.* 1998; **33**:1251–1253.
42. deMontalembert, M., Girot, R., Revillon, Y. *et al.* Partial splenectomy in homozygous beta thalassemia. *Arch. Dis. Child.* 1990; **65**:304–307.
43. Politis, C., Spigos, D. G., Georgiopoulou, P. *et al.* Partial splenic embolization for hypersplenism of thalassemia major: five-year follow-up. *Br. Med. J.* 1987; **294**:665–667.
44. Pinca, A., Di Palma, A., Soriani, S. *et al.* Effectiveness of partial splenic embolization as treatment of hypersplenism in thalassemia major: a 7-year follow-up. *Eur. J. Haematol.* 1992; **49**:49–52.
45. Al-Salem, A. H., Naserullah, Z., Qaisaruddin, S. *et al.* Splenic complications of the sickling syndromes and the role of splenctomy. *J. Pediatr. Hematol. Oncol.* 1999; **21**:401–406.
46. Aquino, V. M., Norvell, J. M., Buchanan, G. R. Acute splenic complications in children with sickle cell-hemoglobin C disease. *J. Pediatr.* 1997; **130**:961–965.
47. Owusu-Ofori, S. & Riddington, C. Splenectomy versus conservative management for acute sequestration crises in people with sickling cell disease. *Cochrane Database Syst. Rev.* 2002; **4**:CD003425.
48. Kar, B. C. Splenectomy in sickle cell disease. *J. Assoc. Phys. India* 1999; **47**:890–893.
49. Svarch, E., Nordet, I., Valdes, J. *et al.* Partial splenectomy in children with sickle cell disease. *Haematologica* 2003; **88**:222–223.
50. DiPaola, J. A. & Buchanan, G. R. Immune thrombocytopenic purpura. *Pediatr. Clin. North. Am.* 2002; **49**:911–928.
51. Mandeiros, D. & Buchanan, G. R. Idiopathic thrombocytopenic purpura: beyond consensus. *Curr. Opin. Pediatr.* 2000; **12**:4–9.
52. Tura, S., Fiacchini, M., Zinzani, P. L., Brusamolino, E., & Gobbi, P. G. Splenectomy and the increasing risk of secondary acute leukemia in Hodgkin's disease. *J. Clin. Oncol.* 1993; **11**:925–930.
53. Dietrich, P. Y., Henry-Amar, M., Cosset, J. M., Bodis, S., Bosq, J., & Hayat, M. Secondary primary cancers in patients continuously disease-free from Hodgkin's disease: a protective role for the spleen? *Blood* 1994; **84**:1209–1215.
54. Brodsky, J., Abcar, A., & Styler, M. Splenectomy for non-Hodgkin's lymphoma. *Am. J. Clin. Oncol.* 1996; **19**:558–561.
55. Morel, P., Dupriez, B., Gosselin, B. *et al.* Role of early splenectomy in malignant lymphomas with prominent splenic involvement (primary lymphomas of the spleen). A study of 59 cases. *Cancer* 1993; **71**:207–215.
56. Yoong, Y., Kurtin, P. J., Allmer, C., Geyer, S. *et al.* Efficacy of splenectomy for patients with mantle cell non-Hodgkin's lymphoma. *Leuk Lymphoma* 2001; **42**:1235–1241.
57. Rubin, M., Yampolski, I., Lambrozo, R. *et al.* Partial splenectomy in Gaucher's disease. *J. Pediatr. Surg.* 1986; **21**:125–128.
58. Fleshnew, P. R., Aufses, A. H., Grabowski, G. A. *et al.* A 27-year experience with splenectomy for Gaucher's disease. *Am. J. Surg.* 1991; **161**:69–75.
59. Zer, M. & Freud, E. Subtotal splenectomy in Gaucher's disease: towards a definition of critical splenic mass. *Br. J. Surg.* 1993; **80**:399.
60. Freud, E., Cohen, I. J., Mor, C. *et al.* Splenic "regeneration" after partial splenectomy for Gaucher disease: histological features. *Blood Cells, Molec. Dis.* 1998; **24**:309–316.
61. Dweck, A., Abrahamov, A., Hadas-Halpern, I. *et al.* Type I Gaucher disease in children with and without enzyme therapy. *Pediatr. Hematol. Oncol.* 2002; **19**:389–397.
62. Weinreb, N. J., Charrow, J., Andersson, H. C. *et al.* Effectiveness of enzyme replacement therapy in 1028 patients with type I Gaucher disease after 2 to 5 years of treatment: a report from the Gaucher registry. *Am. J. Med.* 2002; **113**:112–119.
63. Davidson, R. N. & Wall, R. A. Prevention and management of infections in patients without a spleen. *Clin. Microbiol. Infect.* 2001; **7**:657–660.
64. Horan, M. & Colebatch, J. H. Relation between splenectomy and subsequent infection: a clinical study. *Arch. Dis. Child.* 1962; **37**:398.
65. Ellis, E. F. & Smith, R. T. The role of the spleen in immunity with special references to the post-splenectomy problems in infants. *Pediatrics* 1966; **37**:111.
66. Ellison, E. C. & Fabri, P. J. Complications of splenectomy. *Surg. Clin. North. Am.* 1983; **63**:1313.
67. Holdsworth, R. J., Irving, A. D., & Cuschieri, A. Postsplenectomy sepsis and its mortality rate: actual versus perceived risks. *Br. J. Surg.* 1991; **78**:1031.
68. Bisharat, N., Omari, H., Lavi, I., & Raz, R. Risk of infection and death among post-splenectomy patients. *J. Infect.* 2001; **43**:183–186.
69. Sumaraju, V., Smith, L. G., & Smith, S. M. Infectious complications in asplenic hosts. *Infect. Dis. North Am.* 2001; **15**(2) 551–565.
70. Deodhar, H. A., Marshall, R. J., & Barnes, J. N. Increased risk of sepsis after splenectomy. *Br. Med. J.* 1993; **307**:1408.
71. Castagnola, E. & Fioredda, F. Prevention of life-threatening infections due to encapsulated bacteria in children with hyposplenia or asplenia: a brief review of current recommendations for practical purposes. *Eur. J. Haematol.* 2003; **71**:319–326.
72. Konradsen, H. B., Rasmussen, C., Ejstrud, P., & Hansen, J. B. Antibody levels against *Streptococcus pneumoniae* and

Haemophilus influenzae type B in a population of splenectomized individuals with varying vaccination status. *Epidemiol. Infect.* 1997; **119**:167–174.

73. Eber, S. W., Langendorfer, C. M., Ditzig, M. *et al.* Frequency of very late fatal sepsis after splenectomy for hereditary spherocytosis: impact of insufficient antibody response to pneumococcal infection. *Ann. Hematol.* 1999; **78**:524–528.
74. Gaston, M. H., Verter, J. I., Woods, G. *et al.* Prophylaxis with oral penicillin in children with sickle cell anemia: a randomized trial. *N. Eng. J. Med.* 1986; **314**:1593–1599.
75. White, K. S., Covington, D., Churchill, P. *et al.* Patient awareness of health precautions after splenectomy. *Am. J. Infect. Contr.* 1991; **19**:36–41.
76. Kinnersley, P., Wilkinson, C. E., & Srinivasan, J. Pneumococcal vaccination after splenectomy: Survey of hospital and primary care records. *Br. Med. J.* 1993; **307**:1398–1399.
77. Rasmussen, C., Ejstrud, P., Hansen, J. B., & Konradsen, H. B. Asplenic patients' knowledge of prophylactic measures against severe infections (brief report). *Clin. Infect. Dis.* 1997; **25** (3):738.
78. Wright, J. G., Hambelton, I. R., Thomas, P. W. *et al.* Postsplenectomy course in homozygous sickle cell disease. *J. Pediatr.* 1991; **134**:304–309.
79. Brigden, M. L. & Pattullo, A. L. Prevention and management of overwhelming postsplenectomy infection: an update. *Crit. Care Med.* 1999; **27**:836–842.

35

Biliary atresia

Edward R. Howard

King's College Hospital, London, UK

Introduction

Biliary atresia presents in the neonatal period, occurs with a frequency of between 1 in 8000 and 1 in 16 000 live births and accounts for more than 50% of pediatric liver transplantation.[1] The cause of the disease remains obscure but current evidence suggests that there is more than one etiologic factor. Both the intra- and extrahepatic bile ducts are affected and affected infants present with jaundice and pale stools within the first few weeks of life. The intrahepatic pathology, which has been likened to sclerosing cholangitis,[2] is accompanied by an inflammatory sclerosing lesion of the extrahepatic bile ducts, which results in obstruction of the lumen and, in some cases, complete disappearance of segments of the biliary tract. Death from cirrhotic liver failure occurs within 2 years in untreated cases and biliary atresia represents the most frequent reason for liver transplantation in childhood.

Historical issues

Thomson[3] published the first major review in 1892. He collected 49 cases from the literature and added a further case of his own. He recorded that "the children themselves are either jaundiced at birth, or they become so within the first week or so of life; otherwise they are healthy and well nourished." He concluded that, whatever the etiology of the condition, it was characterized by a progressive destructive inflammatory lesion of the biliary tract. A majority of the affected infants he described died from complications of spontaneous hemorrhage during the first few months of life and the increased risk of bleeding was ascribed to an "impoverishment of the blood". He suggested that the inflammatory component of biliary atresia was secondary to a congenital abnormality of the ducts, which interferes with bile flow and that the inflammation is progressive and can result in a variable pattern of duct occlusion. He also suggested that the obliteration of the ducts becomes complete at an early, but variable period during intrauterine life.

Holmes, in 1916,[4] first suggested that some cases of biliary atresia might be surgically correctable. He reviewed more than 100 case reports and found evidence of residual segments of bile ducts in 16%. Diagnostic confusion is evident in some of the early case reports. Ladd,[5] for example, reported surgical correction in eight out of 20 cases in 1928 but it appears that two were examples of choledochal cysts and two were patients with neonatal hepatitis and hypoplastic bile ducts rather than biliary atresia.

Historically, cases of biliary atresia were described as "correctable" or "non-correctable" depending on the presence or absence of residual patent segments of proximal bile ducts. Successful surgical treatment was uncommon; Hays and Snyder reported in 1963[6] that less than 5% of children with biliary atresia survived beyond early childhood. A variety of ineffective surgical procedures were tried, including partial hepatectomy, the insertion of a variety of tubes into the hepatic parenchyma and the drainage of lymph into the gastrointestinal tract via an anastomosis between the thoracic duct and the esophagus.

More than 85% of biliary atresia is of the "non-correctable" type in which there is occlusion of the hepatic ducts at the porta hepatis. In 1959, radical resection of the extrahepatic biliary tree was proposed after histologic studies had revealed that microscopic ductular structures

Pediatric Surgery and Urology: Long-term Outcomes, Mark Stringer, Keith Oldham, Pierre Mouriquand.
Published by Cambridge University Press.

Table 35.1. Chromosomal abnormalities associated with biliary atresia

• Trisomy 18	– Ikeda *et al.*[10]
• Trisomy 18	– Buffa *et al.*[11]
• Trisomy 17–18	– Alpert *et al.*[12]
• Trisomy 21	– Danks[13]

were present in tissue resected from the porta hepatis. The ductules, which measured up to 300 μm in diameter, were shown to communicate with intrahepatic ducts. Successful drainage of bile was observed after resection of all residual biliary tissue in the porta hepatis and anastomosis of the resected area to a Roux loop of bowel allowed satisfactory transit of bile into the gut (the portoenterostomy operation).[7,8] The operation was shown to be most effective when performed before eight weeks of age. An increasing number of portoenterostomy patients have since survived into adult life.

The chance of long-term survival was further increased by the development of liver transplantation. Failure to achieve satisfactory early bile flow after portoenterostomy, or progression to cirrhotic liver failure later in life, are now recognized indications for transplantation.

Studies of etiology

The etiology of biliary atresia remains unknown, but current evidence suggests that there may be a genetic defect in morphogenesis in approximately 20% of cases. Hypotheses for the remaining 80% have included viral, autoimmune and immune-mediated pathogeneses as well as damage to the biliary tract by toxic monohydroxy bile acids.[9]

Embryologic and genetic factors

There are a few reports of an association with chromosomal abnormalities which have included trisomy 17, 18, and 21 (Table 35.1). Twin studies, however, have not suggested any significant genetic transmission with reports of only two pairs of offspring concordant for biliary atresia,[14,15] compared with 21 discordant pairs.[16]

Reports of a familial incidence of biliary atresia are also unusual and have included two affected siblings in each of ten families, and three affected siblings in each of four families.[15]

A study of human leukocyte antigens (HLA) in 55 children was reported to show a significantly higher frequency of HLA-B12, A9-B5 and A28-B35, and of their disequilibrium values compared with controls.[17] It was concluded that immunogenetic factors may have a role in determining susceptibility to the disease. However, the later studies of Jurado *et al.*[18] and Donaldson *et al.*[19] failed to identify any relationship between biliary atresia and HLA status.

Desmet and Callea[20] observed that the majority of intrahepatic bile ducts affected by epithelial damage and destruction in biliary atresia have a mature tubular shape. However, 20%–25% of cases show features reminiscent of "ductal plate malformation" which is represented by partial or complete persistence of the original embryonic form of the intrahepatic ducts.

Human embryologic studies have shown a striking similarity between the appearances of normal developing bile ducts during the first trimester of pregnancy and the abnormal ductules observed within the residual tissue resected from the porta hepatis during portoenterostomy.[21] These studies demonstrate that at 6 weeks' gestation the biliary epithelium of the ductal plate arises from hepatocyte precursor cells at the hepatic–mesenchymal margin adjacent to the portal vein. At 11 weeks' gestation the common hepatic duct, which arises from the hepatic diverticulum of the foregut, is in communication with the lumen of the ductal plate. Intrahepatic ducts develop towards the periphery of the liver at around 12 weeks and bile first appears at this time. Comparison of the embryologic features at 12 weeks with sections of tissue taken from the porta hepatis of infants with biliary atresia reveals similar histologic features. The histologic appearances in biliary atresia might result from a disruption in the process of remodelling of the ductal plate during this phase of development together with an inflammatory reaction secondary to bile leakage from abnormal ducts.

Evidence for an early gestational origin of biliary atresia has been provided by antenatal ultrasound diagnosis on at least five occasions.[22] Hinds *et al.*[23] reported that nine of 194 cases of atresia had been detected on routine antenatal scanning. At surgery six had type 3 disease, two had type 2, and one had type 1. All nine cases underwent successful portoenterostomy. Furthermore, estimations of gamma-glutamyl transpeptidase (GGT) activity in amniotic fluid samples taken at different points in gestation from 10 000 pregnant women showed low levels of the enzyme between 18 and 20 weeks in three cases. The infants of these three women were found to have biliary atresia.[24] Further support for the relationship of low amniotic GGT levels and biliary atresia was reported by Ben-Ami *et al.*[25] GGT is synthesized in the liver, reaches the gut in bile, and passes into the amniotic fluid during defecation. The observation of low levels of the enzyme in amniotic fluid is consistent with an onset of biliary atresia early in gestation.

Infective factors

Although there were early reports of a possible relationship between biliary atresia and infection with cytomegalovirus (CMV),[26] rubella[27] and Epstein–Barr virus (EBV),[28] the evidence remains confusing. This confusion is illustrated by studies of human papillomavirus (HPV). Drut *et al.*[29] reported evidence of HPV infection in liver biopsies from 16 out of 18 cases of BA compared with no evidence of infection in 30 control cases. In contrast, Domiati-Saad *et al.*[30] showed no association with HPV infection in 19 cases of neonatal hepatitis or BA. These children were also negative for EBV, although three cases were positive for CMV. Jevon and Dimmick[31] also examined bile duct tissue from 12 cases of BA for evidence of CMV infection but all were negative.

Most experimental work on infection has related to the hepatotropic RNA viruses, reovirus and rotavirus. Weanling mice exposed to reo 3 virus develop chronic liver disease and obstructive jaundice[32] and histologic examination of the porta hepatis shows changes with similarities to biliary atresia.[33] Morecki *et al.*[34] reported reovirus antigens in 68% of a group of infants with biliary atresia compared with 8% of age-matched controls, but other studies failed to confirm the results.[35,36] There is also conflicting evidence for the role of reovirus infection from studies using reverse transcriptase polymerase chain reaction (RT-PCR) techniques. Tyler *et al.*[37] detected reovirus RNA in hepatic and/or biliary tissues from 55% of 23 infants with biliary atresia compared with 12%–21% of control cases but these findings were at variance with a previous study.[38]

The case for a viral etiology in biliary atresia remains unproven.

Associated abnormalities

A review of ten major series of biliary atresia showed that an average of 21% had additional abnormalities outside of the hepatobiliary system.[16] The most frequent abnormalities affected the cardiovascular system, the gut (situs inversus) and the spleen (Table 35.2).[39] A variety of splenic malformations have been described which include the polysplenia syndrome,[40] double spleen, and asplenia.[41] The polysplenia syndrome includes multiple spleens, situs inversus, preduodenal portal vein and malformations of the inferior vena cava. Davenport *et al.*[41] reported a 7.5% incidence of the syndrome in 308 cases of atresia and proposed the term "biliary atresia splenic malformation" (BASM). It was noted that four infants with BASM were born to mothers with diabetes mellitus. Fischler *et al.*,[42] in an investigation of 85 cholestatic infants in Sweden, showed that the mothers of biliary atresia patients had a higher mean age and were more commonly treated for gestational diabetes than mothers of patients with other causes of jaundice. Davenport *et al.*[41] suggested that the BASM syndrome might be a subgroup with a separate etiology from the more common cases of biliary atresia without extrahepatic abnormalities and that the insult to the bile duct might occur early in gestation at a time coinciding with the development of the spleen and gut rotation.

Table 35.2. Biliary atresia and associated abnormalities in 251 patients (Carmi *et al.*[39])

30 (59%)	Isolated abnormalities (cardiac, renal, etc.)
15 (29%)	Multiple abnormalities (polysplenia, preduodenal portal vein, situs inversus, etc.)
6 (12%)	Situs inversus alone
Total	51 (20%)

Organ asymmetry in the embryo starts to occur before 30 days' gestation and would be disturbed by suppression of left- or right-sided development. Deletion of the inversin (INV) gene in transgenic mice[43] results in situs inversus and atretic bile ducts. It was suggested that this might imply a role for the inversin gene in normal human bile duct development and that such a gene mutation might support a genetic basis of the BASM syndrome. However, a study of 65 patients with laterality defects did not reveal any mutation of the human inversin gene and the authors concluded that "the absence of mutation in a series of 7 cases with lateralization defects and biliary anomalies (BASM), demonstrates that INV is not frequently involved in such a phenotype in humans."[44]

Presentation and immediate management

Physiologic jaundice (unconjugated hyperbilirubinemia) occurs in up to 90% of healthy neonates and is defined as a temporary inefficient hepatic excretion of bilirubin. Conjugated hyperbilirubinemia (hepatitis syndrome) is always pathological and may be caused by hepatocellular dysfunction secondary to infective, metabolic, drug, and endocrine disorders. The clinical presentation of structural defects such as biliary atresia is similar to the presentation of hepatocellular disease in the young infant and because of the urgent need for surgical correction of atresia the hepatocellular causes of conjugated hyperbilirubinemia such as alpha-1-antitrypsin deficiency, cystic fibrosis and endocrine disorders must be rapidly excluded.[45]

As well as conjugated hyperbilirubinemia and non-pigmented, white stools in biliary atresia patients there may be some hepatomegaly and, in a minority of cases, a range of associated abnormalities that can include cardiac defects, situs inversus and renal problems. Splenomegaly becomes more obvious after the first eight to 12 weeks of life and poor weight gain and growth retardation also occur with increasing age.

It is advised that all infants who remain jaundiced after 14 days of age should have urinalysis for bilirubin and measurement of total and direct bilirubin in serum. Physiologic jaundice has usually disappeared by this time except in a small number of breast fed infants. If conjugated bilirubin is present and the stools are non-pigmented, investigations for biliary atresia should proceed immediately.

It should be emphasized that most infants with biliary atresia are entirely well during the first 4 to 8 weeks of life apart from moderate jaundice. The diagnosis will only be suspected by the demonstration of conjugated hyperbilirubinemia and this must be investigated in an infant with yellow, rather than colourless, urine and pale stools.[46]

Investigations

Early diagnosis is imperative for good results after portoenterostomy (see below) and infective, metabolic, endocrine, and drug-related causes of conjugated hyperbilirubinemia are excluded as quickly as possible so that surgery may be performed within the first 8 to 10 weeks of life. In early infancy the clinical features and biochemical tests of liver function are very similar in hepatocellular disease, hypoplasia of the bile ducts, obstruction of the extrahepatic ducts caused by choledochal cysts, and biliary atresia. Biochemical tests of liver function, such as the intracellular enzymes aspartate aminotransferase (AST), and alanine aminotransferase (ALT), give a measure of the severity of the liver disease but are of little diagnostic help. All four conditions present with jaundice, pale stools and dark urine and may be complicated by bleeding from malabsorption of vitamin K. Ultrasound examination is useful for assessing the structure of the gall bladder and the presence or absence of a choledochal cyst, inspissated bile, or gall stones. Intrahepatic bile duct dilatation is not a feature of biliary atresia and this limits the value of sonography, although an abnormally small or absent gall bladder may be suggestive of the diagnosis. Technetium labelled compounds such as methylbromoiminodiacetic acid (BrIDA), which are taken up by hepatocytes even in the presence of jaundice, are excreted into the biliary tract in high concentrations. No excretion of the isotope within 24 hours suggests a differential diagnosis of severe cholestasis or biliary atresia. The sensitivity of the investigation is increased by the prior administration of a 3-day course of phenobarbitone (5 mg/kg per day).

Percutaneous biopsy of the liver is mandatory and although equivocal histologic findings are present in approximately 13% of cases,[47] this failure rate may be improved by combining the biopsy with a laparoscopy and laparoscopic-guided cholangiography.[48] Alternatively, endoscopic retrograde cholangiography (ERC) may be indicated in an infant who has shown no excretion of isotope from the liver but in whom the histology is doubtful. In an early series of nine cases of neonatal jaundice investigated in this way, normal bile ducts were demonstrated in four and atresia suggested in four.[49] However, one of the latter cases proved to have patent bile ducts at surgery. One examination was a technical failure. Accurate results were therefore achieved in seven out of nine cases (78%). In a larger series, the diagnostic success rate with ERC was 86%.[50] Iinuma *et al.*[51] reported successful visualization of the biliary tract in 43 of 50 ERCPs without complication. Biliary atresia was diagnosed after successful cannulation of the ampulla and opacification of the pancreatic duct or a small residual segment of bile duct. Diagnoses of neonatal hepatitis, biliary hypoplasia or choledochal cyst were achieved after complete imaging of the biliary tract in 14 infants. Biliary atresia was later confirmed at surgery in six of the seven examinations classified as technical failures. A further advantage of ERCP is the ability to observe and aspirate the contents of the duodenum as the presence of bile excludes a diagnosis of atresia.

A firm diagnosis of biliary atresia therefore requires a series of tests, all of which must be completed in a short period of time. A preoperative diagnosis is very important to the surgeon because the lumen of the biliary tract in an infant with either hepatocellular dysfunction or biliary hypoplasia is very small and failure to adequately visualize the bile ducts with intraoperative cholangiography could result in unnecessary surgery.[52]

Pathology and influence on long-term outcome

The liver architecture in biliary atresia is preserved during the first few weeks of life but occlusion of the extrahepatic ducts leads to widening of the portal tracts with edema and increased amounts of fibrous tissue. Proliferation of bile ductules is accompanied by bile stasis within both canaliculi and hepatocytes. In contrast, typical findings in neonatal hepatitis include hepatocellular necrosis with an inflammatory cell infiltrate in the hepatic parenchyma and multinucleate giant cell formation. However, these features are not pathognomonic and may be observed in some cases of biliary atresia, reducing the accuracy of liver biopsy to between 83% and 87%.[47,53] Alpha-1-antitrypsin deficiency is diagnosed in 10%–20% of infants who present with the neonatal hepatitis syndrome and percutaneous liver biopsy in this condition may show features similar to those of biliary atresia. The difficulty with histologic diagnosis of alpha-1-antitrypsin deficiency may be compounded by the absence of PAS-positive inclusions, which are characteristic of this condition in older patients, and urgent phenotyping is therefore essential as part of the investigation of persistent neonatal hyperbilirubinemia. Difficulty in the interpretation of liver biopsies may also occur in infants with biliary hypoplasia. Inflammatory features may be present within the parenchyma and portal tracts but, in contrast to biliary atresia, bile ductules are absent or very sparse. However, the not infrequent syndromic association with vertebral anomalies, cardiovascular defects such as pulmonary stenosis, and a characteristic facial appearance aids the diagnosis of hypoplasia.[54]

The appearances of the extrahepatic bile ducts in biliary atresia vary greatly from case to case and may lead the inexperienced surgeon to an incorrect diagnosis. Abnormal segmental dilatations, for example, may superficially resemble a choledochal cyst. Proximal dilatation of the common hepatic duct may be secondary to an atretic occlusion of the distal common bile duct and although satisfactory bile drainage may be achieved after hepaticojejunostomy, the intrahepatic changes of biliary atresia may still affect the long-term prognosis. Non-communicating segmental dilatations containing clear mucus can also occur at any level of the extrahepatic biliary tract and may be misdiagnosed as a choledochal cyst and hence treated with an ineffectual anastomosis of bile duct to bowel.

The historical classification of "correctable" and "non-correctable" atresia was replaced by a classification devised by the Japanese Society of Pediatric Surgeons more than 25 years ago.[55] The lesions were classified into three principal types:

- type 1: a bile-containing dilatation of a residual segment of proximal bile duct communicating with intrahepatic ducts
- type 2: residual lumen in undilated right and left hepatic ducts communicating with intrahepatic ducts but with atresia of the common hepatic duct
- type 3: complete atresia of the extrahepatic biliary tree including the right and left hepatic ducts

An analysis of 643 cases showed a 10% incidence of type 1 and an 88% incidence of type 3 atresias. Type 2 lesions were rare and made up only 2% of the series.[56] Histologic assessment of the residual biliary tissue found at the porta hepatis may show persisting segments of the right and/or left hepatic ducts, multiple ductules, inflammatory cell infiltrates and fibrosis but even the larger duct remnants show at least partial loss of epithelium. The histologic appearances of the tissue at the porta hepatis have been classified into three main types.[57] In type 1 the bile ducts are replaced completely by fibrous tissue with an inflammatory cell infiltrate and there is a complete absence of ducts and ductules. Type 2 tissue contains small ductules, approximately 50 μm in diameter, which are lined by cuboidal epithelium. In type 3 cases, bile ducts lined by columnar epithelium and bile-containing macrophages are present in more than two-thirds of resected specimens. Three-dimensional reconstruction studies have shown that, during the first few weeks of life, intrahepatic bile ducts are in communication with the residual tissue in the porta hepatis. The terminal portions of these bile ducts are the small ductules observed in tissue resected during the operation of portoenterostomy. The number of intrahepatic ducts decreases progressively with age but this process may be arrested if satisfactory bile drainage can be established within the first few weeks of life.[58]

It has been suggested that satisfactory bile flow may be anticipated after portoenterostomy when histological examination reveals residual ducts at the porta hepatis with diameters greater than 150 μm.[59,60] However, good bile flow can be achieved in cases with much smaller ducts and histologic analysis is not always a good guide to prognosis.[61] No statistically significant difference in bile ductule histology in tissue from the porta hepatis could be identified by Tagge *et al.*[62] who found, in a series of 34 cases, that 43% with residual ducts less than 150 μm in diameter became anicteric compared with 36% of those with ducts over 150 μm.

The response to surgery cannot be predicted from the histology of the hepatic parenchyma. Analyses of hepatic fibrosis, inflammatory change, and giant cell formation have not shown any clear correlation with postoperative bile flow.[63,64] It is disappointing that hepatic fibrosis may even increase after achieving good biliary drainage; this progression has been demonstrated in 70% of long-term jaundice-free patients.[65] The original Japanese classification of bile duct morphology in biliary atresia included many subtypes which recorded the patency or occlusion of the distal common bile duct, the anatomic features of the gall bladder and the appearance of residual tissue at the

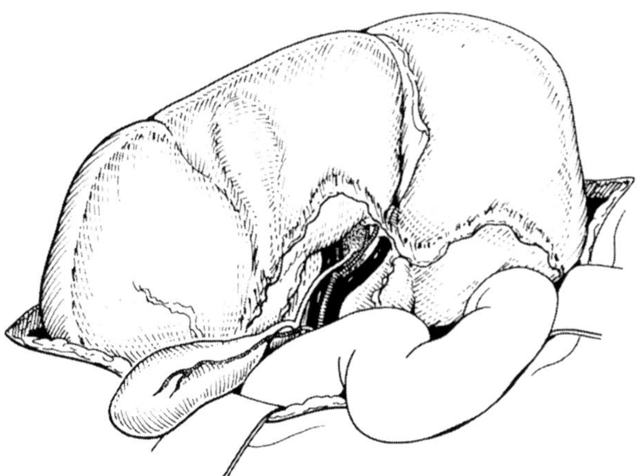

Fig. 35.1. Figures 1–7 illustrate the operation of portoenterostomy. The operation commences with mobilization of the liver to expose the porta hepatis. Reproduced with permission, from Howard ER. *Rob and Smith's Operative Surgery 5th edn – Paediatric Surgery*; Chapman & Hall;1995:551–561).

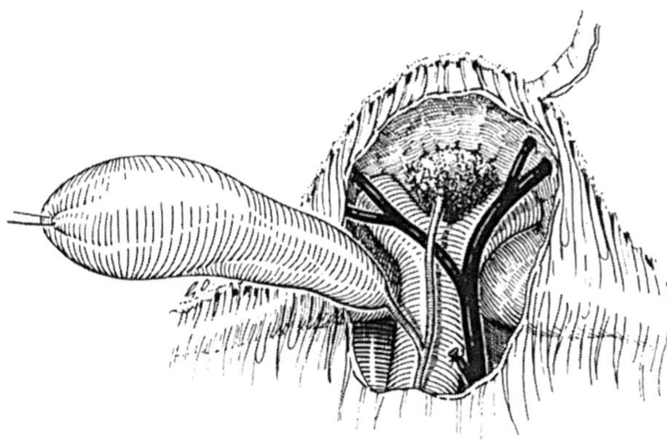

Fig. 35.2. The mobilized gall bladder is used as a guide to the fibrous remnants of the extrahepatic bile ducts.

porta hepatis. Tan *et al.*[66] analyzed the pattern and extent of the obliteration of the extrahepatic bile ducts in 205 cases and classified them into seven types but they found no correlation with long-term prognosis. It is concluded that these subtypes have little prognostic significance.

The macroscopic appearances of the liver, porta hepatis, and portal venous system were recorded and correlated prospectively with subsequent bile flow.[67] After a mean follow-up period of 32 months, 20 infants had a successful outcome compared with ten failures. Statistical analysis revealed that the only significant positive correlation with a successful outcome was the size of the tissue mass at the porta hepatis.

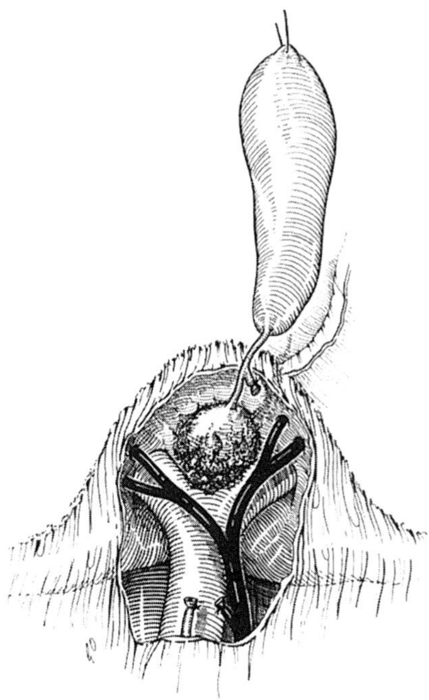

Fig. 35.3. The common bile duct is divided and the hepatic artery and portal vein are exposed.

Surgical techniques

Portoenterostomy

The operation was first devised by Kasai[68] who observed that excision of all residual bile duct tissue from the porta hepatis could result in satisfactory drainage of bile from residual bile ducts. The essential steps in the operation are detailed in Figs. 35.1–35.7. It is important that the porta hepatis is fully visualized during the operation and in many cases this is only achieved by full mobilization of the liver and rotation of its inferior surface. The dissection extends behind the bifurcation of the portal vein and small tributaries of the vein to the caudate lobe are ligated to avoid hemorrhage during resection of the residual bile duct tissue. The biliary tissue at the porta hepatis is excised, together with the gallbladder and common bile duct, in a plane which is parallel with the liver capsule. The capsule itself should be damaged as little as possible as this might cause fibrous occlusion of the ductules at the porta hepatis. A long Roux loop of jejunum is used for the anastomosis at the porta hepatis; cutaneous enterostomies and antireflux valves are no longer in general use as they have not proved effective in the prevention of recurrent cholangitis (see below). Attempts to replace

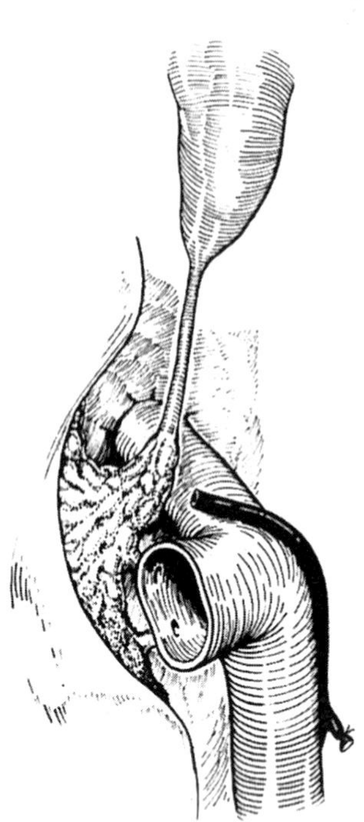

Fig. 35.4. The bifurcation of the portal vein is mobilized with division of tributaries to the caudate lobe.

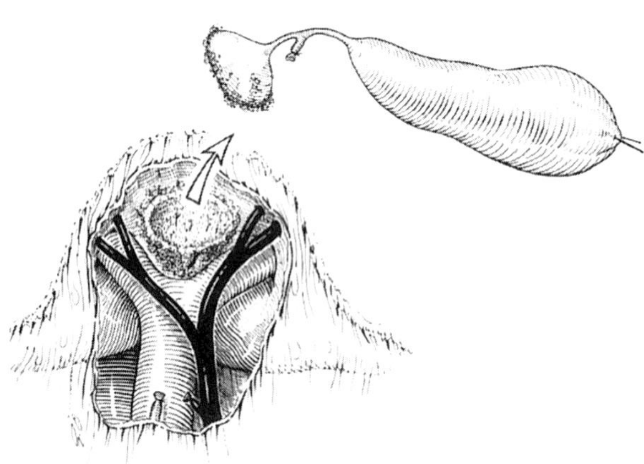

Fig. 35.5. The fibrous tissue in the porta hepatis is divided flush with the capsule of the liver. All tissue within the main divisions of the vessels is removed.

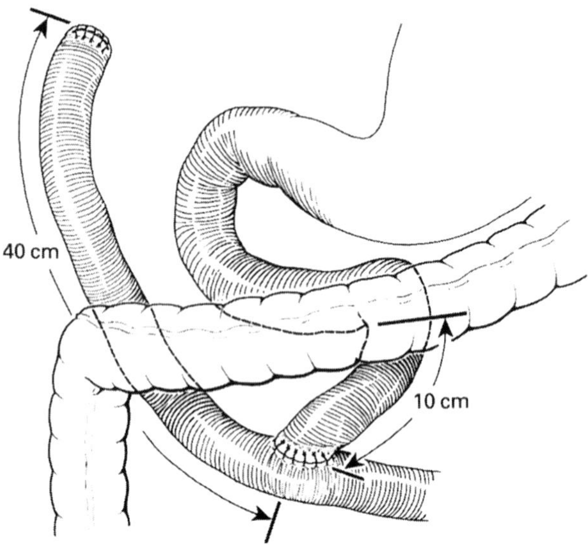

Fig. 35.6. A 40 cm Roux-en-Y loop of jejunum is prepared and passed in a retrocolic manner to the hilum of the liver.

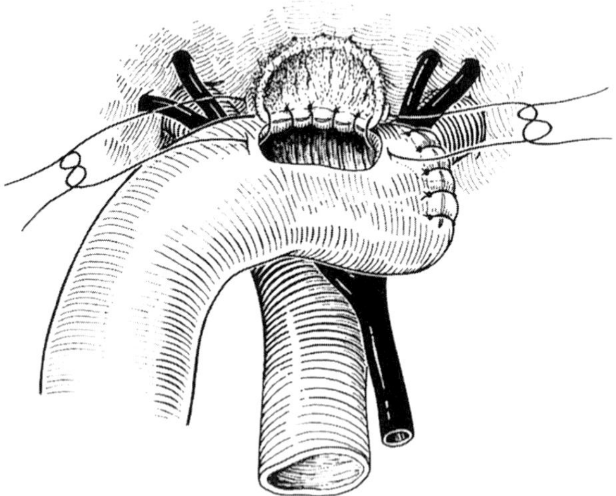

Fig. 35.7. An anastomosis is fashioned between the cut edge of the transected tissue in the porta hepatis and the side of the Roux loop.

the Roux loop with a conduit fashioned from the appendix (porto-appendiceal-duodenostomy), have also proved less effective than the standard operation, and a comparison of the results of the two procedures showed effective bile drainage in 31% of cases treated with an appendiceal conduit and 82% in those with a standard Roux loop of jejunum.[69] Accurate dissection of the porta hepatis remains the most important factor in achieving successful bile drainage.

In common with many other abdominal operations, portoenterostomy has now been performed laparoscopically in children.[70] Four trochar ports were used for access and the Roux-en-Y jejunal anastomosis was performed through the umbilical port. The authors claimed that the technique avoids liver mobilization and the consequent risk of extensive adhesion formation.

Hepaticojejunostomy

In cases of type 1 atresia the remnant of proximal bile duct may be large enough to allow the construction of a conventional hepaticojejunostomy. However, this is possible in only a small minority of cases.

Portocholecystostomy

The gallbladder has been used for biliary drainage after cholangiographic confirmation of the patency of the cystic and distal common bile ducts. Complications are more frequent than after the standard portoenterostomy operation and include bile leaks, gallbladder obstruction, and kinking of the common bile duct.[71,72] However, there does appear to be a reduction in postoperative cholangitis compared with portoenterostomy. A survey of 670 children from the North American Biliary Atresia Registry reported a 35% incidence of cholangitis after portocholecystostomy compared with 55% after other types of reconstruction ($P = 0.02$). The data were collected from more than 100 institutions.[73]

Postoperative management

Fat-soluble vitamins are essential in preventing metabolic and coagulation abnormalities after surgery. Phenobarbitone and cholestyramine are often used to try and maximize bile flow although small prospective randomized controlled trials have not shown any definite advantage.[74,75] Steroids have been suggested to prevent fibrosis at the porta hepatis but there are, as yet, no published controlled trials to prove their efficacy. Reports of the use of steroids in patients who have suffered from either cholangitis or diminishing bile flow have been encouraging. Kasai *et al.*[76] recommended prednisolone 20 mg/day with a gradual reduction over 2 to 3 weeks and Altman and Anderson[77] used 2 mg/kg per day with a reduction over 12 days. Karrer and Lilly,[78] gave 10 mg/kg as an initial dose to 16 patients and discontinued the treatment after 4–7 days. The results were compared with 16 infants who were treated with antibiotics alone. In comparison with the controls, the patients treated with steroids seemed to show significant increases in their daily bile output; reductions in serum alkaline phosphatase and bilirubin levels were also noted. However, interpretation of these results is not straightforward as seven of the children had undergone revisional surgery before starting steroid therapy and the long-term results of the treatment were not given.

Dillon *et al.*[79] reported freedom from jaundice in 76% of 25 portoenterostomies who had been given long-term postoperative oral steroids. Unfortunately, these cases were not part of a randomized trial and similar results have been reported in steroid-free series (see below). A further study comparing 14 infants treated with portoenterostomy and steroids (prednisone 2 mg/kg per day) with 14 who were not given steroids showed a 79% success rate in the former group compared with 21% in the latter.[80] As in the previous report, this was not a randomized trial and treatment depended on surgeon preference.

In summary, a beneficial effect of corticosteroid therapy after portoenterostomy remains unproven.

Long-term complications following surgery

Cholangitis

Early cholangitis

Most surgeons give some form of antibiotic prophylaxis during the perioperative period to prevent attacks of bacterial cholangitis. The antibiotics are continued for a variable length of time but good evidence of any long-term benefit is not clear. Chaudary and Turner,[81] recommended that trimethoprim-sulphamethoxazole (TMP/SMZ) be used for all cases after portoenterostomy and based this advice on the successful treatment of four children, who had suffered repeated attacks of cholangitis. Bu *et al.*[82] compared two groups of infants treated with either TMP/SMZ or neomycin prophylaxis and compared both with a group of prophylaxis-free patients over a period of 14 months. The two treatment regimens were equally effective in reducing the rates of cholangitis compared with the control patients ($P = 0.042$ and 0.011). However, other authors have found no significant benefit from prophylaxis. For example, in one series of 41 infants, nine developed cholangitis, five of whom had received antibiotics and four no prophylaxis.[83] A large multicentre prospective trial will be required to resolve this problem.

Cholangitis, which is believed to be an ascending infection from the bowel affecting partially drained segments of liver, continues to be a major postoperative problem. (It is very rarely a problem after the surgical correction of choledochal cysts in which there is free drainage from all intrahepatic bile ducts.) Episodes of infection occur after portoenterostomy in 30%–60% of cases[84] and can cause at least a transient deterioration in liver function. A wide range of enteric organisms may be identified and include *E. coli*, *Proteus*, and *Klebsiella* spp., *Pseudomonas aeruginosa*, *Acinobacter baumanni* and *Salmonella typhi*.[85] Treatment of acute attacks is empirical and includes the prompt use of wide spectrum antibiotics such as cephalosporins and gentamicin.

Houwen *et al.*[86] reported that the incidence of cholangitis was the most important determinant of successful surgical outcome. A 5-year survival rate of 54% was recorded in patients who suffered cholangitis compared with 91% for patients who remained free of infection.

Prevention of enteric infection by separating the biliary and gastrointestinal tracts has resulted in the development of many types of external biliary diversion.[87] However, the cholangitis rate has been little affected by these procedures and when a group of 12 patients with biliary diversion was compared with a group of 19 who did not have diversion the incidence of cholangitis was almost identical (33% vs. 32%).[84] A difference in cholangitis rates for different operations does not necessarily influence outcome. For example, Tagge *et al.*[62] performed a standard Kasai operation in 32% of 34 cases and a complete diversion of bile in 68%. Although there was a higher incidence of cholangitis in the biliary diversion group, there was no difference in the one-year survival.

Ohi[88] illustrated and evaluated the results of various modified procedures performed throughout Japan between 1981 and 1985. He found that 43% had suffered attacks of cholangitis and that the first attack commonly occurred from one to three months after portoenterostomy. Only 10% developed infection for the first time more than 6 months after surgery. Importantly, 45% of 153 patients who had the original unmodified type of portoenterostomy had at least one attack of cholangitis compared with 41% of those who had modified procedures which included Roux-en-Y loops with tube enterostomies, complete diversion of bile via cutaneous stomas, interposition biliary conduits, and gastric tube reconstructions. One small prospective study investigated the value of an antireflux valve, constructed by intussuscepting a segment of bowel in the Roux-en-Y loop of jejunum; the valve made no significant difference to the incidence of subsequent attacks of cholangitis.[89] Most of these techniques are now of historical interest only as they appear to be of little benefit and they increase the difficulties of transplantation, should this be necessary at a later date. External stomas may also be complicated by excessive electrolyte losses and by bleeding from varices that readily form on the stomal margins.

Patency of the gallbladder and distal common bile duct was observed in 28% of boys and 18% of girls in 904 cases collected by the Biliary Atresia Registry of N. America.[73] This variant of biliary atresia allows the use of the gallbladder as a conduit for biliary drainage (see above). Infants undergoing portocholecystostomy had a 35% incidence of cholangitis compared with 55% for other types of reconstruction. Ohi[88] also reported a relatively low incidence of cholangitis (20%) in his review of this procedure. Unfortunately, portocholecystostomy may be complicated by poor drainage of bile and by kinking of the cystic duct and Ohi did not recommend it as the procedure of choice in spite of the low incidence of subsequent infection.

Late cholangitis

Bacterial cholangitis decreases with age and is less frequent after 2 years.[89] Gottrand *et al.*[90] described four children who presented with infection between seven and 13 years of age. The cases represented 5% of 76 long-term survivors who had become anicteric after surgery. The infections were confirmed from either the histologic appearances of a liver biopsy or by culture of the liver tissue. All four presented with fever, jaundice and abdominal pain and all responded to antibiotic therapy and remained free of jaundice between 4 months and 4 years later.

Occasionally, cholangitis may be precipitated by mechanical obstruction within the Roux loop, caused either by stenosis of an anastomosis or by an intra-abdominal adhesion. Surgical correction of the obstruction led to resolution of cholangitis in three of my own long-term survivors. Late presenting cholangitis should be investigated with a liver biopsy to confirm the diagnosis, and with a liver nuclide excretion scan to confirm the presence or absence of mechanical obstruction in the Roux loop. It is recommended that delayed excretion on the nuclide scan should be investigated by percutaneous cholangiography to give a more accurate visualization of the site of obstruction.

Portal hypertension

Portal hypertension has been demonstrated in 68% of infants with biliary atresia between two and four months of age.[91] Stringer *et al.*[92] found varices in 67% of 61 children during endoscopies performed 2.5 years or more after portoenterostomy and variceal hemorrhage had occurred in 17 (28%). Portal hypertension was more common in children with jaundice than in those who were anicteric (86% vs. 62%) and also occurred more frequently in those who had suffered recurrent cholangitis. Furthermore, the risk of death or transplantation among 134 patients was approximately 50% within 6 years of the initial episode of bleeding from esophageal varices.[93]

Ohi *et al.*[94] documented effective endoscopic obliteration of varices with 5% ethanolamine oleate in all children who completed their course of sclerotherapy; only one of the treated children died from uncontrolled hemorrhage. Complications, however, included three cases of symptomatic esophageal stricture, which responded satisfactorily to simple dilatation. There were no serious bleeding episodes from gastric varices in this report.

Concern with the possible complications of injection sclerotherapy stimulated the development of the technique of variceal ligation, described by Hall *et al.*[95] in six children, two of whom were cases of biliary atresia. Each varix is ligated with an elastic band mounted on a modified gastroscope. The varix is occluded and necrosed by the band and sloughs in 5 to 10 days. Randomized trials in adults have now shown that banding is associated with fewer complications than sclerotherapy and with improved variceal obliteration. A preliminary study by Celinska-Cedro *et al.*[96] has confirmed the efficacy of variceal ligation in 37 children, seven of whom were cases of biliary atresia. Eradication of the varices was achieved in 28 patients after two sessions of ligation with no significant post-treatment complications.

Portosystemic shunting has also been effective in the management of portal hypertension in biliary atresia patients. Valayer[97] reported 14 cases treated in this manner before the advent of sclerotherapy and liver transplantation. Shunting remains a useful, occasional, option in patients with bleeding ectopic varices in regions of the gut other than the esophagus, for example, the stomach or at the sites of surgical anastomoses.

The formation of an intrahepatic portosystemic shunt by creating a passage between the hepatic and portal veins via a transjugular approach was made possible by the introduction of expandable metal stents.[98] The procedure, known as TIPPS (transjugular intrahepatic portosystemic stent-shunt), is associated with complications of shunt thrombosis, encephalopathy, damage to the portal vein and shunt occlusion related to intimal proliferation within the stent which may occur in up to 50% of patients at 12 months.[99] The technique has been used in children after portoenterostomy as young as 2 years.[100] Schweizer *et al.*[101] reported results in seven such cases. However, liver transplantation is now generally regarded as the most effective way of treating severe recurrent variceal bleeding in the esophagus or other parts of the gastrointestinal tract secondary to progressive liver disease from biliary atresia.

Splenomegaly, associated with portal hypertension, is observed in the majority of long-term survivors after portoenterostomy and may be complicated by abdominal pain and distension, thrombocytopenia and leucopenia. Low platelet counts are found in many long-term survivors; the prevalence after 2 and 10 years has been recorded as 43% and 25%, respectively.[102] The platelet count may be low enough to cause severe spontaneous bruising, particularly in the lower limbs. Stellin *et al.*[103] treated a 6-year-old girl by splenic embolization using a percutaneous femoral artery catheter to introduce Gelfoam particles into the splenic artery. The procedure was complicated by abdominal pain, ileus and fever but platelet and white blood cell counts returned rapidly to normal.

Chiba *et al.*[102] confirmed the effectiveness of the procedure in 19 postportoenterostomy children aged between 3 and 13 years of age in whom platelet counts ranged from 26 000 to 110 000/mm^3. Between 45% and 90% of the splenic tissue was embolized with no serious morbidity. Nine of the children were restudied 4 years later by scintigraphy and measurements of platelet counts. In some patients considerable regeneration of splenic tissue had occurred. In seven, the regeneration ranged from 23% to 76% with a mean of 41%, whilst in two cases there was no recovery of splenic volume. The platelet count increased more than fourfold in seven patients but two children showed signs of hypersplenism that required further embolization. A recent study of 32 children with biliary atresia again confirmed the long-term effectiveness of the technique. The average volume of spleen embolized was 70% and hematologic improvements were maintained in 17 out of 24 survivors who did not undergo liver transplantation.[104]

In summary, portal hypertension is a problem in a significant proportion of the survivors of the portoenterostomy operation. Endoscopic sclerotherapy and banding are excellent methods for the control of esophageal varices although portosystemic shunting may be required very occasionally for ectopic varices which have occurred at anastomotic sites within the gut (provided that the patient's liver function is well preserved). Hypersplenism may be controlled with embolization rather than with splenectomy or portosystemic shunting. Complications of portal hypertension occurring in patients with biliary cirrhosis and poor liver function are best treated by liver transplantation.

Intrahepatic cystic change

Large intrahepatic cysts, easily detectable with ultrasonography, may develop in both jaundiced and anicteric long-term survivors. Tsuchida *et al.*[105] reported 29 well-documented cases of whom 12 were males. The cysts were located near the hepatic hilum in 20 cases and at the periphery of the liver in eight.

Cystic change was classified into three types:

type A: non-communicating
type B: communicating with the Roux-en-Y loop at the porta hepatis
type C: multiple cystic dilatations of irregular bile ducts

Clinical symptoms caused by the cysts included cholangitis and jaundice; in 66% of patients these occurred within 4 years of the portoenterostomy operation. Treatment included antibiotics and percutaneous drainage. Cyst-enterostomy was possible in six cases. However, five of the six cases of type C disease developed symptoms between 10 and 28 years after surgery and the prognosis of this group was compromised by repeated infection. The development of this type of cystic change is probably an indication for liver transplantation.

Metabolic problems

The extent to which malabsorption improves after portoenterostomy is related to the adequacy of bile drainage. Maximal bile flow may not be achieved for one year after operation[106] and even then bile salts seem to be excreted preferentially to cholesterol and phospholipid.[107] The latter may take many months to normalize in successful cases. Lipid absorption can be improved by giving milk which contains fat in the form of medium-chain trigylcerides. The consequences of malabsorption are further reduced by regular dietary supplementation with fat-soluble vitamins, particularly D, E and K, and a multivitamin preparation of thiamine, riboflavine, pyridoxine, ascorbic acid, and folic acid.[108]

Bile is important for the intestinal absorption of calcium and magnesium because it is necessary for the absorption of vitamin D[109] but cirrhosis may also interfere with the hydroxylation of vitamin D in the liver. In one study, rickets was found in 23 out of 39 patients (59%) with surgically uncorrected atresia and in four out of 15 (27%) who had undergone surgery. Osteoporosis was also found to develop a little later in both groups. In another report rickets was detected in 32% of long-term survivors older than 3 years.[73] Florid rickets can be corrected rapidly by giving large doses of vitamin D and ensuring that there is adequate calcium and phosphate intake and absorption.

Chronic liver disease may also lead to vitamin E deficiency in young children and this has been associated with a progressive neurologic disorder characterised by loss of tendon reflexes, a reduction in proprioception, abnormal eye movements and intellectual deterioration.[110]

Long-term biliary atresia survivors with severe liver fibrosis or cirrhosis may also suffer effects from poor absorption of soluble vitamins, protein, iron, calcium, zinc, and copper.

Hepatopulmonary syndrome and pulmonary hypertension

In common with other forms of chronic liver disease, hypoxia with cyanosis on standing and exertion, dyspnea and finger clubbing may result from diffuse intrapulmonary shunting and intrapulmonary vascular dilatation in patients with biliary atresia. Valayer[111] has pointed out that this complication, known as hepatopulmonary syndrome, is seen most frequently in the group of patients with an associated polysplenia syndrome and that the condition can be reversed by liver transplantation.

Pulmonary arterial hypertension, which is recognized as a complication of cirrhosis in adults, may also occur in long-term survivors with biliary atresia, as well as in patients with prehepatic venous block, and congenital hepatic fibrosis.[112] Possible etiologic factors include vasoactive substances such as endothelin or prostaglandin F2, which are either not metabolized by the liver, or are secreted by endothelial cells. Moscoso *et al.*[113] reported the sudden death of a 10-year-old boy with pulmonary artery hypertension after a successful portoenterostomy. He had been asymptomatic and had been able to take part in normal sporting activities, such as swimming. At autopsy, the pulmonary arteries showed widespread thickening of the muscular media of the pulmonary arteries as well as proliferation of muscle and fibrous tissue within the subendothelial layer. Fresh fibrin thrombi were seen in some of the small arterioles and right ventricular hypertrophy was severe. The authors suggested that, in view of the asymptomatic nature of the pulmonary hypertension in this case, children with chronic liver disease such as biliary atresia should be followed up with assessments of pulmonary and cardiovascular function, and that liver transplantation might be the only option for those showing increasing vascular resistance in the pulmonary arteries.

Malignant change in the liver

Malignant change in the cirrhotic liver of patients with biliary atresia has been reported on at least 15 occasions, eight at autopsy and seven during hepatic transplantation,[111,114] with an age range of 3 to 16 years. The tumors have included cholangiocarcinoma (2 cases), hepatoma (12 cases) and a single case of hepatoblastoma, and all were associated with advanced biliary cirrhosis. On the basis of these cases, Tatekawa *et al.*[114] advised routine screening of long-term biliary atresia patients with alpha-fetoprotein levels, CT scans and MR imaging.

Six of the seven transplant cases were reported to show no evidence of recurrent tumor. It is likely that more cases will occur as the number of long-term survivors increases.

Long-term outcomes

A baseline for survival of patients with untreated biliary atresia was defined by Hays and Snyder[6] in a review of 41 cases seen at the Los Angeles Children's Hospital between

Table 35.3. The incidence of esophageal varices and bleeding in long-term survivors after portoenterostomy

	Survival numbers	Varices	Bleeding
Tagge *et al.*[62]	34	?	6 (18%)
Stringer *et al.*[92]	61	41 (67%)	17 (28%)
Miga *et al.*[93]	134		39 (29%)
Valayer[111]	80	?	19 (24%)
Laurent *et al.*[119]	40	24 (60%)	15 (37%)
Karrer *et al.*[120]	35	?	20 (55%)
Howard & Davenport[121]	51	21 (41%)	8 (16%)
Totals	435		124 (28.5%)

1947 and 1961, before the introduction of the portoenterostomy procedure. Successful surgical correction had been possible in only one case and the average length of survival for the rest of the infants was only 19 months.

Prolonged survival followed the introduction of the portoenterostomy procedure and an increasing number of long-term outcome studies are now appearing. Unfortunately, as Davenport has pointed out,[115] an accurate comparative analysis of all long-term results is difficult as authors have tended to present their own results in an idiosyncratic manner. More uniformity in reporting is required but it is possible to deduce from the literature that long-term survival depends on a rapid postoperative fall of serum bilirubin into the normal range. It is also clear, however, that the attainment of a normal bilirubin level does not guarantee prolonged survival.

At least 35% of cases suffer postoperative cholangitis but the effect of these infections on long-term survival remains debatable. Three reports[86,87,116] appeared to demonstrate decreased survival after episodes of cholangitis but three other studies failed to confirm this relationship.[62,73,117] Data from King's College Hospital, London, revealed a history of cholangitis in 41% of the ten-year survivors and 36.6% of the 5-year survivors.[117]

The type of biliary drainage technique used in the portoenterostomy operation does not seem to influence the incidence of postoperative bacterial cholangitis. In a review of 1370 cases from the Japanese Biliary Atresia Registry, Nio *et al.*[118] reported no significant differences in the incidence of cholangitis between the various techniques of biliary drainage recommended in the past and stated that since 1999, 96% of Japanese patients have undergone a standard portoenterostomy without modification.[118]

The prevalence of portal hypertension is similar in all of the published long-term results. Endoscopic evidence of esophageal varices is found in 40% to 60% of cases but esophageal bleeding is a problem in only about 28% (Table 35.3).

Table 35.4. Collected 5-year survival figures after portoenterostomy for biliary atresia

	Patient numbers	5-year survival	No jaundice
Tagge *et al.*[62]	34	19 (37%)	7 (20%)
Houwen *et al.*[86]	71	17 (24%)	11 (15%)
Ohi *et al.*[87]	214	52 (24%)	47 (22%)
Howard *et al.*[121]	184	71 (39%)	68 (37%)
Kobayashi *et al.*[122]	132	32 (24%)	17 (13%)
Gauthier *et al.*[123]	69	31 (45%)	23 (33%)
Totals	704	222 (32%)	173 (25%)

Table 35.5. Collected 10-year survival figures after portoenterostomy for biliary atresia

	Patient numbers	10-year survival	No jaundice
Caccia *et al.*[116]	46	13 (28%)	8 (17%)
Valayer[111]	271	80 (30%)	38 (14%)
Karrer *et al.*[120]	98	23 (23%)	19 (19%)
Howard *et al.*[121]	39	17 (43%)	9 (23%)
Nio *et al.*[118]	108	57 (53%)	?
Totals	562	190 (34%)	74 (16%)[a]

[a] Denominator derived from the four series with complete data.

Five-year survival figures after surgery for biliary atresia are shown in Table 35.4. Most of these cases were treated by portoenterostomy but sometimes it is not clear from the text whether or not an occasional case of hepaticojejunostomy is included. The figures are reasonably consistent in the various reports with a range of 24% to 45% and an average survival of 32%. Freedom from jaundice at 5 years is approximately 25%.

The 10-year survival figures reveal that, although the survival rate of 34% is similar to the 5-year figure of 32%, there is a reduction in the proportion of cases who are free of jaundice. At 10 years approximately 16% are anicteric compared with 25% at five years. This figure could be useful when predicting the overall proportion of biliary atresia patients for whom transplantation might eventually be necessary (Table 35.5).

Transplantation after failed portoenterostomy significantly increases the figure for long-term survival. The overall survival in Japan is now 75.3% at 5 years and 66.7% at 10 years.[118] An illustration of the difficulty in comparing published results is provided by the report of Carcellar *et al.*[124] who described the results of portoenterostomy in

Table 35.6. Prognostic studies concerning portoenterostomy

Lawrence *et al.*[61]	Bile drainage not related to histology of porta hepatis
Lopez Gutierrez *et al.*[125]	Bile flow not related to histology of liver or porta hepatis
Lopez Gutierrez *et al.*[126]	Prognosis related to portal and hepatic arterial flow
Kang *et al.*[127]	No relation between hepatic histology at portoenterostomy and development of varices
Trivedi *et al.*[128]	Progressive liver damage associated with increasing levels of serum hyaluronic acid
Davenport & Howard[67]	Macroscopic features at time of surgery related to effective postoperative bile drainage

Table 35.7. Relationship between the age at which portoenterostomy is performed and the restoration of bile flow

Mieli-Vergani *et al.*[64]	(< 8 weeks) 12/14 (86%)	(> 8 weeks) 13/36 (36%)
Houwen *et al.*[86]	(< 11 weeks) 40/59 (68%)	(> 11 weeks) 6/12 (50%)
Nio *et al.*[118]	(< 10 weeks) 241/728 (33%)	(>10 weeks) 157/453 (34%)
Gauthier *et al.*[123]	(< 8 weeks)31/50 (62%)	(> 8 weeks) 52/143 (36%)
Caccia *et al.*[133]	(<10 weeks) 31/48 (65%)	(>10 weeks) 4/16 (25%)
Totals	355/899 = 39%	232/660 = 36%

77 patients at a mean follow-up of 8 years and 8 months. Seventeen (26%) were alive with their native liver and 25 after a transplant and therefore 42 (77%) of the original cohort were alive with a combination of portoenterostomy and transplantation. Unfortunately, it is not possible to compare these Canadian results directly with the previously quoted Japanese series as the method of reporting is so different.

Prognostic factors for long-term survival

Histologic studies of the liver and of atretic remnants of the biliary tract have not revealed any consistent prognostic features for either postoperative bile drainage or long-term survival after portoenterostomy. Some of these attempts to define prognostic criteria are listed in Table 35.6. Davenport and Howard[67] analyzed the macroscopic features of the biliary tract and liver at the time of surgery; each feature was assigned a score. Outcome after surgery was assessed prospectively. Although the size of the portal remnant at the time of surgery was the most accurate prognostic feature, the discriminative power of the scoring system was not high. However, further analysis did show it to be a more accurate indicator of outcome than age of the infant at the time of surgery.

The prognosis following portoenterostomy has also been related to the speed with which the serum bilirubin falls into the normal range. Eighty one patients were separated into two groups 6 months after portoenterostomy, depending on whether or not their serum bilirubin had fallen into the normal range. The positive predictive value of a successful outcome using this categorization was 96% at 2 years and 95% at 5 years. The negative predictive value of failure was 76% and 74%, respectively. The authors also noted that bridging liver fibrosis and episodes of cholangitis were interdependent risk factors for failure after portoenterostomy.[129]

It is generally believed that early operation, under 8 weeks of age, provides the best chance of effective postoperative bile drainage in biliary atresia; some reports have also demonstrated a relationship between early surgery and long-term survival.[73,87,120] Although several major series have shown this relationship it has been less convincing in others. Tagge *et al.*[62] for example, showed that three out of 12 cases who underwent operation before 8 weeks of age were alive at 5 years compared with seven out of nine operated after 12 weeks. Similarly, Volpert *et al.*[130] reported 92 cases, nine of whom underwent portoenterostomy before 30 days of life. Transplantation was required in seven (78%) of these "early" cases at a mean age of 11 months compared with a transplantation rate of 53% at a mean age of 32 months in the children who were treated after 30 days. The possibility of successful surgery in older age groups was also emphasized by Schoen *et al.*[131] who achieved good bile drainage in five of six children over 10 weeks of age, although the significance of these figures is diminished by the small number of older cases available for analysis.

In a large study of all French cases treated between 1986 and 1996, Chardot *et al.*[132] compared the results of portoenterostomy in 380 infants under 90 days of age with 60 older infants and found no significant difference at 10 years. The 5-year survival of the two groups without transplantation was 35% and 25%, respectively, and the 10-year survival 25% and 22%. Valayer[111] emphasized that, of 38 anicteric patients surviving for 10 years, 24 had undergone surgery later than 8 weeks of age. Davenport *et al.*[117] also failed to find a statistically significant difference between age at the time of surgery and survival at 5 years.

In summary, the previous belief in the benefit of early surgery before eight or ten weeks of age appears to have lost some of its significance as larger numbers of cases have become available for analysis (Table 35.7). Further data on the relationship of age at portoenterostomy and long-term survival are clearly needed to solve the apparent discrepancies between some of the published studies.

Table 35.8. Survival rates after liver transplantation for biliary atresia

	Number	Survivors
Beath *et al.*[134]	39	28 (72%)
Martinez *et al.*[135]	32	22 (70%)
Valayer *et al.*[136]	72	62 (86%)
Goss *et al.*[137]	190	154 (80%)
Totals	333	266 (80%)

Table 35.9. Complications in 23 of 80 patients who survived ten years after portoenterostomy without transplantation (Ohi[139])

Increased fatigue	23 (29%)
Pruritus	10 (12.5%)
Abdominal pain	4 (5%)
Hepatopulmonary syndrome	3 (4%)
Jaundice	3 (4%)
Recurrent pyrexia	2 (2.5%)

Liver transplantation

It is now clear that the majority of patients will, sooner or later, require hepatic transplantation after portoenterostomy. A proportion of cases will completely fail to drain bile and will require urgent transplantation in the first year of life. Others, in whom satisfactory bile drainage is established, remain at risk from portal hypertension and progressive liver disease and may become candidates for liver replacement after several years of reasonable health. The outcome after liver transplantation for biliary atresia in four series of patients is shown in Table 35.8. Survival after transplantation is approximately 80%. Future quality-of-life studies in long-term survivors will be increasingly important. Goss *et al.*[137] reported results in 190 cases; 1-, 2- and 5-year actuarial survival rates were 83%, 80%, and 78%, respectively. More recently, Diem *et al.*[138] analyzed 328 transplants and reported survival figures at 1, 5 and 10 years of 87%, 83% and 81%, respectively. In this series the child's age at the time of transplantation was a factor in long-term survival: the long-term survival of those treated before 6 years of age was approximately 85% compared with 100% for older age groups. The improved survival in those over 6 years further supports the policy of recommending portoenterostomy as the primary treatment of choice in young infants with biliary atresia.

Quality-of-life and economic considerations

A review of 80 patients who survived for more than 10 years without transplantation revealed complications affecting quality of life in 23 (29%) (Table 35.9).[139] Forty-four were in school and 34 at work. Four women had given birth to normal children. The comments of Nio *et al.*[140] on the status of 22 patients who survived for more than 20 years were very encouraging. One had died at 28 years of age but 16 had led near normal lives and three of the women had married. One of the latter had borne a normal child. Three patients had required a portosystemic shunt for variceal bleeding and one patient had intrahepatic calculi. Physical growth was judged to be normal in all but one case. Girls had had a normal menarche and secondary sexual characteristics had developed normally in the boys. The overall quality of life was judged to be satisfactory in 16 of the patients but three required occasional hospital admission. The authors stated that progressive liver disease had not been observed in the 21 surviving patients. All of the patients were in employment.

Other measures of the quality of life were supplied by Kobayashi *et al.*[122] who reported satisfactory weights in 28 out of 32 survivors beyond five years and satisfactory heights in 17. Ohi *et al.*[87] reported that 48 out of 52 cases surviving more than 5 years (the oldest of whom was 27 years) were leading normal lives and both growth and development were normal in 49. In Valayer's report,[111] school performance assessed in 26 ten-year survivors was judged to be normal in eight, 1 year below normal in 11, and 2 to 3 years below normal in seven. Twelve of the teenagers showed good sporting ability and professional activity for those in their twenties was said to be "normal."

Karrer *et al.*[120] discussed the quality of life in 30 patients who had survived at least ten years after portoenterostomy, 25 of whom were within the normal expected range for height. Age-appropriate school or employment had been achieved in 75% of cases. One patient was pregnant at the time of the report.

A unique study of the quality of life (QoL) of long-term survivors compared 30 Japanese over 14 years of age with 25 UK patients in the same age range.[141] Blood and liver function tests did not show any significant differences between the two groups. Overall, there were no significant differences in the QoL measures which included functional status, well-being and an overall evaluation of health. Furthermore, there was a very satisfactory comparison with normative population data in both countries. The study confirmed that excellent long-term survival is possible after portoenterostomy in at least a proportion of patients.

Successful pregnancy in patients treated for biliary atresia has now been reported by at least five authors.[87,111,120,142,143] Questionnaires sent to 134 institutions affiliated to the Japanese Biliary Atresia Society included questions on menstrual irregularities, numbers of pregnancies, problems related to pregnancy and delivery, and the health of the baby. Sixteen patients had given birth on 23 occasions (nine delivered once and seven delivered twice). However, only three (19%) had had a problem-free pregnancy. Deterioration of liver function occurred after delivery in six (37.5%), and one of these women required urgent transplantation. Cholangitis required treatment in four (25.0%). Other problems included two abortions, one of which was related to shock from bleeding esophageal varices. A further case of variceal bleeding was treated by endoscopic variceal ligation.[143] In common with other reports, none of the babies of biliary atresia mothers had any liver problem or other congenital abnormality. This large collected series indicates that pregnancy in biliary atresia patients carries a high degree of risk and requires close surveillance.

Barkin and Lilly[144] examined the stresses on parents of children with biliary atresia. Paradoxically, the stresses appeared to be greater in families whose children had undergone successful surgery. Problems included "marital discord" (4), divorce (2), abandonment of the child (1), and unemployment and financial pressures (3). All of the families interviewed had some difficulty coming to terms with the chronic illness. Unfortunately, no comparison was made with families caring for children with other forms of chronic disease. The authors mentioned the existence of a support organization in North America for the families of children with biliary atresia. The Children's Liver Disease Foundation charity in the UK performs a similar role in providing clinical information and support for the families of affected children.

The satisfactory outcome after portoenterostomy in a proportion of children and the low rehospitalization rate suggest that this procedure should continue as first-line treatment of biliary atresia. Shortage of donor organs, complications of immunosuppression, chronic rejection and repeat transplantation remain limiting factors for primary transplantation particularly in children under six years of age. The overall mortality rate of liver transplantation in children over 3 years of age is approximately 20%. Portoenterostomy continues to be the primary treatment for biliary atresia, reserving transplantation for the failures and complications of the procedure.

Summary

- Before the introduction of the portoenterostomy operation, the mortality rate for biliary atresia was virtually 100%.
- The introduction and refinement of portoenterostomy resulted in long-term survival with a good quality of life in approximately 25% of the children.
- Complications in long-term survivors of portoenterostomy include cholangitis, portal hypertension, bleeding esophageal varices, intrahepatic cystic dilatation and cholelithiasis, hypoxia from pulmonary artery pathology, and malignant change in the liver.
- Liver transplantation is a successful mode of treatment for infants who fail to achieve satisfactory bile drainage after portoenterostomy and for complications in long-term survivors, including progressive liver disease and cirrhosis.
- The overall survival for biliary atresia patients treated in combined programmes of portoenterostomy and transplantation is greater than 80%.
- The quality of life in the majority of long-term survivors is very satisfactory and as yet there are no reports of transmission of bilary atresia to the offspring of patients.

REFERENCES

1. Balistreri, W. F., Grand, R., Hoofnagle, J. H. *et al.* Biliary atresia: current concepts and research directions. *Hepatology* 1996; **23**:1682–1692.
2. Hays, D. M. & Kimura, K. *et al.* Biliary atresia: new concepts of management. *Curr. Prob. Surg.* 1981; **18**:546.
3. Thomson, J. *Congenital Obliteration of the Bile Ducts.* Edinburgh:Oliver and Boyd:1892.
4. Holmes, J. B. Congenital obliteration of the bile duct: diagnosis and suggestions for treatment. *Am. J. Dis. Child.* 1916; **11**:405–431.
5. Ladd, W. E. Congenital atresia and stenosis of the bile duct. *J. Am. Med. Assoc.* 1928; **91**:1082–1084.
6. Hays, D. M., Snyder, W. H. Life-span in untreated biliary atresia. *Surgery* 1963; **64**:373–375.
7. Kasai, M. & Suzuki, S. A new operation for 'non-correctable' biliary atresia: hepatic portoenterostomy. *Shuzutsu* 1959; **3**:733–739.
8. Kasai, M. Treatment of biliary atresia with special reference to hepatic portoenterostomy and its modifications. *Prog. Pediatr. Surg.* 1974; **6**:5–52.
9. Jenner, R. E. & Howard, E. R. Unsaturated monohydroxy bile acids as a cause of idiopathic obstructive cholangiopathy. *Lancet* 1975; **2**:1073–1074.
10. Ikeda, S., Sera, Y., Yoshida, M. *et al.* extrahepatic atresia associated with trisomy 18. *Pediatr. Surg. Int.* 1999; **15**:137–138.
11. Buffa, V., Tancredi, F., Pierro, M. *et al.* Case of trisomy of chromosome 18 associated with hypermethioninemia and biliary atresia. *Pediatria (Napoli)* 1972; **80**:159–169.
12. Alpert, L. I., Strauss, L., & Hirschorn, K. Neonatal hepatitis and biliary atresia associated with trisomy 17–18 syndrome. *N. Engl. J. Med.* 1969; **280**:16–20.

13. Danks, D. M. Prolonged neonatal obstructive jaundice. A survey of modern concepts. *Clin. Pediatr.* 1965; **4**:499–510.
14. Khaimin, V. M. Congenital atresia of the bile ducts in twin boys (Russian). *Vopr. Okhr. Materin. Det.* 1969; **14**:184.
15. Smith, B. M., Laberge, J. M., Schreiber, R. *et al.* Familial biliary atresia in three siblings including twins. *J. Pediatr. Surg.* 1991; **26**:1331–1333.
16. Silveira, T. R., Salzano, F. M., Howard, E. R. *et al.* Congenital structural abnormalities in biliary atresia: evidence for etiopathogenic heterogeneity and therapeutic implications. *Acta Paediatr. Scand.* 1991; **80**:1192–1199.
17. Silveira, T. R., Salzano, F. M., Donaldson, P. T. *et al.* Association between HLA and extrahepatic biliary atresia. *J. Pediatr. Gastroenterol. Nutr.* 1993; **16**:114–117.
18. Jurado, A., Jara, P., Camarena, C. *et al.* Is extrahepatic biliary atresia an HLA-associated disease? *J. Pediatr. Gastroenterol. Nutr.* 1997; **25**:557–558.
19. Donaldson, P. T., Clare, M., Constantini, P. K. *et al.* HLA and cytokine gene polymorphisms in biliary atresia. *Liver* 2002; **22**:213–219.
20. Desmet, V. & Callea, F. Ductal plate malformation (DPM) in extrahepatic bile duct atresia (EHBDA). In Ohi, R., ed. *Biliary Atresia.* ICOM Associates Inc. 1991; 27–31.
21. Tan, C. E. L., Driver, M., Howard, E. R. *et al.* Extrahepatic biliary atresia: a first-trimester event? Clues from light microscopy and immunohistochemistry. *J. Pediatr. Surg.* 1994; **29**:808–814.
22. Tsuchida, Y., Kawarasaki, H., Iwanaka, T. *et al.* Antenatal diagnosis of biliary atresia (type 1 cyst) at 19 weeks gestation: differential diagnosis and etiologic implications. *J. Pediatr. Surg.* 1995; **30**:697–699.
23. Hinds, R., Davenport, M., Mieli-Vergani, G. *et al.* Antenatal presentation of biliary atresia. *J. Pediatr.* 2004; **144**:43–46.
24. MacGillivray, T. E. & Scott Adzick, N. Biliary atresia begins before birth. *Pediatr. Surg. Int.* 1994; **9**:116–117.
25. Ben-Ami, M., Perlitz, Y., Shalev, S. *et al.* Prenatal diagnosis of extrahepatic biliary duct atresia. *Prenat. Diagn.* 2002; **22**:583–585.
26. Tarr, P. I., Haas, J. E., & Christie, D. L. Biliary atresia, cytomegalovirus, and age at referral. *Pediatrics* 1996; **97**:828–831.
27. Strauss, L. & Bernstein, J. Neonatal hepatitis in congenital rubella; a histopathological study. *Arch. Pathol.* 1968; **86**:317–327.
28. Weaver, L. T., Nelson, R., & Bell, T. M. The association of extrahepatic bile duct atresia and neonatal Epstein–Barr virus infection. *Acta. Pediatr. Scand.* 1984; **73**:155–157.
29. Drut, R., Drut, R. M., Gomez, M. A. *et al.* Presence of human papillomavirus in extrahepatic biliary atresia. *J. Pediatr. Gastroenterol. Nutr.* 1998; **27**:530–535.
30. Domiati-Saad, R., Dawson, D. B., Margraf, L. R. *et al.* Cytomegalovirus and human herpesvirus 6, but not human papillomavirus, are present in neonatal giant cell hepatitis and extrahepatic biliary atresia. *Pediatr. Dev. Pathol.* 2000; **3**:367–373.
31. Jevon, G. P. & Dimmick, J. E. Biliary atresia and cytomegalovirus infection: a DNA study. *Pediatr. Dev. Pathol.* 1999; **2**:11–14.
32. Phillips, P. A., Keast, D., Papadimitriou, J. M. *et al.* Chronic obstructive jaundice induced by reovirus type 3 in weanling mice. *Pathology.* 1969; **1**:193–203.
33. Morecki, R., Glaser, J. H., & Horwitz, M. S. Etiology of biliary atresia: the role of reo 3 virus. In Daum, F., ed. *Extrahepatic Biliary Atresia.* New York: Marcel Dekker, 1983; 1–9.
34. Morecki, R., Glaser, J. H., Cho, S. *et al.* Biliary atresia and reovirus type 3 infection. *N. Eng. J. Med.* 1982; **307**:481–484.
35. Dussaix, E., Hadchouel, M., Tardieu, M. *et al.* Biliary atresia and reo virus type 3 infection. *N. Engl. J. Med.* 1984; **311**;658–66l.
36. Brown, W. R., Sokol, R. J., Levin, M. R. *et al.* Lack of correlation between infection with reovirus 3 and extrahepatic biliary atresia or neonatal hepatitis. *J. Pediatr.* 1988; **113**:670–676.
37. Tyler, K. L., Sokol, R. J., Oberhaus, S. M. *et al.* Detection of reovirus RNA in hepatobiliary tissues from patients with extrahepatic biliary atresia and choledochal cysts. *Hepatology* 1998; **27**:1475–1482.
38. Steele, M. I., Marshall, C. M., Lloyd, R. D. *et al.* Reovirus 3 not detected by reverse transcriptase-mediated polymerase chain reaction analysis of preserved tissue from infants with cholestatic liver disease. *Hepatology* 1995; **21**:697–702.
39. Carmi, R., Magee, C. A., Neill, C. A. *et al.* Extrahepatic biliary atresia and associated anomalies: etiologic heterogeneity suggested by distinctive patterns of associations. *Am. J. Med. Genet.* 1993; **45**:683–693.
40. Chandra, R. S. Biliary atresia and other structural anomalies in the congenital polysplenia syndrome. *J. Pediatr.* 1974; **85**:649–655.
41. Davenport, M., Savage, M., Mowat, A. P. *et al.* Biliary atresia splenic malformation syndrome: an etiological and prognostic subgroup. *Surgery* 1993; **113**:662–668.
42. Fischler, B., Papadogiannakis, N., & Nemeth, A. Aetiological factors in neonatal cholestasis. *Acta. Paediatr.* 2001; **90**:88–92.
43. Mazziotti, M. V., Willis, L. K., Heuckroth, R. O. *et al.* Anomalous development of the hepatobiliary system in the INV mouse. *Hepatology* 1999; **30**:372–378.
44. Schon, P., Tsuchiya, K., Lenoir, D. *et al.* Identification, genomic organization, chromosomal mapping and mutation analysis of the human INV gene, the ortholog of a murine gene implicated in left–right axis development and biliary atresia. *Hum. Genet.* 2002; **110**:157–165.
45. Mieli-Vergani, G. & Mowat, A. P. Paediatric liver disease: medical aspects. In Millward-Sadler, G. H., Wright, R. Arthur, M. J. P. eds. *Wright's Liver and Biliary Disease*, 3rd edn. London: WB Saunders, 1992; 1189–207.
46. Hussein, M., Howard, E. R., Mieli-Vergani, G. *et al.* Jaundice at 14 days of age: exclude biliary atresia. *Arch. Dis. Child.* 1991; **66**:1177–1179.
47. Davenport, M., Betalli, P., D'Antiga, L. *et al.* The spectrum of surgical jaundice in infancy. *J. Pediatr. Surg.* 2003; **38:**1471–1479.

48. Hay, S. A., Soliman, H. E., Sherif, H. M. *et al.* Neonatal jaundice: the role of laparoscopy. *J. Pediatr. Surg.* 2000; **35**:1706–1709.
49. Wilkinson, M. L., Mieli-Vergani, G., Ball, C. *et al.* Endoscopic retrograde cholangiopancreatography in infantile cholestasis. *Arch. Dis. Child.* 1991; **66**:121–123.
50. Takahashi, H., Kuriyama, Y., Maiae, M. *et al. ERCP in jaundiced infants.* In Ohi, R., ed. *Biliary Atresia.* Tokyo: Professional Postgraduate Services, 1987; 110–113.
51. Iinuma, Y., Narisawa, R., Iwafuchi, M. *et al.* The role of endoscopic retrograde cholangiopancreatography in infants with cholestasis. *J. Pediatr. Surg.* 2000; **35**:545–549.
52. Mason, G. R., Northway, W., & Cohn, R. B. Difficulties in the operative diagnosis of congenital atresia of the biliary ductal system. *Am. J. Surg.* 1966; **112:**183–187.
53. Manolaki, A. G., Larcher, V. F., Mowat, A. P. *et al.* The prelaparotomy diagnosis of extrahepatic biliary atresia. *Arch. Dis. Child.* 1983; **58:**591–594.
54. Alagille, D., Odievre, M., Gautier, M. *et al.* Hepatic ductular hypoplasia associated with characteristic facies, vertebral malformation, retarded physical, mental and sexual development and cardiac murmur. *J. Pediatr.* 1975; **86**:63–71.
55. Hays, D. M. & Kimura, K. *Biliary Atresia: The Japanese Experience.* Cambridge, MA: Harvard University Press, 1980; 22.
56. Ohi, R., Chiba, T., Ohkochi, N. *et al.* The present status of surgical treatment for biliary atresia: report of the questionnaire for the main institutions in Japan. In Ohi, R., ed. *Biliary Atresia.* Tokyo: Professional Postgraduate Services, 1987; 125–30.
57. Gautier, M. & Eliot, N. Extrahepatic biliary atresia: morphological study of 98 biliary remnants. *Arch. Path. Lab. Med.* 1981; **105**:397–402.
58. Kasai, M., Ohi, R., & Chiba, T. Intrahepatic bile ducts in biliary atresia. In Kasai, M., & Shiraki, K. eds. *Cholestasis in Infancy.* Baltimore: University Park Press, 1980; 181–188.
59. Altman, R. P., Chandra, R., & Lilly, J. R. Ongoing cirrhosis after successful porticoenterostomy in infants with biliary atresia. *J. Pediatr. Surg.* 1975; **10**:685–689.
60. Ohi, R., Shikes, R. H., Stellin, G. P. *et al.* In biliary atresia duct histology correlates with bile flow. *J. Pediatr. Surg.* 1984; **19**:467–470.
61. Lawrence, D., Howard, E. R., Tzanatos, C. *et al.* Hepatic portoenterostomy for biliary atresia. *Arch. Dis. Child.*, 1981; **56**:460–463.
62. Tagge, D. U., Tagge, E. P., Drongowski, R. A. *et al.* A long-term experience with biliary atresia. Reassessment of prognostic factors. *Ann. Surg.* 1991; **214**:590–598.
63. Altman, R. P. The portoenterostomy procedure for biliary atresia. *Ann. Surg.* 1978; **188**:357–361.
64. Mieli-Vergani, G., Howard, E. R., Portmann, B. *et al.* Late referral for biliary atresia – missed opportunities for effective surgery. *Lancet* 1989; **1**:421–423.
65. Gautier, M., Valayer, J., Odievre, M. *et al.* Histological liver evaluation 5 years after surgery for extrahepatic biliary atresia: a study of 20 cases. *J. Pediatr. Surg.* 1984; **19**:263–268.
66. Tan, C. E. L., Davenport, M., Driver, M., & Howard, E. R. Does the morphology of the extrahepatic biliary remnants in biliary atresia influence survival? A review of 205 cases. *J. Pediatr. Surg.* 1994; **29**:1459–1464.
67. Davenport, M. & Howard, E. R. Macroscopic appearance at portoenterostomy – a prognostic variable in biliary atresia. *J. Pediatr. Surg.* 1996; **31**:1387–1390.
68. Kasai, M., Kimura, S., Asakura, Y. *et al.* Surgical treatment of biliary atresia. *J. Pediatr. Surg.* 1968; **3**:665–675.
69. Tsao, K., Rosenthal, P., Dhawan, K. *et al.* Comparison of drainage techniques for biliary atresia. *J. Pediatr. Surg.* 2003; **38**:1005–1007.
70. Esteves, E., Clemente Neto, E., Ottaiano Neto, M. *et al.* Laparoscopic Kasai portoenterostomy for biliary atresia. *Pediatr. Surg. Int.* 2002; **18**:737–740.
71. Lilly, J. R. Hepatic portocholecystostomy for biliary atresia. *J. Pediatr. Surg.* 1979; **14**:301–304.
72. Freitas, L., Gauthier, F., & Valayer, J. Second operation for repair of biliary atresia. *J. Pediatr. Surg.* 1987; **22**:857–60.
73. Karrer, F. M., Lilly, J. R., Stewart, B. A. *et al.* Biliary atresia registry, 1976 to 1989. *J. Pediatr. Surg.* 1990; **25**:1076–1081.
74. Vajro, P., Couterier, M., Lemmonier, F. *et al.* Effects of postoperative cholestyramine and phenobarbital administration on bile flow restoration in infants with extrahepatic biliary atresia. *J. Pediatr. Surg.* 1986; **21**:262–265.
75. Nittono, H., Tokita, A., Hayashi, M. *et al.* Ursodeoxycholic acid in biliary atresia. *Lancet* 1988; **1**:528.
76. Kasai, M., Suzuki, H., Ohashi, E. *et al.* Technique and results of operative management of biliary atresia. *World J. Surg.* 1978; **2:** 571–580.
77. Altman, R. P. & Anderson, K. D. Surgical management of intractable cholangitis following successful Kasai procedure. *J. Pediatr. Surg.* 1982; **17:**894–900.
78. Karrer, F. M., Lilly, J. R. Corticosteroid therapy in biliary atresia. *J. Pediatr. Surg.* 1985; **20**:683–695.
79. Dillon, P. W., Owings, E., Cilley, R. *et al.* Immunosuppression as adjuvant therapy for biliary atresia. *J. Pediatr. Surg.* 2001; **36**:80–85.
80. Meyers, R. L., Book, L. S., O'Gorman, M. A. *et al.* High-dose steroids, ursodeoxycholic acid, and chronic intravenous antibiotics improve bile flow after Kasai procedure in infants with biliary atresia. *J. Pediatr. Surg.* 2003; **38**:406–411.
81. Chaudhary, S. & Turner, R. B. Trimethoprim-sulfamethoxazole for cholangitis following hepatic portoenterostomy for biliary atresia. *J. Pediatr.* 1981; **99**:656–658.
82. Bu, L. N., Chen, H. L., Chang, C. J. *et al.* Prophylactic oral antibiotics in prevention of recurrent cholangitis after the Kasai portoenterostomy. *J. Pediatr. Surg.* 2003; **38**:590–593.
83. Lally, K. P., Kenegaye, J., Matsumura, M. *et al.* Perioperative factors affecting the outcome following repair of biliary atresia. *Pediatrics* 1989; **83**:723–726.
84. Burnweit, C. A. & Coln, D. Influence of diversion on the development of cholangitis after hepatoportoenterostomy for biliary atresia. *J. Pediatr. Surg.* 1986; **21**:1143–1146.
85. Wu, E. T., Chen, H. L., Ni, Y. H. *et al.* Bacterial cholangitis in patients with biliary atresia: impact on short-term outcome. *Pediatr. Surg. Int.* 2001; **17**:390–395.

86. Houwen, R. H. J., Zwierstra, R. P., Severijnen, R. S. *et al.* Prognosis of extrahepatic biliary atresia. *Arch. Dis. Child.* 1989; **64**:214–218.
87. Ohi, R., Hanamatsu, M., Mochizuki, I. *et al.* Progress in the treatment of biliary atresia. *World J. Surg.* 1985; **9**:285–293.
88. Ohi, R. Biliary atresia: long-term results of hepatic portoenterostomy. In Howard, E. R. ed. *Surgery of Liver Disease in Children*, Oxford:Butterworth-Heinemann, 1991; 60–71.
89. Ecoffey, C., Rothman, E., Bernard, O. *et al.* Bacterial cholangitis after surgery for biliary atresia. *J. Pediatr.* 1987; **111**:824–829.
90. Gottrand, F., Bernard, O., Hadchouel, M. *et al.* Late cholangitis after successful surgical repair of biliary atresia. *Am. J. Dis. Child.* 1991; **145**:213–215.
91. Kasai, M., Okamoto, A., Ohi, R. *et al.* Changes of portal vein pressure and intrahepatic blood vessels after surgery for biliary atresia. *J. Pediatr. Surg.* 1981; **16**:152–159.
92. Stringer, M., Howard, E. R., & Mowat, A. P. Endoscopic sclerotherapy in the management of esophageal varices in 61 children with biliary atresia. *J. Pediatr. Surg.* 1989; **24**:438–442.
93. Miga, D., Sokol, R. J., Narkewicz, M. R. *et al.* Survival after first esophageal variceal hemorrhage in patients with biliary atresia. *Hepatology* 2002; **26**:498–499.
94. Ohi, R., Mochizuki, I., Komatsu, K. *et al.* (1986) Portal hypertension after successful hepatic portoenterostomy in biliary atresia. *J. Pediatr. Surg.* 1986; **21**:271–274.
95. Hall, R. J., Lilly, J. R., & Stiegmann, G. V. Endoscopic esophageal varix ligation: technique and preliminary results in children. *J. Pediatr. Surg.* 1988; **23**:1222–1223.
96. Celinska-Cedro, D. Teisseyre, M., Woynarowski, M. *et al.* Endoscopic ligation of esophageal varices for prophylaxis of first bleeding in children and adolescents with portal hypertension: preliminary results of a prospective study. *J. Pediatr. Surg.* 2003; **38**:1008–1011.
97. Valayer, J. Portosystemic shunt surgery. In Howard, E. R. ed. *Surgery of Liver Disease in Children*. Oxford:Butterworth-Heinemann. 1991; 171–80.
98. Rossle, M., Richter, G. M., Noldge, G. *et al.* Performance of an intrahepatic portocaval shunt (PCS) using a catheter technique: a case report. *Hepatology* 1988; **8**:1348.
99. Benner, K., Sahagun, G., Meyer, R. A. *et al.* Shunt patency after transjugular intrahepatic portosystemic shunt. *Gastroenterology* 1993; **104**:A876.
100. Kimura, B. T., Hasegawa, T., Oue, T. *et al.* Transjugular intrahepatic portosystemic shunt performed in a 2-year-old infant for uncontrollable intestinal bleeding. *J. Pediatr. Surg.* 2000; **35**:1597–1599.
101. Schweizer, P., Brambs, H. J., Schweizer, M. *et al.* TIPS: a new therapy for esophageal variceal bleeding caused by EHBA. *Eur. J. Pediatr. Surg.* 1995; **5**:211–215.
102. Chiba, T., Ohi, R., Yaoita, M. *et al.* Partial splenic embolization for hypersplenism in pediatric patients with special reference to its long-term efficacy. In Ryoji, O. ed. *Biliary Atresia*, Tokyo:ICOM Associates Inc., 1991; 154–158.
103. Stellin, G., Kumpe, D. A., & Lilly, J. R. Splenic embolization in a child with hypersplenism. *J. Pediatr. Surg.* 1982; **17**:892–893.
104. Nio, M., Hayashi, Y., Sano, N. *et al.* Long-term efficacy of partial splenic embolization in children. *J. Pediatr. Surg.* 2003; **38**:1760–1762.
105. Tsuchida, Y., Honna, T., & Kawarasaki, H. Cystic dilatation of the intrahepatic biliary system in biliary atresia after hepatic portoenterostomy. *J. Pediatr. Surg.* 1994; **29:**630–634.
106. Howard, E. R. & Mowat, A. P. Hepatobiliary disorders in infancy: hepatitis; extrahepatic biliary atresia; intrahepatic biliary hypoplasia. In Thomas, H. C. & McSween, R. N. M. eds. *Recent Advances in Hepatology*. London: Churchill Livingstone, 1984; 153.
107. Lilly, J. R. & Javitt, N. B. Biliary lipid excretion after hepatic portoenterostomy. *Ann. Surg.* 1976; **184**:369–375.
108. Greene, H. L. Nutritional aspects in the management of biliary atresia. In Daum, F., ed. *Extrahepatic Biliary Atresia*. New York: Marcel Dekker, 1983; 133–143.
109. Kobayashi, A., Kawai, S., Utsunomiya, T. *et al.* Bone disease in infants and children with hepatobiliary disease. *Arch. Dis. Child.* 1974; **49**:641–646.
110. Nelson, J. S., Rosenblum, J. L., Keating, J. P. *et al.* Neuropathological complications of childhood cholestatic liver disease. In Daum, F. ed. *Extrahepatic Biliary Atresia*. New York: Marcel Dekker, 1983; 153–157.
111. Valayer, J. Conventional treatment of biliary atresia. *J. Pediatr. Surg.* 1996; **31**:1546–1551.
112. Soh, H., Hasegawa, T., Sasaki, T. *et al.* Pulmonary hypertension associated with postoperative biliary atresia: report of two cases. *J. Pediatr. Surg.* 1999; **34**:1779–1781.
113. Moscoso, G., Mieli-Vergani, G., Mowat, A. P. *et al.* Sudden death caused by unsuspected pulmonary arterial hypertension, 10 years after surgery for extrahepatic biliary atresia. *J. Pediatr. Gastroenterol. Nutr.* 1991; **12**:388–393.
114. Tatekawa, Y., Asonuma, K., Uemoto *et al.* Liver transplantation for biliary atresia associated with malignant tumors. *J. Pediatr. Surg.* 2001; **36**:436–439.
115. Davenport, M. Biliary atresia (letter). *J. Pediatr. Surg.* 2001; **36**:1318.
116. Caccia, G., Dessanti, A., Alberti, D. *et al.* More than 10 years survival after surgery for biliary atresia. In Ohi, R., ed. *Biliary Atresia*. Tokyo:ICOM Associates Inc, 1991; 246–249.
117. Davenport, M., Kereker, N., Mieli-Vergani, G. *et al.* (1997) Biliary atresia: the King's College Hospital experience (1974–95) *J. Pediatr. Surg.* 1997; **32**:1–8.
118. Nio, M., Ohi, R., Miyano, T. *et al.* Five and 10-year survival rates after surgery for biliary atresia: a report from the Japanese Biliary Atresia Registry. *J. Pediatr. Surg.* 2003; **38**:997–1000.
119. Laurent, J., Gauthier, F., Bernard, O. *et al.* Long-term outcome after surgery for biliary atresia. Study of 40 patients surviving for more than 10 years. *Gastroenterology* 1990; **99**:1793–1797.
120. Karrer, F. M., Price, M. R., Bensard, D. D. *et al.* Long-term results with the Kasai operation for biliary atresia. *Arch. Surg.* 1996; **131**:493–496.
121. Howard, E. R. & Davenport, M. The treatment of biliary atresia in Europe – 1969–1995. *Tohuko. J. Exp. Med.* 1997; **181**:75–83.

122. Kobayashi, A., Itabashi, F., & Ohbe, Y. Long-term prognosis in biliary atresia after hepatic portoenterostomy: analysis of 35 patients who survived beyond 5 years of age. *J. Pediatr.* 1984; **105**: 243–246.
123. Gauthier, F., Laurent, J., Bernard, O. *et al.* Improvement of results after Kasai operation: the need for early diagnosis and surgery. In Ohi, R., ed. *Biliary Atresia.* Tokyo:ICOM Associates Inc. 1991; 91–95.
124. Carcellar, A., Blanchard, H., Alvarez, F. *et al.* Past and future of biliary atresia. *J. Pediatr. Surg.* 2000; **35**:717–720.
125. Lopez, Gutierrez. J. C., Vazquez, J., Ros, Z. *et al.* Histopathology of biliary atresia: correlation with biliary flow. *Cir. Pediatr.* 1991; **4**:16–18.
126. Lopez, Gutierrez J. C., Vazquez, J., Prieto, C. *et al.* Portal venous flow as a prognostic factor in biliary atresia. A preliminary study. *Cir. Pediatr.* 1992; **5**:17–9.
127. Kang, N., Davenport, M., Driver, M. *et al.* Hepatic histology and the development of esophageal varices in biliary atresia. *J. Pediatr. Surg.* 1993; **28**:63–66.
128. Trivedi, P., Cheeseman, P., & Mowat, A. P. Serum hyaluronic acid in healthy infants and children and its value as a marker of progressive hepatobiliary disease starting in infancy. *Clin. Chim. Acta.* 1993; **215**:29–39.
129. Wildhaber, B. E., Coran, A. G., Drongowski, R. A. *et al.* The Kasai portoenterostomy for biliary atresia: a review of a 27-year experience with 81 patients. *J. Pediatr. Surg.* 2003; **38**:1480–1485.
130. Volpert, D., White, F., Finegold, M. J. *et al.* Outcome of early hepatic portoenterostomy for biliary atresia. *J. Pediatr. Gastroenterol. Nutr.* 2001; **32**:265–269.
131. Schoen, B. T., Lee, H., Sullivan, K. *et al.* The Kasai portoenterostomy: when is it too late? *J. Pediatr. Surg.* 2001; **36**:97–99.
132. Chardot, C., Carton, M., Spire-Bendelac, N. *et al.* Is the Kasai operation still indicated in children older than 3 months diagnosed with biliary atresia? *J. Pediatr.* 2001; **138**:224–228.
133. Caccia, G., Dessanti, A., & Alberti, D. An 8-year experience on the treatment of extrahepatic biliary atresia: results in 72 cases. In Kasai, M., ed. *Biliary Atresia and its Related Disorders.* Amsterdam: Excerpta Medica, 1983:181–184.
134. Beath, S., Pearmain, G., Kelly, D. *et al.* Liver transplantation in babies and children with extrahepatic biliary atresia: *J. Pediatr. Surg.* 1993; **28**:1044–1047.
135. Martinez Ibanez, V., Iglesias, J., Lloret, J. *et al.* 7 years experience with hepatic transplantation in children. *Cir. Pediatr.* 1993; **6**:7–10.
136. Valayer, J., Gauthier, F., Yandza *et al.* Biliary atresia: results of long-term conservative treatment and of liver transplantation. *Transpl. Proc.* 1993; **25**:3290–3292.
137. Goss, J. A., Shackleton, C. R., Swenson, K. *et al.* Orthotopic liver transplantation for congenital biliary atresia. An 11 year single-centre experience. *Ann. Surg.* 1996; **224:**276–284.
138. Diem, H. V., Evrard, V., Vinh, H. T. *et al.* Pediatric liver transplantation for biliary atresia: results of primary grafts in 328 recipients. *Transplantation* 2003; **75**:1692–1697.
139. Ohi, R. Biliary atresia: long-term outcomes. In Howard, E. R., Stringer, M. D., & Colombani, P. M., eds. *Surgery of the Liver, Bile ducts and Pancreas in Children, 2nd edn.* London:Arnold, 2002; 133–147.
140. Nio, M., Ohi, R., Hayashi, Y. *et al.* Current status of 21 living patients surviving more than 20 years after surgery for biliary atresia. *J. Pediatr. Surg.* 1996; **31:**381–384.
141. Howard, E. R., MacLean, G., Nio, M. *et al.* Survival patterns in biliary atresia and comparison of quality of life of long-term survivors in Japan and England. *J. Pediatr. Surg.* 2001; **36**:892–897.
142. Hadzic, N., Davenport, M., Tizzard, S. *et al.* Long-term survival following Kasai portoenterostomy: is chronic liver disease inevitable? *J. Pediatr. Gastroenterol. Nutr.* 2003; **37**:430–433.
143. Shimaoka, S., Ohi, R., Saeki, M. *et al.* Problems during and after pregnancy of former biliary atresia patients treated successfully by the Kasai procedure. *J. Pediatr. Surg.* 2001; **36**:349–351.
144. Barkin, R. M. & Lilly, J. R. Biliary atresia and the Kasai operation: continuing care. *J. Pediatr.*, 1980; **96**:1015–1019.

36

Choledochal cyst

Takeshi Miyano

Department of Pediatric General and Urogenital Surgery, Juntendo University School of Medicine, Bunkyo-ku, Tokyo, Japan

Introduction

Choledochal cyst is a congenital dilatation of the common bile duct and has the potential to become malignant. It has a hereditary predisposition, which may explain the higher incidence seen in Asia, particularly in Japan, and its familial occurrence in siblings and twins.[1,2] It was first reported by Douglas in 1852[3] and may or may not be associated with congenital dilatation of the intrahepatic bile ducts (Fig. 36.1). Choledochal cyst is almost always associated with an abnormal junction between the pancreatic and common bile duct, i.e., pancreaticobiliary malunion. This allows pancreatic secretions to reflux into the biliary tree, and bile to flow into the pancreatic duct, causing various pathologic changes in the biliary tract, pancreas, and liver.[4,5]

Because concurrent abnormalities of the pancreatic duct and intrahepatic bile ducts are almost always present, the importance of cholangiography in the planning of surgical management cannot be overemphasized. If these anomalies go unnoticed, aberrant pancreatic anatomy might be damaged, causing serious postoperative morbidity. Internal drainage of the choledochal cyst, a procedure popular in the past, has been abandoned for more than a decade now because of a prohibitive incidence of postoperative complications such as recurrent cholangitis, cholelithiasis, and biliary duct cancer.[6] Primary cyst excision with biliary reconstruction to avoid two-way reflux of bile and pancreatic secretions is now the standard surgical treatment of choice.[7]

Surgery for choledochal cyst is generally successful and a satisfactory surgical outcome with low morbidity is expected in the short term. However, on mid- to long-term follow-up, there are increasing reports of post-cyst excision complications, including recurrent cholangitis, intrahepatic bile duct stone formation, relapsing pancreatitis, stone formation in the intrapancreatic residual terminal choledochus, and malignancy.[6–22] Long-term follow-up is mandatory and must be thorough.

Recently, laparoscopic cyst excision and biliary reconstruction techniques have been introduced.[23–26] These advanced laparoscopic techniques are not widely used as yet, and there are no results available for mid- to long-term follow-up.

Classification

There are various types of choledochal cyst. Alonso-Lej *et al.*,[27] Todani *et al.*,[28] and Komi *et al.*[29] each described classifications of choledochal cysts based on anatomy, cholangiography of the hepatic ducts, and the pancreaticobiliary junction. However, we prefer to classify choledochal cysts into groups according to the presence or absence of pancreaticobiliary malunion (Fig. 36.2). Cystic or fusiform types are the most common while other types such as diverticulum of the common bile duct, choledochocele and Caroli's disease are extremely rare in children in the author's experience. Todani *et al.*[30] also reported only cystic or fusiform types in his series of 103 cases.

Protocol for surgical management

Before surgery, the precise anatomy of the entire hepato-biliary-pancreatic tract, including the intrahepatic and

Pediatric Surgery and Urology: Long-term Outcomes, Mark Stringer, Keith Oldham, Pierre Mouriquand.

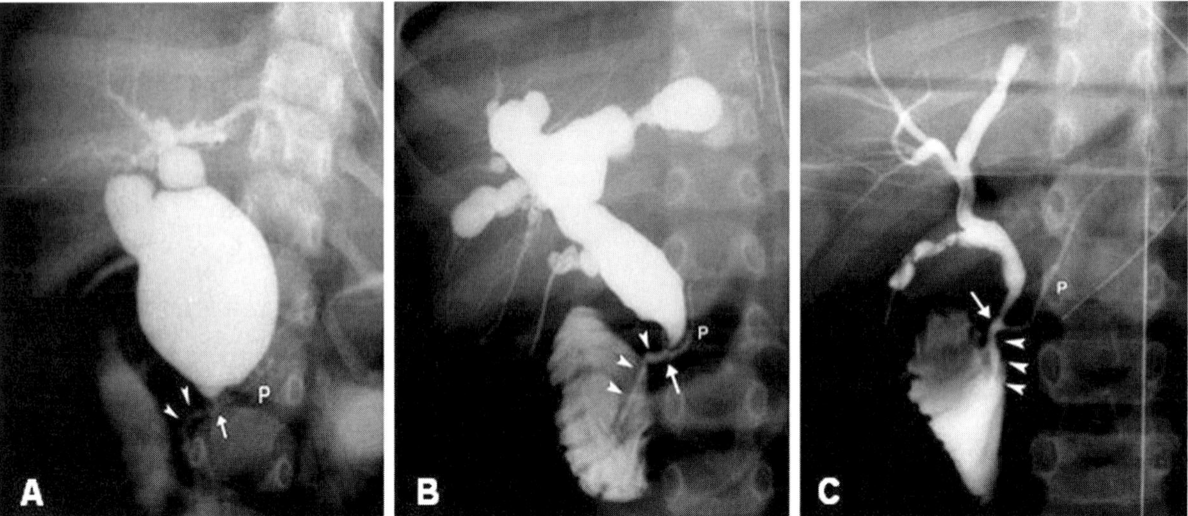

Fig. 36.1. Intraoperative cholangiograms. (a) Cystic choledochal dilatation (b) Fusiform choledochal dilatation (c) Forme fruste choledochal cyst. P: Pancreatic duct. Arrow: Junction between the pancreatic duct and the common bile duct. Arrowheads: long common channel.

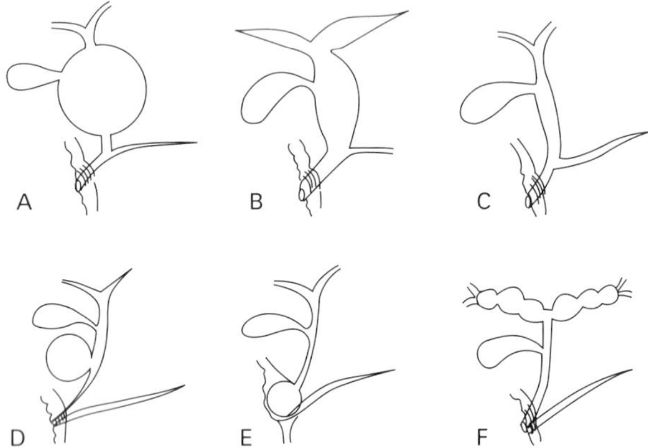

Fig. 36.2. Classification of choledochal cysts. With pancreaticobiliary malunion: (a) Cystic type. (b) Fusiform type (c) Forme fruste. Without pancreaticobiliary malunion: (d) Cystic diverticulum of the common bile duct. (e) Choledochocele (diverticulum of the distal common bile duct). (f) Intrahepatic bile duct dilatation alone (Caroli's disease). (Reproduced from Miyano T, Yamataka A. Choledochal cysts. *Curr. Opin. Pediatr.* 1997; **9**:284.)

extrahepatic bile ducts, and the intrapancreatic duct must be obtained.

Major steps in the surgical management of choledochal cyst are:

(i) cholangiography
(ii) cyst excision
(iii) intraoperative endoscopy
(iv) dissection and excision of the distal common bile duct
(v) adequate excision of the common hepatic duct at the correct level
(vi) hepaticojejunostomy (end-to-end anastomosis)
(vii) roux-en-Y biliary reconstruction

Cholangiography

Recent developments in imaging technology such as the introduction of magnetic resonance cholangiopancreatography (MRCP) and improvements in endoscopic retrograde cholangiopancreatography (ERCP) now allow the anatomy of the hepato-biliary-pancreatic ductal system to be visualized preoperatively in most choledochal cyst cases.[31] Before cyst excision, detailed information about intrahepatic bile duct anomalies such as ductal stenosis, dilatation, and the presence of debris/stones (Fig. 36.3), as well as intrapancreatic bile duct anomalies such as the type of pancreaticobiliary malunion, presence of debris/protein plugs in the common channel (Fig. 36.4(a)), and dilatation of the pancreatic duct must be obtained.

MRCP is generally reliable in children over 3 years old (Fig. 36.4(a)), but if the patient is an infant or younger child, pancreaticobiliary malunion may not be demonstrated clearly. If pancreatitis is present, ERCP is generally contraindicated, so intraoperative cholangiography is then the only option for obtaining information about the entire anatomy of the hepato-biliary-pancreatic duct system.

Cyst excision

There are usually more adhesions between a cystic type choledochal cyst and surrounding vital structures such as the portal vein and hepatic artery compared with a fusiform

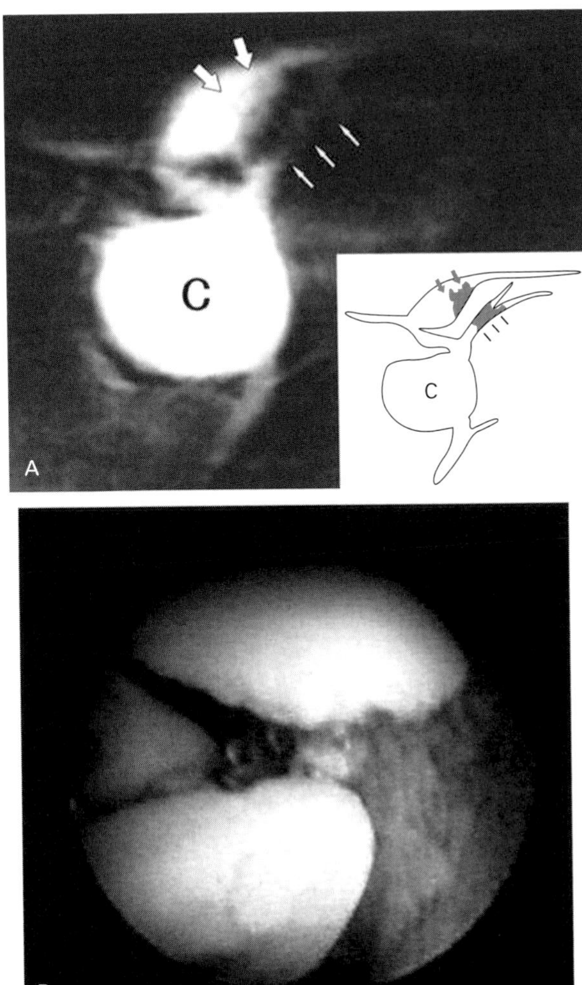

Fig. 36.3. (a) Preoperative MRCP showing extensive debris within dilated intrahepatic bile ducts (large arrows) and non-dilated intrahepatic bile ducts (small arrows). C: choledochal cyst. (b) Intrahepatic bile duct debris seen through the pediatric cystoscope. (Reproduced from Shimotakahara A. *et al. Pediatr. Surg. Int.* 2004; **20**:68.)

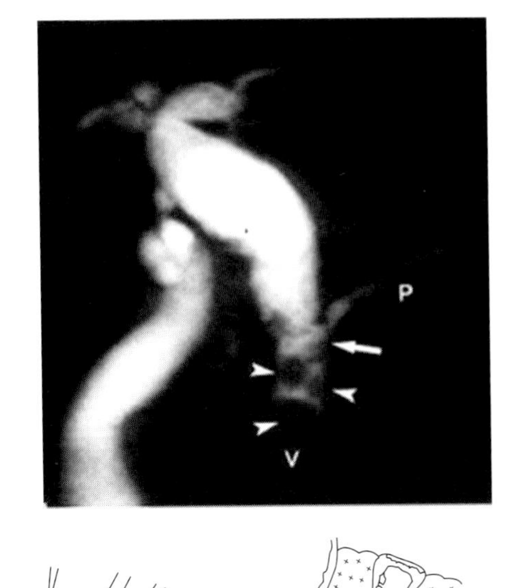

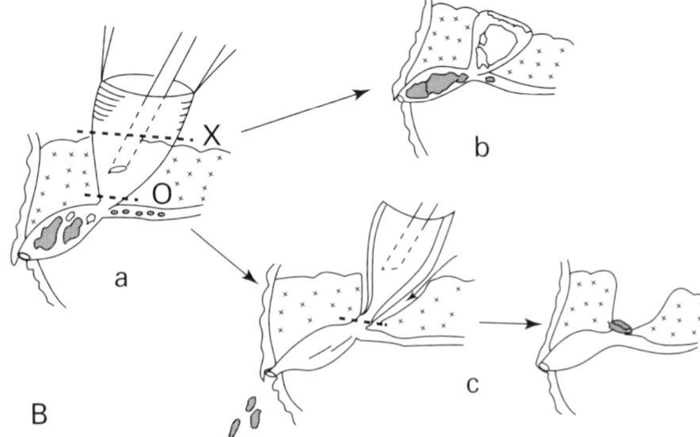

Fig. 36.4. (a) MRCP showing a fusiform choledochal cyst, long common channel, protein plugs (arrowheads), and pancreatic duct (P). V: Papilla of Vater. Arrow indicates junction between the common bile duct and the pancreatic duct. (Reproduced from Miyano, T. & Yamataka, A. Choledochal cysts. *Curr. Opin. Pediatr.* 1997; **9**:285.) (b) a. O is the appropriate level of excision. X is inadequate. b. Incomplete excision leads to residual cyst formation and protein plugs. c. Intraoperative endoscopy allows safe and complete cyst excision and irrigation of the common channel. (From Miyano, T. (2006). Choledochal cyst. In *Pediatric Surgery* (Springer Surgery Atlas Series), ed. P. Puri and M. Hollwarth, Berlin: Springer-Verlag.)

type choledochal cyst, especially if the patient is an older child. In adolescents and adults with a cystic type choledochal cyst, adhesions are often very dense, and great care is required during cyst excision.

Prior to dissection of the cyst, we always open the anterior wall of the choledochal cyst transversely (Fig. 36.5(a)). Because anatomical variants of the common hepatic duct are sometimes associated with a cystic type choledochal cyst, this incision should be made below the middle of the cyst. By opening the cyst anteriorly, the posterior wall of the cyst is visible directly from the inside (Fig. 36.5(b), (d)), and dissection of the choledochal cyst from surrounding tissues is easier than dissecting the cyst *in toto*. If the cyst is extremely inflamed and adhesions are very dense, a mucosectomy (Fig. 36.5(c), (d)) rather than full-thickness dissection should be performed (Fig. 36.5(b), (d)) to minimize the risk of damaging surrounding structures such as the portal vein and hepatic artery.

Compared with the cystic type, adhesions between the extrahepatic duct and surrounding structures are less dense in fusiform choledochal cysts, especially in young children. As a result, the common hepatic duct can be safely dissected free from the portal vein and hepatic artery, after

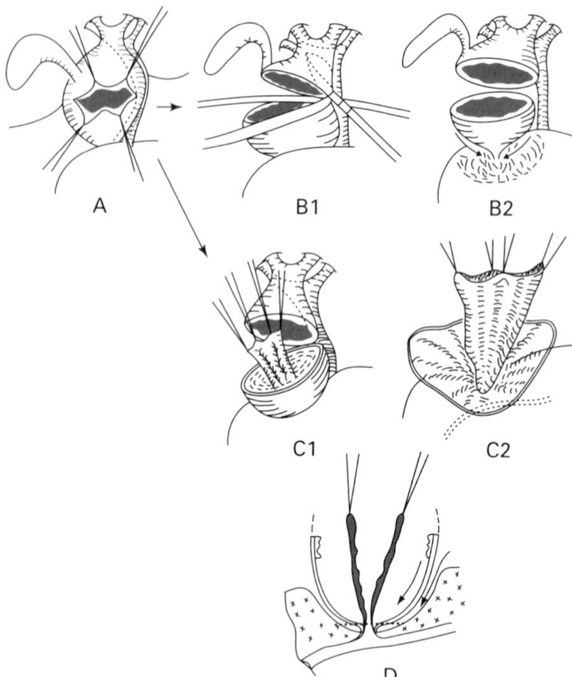

Fig. 36.5. (a) Opening the anterior wall of the choledochal cyst transversely. (b1) The posterior wall of the cyst is visible from the inside and this facilitates dissection of the choledochal cyst. (b2) Full-thickness dissection of the cyst. (C1, C2) If the cyst is extremely inflamed and adhesions dense, mucosectomy should be performed. (d) Arrows indicate the appropriate layer for full-thickness dissection and mucosectomy. (From Miyano, T. (2006). Choledochal cyst. In *Pediatric Surgery* (Springer Surgery Atlas Series), ed. P. Puri and M. Hollwarth, Berlin: Springer-Verlag.)

the anterior wall of the common bile duct is incised as described above.

Intraoperative endoscopy

Before the introduction of intraoperative endoscopy, it was difficult to safely excise the pancreatic portion of a fusiform type choledochal cyst at an adequate level for fear of injuring the pancreatic duct (Fig. 36.4(b)). We began performing intraoperative endoscopy routinely using a neonatal or pediatric cystoscope in 1986.[17] Intraoperative endoscopy allows safe and complete excision of the intrapancreatic portion of a fusiform type choledochal cyst without damaging the pancreatic duct; it also enables the common channel to be irrigated and cleared of any debris or protein plugs. We believe that intraoperative endoscopy reduces the risk of postoperative complications such as recurrent pancreatitis, stone formation, and carcinoma.[17]

Intraoperative endoscopy is also useful for identifying debris in dilated intrahepatic bile ducts, determining the ideal level of resection for the common hepatic duct, and for assessing the severity of any intrahepatic bile duct stenosis. A high incidence (26%) of intrahepatic bile duct debris not usually detected by preoperative radiologic investigations has been reported from the author's institution.[32] Without endoscopy, there is a tendency to overlook debris in the intrahepatic bile ducts noted on preoperative imaging. Furthermore, debris can be present in non-dilated intrahepatic bile ducts, although it is far more common when these ducts are dilated. These facts indicate that intraoperative endoscopic examination of intrahepatic bile ducts is mandatory even if preoperative radiologic investigations have shown no debris or abnormality.

Dissection and excision of the distal common bile duct

A fusiform type choledochal cyst is usually associated with complicated pancreaticobiliary malunion as well as debris/protein plugs in the common channel (Fig. 36.4). Pancreatic duct anomalies are also often present.[27,33] Thus, dissection of the distal common bile duct in a fusiform type choledochal cyst should be performed with great care so as to avoid leaving behind any intrapancreatic portion of the common bile duct and to prevent injury to the pancreatic duct. Intraoperative endoscopy of the distal common bile duct should be performed in all cases, but especially in patients with a fusiform type choledochal cyst.

Fusiform type choledochal cyst is associated with a specific complication shown in Fig. 36.4. If the distal common bile duct is resected along line X (Fig. 36.4(*b*)a), a cyst will gradually reform around the distal duct left within the pancreas, leading to recurrent pancreatitis and/or stone formation or malignancy within the cyst (Fig. 36.4(*b*)b).[33] In contrast, if the distal duct is resected along line O just above the pancreaticobiliary ductal junction, this complication is unlikely to develop (Fig. 36.4(*b*)a). With a cystic type choledochal cyst (Fig. 36.5), the distal common bile duct is often narrow; occasionally, it is so narrow that it cannot be identified and the cyst appears blind-ended. In such cases, mucosectomy or full-thickness cyst excision need only be performed to the level of the pancreaticobiliary junction.

Adequate excision of the common hepatic duct at the correct level

The ideal length of the common hepatic duct required for anastomosis is approximately 10 mm, since a longer common hepatic duct may become kinked leading to bile stasis in the intrahepatic bile ducts. However, the lumen of the common hepatic duct should be inspected before it is shortened, because ductal anomalies such as luminal stenosis, an aberrant duct opening, or a septum may be present. These anatomical variations have been described in the literature and encountered by the author[16,30] and can affect the success of hepaticoenterostomy after cyst excision. Intraoperative endoscopy can also be used to inspect the common hepatic duct and minimize difficulties arising from duct anomalies.[17]

A cystic type choledochal cyst is often associated with stenosis and dilatation of intrahepatic bile ducts. The incidence of postoperative complications such as recurrent cholangitis, stone formation, and anastomotic stricture is increased in patients with intrahepatic bile duct dilatation.[8–10] Surgical correction is required for severe congenital intrahepatic duct stenosis, especially if the proximal intrahepatic bile ducts are very dilated. However, the incidence of late complications secondary to stenosis or dilatation of intrahepatic ducts is generally low, especially in young children.[8] Therefore, excessive surgical intervention may be unnecessary except in cases where there is massive dilatation of peripheral intrahepatic bile ducts with severe downstream stenosis. If intrahepatic bile duct dilatation persists after definitive surgery, careful follow-up is mandatory.

When ductal stenosis is present at the hepatic hilum or at the first branch of the left or right hepatic ducts, surgical dilatation or duct plasty can be performed.[16,34] However, if the stenosis is located more peripherally, treatment is difficult. Large diffusely dilated intrahepatic bile ducts in both lobes cannot be treated but if cholangitis or stone formation affects a localized area of dilated intrahepatic ducts, liver resection may be indicated at a later stage.

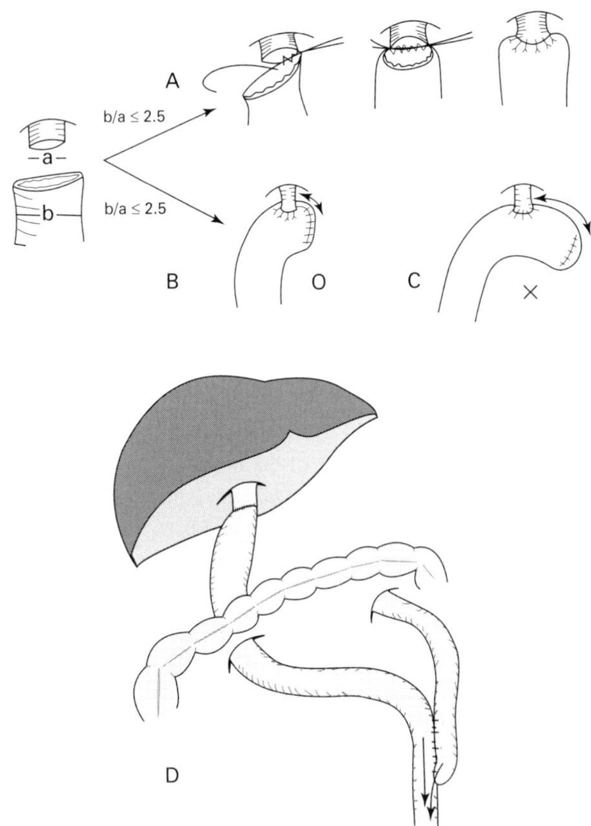

Fig. 36.6. Hepaticojejunostomy. (a) End-to-end anastomosis. (b) End-to-side anastomosis as close as possible to the closed end of the Roux loop. (c) If an end-to-side anastomosis is performed far from the closed end of the Roux loop, elongation of the blind pouch will occur leading to complications. (d) An adequate Roux-en-Y hepatico-jejunostomy. Arrowheads indicate the approximated native jejunum and distal Roux limb. Arrows indicate smooth passage without reflux of small bowel contents. (a)–(c) from Miyano T. (2006). Choledochal cyst. In *Pediatric Surgery* (Springer Surgery Atlas Series), ed. P. Puri and M. Hollwarth, Berlin: Springer-Verlag. (d) from Yamataka A. *et al.* Recommendations for preventing complications related to Roux-en-Y hepatico-jejunostomy performed during excision of choledochal cyst in children. *J. Pediatr. Surg.* 2003; **38**:1831.)

Hepaticojejunostomy (end-to-end anastomosis)

After cyst excision and Roux-en-Y hepaticojejunostomy, a good short-term outcome is expected. However, with time, complications related to Roux-en-Y hepaticojejunostomy in childhood develop often enough to be of concern; they are mostly related to elongation of the blind pouch at the hepaticojejunostomy or at the Roux-en-Y jejunal anastomosis as a result of the child's growth.[35] Based on experience and complications reported in the literature,[6–13] the author's institution developed the following recommendations to prevent complications related to the Roux-en-Y hepaticojejunostomy.[35]

An end-to-end anastomosis at the Roux-en-Y hepaticojejunostomy is recommended if the ratio between the diameters of the common hepatic duct and the proximal Roux-en-Y jejunum at the proposed site of anastomosis is less than or equal to 1 (common hepatic duct): 2.5 (jejunum) (Fig. 36.6(a)) – this prevents elongation of the blind pouch. If an end-to-side anastomosis is unavoidable, the common hepatic duct should be anastomosed as close as possible to the closed end of the Roux loop (Fig. 36.6(b)); if this anastomosis is constructed some distance away from the blind end of the Roux loop (Fig. 36.6(c)), elongation of the blind pouch will occur later in life as the child grows, causing bile stasis in the pouch and intrahepatic bile ducts (especially if they are dilated) and subsequent cholangitis and stone formation. An end-to-end hepaticojejunostomy or a modified end-to-side anastomosis as mentioned above prevents these complications.

Roux-en-Y biliary reconstruction

Some surgeons predetermine the length of the Roux-en-Y jejunal limb (e.g., 30 cm, 40 cm, 50 cm, or 60 cm) without considering the size of the child, which results in an unnecessarily long Roux-en-Y jejunal limb, especially in infants and younger children. Redundancy of the Roux-en-Y limb is likely to occur later in life as the patient grows and may cause bile stasis in the Roux loop itself as well as the intrahepatic bile ducts, leading to cholangitis and/or stone formation. Thus, the length of the Roux-en-Y limb should be individualized so that the Roux-en-Y jejunojejunostomy fits naturally into the splenic flexure after it is returned to the peritoneal cavity (Fig. 36.6(d)). In this way, redundancy of the Roux-en-Y limb can be prevented.

When a jejunojejunostomy and Roux-en-Y limb are used, both the native jejunum and the Roux-en-Y jejunal limb proximal to the jejunojejunostomy should be approximated for up to 8 cm to ensure that both the bile in the Roux-en-Y limb and the contents of the native jejunum flow smoothly down into the distal jejunum (Fig. 36.6(d)). If this approximation is not performed, the jejunojejunostomy tends to be T-shaped, and there may be reflux of jejunal contents into the Roux-en-Y limb, leading to dilatation and biliary stasis in the Roux loop, a situation the author recently encountered in an 18-year-old girl who had had cyst excision and Roux-en-Y hepaticojejunostomy at another hospital 17 years earlier.[36] Biliary stasis in the Roux-en-Y limb in this patient resulted in stone formation in the intrahepatic bile ducts (Fig. 36.7). She required endoscopic removal of intrahepatic bile duct stones and revision of the Roux-en-Y jejunojejunostomy.

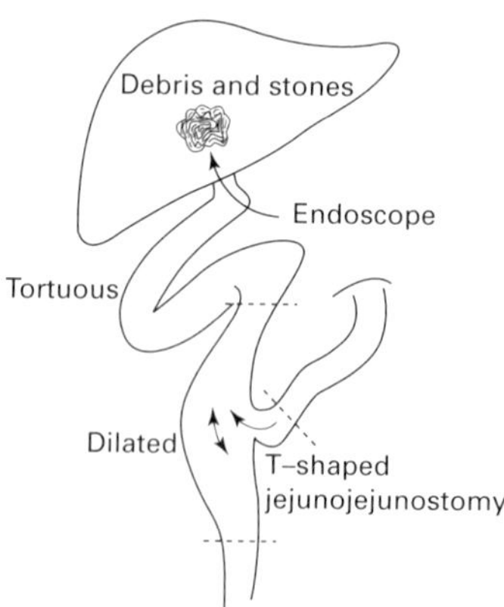

Fig. 36.7. In this case, a flexible endoscope was inserted into the intrahepatic bile ducts and massive debris and multiple biliary stones were removed using an electro hydraulic lithotripsy device inserted through the endoscope. The patient had a tortuous, dilated Roux-en-Y loop and T-shaped jejunojejunostomy, and there appeared to be reflux (arrow) of jejunal contents up the Roux loop. The jejunojejunostomy and the dilated distal part of the Roux loop (between the dotted lines) were revised. (Reproduced from Shima, H. *et al.* Intracorporeal electrohydraulic lithotripsy for intrahepatic bile duct stone formation after choledochal cyst excision: a case report. *Pediatr. Surg. Int.* 2004; **20**:71.)

Short-term outcome

The postoperative course of primary cyst excision with biliary reconstruction is generally uneventful in children, and the short-term outcome is excellent with few exceptions reported in the literature.[6,37–40] Perioperative death due to primary cyst excision is extremely rare in children. The author's institution and affiliated hospitals have performed primary cyst excision with no operative mortality in 176 children with choledochal cyst aged 15 years or less.

Early post excision complications seen occasionally include minor leakage at the hepaticojejunostomy, elevation in pancreatic or hepatic enzymes (asymptomatic in the author's series), and adhesive bowel obstruction. All can usually be managed conservatively and rarely require emergency surgery except for severe adhesive bowel obstruction.[6,8]

The incidence of minor leakage at the hepaticoenterostomy anastomosis has been reported to range from 4 to 14%,[6,41] although this complication was not encountered in the author's series. Leakage is probably a result of severe inflammation in the wall of the common hepatic duct at the anastomosis rather than technical failure, and is therefore more likely in adolescents and adults. Appropriate placement of a Penrose drain is extremely important in keeping the hepaticoenterostomy anastomosis drained postoperatively, thereby helping to prevent abscess formation due to a small bile leak.

After cyst excision, bleeding from the operative site, gastrointestinal bleeding due to peptic ulceration (possibly secondary to Roux-en-Y hepaticojejunostomy), acute pancreatitis, and pancreatic fistula have all been reported[30] but the author has not personally experienced these postoperative complications.

Long-term outcome

Based on the author's experience, the risk of post-cyst excision complications is reduced in patients who undergo cyst

Table 36.1. Type of cyst excision and hepaticoenterostomy and postoperative complication rate for children vs. adults[8]

Type of excision	Number of children	Number of adults
Primary cyst excision	176 (13) [7.4%]	22 (6) [27.3%]
Cyst excision after cystoenterostomy	5 (0) [0%]	9 (5) [55.6%]
Cyst excision after other biliary surgery[a]	19 (5) [26.3%]	9 (6) [66.7%]
Total	200 (18) [9.0%]	40 (17) [42.5%]

Note: Numbers in parentheses indicate number of patients who had post-cyst excision complications, percent in brackets indicate post-cyst excision complication rate.
[a]Percutaneous transhepatic biliary drainage, percutaneous cyst drainage, T-tube drainage, cholecystectomy, choledochotomy or sphincterotomy.

excision as young children (at 5 years of age or less) compared to older children or adults.[8] Many published series of choledochal cysts[6–15,30] include a large number of adults and other patients who had secondary cyst excision after previous cystoenterostomy (no longer recommended). As a result, these reports may not reflect the true incidence of complications after primary cyst excision in children.

This chapter provides a more accurate description of long-term complications after primary cyst excision in children with a choledochal cyst. Thus, data from children are presented separately from adult data and from patients who underwent secondary cyst excision after previous cystoenterostomy or other drainage procedures.

"Cystic"- or "fusiform"-type choledochal cysts

Children vs. adults

The author has reviewed 200 children and 40 adults who had a choledochal cyst excised between 1964 and 1995 and who have been followed up for more than 8 years. Patients were classified as children if they underwent surgery when less than 16 years of age, and as adults if they had a cyst excised at 16 years of age or older. Choledochal cysts were either cystic or fusiform. Complications and their surgical management were of particular interest.

Children

Of the 200 children, 145 were aged 5 years or less at the time of cyst excision; the overall mean age at cyst excision was 4.2 years. One hundred and seventy-six had primary cyst excision, 5 had cyst excision after previous cystoenterostomy, and 19 had cyst excision after other types of biliary surgery (Table 36.1). Of the 200 hepaticoenterostomies, 159 were end-to-side anastomoses (147 Roux-en-Y hepaticojejunostomies, 11 standard hepaticoduodenostomies, and 1 jejunal interposition hepaticoduodenostomy), and 41 were end-to-end Roux-en-Y hepaticojejunostomies. The age at onset of symptoms (abdominal pain and/or jaundice and/or abdominal mass) was 5 years or less in 175 children, and between 6 and 15 years in the remaining 25 children (overall mean 3.0 years). Intraoperative endoscopy was performed in 70 children treated between 1986 and 1995. The mean duration of follow-up was 17.9 years.

Adults

The mean age at cyst excision was 35 years. Of the 40 adults, 22 had primary cyst excision, 9 had cyst excision after previous cystoenterostomy, and 9 had cyst excision after other types of biliary surgery (Table 36.1). Of the 40 hepaticoenterostomies, 38 were end-to-side Roux-en-Y hepaticojejunostomies, and 2 were end-to-end hepaticojejunostomies. Eleven adults were symptomatic as children (less than 16 years of age) and the remaining 29 became symptomatic at a later age (mean 26 years). The mean duration of follow-up was 17.7 years.

The time interval between the onset of initial symptoms and cyst excision was significantly less in children than in adults ($P < 0.0001$: ANOVA). The number of children and adults with post-cyst excision complications was 18/200 (9.0%) and 17/40 (42.5%), respectively (Table 36.1). The complication rate in children was significantly lower than in adults ($P < 0.0001{:}\chi^2$).

Complications after cyst excision in children

Twenty-five complications after cyst excision were seen in 18 children (Table 36.2). Fifteen of the 18 children required surgical intervention (Table 36.3). Intrahepatic bile duct stone formation occurred in three children who had primary cyst excision; two had stones at the porta hepatis, and one had stones at the porta hepatis and in the left lobe of the liver. All three had intrahepatic bile duct dilatation prior to cyst excision that persisted postoperatively. Two of the three children with stones had a stricture at the end-to-side hepaticojejunostomy (aged 7 and 12 years at cyst excision). The remaining child had no anastomotic stricture but there was an abnormally long blind pouch of jejunum at the end-to-side hepaticojejunostomy (Fig. 36.8), bile stasis in dilated intrahepatic bile ducts exacerbated by this long blind pouch was considered to be the cause of stone formation. The two children with strictures presented with ascending cholangitis and the other patient with recurrent epigastric pain. Recurrent ascending cholangitis without intrahepatic bile duct stone formation was seen in the child who was treated at another hospital by cyst excision and a jejunal interposition hepaticoduodenostomy. Revision

Table 36.2. Complications after cyst excision and hepaticoenterostomy: children vs. adults[8]

Complication	Incidence in 200 children	Incidence in 40 adults
Ascending cholangitis	3	9
Intrahepatic bile duct stones	3	5
Intrapancreatic terminal choledochal calculi	3[a]	1
Pancreatic duct calculus	1	1
Stones in the blind pouch of the end-to-side Roux loop	1[a]	0
Bowel obstruction	9	3
Cholangiocarcinoma	0	2
Liver dysfunction	0	1
Pancreatitis	5	5
Total	25 (18)	27 (17)

Note: The numbers in parentheses indicate the number of patients who had post-cyst excision complications (18 children and 17 adults had 25 and 27 complications, respectively).

[a]One patient with intrapancreatic terminal choledochal calculi also had a stone in the blind pouch of an end-to-side hepaticojejunostomy.

Table 36.3. Surgical management of post-cyst excision complications in children vs. adults[8]

Surgical management	Number of children	Number of adults
Revision of hepaticoenterostomy	4[a]	2
Percutaneous transhepatic cholangioscopic lithotomy	1	2
Left hepatic lobectomy	0	1
Excision of residual intrapancreatic terminal choledochus	2[b]	0
Endoscopic sphincterotomy	1	2
Pancreaticojejunostomy (Puestow procedure)	1	0
Exploratory laparotomy for malignancy	0	2
Laparotomy for bowel obstruction	6	1
Total	15	10

[a]One child also required left lateral segmentectomy of the liver.

[b]One child also required excision of the blind pouch of the end-to-side Roux-en-Y hepaticojejunostomy which contained stones.

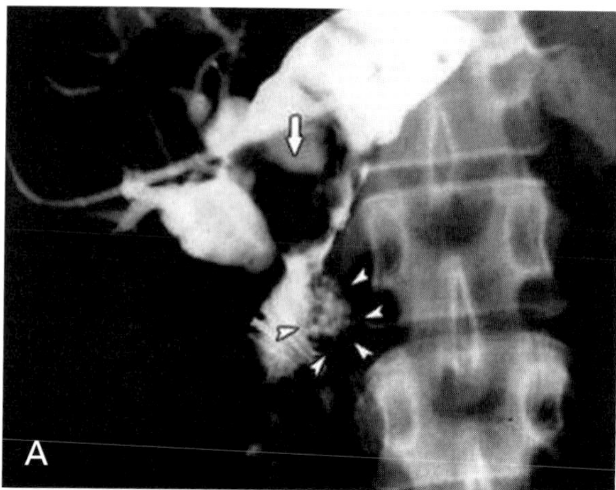

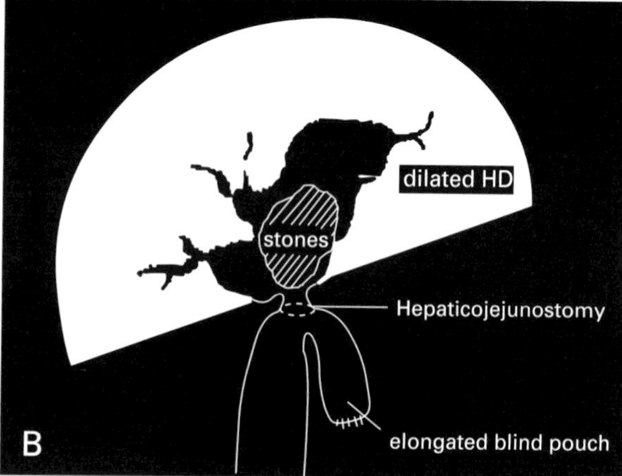

Fig. 36.8. (a) Percutaneous transhepatic cholangiogram. Arrowheads show an elongated blind pouch at the end-to-side hepaticojejunostomy. The arrow shows stones in the dilated intrahepatic bile ducts. (b) Diagram of the findings.

of the hepaticoenterostomy was performed in three cases and percutaneous transhepatic cholangioscopic lithotomy in one. Stone formation in the residual intrapancreatic terminal choledochus developed postoperatively in three children after primary cyst excision (Fig. 36.9).

Pancreatic duct stones developed in one patient 11 years after secondary cyst excision. Four patients presented with recurrent pancreatitis; two had excision of a remnant intrapancreatic terminal choledochus, one had stones removed by endoscopic sphincterotomy, and the remaining patient had a pancreaticojejunostomy. One additional child had pancreatitis without stone formation after primary cyst excision, and was treated medically.

Nine children developed adhesive bowel obstruction. One required revision of the Roux-en-Y hepaticojejunostomy; in this case, cyst excision with hepaticojejunostomy had been performed at another hospital and dense adhesions had formed between the Roux-en-Y limb, the

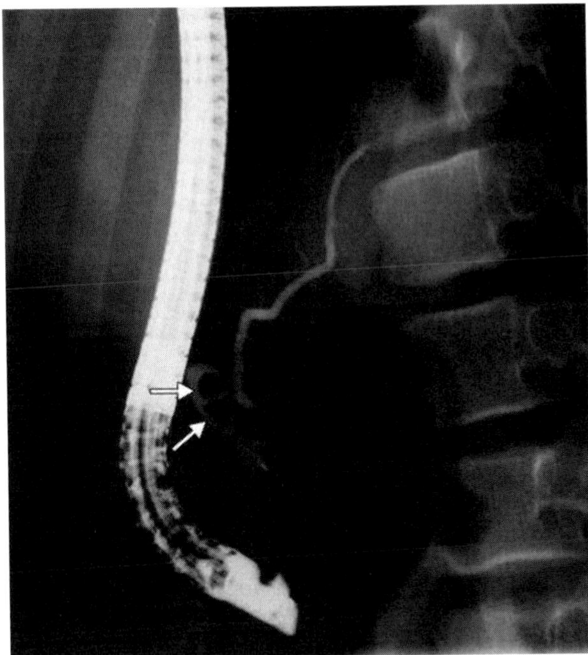

Fig. 36.9. ERCP showing stones (arrow) in the residual intrapancreatic terminal choledochus after excision of fusiform type choledochal cyst. (Reproduced from Yamataka, A. *et al.* Complications after cyst excision with hepaticoenterostomy for choledochal cyst and their surgical management in children versus adults. *J. Pediatr. Surg.* 1997; **32**:1099.)

duodenum, and an abnormally elongated blind pouch of the end-to-side hepaticojejunostomy. After adhesiolysis and excision of the redundant pouch, the end-to-side anastomosis was converted to an end-to-end anastomosis. In the remaining eight patients, six required adhesiolysis and two were treated conservatively.

Stone formation after cyst excision occurred in seven (3.5%) children, all of whom underwent cyst excision at the age of 6 years or more (Table 36.4). One patient had stone formation both in the residual intrapancreatic terminal choledochus and in the blind pouch of the end-to-side hepaticojejunostomy. Neither stone formation nor anastomotic stricture was seen in the 145 children who underwent cyst excision at 5 years of age or less. The incidence of stone formation after cyst excision in children aged 5 years or less was significantly lower than in older children (12.7%) and adults (17.5%) ($P < 0.0001{:}\chi^2$).

It is worth emphasizing that there was neither stone formation, anastomotic stricture, nor cholangitis after cyst excision in the 70 children who had intraoperative endoscopy, and in the 41 children who underwent end-to-end hepaticojejunostomy.

Table 36.4. Stone formation after cyst excision and hepaticoenterostomy: children vs. adults[8]

	145 children aged < or = 5 yr[a]	55 children >5 yr[a]	40 adults >15 yr[a]
Number of patients with stones	0 (0%)[b]	7[c] (12.7%)	7 (17.5%)

Note: Percentages in parentheses indicate the incidence of post-cyst excision stone formation.
[a]Age at cyst excision.
[b]$P < 0.0001$ for children aged < or = 5 yr vs. children aged >5 yr or adults.
[c]One child formed two stones (one in the residual intrapancreatic terminal choledochus and the other in the blind pouch of the end-to-side Roux loop).

Complications after cyst excision in adults

Twenty-five complications were seen after cyst excision in 17 (42.5%) adults (Table 36.2). Ten of these 17 adults required surgical intervention (Table 36.3).

Intrahepatic bile duct stone formation at the porta hepatis occurred in four cases, all of whom had secondary cyst excision after a previous cystoenterostomy. Two of these patients had an anastomotic stricture of an end-to-side hepaticojejunostomy. Intrahepatic bile duct stones developed in the left lobe of the liver in one patient 10 years after secondary cyst excision (Fig 36.10). Four of these five patients also had intrahepatic bile duct dilatation before cyst excision that persisted postoperatively. All five presented with ascending cholangitis. Revision of the hepaticoenterostomy was performed in two, percutaneous transhepatic cholangioscopic lithotomy in two, and left hepatic lobectomy in one.

Stone formation in the residual intrapancreatic terminal choledochus developed in one adult and a pancreatic duct stone in another. The former had undergone secondary cyst excision after cystoenterostomy, and the latter had had primary cyst excision. Both presented with recurrent pancreatitis. Both patients underwent endoscopic sphincterotomy and stone removal.

Two adults died of cholangiocarcinoma at 54 years and 29 years of age, respectively. The former had secondary cyst excision at the age of 48 years after a previous cholecystectomy at the age of 32 years, and developed carcinoma in a dilated intrahepatic bile duct in the left lobe. The other patient underwent primary cyst excision at the age of 25 years, and carcinoma developed within a large remnant intrapancreatic terminal choledochus. Both patients presented with ascending cholangitis and both had an exploratory laparotomy.

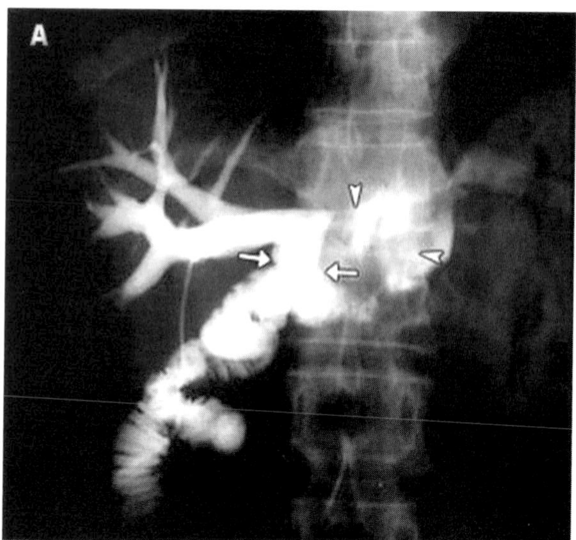

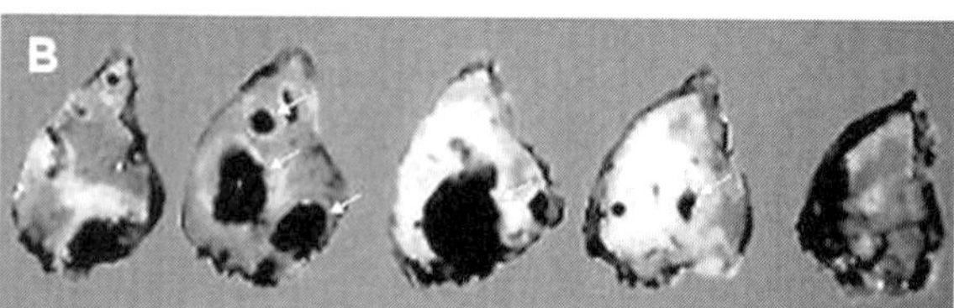

Fig. 36.10. Preoperative cholangiogram and pathologic sections of resected specimen from an adult who required a left lobectomy for hepatolithiasis. (a) Cholangiogram suggests stones (arrowheads) in the left hepatic lobe and a patent hepaticojejunostmy (arrows). (b) Sections of resected left hepatic lobe showing stones in dilated intrahepatic bile ducts (arrows). (Reproduced from Yamataka A. *et al.* Complications after cyst excision with hepaticoenterostomy for choledochal cyst and their surgical management in children versus adults. *J. Pediat. Surg.* 1997; **32**:1100.)

Two adults with intrahepatic bile duct dilatation had ascending cholangitis without stone formation; both had had secondary cyst excision. Three adults had recurrent pancreatitis without stone formation after secondary cyst excision and one further adult had postoperative liver dysfunction. These six subjects were treated medically.

Three adults developed adhesive bowel obstruction, one of whom required laparotomy and adhesiolysis.

Stone formation in intrahepatic bile ducts

In the author's experience, the risk factors for intrahepatic bile duct stone formation are intrahepatic bile duct dilatation, anastomotic stricture, and residual debris in the intrahepatic bile ducts.[32]

Dilated intrahepatic bile ducts

Intrahepatic bile duct dilatation typically improves or resolves after cyst excision, particularly in young children.[39] However, it tends to persist in adolescents and adults. This is because histologic damage to intrahepatic bile ducts appears to be reversible in young children but not in adolescents and adults. Dilatation of peripheral intrahepatic bile ducts in adults is associated with late complications such as stone formation and recurrent cholangitis, and is thus occasionally managed by liver resection, intrahepatic cystoenterostomy, or balloon dilatation of duct stenoses at the time of cyst excision.[18,28,41,42] In contrast, the incidence of late complications is much less in children with intrahepatic bile duct dilatation than in adults, and so similar surgical interventions may be unnecessary, although these children must be followed-up very carefully.

Anastomotic stricture

In the author's series, an anastomotic stricture developed in four patients who had had cyst excision at the ages of 7, 12, 16, and 19 years, respectively. There appears to be an increased incidence of stricture in older children undergoing cyst excision; no anastomotic strictures developed in the 145 children who had cyst excision at 5 years of age or less. Inflammation of the cyst wall tends to be mild in children under 10 years of age and more severe in older patients, indicating that histologic damage to the common hepatic duct at the site of the hepaticoenterostomy is more marked in older children and adults.[39] Bile stasis in dilated intrahepatic bile ducts probably further exacerbates inflammatory changes at the anastomosis. A previous cystoenterostomy is also likely to have caused irreversible histologic damage to the common hepatic duct and intrapancreatic ducts. Our four patients who had an anastomotic stricture either had intrahepatic bile duct dilatation or a previous cystoenterostomy.

Anastomotic leakage secondary to technical problems can cause the development of granulation tissue that may result in an anastomotic stricture. The fate of a hepaticoenterostomy in young children (5 years of age or less at cyst excision) is probably related more to surgical skill than histologic damage to the common hepatic duct. Mortality or serious morbidity secondary to an anastomotic stricture and intrahepatic bile duct stone formation have been widely reported in young children.[9–12,43] Common hepatic ducts are generally larger in older children and adults and the hepaticoenterostomy is usually easier than in young children. However, cyst excision is more difficult in adolescents and adults because of the presence of severe pericyst inflammation, and histologic damage of the common hepatic duct is more marked. Consequently, an anastomotic stricture occurring in older children and adults is more likely to be caused by inflammatory changes rather than surgical inexperience.

Residual debris in the intrahepatic bile ducts

Stones may occasionally develop in dilated intrahepatic bile ducts even when there is no anastomotic stricture or bile duct stenosis.[9,11–13] Choledochal cysts in adults are frequently associated with stones or debris in the biliary tract before surgery.[14,22,44] Debris in the intrahepatic bile ducts is also commonly seen in children at the time of cyst excision.[32] This can sometimes be impacted. Intraoperative endoscopy is beneficial in such cases to ensure that the ducts are cleared of debris. In the author's series, there was no instance of intrahepatic bile duct stone formation in the 70 children who had intraoperative endoscopy. In contrast, in the subjects who developed intrahepatic bile duct stones in our series and in previous reports, intraoperative endoscopy had not been performed.[9–11] Thus, residual debris in the intrahepatic bile ducts at the time of cyst excision is likely to be a risk factor for stone formation after cyst excision.[32]

Stone formation in the intrapancreatic residual choledochus

Stone formation may occur as a result of stasis of pancreatic secretions in the intrapancreatic terminal choledochus (from incomplete excision of the terminal choledochus at the time of cyst excision) or from residual protein plugs/debris within the common channel. Many surgeons divide the distal part of the choledochal cyst just above the pancreatic head during cyst excision, even if the cyst is fusiform. However, by doing this, a large intrapancreatic terminal choledochus, which is the distal end of the choledochal cyst, often ends up being left behind, particularly when the choledochal cyst is fusiform. This problem can also occur in cystic type choledochal cysts in adults, because of the difficulty in excising the distal part of the cyst in the presence of severe pericystic inflammation around the pancreas. To prevent stone formation in the residual intrapancreatic choledochus, complete excision of the distal part of the choledochal cyst should be performed under intraoperative endoscopic control.[33,45]

Malignancy

Although excision of the cyst removes a potential site of malignant change, it does not prevent the development of carcinoma[38] (see also Chapter 20). The relative risk for carcinoma after excision is still higher than that in the general population, although the risk is decreased by approximately 50% by cyst excision.[46] The interval between primary cyst excision and the development of cancer ranges from 1.8 to 25 years.[47] This indicates that the epithelium of the remnant bile duct wall may have already progressed to a precancerous stage at the time of surgery.

There are case reports of cholangiocarcinoma arising from the intrahepatic bile ducts, within the intrapancreatic residual terminal choledochus, and at the hepaticojejunostomy anastomosis.[19–21] The author has had no cases of cholangiocarcinoma in children but two adults have died from cholangiocarcinoma, one after primary cyst excision at the age of 25 years. There is one report of a cholangiocarcinoma developing in the intrapancreatic residual terminal choledochus after primary cyst excision at the age of 14 years.[19]

Chronic bile stasis in the intrahepatic bile ducts may be responsible for the development of carcinoma in intrahepatic bile ducts.[6] Carcinoma in the intrapancreatic residual choledochus could be due to continuous reflux of pancreatic secretions into this segment. If so, complete excision of the intrapancreatic terminal choledochus should reduce this risk.

"Forme fruste" choledochal cyst

Okada *et al.*[48] were the first to report a case of a common pancreaticobiliary channel with minimal dilatation of the common bile duct in 1981 and called it "common channel syndrome." It was later renamed "forme fruste choledochal cyst" by Lilly *et al.*[49] in 1985 who described pancreaticobiliary malunion with little or no dilatation of the common bile duct (Fig. 36.1(c)). The optimal treatment of this condition in adults is controversial[50,51] but, in children, the common bile duct should always be excised because of the long-term risk of bile duct malignancy from pancreaticobiliary reflux associated with the common channel.[52] There are only a few reports on forme fruste choledochal cyst in the English-language literature.[53–55]

We have experience of 17 (6%) cases from a total of 281 choledochal cysts treated by cyst excision between 1965 and 2002 at the author's institute or affiliated hospitals. The maximum diameter of the normal common bile duct in children has been reported to vary from 3 to 6 mm.[56,57] Minimal dilatation of the common bile duct is therefore defined as a maximum diameter of less than 10 mm. Pancreaticobiliary malunion was identified in all 17 of our patients using cholangiography. The mean diameter of the common bile duct was 7.8 mm (range 4 to 10 mm). Age at diagnosis ranged from 1 to 7 years (mean 2.5 years). Presenting symptoms were those of pancreatitis, i.e. abdominal pain associated with an elevated serum amylase, with or without jaundice. Mean age at common bile duct excision was 2.9 years. Fourteen patients had Roux-en-Y hepaticojejunostomy (end-to-end anastomosis in 5; end-to-side in 9), and 3 had hepaticoduodenostomy, using a single layer of 5–0 absorbable sutures. Interrupted sutures were used for both the anterior and posterior walls of the anastomosis in 8 cases, continuous sutures for both walls in 6 cases, and a combination of a continuous suture for the posterior wall and interrupted sutures for the anterior wall in 3 cases.

Histopathology of the excised common bile duct showed mucosal ulceration and/or slough in 35%, fibrosis in 53%, and inflammatory cell infiltration in 41%. The common bile duct in forme fruste choledochal cyst is therefore fragile and inflamed.[48,58] Consequently, hepaticoenterostomy can be difficult and tenuous, with a greater potential for anastomotic complications.[49]

The common channel contained protein plugs/debris in nine cases (54%), identified either by MRCP preoperatively or by endoscopic examination of the common channel intraoperatively. Intrahepatic bile ducts were dilated in 10 cases (59%) on preoperative MRCP and half contained debris. Intraoperative endoscopy was successfully used to remove all debris. Intrahepatic bile duct dilatation resolved in nine of ten cases postoperatively.

All patients are currently well after a mean postoperative follow-up period of 10.8 years (range 3 to 19 years), although one has occasional attacks of mild epigastric pain. No postoperative morbidity (e.g., ascending cholangitis, anastomotic stricture, or pancreatitis) was observed.

The majority of forme fruste choledochal cysts in adults have been found as an incidental finding during investigation of an abnormality of the gall bladder such as a tumor, polyp, or thickening of the wall.[59,60] Simple cholecystectomy without biliary reconstruction is often performed for adult cases.[55] In contrast, the majority of children with forme fruste choledochal cyst present with pancreatitis. A forme fruste choledochal cyst must be considered in a child with recurrent pancreatitis of unknown cause. MRCP or ERCP should confirm or exclude the presence of pancreaticobiliary malunion, which is a pathognomonic feature.

Recent research

Hepaticojejunostomy vs. hepaticoduodenostomy

Primary cyst excision with biliary reconstruction is generally accepted as the treatment of choice for choledochal cyst. The type of biliary reconstruction is based on the personal preference of the surgeon – some use Roux-en-Y hepaticojejunostomy, others hepaticoduodenostomy, and a few use other methods such as jejunal graft interposition hepaticoduodenostomy.[15,16,35,61]

A case of hilar bile duct carcinoma developing 19 years after primary cyst excision and hepaticoduodenostomy at the age of 13 months has recently been reported.[62] The author's institution reviewed 86 children who had primary cyst excision with either Roux-en-Y hepaticojejunostomy (n = 74: end-to-end anastomosis in 58; end-to-side anastomosis in 16) or hepaticoduodenostomy (n = 12) between 1986 and 2002, with special emphasis on postoperative complications related to the type of biliary reconstruction.[63] Forty-six hepaticojejunostomy cases were associated with intrahepatic bile duct dilatation and were excluded in order to focus on the results of biliary reconstruction alone. Hepaticoduodenostomy was not used for biliary reconstruction if intrahepatic bile duct dilatation was present. Thus, 28 children who had hepaticojejunostomy were compared with 12 children who had hepaticoduodenostomy. Mean duration of follow-up was 8.7 years after hepaticojejunostomy and 7.9 years after hepaticoduodenostomy. Differences between the hepaticojejunostomy and hepaticoduodenostomy groups with respect to type of choledochal cyst, age at cyst excision and length of follow-up were not statistically significant. However, the incidence of postoperative complications such as endoscopy-proven bilious gastritis due to duodenogastric reflux of bile (4/12 [33%] of the hepaticoduodenostomy group) and adhesive bowel obstruction (2/28 (7%) of the hepaticojejunostomy group) were significantly different. It would appear that hepaticoduodenostomy is not an ideal biliary reconstructive technique after choledochal cyst excision because of the high incidence of duodenogastric bile reflux. Currently, Roux-en-Y hepaticojejunostomy is the technique of choice in such patients.

Hepaticoenterostomy at the hepatic hilum is used by some surgeons because they consider that a wider anastomosis created by incising the lateral wall of both transected hepatic ducts at the hepatic hilum may prevent anastomotic stricture and may also allow better drainage of bile.[9,64] Although hepaticoenterostomy at the hepatic hilum is appealing technically, it is a more complicated procedure and is indicated in selected cases only such as adolescents with severe inflammation of the common hepatic duct requiring secondary cyst excision, and children with intrahepatic bile duct dilatation and relative stenosis at the porta hepatis.

Prenatally diagnosed choledochal cyst

There are increasing reports on the management of the asymptomatic choledochal cyst detected prenatally. Some pediatric surgeons recommended primary cyst excision soon after birth in such cases or soon after diagnosis in neonates.[65,66] The author's experience is that cyst excision need not be performed hastily in these infants; rather they should be thoroughly assessed and surgery should be planned and performed by experienced, well-trained pediatric surgeons.[66–68] If obstructive jaundice is severe, external biliary drainage is recommended either by percutaneous transhepatic cholangiocatheter or direct percutaneous cyst drainage. Delayed primary cyst excision may then be carried out 1 or 2 months later.

Conclusions

With improvements in diagnostic imaging and prenatal ultrasound screening more cases of choledochal cyst are being detected. The author recommends choledochal cyst excision and hepaticojejunostomy with an end-to-end anastomosis. Intraoperative endoscopy is easy and highly effective in preventing many long-term complications and should be regarded as routine. The key to successful management of a choledochal cyst is early diagnosis and a clean hepatobiliary–pancreatic system. Surgical expertise, a good understanding of the anatomy of the hepatobiliary–pancreatic system, and careful long-term follow-up are also important factors in achieving good long-term outcomes.

REFERENCES

1. Miyano, T. & Yamataka, A. Choledochal cysts. *Curr. Opin. Pediatr.* 1997; **9**:283–288.
2. Lane, G. J. Different types of congenital biliary dilatation in dizygotic twins: a case report. *Pediatr. Surg. Int.* 1999; **15**:403–404.
3. Douglas, A. H. Case of dilatation of the common bile duct. *Monthly. J. Med. Sci.* 1852; **14**:97–99.
4. Babbitt, D. P. Congenital choledochal cyst: new etiologic concepts on anomalous relationships of the common bile and pancreatic bulb. *Ann. Radiol.* 1969; **12**:231–241.
5. Miyano, T., Suruga, K., & Suda, K. Abnormal choledocho-pancreatico ductal junction related to the etiology of infantile obstructive jaundice diseases. *J. Pediatr. Surg.* 1979; **14**:16–25.
6. Todani, T., Watanabe, Y., Toki, A. *et al.* Reoperation for congenital choledochal cyst. *Ann. Surg.* 1987; **207**:142–147.
7. Metcalfe, M. S., Wemyss-Holden, S. A., & Maddern, G. J. Management dilemmas with choledochal cysts. *Arch. Surg.* 2003; **138**:333–333.
8. Yamataka, A., Ohshiro, K., Okada, Y. *et al.* Complications after cyst excision with hepaticoenterostomy for choledochal cyst and their surgical management in children versus adults. *J. Pediatr. Surg.* 1997; **32**:1097–1102.
9. Todani, T., Watanabe, Y., Urushihara, N. *et al.* Biliary complications after excisional procedure for choledochal cyst. *J. Pediatr. Surg.* 1995; **30**:478–481.
10. Ohi, R., Yaoita, S., Kamiyama, T. *et al.* Surgical treatment of congenital dilatation of the bile duct with special reference to late complications after total excisional operation. *J. Pediatr. Surg.* 1990; **25**:613–617.
11. Arima, T., Suita, S., Kubota, M. *et al.* Endoscopic treatment of intrahepatic gallstones after surgery for choledochal cyst. *Pediatr. Surg. Int.* 1995; **10**:218–220.
12. Schier, F., Clausen, M., Kouki, M. *et al.* Late results in the management of choledochal cysts. *Eur. J. Pediatr. Surg.* 1994; **4**:141–144.
13. Chijiwa, K. & Tanaka, M. Late complications after excisional operation in patients with choledochal cyst. *J. Am. Coll. Surg.* 1994; **179**:139–144.
14. Nagorney, D. M., MacIrath, D. C., & Adson, M. A. Choledochal cysts in adults: clinical management. *Surgery* 1984; **96**:656–663.
15. Todani, T., Watanabe, Y., Mizuguchi, T. *et al.* Hepaticoduodenostomy at the hepatic hilum after excision of choledochal cyst. *Am. J. Surg.* 1981; **142**:584–587.
16. Miyano, T., Yamataka, A., Kato, Y. *et al.* Hepaticoenterostomy after excision of choledochal cyst in children: A 30-year experience with 180 cases. *J. Pediatr. Surg.* 1996; **31**:1417–1412.
17. Miyano, T., Yamataka, A., Kato, Y. *et al.* Choledochal cysts: special emphasis on the usefulness of intraoperative endoscopy. *J. Pediatr. Surg.* 1995; **30**:482–484.
18. Ando, H., Ito, T., Kaneko, K. *et al.* Intrahepatic bile duct stenosis causing intrahepatic calculi formation following excision of a choledochal cyst. *J. Am. Coll. Surg.* 1996; **183**:56–60.
19. Yoshikawa, K., Yoshida, K., Shirai, Y. *et al.* A case of carcinoma arising in the intrapancreatic terminal choledochus 12 years after primary excision of a giant choledochal cyst. *Am. J. Gastroenterol.* 1986; **81**:378–384.
20. Yamamoto, J., Shimamura, Y., Ohtani, I. *et al.* Bile duct carcinoma arising from the anastomotic site of hepaticojejunostomy after the excision of congenital biliary dilatation: a case report. *Surgery* 1996; **119**:476–479.
21. Chaudhuri, P. K., Chaudhuri, B., Schuler, J. J. *et al.* Carcinoma associated with congenital cystic dilatation of bile ducts. *Arch. Surg.* 1982; **117**:1349–1351.
22. Deziel, D. J., Rossi, R. L., Munson, J. L. *et al.* Management of bile duct cysts in adults. *Arch. Surg.* 1986; **121**:410–415.
23. Shimura, H., Tanaka, M., Shimizu, S. *et al.* Laparoscopic treatment of congenital choledochal cyst. *Surg. Endosc.* 1998; **12**:1268–1271.

24. Mori, T., Abe, N., Sugiyama, M. *et al.* Laparoscopic hepatobiliary and pancreatic surgery: an overview. *J. Hepatobiliary. Pancreat. Surg.* 2002; **9**:710–722.
25. Tanaka, M., Shimizu, S., Mizumoto, K. *et al.* Laparoscopically assisted resection of choledochal cyst and Roux-en-Y reconstruction. *Surg. Endosc.* 2001; **15**:545–552.
26. Watanabe, Y., Sato, M., Tokui, K. *et al.* Laparoscope-assisted minimally invasive treatment for choledochal cyst. *J. Laparoendosc. Adv. Surg. Tech. A.* 1999; **9**:415–418.
27. Alonso-Lej, F., Rever, W. B., & Pessagno, D. J. Congenital choledochal cyst, with a report of 2, and an analysis of 94 cases. *Int. Abst. Surg.* 1959; **108**:1–30.
28. Todani, T., Narusue, M., Watanabe, Y. *et al.* Management of congenital choledochal cyst with intrahepatic involvement. *Ann. Surg.* 1977; **187**:272–280.
29. Komi, N., Takehara, H., Kunitomo, K. *et al.* Does the type of anomalous arrangement of the pancreaticobiliary ducts influence the surgery and prognosis of choledochal cyst? *J. Pediatr. Surg.* 1992; **27**:728–731.
30. Todani, T. Choledochal cysts. In Stringer, M. D., Oldham, P., Mouriquand, D. E., Howard, E. R. eds. *Pediatric Surgery and Urology: Long Term Outcomes.* London: WB Saunders; 1998; 417–429.
31. Yamataka, A., Kuwatsuru, R., Shima, H. *et al.* Initial experience with non-breath-hold magnetic resonance cholangiopancreatography: a new noninvasive technique for the diagnosis of the choledochal cyst in children. *J. Pediatr. Surg.* 1997; **32**:1560–1562.
32. Shimotakahara, A., Yamataka, A., Kobayashi, H. *et al.* Massive debris in the intrahepatic bile ducts in choledochal cyst: possible cause of postoperative stone formation. *Pediatr. Surg. Int.* 2004; **20**:67–69.
33. Yamataka, A., Segawa, O., Kobayashi, H. *et al.* Intraoperative pancreatoscopy for pancreatic duct stone debris distal to the common channel in choledochal cyst. *J. Pediatr. Surg.* 2000; **35**:1–4.
34. Ando, H., Kaneko, K., Ito, F. *et al.* Operative treatment of congenital stenoses of the intrahepatic bile ducts in patients with choledochal cysts. *Am. J. Surg.* 1997; **173**:491–494.
35. Yamataka, A., Kobayashi, H., Shimotakahara, A. *et al.* Recommendations for preventing complications related to Roux-en-Y hepatico-jejunostomy performed during excision of choledochal cyst in children. *J. Pediatr. Surg.* 2003; **38**:1830–1832.
36. Shima, H., Yamataka, A., Yanai, T. *et al.* Intracorporeal electrohydraulic lithotripsy for intrahepatic bile duct stone formation after choledochal cyst excision: a case report. *Pediatr. Surg. Int.* 2004; **20**:70–72.
37. Lilly, J. R. Total excision of choledochal cyst. *Surg. Gyn. Obst.* 1978; **146**:254–256.
38. Joseph, V. T. Surgical techniques and long-term results in the treatment of choledochal cyst. *J. Pediatr. Surg.* 1990; **25**:782–787.
39. O'Neill, J. A., Jr. Choledochal cyst. *Curr. Prob. Surg.* 1992; **29**:361–410.
40. Stringer, M. D., Dhawan, A., Davenport, M. *et al.* Choledochal cysts: lessons from a 20 year experience. *Arch. Dis. Child.* 1995; **73**:528–531.
41. Warren, K. W., Kune, G. A., Hardy, K. J. *et al.* Biliary duct cysts. *Surg. Clin. North. Am.* 1968; **88**:567–577.
42. Eagle, J. & Salmon, P. A. Multiple choledochal cysts. *Arch. Surg.* 1964; **88**:345–349.
43. Csentino, C. M., Luck, S. R., & Raffensperger, J. G. *et al.* Choledochal duct cyst. Resection with physiological reconstruction. *Surgery* 1992; **112**:740–748.
44. Voyles, C. R., Smadja, C., Shands, W. C. *et al.* Carcinoma in choledochal cysts. *Arch. Surg.* 1983; **118**:986–988.
45. Long, L., Yamataka, A., Segawa, O. *et al.* Coexistence of pancreas divisum and septate common channel in a child with choledochal cyst. *J. Pediatr. Gastroenterol. Nutr.* 2001; **32**:602–604.
46. Kobayashi, S., Asano, T., Yamasaki, M. *et al.* Risk of bile duct carcinogenesis after excision of extrahepatic bile ducts in pancreaticobiliary maljunction. *Surgery* 1999; **126**:939–944.
47. Ng, W. T. In "Letters to the editors". *Surgery* 2000; **128**: 492–494.
48. Okada, A., Nagaoka, M., Kamata, S. *et al.* "Common channel syndrome": anomalous junction of the pancreatico-biliary ductal system. *Z. Kinderchir.* 1981; **32**:144–151.
49. Lilly, J. R., Stellin, G. P., Karrer, F. M. Forme fruste choledochal cyst. *J. Pediatr. Surg.* 1985; **20**:449–451.
50. Aoki, T., Tsuchida, A., Kasuya, K. *et al.* Is preventive resection of the extrahepatic bile duct necessary in cases of pancreaticobiliary maljunction without dilatation of the bile duct? *Jpn J. Clin. Oncol.* 2001; **31**:107–111.
51. Murakami, T., Kodama, T., Takesue, Y. *et al.* Anomalous arrangement of the pancreaticobiliary ductal system without the dilatation of the biliary tract. *Surg. Today* 1992; **22**:276–279.
52. Morishita, H., Kamei, K., Funabiki, T. *et al.* A case of pancreaticobiliary maljunction without bile duct dilatation associated with gallbladder cancer and minute bile duct cancer. *Tando* 1992; **6**:176–183.
53. Miyano, T., Ando, K., Yamataka, A. *et al.* Pancreaticobiliary maljunction associated with nondilatation or minimal dilatation of the common bile duct in children: Diagnosis and treatment. *Eur. J. Pediatr. Surg.* 1996; **6**:334–337.
54. Ando, H., Ito, T., Nagaya, M. *et al.* Pancreaticobiliary maljunction without choledochal cysts in infants and children: Clinical features and surgical therapy. *J. Pediatr. Surg.* 1995; **30**:1658–1662.
55. Tanaka, K., Nishimura, A., Yamada, K. *et al.* Cancer of the gallbladder associated with anomalous junction of the pancreaticobiliary duct system without bile duct dilatation. *Br. J. Surg.* 1993; **80**:622–624.
56. Witcombe, J. B. & Cremin, B. J. The width of the common bile duct in childhood. *Pediatr. Radiol.* 1978; **7**:147–149.
57. Schulman, M. H., Ambrosino, M. M., Freeman, P. C. *et al.* Common bile duct in children: sonographic dimensions. *Radiology* 1995; **195**:193–195.

58. Pushparani, P., Redkar, R. G., & Howard, E. R. Progressive biliary pathology associated with common pancreato-biliary channel. *J. Pediatr. Surg*. 2000; **35**:649–651.
59. Sugiyama, M. & Atomi, Y. Anomalous pancreaticobiliary junction without congenital choledochal cyst. *Br. J. Surg*. 1998; **85**:911–916.
60. Mori, K, Akimoto, R., Kanno, M. *et al*. Anomalous union of the pancreaticobiliary ductal system without dilatation of the common bile duct or tumor: case reports and literature review. *Hepato-Gastroenterology*. 1999; **46**:142–148.
61. Rao, K. L. N., Mitra, S. K., Kochher, R. *et al*. Jejunal interposition hepaticoduodenostomy for choledochal cyst. *Am. J. Gastroenterol*. 1987; **82**:1042–1045.
62. Todani, T., Watanabe, Y., Toki, A., *et al*. Hilar duct carcinoma developed after cyst excision followed by hepaticoduodenostomy. In Koyanagi, Y., Aoki, T., (eds) *Pancreaticobiliary Maljunction*, Tokyo: Igaku tosho shuppan; 2002; 17–21.
63. Shimotakahara, A., Yamataka, A., Yanai, T. *et al*. Roux-en-Y hepaticojejunostomy or hepaticoduodenostomy for biliary reconstruction during the surgical treatment of choledochal cyst; which is better? *Pediatr. Surg. Int*. 2005; **21**:5–7.
64. Lilly, J. R. Surgery of coexisting biliary malformations in choledochal cyst. *J. Pediatr. Surg*. 1979; **14**:643–647.
65. Burnweit, C. A., Birken, G. A., & Heiss, K. The management of choledochal cysts in the new born. *Pediatr. Surg. Int*. 1996; **11**:130–133.
66. Lugo-Vicente, H. L. Prenatally diagnosed choledochal cysts: observation or early surgery. *J. Pediatr. Surg*. 1995; **30**:1288–1290.
67. Lane, G. J., Yamataka, A., Kohn, S. *et al*. Choledochal cyst in the newborn. *Asian J. Surg*. 1999; **22**:310–312.
68. Miyano, T. Congenital biliary dilatation. In Puri P., ed. *Newborn Surgery*, Oxford, UK: Butterworth-Heinemann; 1996; 433–439.

37

Biliary stone disease

Faisal G. Qureshi,[1] Evan P. Nadler,[2] and Henri R. Ford[3]

[1]Division of Pediatric Surgery, Children's Hospital of Los Angeles, CA, USA
[2]New York University School of Medicine, NY, USA
[3]Division of Pediatric Surgery, Children's Hospital of Pittsburgh, University of Pittsburgh School of Medicine, PA, USA

Introduction

Over the past decade, cholelithiasis and choledocholithiasis have been diagnosed with increasing frequency during infancy and childhood.[1–3] The increased rate of diagnosis may be related to a true rise in the incidence of the disease, or, more likely, to an enhanced ability to detect gallstones.[2–4] The prevalence of gallstones in the pediatric population has been reported to be between 0.13% and 0.22%.[5,6] However, in children who undergo an abdominal sonogram for abdominal pain, the incidence of gallstones and sludge has been reported to be as high as 1.9%.[7] The mean age for cholelithiasis in pediatric patients is between 7 and 10 years.[2,7–9] Most authors report a slight preponderance of boys among pre-adolescents with cholelithiasis. However, this trend is completely reversed in the adolescent group.[2,7]

Although underlying hematologic diseases such as sickle cell anemia, hereditary spherocytosis and thalassemia have been implicated as major predisposing factors for childhood cholelithiasis, the majority of gallstones in children are believed to be idiopathic. Several series suggest that only 20% of gallstones are related to hematologic diseases.[8,10,11] Other putative risk factors for childhood cholelithiasis include: total parenteral nutrition; ileal resection; ileal disorders; obesity; family history of gallstones; cystic fibrosis; biliary tract anomalies and medications (birth control pills, cyclosporin, ceftriaxone).[7,8,12–17] Gallstones can be classified as pigment, cholesterol or mixed-type stones. Pigment stones are usually detected during infancy and early childhood, and typically are associated with hemolytic disorders. In contrast, cholesterol and mixed-type stones are more commonly seen in adolescents.[18,19] Because pigmented stones are more radio-opaque than cholesterol stones, plain abdominal radiographs are useful in diagnosing gallstones in up to 50% of children.[20,21]

Children with symptomatic gallstones present most commonly with right upper quadrant pain (75%–85%), followed by nausea or vomiting in 60%. Jaundice is less frequently seen and epigastric tenderness is found in only one-third of the patients. Gallstones can be asymptomatic in up to 17% of children.[7,8] Medical therapy is ineffective in children with symptomatic cholelithiasis; cholecystectomy is the treatment of choice.[11,22] Laparoscopic cholecystectomy (LC) has become standard of care in children.[23]

In this chapter, we will discuss the different aspects of management and the long-term outcomes of biliary stone disease in children.

Management of gallstones in asymptomatic patients

The relatively frequent use of abdominal ultrasound in children with abdominal disorders in recent years has resulted in the diagnosis of gallstones in a large number of "asymptomatic" children. Despite the fact that they comprise up to 17% of children with gallstones, very little information exists regarding the appropriate management of children with asymptomatic cholelithiasis.[7,8] In addition, because these data were collected on patients undergoing workup for abdominal symptoms, the true incidence of asymptomatic gallstones in children is unknown.

In adults, previously asymptomatic patients develop biliary symptoms at a rate of 2% to 4% per year, with relatively

Pediatric Surgery and Urology: Long-term Outcomes, Mark Stringer, Keith Oldham, Pierre Mouriquand.
Published by Cambridge University Press.

little associated morbidity or mortality.[24] The most recent reports studying the natural history of asymptomatic gallstones in children are summarized in Table 37.1. In one study by Bruch *et al.*, 3 of 41 patients underwent cholecystectomy while another 4 developed symptoms but had not undergone cholecystectomy. However, mean follow-up was relatively short (21 months). Although the number of patients in each of the various series is relatively small, based upon the low rate of development of symptoms and the absence of complications, clinical follow-up of patients with asymptomatic gallstones without associated comorbidities is advisable. A similar recommendation can be made for patients with gallbladder sludge as this condition usually resolves spontaneously.[7]

Complications of biliary stone disease in children

Patients with biliary stone disease may develop a number of complications (Table 37.2) which include:

(i) Biliary colic or chronic abdominal pain
(ii) Cholecystitis
(iii) Common bile duct obstruction
(iv) Pancreatitis
(v) Acute cholangitis

Based on several reports, chronic and intermittent abdominal pain are the most common complications of biliary stone disease in children.[7–9] These symptoms usually consist of postprandial right upper quadrant or epigastric abdominal pain, nausea, vomiting, and jaundice. Acute cholecystitis complicates biliary stone disease in 3%–14% of the patients; the diagnosis relies on the clinical findings of acute right upper quadrant abdominal pain, fever, and leukocytosis (Murphy's triad). Patients with cholangitis present with similar findings and jaundice; however, cholangitis complicating biliary stone disease is relatively rare, affecting only 2% of patients.[9]

The incidence of choledocholithiasis in pediatric patients has been reported to be between 0% and 5%.[25,26] However, more recent reports suggest that the incidence may be as high as 18% among patients with gallstones.[8,27] Common bile duct (CBD) stones are found more commonly in patients with hematological disorders and may be related to the smaller size of pigment stones which allow them to pass into the CBD more easily.[28] Gallstone pancreatitis, resulting from the passage of gallstones into the CBD, has been seen in up to 7% of patients with biliary stone disease. The management of CBD stones, biliary stone disease in patients with hematological disorders, and the management and outcomes of patients with gallstone pancreatitis will be discussed in subsequent sections of this chapter.

Table 37.1. Follow-up of children with asymptomatic gallstones

Author	Asymptomatic patients	Follow-up Mean/range (months)	Number that developed symptoms	Complications
Bruch, 2000[96]	41	21 (3–41)	7 (33%)	0
Wesdorp, 2000[7]	16	54 (2–216)	1 (2%)	0
Kumar, 2000[8]	10	114 (12–228)	0 (0%)	0

Table 37.2. Complications of biliary stone disease in children. NA = not available

Author, year and number of patients	Cholecystitis	CBD stones	Pancreatitis
Holcomb, 1999, $n = 100$[23]	7%	2%	5%
Waldhausen, 1999, $n = 121$[2]	4%	7%	7%
Miltenburg, 2000, $n = 132$[9]	14%	NA	4%
Kumar, 2000, $n = 102$[8]	3%	18%	1%
Wesdorp, 2000, $n = 82$[7]	4%	0%	2%
Bruch, 2000, $n = 74$[96]	4%	3%	3%

Safety, efficacy and cost effectiveness of laparoscopic cholecystectomy (LC) in children

With an increasing number of children diagnosed with gallstones, the optimal management must be discussed. Laparoscopic cholecystectomy has now supplanted open cholecystectomy (OC) as the gold standard for management of symptomatic gallstones in adults.[29] Similarly, LC has gained widespread acceptance in the management of symptomatic gallstones in children. Several authors have examined the safety, efficacy and cost effectiveness of this procedure in the pediatric population. Holcomb *et al.* first reported the safety and efficiency of LC for the treatment of acute cholecystitis in five children.[30] These patients had no evidence of complications during the follow-up period of 16 months (range 2–24 months). In this early report, the authors also compared elective LC versus open cholecystectomy (OC) in children. Patients undergoing elective LC had shorter hospital stay, reduced analgesic requirement and decreased total hospital charges. Since that report, several authors have compared LC with OC in children (Table 37.3). As can be seen, postoperative analgesic requirements, length of hospital stay and overall hospital costs are improved in the LC group. Operative time and operative costs are higher in the LC group, but these are offset by the shorter hospital stay. LC has now become the standard of care in managing gallstone disease in children.

Table 37.3. Laparoscopic vs. open cholecystectomy. Comparison of postoperative analgesic requirements, length of hospital stay, hospital costs and complication rates between LC and OC. Only data corresponding to the LC group are presented. NA = not available

	Analgesics	Operative time	Hospital stay	Hospital costs	Complications
Kim, 1995[97]	Decreased	Equal	Shorter	Less	Equal
Al-Salem, 1997[28]	NA	Greater	Shorter	NA	Equal
Jawad, 1998[56]	Decreased	Equal	Shorter	Less	Equal
Luks, 1999[98]	NA	Greater	Shorter	Less	NA

The complication rate of LC in children is 0%–15.5%.[2,23,31] Although this range seems rather wide, it probably reflects the more stringent classification of complications in these reports. For instance, Esposito *et al.* reported 17/110 patients with complications, which included 11 gallbladder perforations, 1 "fall of stones into the abdominal cavity" and 5 trocar site infections.[31] The inclusion of gallbladder perforation and loss of stones into the abdominal cavity as complications of LC may have skewed the data. Most authors report a complication rate of less than 5%, with trocar site infections being most common.[2,28] Patients undergoing urgent LC for acute cholecystitis and especially those patients with sickle cell disease or other significant comorbid conditions have a higher rate of complications.[9,32] Patients with sickle cell disease are prone to respiratory compromise and re-hospitalization with abdominal pain, whilst those with cardiac comorbidity have a higher incidence of multisystem organ failure.[9,33]

Very little information regarding the true rate of bile duct injury following LC in children is known. In two series of over 100 patients each, there were no reports of bile duct injury or the development of a biloma.[23,33]

Diagnosis and treatment of common bile duct stones and gallstone pancreatitis

Although most authors report the incidence of CBD stones to be around 5% among children with biliary stone disease, some suggest that CBD stones may be present in up to 18% of this population.[8,25,26] In patients with hematologic disorders, the incidence approaches 26%, perhaps due to the smaller size of pigment stones that allows them to pass easily into the CBD.[34,35]

Clinical, laboratory and radiographic tools have been used to predict or diagnose CBD stones in adults. However, their utility in diagnosing CBD stones in children is not known. Two retrospective reviews of 182 patients revealed that clinical, laboratory and ultrasound findings were inaccurate in predicting CBD stones in up to 43% of children.[7,27,36] Because these studies were retrospective in nature, a prospective study with stringent criteria will be required to determine whether non-invasive testing and clinical presentation can accurately predict CBD stones.

Endoscopic retrograde cholangiopancreatography (ERCP) and intraoperative cholangiography (IOC)

Endoscopic retrograde cholangiopancreatography has been used both as a diagnostic and therapeutic tool in children with choledocholithiasis from 1 month to 18 years of age with a success rate of up to 95%.[37–40] Reported complication rates are similar to those seen in adults, with post-ERCP pancreatitis occurring in up to 8% of children. The incidence of pancreatitis is even higher in children undergoing therapeutic ERCP. Hemorrhage and perforation are seen in 0.3% to 2% of children undergoing ERCP.[38] A conventional duodenoscope can be used for children above 10 years of age, while a pediatric duodenoscope is used in children under 10 years of age. More recently a small caliber videoduodenoscope for ERCP in very young children and infants has been developed and successfully used for diagnosis and extraction of stones.[41] In patients with biliary stone disease, ERCP has been noted to be safe and efficacious before, during or after laparoscopic cholecystectomy with CBD clearance achieved in 95% of patients.[7,16,27,42] CBD stones were extracted by endoscopic sphincterotomy and the use of a balloon or basket. Newman *et al.* have suggested that preoperative ERCP may be most efficacious if preoperative work-up suggests or demonstrates CBD stones.[36] Concomitant ERCP with LC can increase operative time by 86% and thus may impact on operative costs.[23]

The disadvantages of ERCP include complication rates of up to 8% and the need for general anesthesia in young children.[43] Thus, intraoperative cholangiography (IOC) may be a more appropriate initial step in patients with biliary stone disease and a suspected CBD stone. Holcomb *et al.* performed IOC in 57 patients undergoing LC.[23] These authors reported success in 49 patients, with an overall increase in operative time of 29%. Kumar *et al.* attempted 88 IOCs and reported a 100% success rate without any complication related to the IOC.[8] To determine the role of IOC in children with biliary stone disease, Waldhausen *et al.* performed 63 IOCs in 100 children undergoing LC; 55 had successful studies.[27] CBD stones were found in 18 patients. IOC increased operative time by 35% and did not result in any complications. Preoperative symptoms and/or laboratory findings were inaccurate in predicting CBD stones in 8 patients. Based on these findings, Waldhausen *et al.* concluded that routine IOC in all children undergoing LC was warranted since preoperative work-up was inaccurate. Furthermore, they argued that IOC could help avoid unnecessary ERCP and the obligatory second anesthetic. Callery *et al.* also recommend routine IOC in all children undergoing LC to demonstrate choledocholithiasis and define biliary tract anatomy.[44]

The ideal management of suspected choledocholithiasis in children in the era of laparoscopic cholecystectomy is unknown. Options include preoperative or postoperative ERCP with sphincterotomy and removal of stones; intraoperative ERCP during LC, or IOC during LC with laparoscopic or open common bile duct exploration.[16] Newman *et al.* have suggested that preoperative ERCP should be performed on patients with suspected CBD stones followed by LC.[36] Despite their recommendation, however, 42% of children had negative ERCP and therefore underwent an unnecessary procedure. The high rate of negative ERCP in patients with suspected CBD stones has been documented by other authors.[27,33] Based on these findings, Tagge *et al.* and Shah *et al.* have recommended that children undergoing LC should also undergo IOC with concomitant laparoscopic common bile duct exploration either via the cystic duct or via the CBD if the IOC reveals CBD stones.[33,104] Neither group reported any biliary tract injuries or long-term complications. Preoperative ERCP has been reserved for those children with fulminant pancreatitis, cholangitis, or those with CBD obstruction. Intraoperative ERCP is reserved for those patients whose CBD stones either cannot be managed via laparoscopy, or the surgical endoscopist is unavailable. Postoperative ERCP is reserved for those patients in whom CBD stones are retained or recur after LC (Fig. 37.1). Some authors have suggested that expectant management of small, asymptomatic CBD stones is acceptable, but this approach has not gained widespread acceptance.[45]

Magnetic resonance cholangiopancreatography (MRCP)

Little is known about the utility of MRCP in predicting CBD stones in children. Topal *et al.* have shown that, in adults with a predicted probability of CBD stones of greater than 5%, MRCP can confirm the presence or absence of stones, with an observed sensitivity of 95%, a specificity of 100%, a positive predictive value of 100% and a negative predictive value of 98%.[46] The model used by these authors to predict common duct stones included ultrasonography, which revealed CBD stones or bile duct dilatation, age greater than

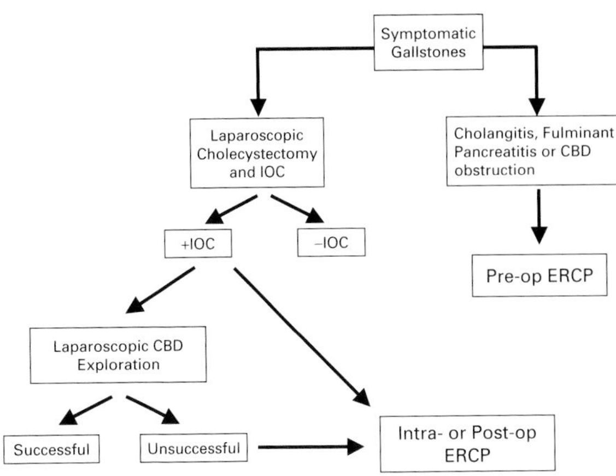

Fig. 37.1. Management of symptomatic gallstones and common bile duct stones in children. IOC = intraoperative cholangiogram, CBD = common bile duct, ERCP = endoscopic retrograde cholangiopancreatography.

60 years, fever, serum alkaline phosphatase level above 670 units/l and serum amylase level above 95 units/l. Although MRCP has been shown to be accurate in predicting pancreatobiliary disease in children, its role in predicting CBD stones in this population is not known at present.[47]

Gallstone pancreatitis

Gallstone pancreatitis occurs in 1%–5% of children with cholelithiasis and is an absolute indication for cholecystectomy (Table 37.2). Affected children should undergo laparoscopic cholecystectomy with IOC following initial supportive care and resolution of the acute bout of pancreatitis. Holcomb *et al.* reported five patients with gallstone pancreatitis who underwent LC and IOC. None of these patients had documented CBD stones.[23] Rescorla and colleagues suggest that children with gallstone pancreatitis should be treated initially with supportive care followed by delayed LC and IOC once laboratory values have normalized. This approach reduced the rate of positive IOC from 63%–75% to 2%–5%, and therefore obviated the need for CBD exploration/ERCP in a significant number of patients in their hands.[11]

Pancreatitis has also been associated with gallbladder sludge. Choi *et al.* reported their experience with biliary disease-related pancreatitis in eight children; six patients had sludge and two had gallstones.[48] All patients with biliary sludge underwent ERCP with sphincterotomy and endoscopic naso-biliary drainage. Three of the six patients with gallbladder sludge subsequently developed recurrent pancreatitis within 3 years, while two patients had a follow-up of less than a year and one patient did not develop any

Table 37.4. Biliary dyskinesia in children. Outcome in children undergoing cholecystectomy for biliary dyskinesia

Author, year	*n*	Ejection fraction	Clinical improvement	Chronic inflammatory changes	Follow-up period (mean or range)
Lugo-Vicente, 1997[99]	12	<20%	92%	10/12	17 months
Dumont, 1999[100]	42	<50%	96%	20/42	21 months
Gollin, 1999[101]	29	<40%	79%	21/29	1–24 months
Al-Homaidhi, 2002[102]	10	<30%	100%	7/10	12.8 months
Wood, 2004[103]	5	<50%	40%	5/5	36 months

recurrence within 2 years. This series suggests that patients with pancreatitis from gallbladder sludge should undergo cholecystectomy. However, most authors argue that gallbladder sludge is rarely associated with significant complications and thus does not warrant routine cholecystectomy in the absence of documented complications.

Synopsis

1. Preoperative clinical, radiographic and laboratory work-up for common bile duct stones may be inaccurate in children.
2. Both diagnostic and therapeutic ERCP can be done in children of all ages but false-negative results can be high.
3. IOC is safe, efficacious and may be performed concomitantly with LC, especially in patients with suspected CBD stones or after biliary pancreatitis; it may serve to prevent unnecessary ERCP in children.
4. No clear role for MRCP in the management of children with biliary stone disease has been established.
5. Patients with gallstone pancreatitis should undergo delayed LC with IOC upon resolution of the acute pancreatitis.

Neonatal and infantile gallstones

Gallstones have been found in up to 0.5% of unselected newborns. Most patients are asymptomatic.[49–53] Associated risk factors include Down syndrome, furosemide therapy, polycythemia, decreased output of bile acids, shortened red blood cell lifespan, phototherapy for jaundice, maternal morphine addiction and nephrocalcinosis.[13,54,55] The large majority of patients, however, have no recognized predisposing factor.[51,52] Symptomatic infants have been treated successfully using a variety of approaches, including open or laparoscopic cholecystectomy, ERCP and common bile duct exploration.[8,30,56,57]

Spontaneous resolution or dissolution occurs in up to 50% of neonates.[51,53,58,59] Occasional fatal complications including perforation, obstruction and peritonitis have been reported.[60] Based on these findings, Jawad *et al.* recommend observation of asymptomatic infants for 3–6 months. If there is failure of resolution or if the stones become calcified, then LC is recommended.[56]

Diagnosis and management of biliary dyskinesia

Biliary dyskinesia is a syndrome characterized by biliary colic without evidence of cholelithiasis or acute cholecystitis. The diagnosis can be aided by demonstrating a decreased gallbladder ejection fraction upon cholecystokinin dimethyl-iminodiacetic acid scanning (CCK-HIDA).[61,62] Although LC is the treatment of choice in adults, the diagnosis, management and outcome in children is less clear. Table 37.4 summarizes the most recent reports on biliary dyskinesia in children. All but one strongly suggest that children with symptoms of biliary colic and evidence of a diminished gallbladder ejection fraction should undergo cholecystectomy.

Hematologic disorders and biliary stone disease

Excess red blood cell hemolysis can overwhelm the bilirubin clearance mechanisms in the liver. The excess bilirubin can coalesce in the gall bladder to form stones or sludge. Although Miltenburg *et al.* reported that 52 (41%) of their 128 children undergoing cholecystectomy had gallstones associated with hemolytic disorders, most authors report an incidence of about 20%.[2,8] The discrepancy may be explained by the increasing rate of cholelithiasis with advancing age.[11] Conditions associated with excessive hemolysis and the development of sludge or stones in the gallbladder include hereditary spherocytosis and sickle cell disease (prevalence up to 43%) as well as the thalassemias (prevalence up to 23%).[11]

Hereditary spherocytosis (HS)

Two areas of controversy exist regarding the management of cholelithiasis in patients with HS. The first is whether HS patients with asymptomatic gallstones should undergo cholecystectomy, and the second, whether the cholecystectomy should be done concomitantly with splenectomy. The role of cholecystectomy in asymptomatic patients has not been clearly delineated, but most authors recommend cholecystectomy in patients who are undergoing splenectomy, especially if they are symptomatic.[11,63,64] Marchetti *et al.* undertook a quality of life analysis in patients with mild HS undergoing splenectomy and cholecystectomy for asymptomatic gallstones and determined that prophylactic splenectomy and cholecystectomy provide a gain in quality-adjusted life expectancy in patients over 6 years of age.[65] This improvement may be further enhanced by using a minimally invasive or laparoscopic approach to perform the splenectomy and cholecystectomy in patients with HS and gallstones.[66,67] The higher incidence of CBD stones in patients with hemolytic disorders also argues in favor of prophylactic cholecystectomy in patients with HS and documented gallstones who are undergoing splenectomy.[35] Currently, there is no role for prophylactic cholecystectomy in patients with normal gallbladders (no gallstones) undergoing splenectomy for HS.[68]

Sickle cell hemoglobinopathies and thalassemias

Laparoscopic cholecystectomy has been safely performed in children with symptomatic gallstones and sickle cell disease (SCD) after receiving packed red blood cell transfusions to achieve a hemoglobin level of 10 g/dl, or exchange transfusion to reduce the concentration of hemoglobin S to a level below 50%.[32,69,70] In addition, simultaneous cholecystectomy and splenectomy have been safely performed in children with SCD.[71] Splenectomy with cholecystectomy was performed in 19 patients for sequestration crises (12), splenic abscess (3) or hypersplenism and infarction (4). Thirteen of the 19 patients had asymptomatic gallstones and postoperative complications occurred in 2 patients. One patient had a wound infection while the other had a hematoma in the splenic bed. On pathologic examination, chronic cholecystitis is often found in gallbladder specimens from children with sickle cell disease and gallstones.

The management of "asymptomatic" gallstones in patients with SCD is more controversial. Because patients with SCD often present with abdominal pain, differentiating between a vaso-occlusive event and biliary colic as the cause is often a daunting task. Parez *et al.* reported that 28% of their patients with asymptomatic gallstones developed clinical manifestations within a follow-up period of 30 months.[72] Given the difficulties in accurately diagnosing the cause of abdominal pain in patients with SCD, the higher rate of development of symptomatic gallstones, and the higher incidence of CBD stones, several authors have recommended prophylactic cholecystectomy in patients with SCD and asymptomatic gallstones.[20,72–75] Others disagree, based on the theoretical increased complication rate in children with SCD undergoing operative procedures.[76] However, given the reported safety and efficacy of laparoscopic cholecystectomy as compared to open cholecystectomy in patients with SCD, prophylactic cholecystectomy is now recommended.[69,77]

The most appropriate management of CBD stones in patients with SCD is unclear. Most authors have recommended that CBD stones be managed by ERCP.[28,78,79] This recommendation may be based on the increased operative time required for CBD exploration and the possible increase in complications. One further area of study in patients with SCD includes the perioperative blood transfusion management. Both aggressive and conservative preoperative blood transfusion regimens have been successfully used in patients with SCD undergoing operative procedures, but no clear directives have been determined.[34,35,80] Further studies will be required to clarify this issue; currently, institution-based protocols should be followed. The laparoscopic approach has not reduced the incidence of acute chest syndrome in children with SCD; therefore, it should be anticipated postoperatively and minimized by careful preoperative management.[81,82,105]

Children with beta-thalassemia have bile stasis, enlarged gallbladders and impaired emptying which may lead to the development of pigment stones.[83] There is a higher rate of gallstones in patients with thalassemia minor and those with coinherited Gilbert's syndrome.[84,85] As in patients with SCD, concomitant cholecystectomy and splenectomy have been successfully performed in patients with beta-thalassemia.[74] Feretis *et al.* suggest that patients with beta-thalassemia undergoing splenectomy should also undergo prophylactic cholecystectomy but this recommendation has not been further studied.[86]

Biliary stone disease and special circumstances

Colon cancer

In the previous edition of this textbook, the association of cholecystectomy with the development of colon carcinoma was discussed. After examining the reports by Ekbom, Zuccato and Mcfarlane *et al.*, the authors concluded that there was a slightly increased risk of colorectal carcinoma in women more than 15 years after cholecystectomy.

However, the increased risk seemed to be related to the presence of gallstones and not the cholecystectomy.[87–89] Despite this reported association, cholecystectomy should not be withheld when indicated.[90]

Transplant

Children undergoing solid organ and bone marrow transplantation develop gallstones at a higher rate than non-transplant patients. This phenomenon may be related to drug therapy (ceftriaxone, cyclosporin, octreotide, and clofibrate), sepsis, parenteral nutrition, or surgical complications.[91] The incidence is probably highest amongst cardiac transplant patients. Sakopoulos and colleagues reviewed their experience with children undergoing cardiac transplant and reported an overall rate of gallstone formation between 3.2% and 8% in infants transplanted under the age of 3 months.[92] Elective cholecystectomy is recommended for all cardiac transplant patients with cholelithiasis, whether they are symptomatic or not.[93]

In a review of 235 children undergoing abdominal ultrasound for jaundice, sepsis or abdominal pain after bone marrow transplant, Safford *et al.* reported the development of gallstones in 20 (8.5%) patients.[94] Only three underwent cholecystectomy for symptoms; spontaneous resolution was reported in five, three remained asymptomatic and nine died from their primary disease. LC should only be offered to symptomatic patients with gallstones following bone marrow transplant. Because patients undergoing renal transplant have a lower incidence of symptomatic gallstones, Melvin *et al.* argue that screening for gallstones and subsequent prophylactic cholecystectomy is not warranted in this population.[95]

Long-term outcomes

The preceding sections have considered the complications of cholelithiasis and choledocholithiasis. In this section, we will review the very limited information available on the long-term outcomes of the management of children with biliary stone disease. Kumar *et al.* reported their experience with 102 children with cholelithiasis managed between 1979 and 1996.[8] Eighty-one patients underwent OC while only seven underwent LC; 82 of 88 patients treated operatively remained asymptomatic after a mean follow-up of 9 years. Six patients had recurrent abdominal pain. Fourteen children in this series were treated non-operatively; nine of these remained symptom-free while five had recurrent vague abdominal pain. Gallstones resolved completely in six of the 14 patients treated non-operatively. Wesdorp *et al.* also reported the long-term follow-up of 50 of 82 children with cholelithiasis or choledocholithiasis detected on abdominal ultrasound using a follow-up questionnaire.[7] A total of 18 out of 34 symptomatic patients undergoing either cholecystectomy or ERCP developed recurrent symptoms after a mean follow-up period of 4.6 years. The operative technique for cholecystectomy (laparoscopic or open) was not reported. However, it was noted that recurrent symptoms occurred more commonly in patients undergoing ERCP alone. Of note, 15 of the 16 asymptomatic patients who did not undergo any invasive therapy remained symptom-free. Holcomb and colleagues published their experience with 100 children undergoing laparoscopic cholecystectomy between 1990 and 1998. They reported a single wound infection as the only surgical complication.[23] The majority of the children in Holcomb's series had no long-term complications. Esposito *et al.* similarly reported longer-term follow-up of 110 symptomatic children undergoing laparoscopic cholecystectomy.[31] There were no serious early or long-term complications after a follow- up of 1–5 years. Only one child underwent an IOC. Based on these reports, children with biliary stone disease undergoing operative or endoscopic management have excellent long-term outcomes.

Summary

1. Biliary stone disease has become more common in children and is often idiopathic.
2. Clinical symptoms, radiographic, and laboratory findings may be inaccurate in predicting the presence of common bile duct stones.
3. Asymptomatic children with gallstones or sludge but without associated comorbidities should be managed expectantly.
4. Laparoscopic cholecystectomy, intraoperative cholangiogram and laparoscopic common bile duct exploration have been found to be safe and effective in children.
5. ERCP is successful in children and can be used preoperatively, intraoperatively or postoperatively to clear the common bile duct of stones. It may be most useful in patients who present with cholangitis.
6. Gallstones can be identified in neonates and infants. Asymptomatic patients should be followed clinically as gallstones may dissolve spontaneously in this age group. In contrast, symptomatic patients should undergo laparoscopic cholecystectomy.
7. Children with biliary colic but with neither stones nor sludge should be investigated for biliary dyskinesia. If

CCK-HIDA shows delayed gallbladder emptying laparoscopic cholecystectomy should be performed.

8. Symptomatic children with hemolytic disorders and documented cholelithiasis should undergo laparoscopic cholecystectomy. Patients with hemolytic disorders who are scheduled for splenectomy, should also undergo concomitant cholecystectomy for asymptomatic gallstones.
9. Limited data indicate that children with biliary stone disease managed appropriately have excellent long-term outcomes.

REFERENCES

1. Lugo-Vicente, H. L. Trends in management of gallbladder disorders in children. *Pediatr. Surg. Int*. 1997; **12**(5–6):348–352.
2. Waldhausen, J. H. & Benjamin, D. R. Cholecystectomy is becoming an increasingly common operation in children. *Am. J. Surg*. 1999; **177**(5):364–367.
3. Bailey, P. V., Connors, R. H., Tracy, T. F., Jr., Sotelo-Avila, C., Lewis, J. E., & Weber, T. R. Changing spectrum of cholelithiasis and cholecystitis in infants and children. *Am. J. Surg*. 1989; **158**(6):585–588.
4. Rescorla, F. J. & Grosfeld, J. L. Cholecystitis and cholelithiasis in children. *Semin. Pediatr. Surg*. 1992; **1**(2):98–106.
5. Colcock, B. P. & Mc, M. J. Cholecystectomy for cholelithiasis; a review of 1356 cases. *Surg. Clin. North Am*. 1955; Lahey Clinic No.:765–771.
6. Palasciano, G., Portincasa, P., Vinciguerra, V. *et al.* Gallstone prevalence and gallbladder volume in children and adolescents: an epidemiological ultrasonographic survey and relationship to body mass index. *Am. J. Gastroenterol*. 1989; **84**(11):1378–1382.
7. Wesdorp, I., Bosman, D., de Graaff, A., Aronson, D., van der Blij, F., & Taminiau, J. Clinical presentations and predisposing factors of cholelithiasis and sludge in children. *J. Pediatr. Gastroenterol. Nutr*. 2000; **31**(4):411–417.
8. Kumar, R., Nguyen, K., & Shun, A. Gallstones and common bile duct calculi in infancy and childhood. *Aust. N Z J. Surg*. 2000; **70**(3):188–191.
9. Miltenburg, D. M., Schaffer, R., 3rd, Breslin, T., & Brandt, M. L. Changing indications for pediatric cholecystectomy. *Pediatrics* 2000; **105**(6):1250–1253.
10. Holcomb, G. W., Jr., O'Neill, J. A., Jr., & Holcomb, G. W., 3rd. Cholecystitis, cholelithiasis and common duct stenosis in children and adolescents. *Ann. Surg*. 1980; **191**(5):626–635.
11. Rescorla, F. J. Cholelithiasis, cholecystitis, and common bile duct stones. *Curr. Opin. Pediatr*. 1997; **9**(3):276–282.
12. Roslyn, J. J., Berquist, W. E., Pitt, H. A. *et al.* Increased risk of gallstones in children receiving total parenteral nutrition. *Pediatrics*. 1983; **71**(5):784–789.
13. Grosfeld, J. L., Rescorla, F. J., Skinner, M. A., West, K. W., & Scherer, L. R., 3rd. The spectrum of biliary tract disorders in infants and children. Experience with 300 cases. *Arch. Surg*. 1994; **129**(5):513–518; discussion 518–520.
14. Bonioli, E., Bellini, C., & Toma, P. Pseudolithiasis and intractable hiccups in a boy receiving ceftriaxone. *N. Engl. J. Med*. 1994; **331**(22):1532.
15. Weinstein, S., Lipsitz, E. C., Addonizio, L., & Stolar, C. J. Cholelithiasis in pediatric cardiac transplant patients on cyclosporine. *J. Pediatr. Surg*. 1995; **30**(1):61–64.
16. Al-Salem, A. H. & Nourallah, H. Sequential endoscopic/laparoscopic management of cholelithiasis and choledocholithiasis in children who have sickle cell disease. *J. Pediatr. Surg*. 1997; **32**(10):1432–1435.
17. Tamary, H., Aviner, S., Freud, E. *et al.* High incidence of early cholelithiasis detected by ultrasonography in children and young adults with hereditary spherocytosis. *J. Pediatr. Hematol. Oncol*. 2003; **25**(12):952–954.
18. Stringer, M. D., Taylor, D. R., & Soloway, R. D. Gallstone composition: are children different? *J. Pediatr*. 2003; **142**(4):435–440.
19. Escobar Castro, H., Garcia Novo, M. D., & Olivares, P. [Biliary lithiasis in childhood: therapeutic approaches]. *Ann. Pediatr. (Barc.)* 2004; **60**(2):170–174.
20. Stephens, C. G. & Scott, R. B. Cholelithiasis in sickle cell anemia: surgical or medical management. *Arch. Intern. Med*. 1980; **140**(5):648–651.
21. Robertson, J. F., Carachi, R., Sweet, E. M., & Raine, P. A. Cholelithiasis in childhood: a follow-up study. *J. Pediatr. Surg*. 1988; **23**(3):246–249.
22. Gamba, P. G., Zancan, L., Midrio, P. *et al.* Is there a place for medical treatment in children with gallstones? *J. Pediatr. Surg*. 1997; **32**(3):476–478.
23. Holcomb, G. W., 3rd, Morgan, W. M., 3rd, Neblett, W. W., 3rd, Pietsch, J. B., O'Neill, J. A., Jr., & Shyr, Y. Laparoscopic cholecystectomy in children: lessons learned from the first 100 patients. *J. Pediatr. Surg*. 1999; **34**(8):1236–1240.
24. Schwesinger, W. H. & Diehl, A. K. Changing indications for laparoscopic cholecystectomy. Stones without symptoms and symptoms without stones. *Surg. Clin. North Am*. 1996; **76**(3):493–504.
25. Friesen, C. A. & Roberts, C. C. Cholelithiasis. Clinical characteristics in children. Case analysis and literature review. *Clin. Pediatr. (Phila.)* 1989; **28**(7):294–298.
26. Reif, S., Sloven, D. G., & Lebenthal, E. Gallstones in children. Characterization by age, etiology, and outcome. *Am. J. Dis. Child*. 1991; **145**(1):105–108.
27. Waldhausen, J. H., Graham, D. D., & Tapper, D. Routine intraoperative cholangiography during laparoscopic cholecystectomy minimizes unnecessary endoscopic retrograde cholangiopancreatography in children. *J. Pediatr. Surg*. 2001; **36**(6):881–884.
28. Al-Salem, A. H., Qaisaruddin, S., Al-Abkari, H., Nourallah, H., Yassin, Y. M., & Varma, K. K. Laparoscopic versus open cholecystectomy in children. *Pediatr. Surg. Int*. 1997; **12**(8):587–590.
29. Warshaw, A. L. Reflections on laparoscopic surgery. *Surgery*. 1993; **114**(3):629–630.

30. Holcomb, G. W., 3rd, Sharp, K. W., Neblett, W. W., 3rd, Morgan, W. M., 3rd, & Pietsch, J. B. Laparoscopic cholecystectomy in infants and children: modifications and cost analysis. *J. Pediatr. Surg.* 1994; **29**(7):900–904.
31. Esposito, C., Gonzalez Sabin, M. A., Corcione, F., Sacco, R., Esposito, G., & Settimi, A. Results and complications of laparoscopic cholecystectomy in childhood. *Surg. Endosc.* 2001; **15**(8):890–892.
32. Al-Mulhim, A. S., Al-Mulhim, F. M., & Al-Suwaiygh, A. A. The role of laparoscopic cholecystectomy in the management of acute cholecystitis in patients with sickle cell disease. *Am. J. Surg.* 2002; **183**(6):668–672.
33. Tagge, E. P., Hebra, A., Goldberg, A., Chandler, J. C., Delatte, S., & Othersen, H. B., Jr. Pediatric laparoscopic biliary tract surgery. *Semin. Pediatr. Surg.* 1998; **7**(4):202–206.
34. Ware, R. E., Schultz, W. H., Filston, H. C., & Kinney, T. R. Diagnosis and management of common bile duct stones in patients with sickle hemoglobinopathies. *J. Pediatr. Surg.* 1992; **27**(5):572–575.
35. Bhattacharyya, N., Wayne, A. S., Kevy, S. V., & Shamberger, R. C. Perioperative management for cholecystectomy in sickle cell disease. *J. Pediatr. Surg.* 1993; **28**(1):72–75.
36. Newman, K. D., Powell, D. M., & Holcomb, G. W., 3rd. The management of choledocholithiasis in children in the era of laparoscopic cholecystectomy. *J. Pediatr. Surg.* 1997; **32**(7):1116–1119.
37. Iinuma, Y., Narisawa, R., Iwafuchi, M. *et al.* The role of endoscopic retrograde cholangiopancreatography in infants with cholestasis. *J. Pediatr. Surg.* 2000; **35**(4):545–549.
38. Fox, V. L., Werlin, S. L., & Heyman, M. B. Endoscopic retrograde cholangiopancreatography in children. Subcommittee on Endoscopy and Procedures of the Patient Care Committee of the North American Society for Pediatric Gastroenterology and Nutrition. *J. Pediatr. Gastroenterol. Nutr.* 2000; **30**(3):335–342.
39. Teng, R., Yokohata, K., Utsunomiya, N., Takahata, S., Nabae, T., & Tanaka, M. Endoscopic retrograde cholangiopancreatography in infants and children. *J. Gastroenterol.* 2000; **35**(1):39–42.
40. Poddar, U., Thapa, B. R., Bhasin, D. K., Prasad, A., Nagi, B., & Singh, K. Endoscopic retrograde cholangiopancreatography in the management of pancreaticobiliary disorders in children. *J. Gastroenterol. Hepatol.* 2001; **16**(8):927–931.
41. Kato, S., Kamagata, S., Asakura, T. *et al.* A newly developed small-caliber videoduodenoscope for endoscopic retrograde cholangiopancreatography in children. *J. Clin. Gastroenterol.* 2003; **37**(2):173–176.
42. De Palma, G. D., Angrisani, L., Lorenzo, M. *et al.* Laparoscopic cholecystectomy (LC), intraoperative endoscopic sphincterotomy (ES), and common bile duct stones (CBDS) extraction for management of patients with cholecystocholedocholithiasis. *Surg. Endosc.* 1996; **10**(6):649–652.
43. Pfau, P. R., Chelimsky, G. G., Kinnard, M. F. *et al.* Endoscopic retrograde cholangiopancreatography in children and adolescents. *J. Pediatr. Gastroenterol. Nutr.* 2002; **35**(5):619–623.
44. Callery, M. P. & Soper, N. J. Laparoscopic management of complicated biliary tract disease in children. *Surg. Laparosc. Endosc.* 1996; **6**(1):56–60.
45. Clements, R. H. & Holcomb, G. W., 3rd. Laparoscopic cholecystectomy. *Curr. Opin. Pediatr.* 1998; **10**(3):310–314.
46. Topal, B., Van de Moortel, M., Fieuws, S. *et al.* The value of magnetic resonance cholangiopancreatography in predicting common bile duct stones in patients with gallstone disease. *Br. J. Surg.* 2003; **90**(1):42–47.
47. Arcement, C. M., Meza, M. P., Arumanla, S., & Towbin, R. B. MRCP in the evaluation of pancreaticobiliary disease in children. *Pediatr Radiol* 2001; **31**(2):92–97.
48. Choi, B. H., Lim, Y. J., Yoon, C. H., Kim, E. A., Park, Y. S., & Kim, K. M. Acute pancreatitis associated with biliary disease in children. *J. Gastroenterol. Hepatol.* 2003; **18**(8):915–921.
49. Wendtland-Born, A., Wiewrodt, B., Bender, S. W., & Weitzel, D. [Prevalence of gallstones in the neonatal period]. *Ultraschall. Med.* 1997; **18**(2):80–83.
50. Brown, D. L., Teele, R. L., Doubilet, P. M., DiSalvo, D. N., Benson, C. B., & Van Alstyne, G. A. Echogenic material in the fetal gallbladder: sonographic and clinical observations. *Radiology* 1992; **182**(1):73–76.
51. St-Vil, D., Yazbeck, S., Luks, F. I., Hancock, B. J., Filiatrault, D., & Youssef, S. Cholelithiasis in newborns and infants. *J. Pediatr. Surg.* 1992; **27**(10):1305–1307.
52. Debray, D., Pariente, D., Gauthier, F., Myara, A., & Bernard, O. Cholelithiasis in infancy: a study of 40 cases. *J. Pediatr.* 1993; **122**(3):385–391.
53. Petrikovsky, B., Klein, V., & Holsten, N. Sludge in fetal gallbladder: natural history and neonatal outcome. *Br. J. Radiol.* 1996; **69**(827):1017–1018.
54. Amin, A., Rejjal, A., McDonald, P., & Nazer, H. Nephrocalcinosis, cholelithiasis, and umbilical vein calcification in a premature infant. *Abdom. Imaging.* 1994; **19**(6):559–560.
55. Aynaci, F. M., Erduran, E., Mocan, H., Okten, A., & Sarpkaya, A. O. Cholelithiasis in infants with Down syndrome: report of two cases. *Acta Paediatr.* 1995; **84**(6):711–712.
56. Jawad, A. J., Kurban, K., el-Bakry, A., al-Rabeeah, A., Seraj, M., & Ammar, A. Laparoscopic cholecystectomy for cholelithiasis during infancy and childhood: cost analysis and review of current indications. *World J. Surg.* 1998; **22**(1):69–73; discussion 74.
57. Farrow, G. B., Dewan, P. A., Taylor, R. G., Stokes, K. B., & Auldist, A. W. Retained common-duct stones after open cholecystectomy and duct exploration in children. *Pediatr. Surg. Int.* 2003; **19**(7):525–528.
58. Jacir, N. N., Anderson, K. D., Eichelberger, M., & Guzzetta, P. C. Cholelithiasis in infancy: resolution of gallstones in three of four infants. *J. Pediatr. Surg.* 1986; **21**(7):567–569.
59. Morad, Y., Ziv, N., & Merlob, P. Incidental diagnosis of asymptomatic neonatal cholelithiasis: case report and literature review. *J. Perinatol.* 1995; **15**(4):314–317.
60. Xanthakos, S. A., Yazigi, N. A., Ryckman, F. C., & Arkovitz, M. S. Spontaneous perforation of the bile duct in infancy: a rare but important cause of irritability and abdominal distension. *J. Pediatr. Gastroenterol. Nutr.* 2003; **36**(2):287–291.
61. Patel, N. A., Lamb, J. J., Hogle, N. J., & Fowler, D. L. Therapeutic

efficacy of laparoscopic cholecystectomy in the treatment of biliary dyskinesia. *Am. J. Surg*. 2004; **187**(2):209–212.

62. Bingener, J., Richards, M. L., Schwesinger, W. H., & Sirinek, K. R. Laparoscopic cholecystectomy for biliary dyskinesia: correlation of preoperative cholecystokinin cholescintigraphy results with postoperative outcome. *Surg. Endosc*. 2004.
63. Holcomb, G. W., Jr., Holcomb, G. W., 3rd. Cholelithiasis in infants, children, and adolescents. *Pediatr. Rev*. 1990; **11**(9):268–274.
64. Flake, A. *Disorders of the Gallbladder and Biliary Tract*. Philadelphia, PA: Lippincott-Raven; 1997.
65. Marchetti, M., Quaglini, S., & Barosi, G. Prophylactic splenectomy and cholecystectomy in mild hereditary spherocytosis: analyzing the decision in different clinical scenarios. *J. Intern. Med*. 1998; **244**(3):217–226.
66. Patton, M. L., Moss, B. E., Haith, L. R., Jr. *et al.* Concomitant laparoscopic cholecystectomy and splenectomy for surgical management of hereditary spherocytosis. *Am. Surg*. 1997; **63**(6):536–539.
67. Yamagishi, S. & Watanabe, T. Concomitant laparoscopic splenectomy and cholecystectomy for management of hereditary spherocytosis associated with gallstones. *J. Clin. Gastroenterol*. 2000; **30**(4):447.
68. Sandler, A., Winkel, G., Kimura, K., & Soper, R. The role of prophylactic cholecystectomy during splenectomy in children with hereditary spherocytosis. *J. Pediatr. Surg*. 1999; **34**(7):1077–1078.
69. Leandros, E., Kymionis, G. D., Konstadoulakis, M. M. *et al.* Laparoscopic or open cholecystectomy in patients with sickle cell disease: which approach is superior? *Eur. J. Surg*. 2000; **166**(11):859–861.
70. Sandoval, C., Stringel, G., Ozkaynak, M. F., Tugal, O., & Jayabose, S. Perioperative management in children with sickle cell disease undergoing laparoscopic surgery. *J. Soc. Laparoendosc. Surgs*. 2002; **6**(1):29–33.
71. Al-Salem, A. H. Should cholecystectomy be performed concomitantly with splenectomy in children with sickle-cell disease? *Pediatr. Surg. Int*. 2003; **19**(1–2):71–74.
72. Parez, N., Quinet, B., Batut, S. *et al.* [Cholelithiasis in children with sickle cell disease: experience of a French pediatric hospital]. *Arch Pediatr*. 2001; **8**(10):1045–1049.
73. Rambo, W. M. & Reines, H. D. Elective cholecystectomy for the patient with sickle cell disease and asymptomatic cholelithiasis. *Am. Surg*. 1986; **52**(4):205–207.
74. Pappis, C. H., Galanakis, S., Moussatos, G., Keramidas, D., & Kattamis, C. Experience of splenectomy and cholecystectomy in children with chronic haemolytic anaemia. *J. Pediatr. Surg*. 1989; **24**(6):543–546.
75. Alexander-Reindorf, C., Nwaneri, R. U., Worrell, R. G., Ogbonna, A., & Uzoma, C. The significance of gallstones in children with sickle cell anemia. *J. Natl. Med. Assoc*. 1990; **82**(9):645–650.
76. Drucker, D. *Cholelithiasis in Children*. Chicago: Mosby Yearbook; 1991.
77. Fall, B., Sagna, A., Diop, P. S., Faye, E. A., Diagne, I., & Dia, A. [Laparoscopic cholecystectomy in sickle cell disease]. *Ann. Chir*. 2003; **128**(10):702–705.
78. Johna, S., Shaul, D., Taylor, E. W., Brown, C. A., & Bloch, J. H. Laparoscopic management of gallbladder disease in children and adolescents. *J. Soc. Laparoendosc. Surgs*. 1997; **1**(3):241–245.
79. Al-Abkari, H. A., Abdulnabi, H. I., Al-Jamah, A. H., & Meshikhes, A. N. Laparoscopic cholecystectomy in patients with Sickle Cell Disease. *Saudi Med. J*. 2001; **22**(8):681–685.
80. Riddington, C. & Williamson, L. Preoperative blood transfusions for sickle cell disease. *Cochrane Database Syst. Rev*. (3):CD003149.
81. Delatte, S. J., Hebra, A., Tagge, E. P., Jackson, S., Jacques, K., & Othersen, H. B., Jr. Acute chest syndrome in the postoperative sickle cell patient. *J. Pediatr. Surg*. 1999; **34**(1):188–191; discussion 191–182.
82. Wales, P. W., Carver, E., Crawford, M. W., & Kim, P. C. Acute chest syndrome after abdominal surgery in children with sickle cell disease: Is a laparoscopic approach better? *J. Pediatr. Surg*. 2001; **36**(5):718–721.
83. Kalayci, A. G., Albayrak, D., Gunes, M., Incesu, L., & Agac, R. The incidence of gallbladder stones and gallbladder function in beta-thalassemic children. *Acta. Radiol*. 1999; **40**(4):440–443.
84. Galanello, R., Piras, S., Barella, S. *et al.* Cholelithiasis and Gilbert's syndrome in homozygous beta-thalassaemia. *Br. J. Haematol*. 2001; **115**(4):926–928.
85. Borgna-Pignatti, C., Rigon, F., Merlo, L. *et al.* Thalassemia minor, the Gilbert mutation, and the risk of gallstones. *Haematologica* 2003; **88**(10):1106–1109.
86. Feretis, C. B., Legakis, N. C., Apostolidis, N. S., Katergiannakis, V. A., & Philippakis, M. G. Prophylactic cholecystectomy during splenectomy for beta thalassemia homozygous in Greece. *Surg. Gynecol. Obstet*. 1985; **160**(1):9–12.
87. Ekbom, A., Yuen, J., Adami, H. O. *et al.* Cholecystectomy and colorectal cancer. *Gastroenterology* 1993; **105**(1):142–147.
88. Zuccato, E., Venturi, M., Di Leo, G. *et al.* Role of bile acids and metabolic activity of colonic bacteria in increased risk of colon cancer after cholecystectomy. *Dig. Dis. Sci*. 1993; **38**(3):514–519.
89. McFarlane, M. J. & Welch, K. E. Gallstones, cholecystectomy, and colorectal cancer. *Am. J. Gastroenterol*. 1993; **88**(12):1994–1999.
90. Rahman, M. I., Gibson-Shreve, L. D., Yuan, Z., & Morris, H. A. Selections from current literature: cholelithiasis, cholecystectomy and the risk of colorectal cancer. *Fam. Pract*. 1996; **13**(5):483–487.
91. Ganschow, R. Cholelithiasis in pediatric organ transplantation: detection and management. *Pediatr. Transpl*. 2002; **6**(2):91–96.
92. Sakopoulos, A. G., Gundry, S., Razzouk, A. J., Andrews, H. G., & Bailey, L. L. Cholelithiasis in infant and pediatric heart transplant patients. *Pediatr. Transpl*. 2002; **6**(3):231–234.
93. Milas, M., Ricketts, R. R., Amerson, J. R., & Kanter, K. Management of biliary tract stones in heart transplant patients. *Ann. Surg*. 1996; **223**(6):747–753; discussion 753–746.

94. Safford, S. D., Safford, K. M., Martin, P., Rice, H., Kurtzberg, J., & Skinner, M. A. Management of cholelithiasis in pediatric patients who undergo bone marrow transplantation. *J. Pediatr. Surg*. 2001; **36**(1):86–90.

95. Melvin, W. S., Meier, D. J., Elkhammas, E. A. *et al*. Prophylactic cholecystectomy is not indicated following renal transplantation. *Am. J. Surg*. 1998; **175**(4):317–319.

96. Bruch, S. W., Ein, S. H., Rocchi, C., & Kim, P. C. The management of nonpigmented gallstones in children. *J. Pediatr. Surg*. 2000; **35**(5):729–732.

97. Kim, P. C., Wesson, D., Superina, R., & Filler, R. Laparoscopic cholecystectomy versus open cholecystectomy in children: which is better? *J. Pediatr. Surg*. 1995; **30**(7):971–973.

98. Luks, F. I., Logan, J., Breuer, C. K., Kurkchubasche, A. G., Wesselhoeft, C. W., Jr., & Tracy, T. F., Jr. Cost-effectiveness of laparoscopy in children. *Arch. Pediatr. Adolesc. Med*. 1999; **153**(9):965–968.

99. Lugo-Vicente, H. L. Gallbladder dyskinesia in children. *Jsls* 1997; **1**(1):61–64.

100. Dumont, R. C. & Caniano, D. A. Hypokinetic gallbladder disease: a cause of chronic abdominal pain in children and adolescents. *J. Pediatr. Surg*. 1999; **34**(5):858–861; discussion 861–852.

101. Gollin, G., Raschbaum, G. R., Moorthy, C., & Santos, L. Cholecystectomy for suspected biliary dyskinesia in children with chronic abdominal pain. *J. Pediatr. Surg*. 1999; **34**(5):854–857.

102. Al-Homaidhi, H. S., Sukerek, H., Klein, M., & Tolia, V. Biliary dyskinesia in children. *Pediatr. Surg. Int*. 2002; **18**(5–6):357–360.

103. Wood, J., Holland, A. J., Shun, A., Martin, H. C. Biliary dyskinesia: is the problem with Oddi? *Pediatr. Surg. Int*. 2004; **20**(2):83–86.

104. Shah, R. S., Blakely, M. L., & Lobe, T. E. The role of laparoscopy in the management of common bile duct obstruction in children. *Surg. Endosc*. 2001; **15**:1353–1355.

105. Kokoska, E. R., West, K. W., Carney, D. E., Engum, S. E., Heiny, M. E., & Rescorla, F. J. Risk factors for acute chest syndrome in children with sickle cell disease undergoing abdominal surgery. *J. Pediatr. Surg*. 2004; **39**:848–850.

38a

Portal hypertension: surgery and interventional radiology

Frédéric Gauthier,[1] Danièle Pariente,[2] and Sophie Branchereau[1]

[1]Division of Surgery, Federation of Paediatrics, Centre Hospitalier Universitaire Bicêtre, France
[2]Division of Radiology, Federation of Paediatrics, Centre Hospitalier Universitaire Bicêtre, France

Gastrointestinal bleeding related to portal hypertension (PH) in children may be life threatening. Therapeutic alternatives used to relieve PH and reduce the risk of bleeding include various types of surgical and radiologic vascular procedures. Shunt surgery, which usually results in total diversion of portal blood flow, was introduced several decades ago. The long-term benefits and complications of this therapy have been critically reviewed in the previous edition of this book.[1] New techniques developed during the 1990s. The transjugular intrahepatic porto-systemic stent shunt (TIPS) is now preferred to surgical shunts for treatment of PH in most cirrhotic patients. The splanchnic-to-left-portal vein bypass (Rex shunt), designed for definitive treatment of portal vein obstruction, results in restoration of physiologic intrahepatic portal blood flow. The less invasive techniques of percutaneous endoluminal dilatation or thrombectomy of the portal vein, with or without placement of a stent, have been used mainly as rescue therapies after failed shunts, TIPS or bypasses; a few attempts have been made to use them as a definitive treatment of portal vein obstruction.

Shunt surgery

Evolution of indications for shunt surgery

Different pathologic conditions cause portal hypertension in children and etiology must be considered when choosing a treatment for PH.[2] In the case of extrahepatic portal obstruction (EHPO), which is either idiopathic or a complication of perinatal thrombosis of the portal vein, liver function is normal or near-normal, and for many years a shunt operation has been considered as the best method of providing lifetime protection against recurrence of bleeding, with an acceptable risk of complications. In the case of chronic liver disease with intrahepatic portal hypertension (IHPO), the choice of treatment depends on the liver function. Children with ongoing cirrhosis (Child-Pugh B or C) are candidates for liver transplantation (LT); there is now evidence that shunt surgery might precipitate liver failure in these patients and it should therefore be avoided. For children in whom LT is not being considered in the near future (Child-Pugh A), alternative treatments include shunt surgery and endoscopic therapy.

Experience of shunt surgery in children

Indications and results of shunt surgery in major series are listed on Table 38a.1.[1,3–14] Although satisfactory results in pediatric patients were reported by adult surgical teams in the 1970s and early 1980s,[3,4] the experience of pediatric surgical teams with shunt surgery was somewhat limited for a number of reasons, including the relative paucity of cases of PH in children and a reluctance to perform such surgery in small children with small vessels.[5] A multicenter study by the American Academy of Pediatrics of 48 patients submitted to shunt surgery could not reach any definite conclusions about long-term results because of the small number of patients and the great variety of shunt procedures.[7] Other series include two important reports from India,[8,12] where some units have employed shunt surgery in preference to sclerotherapy because of the risk of viral transmission from blood transfusion. A long-term follow-up of 162 adults and children treated at a single institution in San Diego stands out as the largest North American experience.[10]

Pediatric Surgery and Urology: Long-term Outcomes, Mark Stringer, Keith Oldham, Pierre Mouriquand.
Published by Cambridge University Press.

Table 38a.1. Results of porto-systemic shunt surgery from 12 pediatric series

Author	Date	Reference	Number of patients	Cirrhotic (%)	Non-cirrhotic (%)	Follow-up	Patency (%)	Died n (%)
Auvert	1975	3	46	30	70	2–15 y	72	0
Bismuth	1980	4	90	42	58	?	94	1 (1 %)
Tocornal	1981	6	23	0	100	?	91	0
Altman	1982	7	48	46	54	?	73	8 (17 %)
Mitra	1993	8	104	0	100	1–14 y	87	1 (1 %)
Maksoud	1994	9	29	?	?	6.5 y (mean)	95	0
Orloff	1994	10	120	0	100	5–10 y	98	0
Losty	1994	11	21	0	100	10–23 y	56	0
Prasad	1994	12	160	0	100	1–15 y	89	4 (2%)
D'Cruz	1995	13	48	?	?	> 18 mths	98	0
Bicêtre	1996	1	190	35	65	0.25–17 y	87	11 (6 %)
Sigalet	2001	14	20	0	100	4.3 y (mean)	100	1 (5 %)

At the Bicêtre Hospital, 190 children (132 with EHPO, 52 with IHPO and 6 with Budd Chiari syndrome) were submitted to shunt surgery between 1977 and 1996. The exact type of operation was determined by the local venous anatomy, but the preference was for some sort of H-type procedure, principally mesocaval using the internal jugular vein.[15,16] The age range at operation was 18 months to 17 years (mean 8 years), with a follow-up ranging from 3 months to 18 years. Shunt failure occurred in 35 patients (18%), of whom 15 (8%) were submitted to a second shunt operation, successful in ten cases. Thus, a total of 165 (87%) patients had a patent shunt at follow-up.

Woven Dacron prostheses have rarely been used in children owing to the risk of thrombosis. Recently, satisfactory results have been achieved with PTFE prostheses in two cases maintained on low dose aspirin therapy followed up for 3 and 4 years, respectively.

Analysis of outcome

Shunt patency

In the postoperative period, patency of the shunt is best assessed by abdominal Doppler ultrasound, while disappearance of esophageal varices is usually demonstrated later, sometimes 3 to 12 months postoperatively. When the shunt cannot be directly visualized by ultrasound, indirect signs of changes in portal flow can be demonstrated, such as diminishing thickness of the lesser omentum and increasing diameter of the inferior vena cava. In cases where doubt remains about the patency of the shunt, non-invasive angiography using CT or MRI can be performed.

From an analysis of the literature, and our own experience at Bicêtre, long-term shunt patency of approximately 80%–90% should be anticipated, provided that local venous anatomy was initially favorable for construction of an appropriate shunt.[2] Patency rates are expected to be higher in older children because of the larger diameter of portomesenteric vessels used for anastomosis. In the Bicêtre series a patent shunt was demonstrated in 40 children (80%) operated on between the ages of 1 and 5 years and in 89% of 125 children operated on after the age of 5 years; this difference was however not significant.[1] Also apparent from larger series is the fact that shunt patency may be achieved in the majority of cases, whatever the technique used. However, splenectomy is not recommended, such as with a central splenorenal shunt,[12] because of the risk of overwhelming post-splenectomy infection. One child died from this complication at the beginning of the Bicêtre experience.

The long-term results of an efficient shunt procedure – the so-called superior mesenteric vein-inferior vena cava shunt described by Santy and Marion in France and by Clatworthy in the USA – were reported in 1975.[3] Forty-six patients, most of them under 10 years of age, were treated by the authors using this procedure. Shunt patency, with no recurrent bleeding, was proven in 72% of cases. Other series, although small, have reported on shunt patency up to the age of 30 years.[11] When considering the larger series,[8,10,12] it is obvious that rebleeding occurs only when a shunt has failed.

In the Bicêtre series,[1] 110 children were last seen at 1–5 years after surgery, 33 at 5–10 years, and 22 more than 10 years later; the oldest patient was seen 26 years after surgery. From the charts of these patients, it appears that, once shunt patency has been confirmed postoperatively, this should be considered a permanent result, since further clinical and abdominal ultrasound examinations seem to show no subsequent evidence of recurrent PH.

Long-term benefits of shunt surgery

Prevention of hemorrhage and control of hypersplenism

In the Bicêtre series, 147 patients (77%) were submitted to fiberoptic esophagascopy at least once during follow-up; among the so-called good results, in 71 cases there was complete disappearance of varices, and in another 60 evidence of a distinct improvement. In 16 patients, varices were unchanged. Among those not submitted to endoscopy, results were still considered to be good in 34 cases because of direct or indirect evidence from abdominal ultrasound scans.

It often takes several months before reduction in size of the spleen and correction of hypersplenism become obvious. Splenomegaly may be present on examination after a successful shunt in cases where the spleen was very large and somewhat fibrous preoperatively. At Bicêtre, 119 children considered as having a patent shunt had a definite reduction in size of their spleen, with no palpable splenomegaly on clinical examination in 55 (46%) of these. Patency of the shunt should be rapidly followed by a rise in platelet count, but normal levels will not be reached for several weeks.

Improved growth

For unclear reasons, a striking improvement in growth may be seen after shunt surgery for EHPO. In an earlier study from the Bicêtre Hospital, 16 children out of a group of 25 in which shunt surgery had been successful had an accelerated growth curve during the first year after porto-systemic shunting.[17] Similar results have been reported recently from an American centre.[18]

Correction of biliary abnormalities

Biliary abnormalities are infrequently associated with EHPO, but in some cases they appear to be related directly to the abnormal venous anatomy since they subside after relief of PH. Intrahepatic and extrahepatic bile duct dilatation was demonstrated by ultrasound scan in 4/132 of the Bicêtre cases of EHPO, and also reported in 5/21 consecutive patients in a prospective study of adults and children with EHPO from India.[19] These morphologic changes are believed to be related to bile duct compression by collateral veins, scar tissue or ischemic injury to ducts. Any element of obstructive jaundice tends to resolve after successful treatment of portal hypertension.[20] Cholelithiasis is also occasionally associated with EHPO, and can be treated by cholecystectomy at the time of the shunt operation or later. In five Bicêtre cases, all but one associated with EHPO, no subsequent complications have developed.

A bridge to liver transplantation

For children awaiting liver transplantation, the development of gastrointestinal bleeding from PH is a serious complication. Before the TIPS era shunt operations were sometimes considered in the pretransplant management of some of these children, in order to avoid the risk of liver failure precipitated by hemorrhage and also to facilitate total hepatectomy. Eight of 410 children submitted to liver transplantation in Bicêtre had previously undergone porto-systemic shunt surgery. The recipient hepatectomy and the transplant procedure itself were smoother than in cases with persistent PH.

Quality of life

Abolition of the bleeding risk after successful porto-systemic shunting provides understandable relief for the child and the parents. This psychological effect is clearly apparent during subsequent conversations with the family. Assessment of quality of life, based on information about scholarship and professional achievement, was available in only 44 Bicêtre cases. Eighteen youngsters out of 37 still at school were considered to be functioning at a lower level than expected, and this is a greater proportion than normal for the general French teenage population. However, the sample is too small to draw any conclusions about potential late effects of porto-systemic shunt operations. With regard to the seven adults for whom equivalent information was available, their activities were as varied as student, lawyer, electrician, travel agent, etc. At least two patients have become pregnant, without adverse effects; one has had two children.

Adverse effects of shunt surgery

Mortality

Death after shunt surgery for PH is rare. In the Bicêtre series 11 children have died, five from shunt-related problems. Splenectomy should be avoided in association with a shunt operation because of the well-recognized risk of overwhelming late sepsis. Death in two of our cases occurred suddenly at home, with no available autopsy findings. Postoperative hemodynamic changes with pulmonary hypertension may have been the cause of death in one of these cases.

Porto-systemic encephalopathy

Porto-systemic encephalopathy (PSE) may be detected clinically or by electroencephalography. Clinical signs may be mild and only detectable by appropriate psychometric tests and/or associated with learning difficulties at school. Parents and patients should be questioned about any disorientation or forgetfulness. Fasting and postprandial blood ammonia levels should be measured regularly.

In a series of 100 adult cirrhotic patients (Child-Pugh class A or B), all with mesocaval interposition shunts, PSE developed in 12%.[21] In a retrospective review of Bicêtre cases in 1985,[22] 9/31 children (29%) treated by porto-systemic shunting for PH complicating cirrhosis presented with at least one episode of PSE, a few days to 11 years postoperatively; this complication was generally triggered by an additional event, namely protein excess, bleeding or intercurrent infection.

In 1980, Warren *et al.*[23] reported a case of severe PSE 21 years after a central splenorenal shunt for EHPO; the patient's condition returned to normal after closure of the shunt (it is not stated whether bleeding recurred or not). A relatively dated study of 16 patients submitted to a porto-systemic shunt in childhood, eight of whom had normal livers, appeared to demonstrate some evidence of neurological impairment 4–19 years later.[24] The degree of late impairment showed some correlation with the duration of shunting. Except for these two reports, follow-up studies have shown no evidence of a long term risk of PSE in EHPO patients.

In 1986 at the Bicêtre Hospital, the long-term effects of shunt procedures in children with EHPO and no associated liver disease were evaluated. Forty-two patients followed up to 24 years postoperatively were assessed, taking into account the impact of neonatal events, surgery, and family situation. Comparison was made with two other groups of children, one with EHPO without a shunt and the other with chronic idiopathic thrombocytopenia who had undergone splenectomy.[25] Although the sample sizes were small, no late neuropsychologic complications were demonstrated in any case by neurologic examination, psychometric testing, and EEG. The level of school performance and employment was normal in 50% of the cases. In another series of 43 EHPO patients,[26] 30 of whom had been treated by a shunt operation, it was stated that none of the 19 survivors showed any obvious evidence of neuropsychiatric disturbance. Two series from India of 160 and 30 EHPO patients, respectively,[12,27] reported no children suffering from late neuropsychiatric sequelae.

Venous complications

Late venous complications, such as leg edema and episodes of phlebitis, may occur after interruption of the inferior vena cava which is undertaken in some shunt operations. Five out of 12 patients who underwent division of the inferior vena cava in one series suffered from these complications[26] as did two of the authors' patients. One of the latter patients presented with a large ovarian cyst during puberty, and the dense venous collateral circulation within the pelvis noted at operation was suspected to be implicated in the ovarian pathology. In children undergoing a mesocaval shunt using an interposed segment of internal jugular vein, the scar on the neck is occasionally a cosmetic concern; use of transverse cervical incisions gives a more satisfactory result.

Hepatopulmonary syndrome

A severe but rare complication of liver disease and porto-systemic shunts is hepatopulmonary syndrome (HPS) whereby systemic venous blood enters the arterial circulation without exposure to alveolar oxygen. The mechanism is not fully understood, but it involves right-to-left shunting of blood via communications between esophageal varices and pulmonary veins (portopulmonary shunts), and/or direct arteriovenous shunts within the lung.[28] Shunting may be demonstrated by technetium-99m-labeled macroaggregated albumin pulmonary scanning.[29]

In a study at the Bicêtre Hospital, 24 children suffering from cirrhosis and another with PH from EHPO had symptoms of pulmonary arteriovenous shunting.[30] They presented at 6 months to 14 years, with cyanosis, dyspnea, or both, and symptoms occurred especially early in children with biliary atresia and polysplenia. Six of these children had previously had a successful porto-systemic shunt. Seven untreated children died 3 months to 8 years after the diagnosis of intrapulmonary shunting. Liver transplantation is the treatment of choice for those children with HPS. Seven out of 11 patients of the latter series are alive with no signs of intrapulmonary shunting. Both survival and post-transplant morbidity are clearly related to the severity of shunting.[31]

Pulmonary arterial hypertension

Another rare but more serious cardiovascular complication of porto-systemic shunt surgery is the occurrence of pulmonary arterial hypertension (PAH). The pathogenesis of PAH is unclear. It appears to result from a combination of factors including recurrent pulmonary microemboli, and plexogenic pulmonary arteriopathy (thought to be a consequence of vasoactive or hepatotoxic substances such as neuro-peptide and serotonin escaping liver metabolism via natural or surgical shunts). Most reported cases of coexistent PAH and PH are in patients with cirrhosis. About 1% of patients with PH due to cirrhosis are believed to suffer from PAH.[28] Such a complication can also develop with biliary atresia and associated polysplenia syndrome, even after a successful Kasai operation.[32]

PAH may rarely complicate PH in the absence of liver disease, either in patients with spontaneous shunts or after surgical shunting[26,33,34]

Clinical manifestations of PAH such as exertional dyspnea, chest pain and fatigue reflect an advanced stage of the disease, with a high risk of right heart failure and sudden death. Therefore, annual echocardiography is recommended to check for the preclinical signs of this serious but rare complication of PH and shunt surgery. In cases of PH due to cirrhosis, liver transplantation should be considered once PAH is detected.[28]

Liver tumors and tumor-like lesions

In experimental studies in rats, portocaval anastomosis promotes the development of hyperplastic nodules or even hepatocellular carcinoma.[35,36] In humans, cases of focal nodular hyperplasia, single or multiple hyperplastic nodular lesions, and even hepatoblastoma, have been reported in association with congenital absence of the portal vein.[37–40] However, as yet there have been no reports of a liver malignancy developing in a previously normal liver after a porto-systemic shunt in childhood.

Shunt failure

Failure of the surgical shunt, related in most cases to the small size and unfavorable pattern of splanchnic veins,[2] is an unfortunate early complication. Further surgery may be limited by the availability of a suitable venous autograft.

Before interventional radiologic techniques were developed, it was presumed that failure was always due to shunt thrombosis, and attempts were made to create an alternative shunt. In the Bicêtre experience this was done in 15 cases between 4 months and 7 years (mean 4.5 years) postoperatively, and was successful in 10 cases.

More recently, we have become convinced that the cause of shunt failure is more often due to stenosis than thrombosis and that a radiologic attempt at recanalization (see below) should be considered before further surgery.

Transjugular intrahepatic porto-systemic shunts (TIPS)

Historical considerations

TIPS procedures were developed by radiologists as a short-term efficient alternative to surgery for the treatment of complications of PH.[41,42] Technical modifications have been introduced in order to facilitate placement of TIPS into the small size vessels of children.[43] However, TIPS have been used infrequently in pediatric patients in comparison to adults.

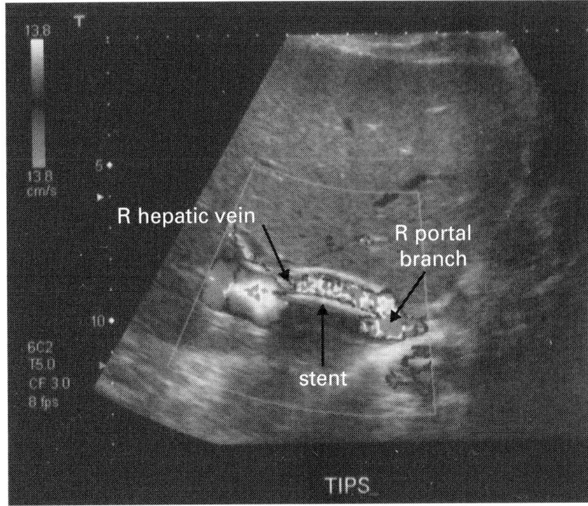

Fig. 38a.1. Successful TIPS: Doppler ultrasonographic appearance.

Assessment of TIPS patency

Routine assessment of the patency of TIPS is performed by repeated clinical examination and Doppler ultrasound (Fig. 38a.1). In patients with evidence of shunt dysfunction, transjugular portal venography allows accurate diagnosis of shunt stenosis or obstruction, and appropriate interventions by balloon dilatation or placement of a new stent if necessary (Fig. 38a.2a–c).

Results of TIPS

Results of TIPS in children from six series[43–48] are shown in Table 38a.2. From detailed analysis of these reports, it appears that patients who survived more than 1 year after TIPS placement without liver transplantation could not escape the need for repeat dilatations. In the Bicêtre experience with 12 patients aged 2 to 15 years, nine procedures were successful, all nine in children over 5 years of age. Recent experience in adults suggests that long-term results could probably be improved in the future by the use of PTFE covered stents.[49,50]

TIPS placement may also improve hepatopulmonary syndrome. Such a case has recently been reported in an 11-year-old girl with biliary atresia and the polysplenia syndrome.[51]

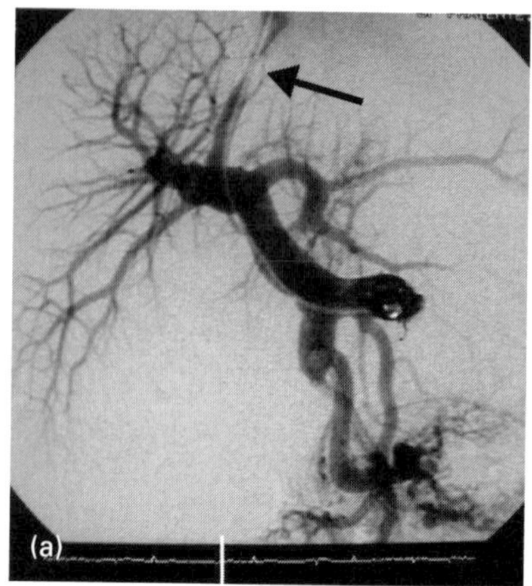
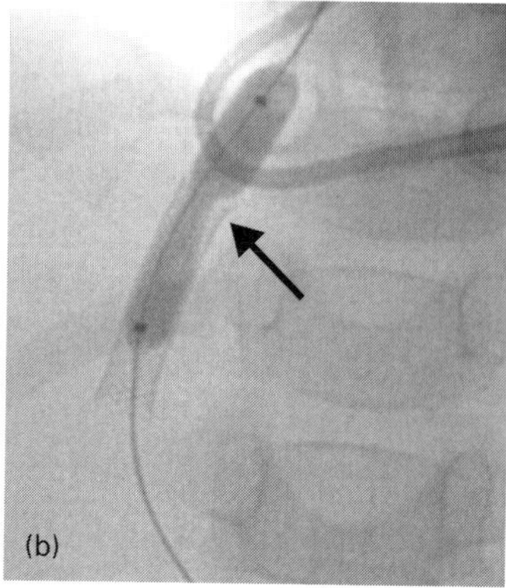
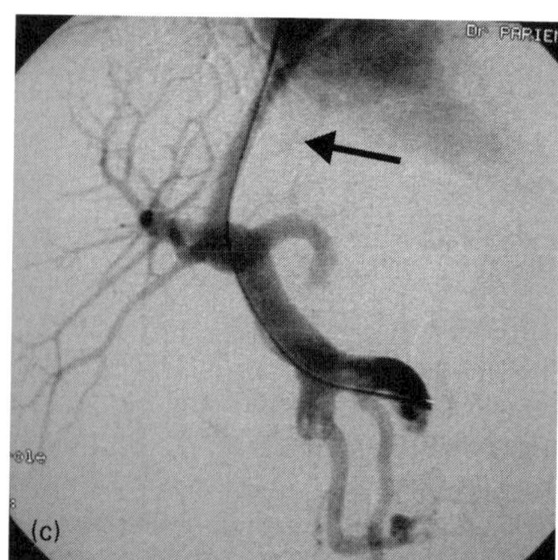

Fig. 38a.2. Stenosis of a TIPS. Treatment by percutaneous balloon dilatation.
(a) Angiogram before dilatation (arrow = stricture zone).
(b) Balloon within stent prosthesis (arrow = stricture zone).
(c) Repeat angiogram after dilatation.

Table 38a.2. Results of TIPS in six pediatric series

Author (year)	Number of patients	Age (years)	Success rate	Longest follow-up	Need for dilatations
Berger *et al.* (1994)[44]	2	10 & 11	2 / 2	1 year	
Johnson *et al.* (1996)[45]	3	6 to 11	3 / 3	Unknown	
Heyman *et al.* (1997)[43]	9	5 to 15	7 / 9	1–800 days	
Hackworth *et al.* (1998)[46]	12	2.5 to 16	11 / 12	2 patent at 1 year	
Huppert *et al.* (2002)[47]	9	3 to 13	9 / 9	75 months	8 / 9
Pozler *et al.* (2003)[48]	5	8 to 18	5 / 5	81 months	5 / 5

Bypass surgery – the Rex shunt

Principle of bypass surgery

The goal of bypass surgery (the so-called "Rex shunt") in cases of portal vein obstruction is to achieve both portal decompression and restoration of physiologic intrahepatic portal blood flow. The operation consists of interposing a conduit, usually a jugular venous autograft, between one of the main veins of the extrahepatic portomesenteric system and the left branch of the portal vein (Fig. 38a.3a–c). This technique was initially developed for the treatment of portal vein thrombosis complicating liver transplantation and was subsequently applied to selected cases of idiopathic or iatrogenic portal vein obstruction with cavernous transformation.[52] Bypass surgery can be considered when two anatomical conditions are fulfilled. First, a large extrahepatic vessel must be available for anastomosis; this is nowadays best assessed by means of CT scan or MR angiography. Second, the left portal vein and its branches within the liver must be patent; this is best assessed by a combination of duplex sonography and wedged hepatic venography.[53]

Results of bypass surgery

Assessment of the results of bypass surgery is based on the same clinical, endoscopic, ultrasonographic and radiologic criteria as after porto-systemic shunt surgery.

Since the first report from De Ville de Goyet *et al.* on bypass surgery in seven cases of portal vein thrombosis after LT,[54] several series with satisfactory results have been published[55–58] (Table 38a.3). Immediate patency of the shunt with relief of symptoms of PH was achieved in all reported cases. Late stenoses in two series were treated successfully by either redoing the shunt or by percutaneous angioplasty.[52,55] In the Bicêtre experience 21 bypass procedures were performed between 1996 and 2003. The indication for surgery was EHPVO in 15 patients aged 2 to 16 years and post-transplantation portal vein thrombosis (PTPVT) in 6 patients aged 1 to 8 years. Initial patency was achieved in 12/15 (80%) patients with EHPVO and in all patients with PTPVT. Two EHPVO patients underwent a successful secondary mesocaval shunt after early (one case) or delayed (one case) failure of the bypass, and one EHPVO patient with early failure of the bypass had an unsuccessful rescue splenorenal shunt. One patient with PTPVT who developed a stenosis of the bypass with secondary

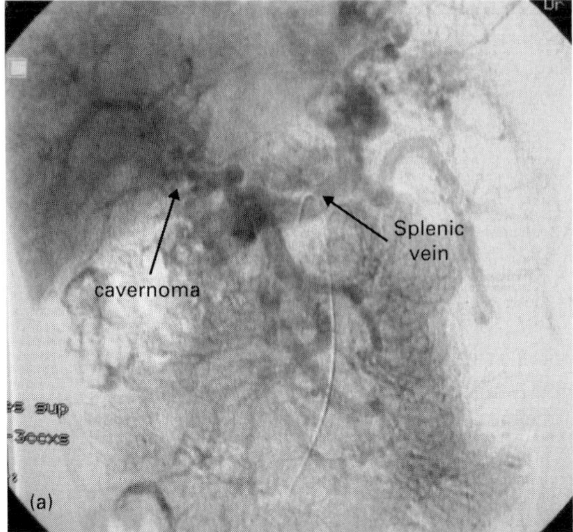

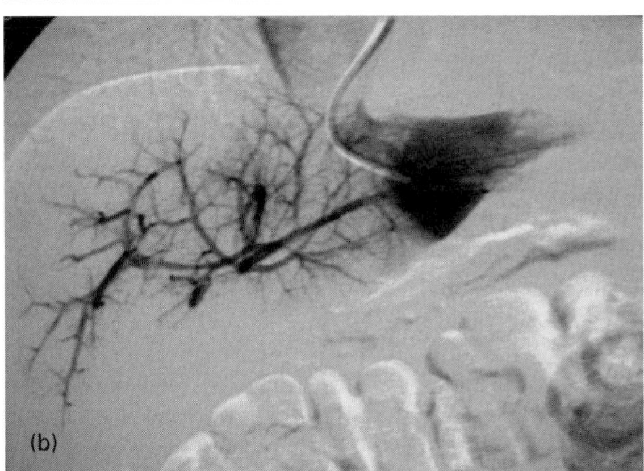

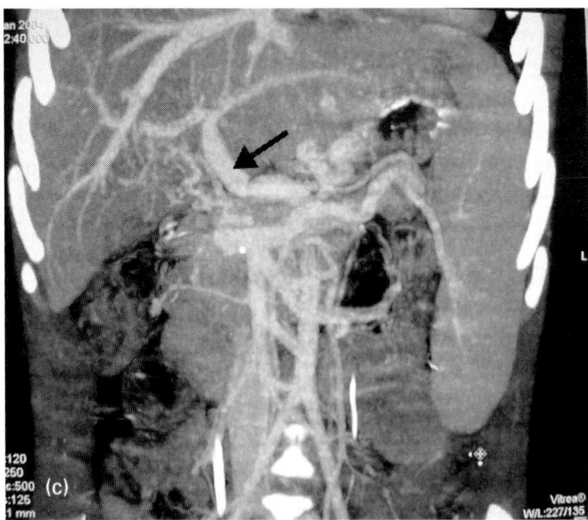

Fig. 38a.3. Portal vein obstruction: splenic vein-to-left portal branch bypass with an internal jugular graft.
(a) Venous phase of selective superior mesenteric angiography.
(b) Wedged hepatic venography.
(c) Postoperative angio-CT-scan. Arrow = jugular venous graft.

thrombosis was successfully treated by percutaneous thrombectomy and placement of a stent. A significant improvement in coagulation factors in the year following successful bypass surgery was reported in one series[56] but this was not seen in our experience. However, a rapid improvement in intrahepatic portal perfusion is usually observed after successful bypass,[57,58] and relief of hepatopulmonary syndrome was described in one case.[57]

Technical variants of bypass surgery

Most reported cases have been superior mesenteric–left portal vein bypasses, but variant techniques may be used, such as the inferior mesenteric–left portal vein bypass reported by Ates *et al.*[59] In the Bicêtre experience the splenic vein or an enlarged pancreatico-duodenal vein were used as the origin of the bypass in seven and two cases, respectively, with a 7/9 (78%) success rate.

Percutaneous radiologic procedures

Percutaneous radiologic procedures have been valuable in a few selected situations.

After failure of a surgical porto-systemic shunt, a femoral vein approach provides an easy route to angioplasty of an anastomotic stenosis or even recanalization of an occluded shunt (Fig. 38a.4). This has been successfully performed in nine out of ten cases in the Bicêtre series.

Percutaneous transhepatic puncture of intrahepatic portal vein branches under ultrasonographic guidance may allow dilatation of a stenosed Rex shunt (two cases) or recanalization of portal vein occlusion complicating liver transplantation; the latter was achieved in 9 out of 20 attempts at Bicêtre with placement of a stent in only two cases. The portal veins remained patent without further dilatation with a follow-up ranging from 1 to 8 years.

In our experience, interventional radiologic techniques were successful in only one out of ten cases of portal vein obstruction affecting the native liver. In this case, a 9-year-old girl presenting with splenomegaly since 5 years of age and high grade esophageal varices, recanalization and angioplasty of the occluded portal vein avoided the need for surgery. Her portal vein has remained widely patent with a follow-up of more than 3 years. One other successful recanalization of an occluded portal vein with a stent has been reported by Cwikiel *et al.*[60]

Conclusions

Extrahepatic portal vein obstruction may be regarded as an exclusively vascular disease. Thus a single vascular operation providing definitive relief of PH should rightfully be regarded as a valuable option. When anatomically feasible,

Table 38a.3. Results of bypass surgery (Rex shunt) from the literature together with two unpublished series from Leeds, UK and Bicêtre, France

Author (year)	Indication	Number of patients	Follow-up	Number of patent shunts at follow-up	Complications	Secondary procedures
de Ville de Goyet (1996)	post-LT PVT	7				
de Ville de Goyet (1999)	EHPVO	11	1–32 months	11	2 stenoses	2 re-do
Bambini (2000)	mixed	5	7–21 months	3	2 stenoses	2 dilatations
Mack (2003)	EHPVO	11		11		
Fuchs (2003)	EHPVO	7	3–28 months	7	0	
Gehrke (2003)	EHPVO	13	6–24 months	13		nil
Stringer (unpublished)	EHPVO	7	2–35 months	7	0	nil
Bicêtre (unpublished)	post-LT PVT	6		6	1 stenosis	stent
Bicêtre (unpublished)	EHPVO	15	6–100 months	11	3 thromboses	3 PS shunts

Abbreviations:
LT = liver transplantation.
EHPVO = extrahepatic portal vein obstruction.
PVT = portal vein thrombosis.
PS = porto-systemic.

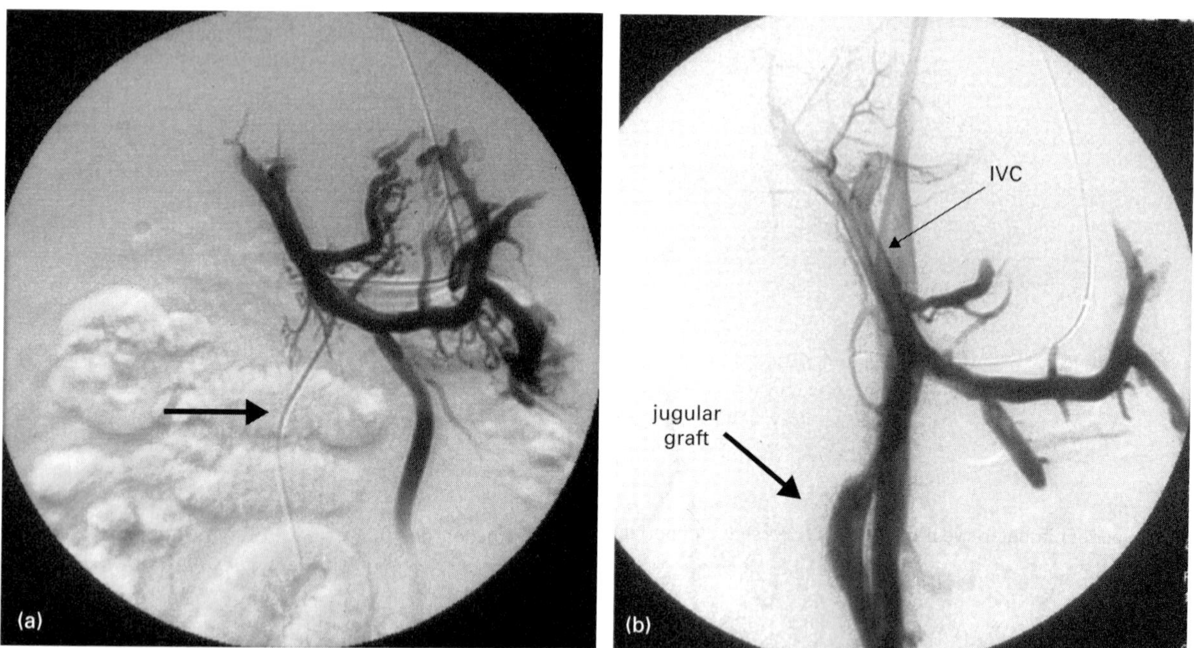

Fig. 38a.4. Failed mesocaval shunt for Budd–Chiari syndrome: percutaneous recanalization 4 years later.
(a) Before dilatation: the femoral venous catheter (arrow) is guided through the occluded venous graft.
(b) After dilatation: patent jugular graft and flow from mesenteric vein to inferior vena cava.

bypass surgery is nowadays the gold standard for treatment of EHPO, since it achieves restoration of physiologic portal blood flow, with a high probability of success. In patients with favorable extrahepatic but unfavorable intrahepatic vascular anatomy, porto-systemic shunt surgery is a useful option, since the long-term risk of adverse effects is low. In patients whose vascular anatomy is diffusely abnormal, Non-vascular surgery and/or endoscopic therapies should be preferred.

With intrahepatic portal vein obstruction, the severity of the liver disease is the dominant factor in deciding the best treatment of PH. In the child with severe liver disease awaiting LT, the goal is to prevent harmful gastrointestinal bleeding. Endoscopic therapy is the usual choice, but TIPS should also be considered, since relief of PH facilitates the transplant hepatectomy. In patients with liver disease but normal or near-normal liver function, LT is too radical and shunt surgery, which is anatomically straightforward with a low risk of PSE, should be considered providing that there is careful long-term screening for cardiovascular complications.

In Budd–Chiari syndrome the true risk is not gastrointestinal bleeding but progressive liver damage.[2] Shunt surgery or TIPS, depending on the general condition and vascular anatomy of the patient, should be planned as soon as possible.

Acknowledgments

The authors wish to express their thanks to Jacques Valayer, now retired, who developed PH surgery in Bicêtre, to their coworkers Jean Marie Hay (retired), Olivier de Dreuzy and Christophe Chardot, to their colleagues in the Hepatology Unit (headed by Olivier Bernard), and in the Radiology Unit of the Federation of Paediatrics in Bicêtre. Special thanks are due to Daniel Alagille, now retired, who believed in surgery and surgeons.

REFERENCES

1. Valayer, J. & Branchereau, S. Portal hypertension: porto-systemic shunts In Stringer M. D., Oldham, K. T., Mouriquand, P. D. E., & Howard, E. R., eds. *Pediatric Surgery and Urology: Long-term Outcomes*. London: W.B. Saunders, 1998: 439–446.
2. Gauthier, F. Surgery for portal hypertension In Howard, E. R., Stringer, M. D., Colombani, P. M., eds. *Surgery of the Liver, Bile Ducts and Pancreas in Children*. London: Arnold, 2002: 315–29.
3. Auvert, J. & Weisgerber, G. Immediate and long-term results of superior mesenteric vein-inferior vena cava shunt for portal hypertension in children. *J. Pediatr. Surg.* 1975; **10**:901–908.
4. Bismuth, H., Franco, D., & Alagille, D. Portal diversion for portal hypertension in children. The first ninety patients. *Ann. Surg.* 1980; **192**:18–24.
5. Clatworthy, H. W., Nahmad, M., & Hollabaugh, R. S. Presinusoidal extrahepatic portal hypertension: a review of thirty-five cases variously treated. *Progr. Pediatr. Surg.* 1978; **1**:125–139.
6. Tocornal, J. & Cruz, F. Portal–systemic shunts for extrahepatic portal hypertension in children. *Surg. Gynecol. Obstet.* 1981; **153**:53–56.
7. Altman, R. P. & Krug, J. Portal hypertension: American Academy of Pediatrics Surgical Section Survey 1981. *J. Pediatr. Surg.* 1982; **17**:567–575.
8. Mitra, S. K., Rao, K. L. N., Narasimshan, K. L. *et al.* Side-to-side lienorenal shunt without splenectomy in noncirrhotic portal hypertension in children. *J. Pediatr. Surg.* 1993; **28**:398–402.
9. Maksoud, J. G. & Goncalves, M. E. P. Treatment of portal hypertension in children. *World J. Surg.* 1994; **18**:251–258.
10. Orloff, M. J., Orloff, M. S., & Rambotti, M. Treatment of bleeding oesophagogastric varices due to extrahepatic portal hypertension: results of portal-systemic shunts during 35 years. *J. Pediatr. Surg.* 1994; **29**:142–154.
11. Losty, P. D., Lyndh, M. J., & Guiney, E. J. Long term outcome after surgery for extrahepatic portal vein thrombosis. *Arch. Dis. Child.* 1994; **71**:437–440.
12. Prasad, A. S., Gupta, S., Kohli, V. *et al.* Proximal spleno-renal shunts for extrahepatic portal venous obstruction in children. *Ann. Surg.* 1994; **219**:193–196.
13. D'Cruz, A. J., Kamath, P. S., Ramachandra, C., Jalihal, A. Non-conventional portal-systemic shunts in children with extrahepatic portal vein obstruction. *Acta. Paediatr. Jpn* 1995; **37**:17–20.
14. Sigalet, D. L., Mayer, S., & Blanchard, H. Portal venous decompression with H-type mesocaval shunt using autologous venous graft: a North American experience. *J. Pediatr. Surg.* 2001; **36**:91–96.
15. Valayer, J., Hay, J. M., Gauthier, F., & Broto, J. Shunt surgery for treatment of portal hypertension in children. *World J. Surg.* 1985; **9**:258–268.
16. Gauthier, F., de Dreuzy, O., Valayer, J., & Montupet, P. H-type shunt with an autologous venous graft for treatment of portal hypertension in children. *J. Pediatr. Surg.* 1989; **24**:1041–1043.
17. Alvarez, F., Bernard, O., Brunelle, F., Hadchouel, P., & Odievre, M. Portal obstruction in children. II: Results of portal-systemic shunts. *J. Pediatr.* 1983; **103**:703–707.
18. Kato, T., Romero, R., Koutouby, R. *et al.* Portal-systemic shunting in children during the era of endoscopic therapy: improved postoperative growth parameters. *J. Pediatr. Gastroenterol. Nutr.* 2000; **30**:419–425.
19. Khuroo, M. S., Yattoo, G. N., Zargar, S. A. *et al.* Biliary abnormalities associated with extrahepatic portal venous obstruction. *Hepatology* 1993; **17**:807–813.
20. Chaudhary, A., Dhar, P., Sarin, S. K. *et al.* Bile duct obstruction due to portal biliopathy in extrahepatic portal hypertension: surgical management. *Br. J. Surg* 1998; **85**:326–329.
21. Paquet, K. J., Mercado, M. A., Kalk, J. F. *et al.* Analysis of a prospective series of 100 mesocaval interposition shunts for bleeding portal hypertension. *Hepatogastro-enterology* 1990; **37**:115–120.
22. Bernard, O., Alvarez, F., Brunelle, F., Hadchouel, P., & Alagille, D. Portal hypertension in children. *Clin. Gastroenterol.* 1985; **14**:33–54.
23. Warren, D., Millikian, W. J., Smith, R. B. *et al.* Non-cirrhotic portal vein thrombosis. *Ann. Surg.* 1980; **192**:341–349.
24. Vorhees, A. B., Chaitman, E., Schneider, S. *et al.* Portal-systemic encephalopathy in the noncirrhotic patient; effect of portal-systemic shunting. *Arch. Surg.* 1973; **107**:659–663.
25. Alagille, D., Cartier, J. C., Chiva, M. *et al.* Long term neuro-psychological outcome in children undergoing

portal–systemic shunts for portal vein obstruction without liver disease. *J. Pediatr. Gastroenterol. Nutr.* 1986; **5**:861–866.

26. Boles, E. T., Wise, E., & Birken, G. Extrahepatic portal hypertension in children: long term evaluation. *Am. J. Surg.* 1986; **151**:734–739.
27. Mohapatra, M. K., Mohapatra, A. K., Acharya, S. K., Sahni, P., & Nundy, S. Encephalopathy in patients with extrahepatic obstruction after lienorenal shunts. *Br. J. Surg.* 1992; **79**:1103–1105.
28. Krowka, M. J. & Cortese, D. A. Pulmonary aspects of chronic liver disease and liver transplantation. *Mayo Clin. Proc.* 1985; **60**:407–418.
29. Teisseyre, M., Szymczak, M., Swiatek-Rawa, E. *et al.* Scintiscaning in diagnostics of hepatopulmonary syndrome in children. *Med. Sci. Monit.* 2001; **7**suppl:255–261.
30. Barbe, T., Losay, J., Grimon, G. *et al.* Pulmonary arterio-venous shunting in children with liver disease. *J. Pediatr.* 1995; **126**:571–579.
31. Egawa, H., Kasahara, M., Inomata, Y. *et al.* Long-term outcome of living related liver transplantation for patients with intrapulmonary shunting and strategy for complications. *Transplantation* 1999; **15**:712–717.
32. Schujtvlot, E. T., Bax, N. M. A., Houwen, R. H. J., & Hruda, J. Unexpected lethal pulmonary hypertension in a (-year-old girl successfully treated for biliary atresia. *J. Pediatr. Surg.* 1995; **30**:589–590.
33. Levine, O. R., Harris, R. C., Blanc, W. A., & Mellins, R. B. Progressive pulmonary hypertension in children with portal hypertension. *J. Pediatr.* 1973; **83**:964–972.
34. Yamaguchi, M., Kumada, K., Okamoto, R., Osawa, K., & Morikawa, S. Pulmonary hypertension associated with portal hypertension in a child. *Pediatr. Surg. Int.* 1991; **6**:47–49.
35. Weinbren, K. & Washington, S. L. A. Hyperplastic nodules after portal anastomosis in rats. *Nature* 1976; **264**:440–442.
36. Preat, V., Pector, J. C., Taper, H. *et al.* Promoting effect of portocaval anastomosis in rat hepatocarcinogenesis. *Carcinogenesis* 1984; **5**:1151–1154.
37. Barton, J. W. III & Relier, M. S. Liver transplantation for hepatoblastoma in a child with congenital absence of the portal vein. *Pediatr. Radiol.* 1989; **20**:113–114.
38. Altavilla, G. & Guariso, G. Focal nodular hyperplasia of the liver associated with portal vein agenesis: a morphological and immunohistochemical study of one case and review of the literature. *Adv. Clin. Path.* 1999; **3**:139–145.
39. Howard, E. R. & Davenport, M. Congenital extrahepatic portocaval shunts – the Abernathy malformation *J. Pediatr. Surg.* 1997; **32**:494–497.
40. Tanaka, Y., Takayanagi, M., Shiratori, Y. *et al.* Congenital absence of portal vein with multiple hyperplastic nodular lesions in the liver. *J. Gastroenterol.* 2003; **38**:288–294.
41. LaBerge, J. M., Ring, E. J., Gordon, R. L. *et al.* Creation of transjugular intrahepatic portal-systemic stent shunts with the wallstent endoprosthesis: results in 100 patients. *Radiology* 1993; **187**:413–420.
42. Rôssle, M., Haag, K., Ochs, A. *et al.* The transjugular intrahepatic portal-systemic stent-shunt procedure for variceal bleeding. *N. Engl. J. Med.* 1994; **330**:165–171.
43. Heyman, M. B., LaBerge, J. M., Somberg, K. A. *et al.* Transjugular portosystemic shunts (TIPS) in children. *J. Pediatr.* 1997; **131**:914–919.
44. Berger, H., Bugnon, F., Goffette, P. *et al.* Percutaneous transjugular intrahepatic stent shunt for treatment of intractable varicose bleeding in paediatric patients. *Eur. J. Pediatr.* 1994; **153**:721–725.
45. Johnson, S. P., Leyendecker, J. R., Joseph, F. B. *et al.* Transjugular portosystemic shunts in pediatric patients awaiting liver transpolantation. *Transplantation* 1996; **27**:1178–1181.
46. Hackworth, C. K., Leef, J. A., Whitington, P. F., Millis, J. M., & Alonso, E. M. Transjugular intrahepatic portosystemic shunt creation in children: initial clinical experience. *Radiology* 1998; **206**:109–114.
47. Huppert, P. E., Goffette, P., Astfalk, W. *et al.* Transjugular intrahepatic portosystemic shunts in children with biliary atresia. *Cardiovasc. Intervent. Radiol.* 2002:484–493.
48. Pozler, O., Krajina, A., & Vanicek, H. Transjugular intrahepatic portosystemic shunt in five children with cystic fibrosis: long-term outcome. *Hepatogastroenterology* 2003; **50**:1111–1114.
49. Bureau, C., Garcia-Pagan, J. C., Otal, P. *et al.* Improved clinical outcome using polytetrafluoroethylene-coated stents for TIPS: results of a randomized study. *Gastroenterology* 2004; **126**:469–475.
50. Rossi, P., Salvatori, F. M., Fanelli, F. *et al.* Polytetrafluoroethylene-covered nitinol stent-graft for transjugular intrahepatic portosystemic shunt creation: 3-year experience. *Radiology* 2004; **23**:820–830.
51. Paramesh, A. S., Husain, S. Z., Shneider, B. *et al.* Improvement of hepatopulmonary sundrome after transjugular intrahepatic portosystemic shunting: case report and review of literature. *Pediatr. Transpl.* 2003; **7**:157–162.
52. De Ville de Goyet, J., Alberti, D., Falchetti, D. *et al.* Treatment of extrahepatic portal hypertension in children by mesenteric-to-left portal vein bypass: a new physiological procedure. *Eur. J. Surg.* 1999; **165**:777–781.
53. John, P. & de Ville de Goyet, J. Wedged hepatic venography in portal cavernomas: an imaging window before mesoportal bypass surgery. *Pediatr. Radiol.* 2003; **3382**:533
54. De Ville de Goyet, J., Gibbs, P., Clapuyt, P. *et al.* Original extrahilar approach for hepatic portal revascularization and relief of extrahepatic portal hypertension related to late portal vein thrombosis after liver transplantation. *Transplantation* 1996; **62**:71–75.
55. Bambini, D. A., Superina, R. A., Almond, P. S., Whitington, P. F., & Alonso, E. Experience with the Rex shunt (mesenterico-left portal bypass) in children with extrahepatic portal hypertension. *J. Pediatr. Surg.* 2000; **35**:13–18.
56. Mack, C. L., Superina, R. A., & Whitington, P. F. Surgical restoration of portal flow corrects procoagulant and anticoagulant deficiencies associated with extrahepatic portal vein thrombosis. *J. Pediatr.* 2003; **142**:197–199.

57. Fuchs, J., Warmann, S., Kardorff, R. *et al.* Mesenterico-left portal vein bypass in children with congenital extrahepatic vein thrombosis: a unique curative approach. *J. Pediatr. Gastroenterol. Nutr.* 2003; **36**:213–216.
58. Gehrke, I., John, P., Blundell, J. *et al.* Meso-portal bypass in children with portal vein thrombosis: rapid increase of the intrahepatic portal venous flow after direct portal hepatic reperfusion. *J. Pediatr. Surg.* 2003; **38**:1137–1140.
59. Ates, O., Hakguder, G., Olguner, M., & Akgur, F. M. Extrahepatic portal hypertension treated by anastomosing inferior mesenteric vein to left portal vein at Rex recessus. *J. Pediatr. Surg.* 2003; **38**:E10–E11.
60. Cwikiel, W., Keussen, I., Larsson, L., Solvig, J., & Kullendorff, C. M. Interventional treatment of children with portal hypertension secondary to portal vein occlusion. *Eur. J. Pediatr. Surg.* 2003; **13**:312–318.

38b

Portal hypertension: Endoscopic treatment

Mark D. Stringer

Children's Liver and GI Unit, St James's University Hospital, Leeds, UK

Introduction

Portal hypertension is not a definitive diagnosis since it is caused by a wide variety of conditions each with a different natural history. Successful management of the child with portal hypertension requires an accurate diagnosis of the underlying cause, and a full understanding of the therapeutic options.

Portal hypertension is defined by an increased hepatic venous pressure gradient (>5 mmHg), the difference between portal venous pressure and free hepatic venous pressure. A hepatic venous pressure gradient of >12 mmHg is necessary for the development of esophageal varices.[1] Submucosal varices in the lower esophagus are particularly prone to rupture. Although the relationship is not linear, the risk of variceal bleeding is increased in larger varices and those with a higher intravariceal pressure and wall tension.[2,3] Wall tension is inversely proportional to wall thickness – a large varix with thin walls (evidenced by "red color signs" on endoscopy) will reach a high wall tension and risk of bleeding at much lower variceal pressures. In cirrhotics, the risk of variceal bleeding is related to the severity of the liver disease (reflected by the Child–Pugh score).

Bleeding from esophageal varices is the commonest cause of serious gastrointestinal hemorrhage in children. For children with chronic liver disease, subsequent prognosis is determined more by underlying liver pathology whereas for those with extrahepatic portal hypertension (who typically have a healthy liver), outcome is dictated by the success of treating portal hypertension.

Indications for surgery

The management of children with variceal bleeding complicating portal hypertension demands multidisciplinary teamwork and the use of a variety of complementary techniques, each of which may be limited by applicability, efficacy and complications. Endoscopic therapy is highly effective and has an established track record, especially in the acute management of bleeding from esophageal varices. However, surgery continues to be an essential element for successful treatment of portal hypertension in many children. The indications for surgery have changed over the years. In the current management of portal hypertension, the following should be considered:

- The Rex shunt (portal vein bypass) should now be regarded as the optimum method of treating children with extrahepatic portal vein obstruction (PVO) and no associated liver disease.[4–6] This shunt, first developed for patients with portal vein thrombosis complicating liver transplantation, consists of a bypass graft between the portomesenteric venous system (typically the superior mesenteric vein) and the left branch of the portal vein, found in the Rex recessus adjacent to the falciform ligament. Autologous jugular vein is the best type of graft. The bypass restores physiologic liver portal blood flow and corrects portal hypertension. The operation requires the presence of an adequate caliber, patent intrahepatic left portal vein and patent, communicating splenic and mesenteric veins. There should be no underlying liver disease. Owing to the variable pattern of portomesenteric venous occlusion both outside[7] and within[4] the liver, this

Pediatric Surgery and Urology: Long-term Outcomes, Mark Stringer, Keith Oldham, Pierre Mouriquand.
Published by Cambridge University Press.

bypass is not anatomically feasible in every child with extrahepatic portal hypertension. Shunt thrombosis is a potential hazard but short-term follow-up studies have shown patency rates in excess of 95% when an autologous vein graft has been used for the bypass.[8]

- Portosystemic shunting has a valuable role in treating bleeding esophageal varices that are unresponsive to endoscopic therapy and in dealing with bleeding from gastrointestinal varices, provided liver function is well preserved. Portosystemic shunting can offer effective primary treatment of extrahepatic PVO for some patients in whom a Rex shunt is not feasible but the decision to operate will depend not only on venous anatomy but also local factors such as surgical and endoscopic expertise and the safety of blood transfusion. Portomesenteric venous anatomy does not permit successful shunt surgery in every child, and shunt thrombosis is a hazard with all types of shunts, especially in small children.[9–12]
- Liver transplantation is the procedure of choice for patients with complications of portal hypertension associated with advanced liver disease. Endoscopic treatment usually provides effective control of variceal bleeding in children awaiting transplant; banding may be safer than sclerotherapy immediately prior to transplantation.[13] Endoscopic therapy does not reduce portal perfusion, precipitate encephalopathy, or add to the technical difficulties of subsequent liver transplantation. Transjugular intrahepatic stent shunt (TIPS) should be considered as a bridge to transplant for endoscopic treatment failures.[14]
- For patients with complications of portal hypertension associated with milder degrees of chronic liver disease, endoscopic therapy, TIPS, or a portosystemic shunt are alternative palliative options. For children with extrahepatic PVO who are either unsuitable for surgery or who have had failed surgery, endoscopic therapy is usually effective.
- Radiologic techniques, portosystemic shunting, and liver transplantation all have a role in managing the spectrum of children with Budd–Chiari syndrome.

This chapter focuses on the long-term outcome of endoscopic therapies for variceal bleeding. A more comprehensive review of portal hypertension in children can be found elsewhere.[15]

Historical background

Endoscopic injection sclerotherapy was introduced by two Swedish surgeons, Crafoord and Frenckner, more than 60 years ago.[16] They described an 18-year-old girl with bleeding esophageal varices, treated by rigid endoscopy and serial intravariceal injections of quinine; variceal obliteration was observed within one month. By 1955, the technique had been successfully applied to children.[17] In the 1980s several large pediatric series were published confirming the efficacy of this treatment.[18,19] In 1988, Stiegmann and Goff introduced endoscopic variceal ligation as an alternative to sclerotherapy.[20]

Techniques

Acute variceal bleeding is managed by a combination of resuscitation, cautious blood transfusion, octreotide infusion, optimization of clotting parameters and, rarely, balloon tamponade.[21] Flexible fiberoptic endoscopy is carried out under general anesthesia with an endotracheal tube in situ within 24 hours of admission. The upper gastrointestinal tract is assessed and varices are graded according to their size and appearance. Large varices are blue and may show "red signs" of recent or impending variceal hemorrhage; these include "cherry red spots" and "varices on varices" (Fig. 38b.1a–c). Portal gastropathy is characterized by mucosal hyperemia and speckling when mild, and mosaic red spots and hemorrhagic lesions when severe.

Two endoscopic techniques are commonly used to treat esophageal varices.

Injection sclerotherapy

Endoscopic injection sclerotherapy (EIS) can be used to treat children of any age with esophageal varices. Varices are injected with a flexible 25G needle inserted through the biopsy channel of the endoscope. Various injection techniques and sclerosants have been used, e.g., intravariceal injection of 5% ethanolamine oleate.[21] Between 1 and 3 ml of sclerosant are injected into each of the major variceal columns in the distal 3 cm of esophagus just above the gastroesophageal junction. Paravariceal injections are occasionally used to stop bleeding from a puncture site. Varices are initially injected every 1–2 weeks and then at monthly intervals until obliterated; injection is deferred for 1 week if there is significant esophageal mucosal ulceration. Oral Ranitidine and Sucralfate are given for up to 2 weeks after each injection session to reduce complications from sclerotherapy-induced ulcers. Antibiotic prophylaxis is recommended for those with damaged/prosthetic heart valves[22] and the immunosuppressed. Variceal obliteration can often be accomplished within six treatment sessions. Day-case endoscopic review is advisable after 6 months and then annually to diagnose and treat recurrent varices.

(a)

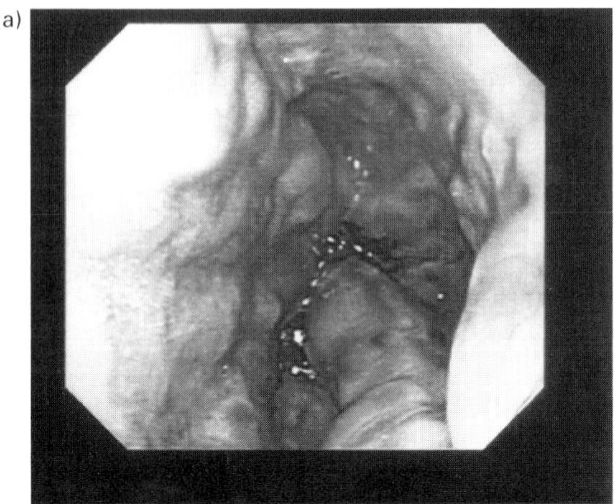

(b)

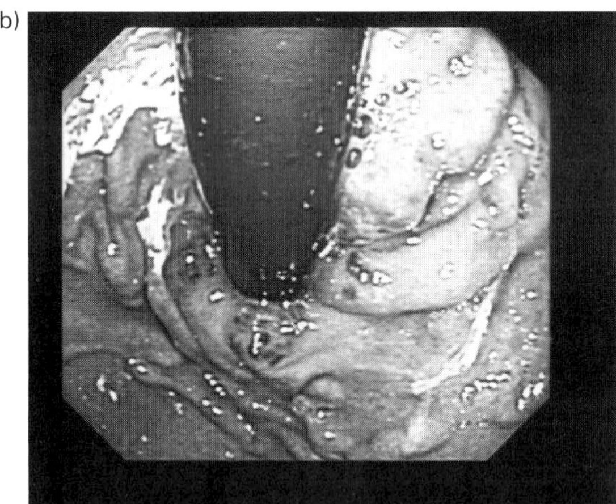

(c)

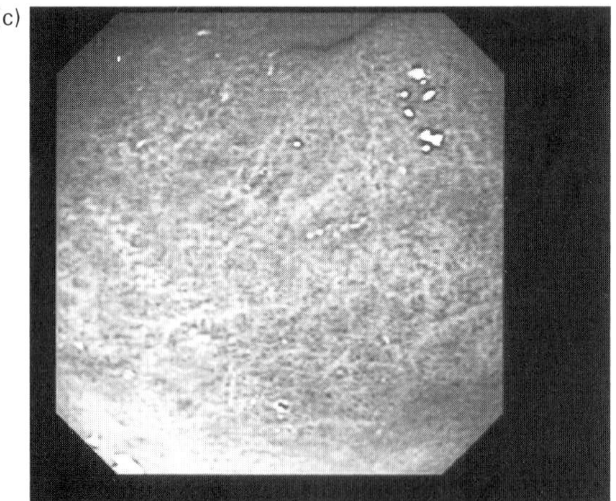

Fig. 38b.1. Endoscopic appearances in children with portal hypertension.
(a) Esophageal varices with red signs indicative of recent or impending variceal hemorrhage.
(b) Fundal varices (contiguous with esophageal varices) showing red signs.
(c) Portal hypertensive gastropathy in the antrum.

Table 38b.1. Most frequent complications of endoscopic injection sclerotherapy

Transient retrosternal discomfort and/or fever
Esophageal ulceration and stricture formation
Bleeding before variceal obliteration (usually from varices or sclerotherapy ulcers)
Recurrent esophageal varices
Worsening portal gastropathy
Bacteremia

Variceal ligation (banding)

In this method, the varix is aspirated into a transparent cylinder fitted to the end of a flexible fiberoptic endoscope and a preloaded elastic band is deployed around the varix. Endoscopic variceal ligation (EVL) leads to strangulation of the varix which then thromboses and sloughs. Treatment begins with ligation of varices in the distal esophagus just above the gastro-esophageal junction, and extends proximally within the distal 5 cm of esophagus. Using a multiband ligating device, up to six bands can be applied at each session, but usually no more than four, one on each of the major variceal columns. Treatment is repeated after 1–2 weeks and then monthly. Following variceal obliteration, patients are endoscoped after 3–6 months and then annually and any recurrent varices treated.

Early results and complications

Injection sclerotherapy

In experienced centers, EIS is a highly effective treatment for esophageal varices. In an early series of 108 children with variceal bleeding, complete sclerosis was achieved in all patients with PVO and in more than 90% of those with chronic liver disease who did not require liver transplantation.[18] In the subgroup of patients with biliary atresia, injection sclerotherapy proved to be effective in controlling esophageal variceal bleeding in 15 out of 16 cases (94%);[23] an average of five to six injection sessions was required during a mean period of 1 year. Similar successful results have been reported by others using injection sclerotherapy for esophageal variceal bleeding in children.[19,24–26]

EIS has a risk of morbidity: the more common complications are listed in Table 38b.1. Transient self-limiting retrosternal discomfort and fever are common after sclerotherapy but a marked or persistent pyrexia requires antibiotic therapy because of the possibility of bacteremia. Gastrointestinal bleeding before variceal obliteration is complete is usually due to a non-thrombosed varix or an

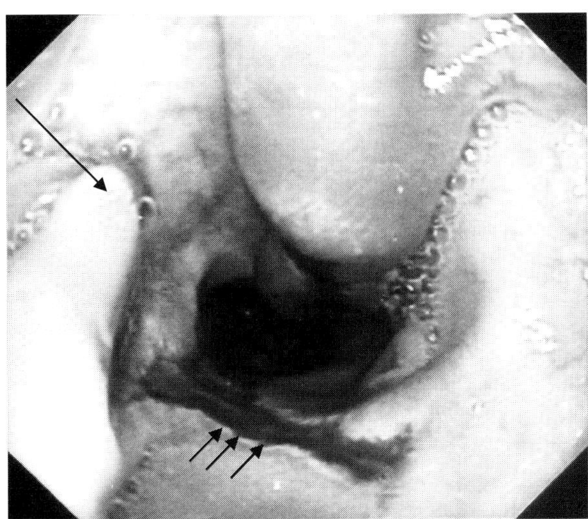

Fig. 38b.2. Endoscopic appearances of the distal esophagus in a 15-year-old girl who was first treated by injection sclerotherapy at 3 years of age. The distal esophagus was relatively rigid with chronic erythematous esophagitis (short arrows) and mucosal tags (long arrow).

esophageal mucosal ulcer; this complication is less likely after the first few injections. Bleeding after variceal obliteration is usually due to other pathology such as peptic ulceration or is from recurrent esophageal or gastric varices. The short-term incidence of recurrent esophageal varices is low (<10%) and most respond to further sclerotherapy.[18] The treatment of small asymptomatic recurrent esophageal varices at review endoscopies reduces this problem.

Injection of sclerosant into the esophageal varix results in venous thrombosis, localized chemical esophagitis and mucosal ulceration.[27] Most sclerotherapy ulcers are asymptomatic and an inevitable temporary consequence of the sclerosant.[28,29] They more often follow frequent or large volume injections,[30] but may additionally be related to the depth of injection. Sclerotherapy ulcers and associated bleeding can be reduced by prophylactic Ranitidine.[31] An esophageal stricture probably arises from a combination of chemical esophagitis, ulceration and acid reflux. Although a 16% incidence of post-sclerotherapy strictures was reported in an early series[18] (all of which responded to simple esophageal dilatation), this complication is now seen in less than 5% of cases in the author's practice and in recent series,[32] probably as a result of using smaller volumes of sclerosant, and prophylactic Ranitidine and Sucralfate.[33]

After injection sclerotherapy, the esophageal mucosa heals leaving residual mucosal tags and the esophageal wall becomes more rigid (Fig. 38b.2). This may lead to esophageal dysmotility and gastroesophageal reflux which can cause intermittent dysphagia and heartburn. Manometric and pH studies after sclerotherapy have demonstrated esophageal dysmotility, reduced lower esophageal sphincter tone, and reduced clearance of refluxed acid.[28,34]

More serious complications, such as distant effects from the passage of sclerosant into systemic veins or tributaries of the portal venous system have been reported, mostly in adults where the disease spectrum is different and patient numbers are vast;[21] these complications are rare in children.[18,35]

Variceal ligation (banding)

EVL is currently the optimum endoscopic method of controlling active bleeding and in preventing rebleeding from esophageal varices. EVL and EIS are similarly effective but EVL offers more rapid eradication (usually within two to four sessions) and is associated with fewer complications. Esophageal ulcers caused by banding are more superficial and resolve quicker than those induced by sclerotherapy and the incidence of esophageal stricture and systemic complications is lower.[36] The safety and efficacy of EVL in children has been confirmed in several studies.[32,37,38] Complications include bleeding before variceal obliteration is complete, esophageal perforation (rare), and recurrent varices. At present, technical difficulties limit the safe use of the technique in small children (<10 kg). EVL and EIS are not mutually exclusive and a combination of both can be particularly useful in some children.

In a prospective study, McKiernan *et al.* (2002) treated 28 patients with a mean age of 11 years (range 0.3–16 years), 68% of whom had intrahepatic portal hypertension.[37] During a median follow-up period of 9 months after variceal obliteration, two children developed bleeding gastric varices requiring surgery, seven were transplanted, and esophageal varices recurred in seven (33% of those at risk). Recurrent varices responded to further ligation.

In a larger study, which has not yet been published in full, Celinska-Cedro *et al.* (2002) reported on 64 children with a mean age of 8.3 ± 4.2 years and a history of bleeding from esophageal varices, 59% of whom had extrahepatic portal hypertension.[38] Children under 2 years of age were excluded. Variceal eradication using EVL was achieved in 91% with an average of 2.3 banding sessions per child. Bleeding before variceal eradication was complete occurred in 22%, and there was one treatment failure. Recurrent varices were found in 18% of patients (with two rebleeds) during a mean follow-up period of 19.9 ± 10.2 months.

One randomized controlled trial of EIS versus EVL in children has been reported. Zargar *et al.* (2002) randomized 49 patients aged between 4 and 14 years with extrahepatic PVO and bleeding from esophageal varices, to EIS ($n = 24$) and EVL ($n = 25$).[32] Acute variceal bleeding was controlled endoscopically in all cases and variceal eradication was achieved in 92% and 96%, respectively. However, band ligation required fewer treatment sessions (a mean of four rather than six) and bleeding before variceal eradication was complete and the incidence of complications were significantly higher (25%) with EIS than with EVL (4%). During a 2-year follow-up period after variceal eradication, recurrent esophageal varices occurred in 10% of the EIS group and 17% of the EVL group but this difference was not statistically significant; recurrent varices were successfully treated endoscopically. Changes in gastric varices and portal hypertensive gastropathy were similar in both groups.

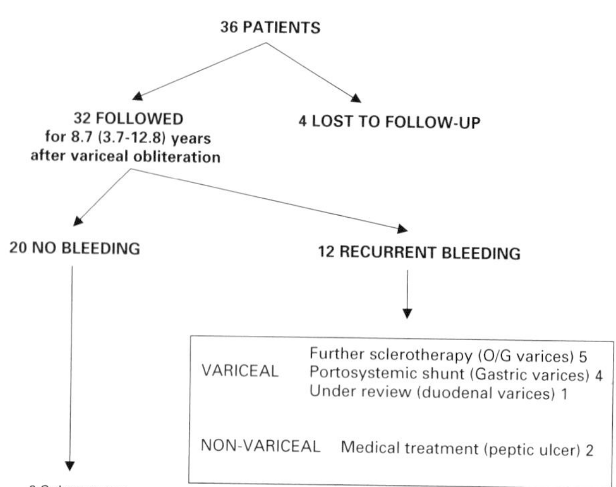

Fig. 38b.3. Summary of long-term outcome after endoscopic injection sclerotherapy for bleeding esophageal varices in children with extrahepatic portal hypertension.[43]

Gastric and ectopic varices

Most gastric varices are fundal and directly contiguous with lower esophageal varices (gastro-esophageal varices). These are often eradicated during endoscopic treatment of esophageal varices. About 10% of patients develop significant gastric varices after endoscopic obliteration of esophageal varices. Bleeding from gastro-esophageal varices may respond to endoscopic treatment but isolated gastric varices, which are not contiguous with the esophagus, pose a much greater threat.[39] Banding of gastric varices is associated with a high incidence of rebleeding but sclerosants such as bovine thrombin and cyanoacrylate have been used successfully in adults with bleeding gastric varices.[40] Concern about potential venous embolization of the latter has so far limited its use in children. It is important to exclude isolated splenic vein thrombosis as a cause of gastric varices, since this may be treated effectively by splenectomy.

Bleeding from intestinal (ectopic) varices is rare but occurs more often in patients with long-standing portal hypertension from PVO than in those with intrahepatic disease.[41] Ectopic varices are most common in the anorectum, duodenum, at sites of previous intestinal anastomoses and around stomas. Anorectal varices and hemorrhoids are found in up to one-third of children with portal hypertension.[42] Bleeding is uncommon and can often be controlled by local measures such as injection sclerotherapy or banding. Bleeding from ectopic varices at other sites should be investigated by endoscopy and angiography. Local resection provides only transient respite and portosystemic shunting or liver transplantation, depending on the underlying pathology, is usually required to control persistent bleeding.

Long-term outcomes

As yet, there are no long-term studies after EVL in children. Although there are concerns that variceal recurrence after EVL may be greater than after EIS, recurrent bleeding in the short term is reported to be uncommon and surveillance endoscopies with appropriate treatment appears to achieve effective control.

The main long-term concerns about EIS have centered around the incidence of subsequent bleeding from recurrent esophageal or gastrointestinal varices and the potential local risks of esophageal sclerosis. These issues are much more pertinent to extrahepatic PVO in which portal hypertension is the dominant problem than to intrahepatic portal hypertension where outcome is more dependent on the underlying liver disease.

Extrahepatic portal hypertension

A study from King's College Hospital reviewed the longer-term outcome of 36 consecutive children with bleeding esophageal varices and PVO.[43] Four patients were lost to follow-up but the remaining 32 (21 males) were reassessed at a mean age of 17.2 (6.8–26.7) years which corresponded to a mean period of 8.7 (3.7–12.8) years since variceal obliteration (Fig. 38b.3). One boy had died from unrelated causes 6 years after successful treatment of his varices.

Recurrent gastrointestinal bleeding occurred in 12 patients but was due to peptic ulceration in two. Five children, including one who defaulted from follow-up, developed melena and/or hematemesis due to recurrent esophago-gastric varices which responded to further sclerotherapy. Four patients required portosystemic shunting for bleeding gastric varices. One 11-year-old boy had had a single minor bleed from duodenal varices. Three of these 12 children had also required a variety of local treatments to control bleeding from anorectal varices.

Esophageal strictures associated with the initial sclerotherapy course did not recur. One patient developed mild dysphagia following injections at surveillance endoscopies and this resolved after a single esophageal dilatation and two others had mild asymptomatic reflux oesophagitis. Six patients required surgery for complications of portal hypertension (bleeding gastric varices in four treated by mesocaval shunt, and splenectomy in two for painful splenomegaly). Of those who had not undergone portosystemic shunting or splenectomy, half had persistent thrombocytopenia ($<100\,000 \times 10^9$/l) and relative leukopenia indicating hypersplenism. No patient developed clinical evidence of pulmonary hypertension.

Data on height and weight were available for 26 patients and were unremarkable except that 9 of 19 boys had heights above the 90th centile. Of 15 patients over 18 years, 12 were in full-time employment and two had had children.

In summary, there were no deaths and minimal long-term morbidity related to sclerotherapy. Recurrent variceal bleeding developed in ten (31%) patients but half of these were effectively controlled by further sclerotherapy. Gastric variceal bleeding not amenable to sclerotherapy necessitated portosystemic shunt surgery in 13% of patients. During a mean follow-up period of almost 9 years, EIS alone proved safe and effective in controlling variceal bleeding from portal hypertension in over 80% of children with PVO in this series.

In a recent study, Zargar *et al.* (2004) from Kashmir, India, followed 59 children with PVO after variceal eradication by EIS.[44] During a mean follow-up of 15 (10.4–20) years, 7(12%) developed recurrent bleeding (esophageal varices, four, gastric varices, two, peptic ulcer, one) after a median of 3 (1–13) years; five of these were treated successfully by further EIS. Esophageal varices recurred in eight (14%), all of whom responded to further sclerotherapy. Two patients with gastric variceal bleeding were unresponsive to sclerotherapy and required shunt surgery. Elective surgery was also needed in six others for reasons related to portal hypertension but not because of recurrent varices or bleeding; portal biliopathy in three and massive splenomegaly in three. One patient died from sepsis after surgery to control gastric variceal bleeding. As in the King's College series, long-term morbidity from EIS itself was minimal.

Of the 32 patients (12 men) who were 25 years or older at the time of review, 20 were married with children, and the eight women had had 15 uneventful pregnancies. However, four had chronic viral hepatitis but it is not certain whether this was acquired through blood transfusion.

The authors concluded that sclerotherapy is not only safe and effective treament for bleeding esophageal varices but it prevented rebleeding in 88% of patients with PVO after variceal eradication. They recommended annual surveillance endoscopy for the first 4 years after variceal eradication.

Paquet and Lazar (1994) reported the long-term outcome of 66 children treated by paravariceal sclerotherapy for bleeding esophagogastric varices in their unit in Germany during a 20-year period.[35] Two-thirds had extrahepatic portal hypertension and there were no late deaths in this group. In contrast, the late mortality was 25% in those with intrahepatic disease, these deaths being largely related to liver failure. Recurrent hemorrhage occurred in 10% of those with portal vein obstruction and was treated by portosystemic shunt surgery.

A relatively small Canadian study of children with extrahepatic portal hypertension and bleeding esophageal varices treated by injection sclerotherapy reported only one recurrent bleed during follow-up periods ranging up to 7 years (and this was in a patient who temporarily defaulted from surveillance) and no bleeding from gastric varices.[45]

Intrahepatic portal hypertension

In children with cirrhosis, long-term outcome is jeopardized not only by complications of portal hypertension but also by deteriorating liver function. Endoscopic treatment of bleeding esophageal varices is usually effective in controlling hemorrhage and, unlike portosystemic shunting, does not reduce portal perfusion or carry the risk of encephalopathy and does not add to the technical difficulties of subsequent liver transplantation. Other therapies such as TIPS may provide a bridge to transplant in selected cases unresponsive to endoscopic therapy.

Finally, the long-term risk of neoplasia from childhood sclerotherapy remains a possibility but, despite the global application of this technique in patients with portal hypertension, there are only a few isolated reports of this potential association in adults.[46] Moreover, recognized risk factors for esophageal cancer have coexisted in these cases and a systematic study using brush cytology failed to support this potential association.[47] Nevertheless, the long-term morbidity of sclerotherapy and band ligation must remain under review.

REFERENCES

1. Garcia-Tsao, G., Groszmann, R. J., Fisher, R. L. *et al.* Portal pressure, presence of gastrovarices and variceal bleeding. *Hepatology* 1985; **5**:419–424.
2. Lebrec, D., DeFleury, P., Rueff, B. *et al.* Portal hypertension, size of esophageal varices, and risk of gastrointestinal bleeding in alcoholic cirrhosis. *Gastroenterology* 1980; **79**:1139–1144.
3. Dawson, J. L. Oesophageal varices: curiosities. *Br. Med. J.* 1983; **286**:826.
4. de Ville de Goyet, J., Alberti, D., Clapuyt, P. *et al.* Direct bypassing of extrahepatic portal venous obstruction in children: a new technique for combined hepatic portal revascularization and treatment of extrahepatic portal hypertension. *J. Pediatr. Surg.* 1998; **33**:597–601.
5. de Ville de Goyet, J., Alberti, D., Falchetti, D. *et al.* Treatment of extrahepatic portal hypertension in children by mesenteric-to-left portal vein bypass: a new physiological procedure. *Eur. J. Surg.* 1999; **165**:777–81.
6. Bambini, D. A., Superina, R., Almond, P. S., Whitington, P. F., & Alonso, E. Experience with the Rex shunt (mesenterico-left portal bypass) in children with extrahepatic portal hypertension. *J. Pediatr. Surg.* 2000; **35**:13–19.
7. Stringer, M. D., Heaton, N. D., Karani, J., Olliff, S., & Howard, E. R. Patterns of portal vein occlusion and their aetiological significance. *Br. J. Surg.* 1994; **81**:1328–1331.
8. Gehrke, I., John, P., Blundell, J., Pearson, L., Williams, A., & de Ville de Goyet, J. Meso-portal bypass in children with portal vein thrombosis: rapid increase of the intrahepatic portal venous flow after direct portal hepatic reperfusion. *J. Pediatr. Surg.* 2003; **38**:1137–1140.
9. Bismuth, H., Franco, D., & Alagille, D. Portal diversion for portal hypertension in children. *Ann. Surg.* 1980; **192**:18–24.
10. Mitra, S. K., Rao, K. L. N., Narasimhan, K. L. *et al.* Side-to-side lienorenal shunt without splenectomy in non-cirrhotic portal hypertension in children. *J. Pediatr. Surg.* 1993; **28**:398–402.
11. Orloff, M. J., Orloff, M. S., & Rambotti, M. Treatment of bleeding oesophagogastric varices due to extrahepatic portal hypertension: results of portal-systemic shunts during 35 years. *J. Pediatr. Surg.* 1994; **29**:142–154.
12. Prasad, A. S., Gupta, S., Kohli, V., Pande, G. K., Sahni, P., & Nundy, S. Proximal splenorenal shunts for extrahepatic portal venous obstruction in children. *Ann. Surg.* 1994; **219**:193–196.
13. Vickers, C. R., O'Connor, H. J., Quintero, G. A., Aerts, R. J., Elias, E., & Neuberger, J. M. Delayed perforation of the esophagus after variceal sclerotherapy and hepatic transplantation. *Gastrointest. Endosc.* 1989; **35**:459–461.
14. Heyman, M. B. & LaBerge, J. M. Role of transjugular intrahepatic portosystemic shunt in the treatment of portal hypertension in pediatric patients. *J. Pediatr. Gastroenterol. Nutr.* 1999; **29**:240–249.
15. Howard, E. R., Stringer, M. D., & Colombani, P. M. *Surgery of the Liver, Bile-Ducts and Pancreas in children.* 2nd edn. Arnold Publishers, London, 2002.
16. Crafoord, C. & Frenckner, P. New surgical treatment of varicose veins of the oesophagus. *Acta Otolaryngol.* 1939; **27**:422–429.
17. Fearon, B. & Sass-Kortsak, A. The management of esophageal varices in children by injection of sclerosing agents. *Ann. Otol. Rhinol. Laryngol.* 1959; **68**:906–915.
18. Howard, E. R., Stringer, M. D., & Mowat, A. P. Assessment of injection sclerotherapy in the management of 152 children with oesophageal varices. *Br. J. Surg.* 1988; **75**:404–408.
19. Paquet, K. J. Ten years experience with paravariceal injection sclerotherapy of esophageal varices in children. *J. Pediatr. Surg.* 1985; **20**:109–112.
20. Stiegmann, G. V. & Goff, J. S. Endoscopic oesophageal varix ligation. Preliminary clinical experience. *Gastrointest. Endosc.* 1988; **34**:113–17.
21. Stringer, M. D. Pathogenesis and management of esophageal and gastric varices. In Howard, E. R., Stringer, M. D., & Colombani, P. M. eds. *Surgery of the Liver, Bile-Ducts and Pancreas in children.* 2nd edn. London: Arnold Publishers, 2002: 314.
22. Sauerbruch, T., Holl, J. & Ruckdeschel, G. Bacteraemia associated with endoscopic sclerotherapy of oesophageal varices. *Endoscopy* 1985; **17**:170–172.
23. Stringer, M. D., Howard, E. R., & Mowat, A. P. Endoscopic sclerotherapy in the management of esophageal varices in 61 children with biliary atresia. *J. Pediatr. Surg.* 1989; **24**:438–442.
24. Yachha, S. K., Sharma, B. C., Kumar, M., & Khanduri, A. Endoscopic sclerotherapy for esophageal varices in children with extrahepatic portal venous obstruction: a follow-up study. *J. Pediatr. Gastroenterol. Nutr.* 1997; **24**:49–52.
25. Patraval, V., Rathi, P., Sawant, P., Vyas, K., & Das, H. Endoscopic sclerotherapy in children with extrahepatic portal venous obstruction. *Trop. Gastroenterol.* 2001; **22**:137–140.
26. Poddar, U., Thapa, B. R., & Singh, K. Endoscopic sclerotherapy in children: experience with 257 cases of extrahepatic portal venous obstruction. *Gastrointest. Endosc.* 2003; **57**:683–686.
27. Evans, D., Jones, D., Cleary, B., & Smith, P. Oesophageal varices treated by sclerotherapy: a histopathological study. *Gut* 1982; **23**:615–620.
28. Reilly, J. J., Schade, R. R., & Van Rhiel, D. S. Esophageal function after injection sclerotherapy: pathogenesis of esophageal stricture. *Am. J. Surg.* 1984; **147**:85–88
29. Sarin, S. K., Nanda, R., Vij, J. C., & Anand, B. S.. Esophageal ulceration after endoscopic sclerotherapy – an accompaniment or a complication? *Endoscopy* 1986; **18**:44–45.
30. Sorenson, T., Burcharth, F., Pederson M. L., & Findahl, F. Oesophageal stricture and dysphagia after endoscopic sclerotherapy for bleeding varices. *Gut* 1984; **25**:473–477.
31. Kumar, A., Mehta, S. R., Joshi, V., Kasthuri, A. S., & Narayanan, V. A. Ranitidine for the prevention of complications following

endoscopic sclerotherapy for esophageal varices. *J. Assoc. Phys. India.* 1993; **41**:584–589.

32. Zargar, S. A., Javid, G., Khan, B. A. *et al.* Endoscopic ligation compared with sclerotherapy for bleeding esophageal varices in children with extrahepatic portal venous obstruction. *Hepatology* 2002; **36**:666–672.
33. Guady, H., Rosman, A., & Korssen, M. Prevention of stricture formation after endoscopic sclerotherapy of esophageal varices. *Gastrointest. Endosc.* 1989; **35**:377–380.
34. Greenholz, S. K., Hall, R. J., Sonheimer, J. M., Lilly, J. R., & Hernandez-Cano, A. M. Manometric and pH consequences of esophageal endosclerosis in children. *J. Pediatr. Surg.* 1988; **23**:38–41.
35. Paquet, K. J. & Lazar, A. Current therapeutic strategy in bleeding esophageal varices in babies and children and long-term results of endoscopic paravariceal sclerotherapy over twenty years. *Eur. J. Pediatr. Surg.* 1994; **4**:165–172.
36. Helmy, A. & Hayes, P. C. Review article: current endoscopic therapeutic options in the management of variceal bleeding. *Aliment. Pharmacol. Ther.* 2001; **15**:575–594.
37. McKiernan, P. J., Beath, S. V., & Davison, S. M. A prospective study of endoscopic esophageal variceal ligation using a multiband ligator. *J. Pediatr. Gastroenterol. Nutr.* 2002; **34**:207–211.
38. Celinska-Cedro, D., Teisseyre, M., Woynarowski, M., Socha, P., & Socha, J. Long-term results of endoscopic variceal ligation of oesophageal varices for prophylaxis of variceal rebleeding in children with portal hypertension. *J. Pediatr. Gastroenterol. Nutr.* 2002; **34**:433 (Abstract).
39. Sarin, S. K. Long-term follow-up of gastric variceal sclerotherapy: an eleven-year experience. *Gastrointest. Endosc.* 1997; **46**:8–14.
40. Binmoeller, K. F. & Borsatto, R. Variceal bleeding and portal hypertension. *Endoscopy* 2000; **32**:189–199.
41. Lebrec, D. & Benhamou, J. P. Ectopic varices in portal hypertension. *Clin. Gastroenterol.* 1985; **14**:105–121.
42. Heaton, N. D., Davenport, M., & Howard, E. R. Incidence of haemorrhoids and anorectal varices in children with portal hypertension. *Br. J. Surg.* 1993; **80**:616–618.
43. Stringer, M. D. & Howard, E. R. Long term outcome after injection sclerotherapy for oesophageal varices in children with extrahepatic portal hypertension. *Gut* 1994; **35**:257–259.
44. Zargar, S. A., Yattoo, G. N., Javid, G. *et al.* Fifteen-year follow up of endoscopic injection sclerotherapy in children with extrahepatic portal venous obstruction. *J. Gastroenterol. Hepatol.* 2004; **19**:139–145.
45. Hassall, E., Berquist, W. E., Ament, M. E., Vargas, J., & Dorney, S. Sclerotherapy for extrahepatic portal hypertension in childhood. *J. Pediatr.* 1989; **115**:69–74.
46. Kokudo, N., Sanio, K., Umekita, N., Harihara, Y., Tada, Y., & Idezuki, Y. Squamous cell carcinoma after endoscopic injection sclerotherapy for esophageal varices. *Am. J. Gastroenterol.* 1990; **85**:861–864.
47. Dina, R., Cassisa, A., Baroncini, D., & D'Imperio, N. Role of esophageal brushing cytology in monitoring patients treated with sclerotherapy for esophageal varices. *Acta Cytol.* 1992; **36**:477–479.

39

Persistent hyperinsulinemic hypoglycemia in infancy

Pascale de Lonlay and Jean-Jacques Robert

Hôpital Necker Enfants Malades, Paris, France

Introduction

Persistent hyperinsulinemic hypoglycemia of infancy (PHHI) is the most important cause of hypoglycemia in early infancy.[1] The inappropriate oversecretion of insulin is responsible for profound hypoglycemia which requires aggressive treatment to prevent severe and irreversible brain damage.[2,3]

The hyperinsulinism can be classified according to three criteria: (i) the time of onset of hypoglycemia, whether in the neonatal period or later in infancy – this also influences the severity of hypoglycemia; (ii) the histologic lesion, whether it is focal or diffuse – these two forms are not clinically distinct but their surgical treatment differs dramatically. A focal lesion is definitively cured by a limited pancreatectomy whereas a diffuse lesion resistant to medical therapy requires a subtotal pancreatectomy with the high likelihood of subsequent diabetes mellitus;[4,5] (iii) the mode of genetic transmission, whether it is sporadic, autosomal recessive, or dominant. Diffuse PHHI is most often caused by a recessive gene (particularly the neonatal form) and only rarely a dominant gene. To date, focal lesions have been sporadic.

Physiology of insulin secretion

Hyperinsulinemic hypoglycemia is due to insulin hypersecretion by the islets of Langerhans. Insulin is the only hormone to lower the plasma glucose concentration, which it does by both inhibiting glucose release from hepatic glycogen and increasing glucose uptake in muscle cells. This explains the two main characteristic findings of neonatal PHHI: the high glucose requirement to correct hypoglycemia and the responsiveness of hypoglycemia to exogenous glucagon. Several pathways are involved in the regulation of insulin secretion by pancreatic β-cells and this helps to explain the effectiveness of the different medical treatments, such as diazoxide, octreotide, calcium-channel blockers and protein restricted diet. Glucose and amino acids stimulate insulin secretion through their metabolism. Glucokinase, the enzyme that initiates glucose metabolism in β-cells, has a high K_m for glucose. Thus, the circulating concentration of glucose directly determines the rate of glucose oxidation. High blood glucose levels increase glucose oxidation and, subsequently, the ATP–ADP ratio, which activates a plasma membrane protein, the sulfonylurea receptor (SUR), and closes an ATP-dependent potassium channel (K_{ATP} channel). This leads to the depolarization of the β-cell membrane, to an influx of extracellular calcium, and the release of insulin from storage granules. Leucine, one of the most potent amino acids to stimulate insulin secretion, acts somewhat indirectly as a positive allosteric effector of glutamate dehydrogenase to increase the rate of oxidation of glutamate. An increased glutamate dehydrogenase activity is responsible for hyperammonemia, an increased alpha ketoglutarate level and, consequently, an increased Krebs cycle activity and β-cell ATP/ADP ratio, with subsequent exaggerated insulin release. Sulfonylureas, such as tolbutamide, stimulate insulin secretion by binding directly to the SUR. Diazoxide inhibits insulin secretion by also binding to the SUR.

Pediatric Surgery and Urology: Long-term Outcomes, Mark Stringer, Keith Oldham, Pierre Mouriquand.
Published by Cambridge University Press.

Clinical presentation and diagnosis of hyperinsulinemic hypoglycemia

The diagnostic criteria for congenital hyperinsulinism include: fasting and post-prandial hypoglycemia (<3 mmol/l) with concomitant hyperinsulinemia (plasma insulin concentrations >3 mU/l), requiring high rates of intravenous glucose infusion (>10 mg/kg/min) to maintain blood glucose >3 mmol/l in cases of neonatal onset; a positive response to the subcutaneous or intramuscular administration of glucagon (plasma glucose concentration increase of 2 to 3 mmol/l following 0.5 mg glucagon); and persistent hypoglycemia throughout the first month of life. In the absence of clearly abnormal insulin levels during hypoglycemia, a search for inappropriately low plasma levels of ketone bodies, free fatty acids and branched chain amino acids after a 4- to 6-hour fast may be helpful.

The diagnosis is usually straightforward in the neonatal period, mostly because of the severity of hypoglycemia occurring within 72 hours of birth and the glucagon responsiveness. The majority of affected newborns are macrosomic. Hypoglycemia is always severe, manifested by seizures in half the cases, with the risk of brain damage. The mean rate of intravenous glucose administration required to prevent hypoglycemia was 17 mg/kg per min in our series. Mild hepatomegaly is frequent. Later in infancy (between 1 and 12 months), hypoglycemia is still manifest by seizures in half the cases and a history of macrosomia is common (mean birth weight 3.6 kg in our series). The characteristics of hypoglycemia are similar but lower rates of intravenous glucose are required to maintain normoglycemia (12–13 mg/kg per min).[4] Hypoglycemia is better tolerated and the diagnosis is often delayed. In older children, between 4 and 8 years of age, the rates of oral or intravenous glucose required to maintain normoglycemia are lower; not all of these children required continuous glucose administration in our series. Macrosomia at birth is usual.

The clinical presentation of hypoglycemia is similar irrespective of the histologic lesion and mode of transmission of the condition. Its severity depends on the age at presentation. Typically, no other symptoms are associated with hypoglycemia. Facial dysmorphism with a high forehead, a large and bulbous nose with short columella, and a smooth philtrum and thin upper lip is frequently observed in all types of hyperinsulinism. A few syndromic hyperinsulinisms have been described, such as hyperinsulinism associated with Usher syndrome type Ic or congenital disorders of glycosylation. Similarly, a few patients with hyperinsulinism and Beckwith–Wiedemann syndrome, Perlman syndrome and Sotos syndrome have been described. Munchausen syndrome by proxy is included in the differential diagnosis.[7]

Medical treatment

Treatment must be rapid and aggressive to prevent irreversible brain damage. It often necessitates a central venous catheter for intravenous glucose in addition to continuous oral feeding via a nasogastric tube. A continuous intravenous glucagon infusion (1 to 2 mg per day) can be added to the intravenous glucose when blood glucose levels are not maintained despite high rates of glucose administration.

At the same time, specific treatments must be given. Oral diazoxide is a first line drug in PHHI and is given at 15 mg/kg per day divided into three doses. This agent is mostly effective in infantile forms (60% of cases in our experience) whereas most neonatal forms are resistant to diazoxide (90% of our cases). Diazoxide efficacy is defined by the normalization of blood glucose levels (>3 mmol/l) measured before and after each meal in patients fed normally with a physiologic overnight fast, after stopping intravenous glucose and any other medications for at least five consecutive days. Two confirmed episodes of hypoglycemia (<3 mmol/l) during such a 24-hour cycle qualifies the patient as diazoxide-unresponsive and he/she must be restarted on continuous drip feeding and/or other measures to reestablish permanent normoglycemia. Diazoxide typically is well tolerated. The most frequent adverse effect is hirsutism, which can occasionally be marked and distressing in young children. Hematologic side effects and troublesome fluid retention are very rare with usual doses.

A trial of octreotide should be given before considering surgery in cases of diazoxide-unresponsiveness. Depending on the author, doses of octreotide have varied from 3–15 mcg/day to 50 mcg/d divided into three or four doses given by subcutaneous injection. High doses can lead to worsening hypoglycemia by suppressing both glucagon and growth hormone secretion. Soon after starting octreotide treatment, many patients experience vomiting and/or diarrhea and abdominal distension but this resolves spontaneously within 7–10 days. Steatorrhea may occur; it is partially responsive to oral pancreatic enzymes and tends to remit after several weeks or months. Gallbladder sludge can also be found and justifies routine abdominal ultrasound scanning. Other drugs such as calcium-channel blockers (e.g., nifedipine) have been proposed but their efficacy has not been fully demonstrated.[8]

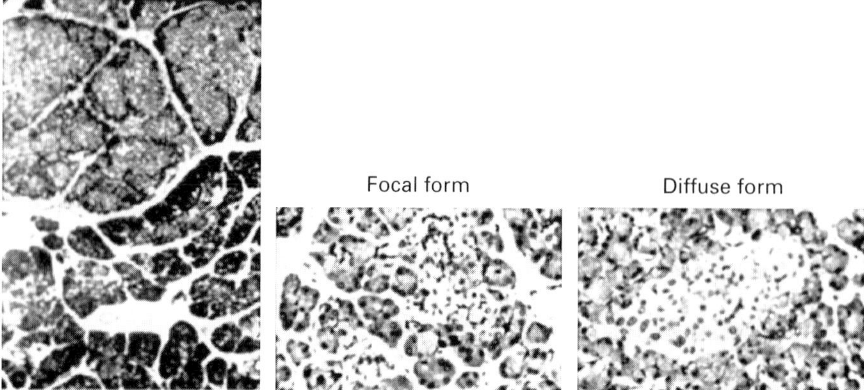

Fig. 39.1. The two histologic types of PHHI.

A restricted protein diet, limiting leucine intake to 200 mg of leucine per meal, is mandatory in the hyperammonemia/hyperinsulinism syndrome, in which it is often effective. When medical or dietary interventions are ineffective, surgical treatment is required. Hitherto, most pediatric surgeons have recommended a 95% subtotal pancreatectomy but this is associated with a high risk of subsequent insulin-dependent diabetes mellitus. There is now strong evidence that the histologic lesions associated with PHHI are of two types, diffuse or focal, which demand very different surgical strategies (Fig. 39.1).

Two histological lesions: distinct surgical treatments

Patients who are treated surgically must be classified according to histologic criteria.[9,10] The focal form of PHHI is due to a focal adenomatous hyperplasia. The lesion measures 2.5 to 7.5 mm in diameter and differs from the true adult-type pancreatic adenoma, which is more clearly defined and has a different topographic distribution. Diffuse PHHI shows abnormal β-cell nuclei throughout the whole pancreas. In the absence of any distinctive clinical feature, and because preoperative pancreatic imaging techniques such as ultrasound, CT scan and magnetic resonance imaging are not able to distinguish focal forms of the disease, pancreatic venous catheterization and pancreatic arteriography have, until recently, been the only preoperative procedures available for localizing the site of insulin secretion.[11,12] They are not performed before 1 month of age in order to exclude patients with transient forms of hyperinsulinism. Nor are they necessary in patients with hyperammonemia or with familial or consaguineous forms of PHHI who are likely to have diffuse disease.

For pancreatic venous sampling (PVS), diazoxide and all other drugs are stopped 5 days before catheterization and a continuous intravenous dextrose infusion is given to prevent hypoglycemia. Plasma glucose is monitored regularly during the night preceding the test. During the investigation the dextrose infusion is adjusted to maintain the glucose concentration between 2 and 3 mmol/l. Percutaneous transhepatic catheterization is undertaken under general anesthesia, without halothane. Venous blood samples are collected from the head, isthmus, body, and tail of the pancreas for measurements of plasma glucose, insulin and C-peptide, as previously described. Patients with a focal lesion have high plasma insulin and C-peptide concentrations in one or several contiguous samples, with low concentrations in the remaining samples. Patients with diffuse disease have high plasma insulin and C-peptide concentrations in all samples.

Recently, the use of [^{18}F]-fluoro-L-DOPA whole-body positron emission tomography (PET) has been evaluated in the detection of hyperfunctional islet pancreatic tissue. An abnormal focal uptake of [^{18}F]-fluoro-L-DOPA is observed within the pancreas of patients with a suspected focal lesion on PVS (subsequently confirmed on histology). In diffuse disease, a generalized uptake of the radiotracer is observed throughout the pancreas. We hope that this new test, an accurate non-invasive technique, will replace PVS for the identification and correct localization of focal lesions in children with PHHI. L-DOPA PET scanning requires all relevant drugs to be stopped four days before. The patient is fasted and a glucose infusion is used to maintain normoglycemia.

Patients considered to have a focal lesion should undergo surgery. Patients with diffuse disease are also operated on if they are resistant to or intolerant of medical treatment. Intraoperatively, a systematic histologic analysis is performed to confirm the pancreatic catheterization findings and to guide the limits of resection in cases of focal disease. Pancreatic biopsies are taken from the head, isthmus, body and tail of the pancreas and immediately examined microscopically. Diffuse lesions are characterized by β cells with large nuclei and abundant cytoplasm in all samples[9,10] (Fig. 39.1). A subtotal pancreatectomy is performed for diffuse lesions. Histologic analysis of focal lesions shows no abnormal β-cell nuclei but a shrunken cytoplasm giving a pattern of crowded β-cells outside the lesion (the appearance of "resting" tissue with a condensed cytoplasm). In such cases, additional samples are taken to localize the lesion, guided by the findings from PVS. The correct localization of focal lesions is crucial. Focal lesions may be found in the head of the pancreas. After partial pancreatectomy, further samples are examined to ensure that the resection margins consist of normal pancreatic tissue. Following partial pancreatectomy, transient hyperglycemia may occur because healthy β-cells located outside the lesion are relatively quiescent because of the previous negative feedback from insulin hypersecretion. It generally takes a few days for patients to recover full glycemic control.

Long-term metabolic outcome

Most of the patients treated medically remain drug dependent for several years, but some who respond well to medical management (diazoxide and/or octreotide) may have a complete clinical remission. Medical treatment can often be discontinued sooner (<16 months) in patients with a probable focal lesion (heterozygous SUR1 mutation) than in those (60 months) with diffuse disease (homozygous SUR1 mutation). This justifies stopping medical treatment once a year under careful supervision to check for signs of a spontaneous recovery. A conservative approach is preferable in patients with PHHI associated with hyperammonemia; they are mostly responsive to diazoxide and to a low leucine diet and have a favorable outcome.

Patients who have undergone surgical treatment are reassessed regularly. Annual investigation of residual insulin secretion, based on pre and postprandial plasma glucose and insulin levels as well as measurement of glycosylated hemoglobin (HbA1c) and an oral glucose tolerance test (OGTT) is mandatory, since diabetes mellitus or glucose intolerance may develop.

Patients with focal PHHI treated by adequate partial pancreatectomy are completely cured without any evidence of residual hypoglycemia.[13,14] None has shown any clinical or biochemical evidence of hypoglycemia during their postoperative recovery or in subsequent years. All have been able to eat a normal diet and none has required further medical treatment, surgery or readmission to hospital (except for reassessment). With a mean follow-up of more than 5 years, and an individual follow-up of up to 15 years, all patients continue to sustain a physiologic overnight fast and have no symptoms of hypoglycemia. Pre- and postprandial plasma glucose levels, HbA1c concentrations and OGTTs remain normal.

In contrast, after subtotal pancreatectomy for diffuse PHHI, residual postoperative hypoglycemia may occur despite extensive surgery and/or insulin-dependent diabetes mellitus may develop.[15] A few patients have suffered recurrent severe hypoglycemia requiring total pancreatectomy, 1 to 10 months after the first operation. Hypoglycemic events recurred shortly after surgery in more than half the cases treated by subtotal pancreatectomy; these episodes were generally much less severe than before surgery, often manifest as biochemical hypoglycemia only, and could be well controlled by the administration of raw corn starch, diazoxide and sometimes octreotide or corticosteroids. However, treatment had to be maintained up to 6 years after surgery. Despite fasting, most of these hypoglycemia patients have shown high plasma glucose levels postprandially and/or during the OGTT. After variable time periods, but mostly between 5 and 15 years of age, they have required insulin treatment. In a few patients, insulin was started in the immediate postoperative period, but it could be discontinued for several months in some. Overall, insulin has been needed in about 90% of the subtotal pancreatectomy patients after 15 years of age. Pancreatic exocrine insufficiency requiring pancreatic enzyme supplements may also be required.

Long-term neurologic outcome

We retrospectively studied the neurodevelopmental outcome of 90 patients with PHHI, 63 of whom were treated surgically and 27 treated medically.[16] Of 54 neonates in this series, 46 were managed surgically (19 had focal disease and 27 had diffuse disease) and 8 medically. Of 36 with infancy-onset hyperinsulinism, 17 were managed surgically (10 had focal adenomatous hyperplasia and 7 had diffuse disease) and 19 medically.

For psychomotor outcome assessment, the patients were categorized into three groups: group 1 normal – development quotient (DQ)/IQ>80 or only one minor disability, one failure at school, psychological, psychomotor or orthophonic support, behavioral disorder, minor neurologic symptom; group 2 – children with intermediate disability – DQ<60/IQ<80, two failures at school or in a special class, or two or more of the above intellectual or motor disorders; group 3 – children with major retardation – DQ/IQ<60, major intellectual or motor disability, attending a special school, major neurologic impairment. Patients were evaluated during the year of surgery or at the time of investigation ($n = 90$), and after 3 years ($n = 59$), 6 years ($n = 38$), and 10 years ($n = 25$).

Psychomotor retardation was found in 26% of the patients, 8% with major retardation (group 3) and 18% with an intermediate disability (group 2). Major retardation was more frequent in neonatal-onset patients (11%) than in those with PHHI onset in infancy (3%). It was also more frequent in patients who had had surgery (10%) than in those who required medical treatment only (4%). Within the operated group, there was no difference between patients with focal and diffuse hyperinsulinism. For patients with intermediate disability, there was no difference related to age at onset of symptoms, medical or surgical treatment, and type of histologic lesion.

Table 39.1 shows selected clinical features of patients with severe and intermediate mental retardation. Of seven patients with severe retardation, six had manifest hyperinsulinism within the first few hours of life; three neonates had repeated seizures and three demonstrated generalized hypotonia. Plasma glucose levels were low in all cases, and before the onset of symptoms in 3. Four of these six patients were rapidly treated in neonatal/intensive care units; hyperinsulinism was not recognized immediately in the other two patients and they presented with hypoglycemic seizures at 5 weeks and status epilepticus at 9 months of age, respectively. The seventh patient presented with repeated brief episodes of loss of consciousness at 5 months of age, after an apparently asymptomatic early infancy. On admission to our unit, before investigations and surgery, all seven patients were judged to be neurologically abnormal with hypotonia and poor eye contact. These patients have now been followed up for 15 months to 15 years. Five started walking between 2 and 4 years of age; the other two do not sit without support at 15 and 24 months of age. Four have associated epilepsy and four have microcephaly. One patient is blind and one has strabismus. Three of these seven patients had focal adenomatous hyperplasia, three had diffuse hyperinsulinism, and one received medical treatment alone.

Among the 12 patients with intermediate disability, seven were found to be hyperinsulinemic in the first 2 days of life, four because of seizures (one status epilepticus), two because of neurologic symptoms and/or cyanosis, and one after a routine blood glucose assay. Five patients first presented between 1.5 and 9 months of age; four had seizures and one lost consciousness. Six patients had an abnormal neurologic examination when first admitted to our unit. The patients are now between 6 and 14 years of age. None of them began to walk late. Seven have epilepsy, four have microcephaly, two have deafness and one has strabismus. Four of this group of patients were treated medically and eight had surgery (four with focal adenomatous hyperplasia and four with diffuse hyperinsulinism).

The patients in groups 2 and 3 did not differ from each other, or from patients in group 1, in terms of gestational age, weight and head circumference at birth, or in the frequency of seizures as first symptoms. The frequency of acute fetal distress tended to increase from group 1 (4%) to group 2(9%) and group 3 (16%), but this was not significantly different. The first neurologic examination in our unit was abnormal in 22% of group 1 patients, 50% of those in group 2, and 100% of those in group 3. Microcephaly was present in 14% of the patients in groups 1 and 2 and 57% of those in group 3. For operated patients, the frequency of hypoglycemic relapses after surgery, either clinical or subclinical (blood glucose monitoring), did not differ significantly between the 3 groups.

Epilepsy developed in 16 patients (18%). Thirteen had neonatal onset and three had infancy-onset hyperinsulinism. This represents 24% and 8% of the neonatal and infancy-onset patients, respectively, but this difference failed to reach statistical significance. Three of these patients were treated by medication alone (11% of all medically managed patients) compared to 13 who underwent pancreatectomy (21% of all surgical patients) but again, this difference was not significant. There was no difference in the frequency of epilepsy between patients with focal (24%) and diffuse (17%) lesions.

Genetic aspects

The estimated incidence of PHHI is 1:50 000 live births, but the incidence may be as high as 1:2500 in countries with substantial inbreeding. In recent years, there have been major advances in our understanding of the molecular mechanisms involved in PHHI. The two histologic forms found in both neonates and infants correspond to distinct molecular entities.

Focal adenomatous hyperplasia is due to hyperplasia of endocrine cells with a loss of the 11P15 maternal allele in the lesion, leading to an unbalanced expression of 11P15 imprinted genes (11P15.5), which include growth factor and tumor suppressor genes responsible for cell proliferation.[13,17] Hypoglycemia in focal hyperinsulinism is due to hemi- or homozygosity of a paternally inherited mutation of the sulfonylurea-receptor (SUR1) or

Table 39.1. Selected clinical characteristics of hyperinsulinemic patients with severe retardation (group 3) and intermediate disability (group 2)

Patient	Year of birth	Age at onset	Type of lesion	First symptom	Abnormal neurology	Age at walking	Microcephaly	Epilepsy	Other symptom
Group 3									
1	1997	12 h	Diffuse	Hypotonia	+	no	+	–	–
2	1984	24 h	Diffuse	Hypotonia	+	24 m	–	+	–
3	1998	1 h	Focal	Screening	+	no	+	–	–
4	1995	20 h	Focal	Seizure	+	no	–	+	Anoxia
5	1990	1 h	Focal	Hypotonia	+	no	+	+	Blindness
6	1983	24 h	Non op.	Hypotonia	+	4 yr	–	–	Strabismus
7	1991	5 m	Diffuse	Coma	+	28 m	+	+	–
Group 2									
8	1988	1.5 m	Focal	Seizure	–	14 m	+	–	Strabismus
9	1985	<24 h	Diffuse	Cyanosis	+	14 m	–	+	–
10	1995	1 h	Diffuse	None	+	13 m	+	–	–
11	1986	<24 h	Diffuse	Seizure	+	21 m	–	+	Deafness
12	1985	28 h	Focal	Seizure	+	15 m	–	+	–
13	1990	25 h	Focal	Seizure	+	16 m	–	+	–
14	1992	24 h	Non op.	Seizure	+	13 m	–	+	–
15	1987	<24 h	Non op.	Hypotonia	–	18 m	+	+	–
16	1988	3 m	Diffuse	Seizure	–	15 m	–	+	Deafness
17	1987	2 m	Focal	Coma	–	16 m	+	–	–
18	1982	9 m	Non op.	Seizure	–	18 m	–	–	–
19	1996	2.5 m	Non op.	Seizure	+	19 m	–	–	–

the inward-rectifying potassium-channel (Kir6.2) genes on chromosome 11P15 (11P15.1). Focal lesions are probably sporadic in origin, as suggested by the somatic molecular abnormality in the pancreas and by the existence of discordant identical twins. However, the coexistence of focal and diffuse forms of hyperinsulinism in the same family cannot be excluded.

Diffuse hyperinsulinism is a heterogeneous disorder involving various genes: the genes encoding the sulfonylurea receptor[18–20] or the inward-rectifying potassium channel[21,22] in recessively inherited hyperinsulinism or, more rarely, dominantly inherited hyperinsulinism (in these cases, hypoglycemia seems less severe); the glucokinase gene[23] or other loci in dominantly inherited hyperinsulinism; and the glutamate dehydrogenase gene when hyperammonemia is associated with hyperinsulinism.[24,25] In the latter, transmission can be sporadic or dominant. More recently, short-chain L-3-hydroxyacyl-CoA dehydrogenase (SCHAD) has been implicated.[26] Other genes could yet be implicated in the pathogenesis of PHHI, specifically genes playing a role in insulin secretion.

The clinical presentation of hyperinsulinism secondary to the potassium channel defect (with focal or diffuse lesions) depends only on the age of onset of hypoglycemia. In contrast, hyperinsulinism associated with hyperammonemia is less severe, even when the onset is in the newborn. Patients with neonatal PHHI responsive to diazoxide probably have a transient form of hyperinsulinism or the hyperinsulinism–hyperammonemia syndrome. Adenoma radically differs from focal PHHI by the lat -onset of hypoglycemia and its histology. Hitherto, its etiology is unknown except in adenomas related to the MEN1 syndrome (when there is a dominant mutation on the MEN1 gene), in those related to menine protein deficiency (a loss of the 11P13 region), and in Bourneville's tuberous sclerosis.

Although considerable progress has been made in both our understanding and management of PHHI, there are still major challenges, such as the development of simpler methods of identifying and localizing focal lesions (i.e., PET scan) and discovering new medical approaches to managing diffuse hyperinsulinism.

Acknowledgments

We wish to acknowledge the contribution of our colleagues to the management of these patients and to progress in the treatment of persistent hyperinsulinemic hypoglycemia of infancy. In particular, we thank Irina Giurgea, Maria Ribeiro, Francis Jaubert, Jacques Rahier, Francis Brunelle, Claire Nihoul-Fékété, and Jean-Marie Saudubray.

REFERENCES

1. Pagliara, A. S., Karl, I. E., Haymond, M., & Kipnis, D. M. Hypoglycemia in infancy and childhood. Part I. *J. Pediatr.* 1973; **82**:365–379.
2. Cornblath, M., Schwartz, R., Aynsley-Green, A., & Lloyd, J. K. Hypoglycemia in infancy: the need for a rational definition. *Pediatrics* 1990; **85**:834–837.
3. Volpe, J. J. Hypoglycemia and brain injury. In Volpe, J. J., ed. *Neurology of the Newborn*. Philadelphia: W.B. Saunders Co.1995, 467–489.
4. De Lonlay-Debeney, P., Poggi-Travert, F., Fournet, J. C. *et al.* Clinical features of 52 neonates with hyperinsulinism. *N. Engl. J. Med.* 1999; **340**:1169–1175.
5. Rahier, J., Fälts, K., Münterfering, H., Becker, K., Gepts, W., & Falkmer, S. The basic structural lesion of persistent neonatal hypoglycaemia with hyperinsulinism: deficiency of pancreatic D cells or hyperactivity of B cells? *Diabetologia* 1984; **26**:282–289.
6. Kukuvitis, A., Deal, C., Arbour, L., & Polychronakos, C. An autosomal dominant form of familial persistent hyperinsulinemic hypoglycemia of infancy, not linked to the sulfonylurea receptor locus. *J. Clin. Endocrinol. Metab.* 1997; **82**:1192–1194.
7. Dershewitz, R., Vestal, B., Maclaren, N., & Cornblath, M. Malicious insulin administration resulting in transient hepatomegaly and hypoglycemia. *Am. J. Dis. Child.* 1976; **130**:998–999.
8. Lindley, K. J., Dunne, M. J., Kane, C. *et al.* Ionic control of B-cell function in nesidioblastosis. A possible therapeutic role for calcium channel blockade. *Arch. Dis. Child.* 1996; **74**:373–378.
9. Sempoux, C., Guiot, Y., Lefevre, A. *et al.* Neonatal hyperinsulinemic hypoglycemia: heterogeneity of the syndrome and keys for differential diagnosis. *J. Clin. Endocrinol. Metab.* 1998; **83**:1455–1461.
10. Rahier, J., Sempoux, C., Fournet, J. C. *et al.* Partial or near-total pancreatectomy for persistent neonatal hyperinsulinaemic hypoglycaemia: the pathologist's role. *Histopathology* 1998; **32**:15–19.
11. Brunelle, F., Negre, V., Barth, M. O. *et al.* Pancreatic venous sampling in infants and children with primary hyperinsulinism. *Pediatr. Radiol.* 1989; **19**:100–103.
12. Dubois, J., Brunelle, F., Touati, G. *et al.* Hyperinsulinism in children: diagnostic value of pancreatic venous sampling correlated with clinical, pathological and surgical outcome in 25 cases. *Pediatr. Radiol.* 1995; **25**:512–516.
13. De Lonlay P., Fournet, J. C., Rahier, J. *et al.* Somatic deletion of the imprinted 11P15 region in sporadic persistent hyperinsulinemic hypoglycemia of infancy is specific of focal

adenomatous hyperplasia and endorses partial pancreatectomy. *J. Clin. Invest.* 1997; **100**:802–807.

14. De Lonlay, P., Fournet, J. C., Touati, G. *et al.* Heterogeneity of persistent hyperinsulinemic hypoglycemia of infancy. A series of 175 cases. *Eur. J. Pediatr.* 2002; **161**:37–48.
15. Leibowitz, G., Glaser, B., Higazi, A. A., Salameh, M., Cerasi, E., & Landau, H. Hyperinsulinemic hypoglycemia of infancy (nesidioblastosis) in clinical remission: high incidence of diabetes mellitus and persistent B-cell dysfunction at long-term follow-up. *J. Clin. Endocrinol. Metab.* 1995; **80**:386–392.
16. Menni, F., de Lonlay, P., Brunelle, F., Nihoul-Fékété, C., Saudubray, J. M., & Robert, J. J. Neurological outcome of hyperinsulinism: a series of 100 patients. *Pediatrics* 2001; **107**:476–479.
17. Verkarre, V., Fournet, J. C., de Lonlay, P. *et al.* Paternal mutation of the sulfonylurea receptor (SUR1) gene and maternal loss of 11P15 imprinted genes lead to persistent hyperinsulinism in focal adenomatous hyperplasia. *J. Clin. Invest.* 1998; **102**:1286–1291.
18. Thomas, P. M., Cote, G. J., Wohllk, N. *et al.* Mutations in the sulfonylurea receptor gene in familial persistent hyperinsulinemic hypoglycemia of infancy. *Science* 1995; **268**:426–429.
19. Kane, C., Shepherd, R. M., Squires, P. E. *et al.* Loss of functional K^+ATP channels in persistent hyperinsulinemic hypoglycaemia of infancy. *Nature Med.* 1996; **2**:1344–1347.
20. Nestorowicz, A., Wilson, B. A., Schoor, K. P. *et al.* Mutations in the sulfonylurea receptor gene are associated with familial hyperinsulinism in Ashkenazi Jews. *Hum. Mol. Genet.* 1996; **5**:1813–1822.
21. Thomas, P., Ye, Y., & Lightner, E. Mutation of the pancreatic islet inward rectifier Kir6.2 also leads to familial persistent hyperinsulinemic hypoglycemia of infancy. *Hum. Mol. Genet.* 1996; **5**:1809–1812.
22. Nestorowicz, A., Inagaki, N., Gonoit, T. *et al.* A nonsense mutation in the inward rectifier potassium channel gene, Kir6.2, is associated with familial hyperinsulinism. *Diabetes* 1997; **46**:1743–1748.
23. Glaser, B., Kesavan, P., Heyman, M. *et al.* Familial hyperinsulinism caused by an activating glucokinase mutation. *N. Engl. J. Med.* 1998; **338**:226–230.
24. Stanley, C. A., Lieu, Y. K., Hsu, B. Y. *et al.* Hyperinsulinemia and hyperammonemia in infants with regulatory mutations of the glutamate dehydrogenase gene. *N. Engl. J. Med.* 1998; **338**:1352–1357.
25. Zammarchi, E., Filippi, L., Novembre, E., & Donati, M. A. Biochemical evaluation of a patient with a familial form of leucine-sensitive hypoglycemia and concomitant hyperammonemia. *Metabolism* 1996; **45**:957–960.
26. Clayton, P. T., Eaton, S., Aynsley-Green, A. *et al.* Hyperinsulinism in short-chain L-3-hydroxyacyl-CoA dehydrogenase deficiency reveals the importance of beta-oxidation in insulin secretion. *J. Clin. Invest.* 2001; **108**:457–465.

Editor's footnote

Surgical aspects

The nomenclature for the extent of pancreatic resection in the literature is confusing – terms such as partial, subtotal and near-total pancreatectomy are not always defined. The extent of resection is best described in relation to anatomical landmarks (Fig. 39.2).[1] These guidelines are important, particularly when evaluating long-term outcomes, to ensure that reference is made to comparable pancreatic resections. However, an autopsy study showed that even these definitions are not precise and generally overestimate the extent of pancreatic resection.[2] Nevertheless, much of the variability is accounted for by the uncinate process and a so-called 95% resection has a reasonable degree of uniformity (Fig. 39.3).

During surgery, care must be taken to avoid injury to the common bile duct which usually lies on the posterior aspect of the head of the gland but may course through the substance of the pancreas.[2] Bile duct injury has been reported by several authors. In one study of 48 patients, there were two intraoperative bile duct injuries and 5 children subsequently required a choledochoduodenostomy for a biliary leak or delayed bile duct stricture.[3] Other complications in this series included major intraoperative bleeding (2), splenic injury (1), wound infection (3) and adhesion

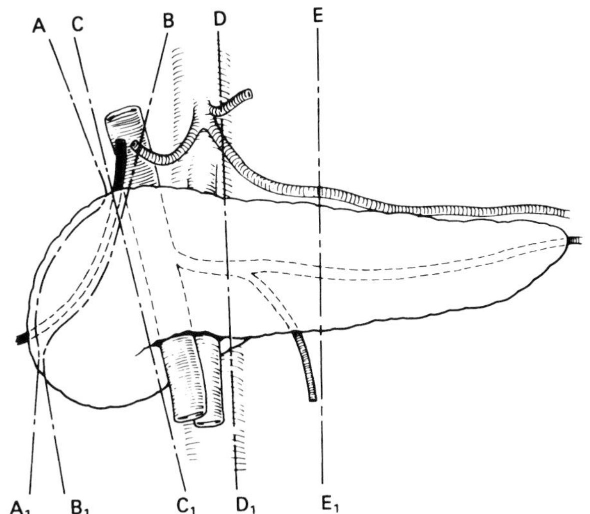

Fig. 39.2. Extent of pancreatic resection: A–A′ = 99%, B–B′ = 95%, C–C′ = 80%, D–D′ = 50%. A 95% resection leaves only pancreatic tissue between the common bile duct and the duodenum and a tiny rim of pancreatic tissue on the concavity of the duodenal wall. After Spitz.[1]

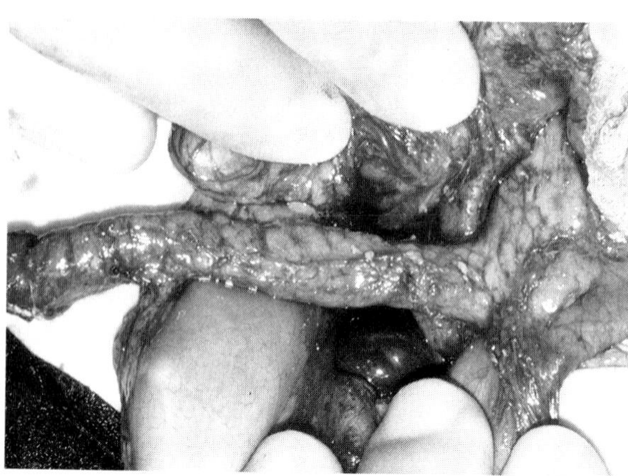

Fig. 39.3. Operative photograph of a 95% pancreatic resection for PHHI in progress. Bipolar diathermy dissection/hemostasis is invaluable.

obstruction (1). Nine of the 48 patients required further pancreatic resection because of continued hypoglycemia.[3]

In recent years, laparoscopic techniques have been developed for successfully treating focal forms of PHHI (Klaas Bax, personal communication).

Temporary feeding difficulties necessitating supplementary tube feeding have been reported in some children after 95% pancreatectomy for PHHI.[4] There are few data on the long-term nutritional status and growth of such patients. Parashar *et al.*[5] recorded normal growth parameters in a group of 11 patients 1–10 years after 95% pancreatectomy, whilst Soliman *et al.*[6] reported growth retardation in a series of seven patients 5 years after 95–98% pancreatectomy.

M. D. Stringer

REFERENCES

1. Spitz, L. Surgery for hyperinsulinaemic hypoglycaemia. In Spitz, L., & Coran, A. G., eds. *Pediatric Surgery* 5th edn, London: Chapman & Hall, 1995:618–622.
2. Reyes, G. A., Fowler, C. L., & Pokorny, W. J. Pancreatic anatomy in children: emphasis on its importance to pancreatectomy. *J. Pediatr. Surg.* 1993; **28**:712–715.
3. McAndrew, H. F., Smith, V., & Spitz, L. Surgical complications of pancreatectomy for persistent hyperinsulinaemic hypoglycaemia of infancy. *J. Pediatr. Surg.* 2003; **38**:13–16.
4. Cade, A., Walters, M., Puntis, J. W., Arthur, R. J., & Stringer, M. D. Pancreatic exocrine and endocrine function after pancreatectomy for persistent hyperinsulinaemic hypoglycaemia of infancy. *Arch. Dis. Child.* 1998; **79**:435–439.
5. Parashar, K., Upadhyay, V., & Corkery, J. J. Partial or near total pancreatectomy for nesidioblastosis? *Eur. J. Pediatr. Surg.* 1995; **5**:146–148.
6. Soliman, A. T., Alsalmi, I., Darwish, A., & Asfour, M. G. Growth and endocrine function after near total pancreatectomy for hyperinsulinaemic hypoglycaemia. *Arch. Dis. Child.* 1996; **74**:379–385.

40

Acute and chronic pancreatitis in children

Pierre Tissières[1] and Claude Le Coultre[2]

[1]Multidisciplinary Paediatric Intensive Care Unit, Bicêtre Hospital, Le Kremlin-Bicêtre, France
[2]Paediatric Surgery Department, Children's Hospital, Geneva, Switzerland

Pancreatitis in children is relatively rare but may be increasing in frequency.[1] Two main patterns of disease exist in children: acute pancreatitis, which accounts for 75% of all cases, is abrupt in onset but usually self-limiting; and chronic pancreatitis, in which pancreatic inflammation and gland destruction are progressive.

Acute pancreatitis

Etiology

Although the pathophysiology and functional consequences of acute pancreatitis in children are identical to those observed in adults, etiology differs significantly (Table 40.1).[1–19] In children, drugs and toxins (12%–18%) and systemic disease (12%–35%) are major causes of acute pancreatitis. Abdominal trauma is another important cause of acute pancreatitis, accounting for between 14% and 29% of cases; it may be related to blunt abdominal trauma, surgical trauma, or, in some instances, to child abuse. Up to 25% of cases are idiopathic,[1–19] although this proportion is less in more recent series.[1] Recurrent acute pancreatitis, characterized by repeated acute episodes, is associated with obstructive disease, such as pancreatic ductal abnormalities, biliary tract obstruction, duplication cyst and biliary lithiasis. Pancreas divisum is the most frequently encountered pancreatic malformation present in as many as 10%–15% of patients undergoing magnetic resonance cholangiopancreatography; this anomaly is associated with 2.5% of acute pancreatitis in children. Acute pancreatitis can occur within the first month of life, but most cases present around the age of 5 years and during adolescence.

Diagnosis

Diagnosis of acute pancreatitis can be difficult and outcome unpredictable at onset, as several local, regional and systemic insults can hamper the diagnosis and affect the prognosis. Most cases of acute pancreatitis are morphologically characterized by edematous interstitial inflammation. Typically, episodes are mild and self-limiting and spontaneous resolution occurs with bowel rest, analgesia and fluid/electrolyte management. However, 10%–20% of cases may progress to more severe disease, classified as severe acute pancreatitis, in which pancreatic inflammation is complicated by necrosis and hemorrhage in the pancreas and surrounding tissues, as well as by remote systemic complications and organ dysfunction. The gold standard of diagnosis is direct inspection at laparotomy and histopathologic examination of surrounding tissues (fat necrosis). However, clinical pointers include the sudden onset of a constant and sharp abdominal pain associated with nausea, vomiting, and fever. In severe cases of necrotizing pancreatitis, ecchymoses in the flank (Grey–Turner's sign) and peri-umbilical (Cullen's sign) region may be observed; and systemic symptoms related to hypovolemic shock and/or organ dysfunction seen. Hyperamylasemia has a high sensitivity within 24 hours of symptoms, but a low specificity. However, the magnitude of hyperamylasemia is not correlated with the severity of disease. The association of hyperamylasemia and a compatible clinical presentation is suggestive of acute pancreatitis. Diagnostic specificity is further improved if there is an associated elevated lipase concentration (99% specificity). Serum lipase levels may remain elevated when the amylase has returned to normal.[20] Other pancreatic enzymes, such as trypsin, elastase, and phospholipase A_2 are elevated in acute

Pediatric Surgery and Urology: Long-term Outcomes, Mark Stringer, Keith Oldham, Pierre Mouriquand.
Published by Cambridge University Press.

Table 40.1. Causes of pancreatitis in children[1–19]

Systemic disease	Systemic lupus erythematosus, Reye syndrome, fulminant liver failure, Henoch–Schönlein purpura, Kawasaki disease, hemolytic-uremic syndrome, renal failure, hyperparathyroidism, Crohn's disease, hypertriglyceridemia, malnutrition, cystic fibrosis, solid organ transplantation, hyperlipoproteinemia (types 1 and 5), α_1-antitrypsin deficiency
Drugs and toxins	Valproic acid, thiazides, furosemide, cimetidine, L-asparaginase, azathioprine, 6-mercaptopurine, cyclosporine A, tacrolimus, didanosine, corticosteroids, estrogen, sulfonamides, tetracycline, erythromycin
Infections	Mumps, *Coxsackie B virus, Epstein-Barr virus, hepatitis A and B virus*, measles, malaria, *Mycoplasma*, rubella, *Influenzae A and B virus*, varicella, *HIV*, scorpion bites
Obstructive disease	Pancreatic ductal abnormalities, biliary tract malformations, pancreas divisum, duplication cyst, pancreatic pseudocyst, biliary lithiasis, tumors, ascariasis
Trauma	Blunt or penetrating abdominal injury, surgical trauma, child abuse
Hereditary pancreatitis	Familial, e.g., cationic trypsinogen gene mutation

pancreatitis. However, these tests are not routinely performed, are expensive and their prognostic significance remains doubtful. C-reactive protein is valuable and a concentration above 150 mg/l has a positive predictive value for severe acute pancreatitis of more than 90%.[21]

A plain abdominal radiograph may reveal signs of an adynamic ileus, a sentinel loop, and the colon cut-off sign at the splenic flexure. Although plain radiography may help in differential diagnosis by, for example, showing evidence of hollow viscus perforation, its use in the diagnosis of pancreatitis and its complications is limited. Abdominal ultrasound examination is non-invasive, inexpensive and repeatable, but is highly operator and technique dependent since most of the gland may be obscured by abdominal gas. Ultrasound is useful in delineating pseudocysts, pancreatic ascites, and vascular thrombosis, as well as guiding paracentesis in cases of proven pancreatitis. Recently, endoscopic ultrasound has become available in children and provides detailed information on pancreatic anatomy, both parenchymal and ductal, the biliary ducts, and the presence of cystic lesions (Fig. 40.1b).[22] Accurate determination of the extent of pancreatic necrosis, and peripancreatic fluid collections, and the diagnosis of acute pancreatitis can be obtained by contrast enhanced abdominal computerized tomography (CT). CT signs of acute pancreatitis include marked glandular enlargement, reduced pancreatic density on precontrast phase images, and extrapancreatic extension of inflammation (Fig. 40.1(a)). The specificity of an admission CT for the diagnosis of acute pancreatitis approaches 100% and its sensitivity is 85%. Importantly, contrast enhanced CT allows the detection and assessment of intra- and extrapancreatic necrosis. A repeat examination (after a delay of 48 hours) may provide dynamic information and help to differentiate between edematous and necrotizing pancreatitis.

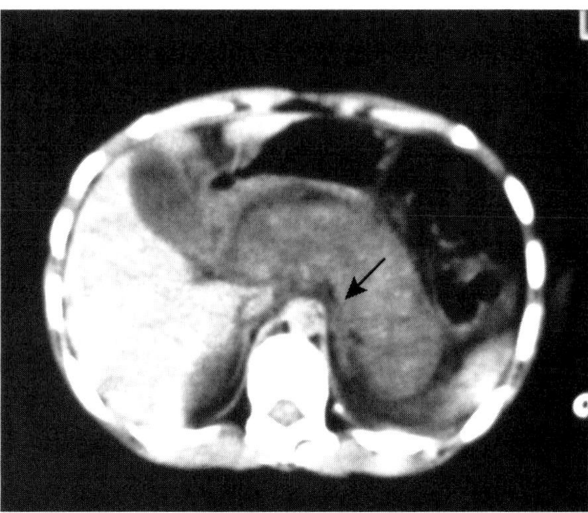

(a)

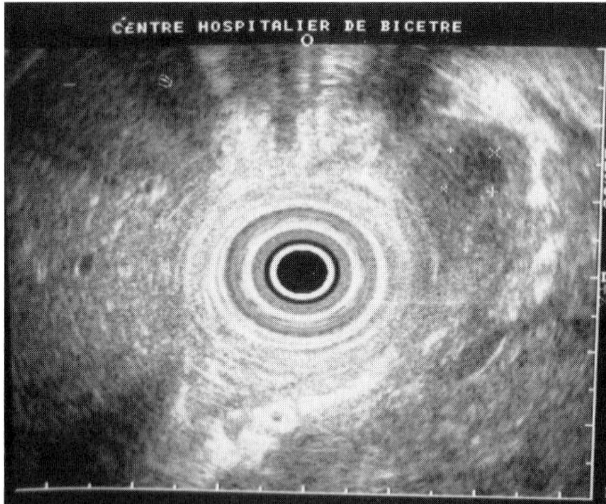

(b)

Fig. 40.1. (a) Contrast enhanced CT scan on admission reveals extensive focal areas of low attenuation indicative of pancreatic necrosis (arrow). (b) Eight days later, endoscopic ultrasound shows a pseudocyst (arrow) localized within a heterogeneous and enlarged pancreatic tail in a 13-year-old boy who had sustained blunt abdominal trauma (with permission of Bicêtre Hospital).

Magnetic resonance imaging is emerging as an alternative to contrast enhanced CT. It allows better determination of necrotic foci but its use remains limited in critically ill patients and it does not permit guided percutaneous paracentesis. In cases of ruptured pseudoaneurysm and subsequent hemorrhage, angiography is preferred, although new generation helical CT scans may give equivalent diagnostic accuracy. Endoscopic retrograde cholangiopancreatography (ERCP) has become an important tool in evaluating relapsing pancreatitis and may be useful in demonstrating obstructing lesions, stones, ductal stricture, duplication cyst, and other anatomic anomalies. However, ERCP may precipitate acute pancreatitis and should largely be avoided in the acute setting. An alternate to ERCP remains guided percutaneous or intraoperative cholangiopancreatography (Fig. 40.2(b)). Magnetic resonance cholangiopancreatography (MRCP) (Fig. 40.2(a)) has the advantage over ERCP in the delineation of the ductal configuration in pancreas divisum because it can show the dominant dorsal pancreatic duct in its entirety, whereas standard ERCP is usually limited to opacifying the ventral duct via cannulation of the major papilla.[23] MRCP cannot detect early side-branch abnormalities of chronic pancreatitis, but can demonstrate dilatation, stricture, pseudocysts, and ductal filling defects, including calculi, mucinous plugs, and sludge.[24]

Early and late complications

In contrast to adults, most fatalities in children are due to concurrent systemic illness primary or secondary associated with acute pancreatitis (Table 40.2). Mortality ranges between 2.5% and 10% and death occurs in one-third of cases early in the course of disease. Systemic complications are mediated by the overspill of pancreatic enzymes and inflammatory cytokines into the systemic circulation, inducing a systemic inflammatory response syndrome (SIRS) and organ dysfunction.[25] In the early phase of severe acute pancreatitis, circulatory failure occurs with a hemodynamic profile mimicking sepsis. Myocardial depression occasionally occurs. Respiratory failure results from both a restrictive process (pleural effusion, limited diaphragmatic excursion due to retroperitoneal inflammation) and acute lung injury, that may lead to the acute respiratory distress syndrome.[26] Metabolic failure is common and associated with an increase in resting energy expenditure (up to 125% of predicted), greater protein catabolism, and hepatic and peripheral insulin resistance with β-cell dysfunction and hyperglucagonemia resulting in hyperglycemia. In some instances, diabetic ketoacidosis and non-acidotic diabetic coma may develop. Local complications typically

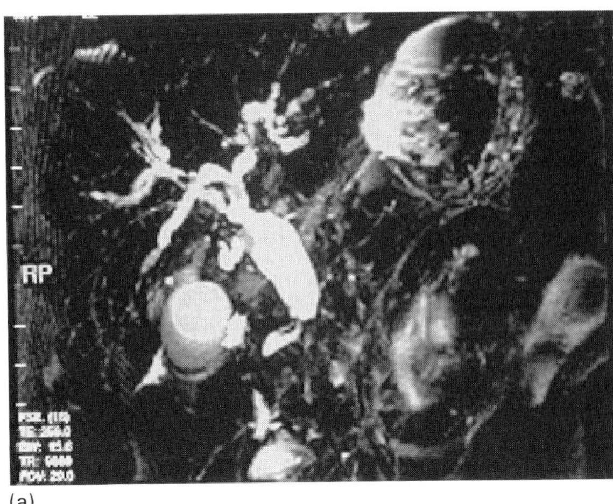

(a)

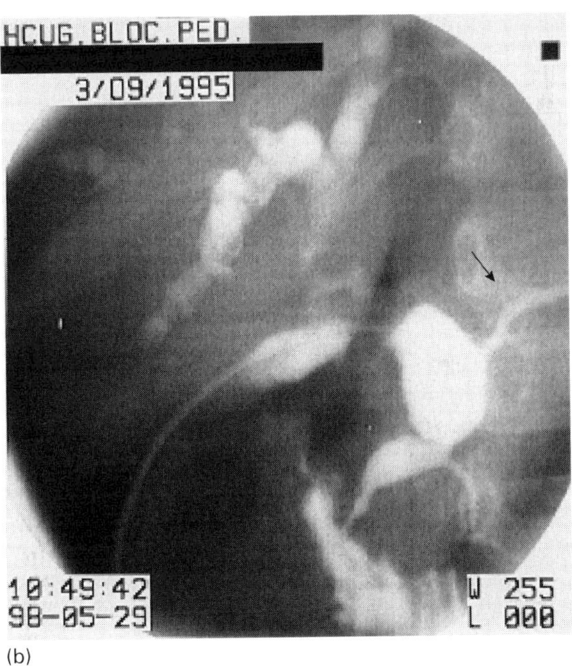

(b)

Fig. 40.2. (a) Projective MRCP image, and (b) peri-operative cholangiogram showing cystic dilatation of the biliary tract in a 2.5-year-old boy with acute pancreatitis secondary to a congenital choledochal cyst. Wirsung's duct is dilated (small arrow) (With permission of the Pediatric Surgical Clinic of the Children's Hospital of Geneva).

Table 40.2. Early and late complications of pancreatitis

	Early complications	Later complications (>2 weeks)
Acute pancreatitis	Capillary leak syndrome Systemic inflammatory response syndrome Circulatory failure Metabolic failure (hyperglycemia, hypocalcemia, hypertriglyceridemia) Pancreatic necrosis Abdominal compartment syndrome Respiratory failure Disseminated intravascular coagulopathy Renal failure Cardiac failure Encephalopathy	Infection of necrosis/pseudocyst (Gram negative, polymicrobial, *Candida*) Disruption of pancreatic duct: – pancreatic ascites – pleural/pericardial fistula – pseudocyst. Viscus perforation Pseudoaneurysm Splanchnic venous thrombosis Bowel infarction
Chronic pancreatitis	Obstructive cholestasis Cholangitis	Pseudocyst/ascites/fistula Pancreatic fibrosis Abscess Pseudoaneurysm Splanchnic vein thrombosis Pancreatic exocrine and endocrine insufficiency

occur after the second week, although severe arterial hemorrhage, intestinal perforation, or infection of pancreatic necrosis may occur earlier. Close monitoring is mandatory, particularly in patients who fail to improve despite intensive supportive care. Repeated abdominal CT or ultrasound scans may identify an acute pseudocyst, necrosis, fistula tract, pseudoaneurysm, pancreatic hemorrhage, or venous thrombosis (portal, splenic, mesenteric). In addition to imaging, diagnostic paracentesis of abdominal fluid collections should be performed if infection is suspected. Bacterial and more specifically fungal infection of devitalized tissues are known to be responsible for up to 80% of deaths from acute pancreatitis. Early diagnosis is crucial, and drainage and/or surgical debridement are mandatory in such cases.

Prognostic indicators

Major determinants of outcome are the extent of pancreatic necrosis, the presence of secondary infection of devitalized tissue, and the severity of systemic insults.[25,27,28] In adults, Ranson and Imrie used clinical and laboratory criteria to provide early stratification of the severity of acute pancreatitis.[29] However, low specificity and sensitivity have limited the practical value of this score in the initial evaluation of acute pancreatitis. Severity scoring systems, such as the Acute Physiology and Chronic Health Evaluation (APACHE) II and the Sequential Organ Failure Assessment (SOFA) score, can be used to predict severity of the systemic insult but these scores have not been specifically evaluated in acute pancreatitis in children. An alternative approach is to use the pediatric logistic organ dysfunction (PELOD) score.[30] Clinical assessment on admission, even when performed by experienced clinicians, fails to identify up to 60% of severe cases. Clinical indicators of severity, irrespective of bacteriologic status and extent of necrosis, rely on remote organ dysfunction. Therefore, repeated and detailed assessment to identify systemic organ failure is mandatory. In adults, Balthazar *et al.* (2002), has established a CT severity scoring system that correlates well with the Ranson score, length of hospital stay, the development of serious complications, and mortality.[31]

Treatment

Medical

Medical management is largely empirical and directed toward maintaining normovolemia, normoglycemia, electrolyte and acid-base balance, as well as the identification and treatment of systemic and local complications. Table 40.3 summarizes the current status of specific therapeutic

Table 40.3. Evidence-based medical treatments in acute pancreatitis[32–40]

Therapy	Results	Level of evidence
Recommended		
Glycemic control	Intensive insulin therapy to maintain blood glucose at or below 110 mg per decilitre reduces morbidity and mortality among critically ill patients[32]	A
Enteral nutrition vs. parenteral nutrition	Early enteral nutrition reduces the rate of septic complications (infected pancreatic necrosis, abscess)[33,34]	A
Somatostatin and octreotide	Antisecretory agents are able to reduce mortality without affecting complications[36]	A
Not recommended		
Antibiotic prophylaxis	Antibiotic prophylaxis do not affect outcome in patient with severe acute pancreatitis[35]	B/C
Gabexate mesilate *(antiprotease)*	Gabexate mesilate does not affect mortality at 90 days, but significantly reduces the incidence of complications[37]	A
Peritoneal lavage	Use of continuous peritoneal lavage in patients with acute pancreatitis is not associated with any significant improvement in mortality or morbidity[38]	A
Lexipafant *(platelet activating factor antagonist)*	Lexipafant does not ameliorate the systemic inflammatory response syndrome in severe acute pancreatitis[39]	A
Loxiglumide *(CCK-1 receptor blockade)*	Loxiglumide decreases the intensity of abdominal pain and serum level of pancreatic amylase and trypsin[40]	A

interventions in acute pancreatitis.[32–40] It should be noted that the evidence-base for these recommendations has been derived from studies in adults.

Surgical

No clear consensus exists on the indications for surgery in acute pancreatitis. In recent years, the treatment of acute pancreatitis has shifted away from early surgical necrosectomy to aggressive intensive medical care with specific criteria for operative intervention. Surgical or percutaneous drainage of intra-abdominal collections is essential if sepsis is suspected. Various surgical techniques have been used to treat severe pancreatitis – these utilize either a transperitoneal or retroperitoneal approach, with or without continuous lavage of the pancreatic compartment. Laparotomy and laparoscopy are both used but have never been compared. One randomized study identified a better prognosis in adult patients undergoing delayed necrosectomy.[41] Percutaneous drainage of infected collections and abscesses should be performed with large gauge drains. No controlled study has specifically evaluated the surgical treatment of sterile pancreatic necrosis but retrospective studies indicate that there is an evolution toward spontaneous recovery in such cases. Early decompressive laparotomy is the mainstay of treatment for acute compartment syndrome complicating acute pancreatitis. In general, surgical treatment of gallstone pancreatitis should be delayed until the pancreatitis has settled unless there is cholangitis or progressive obstructive jaundice.[42]

Outcome

The overall outcome of acute severe pancreatitis is determined by the severity of the associated systemic insult, the development of septic complications, and the presence of comorbidity.[1,19,43,44] Compared to adults, children tend to have a better outcome, even in severe cases. The overall reported mortality is around 10%.[2] In most cases, the long-term outcome after acute pancreatitis in children, including functional recovery, is excellent. However, recurrent episodes may occur if congenital anomalies or obstructing lesions are not diagnosed and treated adequately and in cases of hereditary pancreatitis where the underlying genetic defect may cause progression to chronic pancreatitis. After severe necrotizing pancreatitis in adults, both endocrine and exocrine failure are much more likely.[45]

Chronic pancreatitis

Etiology and diagnosis

Chronic pancreatitis is less frequent than acute pancreatitis in children. In Western countries, idiopathic, familial, and obstructive varieties predominate. Choledochal cyst, enteric duplication (i.e., duodenal, gastric), and pancreas divisum are responsible for most cases of obstructive chronic pancreatitis in children; tumor and pseudocyst are rare causes (Table 40.1). Pancreatic calcification may be seen on a plain abdominal radiograph but is uncommon. Abdominal ultrasound allows the identification of an enlarged and hyperechogenic pancreas, and dilatation of the pancreatic duct and/or biliary tree. ERCP is particularly useful in demonstrating anatomical lesions responsible for obstruction and, additionally, offers the possibility of therapy in selected cases. MRCP is emerging as an accurate and non-invasive complementary diagnostic tool.

Early and late complications

In children, pseudocysts are reported in 11%–27% of all pancreatitis but it is important to distinguish whether it results from acute or chronic pancreatitis (Table 40.2). Spontaneous resolution of a pseudocyst is frequent in children, but may be complicated by abscess formation, hemorrhage, or rupture. A pseudoaneurysm is a rare complication of a pseudocyst; typically this affects the splenic, gastroduodenal, pancreaticoduodenal, gastric or hepatic arteries. Bleeding from a pseudoaneurysm has a 90% mortality if untreated. The pseudoaneurysm may be identified on CT scan or by angiography. Biliary obstruction may result from pancreatic fibrosis, pseudocyst formation or chronic inflammation. Jaundice is found in only half the cases but obstruction may be complicated by cholangitis. Symptomatic duodenal compression is infrequent but may rarely occur with pancreas divisum, pseudocyst, or inflammation of the pancreatic head. Mesenteric vein thrombosis is a severe but also rare complication of acute and chronic pancreatitis in children. Splenic pseudocyst formation has also been described; it results from either extension of a pancreatic pseudocyst into the spleen or direct splenic injury from pancreatic enzymes. Diabetes mellitus is a well-recognized complication of chronic pancreatitis. Exocrine pancreatic insufficiency may impair vitamin metabolism, especially B_{12} and fat-soluble vitamins or lead to disturbances of nutrition and growth.

Treatment

Surgical and endoscopic therapy

Pediatric practice has largely evolved from adult experience. Endoscopic treatment in chronic pancreatitis is limited to selected interventions: sphincterotomy, stone extraction, and insertion of pancreatic/biliary endoprostheses.[46,47] In our experience, pancreatic stones and debris associated with a choledochal cyst can be treated during surgery by removal supplemented by intra-operative endoscopy of Wirsung's duct. Ductal anomalies such as pancreas divisum or a dominant Santorini duct can either be managed conservatively by endoscopic papillotomy of the minor papilla or by accessory duct sphincteroplasty. There are no randomized studies analyzing endoscopic treatment of chronic pancreatitis in children. The principal surgical technique in cases of chronic pancreatitis and a dilated Wirsung duct is the modified Puestow procedure or Roux-en-Y lateral pancreaticojejunostomy, as initially described by Partington and Rochelle.[48] In cases with an inflammatory mass in the head of the pancreas, a proximal pancreatectomy combined with Roux-en-Y pancreaticojejunostomy can be performed without inducing endocrine or exocrine pancreatic insufficiency.[49] The size of Wirsung's pancreatic duct is the principal limitation to pancreatic anastomosis. In selected cases, pancreatoduodenectomy with or without pyloric preservation has been performed. Enteric duplication involving the pancreatic head may be managed by local resection and Roux-en-Y cystenterostomy.[50] Distal pancreatectomy with or without pancreaticojejunostomy is considered in cases involving the tail of the pancreas.

Minimally invasive therapy of complications of pancreatitis

Endoscopic techniques and percutaneous drainage have gained popularity for the treatment of complications of pancreatitis. Pseudocysts and pancreatic abscesses can be drained percutaneously. Although the evidence is not strong, the administration of an octreotide analogue may reduce the duration of drainage.[51] ERCP with transpapillary drainage can be performed in cases where the pseudocyst communicates with the pancreatic duct. Endoscopic transmural cystogastrostomy has yielded good results in adults, although intraperitoneal perforation and bleeding are risks. Pancreatic fistulae can be treated by ERCP with internal drainage of the pancreatic duct proximal to the fistula. In adults, Kozarek *et al.* have reported successful transpapillary drainage of pancreatic pseudocysts associated with a fistula in 9 out of 18 patients.[52]

Outcome

In the long term, surgery for chronic pancreatitis is more often complicated by diabetes mellitus if more than 20%–30% of the gland has been removed. In large adult series, the 5-year probability of diabetes in cases of chronic pancreatitis undergoing surgery is about 20%–40%. In children, pancreatic function seems to be preserved in those undergoing early surgery for chronic pancreatitis associated with pancreatic duct dilatation.[46,49] This is illustrated by DuBay *et al.* who reported 12 children followed up for a median of 15 years after lateral pancreaticojejunostomy: 8 experienced further episodes of pancreatitis but symptoms were severe in only one; 11 were considered to have a good or excellent outcome; all had an improved nutritional status; and none developed diabetes mellitus.[49] In adults, randomized studies comparing proximal pancreaticoduodenectomy with Roux-en-Y pancreaticojejunostomy have shown a significant advantage for the latter in terms of quality of life and preservation of endocrine function in chronic pancreatitis.[53,54] The Puestow procedure results in the relief of pain in at least 80% of children in the short term. However, chronic pain may recur in as many as 25%–50% of patients after 3 to 5 years.[55]

There is a significant mortality and morbidity associated with pancreatic resection for chronic pancreatitis. In one study of 484 adults and children who underwent surgery for chronic pancreatitis during a 20-year period, total pancreatectomy was associated with a 30-day mortality of 5% and a morbidity of 47%, whilst pancreaticoduodenectomy had a mortality of 3% and morbidity of 32%. Both procedures were associated with pancreatic insufficiency, and peptic and anastomotic ulceration. However, 79% of patients were reported to be living normally after surgery.[56] Distal pancreatectomy also has numerous potential complications including splenic devascularization and diabetes mellitus.

Pancreatic exocrine insufficiency is a recognized risk of chronic pancreatitis and is more likely after resectional surgery. Pancreatic enzyme deficiency is known to reduce the absorption of fat-soluble vitamins and vitamin B_{12}. Deficiency of vitamin B_{12} may be found in between one and two-thirds of patients.

Antioxidants have been used in an attempt to treat chronic pancreatitis and delay disease progression by reducing oxidant stress. There is some evidence for benefit from antioxidant therapy in patients with recurrent acute and chronic pancreatitis.[57,58]

Two variants of chronic pancreatitis in children deserve brief additional comment. The first is idiopathic fibrosing pancreatitis which is very rare and tends to present with obstructive jaundice, sometimes mimicking a pancreatic tumor.[59] The diagnosis can be confirmed by percutaneous pancreatic needle biopsy. The jaundice may resolve spontaneously or after a period of endoscopic biliary stenting.[60] Exocrine and endocrine insufficiency are long-term risks but the natural history is not currently well defined. The second variant is hereditary pancreatitis. Comparing the clinical course of hereditary pancreatitis (at least two affected family members) with idiopathic chronic pancreatitis, children with hereditary disease tend to have more complications (pseudocysts, steatorrhea, ascites, portal hypertension, and diabetes) and are more likely to require surgical intervention in the long term.[61,62]

Conclusions

In recent years, the treatment of both acute and chronic pancreatitis has shifted toward a less invasive approach. Early identification of infective complications and initiation of adequate supportive care is the mainstay of therapy in acute pancreatitis. Percutaneous drainage of pancreatic collections has replaced more aggressive techniques. The long-term outcome of acute pancreatitis is related to its underlying cause; obstructive and familial etiologies are more likely to evolve toward relapsing and chronic pancreatitis. The surgical therapy of chronic pancreatitis has changed as a result of advances in minimally invasive procedures. Although not prospectively validated in randomized trials, endoscopic treatment of pseudocyst, pancreatic abscess, pancreatic fistula and biliary stenosis may be advantageous. Surgical drainage procedures for chronic pancreatitis associated with ductal dilatation are effective but resectional procedures may exacerbate the tendency to long-term endocrine and exocrine insufficiency and other metabolic complications.

REFERENCES

1. Werlin, S. L., Kugathasan, S., & Frautschy, B. C. Pancreatitis in children. *J. Pediatr. Gastroenterol. Nutr.* 2003; **37**:591–595.
2. Benifla, M. & Weizman, Z. Acute pancreatitis in childhood: analysis of literature data. *J. Clin. Gastroenterol.* 2003; **37**:169–172.
3. Hendren, W. H., Greep, J. M., & Patton, A. S. Pancreatitis in childhood: experience with 15 cases. *Arch. Dis. Child.* 1965; **40**:132–145.
4. Fonkalsrud, E. W., Henney, R. P., Riemenschneider, T. A. *et al.* Management of pancreatitis in infants and children. *Am. J. Surg.* 1968; **116**:198–203.

5. Moossa, A. R. Acute pancreatitis in childhood. *Progr. Pediatr. Surg.* 1972; **4**:111–127.
6. Buntain, W. L., Wood, J. B., & Wooley, M. M. Pancreatitis in childhood. *J. Pediatr. Surg.* 1978; **13**:143–148.
7. Eichelberger, M. R., Hoelzer, D. J., & Koop C. E. Acute pancreatitis: the difficulties of diagnosis and therapy. *J. Pediatr. Surg.* 1982; **17**:244–54.
8. Forbes, A., Leung, J. W. C., & Cotton, P. B. Relapsing acute and chronic pancreatitis. *Arch. Dis. Child.* 1984; **59**:927–934.
9. Tam, P. K. H., Saing, H., Irving, I. M. *et al.* Acute pancreatitis in children. *J. Pediatr. Surg.* 1985; **20**:58–60.
10. Beshlian, K. & Ryan, J. A. Pancreatitis in teenagers. *Am. J. Surg.* 1986; **152**:133–138.
11. Synn, A. Y., Mulvihill, S. J., & Fonkasrud, E. W. Surgical management of pancreatitis in childhood. *J. Pediatr. Surg.* 1987; **22**:628–632.
12. Ziegler, D. W., Long, J. A., Philippart, A. I. *et al.* Pancreatitis in childhood: experience with 49 patients. *Ann. Surg.* 1988;**207**:257–261.
13. Weizman, Z. & Durie, P. R. Acute pancreatitis in childhood. *J. Pediatr.* 1988; **113**:24–29.
14. Vane, D. W., Grosfeld, J. L., West, K. W. *et al.* Pancreatic disorders in infancy and childhood: experience with 92 cases. *J. Pediatr. Surg.* 1989; **24**:771–776.
15. Haddock, G., Coupar, G., Youngson, G. G. *et al.* Acute pancreatitis in children: a 15-year review. *J. Pediatr. Surg.* 1994; **29**:719–722.
16. Yeung, C. Y., Lee, H. C., Huang, F. Y. *et al.* Pancreatitis in children – experience with 43 cases. *Eur. J. Pediatr.* 1996; **155**:458–463.
17. Jordan, S. C. & Ament, M. E. Pancreatitis in children and adolescents. *Pediatrics* 1977; **91**:211–216.
18. Berney, T., Belli, D., Bugmann, P. *et al.* Influence of severe underlying pathology and hypovolemic shock on the development of acute pancreatitis in children. *J. Pediatr. Surg.* 1996; **31**:1256–1261.
19. Tissieres, P., Simon, L., Debray, D. *et al.* Acute pancreatitis after orthotopic liver transplantation in children: incidence, contributing factors, and outcome. *J. Pediatr. Gastroenterol. Nutr.* 1998; **26**:315–320.
20. Steinberg, W. M., Goldstein, S. S., Davis, N. D. *et al.* Diagnostic assays in acute pancreatitis. *Ann. Intern. Med.* 1985; **102**:576–580.
21. Wilson, C., Heads, A., Shenkin, A., & Imrie, C. W. C-reactive protein, antiproteases and complement factors as objective markers of severity in acute pancreatitis. *Br. J. Surg.* 1989; **76**:177–781.
22. Roseau, G., Palazzo, L., Dumontier, I. *et al.* Endoscopic ultrasonography in the evaluation of pediatric digestive disease: preliminary results. *Endoscopy* 1998; **30**:477–481.
23. Hirohashi, S., Hirohashi, S., Uchida, H. *et al.* Pancreatitis: evaluation with MR cholangio-pancreatography in children. *Radiology* 1997; **203**:411–415.
24. Barish, M. A., Yucel, E. K., & Ferrucci, J. T. Magnetic resonance cholangiopancreatography. *N. Engl. J. Med.* 1999; **341**:258–264.
25. Dugernier, T. L., Laterre, P. F., Wittebole, X. *et al.* Compartmentalization of the inflammatory response during acute pancreatitis. *Am. J. Respir. Crit. Care. Med.* 2003; **168**:148–157.
26. Pastor, C. M., Matthay, M. A., & Frossard, J. L. Pancreatitis-associated acute lung injury. New insight. *Chest* 2003; **124**:2341–2351.
27. Renner, I. G., Savage, W. T. III, Pantoja, J. L. *et al.* Death due to acute pancreatitis: a retrospective analysis of 405 autopsy cases. *Dig. Dis. Sci.* 1985; **30**:1005–1018.
28. de Beaux, A. C., Palmer, K. R., & Carter, D. C. Factors influencing morbidity and mortality in acute pancreatitis; an analysis of 279 cases. *Gut* 1995; **37**:121–126.
29. Ranson, J. H., Rifkind, K. M., Roses, D. F. *et al.* Prognostic signs and the role of operative management in acute pancreatitis. *Surg. Gynecol. Obstet.* 1974; **139**:69–81.
30. Leteurtre, S., Martinot, A., Duhamel, A. *et al.* Validation of the paediatric logistic organ dysfunction (PELOD) score: prospective, observational, multicentre study. *Lancet* 2003; **362**:192–197.
31. Balthazar, E. J. Complications of acute pancreatitis: clinical and CT evaluation. *Radiol. Clin. North. Am.* 2002; **40**:1211–1227.
32. van den Berghe, G., Wouters, P., Weekers, F. *et al.* Intensive insulin therapy in the critically ill patients. *N. Engl. J. Med.* 2001; **345**:1359–1367.
33. Olah, A., Pardavi, G., Belagyi, T. *et al.* Early nasojejunal feeding in acute pancreatitis is associated with a lower complication rate. *Nutrition* 2002; **18**:259–262.
34. Meier, R., Beglinger, C., Layer, P. *et al.* Consensus statement: ESPEN guidelines on nutrition in acute pancreatitis. *Clin. Nutr.* 2002; **21**:173–183.
35. Nathens, A. B., Curtis, J. R., Beale, R. J. *et al.* (2004). Management of the critically ill patient with severe acute pancreatitis. *Crit. Care. Med.*, **32**, 2524–2536.
36. Andriulli, A., Leandro, G., Clemente, R. *et al.* Meta-analysis of somatostatin, octreotide and gabexate mesilate in the therapy of acute pancreatitis. *Aliment. Pharmacol. Ther.* 1998; **12**:237–245.
37. Messori, A., Rampazzo, R., Scroccaro, R. *et al.* Effectiveness of gabexate mesilate in acute pancreatitis. A metaanalysis. *Dig. Dis. Sci.* 1995; **40**:734–738.
38. Platell, C., Cooper, D., & Hall, J. C. A meta-analysis of peritoneal lavage for acute pancreatitis. *J. Gastroenterol. Hepatol.* 2001; **16**:689–693.
39. Johnson, C. D., Kingsnorth, A. N., Imrie, C. W. *et al.* Double blind, randomised, placebo controlled study of a platelet activating factor antagonist, lexipafant, in the treatment and prevention of organ failure in predicted severe acute pancreatitis. *Gut* 2001; **48**:62–69.
40. Shiratori, K., Takeuchi, T., Satake, K. *et al.* Clinical evaluation of oral administration of a cholecystokinin-A receptor antagonist (loxiglumide) to patients with acute, painful attacks of chronic pancreatitis: a multicenter dose-response study in Japan. *Pancreas* 2002; **25**:e1–5.

41. Mier, J., Luque-de Leon, E., Castillo, A. *et al.* Early versus late necrosectomy in severe necrotizing pancreatitis. *Am. J. Surg.* 1997; **173**:71–5.
42. Kelly, T. R. & Wagner, D. S. Gallstone pancreatitis: a prospective, randomized trial of the timing of surgery. *Surgery* 1988; **104**:600–605.
43. Eghtesad, B., Reyes, J. D., Ashrafi, M. *et al.* Pancreatitis after liver transplantation in children: a single-center experience. *Transplantation* 2003; **75**:190–193.
44. Company, L., Saez, J., Martinez, J. *et al.* Factors predicting mortality in severe acute pancreatitis. *Pancreatology* 2003; **3**:144–148.
45. Tzovaras G, Parks RW, Diamond T, Rowlands BJ. Early and long-term results of surgery for severe necrotising pancreatitis. Dig. Surg. 2004; **21**:41–47.
46. Neblett, W. W. & O'Neill, J. A. Surgical management of recurrent pancreatitis in children with pancreas divisum. *Ann. Surg.* 2000; **231**:899–908.
47. Shukri, N., Wasa, M., Hasegawa, T. *et al.* Diagnostic significance of pancreas divisum in early life. *Eur. J. Pediatr. Surg.* 2000; **10**:12–16.
48. Partington, P. F. & Rochelle, R. E. Modified Puestow procedure for retrograde drainage of the pancreatic duct. *Ann. Surg.* 1960; **152**:1037–1042.
49. DuBay, D., Sandler, A., Kimura, K., Bishop, W., Eimen, M., & Soper, R. The modified Puestow procedure for complicated hereditary pancreatitis in children. *J. Pediatr. Surg.* 2000; **35**:343–348.
50. Siddiqui, A. M., Shamberger, R. C., Filler, R. M. *et al.* Enteric duplications of the pancreatic head: definitive management by local resection. *J. Pediatr. Surg.* 1998; **33**:1117–1120.
51. Tissieres, P., Bugmann, P., Rimensberger, P. C. *et al.* Somatostatin in the treatment of pancreatic pseudocyst complicating acute pancreatitis in a child with liver transplantation. *J. Pediatr. Gastroenterol. Nutr.* 2000; **31**:445–447.
52. Kozarek, R. A., Ball, T. J., Patterson, D. J. *et al.* Endoscopic transpapillary therapy for disrupted pancreatic duct and peripancreatic fluid collections. *Gastroenterology* 1991; **100**:1362–1370.
53. Buechler, M. W., Friess, H., Mueller, M. W. *et al.* Randomized trial of duodenum-preserving pancreatic head resection versus pyloric-preserving Whipple in chronic pancreatitis. *Am. J. Surg.* 1995; **169**:65–69.
54. Izbicki, J. P., Bloechle, C., Broering, D. C. *et al.* Extended drainage versus resection in surgery for chronic pancreatitis. A prospective randomized trial comparing the longitudinal pancreaticojejunostomy combined with local pancreatic head excision with the pylorus-preserving pancreatoduodenectomy. *Ann. Surg.* 1998; **228**:771–779.
55. Pegoli Jr, W. Acute and chronic pancreatitis and pancreatic trauma. In Howard, E. R., Stringer, M. D. & Colombani, P. M. *Surgery of the Liver, Bile Ducts and Pancreas in Children*, 2nd edn. London: Arnold, 2002.
56. Sakorafas, G. H., Farnell, M. B., Farley, D. R. *et al.* Long-term results after surgery for chronic pancreatitis. *Int. J. Pancreatol.* 2000; **27**:131–142.
57. Braganza, J. M., Thomas, A., & Robinson, A. Antioxidants to treat chronic pancreatitis in childhood? Case report and possible implications for pathogenesis. *Int. J. Pancreatol.* 1988; **3**:209–216.
58. Uden, S., Bilton, D., Nathan, L. *et al.* Antioxidant therapy for recurrent pancreatitis: placebo-controlled trial. *Aliment. Pharmacol. Ther.* 1990; **4**:357–371.
59. Sylvester, F. A., Shuckett, B., Cutz, E. *et al.* Management of fibrosing pancreatitis in children presenting with obstructive jaundice. *Gut* 1998; **43**:715–720.
60. EL-Matary, W., Casson, D., Hodges, S. *et al.* Successful conservative management of idiopathic fibrosing pancreatitis in children. *Eur. J. Pediatr.* 2006; March 22 E pub.
61. Konzen, K. M., Perrault, J., Moir, C., & Zinsmeister, A. R. Long-term follow-up of young patients with chronic hereditary or idiopathic pancreatitis. *Mayo. Clin. Proc.* 1993; **68**:449–453.
62. Moir, C. R., Konzen, K. M., & Perrault, J. Surgical therapy and long-term follow-up of childhood hereditary pancreatitis. *J. Pediatr. Surg.* 1992; **27**:282–286.

Part V

Urology

41

Introduction

Pierre D. E. Mouriquand

Department of Paediatric Urology/Surgery, Debrousse Hospital, Lyon, France

At the dawn of a new millennium, pediatric urology, like adult urology 30 years ago, has become an independent specialty, covering the vast field of congenital and acquired anomalies of the genitourinary (GU) tract in children. This does not mean that it is an insular field. On the contrary, it has very close links with associated pediatric specialties such as pediatric nephrology, pediatric radiology, pediatric endocrinology, and pediatric oncology. The advent and development of antenatal ultrasonography, a better understanding of the pathophysiology of congenital urine flow impairment, the revolution of minimally invasive surgery and robotics, the promising future of tissue engineering, and the improvements in reconstructive surgery of the lower GU tract, have completely changed the management of congenital GU malformations over the last 25 years.

Before getting to the heart of the matter, one should remember that this leap forward in pediatric urology is a result of the hard work and imagination of several memorable surgeons who, well before anyone else, anticipated this evolution and laid the foundation of pediatric urology. It is impossible to list all these pioneering efforts which began in the mid-nineteenth century in the old world, with some daring and precursory ideas in the field of reconstructive surgery[1–3] and continued in the twentieth century all around the world. However, it would be impossible not to mention here the name of Sir David Innes Williams, who is the genuine father of modern pediatric urology and who had the genius to understand, with a few others, the forthcoming changes in this specialty. Sir David Innes Williams provided a great lesson in humility when, receiving the medal of Honorary Member of the European Society for Paediatric Urology in 1990, he said: "The current generation of pediatric urologists is undiverting all patients that the former generation has previously diverted, but the present generation should not forget that the next generation of pediatric urologists will be undoing again what has just been done."

The Belgian ethnologist Claude Lévi-Strauss,[4] distinguished two civilizations, one that roasts (people from the South) and the other that boils (people from the North), and he described how climate can affect life's habits. The same distinction can apply to medicine, and having had the privilege to work in both climates and cultures – the Latin culture in France and the Anglo-Saxon culture in England – I can sense the pros and cons of each. I have learned five major lessons.

- There may be several acceptable solutions to the same problem and some of these solutions may be entirely contradictory although valid.
- What is true today may well be entirely wrong tomorrow.
- Principles and theories in medicine are only tools which should be used sparingly, should be challenged continuously and should not divert us from our main mission, to help patients feel better. "The temptation to form premature theories upon insufficient data is the bane of our profession"[5] is the essential message that I received from Sir Arthur Conan Doyle who lived only a few blocks from my consulting rooms in London.
- The sheer weight of knowledge might be detrimental to the progress of healthcare. The more controversial information you gain about one subject (for example, vesicoureteric reflux), the more confused you become when trying to make a sensible decision for the nice little girl sitting in front of you in your consulting room. This brings to my mind the excellent article of the former Principal and Vice Chancellor of the University of Strathclyde

Pediatric Surgery and Urology: Long-term Outcomes, Mark Stringer, Keith Oldham, Pierre Mouriquand.

(Glasgow), Sir Graham Hills,[6] who said that knowledge is luggage and it is best to travel light.

- Fashion has brought new methods of scientific evaluation of medical material such as "evidence-based medicine," which may be inadequate to approach many medical situations and might satisfy only statisticians and rationalists. Modeling medical problems might be an erroneous simplification, which may lead to adventurous conclusions and may get things out of proportion. It frequently appears that, when a disease escapes our understanding, there is always someone to create a dogma and an international classification to hide our ignorance. Empirical knowledge derived from follow-up consultations might be as instructive as the most sophisticated methods of investigation. The last decade with its increasing influence of material equipment over intelligence has shown that doctors tend to become technicians dominated by administrators who ignore that medicine is not a science, not a business, but an art. We should never forget this and hope that the Truth does not exist. I can only support the Italian writer Antonio Tabucchi when he said: "I hate answers!".

Here comes the second edition of this textbook focused on the long-term outcomes of our art. This is a lesson of intelligence and humility given by some of the greatest pediatric urologists throughout the world. They provide their own analyses and conclusions about what they think might be the best options for their patients just after the change of millennium. Some contributors are from the North, some from the South, and some from the USA, where they don't boil, they don't roast, they microwave. They should be warmly thanked for their outstanding contributions.

REFERENCES

1. Duplay, S. De l'hypospadias périnéo-scrotal et de son traitement chirurgical. *Arch. Gen. Med.* 1874; **1**:613–657.
2. Thiersch, C. Uber die Entstehungsweise und Operative Behandlung der Epispadie. *Arch. Heitkunde* 1869; **10**:20–25.
3. Cantwell, F. V. Operative technique of epispadias by transplantation of the urethra. *Ann. Surg.* 1895; **22**:689–692.
4. Lévi-Strauss, C. *Le Cru et le Cuit*. Paris: Plon Publishers, 1964.
5. Sir Arthur Conan Doyle. Sherlock Holmes speaking to Inspector McDonald about the murder of John Douglas. In *The Valley of Fear*, chapter 2. London: Penguin Books.
6. Sir Graham Hills. The knowledge disease. *Br. Med. J.* 1993; **307**:1578.

42

Upper tract dilation

Venkata R. Jayanthi and Stephen A. Koff

Division of Urology, The Ohio State University, Columbus, Ohio, USA

Introduction

In former years, the clinical management of upper tract dilation was simple. Because most children with hydronephrosis presented with a mass or a clinical problem such as infection or pain, it was assumed that the cause was an obstruction. Surgical treatment was performed and the outcome was usually satisfactory. The advent of prenatal ultrasonography and the resultant identification of large numbers of asymptomatic upper tract dilation has forced physicians to alter their understanding of the significance of hydronephrosis and to better define obstruction. This is largely because dilation often improves or resolves spontaneously, which questions the necessity of surgical treatment. Whereas in the past only few natural history studies were available, a greater appreciation of the spontaneous resolution of prenatally detected hydronephrosis has been gleaned from multiple studies from various centers around the world.

Any analysis of long-term outcomes of upper tract dilation management must of necessity deal separately with the symptomatic and asymptomatic varieties and must also recognize that dilation involving the kidney alone is different from dilation affecting kidney and ureter together. Accordingly, this chapter will be divided into two sections. The first will deal with pure hydronephrosis and consider the child with dilated renal collecting systems without ureteral dilation. The second portion will examine hydroureteronephrosis and dilation of both the renal collecting system and ureter.

Dilation of the renal collecting system is easily diagnosed on radiographic imaging studies. However, not all upper tract dilation is caused by obstruction. Surgical treatment of hydronephrosis caused by obstruction will benefit and protect the kidneys, whereas surgical treatment of non-obstructive hydronephrosis is unnecessary and ill-advised. The critical management decision for hydronephrosis is therefore a determination of the presence of obstruction.

How does one define and diagnose obstruction?

Although obstruction may intuitively be defined as a significant restriction to urinary flow, it is often quite difficult to determine the presence of such an impediment to flow especially in the neonatal period because the anatomy and function of the kidney is changing rapidly. This is compounded by the fact that there is no useful biochemical marker for unilateral obstruction. Furthermore, the mere presence of hydronephrosis and/or diminished function are invalid indicators of obstruction as many hydronephrotic kidneys will improve spontaneously over time with an increase in renal function and a decrease in hydronephrosis. However, despite this shortcoming, obstruction can be diagnosed clinically by the effect it has on the kidney over time, and thus obstruction may be defined as any restriction to urinary flow that, if untreated, will injure the kidney. This definition is useful clinically but it requires that tests in the infant be performed serially to look for improvement or deterioration in function and anatomy.

Diuretic renography is a commonly used method of diagnosing obstruction. It must be recognized, however, that even with diuretic stimulation slow washout of tracer from the newborn kidney is to be expected and is normal. This delay is caused by a combination of diminished glomerular and tubular function, which causes a poor response

Pediatric Surgery and Urology: Long-term Outcomes, Mark Stringer, Keith Oldham, Pierre Mouriquand. Published by Cambridge University Press.

to diuretics, and a disproportionately large renal pelvis, which functions as a sluggish mixing chamber. Furthermore, the infant renal pelvis is a very compliant structure with a marked increase in volume associated with the sudden fluid load due to diuretic stimulation. This fluid load naturally will necessitate greater time for drainage and thus prolonged "washout curves" even in the absence of obstruction. For these reasons a delayed washout pattern on an isolated renogram is invalid as the sole indicator of obstruction.[1] The diuretic washout pattern should only be considered valid in the newborn period if it demonstrates prompt drainage, thereby excluding obstruction.

The primary role of diuretic renography in the infant should be to measure differential renal function. Serial measurements will help determine if renal function is improving or deteriorating. If serial measurements indicate that the affected kidney is improving quickly and appropriately, it confirms that obstruction does not exist and that there is no need to perform surgery. If sequential measurements indicate that renal function is either deteriorating or failing to improve as expected, then obstruction is likely present and should be corrected surgically.

Ultrasonography has become the standard for identifying hydronephrosis in infancy and, statistically, the degree of pelvic enlargement correlates with the presence of obstruction. However, ultrasonography cannot be used to diagnose obstruction because, in an individual kidney, the degree of hydronephrosis neither indicates the presence or absence of obstruction nor predicts whether the hydronephrosis will improve or worsen. This is especially true in the newborn where hydronephrosis may disappear transiently after birth and fluctuate significantly with time, hydration and bladder fullness. Furthermore, after surgical correction, radiographic studies may show some improvement in upper tract dilation, but in most cases there will not be normalization. This would suggest that the mere presence of hydronephrosis in and of itself is not indicative of obstruction. The only way to use ultrasonography meaningfully in this age group is to obtain serial measurements. Progressive worsening of dilation usually indicates an obstruction, whereas improvement indicates the opposite. The measurement of resistive indices has no role in the diagnosis of obstruction in children.[2]

Contrast-enhanced magnetic resonance (MR) urography is a promising technique that provides differential function values that correlate with nuclear scintigraphy while simultaneously offering detailed anatomical information.[3] As with nuclear renography, however, objective criteria for obstruction are lacking. Captopril renography is another technique which may detect kidneys whose function is seemingly preserved but due to subclinical activation of the renin-angiotensin system.[4,5]

The difficulties in the accurate diagnosis of obstruction is clearly demonstrated by the fact that patients with intermittent flank pain and classic symptomatic UPJ obstruction may have totally normal imaging studies yet obtain symptomatic relief after surgical correction. In contrast, neonates with massive hydronephrosis and markedly delayed drainage may have complete spontaneous normalization with time.

Outcomes analysis

To adequately assess the impact of any therapeutic intervention, one must compare the outcome of the intervention with the natural history of the untreated condition. Herein lies the major historical difficulty in understanding the management of hydronephrosis. Few studies have attempted, or have been able, to define and characterize the natural history of this condition.

When assessing the impact of a therapeutic intervention, one must define a group of parameters which will reflect all aspects of the pathological process. These factors may include (1) clinical parameters, e.g., the relief of symptoms, (2) functional parameters, (3) radiographic parameters, e.g., degree of hydronephrosis and (4) physiological parameters, e.g., transit time, emptying and washout. Unless all parameters are carefully considered pre- and postoperatively, the diagnosis of obstruction, the indications for surgery, the presence of residual obstruction, and the outcome analysis may be subject to misinterpretation.

Hydronephrosis

Clinical improvement

Symptomatic hydronephrosis in children occurs much less commonly than antenatally diagnosed hydronephrosis. There are reports on the development of symptoms in infants with hydronephrosis, but no studies report on the long-term follow-up of symptomatic hydronephrosis in the pediatric population. The long-term follow-up of adults who underwent pyeloplasty many years earlier document the unquestionable effectiveness of surgical correction at relieving symptoms and the durability of that effect.[6,7]

Functional improvement

Several authors have studied the natural history of non-operated newborn hydronephrosis with regard to potential deterioration of renal function. Cartwright reported on 45 patients with "apparent ureteropelvic junction obstruction" and relative renal function greater than 35%.[8] In this study they compared the outcome of 33 patients who were followed non-operatively with 12 who underwent pyeloplasty within the first few months of life. This data demonstrated no difference in differential function between the two groups. Ransley followed 100 patients with antenatally detected hydronephrosis and relative function greater than 40% and only 14 had a decrease in differential function in follow-up.[9] Freedman followed 140 patients with unilateral hydronephrosis and only 5 (3.5%) had a decrease in relative function in extended follow-up.[10] These preceding studies only included patients with good relative function (>35%). Koff, however, followed non-operatively 104 patients with antenatal hydronephrosis and suspected obstruction despite reductions in differential function to as low as 7%.[11] He found that 97 (93%) had stable or improved relative renal function. If differential function was initially low, it rapidly improved. Indeed, even neonates with bilateral hydronephrosis can initially be managed expectantly since two-thirds of such kidneys will have spontaneous improvement in dilation.[12] These studies suggest that the majority of children with antenatally diagnosed hydronephrosis do not have an obstruction and can be safely followed non-operatively. Renal function will usually normalize or improve and deterioration is relatively uncommon occurring in less than 15% of children. Extended observation is required since mean time to maximum improvement of hydronephrosis is up to 2.5 years.[13]

It is against this background of natural history of congenital hydronephrosis that reports on the outcome of pyeloplasty need to be evaluated. Does early surgical correction avert functional loss? Does surgical correction lead to greater ultimate function? King reported on twelve neonates with hydronephrosis who had poorly functioning kidneys preoperatively.[14] Within the first few months of life, all of these children underwent pyeloplasty and there was a mean increase of 154% in the relative differential function on postoperative studies. Similarly, Dowling reported that functional improvement only occurred in children who underwent surgery less than 1 year of age.[15] Koff, however, followed 16 neonates with poorly functioning severely hydronephrotic kidneys non-operatively.[11] Over the course of time, 15 of these children had normalization of relative function. Cartwright noted the same rise in renal function in the first year of life in both non-operated and operated kidneys.[8] These latter reports suggest that hydronephrotic kidneys in newborns tend to show rapid improvement in differential function during the first year of life.

Salem reported that patients with symptomatic UPJ obstruction were more likely to have some improvement in differential function postoperatively, whereas most (80%) who underwent pyeloplasty for antenatally diagnosed hydronephrosis had no improvement in function.[16] There was no correlation between outcome and the ages of the children or the mode of presentation. MacNeily studied the effect of pyeloplasty on seventy-five children who underwent surgery for varying indications.[17] In this study most patients had no change in function with surgery and a greater number had a drop in function than an improvement. Again, these results did not separate those who presented with antenatal hydronephrosis from those who presented with symptomatic upper tract dilation. In fact, the authors commented on "the irrelevance of surgery to the ultimate differential function" that was evidenced by the fact that there was no difference in final relative function between those who had uncomplicated repairs and those who had complications (including those requiring surgery for persistent obstruction). Capolicchio *et al.* did compare children with neonatal hydronephrosis with older children with symptomatic UPJ obstruction and noted the latter did have relatively poorer differential function that did not improve after surgery.[18] Thus looking at large inclusive groups of patients, pyeloplasty does not appear to improve the function of hydronephrotic kidneys which have either near normal renal function or a chronically-fixed decrease in function.

In contrast, if surgery is being performed specifically because there has been a drop in relative function on close follow-up with serial investigations, one can expect the renal function to recover to baseline values and even improve. Chertin *et al.* reviewed 44 patients who were managed expectantly but underwent surgery specifically for functional deterioration.[19] Ninety-five percent had recovery of function to baseline or even improvement. Chandrasekharam *et al.* noted that functional improvement, when it occurs, might take up to one year after surgery.[20] Of prime importance in any observational protocol are close follow-up and good patient compliance. Chertin *et al.* reported on 63 patients with prenatal hydronephrosis that were lost to follow-up.[21] These patients had significantly reduced relative renal function compared to those who were compliant and were followed closely. Several authors have noted, however, that some patients who are followed expectantly do not have recovery of function after surgery.[22–24] In these series, however, the time period between renographic examinations was 6 months or greater. In the first year of life, and specifically during the period of transitional nephrology, close observation using shorter intervals (3 months) is necessary to allow prompt detection of increasing hydronephrosis or of functional deterioration. Waiting 6 months in between studies during this important time period may permit unrecognized obstruction to lead to permanent loss of function.

Two authors have attempted to correlate differential function with renal histologic changes. Elder reported that 21% of those with a good differential function (>40%) had abnormal biopsies, whereas 33% of those with poor differential functions had normal biopsies.[25] Stock showed that those who had poor function preoperatively had abnormal biopsies and that there was no improvement in function in these kidneys postoperatively.[26] These studies illustrate the deficiencies of our present methods of determining relative renal function and on assessing the potential for decreased function to improve. One cannot determine the relative health of a kidney based on a single diagnostic or biopsy study, as even children with normal differential function may have foci of abnormal renal histology. On the other hand, children with poorly functioning kidneys may have normal histology. This suggests that sequential studies are required to determine the presence of obstruction in newborns with unilateral hydronephrosis.

Effect on hydronephrosis and drainage times

Amling *et al.* reported that on the long-term outcome of pyeloplasty in 44 children who had at least 2 years of postoperative imaging available for review.[27] They found that 91% had no change or worsening hydronephrosis at 1 month. There was improvement in only 38% at 6 months and this increased to 81% by 2 years. Only 19% had complete resolution. Salem reported that drainage times as determined by nuclide renography improved to less than 10 minutes in 98%.[16] Thus surgery is effective at improving the radiographic appearance and washout kinetics of the hydronephrotic kidney. However, unless the kidney is clearly proven to be obstructed, the added benefit of surgery is not clear since the same improvement may be observed without surgery.[11]

Operative techniques

Multiple studies have demonstrated that pyeloplasty can correct UPJ obstruction with high rates of success and with minimal morbidity. In the pediatric population, a dismembered repair as described by Anderson and Hynes is preferable to a flap-type of procedure as the obstructing segment is typically stenotic and fibrotic and unsuitable for incorporation into the repair. One may approach the kidney through either the flank or posteriorly. Although the posterior approach may be better tolerated in adults, the differences are minimized in the pediatric population. Furthermore, the flank approach may allow better exposure for massively dilated kidneys or for those with long segment obstruction.

The main controversy with regard to the technique of surgery is whether stents or nephrostomy tubes are helpful. Though stenting clearly is useful in adults in minimizing the risk of postoperative leakage, the rate of urinoma formation after a carefully performed stentless pyeloplasty is quite low. Urine leakage after pyeloplasty is not uncommon and the risk of development of a urinoma can be minimized by leaving a drain for up to a week following cessation of flank drainage.[28] Stents or nephrostomy tubes may be advisable, however, in the presence of active inflammation, after a difficult repair or with a solitary kidney.

Complications of pyeloplasty include extravasation, urinoma, and persistent obstruction. The overall re-operative rate is quite low at approximately 5%.

Pesce *et al.* reported on a novel technique for correction of intermittent UPJ obstruction related to lower pole aberrant vessels.[29] Since, in this situation, the UPJ itself may be inherently normal with obstruction being related to extrinsic compression from the vasculature, they suggested transposition of the vessels away from the UPJ and fixation of these vessels to the anterior pelvis without any formal pyeloplasty being performed. As the vessels no longer would be near the UPJ, the obstruction should be relieved. In their study 10/11 patients had relief of obstruction with vessel transposition alone.

Minimally invasive procedures that initially were described for adults are now being applied to the pediatric population. Endopyelotomy may be performed in either an antegrade or retrograde fashion. The latter, however, may be more problematic in younger children with a greater risk of ureteral injury. Success rates for primary UPJ obstruction are high, approaching 85%, but are not as good as with standard open repair.[30–32] Endopyelotomy, however, has a high rate of success, approaching 100%, after failed open pyeloplasty.[32]

Pyeloplasty, performed via either a laparoscopic or retroperitoneoscopic approach is another minimally invasive technique.[33,34] With these procedures, a repair identical to standard open pyeloplasty is performed with identical success rates. The main disadvantage is the long learning curve necessary to master technically challenging reconstructive and suturing techniques.

These minimally invasive procedures are most useful in older children with symptomatic UPJ obstruction. In the neonatal group, the efficacy of standard surgery, the small incision usually required, the relatively minor pain involved, and the potentially deleterious effects of recurrent obstruction in a developing kidney would argue against any of these endoscopic techniques and for standard repair at this time.

Summary of outcomes of management of upper tract dilation

It is clear that pyeloplasty is very successful in correcting UPJ obstruction. Success rates of greater than 95% can be expected. The main controversy in the management of hydronephrosis pertains to deciding which child will benefit from surgery. Symptomatic UPJ obstruction clearly needs to be corrected. Data on the natural history of antenatally detected hydronephrosis suggest that the majority have non-obstructed upper tract dilation and that careful observation is all that is needed in most. Only a minority of children will have true obstruction as manifested by deterioration in function or worsening of hydronephrosis. For this small group of patients, pyeloplasty is quite efficacious at relieving the obstruction and preserving renal function. Surgery for these children should be performed immediately regardless of patient age once the diagnosis of true obstruction is made.

Hydroureteronephrosis

The management of "obstructed" megaureters has changed markedly over the past 20 years and mirrors the management of ureteropelvic junction "obstruction." More children with hydroureteronephrosis are now being detected antenatally prior to the onset of any clinical problem. One needs to understand the natural history of renal and ureteral dilation to appropriately consider outcomes of surgical intervention. This discussion will not include reflux-induced ureteral dilation or coexisting reflux and obstruction.

Natural history of hydroureteronephrosis

Baskin reported on 25 neonates with antenatally detected hydroureteronephrosis who were followed non-operatively for a mean period of 7 years.[35] Of these children 18 had serial intravenous pyelograms performed with improvement in dilation noted in 12. Serial nuclear renograms were performed in 16 and all had the age-related increases in glomerular filtration rates without any deterioration in differential renal function. Liu similarly followed 53 newborns with dilated ureters, including 14 with bilateral megaureters.[36] After a mean follow-up of 3 years, 34% had resolved while 49% had stable dilation. Only 20% of the children required surgery, for either breakthrough infections or deterioration of function. Cozzi *et al.* followed 21 newborns with non-refluxing megaureters for up to 8 years and only one ultimately required surgical correction.[37] Many of the children in these reports had striking improvement in ureteral dilation over the course of time. Thus the natural history of primary non-reflux-hydroureteronephrosis tends towards spontaneous improvement. McLellan *et al.* demonstrated that gender, laterality, and retrovesical ureteral diameter did not correlate with age at resolution of dilation, although more severe degrees of hydronephrosis did take longer to resolve.[38] At the very least, most will have non-progression of the ureteral dilation. Surgical correction, however, is mandated if there is evidence of deteriorating function, worsening dilation or breakthrough infections.

Operative techniques

Though temporary stenting has been proposed as an option for managing UVJ obstruction in infants, the standard for the surgical correction of the obstructed megaureter involves excision of the stenotic ureteral segment, reduction of caliber of the dilated distal ureter and ureteral reimplantation.[39] The main controversy with megaureter repair is the method of reducing the diameter of the dilated distal ureter. Three main methods have been proposed. Hendren's method involves detubularization of the distal ureter along with excision of a portion of the ureter.[40] The ureter is then retubularized over a 10–12 Fr. catheter. Kalicinski described a modification of Hendren's technique whereby the ureter is tapered over a catheter by the placement of horizontal mattress sutures.[41,42] The excess ureter which has thus been excluded from the lumen of the ureter is not excised but rather folded onto itself. Starr's method involves the placement of Lembert stitches to plicate the ureter over an indwelling catheter.[43] Elegant animal studies by Starr show that, after a period of time, the excess tissue that was plicated will resorb and ultimately the ureter will have a normal histologic appearance. Theoretically, the folding or plication methods are less likely to jeopardize the potentially fragile blood supply of the distal ureter as no tissue is excised. Microangiographic studies done in a minipig model have shown better preservation of the blood supply in the distal ureter after a folding type of repair as opposed to an excisional approach.[44]

Once the ureteral caliber has been reduced, the ureter may be reimplanted into the bladder. The specific method chosen(Leadbetter-Politano, cross-trigonal, extravesical) is not as important as the formation of an adequate length of a detrusor tunnel aimed at a length-to-width ratio of 5:1.

A psoas hitch may be necessary to ensure the creation of a long tunnel. This will also decrease the risk of persistent obstruction due to J-hooking of the ureter at the detrusor hiatus. Temporary stenting is advisable if an excisional repair is performed, as there is a greater risk of leakage of urine outside the bladder. Stenting is not routinely needed if a folding or plication method is used.[45]

The major short-term complication is urinary extravasation. This is more likely with an excisional repair and may be minimized by the placement of a ureteral stent. It may also occur after a plication or folding repair if the vascularity of the distal ureter has been compromised. Long-term complications include reflux or persistent obstruction. Persistent reflux may occur if the detrusor tunnel length was inadequate or if there is retraction of the ureteral orifice. Persistent obstruction is more likely due to angulation of the ureter at its entrance into the bladder. It may also be due to an ischemic stricture in the distal ureter.

Success rates after a carefully performed megaureter repair are quite high, exceeding 95% regardless of which method is used.

Summary of outcomes for hydroureteronephrosis

The management of hydroureteronephrosis is much less controversial than that for hydronephrosis. The consensus of contemporary reports suggest that, in most cases, it represents non-obstructive dilation and therefore careful observation with antibiotic prophylaxis is all that is needed for most children. Should clear demonstration of obstruction occur immediate treatment is required; even massively dilated ureters may be carefully repaired with a high rate of success and with minimal morbidity.

Summary

This brief review has attempted to demonstrate that upper tract dilation is not synonymous with obstruction and that, in fact, the majority of neonates with hydronephrosis and hydroureteronephrosis have non-obstructive dilation. While it is axiomatic that once true obstruction has been diagnosed prompt surgical relief is indicated, the diagnosis of obstruction in young children is fraught with inaccuracy since predictive diagnostic tests do not yet exist and serial measurements of differential function are still imprecise. It is hoped that, as technology and knowledge increase, more specific and sensitive markers of obstruction will develop. Until such occurs, the changing and dynamic nature of postnatal kidney function and development require that functional evaluations must be performed serially in order to ensure an accurate assessment of obstruction in upper tract dilation.

REFERENCES

1. Amarante, J., Anderson, P. J., & Gordon I. Impaired drainage on diuretic renography using half-time or pelvic excretion efficiency is not a sign of obstruction in children with a prenatal diagnosis of unilateral renal pelvic dilatation. *J. Urol.* 2003; **169**(5):1828–1831.
2. Vade, A., Dudiak, C., McCarry, P. *et al.* Resistive indices in the evaluation of infants with obstructive and nonobstructive pyelocaliectasis. *J. Ultrasound Med.* 1999; **18**(5):357–361.
3. Perez-Brayfield, M. R., Kirsch, A. J., Jones, R. A., & Grattan-Smith, J. D. A prospective study comparing ultrasound, nuclear scintigraphy and dynamic contrast enhanced magnetic resonance imaging in the evaluation of hydronephrosis. *J. Urol.* 2003; **170**(4 Pt 1):1330–1334.
4. Homsy, Y. L., Tripp, B. M., Lambert, R. *et al.* The captopril renogram: a new tool for diagnosing and predicting obstruction in childhood hydronephrosis. *J. Urol.* 1998; **160**(4):1446–1449.
5. Bajpai, M., Puri, A., Tripathi, M., & Maini, A. Prognostic significance of captopril renography for managing congenital unilateral hydronephrosis. *J. Urol.* 2002; **168**(5):2158–2161; discussion 2161.
6. Mikkelsen, S. S., Rasmussen, B. S., Jensen, T. M. *et al.* Long-term follow-up of patients with hydronephrosis treated by Anderson–Hynes pyeloplasty. *Br. J. Urol.* 1992; **70**(2):121–124.
7. Notley, R. G. & Beaugie, J. M. The long-term follow-up of Anderson–Hynes pyeloplasty for hydronephrosis. *Br. J. Urol.* 1973; **45**(5):464–467.
8. Cartwright, P. C., Duckett, J. W., Keating, M. A. *et al.* Managing apparent ureteropelvic junction obstruction in the newborn. *J. Urol.* 1992; **148**(4):1224–1228.
9. Ransley, P. G., Dhillon, H. K., Gordon, I. *et al.* The postnatal management of hydronephrosis diagnosed by prenatal ultrasound. *J. Urol.* 1990; **144**(2 Pt 2):584–587; discussion 593–594.
10. Freedman, E. R. & Rickwood, A. M. Prenatally diagnosed pelviureteric junction obstruction: a benign condition? *J. Pediatr. Surg.* 1994; **29**(6):769–772.
11. Koff, S. A. & Campbell, K. D. The nonoperative management of unilateral neonatal hydronephrosis: natural history of poorly functioning kidneys. *J. Urol.* 1994; **152**(2 Pt 2):593–595.
12. Onen, A., Jayanthi, V. R., & Koff, S. A. Long-term followup of prenatally detected severe bilateral newborn hydronephrosis initially managed nonoperatively. *J. Urol.* 2002; **168**(3):1118–1120.
13. Ulman, I., Jayanthi, V. R., & Koff, S. A. The long-term followup of newborns with severe unilateral hydronephrosis initially treated nonoperatively. *J. Urol.* 2000; **164**(3 Pt 2):1101–1105.
14. King, L. R., Coughlin, P. W., Bloch, E. C. *et al.* The case for immediate pyeloplasty in the neonate with ureteropelvic junction obstruction. *J. Urol.* 1984; **132**(4):725–728.

15. Dowling, K. J., Harmon, E. P., Ortenberg, J. *et al.* Ureteropelvic junction obstruction: the effect of pyeloplasty on renal function. *J. Urol.* 1988; **140**(5 Pt 2):1227–1230.
16. Salem, Y. H., Majd, M., Rushton, H. G. *et al.* Outcome analysis of pediatric pyeloplasty as a function of patient age, presentation and differential renal function. *J. Urol.* 1995; **154**(5):1889–1893.
17. MacNeily, A. E., Maizels, M., Kaplan, W. E. *et al.* Does early pyeloplasty really avert loss of renal function? A retrospective review. *J. Urol.* 1993; **150**(2 Pt 2):769–773.
18. Capolicchio, G., Leonard, M. P., Wong, C. *et al.* Prenatal diagnosis of hydronephrosis: impact on renal function and its recovery after pyeloplasty. *J. Urol.* 1999; **162**(3 Pt 2):1029–1032.
19. Chertin, B., Rolle, V., Farkhas, A., & Puri, P. *et al.* Does delaying pyeloplasty affect renal function in children with a prenatal diagnosis of pelvi-ureteric junction obstruction? *BJU Int.* 2002; **90**(1):72–75.
20. Chandrasekharam, V. V., Srinivas, M., Bal, C. S. *et al.* Functional outcome after pyeloplasty for unilateral symptomatic hydronephrosis. *Pediatr. Surg. Int.* 2001; **17**(7):524–527.
21. Chertin, B., Fridmans, A., Knizhnik, M. *et al.* Does early detection of ureteropelvic junction obstruction improve surgical outcome in terms of renal function? *J. Urol.* 1999; **162**(3 Pt 2):1037–1040.
22. Subramaniam, R., Kouriefs, C. & Dickson, A. P. Antenatally detected pelvi-ureteric junction obstruction: concerns about conservative management. *BJU Inte.* 1999; **84**(3):335–338.
23. Cornford, P. A. & Rickwood, A. M. Functional results of pyeloplasty in patients with ante-natally diagnosed pelvi-ureteric junction obstruction. *Br. J. Urol.* 1998; **81**(1):152–155.
24. Palmer, L. S., Maizels, M., Cartwright, P. C. *et al.* Surgery versus observation for managing obstructive grade 3 to 4 unilateral hydronephrosis: a report from the Society for Fetal Urology. *J. Urol.* 1998; **159**(1):222–228.
25. Elder, J. S. *et al.* Renal histological changes secondary to ureteropelvic junction obstruction. *J. Urol.* 1995; **154**(2 Pt 2): 719–722.
26. Stock, J. A., Krons, H. F., Hefferman, J. *et al.* Correlation of renal biopsy and radionuclide renal scan differential function in patients with unilateral ureteropelvic junction obstruction. *J. Urol.* 1995; **154**(2 Pt 2):716–718.
27. Amling, C. L., O'Hara, S. M., Werner, J. S. *et al.* Renal ultrasound changes after pyeloplasty in children with ureteropelvic junction obstruction: long-term outcome in 47 renal units. *J. Urol.* 1996; **156**(6):2020–2024.
28. Homsy, Y., Saad, F., Laberge, I. *et al.* Pyeloplasty: to divert or not to divert? *Urology* 1980; **16**(6):577–583.
29. Pesce, C., Campobasso, P., Costin, L. *et al.* Ureterovascular hydronephrosis in children: is pyeloplasty always necessary? *Eur. Urol.* 1999; **36**(1):71–4.
30. Rodrigues Netto, N. Jr., Ikari, O., Esteves, S. C., & D'Ancona, C. A. Antegrade endopyelotomy for pelvi-ureteric junction obstruction in children. *Br. J. Urol.* 1996; **78**(4):607–612.
31. Figenshau, R. S., Clayman, R. V., Colberg, J. W. *et al.* Pediatric endopyelotomy: the Washington University experience. *J. Urol.* 1996; **156**(6):2025–2030.
32. Capolicchio, G., Homsy, Y. L., Houle, A. M. *et al.* Long-term results of percutaneous endopyelotomy in the treatment of children with failed open pyeloplasty. *J. Urol.* 1997; **158**(4):1534–1537.
33. Yeung, C. K., Tam, Y. H., Sihoe, J. D. *et al.* Retroperitoneoscopic dismembered pyeloplasty for pelvi-ureteric junction obstruction in infants and children. *BJU Inte.* 2001; **87**(6):509–513.
34. Tan, H. L. Laparoscopic Anderson–Hynes dismembered pyeloplasty in children. *J. Urol.* 1999; **162**(3 Pt 2):1045–1047; discussion 1048.
35. Baskin, L. S., Zderic, S. A., Snyder, H. M., & Duckett, J. W. Primary dilated megaureter: long-term followup. *J. Urol.* 1994; **152**(2 Pt 2):618–621.
36. Liu, H. Y., Dhillon, H. K., Yeung, C. K. *et al.* Clinical outcome and management of prenatally diagnosed primary megaureters. *J. Urol.* 1994; **152**(2 Pt 2):614–617.
37. Cozzi, F., Madonna, L., Maggi, E. *et al.* Management of primary megaureter in infancy. *J. Pediatr. Surg.* 1993; **28**(8):1031–1033.
38. McLellan, D. L., Retik, A. B., Bauer, S. B. *et al.* Rate and predictors of spontaneous resolution of prenatally diagnosed primary nonrefluxing megaureter. *J. Urol.* 2002; **168**(5):2177–2180; discussion 2180.
39. Shenoy, M. U. & Rance, C. H. Is there a place for the insertion of a JJ stent as a temporizing procedure for symptomatic partial congenital vesico-ureteric junction obstruction in infancy? *BJU Int.* 1999; **84**(4):524–525.
40. Pfister, R. C. & Hendren, W. H. Primary megaureter in children and adults. Clinical and pathophysiologic features of 150 ureters. *Urology* 1978; **12**(2):160–176.
41. Kalicinski, Z. H., Kansy, J., Kotarbinska, B., & Joszt, W. Surgery of megaureters – modification of Hendren's operation. *J. Pediatr. Surg.* 1977; **12**(2):183–188.
42. Perdzynski, W. & Kalicinski, Z. H. Long-term results after megaureter folding in children. *J. Pediatr. Surg.* 1996; **31**(9): 1211–1217.
43. Starr, A. Ureteral plication. A new concept in ureteral tailoring for megaureter. *Invest. Urol.* 1979; **17**(2):153–158.
44. Bakker, H. H., Scholtmeijer, R. J., & Klopper, P. J. Comparison of 2 different tapering techniques in megaureters. *J. Urol.* 1988; **140**(5 Pt 2):1237–1239.
45. Ehrlich, R. M. The ureteral folding technique for megaureter surgery. *J. Urol.* 1985; **134**(4):668–670.

43

Posterior urethral valves

Peter M. Cuckow

Department of Paediatric Urology, Great Ormond Street Hospital, London, UK

Introduction

Posterior urethral valves are the commonest congenital obstruction of the lower urinary tract,[1] comprising 10% of antenatally diagnosed uropathies with an incidence of up to 1 in 4000.[2,3] This figure will rise if non-viable and terminated fetuses are included and as antenatal diagnosis is refined. Equally, there is a group of boys at the other end of the spectrum, whose lesser urethral obstruction produces no early urinary tract dilatation and who present late, even in adulthood with normal renal function and voiding difficulty.[4] The interpretation of this latter group accounts for much of the variation in incidence and the different spectrum of severity found in different series of valve patients.[4,5]

Posterior urethral obstruction more than any other urinary anomaly, has the capacity to affect the development and function of the whole urinary tract. Our understanding of this problem has evolved over the past decades and has included the identification, classification and treatment of the obstruction; recognition and management of the degrees and types of renal impairment that may be associated with it; the approach to associated vesicoureteric reflux and dilated upper urinary tracts; the function and development of the "valve bladder" (a central issue in our current thoughts about the long-term outcome of posterior urethral valves) and finally the impact on our practice of antenatal diagnosis and the opportunities that it offers not only in the identification but also in the early treatment of posterior urethral valves. With this growing experience and careful follow-up in some centres awareness of the long-term effects of posterior urethral valves has increased and factors in early life that influence them have been identified.[6–8]

Historical aspects

Young classified membranous urethral obstruction in 1919 after analysing clinical and postmortem cases and described three distinct types.[9] His type II are now discounted as non-obstructive folds of superficial muscle and mucosa, between the veru montanum and the bladder neck. The separate existence of types I and III valves has been called into question by careful postmortem dissection[10] and observation of uninstrumented valve urethras.[11] Urethral instrumentation changes the appearance of type III valves (perforated urethral membrane below the veru) to that of type I valves (coapting membranous folds attached to the veru posteriorly and extending to the membranous urethra with a posterior-based perforation) and that previously noted differences may be artefactual. The characteristics of this unified urethral valve are variable but include: attachment posteriorly to the distal part of the verumontanum; a small hole adjacent to the veru; an oblique membrane with the distal attachment lying anteriorly; paramedian parallel reinforcements; distal ballooning with suprapubic pressure; traversing the urethral sphincter.[12] The embryological origins may either be an abnormality of the müllerian duct system or remnants of the cloacal membrane, dating the appearance of the membrane at between the 7th and the 11th week of intrauterine life.[11,12] These revelations have not impacted on the management or clinical outcome of posterior urethral valves.

Pediatric Surgery and Urology: Long-term Outcomes, Mark Stringer, Keith Oldham, Pierre Mouriquand.
Published by Cambridge University Press.

Presentation, imaging, and initial management

Historically one-third of cases presented during the neonatal period, one-third between 1 month and 1 year and one-third over 1 year of age.[6,13,14] An increasing presentation during the neonatal period relates to a greater awareness of the condition, quite apart from antenatal diagnosis (see below).[1,15] The most severe cases may present in the puerperium with respiratory difficulties, limb deformities, Potter's fascies, and distended, palpable urinary tracts, reflecting their severe form of obstruction and oligohydramnios. Nakayama described respiratory insufficiency in 7 of 11 patients presenting within the first week of life. Three died of pulmonary hypoplasia and respiratory failure, a further 2 of renal failure after initial respiratory distress and all were related to oligohydramnios. Of six survivors, 2 required prolonged ventilation and 2 presented with bilateral pneumothoraces.[16] In neonates, obstructive symptoms (straining, poor stream, dribbling, palpable bladder) may be seen in 77% and renal failure predominates.[1,13,17]

Later symptoms and signs within the first year of life are related to (i) infection (septicaemic shock, poor feeding, abdominal pain, positive urine culture) in 78% of boys;[13] (ii) abdominal distension and dribbling in 40%; (iii) failure to thrive in 30%; (iv) palpable kidneys in 25%.[15] In toddlers renal failure becomes less common, voiding symptoms and infection predominate[1] with 50% of the over-fives presenting with enuresis and dribbling.[1,17] This later presentation, indicative of milder forms of valvular obstruction, may be delayed into adulthood.[4]

In common with other anomalies causing fetal urinary tract dilatation, posterior urethral valves are increasingly recognized by routine prenatal screening ultrasound[1–3,15,18,19] and currently 40%–50% of new patients present this way to major units in the UK.[2,18,19] The characteristic findings are bilateral hydronephrosis and a distended thickened bladder, although a dilated prostatic urethra can occasionally be seen. Low amniotic fluid volume and bright renal parenchyma (suggesting dysplasia) are important indicators of severity.[20] The diagnosis is usually only suggested prenatally and postnatal investigation provides confirmation.

Ultrasound is the first postnatal investigation and demonstrates hydroureteronephrosis, a thick-walled bladder and occasionally a dilated posterior urethra. Bright kidneys with loss of cortico-medullary differentiation suggest dysplasia.[21] Micturating cystourethrography provides the definitive diagnosis, however, and is performed via a urethral or suprapubic catheter. It demonstrates the bladder, confirms the urethral pathology and permits assessment of vesicoureteric reflux. Radioisotope renography with MAG3 can be performed after 1 month of age to provide information about renal function and drainage and, combined with indirect radionuclide cystography, is useful in long-term follow-up.[22]

It is an early priority to achieve adequate urine drainage with either a fine urethral catheter (5 to 8Fr infant feeding tube) or a suprapubic catheter. Attention is paid to the fluid, electrolyte, and acid–base balance, and intravenous broad spectrum antibiotics are administered to treat or prevent sepsis. In antenatal cases the initial serum creatinine is related to prenatal placental function and will rise over the next 48 hours to reflect baby's native renal function. Intensive early management usually results in stabilisation but rising creatinine, recurrent urinary infection or doubts over the efficacy of bladder drainage may prompt diversion, usually vesicostomy. Valve ablation is then performed once the child is stable.[8,13]

Mortality

Most early infant mortality in posterior urethral valves is related to pulmonary hypoplasia, a common but by no means inevitable consequence of maternal oligohydramnios probably preventing chest mobility and lung expansion in utero,[2,15,16] whose mortality is up to 63%.[16] Failure to recognize the underlying obstructive uropathy accounts for the previously hidden mortality of posterior urethral valves, which antenatal diagnosis is now revealing.[2,15,16]

Table 43.1 illustrates mortality from early reported series of posterior urethral valves.[1,14,15,17,23,24] It was almost 50% in the 1950s,[24] more than halved by the 1960s,[17,23] and fell to current levels of 0 to 3% for most pediatric urological centers in the 1970s.[1,15,17,25] Most mortality has occurred in boys less than 1 month old at presentation and is due to severe respiratory and/or renal failure, reflecting greater severity with early presentation. Improved mortality and morbidity over recent years is accredited to: (i) earlier diagnosis and referral to specialist pediatric urological centers, with significantly better renal function at initiation of management; (ii) improved instrumentation making management of the valves easier; (iii) improved pre- and post-operative management of the valve patient including intensive care of respiratory, fluid and electrolyte disturbances and the availability and use of more effective antibiotics; (iv) greater experience leading to improved care and the avoidance of unnecessary surgical procedures.[15] To this should be added the advances in the management of renal

Table 43.1. Mortality from early series of posterior urethral valves

Author date	Ellis 1966	Johnston 1971	Williams 1973	Cass 1974	Atwell 1983	Churchill 1983
Number of patients	29	62	172	113	108	207
Period of study	1947–1965	up to 1971	1956–1970	1950–1972	1970–1980	1957–1978
Follow-up			5 yrs 7 m mean	5.4yrs mean	2 to 10 years	
Overall mortality	48%	32%	16.2%	25%	7.4%	
<1 month	71%	50%	*included below*	52%	*included below*	37%
1–3 months	*included below*	*included below*	40.6% (<3 m)	*included below*	13.2%	*included below*
3 months–1 year	33%	27%	8.3%	37.5%	*included below*	13%
> 1 year	0%	17.4%	3.7%	5.5%	1.8%	3%
Early mortality (dates)	73% (<1961)		36% (1956–60) (under 1 yr)	44% (<1961)		25% (<1968)
Recent mortality (dates)	21% (>1961)		20% (1961–65) 15% (1966–70) 0% (>1971)	10% (>1962)		3% (>1968)

failure that allow many patients with severe compromise to survive to transplantation.[26]

Whilst most mortality is close to the first hospital admission, longer follow-up has shown up to 6.4% of boys die in chronic renal failure between 3 and 12 years after presentation.[7,8] Better early management will certainly result in increasing numbers of patients surviving to be recruited into renal replacement programs. Renal dialysis and transplantation themselves carry morbidity and mortality so life expectancy will be significantly reduced in many patients and will be defined when follow-up data extends to several decades.

The urethra

Valve ablation

Before the development of suitably small endoscopes there were many different approaches to infant valve ablation, with varying degrees of success.[27] Perineal urethrostomy was used for endoscopic valve resection fulguration in smaller patients (53% in D. I. Williams' series and in all infants below 5 kg in Scott's series).[13,14,17] The major complication of this was urethral stricture, seen in 19% of patients according to Churchill, and more rarely urethral diverticulum.[15] Williams tried two alternatives: rupturing the valve by sharp withdrawal of a Fogarty balloon catheter (successful in 9 of 10 patients but often associated with periurethral extravasation of urine[28]) and using an insulated crochet hook, developed further by Whitaker, that was passed blindly or with fluoroscopic control to catch the valve leaflets on withdrawal in its uninsulated crook so they could be diathermied.[17,29] Results of the latter technique compare favorably with neonatal endoscopic ablation.[30] Hendren operated on seven valves from above but three patients later suffered from stress incontinence.[4] Percutaneous endoscopic antegrade valve ablation was suggested by Zaontz, and Gibbons has also described endoscopic ablation through vesicostomies.[27] Vesicostomy also enables valve treatment to be deferred until urethral size permits endoscopic ablation.[31]

Better and more miniaturized instrumentation allows the majority of posterior urethral valves to be treated transurethrally. Repeat endoscopy may be required to check the efficacy of valve ablation as re-resection (in up to 11% of cases in Williams' series[17]) is preferable to stricturing or sphincter damage, through over aggressive diathermy. Strictures were reported in around 8% of patients,[17,32] related to the use of the resectoscope and a "dry" urethra when ablation and diversion are combined.[15,31,32] Nowadays, they are a rare occurrence through the use of small 7 to 9Fr cystoscopes and fine (3Fr) bugabee electrodes.[33] Nijman described increasing the size of the transurethral catheter stepwise from 5Fr to 8Fr prior to urethroscopy in small neonates. In his series of 85 patients there were no strictures but three patients had incontinence and one developed a small urethral diverticulum associated with valve ablation (a complication rate of 5%).[33] More precise valve destruction may be achieved by use of the laser.[27]

In the past the narrowing at the level of the bladder neck, seen above the dilated posterior urethra on cystogram, has been wrongly interpreted as obstructive.[14,17,24] Bladder neck incision or plasty was commonly performed (24% of D. I. Williams' patients[17]) until follow-up studies demonstrated the high rates of incontinence.[29]

Sexual function

Sexual function may be impaired due to a higher incidence of undescended testes (12% vs. 0.8% for the male population[34]), impaired function of the posterior urethra and ejaculatory mechanism and the effect of urethral surgery and renal failure on potency. Woodhouse reviewed 21 men aged 19 to 37 and found 20 capable of normal intercourse, 1 with poor erections after starting dialysis, and 1 impotent who was on long-term dialysis.[35] Half of the patients complained of dry or slow ejaculation but retrograde ejaculation was only confirmed in 1 of 7 patients, based on postejaculation urinalysis. All semen samples were fertile and 3 men had fathered children.[35]

The kidney and upper urinary tract

Renal function

Impairment of renal function is found in around 70% of boys at presentation[13,23] and over 80% of boys less than 3 months old.[13,23] After their initial management, 60% of patients recover normal biochemical renal function on short-term follow-up.[13] The glomerular filtration rate is a better predictor of outcome than serum creatinine levels and Scott found only 27% of patients with abnormal values recovered normal renal function at follow-up of up to 10 years.[13] In two studies, nadir serum creatinine levels below 0.8[36] or 1.0 mg%[37] during the first year of life have always been associated with a good outcome (5.8[36] and 6.8[37] years mean follow-up). With nadir levels greater than these 0%[36] to 33%[37] had normal renal function at follow-up. Lopes has more recently demonstrated that a GFR over 80 ml/min per 1.73m^2 at 1 year of age is invariably associated with good long-term renal function.[38]

Longer follow-up studies have shown that between 13 and 28% of patients are in end-stage renal disease between 10 and 15 years-follow-up.[6,8,13,15] Smith found the incidences of chronic and end-stage renal failure were 34% and 10%, respectively, at 10 years of age and 51% and 38% at 20 years of age[8] and using Kaplan–Meier graphs demonstrated a 5 year lag between them. End-stage renal disease peaks during the first year of life and again later in childhood or adolescence.[6,8,13] Parkhouse showed 26% of boys over the age of 18 years in chronic or end-stage renal failure and all but one of these had normal renal function earlier in childhood with a progression to renal failure from 6 to 14 years.[7]

The metanephros appears at 5 weeks' gestation and nephron development has advanced sufficiently for filtration and urine production by 10 weeks, around the time that posterior urethral valves appear.[39] While early renal impairment may be due to dysplasia and the effects of impaired urine flow in utero, factors influencing late progression may include ongoing urine flow impairment, pressure, vesicoureteric reflux, urine infection and hyperfiltration. In many patients these factors are exacerbated by abnormalities of the distal nephron producing a urine concentrating defect and increased urine production. Certainly, the relationship between bladder dysfunction and deteriorating renal function is well established (see below).[40,41]

Dysplasia

Renal dysplasia is a major developmental abnormality and its extent defines the functional potential of the affected kidney. Microscopic evidence of anomalous metanephric development is pathognomonic of dysplasia whose association with posterior urethral valves is well established, but the cause–effect relationship is poorly understood.[42] It may be a primary event, associated with the other anomalies of posterior urethral valves.[42] In the postmortem examination of 30 children with congenital urethral obstruction (27 posterior urethral valves and 3 urethral atresia) Cussen confirmed dysplasia histologically in 37% and it was always associated with ipsilateral reflux.[43] The clinical experience of Johnston and Hoover has also confirmed the coexistence of ipsilateral reflux and dysplasia in kidneys excised for non-function.[44,45] Henneberry and Stephens correlated histological findings in 22 renal units from boys with posterior urethral valves with the position of the ipsilateral ureteric orifice.[46] In this paper the severity of renal dysplasia increased the more lateral the ureteric orifice position, leading the authors to conclude that renal dysplasia is a primary developmental malformation, due to abnormal implantation of the ureteric bud into the metanephric blastema.[46]

Alternatively, Bernstein proposed that dysplasia represents the final expression of fetal renal injury secondary to the abnormal urodynamics of obstruction.[47] This contention is supported by animal work in which early unilateral ureteric obstruction in fetal lamb kidneys produced changes similar to dysplasia seen in the kidneys of a human fetus with urinary tract obstruction.[48] Whichever mechanism is responsible for dysplasia it is clearly an early embryological event that presents a fixed renal deficiency at birth. If the latter mechanism is true, then severity will be related to duration of obstruction (confirmed by prenatal findings[2]) and it is conceivable that its effects could be reduced by decompression before birth.

Reflux

Vesicoureteric reflux is found in between 37% and 67% of boys at diagnosis[14,15,17,23,44] and is more common in the younger patients.[15] Following valve ablation, complete or partial (unilateral) resolution occurs spontaneously in 27% to 55% of patients,[14,15,17,23,44] is also more likely in younger patients (57% of neonates, 44% of infants and 13% > 1 year[15]) and occurs regardless of initial management.[25] Johnston discovered increased mortality with bilateral reflux at diagnosis (57.1% bilateral reflux: 17.4% unilateral: 9% no reflux) which was greater below one month of age (67% bilateral: 20% unilateral: 14% no reflux).[44] Bilateral reflux is significantly associated with poor long-term outcomes (death in renal failure, end-stage or chronic renal failure) in 58% of boys at 11 to 22 years follow-up compared to 22% and 20% for unilateral and no reflux.[6] Reflux to a usefully functioning kidney usually resolves and persistent unilateral reflux is usually associated with non-function.[44,45] The persistence of reflux is also associated with continued bladder dysfunction, supported by the high resolution rate in patients whose urodynamic abnormality is treated with anticholinergics (see below).

Reimplantation for reflux is rarely indicated and management is either expectant or nephroureterectomy.[44] The effects of reflux include pyelonephritis, compromised detrusor and ureteric function, residual urine and high-pressure reflux.[25] Failure of reimplantation with recurrent reflux is reported in up to 67% of patients due to the abnormal valve bladder[23,49] but El Sherbiny *et al.* demonstrated greater success with the use of a psoas hitch.[50] The "STING" has been successfully applied to high-grade unilateral and bilateral reflux.[51] Whilst most kidneys excised for non-function have histological features of dysplasia,[44,45] a few, and all from one series,[52] are more in keeping with an acquired process of inflammation and scarring. Nephroureterectomy for reflux and unilateral non-function is reported in 14% of valve patients[19] and may also improve voiding dynamics by reducing the "false residual" urine.[45] Studies in patients with bilateral reflux demonstrate an inverse relationship between filling detrusor pressure and GFR.[7]

Persistent upper tract dilatation

Almost all infants presenting with posterior urethral valves have significant upper tract dilatation which, in the majority, improves spontaneously after transurethral valve ablation.[14,15,23,53] Where it persists or increases, there has been much debate over correct management, which has varied between complete early reconstruction with ureteric tapering and reimplantation[4] and a much more conservative approach.[8,13,15] Antegrade pressure perfusion studies have shown that true obstruction at the vesicoureteric junction is rare but ureteric drainage is impaired during bladder filling, emptying occurring when the bladder is empty.[53,54] At the same time it was observed that most patients also had polyuria and thickened non-compliant bladders which combination is termed the valve bladder syndrome by Mitchell, who saw it in 16% of severe cases[53] and this has later been confirmed by many authors.[55] Reimplantation in this circumstance leads to recurrent or even worsening upper tract dilatation, whose cause (the bladder and polyuria) had been overlooked.[14,54] Drainage improves spontaneously following valve ablation, even from severely affected systems,[56] and good results from early reconstruction may merely reflect this.[4,57]

Upper tract decompression with ureterostomy was initially used when primary valve ablation was not possible[17] or as a rescue maneuver for patients with severe dilatation, rising creatinine and sepsis.[14,17,58] The latter indication implies selection of a poor prognosis group and Rabinowitz found a high mortality (26%) with dysplasia at postmortem in 67% of cases[58] and Duckett found non-outcome benefit from secondary ureterostomy.[8] The early application of ureterostomy when upper tract dilatation did not improve in Toronto led to a report that renal function and somatic growth were better compared to undiverted patients, in spite of higher initial creatinine levels.[59] This retrospective uncontrolled study led to a general increase in the use of ureterostomy. Few authors have found a similar benefit to somatic growth[55] although most refute the findings[60,61] and subsequent uncontrolled studies have found no difference or worse outcome with ureterostomy.[8,61,62] Ghali used loop ureterostomies in patients with a high creatinine and persistent hydronephrosis after valve ablation and concluded that there was no significant difference in the progression to renal failure, compared with boys treated by primary valve resection alone. They also highlighted the increased surgical morbidity for the patient and suggested that antegrade contrast studies and nephrostomies could help identify the exceptional patients that might benefit.[63]

Vesicostomy may offer effective upper tract drainage in selected severe cases[60] and some have argued its routine use with delayed valve ablation.[31] The results of this are equivalent to series with predominantly primary endoscopic treatment and the price is also increased surgical procedures, so this approach seems hard to justify for most patients.[31]

Urine concentrating ability

Damage to the distal nephron due to increased intraluminal pressures causes impaired urine concentrating ability, polyuria and polydipsia (nephrogenic diabetes insipidus) which may or may not be associated with impaired glomerular function.[7] This increased urine output with an abnormal bladder worsens lower tract symptoms (incontinence) and promotes secondary renal damage. Dinneen studied urinary concentrating ability, urine production and glomerular filtration rates in 51 boys with valves aged 5.4 to 9.9 years.[64] 59% were unable to achieve urine concentrations greater than 800 mOsm overnight and following injection of DDAVP. There were significant ($P < 0.001$) correlations between concentrating ability and GFR and concentrating capacity and 24-hour urine volumes or overnight urine production.[64] Inability to conserve water leads to rapid dehydration with episodes of high fever or gastroenteritis in these boys and they commonly fail to thrive.[64]

Hyperfiltration

The normal response to a reduction in numbers of functioning nephrons, as in renal dysplasia, is to increase the amount of work done by individual nephrons (single nephron GFR) by a combination of nephron hypertrophy and hyperfiltration.[39] The latter is a result of vasodilatation of the afferent arterioles leading to an increase in the glomerular plasma flow and glomerular capillary hypertension. There is a disproportionate increase in glomerular filtration rate as the fraction of afferent blood filtered is increased, hence the term hyperfiltration. In time proteinuria and hypertension develop, coinciding with glomerulosclerosis and decreasing GFR.[65] There is some evidence that a low protein diet, with its reduced solute load, can delay this process,[58] although a recent prospective randomised trial of low protein diet failed to show any difference in the progression of renal failure in children.[66] Proteinuria at 5 years of age has been associated with a poor long-term outcome in 71% of cases followed between 11 and 22 years.[7]

Infection

Persistent urinary tract infection combined with dilated upper urinary tracts was associated with high morbidity and all late mortality in Williams' series.[17] Prophylactic antibiotics are mandatory, although the effect of chronically elevated bladder pressure alone may cause renal scarring with reflux, as demonstrated by animal studies.[67] Circumcision may be an important adjunct in the prevention of infection and some argue that it should be performed routinely at the time of valve resection. Thirteen boys with PUV at our hospital (of which 8 also had VUR) had suffered between two and five UTIs prior to circumcision – requiring between one and three inpatient treatment episodes. Those aged a mean of 8 months at the time of circumcision (mean of 8 months), (80%), suffered no further UTIs (follow-up of 2–17 years) or appeared less susceptible.[68]

The bladder

Continence

Bladder dysfunction, manifested as incontinence, is present in between 13% and 38% of patients following resection of posterior urethral valves.[1,6,13,17,23,29,69,70] Whitaker found only 29% of his 112 boys were fully continent at a mean age of 6.5 years[29] and, among those with previous bladder neck surgery, 88% had either complete or stress incontinence. The risk of incontinence seemed to increase with presentation in infancy for which greater deformation of the sphincter in this age group was blamed, whilst improvement at puberty was attributed to increased urethral resistance with prostatic growth. A postscript on this paper told of the dramatic improvement in five patients treated with imipramine and was the first suggestion of a primary bladder cause.[29] Later, Churchill showed how incontinence improved from 35% to 16% with the abandonment of bladder neck resection.[69]

Attainment of day and night-time continence is delayed in valve patients and was 19% at 5 years, 46% at 10 years and all except 1 at 20 years in Duckett's series.[8] Forty-five percent of 5-year-old boys were incontinent by day in Parkhouse's series and 46% of these had a bad long-term outcomes (death in renal failure, end-stage or chronic renal failure), compared with continent patients of whom only 4% had bad outcomes between 11 and 22 years.[6] The symptom of incontinence, manifesting underlying bladder dysfunction, is strongly related to both upper tract dilatation and poor long-term renal outcome.[37,71,72] Two cohort studies performed at Great Ormond Street Hospital of 42 (aged 1 month to 14 years)[7] and 51 (aged 6 to 9 years) boys[73] have both shown urodynamic abnormalities in 75% of valve patients.

Urodynamic studies

Bauer performed urodynamic studies on eight incontinent patients and described five patterns: normal; myogenic failure (no bladder contractions and voiding by abdominal straining with large residuals); high voiding pressures; uninhibited contractions and small capacity bladders.[74] Normal sphincter EMGs pointed to the bladder as the cause of incontinence. Peters assessed 41 patients urodynamically, of whom 35 were incontinent, and defined three predominant and overlapping abnormalities: (i) hypertonic, low compliance, small capacity bladder (11 patients, mean age 7 years) treated in 3 with anticholinergics and with augmentation in 3; (ii) hyper-reflexic bladder with uninhibited contractions during filling (10 patients, mean age 8.4 years) that appeared to improve with time. This was successfully managed by anticholinergics in 5 of 7 patients, intermittent catheterization in 2 and augmentation in 1; (iii) myogenic failure with overflow and Valsalva voiding (14 patients, mean age 12 years). These were treated by double or triple voiding in 4, α-blockade in 1, clean intermittent catheterization in 3 and bladder augmentation in 2.[71]

An apparent evolution in urodynamic abnormality with age, suggested by Peters' data, is also shown by Holmdahl who compared findings in pre- and postpubertal boys.[75] There was a decrease in instability and the strength of voiding contractions whilst bladder capacity and residual urine increased. Unstable poorly compliant, overdistended bladders changed towards decompensation with time and increased capacity after puberty was attributed to increased prostatic/urethral resistance.[75] Serial assessment of 16 babies during the first 3 years of life revealed initially hypercontractile low capacity bladders after valve ablation.[76] Hypercontractility vanished with time as capacity increased, whilst instability and incomplete bladder emptying remained and it is speculated that these patients later develop abnormalities seen in older age groups.[76] Several authors have since concurred with these findings.[77,78]

De Gennaro *et al.*[78] analysed serial pressure flow traces, comparing findings at 7 years of age to those at 12. Early features of detrusor instability compared to the later finding of impaired detrusor contractility: present in five of six patients studied after puberty. Of these five patients, three had significant residual urine volumes, increased bladder capacities and needed abdominal effort to void. Misseri *et al.* found less myogenic failure in their larger group of boys with urodynamic studies before and after 10 years of age[79] – only 3 of 51 cases and all 3 had started with poor compliance. Both authors agreed that treating bladder dysfunction with anticholinergics was a contributor to detrusor failure.[78,79]

The link between abnormal urodynamic parameters and deteriorating renal function has been illustrated by Lopes in 10-year-olds.[41] Of patients with normal renal function 51% had an abnormal urodynamic study and in 90% this was instability. In those with end-stage renal failure, there was a greater incidence of bladder dysfunction (68%) and poor compliance was more common than instability. Of the nine patients with poor compliance, eight were in end-stage failure, highlighting this as the most dangerous influence on long-term outcome.

Treatment

The wider adoption of urodynamic surveillance has led to increased identification of abnormal bladders and offers the opportunity for treatment and protection of renal function. Strategies include α blockers and double or triple voiding regimens to improve bladder emptying. Aggressive anticholinergic therapy to treat instability and poor compliance is advocated by many authors.[72] A catch is those patients (3 of 37 patients in Misseri's series) in whom reversible bladder failure may actually be precipitated by anticholinergic therapy.[79] Kim showed anticholinergics were effective in the management of incontinence in older boys (echoing Whitaker[29]) and also for resolution of persistent reflux.[80]

In patients with myogenic failure clean intermittent catheterization (CIC) has proved successful,[71,75] although there is normal urethral sensation and it may not be tolerated. Holmdahl *et al.* performed early urodynamic studies and commenced patients on CIC at a median 8 months of age if they had bladder dysfunction with features of poor emptying, high pressures, dilating reflux and renal impairment.[81] Follow-up at 8 years suggested an increase in the GFR and an improvement in both instability and compliance. Renal function deteriorated in the two boys who were not compliant with this regime, although there were no controls to determine the true contribution of catheterization to urodynamic improvement.

Abnormal urodynamic parameters and polyuria are a dangerous combination in many of these patients and no assessment is complete without consideration of 24 hour and particularly night-time urine output.[75] Ransley has advocated the use of a Mitrofanoff conduit for overnight drainage and as an alternative to urethral catheterization in selected patients.[82] Nocturnal urodynamic studies in small boys have shown an improvement in urodynamic parameters with more stable bladders, lower detrusor pressures and greater functional capacities compared to the daytime.[83]

Options for reconstruction include bladder augmentation with the addition of a Mitrofanoff conduit to enable catheterization and overnight drainage if required.[82] A review of 20 patients undergoing augmentation of poorly compliant, unstable bladders with low functional capacities has shown its potential in selected cases.[84] All patients were resistant to anticholinergic therapy and had high 24-hour urine outputs and abnormal GFRs. Augmentation was with ileum,[9] stomach,[7] colon,[2] and ureter[2] and 6 had a simultaneous Mitrofanoff conduit. Upper tract dilatation improved in 17 and stabilized in 3. Seventeen patients became dry day and night, 11 could void spontaneously to completion, 7 could void but catheterized to achieve satisfactory emptying and a further 2 were dependent on catheterization. Three patients required overnight drainage for extreme polyuria.[84]

The bladder after diversion

Duckett believed that the changes in bladder collagen brought about by infravesical obstruction, may heal if the bladder resumes its normal cycling function early.[60] This is best achieved by primary valve ablation and has resulted in better urodynamics and fewer augmentations in later life, whereas upper tract diversion predisposed to small contracted bladders that required later augmentation.[8,60] Certainly 13 patients of the 20 augmented at Great Ormond Street had prior upper diversions.[84] In contrast others have reported marginally better urodynamic and functional outcomes following vesicostomy or pyelostomy perhaps resulting from resting the bladder.[85] Many authors have studied the effect of upper tract diversion on long-term outcomes in recent years. Both Close and Podesta studied long-term bladder function in two groups of patients treated either by ureterostomies with delayed underversion and valve ablation or by primary valve ablation. Urodynamics revealed significant reductions in capacity and compliance and an increase in instability in the diverted groups.[61,62] Jaureguizar found no statistical differences in urodynamic indices following the two treatment strategies[86] and Laird advocated the technique of ureterostomy (in his case a Sober "en T") could preserve bladder cycling and thus long-term function after undiversion.[87] Although it is difficult to come to any firm conclusion about the impact of ureterostomies in the long term, they may represent a surgical challenge both to create and to close with multiple surgical procedures (59 in 6 patients reported by Pinto[88]), so perhaps for this reason they should be avoided. Vesicostomies may permit some bladder filling[60,89] and can be closed successfully with temporary suprapubic catheter drainage[73] making them the diversion of choice in severe cases. Until there is clear evidence to the contrary, there is a strong argument for the vast majority of cases of posterior urethral valves to be treated expectantly following valve ablation.[8,13,60,62]

"Pop off" mechanisms

Any mechanism providing release of pressure in utero may mitigate the effects of posterior urethral valves on the urinary tract. This is well illustrated by seven cases at Great Ormond Street with coexisting urethral duplication – 6 epispadic and 1 a Y-duplication.[90] They presented late with urinary tract infection (mean 5.5 years), urethroscopy confirmed posterior urethral valves and they were treated by valve resection followed by urethroplasty and excision of the duplicated urethra at a later stage. At follow-up (median of 7 years) all had normal renal function, 5 voided normally and in two voiding difficulties were related to coexistent neuropathic bladder.

Hoover and Duckett assessed 12 boys with persistent unilateral reflux into a non-functioning kidney, all had nephrectomy and dysplasia was confirmed in 10. Finding normal serum creatinine in 75%, they speculated that pressure dissipation into the dilated non-functioning upper tract ("pop off") protected the developing contralateral non-refluxing kidney, conferring "excellent" prognosis for renal function.[45] Greenfield described a similar group of patients with normal renal function in 6 of 8 with mean follow-up of 6 years but one 12-year-old was on hemodialysis.[52] The term VURD (valves ureteral reflux dysplasia) syndrome was coined.[91]

Other forms of "pop off" reported include urinary extravasation and huge bladder diverticula.[91] A group of 20 boys with a pop off (9 VURD, 5 large bladder diverticula, 6 urinary ascites or perinephric urinoma) aged 2½ to 8 years were compared with 51 boys presenting without a pop off. One child with a pop off had elevated serum creatinine compared to 39% of children without, of whom 7 (14%) required renal replacement.[91] Five cases with antenatal extravasation of urine (possibly offering an alternative circulation of urine within the body) all had a favorable outcome in terms of renal function.[92]

Twelve patients with the VURD syndrome (6.6% of the valve population) presented to Great Ormond Street in the 1980s. All had persistent unilateral reflux after valve ablation and had had a non-functioning dysplastic kidney removed.[93] Serum creatinine values were normal in 8 of 12 patients during the second year of life but in only 3 of 10 patients after 8 to 10 years' follow-up. In contrast, initial

GFR (during the second year of life in 10 patients) was in the normal range for only 3 of 12 and in 2 of 8 patients reassessed later (5 to 8 years of age). Longer follow-up and using GFR could not confirm preservation of renal function with the VURD syndrome in our patients. Patients with unilateral renal agenesis or nephrectomized in childhood have GFRs in the normal range when followed up to 40 years. None of the data from the VURD syndrome compares favorably with such a control group.[94]

Kaefer suggested a pressure "pop off" was a favorable prognostic sign for ultimate bladder function.[95] Of 63 patients, 71% had one or more (severe reflux, VURD, patent urachus, large diverticula or urinomas) and bladder outcome, judged by clinical and urodynamic parameters, was favorable in 87% at mean follow-up of 6.4 years. Favorable outcome occurred in 55% of bladders without pop off and, of the remainder, 71% had required bladder augmentation. Whitaker had previously noticed a higher rate of preoperative reflux in continent patients and suggested it was due to dissipation of intravesical pressure in utero.[29]

Antenatal diagnosis

Of 42 patients presenting to Great Ormond Street Hospital between 1987 and 1990, 10 (45%) were detected prenatally and 23 (55%) presented acutely within 6 months of birth. All mothers had prenatal scans but 21 of the 23 in whom the uropathy was missed were only scanned before 24 weeks' gestation. In contrast, 12 of the 14 scans performed after 24 weeks were diagnostic. Serum creatinine at presentation was significantly lower in the prenatal group than in patients presenting acutely postnatally and their renal outcomes, assessed at 1 year, were also better.[18] Another study found little outcome benefit from antenatal diagnosis and serum creatinine was higher at presentation in the antenatal group.[19] Reinberg found antenatal diagnosis was associated with a poor outlook. There was a higher incidence of renal failure at presentation (64% compared to 33% in postnatal patients) and progressive renal failure and transient pulmonary failure in 64%, although only high-risk mothers were screened in his population.[62] In both of the latter studies maternal oligohydramnios and postnatal pulmonary insufficiency were associated with poor renal outcome in 80%.[19,62] Hutton demonstrated that gestational age at detection is a predictor of outcome. 53% of patients detected at or before 24 weeks died or were in renal failure at a median follow-up of 3.9 years. Of those detected after 24 weeks only 1 of 11 patients had a poor outcome, whose initial scan at 18 weeks had been technically difficult.[2]

The above studies show that dilatation seen late in pregnancy or postnatally may have been absent on one or more previous scans, probably due to the incomplete nature of the obstruction. The prognosis in these cases is better[2,18] and it is argued that prenatal intervention is unlikely to affect outcome.[19,96] At the other end of the spectrum is a group of patients whose obstruction is complete, causing massive early dilatation, oligohydramnios, severe renal dysplasia and pulmonary hypoplasia with inevitable bad outcome.[82] In between these two groups are patients with lesser dysplasia that may benefit from early relief of the obstruction and increasing amniotic fluid volume by placement of vesicoamniotic shunts. It has been demonstrated in the lamb model of severe fetal nephropathy that pulmonary hypoplasia and renal dysplasia can be ameliorated by timely placement of a vesicoamniotic shunt.[97,98]

Dysplastic fetal kidneys cannot reabsorb sodium from the glomerular filtrate and maintain low urinary osmolarity relative to plasma and this enables their function and outlook to be assessed. Analysis of urine samples aspirated from the fetal bladder has established criteria for a good renal outcome (Na $<$ 100 meq/l, Cl $<$ 90 meq/l and osmolarity $<$ 210 mOsm/l).[99] However, cases are reported where both sonographic evidence of renal dysplasia and unfavorable urine biochemistry have been associated with good postnatal renal function.[100] In one study of 9 patients, 4 fetuses were assigned a poor prognosis after urine sampling. Although all 4 died (2 terminations) renal histology following one neonatal death revealed no evidence of renal dysplasia. Of the 5 fetuses with good predicted outcome, one was terminated and found to have dysplastic kidneys, 3 developed renal failure after birth and 1 is well.[101] The inclusion of other markers such as calcium and B_2 microglobulin has improved both the sensitivity (83%–91%) and specificity (77%–80%) for these tests.[102,103] Fetal urinary B_2 microglobulin levels were the best predictor of renal function during the second year of life in 42 surviving children of 100 prenatally diagnosed uropathies[103] and levels above 13 mg/l have invariably been associated with a fatal outcome.[104]

Results of 57 reported interventions for fetal obstructive uropathy, including 21 vesicoamniotic shunt placements, were reviewed by Elder. There were complications in 44%, including incorrect shunt placement (19%), premature labour (12%), urinary ascites (7%) and chorioamnionitis (5%). Of the patients with associated oligohydramnios 79% died in spite of intervention.[96] A report from the International Fetal Surgery Registry in 1986 included 73 patients in whom vesicoamniotic shunts were placed for fetal obstructive uropathy.[105] Sixty-nine patients required between 2 and 7 attempts at shunt placement, procedure related mortality was 4.8% and 77% of patients with confirmed posterior urethral valves survived.[105]

The San Francisco group retrospectively reviewed 40 fetuses referred for assessment and possible treatment of fetal uropathy.[20] Each was assigned to a good prognosis group if the urine was hypotonic (Na < 100 meq/l, Cl < 90 meq/l and osmolarity < 210 mOsm/l) and ultrasound suggested no dysplasia and to a poor prognosis group if all these criteria were not met. There was a significant difference in outcome between the two groups (87% vs. 30% mortality excluding abortions). Survival was greater in 17 patients selected for intervention for both prognostic groups. All 3 survivors from the poor prognosis group had undergone intervention (11 of 14 untreated fetuses were terminated) and 2 of the 3 subsequently went into renal failure. Amniotic fluid volume was restored in 9 of 17 fetuses with shunting, saving them from respiratory complications.[20] Retrospective analysis of 55 patients presenting for antenatal assessment identified 13 patients with posterior urethral valves.[106] Seven fetuses had urinary electrolytes suggesting a good prognosis. 2 were lost with chorioamnionitis (1 after shunting) and of the remaining 5 all were shunted: 3 had normal renal function, it was mildly impaired in 1 and another had renal failure. Five of the 6 fetuses assessed with poor prognosis died: 2 terminations, 3 pulmonary hypoplasia (2 with a shunt and 1 without), 1 survivor in renal failure after shunting. The authors claimed outcomes for the survivors similar to postnatally presenting patients.[106] Many urologists, however, remained sceptical about the conclusions drawn from this retrospective study.[106] Holmes has subsequently reviewed the results of the whole San Francisco experience of posterior urethral valve interventions.[107] Of 14 fetuses 11 had interventions (six shunts, two bladder marsupializations, two in utero valve ablations and one ureterostomy) and six died (five of premature labour and respiratory failure and one was terminated). Of eight patients followed up to 11 years, five were in chronic or end-stage renal failure and five had urinary diversion. The authors concluded that intervention may not alter prognosis and that the sequelae of the valve diagnosis were not preventable by these interventions. Clarke's meta-analysis also failed to come to any firm conclusions and, in the absence of a prospective trial, it will be hard to rationalize this approach.[108] Freedman found similarly high mortality and three of four survivors required bladder reconstruction.[109]

Possible future interventions include fetal cystoscopy and in utero treatment of the valves[110] and amnioinfusion to allow normal pulmonary development, successful in a fetus with bilateral renal agenesis.[111] Given future advances in renal replacement therapy, the latter theoretically offers a means of salvaging some of the severe cases. Welsh reported cystoscopy in 13 fetuses, for which ten had an intervention (four hydroablation of valves ± nine guide wire ablations).[112] Posterior urethral valves were seen in four of nine cases with postnatal confirmation and they claimed "therapeutic success" in six of ten cases.

Enthusiasm for prenatal intervention is tempered, however, by the difficulty of making an early diagnosis, problems with shunt placement, a high complication rate and fetal loss and an inability to demonstrate benefit over postnatal management alone. The challenge is to identify the patients who will benefit most (probably through fetal urine sampling[102–104]), time intervention correctly (as early as possible) and design a study to assess its efficacy (a prospective randomized trial?).[82] In the meantime, prenatal diagnosis is useful to predict outcome, plan prompt postnatal management in a specialized centre and to enable counseling of parents.[3,102]

Management of renal failure and renal replacement

Advances in the management of chronic renal failure include management of growth and nutrition, and dialysis and transplantation in increasingly younger patients. Reduction of GFR below 25% of the expected means dialysis and transplantation, so management is directed at delaying this as long as possible.

Chronic renal failure profoundly effects somatic growth with most patients below the third percentile for height, weight, and head circumference.[2,113] Treatment strategies include: monitoring fluid and electrolyte balance, particularly potassium and magnesium homeostasis; oral bicarbonate reduced dietary protein to correct chronic metabolic acidosis; low solute high volume formulas to compensate for polyuria; monitoring serum calcium, phosphate and parathormone levels, treating hyperphosphatemia by reduced oral intake and phosphate binders and avoiding aluminium intoxication; treating renal bone disease with activated vitamin D supplements.[113] Administration of recombinant human growth hormone is an effective adjunct in the management of growth retardation.[114]

Dialysis is usually peritoneal via a surgically placed cuffed catheter with hemodialysis via a dual lumen central line reserved for acute situations or where the peritoneum is unavailable. The mortality of infant dialysis is 16%[115] and complications of peritoneal dialysis include peritonitis and protein loss in the dialysate. Ellis reviewed peritoneal dialysis in 21 infants less than 1 year old (starting weight 3.6 ± 1.6 kg) after a mean 10 months. Mortality was 43% but there

Table 43.2. Indicators of prognosis in posterior urethral valves

Age group	Indicator	% poor outcome (follow-up)
Prenatal	Early (<24 week) presentation	53% (3.9yrs)[1]
	Oligohydramnios	80%[2,3]
	B2 microglobulin in fetal urine >13 mg/l	100%[4]
Postnatal	Presentation < 1 month	42%(11–22yrs)[5]
	Bilateral reflux	58%(11–22yrs)[5,6]
1 year of age	Nadir creatinine level > 1.0 mg%	70–100%(6–7yrs)[7,8]
	Glomerular filtration rate	73%(10yrs)[6]
	GFR > 80 ml/min per 1.73 m^2	0% (no renal failure)[9]
5 years of age	Daytime incontinence	46%(11–22yrs)[5]
	Proteinuria	71%(11–22yrs)[5]
10 years of age	Urodynamics	89%[10]
	Poor compliance	67%[10]
	Myogenic failure	23%[10]
	Instability	

1. Hutton, K. A., Thomas, D. F., Arthur, R. J. *et al.* Prenatally detected posterior urethral valves: is gestational age at detection a predictor of outcome? *J. Urol.* 1994; **152**(2):698–701.
2. Reinberg, Y., D. I. & Gonzalez, R. Prognosis for patients with prenatally diagnosed posterior urethral valves. *J. Urol.* 1992; **148**(1):125–126.
3. Jee, L. D., Rickwood, A. M., & Turnock, R. R. Posterior urethral valves. Does prenatal diagnosis influence prognosis? [see comments]. *Br. J. Urol.* 1993; **72**(5):830–833.
4. Lipitz, S., Ryan, G., Samuell, C. *et al.* Fetal urine analysis for the assessment of renal function in obstructive uropathy. *Am. J. Obst. Gynecol.* 1993; **168**(1):174–179.
5. Parkhouse, H. F., Barrett, T. M., Dillon, M. J. *et al.* Long-term outcome of boys with posterior urethral valves. *Br. J. Urol.* 1988; **62**(1):59–62.
6. Scott, J. E. Management of congenital posterior urethral valves. *Br. J. Urol.* 1985; **57**(1):71–77.
7. Connor, J. P. & Burbige, K. A. Long-term urinary continence and renal function in neonates with posterior urethral valves. *J. Urol.* 1990; **144**(5):1209–1211.
8. Warshaw, B. L., Hymes, L. C., Trulock, T. S., & Woodard, J. R. Prognostic features in infants with obstructive uropathy due to posterior urethral valves. *J. Urol.* 1985; **133**(2):240–243.
9. Lopez, Pereira P., M. J., Martinez Urritina, L., Espinosa, *et al.* Posterior urethral valves: prognostic factors. 2003; **91**(7):687–690.
10. Lopez, P. Pereira, M. J., Espinosa, L., Martinez Urritina *et al.* Bladder dysfunction as a prognostic factor in patients with posterior urethral valves. 2002; **90**(3):308–311.

were associated non-renal abnormalities and oliguria in all these nine cases. Of the remainder, four continued to be dialysed and seven had been successfully transplanted.[26]

Comparing results of transplantation in 18 valve patients with 18 with reflux nephropathy and 36 matched controls showed no difference in patient survival, although 5-year graft survival was 50% in the valve patients vs. 73% and 75% in the other two groups.[116] Graft function is also significantly worse in the valve group[116] and urinary infection may be more common. Salomon reported 44 boys with surviving grafts and divided them into two groups dependent on the presence or absence of voiding dysfunction. The mean plasma creatinines were significantly different: 285 and 140, respectively, at 10 years, pointing again to the valve bladder.[117] Reported graft survival rates are 70% at 5 years and 63% at 10 years,[118] no different from the transplant population and our results mirror these.[119] The valve bladder undoubtedly has a role in the function of renal transplants and should be assessed preoperatively with urodynamics to consider augmentation (1 of 7 patients at Great Ormond Street).[119] It is possible, given normal urine volumes after transplantation, that many bladders improve significantly, although postoperative bladder dysfunction has been seen in up to 13% of patients.[118] Excellent results are reported from patients following bladder reconstruction and augmentation prior to transplantation.[120]

Conclusions

Posterior urethral valves are responsible for a constellation of complications throughout the urinary tract whose interaction will determine the long-term outcome for each individual. Today's long-term results are based on the treatment strategies of the 1970s and it will be another 20 years before we see if the significant advances in our understanding have led to any improvement in outcome. Comparison of data from different centers is hampered by differences in their valve populations and local bias in determining treatment, whose efficacy has always been assessed retrospectively. Few if any prospective studies have been performed, although in controversial areas like temporary diversion and fetal intervention they offer the only chance of clarification.

It is clear, however, that dysplasia is a fixed renal deficit, present at birth, whose outcome can only marginally be improved by postnatal management but may possibly be influenced in the future by prenatal intervention. Up to 50% of valve patients have developed renal impairment later in life, regardless of their chosen method of management, and certain criteria have been established to determine those in whom a poor long-term outcome is likely (Table 43.2). The diagnosis of posterior urethral valves implies a commitment to long-term follow-up, with early identification and treatment of bladder dysfunction in particular. Better early management of these patients has increased the number entering renal replacement programs and requires an integrated team approach from obstetricians, pediatricians and nephrologists as well as pediatric urologists.

REFERENCES

1. Atwell, J. D. Posterior urethral valves in the British Isles: a multicenter B. A. P. S. review. *J. Pediatr. Surg* 1983; **18**(1):70–74.
2. Hutton, K. A., Thomas, D. F., Arthur, R. J. *et al.* Prenatally detected posterior urethral valves: is gestational age at detection a predictor of outcome? *J. Urol.* 1994.
3. Thomas, D. F. M. & Gordon, A. C. Management of prenatally diagnosed uropathies. *Arch. Dis. Child.* 1989; **64**:58–63.
4. Hendren, W. H. Posterior urethral valves in boys. A broad clinical spectrum. *J. Urol.* 1971; **106**(2):298–307.
5. Pieretti, R. V. The mild end of the clinical spectrum of posterior urethral valves. *J. Pediatr. Surg.* 1993; **28**(5):701–704.
6. Parkhouse, H. F., Barrett, T. M., Dillon, M. J. *et al.* Long-term outcome of boys with posterior urethral valves. *Br. J. Urol.* 1988; **62**(1):59–62.
7. Parkhouse, H. F. & Woodhouse, C. R. Long-term status of patients with posterior urethral valves. *Urol. Clin. North Am.* 1990; **17**(2):373–378.
8. Smith, G. H., Canning, D. A., Schulman, S. L. *et al.* The long-term outcome of posterior urethral valves treated with primary valve ablation and observation. *J. Urol.* 1996; **155**(5):1730–1734.
9. Young, H. H. & Frantz, W. A. Congenital obstruction of the posterior urethra. *J. Urol.* 1919; **3**:289–365.
10. Robertson, W. B. & Hayes, J. A. Congenital diaphragmatic obstruction of the male posterior urethra. *Br. J. Urol.* 1969; **41**:592–598.
11. Dewan, P. A., Zappala, S. M., Ransley, P. G., & Duffy, P. G. Endoscopic reappraisal of the morphology of congenital obstruction of the posterior urethra. *Br. J. Urol.* 1992; **70**(4):439–444.
12. Dewan, P. A., Ansell, J. S., & Duckett J. W. Congenital obstruction of the male urethra. *Dialogues Pediatr. Urol.* 1995; **18**(8): 6–9.
13. Scott, J. E. Management of congenital posterior urethral valves. *Br. J. Urol.* 1985; **57**(1):71–77.
14. Johnston, J. H. & Kulatilake, A. E. The sequelae of posterior urethral valves. *Br. J. Urol.* 1971; **43**(6):743–748.
15. Churchill, B. M., Fleisher, M. H., Krueger, R. *et al.* Posterior urethral valve management. *Dialogues Pediatr. Urol.* 1983; **6**(6):1–8.
16. Nakayama, D., Harrison, M. R., & deLorimer, A. A. Prognosis of posterior urethral valves presenting at birth. *J. Pediatr. Surg.*, 1986; **21**(1):43–45.
17. Williams, D. I., Whitaker, R. H., Barratt, T. M., & Keeton, J. E. Urethral valves. *Br. J. Urol.* 1973; **45**:200–210.
18. Dinneen, M. D., Dhillon, H. K., Ward, H. C. *et al.* Antenatal diagnosis of posterior urethral valves [see comments]. *Br. J. Urol.* 1993; **72**(3):364–369.
19. Jee, L. D., Rickwood, A. M., & Turnock, R. R. Posterior urethral valves. Does prenatal diagnosis influence prognosis? [see comments]. *Br. J. Urol.* 1993; **72**(5):830–833.
20. Crombleholme, T. M., Harrison, M. R., Golbus, M. S. *et al.* Fetal intervention in obstructive uropathy: prognostic indicators and efficacy of intervention. *Am. J. Obst. Gynecol.* 1990; **162**(5):1239–1244.
21. Cremin, B. J. & Aaronson, I. A. Ultrasonic diagnosis of posterior urethral valve in neonates. *Br. J. Radiol.*, 1983; **56**(667):435–438.
22. Dinneen, M. D., Duffy, P. G., Lythgoe, M. F. *et al.* Mercaptoacetyltriglycine (MAG 3) renography and indirect radionuclide cystography in posterior urethral valves. *Br. J. Urol.* 1994; **74**(6):785–789.
23. Cass, A. S. & Stephens, F. D. Posterior urethral valves: diagnosis and management. *J. Urol.* 1974; **112**(4):519–525.
24. Ellis, D. G., Fonkalsrud, E. W., & Smith, J. P. Congenital posterior urethral valves. *J. Urol.* 1966; **95**(4):549–554.
25. Churchill, B. M., McLorie, G. A., Khoury, A. E. *et al.* Emergency treatment and long-term follow-up of posterior urethral valves. [Review]. *Urol. Clin. North Am.* 1990; **17**(2):343–360.
26. Ellis, E. N., Pearson, D., Champion, B., & Wood, E. G. *et al.* Outcome of infants on chronic peritoneal dialysis. *Adv. Peritoneal Dialysis* 1995; **11**:266–269.
27. Zaontz, R. *et al.* Posterior urethral valves: Update on treatment modalities. *Dialogues Pediatr. Urol.* 1988; **11**(3).
28. Diamond, D. A. & Ransley, P. G. Fogarty balloon catheter ablation of neonatal posterior urethral valves. *J. Urol.* 1987; **137**(6):1209–1211.
29. Whitaker, R. H., Keeton, J. E., & Williams, D. I. Posterior urethral valves: a study of urinary control after operation. *J. Urol.* 1972; **108**:167–171.
30. Deane, A. M., Whitaker, R. H., & Sherwood, T. Diathermy hook ablation of posterior urethral valves in neonates and infants. *Br. J. Urol.* 1988; **62**(6):593–594.
31. Walker, R. D. & Padron, M. The management of posterior urethral valves by initial vesicostomy and delayed valve ablation. *J. Urol.* 1990; **144**(5):1212–1214.
32. Crooks, K. K. Urethral strictures following transurethral resection of posterior urethral valves. *J. Urol.* 1982; **127**(6):1153–1154.
33. Nijman, R. J. & Scholtmeijer, R. J. Complications of transurethral electro-incision of posterior urethral valves. *Br. J. Urol.* 1991; **67**(3):324–326.
34. Krueger, R. P., Hardy, B. E., & Churchill, B. M. Cryptorchidism in boys with posterior urethral valves. *J. Urol.* 1980; **124**(1):101–102.
35. Woodhouse, C. R., Reilly, J. M., & Bahadur, G. Sexual function and fertility in patients treated for posterior urethral valves. *J. Urol.* 1989; **142**:586–588.
36. Warshaw, B. L., Hymes, L. C., Trulock, T. S., & Woodard, J. R. Prognostic features in infants with obstructive uropathy due to posterior urethral valves. *J. Urol.* 1985; **133**(2):240–243.

37. Connor, J. P. & Burbige, K. A. Long-term urinary continence and renal function in neonates with posterior urethral valves. *J. Urol.* 1990; **144**(5):1209–1211.
38. Lopez, Pereira, P., Espinosa, L., Martinez Urrutina, M. J. *et al.* Posterior urethral valves: prognostic factors. 2003; **91**(7):687–690.
39. Chevalier, R. L. Developmental renal physiology of the low birth weight pre-term newborn. *J. Urol.* 1996; **156**:714–719.
40. Ghanem, M. A., Wolffenbuttel, K. P., De Vylder, A., & Nijman, R. J. Long-term bladder dysfunction and renal function in boys with posterior urethral valves based on urodynamic findings. 2004. **171**(6 Pt 1):2409–2412.
41. Lopez, Pereira, P., Martinez Urritina, M. J., Espinosa, L. *et al.* Bladder dysfunction as a prognostic factor in patients with posterior urethral valves. 2002. **90**(3):308–311.
42. Milliken, L. D. & Hodgson, N. B. Renal dysplasia and urethral valves. *J. Urol.* 1972; **108**:960–962.
43. Cussen, L. J. Cystic kidneys in children with congenital urethral obstruction. 1971; **106**(6):939–941.
44. Johnston, J. H. Vesicoureteric reflux in children with posterior urethral valves. *Br. J. Urol.* 1979; **51**:100–104.
45. Hoover, D. L. & Duckett, J. J. Posterior urethral valves, unilateral reflux and renal dysplasia: a syndrome. *J. Urol.* 1982; **128**(5):994–997.
46. Henneberry, M. O. & Stephens, F. D. Renal hypoplasia and dysplasia in infants with posterior urethral valves. *J. Urol.* 1980; **123**(6):912–915.
47. Bernstein, J. Developmental abnormalities of the renal parenchyma – renal hypoplasia and dysplasia. *Pathol. Ann.* **1968**(3):213–247.
48. Beck, A. D. The effect of intra-uterine urinary obstruction upon the development of the fetal kidney. *J. Urol.* 1971; **105**:784.
49. Tejani, A., Butt, K., Glassberg, K. *et al.* Predictors of eventual end stage renal disease in children with posterior urethral valves. *J. Urol.* 1986; **136**(4):857–860.
50. El Sherbiny, M. T., Hafez, A. T., Ghoneim, M. A., & Greenfield, S. P. Ureteroneocystostomy in children with posterior urethral valves: indications and outcome. 2002; **168**(4 Pt 2):1836–1839.
51. Puri, P. & Kumar, R. Endoscopic correction of vesicoureteral reflux secondary to posterior urethral valves. *J. Urol.* 1996.
52. Greenfield, S. P., Hensle, T. W., Berdon, W. E., & Wigger, H. J. Unilateral vesicoureteral reflux and unilateral nonfunctioning kidney associated with posterior urethral valves–a syndrome? *J. Urol.* 1983; **130**(4):733–738.
53. Glassberg, K. I., *et al.* Persistent ureteral dilatation following valve resection. *Dialogues Pediatr. Urol.* 1982; **5**(4).
54. Whitaker, R. H. The ureter in posterior urethral valves. *Br. J. Urol.* 1973; **45**(4):395–403.
55. Glassberg, K. I. Posterior urethral valves: lessons learned over time. 2003; **13**(4):325–327.
56. Noe, H. N. & Jerkins, G. R. Oliguria and renal failure following decompression of the bladder in children with posterior urethral valves. *J. Urol.* 1983; **129**(3):595–597.
57. Decter, R. M., *et al.* The challenge of the thick walled bladder. *Dialogues Pediatr. Urol.* 1990; **13**(8).
58. Rabinowitz, R., Barkin, M., Schillinger, J. F. *et al.* Upper tract management when posterior urethral valve ablation is insufficient. *J. Urol.* 1979; **122**(3):370–372.
59. Krueger, R. P., Hardy, B. E., & Churchill, B. M. Growth in boys and posterior urethral valves. Primary valve resection vs upper tract diversion. *Urol. Clin. North Am.* 1980; **7**(2):265–272.
60. Duckett, J. W. Are valve bladders congenital or iatrogenic? *Br. J. Urol.* 1997; **79**:271–275.
61. Close, C. E., Carr, M. C., Burns, M. W., & Mitchell, M. E. Lower urinary tract changes after early valve ablation in neonates and infants: is early diversion warranted? 1997; **157**(3):984–988.
62. Reinberg, Y., C. I. de & Gonzalez, R. Influence of initial therapy on progression of renal failure and body growth in children with posterior urethral valves. *J. Urol.* 1992; **148**:532–533.
63. Ghali, A. M., El Malki, T., Sheir, K. Z. *et al.* Posterior urethral valves with persistent high serum creatinine: the value of percutaneous nephrostomy. 2000; **164**(4):1340–1344.
64. Dinneen, M. D., Duffy, P. G., Barratt, T. M., & Ransley, P. G. Persistent polyuria after posterior urethral valves. *Br. J. Urol.* 1995; **75**(2):236–240.
65. Brenner, B. M., Meyer, T. W., & Hostetter, T. H. Dietary protein intake and the progressive nature of kidney disease: the role of hemodynamically mediated glomerular injury in the pathogenesis of progressive glomerular sclerosis in aging, renal ablation and intrinsic renal disease. *N. Engl. J. Med.* 1982; **307**:652–660.
66. Kist-vanHolthe-tot-Echten, J. E., Nanta, J., Hop, W. C. *et al.* Protein restriction in chronic renal failure. *Arch. Dis. Child.* 1993; **68**:371–375.
67. Ransley, P. G., Risdon, R. A., & Godley, M. L. High pressure sterile vesicoureteric reflux and renal scarring: an experimental study in the pig and minipig. *Contrib. Nephrol.* 1984; **39**:320.
68. Thiruchelvam, N. & Cuckow, P. M. The role of circumcision in posterior urethral valves. *Br. J. Urol. Int.* 2005; **95**:453–454.
69. Churchill, B. M., Krueger, R. P., Fleisher, M. H., & Hardy, B. E. Complications of posterior urethral valve surgery and their prevention. *Urol. Clin. North Am.* 1983; **10**(3):519–530.
70. Kurth, K. H., Alleman, E. R., & Schroder, F. H. Major and minor complications of posterior urethral valves. *J. Urol.* 1981; **126**(4):517–519.
71. Peters, C. A., Bolkier, M., Bauer, S. B. *et al.* The urodynamic consequences of posterior urethral valves. *J. Urol.* 1990; **144**(1):122–126.
72. Glassberg, K. I. The valve bladder syndrome: 20 years later. *J. Urol.* 2001; **166**(4):1406–1414.
73. Dinneen, M. D. & Duffy, P. G. Posterior urethral valves. [Review]. *Br. J. Urol.* 1996; **78**(2):275–281.
74. Bauer, S. B., Dieppa, R. A., Labib, K., & Retik, A. B. The bladder in boys with posterior urethral valves: a urodynamic assessment. *J. Urol.* 1979; **121**(6):769–773.

75. Holmdahl, G., Sillen, U., Harrison, E. *et al.* Bladder dysfunction in boys with posterior urethral valves before and after puberty. *J. Urol.* 1996; **155**(2):694–698.
76. Holmdahl, G., Sillen, U., Bachelard, M. *et al.* The changing urodynamic pattern in valve bladders during infancy. *J. Urol.* 1995; **153**(2):463–467.
77. Woodhouse, C. R. The fate of the abnormal bladder in adolescence. *J. Urol.* 2001; **166**(6):2396–2400.
78. De Gennaro, M., Capitanucci, M. L., Silven, M. *et al.* Detrusor hypocontractility evolution in boys with posterior urethral valves detected by pressure flow analysis. *J. Urol.* 2001; **165**(6 Pt 2):2248–2252.
79. Misseri, R., Combs, A. J., Horowitz, M. *et al.* Myogenic failure in posterior urethral valve disease: real or imagined? *J. Urol.* 2002; **168**(4 Pt 2):1844–1848.
80. Kim, Y. H., Horowitz, M., Combs, A. J. *et al.* Management of posterior urethral valves on the basis of urodynamic findings. *JK. Urol.* 1997; **158**(3 Pt 2):1011–1016.
81. Holmdahl, G., Sillen, U., Hellstrom, A. L. *et al.* Does treatment with clean intermittent catheterization in boys with posterior urethral valves affect bladder and renal function? *J. Urol.* 2003; **170**(4 Pt 2):1681–1685.
82. Ransley, P. G. Posterior urethral valves: an essay in honour and memory of Herbert Ecstein. In Williams, D. I. & Etker, S., eds *Contemporary Issues in Pediatric Urology in Memoriam Herbert B. Ecstein.* Istanbul: Logos, 1996: 51–55.
83. Holmdahl, G., Sillen, U., Bertilsson, M. *et al.* Natural filling cystometry in small boys with posterior urethral valves: unstable valve bladders become stable during sleep. *J. Urol.* 1997; **158**(3 Pt 2):1017–1021.
84. Kajbafzadeh, A. M., Quinn, F. M., Duffy, P. G., & Ransley, P. G. Augmentation cystoplasty in boys with posterior urethral valves. *J. Urol.* 1995.
85. Kim, Y. H., Horowitz, M., Combs, A. *et al.* Comparative urodynamic findings after primary valve ablation, vesicostomy or proximal diversion. *J. Urol.* 1996; 156:673–676.
86. Jaureguizar, E., Lopez Pereira, P., Martimez Urritia, M. J. *et al.* Does neonatal pyeloureterostomy worsen bladder function in children with posterior urethral valves? *J. Urol.* 2000; **164**(3 Pt 2):1031–1033.
87. Liard, A., Seguier-Lipszyc, E., & Mitrofanoff, P. Temporary high diversion for posterior urethral valves. *J. Urol.* 2000; **164**(1):145–148.
88. Pinto, M. H., Markland, C., & Fraley, E. E. Posterior urethral valves managed by cutaneous ureterostomy with subsequent ureteral reconstruction. *J. Urol.* 1978; **119**(5):696–698.
89. Cendron, M., *et al.* Discussion: temporary cutaneous urinary diversion in children. *Dialogues Pediatr. Urol.* 1995; **18**(12).
90. Quinn, F. M. J. *et al.* Urethral duplication in children with posterior urethral valves. In *Eurpean Society of Paediatric Urology.* London, 1996.
91. Rittenberg, M. H., Hulbert, W. C., & Snyder, H. M. 3rd. Protective factors in posterior urethral valves. *J. Urol.* 1988; **140**(5):993–996.
92. Greenfield, S. P., Hensle, T. W., Berdon, W. E., & Geringer, A. M. Urinary extravasation in the newborn male with posterior urethral valves. *J. Pediatr. Surg.* 1982; **17**(6):751–756.
93. Cuckow, P. M., Dinneen, M. D., Risdon, R. A. *et al.* Long-term renal function in the posterior urethral valves, unilateral reflux and renal dysplasia syndrome. *J. Urol.* 1997; **158**(3 Pt 2):1004–1007.
94. Wikstad, I., Celsi, G., Larsson, L. *et al.* Kidney function in adults born with unilateral renal agenesis or nephrectomized in childhood. *J. Urol.* 1988; **2**(2):177–182.
95. Kaefer, M., Keating, M. A., Adams, M. C., & Rink, R. C. *et al.* Posterior urethral valves, pressure pop-offs and bladder function. *J. Urol.* 1995; **154**:708–711.
96. Elder, J. S., Duckett, J. W., & Snyder, H. M. Intervention for fetal obstructive uropathy: has it been effective? *Lancet* 1987; **2**:1007–1010.
97. Harrison, M. R., Nakayama, D. K., & Noall, R. Correction of congenital hydronephrosis in utero II. Decompression reverses the effect of obstruction on the fetal lung and urinary tract. *J. Pediatr. Surg.* 1982; **17**:965–974.
98. Glick, P. L., Harrison, M. R., & Adzick, N. S. Correction of congenital hydronephrosis in utero IV. In utero decompression prevents renal dysplasia. *J. Pediatr. Surg.* 1987; **19**:649–657.
99. Golbus, M. S., Tilly, R. A., Callen, P. W. *et al.* Fetal urinary tract obstruction: management and selection for treatment. *Semin. Perinatol.* 1985; **9**:91.
100. Silver, R. K., *et al.* Fetal posterior urethral valve syndrome: a prospective application of antenatal prognostic criteria. *Obst. Gynecol.* 1990.
101. Wilkins, I. A., Chitkara, U., Lynch, L. *et al.* The non predictive value of urinary electrolytes: preliminary report of outcomes and correlations with pathologic diagnosis. *Am. J. Obst. Gynecol.* 1987; **157**(3):694–698.
102. Nicolaides, K. H., Cheng, H. H., Snijder, R. J., & Moniz, C. F. Fetal urine biochemistry in the assessment of obstructive uropathy. *Am. J. Obst. Gynecol.* 1992; **166**(3):932–937.
103. Muller, F., Dommergues, M., Mandelbrot, L. *et al.* Fetal urinary biochemistry predicts postnatal renal function in children with bilateral obstructive uropathies. *Obst. Gynecol.* 1993; **82**(5):813–820.
104. Lipitz, S., Ryan, E., Samuell, C. *et al.* Fetal urine analysis for the assessment of renal function in obstructive uropathy. *Am. J. Obst. Gynecol.* 1993; **168**(1):174–179.
105. Manning, F., Harrison, M. R., & Rodeck, C. Catheter shunts for fetal hydronephrosis and hydrocephalus. Report of the International Fetal Surgery Registry. *N. Engl. J. Med.* 1986; **315**(5):337–340.
106. Freedman, A. L., Vates, T. S., Stewart, T. *et al.* Fetal therapy for obstructive uropathy: specific outcomes diagnosis. *J. Urol.* 1996.
107. Holmes, N., Harrison, M. R., & Baskin, L. S. Fetal surgery for posterior urethral valves: long-term postnatal outcomes. 2001; **108**(1): E7.

108. Clark, T. J., Martin, W. L., Divakaran, T. G. *et al.* Prenatal bladder drainage in the management of fetal lower urinary tract obstruction: a systematic review and meta-analysis. *Obstet. Gynecol.* 2003; **102**(2):367–382.
109. Freedman, A. L., Johnson, M. P., Smith, C. A. *et al.* Long-term outcome in children after antenatal intervention for obstructive uropathies. *Lancet* 1999; **354**(9176):374–377.
110. Quintero, R. A., Johnson, M. P., & Romero, R. In-utero percutaneous cystoscopy in the management of posterior urethral valves. *Lancet* 1995; **346**:537–540.
111. Cameron, D., Lupton, B. A., Farquharson, D., Hiruki, T. Amnioinfusions in renal agenesis. *Obst. Gynecol.* 1994; **83**(5):872–876.
112. Welsh, A., Agarwal, S., Kumar, S. *et al.* Fetal cystoscopy in the management of fetal obstructive uropathy: experience in a single European centre. *Prenat. Diagn.* 2003; **23**(13):1033–1041.
113. Seldman, A., Friedman, A., Boinean, F. *et al.* Nutritional management of the child with mild to moderate chronic renal failure. *J. Pediatr.*, 1996; **129**(2):p. s13–s18.
114. Fine, R. N. Recombinant human growth hormone in dialysis patients: update 1995. *Adv. Peritoneal Dialysis*, 1995; **11**:261–265.
115. Bunchman, T. E. Chronic dialysis in the infant less than 1 year of age. *Pediatr. Nephrol.* 1995; **9**(suppl.):s18–s22.
116. Reinberg, Y., Gonzalez, R., Fryd., D. *et al.* The outcome of renal transplantation in children with posterior urethral valves. *J. Urol.* 1988; **140**(6):1491–1493.
117. Salomon, L., Fontaine, E., Guest, G. *et al.* Role of the bladder in delayed failure of kidney transplants in boys with posterior urethral valves. *J. Urol.* 2000; **163**(4):1282–1285.
118. Connolly, J. A., Miller, B., & Bretan, P. N. Renal transplantation in patients with posterior urethral valves: favorable long-term outcome. *J. Urol.* 1995; **154**(3):1153–1155.
119. Dinneen, M. D., Fitzpatrick, M. M., Godley, M. L. *et al.* Renal transplantation in young boys with posterior urethral valves: preliminary report. *Br. J. Urol.* 1993; **72**(3):359–363.
120. McLorie, G. A., *et al.* Outcome of renal transplantation in patients with posterior urethral valves – does bladder reconstruction provide benefit? In *European Society of Paediatric Urology*. London, 1996.

44a

Vesicoureteric reflux: definition and conservative management

Judith H. van der Voort and Kate Verrier Jones

Department of Paediatric Nephrology, University of Wales College of Medicine, Cardiff, UK

Introduction

Vesicoureteric reflux is important because of the association with recurrent urinary tract infection and congenital renal problems and the tendency for renal scarring to develop in some cases. Much of the early data were derived from postmortem material but, in the last 30 years, cases have been identified during life as a result of radiological investigation of children following urinary tract infection and, more recently, because of antenatal screening or family history. Since the advent of antibiotics, the natural history of reflux, urinary tract infection and renal scarring has improved considerably and now it is very rare for a child or young adult to die from urinary tract infection or acute pyelonephritis. Although the prevalence of reflux nephropathy appears to be falling, this remains an important cause of end-stage renal failure in both children and adults. There are interesting differences in natural history and clinical presentation between boys and girls.

Historical aspects

The valvular nature of the vesicoureteric junction was recognized in medieval times, when the pig bladder, filled with water, was used as a football and ligation of the ureters was found to be unnecessary. In the seventeenth century, pathologists observed at post mortem examination that urine flow from bladder to ureters did not normally occur in humans. The role of vesicoureteric reflux as a host factor, causing and maintaining urinary tract infection, was proposed 100 years ago by Sampson.[1] Hodson and Edwards[2] linked vesicoureteric reflux with progressive renal damage by assessing radiological studies carried out in children with recurrent urinary tract infections. Following this and other reports linking vesicoureteric reflux with dilatation of the urinary tract, incomplete bladder emptying, urinary tract infection, and renal damage, it was postulated that surgical correction of covert outflow obstruction by urethral stretching might be beneficial. This approach remained popular for several decades but the long-term benefit has been questioned, and it is rarely carried out now as there is no evidence to support the hypothesis or practice. Subsequently, vesicoureteric reflux was thought to be a congenital abnormality due to incompetence of the ureterovesical valve and attention focused on the vesicoureteric junction. This chapter deals mainly with the natural history and medical management of children with primary vesicoureteric reflux and its sequelae.

Definitions

Vesicoureteric reflux

Vesicoureteric reflux is defined as the retrograde flow of urine from the bladder into the ureter, sometimes extending up into the kidneys. Primary reflux refers to the situation where there are no major, predisposing, anatomical abnormalities. It is thought to be due to a minor structural anomaly or immaturity of the vesicoureteric orifice possibly related to the protein structure within the tissues. Secondary vesicoureteric reflux is associated with outlet obstruction, for example, posterior urethral valves or a neuropathic bladder. In both situations reflux can be unilateral or bilateral.

Pediatric Surgery and Urology: Long-term Outcomes, Mark Stringer, Keith Oldham, Pierre Mouriquand.

Reflux nephropathy

Reflux nephropathy refers to the focal renal scarring seen at one time fairly commonly at postmortem in individuals with recurrent, acute pyelonephritis and vesicoureteric reflux. Wedge-shaped scars can be seen macroscopically as depressed, shrunken fibrosed areas with a characteristic histological appearance. More recently, with the use of antenatal ultrasound scanning, a condition sometimes named "fetal reflux nephropathy" has been recognised. This refers to the renal dysplasia associated with vesicoureteric reflux, present from birth and more common in males.[3] There is ample evidence to demonstrate the development of the classic radiological wedge-like appearance of scars following recurrent infection during childhood, particularly when there are delays in making the diagnosis or starting treatment.[4] Reflux is present in around 50%–80% of these cases.

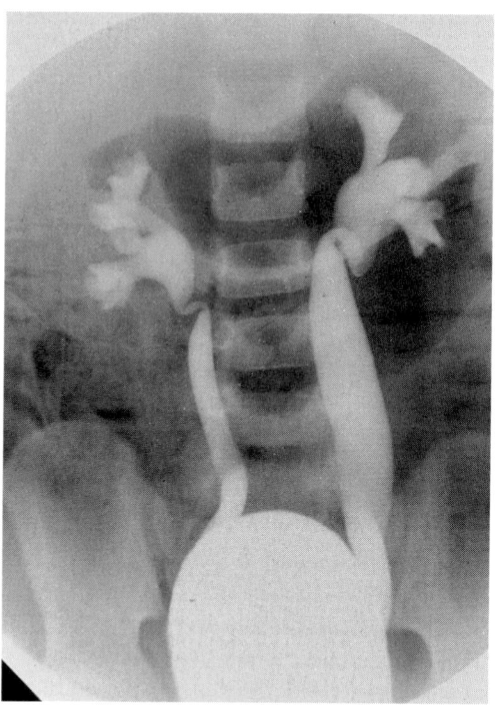

Fig. 44a.1. Micturating cystogram showing bilateral grade 3 vesicoureteric reflux.

Diagnosis and presentation

Reflux is a silent condition in so far as it rarely gives rise to symptoms unless there is some complicating factor such as infection or impaired renal function. It cannot be detected or even suspected by physical examination or by a simple test. Most reflux is detected after radiological screening tests in infants after a urinary tract infection or when diagnosed with hydronephrosis antenatally. Older children with recurrent urinary tract infections and renal scarring also have reflux in a third of cases.[5]

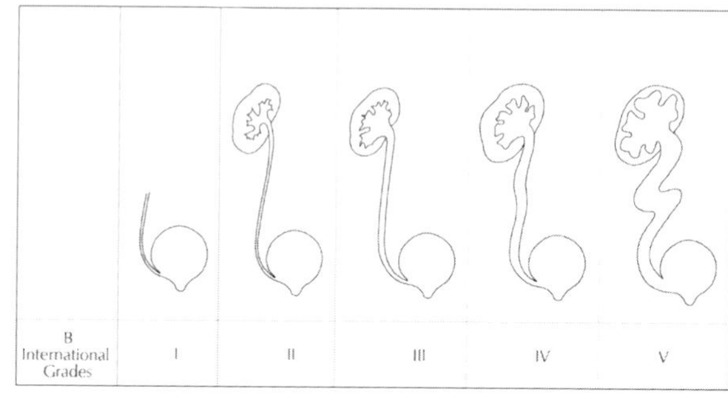

Fig. 44a.2. International reflux grading system shows grades 1 to 5. Grade 1 represents reflux into the lower, undilated ureter, grade 2 indicates reflux up to a non-dilated renal pelvis, grade 3 indicates reflux into a mildly dilated renal pelvis, while grades 4 and 5 represent reflux into grossly dilated systems.

Imaging for reflux

The gold standard for diagnosing vesicoureteric reflux in infants and young children is the micturating cystourethrogram, which gives information about the anatomy of the renal tract as well as the severity of the reflux (Fig. 44a.1). Many centers now use the method and grading system (I to V) described by the International Reflux Study Group (Fig. 44a.2).[6] Intrarenal reflux is defined as the presence of contrast medium in the renal parenchyma during cystography. It is only seen in infants with severe reflux and is almost invariably associated with reflux nephropathy.[7]

Other imaging tests for vesicoureteric reflux

Vesicoureteric reflux can also be diagnosed by indirect cystography using ^{99m}Tc DTPA or MAG3 (Fig. 44a.3.)[8] Vesicoureteric reflux is sometimes, but not always, associated with dilatation of the renal pelvis or ureter visible on ultrasound (Fig. 44a.4). Moderate and severe vesicoureteric reflux can be missed with ultrasound examination and therefore ultrasound cannot be used to exclude reflux. The use of air enhanced sonographic contrast has enabled dynamic studies to detect vesicoureteric reflux

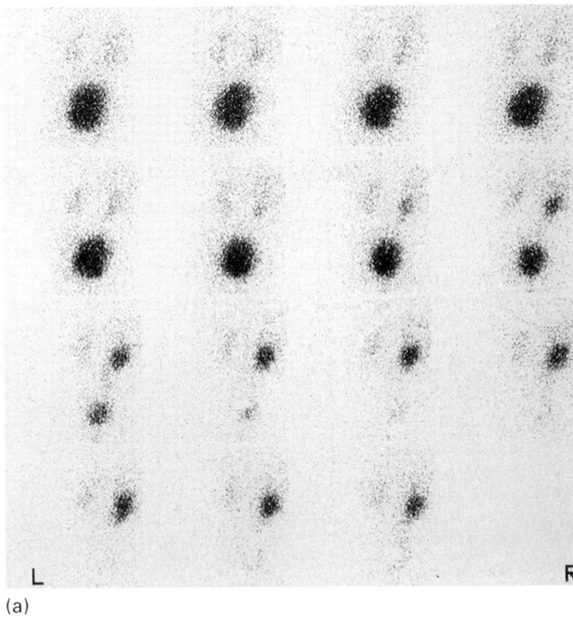

(a)

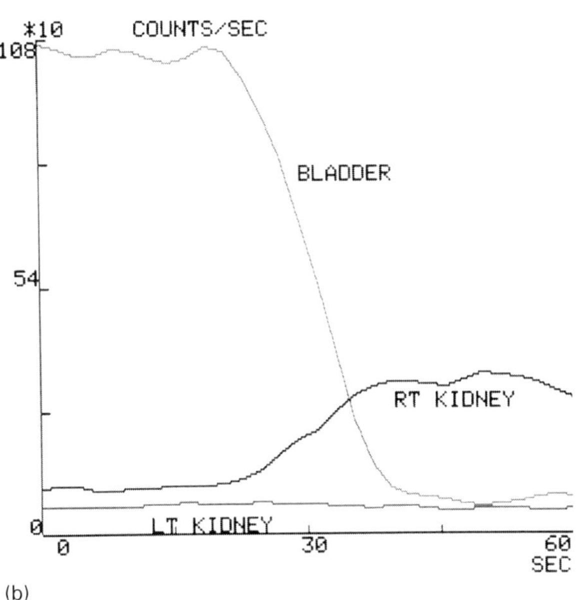

(b)

Fig. 44a.3. MAG 3 Indirect cystogram showing: (a) a sequence of images during micturition. As the count over the bladder falls the count over the right kidney rises; (b) a graph showing the above relationship against time.

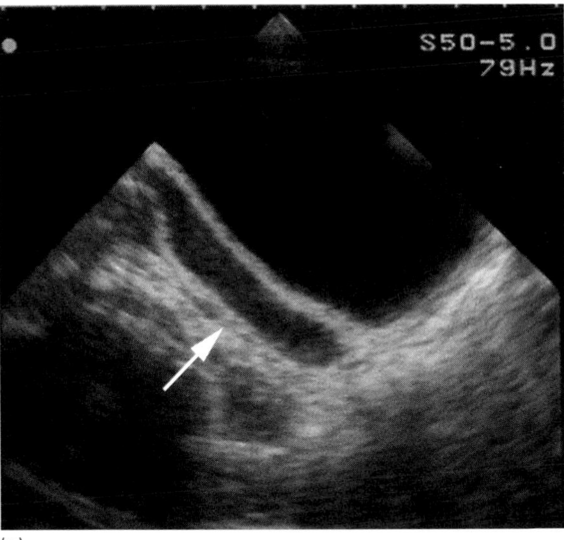

(a)

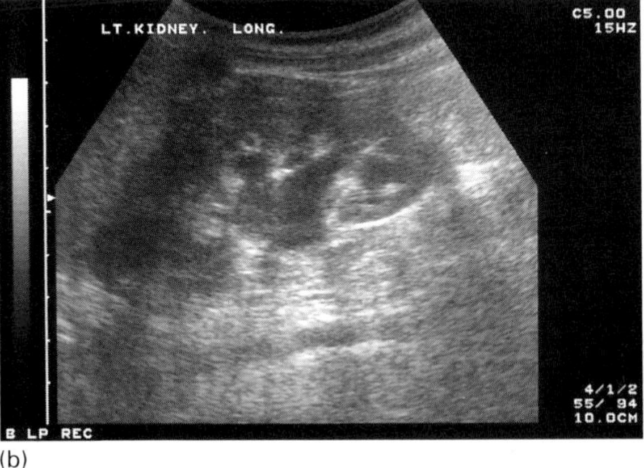

(b)

Fig. 44a.4. Ultrasound scan showing: (a) a dilated ureter below the bladder; (b) a kidney with a dilated renal pelvis from the same child who had recurrent urinary tract infections and VUR.

using ultrasound but this has not been used routinely in clinical practice yet. Similarly, MRI scanning with contrast has been used successfully as a research tool. Although these methods do not involve radiation, they still require bladder catheterization and therefore do not represent a major advance on conventional tests.

Radiological features of reflux nephropathy

Originally, the diagnosis of reflux nephropathy was made using intravenous urography, but the high risk of allergic reactions and the relatively large dose of radiation involved has resulted in a shift towards newer alternative techniques using isotopes or ultrasound.

Intravenous urography

The radiological features were described by Hodson and Edwards,[2] showing areas of cortical thinning overlying clubbed calices. The normal caliceal shape with sharp points due to indentation by renal papillae is lost. These characteristic focal scars occur most often at the upper

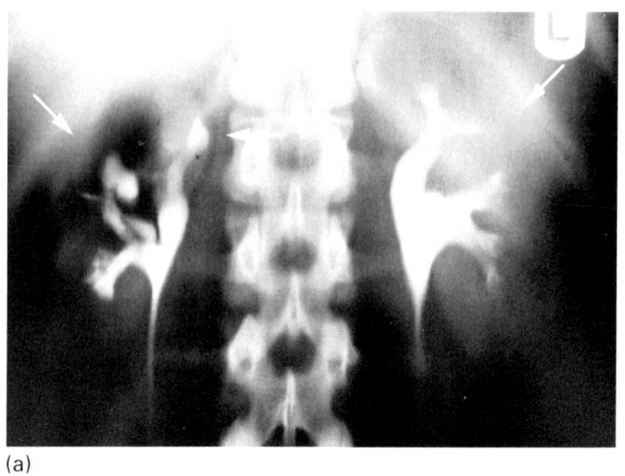
(a)

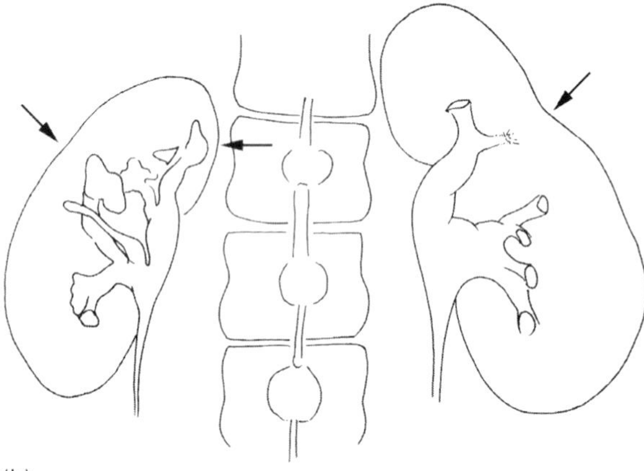
(b)

Fig. 44a.5. Intravenous pyelogram ((a) tomogram, (b) line drawing) showing cortical thinning overlying clubbed calices and reduced renal length on the right.

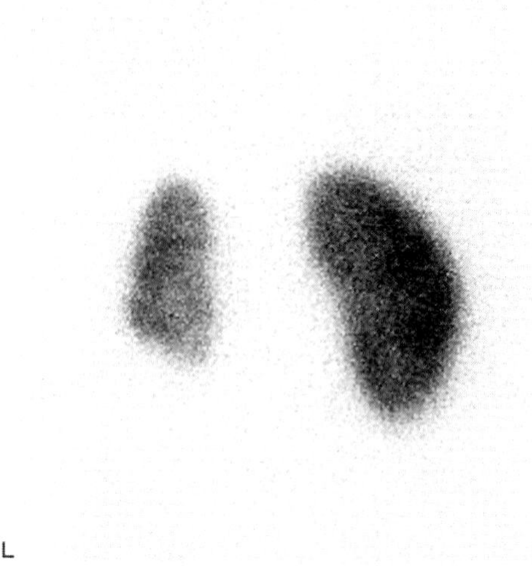

Fig. 44a.6. DMSA isotope scan showing reduced function and focal scarring on the left.

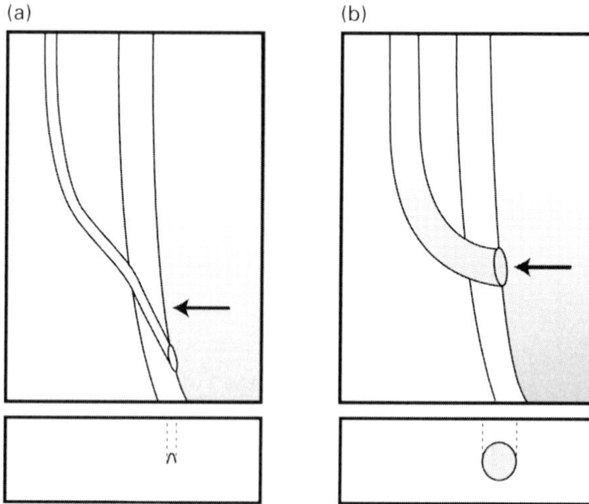

Fig. 44a.7. Diagram to show the insertion of the ureter into the bladder: (a) normal ureter, narrow diameter, entering obliquely through the bladder wall, the view from within the bladder (below) is a crescentic slit; (b) a refluxing dilated ureter with gaping orifice, below.

and lower poles or at the mid-lateral border (Fig. 44a.5). Less commonly there is a small smooth kidney with relatively well-preserved calices, sometimes described as globally scarred.

^{99m}Tc DMSA scan

This is now the preferred test for the detection of renal scarring; however, results are not entirely comparable to the traditional pyelogram. Affected areas of cortex are recognized as areas of poor isotope fixation (Fig. 44a.6). Acute pyelonephritis causes transient changes, which are often indistinguishable from the permanent changes seen with reflux nephropathy. The test must therefore be carried out at least 3 months after resolution of any infection if it is used to assess renal scarring. Permanent renal scarring develops at sites identified during acute infection. It is a very sensitive test and appears to detect some scars that are not seen at intravenous urography or on ultrasound. The DMSA scans in neonates with high grade congenital vesicoureteric reflux often show a reduction in tracer uptake without focal scarring present, sometimes referred to as global scarring or renal hypoplasia. In clinical practice it is often impossible to distinguish between congenital renal hypoplasia and acquired focal scarring.

Ultrasound

Ultrasound is a simple, non-invasive test, which is widely used as a first-line screening test in the investigation of children with renal disease of all types. Unfortunately, it is insensitive in the detection of both vesicoureteric reflux and scarring. Although the clinical significance of minor scars missed on ultrasound scanning is not known and may not be important, there is anecdotal evidence of significant vesicoureteric reflux and scarring having been missed in some cases.[9] Ultrasound is most useful for the exclusion of obstruction and to confirm the presence and normal position of the kidneys. Size can be easily measured; significantly scarred kidneys tend to be smaller than normal kidneys but may not always fall outside the centiles. Acute infection tends to cause swelling and therefore renal measurements and assessment of renal growth should be interpreted with caution.[10]

Etiology of vesicoureteric reflux and reflux nephropathy

Ureterovesical junction

In normal children the competence of the ureterovesical junction is achieved by the relatively long, intramural portion of the ureter, which is compressed during micturition, acting as a valve and preventing the retrograde passage of urine up the ureters as the bladder fills or empties. A shortened submucosal tunnel is associated with lateral displacement of the ureteric opening and an increased risk of vesicoureteric reflux.[11] The length of the intravesical ureter increases with age, resulting in the spontaneous resolution of reflux with time in many cases. The precise reason for this is unknown; however, observations on the dominant inheritance pattern in some families and the quest to identify the gene may give further clues in the foreseeable future.

Reflux and renal scarring

The causal relationship between renal scarring and vesicoureteric reflux is complex and at times the evidence appears conflicting. Scarring sometimes occurs without the presence of vesicoureteric reflux and vesicoureteric reflux can be present without causing scars. The third factor in this equation is urinary tract infection, which is more common in children with both vesicoureteric reflux and scarring.

Bladder sphincter dysfunction and detrusor instability can contribute to reflux. In patients with neurogenic bladders, detrusor contraction against a closed bladder neck creates high bladder pressure, which can cause dilatation of the urinary tract and distortion of the ureteric orifice. This gives rise to secondary reflux and predisposes to inadequate bladder emptying. The use of oxybutinin, an anticholinergic agent has been associated with resolution of symptoms such as incontinence as well as vesicoureteric reflux in children with unstable bladders.[12]

Hodson first showed that reflux was involved in the pathogenesis of renal scarring in studies in children after urinary tract infection.[2] Sterile scar formation was reported in infants with intra-renal reflux but there is a possibility that cystography under high pressure contributed to renal damage.[7]

Ransley and Risdon showed in their experiments that the combination of reflux, intrarenal reflux, and infection could rapidly cause renal scarring in pigs.[13] In later experiments they demonstrated that the early introduction of antibiotics reduced the extent of the damage. They showed that scars developed at the site of compound papillae, which allowed the retrograde passage of infected urine into the collecting ducts.

Prevalence

Prevalence of vesicoureteric reflux

Vesicoureteric reflux is not usually present in humans; the estimated incidence in infants is 2%.[14] There is a biphasic distribution of age at diagnosis of vesicoureteric reflux in children related to the mode of presentation. The first group is recognized following investigation for antenatal hydronephrosis or after genetic counselling. Anderson, Allan, and Abbott (2004) showed that fluctuations in the size of renal pelvis detected antenatally were very strongly associated with vesicoureteric reflux.[15] The antenatal hydronephrosis group is predominantly male, while those diagnosed because of family history show no gender predominance. Neonatal vesicoureteric reflux resolved or improved in 76% of patients by 4 years and the prevalence of vesicoureteric reflux in siblings of index cases also improved over time.[16]

The second group is diagnosed later, after a urinary tract infection and is predominantly female. Infants with antenatally diagnosed hydronephrosis have a diagnosis of vesicoureteric reflux in between 10% and 30%.[17] The prevalence of vesicoureteric reflux ascertained by radiological investigation in children after a diagnosis of urinary tract infection is around 30% in contrast to around 5% of adults.[2,18,1920] The incidence of vesicoureteric reflux amongst black children with urinary tract infection in

America and Africa was only 9%.[21] This may explain the observation that the incidence of urinary tract infection is also lower in black children.

Wettergren found reflux in 10% of asymptomatic infants with bacteriuria in a prospective study near Gothenberg.[22] In contrast, the presence of reflux in a third of schoolgirls with asymptomatic bacteriuria was similar to the prevalence in symptomatic girls.[23] In both these studies vesicoureteric reflux resolved or improved spontaneously.

Smellie followed children with grade III or IV vesicoureteric reflux prospectively for 10 years. A continuing reduction in the severity of the vesicoureteric reflux was observed and based on the negative findings of two consecutive cystograms, vesicoureteric reflux was absent in half of the children four years later.[24] In the long-term follow-up studies from Lenaghan (1972) vesicoureteric reflux disappeared in only 42% of patients, with younger age having a greater chance of cessation and dilatation of ureter reducing this chance.[25] In the Birmingham and International reflux studies the resolution rate was 9% to 15% per year.[26,27] Mild reflux is more likely to resolve or improve than severe reflux.[28] Neonatal reflux associated with prenatally diagnosed hydronephrosis has a high resolution rate, with 76% resolution or improvement in one series.[17]

Prospective screening studies of both siblings and offspring of patients with vesicoureteric reflux showed a prevalence of reflux amongst siblings which varied between 32 and 66%.[29,30] The most severe reflux was found in children less than 2 years of age. Most of these patients were asymptomatic and had no history of abnormal voiding or symptoms of urinary tract infection. Renal scarring was found in 15% of asymptomatic siblings.[31,32] This high rate of transmission from parents to child is consistent with an autosomal dominant mode of inheritance.[14] In some families with reflux there is an association with renal dysplasia, duplex systems, and other congenital renal anomalies.

In two recent studies, involving 99 children with vesicoureteric reflux diagnosed after detection of antenatal hydronephrosis, damage was present from birth and modification of vesicoureteric reflux did not affect renal function. Vesicoureteric reflux improved or resolved spontaneously and this was associated with a low urinary tract infection rate.[3,17] In several studies using conventional imaging techniques, reflux was found in the majority of children with renal scarring.[5,33] More recently, using ^{99m}Tc DMSA, Rushton *et al.*[34] found several children with changes on isotope studies that suggested scarring not accompanied by reflux. It is not clear to what extent the studies using this newer technique are comparable to the original studies with radio-opaque contrast media, which were generally carried out following recurrent urinary tract infections. In schoolgirls with asymptomatic bacteriuria, renal scarring was present in 25% of the study population and reflux was present in 33%. Half of the cases of reflux also had scarring and two thirds of those with renal scarring had vesicoureteric reflux.[23]

It is now recognized that reflux and both focal and global renal damage can be present from birth without recurrent urine infections, particularly males.[35]

Prevalence of scarring

In a large retrospective study, Merrick *et al.* found that the risk of progressive renal damage in a group of children investigated after urinary tract infection was increased 17 times in the presence of vesicoureteric reflux and renal scarring. If either reflux or scarring was present, subsequent urinary tract infection was associated with a similar increase in risk.[8] In their studies, vesicoureteric reflux was an important risk factor, principally when associated with further infection, except in boys under 1 year of age.[36] Reflux has been detected in 60%–85% of children with scarred kidneys.[5,37] In recent studies, renal scarring is present in 10% of patients with acute urinary tract infection, but higher rates of renal scarring were detected in some of the earlier studies and in studies of asymptomatic bacteriuria. This suggests either that management has improved or that cases are now detected earlier, before scarring has developed. The incidence of renal scarring in children with infection and reflux is significantly higher than in children with urinary tract infection generally and has been estimated to be 30%–50% of this population.

Urinary tract infection

The relationship between urinary tract infection, vesicoureteric reflux, and reflux nephropathy is important since these conditions when combined may cause new or progressive renal damage.[38,39] Detailed discussion of urinary tract infection is outside the scope of this chapter.

Recurrent infections occur most often in girls and tend to decrease with time in many cases. In boys, recurrent infections occur mainly in infancy, soon after the presenting infection.[40] It is not clear whether this is due to improvement and eventual disappearance of reflux with time[28] or due to the natural history of urinary tract infection in response to changes in other host factors with increasing age, including the natural improvement of vesicoureteric reflux with time. Following surgical correction of reflux, there is little change in the risk of developing recurrent infection although there is a reduction in the number of episodes of acute pyelonephritis.[26,41]

Iatrogenic infections can occur after catheterization or surgery, when bacteria are introduced into the urinary tract inadvertently and the normal defences are overcome.[42] Disruption of the urothelium and its mucous lining also contribute to the establishment of infection after instrumentation.

Treatment

Prompt treatment of acute infections with broad spectrum antibiotics is thought to minimise renal scarring. This applies particularly to the management of infants and young children with evidence of acute pyelonephritis. Infants in the first 2 months of life and children in whom pyelonephritis is suspected should be treated with intravenous therapy initially. Studies have shown that 3 days of intravenous treatment followed by oral therapy is as effective as a 10-day course of intravenous therapy.[43] A 3- to 5-day course for a lower urinary tract infection is proven to be as effective as a conventional 7- to 10-day course.[44]

Prophylaxis

The use of prophylactic antibiotics in children at risk of recurrent urinary tract infections, including those with vesicoureteric reflux, is common. The aim is to prevent reinfection and thus to prevent renal scarring. A recent systematic review has shown that the evidence for the effectiveness of this approach is weak and there is no evidence that this approach can reduce the incidence of renal scarring although there is a strong clinical impression that prophylaxis reduces the rate of reinfection. Properly powered, randomised trials are needed to determine the efficacy of prophylaxis in susceptible children, assessing both the incidence of urinary tract infections and of renal scarring.[45] In spite of the lack of evidence, guidelines of the Royal College of Physicians of London recommend the use of antibiotic prophylaxis in children with reflux to prevent renal scarring and this is common practice.[46] Views differ on the optimal duration of this therapy; practice varies from 2 to 5 years, or until reflux subsides.

The use of prophylaxis to cover surgical procedures such as cystoscopy and catheterization for micturating cystography is also important. In the absence of prophylaxis the risk of infection is up to 20%.[42] These infections are occasionally severe and have the potential to cause renal damage. Oral trimethoprim has been used successfully for micturating cystography but urologists often favor the use of gentamicin and ampicillin for surgical procedures, particularly in children with abnormal urinary tracts.

Investigation following urinary tract infection

In 1991 the Royal College of Physicians (London) produced guidelines on the diagnosis and management of urinary tract infection in children.[46] There was a consensus statement on the minimum level of investigation for children with straightforward infection. Tests were aimed at recognizing or excluding obstruction, reflux, and renal scarring in those children at greatest risk of developing renal damage so that cases could be selected for long-term prophylactic antibiotics or surgery.

It was recommended that all children should have an ultrasound scan to exclude obstruction, but in addition children under 7 years should have a DMSA scan after an infection free period of at least 3 months, to look for renal scarring and infants (under 1 year) should have, in addition, a cystogram to exclude reflux. Other tests should be undertaken if indicated on clinical grounds or following the detection of an abnormality on these screening tests. They recommended that, after reflux and renal damage have been excluded, prophylactic antibiotics may be discontinued.

While this approach represented expert opinion at that time, the rigorous approach to guideline development used now was lacking. Some doctors have questioned the clinical and economic value of this extensive screening program.[47,48] It might be more appropriate to do fewer investigations, perhaps ultrasound alone, in those children with mild illness and no clinical evidence of renal involvement.[49] A plain abdominal film may be carried out in selected cases to identify renal calcification, stones and spinal abnormalities. Occasionally, it may be used to confirm or exclude suspected constipation.[50]

Long-term outcome of vesicoureteric reflux and renal damage

In addition to the acute inflammation caused by urinary tract infection there are several patterns of permanent renal damage associated with the presence of reflux, which have been described earlier.

Chronic pyelonephritis, renal scarring, or reflux nephropathy

Chronic pyelonephritis is the pathological description of permanent renal damage found in children and adults following upper tract infection. In early studies, before antibiotics became available, these changes were described at post mortem examination in children and adults who had suffered from long-standing upper tract infection and there was a close relationship between the development of recurrent acute pyelonephritis and the development of chronic pyelonephritis. Often the two conditions coexisted. Weiss and Parker described children with recurrent infection, failure to thrive, chronic renal failure and metabolic bone disease. They also described women with recurrent infection, hypertension, eclampsia, spontaneous abortion, small for dates infants, anemia, proteinuria, and neurological complications of hypertension who had evidence of chronic pyelonephritis after death.[51]

Because renal scars were seen most often in children and adults with reflux, the term reflux nephropathy was introduced to reflect the common association and the presumed causal relationship. However, pyelonephritic scarring or chronic pyelonephritis can be found without reflux and might be a more accurate term in cases where infection is felt to play an important role. When damage has developed as a result of other risk factors such as renal stones or obstruction, this term is inappropriate. Risk factors in addition to the presence of reflux and intrarenal reflux for the acquisition of reflux nephropathy are severe or recurrent infections, young age, delay in starting treatment, and the presence of existing scars.

The presence of major urological anomalies such as obstruction, renal calculi and neurogenic bladder are less common but more serious risk factors for renal damage. These conditions interfere with the normal mechanisms of urinary drainage and are associated with frequent infections. Other congenital anomalies such as duplex, horseshoe, and ectopic kidneys are associated with an increased incidence of reflux and obstruction. Presumably, when scarring develops in these children it is because of the presence of reflux or obstruction rather than as a direct consequence of the unusual anatomy.

Small kidneys and congenital renal dysplasia

Congenital renal dysplasia and acquired renal damage are often impossible to distinguish on clinical grounds. Both are commonly associated with vesicoureteric reflux. It is possible that small smooth kidneys with refluxing ureters were congenitally small due to renal dysplasia or hypoplasia and later develop infection because of vesicoureteric reflux, which is often present.[35] There may be a causal relationship between ureteric and renal mal-development with renal hypoplasia with renal hypoplasia and reflux as outcomes. It seems likely that displacement of the ureteric bud may adversely influence renal development and nephron formation. Alternatively, high pressures transmitted to the developing kidney in utero may interfere with renal development particularly if it is severe enough to produce functional obstruction.[52]

Long-term outcome of reflux nephropathy

There are several long-term follow-up studies of children who presented with acute urinary tract infection and found subsequently to have reflux and renal scarring and who have now been followed into adult life.[53–55] There are also long-term follow-up studies of children, mainly girls, with asymptomatic bacteriuria, many of whom had reflux and scarring.[30,56] In addition there are data on children with reflux nephropathy who had ureteric reimplantation over a decade ago. These groups of children, now adults, have provided much valuable information on the natural history of reflux nephropathy and the progression of renal damage.[57]

Renal function in reflux nephropathy

Scarred areas of kidney are non-functional and unable to filter the blood and produce urine. Total renal function may remain normal or near normal until renal damage is severe because compensatory hypertrophy of the opposite kidney.[37] When both kidneys are affected, healthy islands of renal tissue mask the real extent of renal damage. In a long-term follow-up study, children with urographic renal scarring were compared with matched subjects 16 to 26 years after the first urinary tract infection in childhood. The GFR two decades after the first recognized urinary tract infection was well preserved, although a significant reduction of individual renal GFR in the unilaterally scarred kidney was found. In patients with bilateral scarring, a significant fall in GFR occurred.[56] A long-term follow-up study of patients with chronic pyelonephritis over the age of 18 years had a good prognosis if their creatinine was below 90 micromol/l.[58] Others have shown that reflux nephropathy is associated with a variety of markers for renal damage including NAG, beta 2 microglobulin and proteinuria.

Progressive scarring

In spite of the large volume of data linking urinary tract infection, vesicoureteric reflux and scarring, the majority of renal scars in any series are present at the time of presentation and relatively few new scars develop during the follow-up period.[59,60] This applies to children treated both medically and surgically. Even when no treatment was given, as in the Cardiff–Oxford bacteriuria survey,[30] very few new scars developed over 4- and 10-year follow-up periods and no child with normal kidneys at the start developed scarring. Similarly, in a large Swedish study, new scars only developed occasionally, exclusively in children who had already been identified as having damaged kidneys at the start. Smellie *et al.* in 1985 described the development of new scars in 74 infants and children gathered over a wide geographical area and time frame.[4] She observed that diagnosis and effective treatment had been delayed in 45 children and 58 experienced recurrent infections after their first radiological investigation and before the introduction of prophylaxis. Vesicoureteric reflux was detected in all but 15 children and in half of those without vesicoureteric reflux the cystogram had been delayed for over 2 years from presentation. New scars occurred most often in the youngest children but were also documented in children of up to 9 years. Progression of existing scars occurred slightly later.

Progression of renal disease

Following the development of serious renal damage due to reflux nephropathy the patient is at increased risk of progressive renal damage due to hyperfiltration. This is a secondary event and is the final common pathway to the development of renal failure occurring in kidneys damaged by a variety of causes. A 10–35-year follow-up study of 226 adults with childhood vesicoureteric reflux showed 17 adults had hypertension and/or raised plasma creatinine, 16 with scarred kidneys and predictable deterioration because of scar type, blood pressure or creatinine levels in childhood. No new scars developed after puberty. Those with vesicoureteric reflux but no scarring did not suffer serious consequences as adults.[54]

Proteinuria

Once scarring has occurred, the long-term prognosis for renal function depends on the severity of the initial damage and the presence and degree of proteinuria which correlates well with the presence of focal and segmental glomerulosclerosis. The course of progression to end-stage renal failure is slow, but inevitable over 5–20 years once proteinuria has become established. In an adult population with reflux nephropathy, Zhang and Bailey found that proteinuria gradually increased from 8.5% at presentation to 31% after 14 years of follow-up.[61] Hyperperfusion and hyperfiltration, resulting from the reduced renal mass is thought to be the underlying cause of these glomerulosclerotic lesions. Compensatory hypertrophy of undamaged parenchyma masks the effect of reflux nephropathy on kidney function and kidney size until late in the disease process and the presence of proteinuria is the first sign of the severe and progressive nature of this condition in many cases.

Hypertension

Hypertension may develop in children with either unilateral or bilateral renal scarring, although it occurs much more often in the latter. Goonasekera *et al.* found raised blood pressure in 14% of patients with reflux, urinary tract infection and scarring on 15-year follow-up.[62] Although the plasma renin activity was raised in patients with reflux nephropathy, and this is thought to be the mechanism in the majority of cases, this did not predict the development of future hypertension reliably. Jacobson *et al.* found that in 30 patients with focal renal scarring, there was an additional risk of 13% after 27 years of follow-up,[60] whereas Zhang and Bailey found hypertension in 38%.[61] In contrast, a study by Wennerstrom evaluating 57 children with renal scarring from a cohort of 1221 consecutive children with first urinary tract infection, found no significant differences in blood pressure with a matched group without scarring.[63] In a large group of British children with significant hypertension, renal scarring accounted for 14% and this was the commonest single cause.[64]

Renal failure

Reflux nephropathy is an important cause of end-stage renal failure in children and adults. The incidence of reflux nephropathy as a cause of end-stage renal disease varies widely, either because of differences in definition or management. A report from 12 European registries found that 21% of all end-stage renal disease in children under 19 years of age was due to reflux nephropathy.[65] It is responsible for 22% of pediatric cases of end-stage renal failure in Great Britain[64] and 9.6% in France.[66] In Sweden there were no new cases of end-stage renal disease caused by reflux nephropathy in an 8-year period.[67] Renal insufficiency in an adult population in New Zealand with reflux nephropathy correlated well with the degree of parenchymal scarring and developed in 24% of patients over 14 years.[61] In an adult population, 37% of adults with reflux nephropathy and/or vesicoureteric reflux showed a deterioration of renal function of whom 14% developed end-stage renal failure.[68]

Deterioration of renal function, once started, occurs even when urinary tract infections are successfully prevented or treated and hypertension satisfactorily controlled. There is good evidence that repair of reflux at this stage does not change the progression of the development of renal failure.[69] GFR starts dropping at a late stage when hypertrophy of the rest of the kidney and contralateral kidney cannot compensate for the loss of renal tissue due to renal scarring, or when, through hyperfiltration, the previously normal kidney tissue starts to decompensate. The rate of functional decline of scarred kidneys correlates with protein excretion and the percentage of segmentally sclerosed glomeruli, and may be slowed by ACE inhibitors or possibly by a low protein diet.

Pregnancy

Pregnancy is a period of physiological stress and consequently many conditions which cause little trouble outside pregnancy can cause quite serious problems for a few months. Urinary tract infection, vesicoureteric reflux and reflux nephropathy are closely linked and each is associated with specific problems in pregnancy, which affect both mother and foetus.

Urinary tract infection in pregnancy

During pregnancy many women with a past history of urinary tract infection or asymptomatic bacteriuria develop symptomatic upper tract infection. Although the incidence of urinary tract infection is not significantly greater than for non-pregnant, sexually active women, changes in the physiology of the urinary tract with dilatation of the ureters starting in the mid-trimester and changes in receptor expression under hormonal influence combine to put all pregnant women at increased risk of acute pyelonephritis.

Acute pyelonephritis during pregnancy is associated with anemia and premature labour. Women with evidence of previous susceptibility to urinary tract infection, including those with reflux or renal scarring are particularly vulnerable.[70]

The presence of reflux persisting into adult life is thought by some to be a special risk factor for urinary tract infection during pregnancy. But the observation that the incidence of infection is influenced little by ureteric reimplantation does not commend this operation as the solution to recurrent infections. However, in an Australian series women who had undergone reimplantation had slightly fewer infections than those with persisting reflux.[71]

Hypertension, edema, and proteinuria in pregnancy

During pregnancy, women with reflux nephropathy are at increased risk of hypertension and proteinuria.[70] Unlike true pre-eclampsia which affects the first pregnancy most severely, these complications, when they occur secondary to reflux nephropathy, tend to affect all pregnancies, or to become worse with successive pregnancies. It has also been shown that affected women are more likely to require obstetric intervention such as Cesarean section or forceps delivery.[72] Pregnancy in women with reflux nephropathy and impaired renal function has been shown to accelerate deterioration of GFR in some cases but others have undergone successful pregnancies without evidence of deterioration.[73,74] It has been postulated that inadequate management of hypertension may play an important part in the deterioration in some of these women.[74] The Cardiff–Oxford bacteriuria study group followed schoolgirls with asymptomatic bacteriuria until pregnancy and childbirth. The women with renal scarring had a 3.3-fold increased relative risk of hypertension and a 7.6-fold increased risk of hypertension with proteinuria.[75]

Prevention of reflux nephropathy

In spite of the enormous amount of data that has been acquired through observation of the natural history and prospective studies, there is still no clear indication of the best way to manage children with reflux to minimize illness from acute infection and prevent renal scarring. However, when the results of modern treatment are compared with some of the early descriptions of pyelonephritis in children in the preantibiotic era and studies from 30 years ago, it is clear that the morbidity has been significantly reduced.[76,77] However, this may be due as much to the general improvement in diagnosis of infectious illness, the widespread availability of effective antibiotics, and management of sick children generally, as to any specific measures such as ureteric reimplantation and long-term low dose prophylaxis.

Medical management

In the study reported by Edwards *et al.* (1977), renal scarring was present in 17 out of 75 children and progressed in only 2 patients treated medically.[28] As a result they questioned the view expressed at the time that surgical correction was essential and attributed the good results to their management. Studying Edwards' patients further, Smellie[78] demonstrated that impaired kidney growth was not associated directly with the presence of vesicoureteric reflux. However, significant associations were found between poor renal growth and renal scarring and infection independently. Normal growth could be expected in unscarred, uninfected kidneys, whatever the severity of reflux.

Vesicoureteric reflux can be present for a prolonged period of time without causing any damage or deterioration of renal function, and even severe reflux and reflux persisting into adult life can be associated with radiologically normal kidneys. Berg *et al.* (1992) found that children with recurrent episodes of acute pyelonephritis over a period of 1 to 23 years developed scars in 37 out of 105 normal kidneys of which 22 had grade III reflux or worse.[79,80] In a 5-year follow-up study, Arant reported on 59 children under five who received "optimal medical therapy." In children with mild or moderate reflux, scars developed in 10% of normal kidneys without reflux or with grades 1 and 2. In radiologically normal kidneys drained by grades 3 and 4, scarring developed in 28%.[81]

When girls with asymptomatic bacteriuria were followed up prospectively, very few developed new scars even though the treatment group received only intermittent therapy and the control group received no treatment.[82] These observations raise the possibility that prophylaxis may not be necessary or effective in the prevention of progressive scarring if children have access to good services for prompt diagnosis and treatment. In the presence of strongly held views it is now difficult, but still essential, to conduct the necessary clinical trials to establish the superiority or otherwise of long-term low dose prophylaxis over intermittent treatment of acute infections in children with vesicoureteric reflux.

Both the United States and European limbs of the International Reflux Study in Children found no numerical difference in terms of development of new scars, progression of existing scars and renal growth between children treated medically or surgically with grade 3 or 4 reflux after 5 years' follow-up.[41,59] Renal scarring was present in between 49% and 67% of patients at entry in the study. Neither treatment was able to protect kidneys fully from new scar development and new scarring continued to occur during the entire 5-year follow-up period in both treatment limbs. The new scar formation or progression of existing scars mainly developed in kidneys drained by refluxing ureters. Only 5% of children with normal kidneys developed scars, of whom the majority were over 2 years of age. Centers recruiting large numbers of patients for the study had a lower risk of scar formation, progression or recurrence of urinary tract infection, which suggests that other, local factors influence the outcome. Urinary tract infections were less likely after either treatment modality. Surgical correction did not alter the recurrence rate of urinary tract infection, compared to medical treatment, but recurrent acute pyelonephritis was less likely.[27]

Problems with medical management are compliance and breakthrough infections. Parental co-operation and compliance with giving antibiotics to their child on a daily basis is low.[83] Collecting urine samples whenever the child is unwell seems to be difficult for general practitioners.[84] However, reasons given by some parents for the lack of compliance were failure to understand reasons for prophylaxis. By increasing knowledge and understanding, it may be possible to improve the working relationship between carers and health professionals. There is a need to improve awareness of the possibility of urinary tract infection as a cause of fever in very young children, thus reducing the delay before treatment is started. Early identification of vesicoureteric reflux and the introduction of prophylaxis may prevent some cases of renal scarring, but evidence supported by randomized controlled trials is badly needed.

Medical vs. surgical treatment

Ureteric reimplantation was introduced over 30 years ago as a form of treatment to reduce recurrent infection and prevent the acquired renal damage that tends to occur in these children. However, long-term follow-up studies such as those by Smellie (1998) and studies on children with asymptomatic bacteriuria, showed that new renal scars were not common once these children had been diagnosed and investigated.[28,82] Consequently, the value of surgical correction of reflux, a self-limiting condition, was later questioned. It is clear that renal damage, once established, cannot be restored by surgery. A systematic review has summarized the available evidence of surgery combined with antibiotics compared to prophylactic antibiotic treatment only in children with vesicoureteric reflux. Eight trials were identified involving 859 children showing no significant difference in the risk of urinary tract infection after 1–2 and 5 years, although surgery reduced the incidence of febrile urinary tract infections by 60%. However, this reduction was not associated with a concomitant significant reduction in risk of new or progressive renal damage at 5 years.[85] No trials have compared surgery alone with antibiotic prophylaxis or surgery with no treatment. One small trial found no difference between prophylactic antibiotics and no treatment, but the small patient numbers do not exclude a difference between groups. Postoperative obstruction to the urinary tract was reported in 6.6% of children in one trial, but otherwise adverse events were not well reported. Although there is a well-established association between vesicoureteric reflux, urinary tract infection and renal scarring, there is no evidence from randomised controlled trials that this is a modifiable risk factor. At present, adding surgery to prophylactic antibiotic treatment does not show an additional benefit apart from reducing febrile urinary tract infections. The use of prophylactic antibiotics in children with vesicoureteric reflux needs further evaluation in a placebo-controlled trial. A 10-year prospective study of renal growth in children with severe vesicoureteric reflux did not show a difference between medical or surgical management.[86]

Adult patients with vesicoureteric reflux can experience loin pain when their bladders are full or have frequent attacks of pyelonephritis. If conservative management has failed, antireflux surgery should be considered. The loin pain symptoms will be effectively eliminated in some cases. Antireflux surgery is not indicated for arresting renal function deterioration.[87]

Screening for reflux

In view of the disappointing results of the large controlled studies of surgical vs. medical treatment in children with reflux and urinary tract infections, attention has focused on detecting vesicoureteric reflux before the first urinary tract infection has occurred, and reducing the risk of urinary tract infection with prophylactic antibiotics. Antenatal screening for hydronephrosis and family counseling have made the detection of reflux possible soon after birth. Reports of good outcome in this group are difficult to interpret as relatively little is known about the natural history. The role of screening and treatment in this patient group remains controversial and a randomized trial is needed to give the necessary guidance to their management.

Screening in children with urinary tract infection

Most cases of reflux have in the past been detected following proven urinary tract infection. In this situation, it is customary to recommend that children undergo certain radiological investigations[46] and these tests are in effect screening tests for reflux and reflux nephropathy, since they are in most cases not done directly to address ongoing symptoms. The observation in several studies that there are scars in up to 25% of cases at presentation[88] and that relatively few new scars develop in children under medical supervision suggests that most of the renal damage has developed before, or at the time of, the presenting infection.[89] In Sweden, where there is a high level of awareness of the risk of urinary tract infection in infancy, the prevalence of renal scarring after presentation with a urinary tract infection is only 7%. This raises the possibility that extensive screening at a late stage, as practiced in the UK, will not alter the course of the disease significantly. The observation by Jadresic *et al.* (1993) that the number of urine samples sent from young children in general practice varied ten fold between practices and that the number of cases diagnosed depended on the number of samples sent to the laboratory, suggests that there are many undiagnosed infections in this age group.[90] Van der Voort (1997) showed that there is considerable difficulty in collecting urine from infants in primary care[84] and that children with renal scars had consulted their doctors more than twice as often as controls in early childhood although there was no record that urine was examined.[91] This may explain why so many children have renal scars when they are first diagnosed and why so little impact on the natural history is achieved by the accepted forms of screening and treatment following proven infection.

Screening before urinary tract infection

Antenatal diagnosis of hydronephrosis can be due to reflux in utero and can be further investigated after birth. The knowledge of the presence of reflux gives the opportunity to advise and educate the family and carers, to closely monitor progress, to be vigilant for the development of infection and when necessary to treat the patient. In some centers antibiotic prophylaxis has been used in this situation to prevent urinary tract infections. The screening method will only identify a proportion of babies with reflux and at present there is insufficient evidence to know if prognosis of these infants has been altered by screening. Screening of siblings of index cases will identify some infants with vesicoureteric reflux before developing urinary tract infection, especially if reflux is identified in the asymptomatic newborn. The acceptability amongst parents is good,[92] the complication rate is low provided steps are taken to ensure that these infants do not develop iatrogenic infection in relation to catheterization. At present, there is insufficient evidence that this early detection of reflux and prevention of infection-mediated disease using prophylactic antibiotics will alter the course of the disease and reduce the amount of damage to the kidney.

A non-invasive screening test for reflux

When ultrasound first became available, it was anticipated that it would provide a major step forward in the diagnosis of reflux and renal scarring. In spite of extensive research it has proved to be inadequate in both these tasks, and at times has given false reassurance to the unwary. Indirect cystography, although not requiring catheterization, is not effective as a diagnostic tool in infants and requires venepuncture and exposure to radiation.

Attempts to find a biochemical test for reflux have also proved disappointing, and although several candidate tests have been identified none has proved sufficiently sensitive to be worth developing in clinical practice. The urinary enzyme *N*-acetyl-beta-glucosaminidase (NAG) has been measured in the urine, where it appears when tubular damage has occurred. The level of NAG was only related to the most severe forms of reflux and is thus clinically not useful.[93] Other enzymes such as pyruvate kinase, hexokinase and phosphofructokinase, that have much greater activity in the distal nephron, have also been evaluated but not found to be clinically useful.

Vaccines

Another possibility to reduce the risk of renal damage is the use of a vaccine to immunise infants against the development of invasive *E. coli* infection using one or more bacterial components. Roberts *et al.* used a formalin-killed P-fimbriated *E.coli* vaccine in monkeys, but this did not protect against colonisation or time of bacteriuria after artificial infection. It gave limited protection against renal dysfunction and scarring.[94] Because of the large number of different organisms and strains causing urinary tract infection an effective vaccine remains elusive.

REFERENCES

1. Sampson, J. Ascending renal infection with special reference to the reflux of urine from the bladder into the ureters as an aetiological factor in its causation and maintenance. *Bull. Johns Hopkins Hosp.* 1903; **14**:334–350.
2. Hodson, C. J. ED. Chronic pyelonephritis and vesicoureteric reflux. *Clin. Radiol.* 1960; **2**:219–231.
3. Arena, F., Romeo, C., Cruccetti, A. *et al.* Fetal vesicoureteral reflux: neonatal findings and follow-up study. *Pediatr. Med. Chir.* 2001; **23**(1):31–34.
4. Smellie, J. M., Ransley, P. G., Normand, I. C., Prescod, N., & Edwards, D. Development of new renal scars: a collaborative study. *Br. Med. J. (Clin. Res. Ed.)* 1985; **290**(6486):1957–1960.
5. Smellie, J. M., Hodson, C. J., Edwards, D. & Normand, I. C. Clinical and radiological features of urinary infection in childhood. *Br. Med. J.* 1964; **5419**:1222–1226.
6. Lebowitz, R. L., Olbing, H., Parkkulainen, K. V., Smellie, J. M., & Tamminen-Mobius, T. E. International system of radiographic grading of vesicoureteric reflux. *International Reflux Study in Children. Pediatr. Radiol.* 1985; **15**(2):105–109.
7. Rolleston, G. L., Maling, T. M., & Hodson, C. J. Intrarenal reflux and the scarred kidney. *Arch. Dis. Child.* 1974; **49**(7):531–539.
8. Merrick, M. V., Notghi, A., Chalmers, N., Wilkinson, A. G., & Uttley, W. S. Long-term follow up to determine the prognostic value of imaging after urinary tract infections. Part 2: Scarring. *Arch. Dis. Child.* 1995; **72**(5):393–396.
9. Smellie, J. M. & Rigden, S. P. Pitfalls in the investigation of children with urinary tract infection. *Arch. Dis. Child.* 1995; **72**(3):251–285; discussion 255–8.
10. Smellie, J. M., Rigden, S. P., & Prescod, N. P. Urinary tract infection: a comparison of four methods of investigation. *Arch. Dis. Child.* 1995; **72**(3):247–50.
11. Hutch, J. Theory of maturation of the intravesical ureter. *J. Urol.* 1961; **86**:534.
12. Koff, S. A. & Murtagh, D. S. The uninhibited bladder in children: effect of treatment on recurrence of urinary infection and on vesicoureteral reflux resolution. *J. Urol.* 1983; **130**(6):1138–1141.
13. Ransley, P. G. & Risdon, R. A. Reflux and renal scarring. *Br. J. Radiol.* 1978; **51**(Suppl. 14):1–35.
14. Report of a meeting of physicians at the Hospital for Sick Children, Gt Ormond Street. Vesicoureteric reflux: all in the genes? *Lancet* 1996; **348**:725–728.
15. Anderson, N. G., Allan, R. B., & Abbott, G. D. Fluctuating fetal or neonatal renal pelvis: marker of high-grade vesicoureteral reflux. *Pediatr. Nephrol.* 2004; **19**(7):749–753.
16. Kenda, R. B., Zupancic, Z., Fettich, J. J., & Meglic, A. A follow-up study of vesico-ureteric reflux and renal scars in asymptomatic siblings of children with reflux. *Nucl. Med. Commun.* 1997; **18**(9):827–831.
17. Upadhyay, J., McLorie, G. A., Bolduc, S., Bagli, D. J., Khoury, A. E., & Farhat, W. Natural history of neonatal reflux associated with prenatal hydronephrosis: long-term results of a prospective study. *J. Urol.* 2003; **169**(5):1837–1841; discussion 1841; author reply 1841.
18. Cascio, S., Chertin, B., Yoneda, A., Rolle, U., Kelleher, J., & Puri, P. Acute renal damage in infants after first urinary tract infection. *Pediatr. Nephrol.* 2002; **17**(7):503–505.
19. Marild, S., Hellstrom, M., Jodal, U., & Eden, C. S. Fever, bacteriuria and concomitant disease in children with urinary tract infection. *Pediatr. Infect. Dis. J.* 1989; **8**(1):36–41.
20. Arze, R. S., Ramos, J. M., Owen, J. P. *et al.* The natural history of chronic pyelonephritis in the adult. *Quart. J. Med.* 1982; **51**(204):396–410.
21. Skoog, S. J. & Belman, A. B. Primary vesicoureteral reflux in the black child. *Pediatrics* 1991; **87**(4):538–543.
22. Wettergren, B. & Jodal, U. Spontaneous clearance of asymptomatic bacteriuria in infants. *Acta Paediatr. Scand.* 1990; **79**(3):300–304.
23. McLachlan, M. S., Meller, S. T., Jones, E. R. *et al.* Urinary tract in schoolgirls with covert bacteriuria. *Arch. Dis. Child.* 1975; **50**(4):253–8.
24. Smellie, J. M., Jodal, U., Lax, H., Mobius, T. T., Hirche, H., & Olbing, H. Outcome at 10 years of severe vesicoureteric reflux managed medically: report of the International Reflux Study in Children. *J. Pediatr.* 2001; **139**(5):656–663.
25. Lenaghan, D., Whitaker, J. G., Jensen, F., & Stephens, F. D. The natural history of reflux and long-term effects of reflux on the kidney. *J. Urol.* 1976; **115**(6):728–730.
26. Prospective trial of operative versus non-operative treatment of severe vesicoureteric reflux in children: five years' observation. Birmingham Reflux Study Group. *Br. Med. J. (Clin. Res. Ed.)* 1987; **295**(6592):237–241.

27. Smellie, J. M., Tamminen-Mobius, T., Olbing, H. *et al.* Five-year study of medical or surgical treatment in children with severe reflux: radiological renal findings. The International Reflux Study in Children. *Pediatr. Nephrol.* 1992; **6**(3):223–230.
28. Edwards, D., Normand, I. C., Prescod, N., & Smellie, J. M. Disappearance of vesicoureteric reflux during long-term prophylaxis of urinary tract infection in children. *Br. Med. J.* 1977; **2**(6082):285–288.
29. Kenda, R. B. & Fettich, J. J. Vesicoureteric reflux and renal scars in asymptomatic siblings of children with reflux. *Arch. Dis. Child.* 1992; **67**(4):506–508.
30. Aggarwal, V. K., Verrier, Jones K., Asscher, A. W., Evans, C., & Williams, L. A. Covert bacteriuria: long term follow up. *Arch. Dis. Child.* 1991; **66**(11):1284–1286.
31. Kenda, R. B. & Zupancic, Z. Ultrasound screening of older asymptomatic siblings of children with vesicoureteral reflux: is it beneficial? *Pediatr. Radiol.* 1994; **24**(1):14–16.
32. Connolly, L. P., Treves, S. T., Zurakowski, D., & Bauer, S. B. Natural history of vesicoureteral reflux in siblings. *J. Urol.* 1996; **156**(5):1805–1807.
33. Savage, D. C., Wilson, M. I., McHardy, M., Dewar, D. A., & Fee, W. M. Covert bacteriuria of childhood. A clinical and epidemiological study. *Arch. Dis. Child.* 1973; **48**(1):8–20.
34. Rushton, H. G. The evaluation of acute pyelonephritis and renal scarring with technetium 99m-dimercaptosuccinic acid renal scintigraphy: evolving concepts and future directions. *Pediatr. Nephrol.* 1997; **11**(1):108–120.
35. Wennerstrom, M., Hansson, S., Jodal, U., & Stokland, E. Primary and acquired renal scarring in boys and girls with urinary tract infection. *J. Pediatr.* 2000; **136**(1):30–34.
36. Merrick, M. V., Notghi, A., Chalmers, N., Wilkinson, A. G., & Uttley, W. S. Long-term follow up to determine the prognostic value of imaging after urinary tract infections. Part 1: Reflux. *Arch. Dis. Child.* 1995; **72**(5):388–392.
37. Verrier, Jones, K., Asscher, A. W., Verrier, Jones, E. R., Mattholie, K., Leach, K., & Thomson, G. M. Glomerular filtration rate in schoolgirls with covert bacteriuria. *Br. Med. J.* (*Clin. Res. Ed.*) 1982; **285**(6351):1307–1310.
38. Smellie, J. M., Poulton, A., & Prescod, N. P. Retrospective study of children with renal scarring associated with reflux and urinary infection. *Br. Med. J.* 1994; **308**(6938):1193–1196.
39. Orellana, P., Baquedano, P., Rangarajan, V. *et al.* Relationship between acute pyelonephritis, renal scarring, and vesicoureteral reflux. Results of a coordinated research project. *Pediatr. Nephrol.* 2004; **19**(10):1122–1126.
40. Winberg, J., Bergstrom, T., & Jacobsson, B. Morbidity, age and sex distribution, recurrences and renal scarring in symptomatic urinary tract infection in childhood. *Kidney Int.* (Suppl.) 1975; **4**:S101–S106.
41. Weiss, R., Duckett, J., & Spitzer, A. Results of a randomized clinical trial of medical versus surgical management of infants and children with grades III and IV primary vesicoureteral reflux (United States). The International Reflux Study in Children. *J. Urol.* 1992; **148**(5 Pt 2):1667–1673.
42. Hallett, R. J., Pead, L., & Maskell, R. Urinary infection in boys. A three-year prospective study. *Lancet* 1976; **2**(7995):1107–1110.
43. Benador, D., Neuhaus, T. J., Papazyan, J. P. *et al.* Randomised controlled trial of three day versus 10 day intravenous antibiotics in acute pyelonephritis: effect on renal scarring. *Arch. Dis. Child.* 2001; **84**(3):241–246.
44. Michael, M., Hodson, E. M., Craig, J. C., Martin, S., & Moyer, V. A. Short compared with standard duration of antibiotic treatment for urinary tract infection: a systematic review of randomised controlled trials. *Arch. Dis. Child.* 2002; **87**(2):118–123.
45. Williams, G., Lee, A., & Craig, J. Antibiotics for the prevention of urinary tract infection in children: a systematic review of randomized controlled trials. *J. Pediatr.* 2001; **138**(6):868–874.
46. Guidelines for the management of acute urinary tract infection in childhood. Report of a Working Group of the Research Unit, Royal College of Physicians. *J. Roy. Coll Phys. Lond.* 1991; **25**(1):36–42.
47. Stark, H. Urinary tract infections in girls: the cost-effectiveness of currently recommended investigative routines. *Pediatr. Nephrol.* 1997; **11**(2):174–177; discussion 180–1.
48. Chambers, T. An essay on the consequences of childhood urinary tract infection. *Pediatr. Nephrol.* 1997; **11**(2):178–179.
49. Deshpande, P. V. & Jones, K. V. An audit of RCP guidelines on DMSA scanning after urinary tract infection. *Arch. Dis. Child.* 2001; **84**(4):324–327.
50. Blethyn, A. J., Jenkins, H. R., Roberts, R., & Verrier Jones, K. Radiological evidence of constipation in urinary tract infection. *Arch. Dis. Child.* 1995; **73**(6):534–535.
51. Weiss, S. P. F. Vascular changes in pyelonephritis and their relation to arterial hypertension. *Trans. Assoc. Am. Phys.* 1938; **53**:60.
52. Risdon, R. A. The small scarred kidney in childhood. *Pediatr Nephrol* 1993; **7**(4):361–4.
53. Jacobson, S. H., Eklof, O., Lins, L. E., Wikstad, I., & Winberg, J. Long-term prognosis of post-infectious renal scarring in relation to radiological findings in childhood – a 27-year follow-up. *Pediatr. Nephrol.* 1992; **6**(1):19–24.
54. Smellie, J. M., Prescod, N. P., Shaw, P. J., Risdon, R. A., & Bryant, T. N. Childhood reflux and urinary infection: a follow-up of 10–41 years in 226 adults. *Pediatr. Nephrol.* 1998; **12**(9):727–736.
55. Martinell, J., Lidin-Janson, G., Jagenburg, R., Sivertsson, R., Claesson, I., & Jodal, U. Girls prone to urinary infections followed into adulthood. Indices of renal disease. *Pediatr. Nephrol.* 1996; **10**(2):139–142.
56. Wennerstrom, M., Hansson, S., Jodal, U., Sixt, R., & Stokland, E. Renal function 16 to 26 years after the first urinary tract infection in childhood. *Arch. Pediatr. Adolesc. Med.* 2000; **154**(4):339–345.
57. Goonasekera, C. D., Gordon, I., & Dillon, MJ. 15-year follow-up of reflux nephropathy by imaging. *Clin. Nephrol.* 1998; **50**(4):224–231.
58. Goodship, T. H., Stoddart, J. T., Martinek, V. *et al.* Long-term follow-up of patients presenting to adult nephrologists with

chronic pyelonephritis and 'normal' renal function. *Quart. J. Med.* 2000; **93**(12):799–803.

59. Olbing, H., Claesson, I., Ebel, K. D. *et al.* Renal scars and parenchymal thinning in children with vesicoureteral reflux: a 5-year report of the International Reflux Study in Children (European branch). *J. Urol.* 1992; **148**(5 Pt 2):1653–1656.
60. Jacobson, S. H., Eklof, O., Eriksson, C. G., Lins, L. E., Tidgren, B., & Winberg, J. Development of hypertension and uraemia after pyelonephritis in childhood: 27 year follow up. *Br. Med. J.* 1989; **299**(6701):703–706.
61. Zhang, Y. & Bailey, R. R. A long term follow up of adults with reflux nephropathy. *N Z Med. J.* 1995; **108**(998):142–144.
62. Goonasekera, C. D., Shah, V., Wade, A. M., Barratt, T. M., & Dillon, M. J. 15-year follow-up of renin and blood pressure in reflux nephropathy. *Lancet* 1996; **347**(9002):640–643.
63. Wennerstrom, M., Hansson, S., Hedner, T., Himmelmann, A., & Jodal, U. Ambulatory blood pressure 16–26 years after the first urinary tract infection in childhood. *J. Hypertens.* 2000; **18**(4):485–491.
64. Gill, D. G., Mendes, de Costa, B., Cameron, J. S., Joseph, M. C., Ogg, C. S., & Chantler, C. Analysis of 100 children with severe and persistent hypertension. *Arch. Dis. Child.* 1976; **51**(12):951–956.
65. van der Heijden, B. J., van Dijk, P. C., Verrier-Jones, K., Jager, K. J., & Briggs, J. D. Renal replacement therapy in children: data from 12 registries in Europe. *Pediatr. Nephrol.* 2004; **19**(2):213–221.
66. Habib, R., Broyer, M., & Benmaiz, H. Chronic renal failure in children; causes, rate of deterioration and survival data. *Nephron* 1973; **11**:209–220.
67. Esbjorner, E., Berg, U., & Hansson, S. Epidemiology of chronic renal failure in children: a report from Sweden 1986–1994. Swedish Pediatric Nephrology Association. *Pediatr. Nephrol.* 1997; **11**(4):438–442.
68. el-Khatib, M. T., Becker, G. J., & Kincaid-Smith, P. S. Reflux nephropathy and primary vesicoureteric reflux in adults. *Quart. J. Med* 1990; **77**(284):1241–1253.
69. Smellie, J. M., Barratt, T. M., Chantler, C. *et al.* Medical versus surgical treatment in children with severe bilateral vesicoureteric reflux and bilateral nephropathy: a randomised trial. *Lancet* 2001; **357**(9265):1329–1333.
70. Verrier Jones, K. Urinary tract infection. In Catto, G., ed. *Pregnancy and Renal Disorders.* Dordrecht: Kluwer, 1988:1–40.
71. el-Khatib, M., Packham, D. K., Becker, G. J., & Kincaid-Smith, P. Pregnancy-related complications in women with reflux nephropathy. *Clin. Nephrol.* 1994; **41**(1):50–55.
72. Sacks, S. H., Verrier, Jones K., Roberts, R., Asscher, A. W., & Ledingham, J. G. Effect of symptomless bacteriuria in childhood on subsequent pregnancy. *Lancet* 1987; **2**(8566):991–994.
73. Becker, G. J., Ihle, B. U., Fairley, K. F., Bastos, M., & Kincaid-Smith, P. Effect of pregnancy on moderate renal failure in reflux nephropathy. *Br. Med. J.* (*Clin. Res. Ed.*) 1986; **292**(6523):796–798.
74. Martinell, J., Jodal, U., & Lidin-Janson, G. Pregnancies in women with and without renal scarring after urinary infections in childhood. *Br. Med. J.* 1990; **300**(6728):840–844.
75. Cardiff–Oxford bacteriuria group. Long-term effects of bacteriuria on the urinary tract in schoolgirls. *Radiology* 1979; **132**:343–350.
76. Stansfeld, J. M. Relapses of urinary-tract infections in children. *Br. Med. J.* 1966; **5488**:635–637.
77. Stansfeld, J. M. Clinical observations relating to incidence and aetiology of urinary-tract infections in children. *Br. Med. J.* 1966; **5488**:631–634.
78. Smellie, J. M., Edwards, D., Normand, I. C., & Prescod, N. Effect of vesicoureteric reflux on renal growth in children with urinary tract infection. *Arch. Dis. Child.* 1981; **56**(8):593–600.
79. Berg, U. B. Long-term followup of renal morphology and function in children with recurrent pyelonephritis. *J. Urol.* 1992; **148**(5 Pt 2):1715–1720.
80. Jakobsson, B., Soderlundh, S., & Berg, U. Diagnostic significance of ^{99m}Tc-dimercaptosuccinic acid (DMSA) scintigraphy in urinary tract infection. *Arch. Dis. Child.* 1992; **67**(11):1338–1342.
81. Arrant, B. Medical management of mild and moderate vesicoureteric reflux: follow-up studiesof infants and young children. A preliminary report of the Southwest Pediatric Nephrology Study Group. *J. Urol.* 1992; **148**:1683–1687.
82. Long-term effects of bacteriuria on the urinary tract in schoolgirls. *Radiology* 1979; **132**(2):343–350.
83. Smyth, A. R. & Judd, B. A. Compliance with antibiotic prophylaxis in urinary tract infection. *Arch. Dis. Child.* 1993; **68**(2):235–236.
84. van der Voort, J., Edwards, A., Roberts, R., & Verrier, Jones K. The struggle to diagnose UTI in children under two in primary care. *Fam. Pract.* 1997; **14**(1):44–48.
85. Wheeler, D., Vimalachandra, D., Hodson, E. M., Roy, L. P., Smith, G., & Craig, J. C. Antibiotics and surgery for vesicoureteric reflux: a meta-analysis of randomised controlled trials. *Arch. Dis. Child.* 2003; **88**(8):688–694.
86. Olbing, H., Hirche, H., Koskimies, O. *et al.* Renal growth in children with severe vesicoureteral reflux: 10-year prospective study of medical and surgical treatment: the International Reflux Study in Children (European branch). *Radiology* 2000; **216**(3):731–737.
87. Kohler, J., Thysell, H., Tencer, J., Forsberg, L., & Hellstrom, M. Conservative treatment and anti-reflux surgery in adults with vesico-ureteral reflux: effect on urinary-tract infections, renal function and loin pain in a long-term follow-up study. *Nephrol. Dial. Transpl.* 2001; **16**(1):52–60.
88. Arant, B. S., Jr. Vesicoureteric reflux and renal injury. *Am. J. Kidney Dis.* 1991; **17**(5):491–511.
89. Ataei, N., Madani, A., Esfahani, S. T. *et al.* Screening for vesicoureteral reflux and renal scars in siblings of children

with known reflux. *Pediatr. Nephrol.* 2004; **19**(10):1127–1131.

90. Jadresic, L., Cartwright, K., Cowie, N., Witcombe, B., & Stevens, D. Investigation of urinary tract infection in childhood. *Br. Med. J.* 1993; **307**(6907):761–764.
91. Van, Der Voort, J. H., Edwards, A. G., Roberts, R., Newcombe, R. G., & Jones, K. V. Unexplained extra visits to general practitioners before the diagnosis of first urinary tract infection: a case-control study. *Arch. Dis. Child.* 2002; **87**(6):530–532.
92. Aggarwal, V. K., Verrier, Jones K. Vesicoureteric reflux: screening of first degree relatives. *Arch. Dis. Child.* 1989; **64**(11):1538–1541.
93. Williams, M. A., Jones, D., & Noe, H. N. Urinary *N*-acetyl-beta-glucosaminidase as a screening technique for vesicoureteral reflux. *Urology* 1994; **43**(4):528–530.
94. Roberts, J. A., Kaack, M. B., Baskin, G., & Svenson, S. B. Vaccination with a formalin-killed P-fimbriated *E. coli* whole-cell vaccine prevents renal scarring from pyelonephritis in the non-human primate. *Vaccine* 1995; **13**(1):11–16.

44b

Vesicoureteric reflux: surgical treatment

David Gough†

†Formerly Department of Paediatric Urology, Royal Manchester Children's Hospital, UK

There is a world of difference between a good Physician and a bad Physician but not much difference between a good Physician and no Physician at all

Although reflux of urine from the bladder to the ureter and its diagnosis by means of cystography were well known in the early part of the twentieth century, it was not until 1952 that any systematic attempt was made to correct this condition.[1]

The association of urinary infection with reflux and "reflux nephropathy" in children was established in 1960 and may have been partly responsible for the birth of pediatric urology as reimplantation of the ureters was the most frequently performed major operation in children's surgery, and many surgeons operated on such patients on a weekly basis. Reimplantation of the ureter was indeed very fashionable during the period 1960–1985 but it then began to fall in to some disfavor as new insights and new treatments developed.[2] There is, however, a large population of patients who have been subjected to surgery for vesicoureteric reflux and patients continue to receive treatment for this condition.

Discussing the long-term effects of surgical treatment for vesicoureteric reflux (VUR) is not easy as most of the early articles were concerned with technique and short-term results, with very few authors willing, or able, to undertake the huge task of long-term follow-up.

What will become apparent in this review is that the effects of treatment have infrequently been clearly studied against controlled groups of patients, nor have the effects of the disease process in isolation been clearly outlined.

Furthermore, it was assumed that vesicoureteric reflux was in itself a phenomenon that had a unified cause and was always associated with ascending urinary tract infection.

We now know that there is a spectrum of causes of vesicoureteric reflux which may be:

- congenital due to anatomical abnormalities of the VU junction
- secondary to abnormal bladder behavior such as dyssynergia, infrequent voiding or an overactive bladder
- combinations of the above.

The complexities of urinary tract function and the pathophysiological effects of reinfection cannot be simplified down to the simple concept of vesicoureteric reflux that requires surgical correction. Understanding the bladder is probably more important, and therefore, when we discuss the long-term outcomes of reflux, there can be no certainty unless we discuss:

- the long-term outcome of the underlying cause in the bladder
- the long-term outcome on the condition of the upper tracts
- the effects that treatment may have; beneficially or adversely;

and the long-term outcomes and complications of:

- medical treatment
- surgical treatment
- endoscopic treatment with any of the substances currently available, all of which have their long-term hazards
- minimally invasive therapy.

Even with new depths of understanding, we remain perplexed by the role of voiding abnormalities and the fine balance between the psyche, the sphincter, and detrusor function. Despite years of study, we remain in a quandary when faced with a patient who suffers vesicoureteric reflux,

Pediatric Surgery and Urology: Long-term Outcomes, Mark Stringer, Keith Oldham, Pierre Mouriquand.
Published by Cambridge University Press. © Cambridge University Press, 2006.

unsure whether to treat the reflux surgically, medically, or endoscopically.

Antenatal diagnosis of hydronephrosis has increased our understanding of the role of embryological development in producing abnormalities that were so often regarded as acquired, and has also raised doubts as to whether any of the upper tract effects of VUR are indeed preventable when we observe the damage apparently caused to the upper tract during development.[3]

There are still areas of darkness in our knowledge. Why is it for example, that the majority of children who seem to have reflux diagnosed antenatally are male, yet the incidence of reflux is much greater in females who present later in childhood. This might suggest that, in females, most if not all of the pathology is acquired, and the speculation is that it is high voiding pressures in the newborn male which are responsible for the persistence of reflux and its rapid resolution as the bladder matures.

We will continue to argue about the etiology of reflux nephropathy and its possible causation by hypersensitivity responses to infection early in life, and the fact that some may see antireflux surgery as "shutting the door after the horse has bolted."

Yet thousands of children throughout the world have had treatment for VUR and thousands more will undergo a procedure which, although designed to improve their health, will occasionally harm them.

Surgical treatment for VUR is not confined to open surgical treatment and in 1984 O'Donnell and Puri first brought to our attention the use of injection treatment performed endoscopically as a day patient for reflux. Latterly, there have been attempts, mostly successful, to treat vesicourerteric reflux with laparoscopic techniques using gas insufflation of the bladder.[4]

In addition, many different operations are performed for VUR each year with certain possible complications. In looking therefore at the long-term outcome from surgery it is necessary to take into account:

- the long-term complications of each operation
- the effectiveness of each operation
- how treatment has modified the effects on renal function or renal growth
- whether it has affected the patient's overall well-being

Successful surgery for primary reflux and good postoperative management in a patient with unscarred kidneys and no voiding abnormalities is likely to give both excellent short- and long-term results, with the potential for lower tract infections resolving with time and antibiotic prophylaxis.

On the other hand, an obstructive complication which goes unrecognized in a patient with renal scarring in the contralateral kidney will cause serious long-term effects of hypertension and possibly even renal failure.

Trying to treat incontinence and urinary infection by antireflux surgery in the infrequent voider is not likely to be helpful and will clearly affect the results of the outcome of treatment and reputation of not only the surgery but also the surgeon.

Injection treatment

Injection treatment for VU reflux

It was in 1984 that O'Donnell and Puri first reported the systematic use of injection treatment for reflux in children. In the last 20 years this procedure has been widely adopted for the primary treatment of vesicoureteric reflux in children both for primary cases and for secondary cases related to neuropathic bladder, urethral valves, or duplex systems.[5–7]

The initial procedure consisted of the endoscopic injection of polytetrafluoroethylene (PTFE) paste suspended in glycerine. Injection was into the lamina propria just behind the ureteric opening and was shown to be very effective in a number of clinical studies.

The initial problem with PTFE was the difficulty with injection as it was an extremely viscous substance and required special instrumentation to deliver the paste into the bladder.

The theoretical concerns about safety and the difficulty of injection led to the development of other substances for the same purpose. Bovine collagen was one of the first alternatives to PTFE and had a history of usage in cardiac surgery and soft tissue substitution. Cross-linked bovine collagen was a soluble and purified preparation of bovine collagen further stabilised by the addition of 0.0075% glutaraldehyde to effect fibril cross-linking. It caused minimal tissue reaction locally when injected and was much more easy to inject through a 25-gauge needle with standard endoscopic equipment. It was promising in the short term but seemed to "fail" quite quickly in a significant number of patients who had effective initial cure.[8,9]

In one study of 92 ureters treated with bovine collagen, 63% were cured at a month after one treatment and there was a 75% cure after multiple injections.[8] Simple systems had a higher cure rate than duplex systems and dilating reflux had cure rates of only 40%. Of the 68 ureters evaluated at 1 year, 64.7% were cured. If one looked at the "long-term" cure rates at 1 year nearly 25% of the patients had a recurrence of the reflux and similar results were noted in other studies using collagen.[9,10] Interdermal testing was recommended prior to the injection of bovine collagen and then, with the anxieties about bovine tissues that existed in Europe, the substance seems to have fallen into disfavor.

Deflux is another biocompatible material consisting of microspheres of dextranomas mixed in a 1% high molecular weight sodium hyaluanon solution. The dextran microspheres are made from cross-linked dextran polymers with a network configuration. This net will act as a carrier, which recruits cells from surrounding tissues. Results of the use of this material and the treatment of VUR showed very similar results with early studies confirming 72% success rate with resolution of VUR at 3 months and a 10% failure rate of successful treatment when followed for 1 year.[11] This material would seem to be a promising alternative to Teflon™ as it is much easier to inject and has apparently a lower long-term failure rate after initial successful treatment.

Particulate silicone injections (Macroplastique™) have been used in several studies to correct vesicoureteric reflux with similar early success rates, and again some concerns about the longevity of the treatment success has been raised.[12]

Stranger still was the harvesting of the patient's chondrocytes and then injecting them after growth in vitro as a bulking agent for the treatment of vesicoureteric reflux by endoscopic injection. This complex procedure does not seem to have caught the imagination of many practitioners.[13]

Concerns therefore about injection treatment for reflux center on the possible long-term effects of the injected substance or the recurrence of reflux, or at a more basic level whether treatment modifies the natural history of the condition at all.

Potential problems with injectables

Silicone

Distant particle migration is reported more often with solid plastic implants than with injectable biomaterials: solid plastic implants such as breast prosthesis,[14] penile prosthesis,[15] artificial sphincters,[16] and hemodialysis tubing.[17] The question is whether this migration is of any significance or not.

PTFE

Distant PTFE migration following periurethral injection in humans has been documented in only three cases during the last 30 years. One was found in a boy 6 years old in whom pulmonary granulomas surrounding PTFE particles were found at an autopsy following accidental death.[18] Another autopsy documented case of pulmonary PTFE particles has been reported,[19] as has one case of apparent pneumonitis with pathological documentation of PTFE particles.[20]

Only one report is currently available that documents particle migration following subureteric injection of PTFE paste.[18] Here, 1 hypogastric ganglia out of 7 patients who were examined was found to have particles. In that instance the injection had been outside the bladder musculature and reflux persisted. In one major study, Kaplan also used Teflon™ to correct VUR in 220 ureters in 117 patients. The longest follow-up was 5 years in 20 patients. His initial 25 cases were studied extensively following sting using ultrasound scans, nuclear cystograms, tomography, and magnetic resonance scans, and there was no evidence of change in local lymph nodes or the emergence of any retroperitoneal or intraperitoneal masses. Also, in those patients in whom sting was unsuccessful and who underwent subsequent open reimplantation, there was no evidence of spread of PTFE into regional lymph nodes sampled at the time of surgery. Histology of the injection site shows that the PTFE was encapsulated in a fibrous sheath. Foreign body giant cells lay within the sheath but there was no evidence of metastasis of the cells.[21]

In summary, the experimental results with migration reported by Malizia *et al.* and Rames and Aaronson have not been supported by the extensive worldwide clinical experience with the use of PTFE paste. No long-term morbidity has been reported to date with the use of PTFE paste to treat urinary incontinence or to correct reflux despite widespread application.

During the last 35 years, 4 patients have been found to have a malignancy adjacent to a PTFE implant:

- a case of fibrosarcoma adjacent to PTFE or aortograft implanted 10 years earlier[22]
- a chondrosarcoma of the vocal chord (a very rare lesion) in a patient who had a PTFE implant 5 years earlier[23]
- carcinoma adjacent to PTFE implant[24]
- vaginal and uterine rhabdomyosarcoma in a patient 10 months following periurethral PTFE injection.

  In none of these cases was there a definite causal relationship to the PTFE implant[25]

These long-term risks, and the potential long-term hazards from obstruction, have dogged the use of this substance with such intensity that even its original proponents have now switched to other injectables.

Long-term hazards with silicone injections

There has been controversy over the alleged association between silicone implants and connective tissue disorders and lymphomas and this was at a time when silicone microspheres were being injected for the control of reflux.

Silicone is widely used in a medical and non-medical environment and is found, for instance, in food additives, deodorants, drinking water, iv tubing, slow release hormone implants, infant bottle teats, and Dimethicone which is widely used for infant colic.[26] Most of the work with regard to silicone in medical circumstances relates to the use of silicone-breast implants and the initial studies that linked breast implants to connective and muscle disorders have not been substantiated.[27] As with other substances in regular usage, opinion waxes and wanes and more recent publications still suggest that there may be some safety concerns about breast implants but the majority of plastic surgeons and urologists regularly insert silicone-based implants into patients.[28] The initial enthusiasm for silicone injection has waned apparently due to a higher long-term failure rate to control the reflux than with other substances.

Long-term hazards with collagen injections

The use of bovine collagen for antireflux surgery has largely been superseded by other substances because of the

- need to check for sensitivity to the bovine collagen with a preliminary injection
- concerns about diseases transmitted between bovine species and humans which are still ongoing at the time of writing. No reported instances of such disease has been encountered.

Deflux has so far not encountered any threats to long-term usage, but these are early days.

Surgical treatment

Is one type of operation superior to another in the long term? There is today a renewed interest in the extravesical methods of treatment, which might lead to earlier discharge from hospital, less catheterization and lower treatment costs. However, "quality treatment" is not always to be equated with an early discharge home and the complication and readmission rates of procedures designed for shorter periods of hospital stay need to be assessed in the overall cost–benefit analysis.

There are variations on these themes such as "Firlit's description of Hodgson's technique in the modified Gil–Vernet procedure!"[29]

There are also endoscopic operative treatments such as modification of the Gil–Vernet procedure and laparoscopic versions of the Cohen procedure.

The two operations performed most commonly are undoubtedly the Cohen[30] and the Leadbetter–Politano[31], both of which have been the subject of comparative studies. The Cohen technique shows lower failure and complication rates in almost every study. Complication rates in the Leadbetter–Politano procedure of 3.4%–12% and in the Cohen procedure 2.2%–3% are reflected in a number of studies.[32,33] More recently, the International Reflux Study in Children IRSC, report from Europe showed that in 237 refluxing units there were ten re-operations for obstruction, one after a Cohen procedure and four after a Leadbetter–Politano procedure and three of these ureters had been transplanted through an intestinal loop transperioneally and thence to the bladder. This is a well-known but preventable complication of the Leadbetter–Politano procedure and raises distinct questions about overall operative safety.[34]

There is little doubt that the choice of patients for operation is not the only factor in the long-term outcome, the choice of surgeon and operative procedure also has an impact. The best results come from those units performing large numbers of operations, those with senior surgeons involved in the operations, and those where specialist pediatric urologists are involved in the surgical care.[35]

The important factors in successful reimplantation surgery are those initially suggested by Paquin.[36] These include:

- submucosal tunnel length five times the diameter of the ureter
- straightening of the ureter and having a smooth passage into the bladder through the bladder wall
- reimplantation of a vascularised ureter without hematoma formation.

What seems to matter little is whether you:

- evert the anastomosis like a nipple
- use the mucosal cuff around the ureter to suture to the new hiatus
- resect the lower portion of the ureter and anastomose this into the bladder

These features were stressed by Glenn and Anderson in describing their own version of the ureteric reimplantation which advances the ureter onto the ipsilateral trigone.[37]

The trigonoplasty (Gil–Vernet) operation seems to have a limited place in the treatment of primary reflux in children.[38] It is apparently at its most effective in treating milder grades of reflux, but these also respond well to injection treatment or non-operative approaches. The originator of this technique had a failure rate of treatment approaching 6%, and a more recent report suggests that it works poorly in those patients most likely to come to reimplantation; those with a patulous orifice, associated paraureteric diverticulae, or a large ureter.[39] There are no reports of short-term bladder disturbance except for dysuria which is also frequently associated with other intravesical operations. The long-term success rate and complications are presumably similar to the original description. Obstruction to ureteric drainage does not, it seems, feature as a complication.

The extravesical approach to antireflux surgery typified by the Litch–Gregoir procedure,[40,41] is attractive in so far as it is effective and can lead to relatively comfortable catheterless surgery. One major disadvantage of this operation is the potential damage to bladder function; this has been noted in the short term yet so far seems absent from long-term results. Some of the published results also suggest treatment for reflux is less likely to be successful in those patients with grade 4 or 5 reflux. A recent study suggested a 100% success rate for antireflux surgery in patients with grade 1–3 reflux but 92% in grade 4 and 67% in grade 5 using this technique.[42] The combined results of treatment of grade 4 and 5 reflux showed a success rate of 85%.

Further modifications of the Litch–Gregoir procedure can be effective it seems, in abolishing surgical complications such as postoperative reflux or obstruction;[29] but again the majority of patients in this study had grade 1–3 reflux and there were only 27 patients with grade 4–5 reflux. The excellent results reported from other studies also tend to gloss over the problems that may occur with bladder function following bilateral procedures.[29,43]

There have been reports of voiding dysfunction and retention of urine following surgery with patients needing vesical diversion or Mitrofanoff-type drainage procedures for intermittent catheterization. This is presumably due to neuropathic damage to the detrusor function from an incision in the detrusor muscle.[44] One study had an incidence of voiding abnormalities requiring intermittent catheterisation of 26%. Incisions in this area of the bladder have been implicated by others as causing denervation patterns in the detrusor muscle.[45] The attraction of this operation is therefore diminished for patients with grades 4 and 5 reflux, and those with some abnormality of the orifice such as a diverticulum. It runs the risk in bilateral cases of causing temporary or permanent voiding dysfunction. Complications such as continuing postoperative reflux are certainly not better than with other methods of repair.

Complications and late effects of surgery

- Obstruction after ureteric reimplantation may be early, late, symptomatic or silent.
- Postoperatively, it is associated with hypertension or reduction in urine output and may need urgent treatment in the form of upper tract drainage by nephrostomy.
- Early presentation may be secondary to hematoma compression which will resolve.
- There may be stenosis at the mucosal level or progressive intramural fibrosis secondary to ischemia of the reimplant. If this occurs it would persist after 3 months and need reoperation.
- In some operations there may be angulation of the ureter at the new bladder hiatus which may cause variable obstruction during bladder filling and require corrective surgery.
- Unrecognized bladder neuropathy may be the underlying cause of ongoing problems. Careful history of the voiding pattern is necessary before reimplantation surgery and formal investigation with cystometry if abnormal or incomplete voidings are suspected or if the patient suffers urinary incontinence.
- Obstructive complications significantly and adversely affect the long-term results of reimplantation surgery. Some renal damage usually results, increasing the long-term complications of hypertension and it has the potential to cause serious permanent renal impairment.

Obstruction is one of the most feared surgical outcomes of antireflux surgery. It may occur early or late after the reimplantation and may cause long-term complications such as hypertension and renal scarring (see later).

Some degree of ureteric dilatation is normal in the early postoperative phase as tissue edema causes pressure on the ureter lumen. Mild hydronephrosis and hydroureter is commonly seen in the first week or two following surgical treatment; it gives rise to no symptoms or abnormal signs and is not associated with complications.

Symptoms of loin pain or signs of hypertension or reduced urine output are much less common and more serious. They suggest the presence of a significant obstruction. Hydronephrosis and hydroureter under these circumstances should be investigated and treated, based on clinical and radiological findings in association with urgent diuresis renography.

If a decision is taken to drain the upper tracts temporarily, there should be resolution after 6–12 weeks. If there is not, there is an intrinsic abnormality of the reimplant needing reoperation; nephrostomy tube drainage should diminish and an antegrade study confirm successful resolution of the problem. Careful management of fluid input and treatment of hypertension can see the patient through a temporary obstruction due to edema or hematoma.[46]

A patient with reflux nephropathy had undergone reimplantation of the ureters and had a brief period of anuria associated with loin pain and hypertension.

The symptoms resolved but the renographic trace remained abnormal. Despite the finding of hydronephrosis and hydroureter, as the patient was then asymptomatic, a conservative approach was undertaken, but there was a marked deterioration in the function of the right kidney after 4 months.

At reoperation no specific obstruction was found. This case illustrates a serious complication of antireflux surgery, which could have been managed by temporary percutaneous upper tract drainage while the obstruction at the reimplantation site resolved.

It might be argued that temporary ureteric stenting in the early postoperative period could have overcome this particular complication. However, as obstruction can continue for several weeks and stents are nearly always removed by 7–10 days, this is unlikely to be the answer. Meticulous hemostasis and attention to surgical detail are more likely to be helpful.

After an intravesical–extravesical approach such as a Leadbetter–Politano reimplant, other symptoms might suggest the need for early reoperation, especially where there is intestinal obstruction or ileus and surgical damage to the intestine is suspected. It is not unknown for the ureter to travel transperitonealy through a loop of intestine, and then enter the bladder totally transfixing the intestine on the way to the new reimplant site. This complication is unlikely to escape early detection or to respond to conservative management.

Other forms of urinary tract obstruction after surgery are due to devascularization of the ureter with ischemia and scarring, or compression of the reimplant at some point due to hematoma or kinking of the entry through the bladder wall, as when there is hooking of the ureter over the superior vesical pedicle. All these are well-known complications and more frequently seen after the Leadbetter–Politano type procedure, and are rare with a Cohen or other advancement techniques such as Glenn–Anderson.

Chronic or progressive hydronephrosis after reimplantation should raise the possibility in the surgeon's mind of an underlying neuropathic bladder, as should persistence of VU reflux.

All patients who have had antireflux surgery should then be followed long term even if the upper tracts are unscarred and the patient is asymptomatic. Half the patients with obstruction will have no symptoms and may present many years later.[47]

It is the author's current view that a urinary tract ultrasound every 1–2 years should be the minimum and a mandatory part of the patient's long-term management to exclude silent obstruction whilst in periods of growth in childhood. Thereafter, obstruction seems to occur but rarely, except of course during pregnancy when the gravid uterus changes the anatomy in the pelvis significantly.

If urinary infection or loin pain supervene between outpatient visits, then some form of urinary obstruction should be excluded with initial ultrasound. If hydronephrosis is increasing, renography and cystometry should be undertaken to define the impairment of upper tract drainage and to exclude bladder neuropathy.

The incidence of obstruction after reimplantation should be no more than 1%–2% in the best hands but it is associated with a high incidence of permanent damage to the upper tract.[42 48]

The causes of long-term obstruction are usually fibrosis in the reimplant, but kinking as it enters the bladder occurs in about 20%.

The author has treated patients with megaureters who have had silent progressive obstruction and one presenting 2 years later with a urinary infection and the finding of hydronephrosis hydroureter following a Cohen reimplantation. In this patient the ureter took a 90° bend at the vesical hiatus and a further reimplant resolved the problem. Reoperation and reimplantation is usually successful in resolving the obstruction and can normally be dealt with successfully by an intravesical procedure.[49]

- Postoperative reflux is found frequently after reimplantation surgery.
- It should be rare in the operated side and is relatively trivial (grade 1–3) in the non-operated side if it occurs.
- Repeated cystography is not necessary more than 6 months after the surgical appraisal, since the majority of reflux found on postoperative studies should be treated conservatively, as there is such a high spontaneous resolution rate.
- For those in whom a recurrence or worsening of the reflux is apparent, then a strong suspicion of neuropathic bladder should be entertained and investigated accordingly.
- In the absence of unrecognized neuropathic bladder, persistent reflux seldom causes adverse long-term clinical effects and a "late cure" can be expected.

This is a very disappointing complication both for the patient and family and for the doctor and is more prevalent than many admit. The recorded incidence will depend on how frequently postoperative cystography is performed, but may also relate to the way that the cystogram is performed and to its timing.

It is well recognized that the reflux may be contralateral following unilateral reimplant or may involve the reimplanted ureter. Ahmed and Tann found contralateral reflux in 12.3% of their patients when the postoperative cystogram was performed 3 months after reimplant.[50]

The encouraging feature in these patients was that there seemed to be few if any symptoms related to the contralateral reflux, and an improvement occurred in all but one of the patients.

Hoenig *et al.* found that, after unilateral reimplantation, there was a 17%–21% incidence of contralateral reflux, depending on whether the original technique had been a Glenn–Anderson or a Cohen reconstruction. Reflux revolved in 61% of these patients; 26 were followed conservatively and 13% underwent surgical treatment. It was noted that patients could have resolution of the reflux as late as 9 years postoperatively.[51] A very high and late spontaneous cure rate, approaching 100%, was also reported by Laurenti *et al.*[52]

The European results from the recent international reflux study in children (IRSC) showed that where frequent postoperative cystography is performed, then a high incidence of vesicoureteric reflux on subsequent cystography is to be expected. Approximately half the patients in the IRSC study had reflux on one or more occasions during follow-up when all the cystograms were taken into consideration. Contralateral long-term reflux was, however, present in 18% but usually of grade 1–3 and in this age group it should be benign and undergo spontaneous cure.[51] On the other hand, high grade persistent reflux of grade 4 or 5 is not likely to undergo spontaneous cure. The IRSC study showed, however, that if the early cystogram at 6 months postoperatively was normal, there was an excellent prognosis. If the early cystogram did show reflux on either the operated or the non-operated side, the majority of patients had a negative cystogram at some point thereafter. It does not seem necessary therefore, to go on performing cystography frequently after reimplantation surgery, to continue to check the result.

When reflux is found on the postoperative cystogram, or appears recurrent and symptomatic, it may be necessary to exclude occult neuropathic bladder as Mesrobian *et al.*[49] found this in 6% of 69 cases.

A simple history of voiding patterns and questioning for voiding frequency and incontinence are usually all that is necessary in conjunction with the radiological and clinical examination preoperatively, but patients who are suspected of having a neuropathic bladder on these grounds will require cystometry as a precautionary measure before deciding on reimplantation surgery.

Other causes of failure of the reimplantation are retraction of the reimplanted ureter into a shorter tunnel or too short a reimplant. If it is necessary to repeat the reimplantation, the overall success rate of reoperation is 70% from an intravesical procedure.[49]

Diverticulum formation

This has been reported as a complication of the transverse advancement technique. In 304 patients reported by Ahmed and Tan[50] there was a 17% incidence of diverticulum formation. Fortunately, the majority of these are relatively small and benign and cause few symptomatic complications. Large diverticulae, however, greater than 1 cm, were associated with significant postoperative infective complications and persistence. Large diverticulae causing repeated infection need surgical treatment because they interfere with successful long-term outcome.

Some quite complex diverticulae patterns can be seen on postoperative cystography. In the long term these have caused few symptoms in the author's experience. They have disappeared spontaneously with growth and have not been seen endoscopically after radiological resolution. Their recurrence seems more frequent after the Cohen reimplantation than after other techniques.

Pyelonephritis

A number of studies have tried to untangle the web of reflux, infection, and renal scarring, and it is not yet clear what precise role reflux plays in the clinical picture. Reflux is absent in nearly half the patients who present with clinical pyelonephritis, and nearly half the patients who show signs on DMSA scanning in the acute episode do not have scarring or permanent change on subsequent studies (Postlethwaite, pers. commun.). It has been clear for many years that stopping reflux does not necessarily stop infection. Pyelonephritis is a cause of both acute and chronic histological changes in the kidney and it certainly causes a severe clinical illness. A strong link has been demonstrated between the presence of high grade VUR and the risk of pyelonephritis and scarring. A Swedish study started with a group of children who had normal kidneys and who suffered further urinary tract infections.[55] There were 37 in which upper tract change occurred, and 22 of these had gross VUR indicating a strong relationship between high grade reflux, pyelonephritis and long-term upper tract damage. Repeated upper tract imaging and creatinine clearance studies are not easy in small children, but it is easy to test for proteinuria, which is the main marker for decreasing renal function.[56]

Treatment does seem to have some part to play in the management of infection and in the prevention of upper tract changes. For example, in one study, when mechanical methods of treatment such a double micturition were used in combination with intermittent chemotherapy in reflux patients, the incidence of further renal scarring was 21%.[57] This figure applied to normal kidneys. In patients who presented with upper tract changes there was a 66% incidence of upper tract deterioration on follow-up using this regime alone.

Studies have shown a probable role for surgery in the management of symptomatic upper tract infections associated with high grade reflux. Weis *et al.*[58] reported that the incidence of symptomatic pyelonephritis was reduced in patients having surgical has opposed to medical treatment.

However, despite the clear association between pyelonephritis, gross VUR and long-term progressive renal damage, there is no clear consensus on whether reimplantation of the ureters has a significant effect on renal function. Some studies strongly support the positive effects of reimplantation surgery on the upper tract showing that renal growth accelerates,[59] and that renal function is measured by creatinine clearance and the glomerular filtration rate (GFR) shows significant improvement.[60] In the latter study there were 56 children between the ages of 2 and 15 years with scarred kidneys who had a GFR of less than 90 ml min^{-1} per 1.73 m^2 at presentation. Thirty-two patients had a bilateral reimplant for bilateral scarring and the GFR improved in 75% with individual GFRs improving in 81% of the 42 kidneys after operation. Children under the age of 2 years were excluded from this study because the GFR normally improves spontaneously during the first 2 years of life, and the best results were seen in children with GFRs greater than 30 ml min^{-1} per 1.73 m^2 at presentation.

Renal tubular acidosis has been suggested as a cause of somatic growth failure in children with reflux and scarring, but there has never been a suggestion that antireflux surgery can correct this aspect of renal impairment.[61]

It has been stated that small or scarred hyperplastic kidneys which provide less than 15% of the overall renal function can improve and do have growth potential.[62] The author's experience has been, however, that DMSA relative function declines progressively in such kidneys owing to compensatory hypertrophy in the contralateral organ, if that was normal at the outset.

Urinary tract infection

The IRSC report published in 1992 confirmed that just over one-third of patients continue to have urinary tract infections postoperatively.[63] This is comparable to the incidence of urinary infection in those patients treated medically. The incidence of pyelonephritic episodes can, however, be shown to be halved in patients subjected to surgery in this study.

Ahmed and Tan[50] found that 52 out of 169 patients (31%) had at least one urinary tract infection 6 months to 7 years postoperatively. The same 31% incidence after reimplantation was found by Waxman *et al.*[64] There seemed to be few if any, specific features that indicate which patients will develop urinary infection, yet in the author's experience it is very rare in boys after successful surgery. This was confirmed in another long-term study where the recurring incidence of pyelonephritis after reimplantation was found to be 27% in women and 9.5% in men.[65] Whether or not this type of urinary infection has any effect on renal growth after antireflux surgery is debatable, but renal growth should be normal in a normal kidney although the kidneys already scarred have a significant risk of developing further change in the long term.[65]

The IRSC data have confirmed those from other studies and show an incidence of apparent new scar formation after surgical or medical treatment is started. Surgery seems to protect these patients from new scar formation 2 years after the institution of treatment compared with medical treatment after which late scars were more frequently seen. Part of the difficulty in assessing the long-term effects of surgical treatment is knowing what the natural history of the disease would have been without any treatment at all; but there is evidence to suggest that repeated clinical pyelonephritis occurs in more than 50% of children if their vesicoureteric reflux remains untreated.[66]

Yet when the long-term effects of antireflux surgery are compared with medical treatment, as in the Birmingham reflux study, there does not seem to be any statistically significant difference in the incidence of urinary infection, which occurs in both patient treatment groups.[67]

Long-term outlook for infective complications

Between 4% and 7% of women will develop bacteriuria in pregnancy, and 20%–40% will have a symptomatic urinary tract infection if left untreated. It is apparent therefore, that as many as 3% of all pregnancies will be complicated by a symptomatic urinary tract infection in the mother.

It has been suggested that the successful treatment of VUR would protect patients in pregnancy from urinary tract infection, yet a study published in 1995 gave some alarming figures.[68] There was a dramatic increase in the number of symptomatic infections in young women who began to engage in sexual activity, and a huge increase in the number of symptomatic and serious urinary tract infections during pregnancy in women who had had antireflux surgery. At the onset of sexual activity, urinary infections occurred in 75% of young women who had previously had a reimplantation of the ureters, and in one-third of these they suffered pyelonephritis. Yet in a group of patients who had VUR with no operation, severe pyelonephritis occurred in only 2%. During pregnancy, 5% of women who had had a reimplantation were hospitalised with pyelonephritis, with some needing upper tract drainage procedures secondary to obstruction. This single report asserts a quite dramatic increase in serious obstructive-type hydronephrosis and infection during pregnancy, and will be a depressing consequence for antireflux surgery should the findings be confirmed by others. All the patients had a Leadbetter–Politano reimplant with a new hiatus for the ureter in the bladder muscle, and it may be that this particular operation has a predilection for causing this type of complication. Well over 1000 patients have been subjected to antireflux surgery by the Cohen technique in the Manchester area of the United Kingdom without the type of experience that the above authors report.

A more recent study suggested that 28% of patients who had had antireflux surgery developed a urinary tract infection in pregnancy and there was a 2% incidence of transgestational ureteric obstruction that required drainage. This was less dramatic than the above experience, yet still gave rise to concern that antireflux surgery may have hazardous effects during pregnancy in a small percentage of patients.[62] One has to observe again, however, that the patients had surgery by the Leadbetter–Politano technique in more than 90% of patients.

The same Leadbetter–Politano operation was performed in the other paper, which suggested a significant incidence of symptomatic urinary tract infection in girls in the long term.[69]

Renal scarring

Urinary tract infection occurs in 3% of the childhood population, one-third of the patients on investigation are found to have vesicoureteric reflux, with one-third of these having scarring at presentation. In the antenatal group, approximately one-third have upper tract change of significance at birth, and those presenting in the first year of life have a high incidence of upper tract scarring.[3]

The long-term effects of antireflux surgery are dominated by the long-term effects of the reflux nephropathy, which can be progressive even when surgical treatment has been undertaken. Yet scars do not improve, and in general patients deteriorate as time goes by rather than get better. The early adverse signs are the development of proteinuria or hypertension, even with stable upper tract change.

The incidence of hypertension in patients with renal scarring after antireflux surgery is the same in those having medical or other forms of treatment; it is likely to be around 20%.[70]

All such patients will therefore be candidates for long-term follow-up of their upper tract function. Most new scars occur in the first year or two following surgical treatment. What causes the new scars is difficult to determine, because 40% of those children in the IRSC study who developed a new scar did not, on careful follow-up, show any evidence of clinical urinary tract infection. Nearly all the new scars and progression occurred in the first 2 years of study. This suggests that methods of diagnosis of scarring were not good enough, and that these might reflect events initiated in the kidney at or before the clinical study and treatment started. Most patients had diagnosis of scarring on IVU and we now know that DMSA scanning is far more sensitive at picking up permanent upper tract change or progressive changes.

Any obstruction in the urinary system following reimplantation will have a very significant effect on upper tract scarring. Of new scars in the surgical section of the IRSC study, 30% were secondary to obstruction following reimplantation.[34]

The incidence of chronic renal failure in the population of patients treated for reflux must depend on the severity of the initial nephropathy. Those with severe bilateral scarring will have an incidence of hypertension at 20 years in excess of 25% and at least 10% of such patients will progress to end-stage renal failure.

Calculus formation seems to occur in approximately the same number of patients as those in the general population and may be symptomatic or silent.[65]

The underlying philosophy?

The basic tenet for the last 40 years has been that vesicoureteric reflux is associated with recurrent urinary tract infections in children and that these recurrent urinary tract infections lead in a third of patients to upper tract damage, and that, though reflux itself may undergo spontaneous cure, while it is persisting, there is a risk of progressive upper tract change. Inherent in this belief has been the concept that:

- reflux could and should be abolished
- infection could and should be prevented

and that a corollary would be that the long-term disease process would be modified.

It was also inherent in this belief that medical or surgical treatment had the capacity to do this with minimal complications and that treatment was always indicated. The last 40 years has taught us that it is certainly possible to harm children by the use of clumsy or inappropriate surgery and that it is also possible to harm children by injecting substances into them or by giving them long-term medication.

What the last 40 years has not taught us very well was whether or not our interventions significantly modified the disease process in a beneficial way.

Only one published trial involved a long-term study where treatment with antibiotics was randomized with no therapy. This failed to show any difference between the outcome for the risk of urinary tract infection or upper tract injury in either group.[53]

In a recent review article that reviewed all the randomized prospective trials we find the statement:

> 'the combined evidence from available randomised controlled trials of interventions in children with vesico-ureteric reflux does not provide compelling reasons why the current practice of diagnosing and treating children with vesico-ureteric reflux confers important health benefits'.[54]

Perhaps we are unable to modify the process of upper tract change and the predisposition to infection that occurs in patients with reflux.

We must therefore look at the long-term hazards of upper tract damage in causing hypertension and perhaps other problems during pregnancy. What if our treatment had the propensity to increase this risk. An unsuccessful reimplant complicated by obstruction increases the risk of scarring and perhaps hypertension in pregnancy or early adult life. What if our surgery causes more problems in pregnancy than patients who have not had treatment.

Much has been made of both the early and late failure of injection treatment to control reflux, but perhaps this is not important as the long-term effects of persisting reflux may not be very sinister.

If this is so, then there is questionable benefit from early treatment by injection and by injection therapy. One must be more concerned about the long-term hazards of the injectable substance, and with some of the substances we do not yet have that information as they have only been in use for less than a decade. Most of the anxiety has been expressed with regard to PTFE and what evidence there is suggests that very little long-term harm will come to patients from the use of this substance as it is such a frequently used medical material, yet we still have to await potential long-term outcomes of this treatment. The use of bovine collagen and silicone has largely been superseded by the use of Deflux™ and as yet very little long-term evidence has come from its use.

Yet, the benefits of injection treatment still remain questionable as the incidence of urinary tract infections in treated and untreated groups seem similar.

If the benefits of injection treatment remain questionable, then so do the results and benefits of surgery. What is clear from the trials that have been performed is that surgery can be beneficial for patients who have:

- normal bladder function
- significant anatomical abnormalities of the vesicoureteric junction
- and who suffer pain or repeated pyelonephritis.

Surgery seems to have to confer little benefit apart from those two events in the patient's life.

We know that dysfunctional voiding syndromes or detrusor instability or infrequent voiders may also suffer from vesicoureteric reflux and repeated positive urine tests, if not repeated urinary infections. The natural history of these conditions in childhood seem lengthy with approximately half the patients continuing with symptoms after a mean of 5 years. It would be important to recognize the fact that these patients have a "cause" of their reflux and until this cause is abolished, then simple surgical or medical treatment of the reflux itself will confer little symptomatic or practical benefit to the patient.

What is clear from all this endeavor is that there is the world of difference between good treatment for reflux and bad treatment for reflux but not much difference between good treatment and no treatment at all.

REFERENCES

1. Hutch, J. A. Vesico-ureteric reflux in the paraplegic: cause and correction. *J. Urol.* 1952; **68**:457–463.
2. Williams, D. I. The history of paediatric urology: personal recollections 1948–1978. BJU Int. (Suppl.) 2003; **92**:1–3.
3. Jewkes, F., Sheridan, M., & Gough, D. C. S. Reflux nephropathy in the first year of life: the role of infection. *Pediatr. Surg. Int.* 1991; **6**: 214–216.
4. O'Donnell, B. & Puri, P. Treatment of vesico-ureteric reflux by endoscopic injection of Teflon. *Br. Med. J.* 1984; **289**:7–9.
5. Puri, P. & Guiney, E. J. Endoscopic correction of vesico-ureteric reflux secondary to neuropathic bladder. *Br. J. Urol.* 1986; **58**:504–506.
6. Puri, P. & Kumar, R. Endoscopic correction of vesico-ureteric reflux secondary to posterior urethral valves. *J. Urol.* 1996; **156**:680–682.
7. Dewan, P. A. & O'Donnell, B. Polytef paste injection of refluxing duplex ureters. *Eur. Urol.* 1991; **19**:35–38.
8. Frey, P., Berger, D., Jenny, P., & Herzog, B. Subureteral collagen injection for the endoscopic treatment of vesico-ureteric reflux in children: follow up study of 97 treated ureters and histological analysis of collagen implants. *J. Urol.* 1992; **148**:718–723.

9. Cendron, M., Leonard, M., Gearhart, J. P., & Jeffs, R. D. Endoscopic treatment of vesico-ureteric reflux using cross-linked bovine dermal collagen. *Pediatr. Surg. Int.* 1991; **6**:295–300.
10. Frey, P., Jenny, P., & Herzog, B., Endoscopic subureteric collagen injection (SCIN): a new alternative treatment for vesicoureteric reflux in children. *Pediatr. Surg. Int.* 1991; **6**:287–294.
11. Lackgren, G. & Stenberg, A. A new bioimplant for VUR treatment. *Dialog Pediatr. Urol.* 1994; **17**:2.
12. Azmy, A. Clinical experience with Macroplastique for correction of vesico-ureteric reflux in children. Abstract at International Congress of Endoscopic Pediatric Urology, Basel, Switzerland, 1993.
13. Atala, A., Cima, L. G., Kim, W. *et al.* Injectable alginate ceded with chondro sites as a potential for vesico-ureteric reflux correction. *J. Urol.* 1993; **150**:745.
14. Tabatoski, K., Elson, C. E., & Johnson, W. W. Silicone lymphadenopathy in a patient with a mammary prosthesis: fine needle aspitation cytology, histology and analytical electron microscopy. *Acta Cytol.* 1990; **34**:10.
15. Barret, D. M., O'Sullivan, D. C., Malizia, A. A., Reinmann, H. M., & Abel Aleff, P. C. Particle shedding and migration from silicone genito-urinary prosthetic devices. *J. Urol.* 1991; **146**: 319–322.
16. Kossovosky, N., Cole, P., & Zackson, D. A. Giant cell myocarditis associated with silicone: an unusual case of biomaterial pathology discovered at autopsy using X-ray energy spectroscopic techniques. *Am. J. Clin. Pathol.* 1981; **107**:611.
17. Bowen, J. H., Woodard, B. H., Barton, T. K., Ingram, P., & Shelbourne, J. D. Infantile pulmonary hypertension associated with a foreign body vasculitis. *Am. J. Clin. Pathol.* 1981; **75**:609.
18. Peters, C. A. Why use Teflon in children? *Dialog. Pediat. Urol.* 1991; **14**:4–5.
19. Mittleman, R. E. & Marracini, J. V. Pulmonary Teflon granuloma following periurethral Teflon injection for urinary incontinence. *Arch. Patheol. Lab. Med.* 1983; **107**:611–612.
20. Claes, H., Stroobants, D., Van der Meerbeek, J. *et al.* Pulmonary migration following polytetrafluoroethylene injection for urinary incontience. *J. Urol.* 1989; **142**:821–822.
21. Kaplan, W. E. Endoscopic injection of Teflon: a US perspective. *Dialog. Pediatr. Urol.* 1991; **14**:3–4.
22. Montgomery, R. Polytetrafluoroethylene. In Clayton, G. D. & Clayton, F. E., eds. *Patty's Industrial Hygiene and Toxicology*, Vol 3C, NY: John Wiley & Sons, 1982; 4308–4310.
23. Hakky, M., Kolbusz, R., & Reyes, C. V. Chondrosarcoma of the larynx. *Ear. Nose Throat J.* 1989; **68**:60–62.
24. Lewy, R. B. Experience with vocal cord injection. *Ann. Otol. Rhinol. Laryngol.* 1976; **85**:440–450.
25. Lockhart, J. L., Walker, R. D., Vorstman, B., & Politano, V. A. Periurethral polytetrafluoroethylene injection following urethral reconstruction in female patients with urinary incontinence. *J. Urol.* 1988; **140**:51.
26. Collis, N., Khoo, C. T., & Sharp, D. T. 477 Media are too eager to link Silicone to disease. *Br. Med. J.* 1998; **316**:477.
27. Kmietowicz, Z. Breast implants deemed safe – again. *Br. Med. J.* 1998; **317**:230.
28. Moynihan, R. Safety concerns about breast implants persist. *Br. Med. J.* 2003; **327**:947.
29. Waxman, J., Gilbert, A., & Sheldon, C. A. Results of the renewed extravesical reimplant for surgical correction of vesico-ureteral reflux. *J. Urol.* 1992; **148**:359–361.
30. Cohen, S. J. Ureterozystoneostomie: eine neue antireflux technik. *Aktuelle Urol.* 1975; **6**:1–7.
31. Politano, V. A. & Leadbetter, F. An operative technique for the correction of vesico-ureteric reflux. *J. Urol.* 1958; **79**:932–934.
32. Burbige, K. A. Ureteral reimplantation: a comparison of the results with cross trigonal and Politano–Leadbetter techniques in 120 patients. *J. Urol.* 1991; **146**:1352–1353.
33. Carpentier, P. J., Bettink, P. J., Hop, W. C. J., & Schroder, F. H. Reflux: a retrospective study of 100 ureteric reimplantations by the Politano–Leadbetter method and 100 by the Cohen technique. *Br. J. Urol.* 1982; **54**:230–233.
34. Hjalmas, K. Lohr, G., Tamminen-Mobius, T. *et al.* Surgical results in the International Reflux Study in Children (Europe). *J. Urol.* 1992; **148**:1657–1661.
35. Smellie, J. M. Commentary: management of children with severe vesico-ureteric reflux. *J. Urol.* 1992; **148**:1676–1678.
36. Paquin, A. J., Jr. Ureterovesico anastomosis: the description and evaluation of a technique. *J. Urol.* 1959; **82**:573–575.
37. Glenn, J. F. & Anderson, E. E. Distal tunnel reimplantation. *J. Urol.* 1967; **97**:623–626.
38. Gill-Vernet, J. M. A new technique for surgical correction of vesico-ureteric reflux. *J. Urol.* 1984; **131**:456–458.
39. De Gennaro, M., Appetito, C., Lais, A. *et al.* Effectiveness of trigonoplasty to treat primary vesico-ureteric reflux. *J. Urol.* 1991; **146**:636–638.
40. Litch, R., Jr., Howerton, L. W., & Davis, L. A. Ureteric reflux: its significance and correction. *Am. Surg.* 1962; **55**:633–636.
41. Gregoir, W. & Van Regemorter, G. V. Le reflux vésico-urétéral congénital. *Urol. Int.* 1964; **18**:122–126.
42. Houle, A. M., McLorie, G. A., Heritz, D. M. *et al.* Txtravesical nondismembered ureteroplasty with detrussorraphy: a renewed technique to correct vesico-ureteric reflux in children. *J. Urol.* 1992; **148**:704–707.
43. Zaontz, M. R., Maisels, M., Sugar, E. C., & Firlit, C. F. Detrussorraphy: extravesical advancement with correction of vesico-ureteric reflux in children. *J. Urol.* 1987; **138**:947–949.
44. Fung, L. C. T., McClorie, G. A., Jain, U., Khoury, A. E., & Churchill, B. M. Voiding efficiency after ureteral reimplantation: a comparison of extravesical and intravesical techniques. *J. Urol.* 1995; **153**:1972–1975.
45. Hollowell, J. G., Hill, P. D., Duffy, P. G., & Ransley, P. G. Bladder function in exstrophy and epispadias. *Lancet* 1991; **338**:926–928.
46. Garratt, R. A. & Shluetter, D. P. Complications of antireflux operations: causes and management. *J. Urol.* 1973; **109**:102–104.
47. Weiss, R. M., Schiff, M., Jr., & Lytton, B. Late obstruction after ureteroneocystostomy. *J. Urol.* 1971; **106**:144–148.

48. Starzl, T. E., Marchioro, T. L., Porter, K. A. *et al.* Renal homo transplantations: late function and complications. *Ann. Intern. Med.* 1964; **61**:470–475.
49. Mesrobian, H. J., Kramer, S. A., & Kelalis, P. P. Re-operative ureteroneocystostomy: a review of 69 cases. *J. Urol.* 1985; **133**:388–390.
50. Ahmed, S. & Tan, H. Complications of transverse advancement ureteral reimplantation: diverticulum formation. *J. Urol.* 1982; **127**:970–973.
51. Hoenig, D. M., Diamond, D. A., Rabinowitz, R., & Caldamone, A. A. Contralateral reflux after unilateral reimplantation. *J. Urol.* 1996; **156**:196–197.
52. Laurenti, C., De Dominicis, C., Iori, F. *et al.* Unilateral primary vesico-ureteric reflux: uni or bilateral reimplantation? *J. d'Urol.* 1989; **95**:213–215.
53. Reddy, P. P., Evans, M. T., Hughes, P. A. *et al.* Antimicrobial prophylaxis in children with vesico-ureteral reflux: a randomised prospective study of continuous therapy versus intermittent therapy versus surveillance. 1997; *Proc. AAP. Paediatr. Suppl.*
54. Wheeler, D., Vimalachandra, D., Hodson, E. M., Roy, L. P., Smith, G., & Craig, J. C. Antibiotics and surgery for vesico-ureteric reflux: a meta-analysis of randomised controlled trials. Arch. Dis. Child. 2003; **88**:688–694.
55. Berg, U. B. Long term follow-up of renal morphology and function in children with recurrent pyelonephritis. *J. Urol.* 1992; **148**:1715–1720.
56. Bailey, R. R., Lynne, K. L., & Smith, A. H. The long term follow up of infants with gross vesico-ureteric reflux. *J. Urol.* 1992; **148**:1709–1711.
57. Lenaghan, D., Whittaker, J. G., Jensen, F., & Stephens, F. D. The natural history of reflux and the long term effects of reflux in the kidney. *J. Urol.* 1976; **115**:728–730.
58. Weiss, R., Duckett, J., Spitzer, A., on behalf of the IRSC. Results of a randomised trial of medical versus surgical management of infants and children with grades III and IV primary vesico-ureteric reflux (United States). *J. Urol.* 1992; **148**:1667–1673.
59. Atwell, J. D. & Vijay, M. R. Renal growth following reimplantation of the ureters for vesico-ureteric reflux. *Br. J. Urol.* 1978; **50**:367–370.
60. Scott, D. J., Blackford, H. N., Joyce, M. R. L. *et al.* Renal function following surgical correction of vesico-ureteric reflux in childhood. *Br. J. Urol.* 1986; **58**:119–124.
61. Guizar, J. M., Kornhauser, C., Malacara, J.M., Sanders, G., & Zamara, J. Renal Tubular acidosis in children with vesico-ureteric reflux. *J. Urol.* 1996; **156**:193–195.
62. Bauer, S. B., Willscher, M. K., Zammuto, P. J., & Retik, A. B. Dilemma of small pyelonephritic kidney associated with vesicoureteral reflux. *Urology* 1980; **15**:466–470.
63. Jodahl, U., Koskimies, O., Hanson, E. *et al.* Infection pattern in children with vesico-ureteric reflux randomly allocated to operation or long term antibacterial prophylaxis. *J. Urol.* 1992; **148**:1650–1652.
64. Waxman, J., Anderson, E. E., & Glenn, J. F. Management of vesico-ureteric reflux. *J. Urol.* 1978; **119**:814–817.
65. Mor, Y., Liebovitch, I., Zalts, R., Lotan, D., Jonas, P., & Ramome, J. Analysis of the long-term outcome of surgically corrected vesico-ureteric reflux. *BJUI* **92**:97–100.
66. Govan, D. E. & Palmer, J. M. Urinary tract infection in children: the influence of successful antireflux operations in morbidity from infection. *J. Urol.* 1969; **44**:677–679.
67. Birmingham Reflux Study Group. Prospective trial of operative versus non-operative treatment of severe vesico-ureteric reflux in children; five years observation. *Br. Med. J.* 1987; **295**:237–241.
68. Mansfield, J. T., Snow, B. W., Cartwright, P. C., & Wadsworth, K. Complications of pregnancy in women after childhood reimplantation for vesico-ureteric reflux: an update with 25 years follow up. *J. Urol.* 1995; **154**:787–790.
69. Cooper, A. & Atwell, J. A long term follow up of surgically treated vesico-ureteric reflux in girls. *J. Pediatr. Surg.* 1993; **28**:1034–1036.
70. Jacobson, S. H., Eklof, O., Eriksson, C. G. *et al.* Development of hypertension and uraemia in childhood:27 years follow up. *Br. Med. J.* 1989; **299**:703–706.

45

Genitoplasty in exstrophy and epispadias

Christopher R. J. Woodhouse

The Institute of Urology and The Hospital for Children, Great Ormond Street, London, UK

There is a spectrum of congenital anomalies of the lower urinary tract and pelvis covered by the term "exstrophy/epispadias." At the worst end is cloacal exstrophy and at the most minor end is an epispadiac position of an otherwise normal urethra (Fig. 45.1). In males and females with an incompletely closed pubic ring the genitalia have a characteristic deformity called epispadias. The reconstruction of this anomaly is the same, regardless of the degree of bladder anomaly, although, especially in males, the system of bladder emptying may influence the surgical decisions. The extent of surgery required depends on the functional consequences of the deformity. Although chordee correction is commonly performed as a part of the reconstruction in infancy, further surgery after puberty is often needed to allow intercourse to take place.

Exstrophy is not, on its own, a lethal condition. The surgery and subsequent complications may be. In 1926 Dr. Charles Mayo, cofounder of the Clinic, published a paper on his experience of 66 cases of exstrophy. He recorded that 72% were still alive but he was not optimistic that the long-term results would be good, as most were still under 10 years old. Historically, 67% of patients would be dead by the age of 20, though his oldest survivor was 73.[1] It was not until after the Second World War that a combination of therapeutic advances conferred a more normal lifespan on exstrophy patients. Between 1986 and 1999 there were no deaths of exstrophy patients in the first year of life, in one US state.[2] As they lived longer and more normal lives, the problems of sexuality and fertility became apparent. Papers in the 1950s and 1960s began to record the sexual and fertility outcomes and later identified the anatomical basis for the problems.

Male and female exstrophy babies are born with a full potential for intercourse and fertility. The questions are whether or not that potential can be realized by proper reconstruction and whether or not it can survive the surgery involved. It is an unfortunate fact that an adult who is infertile is likely to have become so through the complications of infection or surgery.

Anatomy of the male genitalia

The anatomy of the exstrophy pelvis has been investigated clinically, by cavernosography, computed tomography (CT), magnetic resonance imaging (MRI), by experimental models, and by dissection.[3–11]

The pelvic ring is open anteriorly. The pubic bone is poorly formed and 30% shorter than normal.[10] The two halves of the pelvis are rotated downwards by 12 degrees so that the inferior pubic ramus (to which the corpora are attached) is parallel with the floor when the patient is standing upright (Fig. 45.2).[4]

Neonatal osteotomy does change this orientation to a certain degree, even though the symphysis is not completely closed. However, the pelvic floor remains flatter than in normal babies in the coronal plane (103 vs. 80 degrees), but is the same when seen in the sagittal plane.[12]

The penis is short and broad. It is short because the corpora are short and not because a large part is buried in the

Pediatric Surgery and Urology: Long-term Outcomes, Mark Stringer, Keith Oldham, Pierre Mouriquand.
Published by Cambridge University Press.

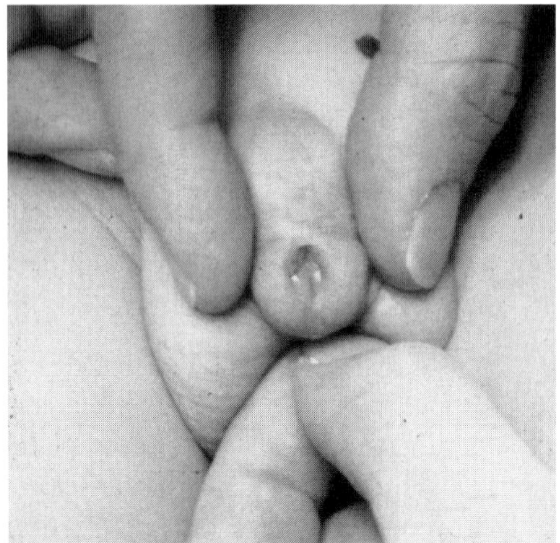

Fig. 45.1. Clinical photograph of a boy with a minor, distal, epispadias.

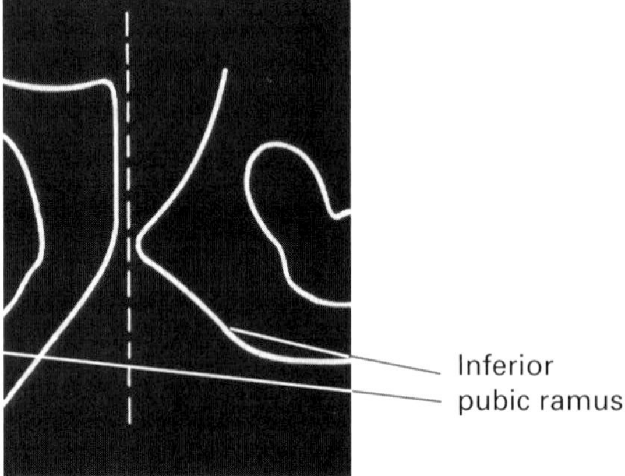

Fig. 45.2. Diagram of the anterior pelvis to show the orientation in normal males (left) and in exstrophy males (right). Note that the inferior pubic ramus is parallel to the floor when the exstrophy male is standing.

pelvis, though the penis is longer if the divarication of the pubic bones is 3 cm or less. There is some experimental evidence that the visible portion of the penis would be longer if the pelvic ring were closed.[8] MRI shows that normal corpora are 60% longer than those of exstrophy (mean of 16.1 cm compared to 10.1 cm). Most of the deficiency is in the anterior or exophytic part (12.3 cm for normal men and 6.9 cm for exstrophy men). The posterior parts of the corpora are of nearly normal length (3.9 cm compared to 3.2 cm). The mean corporeal diameter is 1.4 cm in exstrophy and 1.0 cm in normals.

The prostate is a flat, open plate at birth. With reconstruction, some effort is made to close it, but in adulthood it has been shown never to make a complete ring. The veru montanum is in the normal position and is a useful landmark in adult surgery. The urethra remains anterior to the prostate. Nonetheless, it is of normal size as measured by MRI. At a mean age of 25 years, the volume has been found to be 20.7 ml[3] which is normal for age.

The urethra is also an open plate. With reconstruction it is rolled into a tube. Current practice is to transfer it to the ventrum of the penis. However, until about 1980 it was left on the dorsum. The urethral position will have an impact on the choice of surgical technique used to correct chordee persisting into adult life.

The glans is of normal bulk but is also open and has been likened to a Scottish kipper. Surgical dissection in adults suggests that there is some erectile tissue running along the proximal two-thirds of the ventral aspect, corresponding to the corpus spongiosum.

The fate of the bulbospongiosus muscle is unknown. Logic would suggest that it is present in some form. In the neonate it may be too small to identify and could be destroyed in the initial reconstruction. In adults who happen to have had little reconstruction in childhood, a thin layer of muscle can be found at the base of the penis running from the urethral plate to the pubis on either side. This might represent the bulbo-spongiosus, but it does not encircle the urethra and is unlikely to contribute anything to ejaculation.

The position of the pubic hair depends on the type of primary reconstruction. With the older "W" closure, the hair lies laterally with a large central area of baldness. The mons pubis is absent and this combination may emphasise the penile anomaly (Fig. 45.3). On occasion, the erect penis may retract into the defect like the undercarriage of an old aeroplane. With a successful osteotomy and a midline skin closure, the distribution of hair is normal.

Clinical experience shows that the testes, epididymis, and vasa are normal, though no formal investigation has been done to confirm these data. However, in patients who have been investigated for azoospermia, an obstruction at the level of the prostate has usually been identified. The testes of infants born with cloacal exstrophy are normal on histological examination.[13]

Appearances in adult males

The adult epispadiac penis is short and broad (Fig. 45.4). The abnormalities may be exaggerated by the recession

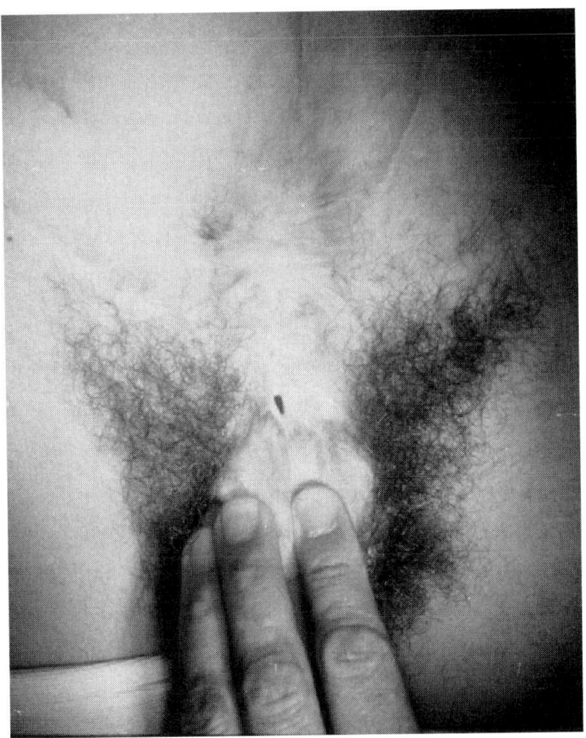

Fig. 45.3. Clinical photograph to show the distribution of pubic hair in exstrophy.

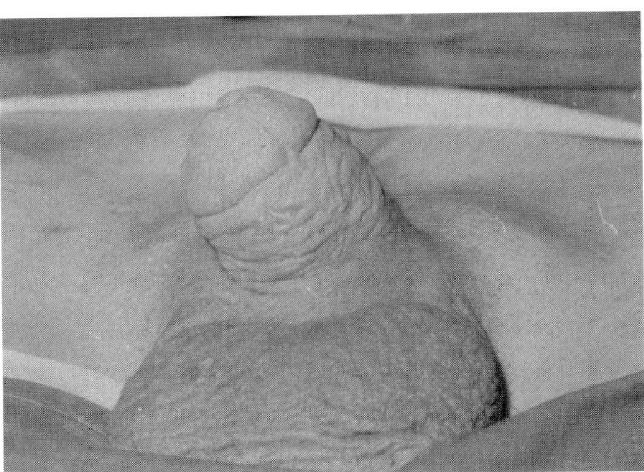

Fig. 45.4. Clinical photograph to show a normal flaccid penis in exstrophy.

of the supra pubic area, absence of the mons pubis and the normal size of the scrotum (Fig. 45.3).

Modern reconstruction in infancy attempts a midline closure of the abdominal wall defect so that the pubic hair grows as a normal triangular escutcheon. There is a much more normal penile appearance with a normal "angle of dangle" in more than half of boys.[14] This is particularly important in childhood, when the penis can have a near normal appearance, which should encourage proper sexuality.[15] Transfer of ventral skin to the dorsum may prevent recurrence of dorsal chordee.[16] However, there is an ever-present danger that radical penile surgery on the penis in infancy will cause ischemia. In a series of 42 infants having complete penile disassembly, ischemic changes in the glans were noted in five, two of whom lost half of the glans as a result. Fortunately, in this series, 81% ended up with a straight penis, 19% had a downward angle and all had erections.[17]

Erectile function in males

The mechanism of erection appears to be normal and so the nerve and blood supply are, presumably, intact. However, the natural erection of an epispadiac penis results in a dorsal chordee, which brings the penis tightly against the abdominal wall (Fig. 45.5).[4] Cavernosogram shows that the site of maximum curvature is more proximal than clinical examination might suggest and is at the point where the corpora emerge from the perineum (Fig. 45.6). The degree of chordee is variable and in some is mild enough to allow intercourse, either in the normal position or in one that brings the penis into closer apposition with the introitus.

Recognition of this anomaly has led to a modification of the primary reconstruction so that serious chordee now is seldom seen in adults. However, it seems likely that infantile surgery is responsible for the more complex erectile deformities that are occasionally found. The simplest of these is overcorrection so that there is sharp downward chordee on erection.

If one of the corpora is damaged, it fails to fill properly and acts as a bowstring on its normal pair. The erection then deviates to one side (Fig. 45.7). If both corpora are damaged, the penis is small, lies higher on the pubis than normal, and may have a limited erection (Fig. 45.8). On cavernosography, the corpora appear to have no attachment to the inferior pubic rami. Erection is very limited and the penis unstable.

In one case in my experience the corpora were so damaged (elsewhere) that, in adulthood, there is no visible and hardly any palpable penis. These problems are still seen, especially in patients operated on outside subspecialist centers: in an update of the Mainz experience, penile

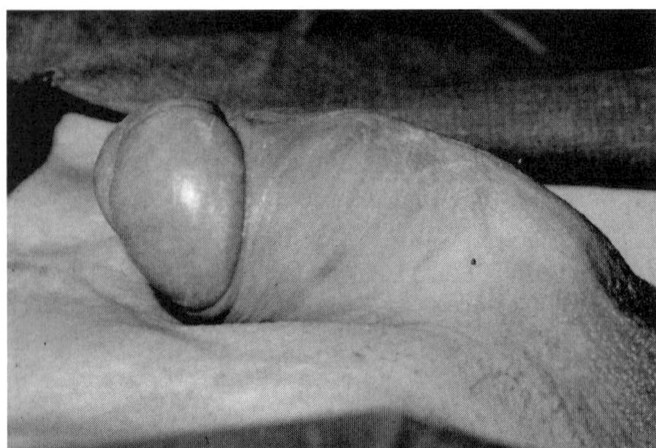

Fig. 45.5. Clinical photograph to show an erect penis in exstrophy. Note that, in addition to dorsal chordee, the penis is partly retracted into the recessed mons.

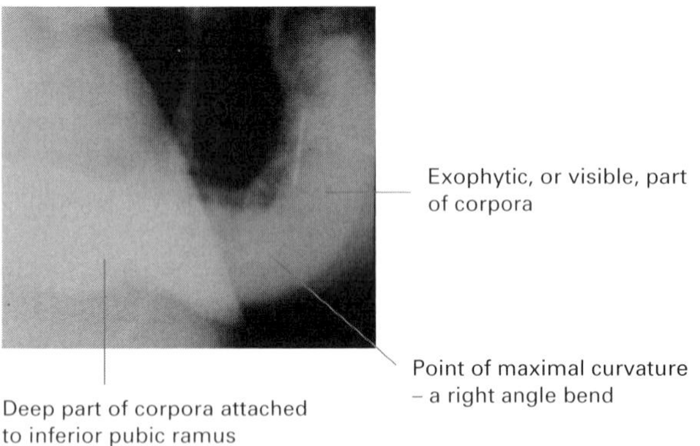

Fig. 45.6. Cavernosogram in a man with exstrophy and dorsal chordee.

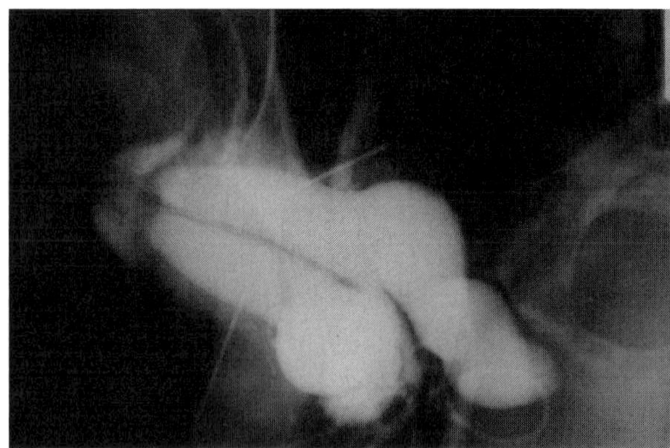

Fig. 45.7. Cavernosogram of a patient with exstrophy showing deviation to the right on erection.

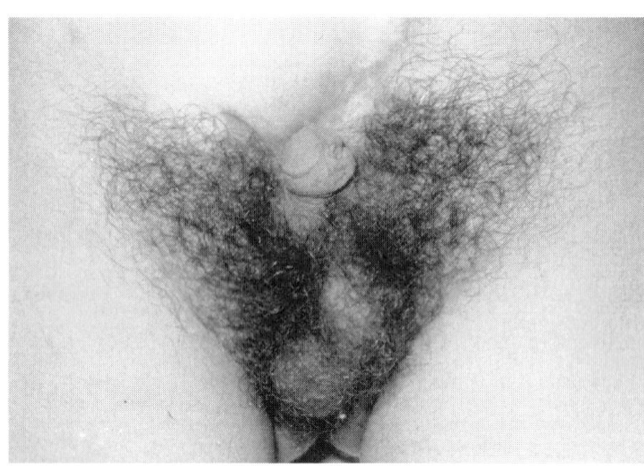

Fig. 45.8. Clinical photograph showing a rudimentary penis. Cavernosogram showed that the corpora were incomplete and had no attachment to the inferior pubic rami. Note that the penis lies higher on the mons than usual.

Table 45.1. Incidence of erectile deformities in exstrophy and epispadias

Dorsal chordee	77%
Unilateral rudimentary corpus	9%
Bilateral rudimentary corpus	14%

deviation was seen in 11 of 32 patients born after 1968. One boy had lost his penis through postoperative ischemia.[18]

The evidence suggests that the corpora are of equal size at birth and are damaged in the primary (and revision) reconstructive surgery.[17,19] The distribution of erectile deformities currently seen in adults is shown in Table 45.1.

Awareness of the erectile problems has led to much better reconstruction in infancy, so that erectile deformity in adults is becoming rare. Even by 1986, more than a half of adults (24 of 44) had a normal angle of erection on reaching adulthood.[14]

Penile reconstruction: length

The common complaint of the adult with epispadias is that the penis is too short. As with a more normal penis, true lengthening is not possible because new corporeal erectile tissue cannot be created. Therefore, longer functioning length can only be made by exposing as much as possible of the existing corpora. Whatever the results in children, pelvic osteotomy in adults seems a

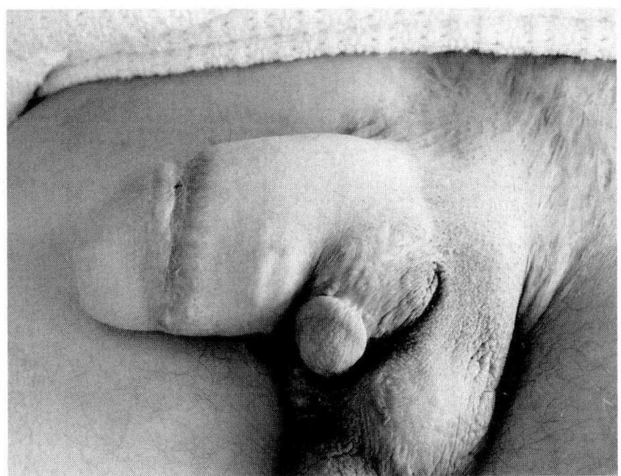

Fig. 45.9. Exstrophy patient with a phalloplasty (above) grafted onto the natural penis (below). With permission from Mr. David Ralph.

rather drastic procedure in an adult just to gain penile length.

Increase in the length of the visible penis can only be achieved by making the best use of the corpora distal to their attachment to the inferior pubic ramus. The horizontal plane in which the rami lie means that penile lengthening can only be achieved by completely detaching the corpora from the ramus. Although a technique has been described with a good result in 9 of 11 children, the risk of devascularizing the corpora has prevented its regular use.[20]

In some adolescents there is still some attachment of the corpora to the body of the pubis, release of which may give a little extra length. There is also some "concertina-ing" of the corpora that can be freed. The results of what amounts to the unpicking of scar tissue is variable. My results have been disappointing but "considerable lengthening" was reported by Hendren.[21] There is no reliable means of giving true functional added length to the adolescent epispadiac penis.

A technique has been described to make a phallus from a skin flap, using the technique for female to male gender reassignment, and to "piggy-back" it onto the natural penis (Fig. 45.9). The exstrophy man then has his own sexual satisfaction from his natural penis and can penetrate his partner's vagina with the reconstructed part. The results in patients are reported to be good with very careful selection.[22] In my own very limited experience of the procedure, the appearance is odd and it can be justified only in those with a very rudimentary natural penis.

Penile reconstruction: chordee

Correction of chordee is a most important procedure, which allows the best use of the existing penis for intercourse. Ideally, this should be achieved in infancy. Release of the urethral plate and chordee and partial detachment of the corpora from the pubis are considered essential steps.[23] However, it is rare for the correction to be achieved in a single stage, the mean being 1.6 operations (range 1–4).[14] A normal appearance with minimal scarring is of paramount importance to children and adolescents.[24,25]

Some of the techniques do give slight increase in length but nothing that makes the adult penis look normal.[26] The principles of reconstruction for chordee are to clear any restricting scar tissue from the dorsum and then either to lengthen the concave aspect or shorten the convex one. Which of these last two is chosen depends mainly on the position of the urethra. If the urethra is a good, complete tube lying on the dorsum, lengthening of the dorsal concave aspect will almost certainly mean that the urethra will ultimately be too short. Urethroplasty will therefore be necessary as a second stage. This seems to be rather a high price to pay for the few millimetres of total lengthening that may be achieved. A ventral Nesbit's procedure gives good correction with minimal shortening. If the urethra has been moved to the ventrum, both options are reasonable.

To lengthen the concave side, the tunica albuginea are incised transversely on the dorsum and the corpora are straightened. This leaves an elliptically shaped defect in each. Ideally, the defects should be closed by rotating the corpora towards each other so that they can be sutured together face to face. This Cantwell Ransley technique works very well in children and adolescents but the follow-up is short.[15,27,28] In adults, the corpora may be so far apart that the technique causes a new deformity of the penis in the shape of an hour-glass.

Alternatively, the defect may be filled with an elliptical patch. This technique was originally described using lyophilized human dura, which is no longer thought to be safe. Autologous material such as tunica vaginalis or rectus sheath has been used but with uneven results. Recently, the present author has been using pigskin in the form of Pelvicol®. The initial results have been good but follow-up is very short (C. R. J. Woodhouse, unpublished data). The reconstruction should include the correct positioning of the pubic hair-bearing skin.

An interesting comparison of the two techniques for the reconstruction of infants has come from Ransley's own unit. Originally, he used a staged repair, later augmented with a dural implant. In the second half of his series he used a corporeal rotation (the Koff technique)[29] and then the cavernocavernostomy (Cantwell–Ransley). The cosmetic result was judged to be acceptable in 40% of the earliest patients, rising to 84% in those having the Cantwell–Ransley procedure. Similarly, 50% of the early patients required radical revision, usually using the Cantwell–Ransley procedure. Obviously, follow-up was very short for the more recent procedures (4 years compared to 9 years). Furthermore, all of the patients were operated on in infancy (3 to 4.8 years) and it is possible that there will be some deterioration with age. In children it may be difficult to assess the angle of erection and its suitability for intercourse.[27]

In boys with isolated epispadias, the abnormality of the penis may be much less severe and the results of reconstruction correspondingly better. Indeed, in a few cases the abnormality may only consist of a urethra which happens to lie on the dorsum of the penis with no other abnormality. The condition is rare. In one series, ten of 45 patients were said to have a completely normal penis after reconstruction. The techniques of reconstruction were the same as those used for exstrophy boys, principally the Cantwell–Ransley operation. All eventually had a good angle of dangle.[30]

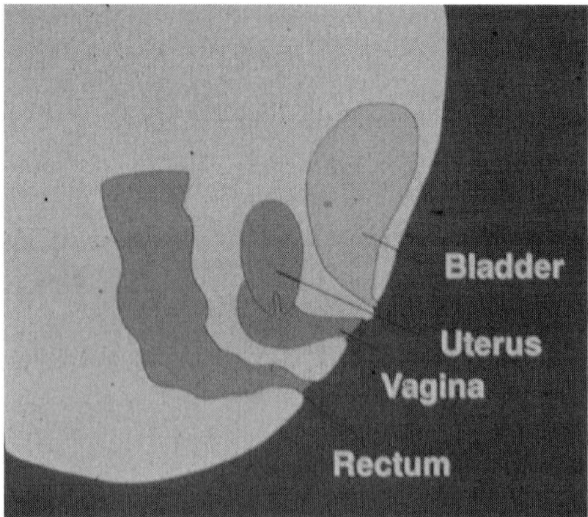

Fig. 45.10. Diagram of the sagittal section of the female pelvis in exstrophy to show the anterior displacement of the organs.

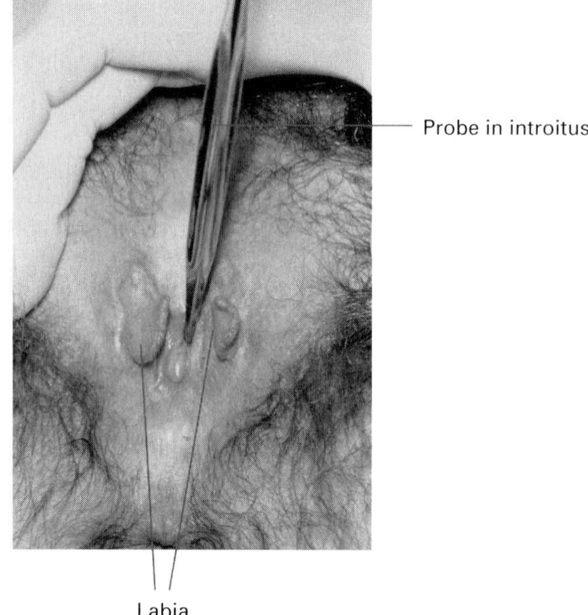

Fig. 45.11. Clinical photograph of the perineum in a female with exstrophy.

Anatomy of the female genitalia

The pelvis has the same orientation as in the male. The ovaries and uterus are normal. However, the supports of the uterus are deficient so that even in the nulliparous female the cervix is low and close to the introitus. With pregnancy a combination of poor ligaments and deficient pelvic floor allows frank prolapse and, in about 50%, a procedentia. It will be interesting to see if the successful osteotomy that now is performed will improve the uterine support. Although MRI appearances of the pelvis after osteotomy have been reported for boys, there is no report on females. If extrapolation can be made from the male appearances, the pelvic floor remains deficient with lateral deviation of the levator ani. The levator hiatus is twice as wide as in normals.[11,12]

In the perineum it could be said that each orifice is displaced anteriorly. If there is a urethra, it is almost on the anterior abdominal wall. The anus is in the position of the normal vaginal introitus.[12] The vagina lies almost horizontally, parallel to the floor when the girl is upright (Fig. 45.10). It is shorter than normal, being seldom more than 5 or 6 centimetres in length but of normal caliber.[31] The introitus is narrow, not because of a hymen but from a substantial bulk of tissue which appears to be a continuation of the posterior vaginal wall (Fig. 45.11). For most girls this tissue will have to be incised or even reconstructed before intercourse is possible. The labia are poorly formed and do not fuse anteriorly to form a fourchette. The clitoris is bifid (Fig. 45.12). The distribution of pubic hair is the same as that seen in males.

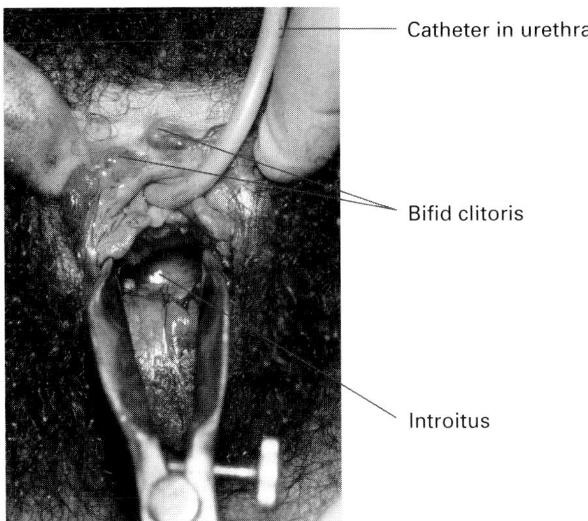

Fig. 45.12. Clinical photograph of the introitus in exstrophy after episiotomy.

Reconstruction of the female genitalia

The object of the genital reconstruction is to open the introitus, to unite the two halves of the clitoris and to fuse the anterior ends of the labia to make a fourchette. It is not possible to move the vagina posteriorly to its usual anatomical position, but labial and pubic reconstruction does disguise the abnormality very well. The main data for this review come from the 42 adult female patients with classical exstrophy who attend the author's adolescent urology clinic. The women were born between 1953 and 1980 and were aged 18 to 45 at the time of assessment.[31] Similar techniques have been reported by Stein *et al.*[32]

The method of surgical reconstruction has evolved over the last 15 years. Early in the series there was less emphasis on the closure of the labia anteriorly, and a number of vaginoplasties were thought to be necessary. Although the parts of the reconstruction are described separately, they are usually performed together.

Vaginoplasty

In spite of the very narrow introitus, the vagina above is of normal caliber. The introitus has been opened in 30 patients. An episiotomy is made posteriorly from the introitus until a two- to three-finger opening has been created (Fig. 45.12). It is usually possible to close the vaginal mucosa to the perineal skin directly. In two cases a primary closure was not achieved and a flap of mucosa from the medial aspect of the labia was rotated on each side to close the defect.

Vulvoplasty

The two halves of the clitoris (assuming that they can be identified), and the anterior ends of the labia are united to make a fourchette. No attempt is made to move the vagina posteriorly to its usual anatomical position.

A diamond-shaped area of skin/mucosa is outlined anterior to the labia and extended down onto the anterior ends of each labus and hemiclitoris. This diamond and the underlying fatty tissue are excised. The defect is then closed longitudinally with fine absorbable sutures.

Anterior fusion of the labia and clitoris has been performed in 15 cases. Primary healing was achieved in all patients with a cosmetic result that was acceptable at least to the surgeon.

Procedentia repair

The defective pelvic floor, open pelvic ring, and poor uterine supports make prolapse common. In a postal survey to which 34 women responded, vaginal and uterine prolapse was reported by 29%, occurring at a mean age of 16 years. Seven of my patients have had a total procedentia, one of whom had never had intercourse or a pregnancy.[33] It may be found in up to 50% of patients after pregnancy.

Several techniques have been reported for the repair of this difficult condition. Hohenfellner advocates fixation of the uterus to the anterior abdominal wall in childhood. This is said to prevent prolapse but still allow normal pregnancy.[32] Two women were able to have normal pregnancies without prolapse, while one of two women who did not have a fixation had "slight prolapse" after delivery. All deliveries were by Cesarean section. This "prophylactic surgery" may well be helpful. However, once prolapse has occurred, I have not found an anterior fixation to be an effective repair.

Although hysterectomy or partial hysterectomy has been advocated in occasional patients,[34] in the present author's view the uterus should not be removed as it is the only solid organ in the pelvis that has any hope of holding up the pelvic floor.

For the repair of procedentia, the most successful procedure is the Gortex wrap. The sacral promontory is exposed. A strip of Gortex is sutured to the periosteum. The end is passed around the cervix through the base of the broad ligament and brought back to the sacrum. This procedure has

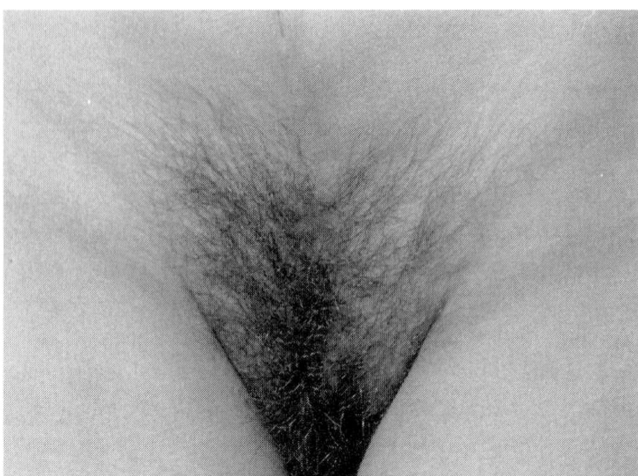

Fig. 45.13. Clinical photograph of the mons in exstrophy after reconstruction.

been successful in all cases with follow-up to a maximum of 6 years.[35]

Monsplasty (both sexes)

It is most important, either in infancy or in adolescence, to rotate hair-bearing flaps of skin and fat to cover the midline defect. The flaps may be based laterally or inferiorly. If there is too little skin available, larger flaps can be created by the use of skin expanders.[36] The only problem with the use of tissue expanders (or using flaps under tension) is that the number of hair follicles is not increased. Thus, although good skin cover is achieved, the pubic triangle can look a little "bald." In one of my cases there was partial necrosis of the skin flaps so that the mons lost most hair-bearing potential.

The scarred and non-hairy skin from the midline is excised. This excision may be continuous with that from the anterior end of the labia. The flaps of hair-bearing skin, including all of the subcutaneous fat are then mobilized and rotated to fill the defect. In females the defect left by repositioning of the flaps can be primarily closed (Fig. 45.13).

Timing of genital reconstruction

It would seem ideal to complete all reconstruction in infancy or early childhood. In males this allows an apparently normal appearance during the childhood years when boys are exploring their bodies and comparing it with their fellows.[15] The only caveat is that the penis is very small and care must be taken not to damage the corpora or the delicate innervation; some of the complex erectile deformities seen in adolescence must be due to surgical damage. In following a large series from Great Ormond Street of complete early reconstructions, four of seven adolescents were reported to have normal intercourse.[27] In females, the reconstruction is comparatively easy and should be an integral part of the definitive reconstruction.

It is more difficult to decide on timing when boys are found to have erectile deformity in the teenage years. Technically, it is possible to achieve correction in post pubertal boys and to establish normal intercourse.[19,37] However, it seems wrong to perform cosmetic surgery on teenagers unless they themselves see the need for it. It is therefore better to do the surgery at a time when they are actively exploring their sexuality but before several failures have dented the self-confidence.

Male sexual function

The more deeply sexuality is investigated, the more complex the definition of "satisfaction" becomes. Studies to date have been confined to the simple questioning about erections, orgasm, penetration, and fertility. In general, patients have given encouraging answers, which surgeons have been anxious to accept. It seems probable that questioning in greater depth would reveal a good deal of latent anger and dissatisfaction. Should that be the case, considerable care would be needed in management as, in the present state of our knowledge, little improvement can be made by surgery. If we accept the superficial data that is available, it is possible to say that patients are able to have sexual intercourse and to form long-term stable relationships.

Erections

It has already been noted that erectile deformity is universal unless corrective surgery is performed. Nonetheless, there are anecdotal examples of men who have had no surgery of any type (even a bladder closure) who have married and, apparently, fathered children: an example of the triumph of love over adversity if ever there was one.

With or without surgical correction, libido appears to be normal at least to superficial questioning. The ability to have erections appears to be normal. There is no cross-circulation between the corpora, unless a Cantwell–Ransley procedure has been done.

Orgasm is much more difficult to investigate as it lacks an objective definition. A man may not know whether he is having orgasms until he has definitely experienced one. It is reported that virtually all patients have orgasm.

Ejaculation cannot, by definition, be normal. It is a process that depends on the forceful expulsion of a bolus of semen from the prostatic urethra augmented by contraction of the bulbospongiosus. As exstrophy patients do not have an encircling prostate or a bulbospongiosus muscle, they cannot achieve a forceful ejaculation. Most men report that some semen dribbles out with orgasm but others say that there is a regular discharge of semen from the meatus unrelated to sexual activity. If men are asked for a semen sample for analysis, few can produce more than 1 ml, though volumes up to 5 ml have been reported.[38] In a review of current literature I found that ejaculation was reported in 101 of 134 men (75%).[39]

In isolated epispadias, ejaculation appears to be more normal, though I still doubt if it can have the same force as in a normal man unless the abnormality is very distal. In one series 17 of 29 adults were said to have normal ejaculation. Three men had fathered about six children (details incomplete) but three had required some form of artificial insemination, in one case using sperm retrieved from the bladder.[30]

It has been suggested that men who underwent early diversion are better able to ejaculate than those who were reconstructed. Most authors who have specifically addressed this problem give results that appear to support this conclusion. For example, in a German series all of five unreconstructed patients had normal ejaculation while 83% of 23 reconstructed patients had only a post-orgasmic dribble and the rest had no ejaculate.[40] In an updated review of the same series, it was even stated that no patient who had had genital (as opposed to bladder) reconstruction could ejaculate properly and none were fertile.[18]

However, the opposite view is taken in Baltimore. Twelve of 16 patients had satisfactory ejaculation. Their previous surgery was not given but it was implied that they had been reconstructed and, furthermore, that cystectomy was a cause of infertility.[41]

In reviewing the literature, I have found that neither view is supported. About 75% of both groups have some form of ejaculation. In several papers it is not possible to discover what surgery has been done or the power of the ejaculation.

Female sexual function

Even in normal women, sexual function has been little studied. An objective measure of successful female sexual function, equivalent to erection or ejaculation, is difficult to define. Most series are confined to expressions of the patients' global satisfaction. The results of vaginal reconstruction appear to be satisfactory in the sense that most patients do not request further cosmetic surgery and most engage in sexual intercourse. In Stein's series 12 of 13 adult women were said to be satisfied with the appearance. All had intercourse but three found it to be unpleasant in an unspecified way.[40] In the postal series of patients operated in Baltimore, only 16 (of an initial target of 83) answered the questions on sexual activity. All had appropriate sexual desire. Ten patients were sexually active with a mean age of debut of 19.9 years. Seven had orgasms. Three always had dyspareunia.[34]

Marriage

My own patients report few casual sexual partners and there are obvious difficulties for exstrophy males in establishing a relationship based on sex alone. Stable partnerships with normal girls seem to be the rule in Europe, though in the United States random, short-term relationships have been reported.[41] Combining Stein's series with my own, 49 of 66 patients for whom full information was available had cohabited. I have one man who is homosexual and another with doubts about his gender identity.[40,42]

Fertility

Although there has been no formal study, it seems likely that females with exstrophy have normal fertility unless surgery has caused tubal obstruction or some other genital complication.

Males are probably born with normal testes and so with normal fertility potential. A combination of surgery, recurrent infection, and the erectile deformities leads to a high rate of infertility.

At the simplest level, the problem may just be the difficulty in getting the sperm to the partner's cervix. If the semen analysis is reasonable, men may be taught to use a syringe to transfer their own semen to the vaginal vault at the fertile point in their partner's cycle.

More often, the problem is of obstructive azoospermia at the level of the prostate. When available, such infertility may be treated by the harvesting of sperm from the epididymis and subsequent ICSI. Occasionally, there is azoospermia or severe oligozoospermia due to recurrent, bilateral, epididymo-orchitis. Treatment of this problem is difficult in all patients, though harvesting and concentration of sperm for ICSI may still be possible.[43]

A successful case of twin pregnancy has been reported with testicular sperm extraction from a man born with exstrophy.[44] There are probably other cases within large series of male factor infertility management.

In a review of the literature from 1974 to 1998 I found that about a half of the men who wished to have children were successful. Whatever may be said about ejaculatory function, fertility was definitely better in boys who had had an early diversion rather than reconstruction.[45]

Fertility in females born with exstrophy should be normal unless the Fallopian tubes have become obstructed by surgery.

Pregnancy and delivery

With modern obstetric care, pregnancy and delivery should be uncomplicated except for the risk of prolapse. The incidence of prolapse is high and presumably is increased by pregnancy and vaginal delivery. Women must be advised of the risk, but as it occurs even in nulliparous women with exstrophy, it does not seem to be a reason, on its own, to avoid pregnancy. In a combined series of patients 43 pregnancies in 28 women were identified. Four ended in spontaneous and four in therapeutic abortion. There were 34 live births and one intrauterine death of twins.[26,34]

Inheritance

The risk of inheriting exstrophy from an affected parent is uncertain. At Great Ormond Street, no cases of exstrophy were found in 162 siblings of 102 exstrophy children, though there was a slightly increased incidence of relatives with neural tube defects. Review of the literature suggested that the risk in siblings was less than 1%.[46] A postal survey gave a 1:70 risk of an exstrophy patient being the parent of an exstrophy baby.[47]

More recently, 18 familial cases from 682 index patients have been reported. The series included two cousins, a mother and a son in a large interconnected family.[48] It would seem that the risk of an affected baby is greater in relatives of index patients than in the normal population. Further work is needed to define the risk and mode of inheritance.

Sexual health and contraception

Exstrophy patients have sexually transmitted diseases just like other adolescents. I have seen gonorrhea, viral warts, and fracture of the penile shaft. Treatment is the same as in the rest of the population. The patient with fractured penile shaft was delayed in presentation and there was no spontaneous healing. The defect in the corpus was closed surgically.

Barrier contraception in males is difficult as conventional condoms do not stay in position. It is sometimes possible to buy, in sex shops, condoms that cover only the head of the penis. Great care is needed in their use.

In females, the introitus must nearly always be opened at surgery before tampons can be used or intercourse take place. I have encountered one girl who became pregnant before her introital reconstruction, presumably because the cervix was just inside the introitus, which was wide enough for semen to leak in from the perineum. Most conventional forms of contraception are satisfactory. Because of the proximity of the cervix to the introitus, contraception based on withdrawal is even less safe than usual.

Quality of life

In recent years I have noticed that there is an increasing dissatisfaction with the size of the penis. It is important to raise exstrophy children in the knowledge that they are normal human beings and can aspire to all the normal attributes of adult life. As the majority of men, even with a very abnormal penis, can have a sexual function that appears to give them pleasure, it would be wrong to embark on surgery to try to enlarge the penis unless there is a very specific abnormality that is amenable to surgical correction. Operations on the genitalia are not good treatment for conditions of the mind.

There is a great difficulty in the assessment of quality of life in adults born with exstrophy. It was pointed out many years ago that exstrophy patients have their own special concerns.[24] Several studies have shown that the patients have a good quality of life and are high achievers.

However, the instruments used to measure quality of life appear not to be measuring the domains or items that the exstrophy patient considers important. Thus the inventories of psychological or physical health may show that they are completely normal while semi-structured interview and interpretive phenomenological analysis shows consistent areas of concern unconsidered by parents or doctors.[25] There is a great wish to be normal, which means voiding and making a noise while so doing. Many of the measures put in place to help the integration of exstrophy adolescents into normal social life effectively emphasize their abnormality and may be counter-productive.[25]

Sexual problems can be helped by sympathetic counseling. However, it is essential to have a group of psychologists who understand both sexual problems and the abnormalities of exstrophy.[41]

Erectile dysfunction is treated along conventional lines. To date, it has been a rare problem in my clinic. Patients who use prostaglandin E_1 must inject each corpus separately as there is no cross-circulation between them. There have been no reports of the use of sildenafil, but there seems to be no reason why it should not work in exstrophy patients with appropriate diagnoses.

Conclusions

All of the abnormalities in the exstrophy and epispadias complex are difficult to reconstruct. To produce an adult who is continent, can void, has normal sexual function, and is fertile is a surgical triumph.

The greater knowledge that has been gathered in the last 20 years about the long-term sexual outcomes has considerably modified the techniques of reconstruction in infancy. The genital reconstructions that used to be common in an adolescent unit are now uncommon. The biggest source of patients requiring such surgery is from pediatric surgical units with little experience of exstrophy. This, on its own, seems a good argument for concentrating the care of children with rare conditions in a very small number of specialist units.

In looking at the literature, it is sad to note that all of the evidence on which we base our care is little more than anecdotal. In the standard categorization of evidence, none is better than grade III and most is grade IV. Even so, many respected authorities have worked very hard to improve the results of exstrophy reconstruction: it is only necessary to look at the continence results from the work of Trendelenberg onwards. Not all surgical techniques require a double-blind randomized controlled trial.[49]

REFERENCES

1. Mayo, C. H. & Hendricks, W. A. Exstrophy of the bladder. *Surg. Gynecol. Obst.* 1926; **43**:129–134.
2. Forrester, M. B. & Merz, R. D. First year mortality rates for selected birth defects, Hawaii, 1986–1999. *Am. J. Med. Genet.* 2003; **119**(A):-311.
3. Johnston, J. H. Lengthening of the congenital or acquired short penis. *Br. J. Urol.* 1974; **46**:685–687.
4. Woodhouse, C. R. J. & Kellett, M. J. Anatomy of the penis and its deformities in exstrophy and epispadias. *J. Urol.* 1984; **132**:1122–1124.
5. Schillinger, J. F. & Wiley, M. J. Bladder exstrophy penile lengthening procedure. *Urology* **1984**; **24**:434–437.
6. Hurwitz, R. S., Woodhouse, C. R. J., & Ransley, P. G. The anatomic course of the neurovascular bundles in epispadias. *J. Urol.* 1986; **136**:68–70.
7. Schlegel, P. N. & Gearhart, J. P. Neuroanatomy of the pelvis in an infant with cloacal exstrophy: a detailed microdissection with histology. *J. Urol.* 1989; **141**:583–585.
8. McClorie, G. A., Bellemore, M. C., & Salter, R. B. Penile deformity in bladder exstrophy: correlation with closure of the pelvic defect. *J. Pediatr. Surg.* 1991; **26**:201–203.
9. Gearhart, J. P., Yang, A., Leonard, M. P., Jeffs, R. D., & Zerhouni, E. A. Prostate size and configuration in adults with bladder exstrophy. *J. Urol.* 1993; **149**:308–310.
10. Sponsellar, P. D., Gearhart, J. P., & Jeffs, R. D. Anatomy of the pelvis in the exstrophy complex. *J. Bone Joint Surg.* 1995; **77**:117–119.
11. Stec, A. A., Pannu, H. K., Tadros, Y. E., Sponsellar, P. D., Fishman, E. K., & Gearhart, J. P. Pelvic floor anatomy in classic bladder exstrophy using 3-dimensional computerised tomography: initial insights. *J. Urol.* 2001; **166**:1444–1449.
12. Halachmi, S., Farhat, W., Konen, O., *et al.* Pelvic floor magnetic resonance imaging after neonatal single stage reconstruction in male patients with classic bladder exstrophy. *J. Urol.* 2003; **170**:1505–1509.
13. Mathews, R. I., Perlman, F., Marsh, D. W., & Gearhart, J. P. Gonadal morphology in cloacal exstrophy. *Br. J. Urol. Inter.* 1999; **84**:99–100.
14. Mesrobian, H.-G. J., Kelalis, P. P., & Kramer, S. A. Long term follow up of the cosmetic appearance and genital function in boys with exstrophy: review of 53 patients. *J. Urol.* 1986; **136**:256–258.
15. Perovic, S., Scepanovic, D., & Sremcevic, D. Epispadias surgery: the Belgrade experience. *Br. J. Urol.* 1992; **70**:674–677.
16. Pippi Salle, J. L., Jednak, K., Cappolichio, G., Franca, I. M., Labbie, A., & Gosalbez, R. A ventral rotational skin flap to improve cosmesis and avoid chordee recurrence in epispadias repair. *Br. J. Urol. Int.* 2002; **90**:918–923.
17. Hammouda, H. M. Results of complete disassembly for epispadias repair in 42 patients. *J. Urol.* 2003; **170**:1963–1965.
18. Stein, R., Hohenfellner, K., Fisch, M. *et al.* Social integration, sexual behaviour and fertility in patients with bladder exstrophy: a long term follow up. *Eur. J. Pediatr.* 1996; **155**:678–683.
19. Woodhouse, C. R. J. The management of erectile deformity in exstrophy and epispadias. *J. Urol.* 1986; **135**:932–936.

20. Kelley, J. H. & Eraklis, A. J. A procedure for lengthening the phallus in boys with exstrophy of the bladder. *J. Pediatr. Surg.* 1971; **6**:645–649.
21. Hendren, W. H. Penile lengthening after previous repair of epispadias. *J. Urol.* 1979; **121**:527–534.
22. Sadove, R. C., Sengezer, M., McRoberts, J. W., & Wells, M. D. One stage total penile reconstruction with a free sensate osteocutaneous fibula flap. *Plast. Reconstruc. Surg.* 1993; **92**:1314–1325.
23. Snyder, H. M. Epispadias and exstrophy. In Whitfield, H. N., ed. *Rob and Smith's Operative Surgery: Genito Urinary Surgery.* Oxford: Butterworth-Heinemann, 1993; 786–813.
24. Feinberg, T., Lattimer, J. K., Jeter, K., Langford, W., & Beck, L. Questions that worry children with exstrophy. *Pediatrics* 1974; **53**:242–246.
25. Wilson, C., Christie, D., & Woodhouse, C. R. J. The ambitions of adolescents born with exstrophy: a structured survey. *Br. J. Urol. Int.* 2004; **94**:607–612.
26. Woodhouse, C. R. J. Sexual and reproductive consequences of congenital genitourinary anomalies. *J. Urol.* 1994; **152**:645–651.
27. Kajbafzadeh, A. M., Duffy, P. G., & Ransley, P. G. The evolution of penile reconstruction in epispadias repair: a report of 180 cases. *J. Urol.* 1995; **154**:858–861.
28. Borzi, P. A. & Thomas, D. F. M. Cantwell–Ransley epispadias repair in male epispadias and bladder exstrophy. *J. Urol.* 1994; **151**:457–459.
29. Koff, S. A. & Eakins, M. The treatment of penile chordee using corporeal rotation. *J. Urol.* 1984; **131**:931–932.
30. Mollard, P., Basset, T., & Mure, P. Y. Male epispadias. *J. Urol.* 1998; **160**:55–59.
31. Woodhouse, C. R. J. & Hinsch, R. The anatomy and reconstrction of the adult female genitalia in classical exstrophy. *Br. J. Urol.* 1997; **79**:618–622.
32. Stein, R., Fisch, M., Bauer, H., & Hohenfellner, R. Operative reconstruction of the external and internal genitalia in female patients with bladder exstrophy or incontinent epispadias. *J. Urol.* 1995; **154**:1002–1007.
33. Woodhouse, C. R. J. The gynaecology of exstrophy. *Br. J. Urol. Int.* 1999; **83**(Suppl. 3):34–38.
34. Mathews, R., Gan, M., & Gearhart, J. P. Urogynaecological and obstetric issues in women with the exstrophy epispadias complex. *Br. J. Urol. Int.* 2003; **91**:845–849.
35. Farkas, A. G., Shepherd, J. E., & Woodhouse, C. R. J. Hysterosacropexy for uterine prolapse with associated urinary tract abnormalities. *J. Obst. Gynaecol.* 1993; **13**:358–360.
36. Marconi, F., Messina, P., & Pavanello, P. Cosmetic reconstruction of the mons veneris and lower abdominal wall by skin expansion as the last stage of surgical treatment of bladder exstrophy. *Plast. Reconstruc. Surg.* 1993; **91**:551–555.
37. Audry, G., Grapin, C., & Loulidi, S. Genital prognosis of boys with bladder exstrophy or epispadias with incontinence apropos of 14 cases. *Ann. d'Urol.* 1991; **25**:120–124.
38. Silver, R. I., Yang, A., Ben-Chaim, J., Jeffs, R. D., & Gearhart, J. P. Penile length in adulthood after exstrophy reconstruction. *J. Urol.* 1997; **157**:999–1003.
39. Woodhouse, C. R. J. Sexual function in congenital anomalies. In Carson, C. C., Kirby, R. S., & Goldstein, I., eds. *Textbook of Erectile Dysfunction.* Oxford: Isis Medical Media, 1999; 613–625.
40. Stein, R., Stockle, M., Fisch, M., & Hohenfellner, R. The fate of the adult exstrophy patient. *J. Urol.* 1994; **152**:1413–1416.
41. Ben-Chaim, J., Jeffs, R. D., Reiner, W. G., & Gearhart, J. P. The outgcome of patients with classic exstrophy in adult life. *J. Urol.* 1996; **155**:1251–1252.
42. Woodhouse, C. R. J. Exstrophy. In *Long-term Paediatric Urology.* Oxford: Blackwell Scientific, 1991; 127–150.
43. Bastuba, M. D., Alper, M. M., & Oates, R. D. Fertility and the use of assisted reproductive techniques in the adult male exstrophy/epispadias patient. *Fertil. Steril.* 1993; **60**:733–736.
44. Lai, R., Perra, G., Usai, V. *et al.* Twin pregnancy achieved through TESE in an adult male exstrophy. *J. Assist. Reprod. Genet.* 2002; **19**:245–247.
45. Woodhouse, C. R. J. Sexual function in boys born with exstrophy, myelomeningocoele and micropenis. *Urology* 1998; **52**:3–11.
46. Ives, E., Coffey, R., & Carter, C. O. A family study of bladder exstrophy. *J. Medi. Geneti.* 1980; **17**:139–141.
47. Shapiro, E., Lepor, H., & Jeffs, R. D. The inheritance of the exstrophy/epispadias complex. *J. Urol.* 1984; **132**:308–310.
48. Messelink, E. J., Aronson, D. C., Knuist, M., Heij, H. A., & Vos, A. Four cases of bladder exstrophy in two families. *J. Med. Geneti.* 1994; **31**:490–492.
49. Smith, G. C. S. & Pell, J. P. Parachute use to prevent death and major trauma related to gravitational challenge: systematic review of randomised controlled trials. *Br. Med. J.* 2003; **327**:1459–1461.

46

Feminization (surgical aspects)

Justine M. Schober

Department of Urology, Hamot Medical Center, Erie, PA

Introduction

Genitoplasty has been the traditional treatment for various forms of ambiguous genitalia and genotypical abnormalities. These conditions represent a spectrum of clitorophallic size and form, as well as vaginal position, size, and location. In some cases, complete absence of the genitalia must also be considered. Careful consideration of anticipated gender and function outcomes must be weighed before choosing some form of feminizing genitoplasty. Through the years, techniques, timing, and materials for genitoplasty have evolved, whereas surgical goals have remained unchanged.

The immediate goal is to provide the external genitalia with an esthetic and feminine appearance. The long-term goals are to produce a functional vagina of sufficient size for comfortable sexual intercourse, to retain sexually sensitive tissue to allow orgasm and, if internal genitalia permit, to preserve fertility potential. The surgeon's intent is to facilitate the patient's positive psychosocial adjustment throughout the patient's life. Sometimes, a completely satisfactory solution is not possible.

Even though techniques have advanced through the years, these demanding repairs and reconstructions are not without significant complications, necessitating careful multidisciplinary follow-up. Though genitoplasty presents many immediate problems and considerations, the most challenging are the long-term surgical outcomes. Many surgeons consider creating presentable external female genitalia with a sizable vagina an adequate outcome, but cosmetic appearance and passive sexual function is only one measure of success. Because scant knowledge exists, little is known about how adults adjust to genitoplasty or whether the genitoplasty expresses their sexual preference. In children and infants who have undergone genitoplasty, what path they would have chosen, given full knowledge of their condition and having been allowed to choose later in life, is unknown. In addition, needs regarding vaginoplasty follow-up care for screening of sexually transmitted diseases and dysplasia have yet to be established.

Unless a clear health risk is identified, no absolute indications exist for genitoplasty. Indeed, some members of the Intersex Society of North America advocate preservation of an intersex appearance and identity.

Issues surrounding genitoplasty are complicated by the highly individualized needs and desires that vary according to the patient's stage in life. These may vary with specific diagnosis, as well as the effect of the intersex condition on masculinization of brain, behavior, and bodily appearance. Expectations and choices also vary with cultural or parental expectations. If surgery is elected, two very different guidelines for timing have emerged, each with its own advantages and disadvantages.

Early feminizing genitoplasty

When feminizing genitoplasty is performed during the patient's infancy, the surgery confers an early physical appearance that is consistent with sex of rearing. Also, the early intervention may cause less psychological trauma than if performed later in life. The disadvantages include the inability to obtain the patient's informed consent and the high likelihood of revision surgery, especially if the assigned gender conflicts with the patient's identity. Also, no evidence exists that early surgery provides a better outcome than surgery performed later in life.

Pediatric Surgery and Urology: Long-term Outcomes, Mark Stringer, Keith Oldham, Pierre Mouriquand.
Published by Cambridge University Press.

Table 46.1. History of surgery on the clitoris

1939	Ombrédanne[1]
	• Overlap the undiminished clitoris with skin flaps.
1957	Stefan and Pinsker[2]
	• Obliterate the corpora with mattress sutures without disturbing the neurovascular bundle.
	• Reduce glans circumference.
	• Bury the glans under the skin.
1961	Lattimer[3]
	• Submerge the clitoris without removing corporal tissue.
	• Reduce the glans circumferencially by trimming the corona.
1961	Schmid[4]
	• Amputate the corpora, leaving the glans on a vascular pedicle with dorsal nerve intact.
1965	Pellerin[5]
	• Relocate the corpora inferior to pubic arch.
1966	Gross *et al.*[6]
	• Remove all tissue of the corpora and glans.
	• Transecting suspensory ligament and also removing corpora as they divide beneath the pubis.
1970	Randolph and Hung[7]
	• Replace the corpora beneath the pubis posteriorly.
	• Reconstruction suturing shaft to periosteum of lower border of pubis of mons veneris to cover clitoris.
1973	Spence and Allen[8]
	• Excise the entire clitoral shaft preserving glans.
	• Suture the stump of glans to undersurface of the pubis.
1974	Kumar *et al.*[9]
	• Preserve neurovascular bundle with partial excision of the corpora.
	• Reduce glans by excision along dorsal coronal margin, preserving ventral glans and frenulum.
	• Approximate glans to the crura clitoris.
1981	Mollard *et al.*[10]
	• Resect the fused portion of corpora preserving the neurovascular bundle.
	• Approximate the two. (Glans shrinks postoperatively, so reduction is unnecessary; ventral frenular blood supply is preserved.)
1982	Mininberg[11]
	Leave the glans clitoris with a portion of prepucial tissue intact circumferentially. Neurovascular bundle is preserved with excision of a portion of the corpora. Glans and prepuce are then capped onto the residual corpora.
1983	Kogan *et al.*[12]
	• Incise tunica with intact neurovascular supply to glans proximal and distal suture ligation of corpus cavernosum.
	• Wedge reduction of glans.
1989	Passerini-Glazel[13]
	• Partial excision of the clitoral corpora with neurovascular preservation. The glans is reduced by cutting out two lateral triangular wedges along its outer circumference and then submerged beneath created labia minora. The urethra is opened and the urethral flap is sutured to the clitoris to create a mucosa lining below the clitoris. Distal portion of mucocutaneous plate is converted to a cylinder whose inter surface is mucocutaneous.
1993	Sagehashi[14]
	• Separate all corporal tissue carefully from a designed "lump" of glans without damage to the neurovascular bundle.
	• Affix preserved glandular tissue to pubic bone.

Delayed feminizing genitoplasty

When feminizing surgery is delayed until adolescence, one advantage is that the patient can provide informed assent/consent. Later surgery might spare multiple revisions and loss of functional/sensitive tissue as identity can generally be clearly established, thus avoiding inappropriate surgical gender assignment. Disadvantages with waiting until adolescence include submitting an adolescent/child to a period when genitals may not be consistent with gender of rearing. Also, the surgery is performed during a time when the adolescent is very aware of the surgery, potentially heightening anxiety. Many surgeons have noted that surgery is technically more difficult because the distance that the vaginal sinus must be mobilized is much greater in adolescents than in infants and children. No studies have been performed to assess whether a "better" outcome is obtained by those who choose to have later surgery.

After many years of genitoplasty experience and technique revisions, certain problems can be anticipated and must be closely monitored during follow-up. When available, the long-term outcome in each procedure is reviewed; however, these procedures were performed with vastly different materials and offered a wide range of success.

Surgery on the clitoris

To evaluate the status of patients whose procedures span more than 50 years of evolving surgery on the clitoris (clitorectomy to clitoroplasty), the surgeries, as well as the surgeons' attitudes, must be understood (Table 46.1).[1–14]

In the 1950s, opinions were repeatedly quoted that the clitoris was unnecessary for normal sexual function. The basis was an unpublished personal communication of P.H. Gulliver who held that women of certain African tribes underwent ceremonial excision of the clitoris, but continued to exhibit normal sexual response and function. In 1955, a second report by Hampson, strengthened this belief.[15] He described six women, five of whom noted sexual gratification after clitorectomy; none of whom experienced orgasm before clitorectomy.

Several other authors, including Ombrédanne,[1] Stefan *et al.*,[2] Lattimer,[3] Pellerin,[5] and Randolph *et al.*[7] recognized the clitoris as an erotically important sensory organ that was worth saving. Instead of burying or submerging the nearly intact glans and corpora, they proposed to create a more feminine appearance, without loss of the sensory/erectile tissue. To avoid painful bowstring erections, they supported the removal of some corporal tissue. This was followed by the revisions of Schmid,[4] who was the first to report excision of corpora, while leaving the glans on a neurovascular pedicle to preserve some sensation.

Many revisions followed, most notably those by Spence and Allen,[8] Kumar *et al.*,[9] Mollard *et al.*,[10] Mininberg,[11] Kogan *et al.*,[12] Passerini-Glazel,[13] and Sagehashi.[14]

All of the above techniques address, to some extent, the more feminine contour and appearance of the body, with an attempt at sensory preservation of the clitoris. When the neurovascular bundle was preserved, Gearhart *et al.*[16] were the first to attempt to establish some objective, postsurgical measure of sensory innervation of the clitoris. Six patients were tested after phallic reduction; the authors demonstrated preservation of electromyographical response in all six.

In 1996, Chase [17] reported that a member of the Intersexual Society of North America (ISNA) underwent postoperative pudendal evoked potentials and demonstrated normal latency, but complete absence of sensation and orgasm.

Recently, fetal and cadaveric studies have elucidated our understanding of the external and internal anatomy of the clitoris and anatomic relationships of the urethra and clitoris.[18] Baskin's anatomic studies of the human clitoris have expanded our understanding of the nerve distribution and supply.[19]

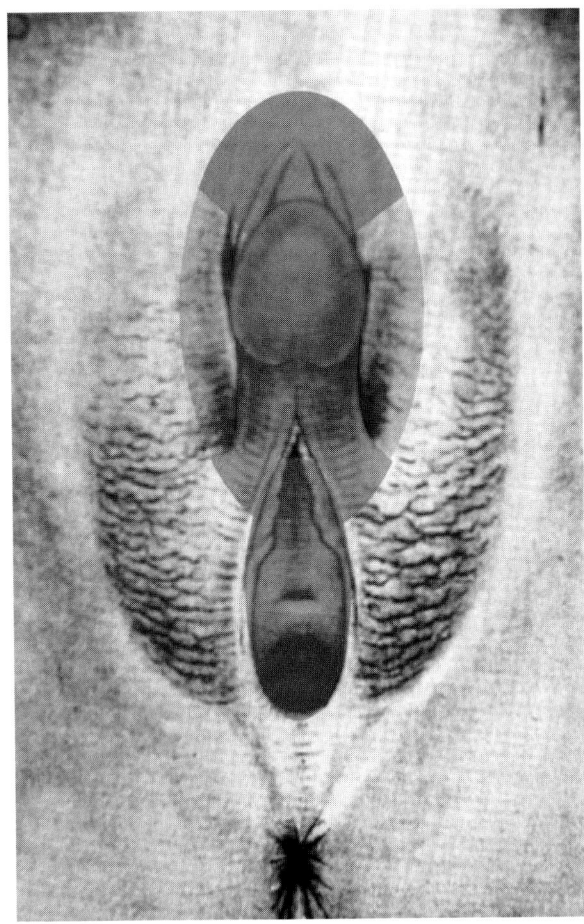

Fig. 46.1. Genital sensitivity ratings for sexual intensity depicted by intensity of blue shaded areas (see colour plate section).

The tunica of the corporeal body of the clitoris is densely innervated via the pudendal nerve. As the nerve passes under the pubic bone, it becomes the cavernosa or dorsal nerve of the clitoris. The glans clitoris forms a cap at the distal end with its highest nerve density dorsally; nerve branches are absent at the 12 o'clock position. Dorsally perforating branches innervate the glans.

Pfaff detailed these receptive fields in the rat.[20] However, little knowledge existed regarding these areas in the human female. The first study by Baskin *et al.*,[19] which detailed nerve density, lends support to observed genital sensitivity patterns in women. Initial studies by Schober and Meyer-Bahlburg indicate that highly sensitive areas (Figs. 46.1, 46.2) correspond with areas of nerve density

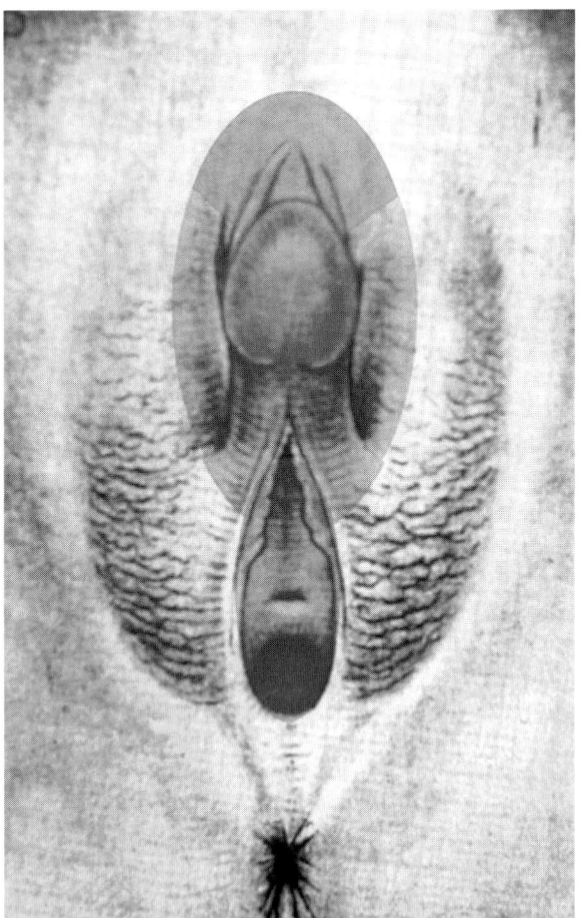

Fig. 46.2. Genital sensitivity ratings, shown as shades of red, for ease of orgasm (see colour plate section).

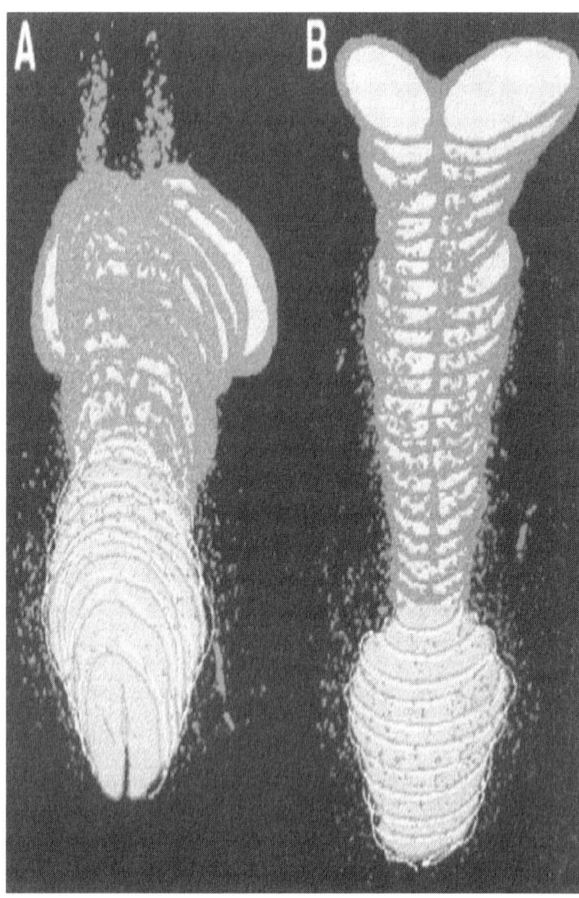

Fig. 46.3. Innervation of the clitoris, shown overlying the corpora and glans. (see colour plate section) (Figure used with permission from *J. Urol.* and Lawrence Baskin.)

reported by Baskin (Figs. 46.3, 46.4).[19,21] Zones of highest sensitivity were noted on and above the clitoris. Respecting and preserving these areas during surgery may decrease risks of loss of sensation (Fig. 46.5).

An intimate relationship exists between the perineal urethra and surrounding clitoral erectile tissue.[18] Partial or total urethrectomy, urethral or vaginal suspension procedures, and partial or total vaginectomy may disrupt this relationship. In feminizing genitoplasty, the mobilization of the genital sinus and separation of the genital sinus from the urethra are examples of maneuvers that may interrupt the innervation as demonstrated by some of these newer studies. Support from the bulbs of the clitoris may also impact vaginal structure and function by maintaining the vagina's rigidity on the anterior wall, thus facilitating intromission. Therefore, the impact of surgery on internal or proximal structures from excision of portions of the clitoris must be carefully considered.

Feminizing genitoplasy has divided into two surgical components: (i) clitoroplasty and (ii) vaginoplasty. Each progresses in critical steps and each is associated with individualized, inherent risks.

Clitoroplasty proceeds in three distinct surgical stages: (i) separation of the glans from prepucial and shaft skin; (ii) excision of a portion of the shaft or erectile tissue; and (iii) excision of a portion of the glans (Figs. 46.6–46.8).[22–24]

Success of clitoroplasty is judged upon three criteria: appearance, sensitivity, and requirements for modification. Three prominent studies detail such outcomes. In 1999, Alizai was the first to review 14 CAH girls (mean age 13.1 yrs). Five of these 14 had notable clitoral atrophy; one of the 14 had an unsightly clitoris. These results were quite surprising, with a revelation that risks were higher than expected and that risks to genital sensitivity might be anticipated.[25]

Repeated modification to achieve an "ideal" clitoral appearance was reported by Creighton,[26] with further

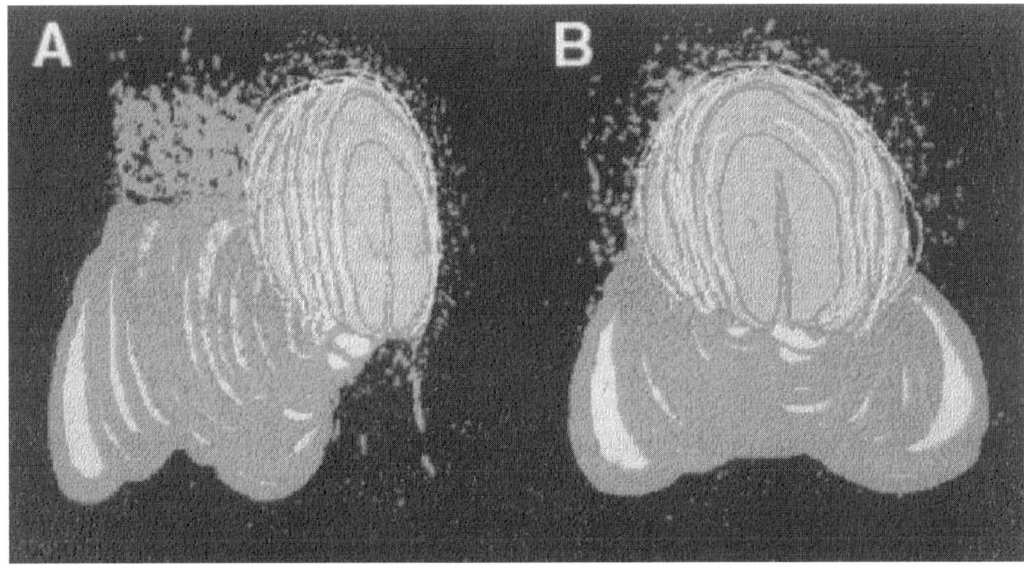

Fig. 46.4. Innervation of the clitoris, depicting major areas of distribution dorsally and laterally (see colour plate section). (Figure used with permission from *J. Urol.* and Lawrence Baskin.)

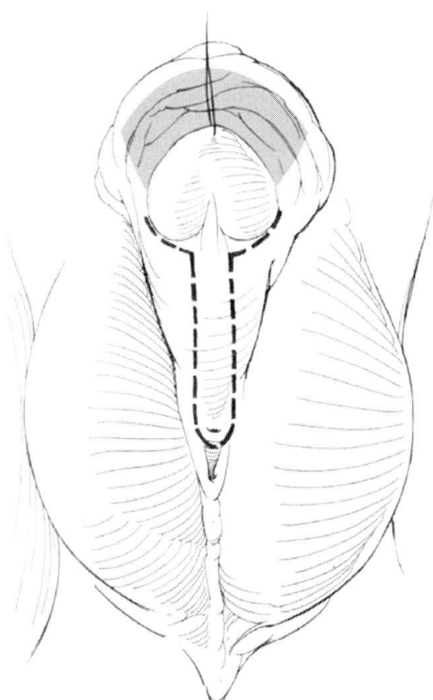

Fig. 46.5. Surgical design preserving sensitivity, with incision lines ventrally away from major innervation. Dashed line designates line of incision.

elucidation of the risk to sensitivity.[27] She reported outcomes after clitoroplasty in 38 subjects, including 21 with CAH; 1, ambiguous genitalia; and 11, cloacal anomalies. From this group, 31 had clitoral reduction; 2, clitoral recession; 2, total clitoral excision; and 3, other clitoral surgery. Twenty-six percent underwent repeated clitoral surgery. Specifically addressing tactile sensitivity after clitoroplasty, she found sensation of the clitoris, but not the vagina, was impaired in adults who underwent genitoplasty. Highly abnormal hot, cold and vibratory sensations were demonstrated by a GenitoSensory Analyzer (GSA Medoc Ltd.).[27]

Vaginoplasty or vaginal construction

Vaginal construction

No settled opinion stands out as to the correct management of vaginal atresia or agenesis. A very long history exists of surgery employing a myriad of native and exogenous materials for construction of the vagina. Each surgery has improved after thoughtful trial and error. Several types of repair have documented success in creation of a vagina (Table 46.2).[13,22,28–54]

Considering the long-term outcome of the vaginoplasty, two criteria of success were utilized to evaluate the literature. These were maintaining: (i) size (depth and width) of the vagina and (ii) ability to perform coitus. Each material/repair was separately considered: vaginal tract without skin graft, split-thickness skin graft, skin flap, bowel segment, amnion, peritoneum, and bladder mucosa. Some of the unique advantages and disadvantages of each are

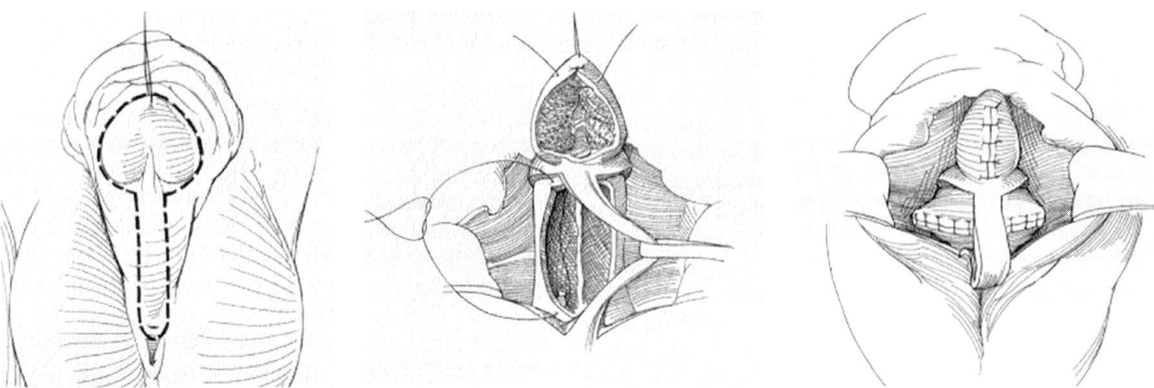

Fig. 46.6. Initial step for clitoral reduction surgery, showing separation of the glans from prepucial and shaft skin. This procedure is aimed to preserve the neurovascular bundle and clitoral erectile mechanism.

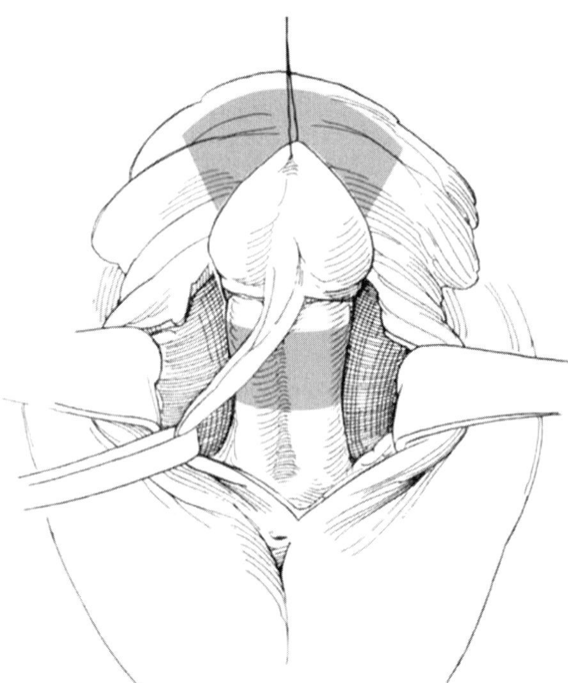

Fig. 46.7. Surgical steps for clitoral and corpora reduction. Illustration depicts excision of a portion of the glans and reduction of the corpora by excision of a central section.

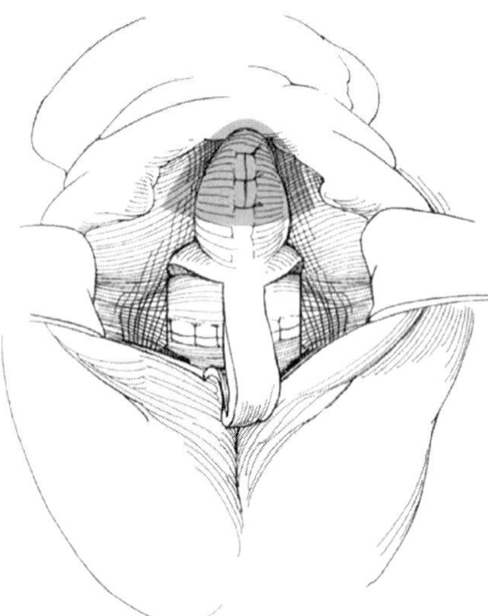

Fig. 46.8. The reanastomosis of borders of the resected areas is done avoiding ligation of the blood supply at any point to preserve potential for sexual sensitivity and function.

described and long-term follow-up included, when available.

Techniques utilized for vaginoplasty were even more variable than those used for clitoroplasty.[55] Perhaps this evolved because no specific surgery emerged as the perfect solution for augmentation or complete construction of the vagina.

The risks for surgical vaginoplasty were different for high and low confluence of the urethra and vagina. The two most common surgical techniques for low confluence involved cut back vaginoplasty and posterior flap vaginoplasty.[22] These probably carried lesser risks and complications than surgery for high confluence; however, no specific long-term outcomes were published for these procedures.

Posterior omega flap

For both low confluence and in some instances, high confluence, a new technique modification for the creation of longer and larger vaginal segments has been described. This modification takes advantage of the rich subcutaneous vasculature to maintain a wider flap. Twenty-eight girls (age range 5 months to 17 years), all of whom had the salt-losing

Table 46.2. Surgical revisions and materials used in vaginoplasty

1817	Dupuytren[28] • Dissect a pouch to epithelialize – no mold used.
1892	Siriecieke[??] • Attempts to line vagina with rabbit intestinal graft.
1898	Abbe[30] • First to use skin over a mold for creation of vagina.
1904	Baldwin[31] • Uses intestinal segments. The sigmoid was used first, later the double loop of ileum was used. Two weeks postop, a spur between the loops was crushed to establish a single barrel canal. Twenty-four percent mortality rate noted later.
1911	Schubert[32] • Uses sigmoid for vaginoplasty.
1921	Graves[33] • Uses labia minora as the donor tissue with pedunculated flaps.
1932	Masson[34] • Uses intestinal segments. (In 14% [2/14] of cases, surgical deaths resulted from sepsis.)
1938	Frank[35] • Applies simple pressure; dilation for two to four hours per day for four+ months using penile-shaped Pyrex tubes.
1938	McIndoe and Bannister[36] • Uses free grafts. • Uses thin, split thickness skin graft in one piece; continuous dilatation over a wound until the contractile phase is over.
1938	Wharton[37] • Creates perineal pouch with subsequent spontaneous epithelialization.
1948	Counsellor[38] • Dissects space between bladder and rectum; epithelialization occurs without the use of a skin graft.
1952	Schmid[39] • Uses sigmoid for vaginoplasty.
1954	Jones and Jones[40] • Simple incision perineal skin over urogenital sinus.
1960	Sheares[41] • Posteriorly based flap lines posterior vagina; soft mold worn through epithelialization of the anterior vagina.
1961	Pratt[42] • Revisited bowel vaginoplasty using a sigmoid loop.
1964	Forunoff *et al.*[43] • Uses skin flap; flap is in shape of inverted U, with the apex near the opening of vagina or sinus.
1964	Williams[44] • Marsupialization of a U-shaped perineal incision. The labia are each separated into two layers. The inner layers are joined in the midline and pouch created and directed inward.
1969	Davydov[45,46] • Creates vagina using pelvic peritoneum.
1980	Hendren and Donahoe[47] • First to use bilateral rotated buttocks flaps and labial flaps to repair difficult urethrovaginal fistulas.
1986	Ashworth *et al.*[48] • Places amnion over the vaginal mold. Approximated labia holds the mold in place. Performs vaginal dilatation after the mold is removed.
1988	Claret *et al.*[49] • Uses bladder mucosa over an inflatable mold.
1989	Passerini-Glazel[13] • All native tissue by flaps. This one-stage procedure uses phallic shaft skin to create an inner labia and fold with lateral labia majora. Uses a wide inverted U flap for introitus for less outlet stenosis.
1991	Johnson *et al.*[50,51] • Uses tissue expanders in the labia to create an elastic and large skin flap. • Free flap vaginoplasty; skin flap attached to its original blood supply to a place remote from the original skin flap.
1992	Pena[52] • Uses transanorectal approach.
1994	Jackson and Rosenblatt[53] • Uses Interceed® absorbable adhesion barrier; nonadherent gelatinous layer between cavity and mold allows epithelialization without adherence to stent.
1997	Pena[54] • Uses total urogenital sinus mobilization.
1998	Rink and Adams[22] • Uses posterior sagittal pararectal approach to the urogenital sinus without colostomy from a prone approach.

form of CAH, were followed. The estimated follow-up was 1 to 4 years. Six patients required reoperation; one for urethral stricture and five to reduce scrotalized labia. Two children required ongoing dilations.[56]

To treat high confluence of the vagina and urethra, at least three surgical options exist: (i) high vaginal sinus mobilization; (ii) total urogenital sinus mobilization; and (iii) creation of a neovagina utilizing McIndoe split-thickness skin graft or sterilized amnion, full thickness skin flaps, peritoneum, small intestine, or colon vaginoplasty.

Outcomes after these varied procedures have a more obvious visual/functional failure potential than the surgical procedures for low confluence of the vagina. Though the seminal reviews were not highly detailed regarding specific surgical methods, they demonstrate a trend toward multiple surgical revisions. The first review by Alizai summarized vaginoplasty outcomes in 14 girls with a diagnosis of CAH (mean age 13.1 yrs).[25] Ninety-three percent (13/14) required additional vaginal surgery. Reasons included stenosis of the introitus in 43% (6/14) and persistent urogenital sinus with or without fibrosis in 50% (7/14). A later study by Bailez *et al.* reviewing outcomes after vaginoplasty disclosed that 79% (22/28) of girls required further surgery.[57] Their mean age at second surgery was 18.3 years (range, 13 to 23 years). Of 22 reoperative patients, 17 underwent two procedures and five, three procedures. Minto and Creighton reviewed outcomes on 28 subjects after vaginoplasty. Sixty-four percent (18/28) had vaginal surgery at a mean age of 9.2 years; 39% (7/28) had a second vaginal surgery; and 11% (2/7) of these, a third had vaginal surgery.[26] Very little data on functional outcome were available. Risk of selection bias (only those patients with problems presenting to a GYN clinic) was also possible and may have influenced outcomes evidence.

Total urogenital sinus mobilization

Establishing the separation of the urethral opening from the vaginal opening on the perineum has been a problem with significant complications of stenosis of the vagina, vaginal atresia, and urethrovaginal fistula, probably secondary to devascularization during separation and movement of the vagina to a more posterior position on the perineum. Dissecting the plane between urethra and vagina (anterior to the vagina) has been theorized to be responsible. Pena's technique for mobilization of the entire urethral vaginal complex allowed separation with better placement without dissection between the two. Originally described in 1994, this technique was popularized by Pena in 1997. Good short-term outcomes have been reported by Kropp and Cheng with seven female patients who have a mean follow-up of 16 months (range 5 to 24 months); all had good cosmesis, no prolapse, and urinary continence. A modified version of this surgery that included a posterior perineal flap was reported by Jenak, Ludwikowski, and Gonzalez.[58] Long-term follow-up has not been established, but short-term outcomes in 4/6 girls demonstrated good vaginal caliber at mean 3.7 months (range 1 to 9 months).[59]

The posterior sagittal approach

Visualization of the urogenital sinus during perineal dissection, especially in high confluence, has always been difficult. Posterior or prone approaches have been utilized, splitting of the rectum for better visualization, as well as pararectal dissection. Protective colostomy was necessary when the anus was either bivalved or split anteriorly. In 1992, Pena first reported meticulous reconstruction of the rectum.[52] No long-term follow-up was available. Benedetto reported a technique that opened the anterior rectal wall in the midline (1997).[60] A series of eight patients undergoing this technique was reported by Braz (1999). All had good fecal continence; 87% (7/8), urinary continence; and 12.% (1/8), were sexually active.[61] Neither detailed nor long-term outcomes was available.

Posterior sagittal pararectal

For patients who had high confluence of the vagina to urethra, a modification through a prone approach was reported by Rink in 1998.[22] This technique was beneficial for obtaining exposure without rectal splitting or temporary colostomy. Follow-up ranged from 6 months to 5 years for eight patients, aged 6 months to 25 years. Four patients required initial dilatations with only one of the four requiring dilation after six months. One patient was reported to have successful intercourse.[22]

Vaginal tract without skin graft

Dupuytren introduced this procedure in 1817.[28] A perineal pouch or space was dissected between bladder and rectum. Later, Wharton[37] and Counsellor[38] used a mold to hold the pouch open, allowing spontaneous epithelialization that took 3 to 6 months.

In a review by Cali and Pratt in 1968,[62] 20% (5/25) of patients experienced complete failure of the procedure, whereas 29% (5/17) had partial or complete stenosis after 10 years. However, 76% (13/17) reported satisfactory sexual function. The authors calculated a 46% failure rate. In the same study, a subsequent patient survey indicated that when no skin graft was used, a mold had to be utilized for several hours per day for an average of more than 3 years, and indefinitely in some cases. Twenty-five percent of patients used lubricants.

In one case, dura mater was utilized at the top of the mold. A squamous cell cancer was later found in this patient.[63]

Though this procedure fell out of vogue, it was resurrected in 1994 by Jackson and Rosenblatt, who used an absorbable adhesion barrier (Interceed®) over a mold in four patients.[53] (They had intended to use a piece of amnion, but it was contaminated.) They proceeded as in a typical Counsellor procedure and reported success in all the patients, all with a satisfactory-sized vagina (6–12 cm). None of the patients reported discomfort with intercourse and none required lubricant. These patients also required a mold for 3 to 6 months after surgery and most continued to wear the mold for 15 minutes, three times a day. One advantage of the procedure was that no scar occurred from harvesting a graft or flap. Montoyama demonstrated normal vaginal epithelium in about one-half of the vagina canal one month postoperatively, and the entire vaginal canal covered with vaginal epithelium 2 months postoperatively in ten patients. No patients required lubricants or dilator use.[64]

Split-thickness skin graft vaginoplasty

Transperineal procedures employ a surgical cut, resulting in a space between bladder and rectum, followed by placement of a split-thickness skin graft covered mold. This evolved from the Wharton technique and was later described by Abbe,[30] and McIndoe and Bannister.[36] Popularized by Counsellor,[38] the technique had the advantage of low morbidity and mortality, since all surgery took place external to the peritoneal cavity.

The major disadvantage was the necessity for persistent and regular dilatation of the tract, because the channel might close up. This most commonly occurred at the vault or "top" area. A risk of fistula of the bladder or rectum existed from wearing the solid mold after surgery, but has decreased with the use of newer, softer, and inflatable molds.[65] This type of skin graft had a tendency to be dry and required lubrication.

McIndoe[66] reported an immediate success rate of 89%. Most patients were 19 to 24 years old at the time of surgery. Long-term (10-year) follow-up of six patients revealed four successful vaginoplasties, one partial failure, and one complete failure.

In 1989, Buss and Lee[67] surveyed 50 intersexuals (mean age 20 years, range 16 to 34 years) and had 47 responders. The mean follow-up was 6.5 years. Forty-three patients were satisfied with the operative result and were able to experience functional intravaginal intercourse without a subsequent surgical procedure. Eighty-five percent (40/47) rated vaginal function and sexual response as "satisfactory" or "good." A few noted inadequate lubrication.

Cali and Pratt[62] recognized the paucity of long-term follow-up information and so concentrated on 113 patients (mean age at surgery, 22.6 years) who were 1 to 37 years post-McIndoe operation. They reported 42% (48/114) had some contracture of the vagina; however, 90% (84/93) expressed satisfaction with sexual function. They examined a second group of patients who underwent the McIndoe procedure, and at the 10-year follow-up, 51% (36/71) showed some vaginal contraction. Only 85% (60/71) responded to questions about coitus; 79% (56/71) noted that it was satisfactory. Many observed that the vagina became shorter over the years. About one-quarter of these patients used lubricants. In this procedure, scarring was noted to be in depth rather than in width and varied from slight scarring to complete stenosis, in 18% (13/71) of patients.

In 1996, Alessandrescu provided a retrospective review of 201 cases (average age at surgery 20.5 years) treated with modified Abbe–McIndoe vaginoplasty.[68] A 3- to 16-year follow-up noted 1%, rectal perforation; 4%, graft infection; and 5.5%, graft site infection. Eighty-four percent of patients gave an anatomic evaluation rate of "good"; 10%, satisfactory; and 6.5%, unsatisfactory. One hundred and fifty-six patients rated sexual satisfaction: 112 (71.8%) noted no dyspareunia and adequate lubrication, as well as vaginal orgasms. Twenty-three percent were able to have intercourse, but no orgasm. During postoperative care, the use of vacuum expandable condom molds may improve outcomes and patient comfort.

Skin flap vaginoplasties

To overcome a shortage of skin in the vaginal perineal area, skin flaps were moved on a pedicle or base to the needy area. These full-thickness skin flaps included a pudendal thigh, fasciocutaneous flap,[69,70] a rectus abdominus flap,[51] labial flap, and buttocks flaps.[47,71] Much later, tissue expanders were used in the labia to produce a much larger flap.[50] The Hendren vaginoplasty featured combinations of flaps from buttocks and labia for difficult high urovaginal sinus repairs.[47] The Passerini–Glazel[13] procedure, probably the most esthetic and well-refined repair, may be a variant of the Williams[44] repair or Sheares,[41] posterior based flap, in which skin flaps pulled down from the reduced phallic shaft created both the labial minora and majora.

On review of the literature, very little information is available on long-term outcomes of patients who have undergone this type of vaginoplasty. The reported advantages included lack of hair in vagina, as well as a wider introitus, with less need for dilatation. These repairs were especially favorable in low vaginal atresia. The disadvantage included scarring from the harvest site, especially the buttocks, thigh, and vulva.

Newman *et al.*[72] reviewed 79 children with ambiguous genitalia who received female gender assignment. For 25% (20/79), the mean follow-up was eight years (range 1 to 24 years). Twelve of 20 children underwent only clitoral surgery. Ten of 12 had highly satisfactory, social, psychologic, and sexual function. One experienced pain with orgasm and one, dyspareunia. Eight of 20 classified sexual function as satisfactory to poor.

In the same study, three of 20 complained of uncomfortable hair growth at the introitus. In those children having "pull-through" vaginoplasty, 8/14 suffered severe vaginal stenosis that required secondary vaginal operations. Almost all of the above patients had absence of the mucous apparatus at the introitus. Two of four patients with thigh flap vaginoplasties continued to experience problems with vaginal size.

In 2000, Li reported a series of 12 patients treated with pudendal thigh flaps.[73] One patient had unilateral necrosis of a flap and rectovaginal fistula. All others had good outcomes. In 2003, Selvaggi reported the outcome of two patients who had pudendal thigh faciocutaneous flap neovaginoplasty. The first patient had a very good outcome. The second had recurrent severe stenosis at the anastamosis to the uterus.[73a] Wu reported on five patients with 6 months' to 24 months' follow-up who had skin flaps created from tissue expanders in the labia minora with a bipedicle flap.[74] All patients had good outcomes; 80% (4/5) were sexually active. Wierrani and Gronberg used deepithelialized dermis from the labia majora for vaginoplasty and reported optimal cosmetic and function results in 17 patients over 16 years.[75]

Bowel segment vaginoplasty

The use of bowel for vaginoplasty was first attributed to Baldwin in 1904.[31] Using a small segment of ileum, he sealed one end and moved it on its vascular supply to the pelvis, stitching the open end around the vaginal entrance. Complications included bowel obstruction and infections. Several mortalities were reported and the method was abandoned. It was subsequently resurrected by Pratt in the 1960s.[42] Pratt used sigmoid, as did later surgeons, with the Ober–Meinrenken and Schubert–Schmidt procedures.[23,39,76]

The advantages are minimal shrinkage, natural elasticity, and lubrication. The disadvantages include prolapse, outlet stenosis, and unless douching was performed on a regular basis, continual discharge with inspissation of the secretions. Other disadvantages include bleeding and paraumbilical discomfort with intercourse.

In 1985, Alexandrov[77] reported long-term success in 82% (128/156) of patients. In reviews by Cali and Pratt,[62] ten patients with a Baldwin (ileum) type repair were followed for a mean of 20.7 years; eight patients had good vaginal depth and width; all reported satisfactory coitus. One patient, a nun, requested the vaginoplasty be removed because of a prolapse. Only one patient with sigmoid vaginoplasty was followed for 15 years. This patient had good vaginal size and satisfactory coitus.

In a 1994 review, Hendren and Atala[78] reported on patients whose vagina was reconstructed with bowel during infancy and childhood from 1964 to 1993. Ten patients are now adults and sexually active. Twenty-five percent (16/65) patients experienced eversion prolapse of the vagina that required simple trimming.

Martinez-Mora[79] reported 19 sigmoid vaginoplasties, 18 with total success over a follow-up ranging from 1 to 15 years. Coitus and orgasm were reported to be "normal" in all patients.

In a 2002 study, Graziano reported her impression that less risk of stenosis of bowel vaginoplasty occurred if surgery was performed after puberty.[80] However, weekly dilatations for the first 6 months to one year were required. Follow-up ranged from 6 to 12 years. All patients were sexually active without dyspareunia and did not require lubrications.

Parsons and Gearhart (2002) also reported a long-term follow-up of vaginal reconstruction using sigmoid colon.[81] Of 28 patients, mean age at surgery was 16 years (range, 6 to 21 years) and mean follow-up, 6.2 years (range, 2 months to 15 years). Introital stenosis was reported in 14% (4/28). These had dilatation of the cutaneous junction while they were under general anesthesia, followed by a regular dilatation protocol, with no subsequent recurrence of stenosis. Mucosal prolapse occurred in 14% (4/28) within 4 weeks of surgery. Of 14 adult heterosexually active patients, 79% (11/14) were very satisfied with sexual development and function; 21% (3/14) were comfortable. None reported dyspareunia. All believed that adolescence was the appropriate time for surgery.

Regarding sigmoid vaginoplasty, the most detailed long-term outcome was presented by Communal *et al.*, who reviewed 16 patients, mean age 18 (range 17 to 22 years), with Mayer–Rokitansky–Kuster–Hauser syndrome.[82] Fourteen underwent sigmoid neovaginoplasty as a first attempt, two after failed vaginoplasty. Follow-up averaged 2 years, range 1 month to 8 years. Physical examination revealed that 12.5% (2/16) had stenosis of the colovestibular anastomosis and 25% (4/16), moderate graft shrinkage. Eleven responded to a questionnaire that combined Rosen's FSFI (female sexual function index) with additional surgery specific items. These patients scored normally regarding global sexual satisfaction, desire, arousability, pleasure, and lubrication, but had lower scores in the comfort domains. Specifically, 27% (3/11) did not attempt vaginal intercourse, 27% (3/11) had superficial dyspareunia; 27% (3/11) had abdominal pain with vaginal penetration; 10% (1/11) vaginal dryness. All patients reached orgasm at least half of the time. Infertility caused anxiety. However, their self esteem as a "woman" and as a "lover" was good. Those who did not attempt sexual intercourse felt less experienced as a lover, but strongly as a woman. Seventy-two percent (8/11) of patients had sexual intercourse at least once a week. They ranked their daily discomfort as moderate because of discharge from the vagina, which required them to use one to two pads daily.

Laparoscopically assisted techniques for sigmoid vaginoplasties have been reported. No long-term follow-up is currently available.[83]

Amnion vaginoplasty

In 1973, Trelford *et al.* was the first to demonstrate the use of amnion as a surgical dressing.[84] In 1986, Ashworth *et al.*[48] reported on a series of 15 patients who had amnion vaginoplasty. The patients' mean age was 19.3 years (range 14 to 28 years). To accomplish this surgery, a perineal space was dissected or an existing strictured space enlarged. Human amnion was prepared by stripping it from the chorion, rinsing it, and storing it at 4 °C in crystalline penicillin (50 000 U per 100 ml). The amnion was then cultured. If sterile, it was draped with the mesenchymal surface outermost over a mold and inserted into the vagina. At 5 to 7 days, the mold was replaced with second piece of amnion. (In one patient, a third piece was used.) Patients continued to use a dilator lubricated with dienestrol cream three times a day for 15 minutes and were able to begin intercourse after 4 to 6 weeks. Improvement was recorded in all patients. Initial epithelialization was excellent; however, some contracture was evident in all patients at 3 month follow-up. Total follow-up reported was only 12 months.[48]

Because amnion does not express histocompatibility antigens, immune rejection is not a problem.[85] Amnion appears to have an antibacterial effect; enzymes such as lysozyme may be bacteriocidal. Tancer *et al.*,[86] Dino *et al.*,[87] and Dhall[88] identified vaginal epithelium by biopsy at 8 to 10 weeks' postoperatively. No long-term follow-up results were available.

Peritoneum vaginoplasty

Use of peritoneum was initially reported in the Russian literature in 1969 and was first referred to as the Davydov method.[45] This was a combined abdominal-peritoneal approach to vaginoplasty. The undersurface of a cylinder of peritoneum was dissected in the abdominal cavity and brought down into a freshly created neovaginal space. A purse-string was used to close the top and circumferencial sutures to attach the peritoneum to vulvovaginal skin. Davydov reported good short-term and long-term results.[46] Martinez-Mora *et al.*[79] supported these conclusions. Their results indicated no contracture of the vagina at 1 to 2 years in four patients, three of whom have normal coitus. (The fourth was only 16 years old and not yet sexually active.)

Reports of laparoscopic dissection of a pelvic peritoneal sleeve and peritoneal tube of Douglas' pouch with suture to introital mucosal flaps were encouraging, but no long-term follow-up is currently available.[89]

Bladder mucosa vaginoplasty

This method was first described by Claret *et al.* in 1988.[49] The graft was obtained by filling the bladder with saline and opening the bladder muscle down to mucosa. The mucosa was then harvested, closing bladder muscle only. The mucosa was then applied over an inflatable mold and inserted into a freshly dissected perineal space. Martinez-Mora *et al.*[79] reported good results in a patient who failed both split skin graft and sigmoid vaginoplasty. No long-term outcome results are available.

Other tissues

Scalp, buccal mucosa, and fetal skin have been used in vaginal construction. No long-term follow-up is available.[90–92]

Tumors and diseases of exogenous tissue used in genitoplasty

When exogenous tissue is used, tissue dysplasia may be expected because the tissue is suddenly subjected to new contacts or stresses. Skin grafted to form vagina loses hair follicles and sweat glands. A reduction in the number of elastic fibers and hyperplasia of epithelial cells occurs. Grafts accumulate large amounts of glycogen,[93] which is typical of vaginal mucosa, but almost never occurs in normal skin. Tumors associated with the exogenous tissue still have the potential to express the expected tumor or

Table 46.3. Documented cases of cancer of the neovagina

Series	Tumor type	Transplanted tissue
Ritchie[94]	AC	Ileum
Lavand-Homme[95]	AC	Ileum
Adryjowicz *et al.*[96]	AC	Cecum
Ursic-Vrscaj *et al.*[97]	AC	Sigmoid
Jackson[98]	SCC	STD
Barclay[99]	SCC	STD
Ramming *et al.*[100]	SCC	STD
Duckler[101]	SCC	STD
Hopkins and Morley[102]	SCC	STD
Gallup *et al.*[103]	SCC	STD
Hiroi *et al.*[104]	AC	Sigmoid
Steiner *et al.*[63]	SCC	Dura mater
Harder *et al.*[105]	SCC	Penile skin
Schult *et al.*[106]	SCC	(none) Phallus phantom

AC = adenocarcinoma.
SCC = squamous cell carcinoma.
STD = split-thickness (thigh) dermal.

inflammatory change, as in the tissue's natural environment. Such problems must be anticipated and monitored in long-term follow-up of the patient with feminizing genitoplasty.

Carcinoma of the neovagina is a very rare malignancy. Fourteen cases have been reported (Table 46.3).[63,94–106] Cancer appears to be related to the type of transplanted tissue. All recorded cases of squamous cell carcinoma are related to split-thickness skin graft or McIndoe variations and all adenocarcinomas to intestinal grafts. No malignancies have been reported in vaginas made from amnion or peritoneum.

Development of these tumors occurs from 8 to 30 years postsurgery, reflecting a younger age range than carcinoma of the natural vagina. Peak incidence for carcinoma of vagina is 65 years of age, whereas carcinoma of the neovagina has been documented in patients between the ages of 25 and 53 years.

In almost every case, cancer of the neovagina presents with a bloody or clear vaginal discharge or postcoital bleeding. As is common with primary vaginal carcinomas, all lesions occur in the posterior vaginal vault. Invasive vaginal cancer tends to be undifferentiated and development of squamous pearls is unusual. In contrast, cancer of the neovagina presents with squamous lesions that typically represent mature squamous cell carcinoma, with pearl formation. Carcinoma of the neovagina is distinct in its occurrence in a young population and histopathologic cell type, but the risk of development after reconstruction is no greater than the reported incidence of vaginal cancer.

Disease survival is significantly related to the stage of disease at diagnosis, just as with carcinoma in a natural vagina.[107] The first four reported patients with cancer of the neovagina were treated with primary radiation therapy. Three developed recurrence, suggesting a high percentage of failure with radiation as a primary treatment modality. The last ten most recent cases were treated with primary surgical therapy; one has recurred.[107]

Ulcerative colitis in the neovagina has also been reported from a colonic vaginoplasty.[108] Syed reported review of 18 children after colovaginoplasty with mean follow-up of 5 years, range 1.5 to 8 years.[109] Three of 18 developed severe vaginal discharge and bleeding two to seven years after colovaginoplasty. Examination showed erythema, edema, ulceration, and bleeding. Treatment was with short chain fatty acids, two did not respond and were treated with steroid enemas and mesalazine. One required surgical reduction.

Discussion

Ambiguous genitalia in the newborn demand an urgent, exacting diagnosis. Tests are available to detect biochemical derangements and chromosomal genotypic patterns, as well as define internal genital anatomy. Yet, even with this abundance of objective information, sexual assignment and choices for treatment remain very difficult decisions. Surgeons have advanced techniques during the last 50 years to the point where they can reliably externally feminize a child. Several tissues can now be used to build a vagina, with variable success. Sexual outcomes remain indeterminate. Some argue that surgery in an infant maximizes a child's social adjustment and acceptance by the family. The needs of parents to have a presentable child can be satisfied. In doing so, can we truly promote the best interest of the adult patient in terms of psychosocial and functional outcomes? This knowledge is still obscured and much remains to be discovered.

Obviously, problems exist that surgeons, despite the most technically perfect surgeries, cannot address. Success in psychosocial adjustment is the true goal of sexual assignment and genitoplasty. The psychosocial long-term outcomes represent the most necessary information to determine if we are successful in treating patients with ambiguous or absent genitalia. However, in conditions other than CAH and MRKH, outcomes are generally unavailable. We need to evaluate these patients, understand their problems, and determine what they want. The present author, through personal communication with three societies of intersexual patients (Hermaphrodite

Table 46.4. Some support groups

Support groups	Telephone number
AIS Support Group	
UK	(0) 1623 661749
USA	(619) 569–5254
Ambiguous Genitalia Support Group	
USA	(209) 369–0414
Intersex Society of North America (ISNA)	
USA	(707) 775–3121
Hermaphrodite Education and Listening Post (HELP)	
USA	(904) 757–5734

Education and Listening Post, Intersex Society of North America, AIS Support Group) (Table 46.4) concludes that certain desires became an obvious and common thread of all the groups.

Truth

Patients believe everyone's interests are best served when information is not withheld. They can deal better with truth and have less difficulty with issues of trust with doctors and parents when truthful information is initially provided.

Counseling

Counseling must be available and must be consistent and long term.

Surgery

Early surgery makes parents and doctors more comfortable, but counseling makes people comfortable too, and is not irreversible. Patients wonder if thinking that surgery will improve the psychological outcome for the intersexual child is logical reasoning mistaken for accurate reasoning. They question if surgery could potentiate impairment of sexual function in adulthood. It may be illusory, but patients believe that the ability to choose for oneself may favorably affect the results of surgery. Surgery must be based on truthful disclosure and support and permit decision-making by parents and patient.

Parental acceptance

Parents need understanding and counseling as their guidance is a strong determinant of how well their child will adjust. This issue must be independent of whether the child receives surgery.

Professional societies

Patients and parents need to be aware of, and have access to, the societies for persons with their particular problems. Patients feel almost universally relieved to know others with similar problems.

Simply understanding and performing good surgery is insufficient. We must also know when to appropriately perform or withhold surgery. Our ethical duty as surgeons is to do no harm and to serve the best interests of our patient. Sometimes, this means admitting that a "perfect" solution may not be attainable.

Acknowledgments

The author acknowledges the staff of Lake Erie Research Institute and Hamot Medical Center, Erie, PA, for editing and typing this book chapter.

REFERENCES

1. Ombrédanne L. In *Les Hermaphrodites et la Chirurgie*. Paris: Masson, 1939.
2. Stefan, H. & Pinsker, P. Surgical reconstruction of the external genitalia in female pseudohermaphroditis. *Vojen zdrav Listy* 1957; **26**:391.
3. Lattimer, J. K. Relocation and recession of the enlarged clitoris with preservation of the glans: an alternative to amputation. *J. Urol.* 1961; **80**:113–116.
4. Schmid, M. A. Plastic correction of the external genitalia in a male pseudohermaphrodite. *Arch. Klin. Chic.* 1961; **298**: 977.
5. Pellerin, D. La reimplantation du clitoris: resection plastique du pseudo-hermaphroditism feminin. *Mem. Acad. Chir. (Paris)* 1965; **91**:965–968.
6. Gross, R. E., Randolph, J., & Crigler, J. F. Jr. Clitorectomy for sexual abnormalities: indications and technique. *Surgery* 1966; **59**(2):300–308.
7. Randolph, J. G. & Hung, W. Reduction clitoroplasty in females with hypertrophied clitoris. *J. Pediatr. Surg.* 1970; **5**:224–231.
8. Spence, J. M. & Allen, T. D. Genital reconstruction in the female with the adrenogenital syndrome. *Br. J. Urol.* 1973; **45**:126–130.
9. Kumar, H., Kiefer, I. E., Rosenthal, I. E., & Clark, S. S. Clitoroplasty: experience during a 19-year period. *J. Urol.* 1974; **111**:81–84.
10. Mollard, P., Juskiewenski, S., & Sarkissian, J. Clitoroplasty in intersex: a new technique. *Br. J. Urol.* 1981; **53**:371–373.
11. Mininberg, D. T. Phalloplasty in congenital adrenal hyperplasia. *J. Urol.* 1982; **128**:355–356.
12. Kogan, S. J., Smey, P., & Levitt, S. B. Subtunical total reduction clitoroplasty: a safe modification of existing techniques. *J. Urol.* 1983; **130**:746–748.

13. Passerini-Glazel, G. A new 1-stage procedure for clitorovaginoplasty in severely masculinized female pseudohemophrodites. *J. Urol.* 1989; **142**:565–568.
14. Sagehashi, N. Clitoroplasty for clitoromegaly due to adrenogenital syndrome without loss of sensitivity. *Plast. Reconstr. Surg.* 1993; **91**:950–955.
15. Hampson, J. G. Hermaphroditic genital appearance, rearing and eroticism in hyperadrenocorticism. *Bull. Johns Hopkins Hosp.* 1955; **96**:265.
16. Gearhart, J. P., Burnett, A., & Owen, J. H. Measurement of pudendal evoked potentials during feminizing genitoplasty: technique and applications. *J. Urol.* 1995; **153**:486–487.
17. Chase, C. Letter of response. *J. Urol.* 1996; **156**:1139–1140.
18. O'Connell, H. E., Hutson, J. M., Anderson, C. R., & Plenter, R. J. Anatomical relationship between urethra and clitoris. *J. Urol.* 1998; **159**:1892–1897.
19. Baskin, L. S., Erol, A., Li, Y. W., Liu, W. H., Kurzrock, E., & Cunha, G. R. Anatomical studies of the human clitoris. *J. Urol.* 1999; **162**:1015–1020.
20. Pfaff, D. W. In *Estrogens and Brain Function: Neural Analysis of a Hormone-controlled Mammalian Reproductive Behavior*. New York: Springer-Verlag, 1980.
21. Schober, J. M. Genital sensitivity mapping. AUA Presidential lecture presented at The Society of Pelvic Surgeons April 2003 and at the Society of GURS, October 31, 2003.
22. Rink, R. C. & Adams, M. C. Feminizing genitoplasty: state of the art. *World J. Urol.* 1998; **16**:212–218.
23. Passerini-Glazel, G. Feminizing genitoplasty. *J. Urol.* 1999; **161**:1592–1593.
24. Passerini-Glazel, G. A new 1-stage procedure for clitorovaginoplasty in severely masculinized female pseudohermaphrodites. *J. Urol.* 1989; **142**:565–568, 572.
25. Alizai, N. K., Thomas, D. F., Lilford, R. J., Batchelor, A. G., & Johnson, N. Feminizing genitoplasty for congenital adrenal hyperplasia: what happens at puberty? *J. Urol.* 1999; **161**: 1588–1591.
26. Minto, C. L., Liao, L. M., Woodhouse, C. R., Ransley, P. G., & Creighton, S. M. The effect of clitoral surgery on sexual outcome in individuals who have intersex conditions with ambiguous genitalia: a cross-sectional study. *Lancet* 2003; **361**:1252–1257.
27. Crouch, N. S., Minto, C. L., Liao, L. M., Woodhouse, C. R. J., & Creighton, S. M. (in press). Genital sensation following feminizing genitoplasty for CAH: a pilot study. *BJU Int.* 2004; **93**(1): 135.
28. Dupuytren, G. (1817). Cited in Judin, *S. Surg. Gynec. & Obst.* 1927; **44**: 530.
29a. Early attempts at vaginal surgery. *AIS Review* ALIAS no. 4, July 4, 1996.
29b. Alexandrov, M. S. Obrazovanie iskustvennogo vlagalishchaiz sigmovidnoi kishki. *Medgiz*, Moskova, 1955, p. 185.
30. Abbe, R. A new method of creating a vagina in a case of congenital absence. *Med. Rec.* 1898; **54**:836–838.
31. Baldwin, J. F. The formation of an artificial vagina by intestinal transplantation. *Ann. Surg.* 1904; **40**:398.
32. Schubert, G. *Zentralbl. Gynäk* 1911; **35**:1017.
33. Graves, W. P. Methods of constructing an artificial vagina. *Surg. Clin. North Am.* 1921; **1**:611.
34. Masson, J. C. Congenital absence of the vagina and its treatment. *Am. J. Obstet. Gynec.* 1932; **24**:583.
35. Frank, R. T. The formation of an artificial vagina without operation. *Am. J. Obstet. Gynec.* 1938; **35**:1053–1055.
36. McIndoe, A. H. & Bannister, J. B. An operation for the cure of congenital absence of the vagina. *J. Obstet. Gynaecol. Br. Emp.* 1938; **45**:490–494.
37. Wharton, L. R. A simplified method of constructing a vagina. *Ann. Surg.* 1938; **107**:842.
38. Counsellor, V. S. Congenital absence of the vagina *J. Am. Med. Assoc.* 1948; **136**:861.
39. Schmid, H. H. Construction of artificial vagina using the flexure. *Zentralbl. Chir.* 1952; **77**:2119.
40. Jones, H. W. Jr. & Jones, G. E. S. The gynecological aspects of adrenal hyperplasia and allied disorders. *Am. J. Obstet. Gynec.* 1954; **68**:1330.
41. Sheares, B. H. Congenital atresia of the vagina – a new technique for tunneling the space between the bladder and rectum and construction of a new vagina by a modified Wharton technique. *J. Obstet. Gynaecol. Br. Emp.* 1960; **67**:24–31.
42. Pratt, J. H. Sigmoidovaginostomy: a new method of obtaining satisfactory vaginal depth. *Am. J. Obstet. Gynecol.* 1961; **81**:535–545.
43. Fortunoff, S., Lattimer, J. K., & Edson, M. Vaginoplasty technique for female pseudohermaphrodites. *Surg. Gynecol. Obstet.* 1964; **118**:545–548.
44. Williams, E. A. Congenital absence of the vagina: a simple operation for its relief. *Br. J. Obstet. Gynaecol.* 1964; **4**:511–512.
45. Davydov, S. N. & Zhvitiashvili, O. D. Formation of vagina (colpopoiesis) from peritoneum of Douglas pouch. *Acta Chir. Plast.* 1974; **16**:35–41.
46. Davydov, S. N. Modifizierte Kolpopoese aus Peritoneum der Excavatio rectouterina. *Ginekologiia, Moskau*, 1969; **45**:55–57.
47. Hendren, W. D. & Donahoe, P. K. Correction of congenital abnormalities of the vagina and perineum. *J. Pediatr. Surg.* 1980; **15**:751–763.
48. Ashworth, M. F., Morton, K. E., Dewhurst, J., Lilford, R. J., & Bates, R. G. Vaginoplasty using amnion. *Obstet. Gynec.* 1986; **67**:443–446.
49. Claret, I., Castañón, M., Rodo, J. *et al.* Neovagina con injerto libre do mucosa vesical (técnica original de Claret). Libro de Actas del XXVIII Congreso de la Sociedad Española de Cirugía Pediátrica, Lloret de Mar, Spain, June 15–19, p. 40y video, 1988.
50. Johnson, N., Batchelor, A., & Lilford, R. J. Experience with tissue expansion vaginoplasty. *Br. J. Obstet. Gynaecol.* 1991; **98**:564–568.
51. Johnson, N., Batchelor, A., & Lilford, R. J. The free-flap vaginoplasty: a new surgical procedure for the treatment of vaginal agenesis. *Br. J. Obstet. Gynaecol.* 1991; **98**:184–188.
52. Pena, A., Filmer, B., Bonilla, E., Mendez, M., & Stolar, C. Transanorectal approach for the treatment of urogenital sinus: preliminary report. *J. Pediatr. Surg.* 1992; **27**:681–685.

53. Jackson, N. D. & Rosenblatt, P. L. Use of Interceed® absorbable adhesion barrier for vaginoplasty. *Obstet. Gynec.* 1994; **84**:1048–1050.
54. Pena, A. Total urogenital mobilization–an easier way to repair cloacas. *J. Pediatr. Surg.* 1997; **32**:263–268.
55. Schober, J. M. Feminizing genitoplasty for Intersex. In Stringer, M. D., Oldham, K. T., Mouriquand, P. D. E., & Howard, E. R., eds. *Pediatric Surgery and Urology: Long-Term Outcomes.* London: W.B. Saunders Co., 1st edn, 1998, Ch. 44, 549–558.
56. Freitas Filho, L. G., Carnevale, J., Melo, C. E., Laks, M., & Calcagno, Silva, M. A posterior-based omega-shaped flap vaginoplasty in girls with congenital adrenal hyperplasia caused by 21-hydroxylase deficiency. *BJU Int.* 2003; **91**:263–267.
57. Bailez, M. M., Gearhart, J. P., Migeon, C., & Rock, J. Vaginal reconstruction after initial construction of the external genitalia in girls with salt-wasting adrenal hyperplasia. *J. Urol.* 1992; **148**:680–684.
58. Jenak, R., Ludwikowski, B., & Gonzalez, R. Total urogenital sinus mobilization: a modified perineal approach for feminizing genitoplasty and urogenital sinus repair. *J. Urol.* 2001; **165**:2347–2349.
59. Ludwikowski, B., Oesch Hayward, I., & Gonzalez, R. Total urogenital sinus mobilization: expanded applications. *BJU Int.* 1999; **83**:820–822.
60. Di Benedetto, V., Gioviale, M., Bagnara, V., Cacciaguerra, S., & Di Benedetto, A. The anterior sagittal transanorectal approach: a modified approach to 1-stage clitoral vaginoplasty in severely masculinized female pseudohermaphrodites – preliminary results. *J. Urol.* 1997; **157**:330–332.
61. Braz, A. Posterior sagittal transanorectal approach in patients with ambiguous genitalia: report of eight cases. *Pediatr. Surg. Int.* 1999; **15**:108–110.
62. Cali, R. W. & Pratt, J. H. Congenital absence of the vagina. Long-term results of vaginal reconstruction in 175 cases. *Am. J. Obstet. Gynec.* 1968; **100**:752–763.
63. Steiner, E., Woernle, F., Kuhn, W. *et al.* Carcinoma of the neovagina: case report and review of the literature. *Gynecol. Oncol.* 2002; **84**:171–175.
64. Motoyama, S., Laoag-Fernandez, J. B., Mochizuki, S., Yamabe, S., & Maruo, T. Vaginoplasty with Interceed absorbable adhesion barrier for complete squamous epithelialization in vaginal agenesis. *Am. J. Obstet. Gynecol.* 2003; **188**:1260–1264.
65. Adamson, C. D., Naik, B. J., & Lynch, D. J. The vacuum expandable condom mold: a simple vaginal stent for McIndoe-style vaginoplasty. *Plast. Reconstr. Surg.* 2004; **113**:664–666.
66. McIndoe, A. Discussion of treatment of congenital absence of vagina with emphasis on long-term results. *Proc. Roy. Soc. Med.* 1959; **52**:952–954.
67. Buss, J. G. & Lee, R. A. McIndoe procedure for vaginal agenesis: results and complications. *Mayo Clin. Proc.* 1989; **64**:758–761.
68. Alessandrescu, D., Peltecu, G. C., Buhimschi, C. S., & Buhimschi, I. A. Neocolpopoiesis with split-thickness skin graft as a surgical treatment of vaginal agenesis: retrospective review of 201 cases. *Am. J. Obstet. Gynecol.* 1996; **175**:131–138.
69. Wee, J. T. & Joseph, V. T. A new technique of vaginal reconstruction using neurovascular pudendal-thigh flaps: a preliminary report. *Plast. Reconstr. Surg.* 1989; **83**:701.
70. Gleeson, N. C., Baile, W., Roberts, W. S. *et al.* Pudendal thigh fasciocutaneous flaps for vaginal reconstruction in gynecologic oncology. *Gynecol. Oncol.* 1994; **54**:269–274.
71. Dumanian, G. A. & Donahoe, P. K. Bilateral rotated buttock flaps for vaginal atresia in several masculinized females with adrenogenital syndrome. *Plast. Reconstr. Surg.* 1992; **90**:487–491.
72. Newman, K., Randolph, J., & Anderson, K. The surgical management of infants and children with ambiguous genitalia. Lessons learned from 25 years. *Ann. Surg.* 1992; **215**:644–653.
73. Li, S., Liu, Y., & Li, Y. [Twelve cases of vaginal reconstruction using neurovascular pudendal-thigh flaps]. [Chinese] *Chung-Hua Fu Chan Ko Tsa Chih* [Chin. J. Obst. Gynec.] 2000; **35**:216–218.

73a. Selvaggi, G., Monstrey, S., Depypere, H. *et al.* Creation of a neovagina with use of a pudendal thigh fasciocutaneous flap and restoration of ureterovaginal continutiy. *Fertil. Steril.* 2003; **80**(3):607–611.

74. Wu, J., Hong, Y., Li, S. F., & Hu, Z. Q. [Labia minora skin flap vaginoplasty using tissue expansion]. [Chinese] *Zhonghua Zheng Xing Wai Ke Za Zhi* 2003; **19**:18–20.
75. Wierrani, F. & Grunberger, W. Vaginoplasty using deepithelialized vulvar transposition flaps: the Grunberger method. *J. Am. Coll. Surg.* 2003; **196**:159–162.
76. Goligher, J. C. The use of pedicled transplants of sigmoid or other parts of the intestinal tract for vaginal construction. *Ann. Roy. Coll. Surg. Engl.* 1983; **65**:353–355.
77. Alexandrov, M. S. Obrazovanic iskustvennogo vlagalishcha iz sigmovidnoi kishki. *Medgiz* Moskva 1955: 185.
78. Hendren, W. H. & Atala, A. Use of bowel for vaginal reconstruction. *J. Urol.* 1994; **152**:752–757.
79. Martinez-Mora, J., Isnard, R., Castellvi, A., & Lopez Ortiz, P. Neovagina in vaginal agenesis: surgical methods and long-term results. *J. Pediatr. Surg.* 1992; **27**:10–14.
80. Graziano, K., Teitelbaum, D. H., Hirschl, R. B., & Coran, A. G. Vaginal reconstruction for ambiguous genitalia and congenital absence of the vagina: a 27-year experience. *J. Pediatr. Surg.* 2002; **37**:955–960.
81. Parsons, J. K., Gearhart, S. L., & Gearhart, J. P. Vaginal reconstruction utilizing sigmoid colon: Complications and long-term results. *J. Pediatr. Surg.* 2002; **37**:629–633.
82. Communal, P. H., Chevret-Measson, M., Golfier, F., & Raudrant, D. Sexuality after sigmoid colpopoiesis in patients with Mayer–Rokitansky–Kuster–Hauser syndrome. *Fertil. Steril.* 2003; **80**:600–606.
83. Ota, H., Tanaka, J., Murakami, M. *et al.* Laparoscopy-assisted Ruge procedure for the creation of a neovagina in a patient with Mayer–Rokitansky–Kuster–Hauser syndrome. *Fertil. Steril.* 2002; **73**:641–644.

84. Trelford, J. D., Hanson, F. W., & Anderson, D. G. Amniotic membrane as a living surgical dressing in human patients. *Oncology* 1973; **28**:358–364.
85. Akle, C. A., Adinolfi, M., Welsh, K. I. *et al.* Immunogenicity of human amniotic epithelial cells after transplantation into volunteers. *Lancet* 1981; **ii**:1003.
86. Tancer, M. L., Katz, M., & Veridiano, N. P. Vaginal epithelialization with human amnion. *Obstet. Gynecol.* 1979; **54**: 345.
87. Dino, B. R., Eufemio, G. G., & de Villa, M. S. Human amnion: the establishment of an amnion bank and its practical applications in surgery. *J. Philipp. Med. Assoc.* 1966; **42**:357.
88. Dhall, K. Amnion graft for treatment of congenital absence of the vagina. *Br. J. Obstet. Gynaecol.* 1984; **91**:279.
89. Langebrekke, A., Istre, O., Busund, B., Sponland, G., & Gjonnaess, H. Laparoscopic assisted colpoiesis according to Davydov. *Acta Obstet. Gynecol. Scand.* 1998; **77**:1027–1028.
90. Hockel, M., Menke, H., & Germann, G. Vaginoplasty with split skin grafts from the scalp: optimization of the surgical treatment for vaginal agenesis. *Am. J. Obstet. Gynecol* 2003; **188**:1100–1102.
91. Lin, W. C., Chang, C. Y., Shen, Y. Y., & Tsai, H. D. Use of autologous buccal mucosa for vaginoplasty: a study of eight cases. *Hum. Reprod.* 2003; **18**:604–607.
92. Dong, Y. & Ma, X. M. [Fetal skin used in vaginoplasty: (report of 11 cases)]. [Chinese] *Chung-Hua i Hsueh Tsa Chih* [*Chin. Med. J.*]. 1985; **65**:117–118.
93. Whitacre, F. E. & Wang, Y. Y. Biological changes in squamous epithelium transplanted to the pelvic connective tissue. *Surg. Gynec. Obstet.* 1944; **79**:192.
94. Ritchie, R. N. Primary carcinoma of the vagina following a Baldwin reconstruction operation for congenital absence of the vagina. *Am. J. Obstet. Gynec.* 1929; **18**:794.
95. Lavand-Homme, P. Late carcinoma of the artificial vagina formed from the rectum. *Brux. Med.* 1938; **19**:14.
96. Adryjowicz, E., Qizilbash, A. H., DePatrillo, A. D., O'Connell, G. J., & Taylor, M. H. Adenocarcinoma in a cecal neovagina – complication of irradiation: report of a case and review of literature. *Gynec. Oncol.* 1985; **21**:235–239.
97. Ursic-Vrscaj, M., Lindtner, J., Lamovec, J., & Novak, J. Adenocarcinoma in a sigmoid neovagina 22 years after Wertheim–Meigs operation. Case report. *Eur. J. Gynecol. Oncol.* 1994; **15**:24–28.
98. Jackson, G. W. Primary carcinoma of an artificial vagina. *Obstet. Gynec.* 1959; **14**:534–536.
99. Barclay, D. L. Personal experience cited by Cali, R. W. and Pratt, J. H. Congenital absence of the vagina. *Am. J. Obstet. Gynec.* 1968; **100**:752–763.
100. Ramming, K. P., Pilch, Y. H., Powell, R. D., & Ketcham, A. S. Primary carcinoma in an artificial vagina. *Am. J. Surg.* 1970; **120**:108–112.
101. Duckler, L. Squamous cell carcinoma developing in an artificial vagina. *Obstet. Gynec.* 1972; **40**:35–38.
102. Hopkins, M. P. & Morley, G. W. Squamous cell carcinoma of the neovagina. *Obstet. Gynec.* 1987; **69**:525–527.
103. Gallup, D. G., Castle, C. A., & Stock, R. J. Recurrent carcinoma in situ of the vagina following split-thickness skin graft vaginoplasty. *Gynecol. Oncol.* 1987; **26**:98–102.
104. Hiroi, H., Yasugi, T., Matsumoto, K. *et al.* Mucinous adenocarcinoma arising in a neovagina using the sigmoid colon thirty years after operation: a case report. *J. Surg. Oncol.* 2001; **77**:61–64.
105. Harder, Y., Erni, D., & Banic, A. Squamous cell carcinoma of the penile skin in a neovagina 20 years after male-to-female reassignment. *Br. J. Plast. Surg.* 2002; **55**:449–451.
106. Schult, M., Hecker, A., Lelle, R. J., Senninger, N., & Winde, G. Recurrent rectoneovaginal fistula caused by an incidental squamous cell carcinoma of the neovagina in Mayer–Rokitansky–Kuster–Hauser syndrome. *Gynecol. Oncol.* 2000; **77**:210–212.
107. Peters, W. A. 3rd, Kumar, N. B., & Morley, G. W. Carcinoma of the vagina. Factors influencing treatment outcome. *Cancer* 1985; **55**:892–897.
108. Hennigan, T. W. & Theodorou, N. A. Ulcerative colitis and bleeding from a colonic vaginoplasty. *J. Roy. Soc. Med.* 1992; **85**:418–419.
109. Syed, H. A., Malone, P. S., & Hitchcock, RJ. Diversion colitis in children with colovaginoplasty. *BJU Int.* 2001; **87**:857–860.

47

Hypospadias

Laurence S. Baskin

Department of Urology, UCSF Children's Medical Center,
University of California, San Francisco, USA

Introduction

The treatment of hypospadias has a long and colorful history dating back to AD 100–200, when Heliodorand Antyl is credited with the first surgical management. Since that time, the study of hypospadias has evolved into a subspecialty within pediatric urology, hypospadiology.

In Western civilization the incidence of hypospadias is reported to be increasing.[1,2] A leading hypothesis which is under investigation is maternal exposure to environmental pollutants or endocrine disruptors.[3,4]

Modern techniques have evolved from the myriad of operations described by the pioneers of hypospadias surgery. An understanding of these techniques is germane to present-day practice. We have now come full circle to accept the multistep operations for severe hypospadias and redo surgery which historically had been the procedure of choice.[5–9] It is no longer taboo to consider a two-stage approach as opposed to repairing all hypospadias with a single operation.[10,11]

Historically, the first stage of hypospadias surgery consisted of penile straightening. This was followed by a second-stage urethroplasty using various techniques such as ventral skin tubes (Thiersch-Duplay, flip flaps, Mathieu, Ombredanne and Beck) or urethral mobilization (Beck–Hacker).[12–15] Alternatively, Dennis Browne buried a strip of epithelium for subsequent tubularization.[16] Blair and Byars championed the vertical split of the dorsal hood rotated to the ventrum and advanced onto a split glans for subsequent tubularization.[17] This was the most popular repair and is similar to the two-stage approach advocated today.[18]

Modern techniques

One-stage repairs were first advocated in 1961 using a free graft of preputial skin as described by Devine and Horton.[19] An understanding of the axial nature of the preputial blood supply led to the prepuce being used as a vascularized tube in a one-stage urethroplasty.[20] Hodgson and Asopa described the use of a rotated inner-face island as a patch or a tube with the outerface for skin cover.[21,22] Duckett described the use of the inner prepuce separated from the outer preputial skin, while Standoli used the island tube from the outer prepuce.[10,23]

The description of intraoperative artificial erection in 1974, has allowed confirmation that penile straightening procedures are effective.[24] A better understanding of penile anatomy (Fig. 47.1) has led to preservation of the urethral plate and nerve sparing techniques for the correction of penile curvature (Fig. 47.2).[25–28] Preservation of the urethral plate resulted in vascularized flaps being used in an onlay fashion (Fig. 47.3) with tube repairs following out of fashion.[25,29] Subsequently, preservation of the urethral plate has led to the Snodgrass modification or the tubularized incised urethroplasty. (Fig. 47.4).[30,31]

Optical magnification, delicate instruments and fine sutures have all contributed to better results. Today in the USA the majority of hypospadias surgery is performed between the age of 6 months and 1 year as a day surgical procedure.[32]

Evaluation techniques

The goal of hypospadias surgery is to restore the urethral meatus to its normal position on the glans, to correct penile

Pediatric Surgery and Urology: Long-term Outcomes, Mark Stringer, Keith Oldham, Pierre Mouriquand.
Published by Cambridge University Press.

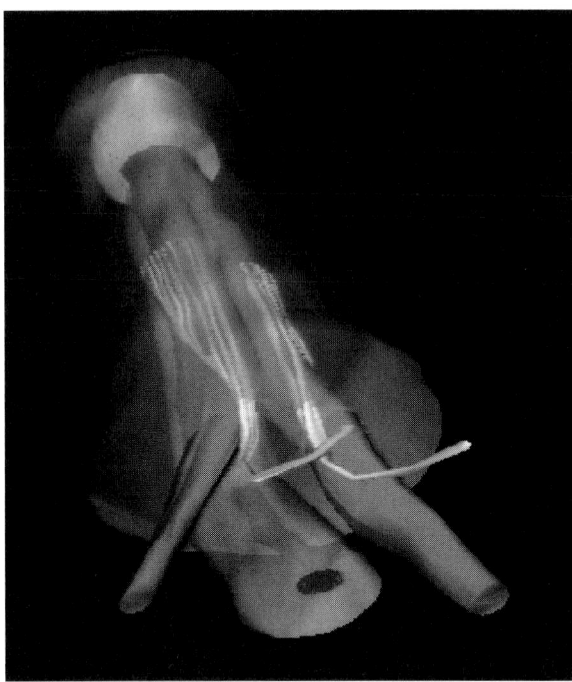

Fig. 47.1. Penile neuroanatomy. 3-D reconstruction of the male human fetal penis depicting the relationship of the dorsal nerves, corporal and crural bodies, urethra and glans (see colour plate section).

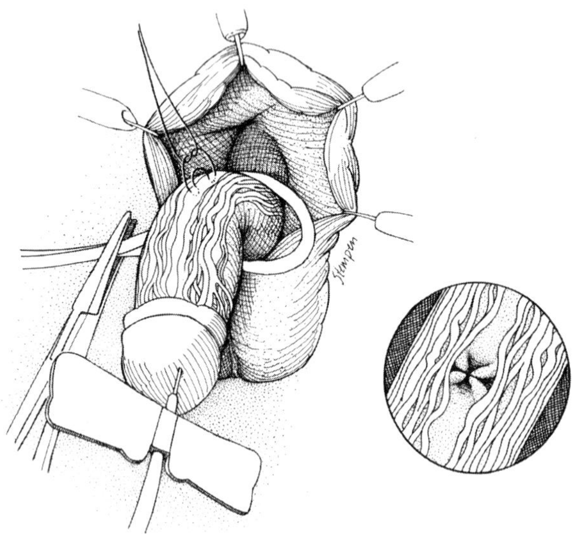

Fig. 47.2. Midline dorsal plication technique for the correction of penile curvature. Two permanent sutures are placed at the point of maximum curvature at the nerve-free 12 o'clock position.

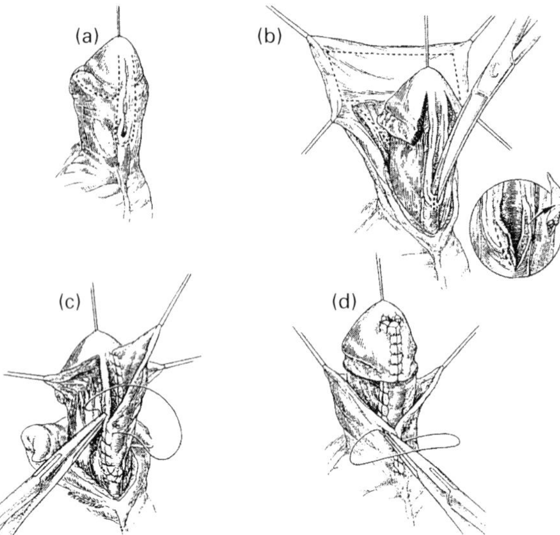

Fig. 47.3. The onlay island flap hypospadias procedure. The urethral plate is preserved in the process of penile degloving (a). The urethroplasty is formed from the excess dorsal prepuce based on this axial blood supply to the foreskin (b). The onlay technique decreases diverticulum and stenosis complications (c), (d).

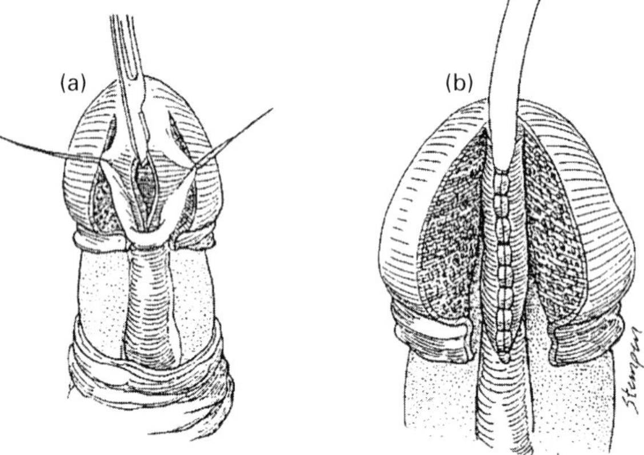

Fig. 47.4. Snodgrass modification. The urethral plate is preserved. A midline incision (a) allows primary tubularization urethroplasty (b). Secondary coverage is provided by a de-epithelialized prepucial pedicle graft.

curvature and create a urethra that allows urination with a controlled stream. These goals must be accomplished with attention to cosmesis. Results of hypospadias surgery can be analyzed by both subjective and objective criteria. Objective criteria includes functional status as measured by uroflow. Subjective criteria are more difficult to define, but certainly include cosmesis, sexual function, psychosocial

Table 47.1. Complications of hypospadias

Urethrocutaneous fistulas
Meatal stenosis
Residual curvature
Torsion
Stricture
Suture tracts
Diverticulum
Subcutaneous cysts
Hairy urethra
Retrusive meatus
Splayed urinary stream
Balanitis xerotica obliterans
Patients with multiple failures
Erectile function
Ejaculatory function
Cosmesis

adjustment and body image. Digital photography has been used in an attempt to provide objectivity to the cosmetic appearance after hypospadias surgery.[33] Objective photographic analysis can also be used to assess postoperative surgical outcomes of specific operations and/or new techniques.

Objective criteria are easier to quantify whereas subjective criteria require patient and/or physician interviews, both of which may be unreliable. Evaluation of the long-term outcome of hypospadias is unique in that the majority of hypospadias surgeons have modified their techniques over time. This renders outcome data somewhat obsolete as compared with current surgical preference. Nevertheless, much can be learned from the reports of prior hypospadiologists.

Hypospadias complications

Long-term hypospadias complications are listed in Table 47.1. As noted previously, these complications fall into two categories; objective and subjective.

Urethrocutaneous fistulas

Urethral cutaneous fistulas are the most common complication of hypospadias surgery. For most one-stage repairs the reported rate is between 10% and 15%. This may be lower than the actual incidence since small fistula often do not become apparent until well after toilet training. The incidence of fistula has been used to evaluate the effectiveness of surgical procedures.[34] Closure of a simple fistula is 90% successful as a day surgical procedure without diversion.[35] Some fistulas, however, are secondary to distal obstruction or meatal stenosis requiring an extensive revision. A child with a repair that does not have a fistula in early follow-up may be considered a success. At long-term follow-up, however, subsequent fistulization may occur if a stricture or urethral diverticulum develop requiring extensive revision. Outcome studies based solely on fistula incidence may therefore be misleading.

Strictures

Strictures after hypospadias repair result from technical problems at the initial repair. Proximal anastomotic strictures may result from either a luminal calibration miscalculation, resulting in a narrow neourethral or an anastomotic overlap. The overlap problem can be avoided by lateral fixation of the oblique anastomoses to the tunica albuginea. In the late case, a meatal stricture can result from chronic balanitis xerotica obliterans (BXO). This reaction is located either at the meatus or may extend into the more proximal urethroplasty. This may be due to a poorly vascularized meatoplasty, such as from free skin grafts or random based flaps especially the Mathieu procedure.[36] The most likely cause for meatal stenosis is vascular compromise of the urethra at the apex of the meatus. It may be secondary to an inadequate glans channel that compresses the vascularity of the pedicle. Once a stricture has developed, it may be repaired by excision and reanastomosis, a patch graft (buccal or skin), or a flap.[37] Long-term success treating strictures secondary to hypospadias surgery with optical internal urethrotomy have not been encouraging.[38]

Diverticulum

Urethral diverticula occur secondary to distal obstruction such as meatal stenosis or more commonly a diffuse diverticulum due to excessive width of the onlay flap or preputial tube creating too large a neourethra. This complication is more common with flap repairs and interim reports using the technique of primary tubularization with and without the Snodgrass modification have not shown diverticulum to be a common complication.[39,40]

When present, reduction of a diverticulum may be necessary and should be done in a longitudinal fashion. Most often, a circumcising incision is used, and the penile skin is dropped to the penoscrotal junction, which allows for the

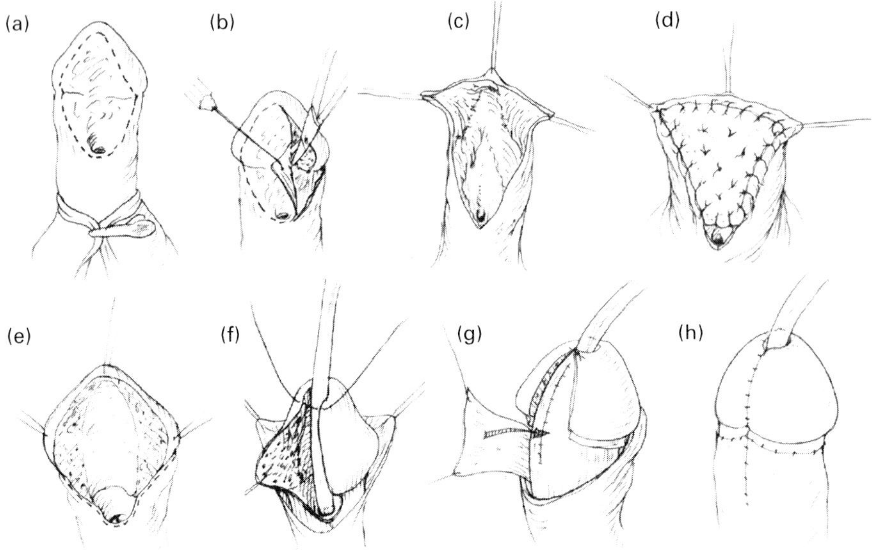

Fig. 47.5. Bracka two-stage hypospadias modification. In the first stage the scar tissue is excised and replaced by a buccal mucosa free graft. After 6 months the buccal mucosa is tubularized into a new urethra. Schematic two-stage Bracka buccal hypospadias repair. First stage: (a) patient with a midshaft hypospadias and a paucity of available skin after multiple previous hypospadias repairs; (b) resection of scar tissue; (c) mobilization of glans wings; (d) buccal free graft quilted into the resected scar. Second stage after 6 months of healing: (e) exposure of glans mesenchyme and trimming of buccal graft for subsequent urethroplasty; (f) urethroplasty; (g) secondary de-epithelialized pedicle coverage of the urethroplasty; (h) two-layer glansplasty and completed repair.

longitudinal repair of the diverticulum without overlying suture lines. Often, an excess amount of subcutaneous skin is present secondary to the urethral diverticulum. Some of this tissue can be used for a second layer to cover the suture line; however, it is reasonable to remove excess subcutaneous tissue with the diverticulum tissue to prevent a bulky repair. Care must be taken to evaluate the caliber of the neourethra with bougie-a-boules at the time of urethral construction and to aggressively trim excess skin to avoid this complication of preputial flap urethroplasty.

Hairy urethra

Urethral hair may grow if hair-bearing skin from the scrotum or proximal penis is used for the urethroplasty. Free grafts from hair-bearing areas of the groin may also lead to intraurethral hair. This hair may not cause a problem other than a meatal beard, which needs a trim now and then. However, in some cases, the hair may contribute to stone formation and encrustation, which can be cleaned out by urethroscopy or in severe cases removal of the hair-bearing skin with substitution urethroplasty.[41] Every effort should be made now to construct a neourethra from tissue that is non-hair bearing. However, there are many older cases with hair causing little problems.

Retrusive meatus and normal location

The urethral meatus may heal after hypospadias surgery in such a way that it retracts and deflects the urinary stream downward. An argument has been made that a coronal or subcoronal meatus is an acceptable outcome for hypospadias repair.[42] We would respectfully disagree, accepting the standard of a slit-like meatus on the ventral aspect of the distal glans.[43]

The problem of the retrusive meatus is more common in the older types of hypospadias repair when the meatus was left in the subcoronal position. A splaying of the stream is the usual complaint often requiring sitting to void. It may be corrected by a Mustarde-type flap and glans channel or a Mathieu flip–flap procedure. However, long-term results with these as secondary procedures are not effective.[44] A more definitive technique is the two-stage approach described by Bracka using either penile skin or buccal mucosa at the first stage followed by secondary closure in 6 months (Fig. 47.5).[7,9,45]

Balanitis xerotica obliterans and lichen sclerosis

On occasions, thickening of the skin urethra, especially around the meatus, has become a late problem. Biopsies in certain instances have shown balanitis xerotica obliterans or lichen sclerosis.[7,41] Steroids may be temporarily helpful. We recommend excising the balanitis xerotica obliterans and/or lichen sclerosis tissue and redoing the urethroplasty. In cases where local skin flaps are not available buccal mucosa free grafts have been useful as urethral replacement.[46]

Residual curvature

Before the use of the artificial erection, residual curvature was much more common.[24] This problem is corrected by mobilizing a sleeve of urethra and overlying skin down to the penoscrotal junction. Any residual scar tissue is resected until the artificial erection shows a straight penis. Slight ventral chordee can be repaired with dorsal suture plication with a permanent suture (Fig. 47.2).[25,26,47]

Rarely, extensive scarring of the ventrum of the penis requires excision of the tunica albuginea with replacement grafts of dermis or tunica vaginalis.[48] If dermal grafts are to be used, care should be taken to be certain that all epidermal elements are removed; otherwise, dermal cysts can develop.[49]

Once the penis is straight, an additional length of neourethra will likely be required to extend the urethra to the glans tip. Preferably, adjacent penile skin is used as a flap. Otherwise, a free graft will be required. Our current preference is for buccal mucosa in a two stage approach as described by Bracka.[9,45]

Patients with multiple failures

There are patients who have had multiple hypospadias repairs that have failed who have been categorized as hypospadias cripples. This term should be abandoned for the patient's sake. These unfortunate outcomes occur even in skilled hypospadiologists' hands. It is often necessary in these patients to discard the problem-plagued urethra created previously and start anew. The penis may be further straightened if needed. In some cases, it may be appropriate to place a meshed STSG and come back later for tubularization[44,50] or place a free graft of buccal or skin onto the area where the scarred urethra has been resected.[7,9] In the past we have used bladder mucosa for the neourethra[51] since the long-term results with free skin grafts have not been as successful as previously reported.[52] Unfortunately bladder mucosa grafts were complicated by eversion of the bladder mucosa at the meatus occurring in up to 30% of the patients.[51] Meatal dilatation on a daily basis could not avoid this problem. More recently we have been pleased with buccal mucosa grafts as a urethral replacement for these difficult patients[53] and presently advocate the two-stage approach of Bracka.[9,45]

Hypospadias outcomes

Reviews from older series

To better assess the functional results of hypospadias surgery, flow rates and the characteristics of the urinary stream have been analyzed. Johanson reviewed the results of 220 cases treated by the Dennis Browne technique. All 220 cases had a straight erection, a formed stream with normal flow rates and a urethra that had developed along with the penis.[54] One hundred and forty-two cases had reached an age where it was appropriate to ask about sexual function, and by history had normal ejaculate. The fact that all patients had a straight penis with normal function is admirable by any standards. However, 144 of the 220 patients had the meatus proximal to the glans, contrary to the standard of an apical meatus for hypospadias surgery performed today.

When the long-term results are evaluated by physicians other than the surgeon, the results as measured by a straight penis and a terminal urethra in a good position on the glans are not as satisfactory as one might expect.[7,54–59] For example, Sommerlad in 1975 evaluated 113 patients who were 17 years or older; 60 treated before 1958 were examined at long-term follow-up, and of these, 30 had Dennis Browne urethroplasties with 27 having a meatus in the middle third or proximal on the penile shaft.[57] Patients with less severe hypospadias treated with the Ombredanne procedure fared better, although the meatus was rarely terminal in position (6 of 60). Ten of the sixty had penile curvature on erection. Approximately one quarter had difficulty in standing to urinate and two-thirds had a stream that splayed. Long-term follow-up from patients operated at Great Ormond Street in the 1950s and 1960s had similar outcomes.[56] In another extensive series from the UK, Bracka reported 213 patients in the age range of 15–24 years.[7] Two-thirds of the repairs were "ventralizing" in nature with either the Dennis Browne or Ombredanne technique and one-third were "terminalizing" repairs of Broadbent, Mustarde or the Cloutier type. The long-term results of these patients mirrored that of Sommerlad[57] and Kenawi[56] with close to one-half requesting further surgery. Bracka's study noted a high level of adult dissatisfaction regarding the quality of the repair, both in terms of function and esthetics.[7] Patient interview also revealed physician criticism in respect of inadequate guidance in terms of recommendations for follow-up. Bracka's assessment is that all patients with hypospadias should be followed into adulthood to assess satisfaction.[7,59]

Follow-up in the very severe hypospadias has been disturbing in one report.[60] In a long-term review of 42 patients with severe posterior hypospadias followed into adulthood, 13 (30%) still had complex problems with sexual ambiguity; most with micro penis, small testes, no palpable prostate and gynecomastia.[60] Six cases were shown to have Reifenstein's syndrome with severe androgen receptor defects. Prospective assessment of androgen receptor levels have not successfully identified these patients.[61] More recent reports are encouraging, however, with more sophisticated molecular biology.[62,63]

Reviews from more recent techniques

The most significant advance in hypospadias surgery over the last 10 years has been the Snodgrass modification for primary tubularization urethroplasty (Fig. 47.4).[30,31,64] Interim reports of the success of the tubularized incised plate urethroplasty are favorable.[40,64,65] The concern for strictures and meatal stenosis has been unfounded. Recreating spongiosal support without the need for vascularized skin flap augmentation should also reduce the incidence of diverticulum. The enthusiasm for the Snodgrass modification seems justified but awaits final confirmation as these children pass through puberty and teenage years.

Systematic long-term studies on children who have undergone single-stage repairs using vascularized preputial pedicle flaps have been reported. Two groups have described the functional evaluation of hypospadias surgery as measured by uroflowmetry in children undergoing distal and proximal hypospadias repairs that were performed in the late 1980s. Jayanthi *et al.* reported on eighty patients with a mean follow-up of 28 months, range 0.5 to 76, average of 5.4 years.[66] Of the 65 patients who had a tubularized island flap repair, 42 or 69% had normal flows. In contrast, 13 of 15 or 87% of the patients who underwent an onlay island flap procedure had normal flows. Eight of the 13 patients who had strictures dilated or excised after hypospadias also had normal flows, whereas 15 of 16 who underwent fistula repair subsequently were recorded to have normal flows. The authors concluded that the neourethra is functionally equivalent to a normal urethra in most boys using preputial island flaps. Garibay *et al.* in Detroit reported similar findings in 32 patients after onlay island flap procedures.[67] In this study 5 asymptomatic patients had abnormal flows and were subsequently found to have strictures.

In contrast, the tubularized island flap urethroplasty even in experienced hands suffers from a high complication rate of approximately 40 %.[68] This procedure has essentially been abandoned in favor of the more reliable onlay flap and the Snodgrass modification of tubularization of the urethral plate.

Van der Werff reported long-term follow-up of his repair and the Dennis Browne repair based on physical examination and urodynamic data.[69,70] Special attention was paid to the functional outcome (spraying, dribbling, urinary deviation), findings at physical examination (curvature, skin surplus, stenosis, fistula, torsion, etc.) and the correlation between complaints on function and physical abnormalities. The authors were able to evaluate long-term 32% of 567 patients. For primary repairs, spraying was encountered infrequently: between 8 and 12%. Postmicturitional dribbling was reported by 16% of patients treated with vdMI repairs, 24% of the vdMII operations and after 30% of the Dennis Browne repairs. Deviation of urinary stream was mentioned by 32% of the vdMI patients, 18% of the vdMII patients and 21% of the Dennis Browne repairs. There was no correlation between the findings at physical examination and the functional complaints confirming the importance of functional studies in the follow-up of patients with hypospadias.[69,70]

In distal hypospadias repairs performed by the MAGPI technique, Macmillan *et al.*, using electronic video photography recorded high-speed pictures of urinary streams documenting normal function.[71] In a more subjective study, Park *et al.* evaluated 90 of 100 consecutive patients undergoing the MAGPI procedure at a mean of 5.7 years after surgery.[72] Ninety-nine percent of the parents expressed a high level of satisfaction with the outcomes based on a telephone survey that assessed cosmesis, function and overall outcome. Six of the 100 required more than one operation.

Adults undergoing redo surgery for hypospadias have not fared as well as the reported success of young children.[73,74] This is especially true when attempting one stage salvage-type procedures. This may be secondary to multiple prior surgeries resulting in ischemic poor quality tissue. Buccal mucosa has been used successfully in this situation.[75]

The two-stage approach for either primary or secondary hypospadias is now an acceptable if not preferred alternative.[9,45]

Psychosocial adjustment

Mureau *et al.* have published three articles on the long-term results of patients undergoing hypospadias repair.[76–79]

The first paper evaluated the psychosocial adjustment of patients over 18 who had undergone hypospadias repair between 1967 and 1990.[77] This group was compared to age matched patients who underwent surgical repair for an inguinal hernia. The authors conducted an extensive psychosocial adjustment, sexual function and genital appraisal via semi-structured interviews with preformed questions. The results of the study are important, although as previously noted the surgical techniques for hypospadias repair have changed. The two groups consist of 73 hypospadias patients randomly selected from 423 consecutive patients compared to 50 controls. The authors found that more hypospadias patients (33%) compared to controls (12%) had been inhibited in seeking sexual contacts. Hypospadias patients had a more negative genital appraisal than comparison subjects, but failed to identify a difference in sexual adjustment. Most importantly, 37% of the patients desired further functional or cosmetic penile improvement after being contacted for the study. In the final outcome, however, the majority of hypospadias patients experienced a normal adult sex life. They were reluctant to seek advice for their problems. The authors therefore recommend that patients who have hypospadias repair as young children be followed through adolescence and offered support and improved cosmesis.

In their second paper, Mureau *et al.* discussed the psychosocial adjustments of children and adolescents ages 9–18 after more recent types of hypospadias surgery.[78] Of the 116 patients approximately one-half had their meatus out to its normal position on the glans, and the other half had ventralizing procedures bringing the meatus further out on the penile shaft, but not in its normal position. These 116 patients were compared to 88 controls treated for inguinal hernias without concomitant genital surgery. Again, a semistructured interview was used consisting of five parts with preformulated questions looking at psychosocial adjustment, sexual behavior and genital appraisal. The results showed that the hypospadias patients had a more negative genital appraisal and anticipated more ridicule by a partner because of their penile appearance when compared to control subjects, but they did not show problems with psychosexual adjustment. No significant impact of the type of repair, meatal location, number of operations or the age at final surgery was noted. As in their first study looking at men greater than 18 years who had undergone hypospadias repair, 38% of these children and adolescents desired further functional or cosmetic penile improvement. The conclusion of this study was similar to their first study; hypospadias patients are reluctant to seek advice for their condition and therefore should be followed through adolescence. They also concluded that hypospadias procedures can be performed at any age without negatively affecting the psychosexual adjustment, contrary to our current recommendation.[32]

Mureau *et al.*'s final paper looked at the satisfaction of penile appearance after hypospadias surgery.[77] In this study the authors looked at 60 boys who had surgery between 1980 and 1992 with half of them undergoing operations for distal hypospadias and the other half for proximal. The techniques for proximal hypospadias repair were reported as the Duckett island flap versus a similar technique described by Perovic. The techniques for distal hypospadias were MAGPI, glans approximation, urethral advancement or the Mathieu. Of this group of 60 patients, the authors were able to examine 35. After a careful comparison between those who were able to be examined and those who were non-responders to their survey, they concluded that the groups were similar, ruling out a major selection bias. The authors found that there was hardly any agreement on satisfaction with appearance between the patient (parent) and the surgeon, the patients being less satisfied than the surgeon. There was also no correlation between penile satisfaction and penile length, this being measured against normative data. Patients with a retracted meatus were less satisfied with their meatal position than those who had the meatus positioned in the terminal position on the glans. Of the 35 patients who were examined, four of them underwent repeat surgery after being interviewed for the study. The authors conclude that hypospadias surgeons should explicitly ask patients (parents) if they are satisfied after their surgery and that they should be followed through adolescence.

One must recognize that these studies reported by Mureau are in boys and men in the Netherlands, a nation that rarely circumcises their boys. The dissatisfaction with appearance may reflect their circumcised status after hypospadias repair. Likewise, results in men older than 18 years reflect outdated techniques while those in 12–18-year-olds with the more modern terminal meatus are too young to fairly assess psychosexual discord. Although these are interesting studies, they should not deter us from the goals of cosmetic and functional perfection.

The need for follow-up into teenage years is echoed by Bracka in his series of 213 postpubertal patients who had hypospadias repaired in infancy.[7] Bracka noted a high level of dissatisfaction regarding the quality of their repairs both in terms of function and esthetics. There was also criticism from the patients of inadequate guidance in respect penile reconstructive surgery.

Adult follow-up was also suggested from a more recent Italian study evaluating the incidence of hypospadias and its effects on psychosexual development.[80] Severity of disease influences a more negative genital appraisal and the number of operations is correlated only with more difficulty in initiating contact with the opposite sex.

Long-term follow-up also exist in adults who have a 46,XY karyotype and presented as infants or children with genital ambiguity, including a small phallus and perineoscrotal hypospadias, reared as both males and females.[81] Long-term medical, surgical and psychosexual outcome was assessed by a written questionnaire, interview and physical examination. Thirty-nine (72%) of 54 eligible patients participated. The cause underlying genital ambiguity of participants included partial androgen insensitivity syndrome ($n = 14$; 5 men and 9 women), partial gonadal dysgenesis ($n = 11$; 7 men and 4 women), and other intersex conditions. Men had significantly more genital surgeries (mean: 5.8) than women (mean: 2.1), and physician-rated cosmetic appearance of the genitalia was significantly worse for men than for women. The majority of participants were satisfied with their body image, and men and women did not differ on this measure. Most men (90%) and women (83%) had sexual experience with a partner. Men and women did not differ in their satisfaction with their sexual function. The majority of participants were exclusively heterosexual, and men considered themselves to be masculine and women considered themselves to be feminine. Finally, 23% of participants (five men and four women) were dissatisfied with their sex of rearing determined by their parents and physicians. The authors concluded that either male or female sex of rearing can lead to successful long-term outcome for the majority of cases of severe genital ambiguity in 46,XY individuals although one-quarter of the patients had sexual identity problems.

Personal conclusions

1. Hypospadias should be repaired within the first year of life, preferably at 4–6 months of age. Pain control and catheters seem better tolerated and the baby's lack of mobility simplifies postoperative care.
2. A terminal slit-like meatus should be the goal with or without preservation of the foreskin depending on parental preference.
3. Preservation of the urethral plate creates the best possible chance to recreate normal urethral anatomy by incorporating the abortive spongiosum into the repair.
4. Midline dorsal plication is safe and effective for the correction of penile curvature in the majority of patients. (Placing more than two rows of sutures is a sign that another technique such as dermal grafting is indicated.)
5. In the small percentage of patients who require resection of the urethral plate a two-stage approach is generally warranted.
6. Vascularized pedicle onlay flaps are successful in primary and redo hypospadias surgery.
7. De-epithelialized vascular flaps should be used as a second layer for all urethroplasties.
8. Patients with a paucity of skin are best managed with the Bracka two-stage buccal repair.
9. Coronal fistulas require a redo glansplasty.

Conclusions

Osler (1919) said, "If you have the good fortune to command a large clinic, remember that one of your chief duties is the tabulation and analysis of the carefully recorded experience."

It took the first 10 years to learn the old and develop the new. The learning curve is slow and tedious. The last 30 years of growth, change and refinement are based on experience following these boys into adulthood and seeing those mistakes of the past. We are fully convinced we have come a long way in simplifying hypospadiology. Reproducibility in the hands of others is essential. It is critical that we follow our children with hypospadias through puberty so that we can continue to refine our techniques.

REFERENCES

1. Paulozzi, L., Erickson, D., & Jackson, R. Hypospadias trends in two US surveillance systems. *Pediatrics* 1997; **100**:831–834.
2. Paulozzi, L. J. International trends in rates of hypospadias and cryptorchidism. *Environ, Health Perspect*, 1999; **107**:297–302.
3. Baskin, L. S., Colborn, T., & Himes, K. Hypospadias and endocrine disruption: is there a connection? *Environm. Health Perspect.* 2001; **109**:1175–1183.
4. North, K. & Golding, J. A maternal vegetarian diet in pregnancy is associated with hypospadias. *The ALSPAC Study Team. Avon Longitudinal Study of Pregnancy and Childhood. BJU Int.* 2000; **85**:107–113.
5. Greenfield, S. P. Two-stage repair for proximal hypospadias: a reappraisal. *Curr. Urol. Rep.* 2003; **4**:151–155.
6. Greenfield, S. P., Sadler, B. T., & Wan, J. Two-stage repair for severe hypospadias. *J. Urol.* 1994; **152**:498–501.
7. Bracka, A. A long-term view of hypospadias. *Br. J. Plast. Surg.* 1989; **42**:251–255.
8. Titley, O. G. & Bracka, A. A 5-year audit of trainees experience and outcomes with two-stage hypospadias surgery. *Br. J. Plast. Surg.* 1998; **51**:370–375.

9. Bracka, A. Hypospadias repair: the two-stage alternative. *Br. J. Urol.* 1995; **76**Suppl 3:31–41.
10. Duckett, J. Transverse preputial island flap technique for repair of severe hypospadias. *Urol. Clin. North Am.* 1980; **7**:423–431.
11. Duckett, J. W. The current hype in hypospadiology. *Br. J. Urol.* 1995; **76**Suppl 3:1–7.
12. Thiersch, C. Ueber die Entstehungsweise und operative Behandlung der epispadie. *Arch. Heitkunde* 1869; **10**:20.
13. Mathieu, P. Traitement en un temps de l'hypospadias balanique et juxtablalanique. *J. Chir.* 1932; **39**:481.
14. Ombredanne, L. *Precis Clinique et Operation de Chirurgie Infantile* Paris: Masson, 1932.
15. Beck, C. Hypospadias and its treatment. *Surg. Gynecol. Obstet.* 1917; **24**:511–532.
16. Browne, D. An operation for hypospadias. *Lancet* 1936; **1**:141.
17. Byars, L. Technique of consistently satisfactory repair of hypospadias. *Surg. Gynecol. Obstet.* 1955; **100**:184–190.
18. Retik, A. B., Bauer, S. B., Mandell, J., Peters, C. A., Colodny, A., & Atala, A. Management of severe hypospadias with a two-stage repair. *J. Urol.* 1994; **152**:749–51.
19. Devine, C. Jr. & Horton, C. A one-stage hypospadias repair. *J. Urol.* 1961; **85**:166–172.
20. Salmon, M. *Arteries de la peau*. Paris: Masson, 1936; 174–179.
21. Hodgson, N. A one-stage hypospadias repair. *J. Urol.* 1970; **104**:281–284.
22. Asopa, H., Elhence, I., Atria, S., & Bansal, N. One-stage correction of penile hypospadias using a foreskin tube. A preliminary report. *Int. Surg.* 1971; **55**:435–440.
23. Standoli, L. One-stage repair of hypospadias: preputial island flap technique. *Ann. Plast. Surg.* 1982; **9**:81–88.
24. Gittes, R. & McLaughlin, A. I. Injection technique to induce penile erection. *Urology* 1974; **4**:473–475.
25. Baskin, L. S., Erol, A., Li, Y. W., & Cunha, G. R. Anatomical studies of hypospadias. *J. Urol.* 1998; **160**:1108–1015.
26. Baskin, L. S., Erol, A., Li, Y. W., & Liu, W. Anatomy of the neurovascular bundle: is safe mobilization possible? *J. Urol.* 2000; **164**:997–980.
27. Yucel, S. & Baskin, L. S. Identification of communicating branches among the dorsal, perineal and cavernous nerves of the penis. *J. Urol.* 2003; **170**:153–158.
28. Erol, A., Baskin, L. S., Li, Y. W., & Liu, W. H. Anatomical studies of the urethral plate: why preservation of the urethral plate is important in hypospadias repair. *BJU Int.* 2000; **85**:728–734.
29. Baskin, L. S., Duckett, J. W., Ueoka, K., Seibold, J., & Snyder, H. D. Changing concepts of hypospadias curvature lead to more onlay island flap procedures. *J. Urol.* 1994; **151**:191–196.
30. Snodgrass, W. Tubularized, incised plate urethroplasty for distal hypospadias. *J. Urol.* 1994; **151**:464–465.
31. Snodgrass, W., Koyle, M., Manzoni, G., Hurwitz, R., Caldamone, A., & Ehrlich, R. Tubularized incised plate hypospadias repair for proximal hypospadias. *J. Urol.* 1998; **159**:2129–2131.
32. American Academy of Pediatrics. Timing of elective surgery on the genitalia of male children with particular reference to the risks, benefits, and psychological effects of surgery and anesthesia. *Pediatrics* 1996; **97**:590–594.
33. Baskin, L. S. Hypospadias: a critical analysis of cosmetic outcomes using photography. *Br. J. Urol. Int.* 2001; **87**:534–539.
34. Retik, A. B., Keating, M., & Mandell, J. Complications of hypospadias repair. *Urol. Clin. North Am.* 1988; **15**:223–236.
35. Hayashi, Y., Mogami, M., Kojima, Y. *et al.* Results of closure of urethrocutaneous fistulas after hypospadias repair. *Int. J. Urol.* 1998; **5**:167–169.
36. Emir, L. & Erol, D. Mathieu urethroplasty as a salvage procedure: 20-year experience. *J. Urol.* 2003; **169**:2325–2326; author reply 2326–2327.
37. Scherz, H. C., Kaplan, G. W., Packer, M. G., & Brock, W. A. Post-hypospadias repair urethral strictures: a review of 30 cases. *J. Urol.* 1988; **140**:1253–1255.
38. Hsiao, K. C., Baez-Trinidad, L., Lendvay, T. *et al.* Direct vision internal urethrotomy for the treatment of pediatric urethral strictures: analysis of 50 patients. *J. Urol.* 2003; **170**:952–955.
39. Jayanthi, V. R. The modified Snodgrass hypospadias repair: reducing the risk of fistula and meatal stenosis. *J. Urol.* 2003; **170**:1603–1605; discussion 1605.
40. Cheng, E. Y., Vemulapalli, S. N., Kropp, B. P. *et al.* Snodgrass hypospadias repair with vascularized dartos flap: the perfect repair for virgin cases of hypospadias? *J. Urol.* 2002; **168**:1723–1726; discussion 1726.
41. Barbagli, G., Palminteri, E., Bracka, A., & Caparros Sariol, J. Penile urethral reconstruction: concepts and concerns. *Arch. Esp. Urol.* 2003; **56**:549–556.
42. Fichtner, J., Filipas, D., Mottrie, A. M., Voges, G. E., & Hohenfellner, R. Analysis of meatal location in 500 men: wide variation questions need for meatal advancement in all pediatric anterior hypospadias cases. *J. Urol.* 1995; **154**:833–834.
43. Genc, A., Taneli, C., Oksel, F., Balkan, C., & Bilgi, Y. Analysis of meatal location in 300 boys. *Int. Urol. Nephrol.* 2001; **33**:663–664.
44. Secrest, C. L., Jordan, G. H., Winslow, B. H. *et al.* Repair of the complications of hypospadias surgery. *J. Urol.* 1993; **150**:1415–1418.
45. Bracka, A. A versatile two-stage hypospadias repair. *Br. J. Plast. Surg.* 1995; **48**:345–352.
46. Baskin, L. S. & Duckett, J. W. Buccal mucosa grafts in hypospadias surgery. *Br. J. Urol.* 1995; **76**Suppl 3:23–30.
47. Mingin, G. & Baskin, L. S. Management of chordee in children and young adults. *Urol. Clin. North Am.* 2002; **29**:277–284, v.
48. Baskin, L., Duckett, J., & Lue, T. Penile curvature. *Urology* 1996; **48**:347–356.
49. Devine, C., Jr. & Horton, C. Use of dermal graft to correct chordee. *J. Urol.* 1975; **113**:56–58.
50. Angermeier, K. W., Jordan, G. H., & Schlossberg, S. M. Complex urethral reconstruction. *Urol. Clin. North Am.* 1994; **21**:567–581.
51. Keating, M. A., Cartwright, P. C., & Duckett, J. W. Bladder mucosa in urethral reconstructions. *J. Urol.* 1990; **144**:827–834.
52. Hendren, W. H. & Keating, M. A. Use of dermal graft and free urethral graft in penile reconstruction. *J. Urol.* 1988; **140**:1265–1269.

53. Duckett, J., Coplen, D., Ewalt, D., & Baskin, L. Buccal mucosa in urethral reconstruction. *J. Urol* 1995; **153**:1660–1663.
54. Johanson, B. & Avellan, L. Hypospadias. A review of 299 cases operated 1957–69. *Scand. J. Plast. Reconstr. Surg.* 1980; **14**:259–267.
55. Farkas, L. G. & Hynie, J. After effects of hypospadias repair in childhood. *Postgrad. Med.* 1970; **47**:103–105.
56. Kenawi, M. Sexual function in hypospadias. *Br. J. Urol.* 1975; **47**:883–890.
57. Sommerlad, B. C. A long-term follow-up of hypospadias patients. *Br. J. Plast. Surg.* 1975; **28**:324–330.
58. Svensson, J. & Berg, R. Micturition studies and sexual function in operated hypospadiacs. *Br. J. Urol.* 1983; **55**:422–426.
59. Bracka, A. Sexuality after hypospadias repair. *BJU Int.* 1999; **83** Suppl **3**:29–33.
60. Eberle, J., Uberreiter, S., Radmayr, C., Janetschek, G., Marberger, H., & Bartsch, G. Posterior hypospadias: long-term followup after reconstructive surgery in the male direction. *J. Urol.* 1993; **150**:1474–1477.
61. Gearhart, J. P., Linhard, H. R., Berkovitz, G. D., Jeffs, R. D., & Brown, T. R. Androgen receptor levels and 5 alpha-reductase activities in preputial skin and chordee tissue of boys with isolated hypospadias. *J. Urol.* 1988; **140**:1243–1246.
62. Klocker, H., Kaspar, F., Eberle, J., Uberreiter, S., Radmayr, C., & Bartsch, G. Point mutation in the DNA binding domain of the androgen receptor in two families with Reifenstein syndrome. *Am. J. Hum. Genet.* 1992; **50**:1318–1327.
63. Albers, N., Ulrichs, C., Gluer, S. *et al.* Etiologic classification of severe hypospadias: implications for prognosis and management [see comments]. *J. Pediatr.* 1997; **131**:386–392.
64. Snodgrass, W., Koyle, M., Manzoni, G., Hurwitz, R., Caldamone, A., & Ehrlich, R. Tubularized incised plate hypospadias repair: results of a multicenter experience. *J. Urol.* 1996; **156**:839–841.
65. Hammouda, H. M., El-Ghoneimi, A., Bagli, D. J., McLorie, G. A., & Khoury, A. E. Tubularized incised plate repair: functional outcome after intermediate followup. *J. Urol.* 2003; **169**:331–333; discussion 333.
66. Jayanthi, V. R., McLorie, G. A., Khoury, A. E., & Churchill, B. M. Functional characteristics of the reconstructed neourethra after island flap urethroplasty [see comments]. *J. Urol.* 1995; **153**:1657–1659.
67. Garibay, J. T., Reid, C., & Gonzalez, R. Functional evaluation of the results of hypospadias surgery with uroflowmetry. *J. Urol.* 1995; **154**:835–836.
68. Elbakry, A. Complications of the preputial island flap-tube urethroplasty. *BJU Int.* 1999; **84**:89–94.
69. van der Werff, J. F., Boeve, E., Brusse, C. A., & van der Meulen, J. C. Urodynamic evaluation of hypospadias repair. *J. Urol.* 1997; **157**:1344–1346.
70. van der Werff, J. F. & Ultee, J. Long-term follow-up of hypospadias repair. *Br. J. Plast. Surg.* 2000; **53**:588–592.
71. MacMillan, R. D., Churchill, B. M., & Gilmour, R. F. Assessment of urinary stream after repair of anterior hypospadias by meatoplasty and glanuloplasty. *J. Urol.* 1985; **134**:100–102.
72. Park, J. M., Faerber, G. J., & Bloom, D. A. Long-term outcome evaluation of patients undergoing the meatal advancement and glanuloplasty procedure [see comments]. *J. Urol.* 1995; **153**:1655–1656.
73. Amukele, S. A., Lee, G. W., Stock, J. A., & Hanna, M. K. 20-year experience with iatrogenic penile injury. *J. Urol.* 2003; **170**:1691–1694.
74. Hensle, T. W., Tennenbaum, S. Y., Reiley, E. A., & Pollard, J. Hypospadias repair in adults: adventures and misadventures. *J. Urol.* 2001; **165**:77–79.
75. Hensle, T. W., Kearney, M. C., & Bingham, J. B. Buccal mucosa grafts for hypospadias surgery: long-term results. *J. Urol.* 2002; **168**:1734–1736; discussion 1736–1737.
76. MacKinnon, A. E. Upper renal tract anomalies in patients with hypospadias [letter]. *J. Pediatr. Surg.* 1990; **25**:1309.
77. Mureau, M. A., Slijper, F. M., Slob, A. K., Verhulst, F. C., & Nijman, R. J. Satisfaction with penile appearance after hypospadias surgery: the patient and surgeon view. *J. Urol.* 1996; **155**:703–706.
78. Mureau, M. A., Slijper, F. M., Nijman, R. J., van der Meulen, J. C., Verhulst, F. C., & Slob, A. K. Psychosexual adjustment of children and adolescents after different types of hypospadias surgery: a norm-related study. *J. Urol.* 1995; **154**:1902–1907.
79. Mureau, M. A., Slijper, F. M., van der Meulen, J. C., Verhulst, F. C., & Slob, A. K. Psychosexual adjustment of men who underwent hypospadias repair: a norm-related study. *J. Urol.* 1995; **154**:1351–1355.
80. Mondaini, N., Ponchietti, R., Bonafe, M. *et al.* Hypospadias: incidence and effects on psychosexual development as evaluated with the Minnesota Multiphasic Personality Inventory test in a sample of 11,649 young Italian men. *Urol. Int.* 2002; **68**:81–5.
81. Migeon, C. J., Wisniewski, A. B., Gearhart, J. P. *et al.* Ambiguous genitalia with perineoscrotal hypospadias in 46,XY individuals: long-term medical, surgical, and psychosexual outcome. *Pediatrics* 2002; **110**:e31.

48

Bladder exstrophy

Thomas E. Novak and John P. Gearhart

Brady Urological Institute, The Johns Hopkins Hospital, Baltimore, MD, USA

Introduction

The epispadias/exstrophy complex encompasses a spectrum of rare midline defects in the pelvis and genitalia. Classic bladder exstrophy is a severe congenital malformation affecting approximately 1 in 40 000 live births. Although the exact etiology remains unknown, current evidence seems to implicate poor mesenchymal ingrowth with subsequent deleterious effects on the timing and position of rupture of the cloacal membrane.

The birth of a child with bladder exstrophy marks the start of a lifelong journey. The severity of the defect promises an extensive surgical undertaking that starts most frequently during the first days of life and often extends through adolescence. Components of surgical correction include: closure of the bladder, posterior urethra, pelvis and abdominal wall at birth, genital reconstruction, and some form of continence procedure. The approach pioneered at the senior author's institution addresses these components in a modern, staged fashion.[1] Alternatively, there are also proponents of complete primary closure, which attempts to address all components in a single operation.[2] However, recent data from the American Academy of Pediatrics reveals inferior continence rates when this technique is used. Longer follow-up is needed to ascertain the applicability of this repair, as the associated complications are not insignificant.[3,4]

With respect to outcomes, the goals of reconstruction in the exstrophy patient are urinary continence and satisfactory genital cosmesis and function. Although most children prefer to achieve continence with voiding per urethra, some will accomplish this same outcome with intermittent catheterization.

Initial bladder and posterior urethral closure

When considering long-term outcomes in exstrophy patients, the importance of a secure primary closure cannot be overstated. Successful initial closure requires meticulous template dissection with firm, tension-free abdomino-pelvic closure, followed by adequate fixation and immobilization postoperatively. The success of the primary closure is paramount in subsequent bladder growth, and ultimately, capacity is the primary determinant of continence after bladder neck reconstruction.[5]

Closure of the pelvic diastasis is a critical element of the primary closure. Reapproximation of the symphysis pubis decreases tension on the abdominal wall closure and returns the bladder neck to a position deep within the pelvic inlet where it is better supported by the levator complex. From a purely orthopedic standpoint, there is no indication to close the diastasis, as this alone imparts no long-term disability to these patients.[6] Secure reapproximation of the pubic diastasis is incumbent upon the malleability of the pelvis, the timing of the closure, and the degree of pubic separation. An examination under anesthesia is an important adjunct to surgical planning. At this time, manual medial rotation of the greater trochanters will give the surgeon some insight as to whether an osteotomy is necessary. In general, when closure is anticipated within 72 hours of birth, the persistence of maternal relaxin allows for sufficient malleability such that osteotomy is seldom needed. Osteotomy is usually required when primary closure is performed beyond 72 hours, at the time of repeat closure for dehiscence or prolapse, in the face of a wide pubic diastasis, and in the special circumstances of cloacal exstrophy closure and combined primary closure with epispadias repair.

Pediatric Surgery and Urology: Long-term Outcomes, Mark Stringer, Keith Oldham, Pierre Mouriquand.

Pelvic osteotomy in conjunction with primary abdominal and posterior urethral closure is a formidable undertaking and requires coordination between the pediatric urologist and orthopedic surgeon. The most common approach to pelvic osteotomy in exstrophy is the combined anterior innominate/vertical iliac osteotomy.

This technique, as described by Sponseller, has replaced posterior iliac osteotomy as the technique of choice at the senior author's institution. A detailed description of the technique is available elsewhere.[7] In comparison with the formerly accepted posterior approach, perceived benefits of the combined anterior approach are: (i) there is no need to prone and turn the patient as both osteotomy and closure are performed in the supine position, (ii) placement of intrafragmentary pins and external fixation is possible under direct vision, (iii) there is less blood loss, and (iv) the cosmetic result is superior.[8]

Meldrum *et al.* recently reported the impact of osteotomy and immobilization on the success of bladder and abdominal wall closures.[9] In patients referred for reclosure who underwent primary closure elsewhere prior to 72 hours of life, the success rates of patients closed with and without osteotomy were 58% and 39%, respectively. The highest success rates of primary closure (98%) were noted in children closed with osteotomy followed by 6–8 weeks of external fixation and modified Buck's traction. An equally high success rate was noted in patients undergoing secondary closure with the same treatment. The use of spica casting and mummy wrapping for immobilization were associated with high failure rates regardless of osteotomy status or setting of closure (i.e., timing, primary vs. secondary). Moreover, these techniques are associated with a higher complication rate, specifically pressure necrosis and ulcer formation.

Long-term (3-year) follow-up of a group of 36 patients who underwent the combined anterior osteotomy from Gearhart *et al.* demonstrated excellent efficacy with minimal morbidity.[8] Only three patients in this series suffered osteotomy, related complications – two patients with transient femoral nerve palsies and one with a superficial pin infection. The effect of osteotomy on abdominal wall closure is highlighted by the fact that none of the 36 patients in this group suffered an abdominal wall dehiscence, despite the fact that 50% were repeat closures.

Okubadejo and colleagues further examined the incidence and type of orthopedic complications in exstrophy patients.[10] Collectively, 26 complications were identified in the 624 reviewed patients (4%). They categorized the complications into five groups. Neurologic complications at the osteotomy site were the most common and were identified in 13 patients. Five bony complications were reported at the osteotomy site, and included non-union, delayed union, joint pain and leg length discrepancy. Traction injuries were reported in four patients. Early deep infection and late plate infection were reported in 2 patients each, respectively. Orthopedic pin care with hydrogen peroxide and antibiotic ointment is an important adjunct to wide-spectrum antibiotics in preventing infection.

A partial recurrence of the pubic diastasis is observed in the majority of patients, but tends to be greatest in those patients who are closed in infancy. Kantor *et al.* reported long-term orthopedic outcomes in a small series of 20 children with bladder exstrophy, 14 of whom had osteotomy. This group noted no long-term orthopedic clinical sequelae in these patients. This finding was irrespective of history of osteotomy or the presence of a recurrent diastasis.[6]

Bladder and posterior urethral closure

A detailed description of closure of the bladder and posterior urethra is available elsewhere.[11] A few technical points merit emphasis, however. The success of the primary closure hinges on the adequate mobilization of the bladder template, minimization of tension on the intrapubic stitch, proper placement of drainage tubes, and appropriate immobilization postoperatively.

Mobilization begins superiorly with reflection of the peritoneum off the eventual dome surface and ligation of the umbilical vessels. Laterally, the template is separated from the rectus fascia on each side. This dissection is carried caudally towards the urogenital diaphragm. Radical dissection of these fibers off the posterior urethra and bladder neck is a critical maneuver. On closure of the pelvis and abdominal wall, this allows the bladder and posterior urethra to seat deep in the pelvis where the levator complex will provide additional support to the outlet of the bladder.

The posterior urethra is closed over a 12F sound, which is passed in and out of the bladder outlet several times during the case to ensure patency. The ultimate goal is to provide enough outlet resistance at the time of closure to stimulate vesical growth and prevent prolapse without subjecting the upper tracts to undue pressures.

The tension to which the intrapubic stitch is subjected is a product of the adequacy of the closure and the intra-abdominal pressure. The senior author's practice of using a No. 2 nylon figure-of-eight suture is derived from work by Sussman *et al.*, who demonstrated superior load to failure ratio using this technique in a porcine model.[12] A second No. 1 nylon at the insertion of the rectus into the pubis provides additional strength to the closure. The role of osteotomy in decreasing this tension has been discussed. Factors influencing intra-abdominal pressure include: bowel-distension, proper placement and function of drainage tubes, and pain control. All of these children have a nasogastric tube placed intraoperatively in anticipation of a postoperative ileus. This is left in place until definitive return of bowel function. Anectdotally, it seems that children undergoing osteotomy have a longer delay in their return of bowel function. One possible explanation is increased blood loss into the retroperitoneum in these patients.

Urinary drainage tubes allow for maximal healing in a dry, decompressed environment. The proper placement of these tubes is a critical step in the primary closure. The bladder is drained with a 10 Fr Malecot catheter. The ureters are drained with 3.5 Fr stents. Confirmation of stent placement in the renal pelves with retrograde opacification and a portable film is advised. Sewing these tubes on both sides of the bladder with absorbable suture and at the skin with a non-absorbable monofilament provides extra security to their placement. Early tube displacement or malfunction can be a catastrophic event for these infants. The urethra is not routinely stented in order to avoid pressure necrosis and accumulation of secretions around an indwelling catheter which could serve as a nidus for infection.

The most secure closure can be jeopardized by inadequate postoperative immobilization techniques. The authors recommend 4 weeks of modified Bryant's traction for patients who are closed without osteotomy and 4–6 weeks of light Buck's traction in the setting of combined osteotomy. Maintaining these children in these positions for up to 6 weeks is a challenge and requires cooperation from parents, nurses, anesthetists and surgeons. Around the clock antispasmodics are recommended in addition to analgesics and light sedatives. Twice daily rounds by the pediatric pain service at our institution help to establish and then maintain a comfort zone that will allow the child to endure this treatment. In the senior author's experience, children who are particularly active despite our best efforts inevitably become quiescent.

The long period of immobilization that follows requires patience. This is difficult for some parents, many of whom have temporarily relocated here, possibly away from their spouses and other children. The role of a good support staff cannot be understated here. During this time, it is important to remain vigilant with respect to frequent examination of the incision and superficial wound and pin care. Broad-spectrum antibiotics are continued throughout this time period.

At 4–6 weeks, the ureteral stents are sequentially removed. The suprapubic catheter is clamped and postvoid residual volumes are measured. After 24–48 hours of voiding trials, an ultrasound is obtained. All of these children will reflux, and a mild amount of upper tract dilatation is inevitable. In children with small postvoid volumes and only minimal to mild hydronephrosis, a urine culture is obtained and the suprapubic catheter is removed. In children with large postvoid residual volumes or moderate to severe hydronephrosis, we will perform cystoscopy with dilation of the outlet and perhaps intermittent catheterization. In children who undergo osteotomy, cystoscopy can be coordinated with removal of the external fixator.

Failure of the primary closure is associated with poor long-term outcomes. This effect appears compounded with each subsequent failed closure. Gearhart *et al.* reviewed 23 patients who had undergone at least two prior exstrophy closures. Only 6 of these patients achieved a bladder capacity sufficient to perform bladder neck reconstruction, and only three of these eventually achieved continence per urethra.[13]

Occasionally, the preliminary examination under anesthesia will reveal a bladder template that is inadequate for closure. This is most frequently secondary to a diminutive template that is less than 3 cm wide in diameter or does not accommodate two fingers of the examining surgeon. In this situation, it is prudent to allow the child to grow for a period prior to performing a delayed primary closure. Consideration can be given for genital reconstruction at the same time. Dodson *et al.* recently reviewed outcomes in 19 such patients. Delayed primary closure was performed at a mean of 13 months after birth (range 6 months to 24 months). Nine of the 19 patients achieved continence after reaching a bladder capacity sufficient for bladder neck reconstruction, while an additional 4 patients were continent with intermittent catheterization after augmentation cystoplasty. Three patients in this group were too young for a continence procedure at the time of the publication.[14]

The preceding comments on primary closure reflect the senior author's personal experience. There are a few centers where ureterosigmoidostomy remains the primary surgical therapy for bladder exstrophy. One large long-term study reported nearly 95% continence with no development of malignancy in 115 patients over 25 years.[15] The senior author's personal experience with approach has been limited to undiversions in patients who were either incontinent or suffering from other associated complications.

Following a successful primary closure, the child enters into an incontinent interval spanning from the day of discharge to the time at which a continence procedure is performed. This length of time varies based on the child's maturity level and desire to achieve continence as well as the rate of bladder growth. Treatment during this time consists of prophylactic antibiotics and routine surveillance of the upper and lower urinary tracts.

As mentioned previously, a mild amount of hydronephrosis is evident in all children after primary closure secondary to vesicoureteral reflux. Ultrasounds are obtained every 4–6 months after discharge. Significant changes in the degree of hydronephrosis should prompt visual inspection of the bladder outlet with cystoscopy. Febrile episodes or other suggestion of pyelonephritis warrant the same.

Lower urinary tract surveillance consists of routine urine cultures and cystoscopies. Urine cultures are recommended approximately every 2 months. Acute or chronic bacteruria may incite postinflammatory scarring which is detrimental to bladder growth. Continuous prophylactic antibiotics are recommended. Starting at 2 years of age, annual cystoscopy with gravity cystogram should be performed under anesthesia. This allows for visual inspection and calibration of the outlet if necessary, as well as an objective measure of bladder growth. Ideally, we expect incremental growth each year. Rarely, a patient's bladder will fail to progress despite a good closure, and clinical judgment is required to balance the future hopes of functional closure against the potential for upper tract deterioration.

Urethral and penile reconstruction

During the incontinent interval, the second phase of reconstruction addresses the male genitalia. The female genitalia are reconstructed at the time of primary closure. Primary closure of the exstrophic male results in the creation of complete male epispadias. Epispadias repair takes place around 6–10 months of age: long before any continence procedure is performed. This rationale is based on work from Gearhart *et al.*, who demonstrated a median increase in bladder capacity of 55.5 ml within 22 months of epispadias repair in males with classic exstrophy.[16] Intramuscular injection of testosterone (2 mg/kg) stimulates phallic growth when given at 5 and 2 weeks prior to the operation.[17]

When considering genitoplasty, it is important to differentiate between cosmetic and functional outcomes. The definition of "acceptable" cosmesis is subjective and is likely to vary depending on whether you are asking the patient, the parent, or the surgeon. That being said, the cosmetic goal of male genitoplasty in the exstrophy patient is to restore the proper anatomic position of the corporeal bodies and glans penis with respect to the urethra while achieving the greatest length and minimizing dorsal chordee. From a functional standpoint, the reconstructed penis and urethra should be capable of voiding, intercourse and ejaculation.

Because the long-term outcomes of epispadias repair are discussed elsewhere, remarks here will remain limited to the senior author's personal experience. The use of the Young repair of epispadias was abandoned at Johns Hopkins after a review of 78 patients demonstrated a frequently tortuous urethra, which was difficult or impossible to catheterize, and an unacceptably high fistula rate of 36%. The modified Cantwell–Ransley repair was adopted and results are available on a total of 129 boys (106 primary and 23 secondary repairs). The incidence of urethrocutaneous fistula has declined dramatically to only 15%. Fistulae were noted with equal frequency in patients in whom paraexstrophy flaps were used and those in whom the mucosal plate was left intact. Anastomotic stricture was noted in 2 boys and 4 suffered minor skin separation. With respect to tortuosity, catheterization with cystoscopy has been performed in 60 patients and revealed an easily negotiable channel in all.[18,19]

The combination of epispadias repair with either secondary closure or bladder neck reconstruction is feasible and appropriate in select patients.[20,21] Data is available from small retrospective series documenting comparable complication rates for epispadias repair performed alone and in combination with either closure or bladder neck repair. Each of these operations is technically challenging in their own right, and their combination poses an obviously formidable task.

Bladder neck reconstruction: Johns Hopkins' experience

The timing of bladder neck reconstruction is based on consideration of two variables: the child's maturity level and their bladder capacity. The child's attitude has significant impact on outcome. They must demonstrate some motivation to achieve continence. Without this, the postoperative course, particularly voiding trials, are likely to be difficult, as this requires patience and active participation from the child. The impact of bladder capacity on the timing and success of bladder neck reconstruction has been recognized, but may have been underestimated in the past. Previously, a capacity of 60 ml was considered sufficient to proceed with bladder neck reconstruction. However, new data by Chan *et al.* reported better outcomes in patients with capacities greater than 85 ml. The mean patient age at the time of bladder neck reconstruction in the Chan group was 4 years.[5]

The senior author uses the modified Young–Dees–Leadbetter technique for bladder neck reconstruction. A few technical points of this operation merit emphasis. The basic components of the operation include:

(i) cephalo-trigonal reimplantation of the ureters,[22] (ii) creation of a mucosal lined tube supported by a muscular funnel at the bladder outlet, and (iii) anterior suspension of the vesicourethral angle. The goals of the operation are to create an outlet with enough resistance to promote storage, while preserving as much capacity as possible and protecting the upper tracts from high-pressure emptying. Intraoperative urodynamics may be helpful in assessing the adequacy of the outlet, but are not necessary. A simple maneuver involves gravity manometry. Absence of leakage at 50 cm of H_2O is indicative of an adequate repair. Retrospective studies have demonstrated that closure pressures of 70–100 cm H_2O are required to prevent leakage when bladder pressure is raised to 50 cm H_2O intraoperatively.[23]

Although the literature details several alternative methods to bladder neck reconstruction, most are simply variants of the original technique described by Hugh Hampton Young in 1922.[24] With early reports of continence in the complete repair being low, this time proven outlet repair has maintained its prominence. Most technical modifications focus on the manner in which the outlet is created. The type of outlet procedure, however, is probably not as important as the ability of the remaining bladder muscle to adapt to increasing volumes of urine at low pressure without the development of instability.

At the time of reconstruction, ureteral stents and a suprapubic catheter are secured both internally and externally. An 8 Fr urethral stent is used intraoperatively to guide closure, but is removed at the conclusion of the case. Urethral instrumentation is strictly avoided for the next 3 weeks. Broad-spectrum antibiotics are administered intravenously during the first week and then converted to prophylactic oral dosing prior to discharge. Around the clock antispasmotdics are important adjuncts to narcotics for analgesia. Three weeks after the repair, the ureteral stents are removed. At this time, the suprapubic tube is clamped and a voiding trial is conducted. If the child fails to void, the child is taken to the operating room where the outlet is inspected and calibrated. An 8 Fr Foley catheter is left in place for 3–5 days. At that time, the catheter is removed and the voiding trial is repeated. Some patients require several iterations of cystoscopy with catheter placement prior to a successful voiding trial. Depending on the appearance of the outlet and the ease of catheter placement, a period of intermittent catheterization may be required. The suprapubic catheter is left in place until the child successfully empties from below or the parent demonstrates the ability to perform intermittent catheterization. The senior author has found it beneficial to actually have the parents enter the operating room and perform this for the first time while the child is anesthetized. If the residual volume after urethral voiding is high, the suprapubic tube may be left in for an extended period of time during which a voiding diary should be maintained. The initial period of clamping is one hour. This interval is then advanced as tolerated by the patient.

Following bladder neck reconstruction, the child's detrusor is subjected to the unfamiliar environment of urine storage. There is a period of adjustment during which the child develops both the spinal and cortical pathways that allow for unconscious urine storage and volitional emptying of their bladder. This adjustment takes time and patience. In a large series from the senior author's institution, the mean intervals to complete daytime and nocturnal continence were 14 months and 22 months, respectively.[5]

Complications of bladder neck reconstruction are divided temporally. The most common early complication is bladder outlet obstruction requiring intermittent catheterization or prolonged suprapubic catheter drainage. Other early complications include the development of urinary tract infection or bladder stones. Late complications include upper tract deterioration and failure to achieve continence. The rate of secondary procedures to address these complications is high.[25]

There are not many series that report long-term outcomes of bladder neck reconstruction in exstrophy patients. Chan *et al.* reviewed clinical data from 65 patients with bladder exstrophy who underwent all phases of reconstruction at the senior author's institution between 1975 and 1998. The average age of bladder neck reconstruction in these patients was 4 years. The median capacity at the time of operation was 85 ml. Day and night continence was achieved in 77% (50/65) of these patients. An additional 14% achieved social continence with greater than 3-hour dry periods during the day, but experienced occasional nocturnal wetness.[5]

Bladder neck reconstruction: other institutions' experience

Mollard *et al.* reported satisfactory continence in 69% of 73 patients who underwent modified Young–Dees–Leadbetter bladder neck reconstruction.[26] This continence rate was irrespective of the number of procedures that it took to achieve that outcome. Nine years later, Mouriquand *et al.* reported on 80 patients who included Mollard's original cohort with some new additions and extended mean follow-up of 11 years. The more recent report documented outcome strictly following one procedure on the bladder neck. Dry intervals greater than 3 hours were noted in

45% of these patients. Of note, most of the males in this group were closed later in childhood and underwent bladder neck repair prior to penile and urethral reconstruction. The capacities at the time of reconstruction were not reported in this group, but other reports would suggest that urethroplasty promotes bladder growth and should be performed prior to bladder neck reconstruction. This practice was subsequently adopted by this group in more recent years, however, and may ultimately affect their continence rates.[25]

Lottman *et al.* presented long-term follow-up from Cendron's exstrophy patients who underwent complete reconstruction. Continence was achieved in 65% of these patients with a mean follow-up of 12 years. Males in this group fared better, with continence rates of 71% vs. females at 53%.[27] Recently, however, Grady and Mitchell reported only 20% long-term continence with complete single stage reconstruction in infancy.[28] Baka-Jakubiak reported excellent results in 73 males undergoing combined penile/urethral and bladder neck reconstruction. This cohort included 36 patients with classic bladder exstrophy, of whom 75%[27/36] achieved continence.[29]

Failed bladder-neck reconstruction

The importance of capacity in outcome following bladder-neck reconstruction is well documented. This concept is fundamental to modern staged reconstruction. The combination of osteotomy with secure primary closure followed by genital and urethral reconstruction for males at approximately one year of age provide the optimal conditions for bladder growth in these children. Failure at any stage can jeopardize the ultimate goal of continence per urethra.

Most children achieve urinary continence, as defined by a 3-hour dry interval, by 1–2 years following bladder-neck reconstruction. As previously noted, improving continence during this time is a reflection of increasing bladder growth in response to the new outlet resistance and coordination of pathways of volitional control, which are obviously delayed in these children who have spent their lives incontinent. It was previously suggested that male patients who remained incontinent would benefit from prostatic growth during puberty. This was subsequently challenged by an MRI evaluation of prostate size and configuration, which found no anatomical basis to support the notion that postpubertal prostate enlargement makes a significant contribution to bladder outlet resistance.[30]

Bladder neck reconstruction fails for one of two reasons: (i) outlet incompetence, or more commonly, (ii) failure of bladder growth. Patients who do not achieve continence during the two years following their bladder-neck reconstruction are unlikely to do so with further observation. Alternative approaches at this point include the following:

- repeat Young–Dees–Leadbetter bladder-neck reconstruction with or without bladder augmentation
- tubularization of the remaining bladder into a neourethra with augmentation colocystoplasty[31]
- insertion of an artificial urinary sphincter device[32]
- transurethral submucosal injection of urethral bulking agent
- transection or reconstruction of bladder neck with bladder augmentation and creation of a catheterizable abdominal stoma[33]
- urinary diversion as a last resort.

Like most reconstructive genitourinary surgery, the best hope for successful outcome with bladder-neck reconstruction lies in the first operation. That being said, it is feasible to attempt repeat bladder-neck reconstruction in the proper setting. Patients particularly suited for this endeavor include those with a patulous bladder neck who have an adequate bladder capacity. A report from the senior author's institution documented continence and voiding per urethra in 6/7 patients who had undergone repeat Young–Dees–Leadbetter bladder-neck reconstructions without bladder augmentation.[34] These patients are exceptional with respect to the fact that most failures of bladder-neck reconstruction require augmentation cystoplasty. If there is any question with regard to the adequacy of capacity, an augmentation is warranted.

Patients with minimal to mild stress urinary incontinence and acceptable bladder capacities may benefit from injection of submucosal bulking agents in the proximal urethra/bladder neck. Ben-Chaim *et al.* used bovine collagen for this purpose in 15 patients following Young–Dees–Leadbetter bladder-neck reconstruction. Repeat injections were necessary in 10 of the 15 patients at a mean interval of 12 months. After a mean follow-up of 26 months (range 9–84 months), improvement was noted in 8 of the patients. Four of these patients noted the improvement as significant. Repeated injections were noted to be beneficial in 9/10 patients.[35] Transurethral collagen injection is safe and carries minimal morbidity. The procedure is performed with anesthesia in an outpatient setting and takes less than 15 minutes to perform. Transurethral collagen injection after failed bladder-neck reconstruction has a reasonable success rate in patients with minimal symptoms. Long-term maintenance procedures are likely necessary with this approach. Recently, the authors have replaced the use of collagen with Deflux. Although the data is not mature, results have improved considerably.

The artificial urinary sphincter has been used in patients

with exstrophy. Some authors have reported excellent continence rates.[32] The senior author has not enjoyed this same success. The principal concern is that of cuff erosion. The blood supply to the bladder-neck following multiple operations is very often tenuous in the young patient. This is reflected in the dense scar that is encountered when attempting to repeat a bladder-neck reconstruction in this setting. This environment is not conducive to artificial sphincter placement. Older children or adolescents are better suited for this operation. They have more vascularized local tissue and mature omentum for interposition between the cuff and bladder neck or proximal urethra.

Augmentation cystoplasty with repeat bladder-neck reconstruction without a catheterizable stoma is technically a possible alternative for those who fail primary bladder-neck reconstruction. Two problems exist which make this a less attractive option: (i) the bladder may be so small that repeat bladder-neck reconstruction leaves little template to complete the ureteral reimplantation or augmentation, and (ii) reliable intermittent catheterization through a reconstructed urethra and bladder neck can be extremely difficult.

Because methods of bladder augmentation and continent urinary diversions are detailed in other chapters, comments here are limited to the approach to a small bladder with a history of failed bladder-neck reconstruction. Ultimately, the decision of whether to augment the existing template versus removing the bladder and replacing it entirely depends on several factors. These include the size of the template after opening the bladder, the competence of the bladder neck, and the type of continence mechanism that will be employed.

If the bladder template is generous, repeat bladder-neck reconstruction with augmentation and catheterizable abdominal stoma is a reasonable alternative. This gives the child some hope of voiding per urethra with the assurance that catheterization through the abdominal stoma is possible if necessary. A smaller template may only accommodate augmentation. This is preferred over cystectomy, because the bladder muscle provides better support for the ureteral reimplants. If this is the case, consideration must be given to transaction of an incompetent bladder neck above the verumontanum. A diminutive template, incapable of supporting either reimplantation or augmentation, should be removed. This is followed by creation of a continent cutaneous catheterizable reservoir or possibly a conduit. Ureterosigmoidostomy has historic relevance as a means of continent diversion and remains popular in Europe today. Continence rates are high in patients with normal anal manometry. Ureterosigmoidostomy is associated with the risk of upper tract deterioration and potential for delayed development of malignancy at the ureterocolonic anastomosis.

Surer *et al.* reported a retrospective review of 91 patients who underwent augmentation cystoplasty with continent catheterizable abdominal stoma creation. Eighty of these patients had classic bladder exstrophy with the remainder having either cloacal exstrophy or complete epispadias. The mean patient age and bladder capacity at the time of surgery were 8 years and 77 cubic centimeters respectively. With respect to technique, augmentation was most commonly performed with either ileum (41 patients, 45%) or sigmoid colon (30 patients, 33%). Stomal construction utilized appendix in the majority of cases (67 patients, 74%). Bladder-neck transection was performed in 59 patients (64%). With respect to outcome, 85 of these patients (93%) achieved continence with intermittent catheterization. Bladder stones and stomal stenosis were the most commonly reported complications, identified in 24 (26%) and 21 (23%) patients, respectively.[33]

Psychosocial issues

A review of long-term outcomes in bladder exstrophy must include an assessment of the patient's self-image and ability to socially integrate into society. Elements of this social integration include education, employment, and the formation of interpersonal relationships. The continence status and sexual and reproductive function of these patients obviously weigh heavily in this equation.

With respect to sexual function in exstrophy patients, we must consider both the physiologic and mechanical ability to achieve intercourse as well as the patient's perception of their genitalia as acceptable and their willingness to enter into a sexual relationship. The genital defect is less severe and reconstruction is more successful in female exstrophy patients. Not surprisingly, females tend to fare better in all of the aforementioned aspects of sexual health. Stein *et al.* reported 16/17 females over age 18 were satisfied with the appearance of their genitalia and that all were sexually active.[37] At our institution, four women participated in a survey of 20 adult patients with bladder exstrophy who had undergone reconstruction. All four of the women had been involved in sexual intercourse with full partner satisfaction. Three of the four had experienced orgasm. With the use of osteotomy, the mons pubis and bifid clitoris can be recreated at the time of primary closure.[38]

The male genital reconstruction is more complex. Loss of the glans or a corporal body are fortunately rare, but devastating complications. The vast majority of men with exstrophy have normal libido and experience normal physiologic erections. The most common structural defects are penile shortening and dorsal chordee. These issues may be addressed at some point during post-pubertal adolescence. This usually entails some degree of corporal plication or tunical release with grafting. In a series from the senior author's institution, 15/16 adult males experienced normal physiologic erections, but only 8 of the 15 described them as satisfactory. Of the remaining seven, six were unsatisfied based on lack of length and one from dorsal chordee. Twelve of the men reported satisfactory orgasm. Ten of the men had engaged in intercourse with 90% partner satisfaction.[38] Stein *et al.* reported normal erections in 34/35 male patients. Of the 32 who had undergone genital reconstruction, penile deviation was noted in 11 men, but was considered distressing in only 2.[37]

Nearly 70% of respondents or their parents reported concern about sexual function or disfigurement in the Ben–Chiam series. The mechanics of sexual intercourse and the appearance and adequacy of their genitalia were sources of anxiety for these patients and viewed as a barrier to relationships. Not surprisingly, Ben–Chaim also observed a delay in initiation of sexual activity until early adulthood.[38]

A review of the literature reveals 45 women with bladder exstrophy who have delivered 49 offspring. The most common complication of pregnancy in these patients is cervical and uterine prolapse.[39] Some have recommended prophylactic anterior fixation of the uterus during the course of urinary reconstruction. Cesarean section should be considered in all exstrophy deliveries, but is clearly recommended in those with functional bladder-neck closures. The vast majority of males with exstrophy are infertile without assisted reproductive techniques. The etiology in these men is usually obstructive. Etiologies include iatrogenic injury to the verumontanum during functional bladder-neck reconstruction, retrograde ejaculation, recurrent epididymitis secondary to reflux of urine into the ejaculatory ducts, and lack of bulbocavernosal muscle in forward propulsion of semen. This is evident in the Stein series. None of the 32 men who had undergone reconstruction reported normal ejaculation and none had fathered children. This is in contrast to the 3 men who were not reconstructed, all of whom reported normal ejaculation and two who had fathered 4 children.[37] Of the 16 men in the Ben–Chaim series, 10 reported ejaculate of a few cubic centimeters of fluid, 3 ejaculated only a few drops and 3 had no ejaculate. Four of these patients had semen analysis with an average volume of 0.4 ml.[3] Three of the patients were azoospermic and one was oligospermic.[38]

The psychological effects of a major congenital genitourinary malformation such as bladder exstrophy can be devastating. Our best surgical efforts mean little if the child is destroyed from a psychosocial standpoint in the process. A child psychologist is an integral part of the team at the senior author's institution and spends hours with these children helping them to overcome their fears and adjust to their deficiencies. Into adolescence and adulthood, urinary continence and genital cosmesis are major factors in the psyche of the patient. In a study out of Norway, Diseth and colleagues reported on long-term mental health and psychosocial functioning in 22 patients with exstrophy and epispadias. They reported that 50% of their patients met criteria for a psychiatric diagnosis. Parental warmth, urinary continence and genital appraisal were identified as predictors of mental health.[40] Feitz and colleagues reported a more positive result in a similar sized study in which only 18% reported clinical levels of psychological stress.[41]

Future directions

Determinants of continence remain the major focus in the exstrophy literature. At the clinical level, the success of the primary closure is the primary determinant of capacity, and capacity is the ultimate determinant of continence. At an ultrastructural level, however, the exstrophic bladder is clearly abnormal, as evidenced by higher collagen to smooth muscle ratios.[42–44] Future intervention at this level may hold the best answer for these children. Recent basic science investigations in the senior author's laboratory into the detrusor's intracellular make-up has shown a clear decrease in the number of caveoli on cell membranes taken from bladders which do not grow after bladder-neck reconstruction.[45] This may prove to be an intracellular marker of inherent detrusor dysfunction prior to attempts at continence surgery.

Finally, the field of embryologic stem cell research and tissue engineering is growing at a rapid pace. While we continue to search for ways to preserve the native bladder, the development of an ideal bladder substitute with this technology may one day dramatically change our surgical approach to children with bladder exstrophy.

REFERENCES

1. Gearhart, J. P. & Jeffs, R. D. State of the art reconstructive surgery for bladder exstrophy at the Johns Hopkins Hospital. *Am. J. Dis. Child.* 1989; **143**:1475–1479.
2. Grady, R. W., Carr, M. C., & Mitchell, M. E. Complete primary closure of bladder exstrophy, epispadias and bladder exstrophy repair. *Urol. Clin. North Am.* 1999; **26**:95.

3. Gearhart, J. P. Complete repair of bladder exstrophy in the newborn: complications and management. *J. Urol.* 2001; **165**:2431–2433.
4. Hussman, D. & Gearhart J. P. Presented at the American Academy of Pediatrics, November 2003.
5. Chan, D. Y., Jeffs, R. D., & Gearhart, J. P. Determinants of continence in the bladder exstrophy population: predictors of success? *Urology* 2001; **57**:774–777,
6. Kantor, R., Salai, M., & Ganel, A. Orthopaedic long-term aspects of bladder exstrophy. *Clin. Orthop.* 1997; **335**:240–245.
7. Sponseller, P. D., Gearhart, J. P., & Jeffs, R. D. Anterior innominate osteotomies for failure or last closure of bladder exstrophy. *J. Urol.* 1991; **146**:137.
8. Gearhart, J. P., Forschner, D. C., Sponseller, P. D., & Jeffs, R. D. A new combined vertical and horizontal pelvic osteotomy approach for the initial and secondary repair of bladder exstrophy. *J. Urol.* 1996; **155**:689–694.
9. Meldrum, K. K., Baird, A. D., & Gearhart, J. P. Pelvic and extremity immobilization after bladder exstrophy closure: complications and impact on success. *Urology* 2003; **62**:1109–1113.
10. Okubadejo, G. O., Sponseller, P. D., & Gearhart, J. P. Complications in orthopedic management of exstrophy. *J. Pediatr. Orthop.* 2003; **23**:522–528.
11. Gearhart, J. P. Exstrophy, epispadias and other bladder abnormalities. In Walsh, P. C. *et al.* (eds.), *Campbell's Urology*. Philadelphia: W.B. Saunders, 2002:2136.
12. Sussman, J., Sponseller, P. D., Gearhart, J. P. *et al.* A comparison of methods of repairing the symphysis pubis in bladder exstrophy by tensile testing. *BJU Int* 1997; **79**:979.
13. Gearhart, J. P., Ben-Chaim, J., Sciortino, C. *et al.* The multiple failed exstrophy closure: strategy for management. *Urology* 1996; **47**:240–244.
14. Dodson, J. L., Surer, I., Baker, L. A., Jeffs, R. D., & Gearhart, J. P. The newborn exstrophy bladder inadequate for primary closure: evaluation, management, and outcome. *J. Urol.* 2001; **165**:1656–1659.
15. Stein, R., Fisch, M., Stockle, M., & Hohenfellner, R. Urinary diversion in bladder exstrophy and incontinent epispadias: 25 years of experience. *J. Urol.* 1995; **154**:1177–1181.
16. Gearhart, J. P. & Jeffs, R. D. bladder exstrophy: increase in capacity following genital reconstructive surgery. *J. Urol.* 1989; **142**:525–529.
17. Gearhart, J. P. & Jeffs, R. D. The use of parenteral testosterone therapy in genital reconstructive surgery. *J. Urol.* 1988; **138**:1077–1080.
18. Gearhart, J. P., Sciortino, C., Ben-Chaim, J., & Jeffs, R. D. The Cantwell–Ransley epispadias repair: lessons learned. *Urology* 1995; **46**:92–96.
19. Gearhart, J. P., Leonard, M. P., Burgers, J. K., & Jeffs, R. D. The Cantwell–Ransley technique for repair of epispadias. *J. Urol.* 1992; **148**:851–855.
20. Gearhart, J. P., Mathews, R. I., Taylor, S., & Jeffs, R. D. Combined bladder closure and epispadias repair in the reconstruction of bladder exstrophy. *J. Urol.* 1998; **160**:1182–1185.
21. Surer, I., Baker, L. A., Jeffs, R. D., & Gearhart, J. P. Combined bladder neck reconstruction and epispadias repair for exstrophy-epispadias complex. *J. Urol.* 2001; **165**:2425–2427.
22. Canning, D. A., Gearhart, J. P., Peppas, D. S., & Jeffs, R. D. The cephalotrigonal reimplant in bladder neck reconstruction for patients with exstrophy or epispadias. *J. Urol.* 1993; **150**:156–159.
23. Gearhart, J. P., Williams, K. A., & Jeffs, R. D. Intraoperative urethral pressure profilometry as an adjunct to bladder neck reconstruction. *J. Urol.* 1986; **136**:1055–1058.
24. Young, H. H. An operation for cure of incontinence associated with epispadias. *J. Urol.* 1922; **7**:1.
25. Mouriquand, P. D. E., Bubanj, T., Feyaerts, A. *et al.* Long-term results of bladder neck reconstruction for incontinence in children with classical bladder exstrophy or incontinent epispadias. *BJU Int.* 2003; **92**:997–1002.
26. Mollard, P., Mouriquand, P. D. E., & Buttin, X. Urinary continence after reconstruction of classic bladder exstrophy. *Br. J. Urol.* 1994; **73**:298–302.
27. Lottman, H., Melin, Y., Lombrail, P. *et al.* Reconstruction of bladder exstrophy: retrospective study of 57 patients with evaluation of factors in favor of acquisition of continence. *Ann. Urol.* 1998; **32**:233.
28. Mitchell, M. E. & Grady, R. W. presented at the American Academy of Pediatrics, November 2003.
29. Baka-Jakubiak, M. Combined bladder neck, urethral and penile reconstruction in boys with the exstrophy-epispadias complex. *BJU Int.* 2000; **86**(4): 513–518.
30. Gearhart, J. P., Yang, A., Leonard, M. P., Jeffs, R. D., & Zerhouni, E. A. Prostate size and configuration in adults with bladder exstrophy. *J. Urol.* 1993; **149**:308–311.
31. Arap, S., Martins, G. A., Menezes, D. E., & Goes, G. Initial results of the complete reconstruction of bladder exstrophy. *Urol. Clin. North Am.* 1980; **7**:477–484.
32. Decter, R. M., Roth, D. R., Fishman, I. J. *et al.* Use of the AS800 device in exstrophy and epispadias. *J. Urol.* 1988; **140**:1202–1206.
33. Surer, I., Ferrer, F. A., Baker, L. A., & Gearhart, J. P. Continent urinary diversion and the exstrophy–epispadias complex. *J. Urol.* 2003; **169**:1102–1105.
34. Gearhart, J. P., Canning, D. A., & Jeffs, R. D. Failed bladder neck reconstruction: options for management. *J. Urol.* 1991; **146**:1082–1087.
35. Ben-Chaim, J., Jeffs, R. D., Peppas, D. S., & Gearhart, J. P. Submucosal bladder neck injections of glutaraldehyde cross-linked bovine collagen for treatment of urinary incontinence in patients with exstrophy/epispadias complex. *J. Urol.* 1995; **154**:862–866.
36. Frimberger, D., Lakshmanan, Y., & Gearhart, J. P. Continent urinary diversions in the exstrophy complex: why do they fail? *J. Urol.* 2003; **170**:1338–1342.
37. Stein, R., Hohenfellner, K., Fisch, M., Stockle, M., Beetz, R., & Hohenfellner, R. Social integration, sexual behavior and fertility in patients with bladder exstrophy – a long term follow up. *Eur. J. Pediatr.* 1996; **155**:678–683.

38. Ben-Chaim, J., Jeffs, R. D., Reiner, W. G., & Gearhart, J. P. The outcome of patients with classic bladder exstrophy in adult life. *J. Urol.* 1996; **155**:1251–1252.
39. Krisiloff, M., Puchner, P. J., Tretter, W. *et al.* Pregnancy in women with bladder exstrophy. *J. Urol.* 1978; **119**:478.
40. Diseth, T. H., Bjordal, R., Schultz, A., Stange, M., & Emblem, R. Somatic function, mental health, and psychosocial functioning in 22 adolescents with bladder exstrophy and epispadias. *J. Urol.* 1998; **159**:1684–1689.
41. Feitz, W. F., Vangrunsven, V. J., & Froeling, F. M. Outcome analysis of the psychosexual and socioeconomic development of adults born with bladder exstrophy. *J. Urol.* 1994; **152**:1417.
42. Mathews, R. I., Gosling, J., & Gearhart J. P. Ultrastructure of the bladder in classic bladder exstrophy – correlation with development of continence. *J. Urol.* 2004; **172**(4 pt 1):1446–1449.
43. Peppas, D. S., Tchetgen, M., Lee, B. R. *et al.* A quantitative histological analysis of the bladder in classical bladder exstrophy in various stages of reconstruction using color morphometry. In Gearhart, J. P. & Mathews, R. I., eds. *The Exstrophy–Epispadias Complex: Research Concepts and Clinical Applications.* New York: Kluwer Academic/Plenum Publishers, 1999.
44. Lee, B. R., Perlman, E. J., Partin, A. W. *et al.* Evaluation of smooth muscle and collagen subtypes in normal newborns and those with bladder exstrophy. *J. Urol.* 1996; **156**:203.
45. Gearhart, J. P. pers. commun.

49

Surgery for neuropathic bladder and incontinence

Prasad Godbole[1] and Duncan T. Wilcox[2]

[1]Department of Paediatric Urology, Sheffield Children's NHS Trust, UK
[2]Pediatric Urology, University of Texas, Dallas, TX, USA

Introduction

Children with a neuropathic bladder may have bladder characteristics ranging from a high pressure non-compliant small capacity bladder with a high outlet resistance (unsafe), on the one hand, to a compliant low pressure capacious bladder with low outflow resistance (safe), on the other. Most children will demonstrate a mixed picture, and bladder and outflow characteristics may change with time thereby necessitating regular surveillance.

The aims of management of these children are:(i) preservation of renal function (ii) attaining urinary continence and therefore (iii) enabling social integration and improvement in quality of life. These aims can be achieved with a container (reservoir), which is capacious and low pressure, adequate outflow resistance (bladder neck and sphincter muscle complex) and a conduit to keep the reservoir empty at regular intervals (urethra, Mitrofanoff conduit).

This chapter concentrates on the long-term outcomes of the various treatment options that have been used and will not describe the technical aspects for which the reader is referred to several excellent texts on the subject.[1–3]

The treatment modalities described include non-surgical (CIC and pharmacotherapy) surgery of the outlet (bladder-neck procedures, minimally invasive procedures and sphincters), surgery of the reservoir (augmentation cystoplasty), continent catheterizable conduits (Mitrofanoff principle), and urinary diversion (vesicostomy, refluxing ureterostomy, and ileal conduit).

Non-surgical methods

Clean intermittent urethral catheterization (CIC)

This technique initially described by Lapides *et al.*[4] allows children or their carers to ensure low pressure emptying of the bladder at periodic intervals with the use of a well-lubricated catheter or a hydrophilic catheter, thereby protecting the upper tracts. It requires attention to detail and compliance on the part of patients and carers alike. Although technically easy at a younger age, it may become difficult for children to self-catheterize urethrally as they grow older. This is most obvious in children with spinal dysraphism, who may be wheelchair bound and unable to get adequate access to their perineum. In boys, negotiating the longer urethra may be difficult and not well accepted. CIC may pose a risk of trauma, false passage, urethritis, and discomfort in those with a sensate urethra.

Wolraich *et al.*[5] report their review of 49 children up to 4 years following institution of CIC for neuropathic bladder. Of these 49% were continent with CIC and anticholinergics or alpha-adrenergics or both. Sixty-five percent remained infection free. Eight children developed reflux during therapy. Nine children had reflux prior to CIC; this improved in one after CIC. A further 5-year follow-up study of this same cohort of patients revealed stable upper tracts, low infection rates, unchanged or improved reflux in most patients, and maintained renal function.[6] Cass *et al.*[7] in their follow-up of 84 children had 63% of children who remained incontinent. Pre-existing reflux deteriorated in 25%, ceased in 35% and was unchanged in 40%. Upper tract dilatation

Pediatric Surgery and Urology: Long-term Outcomes, Mark Stringer, Keith Oldham, Pierre Mouriquand.
Published by Cambridge University Press.

remained stable in the majority of instances and improved in 12.5%. Plunkett *et al.*[8] in their 5-year experience of 98 children have a similar experience. They did not demonstrate any new bouts of pyelonephritis, despite only 21% of children having a sterile urine. Complications of this technique were low and relatively minor. Bacteriuria is unavoidable and has a reported incidence of between 7.5% and 79%[7–9] but with normal upper tracts is usually of no significance. Kass *et al.*[10] reviewed 255 children managed by CIC over a 10-year period and documented bacteriuria in 56%. Febrile urinary tract infections, however, occurred in only 11% and new renal damage in 2.6%. In the absence of pre-existing reflux, new reflux, hydronephrosis, or fresh scars did not develop. Reflux improved in 50% of those with mild pre-existing reflux. Pyelonephritis, however, occurred in 60% of children with pre-existing high grade reflux, which tended to persist despite CIC. There was no correlation between state of the bladder and grade of reflux. Studies have not demonstrated any positive effect of cranberry juice[11] or antibiotic prophylaxis such as nitrofurantoin[12] or the type of catheter used[13] on the incidence of bacteriuria.

In summary, CIC forms the mainstay of management of children with a neuropathic bladder. It maintains renal function, stabilizes upper tract dilatation, and improves vesicoureteric reflux in a significant number of children. Although a majority of children will have bacteriuria, symptomatic urinary tract infections are relatively infrequent and in the absence of significant preexisting reflux, fresh renal scarring is unusual. CIC itself does not necessarily guarantee continence and usually requires the addition of pharmacotherapy in the form of anticholinergics, alpha adrenergics, or surgery.

Suprapubic diversion

In the authors' experience there are certain children who are initially adverse to the concept of CIC or catheterizing via a Mitrofanoff channel. These children may benefit from a period of suprapubic diversion via a suprapubic tube or suprapubic button. A 12 Fr suprapubic tube can be inserted under general anesthesia and can then be changed every 3 months at home by the community team. The suprapubic catheters are fitted with a flip–flow valve which allows children to empty their bladders at regular intervals. In the authors' experience, children seem to be more compliant with this regime and make a smoother transition towards the formation of a Mitrofanoff stoma.

The use of suprapubic button vesicostomy may be favored by some children for esthetic reasons. This may be by initial placement of a suprapubic tube or primary open placement of the button. The button used is a 14Fr McKey gastrostomy button, which can be changed at periodic intervals. This technique has shown good results in those children with a large capacity compliant bladder as an alternative to a Mitrofanoff channel.[14]

Pharmacotherapy

Pharmacotherapy is aimed at reducing the intravesical pressure and improving compliance or increasing the bladder outlet resistance. The former is attained by the use of anticholinergics in the form of oxybutinin (oral or intravesical) and more recently tolteridine. Bladder neck outlet resistance can be improved by the use of sympathomimetics such as ephedrine. Pharmacotherapy is usually combined with CIC to obtain a low pressure compliant reservoir but cannot guarantee continence. There is very limited data available on the long-term follow-up of children being treated with pharmacotherapy alone or with CIC. Ferrara *et al.*[15] in their review of 101 children demonstrated that oral and intravesical oxybutinin both have side effects, and that these are more frequent in children taking oral oxybutinin. Side effects with oral oxybutinin included dry mouth, fever, and facial flushing. Intravesical oxybutinin had a much lower tendency to cause side effects and included hallucinations, cognitive impairment, and drowsiness. Buyse *et al.* demonstrated a significantly lower concentration of the active metabolite of oxybutinin–*N*-desethyl-oxybutinin following intravesical oxybutinin compared to oral oxybutinin due to reduced first metabolism with intravesical oxybutinin and attribute fewer systemic side effects as a result.[16] However, Palmer *et al.* in their experience of intravesical oxybutinin administration to 23 children over a 5-year period demonstrated that 7/23 (30.3%) experienced side effects in the form of facial flushing, dizziness, and agoraphobia necessitating discontinuation of treatment.[17]

Painter *et al.*[18] reviewed 30 children at up to 26 months' duration of treatment with intravesical oxybutinin. They report significant increases in total bladder capacity, mean safe capacity, and mean age-adjusted safe capacity. Of these children, 10% achieved continence and 65% had improved continence with decreased use of sanitary pads. Amark and colleagues[19] in their review of 39 children at up to 5 years demonstrated improved continence and urodynamic parameters in all children. There was an increased incidence of asymptomatic bacteriuria and decreased frequency of urinary tract infections. Kaplinsky *et al.*[20] followed up 28 children for a maximum of 67 months (mean 35 months). Intravesical oxybutinin had to be discontinued in 25% due to side effects. Of the remaining 21, day and night continence was achieved in 57%, 5 achieved daytime continence between catheterizations and there was no change in 4. There was significant improvement in urodynamic parameters in the 21 children who achieved continence. All the above studies demonstrated that intravesical oxybutinin is a useful alternative in those children who have side effects from oral oxybutinin. There is an improvement in urodynamic parameters and continence, and the treatment is well tolerated in most instances.

More recently, oral administration of tolterodine has been shown to be effective in those children who are intolerant to oxybutinin but long-term outcomes are still awaited. Bolduc *et al.*[21] reviewed 34 children who were crossed over from oxybutinin to tolterodine as a result of side effects. All children had been followed up for at least 1 year. Of these, 59% reported no side effects, 6 had the same side effects which were tolerable and 8 patients discontinued treatment due to side effects. The efficacy of tolterodine was comparable with that of oxybutinin as reported by questionnaire and voiding diaries. Injection of botulinum A toxin in the detrusor muscle at multiple sites has been shown to be effective in detrusor hyperreflexia associated with neurogenic bladder in the short term and may be an alternative to anticholinergics[22] but has the disadvantage of requiring anesthesia for administration.

A comparison between CIC and CIC with pharmacotherapy is shown in Table 49.1.

Table 49.1. A comparison of CIC alone and CIC with pharmacotherapy in children with neurogenic bladder dysfunction

	CIC	Pharmacotherapy with CIC
Continence	Variable – up to 49% in various series[5–7]	Variable – up to 57% in various series[18–20]
UTI	Decreased incidence of febrile UTI	Decreased incidence of febrile UTI
Reflux and upper tracts	Stable upper tracts and resolution of mild reflux in majority	Stable upper tracts and resolution of mild reflux in majority
Complications	Non-compliance Urethral trauma, infection	Side effects of anticholinergic medication

Surgery of the bladder outlet

Surgery of the outlet resistance

The aim of this surgery is to increase outlet resistance sufficiently to create continence, but ideally allowing the patient to void. This balance is, as we report, extremely difficult to achieve; consequently, there are multiple procedures described.

Bladder neck reconstruction

Bladder neck procedures

The aim of any bladder neck procedure is to increase the outlet resistance, at the same time maintaining the ability to catheterize urethrally if necessary. These procedures may be divided into those that alter the anatomy of the bladder neck itself (Kropp,[23] Pippe–Salle,[24] Young,[25] Dees,[26] and Leadbetter[27]) or alter the configuration of the bladder neck and outlet externally (periurethral slings, bladder-neck suspension).

Kropp, Pippe–Salle

Bladder neck procedures may be performed concomitantly with an augmentation cystoplasty and a continent catheterizable conduit if the child is not catheterizing urethrally. In selected cases they may be performed in isolation if augmentation is deemed not necessary, or may be performed following a previous augmentation cystoplasty. Kropp *et al.*,[28] in their review of the first 25 patients of urethral lengthening, encountered late complications including catheterization difficulties, vesicoureteric reflux, febrile urinary tract infection, calculi, and peritonitis. Nineteen patients required reoperation but this was due to failure to recognize the need for a low pressure high capacity reservoir. Twenty of their 25 patients were continent and the continence mechanism did not require revision. In their further review of children who had undergone the Kropp urethral lengthening from 1982 to 1995, 72% of children had no catheterization problems.[29] Problems were managed easily by change to a coude catheter and by avoiding overdistention in the majority of patients. Mollard *et al.*[30] reviewed 22 of their female patients undergoing Kropp urethral lengthening. At a follow up of between 6 and 11 years, 86% were dry with no difficulty of catheterization. Similar results have been documented by Snodgrass *et al.*[31] and Belman *et al.*[32] Kropp reviewed 23 patients by urodynamic evaluation at a mean of 43.1 months (4–89) following the lengthening procedure and found that submucosal tunnel pressures remained significantly greater than bladder pressures at the time of first and peak cystoplasty contractions, thereby accounting for the continence mechanism.[33]

In a multicenter UK study of the outcome of the Pippe–Salle procedure for neuropathic incontinence in 28 patients (16 girls and 12 boys), 61% were continent day and night, results being much better in girls than boys (13/16 and 5/12, respectively).[34] At a mean follow-up of 29.3 months, Salle *et al.*[35] achieved continence in 12/18 (72%) patients, 13 of whom had a concomitant augmentation. Two patients developed a urethrovesical fistula. The Pippe–Salle procedure is reported to be easier to perform and may preserve a pop off mechanism in cases of overdistention of the bladder.[36]

Young–Dees–Leadbetter

The Young–Dees–Leadbetter reconstruction was originally described for incontinence in the exstrophy–epispadias complex. Donnahoo *et al.*[37] reviewed their experience of 38 patients with neurogenic incontinence undergoing this procedure either primarily (24), secondarily (6) or with a silicone sheath periurethral placement (8). Continence was achieved in 68%, while 11 patients required further surgery to achieve continence. Patients with silicone sheath placement despite initial good results subsequently developed incontinence due to sheath erosion. A majority of patients in this series required an augmentation cystoplasty to attain continence. A similar experience was noted by Reda[38] who had a 100% continence rate with this technique when combined with an augmentation cystoplasty.

Bladder neck closure

Bladder neck closure with a continent diversion may be considered as an alternative where previous reconstructive efforts have been unsuccessful. Hoebeke *et al.*[39] reviewed 17 children (10 myelomeningocele) at a mean of 35 months following bladder neck closure and continent diversion. All patients were completely dry and patient satisfaction was high, although stomal complications were noted in 8 patients. Secondary leakage by recanalization has however been reported.[40] Nguyen *et al.*[41] report the long-term outcome of bladder neck closure and continent diversion in children with severe urinary incontinence. They demonstrated early urethral fistula in 40% of children needing further surgery. At a mean follow-up of 5.4 years (1 – 12), 85% are dry and the main complications were stomal stenosis in 30% and bladder stones in 40% of children.

Slings

Several techniques have been described to alter the configuration of the bladder outlet externally. While a facial sling for treating intractable urinary incontinence in girls is often successful, its effectiveness in boys remains unclear. Diamond and colleagues[42] reviewed 7 boys with neurogenic incontinence who had a follow-up of 1 to 9 years. All were dry in the first 3 months postoperatively. However, at last follow-up only 1 remains dry, 3 have night-time wetting, 2 have stress incontinence and one has day and night wetting needing bladder neck closure. A 60% continence rate has been reported at medium-term follow-up with the circumferential bladder neck cinch.[43] A long-term follow-up study of the use of periurethral Goretex®(PTFE) slings have shown them to be unreliable due to erosion of the sling despite initial good short-term results.[44] In all the above series, the upper tracts remained stable. Bladder neck suspension in pubertal girls has been described with comparable success.[45]

Bulking agents

Injection of bulking agents may be used primarily along with an augmentation procedure or for persistent incontinence following previous surgery. A recent long-term study of endourethral bulking agents for urinary incontinence for children with a neurogenic bladder has shown a significant improvement in the short term in most children but a deterioration and persistent incontinence on longer follow-up.[46] A similar experience has been reported by Kassouf *et al.*[47] and Guys *et al.*[48] in their series. Early experience of deflux as the bulking agent (dextran/hyaluronic acid copolymer) has been encouraging in incontinence of both neurogenic and structural origin.[49] Lottman *et al.* in their prospective study of 16 children with neuropathic bladder have demonstrated improvement in continence status in 57% of children in the medium term after injection of deflux.[50] The advantage of this technique is that it is minimally invasive and does not preclude further surgery at the bladder neck.

The artificial urinary sphincter (AUS)

The AUS (AMS 800) is most frequently used in cases of neuropathic bladder in children or those with bladder exstrophy. Continence rates in children with neuropathic bladder approaches 90% in the long term with the use of AUS.[51,52] Children are able to void spontaneously or catheterize urethrally or both.[52] Children with bladder exstrophy have not shown to do as well as those with neuropathic bladder.[51] Problems associated with AUS include mechanical failure (leakage, tube kink, and pump malfunction), surgical complications (erosion, infection, and malplacement), functional sphincter revisions (change in cuff size, pump repositioning, and bulbar cuff placement) in up to a third of cases.[51,52] Upper tract dilatation and detrusor instability has been noted requiring anticholinergics and augmentation in up to a third of cases.[53,54] Overall, the 10-year survival rate of the AMS 800 is reported to be around 79% and is not related to age at insertion, sex, model, previous bladder neck surgery, augmentation, or intermittent catheterization.[51] However, Spiess *et al.*[55] report a 8–9-year survival rate of the AMS 800 in their experience with a continence rate of just over 60% in their review of 30 boys with spina bifida followed up for a mean of 6.5 years. They therefore question the role of AUS vs. bladder neck reconstruction in these children.

Gonzalez and colleagues performed a critical review of the literature and compared the outcomes of each technique for the surgical treatment of children with neurogenic sphincter incontinence.[56] The results of each technique were compared in seven objective categories, including continence (defined as complete dryness for 4 hours between voidings or catheterizations), the need for intermittent catheterization, effects on bladder compliance, the need for bladder augmentation, upper tract changes, other complications and the revision rate. They found that the long-term results of the AUS were superior and reproducible in terms of continence, volitional voiding and avoidance of bladder augmentation. Revision rates of various procedures were similar but the incidence of complications was highest with the Kropp procedure. They support the AUS as first-line surgical management of neurogenic sphincter incontinence. However, there is limited long-term published data with regard to various bladder neck slings, reconstruction, injection, suspension, and urethral lengthening procedures.

A comparison of the various bladder neck procedures is shown in Table 49.2.

Table 49.2. Comparative outcomes of various bladder neck procedures in children with neurogenic bladder dysfunction

	Urethral voiding[a]	Continence with cystoplasty	Complications
Bladder neck procedures			
Kropp	no	Up to 80%[28,29]	Difficult catheterization (14–28%[29–30])
Pippe–Salle	acts as pop-off valve	70%[34,35]	"
Young–Dees–Leadbetter	yes	60–70%[37]	"
Bladder neck closure	no	85%[41]	Urethrovesical fistula (up to 40%[40–41]), bladder stones[41]
Bladder neck slings	yes	60%[43]	Erosion, infection[44]
Bulking agents	yes	Up to 57%[49,50]	Minimum, but high failure rate[46–48]
Artificial Urinary Sphincter	yes	90%[51,52]	Erosion, mechanical, upper tracts deterioration (up to 30%[51–54])

[a] Majority will require catheterization for emptying.

Surgery to create the reservoir

The main aim of an augmentation cystoplasty is to produce a large capacity compliant low pressure bladder. The ileum is the most common segment used, although the sigmoid may be used in cases where the mesentery of the ileum is too short to reach the pelvis, e.g. with exaggerated lumbar lordosis. Although detubularized, the bowel may exhibit neuropathic properties and may be hypercontractile and still generate significant pressures following augmentation.[57] This is more so in the case of colonic segments as opposed to ileal segments.[57] Following a cystoplasty, most patients rely on catheterization to empty the bladder either via the urethra or via a continent catheterizable stoma. Most of the complications described arise as a result of contact of intestinal epithelium to urine.

Concern about potential complications has led to an interest in alternative methods for cystoplasty. Techniques such as ureterocystoplasty, autoaugmentation, seromuscular augmentation, alloplastic replacement, and bioprosthetic materials have been considered. These techniques avoid inclusion of the intestinal epithelium in the urinary tract while creating a compliant bladder of adequate capacity.

Ileal/colocystoplasty

With the exception of gastrocystoplasty, most of the other cystoplasties show similar problems in the longer term. These are: (i) mucus formation; (ii) stone; (iii) infections; (iv) metabolic and acid–base; (v) malignancy; (vi) rupture of neobladder.

Mucus formation is a common problem after intestinal cystoplasty. Mucus can be dealt with by using an appropriately sized catheter for drainage and bladder washouts as necessary. Mucus does not seem to be a major problem in those children who are able to void spontaneuosly. Mucus can prevent drainage and emptying of the reservoir thereby making it more prone to calculi, infection and rupture.

Stone formation can occur in up to 20% of individuals and is uncommon in the first 6 months following cystoplasty.[58] It increases in frequency after 2 years.[59] Mathoera *et al.*[60] reported a 16% incidence of calculi at a median follow-up of 4.9 years in 89 patients following augmentation cystoplasty. The incidence was higher in girls and in those with catheterization problems or retention. Mucus may trap organisms thereby acting as a nidus for calculi formation. Close surveillance is therefore necessary as, although most calculi are symptomatic and present as a symptomatic urinary tract infection or hematuria, some may be asymptomatic.[58] Treatment can be either by ESWL or percutaneous vesicolithotomy, but open vesicolithotomy is the safest and most dependable way of removing the entire stone burden.

Up to 20% of children with an augmentation cystoplasty will have a symptomatic urinary tract infection.[61] Gough *et al.* demonstrated an improvement in vesicoureteric reflux, upper tract dilatation, and incidence of symptomatic urinary tract infections following augmentation cystoplasty.[61] Bacteriuria with mixed growth of a urine specimen is common[62] and requires no treatment but an isolated pure growth in an unwell child should prompt full treatment and investigation.

The isolated intestinal patch absorbs chloride and hydrogen ions and can cause hyperchloremic metabolic acidosis. This may be overt or covert and therefore requires close observation. Chronic acidosis can be compensated by respiratory hyperventilation. However, decompensation may occur if there is respiratory compromise such as acute asthma. Furthermore, chronic acidosis may cause mobilization of calcium from bone in an effort to buffer the hydrogen ions thereby leading to demineralization of the bony skeleton. Several long-term studies have shown a decrease in linear growth and bone demineralization in children following augmentation cystoplasty.[63,64] However, Woodhouse *et al.*[65] in their long-term review of children following enterocystoplasty (16.8 years) demonstrated normal growth in 85%. These children remained on, or reached, a higher centile following surgery compared to their precystoplasty centiles. Fifteen percent were in a lower position with a similar trend of their weight centiles following surgery. They conclude that this was not secondary to the enterocystoplasty but rather a non-specific phenomenon. Provided the kidneys were normal at the outset, metabolic acidosis was not found to be a significant feature.[63] If present, early treatment with sodium bicarbonate is essential.

Although there are case reports linking the development of malignancy in an augmented bladder, this is a rare occurrence.[66] However, more cases are likely with longer-term follow-up. With this in mind, in the UK a central registry for children undergoing augmentation cystoplasty has been recommended.[67] In experimental studies, histological changes of hyperplasia or metaplasia occurred along the anastomotic line.[68] Vajda *et al.*[69] were unable to find any histological changes of malignancy in their patients following colocystoplasty or gastrocystoplasty at 10 years follow-up but found a premalignant lesion at 13 years' follow-up. Therefore, surveillance is advisable after the first 7–10 years following an augmentation.

Rupture of the augmented bladder is an unusual complication and occurs most commonly as a result of external trauma to an overdistended bladder. This is most commonly seen in the peripubertal age, where compliance with the catheterization regime declines and it is not uncommon for the adolescent to have waited more than 12 hours to catheterise. Diagnosis may be difficult as a result of altered sensation. Gough *et al.*[70] reported a rupture incidence of 10.3% in 39 children who underwent a clam ileocystoplasty. Prolonged drainage and antibiotics in most cases allow the small perforation to heal; however, surgical exploration may be necessary in some instances, especially if the leak is intraperitoneal. There is no evidence to suggest that placing the augment extraperitoneally may reduce the incidence of rupture but it is the authors' preferred technique where feasible as it may avoid an intraperitoneal leak if rupture should occur.

Few studies exist on the long-term urodynamic evaluation of children with a neurogenic bladder and an enterocystoplasty. Quek *et al.* in their combined series of 26 patients including adults and children 4–13 years following enterocystoplasty demonstrated a significant increase in bladder capacity and a decrease in detrusor pressure. Of their patients, 96% showed an improvement or complete resolution of their urinary incontinence. They conclude that an augmentation cystoplasty provides durable clinical and urodynamic improvement in patients with a neurogenic bladder.[71]

Gastrocystoplasty

The potential advantages of gastrocystoplasty are decreased chloride absorption, mucus production and urinary infection and a low incidence of stone formation and perforation. Although the use of stomach may be beneficial in patients with chronic renal failure, experimental studies have failed to demonstrate any beneficial effect in the face of an acid load.[72]

The use of stomach has become controversial in pediatric lower urinary tract reconstruction. Dezoor *et al.*[73] report urinary continence in 89% of cases at a median follow up of 9.8 years following gastrocystoplasty. Upper tract dilatation was stable in 91%. No patient had chronic metabolic alkalosis. Patch contraction and ureteral obstruction necessitated major surgery in 6 cases. Febrile urinary tract sepsis occurred in 20% and 36% had asymptomatic bacteriuria. In animal studies, seromuscular gastrocystoplasty has been shown to be feasible allowing ingrowth of urothelium to line the gastric patch and increased urinary pH compared to conventional gastrocystoplasty.[74] The hematuria dysuria syndrome has been described in up to 25% of children and can usually be controlled by proton pump inhibitors. However, in some instances, conversion to an alternative form of cystoplasty is required.[75] The incidence of this syndrome has been shown to be lowest in those children who have an insensate urethra and are continent,[76] although this may be because they do not feel the acid burn. The findings of Mingin *et al.*[77] from their series demonstrated a significantly higher incidence of late complications with gastrocystoplasty as compared to other forms of cystoplasty (36% vs. 21.8%). Long-term follow-up in the majority of patients demonstrated significant increase in capacity and increased compliance. Although malignancy following gastrocystoplasty in children has not been documented, experimental studies have shown DNA-ploidy abnormalities along the anastomosis line on flow cytometry studies.[78] No significant adverse effect has been demonstrated with concomitant AUS insertion.[79]

Autoaugmentation

In an attempt to improve bladder compliance and capacity without the use of an intestinal patch, detrusorectomy autoaugmentation has been attempted. The exposed mucosa may be covered with demucosalized detubularised patch of intestine. Although this technique has been shown to improve these parameters in some instances in the short term,[80] on longer-term follow-up, this technique has not been shown to be useful with respect to continence and urodynamic parameters. MacNeily *et al.*[81] reviewed 17 patients who underwent this technique at a median of 75 months (4–126). Worsening upper tract dilatation developed in 5, 4 of whom required an enterocystoplasty. Twelve were considered failures on the basis of significant upper tract deterioration and ongoing incontinence; 93% had no improvement in their urodynamic parameters. Similar results were noted by Marte *et al.*[82] and Malone *et al.*[83] in their series of 11 and 9 patients followed up for a mean of 6.6 years and 5 years, respectively. Experimental studies by Rivas *et al.*[84] have demonstrated a lower bladder rupture volume and pressure with detrusor myotomy compared to ileocystoplasty and native bladders. Gonzalez *et al.*[85] in their experience of seromuscular colocystoplasty lined with urothelium (after detrusorectomy) in 16 patients demonstrated an increase in bladder capacity between 1.4- and 10-fold and a decrease in mean end filling pressures by up to 50%. Similar results were obtained by Lima *et al.*[86] using a similar technique in 10 patients at nearly 4 years' follow-up. Early results from these series did not demonstrate problems with mucus production or electrolyte abnormalities although follow-up is short.

Ureterocystoplasty

A ureterocystoplasty offers the advantage of using urothelium to increase the capacity of the bladder. This is ideally suited for those children with a non-functioning kidney with a megaureter and can be combined with an ipsilateral nephrectomy. There is a potential of devascularizing the ureter due to detubularization of the ureter all the way down to the hiatus thereby compromising the vascular supply. It is now recommended that the last 3 cm of the ureter is not detubularized to avoid this complication.[87] Ureterocystoplasty in the presence of a megaureter but a functioning kidney can be performed along with a transureteroureterostomy.[88,89] A recent multicenter study of ureterocystoplasty compared the rate of reaugmentation and the presence or absence of vesicoureteric reflux, presence of a single or double collecting system, diameter of the megaureter and the compliance of the bladder.[90] They recommend a ureterocystoplasty only in bladders of marginal compliance and where the ureter measures at least 1.5 cm. In the rest of the cases they have shown a high secondary or reaugmentation rate (82%–91%) as a result of persistent poor compliance and capacity secondary to ureterocystoplasty. Pascual *et al.*[89] and Landau *et al.*[91] report good medium-term results with ureterocystoplasty with 4-hour continence rates and improvement in bladder capacity and other urodynamic parameters in up to 90%.

The authors prefer an ileal clam cystoplasty. Children who intend to catheterise urethrally are commenced on a strict regime of CIC prior to surgery. The authors' personal series has shown that augmentation cystoplasty on its own combined with CIC can attain continence rates of up to 70% without the need for any bladder neck procedure.[92]

Continent catheterizable conduits

Mitrofanoff conduit

The Mitrofanoff conduit is the most commonly performed continent catheterizable conduit in patients with a neuropathic bladder. It is the technique of choice in children who are unable to catheterize urethrally as a result of their physical habitus, reluctance to catheterize urethrally or manual dexterity. The appendix if available is the most commonly used conduit followed by ileum (Yang–Monti ileovesicostomy), bladder tube (continent vesicostomy) or non-refluxing ureter. Most stomas are created on the lower abdominal wall; however, umbilical stomas may sometimes be necessary for the child to get easier access. Creation of a Mitrofanoff channel is usually performed concomitantly with an augmentation cystoplasty in children with neuropathic bladder and occasionally with the Malone antegrade continence enema (MACE) procedure.

Long-term follow-up of the Mitrofanoff channel has shown its robustness in the ability to be catheterized. High continence rates have been achieved when combined with an augmentation cystoplasty and bladder neck procedure. However, this channel is not without problems. In Mitrofanoff's own series[93] with 20 years follow-up, stomal stenosis was the most frequent complication requiring revisional surgery. Urinary tract infection, bladder calculi, urine leakage, and progressive bilateral upper tract dilatation were the other noted complications. However, in this series, concomitant bladder augmentation was very rarely performed. Since 1984, apart from stomal stenosis, very few complications have been noted. Several other long-term series demonstrate stomal stenosis to be the most significant complication in 10 to 30% of patients.[94–96] Some authors have found this to be more significant in those with an umbilical stoma than a stoma sited on the lower abdominal wall[97] Other problems include kinking of the channel, long stenosis of the channel, and difficulty in catheterization. A comparative study of the appendico-vecisostomy and the ileovesicostomy demonstrated the ileovesicostomy to be more problematic than the apppendicovesicostomy with regard to ease of catheterization.[98] Pouch formation has been known to occur with the ileovesicostomy adding to the difficulty in catheterization. The incidence of stone formation and urinary tract infection is low in those children who are compliant with the catheterization regime. In a small subset of children who do not require an augmentation, Rink and colleagues have shown the efficacy of the continent vesicostomy as an alternative to appendix or the ileum as a means of urinary diversion.[99] The continent catheterizable conduit has a high continence rate (>90%) but requires revision in a significant proportion of children.

Diversions in the neuropathic bladder

Although achieving continence and preserving function of the upper tracts is the main aim of the aforementioned procedures, success depends on long-term compliance of the patients and their carers. There may be a select group of patients in whom this aim cannot be achieved. It is in this group of children that urinary diversion may be considered. The most commonly performed diversions are: (i) vesicostomy; (ii) refluxing ureterostomy; (iii) ileal conduit.

Vesicostomy

The use of cutaneous vesicostomy in children with myelodysplasia has been well documented. Hutcheson *et al.*[100] reviewed their experience of 23/350 patients with myelodysplasia who had a permanent vesicostomy. At 13 years' follow-up, upper tract dilatation had resolved in all. Two patients required revision. Thirty-three percent had recurrent upper tract calculi. The authors conclude that permanent vesicostomy is a suitable alternative in selected cases of children with myelodysplasia. Temporary cutaneous vesicostomy has also been described for deteriorating upper tracts, failure of CIC and recurrent infections in children with neuropathic bladder.[101] Undiversion in these children has not shown to have any long-term harmful effects on the bladder.[102]

Refluxing ureterostomy

In children with gross vesicoureteric reflux, a dilated ureter and upper tract deterioration, a cutaneous ureterostomy has been demonstrated to be useful as a permanent form of urinary diversion. Sarduy *et al.*[103] in their review of 59 children managed by cutaneous ureterostomy found this to be a safe, quick and effective method of decompressing the kidney. Chronic bacteriuria was common but pyelonephritis was rare. They recommend this technique for long-term use in selected children with dilated ureters. This technique may be used as a temporary method in cases of neuropathic bladder with deteriorating upper tracts due to gross reflux, the ureterostomy acting as a pop-off mechanism.

Ileal conduit

Previously the ileal conduit had been used in children for diversion of urine from the neurogenic bladder to prevent deterioration of the upper urinary tracts and to manage urinary incontinence. Cass *et al.*[104] reviewed 139 children with ileal conduits who were followed up for up to 22 years and found a high incidence of complications, over half of which required surgical correction. Upper tract deterioration occurred in 16.5% of 50 children who were followed up for a mean of 13.3 years. In a review of their experience by Shapiro *et al.*,[105] stomal stenosis and ureteroileal or other intrinsic obstructions requiring ileal loop revisions were frequent and occurred as late as 13 years postoperatively. However, of the 144 renal units followed, 76% improved or were stable and 70% of normal kidneys remained normal after more than 10 years of diversion. Colonic conduits have been described for urinary diversion in children with a neurogenic bladder. Stein *et al.*[106] reviewed their experience of 105 patients (76 with neurogenic bladder). At a mean follow-up of 16.3 years, early and late stenosis at the ureterocolic anastomosis occurred in 7.6% and stomal stenosis in 15.5% of cases. Renal calculi developed in 8.2% of children. There was deterioration in function in 8 renal units which were removed. Ileal conduit/colonic conduit urinary diversion may be considered in those individuals in whom standard techniques have failed or are not suitable. Close and prolonged follow-up is necessary.

The future

The clinical complications arising as a result of enterocystoplasty are due to the exposure of the epithelial lining of the intestine to urine. A number of alternative approaches are being developed to find a practical and functional substitute for native bladder tissue. These include a composite enterocystoplasty where the demucosalized intestine is lined by in vitro propagated urothelial cells to a synthetic substitute to augment the urinary tract. Until such time as an entirely urothelial bladder substitute is available, bladder reconstruction and achieving continence will remain a technical challenge to pediatric urologists.

REFERENCES

1. Belman, A., King, L. R., & Kramer, S. A., eds. *Clinical Pediatric Urology*. 4th edn. Philadelphia: W.B. Saunders, 2003.
2. Gearhart, J. P., Rink, R. C., & Mouriquand, P. D. E., eds. *Pediatric Urology*. 1st edn. Philadelphia: W.B. Saunders, 2001.
3. Frank, J. D., Gearhart, J. P., & Snyder, H. M., eds. *Operative Pediatric Urology*. 2nd edn. Edinburgh: Churchill Livingstone, 2001.
4. Lapides, J., Diokno, A. C., Lowe, B. S., & Kalish, M. D. Follow up on unsterile, intermittent self-catheterization. *J. Urol.* 1974; **111**:184.
5. Wolraich, M. L., Hawtrey, C., Mapel, J., & Henderson, M. Results of clean intermittent catheterization for children with neurogenic bladders. *Urology* 1983; **22**(5):479.
6. Lyn-Dyken, D. C., Wolraich, M. L., Hawtrey, C. E., & Doja, M. S. Follow-up of clean intermittent catheterization for children with neuropathic bladders. *Urology* 1992; **40**(6):525.
7. Cass, A. S., Luxenberg, M., Gleich, P., Johnson, C. F., & Hagen, S. Clean intermittent catheterisation in the management of the neurogenic bladder in children. *J. Urol.* 1984; **132**(3):526.
8. Plunkett, J. M. & Braren, V. Five year experience with clean intermittent catheterization in children. *Urology* 1982; **20**(2):128.
9. Schlager, T. A., Dilks, S., Trudell, J., Whittam, T. S., & Hendley, J. O. Bacteruria in children with neurogenic bladder treated with intermittent cathetrization: natural history. *J. Pediatr.* 1995; **126**(3):490.
10. Kass, E. J., Koff, S. A., Diokno, A. C., & Lapides, J. The significance of bacilluria in children on long term intermittent catheterizatioin. *J. Urol.* 1981; **126**(2):223.
11. Schlager, T. A., Anderson, S., Trudell, J., & Hendley, J. O. Effect of cranberry juice on bacteruria in children with neurogenic bladder receiving intermittent catheterization. *J. Pediatr.* 1999; **135**(6):698.
12. Schlager, T. A., Anderson, S., Trudell, J., & Hendley, J. O. Nitrofurantoin prophylaxis for bacteruria and urinary tract infection in children with neurogenic bladder on intermittent catheterization. *J. Pediatr.* 1998; **132**(4):704.
13. Schlager, T. A., Clark, M., & Anderson, S. Effect of a single use sterile catheter for each void on the frequency of bacteruria in children with neurogenic bladder on intermittent catheterization for bladder emptying. *Pediatrics* 2001; **108**(4):E71.
14. Heineman, J., Gasgarth, M., & Cuckow, P. M. Experience with the vesicostomy button. Presented at the Annual European Society of Pediatric Urology Meeting, Istanbul, 1999.
15. Ferrara, P., D'Aleo, C. M., Tarquini, E., Salvatore, S., & Salvaggio, E. Side-effects of oral or intravesical oxybutinin chloride in children with spina bifida. *BJU Int.* 2001; **87**(7):674.
16. Buyse, G., Waldeck, K., Verpoorten, C., Bjork, H., Casaer, P., & Andersson, K. E. Intravesical oxybutinin for neurogenic bladder dysfunction: less systemic side effects due to reduced first pass metabolism. *J. Urol.* 1998; **160**(3 Pt 1):892.
17. Palmar, L. S., Zebold, K., Firlit, C. F., & Kaplan, W. E. Complications of intravesical oxybutinin chloride therapy in the pediatric myelomeningocoele population. *J. Urol.* 1997; **157**(2):638.
18. Painter, K. A., Vates, T. S., Bukowski, T. P. *et al.* Long-term intravesical oxybutinin chloride therapy in children with myelodysplasia. *J. Urol.* 1996; **156**(4):1459.
19. Amark, P., Bussman, G., & Eksborg, S. Follow-up of long-time treatment with intravesical oxybutinin for neurogenic bladder in children. *Eur. Urol.* 1998; **34**(2):148.
20. Kaplinsky, R., Greenfield, S., Wan, J., & Fera, M. Expanded follow up of intravesical oxybutinin chloride use in children with neurogenic bladder. *J. Urol.* 1996; **156**(2):753.
21. Bolduc, S., Upadhyay, J., Payton, J. *et al.* The use of tolterodine in children after oxybutinin failure. *BJU Int.* 2003; **91**(4):398.
22. Schulte-Baukloh, H., Michael, T., Schobert, J., Stolze, T., & Knispel, H. H. Efficacy of botulinum-a toxin in children with detrusor hyperreflexia due to myelomeningocoele: preliminary results. *Urology* 2002; **59**(3):325.
23. Kropp, K. A. & Angwafo, F. F. Urethral lengthening and reimplantation for neurogenic incontinence in children. *J. Urol.* 1986; **135**:533–536.

24. Pippe Salle, J. L., De, Fraga, J. C. S., & Amarante, A. Urethral lengthening with anterior bladder flap for urinary incontinence: new approach. *J. Urol.* 1994; **152**:803–806.
25. Young, H. H. Exstrophy of the bladder: the first case in which a normal bladder and urinary control have been obtained by a plastic operation. *Surg. Gynecol. Obstet.* 1942; **74**:729.
26. Dees, J. E. Congenital epispadias with incontinence. *J. Urol.* 1949; **62**:513.
27. Leadbetter, W. H. Jr. Surgical correctioin of total urinary incontinence. *J. Urol.* 1964; **91**:261.
28. Nill, T. G., Peller, P. A., & Kropp, K. A. Management of urinary incontinence by bladder tube lengthening and submucosal reimplantation. *J. Urol.* 1990; **144**(2 Pt 2):559–561.
29. Waters, P. R., Chehade, N. C., & Kropp, K. A. Urethral lengthening and reimplantatioin: incidence and management of catheterisation problems. *J. Urol.* 1997; **158**(3 Pt 2):1053–1056.
30. Gauriau, L., Mure, P., & Mollard, P. [Urethral lengthening (the Kropp technic) in neurologic urinary incontinence in children and adolescents. Results of a series of 22 cases] *J. Urol.* (Paris). 1997; **103**(1–2):10–12.
31. Snodgrass, W. A simplified Kropp procedure for incontinence. *J. Urol.* 1997:**158(3** Pt 2):1049–1052.
32. Belman, A. B. & Kaplan, G. W. Experience with the Kropp anticontinence procedure. *J. Urol.* 1989; **141**(5):1160–1162.
33. Parres, J. A. & Kropp, K. A. Urodynamic evaluation of the continence mechanism following urethral lengthening–reimplantation and enterocystoplasty. *J. Urol.* 1991; **146** (2 Pt 2):535–538.
34. Hayes, M. C., Bulusu, A., Terry, T., Mouriquand, P. D., & Malone, P. S. The Pippe–Salle urethral lengthening procedure; experience and outcome from three United Kingdom centres. *BJU Int.* 1999; **84**(6):701–705.
35. Salle, J. L., McLorie, G. A., Bagli, D. J., & Khoury, A. E. Modifications of and extended indications for the Pippe–Salle procedure. *World J. Urol.* 1998; **16**(4):279–284.
36. Mouriquand, P. D. E., Sheard, R., Phillips, N., Sharma, S., & Vandeberg, C. The Kropp–Onlay procedure (Pippe–Salle procedure): a simplification of the technique of urethral lengthening. Preliminary results in eight patients. *Br. J. Urol.* 1995; **75**:656–662.
37. Donnahoo, K. K., Rink, R. C., Cain, M. P., & Casale, A. J. The Young–Dees–Leadbetter bladder neck repair for neurogenic incontinence. *J. Urol.* 1999; **161**(6):1946–1949.
38. Reda, E. F. The use of the Young–Dees–Leadbetter procedure. *Dialog. Pediatr. Urol.* 1991; **14**(4):7–8.
39. Hoebeke, P., De Kuper, P., Geominne, H., Van Laecke, E., & Everaert, K. Bladder neck closure for treating pediatric incontinence. *Eur. Urol.* 2000; **38**(4):453–456.
40. Jayanthi, V. R., Churchill, B. M., McLorie, G. A., & Khoury, A. E. Concomitant bladder neck closure and Mitrofanoff diversion for the management of intractable urinary incontinence. *J. Urol.* 1995; **154**:886–888.
41. Nguyen, H. T. & Baskin, L. S. The outcome of bladder neck closure in children with severe urinary incontinence. *J. Urol.* 2003; **169**(3):1114–1116.
42. Nguyen, H. T., Bauer, S. B., Diamond, D. A., & Retik, A. B. Rectus fascial sling for the treatment of neurogenic sphincteric incontinence in boys: is it safe and effective? *J. Urol.* 2001; **166**(2):658–661.
43. Bugg, C. E., Jr. & Joseph, D. B. Bladder neck cinch for pediatric neurogenic outlet deficiency. *J. Urol.* 2003; **170**(4 Pt 2):1501–1503.
44. Godbole, P. & MacKinnon, A. E. Expanded PTFE bladder neck slings for incontinence in children: the long-term outcome. *BJU Int.* 2004; **93**(1):139–141.
45. Freedman, E. R., Singh, G., Donnell, S. C., Rickwood, A. M., & Thomas, D. G. Combined bladder neck suspension and augmentation cystoplasty for neuropathic incontinence in female patients. *Br. J. Urol.* 1994; **73**(6):621–624.
46. Godbole, P., Bryant, R., MacKinnon, A. E., & Roberts, J. P. Endourethral injection of bulking agents for urinary incontinence in children. *BJU Int.* 2003; **91**(6):536–539.
47. Kassouf, W., Capolicchio, G., Berardinucci, G., & Corcos, J. Collagen injection for the treatment of urinary incontinence in children. *J Urol* 2001; **165**(5):1666–1668.
48. Guys, J. M., Simeoni-Alias, J., Fakhro, A., & Delarue, A. Use of polydimethylsiloxane for endoscopic treatment of neurogenic urinary incontinence in children. *J Urol* 1999; **162**(6):2133–2135.
49. Caione, P. & Capozza, N. Endoscopic treatment of urinary incontinence in pediatric patients: 2-year experience with dextranomer/hyaluronic acid copolymer. *J. Urol.* 2002; **168**(4 Pt 2): 1868–1871.
50. Lottmann, H. B., Margaryan, M., Bernuy, M. *et al.* The effect of endoscopic injections of dextranomer based implants on continence and bladder capacity: a prospective study of 31 patients. *J. Urol.*. 2002; **168**(4 Pt 2): 1863–1867.
51. Hafez, A. T., McLorie, G., Bagli, D., & Khoury, A. A single-centre long-term outcome analysis of artificial urinary sphincter placement in children. *BJU Int.* 2002; **89**(1):82–85.
52. Herndon, C. D., Rink, R. C., Shaw, M. B. *et al.* The Indiana experience with artificial urinary sphincters in children and young adults. *J. Urol.* 2003; **169**(2):650–654.
53. Kryger, J. V., Leverson, G., & Gonzalez, R. Long-term results of artificial urinary sphincters in children are independent of age at implantation. *J. Urol.* 2001; **165**(6 Pt 2):2377–2379.
54. Castera, R., Podesta, M. L., Ruarte, A., Herrera, M., & Medel, R. 10-year experience with artificial urinary sphincter in children and adolescents. *J. Urol.* 2001; **165** (6 Pt 2):2373–2376.
55. Spiess, P. E., Capolicchio, J. P., Kiruluta, G., Salle, J. P., Berardinucci, G., & Corcos, J. Is an artificial sphincter the best choice for incontinent boys with spina bifida? Review of our long term experience with the AS-800 artificial sphincter. *Can. J. Urol.* 2002; **9**(2):1486–1491.
56. Kryger, J. V., Gonzalez, R., & Barthold, J. S. Surgical management of urinary incontinence with neurogenic sphincteric incontinence. *J. Urol.* 2000; **163**(1):256–263.
57. McInerney, P. D., DeSouza, N., Thomas, P. J., & Mundy, A. R. The role of urodynamic studies in the evaluation of patients

with augmentation cystoplasties. *Br. J. Urol.* 1995; **76**(4): 475–478.

58. Nurse, D. E., McInerney, P. D., Thomas, P. J., & Mundy, A. R. Stones in enterocystoplasties. *Br. J. Urol.* 1996; **77**:684–687.
59. Palmer, L. S., Franco, I., & Kogan, S. J. Urolithiasis in children following augmentation cystoplasty. *J. Urol.* 1993; **50**:726–729.
60. Mathoera, R. B., Kok, D. J., & Mijman, R. J. Bladder calculi in augmentation cystoplasty in children. *Urology* 2000; **56**(3):482–487.
61. Krishna, A. & Gough, D. C. Evaluation of augmentatioin cystoplasty in childhood with reference to vesico-ureteric reflux and urinary infection.
62. Woodhouse, C. R. J. The infective, metabolic and histological consequences of enterocystoplasty. *Eur. Urol. Update* 1994; **3**:10–15.
63. Hafez, A. T., McLorie, G., Gilday, D. *et al.* Long-term evaluation of metabolic profile and bone mineral density after ileocystoplasty in children. *J. Urol.* 2003; **170** (4 Pt 2):1639–1641.
64. Vajda, P., Pinter, A. B., Harangi, F., Farkas, A., Vastyan, A., & Oberritter, Z. Metabolic findings after colocystoplasty in children. *Urology* 2003:**62**(3):542–546.
65. Gerharz, E. W., Preece, M., Dufy, P. G., Ransley, P. G., Leaver, R., & Woodhouse, C. R. Enterocystoplasty in childhood: a second look at the effect on growth. *BJU Int.* 2003; **91**(1):79–83.
66. Lane, T. & Shah, J. Carcinoma following augmentation ileocystoplasty. *Urol. Int.* 2000; **64**(1): 31–32.
67. Shaw, J. & Lewis, M. A. Bladder augmentation surgery – what about the malignant risk? *Eur. J. Pediatr. Surg.* 1999; **9** Suppl 1:39–40.
68. Little, J. S., Jr., Klee, L. W., Hoover, D. M., & Rink, R. C. Long-term histopathological changes observed in rats subjected to augmentation cystoplasty. *J. Urol.* 1994; **152** (2 Pt 2): 720–724.
69. Vajda, P., Kaiser, L., Magyarlaki, T., Farkas, A., Vastyan, A. M., & Pinter, A. B. Histological findings after colocystoplasty and gastrocystoplasty. *J. Urol.* 2002; **168**(2):698–701.
70. Krishna, A., Gough, D. C., Fishwick, J., & Bruce, J. Ileocystoplasty in children: assessing safety and success. *Eur. Urol.* 1995:**27**(1):62–66.
71. Quek, M. L. & Ginsberg, D. A. Long-term urodynamics followup of bladder augmentation for neurogenic bladder. *J. Urol.* 2003; **169**(1):195–198.
72. De Freitas, Filho, L. G., Carnevale, J., Leao, J. Q., Schor, N., & Ortiz, V. Gastrocystoplasty and chronic renal failure: an acid-base metabolism study. *J. Urol.* 2001; **166**(1):251–254.
73. DeFoor, W., Minevich, E., Reeves, D. *et al.* Gastrocystoplasty: long-term follow up. *J. Urol.* 2003; **170**(4 Pt 2): 1647–1649.
74. Vastyan, A. M., Pinter, A. B., Farkas, A. P. *et al.* Seromuscular gastrocystoplasty in dogs. *Urol. Int.* 2003; **71**(2):215–218.
75. Leonard, M. P., Dharamsi, N., & Williot, P. E. Outcome of gastrocystoplasty in tertiary paediatric urology practice. *J. Urol.* 2000; **164**(3 Pt 2):947–950.
76. Chadwick Plaire, J., Snodgrass, W. T., Grady, R. W., & Mitchell, M. E. Long-term follow up of the hematuria-dysuria syndrome. *J. Urol.* 2000; **164** (3 Pt 2): 921–923.
77. Mingin, G. C., Stock, J. A., & Hanna, M. K. Gastrocystoplasty: long term complications in 22 patients. *J. Urol.* 1999; **162** (3 Pt 2): 1122–1125.
78. Close, C. E., Tekgul, S., Ganesan, G. S., True, L. D., & Mitchell, M. E. Flow cytometry analysis of proliferative lesions at the gastrocystoplasty anastomosis. *J. Urol.* 2003; **169**(1):365–368.
79. Abdel-Azim, M. S. & Abdel-Hakim, A. M. Gastrocystoplasty in patients with an areflexic low compliant bladder. *Eur. Urol.* 2003; **44**(2):260–265.
80. Perovic, S. V., Djordjevic, M. L., Kekic, Z. K., & Vukadinovic, V. M. Bladder autoaugmentation with rectus muscle backing. *J. Urol.* 2002; **168**(4 Pt 2):1877–1880.
81. MacNeily, A. E., Afshar, K., Coleman, G. U., & Johnson, H. W. Autoaugmentation by detrusor myotomy: its lack of effectiveness in the management of congenital neuropathic bladder. *J Urol* 2003; **170**(4 Pt 2):1643–1646.
82. Marte, A., Di Meglio, D., Cotrufo, A. M., Di Iorio, G., De Pasquale, M., & Vessella, A. A long term follow up of autoaugmentatioin in myelodysplastic children. *BJU Int.* 2002; **89**(9):928–931.
83. Potter, J. M., Duffy, P. G., Gordon, E. M., & Malone, P. R. Detrusor myotomy: a 5-year review in unstable and non compliant bladders. *BJU Int.* 2002; **89**(2):932–935.
84. Rivas, D. A., Chancelloe, M. B., Huang, B., Epple, A., & Figueroa, T. E. Comparison of bladder rupture pressure after intestinal bladder augmentatioin (ileocystoplasty) and myotomy (autoaugmentation). *Urology* 1996; **48**(1):40–46.
85. Gonzalez, R., Buson, H., Reid, C., & Reinberg, Y. Seromuscular colocystoplasty lined with urothelium: experience with 16 patients. *Urology* 1995; **45**:124.
86. Lima, S. V. C., Araujo, L. A. P., Vilar, F. O., Kummer, C. L., & Lima, E. C. Nonsecretory sigmoid cystoplasty: experimental and clinical results. *J. Urol.* 1995; **153**:1651.
87. Adams, M. C., Brock, J. W. 3rd, Pope, J. C. 4th, Rink, R. C. Ureterocystoplasty: is it necessary to detubularize the distal ureter? *J. Urol.* 1998; **160**(3 Pt 1):851–853.
88. Tekgul, S., Oge, O., Bal, K., Erkan, I., & Bakkaloglu, M. Ureterocystoplasty: an alternative reconstructive procedure to enterocystoplasty in suitable cases. *J. Pediatr. Surg* 2000; **35**(4):577–579.
89. Pascual, L. A., Sentagne, L. M., Vega-Perogorria, J. M., de Badiola, F. I., Puigdevall, J. C., & Ruiz, E. Single distal ureter for ureterocystoplasty: a safe first choice tissue for bladder augmentation. *J. Urol.* 2001; **165**(6 Pt 2):2256–2258.
90. Husmann, D. A., Snodgrass, W. T., Koyle, M. A. *et al.* Ureterocystoplasty: indications for a successful augmentation. *J. Urol.* 2004; **171**(1):376–380.
91. Landau, E. H., Jayanthi, V. R., Khoury, A. E. *et al.* Bladder augmentation: ureterocystoplasty versus ileocystoplasty. *J. Urol.* 1994; **152**(2 Pt 2): 716–719.
92. Kufeji, D., Kelly, J., & Wilcox, D. Is bladder neck surgery necessary to axchieve continence in a child with a neuropathic bladder? *BJU Int.* 2003; **91**(1):4.

93. Liard, A., Seguier-Lipszyc, E., Mathiot, A., & Mitrofanoff, P. The Mitrofanoff procedure: 20 years later. *J. Urol.* 2001; **165**(6 Pt 2): 2394–2398.
94. McAndrew, H. F. & Malone, P. S. Continent catheterizable conduits: which stoma, which conduit and which reservoir? *BJU Int.* 2002; **89**(1):86–89.
95. Harris, C. F., Cooper, C. S., Hutcheson, J. C., & Snyder, H. M. 3rd. Appendicovesicostomy: the mitrofanoff procedure – a 15-year perspective. *J. Urol.* 2000; **163**(6):1922–1926.
96. Fishwick, J. E., Gough, D. C., & O'Flynn, K. J. The Mitrofanoff procedure: does it last? *BJU Int.* 2000; **85**(4):496–497.
97. De Ganck, J., Everaert, K., Van Laecke, E., Oosterlinck, W., & Hoebeke, P. A high easy to treat complication rate is the price of a continent stoma. *BJU Int.* 2002; **90**(3):240–243.
98. Narayanswamy, B., Wilcox, D. T., Cuckow, P. M., Duffy, P. G., & Ransley, P. G. The Yang–Monti ileovesicostomy: a problematic channel? *BJU Int.* 2001; **87**(9):861–865.
99. Cain, M. P., Rink, R. C., Yerkes, E. B., Kaefer, M., & Casale, A. J. Long-term follow up and outcome of continent catheterizable vesicostomy using the Rink modification. *J. Urol.* 2002; **168**(6):2583–2585.
100. Hutcheson, J. C., Cooper, C. S., Canning, D. A., Zderic, S. A., & Snyder, H. M. 3rd. The use of vesicostomy as permanent urinary diversion in the child with myelomeningocoele. *J. Urol.* 2001; **166**(6):2351–2353.
101. Connolly, B., Fitzgerald, R. J., & Guiney, E. J. Has vesicostomy a role in the neuropathic bladder? *Z. Kinderchir.* 1988; **43** Suppl 2:17–18.
102. Snyder, H. M. 3rd, Kalichman, M. A., Charney, E., & Duckett, J. W. Vesicostomy for neurogenic bladder with spina bifida: follow up. *J Urol.* 1983; **130**(4):724–726.
103. Sarduy, G. S., Crooks, K. K., Smith, J. P., & Wise, H. A. 2nd. Results in children managed by cutaneous ureterostomy. *Urology* 1982; **19**(5):486–488.
104. Cass, A. S., Luxenberg, M., Gleich, P., & Johnson, C. F. A 22-year follow up of ileal conduits in children with a neurogenic bladder. *J. Urol.* 1984; **132**(3):529–531.
105. Shapiro, S. R., Lebowitz, R., & Colodny, A. H. Fate of 90 children with ileal conduit urinary diversion a decade later: analysis of complicatioins, pyelography, renal function and bacteriology. *J. Urol.* 1975; **114**(2):289–295.
106. Stein, R., Fisch, M., Stockle, M., Demirkesen, O., & Hohenfellner, R. Colonic conduit in children: protection of the upper urinary tract 16 years later? *J. Urol.* 1996; **156**(3):1146–1150.

50

Non-neuropathic bladder–sphincter dysfunction

Göran Läckgren[1] and Tryggve Nevéus[2]

[1]Section of Urology, University Children's Hospital, Uppsala, Sweden
[2]Department of Pediatrics, University Children's Hospital, Uppsala, Sweden

Background

Bladder dysfunction and nocturnal enuresis are the most common urological disorders in children.[1–4] The development of continence and voluntary voiding requires maturation of the neural system and the establishment of sound micturition habits. While the conscious sensation of bladder fullness is usually gained during the second year of life, the ability to void and also to inhibit voiding develops 1–2 years later. Consequently, most healthy children become dry during this period of life.[5] By 4 years of age 75% of all children have attained bladder control and can consciously start, postpone or interrupt voiding. Nocturnal dryness is generally achieved later than daytime bladder control.

Healthy schoolchildren void 3–7 times/day, and most of them empty their bladders completely, without residual urine.[2,6] There is, however, a substantial minority of at least 20% of 7-year old children who have signs of incomplete bladder control, i.e., symptoms of either "non-neuropathic bladder–sphincter dysfunction" or nocturnal enuresis.[6,7–12]

When taking a history in incontinent children over 5 years of age, the severity, frequency and timing of wetting episodes should be described, as well as whether the accidents are preceded by urgency or associated with holding maneuvers.[13] Bowel function should also be assessed. The use of a bladder diary is strongly recommended, since it is the only method of recording incontinent episodes as well as times of micturition, voided volumes, pad usage as well as fluid intake, the degree of urgency and the degree of incontinence.[14,15] The recordings, when used for diagnostic purposes, should be done in natural conditions, with the child drinking and voiding spontaneously. With this structured approach, the diagnosis of any kind of bladder emptying problem and /or incontinence can usually be made with confidence.[2,4]

Because there are few detailed published studies of symptoms of bladder disturbance in different age groups, it is difficult to speculate about the natural history of bladder dysfunction and enuresis in childhood. The aim of this chapter is to discuss voiding abnormalities in childhood and to speculate about the long-term outcome of children with bladder dysfunction or nocturnal enuresis.

Classification of bladder dysfunction in childhood

There is a definitive need for common definitions and a revised general terminology in this area.[15] In 1998 a standardized definition of lower urinary tract dysfunction in children was approved by the International Children's Continence Society (ICCS).[16] This is currently under the process of revision, and the wording of the present chapter tries to follow the new evolving recommendations.[3,14]

Thus, the old concept of "detrusor instability" is replaced by detrusor overactivity and "unstable bladder" has been replaced by overactive bladder (OAB). The distended, weakly contracting "lazy bladder" with residual urine will be called detrusor underactivity (DUA), and the presence of sphincter contractions during the voiding phase (earlier called "detrusor–sphincter dyscoordination") will now be named dysfunctional voiding. Incontinence is

Pediatric Surgery and Urology: Long-term Outcomes, Mark Stringer, Keith Oldham, Pierre Mouriquand.
Published by Cambridge University Press.

Table 50.1. Treatment of bladder dysfunction in childhood

In all children (>5 years of age) with symptoms of disturbed bladder control the most important diagnostic steps also serve as the first steps of therapy. These can be done by any primary care physician:

- a careful history
- micturition charts – including fluid intake
- bowel control.

Information to the parents and the child. In many children a simple bladder training with timed micturition and awareness of the "voiding-process" by the parents is enough therapy. When referred to specialists, the following primary diagnostic steps should be added:

- flowmetry
- residual urine.

In children not responding to the first steps of treatment (including urotherapy and/or pharmacological treatment) further investigations to search for an organic cause of bladder dysfunction is indicated. This may include:

Radiological investigation of the urinary tract:

cystometry

cystoscopy

MRI of the spine.

any involuntary loss of urine at a socially unacceptable time and place, in a child past the age of bladder control. Enuresis means wetting while asleep, regardless of underlying cause. Urgency is best described as the sudden, urgent need to void, and is the hallmark of uninhibited detrusor contractions. When combined with incontinence and an increased voiding frequency (>seven times per day) the syndrome is denoted overactive bladder or urge incontinence.

There are three distinct clinical patterns of bladder dysfunction with possible evolvement from one pattern into another. The first is the overactive bladder or urge syndrome and urge incontinence with normal micturation; the second is dysfunctional voiding with staccato or fractionated micturition. The final step is detrusor underactivity with large residual urine volumes in a bladder with weak detrusor contractions. This latter condition is often complicated by recurrent UTIs and/or vesicoureteral reflux (VUR).

If there is a direct relationship between these three "non-neurogenic bladder–sphincter dysfunctions" it is not clear, but it is likely that some of the patients with dysfunctional voiding may end up with detrusor underactivity which may continue into adulthood.[4,17,18]

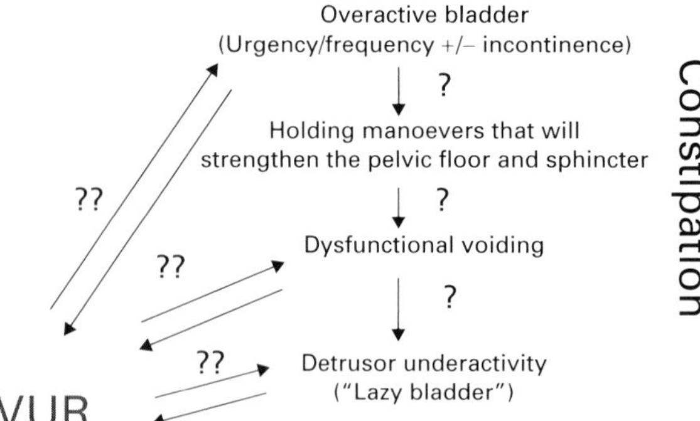

Fig. 50.1. Possible flowchart of "bladder dysfunction" in childhood.

Epidemiology

Nocturnal enuresis ranks high among common childhood disorders, affecting approximately 10% of 7-year-olds.[10,19] However, the prevalence data reported for "non-neuropathic bladder-sphincter dysfunction" are often difficult to interpret, since several different definitions and classifications have been used. The term has been used for all sorts of bladder malfunction between the extremes of simple urgency symptoms and severe cases of bladder dysfunction that may affect the upper urinary tract.

Several surveys of incontinence in different age groups of children have recently been published.[7–9,12,20] In a study on 3556 7-year-old Swedish schoolchildren, Hellström *et al.* found that 26% had at least one symptom suggesting incomplete bladder control, including nocturnal enuresis. Daytime wetting was seen in 6% of the girls and 2.0% of the boys, nocturnal enuresis without daytime incontinence in 2.3% of the girls and 7.0% of the boys, and combined day- and night-time wetting in 2.3% of the girls and 2.0% of the boys.[8] Similar prevalence figures in young schoolchildren have been found by other investigators in different countries.[7–9,12]

Bakker *et al.* examined micturition problems and voiding habits in a slightly older population of 4332 schoolchildren aged 10–14 years and found daytime wetting with or without enuresis in 8% and only 1% with isolated nocturnal enuresis.[7]

Although there are many studies describing the prevalence of urinary incontinence in women and men in various age groups,[21–24] the prevalence of bladder dysfunction and/or incontinence in adolescents or young men and women has not been studied in detail.

Enuresis

Older notions about psychological causes behind this psychologically distressing condition have now been abandoned in favor of endocrinological, urological and sleep-related mechanisms. The emerging consensus is that the enuretic child wets his or her sheets because of a combination of, on the one hand (i) nocturnal polyuria and/or (ii) nocturnal detrusor hyperactivity, and on the other (iii) high arousal thresholds. Proof of the first mechanism came with the pioneer studies by a Danish group who showed that a subgroup of enuretic children produce large amounts of dilute urine at night due to a relative lack of the antidiuretic hormone vasopressin. [25] Detrusor hyperactivity is implicated indirectly by the large overlap between nocturnal enuresis and urge incontinence[8] and has been demonstrated directly in cystometric studies.[26] Finally, the formerly controversial "disorder of arousal" theory, i.e., that enuretic children sleep more "deeply" than their night-dry peers, has been corroborated elegantly using graded arousal stimuli during well-defined sleep stages.[27]

Consequently, enuresis is a heterogenous disorder and different children need different treatments. Two therapies have emerged as safe and reasonably successful first-line alternatives: the vasopressin analogue desmopressin[28] and the enuresis alarm.[29] The former, taken at bedtime, reduces nocturnal polyuria by antidiuretic action, while the latter is an apparatus that addresses the underlying disorder of arousal by waking the child at the moment of micturition. Anticholinergic, detrusor-relaxant drugs such as oxybutynin or tolterodin are probably useful as a second-line treatment in children suffering from enuresis due to detrusor hyperactivity, but this has not, as yet, been substantiated by randomized, controlled studies.[30]

Urge-incontinence and overactive bladder

As mentioned above, this disturbance is characterized by a recurrent, strong need to void, regardless of bladder filling. It is often associated with an increased voiding frequency (>7 times/day).[2,17,31] The urine flow is however normal and there is no residual urine. Simple urge is a "symptom" that most schoolchildren can recognize and Nevéus *et al.* found that 35% of 7–10-year-old children recognized urge symptoms.[10] It is thus more or less a variant of normality and only the severe forms with urgency/frequency, often combined with wetting, may be treated with urotherapy and/or anticholinergics. These children void with normal sphincter relaxation and they have a normal, but sometimes high pressure bladder emptying. The term "overactive bladder" has today been accepted as the descriptive term for urge and urge incontinence.[14,32] Urge symptoms seem to peak at age 6–9 years and diminish towards puberty with an assumed spontaneous cure rate of at least 14% per year.[7,17,33]

In childhood it is common that urge symptoms may be provoked by physical activity, but this is not stress incontinence but a sign of an overactive bladder. Stress incontinence occurs at exertion and is caused by an underactive or damaged sphincter. The condition is very rare in neurologically healthy children but common in children with neurogenic bladder.

Mixed incontinence is due to the combination of overactive detrusor and sphincter deficiency. This is also rare in children not suffering from neurogenic bladder.

A special group of children with symptoms of urgency and holding maneuvers are those with "voiding postponement."[34] The child postpones the voiding until overwhelmed by urgency, then makes a rush to the toilet but often too late so that there is some urge incontinence on the way. A recent study, comparing a cohort of children with "classical" urge syndrome to another group considered to have voiding postponement, has reported a significantly higher frequency of clinically relevant behavioral symptoms in the postponers than in children with urge syndrome. The authors conclude that their findings "support the entity of voiding postponement as an acquired or behavioural syndrome."

Dysfunctional voiding

Dysfunctional voiding (detrusor–sphincter dyscoordination in earlier terminology) is defined as intermittent voiding due to contractions of the sphincter and the pelvic floor muscles, in neurologically normal individuals, often girls 6–12 years of age. The cause of the dysfunctional voiding and also the urge syndrome is believed to lie in the persistence of an immature bladder control.[35] In response to the uninhibited contractions during toilet training most children may "learn" to contract the sphincter to avoid wetting,[4,36,37] and many of these girls evolve a form of urge-syndrome as they learn to suppress the urge and voiding by sphincter contractions and different holding maneuvers like squatting (Vincent's sign).[37,38]

These patients void in small portions with a staccato or fractionated (interrupted) uroflow curve, leaving residual urine in the bladder. This disorder, as well as voiding postponement, is often combined with constipation and encopresis.[39,40]

Detrusor underactivity ("lazy bladder syndrome")

The term lazy bladder has been used to characterize particularly girls with infrequent voiding and poor detrusor function (detrusor underactivity). It affects somewhat older girls (>10 years of age). The girls have learned to suppress the urge to void and they empty their bladders 1–3 times a day.[6,41] The detrusor becomes decompensated and the bladder capacity is increased and it empties poorly. This syndrome most often presents as chronic or recurrent UTI, with or without incontinence and often vesicoureteral reflux. A characteristic finding is that the child has to strain and often use the abdominal muscles to start and maintain micturition. Postvoid residual is always present but may vary considerably in the same patient. Detrusor underactivity may, in some children, be the end point of a pathogenetic cascade, starting with urge syndrome due to idiopathic overactive bladder (probably genetically determined), continuing with dysfunctional voiding with sphincter overactivity (in an attempt to keep dry), and ending up with increasing residual urine volumes distending the bladder with subsequent loss of detrusor contractile force.[42]

Complications

The most important complications to dysfunctional voiding and detrusor underactivity ("lazy bladder") are incontinence, recurrent urinary tract infection and, in many cases, vesicoureteral reflux.

Urinary tract infections and other bladder-related problems are common not only among children with daytime incontinence, but also bedwetters or former bedwetters.[43]

Regular and complete voidings are the most efficient ways to prevent urinary infection that may induce a temporary detrusor overactivity and more importantly girls with asymptomatic bacteriuria (ABU) have symptoms of an overactive bladder, such as urgency and incontinence, in a high percentage.[40,44] Bladder dysfunction may, in some cases, be the cause of vesicoureteral reflux (VUR) in girls, and the VUR may aggravate and perpetuate the dysfunctional bladder.[36,45–47] It is generally considered that conservative treatment of reflux in a patient with non-neuropathic bladder–sphincter dysfunction will be unsuccessful as long as the dysfunction persists. Therefore, rehabilitation of the bladder is important in the treatment of VUR in these patients. The presence of reflux in those patients(mainly girls) may also be the cause of bladder dysfunction and not the result. The anomaly of the ureteric entrance may in some children affect the trigone and the detrusor and thus a non-invasive early treatment of VUR may, in many cases, enhance the cure of bladder dysfunction.[47,48]

It may also be noted that some children with secondary incontinence and urge syndrome or dysfunctional voiding may be victims of child abuse. This may be difficult to prove but should be kept in mind. A significant proportion of adult women with complex urinary symptoms have reported sexual abuse as a child.[17]

Treatment

Urotherapy has been defined as "non-surgical, non-pharmacological treatment for lower urinary tract function of neurogenic and non-neurogenic bladders.[41,49–51]

It is a cognitive-behavioral training, teaching children to recognize and employ their cerebral centers to achieve command over their lower urinary tract. It includes information about normal bladder function and explanations on why the child with bladder dysfunction deviates from the normal. Instruction about what to do about it, and support and encouragement to go through with the training program are essential ingredients in urotherapy.

Urotherapy also includes pelvic floor training, biofeedback (in particular during uroflow), behavioral modification (advice for regular habits regarding meals, drinks, voiding, defecation, and sleep), electrical neurostimulation, and clean intermittent catheterization (instruction and follow-up of CIC in patients with neurogenic bladder and non-neurogenic underactive detrusor).[31,52]

Urotherapy cures about 75% of children with overactive bladder and dysfunctional voiding.[49] However, the non-responders to bladder training and/or anticholinergics should be referred to specialized centers for further urodynamic investigations and eventually biofeedback training.[35,42]

Defecation and voiding are closely linked and the dysfunction of one cannot be properly evaluated without consideration of the other. Thus many of the children with bladder dysfunction also have constipation and therefore an active treatment of the constipation should be included in the urotherapy. In a recent study[53] daytime wetting was strongly associated with fecal incontinence, whereas fecal incontinence and nocturnal enuresis lacked a significant association.

Table 50.2. Treatment

I. Urge and urge incontinence
Girls and boys 5–10 years.

- "Information" about the good prognosis and the maturation of the bladder function and the high "spontaneous cure rate" (15%–20% per year)
- Simple bladder training with "timed micturitions"
- In severe cases controlled by urotherapist
- Add Oxybutynin or Tolteridin in children with frequency and/or incontinence

Most of the children with the urge syndrome have a good prognosis. Early recognition and information is essential.

Table 50.3. Treatment

Dysfunctional voiding
Mainly schoolgirls >6 years of age

- Information – learn how to void
- Urotherapy
- Careful follow-up with regular control-visits and control of flow and residual urine
- Treatment of constipation
- Antibiotic prophylaxis

75% are cured by urotherapy. Early recognition and treatment essential for the outcome.

Table 50.4. Treatment

III. Detrusor underactivity ("lazy bladder")
A severe condition mainly affecting schoolgirls >9 years of age

- Urotherapy
- Careful follow-up with regular control-visits and control of flow and residual urine
- Treatment of constipation
- Sometimes biofeedback-training
- Antibiotic prophylaxis
- In girls with the more severe emptying difficulties
  - Electrostimulation or
  - CIC

In all children with signs and symptoms of detrusor underactivity a long-term follow-up into adulthood is mandatory.

Pharmacological treatment, i.e., Desmopressin, can be used in nocturnal enuresis. There are numerous controlled studies on the efficacy and safety of Desmopressin in children showing clinical good results with 50%–70% full response.[3,19,54] Some children have nocturnal enuresis in combination with an overactive bladder where Desmopressin can be used in combination with anti-cholin ergic or anti-muscarinic drugs. Regarding the pharmacological treatment of overactive bladder, oxybutynin and tolteridin have been used and studied and have good tolerability and efficacy particularly in children with urge incontinence combined with frequency.[6,32,55] In almost all patients the pharmacological treatment should be combined with urotherapy.

Outcome measures for enuresis and "non-neuropathic bladder–sphincter dysfunction"

Assessment of treatment outcome should be based on pretreatment baseline registration of the frequency of incontinent episodes, of bedwetting and/or day wetting. The outcome of different treatment regimens should be given as percentage reduction of the wetting episodes compared to baseline, and grouped as full response, response, partial response, or non-response to therapy. It should be clear that no therapy is fully successful until the child can stay dry after discontinuing treatment.[3,7]

The definition of immediate result of treatment:

- non-response: <50% reduction of wet episodes
- partial response: 50% to 89% reduction.
- response: >90% reduction.
- full response: 100% or less than one incontinent episode per month.

Post-treatment evaluation of surgical or medical therapy of incontinence should be conducted no less often than 1, 6 and 12 months after treatment. The definitions of the long-term result of treatment:

- relapse: more than one accident per month
- continued success: no relapse in 6 months after treatment
- complete success: no relapse in two years after treatment

Evaluation should be done at yearly intervals thereafter and continued as long as possible, preferably for at least 5 years. Questionnaires and frequency–volume charts, used in the diagnosis of incontinence, are the most important tools in reporting on outcome and results of therapeutic interventions.

Long-term follow-up studies

The prevalence of urinary incontinence in adulthood has been extensively studied in different epidemiological reports but most of them concern adult women and only a few studies of young women from late adolescence have been included.[16,56,57] It has been shown that the proportions of types of incontinence differ by age. A survey of older women suggests that mixed incontinence predominates.[21] A survey of young and middle-aged women suggests that pure stress incontinence predominates in that age group.[23,28,58] In a study by Hannested *et al.*[22] the entire age range was included and it demonstrates a fairly regular increase in prevalence of mixed incontinence across the age range, and a regular decrease in prevalence of stress incontinence.

Several different risk factors for future urinary incontinence have been studied,[58–60] but in only a few the bladder dysfunction and/or nocturnal enuresis in childhood have been included as a possible risk factor. Thus, these factors deserve more attention and children should be followed over many years into adulthood. Such a controlled study design is necessary because the effect of childhood incontinence may only become clear years later when the patient is older.

The prevalence of nocturnal enuresis in adolescence and adulthood have been well studied, but the prevalence of daytime wetting or combined daytime and nocturnal wetting in childhood has been poorly investigated and no true longitudinal cohort studies have been published.

Enuresis: long-term outcome without treatment

The prevalence of nocturnal enuresis at the age of 5, 7 and 10 years is approximately 25, 10 and 5%, respectively.[10,61–63] A small percentage of teenagers still wet their beds.[64] There are no major ethnic or geographic differences in this regard.

The often quoted study by Forsythe and Redmond indicates a spontaneous resolution rate of 15% per year from the age of 5 to 19.[65] The problem here is that this is almost the only estimation we have, since nowadays, fortunately, enuretic children are not left untreated. The short observational study by Monda and Husman, however, supports the findings by Forsythe.[66] Although enuresis tends to improve with age, there are still as many as 0.5% of the adult population who experience more or less frequent nocturnal accidents.[67]

Accordingly, a wait-and-see attitude towards a 5-year-old child with enuresis is warranted, but not with a teenager. The chance that the latter will "grow out of" his or her problem within a year or two is not high.

Long-term outcome with treatment

The efficacy and safety of desmopressin has been evaluated in a large number of trials.[28,54,68] It is clear that the frequency of nocturnal accidents is reduced in a majority of patients, but the proportion of children becoming completely dry is less than 50%.[54] Desmopressin may be regarded as symptomatic treatment in children with enuresis due to polyuria, and relapse is the rule after cessation of treatment: the research community is divided as regards its possible curative effects.

Fortunately, desmopressin has been shown to be remarkably safe, even for long-term treatment.[19,69,70] As long as the drug is not combined with excessive fluid intake, no short- or long-term safety concerns have as yet emerged.

The enuresis alarm is successful in between 50% and 80% of children.[71–73] Motivation, information, and follow-up are the major determinants for treatment success. The majority of children successfully treated with the alarm can be considered cured, but approximately 20% relapse after treatment and may need additional sessions.[74] The risks of treatment are nil, but the therapy puts great stress on the family and may be remembered many years afterwards.[75] There are no physical risks or adverse somatic consequences entailed with bedwetting *per se*, although underlying detrusor hyperactivity may certainly cause morbidity via urinary tract infections.

Long-term outcome of bladder dysfunction in childhood

Our knowledge of the future outcome of children with bladder dysfunction is based on a few studies that have followed a population into adolescence, but no particular group of patients have been followed into adulthood. Longitudinal study designs are needed to estimate incidence of voiding dysfunction in adolescence and adulthood and to describe the course of the condition and its different forms.

The urge syndrome is calculated to decrease by 14% per year[7,8,17] and thus most of the children with urge symptoms are cured spontaneously (particularly boys). Furthermore, an active "bladder training" in school-age children may add to the low incidence of urinary problems in late adolescence.[7,18,32] Swithinbank completed a prospective longitudinal study in 1176 British schoolchildren using a questionnaire at 11–12 years and again at 15–16 years. The authors noted a significant steady decrease in the prevalence of urinary symptoms with age. Enuresis decreased from 5% in the 11–12-year-olds to 1% in 15–16-year-olds and daytime symptoms and/or wetting decreased from 12% to 3% in 15–16-year-olds.[76]

Hellström *et al.* performed a follow-up study of 3556 Swedish schoolchildren[33] 10 years later (when they had reached the age of 17 years). A new questionnaire was sent to 1096 randomly selected adolescents from the total group and, in addition, all the children who had reported symptoms (imperative urge, day wetting, emptying difficulties, or bedwetting) were contacted. Of the 151 girls with symptoms at 7 years of age, only 16 still had bladder dysfunction (i.e., 20% cure rate/year), most of them with signs and symptoms of "dysfunctional voiding."

In the 208 boys with symptoms at 7 years of age (of whom 194 had nocturnal enuresis), only 8 still had symptoms of whom 4 still were bedwetting and the remainder had some urge and emptying difficulties (i.e., 25% cure rate/year).

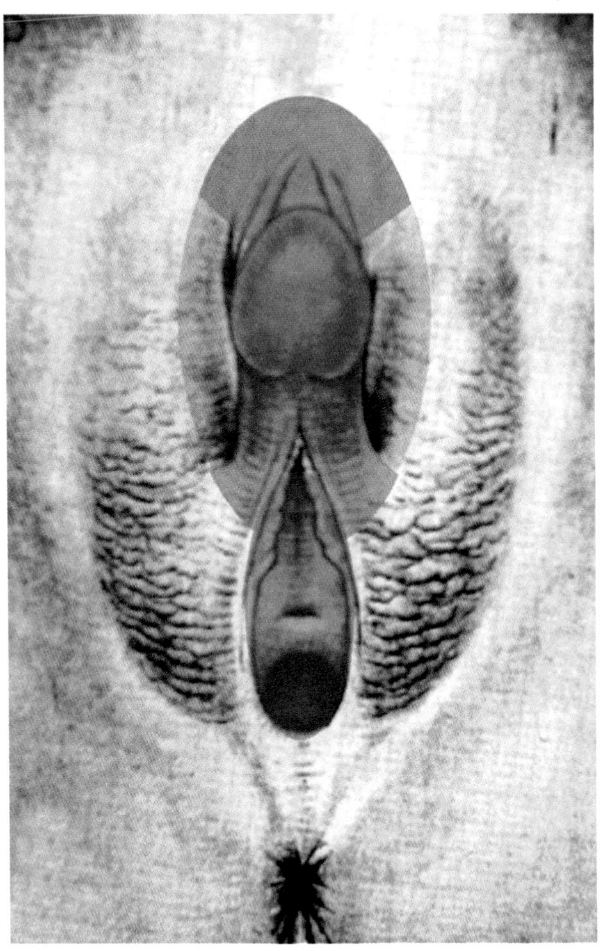

Plate 1 Genital sensitivity ratings for sexual intensity depicted by intensity of blue shaded areas (see Fig. 46.1).

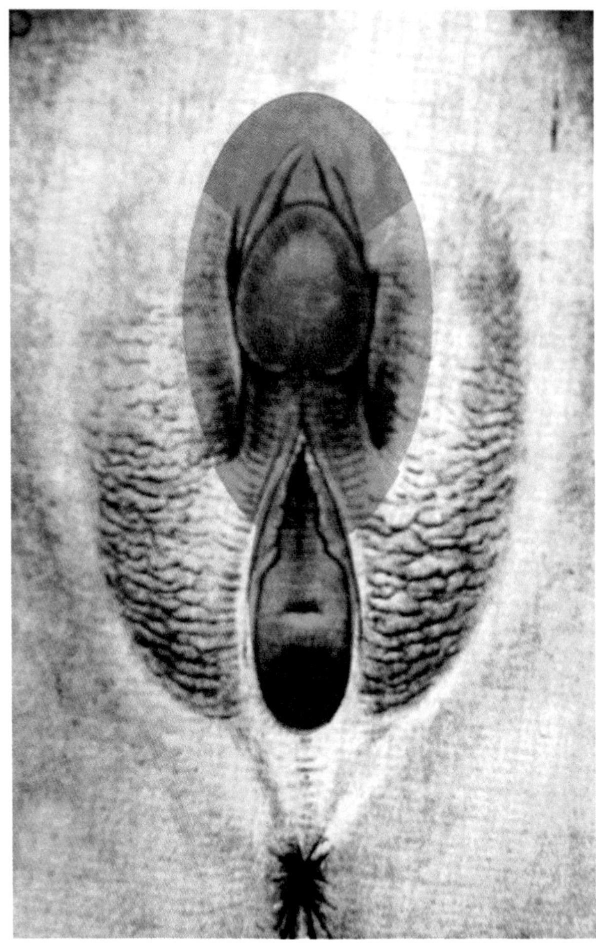

Plate 2 Genital sensitivity ratings, shown as shades of red, for ease of orgasm (see Fig. 46.2).

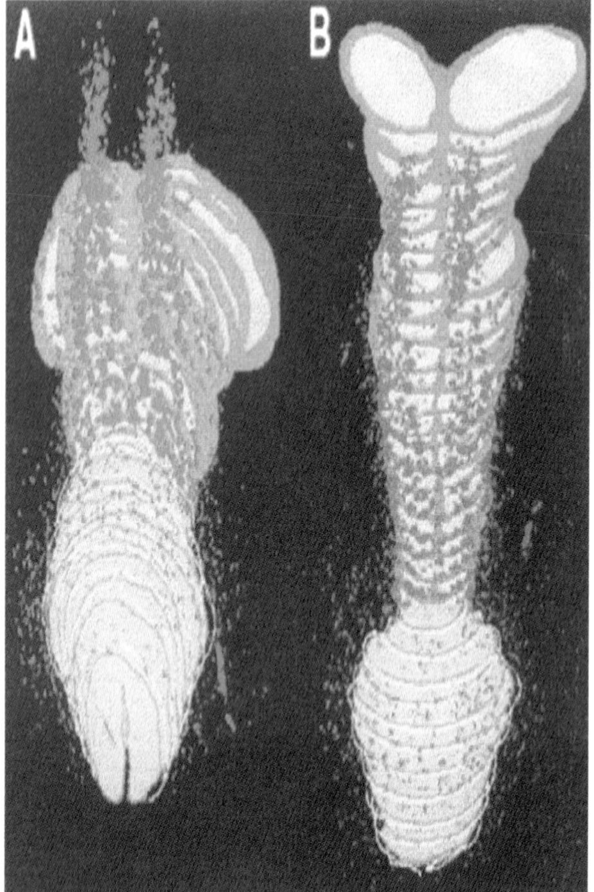

Plate 3 Innervation of the clitoris, shown overlying the corpora and glans. (Figure used with permission from *J. Urol.* and Lawrence Baskin.) (see Fig. 46.3.)

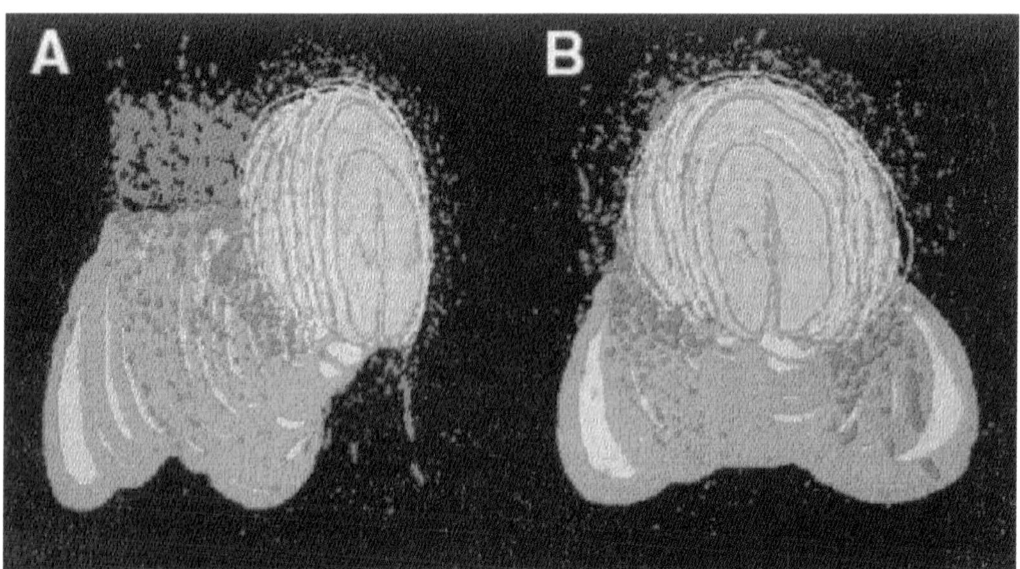

Plate 4 Innervation of the clitoris, depicting major areas of distribution dorsally and laterally. (Figure used with permission from *J. Urol.* and Lawrence Baskin.) (see Fig. 46.4.)

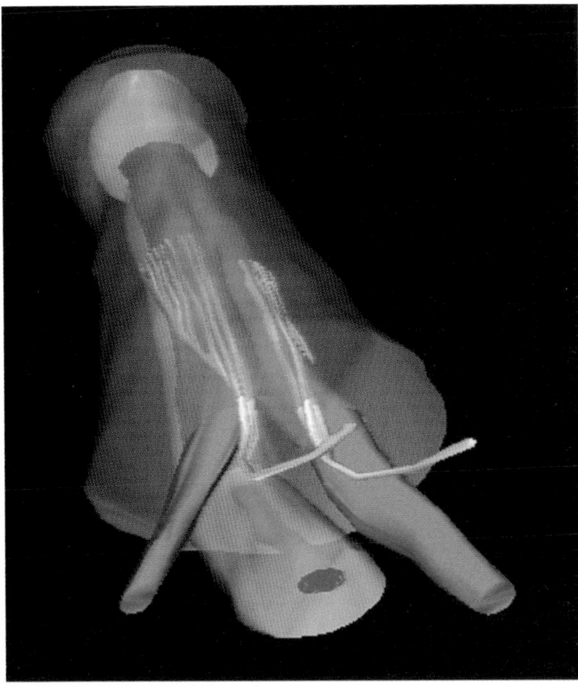

Plate 5 Penile neuroanatomy. 3-D reconstruction of the male human fetal penis depicting the relationship of the dorsal nerves, corporal and crural bodies, urethra and glans (see Fig. 47.1).

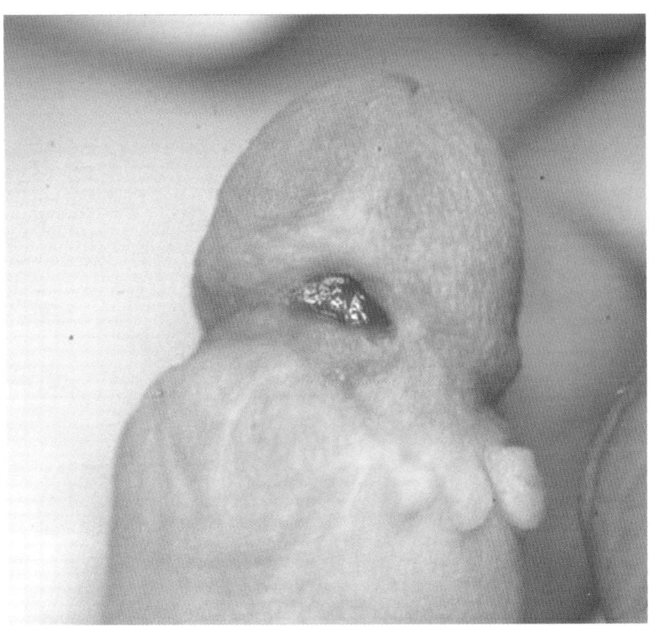

Plate 7 Urethrocutaneous fistula following circumcision, probably due to diathermy around the frenular artery. Note the prominent cross-hatching of the circumcision scar and poor cosmetic result (see Fig. 52.2).

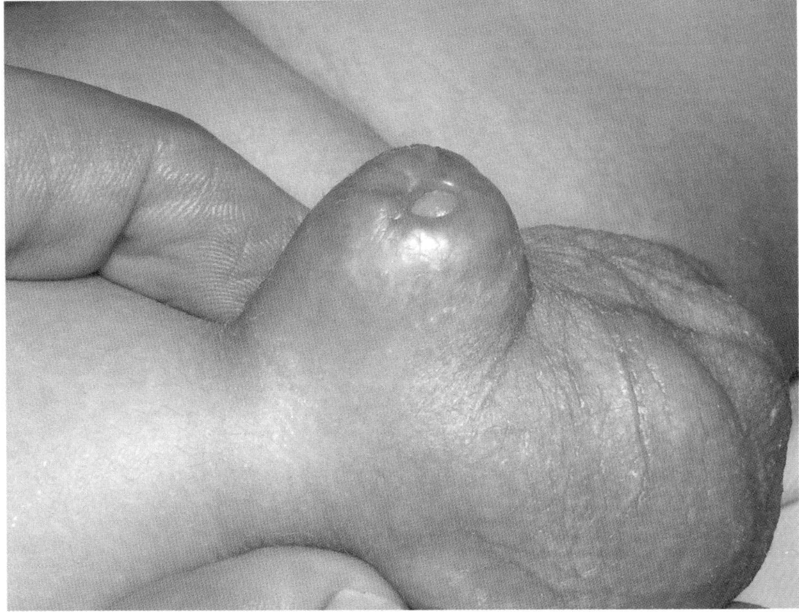

Plate 6 Recurrent phimosis due to contraction of the circumcision scar, concealing the glans (see Fig. 52.1).

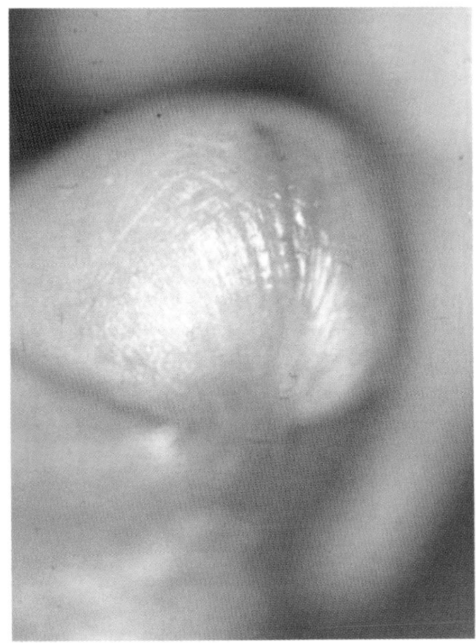

Plate 8 Normal slit-like urethral meatus (see Fig. 52.3).

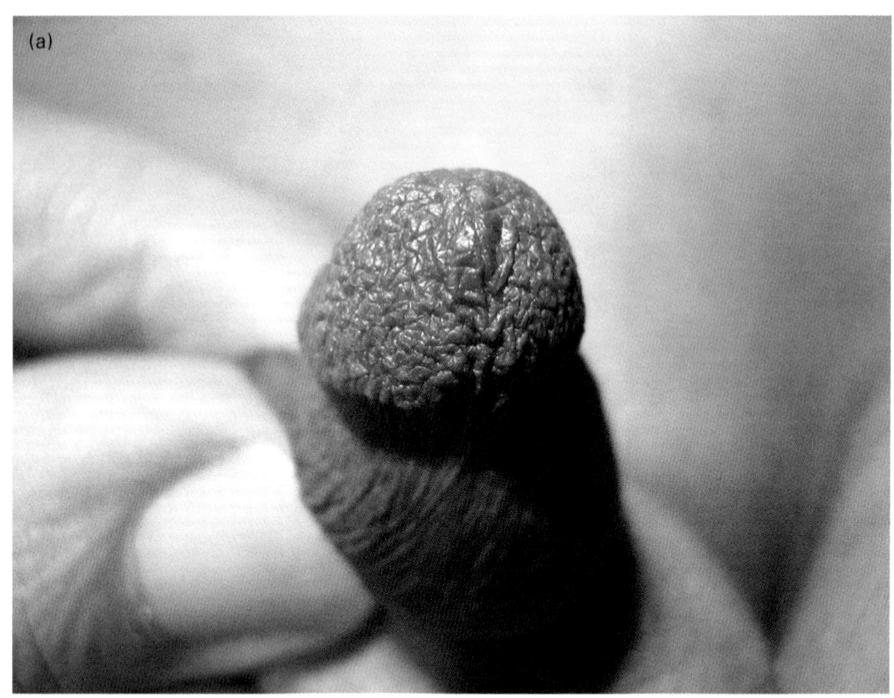

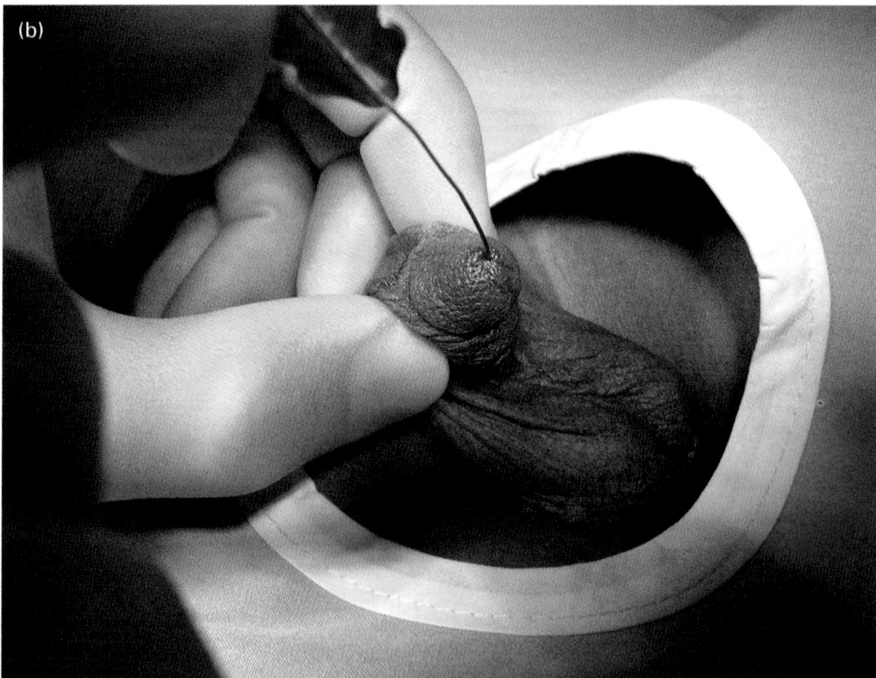

Plate 9 (a) and (b). Reduction of the meatal caliber in meatal stenosis so only a fine lachrymal probe can pass (see Fig. 52.4).

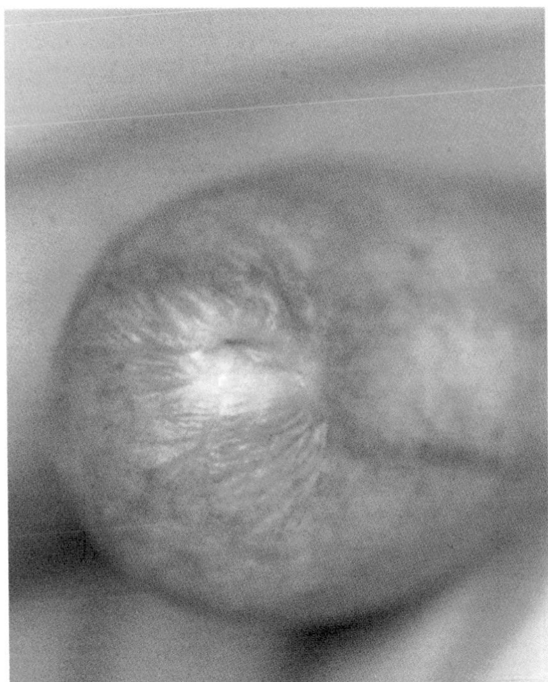

Plate 10 The sclerotic prepucial tip, which is characteristic of BXO (see Fig. 52.6).

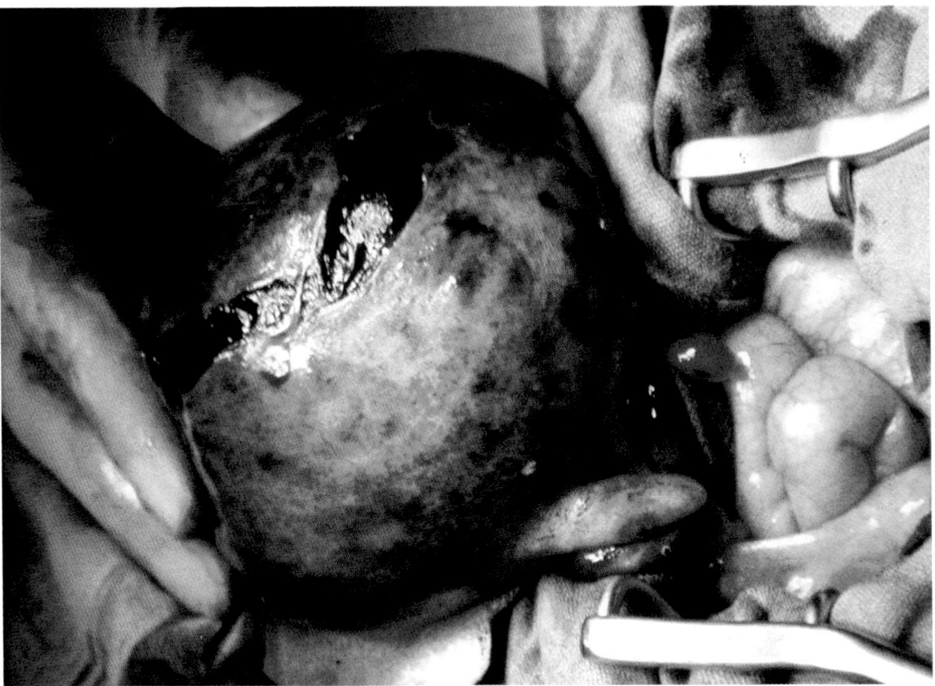

Plate 11 Acute abdomen in a 12-year-old girl. Ultrasound: left heterogeneous ovarian mass 11 × 13 cm. AFP: 123 mg/ml (N<10). Photo 1: Pfannenstiel incision in emergency: the torsed tumor is ruptured. Adenexectomy. No peroperative sign of malignancy. Histology: immature teratoma. The patient is lost to follow-up. 27 months later, new hospitalization for right subcostal pain: abdominal X-ray: numerous calcifications in the right liver lobe. AFP: 69400 (see Fig. 56.1).

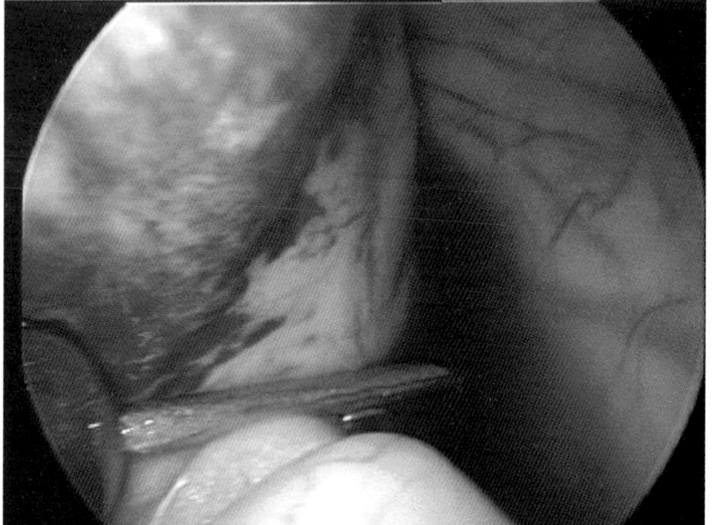

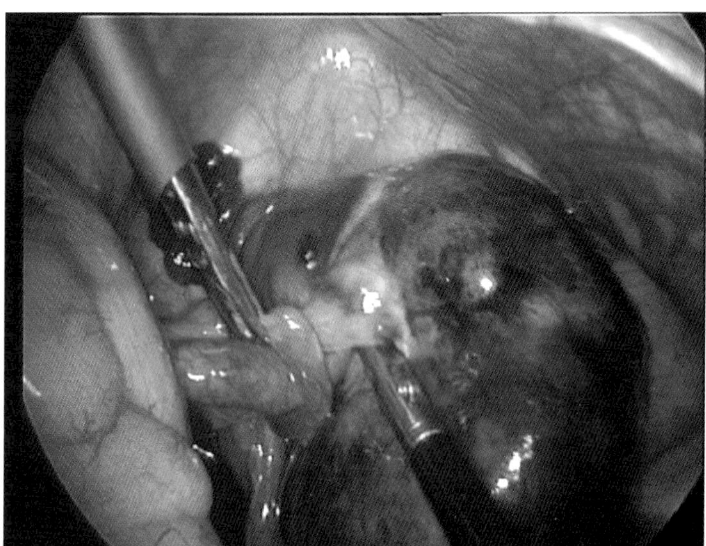

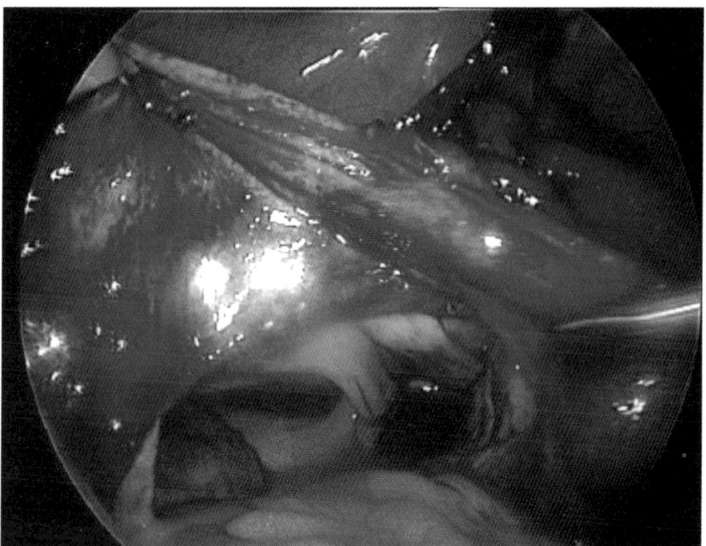

Plate 12 Illustration of new management of adnexal torsion. Acute abdomen in a 13-years-old girl. Ultrasound: torsion of the right adnexa with a 10 cm heterogeneous mass. Marker level: normal. Emergency laparoscopy: view at the beginning. Photo 1: total abdominal exploration (negative in this case) and aspiration of peritoneal ascites in the pouch of Douglas (negative cytology). Photo 2: laparoscopic detorsion with improvement in appearance of ovary, allowing immediate laparoscopic cystectomy. Photo 3: cystectomy by stripping technique after puncture of the cystpuncture, extraction in a bag, and oophoropexy of the ipsilateral ovary. Histology: mucinous cystadenoma (see Fig. 56.2).

From the randomized group, 21 teenagers had symptoms of whom 14 reported them as new.

It was concluded that symptoms of bladder disturbances occurred at a low frequency in children aged 17 years and they were only mild or moderate.

Similar prevalence was found in studies from other countries.[7,9,12] This clearly shows that most of the minor "bladder problems" tend to disappear with time and few of the children with symptoms and signs of an overactive bladder will have problems continuing into adulthood.

However, some of these children with urge incontinence may very well turn into "dysfunctional voiders" later in childhood and the fate of these children in adulthood is not well known. In a recent follow-up study on girls with severe dysfunctional problems and incontinence in adolescence Yang *et al.*[76] found that[77] (30%) of the girls ([27] patients) still suffered from the same problems in adulthood. However, 30% were cured with "conservative" treatment and 30% were lost to follow-up, but still had unresolved problems. The patients in this study comprised a group of 27 children with severe bladder dysfunctional problems and may indicate that the natural course in this group of children may be worse than had previously been expected.[42] There is a lack of the identification of prognostic risk factors and further prospective studies are needed to identify the children at risk. In a Danish study[78] 2613 women aged 30–59 years were randomly selected and responded to a questionnaire. They found that childhood bedwetting was associated with prevalent urge incontinence and also incontinence during sleep as a sign of a persisting overactive bladder. Kuh *et al.* found that childhood enuresis and/or childhood day-time incontinence is over-represented among middle-aged woman who suffer from urge incontinence.[62] Detrusor hyperactivity supposedly may persist even after the patient has become continent.

Moore *et al.*[79] studied a group of adults with idiopathic "detrusor instability" and found that a significant number had suffered from bedwetting as children (63% of men and 38% of women), probably those patients who suffered from detrusor-dependent enuresis and also had daytime urge symptoms. However, this is only speculation and the only way to show the future outcome of these children is to perform controlled prospective studies to find the natural course of bladder dysfunction in childhood.

Thus, the long-term outcome of these conditions is not well known and one can only speculate about the future outcome of girls with childhood bladder dysfunction and deduce the outcome from recent retrospective, interview studies on incontinent adult men and women. Today, in the Western world, nocturnal enuresis and daytime wetting are beginning to be recognized as disorders that can be cured if they are properly diagnosed and treated. However, even in developed countries, the problem is often neglected and parents do not seek help. Therefore, correct treatment may be delayed and in particular the more severe cases with bladder dysfunctions may persist in the long term.[77,80]

The psychological consequences of untreated or unsuccessfully treated nocturnal enuresis and/or bladder dysfunction should, however, not be underestimated. Enuretic children have been shown to have significantly lower self-esteem than unaffected children and children with combined daytime wetting and enuresis even more so – differences that disappear when the children became dry.[81] We can only speculate about the long-term social effects of this, but the impact of chronic low self-esteem in a growing individual may be considerable. Thus it is very important to recognize enuresis and bladder dysfunction in children over the age of 5 years and provide a correct diagnosis leading to information and treatment for the child.

REFERENCES

1. Abidari, J. M. & Shortliffe, L. M. D. Urinary incontinence in girls. *Urol. Clin. N. Am.* 2002; **29**:661–675.
2. Bloom, D. A., Faerber, G., & Bomalaski, M. D. Urinary incontinence in girls. Evaluation, treatment, and its place in the standard model of voiding dysfunctions in children. *Urol. Clin. North. Am.* 1995; **22**(3):521–38.
3. Hjalmas, K., Arnold, T., Bower, W. *et al.* on behalf of the International Children's Continence Society (ICCS). Nocturnal enuresis: an international evidence based management strategy. *J. Urol.* 2004; **171**:2545–2561.
4. Rushton, G. Wetting and functional voiding disorders. *Urol. Clin. North Am.* 1995; **22**:75–93.
5. Bloom, D. A., Sweley, W. M., Ritchey, M. L., & McGuire, E. J. Toilet habits and continence in children: an opportunity sampling in search of normal parameters. *J. Urol.* 1993; **149**:1087–90.
6. Mattsson, S. Urinary incontinence and nocturia in healthy schoolchildren. *Acta Pediatr*. 1994; **83**:950–4.
7. Bakker, E., van Sprundel, M., Van der Auwera, J. C., van Goold, J. D., & Wyndaele, J. J. Voiding habits and wetting in a population of 4,332 Belgian schoolchildren aged between 10 and 14 years. *Scand. J. Urol. Nephrol.* 2002; **36**(5):354–362.
8. Hellstrom, A. L., Hanson, E., Hansson, S., Hjalmas, K., & Jodal, U. Micturition habits and incontinence in 7-year-old Swedish school entrants. *Eur. J. Pediatr.* 1990; **149**:434–437.
9. Kajiwara, M., Inoue, K., Usui, A., Kurihara, M., & Usui, T. The micturition habits and prevalence of daytime urinary incontinence in Japanese primary school children. *J. Urol.* 2004; **171**(1):403–407.
10. Nevéus, T., Hetta, J., Cnattingius, S. *et al.* Depth of sleep and sleep habits among enuretic and incontinent children. *Acta Pædiatr.* 1999; **88**:748–752.
11. Sureshkumar, P., Bower, W., Craig, J. C., & Knight, J. F. Treatment of daytime urinary incontinence in children: a system-

atic review of randomized controlled trials. *J. Urol.* 20003; **170**(1):196–200, discussion 200.
12. Sureshkumar, P., Craig, J. C., Roy, L. P., & Knight, J. F. Daytime urinary incontinence in primary school children: a population-based survey. *J. Pediatr.* 2000; **137**(6):814–818.
13. Meadow, S. R. Day wetting. *Pediatr. Nephrol.* 1990; **4**:178–184.
14. Abrams, P., Cardozo, L., Fall, M. *et al.* The standardisation of terminology of lower urinary tract function: report from the Standardisation Sub-committee of the International Continence Society. *Neurourol. Urodyn.* 2002; **21**:167–178.
15. Hjälmås, K. Urinary incontinence in children: suggestions for definitions and terminology. *Scand. J. Urol. Nephrol.* Suppl., 1992; **141**:1.
16. Cheater, F. M. & Castleden, C. M. Epidemiology and classification of urinary incontinence. *Clin. Obstet. Gynaecol.* 2000; **14**:183.
17. Nijman, R. Classification and treatment of functional incontinence in children. *Br. J. Urol.* 2000; **85** Suppl. 3:43–46.
18. Swithinbank, L. V., Brookes, S. T., Shepherd, A. M., & Abrams, P. H. The natural history of urinary symptoms during adolescence. *Br. J. Urol.* Suppl. 1998; **81**:90.
19. Knudsen, U. B., Rittig, S., Nørgaard, J. P., Lundemose, J. B., Pedersen, E. B., & Djurhuus, J. C. Long-term treatment of nocturnal enuresis with desmopressin. A follow-up study. *Urol. Res.* 1991; **19**(4):237–240.
20. Hansen, A., Hansen, B., & Dahm, T. L. Urinary tract infection, day wetting and other voiding symptoms in seven- to eight-year-old Danish children. *Acta Paediatr.* 1997; **86**(12):1345–1349.
21. Hampel, C., Wienhold, D., Benken, N., Eggersmann, C., & Thurhoff, J. W. Definition of overactive bladder and epidemiology of urinary incontinence. *Urology* 1997; **50**:4.
22. Hannestad, Y. S., Rortveit, G., Sandvik, H., & Hunskaar, S. A community-based epidemiological survey of female urinary incontinence: the Norwegian EPINCONT study. *J. Clin. Epidemiol.* 2000; **53**:1150.
23. Stewart, W., Herzog, A. R., Wein, A. *et al.* Prevalence of overactive bladder in the US: results from the NOBLE program. 2nd International Consultation on Incontinence, abstract no 79, Paris 2001.
24. Swithinbank, L. V., Donovan, J. L., Du Heaume, J. C. *et al.* Urinary symptoms and incontinence in women: relationships between occurrence, age, and perceived impact. *Br. J. Gen. Pract.* 1999; **49**:897.
25. Rittig, S., Knudsen, U. B., Nørgaard, J. P., Pedersen, E. B., & Djurhuus, J. C. Abnormal diurnal rhythm of plasma vasopressin and urinary output in patients with enuresis. *Am. J. Physiol.* 1989; **256**:F664–F671.
26. Yeung, C. K., Chiu, H. N., & Sit, F. K. Bladder dysfunction in children with refractory monosymptomatic primary nocturnal enuresis. *J. Urol.* 1999; **162**(3 Pt 2):1049–1055.
27. Wolfish, N. M., Pivik, R. T., & Busby, K. A. Elevated sleep arousal thresholds in enuretic boys: clinical implications. *Acta Pædiatr.* 1997; **86**:381–384.
28. Tuvemo, T. DDAVP in childhood nocturnal enuresis. *Acta Pædiatr. Scand.* 1978; **67**:753–755.
29. Wille, S. Comparison of desmopressin and enuresis alarm for nocturnal enuresis. *Arch. Dis. Child.* 1986; **61**:30–33.
30. Lovering, J. S., Tallett, S. E., & McKendry, B. I. Oxybutynin efficacy in the treatment of primary enuresis. *Pediatrics* 1988; **82**; 104–106.
31. Hjälmås, K., Hoebeke, P. B., & dePaepe, H. Lower urinary tract dysfunction and urodynamics in children. *Eur. Urol.* 2000; **38**:655.
32. Hjalmas, K., Hellstrom, A. L., Mogren, K., Lackgren, G., & Stenberg, A. The overactive bladder in children: a potential future indication for tolterodine. *BJU Int.* 2001; **87**:569–574.
33. Hellstrom, A., Hanson, E., Hansson, S., Hjalmas, K., & Jodal, U. Micturition habits and incontinence at age 17 -reinvestigation of a cohort studied at age 7. *Br. J. Urol.* 1995; **76**(2):231–234.
34. Lettgen, B., von Gontard, A., Olbing, H., Heiken-Löwenau, C., Gaebel, E., & Schmitz, I. Urge incontinence and voiding postponement in children: somatic and psychosocial factors. *Acta Pædiatr.* 2002; **91**:978–984.
35. Hoebeke, P., Van Laecke, E., Van Camp, C., Raes, A., & Van De Walle, J. One thousand video-urodynamic studies in children with non-neurogenic bladder sphincter dysfunction. *BJU Int.* 2001; **87**:575–580.
36. Allen, T. D. Vesicoureteral reflux as a manifestation of dysfunctional voiding. In Hodson, J. & Kincaid-Smith, P. eds. *Reflux Nephropathy.* Chapter 18, New York: Masson Publishing Co, 1979:171–180.
37. Bauer, S. B. Special considerations of the overactive bladder in children. *Urology* 2002; **60**(5 Suppl 1):43–48; discussion 49.
38. Chiozza, M. L. Dysfunctional voiding. *Pediatr. Med. Chir.* 2002; **24**(2):137–140.
39. von Gontard, A. *Enkopresis: Erscheinungsformen – Diagnostik – Therapie.* Stuttgart: Kohlhammer Verlag, 2004.
40. Hansson, S. Urinary incontinence in children and associated problems. *J. Urol. Nephrol.* Suppl. 1992; **141**:47–55.
41. Hoebeke, P., Renson, C., Raes, A., Vanlaecke, E., & Van de Walle, J. Pelvic floor spasms in children: an unknown condition responding well to pelvic floor therapy. *BJU Int.* 2003; **91** Suppl 1:19.
42. Hobeke, P. New insights in diagnosis and treatment of non-neuropathic bladder-sphincter dysfunction in children. *Thesis. Gent*. 1998.
43. Hellstöm, A.-L., Hanson, E., Hansson, S., Hjälmås, K., & Jodal, U. Association between urinary symptoms at 7 years old and previous urinary tract infection. *Arch. Dis. Child.* 1991; **66**:232–234.
44. Hansson, S., Hjalmas, K., Jodal, U., & Sixt, R. Lower urinary tract dysfunction in girls with untreated asymptomatic or covert bacteriuria. *J. Urol.* 1990; **143**:333–335.
45. Koff, S. A. Relationsship between dysfunctional voiding and reflux. *J. Urol.* 1992; **148**:1703–1705.
46. Sillén, U., Hjälmås, K., Aili, M., Bjure, J., Hansson, E., & Hansson, S. Pronunced detrusor hypercontractility in infants with gross bilateral reflux. *J. Urol.* 1992; **148**:598.
47. Snodgrass, W. Relationship of voiding dysfunction to urinary tract infection and vesicoureteral reflux in children. *Urology* 1991; **38**:341–344.

48. Läckgren, G. & Stenberg, A. Bladder dysfunction and VUR. Result of endoscopic treatment with Deflux. Abstract. ICCS Hongkong, 2002.
49. Hellstrom, A. L., Hjalmas, K., & Jodal, U. Rehabilitation of the dysfunctional bladder in children: method and 3-year follow-up. *J. Urol.* 1987; **138**:847–849.
50. Hobeke, P., Van de Walle, J., Theunis, M., De Paepe, H., & Oosterlinck, Renson, C. Outpatient pelvic floor therapy in girls with daytime incontinence and dysfunctional voiding. *Urology* 1996; **48**:923–927.
51. Vijverberg, M. A., Elzinga-Plomp, A., Messer, A. P., Van Gool, J., & de Jong, T. P. Bladder rehabilitation, the effect of a cognitive training programme on urge incontinence. *Eur. Urol.* 1997; **31**:68–72.
52. Kuh, D., Cardozo, L., & Hardy, R. Urinary incontinence in middle aged women: childhood enuresis and other lifetime risk factors in a British prospective cohort. *J. Epidemiol. Commun. Health* 1999; **53**(8):453–458.
53. Soderstrom, U., Hoelcke, M., Alenius, L., Soderling, A. C., Hjern, A. Urinary and faecal incontinence: a population-based study. *Acta Paediatr*. 2004; **93**(3):386–389.
54. Hjälmås, K., Hanson, E., Hellström, A.-L., Kruse, S., & Sillén, U. Long-term treatment with desmopressin in children with primary monosymptomatic nocturnal enuresis: an open multicentre study. Swedish Enuresis Trial (SWEET) Group. *Br. J. Urol.* 1998; **82**(5):704–709.
55. Reinberg, Y., Crocker, J., Wolper, J., & Vandersten, D. Therapeutic efficacy of extended release oxybutynin chloride, and immediate release and long acting tolterodine tartrate in children with diurnal urinary incontinence. *J. Urol.* 2003; **169**:317–319.
56. Hunskaar, S. One hundred and fifty men with urinary incontinence. I. Demography and medical history. *Scand. J. Prim. Health Care* 1992; **10**:21.
57. Hunskaar, S., Burgio, K., Diokno, A., Herzog, A. R., Hjalmas, K., & Lapitan, M. C. Epidemiology and natural history of urinary incontinence inwomen. *Urology* 2003; **62**:16–23.
58. Samuelsson, E., Victor, A., Tibblin, G. A population study of urinary incontinence and nocturia among women aged 20–59 years. Prevalence, well-being and wish for treatment. *Acta Obstet. Gynecol. Scand.* 1997; **76**:74.
59. Yarnell, J. W., Voyle, G. J., Richards, C. J., & Stephenson, T. P. The prevalence and severity of urinary incontinence in women. *J. Epidemiol. Commun. Health* 1981; **35**:71.
60. Kalo, B. B. & Bella, H. Enuresis: prevalence and associated factors among primary school children in Saudi Arabia. *Acta. Pædiatr.* 1996; **85**:1217–1222.
61. Laberge, L., Tremblay, R. E., Vitaro, F., & Montplaisir, J. Development of parasomnias from childhood to early adolescence. *Pediatrics* 2000; **106**:67–74.
62. van der Wal, M. E., Pauw-Plomp, H., & Schulpen, T. W. Bedplassen bij Nederlandse, Surinaamse, Marokkanse en Turkse kinderen van 3–4, 5–6 enl 11–12 jaar. *Ned. Tijdschr. Geneeskd.* 1996; **140**(48):2410–2414.
63. Marugan de Miguelsanz. J. M., Lapena Lopez de Armentia, S., Rodriguez Fernandez, L. M. *et al.* Analisis epidemiologico de la secuencia de control vesical y prelvalencia de enuresis nocturna en ninos de la provincia de leon. *An. Esp. Pediatr.* 1996; **44**(6):561–567.
64. Forsythe, W. I. & Redmond, A. Enuresis and spontaneous cure rate: study of 1129 enuretics. *Arch. Dis. Child.* 1974; **49**:259–263.
65. Monda, J. M. & Husmann, D. A. Primary nocturnal enuresis: a comparison among, observation., imipramine, desmopressin acetate and bed-wetting alarm systems. *J. Urol.* 1995; **154**(2 Pt 2):745–748.
66. Hirasing, R. A., van Leerdam, F. J., Bolk-Bennink, L., & Janknegt, R. A. Enuresis nocturna in adults. *Scand. J. Urol. Nephrol.* 1997; **31**(6):533–536.
67. Aladjem, M., Wohl, R., Boichis, H., Orda, S., Lotan, D., & Freedman, S. Desmopressin in nocturnal enuresis. *Arch. Dis. Child.* 1982; **57**:137–140
68. Fjellestad-Paulsen, A., Laborde, K., Kindermans, C., & Czernichow, P. Water-balance hormones during long-term follow-up of oral DDAVP treatment in diabetes insipidus. *Acta Pædiatr.* 1993; **82**(9):752–757.
69. Läckgren, G., Nevéus, T., Lilja, B., & Stenberg, A. Desmopressin in the treatment of severe nocturnal enuresis in adolescents – a 7-year follow-up study. *Br. J. Urol.* 1998; **81**(Suppl 3):17–23.
70. Berg, I. B., Forsythe, W. I., & McGuire, R. Response of bed wetting to the enuresis alarm: influence of psychiatric disturbance and maximum functional bladder capacity. *Arch. Dis. Child.* 1982; **57**:394–396.
71. Bollard, J. & Nettelbeck, T. A comparison of dry-bed training and standard urine-alarm conditioning treatment of childhood bedwetting. *Beh. Res. Ther.* 1981; **19**(3):215–226.
72. Devlin, J. B. & O'Cathain, C. Predicting treatment outcome in nocturnal enuresis. *Arch. Dis. Child.* 1990; **65**(10):1158–1161.
73. El-Anany, F. G., Maghraby, H. A., Shaker, S. E., & Abdel-Moneim, A. M. Primary nocturnal enuresis: a new approach to conditioning treatment. *Urology* 1999; **53**(2):405–409.
74. Bengtsson, B. Sök hjälp tidigt för barn med enures. Råd från vuxna som haft svår nattväta som barn. *Läkartidningen* 1997; **94**(4):245–246.
75. Swithinbank, L. V., Carr, J. C., & Abrams, P. H. Longitudinal study of urinary symptoms in children. *Scand. J. Urol. Nephrol.* Suppl. 1994; **163**:67.
76. Yang, C. C. & Mayo, M. E. Morbidity of NNBSB syndrome. *Urology* 1997; **49**:445–448.
77. Foldspang, A. & Mommsen, S. Adult female urinary incontinence and childhood bedwetting. *J. Urol.* 1994; **152**(1):85–88.
78. Moore, K. H., Richmond, D. H., & Parys, B. T. Sex distribution of adult idiopathic detrusor instability in relation to childhood bed-wetting. *Br. J. Urol.* 1991; **68**:479–482.
79. Holst, K. & Wilson, P. D. The prevalence of female urinary incontinence and reasons for not seeking treatment. *N. Z. Med. J.* 1988; **101**:756.
80. Hägglöf, B., Andrén, O., Bergström, E., Marklund, L., & Wendelius, M. Self-esteem before and after treatment in children with nocturnal enuresis and urinary incontinence. *Scand. J. Urol. Nephrol.* 1997; **31**(Suppl. 183):79–82.
81. Schulman, S. L., Quinn, C. K., Plachter, N., & Kodman-Jones, C. Comprehensive management of dysfunctional voiding. *Pediatrics* 1999; **103**(3):E31.

51

Undescended testes

John M. Hutson

Department of General Surgery, Royal Children's Hospital, Parkville, Victoria, Australia

Since ancient times, it has been recognized that the testis needs to be fully descended in the scrotum for normal functioning. Indeed, the testis derives its name from the Latin word "witness," following the custom in Roman times to hold the testicles when taking an oath.[1] Hence, one of the primary concerns of surgeons has been the development of surgical procedures to place an undescended testis into the scrotum. In recent years there have been rapid changes in attitudes to long-term outcomes: not that long ago, success of surgery was measured by such crude criteria as cosmetic result or survival, which could be determined immediately. However, now the profession and the community require and expect a much higher standard, such that at present the yardstick for success in the management of undescended testes is normal fertility and a low risk of malignancy in adult life. Community attitudes, and knowledge about long-term outcomes, are changing rapidly, as evidenced by the fact that standard texts only 25 years ago did not contain any significant information about long-term malignancy risks.[2]

Etiology of the undescended testis

Most undescended testes are probably caused by abnormal migration of the gubernaculum during the inguinoscrotal phase of testicular descent. Testicular descent normally begins at about 10 weeks of gestation, shortly after the onset of sexual differentiation. Two morphological steps in descent can be identified: initial relative movement of the testis (compared with the ovary) from the urogenital ridge to the inguinal region, known as transabdominal descent; and migration from the inguinal canal to the scrotum, known as inguinoscrotal descent.[3] During the first phase, which occurs at approximately 10–15 weeks of gestation, the gubernaculum or genito-inguinal ligament enlarges in the male, but not in the female. The enlarged gubernacular fold effectively anchors the testis near the inguinal region while the embryo is enlarging. This prevents the testis from moving away from the inguinal region as the ovary tends to do. In the second phase of descent, at between 28 and 35 weeks, the gubernaculum migrates from the inguinal canal across the pubic bone and into the scrotum. The end of the gubernaculum is gelatinous mesenchyme while the proximal gubernaculum is hollowed out by a peritoneal diverticulum, the processus vaginalis which contains the testis. The cremaster muscle develops in the outer rim of the gubernaculum outside the peritoneal diverticulum. The gubernaculum is supplied by the genitofemoral nerve, both before, during and after migration to the scrotum.[4]

Normal testicular descent is controlled by hormones. There is controversy about which hormones modulate the first and second stage.[5] Androgens have some role in the first phase, by stimulating regression of the cranial suspensory ligament, which then allows the testis to descend. But it does not appear to have a role in stimulating enlargement of the gubernaculum. The second phase of descent is controlled by androgen, but its action on the gubernaculum appears to be indirect. The primary hormone controlling descent is now known to be insulin-like hormone 3 (INSL3) which is produced by Leydig cells (as well as androgen).[6] Mullerian inhibiting substance/anti-Mullerian hormone appears to be a secondary factor.[7] Recent evidence suggests that the direction of gubernacular migration may be controlled by androgen indirectly via the genitofemoral nerve. A neurotransmitter released from the nerve,

Pediatric Surgery and Urology: Long-term Outcomes, Mark Stringer, Keith Oldham, Pierre Mouriquand.

Table 51.1. Etiology of cryptorchidism

Unknown
Mechanical failure of gubernacular migration
Hormone deficiency syndrome (T, Insl3, MIS)
Placental dysfunction (hCG deficiency)
Abdominal wall defects
Posterior urethral valve (prune belly syndrome)
Spina bifida/cerebral palsy
Chromosomal defects
Multiple malformation syndromes

calcitonin gene-related peptide (CGRP), is implicated in normal testicular descent of rodents and in rodent models with undescended testes.[8]

One cause of abnormal inguinoscrotal migration of the gubernaculum may be a lack of CGRP released from the genitofemoral nerve. Alternatively, the nerve may be abnormally sited so that migration is stimulated in an ectopic direction (e.g., perineal testis).[9]

There are numerous causes for undescended testes (Table 51.1), as normal descent is multiphasic, with different morphology, hormones, and anatomical regulators. Rare hormonal deficiency syndromes of testosterone (e.g., partial androgen insensitivity) or Mullerian inhibiting substance (e.g., persistent Mullerian duct syndrome) do cause undescended testes, but in most children these are not present. Deficiency of INSL3 as a cause of cryptorchidism has not been identified.[10] It is presumed that, in the common variety of undescended testis, there is a mechanical failure of gubernacular migration. This could be secondary to transient androgen deficiency in the third trimester, perhaps caused by placental insufficiency, CGRP deficiency within the genitofemoral nerve, or anatomical defects within the nerve itself. Also, the gubernaculum may have an intrinsic defect preventing it from responding to normal trophism by migration to the scrotum. Various mechanical causes, such as abdominal wall defects or massive prenatal bladder distension, can cause undescended testis. In addition, there are various chromosomal and multiple malformation syndromes, as well as neurological abnormalities, causing cryptorchidism.

The multitude of putative causes of cryptorchidism may produce different long-term outcomes. Also, a significant percentage of undescended testes may be acquired during early childhood, and are not present from birth. This controversial view has profound implications for long-term prognosis and is discussed more later. From a clinical perspective, most of the identified specific causes of undescended teste are rare by comparison with the common idiopathic variety. A simple mechanical failure of gubernacular migration is suspected, either because of an intrinsic mechanical defect or from secondary hormonal deficiency. It is this latter common form of undescended testis that prognostications should be centered around.

Classification of cryptorchidism

Undescended testis can be classified by etiology or position. The first phase of "descent" requires passive anchoring of the testis as the embryo grows and, consequently, intra-abdominal impalpable testes are uncommon. Most testes are palpable in the groin and might be called inguinal. The most common position for an undescended testis is just above and lateral to the external inguinal ring outside the abdominal musculature in the superficial inguinal pouch, described by Denis Browne.[11] There is controversy about whether such a testis is truly ectopic or is merely displaced into a position of lower pressure. Truly ectopic testes in the femoral region, perineum, or prepenile regions are quite rare.

Recent evidence suggests that some undescended testes present later in childhood, after being apparently normal in infancy. In the past, these testes were often called retractile.[12] More recently, some have been classified as ascending testes, which are defined as testes which descend late into the scrotum, in the first 3 months postnatally, but then ascend out of the scrotum again later in childhood.[13] Both ascending testes and severe retractile testes may represent acquired abnormality. In a recent study,[14] dissection within the spermatic cord in these children has revealed the presence of a fibrous string deep to the cremaster muscle and fascia. Transection of this fibrous string has allowed adequate elongation of the vas deferens and gonadal vessels for scrotal placement of the testis. Histological examination of the fibrous string has revealed residual peritoneal cells consistent with incomplete obliteration of the processus vaginalis. It has been proposed that cryptorchidism presenting later in childhood is not only acquired, but may be common, and secondary to incomplete disappearance of the processus vaginalis. Although this diagnosis remains controversial, it has the potential to confound previous long-term outcome studies, which may include an amalgam of congenital and acquired cryptorchid testes.

Current treatments

Current management of cryptorchidism is based on the premise that secondary testicular degeneration caused by

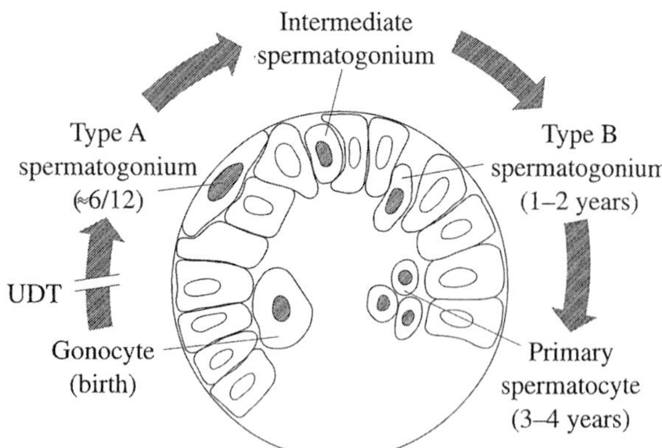

Fig. 51.1. Schematic of germ cell maturation in the postnatal human testis, showing where UDT causes delay and/or disruption of development.

high temperature can be prevented by early intervention.[15] The intra-abdominal core temperature is 3–4 degrees higher than the temperature of the scrotal testis.[16] Recent evidence shows that early postnatal germ cell development is deranged in the undescended testis (Fig. 51.1).[17,18]

Previously, it was well known that after puberty, the intra-abdominal testis suffered irreversible azoospermia, both in animals[19] and in humans.[15] Macroscopic atrophy in school-age children with cryptorchidism then became the criterion for intervention. Light microscopic changes in undescended testes can be identified in the third and fourth years.[20,21] Tubular dysplasia on electron microscopy can be identified in the second year of life.[22] Degeneration of testicular germ cells in the first 6–12 months[23] along with physiological derangements in hormone production by the undescended testis in the first year,[24–26] suggest that intervention must be very early if it is to prevent damage.

Although the evidence for early degeneration, presumed secondary, is substantial, the timing for surgery remains controversial, because previous studies looking at outcome have not demonstrated an association with age. A more detailed account of these studies is given later.

Despite the lack of evidence in humans that early surgery will prevent testicular degeneration, in animal models early surgery does prevent such degeneration.[27–30] However, a difficulty in extrapolation from the experimental rat arises because testicular descent in rats does not occur until puberty, in contrast to prenatal descent in humans. Orchidopexies in rats therefore, need only be done at puberty to demonstrate an effect of "early" surgery. This could be interpreted as suggesting that surgery should be done soon after the time of normal scrotal occupancy by the testis, which is puberty in rats or the neonatal period in humans.

The author now recommends orchidopexy at 6 months of age. Orchidopexy in small infants can be challenging, but in specialized pediatric surgical centers, operation at 6–12 months of age is quite satisfactory and does not appear to increase the risk of complications.[31] All newborn males should be examined carefully for the presence of testes within the scrotum. Those children in whom the testes are not located obviously at the bottom of the scrotum should be reviewed at 12 weeks of age. During that time, about half the cryptorchid testes will descend spontaneously. These children need no immediate intervention, but do require regular annual follow-up to ensure that they do not develop acquired ascending testes. In cases where the testes remain out of the scrotum at 12 weeks, referral for orchidopexy should occur soon after, with the exact timing of surgery dependent on the local circumstances and expertise of the surgeon. Testes that are in the scrotum at 3 months of age, but which do not have a completely dependent position, also should be followed carefully during childhood, to make sure they do not develop acquired maldescent.

The author's own choice of therapy is day surgical correction, with routine orchidopexy and mobilization of the inguinal testis, and surgical placement of the testis within the scrotum. Children presenting later in childhood with an apparent acquired undescended testis may be managed by a similar surgical approach or, alternatively, by using a scrotal approach as described by Bianchi and Squire.[32]

It is not the author's own policy to use hormonal therapy with either human chorionic gonadotrophin (hCG) or luteinizing hormone releasing hormone (LHRH), but these therapies remain in wide use throughout Europe and the USA. Various protocols are described to which the reader is referred.[33–36] Two simple protocols include intramuscular hCG administration at 100 IU twice a week for 3–4 weeks; alternatively, LHRH can be given as a spray at 100 μg in each nostril six times a day for 3–4 weeks.

The major dilemma in predicting long-term outcome for orchidopexy is that recent biological studies suggest that testicular function will be preserved only when surgery is done in infancy. As can be seen from Fig. 51.2, the recommended age for intervention has been falling progressively since the 1950s, and it has only been in the 1980s or 1990s that the recommended age lies within what would be regarded now as the correct range. If extrapolation from animal models and the current biological evidence acquired from human studies is correct, it means that we cannot predict optimal outcomes until children who have been operated on in the last 10–15 years have reached adult life. By contrast, adults operated on in a previous generation have had what is now regarded as inferior treatment,

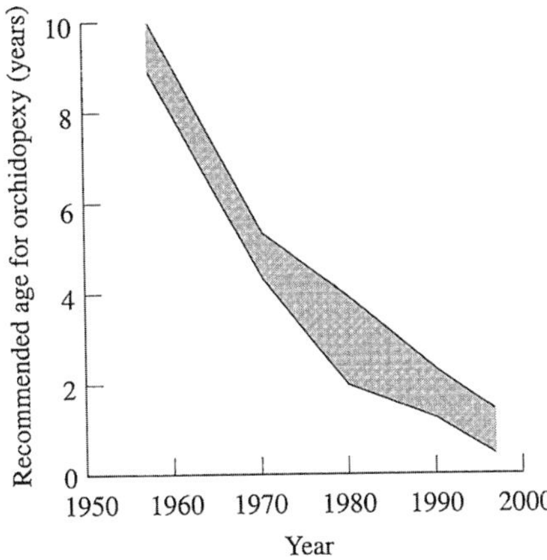

Fig. 51.2. Schematic graph of recommended age for orchidopexy (for congenital UDT) vs. age, showing a rapid fall in recent decades. Currently, orchidopexy is performed around 6 months of age in most pediatric centers.

and so the studies to be reported in the rest of this review need to be considered with some circumspection.

Early complications of surgery

The risk of complications after orchidopexy should be less than 5%, in experienced hands.[31] Atrophy of the testis after intraoperative damage to the testicular vessels is a serious but uncommon complication after orchidopexy. Infants who have a concomitant incarcerated or strangulated hernia are most at risk. Damage to the vas deferens with possible occlusion of the lumen may occur, but is not frequently reported because of difficulty in diagnosis. The use of diathermy or electrocautery has reduced the risk of hemorrhage from poor hemostasis.

With orchidopexy now frequent in infancy, the most common complication is wound infection. Both inguinal and scrotal incisions are at risk of sepsis in infants, but usually they respond to simple treatment. Secondary ascent of the testis out of the scrotum may occur after infection, poor mobilization, or inadequate fixation within the scrotum. Postoperative lymphedema of the testis resolves spontaneously after a few months.

Long-term outcomes

Testicular size and position

Orchidopexy results in an intrascrotal testis of reasonable size in most boys. In a review of 135 testes in 121 boys, 85% of the testes were intrascrotal at long-term follow-up after surgery at 6 years of age.[37] Testes initially beyond the inguinal canal were larger than those within the canal or abdomen. The latter had a higher incidence of persisting abnormality following orchidopexy, particularly failure of the testes to reach the scrotum, inadequate growth, or atrophy of the testes. Complete infarction of the testis occurred in approximately 3% of patients with an impalpable undescended testis. In another 15%–20% of patients with a high intra-abdominal testis, significant atrophy occurred requiring subsequent excision. Puri and Sparnon[38] found a significant correlation between the initial position of the testis and subsequent volume, in a group of 159 children operated on at approximately 9.8 years of age. Nineteen abdominal testes had an average testicular volume in adult life of 4.9 ml, compared with 9.8 ml in canalicular testes and 17 ml, in superficial inguinal pouch testes (Table 51.2).

Table 51.2. Testicular volumes after orchidopexy

Series	Patient numbers	Age at operation (y)	Testicular volume (ml)
Cortes *et al.*[83]	11	3–7 10–12	No difference between groups
Puri and Sparnon[38]	159	10 (7–13.6)	4.9 ± 3.5 abdominal (19) 9.8 ± 5.4 canalicular (36) 17.0 ± 4.9 SIP (119)
Schreiber *et al.*[39]	54	–	18.6 ± 4.0 normal 17.6 unilat. UDT 16.0 ± 4.9 bilat. UDT

SIP, superficial inguinal pouch. Numbers in parentheses in testicular volume column refer to testes.

Most authors have found that, in adults, testicular volume after childhood orchidopexy is slightly lower than normal,[39] although volume at operation has proven to be a poor predictor of germ cell count.[40] Reduced testicular volume is more marked in those with a past history of bilateral orchidopexy.[41,42] The highest incidence of testicular atrophy appears to occur after combined herniotomy and orchidopexy in infants presenting with a strangulated hernia. Exact figures are scarce, but the author's own anecdotal experience is that this difficult dissection may compromise the testicular vessels much more than routine orchidopexy. However, the overall risk of subsequent testicular atrophy with surgery in infancy appears to be low, as long as the surgeon has been trained in the surgery of infancy.[31]

Preoperative and postoperative gonadal position was documented in 1209 cryptorchid testes in 961 boys.[21] Only one-third of all "impalpable" testes were found in the abdomen, while a third were in the inguinal canal. Seven

Table 51.3. Paterniity after orchidopexy

Series	Patient numbers	Age at operation (y)	Successful paternity (%)	
			Unilateral	Bilateral
Gilhooly *et al.*[47]	145	NK	80	48
Cendron *et al.*[48]	40	7.0	87	33
Kumar *et al.*[49]	56	7–18	84	60
Lee[44]	467	NK	88	59
Lee and Coughlin[46]	408	NK	90	65 ($P < 0.001$)

Table 51.4. Semen analysis after orchidopexy

Series	Patient numbers	Age at operation (y)	Normal semen analysis (%)	
			Unilateral	Bilateral
Singer *et al.*[60]	25	6.2	70	40
Puri and O'Donnell[84]	142	7–13	74	30
Bremholm-Rasmussen *et al.*[41]	45	No surgery	NK	33
Okuyama *et al.*[56]	167	2–5	95	24
" " "	43	9–12	86	20
Grasso *et al.*[54]	91	14–29	17	NK
Cortes and Thorup[55]	90	13	NK	0
Mandat *et al.*[58]	135	3–15	53	26
Lee[44]	NK	NK	57	25
Mayr *et al.*[57]	46	2–12	46	32
Cortes *et al.*[53]	146	≤ 12	83	19

percent of impalpable testes were absent. Nearly all (96%) testes reached the scrotum, including 69% of initially intra-abdominal testes and 94% of canalicular testes. The authors concluded that even high testes can have a good result, contrary to common belief. In a selected group of 77 ascending testes, 38 were following previous herniotomy and 39 occurred spontaneously.[43] The final gonadal position was "excellent" in all but 6 instances.

Fertility and subsequent paternity

One way to assess long-term outcome for fertility is to document successful paternity (Table 51.3). Lee[44] in an extensive review of the literature, noted that 15%–20% of normal married couples are infertile, and in a quarter to a third of these, the abnormality is identified in the male.[45] Summarizing a large number of other studies, Lee found that 81.4% of married men with a past history of unilateral undescended testis had offspring. This compared with 50.8%, of married men with offspring who had a previous history of bilateral undescended testes. Lee compared these figures in the literature with the early results of his own follow-up study from Pittsburgh, where over 450 men are still being followed up for long-term outcome from undescended testes. Forty-four out of 66 men with bilateral undescended testes were married, and of those 19 (44%) already had children. Four hundred and seven men were being followed up with unilateral undescended testes, of whom 303 were married, and of these 66% had children.

In a recent update of his figures, Lee[46] found severely compromised paternity rates in adulthood in men born with bilateral cryptorchidism (65.3%) compared to those who were formerly unilaterally cryptorchid (89.7%) or control men (93.2%). Similar results were found 20 years ago by Gilhooly *et al.*[46] He reviewed 45 men with a history of bilateral undescended testes, of whom 73% were attempting conception. Of these, 48% had been successful. This compared with 100 men with a unilateral undescended testis, of whom 90% were attempting conception and 80% had been successful. In a 1989 study, Cendron *et al.*[48] followed up 40 men operated on between 1950 and 1960 when the operation was performed at a mean age of 7 years. Twenty-three out of 30 men with a past history of a unilateral undescended testis had attempted paternity, with an 87% success rate, compared with 3/9 men with bilateral undescended testes attempting paternity and a success rate of only 33%.

In a different approach, Kumar *et al.*[49] reviewed 56 men undergoing orchidopexy between 1950 and 1975; they recorded the age of the man at the birth of his first child, and found only very late treatment affected fertility adversely. However, only 3/113 orchidopexies were done at less than 6 years of age.

Semen analysis

Numerous studies have addressed the outcome for orchidopexy by semen analysis (Table 51.4). Because of their logistic difficulties, none of these studies has huge numbers of patients, with most having between 50 and 150 men enrolled. The age at initial orchidopexy varies from 1.5 to 29 years (!), but most series have an average age for operation of 5–10 years.

Lee[44,46] found that men with a past history of bilateral undescended testes were reported as having a wide range of subnormal sperm counts. Some papers reported a 44% incidence of abnormality, compared with others ranging right up to 100% abnormal. However, in all reports at least half the patients were azoospermic. On average, only 25% with a past history of bilateral undescended testes were reported as having normal sperm counts. This compares with those men with a past history of a unilateral undescended testis, where 20%–69% were reported as having subnormal counts, and 57% were found to have normal sperm counts. Not surprisingly, the results of the semen analysis appear worse than the success rates reported above for paternity. A number of factors are likely to account for this, including the fact that the time taken to achieve paternity has not been calculated, let alone the genetic proof of paternity. Also, it is hard to assess the importance of the deliberate redundancy of biological factors in the semen analysis.

Lee reported that, on his review of the literature,[44] there was no proven effect of decrease in age (at operation) on outcome, and no proven effect of location of the testis on outcome. Similarly, Gracia *et al.*[50] found that, in 251 men with a history of undescended testis, the sperm quality was independent of the age of surgery or testicular location, but was influenced only by whether the cryptorchidism was unilateral or bilateral. Interpretation of such pessimistic conclusions about surgical benefit, however, should be guarded, since these reports described the outcome of operations done 30 years ago.

By contrast, some studies, such as Taskinen *et al.*[51] report significantly better results. They have reviewed 31 men operated on at ages between 10 months and 12 years. Normal semen analysis was found in 90% of those with a unilateral undescended testis, compared with 50% of those with bilateral undescended testes. In particular, those men undergoing surgery before 4 years of age were found to have no abnormalities on semen analysis. Hormone levels were recorded and serum FSH levels were found to be elevated in those with severe testicular damage.

An improved fertility outcome with younger age at surgery may not be obvious with the present long-term follow-up results, but it is anticipated by recent pediatric studies. McAleer *et al.*[52] reviewed 355 testicular biopsies in 226 children coming to orchidopexy at between 6 months and 16 years of age. They calculated the fertility index as the mean number of spermatogonia per cross-section of the tubule (S:T ratio) in 50 tubules, and compared these with age-matched controls. They found that those undergoing surgery at less than one year had a normal fertility index, while those coming to operation beyond one year had a decrease in fertility index compared with controls. The contralateral descended testes had a normal fertility index for operation age up to 6 years, but beyond that time they became abnormal. Huff *et al.*[17] and Hadziselimovic and Herzog[18] summarized their results of germ cell development in undescended testes and showed loss of the germ cells during the first year of life with defective or delayed transformation of neonatal gonocytes into type A spermatogonia. Also, delayed or defective transformation of type A spermatogonia to primary spermatocytes was seen at 3–5 years of age. The contralateral testes showed some changes but much less severe than in the undescended testes. They concluded that these results were consistent with hypogonadotrophic hypogonadism, although equally they could indicate relatively normal testes initially undergoing secondary degeneration.

Cortes *et al.*[53] recently reviewed 1335 boys with cryptorchidism who underwent orchidopexy and biopsy for undescended testes below 12 years of age. One hundred and forty-six of these underwent detailed assessment in adult life. Lack of germ cells in the original biopsy was found from 18 months, and increased with age. Normal sperm counts were found in 19% (14/75) and 83% (54/65) of men who had undergone bilateral or unilateral orchidopexy, respectively.

When surgery is delayed to adolescence or beyond[54] azoospermia or oligospermia is likely. In 91 men with unilateral undescended testes having surgery at between 14 and 29 years, 83% were subsequently found to be oligo- or azoospermic. Cortes and Thorup[55] reviewed 90 boys with an average age of 13 years, undergoing bilateral orchidopexy with biopsy. Seventy-three of these were followed up at an average age of 25.6 years. The fertility index on initial biopsy (percentage of tubular cross-sections with spermatogonia) was correlated with the subsequent maximum sperm density and the volume of the testes, and inversely correlated with the serum FSH level. They found that those testes that were in the superficial inguinal pouch had significantly better outcomes than those that were intracanalicular or abdominal.

Okuyama *et al.*[56] compared 167 men operated on at 2–5 years of age, with 43 operated on at 9–12 years of age. Of those having surgery early in childhood, 95% had normal semen analysis with a unilateral undescended testis, and 24% had a normal sperm count with bilateral undescended testes. This compared with 86% with normal sperm counts in those having surgery in later childhood for a unilateral UDT, and 20% normal sperm counts with bilateral undescended testes. They concluded that operation did not reverse the poor fertility in bilateral undescended testes, and that the contralateral testis in those with a history of a unilateral undescended testis had poor function.

Bremholm-Rasmussen *et al.*[41] reviewed 45 men who had bilateral undescended testes that were never treated by surgery but descended spontaneously after 10 years of age. Clinically, they fell into two groups. In the first group, the testis was in the superficial inguinal pouch and it could be manipulated into the scrotal neck but immediately retracted. The second group had suprascrotal testes which could be manipulated to the middle of the scrotum, but

Table 51.5. Relative risk of testicular malignancy in cohort studies

Series	Number of cancer patients	Number with previous UDT	UDT/cancer (%)	UDT in population (%)	Relative risk
Gilbert and Hamilton[62]	>7000	840	11	0.23	48
Campbell[63]	1422	165	11.6	0.23	50.4

UDT, undescended testis.

then retracted. Such testes would be regarded as retractile or ascending in many series. At 18 years of age they underwent semen analysis, and only 33% were found to have normal values. Forty-seven percent had azoospermia or oligospermia, and a large number had increased FSH levels. Perhaps these patients can be regarded as having acquired maldescent and being equivalent to the subgroup of adolescents whose undescended testes were known in the past to descend spontaneously at puberty. Their poor sperm counts in adult life suggest that, even later in childhood, 5–10 years of non-scrotal position does cause secondary degeneration of the testes.

Mayr *et al.*[57] reviewed 46 men undergoing operation at between 1.5 and 12 years of age. Eleven out of 24 with a unilateral undescended testis had normal sperm counts. By contrast, only 7/22 men with bilateral undescended testes had normal sperm counts; 13% of these had azoospermia. They found there was no correlation between semen analysis and either the age at surgery or the spermatogonia/tubule ratio. They found that there was a correlation between the initial gonadal position and both subsequent sperm counts and FSH levels, with retractile and high scrotal testes having significantly better outcomes than intra-abdominal or inguinal testes.

Mandat *et al.*[58] reviewed 135 men who underwent surgery at between 2.5 and 15 years of age. They grouped them by age at operation: before 6 years of age; at 6–10 years of age; and over 10 years. The position of the gonad was recorded as either abdominal, canalicular or inguinal. The percentage of men with normal sperm counts decreased with increasing age at surgery for the 112 men with a unilateral undescended testis. In addition, the number of sperm also decreased with increasing age in this group. The number of men with bilateral undescended testes was too small to see any age effect. The effect of early operation was more clearly seen when the men were classified into those with gonads in a similar position, where it could be seen that early age was a significant advantage for testes in a similar position. Mandat and colleagues concluded that surgery would be optimal at 1–2 years of age in the hope of preventing this secondary degeneration.

Urry *et al.*[59] looked at the effect of orchidopexy on the development of antisperm antibodies in adult life. Fifty-five men were reviewed by semen analysis for the presence of antisperm antibodies. In the context of an infertility clinic, it was known already that 66% of men with a past history of undescended testes had antibodies, compared with only 2.8% of controls. In their group of 55 men, antibodies were present in 52% after orchidopexy. Antibodies were present when orchidopexy was done at an average age of 11 years. By contrast, when orchidopexy was done at an average age of 8.6 years, antibodies were not present subsequently. It is difficult to interpret these results, but it might be an indicator that testicular degeneration which persists into adolescence allows the patient to be exposed to a testis with a deficient blood–testis barrier, which would then allow autoimmunization against sperm antigens to occur.[60]

Malignancy follow-up studies

In a review of neoplasia in men with previous cryptorchidism, Whitaker[61] reported that Percival Pott knew in 1777 that there was an increased risk of malignancy in the undescended testis. Since that time, however, the relative risk of malignancy related to different forms of cryptorchidism has remained uncertain (Table 51.5). In 1940, Gilbert and Hamilton[62] reviewed records from the US Bureau of Census and found over 7000 cases of testicular malignancy. Review of their past histories revealed 840, or 11%, of the total, who had had previous undescended testis. They related this incidence to over nine million military recruits, of whom 22 665 had undescended testes, an incidence of 0.23%. They concluded therefore, that the relative risk of malignancy in a person with undescended testis was 48-fold. In a similar study, Campbell[63,64] reviewed 1422 patients with testicular tumors, of whom 165 (11.6%) had a history of undescended testis. Using the same population statistics for undescended testis, this gave a relative risk of 50-fold. One difficulty with these studies was the potential bias in the number of patients in the population with undescended testis: the use of adult army recruits introduced

Table 51.6. Relative risk of subsequent malignancy after cryptorchidism

Series	Number of men with previous UDT	Number who developed cancer (95% CI)	Number in population expected to develop cancer	Relative risk (95% CI)
Giwercman *et al.*[65]	506	6	1.3	4.7
" "	–	(2.2–13.1)	–	(1.7–10.2)
Campbell[63]	1413	22	0.07%	22
Benson *et al.*[66]	224	2	<1	11.4
" "	–	–	–	(1.4–41.1)

significant bias as many patients with undescended testis may have been excluded. The relative risk of malignancy would therefore be overestimated if a smaller estimate of the frequency of undescended testis was used as a base.

Using a different approach, Campbell[63] also looked at 1413 men with a past history of undescended testis, and attempted to determine the number who later developed cancer (Table 51.6). He found 22 who developed testicular tumors (1.56%). This was compared with an expected population frequency of 0.07% for testicular tumors. The relative risk of testicular cancer after undescended testis was therefore calculated at 22-fold. By contrast, much more recent cohort studies have found a much lower relative risk of testicular cancer because the population frequency of testicular cancer has increased. In 1987, Giwercman *et al.*[65] reviewed 506 men with a previous history of undescended testis, of whom 6 developed testicular tumors, compared with an expected 1.3; the relative risk was calculated at 4.7. Benson *et al.*[66] reviewed 224 men with undescended testis, 2 of whom later developed cancer when none would have been expected; they calculated a relative risk of cancer after undescended testis of 11.4.

A large number of case-control studies have been done to determine the relative risk of cancer after cryptorchidism (Tables 51.6, 51.7). For example, Morrison reviewed 596 men with testicular cancer and found that 17 (2.85%) had a previous history of undescended testis. In 602 controls, only 2 had developed a testicular tumor, giving a relative risk of 8.8. Case-control studies potentially have greater problems with bias or misclassification, depending on how the patients are selected. For example, Schottenfeld *et al.*[68] reviewed 190 men with testicular tumors, of whom 22 (11.6%) had a past history of undescended testis. They compared this group with 166 patients with lymphoma, of whom 6 had a history of undescended testis, giving a relative risk of 3.49. When they used population controls, they found a relative risk of 2.53. Overall, using modern estimates of the incidence of testicular cancer and undescended testis in the developed world, the relative risk of testicular cancer is probably in the order of 5–10 times. Such cohort studies, using cancer prediction rates based on the general population, underestimate the risk by about 10% because such population figures already contain men who have testicular cancer and cryptorchidism.

Table 51.7. Relative risk of testicular malignancy in case-control studies

Series	Number of cancer patients with UDT	Number of controls with cancer	Relative risk (95% – CI)
Morrison[67]	17/596 (2.85%)	2/602 (0.33%)	8.8 (2.3–56.3)
Henderson *et al.*[85]	10/131 (7.6%)	2/131 (1.53%)	5.0
Schottenfeld *et al.*[68]	22/190 (11.6%)	6/166 (3.6%) (hospital)	3.49 (1.34–8.10)
" "	–	7/142 (4.9%) (population)	2.53 (1.02–5.68)
Pottern *et al.*[86]	25/271 (9.2%)	7/259 (2.7%)	3.7 (1.6–8.6)
Strader *et al.*[87]	40/333 (12%)	15/670 (2.2%)	5.9 (3.9–10.2)

UDT, undescended testis.

The relative risk of testicular cancer with regard to the site of the undescended testis or the age of the boy at operation is not known.[67–70] Great points of controversy at present are whether or not early surgery will reduce the risk of malignancy, and whether testicular biopsy or suture at the time of orchidopexy increases the risk of neoplasm.[71] No studies so far on rates of malignancy have demonstrated an effect of operation at a younger age. However, this is not surprising, given the long lag-time to the development of cancer, which means that we can look only at treatments that were used 30–40 years ago and cannot investigate the outcomes of current treatments.

Recent case-control studies from Denmark show a strong association between low socioeconomic class and undescended testis, and a slight trend of both undescended testis and subsequent malignancy to be more common in firstborn sons and sons of older women.[72] None of the epidemiological studies reported have found an explanation for the increase in testicular malignancy during the last 30 years.[73]

Carcinoma *in situ*

Giwercman *et al.*[74] reviewed 500 men between the ages of 20 and 30 years with a past history of undescended testis, and offered them a biopsy for screening for carcinoma *in situ* (CIS). Three hundred agreed to biopsy, 5 of whom proved positive for CIS (1.7%; 95% confidence interval 0.05–3.9%). The authors concluded that, along with other evidence, the prevalence of CIS in men with a past history of undescended testis was 2%–3%. In a number of publications[75–77] they have built a strong case for the CIS cell being a precursor to malignancy approximately 5–10 years ahead of the clinical disease. They have gone so far as to recommend that all older adolescents and young adults with a past history of undescended testis should have their testes biopsied to determine whether CIS is present.

It has been suggested by Giwercman *et al.*[76] that the CIS cell is an abnormal fetal gonocyte, and that a mutation may have occurred in the fetal gonocyte during early embryogenesis and prior to migration of the gonocytes from the yolk sac to the urogenital ridge. An alternative explanation is provided by the detailed studies of Huff *et al.*[17,18] By examining semithin sections of testicular biopsies taken at orchidopexy in early infancy, they have shown that the first anomaly visible in an undescended testis is hypoplasia of the Leydig cells at about 1 month of age. At 3–6 months of age, failure of the fetal gonocyte to transform into a type-A spermatogonium can be demonstrated, but the total number of germ cells remains satisfactory for at least 7 months. The untransformed gonocytes then appear to degenerate, leading to a fall in the total number of germ cells. They postulated that this was likely to be evidence of hypogonadotrophic hypogonadism and suggested the use of hCG treatment to overcome the gonadotrophin deficiency. They emphasized the point that has been appreciated only in recent years, that the testis is not quiescent in early infancy, but is in fact demonstrating active and possibly crucial germ cell development.

The present author's own experimental work has suggested that gonocyte transformation does not require androgens, as this is normal in an animal model with androgen receptor mutation and is not stimulated in organ culture by addition of androgens. Further, recent laboratory work has shown that the neonatal germ cell demonstrates histochemical markers similar to the fetal gonocyte[78] and this may be the cell which degenerates and leads to the CIS cell later in childhood. CIS cells are known to be absent in the early infant testis, except in those children with a primary dysplasia of the testis and genital anomaly. However, in an undescended testis it is quite likely that the CIS cell occurs as a secondary phenomenon following degeneration of neonatal gonocytes which have failed to transform into type A spermatogonia.

Implications for future management

Current management of undescended testes is based on the dual aims of reducing infertility and preventing malignancy. Although occasionally a primary abnormality in the testis has either been demonstrated or postulated (e.g., epididymal anomalies), it would appear best to assume that, in nearly all children, secondary germ cell deficiency or dysplasia leads to infertility and malignancy. Since the germ cell abnormality is demonstrated within the first 6–12 months of life, orchidopexy at this time has been recommended in the author's unit. It will, however, be a long time before follow-up studies of fertility and malignancy risks reflect this change in management. In the meantime, reassurance is needed that such early management is appropriate. One possible way this might be achieved is by the use of the serum Mullerian inhibiting substance (MIS) assay. MIS is secreted throughout childhood, and levels fall at puberty.[79–80] There is a peak of secretion at between 6 and 12 months of age, which has been postulated to be related to gonocyte transformation.[81] As measurable MIS from the serum does not require priming by prior hCG injection, pre- and postoperative serum MIS levels may be a useful determinant of whether early surgery is preventing or reversing any secondary damage to the testis, long before the final outcome can be known.

Although it is currently controversial, all boys need careful examination on the day of birth, to identify those in whom the testes have not reached the scrotum. This is relatively easy to determine because of the lax scrotum. Those children with a testis out of the scrotum should be re-examined at 12 weeks, by which time "late descenders" would have reached the scrotum. In the latter group, no intervention is required, but they do need annual review to determine whether they have developed an ascending testis. Those with a persisting undescended testis at 12 weeks can be referred for orchidopexy, which probably will be done at between 6 and 12 months. One criterion for intervention for ascending testis is when the testis can no longer reside spontaneously in the scrotum. The authors recommend manipulation of the testis into the scrotum if it is found in the groin. One should then wait a few minutes to see whether it can remain there without being held. A testis which can be manipulated only to the top or middle of the scrotum is abnormal, but does not need intervention until such time as it cannot reach the scrotum at all without being held under traction.

A further screening of boys needs to be carried out at between 5 and 7 years, to diagnose an acquired undescended testis before it has been present for too long. All boys should be examined at some time around school entry, and those whose testes are normally descended at the bottom of the scrotum need no further review. Those where the testis is obviously undescended (presumed acquired) can be referred for orchidopexy, which can be done by either an inguinal or a scrotal approach. Many testes in boys this age might be thought to be retractile. If the testis is sitting high but can remain within the scrotum, then no intervention is required. However, these boys need annual review, as a significant number may need surgery later as the position of the testes becomes more abnormal with increasing age. The criterion for referral is the same as given above for ascending testis: intervention should be initiated once the testis cannot reach the scrotum and remain there without being held.

Using these criteria for management, the risks to fertility and the possibility of cancer can be reduced to the lowest possible level, allowing for intrinsic abnormalities in the epididymis which have been identified in at least 10% of undescended testes.[82]

REFERENCES

1. Short, R. V. The testis: the witness of the mating system, the site of mutation and the engine of desire. *Acta Paediatr. Suppl.* 1997; **422**:3–7.
2. Scorer, C. G. & Farrington, G. H. *Congenital Deformities of the Testis and Epididymis.* London: Butterworth, 1971.
3. Hutson, J. M. & Donahoe, P. K. The hormonal control of testicular descent. *Endocr. Rev.* 1986; **7**:270–283.
4. Hutson, J. M., Hasthorpe, S., & Heyns, C. F. Anatomical and functional aspects of testicular descent and cryptorchidism. *Endocr. Rev.* 1997; **18**:259–280.
5. Nef, S. & Parada, L. F. Hormones in male sexual development. *Genes Dev.* 2000; **14**:3075–3086.
6. Nef, S. & Parada, L. F. Cryptorchidism in mice mutant for Insl3. *Nat. Genet.* 1999; **22**:295–299.
7. Kubota, Y., Temelcos, C., Bathgate, R. A. D. *et al.* The role of insulin 3 testosterone, MIS and relaxin in rat gubernaculum growth. *Hum. Molec. Reprod.* 2002; **8**:900–905.
8. Hrabovszky, Z., Farmer, P. J., & Hutson, J. M. Does the sensory nucleus of the genitofemoral nerve have a role in testicular descent? *J. Pediatr. Surg.* 2000; **35**:96–100.
9. Clarnette, T. D. & Hutson, J. M. Exogenous calcitonin gene-related peptide can change the direction of gubernacular migration in the mutant trans-scrotal rat. *J. Pediatr. Surg.* 1999; **34**:1208–1212.
10. Baker, L. A., Nef, S., Nguyen, M. T., Stapleton, R., Pohl, H., & Parada, L. F. The Insulin-3 gene: lack of genetic basis for human cryptorchidism. *J. Urol.* 2002; **167**:2534–2537.
11. Browne, D. The diagnosis of undescended testis. In Nixon, H. H., Waterston, D., & Wink, C. A. S. (eds.), *Selected Writings of Sir Denis Browne.* London: Trustees of the Sir Denis Browne Memorial Fund, 1983:92–97.
12. Wyllie, G. G. The retractile testis. *Med. J. Austral.* 1984; **140**:403–405.
13. Clarnette, T. D. & Hutson, J. M. Is the ascending testis actually 'stationary'? *Pediatr. Surg. Int.* 1997; **12**:155–159.
14. Clarnette, T. D., Rowe, D., Hasthorpe, S., & Hutson, J. M. Incomplete disappearance of the processus vaginalis as a cause of ascending testis. *J. Urol.* 1997; **157**:1889–1891.
15. Zorgniotti, A. A. *Temperature, and Environmental Effects on the Testis.* New York: Plenum, 1991:1–335.
16. Mieusset, R., Fonda, P. J., Guitard, J. *et al.* Increase in testicular temperature in case of cryptorchidism in boys. *Fertil. Steril.* 1993; **59**:1319–1321.
17. Huff, D. S., Fenig, D. M., Canning, D. A., Carr, M. C., Zderic, S. A., & Snyder, H. M. III. Abnormal germ cell development in cryptorchidism. *Horm. Res.* 2001; **55**:11–17.
18. Hadziselimovic, F. & Herzog, B. Importance of early postnatal germ cell maturation for fertility of cryptorchidism males. *Horm. Res.* 2001; **55**:6–10.
19. Kort, W. J., Hekking-Weijma, I., & Vermeij, M. Artificial intraabdominal cryptorchidism in young adult rats leads to irreversible azoospermia. *Eur. Urol.* 1990; **18**:302–306.
20. Schindler, A. M., Diaz, P., Cuendet, A. *et al.* Cryptorchidism: a morphological study of 670 biopsies. *Helv. Paediatr. Acta* 1987; **42**:145–158.
21. Saw, K. C., Eardley, I., Dennis, M. J. S. *et al.* Surgical outcome of orchidopexy. 1: Previously unoperated testes. *Br. J. Urol.* 1992; **70**:90–94.
22. Hadiziselimovic, F., Herzog, B., & Seguchi, H. Surgical correction of cryptorchidism at 2 years: electron microscopic and morphometric investigations. *J. Pediatr. Surg.* 1975; **10**:19–26.
23. Kogan, S. J. Testis and andrology. *Curr. Opin. Urol.* 1992; **2**:409–413.
24. Gendrel, D., Roger, M., & Job, J.-C. Plasma gonadotropin and testosterone values in infants with cryptorchidism. *J. Pediatr.* 1980; **97**:217–220.
25. Job, J.-C., Toublanc, J. E., Chaussin, J. L. *et al.* Endocrine and immunological findings in cryptorchid infants. *Horm. Res* 1988; **30**:167–172.
26. Yamanaka, J., Metcalfe, S. A., Hutson, J. M. *et al.* Testicular descent. II. Ontogeny and response to denervation of calcitonin gene-related peptide receptors in neonatal rat gubernaculum. *Endocrinology* 1993; **132**:1–5.

27. Juenemann, K. P., Kogan, B. A., & Abozeid, M. H. Fertility in cryptorchidism: an experimental model. *J. Urol.* 1986; **136**:214–216.
28. Kogan, B. A., Gupta, R., & Juenemann, K. P. Fertility in cryptorchidism: further development of an experimental model. *J. Urol.* 1987; **137**:128–131.
29. Kogan, B. A., Gupta, R., & Juenemann, K. P. Fertility in cryptorchidism: improved timing of fixation and treatment in an experimental model. *J. Urol.* 1987; **138**:1046–1047.
30. Patkowski, D., Czernik, J., & Jelen, M. The natural course of cryptorchidism in rats and the efficacy of orchidopexy or orchidectomy in its treatment before and after puberty. *J. Pediatr. Surg* 1992; **27**:870–873.
31. Wilson-Storey, D., McGenity, K., & Dickson, J. A. S. Orchidopexy: the younger the better? *J. Roy. Coll. Surg. Edin.* 1990; **35**:362–364.
32. Bianchi, A. & Squire, B. R. Transscrotal orchidopexy: orchidopexy revisited. *Pediatr. Surg. Int.* 1989; **4**:189–192.
33. Giannopoulos, M. F., Vlachakis, I. G., & Charissis, G. C. Thirteen years' experience with the combined hormonal therapy of cryptorchidism. *Horm. Res.* 2001; **55**:33–37.
34. Rajfer, J., Handelsman, D. J., Swerdloff, R. S. *et al.* Hormonal therapy of cryptorchidism: a randomized, double-blind study comparing human chorionic gonadotropin and gonadotropin-releasing hormone. *N. Engl. J. Med.* 1986; **314**:466–470.
35. Wit, J. I. M., Delemarre-Van de Waal, H. A., Bax, N. M. A. *et al.* Effect of LHRH treatment on testicular descent and hormonal response in cryptorchidism. *Clin. Endocrinol.* 1986; **24**:539–548.
36. de Muinck Keizer-Schrama, S. M. P. F., Hazebroek, F. W. J., Drop, S. L. S. *et al.* Double-blind, placebo-controlled study of luteinising-hormone-releasing-hormone nasal spray in treatment of undescended testes *Lancet* 1986; **i**:876–879.
37. Adamsen, S. & Borjesson, B. Factors affecting the outcome of orchiopexy for undescended testes. *Acta Chir. Scand.* 1988; **154**:529–533.
38. Puri, P. & Sparnon, A. W. Relationship of primary site of testis to final testicular size in cryptorchid patients. *Br. J. Urol.* 1990; **66**:208–210.
39. Schreiber, K., Menardi, G., Marberger, H. *et al.* Late results after surgical treatment of maldescended testes with special regard to exocrine and endocrine testicular function. *Eur. Urol.* 1981; **7**:268–273.
40. Noh, P. H., Cooper, C. S., Snyder, H. M. III, Zderic, S. A., Canning, D. A., & Huff, D. S. Testicular volume does not predict germ cell count in patients with cryptorchidism. *J. Urol.* 2000; **163**:593–596.
41. Bremholm-Rasmussen, T., Ingerslev, H. J., & Hostrup, H. Bilateral spontaneous descent of the testis after the age of 10: subsequent effects on fertility. *Br. J. Surg.* 1988: **75**:820–823.
42. Werder, L. A., Illig' R., Torresani, F. *et al.* Gonadal function in young adults after surgical treatment of cryptorchidism. *Br. Med. J.* 1976; **2**:1357–1359.
43. Eardley, I., Saw, K. C., & Whitaker, R. H. Surgical outcome of orchidopexy. II: Trapped and ascending testes. *Br. J. Urol.* 1994; **73**:204–206.
44. Lee, P. A. Consequence of cryptorchidism: relationship to etiology and treatment. *Curr. Prob. Pediatr.* 1995; **25**:232–236.
45. Bhasin, S., de Kretser, D. M., Baker, H. W. G. Pathophysiology and natural history of male infertility. *J. Clin. Endocr. Metab.* 1994; **79**:1525–1529.
46. Lee, P. A. & Coughlin, M. T. Fertility after bilateral cryptorchidism. Evaluation by paternity, hormone and semen data. *Horm. Res.* 2001; **55**:28–32.
47. Gilhooly, P. E., Meyers, F., & Lattimer, J. K. Fertility prospects for children with cryptorchidism. *Am. J. Dis. Child.* 1984; **139**:940–943.
48. Cendron, M., Keating, M. A., Huff, D. S. *et al.* Cryptorchidism, orchiopexy and infertility: a critical long-term retrospective analysis. *J. Urol.* 1989; **142**:559–572.
49. Kumar, D., Bremner, D. N., & Brown, P. W. Fertility after orchiopexy for cryptorchidism: a new approach to assessment. *Br. J. Urol.* 1989; **64**:516–520.
50. Gracia, J., Sanchez Zalabardo, J., Sanchez Garcia, J., Garcia, C., & Ferrandez, A. Clinical, physical, sperm and hormonal data on 251 adults operated on for cryptorchidism in childhood. *BJU. Int.* 2000; **85**:1100–1103.
51. Taskinen, S., Hovatta, O., & Wikstrom, A. Early treatment of cryptorchidism, semen quality and testicular endocrinology. *J. Urol.* 1996; **156**:82–84.
52. McAleer, I. M., Packer, M. G., Kaplan, G. W. *et al.* Fertility index analysis in cryptorchidism. *J. Urol.* 1995; **153**:1255–1258.
53. Cortes, D., Thorup, J. M., & Visfeldt, J. Cryptorchidism: aspects of fertility and neoplasms. *Horm. Res.* 2001; **55**:21–27.
54. Grasso, M., Buonaguidi, C., Lania, F. *et al.* Postpubertal cryptorchidism: review and evaluation of the fertility. *Eur. Urol.* 1991; **20**:126–128.
55. Cortes, D. & Thorup, J. Histology of testicular biopsies taken at operation for bilateral maldescended testes in relation to fertility in adulthood. *Br. J. Urol.* 1991; **68**:285–291.
56. Okuyama, A., Nonomura, N., Nakamura, M. *et al.* Surgical management of undescended testis: retrospective study of potential fertility in 274 cases. *J. Urol.* 1989; **142**:749–751.
57. Mayr, J., Pusch, H. H., Schimpl, G. *et al.* Semen quality and gonadotropin levels in patients operated upon for cryptorchidism. *Pediatr. Surg. Int.* 1996; **11**:354–358.
58. Mandat, K. M., Wieczorkiewicz, B., Gubala-Kacala, M. *et al.* Semen analysis of patients who had orchidopexy in childhood. *Eur. J. Pediatr.* 1994; **4**:94–97.
59. Urry, R. I., Carrell, D. T., Starr, N. T. *et al.* The incidence of antisperm antibodies in infertility patients with a history of cryptorchidism. *J. Urol.* 1994; **151**:381–388.
60. Singer, R., Dickerman, Z., Sagiv, M. *et al.* Endocrinological parameters and cell-mediated immunity postoperation for cryptorchidism. *Arch. Androl.* 1988; **20**:153–157.
61. Whitaker, R. H. Neoplasia in cryptorchid men. *Semin. Urol.* 1988; **6**:107–109.

62. Gilbert, J. B. & Hamilton, J. B. Studies in malignant testis tumours. III: Incidence and nature of tumours in ectopic testes. *Surg. Gynecol. Obst*. 1940; **761**:731–733.
63. Campbell, H. E. Incidence of malignant growth of the undescended testicle. *Arch. Surg.* 1942; **44**:353–369.
64. Campbell, H. E. The incidence of malignant growth of the undescended testicle: a reply and re-evaluation. *J. Urol.* 1959; **61**:663–668.
65. Giwercman, A., Grindsted, J., Hansen, B. *et al.* Testicular cancer risk in boys with maldescended testis: a cohort study. *J. Urol.* 1987; **138**:1214–1276.
66. Benson, R. C., Beard, C. M., Kelalis, P. P. *et al.* Malignant potential of the cryptorchid testis. *Mayo Clin. Proc.* 1991; **66**:372–378.
67. Morrison, A. S. Cryptorchidism, hernia and cancer of the testis. *J. Natl. Cancer Inst*. 1976; **56**:731–733.
68. Schottenfeld, D., Warshauer, M. E., Sherlock, S. *et al.* The epidemiology of testicular cancer in young adults. *Am. J. Epidemiol.* 1980; **112**:232–246.
69. Pike, M. C., Chilvers, C., & Peckham, M. J. Effect of age at orchidopexy on risk of testicular cancer. *Lancet* 1986; **i**:1246–1248.
70. Chilvers, C., Dudley, N. E., Gough, M. H. *et al.* Undescended testis: the effect of treatment on subsequent risk of sub-fertility and malignancy. *J. Pediatr. Surg*. 1986; **21**:691–696.
71. Woodhouse, C. R. J. Prospects for fertility in patients born with genitourinary anomalies. *J. Urol*. 2001; **165**:2354–2360.
72. Moller, H. & Skakkebaek, N. E. Risks of testicular cancer and cryptorchidism in relation to socio-economic status and related factors: case-control studies in Denmark. *Int. J. Cancer* 1996; **66**:287–293.
73. Brown, L. M., Pottern, L. M., & Hoover, R. N. Testicular cancer in young men: the search for causes of the epidemic increase in the United States. *J. Epidemiol. Commun. Hlth.* 1987; **41**:349–354.
74. Giwercman, A., Bruun, E., Frimodt-Moller, C. *et al.* Prevalence of carcinoma-in-situ and other histopathological abnormalities in testes of men with a history of cryptorchidism. *J. Urol.* 1989; **142**:998–1002.
75. Giwercman, A., Muller, J., & Skakkebaek, N. E. Cryptorchidism and testicular neoplasia. *Horm. Res.* 1988; **30**:157–163.
76. Giwercman, A., Muller, J., & Skakkebaek, N. E. Carcinoma-in-situ of the testis: possible origin, clinical significance and diagnostic methods. *Rec. Cancer. Res.* 1991; **123**:27–36.
77. Giwercman, A., Lundgaard Hansen, L., & Skakkebaek, N. E. Initiation of sperm production after bilateral orchidopexy: clinical and biological implications. *J. Urol.* 2000; **163**:1255–1256.
78. Hasthorpe, S., Farmer, P., Smith, M. *et al.* Typing of the alkaline phosphatase isoenzyme expressed in neonatal testis and cellular localization using the G-5-2 monoclonal antibody. *Biol. Reprod*. 1997;
79. Baker, M. L., Metcalfe, S. A., & Hutson, J. M. Serum levels of Mullerian inhibiting substance in boys from birth to 18 years, as determined by enzyme immunoassay. *J. Clin. Endocr. Metab.* 1990; **70**:11–15.
80. Lee, M. M. & Donahoe, P. K. Mullerian inhibiting substance: a gonadal hormone with multiple functions. *Endocr. Rev.* 1993; **14**:152–164.
81. Zhou, B., Watts, L. M., & Hutson, J. M. Germ cell development in neonatal mouse testes *in vitro* requires mullerian inhibiting substance. *J. Urol.* 1993; **150**:1–4.
82. Johansen, T. E. B. Anatomy of the testis and epididymis in cryptorchidism. *Andrologia* 1987; **19**:565–569.
83. Cortes, D., Thorup, J. M., & Lindinverg, S. Fertility potential after unilateral orchiopexy: an age independent risk of subesquent infertility when biopsies at surgery lack germ cells. *J. Urol*. 1996; **156**:217–220.
84. Puri, P. & O'Donnell, B. Semen analysis of patients who had orchidopexy at or after seven years of age. *Lancet* 1988; **11**: 1051.
85. Henderson, B. E., Benton, B., Jing, J. *et al.* Risk factors for cancer of the testis in young men. *Int. J. Cancer* 1979; **23**:598–602.
86. Pottern, L. M., Brown, L. M., Hoover, R. N. *et al.* Testicular cancer risk among young men: role of cryptorchidism and inguinal hernia. *J. Natl. Cancer Inst*. 1985; **74**:377–381.
87. Strader, C. H., Weiss, N. S., Dating, J. R. *et al.* Cryptorchidism, orchiopexy, and the risk of testicular cancer. *Am. J. Epidemiol.* 1988; **127**:1013–1018.

52

Circumcision

Peter M. Cuckow

Department of Paediatric Urology, Great Ormond Street Hospital, London, UK

Introduction

Circumcision is the most commonly performed operation in males and is among the oldest, with evidence of its practice in Egyptian mummies – long before Abraham's pact with God introduced ritual circumcision to the Jewish nation in 1713 BC.[1] Ritual circumcision is also practiced among Moslems, Aboriginals, and certain African tribes. Hot, dry climates and poor hygiene predispose to balanitis, so circumcision has conferred some medical benefit to these cultures,[2] a fact that did not escape desert troops in the Second World War and led to an increase in circumcision in Western cultures. On the other hand, its identification with Jewish culture has resulted in an avoidance of circumcision in many central European countries since the War. Currently, it is estimated that one-sixth of the world's population is circumcised.[3]

Religious considerations apart, the variable incidence of circumcision betrays marked differences in cultural and medical attitudes towards the foreskin. Currently, in England the majority of circumcisions are performed for medical reasons (about 21 000 annually in children),[3] and it is estimated that 1 in 15 boys are circumcised before their fifteenth birthday. This is significantly less than the 24% rate reported in the 1950s,[4] although more stringent criteria for medical circumcision could undoubtedly effect a further reduction.[5] In Scandinavian countries the rate is the lowest amongst Western cultures[6] in contrast to the United States where routine neonatal circumcision has become the norm and 90% of males are circumcised shortly after birth in some areas.[7] Medical arguments to support this practice have arisen long after its establishment as the cultural, emotional and anatomical "norm."

Development and function of the foreskin

The fetal foreskin is an outgrowth of the epidermis on the penile shaft proximal to the glans, which is completely enveloped by 16 weeks' gestation. The epithelium on its inner surface fuses with that of the developing glans, and these separate later at a variable rate as desquamation of each layer occurs. At birth, only 4% of foreskins are retractile, although the tip of the glans may be revealed in a further 54%. The normal foreskin remains unretractile in 80% of boys at 6 months, 50% at 1 year, 20% at 2 years and 10% by the age of 3.[8] Continued separation of the glanular adhesions and loosening of the prepuce continues so that only 1% are non-retractable at 16 years and adhesions persist in only 3%.[9] In most older boys with a non-retractile foreskin, pathological secondary narrowing or "true phimosis" has developed, characterized clinically by scarring at the tip of the foreskin and associated with histological features of balanitis xerotica et obliterans (BXO) in up to 95% of cases.[10]

The function of the foreskin remains largely a matter of speculation. The high incidence of meatal ulceration after neonatal circumcision, and the obvious differences in texture of the glanular epithelium of a circumcised penis, reflect its protective role of the sensitive glans and meatus, particularly in a diaper-wearing age group.[8] During sexual intercourse the mobility of the penile shaft within an intact prepuce reduces friction, but meaningful research into this has proved impossible.[11]

Pediatric Surgery and Urology: Long-term Outcomes, Mark Stringer, Keith Oldham, Pierre Mouriquand.
Published by Cambridge University Press.

Indications for circumcision

The medical indications for circumcision are few. Balanitis is a self-limiting condition that occurs in fewer than 4% of preschool boys, responds to bathing, recurs in only 20%, and very rarely gives rise to long-term changes in the foreskin.[12] Circumcision may rarely be indicated in a recurrent case. Paraphimosis, or trapping of the foreskin proximal to the coronal sulcus resulting in edema and swelling of the distal penis, can usually be reduced by traction on the foreskin following a period of compression to reduce the edema.[13] It does not imply an abnormal foreskin and circumcision can be avoided.[13] Ballooning, due to turbulence within a non-retractile foreskin, can be prevented by easing the foreskin back gently during micturition and will resolve as it becomes fully retractable, with no long-term problems.[13] The only absolute indication for circumcision is BXO, which is rare under 5 years of age.[10,14] Contraindications for circumcision include a generalized medical condition, in particular a bleeding diathesis, and penile abnormalities such as hypospadias and buried penis.[3,15,16]

Prophylactic circumcision is advocated in the USA in particular, to avoid problems in the future life of the child. The innocent foreskin has been variously blamed for an increased incidence of sexually transmitted disease, HIV infection, and cervical and penile cancer, although the population-based studies on which these arguments rest are not conclusive.[17,18] The foreskin is not itself an abnormal piece of tissue,[19] and there is little doubt that attention to personal hygiene, safer sexual practices and monogamy would greatly reduce, if not eradicate, these diseases.[2,8]

Ginsberg and McCracken[20] first alerted us to the predominance of uncircumcised boys in a cohort of infants with urinary tract infection, and Wiswell and Roscelli[21] subsequently documented a tenfold increased incidence of urinary tract infection in uncircumcised compared with circumcised infants during the first month of life. It is estimated that 100 prophylactic circumcisions would be needed to prevent one urinary tract infection; and, given a rate of renal scarring of 1 per every 5–10 febrile urinary infections, up to 1000 circumcisions to prevent one renal scar.[22] Balanced against this, all of these boys would be exposed to the complications of circumcision (see below). Where an existing urinary anomaly has already been found, there remains a strong argument for circumcision.[17] Preventative hygienic measures to reduce foreskin colonisation by uropathogenic organisms have yet to be studied formally.[19]

It is important to note that circumcision does not eliminate penile problems. Herzog and Alvarez[23] documented a significant incidence of balanitis in circumcised boys (3% compared to 6% in the uncircumcised). A birth cohort of 500 boys in New Zealand actually revealed a higher rate of minor penile problems in circumcised boys.[24] Equally, urinary infection and penile cancer are also found in the circumcised, although less commonly.[17,25]

Techniques

The aim of circumcision is to remove sufficient shaft and inner preputial skin to leave the glans uncovered, while retaining enough to cover the length of the penile shaft.

Neonatal circumcisions are usually performed with the aid of a clamp device without general anesthetic. The Gomco and Plastibel devices are most commonly employed in the United States.[15,16,27] For both, the foreskin is fully retracted, usually with a dorsal slit, and the congenital glanular adhesions are separated. With the Gomco clamp, an appropriately sized steel bell is placed over the glans and the foreskin is replaced over it. The clamp is assembled and the foreskin crushed circumferentially, providing hemostasis after the redundant tissue is excised and the clamp removed. An appropriately sized Plastibel is also placed over the glans and the foreskin similarly retracted back over it. Following this, a strong ligature is tied around the foreskin into a groove in the device and the redundant tissue is excised. The Plastibel is left *in situ* and drops off after a mean of 9 days,[28] when the skin edge necroses and separates from the ligature. The Mogen clamp is commonly used in Jewish ritual circumcision.[29] The foreskin is pulled through the slit in the clamp, which is closed distal to the glans, allowing excess skin to be removed before the glans is uncovered and a dressing applied. In a similar technique to this, bone-cutting forceps are used instead to crush the foreskin prior to its excision.

Circumcision in older children is usually performed under general anesthetic with the addition of a regional anesthetic block.[30] A freehand or sleeve technique is normally used, although larger sizes of circumcision clamps and Plastibels are available for use in older boys, with comparable results.[28] The sleeve technique involved two circular incisions, one in the mucosa proximal to the glans and the other on the shaft skin just below the level of the corona with the foreskin pulled forward. The sleeve of foreskin is excised and hemostasis achieved with absorbable ties or bipolar diathermy before anastomosing skin to mucosa with an absorbable suture. For the freehand technique, a dorsal slit is made and circumcision is completed anteriorly with scissors, leaving a cuff of inner preputial skin to

Table 52.1. Complications of neonatal circumcision in five US studies

	Speert[1]	Patel[26]	Gee and Ansell[23]	Wiswell and Geschke[27]	Wiswell *et al.*[32]
Country (and year)	USA (1953)	Canada (1966)	USA (1976)	USA (1989)	USA (1983)
Type of study	Retrospective over 19 y	Questionnaire and examination 6 mo-2y	Retrospective over 10 y	Armed forces retrospective study	Armed forces retrospective study
Number of patients	10 802	100	5882	100 157	476 (mean age 2.9y)
Hemorrhage	0.037% (4)	4% (moderate)	1.07%	0.083% (surgery in 0.03%)	0.9%
Difficulty with micturition	?	?	0.02% (retention)	?	?
Infection	0.009% (1)	8%	0.42%	0.07% (bacteremia in 0.008%)	0.2%
Meatal ulcer	?	31%	?	0%	?
Meatal stenosis	?	8%	?	0%	?
Serious other complications	0.009% (excessive skin removed)	1% (recurrent phimosis)	0.2% dehiscence 0.02% glans injury 0.05% excess skin Removed 0.13% inappropriate circ. (hypospadias)	0.02% UTI 0.007% dehiscence 0.001% circumcised hypospadias 0.001% urethral injury 0.01% pneumothorax	0.2% aspiration pneumonia 0.4% malignant hyperpyrexia
Inadequate circumcision	?	4%	?	0.015% too little/ too much skin excised	?
Reoperation rate	0.037%	>2%	0.43%	0.052% (potentially from the data)	
Complication rate	0.06%	>35%	1.9%	0.19%	1.7%

Table 52.2. Complications of circumcision in older children

	MacCarthy *et al.*[4]	Leitch[2]	Fraser *et al.*[28]	Stenram *et al.*[6]	Griffiths *et al.*[30]	Cuckow *et al.*[34]
Country (and year)	UK (1952)	Australia (1970)	UK (1981)	Sweden (1986)	UK (1985)	UK (1993)
Type of study	Patient visit at age 4 y	Retrospective	Prospective randomized trial	5 y follow-up	Prospective	Prospective audit
Number of patients	585	200	100	117	140	50
Age group	0–4 y	2.3 y (mean)	4.7 y (mean)	0–10 y	4.3 y (mean)	6.6 y (mean)
Hemorrhage	1.5	7	20	6	1.4 readmitted	6
Difficulty with micturition (%)	0.2 (retention)	?	43	?	0.7 (retention)	14
Infection (%)	1.4	0.5	7	0.8	4.3	12
Meatal ulcer	?	4	?	?	?	?
Meatal stenosis (%)	?	1.5	?	11	2.8	?
Inadequate circumcision (%)	??	1	1	1.7	0.7	6 (poor cosmesis)
Reoperation rate	1.2	3.5	1	1.7	3.6	6
Overall complication rate (%)	5.5	15.5	29	19.6	15	40 (anesthetic comps. included)

be anastomosed to the shaft skin. Hemostasis and closure are achieved in the same way.

Complications

There are few prospective and long-term studies of the complications of circumcision. It is often performed by a junior surgeon,[2] and in the USA is rarely performed by a surgeon at all.[15] The assumed unimportance of the foreskin has led to an underestimate of the importance of the complications of circumcision.

In the UK, between 1942 and 1947 there were an average of 16 deaths a year reported following circumcision in those under 5 years. Causes of death included anesthesia, hemorrhage, and systemic infection. There were two deaths attributable to circumcision in Australia between 1960 and 1966,[2] and more recent reviews suggest that it is now extremely uncommon.[3,15] Outside modern medical practice, there is still a significant mortality, as the experience with the results of ritual circumcision in one African tribe attests.[31]

The tables summarize the complications of circumcision from reported Western series. Table 52.1 relates to routine neonatal circumcision. Three of these studies contain impressively large numbers of patients with low overall complication rates of 0.06–1.9%.[1,27] The performance of procedures in many different centers by unidentified practitioners, the use of retrospective data collection from hospital records, and lack of follow-up in these studies does call into question the validity of the oft-quoted complication rate of 0.06% from Speert's series.[1] There is one prospective study of 100 patients that is limited to one center and a known group of operators, and this involved direct patient/parent contact.[26] This showed a significantly higher complication rate of over 35%. Further comparison is provided in a second study by Wiswell, who identified an increased complication rate of 1.7% in boys circumcised later in life, compared with 0.19% in his series of neonatal circumcisions using the same method of inquiry.[27,32] Many of these patients had developed a medical indication for the procedure, required general anesthetic, and were circumcised by a different technique, although he used these data to further justify the timing of the operation in the neonatal period.[32]

Comparison with clamp-type circumcisions has revealed an increase in infection around retained Plastibel devices and greater bleeding with the Gomco device that relies on skin crushing alone for hemostasis.[33] One study comparing Plastibel to freehand circumcision did not support this increased infection rate and failed to show an appreciable difference in older boys.[28]

Table 52.2 shows a European and Australian experience of circumcisions performed for medical reasons in older boys over the same time period. While numerically smaller, these studies reflect the practice of individual surgeons or groups of surgeons, and their design has been either prospective or retrospective with some patient contact. There are significant differences in complication rates between them and the neonatal group, although the closer agreement with Patel's neonatal series suggests that differences may be more related to the type of study than to the timing or technique of operation. Even within these series there is great variation, alluding to the subjectivity

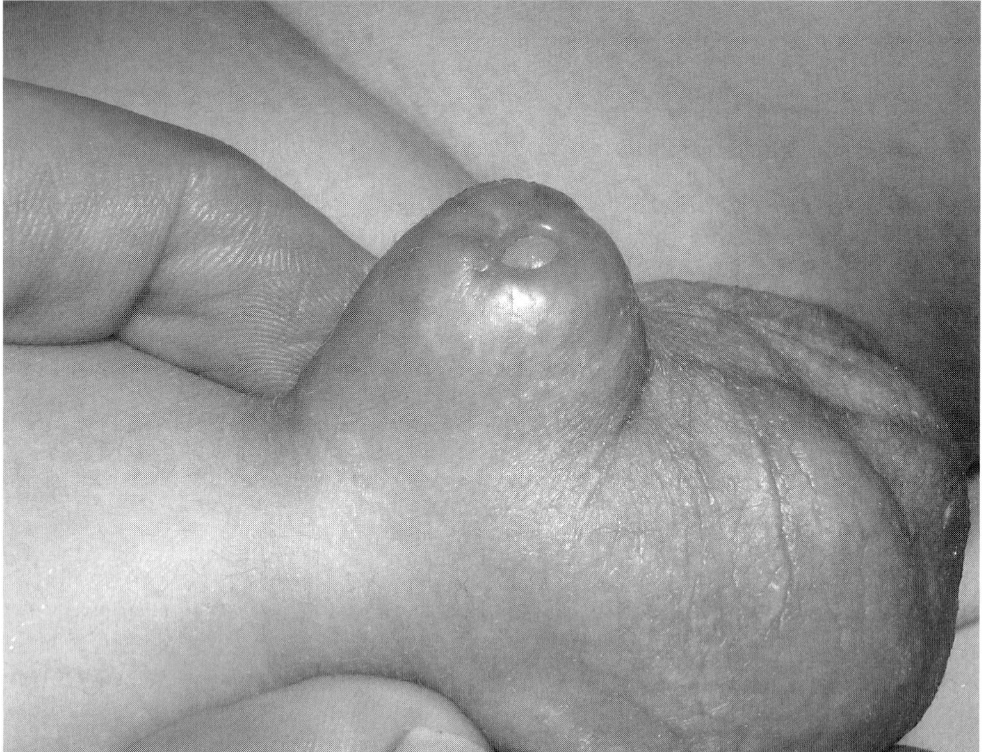

Fig. 52.1. Recurrent phimosis due to contraction of the circumcision scar, concealing the glans (see colour plate section).

of the assessment of complications, which have never been standardised. Thus, hemorrhage varies from 1.4% to 20%, requiring readmission and operation[30,34] but retention requiring a catheter is reported in only 0.2–0.7%.[4,30] Minor infection is common if looked for and results in visits to the family doctor and antibiotic prescription in up to 45% of cases,[34] although it is rarely the cause of long-term problems. The literature contains reports of necrotizing fasciitis, Fournier's gangrene, meningitis, and tetanus following circumcision.[3,15] Such severe sepsis is rare but when encountered may result in death.[35,36] As one might expect, the reoperation rate was highest (14.5%) in the prospective study with the longest follow-up (5 years) and was mostly for the correction of meatal stenosis.[6]

Long-term outcomes

Poor long-term results from circumcision can be subdivided into:

- skin complications: the removal of too much or too little skin, or unsatisfactory skin healing;
- irreversible damage to the penis, glans and erectile mechanism;
- inappropriate circumcision of an abnormal penis (buried penis or hypospadias), compromising reconstruction;
- trauma to the sensitive glans and urethral meatus following their exposure.

Skin complications

Leaving too much of the inner mucosal layer of foreskin followed by cicatrisation at the suture line is a cause of recurrent phimosis or burying of the penis and requires recircumcision[28,37] (Fig. 52.1). The amount of foreskin to be retained after circumcision is set out precisely in Jewish law,[38] but away from this there is considerable variation in opinion as to what constitutes an adequate or "normal" circumcision. Certainly, incomplete or inadequate circumcision is unsightly and often associated with the use of a circumcision clamp. Significant numbers of revision circumcisions are performed in centers where neonatal circumcision is practised, notably Atlanta where 46 were performed in 2 years.[39] In spite of this, large neonatal series often omit this complication.[1,27,33] Among Leitch's 200 consecutive circumcisions, 19 were revisions following an inadequate initial procedure,[2] and McCarthy *et al.* reported revising 1% of cases following freehand circumcision.[4]

Excessive loss of skin can occur with circumcision clamps and results in a denuded penile shaft.[40] This can also be due to local infection and diathermy injury.[3,15] In neonatal circumcision, healing can be achieved by secondary intention through granulation with satisfactory long-term appearance.[29] In older patients, skin grafting gives excellent functional and cosmetic results. Burying the shaft in a scrotal tube is another option, although the cosmetic results using this hair-bearing skin are questionable.[3,33,40]

Glanular adhesions with the inner preputial skin due to reformation or failure to divide them properly at circumcision are well recognized[15,53] and have a tendency to separate spontaneously with time. Adhesion of circumcision scar to a traumatized or ulcerated glans edge may result in a more permanent adhesion or skin-bridge, beneath which smegma accumulates and which can cause pain and deformity.[15] This was seen in around 2% of patients in Ponsky's study of 254 boys following neonatal circumcision[53] and requires surgical release. Epidermal inclusion cysts are also reported,[29] and penile lymphedema, the etiology of which is unclear, is seen extremely rarely.[3,35]

The assessment of cosmetic results is very subjective. A questionnaire sent to the parents of 50 circumcised boys found that 26% found its appearance to be normal, 53% acceptable and 21% slightly scarred with no complaints of a bad result. Surgeons appraising the same patients offered a revision circumcision in three for a poor cosmetic result.[3] Certainly, the skin–mucosal junction may be scarred and unsightly, particularly where sutures produce a cross-hatching effect (see Fig. 52.2). There are no current reviews of this aspect of circumcision and undoubtedly many men put up with poor cosmetic results without complaint.

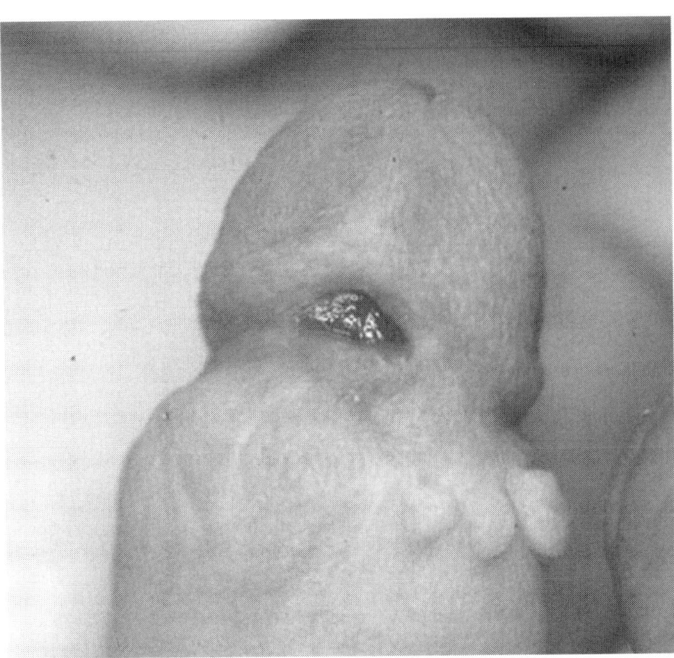

Fig. 52.2. Urethrocutaneous fistula following circumcision, probably due to diathermy around the frenular artery. Note the prominent cross-hatching of the circumcision scar and poor cosmetic result (see colour plate section).

Major penile injury

Amputation of part or all of the glans is rare but may arise when it is caught in the jaws of a circumcision clamp.[39,40] The excised portion may be grafted back on the penis (with reported success),[39,40] or the glans can be repaired.[41] Pressure necrosis is also seen with the Plastibel if too small a bell is selected.[33] Urethral damage is caused by overzealous hemostasis with diathermy on the ventral surface of the penis in the region of the frenular artery (Fig. 52.2). It can also be caught up in a Gomco or Plastibel clamp, leading to a subcoronal fistula, which requires secondary repair.[54]

Corporal fibrosos and total ablation of the penis are fortunately very rare occurrences and are often sequelae of the use of monopolar diathermy alone or in combination with a metal clamp such as the Gomco.[42–44] In some patients, complex reconstruction is possible and reasonable results have been reported.[43,44] Otherwise, gender reassignment, staged genital reconstruction and hormonal manipulation at puberty is advocated by Gearhart and Rock.[42] Two of their four patients are sexually active following their reconstructions and the other two are awaiting the start of estrogen therapy at 11 years and their subsequent vaginoplasty at 15 years of age. All individuals and their families have had counseling and require help to come to terms with the consequences of this disastrous injury and its management.[42]

Although only reported in adults, failure of the erectile mechanism very rarely occurs following intracorporeal injection of local anesthetic agents, or may be a sequence of more serious penile injury.[15]

Inappropriate circumcision

Circumcision should be avoided in hypospadias, where the foreskin is required for reconstruction. While perhaps more understandable in the intact prepuce megameatus variant of hypospadias,[45] which may appear normal to the untrained eye, inappropriate circumcision has been reported in 36% of hypospadii from one series of neonatal circumcisions.[33] This relates probably to its performance

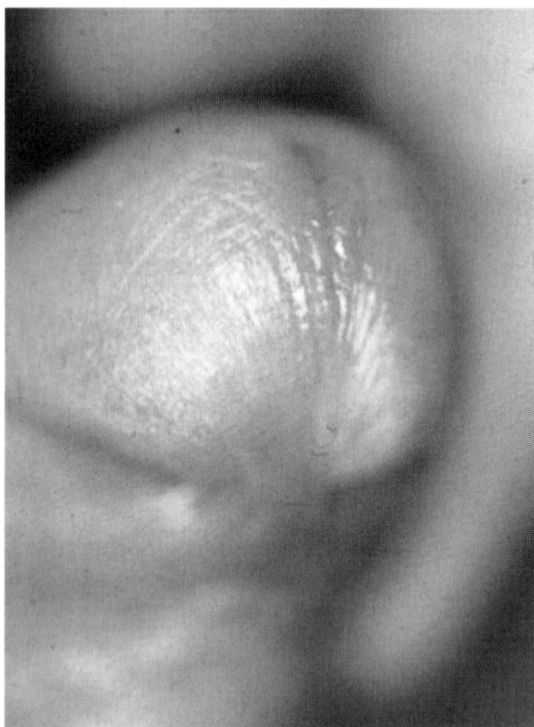

Fig. 52.3. Normal slit-like urethral meatus (see colour plate section).

by non-urologists, e.g., pediatricians, gynecologists, junior residents, and midwives.

Buried penis, an anomaly comprising insufficient shaft skin, abundant inner preputial skin, phimosis retaining the penis within abdominal wall fat, and abnormal tethering of the corporal bodies, is a contraindication to circumcision.[16] Removal of the usual amount of interpreputial skin in these cases leaves skin deficiency. Leaving enough inner preputial skin to cover the penile shaft simply results in recurrent burying of the penis if only a circumcision is performed. A more complex procedure is required to release the corporal bodies and obtain a satisfactory result.[48,55]

Meatal ulceration and stenosis

The urethral meatus is arguably the most sensitive area of the penis, and close inspection reveals the normal eversion of urethral mucosa at this point (Fig. 52.3). Meatal ulceration has been documented in 20% of infants 2–3 weeks after circumcision,[47] and Patel's prospective study revealed this problem in 31%.[26] It is thought to be due to chemical and physical irritation within the wet ammoniacal diaper,[47,48] which is borne out by a lower incidence in older boys – 4% with circumcision performed at a mean age of 2 years 4 months[2] – and offered as a reason to postpone circumcision until after potty training.[49] The natural history of meatal ulceration is either resolution or progression to chronic scarring and meatal stenosis, which is reported in 1.5%–11% of patients after circumcision in those series with sufficient follow-up.[2,6,26,30] This comprised almost 26% of Patel's and 38% of Leitch's patients with early meatal ulceration.[2,26] In addition, Persad *et al.*[48] have proposed that the relative ischemia of the meatus that follows division of the frenular artery is highly significant in the pathogenesis of meatal stenosis. Berry and Cross[48] calibrated the urethral meatus in children and adults: 60% of circumcised men had a meatus of 20F or less, compared with only 25% of uncircumcised men. These differences were more significant with earlier circumcision. In circumcised infants of 12–18 months, only 30% had a meatal caliber greater than or equal to 14F, compared with 53% of those uncircumcised, whereas meatal size was the same in infants under 1 year of age. It appears from these data that meatal stenosis develops some time after circumcision, accounting for its absence as a complication in many series, and will be detectable in at least a subclinical form in most patients. Persad *et al.*[48] reviewed the symptoms of 12 patients presenting between 4 months and 8 years after circumcision, finding pain at the initiation of micturition in them all, a narrow high-velocity stream in 8 cases, spillage of urine around the toilet bowl in 6 cases and urethral bleeding in one case. Clinical examination showed a pinhole meatus with a filmy membrane covering its lower margins (Fig. 52.4(a) and 52.4(b)). There was no history or clinical features of balanitis xerotica et obliterans. Meatotomy – opening the ventral aspect of the meatus proximally in the midline and suturing inner epithelium to outer skin with absorbable sutures – was effective in all cases, and there was no recurrence after a mean follow-up of 13 months.

Rarely the bladder and upper tracts are secondarily affected by meatal stenosis, leading to bladder hypertrophy that may ultimately produce upper urinary tract dilatation and sepsis.[49] Figure 52.5 demonstrates a case of meatal stenosis in a 7-year-old boy who presented several years after circumcision with a long history of difficulty in micturition and a poor urinary stream that progressed to chronic urinary retention. The cystourethrogram, performed via a suprapubic catheter, showed a grossly dilated urethra and trabeculated bladder resulting from chronic meatal stenosis. The upper tracts were not involved and he was treated successfully by meatotomy. With this picture and the high bladder pressures needed to produce effective micturition, it is not surprising that these patients complain of urethral pain.[48]

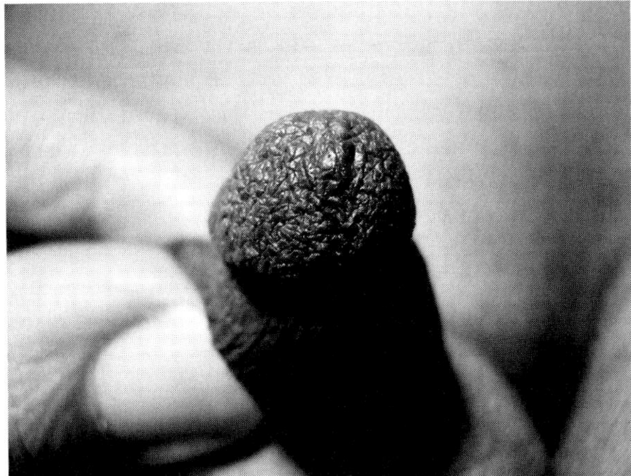

(a)

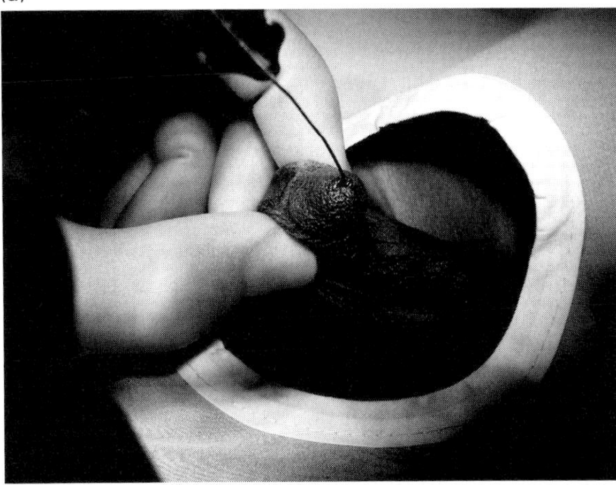

(b)

Fig. 52.4. (a) and (b). Reduction of the meatal caliber in meatal stenosis so only a fine lachrymal probe can pass (see colour plate section).

Balanitis xerotica et obliterans

Otherwise known as lichen sclerosus et atrophicus, BXO is characterized by tight phimosis with a sclerotic whitish ring at the tip of the prepuce and characteristic lesions on the glans. It is occasionally associated with meatal stenosis, perhaps representing a cause of meatal stenosis following circumcision.[30] Frank *et al.*[50] have demonstrated that 10/12 boys with meatal and submeatal stenosis had previously been circumcised for BXO, although this is at variance with the clinical impression of Persad *et al.*[48] for whose 12 patients BXO was not a known precursor of meatal stenosis.

BXO is the truest indication for medical circumcision[13] and is clinically recognized by its sclerotic preputial orifice

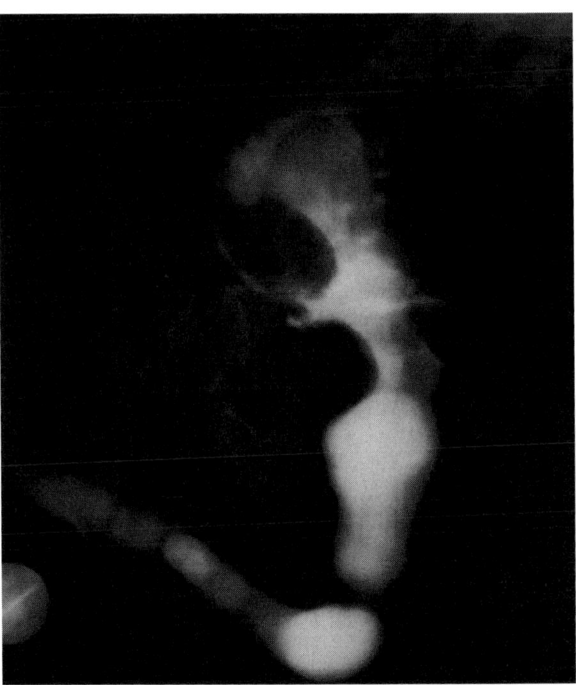

Fig. 52.5. A cystogram in a patient with chronic, severe meatal stenosis with secondary changes in the bladder.

(Fig. 52.6). Complete removal of the foreskin can remove all the affected tissue[14] and glanular lesions appear to regress spontaneously following circumcision. There were no recurrences or long-term complications in 10 children followed up to 5 years.[14]

Religious circumcision

Although performed in the community by Mohels, admissions to hospital following Jewish circumcision of 8-day-old infants reveals a similar spectrum of complications, although the exact rate is unknown.[29,41,51] If the circumcision dressing is too tight, urinary retention, infection, and septicemia may ensue.[39,41] Its use probably explains the increased incidence of urinary tract infection in Jewish boys, which is highest in this group during the 12 days after circumcision.[52] Severe penile injury is related to inexperienced Mohels,[29] and recircumcision is required when too much skin is left.[38] An extreme view from another culture is presented by Crowley and Kessner,[31] who found a mortality of 9% among 45 consecutive youths presenting with severe complications of ritual circumcision amongst the Xhosa people of South Africa.

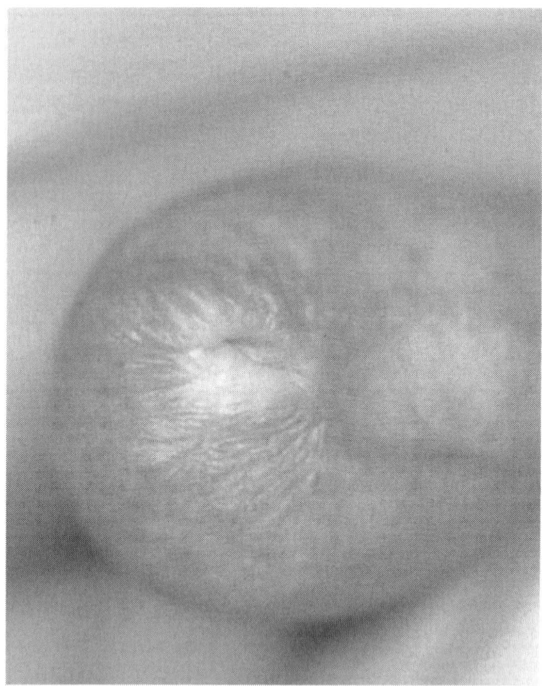

Fig. 52.6. The sclerotic prepucial tip, which is characteristic of BXO (see colour plate section).

Preputial plasty

If the complications of possessing a foreskin are related to its non-retractability and poor hygiene, then there are alternative surgical procedures. Preputial plasty has been used in Europe to produce a retractable yet intact foreskin. There are various techniques, the simplest consisting of a short dorsal incision at the narrowest point of the prepuce.[34] The foreskin is retracted and the congenital adhesions freed. The narrowed distal prepuce produces a constricting band on the shaft of the penis, and this is divided by a dorsal longitudinal incision to the level of Buck's fascia. The resulting defect allows widening of the prepuce at this point and is sutured transversely with absorbable sutures. The foreskin is then checked for mobility and the parents encouraged to commence regular retraction within days of the operation.

Comparing 50 patients undergoing this preputial plasty with 50 undergoing circumcision, there was considerably less short-term morbidity. The minimal dissection required, and in particular avoidance of the ventral aspect of the penis and the frenular artery, results in greater post-operative comfort and elimination of bleeding as a serious complication. There were also fewer consultations with the patient's general practitioner after surgery, and parents were pleased with the operation. Success of preputial plasty depends on early mobilization of the foreskin, which is possible without discomfort in around 90% of boys within 2 weeks of surgery. This prevents contraction of the suture line and scarring that leads to secondary or true phimosis, and was the reason for circumcision in 4% of patients. 70% of parents judged the appearance of the penis to be normal after this procedure, and the long-term results also appear excellent, although they warrant more formal appraisal.[34] Certainly no case of meatal stenosis has been reported following this procedure.[48]

Conclusions

Circumcision and its indications remain a hot discussion topic in both the medical and the lay literature. Arguments are laced with subjectivity, emotion, religious fervour and too little scientific study. There are significant short-term complications of the operation whichever timing, technique or setting is employed, and these are underestimated by many of the studies cited. Major injury to the penis, although fortunately rare, will have a profound effect on the boy's life and, more frequently, loss of protection of the urinary meatus is a potent cause of long-term problems. Avoidance of these is simple – avoidance of circumcision. While most arguments for circumcision are found lacking under scrutiny, congenital urological anomalies diagnosed antenatally may provide the only indication for prophylactic neonatal circumcision to help protect against urinary tract infection. It is true to say that the long-term effects of this procedure are yet to be fully assessed over 3000 years since it was first performed.

Acknowledgment

Marie-Klare Farrugia, Research Registrar in Urology, The Institute of Child Health.

REFERENCES

1. Speert, H. Circumcision of the newborn: appraisal of its current status. *Obstet. Gynecol.* 1953; **2**:164–172.
2. Leitch, I. O. W. Circumcision: a continuing enigma. *Austral. Pediatr. J.* 1970; **6**:59.
3. Williams, N. & Kapila, L. Complications of circumcision. *Br. J. Surg.* 1993; **80**:1231–1236.
4. McCarthy, D., Douglas, J. W. B., & Mogford, C. Circumcision in a national sample of 4-year-old children *Br. Med. J.* 1952; **ii**:755–756.

5. Rickwood, A. M. K. & Walker, J. Is phimosis overdiagnosed and are too many circumcisions performed in consequence? *Ann. Roy. Coll. Surg. Engl.* 1989; **71**:275–277.
6. Stenram, A., Malmfors, G., & Okiman, L. Circumcision for phimosis: a follow-up study. *Scand. J. Urol. Nephrol.* 1986; **20**:89–92.
7. O'Brien, T. R., Calle, E. E., & Poole, W. K. Incidence of neonatal circumcision in Atlanta, 1985–1986. *South. Med. J.* 1995; **88**:411–415.
8. Gairdner, D. The fate of the foreskin. *Br. Med. J.* 1949; **2**:1433–1437.
9. Øster, J. Further rate of the foreskin. *Arch. Dis. Child.* 1986; **43**:200–203.
10. Rickwood, A. M. K., Hemalthala, V., Batcup, G., & Spitz, L. Phimosis in boys. *Br. J. Urol.* 1980; **52**:147–150.
11. Harnes, J. R. The foreskin saga. *J. Am. Med. Assoc.* 1971; **217**:1241–1242.
12. Escala, J. M. & Rickwood, A. M. K. Balanitis. *Br. J. Urol.* 1989; **63**:196–197.
13. Anonymous. Medical indications for childhood circumcision. *Drug Ther. Bull.* 1993; **31**:99–100.
14. Mueli, M., Briner, J., Hanniman, B., & Sacher, P. Lichen sclerosus et atrophicus causing phimosis in boys: a prospective study with 5-year follow-up after complete circumcision. *J. Urol.* 1994; **152**:987–989.
15. Kaplan, G. W. Complications of circumcision. *Urol. Clin. N. Amer.* 1983; **10**:543–549.
16. Alter, G. J., Horton, C. E., & Horton, C. E., Jr. Buried penis as a contraindication for circumcision. *J. Am. Coll. Surg.* 1994; **178**:487–490.
17. Koo, H. P. & Duckett, J. W. Circumcision quo vadis? In: Williams, D. I., & Etker, S. (eds), *Contemporary Issues in Paediatric Urology, in Memoriam Herbert B. Eckstein.* Istanbul: Logos, 1996: 149–154.
18. Schoen, E. J. Report of the task force on circumcision. *Pediatrics* 1990; **84**:388.
19. Winberg, J., Bollgren, I., Gothefors, L., Herthelius, M., & Tullus, K. The prepuce: a mistake of nature? *Lancet* 1989; **i**:598–599.
20. Ginsberg, C. M. & McCracken, G. H. Urinary tract infections in young infants. *Pediatrics* 1982; **69**:409–412.
21. Wiswell, T. E. & Roscelli, J. D. Corroborative evidence for the decreased incidence of urinary tract infections in circumcised male infants. *Pediatrics* 1986; **78**:96–99.
22. Craig, J. C., Knight, J. F., Sureshkumar, P., Mantz, E., & Roy, L. P. Effect of circumcision on incidence of urinary tract infection in preschool boys. *J. Pediatr.* 1996; **128**:23–27.
23. Herzog, L. W. & Alvarez, S. R. The frequency of foreskin problems in uncircumcised children. *Am. J. Dis. Child.* 1986; **140**:254–256.
24. Fergusson, D. M., Lawton, J. M., & Shannon, F. T. Neonatal circumcision and penile problems: an 8 year longitudinal study. *Pediatrics* 1985; **75**:901–903.
25. Wiswell, T. E., Smith, F. R., & Bass, J. W. Decreased incidence of urinary tract infections in circumcised male infants. *Pediatrics* 1985; **75**:901–903.
26. Patel, H. The problem of routine circumcision. *Can. Med. Assoc. J.* 1966; **95**:576–581.
27. Wiswell, T. E. & Geschke, D. W. Risks from circumcision during the first month of life compared with those of uncircumcised boys. *Pediatrics* 1989; **83**:1011–1015.
28. Fraser, I. A., Allen, M. J., Bagshaw, P. F., & Johnstone, M. A. randomised trial of childhood circumcision with the Plastibel device compared to a conventional dissection technique. *Br. J. Surg.* 1981; **68**:593–595.
29. Shulman, J., Ben-Hur, N., & Neuman, Z. Surgical complications of circumcision. *Am. J. Dis. Child.* 1964; **107**:149–154.
30. Griffiths, D. M., Atwell, J. D., & Freeman, N. V. A prospective study of the indications and morbidity of circumcision in children. *Eur. Urol.* 1985; **11**:184–187.
31. Crowley, I. P. & Kessner, K. M. Ritual circumcision (Umkhwetha) amongst the Xhosa of the Ciskei. *Br. J. Urol.* 1990; **66**:318–321.
32. Wiswell, T. E., Tencer, H. L., Welch, C. A., & Chamberlain, J. L. Circumcision in children beyond the neonatal period. *Pediatrics* 1993; **92**:791–793.
33. Gee, W. F. & Ansell, J. S. Neonatal circumcision: a ten-year overview with comparison of the Gomco clamp and Plastibel devices. *Pediatrics* 1976; **58**:824.
34. Cuckow, P. M. & Mouriquand, P. D. E. Saving the normal foreskin. *Br. Med. J.* 1993; **306**:459–460.
35. Fredman, R. M. Neonatal circumcision: a general practitioner survey. *Med. J. Austral.* 1969; **1**:117–120.
36. Cleary, T. G. & Kohl, S. Overwhelming infection with group B beta haemolytic streptococcus associated with circumcision. *Pediatrics* 1979; **64**:301–303.
37. Redman, J. F., Scriber, L. J., & Bissada, N. K. Postcircumcision phimosis and its management. *Clin. Pediatr.* 1975; **14**:407–409.
38. Sotolongo, J. R., Hoffman, S., & Gribetz, M. E. Penile denudation injuries after circumcision. *J. Urol.* 1985; **133**:102–103.
39. Horrowitz, S. J. & Glassberg, K. I. Circumcision: successful glanular reconstruction and survival following traumatic amputation (abstract). American Academy of Pediatrics Annual Meeting, New Orleans, 1995.
40. Gluckman, G. R., Stoller, M. L., Jacobs, M. M., & Kogan, B. A. Newborn penile glans amputation during circumcision and successful reattachment. *J. Urol.* 1995; **153**:778–779.
41. Menahem, S. Complications arising from ritual circumcision: pathogenesis and possible prevention. *Israeli J. Med. Sci.* 1981; **17**:45–48.
42. Gearhart, J. P. & Rock, J. A. Total ablation of the penis after circumcision with electrocautery: a method of management and long term follow-up. *J. Urol.* 1989; **142**:799–801.
43. Azmy, A., Boddy, S. A., & Ransley, P. G. Successful reconstruction following circumcision with diathermy. *Br. J. Urol.* 1985; **57**:587–588.
44. Stefan, H. Reconstruction of the penis after necrosis due to circumcision burn. *Eur. J. Pediatr. Surg.* 1995; **4**:40–43.
45. Duckett, J. W. & Keating, M. A. Technical challenge of the megameatus intact prepuce hypospadias variant: the pyramid procedure. *J. Urol.* 1989; **141**:1407.

46. Joseph, V. T. A new approach to the surgical correction of buried penis. *J. Pediatr. Surg.* 1995; **30**:727–729.
47. MacKenzie, A. R. Meatal ulceration following circumcision. *Obstet. Gynecol.* 1966; **28**:221–223.
48. Persad, R., Sharma, S., McTavish, J., Imber, C., & Mouriquand, P. D. E. Clinical presentation and pathophysiology of meatal stenosis following circumcision. *Br. J. Urol.* 1995; **75**:91–93.
49. Berry, C. D. & Cross, R. R. Urethral meatal calibre in circumcised and uncircumcised males. *Am. Med. Assoc. J. Dis. Child.* 1956; **92**:152–156.
50. Frank, J. D., Pocock, R. D., & Stower, M. J. Urethral strictures in childhood. *Br. J. Urol.* 1998; **62**:590–592.
51. Schlosberg, C. Thirty years of ritual circumcision. *Clin. Pediatr.* 1971; **10**:205–209.
52. Cohen, H. A., Drucker, M. M., Vainer, S. *et al.* Postcircumcision urinary tract infection. *Clin. Pediatr.* 1992; **31**:322–324.
53. Ponsky, L. E., Ross, J. H., Knippper, N., & Kay, R. Penile adhesions after neonatal circumcision. *J. Urol.* 2001; **165**(3):915.
54. Baskin, L. S., Canning, D. A., Snyder, H. M. III & Duckett, J. W. Jr. Surgical repair of urethral circumcision injuries. *J. Urol.* 1997; **158**(6): 2269–2271.
55. Smeulders, N., Wilcox, D. T., & Cuckow, P. M. Surgical correction of the buried penis – an anatomical approach. *BJU Int.* 2000; **86**:523–526.

53

The single kidney

Adrian S. Woolf

Nephro-Urology Unit, UCL Institute of Child Health, London, UK

Introduction

This review covers three clinical scenarios which feature the single kidney. The first category concerns patients who are born with only one kidney: they have congenital solitary functioning kidney, either caused by unilateral renal agenesis or regression of a malformed rudiment. After addressing the definition, incidence and diagnosis of this disorder, three aspects will be discussed: the putative developmental etiologies of this disorder; the occasional familial nature of the disorder suggesting a genetic basis to the disorder, and the long-term outcome of these individuals in terms of risk of subsequent disease in the kidney and the occurrence of hypertension (the "renal prognosis").

The second category concerns patients who, in childhood or adulthood, have had either a unilateral nephrectomy or a subtotal nephrectomy for intrinsic renal disease. The latter subgroup have had one kidney and a fraction of the contralateral organ removed and are said to have a "remnant kidney." I will discuss the clinical evidence which addresses the renal prognosis of these individuals. The third category concerns the renal prognosis of the single kidney in otherwise healthy renal transplant donors.

Renal agenesis and the congenital single kidney

Definition

Renal agenesis implies the total absence of the kidney and can be considered as part of the spectrum of renal malformations which also include: (i) renal hypoplasia, a disorder in which the kidney is small and contains fewer nephrons than normal; (ii) renal dysplasia in which the kidney contains undifferentiated tissue; (iii) the multicystic dysplastic kidney in which the dysplastic organ contains massive cysts and; (iv) renal aplasia which describes a tiny dysplastic organ.[1,2]

Unilateral renal agenesis is often associated with absence of the ipsilateral ureter and bladder trigone. On occasion, the ipsilateral adrenal gland or gonad may also be missing. With the advent of fetal renal ultrasound scanning, it has become clear that a solitary kidney may result from in utero or postnatal regression of a contralateral multicystic dysplastic kidney.[3] In addition, small dysplastic, non-functional, kidneys (i.e., "renal aplasia") can regress in a similar manner.[4] This process is perhaps explained by the excess of programmed cell death, or apoptosis, which has been recorded in these organs.[5]

Clinical diagnosis

Isolated, non-syndromic, renal agenesis is usually clinically silent. Therefore its incidence is probably underestimated. The complete absence of a kidney can only be definitively diagnosed by direct inspection at laparotomy or autopsy. While commonly used renal ultrasound scanning cannot exclude the presence of a tiny contralateral aplastic kidney, this would be the most common imaging technique. While intravenous pyelography and isotope renography would also fail to detect an aplastic contralateral organ, these techniques do have the advantage of detecting an ectopic contralateral organ (e.g., a pelvic kidney) which might be missed on ultrasound imaging.

Pediatric Surgery and Urology: Long-term Outcomes, Mark Stringer, Keith Oldham, Pierre Mouriquand.

Incidence of solitary kidney and contralateral renal agenesis

In a study of 9200 autopsies, unilateral renal agenesis was found in seven subjects.[6] In contrast, a radiological study made this diagnosis in 0.3% of a control population of 682 adults.[7] Bilateral renal agenesis presents with Potter's sequence (oligohydramnios and lung hypoplasia) and is an order of magnitude less common than unilateral agenesis. Bilateral disease occurs in 0.1–0.3 per 1000 births.[8–10] Interestingly, one group reported an excess of bilateral cases born in the spring, similar to neural tube defects.[9]

Urinary tract malformations associated with the congenital single kidney

Malformations associated with the solitary renal tract are not uncommon. For example, Atiyeh and colleagues[11] reviewed 16 pediatric patients with unilateral renal agenesis: of ten who had a micturating cystourethrogram, nine had anomalies of the single kidney with vesicoureteric reflux being the commonest abnormality. Other diagnoses were pelviureteric obstruction, megaureter, ureterovesical obstruction, ectopic ureter with partial obstruction, and hypoplasia.[11] It is worth noting that some of these anomalies would not have been reliably detected on ultrasound scanning or even intravenous pyelography. Moreover, since vesicoureteric reflux can regress during childhood, it is difficult (or impossible) to be sure that a solitary kidney detected in later childhood or adulthood has indeed been connected to a normal urinary tract throughout life.

The developmental anatomy of renal agenesis

The adult mammalian kidney is derived from two components:[1,2] (i) the mesonephric duct epithelium and its outgrowth, the ureteric bud, which forms the branching collecting ducts and epithelia of the renal pelvis, ureter and trigone; (ii) the renal mesenchyme, a segment of intermediate mesoderm which differentiates to form the nephrons (glomeruli, proximal tubule and loop of Henle). In humans the metanephros appears at 5 weeks after conception and the first layer of glomeruli form by 9 weeks. Nephrogenesis continues in the cortex of the fetal kidney until the 34th week of gestation.

In 1927 Boyden demonstrated that ablation of the mesonephric duct in an animal model caused failure of metanephric development, presumably because the ureteric bud did not grow to induce the renal mesenchyme.[12] In 1932 the same investigator examined a 10 mm human embryo with renal agenesis: the ureteric bud had apparently failed to branch from the mesonephric duct, hence the normal reciprocal inductive interaction with the renal mesenchyme could not occur.[13] Others have postulated that an aberrant position of the ureteric bud can give rise to less severe malformations such as renal dysplasia.[14] Of note, the prenatal obstruction of the ureter can generate renal dysplasia but not renal agenesis.[15]

The molecular etiologies of renal agenesis: clues from animal models

Over 40 years ago Clifford Grobstein used organ culture experiments to demonstrate that the renal mesenchyme and ureteric bud fail to differentiate if cultured separately but if recombined they form a kidney in vitro.[16] He concluded that reciprocal interactions, or induction events, are required for normal kidney development. We now know that cell proliferation, survival, and differentiation in normal nephrogenesis are controlled by the expression of genes which encode four classes of molecules: (i) transcription factors which regulate the expression of other genes; (ii) locally acting growth factors; (iii) survival factors; and (iv) cell–cell and cell–matrix adhesion molecules.[1,2] Some of these molecules may act as the inductive signals postulated by Grobstein.

Mutations of genes in mice result in renal agenesis because of the failure of induction of the renal mesenchyme, e.g., the WT1 gene[17] or the failure of ureteric bud outgrowth from the mesonephric duct, e.g., RET gene[18] and PAX2 gene.[19] Animal studies also show that it may be necessary to ablate two related nephrogenesis genes to produce renal agenesis, e.g., the HOX[20] and the retinoic acid receptor[21] families. The experimental genetic ablation of the BCL2 survival factor[22] provides a loose animal analogy to the involution of human aplastic/dysplastic kidneys.[3,4] Here, the affected mice have fulminant apoptosis during nephrogenesis and are born with hypoplastic kidneys.[22]

Finally, teratogens such as drugs can cause various renal malformations in animals and in these cases the period of exposure to the insult determines the final effect on the developing excretory system. Glucose has been implicated as a teratogen that can cause renal agenesis in humans.[23]

Familial renal agenesis: a genetic basis for human disease

Stephens[24] found no familial cases in a review of over 200 individuals with congenital solitary kidney. However, in 1974 Cain *et al.* cited 12 previous reports and described a new kindred with two consecutive male infants: the first had bilateral renal agenesis while the second had agenesis on one side and renal dysplasia in the contralateral system.[25] Other reports of familial bilateral renal agenesis followed.[9,10,26,27] McPherson and colleagues emphasised that dysplasia and absence of a kidney can be inherited within single kindreds in a probable autosomal dominant manner, and that both disorders could occur in the same patient.[28] Roodhoft and coworkers[7] found that siblings and parents of patients with unilateral or bilateral agenesis had an approximately tenfold higher incidence of congenital solitary kidney compared with controls. Murugasu *et al.*[29] and Arfeen *et al.*[30] described kindreds with congenital single kidney with a probable autosomal dominant inheritance.

Syndromes associated with renal agenesis

Numerous human syndromes include unilateral or bilateral renal agenesis. These include those associated with chromosomal anomalies such as 4p- syndrome and partial trisomy 22.[27] Other syndromes include: branchio-oto-renal syndrome, cerebro-oculo-facio-skeletal syndrome, Di George syndrome (cardiac, face, thymus and parathyroid defects), Fraser syndrome (cryptophthalmos and syndactyly), Goldenhar syndrome (oculo-auriculo-vertebral dysplasia), Kallmann's syndrome (olfactory bulb agenesis and infertility), Mayer–Rokitansky–Kuster–Hauser syndrome (aplasia of the female genital tract), renal agenesis with duplicated uterus and/or cervix and the thymic–renal–anal–lung syndrome.[1,2]

Several syndromes are of especial note because they are familial and the genetic bases are being unravelled. The branchio-oto-renal syndrome is an autosomal dominant condition with a genetic locus linked to chromosome 8. The affected individuals have renal, ear and neck malformations and some familes have a mutation of the Eyes-Absent 1 (EYA1) gene which codes for a transcription factor-like molecule.[31] Hepatocyte nuclear factor 1β (HNF1β) is another transcription factor gene which is mutated in humans with congenital solitary functioning kidney; other family members can have renal dysplasia or hypoplasia, and some affected individuals develop diabetes requiring insulin therapy; the gene expressed in the developing kidney and pancreas.[32,33] In the X-linked Kallmann's syndrome the mutated gene is called KAL and it encodes a putative cell-signalling molecule that is expressed in the developing excretory and nervous systems.[34] In Kallmann's syndrome renal agenesis can be uni- or bilateral and there is apparently no left- or right-hand bias for the solitary kidney.[35] Recently, Fraser syndrome was reported to be caused, at least in some families, by mutations of a gene called FRAS1, which codes for a protein which coats embryonic kidney epithelia and mediates interactions with surrounding mesenchyme.[36]

No cases of human solitary kidney or bilateral agenesis have yet been associated with mutations of the mouse nephrogenesis genes such as PAX2, WT1 or BCL2 genes; however, families have been described with congenitally small kidneys and PAX2 mutations and there are other kindreds with renal agenesis and gut anomalies that resemble mice with RET mutations.

Hyperfiltration damage: theory and practice

After nephrectomy, it is the normal response of the remaining kidney to hypertrophy (i.e., the size of its cells increases). The glomeruli increase in size and the glomerular filtration rate remarkably approach the level of excretory function for two organs.[37] There is no convincing evidence that new nephron units can be generated in mammals in response to such an injury when it occurs after birth, although it has been considered possible, particularly in young animals, that some hyperplasia (increase of cell numbers) is involved in addition to hypertrophy. This response can be seen as compensatory and thus positive for the health of the patient or experimental animal: the total renal excretory capacity tends to be maintained. The stimulus for this hypertrophic response is unknown but it follows a rapid increase in renal blood flow in response to contralateral nephrectomy. Thus far no intrarenal or circulating "renotrophic" factor, which might rise in response to uninephrectomy, has been convincingly isolated. It is fascinating that "renal hypertrophy," as assessed by the size of the single kidney, has also been documented to occur before birth.[38,39] In these cases the increase in size cannot be linked to an increased functional need performed by the single kidney because the fetal circulation is effectively dialysed across the placental barrier. Recently, it was reported that fetal uninephrectomy in sheep, when performed two-thirds of the way through gestation, at a time when nephrogenesis is ongoing, leads to a compensatory 45% increase of nephron numbers in the solitary kidney.[40]

Hostetter and colleagues drew attention to the observation that hyperfiltration in remnant nephrons (i.e., increased single nephron glomerular filtration rate) was "a potentially adverse response to renal ablation."[41] Rats with subtotal renal ablation developed glomerulosclerosis and progressive renal damage. This group of investigators demonstrated that hyperfiltration was associated with an elevation of glomerular capillary hydrostatic pressure and, if this could be ameliorated by drugs like angiotensin-converting enzyme inhibitors which dilate the efferent glomerular arteriole, then the progressive injury could be minimized. O'Donnell and coworkers performed unilateral nephrectomy in both immature and adult rats; the younger animals developed focal glomerulosclerosis after a period of greater compensatory renal growth while the adult rats experienced a rise of glomerular capillary hydrostatic pressure but had no evidence of glomerulosclerosis.[42] Similarly, other workers found that: (i) rats are more prone to develop proteinuria and reductions in glomerular filtration rate if uninephrectomy was performed in infancy vs. adulthood;[43] (ii) nephron supply is a major determinant of long-term allograft outcome in rats.[44] However, even healthy rats tend to develop some proteinuria with aging and therefore some investigators have questioned the relevance of these animal studies to clinical practice. On the other hand, Moritz *et al.*[45] reported that fetal uninephrectomy in sheep led to postnatal hypertension associated with a decreased glomerular filtration rate. These animal studies suggest that reduced nephron number leads to progressive glomerular damage and have major implications for human diseases including the human solitary and remnant kidney.

Prognosis of the congenital solitary functioning kidney

In a review of 586 renal biopsies, 29 individuals had a diagnosis of focal segmental glomerulosclerosis: of this group, 5 (17%) had unilateral renal agenesis.[6] In 1984 Thorner and colleagues reported on two children with congenital solitary kidneys who had persistent proteinuria, renal impairment and glomerular sclerosis.[46] One had a single pelvic kidney with no vesicoureteric reflux, while the other had a single hypertrophied kidney in the normal location and also did not have vesicoureteric reflux. Another report described four children with congenital single kidney who had proteinuria.[47] These studies suggest that progressive glomerular damage can be associated with the congenital solitary kidney but do not provide an estimate of the risk of an individual with a congenital solitary kidney developing renal disease. Kiprov reviewed 9200 autopsies and found unilateral renal agenesis in seven subjects, two of whom developed end-stage renal disease due to focal segmental glomerulosclerosis.[6] Of interest is a report by Arfeen and colleagues of a 22-year-old woman with a congenital solitary kidney who was found to have proteinuria during pregnancy. A renal biopsy showed that occasional glomeruli had segmental sclerosis and over the next 10 years her glomerular filtration rate fell from 88 ml/min to levels which required the initiation of dialysis. Two of her four children were also found to have a single kidney and proteinuria, and one affected offspring had a daughter with a single kidney but no proteinuria.[30] In addition, oligomeganephronia can be associated with progressive renal failure and proteinuria.[48] In this disorder there is a severe reduction of nephron number at birth and these nephrons are considerably larger than normal. They are clearly subject to hyperfiltration and it is possible that the poor renal prognosis is determined by "hyperfiltration damage."

Argueso *et al.*[49] reviewed the prognosis of 157 adult patients (mean age at diagnosis was 37 years) with unilateral "renal agenesis" and a normal contralateral kidney, i.e., there was compensatory hypertrophy, no vesicoureteric reflux, no parenchymal scarring and no hydronephrosis. In the whole study population, by the end of the study 27% had died, a survival rate similar to that of age- and sex-matched life tables; however, six had died of renal failure; of 37 tested in life, 19% had proteinuria (>150 mg/day); of 47 tested in life, hypertension developed in 47%; of 32 tested with creatinine clearance in life, 13% had decreased renal function. In a recent study,[50] it was found that, compared with age-, height- and weight-matched controls, children with congenital solitary kidney had mildly elevated blood pressure, as assessed by 24 ambulatory monitoring, e.g., the average daytime systolic pressure was elevated by about 4 mmHg, and the diastolic pressure by about 2 mmHg.

It could be argued that several of the above reports studied populations biased to have disease e.g., because they comprised referrals to a specialist clinic rather than to a primary care setting. There has not been a long-term follow-up (into late adulthood) of a large cohort of pediatric patients diagnosed, using a non-biased screening method, with congenital solitary kidney; certainly, if renal morbidity occurs, it tends to do so later in life, rather than in childhood. On the other hand, these reports do establish the fact that potentially important renal disease can occur in the congenital solitary kidney. It is possible to interpret these outcomes in several ways. First, it is possible that unilateral renal agenesis predisposes to the development of hyperfiltration and glomerular sclerosis in the normal congenital single kidney. Second, an alternative explanation would be that the single kidney was not, in fact, normal. As discussed above, the congenital solitary kidney is often attached to a structurally abnormal lower urinary tract and these abnormalities (e.g., vesicoureteric reflux) would not always be detected by ultrasound scanning or intravenous urography.[11,51] Importantly, a renal biopsy is only performed when significant proteinuria is detected and hence the histology of the solitary kidney at birth is never known. Third, it is conceivable that both the renal agenesis and the glomerulosclerosis are the direct result of another, unknown, a primary event. For example, a yet-to-be defined mutation might perturb both kidney development causing the agenesis and also predispose to glomerulosclerosis. In this context, heterozygous mutations of the WT1 gene cause glomerulosclerosis in the Denys–Drash syndrome in children whereas homozygous mutations cause renal agenesis in mice.

Nephrectomy for renal disease

Renal prognosis after unilateral nephrectomy for renal disease

In a retrospective study Zucchelli drew attention to the occurrence of focal glomerulosclerosis in seven male patients who, as young adults, had nephrectomies for unilateral renal disease such as obstruction or nephrolithiasis.[52] None had systemic hypertension. Of these, four had a renal biopsy showing focal segmental glomerulosclerosis. Renal excretory function and the modest levels of proteinuria (441–1450 mg/day) were unchanged after a further 7 years of follow-up. Another study confirmed that renal excretory function, as assessed by creatinine clearance, was stable after mean follow-up of 23 years in 27 individuals who had undergone unilateral nephrectomy in childhood for hydronephrosis, Wilms' tumor, renal dysplasia or kidney trauma.[53] Another study reported a minimal decline in glomerular filtration rate with time during the follow-up of 36 patients with either unilateral renal agenesis or childhood nephrectomy for hydronephrosis followed for 7–47 years. Having said this, only one individual was found to have a glomerular filtration rate (slightly) lower than normal age-matched range.[54]

One problem with these studies is that it was sometimes unclear whether disease had been rigorously excluded from the remaining kidney at the time of the nephrectomy. In other words, did these patients really have unilateral and not bilateral disease? Argueso and colleagues reported on the prognosis of 30 children with solitary kidney after unilateral nephrectomy for obstruction, vesicoureteric reflux or Wilms' tumor after a median follow-up of 25 years.[55] These authors excluded from analysis those children with evidence of scars or vesicoureteric reflux into the opposite (unoperated) kidney. At follow-up 8 had proteinuria (<1.5 g/day), 9 had renal insufficiency (10–83 ml/min/1.73 m^2) and 3 had systemic arterial hypertension ($>160/95$ mm Hg). Lent and Harth (1994) reported on 39 patients with unilateral nephrectomy after a follow-up of 2–23 years.[56] The initial diagnoses were evenly distributed between nephrolithiasis, tumors or pyelonephritis. The investigators excluded patients with disease of the remaining kidney or who initially had proteinuria >150 mg/day. Qualitative glomerular proteinuria was found in 32 using microelectrophoresis but only 4 had a rise in absolute values to over 150 mg/day.

Another long-term study was recently published by Ohishi and coworkers regarding 21 patients who had undergone nephrectomy in adulthood for unilateral disease. After an average follow-up for 27 years the mean creatinine clearance sustained by the solitary kidney was 88 ml/min/1.73 m^2, or 93% of that expected for a normal age-matched individual! Protein excretion was not significantly raised (214 vs. 119 mg/day) and age at nephrectomy, length of time with a single kidney or sex had little influence on current renal status. Six developed de novo hypertension and tended to have a positive family history of raised blood pressure more often than those with normotension.[57]

Thus it appears to be highly unusual to develop progressive kidney damage of any significance after nephrectomy for unilateral disease in adulthood. On the other hand, there may be a small risk if a similar operation is performed in children. However, even in those cases the question of occult renal disease at the time of nephrectomy must remain open: vesicoureteric reflux might have regressed by the time a micturating cystogram was performed, we know that intravenous urography is less sensitive than the modern renal isotope scans (e.g., DMSA) at detecting renal scars, and tissue for renal histology of the contralateral kidney is clearly not reported or available at the time of nephrectomy for alleged unilateral renal disease.

Renal prognosis after subtotal nephrectomy: the human remnant kidney

Based on experiments in rats, it is possible that humans with subtotal nephrectomy (e.g., single nephrectomy plus partial contralateral nephrectomy) would be susceptible to progressive renal damage.[40] The following reports suggest that subtotal nephrectomy generally has a good renal prognosis in humans. Rutsky and coworkers reported on a 10-year follow-up of an individual with three-quarters renal ablation after vascular trauma. Creatinine clearance increased from 16 to 53 ml/min and remained stable but daily urine excretion rose from 90 to a modest level of 400 mg, the upper end of the normal range.[58] Lhotta and colleagues reported on six patients who underwent enucleation for carcinoma in solitary kidneys: four had previously had a nephrectomy and two had an atrophic non-functioning kidney. None showed progressive deterioration of function or proteinuria over 10–23 months but two subjects had a rise in systemic blood pressure.[59] Foster collected the records of patients with surgical resection resulting in a remnant kidney.[60] All had resection for renal carcinoma and one for tuberculosis. Six patients were observed for at least 10 years, and 6 for 5–7 years: all had stable plasma creatinine levels. Moreover, the two longest surviving patients had pregnancies with no change in renal function. Only one patient had evidence of a progressive rise in plasma creatinine. In a retrospective analysis of 109 cases after nephrectomy for carcinoma only one individual had severe renal impairment after semitotal nephrectomy: in others the progressive impairment could be explained by concomitant renal disease.[61]

While these studies suggest a good renal prognosis in the human remnant kidney, another report suggests a somewhat different story. Novick evaluated 14 patients with a solitary kidney 5–17 years after partial nephrectomy for carcinoma.[62] Twelve had stable renal function but two developed renal failure and nine had proteinuria, which in four was >900 mg/day. None had systemic hypertension. The extent of the proteinuria was proportional to length of follow-up and inversely correlated to amount of remaining renal tissue. The four patients with the most marked proteinuria had renal biopsies and focal segmental glomerulosclerosis was demonstrated in three and global sclerosis in the other patient.

Thus, compared to a simple nephrectomy for disease or transplant donation (see below), there appears to be some evidence which indicates that there is a small but significant risk of developing proteinuria and progressive renal dysfunction after subtotal nephrectomy. At present, we do not know how to predict which patients will deteriorate and long-term follow-up regarding protein excretion and plasma creatinine is warranted in these patients.

Transplant kidney donation

A relatively early study in this population by Hakim and colleagues assessed 52 donors who had been nephrectomized 10 years previously.[63] They found no significant decline of renal function as assessed by levels of serum creatinine or creatinine clearance. There was, however, a higher incidence in mild proteinuria of less than 1 g/day and additionally there was an increase of systemic hypertension in male donors. It was suggested that these results might indicate that a modest degree of hyperfiltration damage had occurred.

Talseth and coworkers examined 68 kidney donors who had their nephrectomies 9–15 years previously.[64] Although 15% were hypertensive, it must be realized that the incidence of high blood pressure in the general population is of this order of magnitude. Twenty-six individuals had a urinary albumin excretion over 10 mg/min or a total daily excretion over 185 mg. However, only four had proteinuria over 400 mg/day and of these three individuals had intercurrent disease. It was found that the compensatory rise in glomerular filtration rate was inversely proportional to age at nephrectomy. In contrast, other studies suggested an increased incidence of proteinuria and hypertension in donors 9–18 years after unilateral nephrectomy.[65]

In 1989 Fotino published a review of 25 studies of long-term follow-up of kidney transplant donors.[66] Based on these studies it was concluded that the raised glomerular filtration rate of the remaining kidney was stable for decades. While some donors did develop mild non-progressive proteinuria, there appeared no definitive evidence that they suffered an undue rise of systemic blood pressure. Since then, several other reports have been published. For example, Goldfarb *et al*[67] reported outcomes 25 years after donor nephrectomy; they noted that, although blood pressure tended to rise, levels remained in the normal range and were similar to that expected for an age-matched population. There was a modest increase in protein excretion rates in male vs. female donors. Eberhard *et al.*[68] monitored living related kidney donors an average of 11 years after donation; 7 of 29 developed microalbuminuria and, even though all donors were considered normotensive before donation, just over a quarter proved to be hypertensive (>130/80, as assessed by 24-hour blood pressure monitoring).

Therefore, there appears to be little evidence that donation of a kidney has an adverse effect on excretory function of the remaining kidney over a period of up to three decades, at least when compared to the modest loss of excretory function which occurs in the normal aging kidney. On the other hand, there is mixed evidence that hypertension may be greater than expected, compared to appropriate controls. It should also be remembered that the populations described above are predominantly adult and it is conceivable that the reaction of the remaining kidney from an individual who donated in childhood might be different; however, it is currently rare to donate a kidney in early childhood.

Acknowledgment

ASW acknowledges grant support from the Kidney Research Aid Fund.

REFERENCES

1. Risdon, R. A. & Woolf, A. S. Developmental defects and cystic diseases of the kidney. In Jennette, J. C., Olson, J. L., Schwartz, M. M., & Silva, F. G., eds. *Heptinstall's Pathology of the Kidney.* 5th edn. Philadelphia-New York, USA: Lippincott-Raven, 1998:1149–1206.
2. Woolf, A. S., Welham, S. J. M., Hermann, M. M., & Winyard, P. J. D. Maldevelopment of the human kidney and lower urinary tract: an overview. In Vize, P. D., Woolf, A. S., & Bard, J. B. L., eds. *The Kidney: From Normal Development to Congenital Disease.* The Netherlands: Elsevier Science/Academic Press, 2003:377–393.
3. Dungan, J. S., Fernandez, M. T., Abbitt, P. L., Thiagarajah, S., Howards, S. S., & Hogge, W. A. Multicystic dysplastic kidney: natural history of prenatally detected cases *Prenat. Diagn.* 1990; **10**:175–182.
4. Hiraoka, M., Tsukahara, H., Ohshima, Y., Kasuga, K., Ishihara, Y., & Mayumi, M. Renal aplasia is the predominant cause of congenital solitary kidney. *Kidney Int.* 2002; **61**:1840–1844.
5. Winyard, P. J. D., Nauta, J., Lirenman, D. S. *et al.* Deregulation of cell survival in cystic and dysplastic renal development. *Kidney Int.* 1996; **49**:135–146.
6. Kiprov, D. D., Calvin, R. B., & McLuskey, R. T. Focal and segmental glomeruloscerosis and proteinuria associated with unilateral renal agenesis. *Lab. Invest.* 1982; **46**:275–281.
7. Roodhooft, A. M., Birnholz, J. C., Holmes, L. B. Familial nature of congenital absence and severe dysgenesis of both kidneys. *N. Engl. J. Med.* 1984; **310**:1341–1345.
8. Potter, E. L. Bilateral renal agenesis. *J. Pediatr. 1946*; **29**:68–76.
9. Carter, C. O., Evans, K., & Pescia, G. A familial study of renal agenesis. *J. Med. Genet.* 1979; **16**:176–188.
10. Bankier, A., De Campo, M., Newell, R., Rogers, J. G., & Danks, D. M. A pedigree study of perinatally lethal renal disease. *J. Med. Genet.* 1985; **22**:104–111.
11. Atiyeh, B., Husmann, D., & Baum, M. Contralateral renal abnormalities in patients with renal agenesis and noncystic renal dysplasia. *Pediatrics* 1993; **91**:812–815.
12. Boyden, E. A. Experimental obstruction of the mesonephric ducts. *Proc. Soc. Exp. Biol. Med.* 1927; **24**:572–576.
13. Boyden, E. A. Congenital absence of the kidney. An interpretation based on a 10 mm human embryo exhibiting unilateral renal agenesis. *Anat. Rec.* 1932; **52**:325–349.
14. Mackie, C. G. & Stephens, F. D. Duplex kidneys: a correlation of renal dysplasia with position of the ureteric orifice. *J. Urol.* 1975; **114**:274–280.
15. Woolf, A. S. Congenital obstructive nephropathy gets complicated. *Kidney Int.* 2003; **63**:761–763.
16. Grobstein, C. Morphogenetic interaction between embryonic mouse tissues separated by a membrane filter. *Nature* 1953; **172**:869–870.
17. Kreidberg, J. A., Sariola, H., Loring, J. M. *et al. WT-*1 is required for early kidney development. *Cell* 1993; **74**:679–691.
18. Schuchardt, A., D'Agati, V., Larsson-Blomberg, L., Costantini, F., & Pachnis, V. Defects in kidney and enteric nervous system of mice lacking the tyrosine kinase receptor Ret. *Nature* 1994; **367**:380–383.
19. Torres, M, Gomex-Pardo, E., Dressler, G. R., & Gruss, P. *Pax-2* controls multiple steps of urogenital development. *Development* 1995; **121**:4057–4065.
20. Davis, A. P., Witte, D. P., Hsieh-Li, H. M., Potter, S. S., & Capecchi, M. R. Absence of radius and ulna in mice lacking hoxa-11 and hoxd-11. *Nature* 1995; **375**:791–795.
21. Mendelsohn, C., Lohnes, D., Decimo, D. *et al.* Function of the retinoic acid receptors (RAR) during development. *Development* 1994; **120**:2749–2771.
22. Veis, D. J., Sorenson, C. M., Shutter, J. R., & Korsmeyer, S. J. Bcl-2-deficient mice demonstrate fulminant lymphoid apoptosis, polycystic kidneys and hypopigmented hair. *Cell* 1993; **75**:229–240.
23. Novak, R. W. & Robinson, H. B. Coincident DiGeorge anomaly and renal agenesis and its relation to maternal diabetes. *Am. J. Med. Genet.* 1994; **50**:311–312.
24. Stevens, A. R. Pelvic single kidneys. *J. Urol.* 1937; **37**:610–618.
25. Cain, D. R., Griggs, D., Lackey, D. A., & Kagan, B. M. Familial renal agenesis and total dysplasia. *Am. J. Dis. Child.* 1974; **128**:377–380.
26. Pashayan, H. M., Dowd, T., & Nigro, A. V. Bilateral absence of the kidneys and ureters. *J. Med. Genet.* 1977; **14**:205–209.
27. Schinzel, A., Homberger, C., & Sigrist, T. Bilateral renal agenesis in 2 male sibs born to consanguineous parents. *J. Med. Genet.* 1978; **15**:314–316.
28. McPherson, E., Carey, J., Kramer, A. *et al.* Dominantly inherited renal adysplasia. *Am. J. Med. Genet.* 1987; **26**:863–872.
29. Murugasu, B., Cole, B. R., Hawkins, E. P., Blanton, S. H., Conley, S. B., & Portman, R. J. Familial renal adysplasia. *Am. J. Kidney Dis.* 1991; **18**:490–494.
30. Arfeen, S., Rosborough, D., Luger, A. M., & Nolph, K. D. Familial unilateral renal agenesis and focal and segmental glomerulosclerosis. *Am. J. Kidney Dis.* 1993; **21**:663–668.
31. Rodriguez-Soriano, J. Branchio-oto-renal syndrome. *J. Nephrol.* 2003; **16**:603–605.
32. Bingham, C., Ellard, S. Cole, T. R. P. *et al.* Solitary functioning kidney and diverse genital tract malformations associated with hepatocyte nuclear factor-1β mutations. *Kidney Int.* 2002; **61**:1243–1251.
33. Kolatsi-Joannou, M., Bingham, C., Ellard, S. *et al.* Hepatocyte nuclear factor 1β: a new kindred with renal cysts and diabetes, and gene expression in normal human development. *J. Am. Soc. Nephrol.* 2001; **12**:2175–2180.
34. Duke, V. M., Winyard, P. J. D., Thorogood, P., Soothill, P., Bouloux, P. M. G., & Woolf, A. S. *KAL*, a gene mutated in Kallmann's syndrome, is expressed in the first timester of human development. *Mol. Cell. Endocrin.* 1995; **110**:73–79.
35. Kirk, J. M. W, Grant, D. B., Besser, G. M. *et al.*. Unilateral renal aplasia in X-linked Kallmann's Syndrome. *Clin. Genet.* 1994; **46**:260–262.
36. McGregor, L., Makela, V., Darling, S., M. *et al.* Fraser syndrome and mouse blebbed phenotype caused by mutations in

FRAS1/Fras1 encoding a putative extracellular matrix protein. *Nat. Genet.* 2003; 34:203–208.

37. Fine, L. G., Kurtz, I., Woolf, A. S. *et al.* Pathophysiology and nephron adaptation in chronic renal failure. In Schrier, R. W. & Gottschalk, C. W., eds. *Diseases of the Kidney*, Boston: Little and Brown, 1992:2703–2742.
38. Mandell, J., Peters, C. A., Estroff, J. A., Allred, E. N., & Benacerraf, B. R. Human fetal compensatory renal growth. *J. Urol.* 1993: **150**:790–792.
39. Glazebrook, K. N., McGrath, F. P., & Steele, B. T. Prenatal compensatory renal growth: documentation with US. *Radiology* 1993; **189**:733–735.
40. Douglas-Denton R., Moritz, K. M., Bertram, J. F., & Wintour, E. M. Compensatory renal growth after untilateral nephrectomy in the ovine fetus. *J. Am. Soc. Nephrol.* 2002; **13**:406–410.
41. Hostetter, T. H., Olson, J. L., Rennke, H. G., & Brenner, B. M. Hyperfiltration in remnant nephrons: a potentially adverse response to renal ablation. *Am. J. Phys.* 1981; **241**:F85–F93.
42. O'Donnell, M. P., Kasiske, B., Raij, L., & Keane, W. F. Age is a determinant of the glomerular morphologic and functional responses to chronic nephron loss. *J. Lab. Clin. Med.* 1985; **106**:308–313.
43. Celsi, G., Bohman, S.-O., & Aperia, A. Development of focal glomeruloscerosis after unilateral nephrectomy in infant rats. *Pediatr. Nephrol.* 1987; **1**:290–296.
44. Mackenzie, H. S., Tullius, S. G., Heemann, U. W. *et al.* Nephron supply is a major determinant of long-term allograft outcome in rats. *J. Clin. Invest.* 1994; **94**:2148–2152.
45. Moritz, K. M., Wintour, E. M., & Dodic, M. Fetal uninephrectomy leads to postnatal hyspertension and compromised renal function. *Hypertension* 2002; **39**:1071–1076.
46. Thorner, P. S., Arbus, G. S., Calermajer, D. S., & Baumal, R. Focal segmental glomerulosclerosis and progressive renal failure associated with a unilateral kidney. *Pediatrics* 1984; **73**:806–810.
47. Gutierrez-Millet, V., Nieto, J., Praga, M. *et al.* Focal glomerulosclerosis and proteinuria in patients with solitary kidneys. *Ann. Intern. Med.* 1986; **146**:705–709.
48. Nomura, S. & Osawa, G. Focal glomerular sclerotic lesions in a patient with unilateral oligomeganephronia and agenesis of the contralateral kidney: a case report. *Clin. Nephrol.* 1990; **33**:7–11.
49. Argueso, L. R., Ritchey, M. L., Boyle, E. T. Jr, Milliner, D. S., Bergstralh, E. J., & Kramer, S. A. Prognosis of patients with unilateral renal agenesis. *Pediatr. Nephrol.* 1992; **6**:412–416.
50. Mei-Zahav, M., Koizets, Z., Cohen, I. *et al.* Ambulatory blood pressure monitoring in children with a solitary kidney – a comparison between unilateral renal agenesis and nephrectomy. *Blood Pressure Monitoring* 2001; **6**:262–267.
51. Cascio, S., Paran, S., & Puri, P. Associated urological anomalies in children with unilateral renal agenesis. *J. Urol.* 1999; **162**:1081–1083.
52. Zucchelli, P., Cagnoli, L., Casanova, S., Donini, V., & Pasquali, S. Focal glomerulosclerosis in patients with unilateral nephrectomy. *Kidney Int.* 1983; **24**:649–655.
53. Robitaille, P., Mongeau, J.-G., Lortie, L., & Sinnasammy, P. Long term follow-up of patients who underwent unilateral nephrectomy in childhood. *Lancet* 1985; **1**:1297–1299.
54. Wikstad, I., Celsi, G., Larsson, L., Herin, P., & Aperia, A. Kidney function in adults born with unilateral agenesis or nephrectomised in childhood. *Pediatr. Nephrol.* 1988; **2**:177–182.
55. Argueso, L. R., Ritchey, M. L., Boyle, E. T., Milliner, D. S., Bergstralh, E. J., & Kramer, S. A. Prognosis of children with solitary kidney after unilateral nephrectomy. *J. Urol.* 1992; **148**:747–751.
56. Lent, V. & Harth, J. Nephropathy in remnant kidneys: pathological proteinuria after unilateral nephrectomy. *J. Urol.* 1994; **152**:312–316.
57. Ohishi, A., Suzuki, H., Nakamoto, H. *et al.* Status of patients who underwent uninephrectomy in adulthood more than 20 years ago. *Am. J. Kidney Dis.* 1995; **26**:889–897.
58. Rutsky, E. A., Dubovsky, E. V., & Kirk, K. A. Long term follow-up of a human subject with a remnant kidney. *Am. J. Kidney Dis.* 1991; **18**:509–513.
59. Lhotta, K., Eberle, H., Konig, P., & Dittrich, P. Renal function after tumour enucleation in a solitary kidney. *Am. J. Kidney Dis.* 1991; **17**:266–270.
60. Foster, M. H., Sant, G. R., Donohoe, J. F., Harrington, J. T. Prolonged survival with a remnant kidney. *Am. J. Kidney Dis.* 1991; **17**:261–265.
61. Grossman, H. B., Sommerfield, D., Konnak, J. W., & Bromberg, J. Long-term assessment of renal function following nephrectomy for stage I renal carcinoma. *Br. J. Urol.* 194; **74**:279–282.
62. Novick, A. C., Gephardt, G., Guz, B., Steinmuller, D., & Tubbs, R. R. Long-term follow up after partial removal of a solitary kidney. *N. Engl. J. Med.* 1991; **325**:1058–1062.
63. Hakim, R. M., Goldszer, R. C., & Brenner, B. M. Hypertension and proteinuria: long-term sequelae of uninephrectomy in humans. *Kidney Int.* 1984; **25**:930–936.
64. Talseth, T., Fauchald, P., Skrede, S. *et al.* Long-term blood pressure and renal function in kidney donors. *Kidney Int.* 1986; **29**:1072–1076.
65. Watnick, T. J., Jenkins, R. R., Rackoff, P., Baumgarten, A., & Bia, M. J. Microalbumin and hypertension in long-term renal donors. *Transplant* 1988; **45**:59–65.
66. Fotino, S. The solitary kidney: a model of chronic hyperfiltration in humans. *Am. J. Kidney Dis.* 1989; **13**:88–98.
67. Goldfarb, D. A., Matin, S. F., Braun, W. E. *et al.* Renal outcome 25 years after donor nephrectomy. *J. Urol.* 2001; **166**:2043–2047.
68. Eberhard, O. K., Kliem, V., Offner, G. *et al.* Assessment of long-term risks for living related kidney donors by 24-h blood pressure monitoring and testing for microalbuminuria. *Clin. Transpl.* 1997; **11**:415–419.

54

Multicystic kidney

Gianantonio M. Manzoni[1] and Anthony A. Caldamone[2]

[1]Division of Urology, Ospedale di Circol e Fondazione Macchi, Varese, Italy
[2]Division of Pediatric Urology, Hasbro Children's Hospital

Although multicystic kidney (MCK) is a common renal anomaly, the management of this entity remains controversial. Much of the controversy stems from a lack of long-term data on its natural history. Only recently have efforts been made to follow the MCK and accumulate long-term data on its natural history. The results of these efforts may have a significant impact on management.

Schwartz is credited with the first description of an MCK in a 7-month-old child.[1] In addition to describing the kidney as having been replaced by multiple cysts in a "bunch of grapes" arrangement, he also reported the ureter to be atretic. Spence's classic article appeared in 1955, in which he further described the MCK, distinguishing it from other forms of renal cystic disease.[2]

This chapter reviews the presentation of MCK and looks at the available long-term data in an attempt to arrive at a management protocol.

Presentation and diagnosis

The classic presentation of MCK was either a palpable mass in a newborn or infant or an incidental finding at autopsy. Pathak and Williams, in a series of 22 cases, reported that eight cases presented with an abdominal mass, seven had vomiting, and three had failure to thrive.[3] With the advent of prenatal ultrasonography, many more asymptomatic lesions are being identified. A review of data accumulated by the National Multicystic Kidney Registry in the USA indicated that 72% of registered cases were discovered on prenatal ultrasound (J. Wacksman, personal communication).

The diagnosis of MCK can be strongly suggested, if not made definitely, by prenatal ultrasound.[4,5] The classic picture of multiple fluid-filled cysts of varying size, randomly arranged with no communication, separated by echodense stroma, is often pathognomonic for MCK (Fig. 54.1). A hydronephrotic variant of MCK, however, may present the ultrasonographer with some concern (Fig. 54.2). In 1975, Felson and Cussen[6] described a pattern in which cysts were located peripherally around a hydronephrotic renal pelvis, with evidence of communication between cysts and pelvis. They also noted some function between the cysts radiographically. The existence of this type of variant of the MCK lends credence to the embryological theory that MCK and obstructed hydronephrotic kidney are on a spectrum of disease. The duration, extent, and timing of the obstruction dictates the outcome (i.e., MCK or hydronephrosis).

Unilateral multicystic kidney dysplasia (UMCK) is the second most common urinary tract abnormality diagnosed antenatally. While the isolated unilateral form UMCK has a good prognosis, a poor outcome must be expected only when it is associated with other complex abnormalities.[7] Bilateral MCK has been reported in 7%–23% of all cases and usually results in an absence of renal function, incompatible with extrauterine life.[8]

In a recent Canadian review of 54 cases Aubertin[4] reported that chromosomal abnormalities may be present in a low proportion (3%) and an amniocentesis is only recommended if associated anomalies are identified. Careful examination of the contralateral kidney is mandatory since up to 33% of genitourinary tract abnormalities may be present and interestingly, a positive family history of structural renal anomalies was found in 20% of the cases. Among non-renal anomalies (16%) congenital heart defects seem to be the most frequent (7%), therefore a careful assessment

Pediatric Surgery and Urology: Long-term Outcomes, Mark Stringer, Keith Oldham, Pierre Mouriquand.
Published by Cambridge University Press.

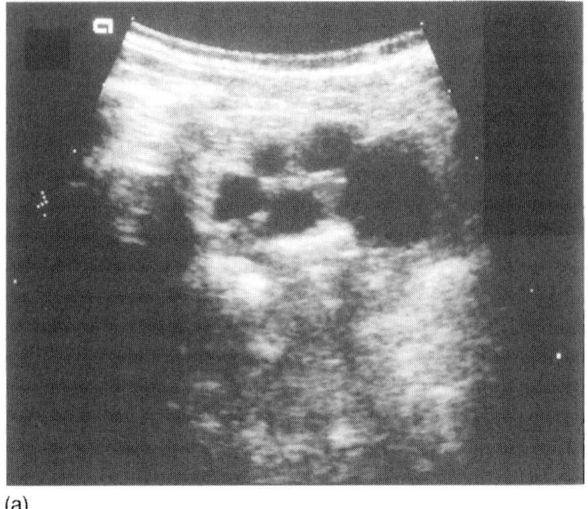

(a)

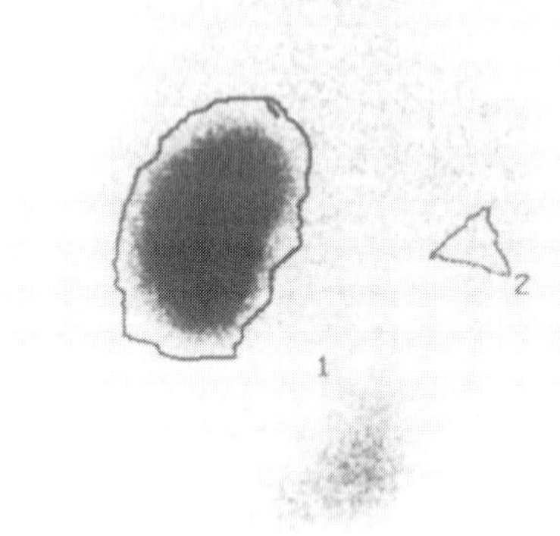

(b)

Fig. 54.1. (a) Ultrasound scan of a newborn male with a history of prenatal hydronephrosis. This shows the typical MCK appearance with cysts of various sizes, without communication and separated by dysplastic parenchyma. (b) DMSA nuclear scan, showing no uptake of tracer in the area of the right kidney.

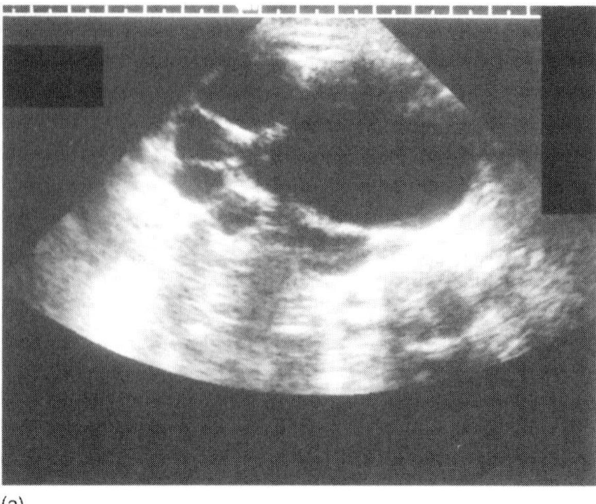

(a)

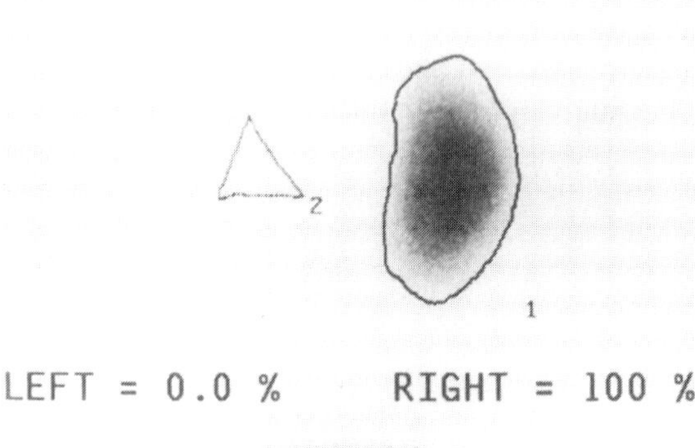

(b)

Fig. 54.2. (a) Ultrasound scan of a hydronephrotic variant of a multicystic kidney. (b) DMSA nuclear scan.

of the fetal heart is always required. Complete prenatal involution of the MCK was documented in two cases.

Ultrasound should be followed by a functional assessment in the renal unit. Virtually any radionuclide agent will determine whether there is functional renal tissue, but the most sensitive are dimercaptosuccinic acid (DMSA) or MAG3. Most often the renal scan will show a deficient area in the appropriate renal fossa on both early and delayed images. If one is dealing with the hydronephrotic variant, however, there may be a small percentage of function seen on the delayed images. Wacksman[9] has pointed out that accuracy in the preoperative diagnosis of MCK is close to 100%, with 97 of the initial 98 patients registered in the United States Multicystic Kidney Registry, who underwent nephrectomy, correctly diagnosed with ultrasound and renal scan. If further assessment is necessary, especially in cases where the ultrasound demonstrates a hydronephrotic pattern or there is function on renal nuclear scan, one can either place a percutaneous nephrostomy tube and later assess for function or surgically explore the kidney with a biopsy. Minevich *et al.*[10] recently reported 4 children who had a presumptive diagnosis of MCK who on follow-up had enlargement of the renal unit which led to exploration. The enlarged renal units were

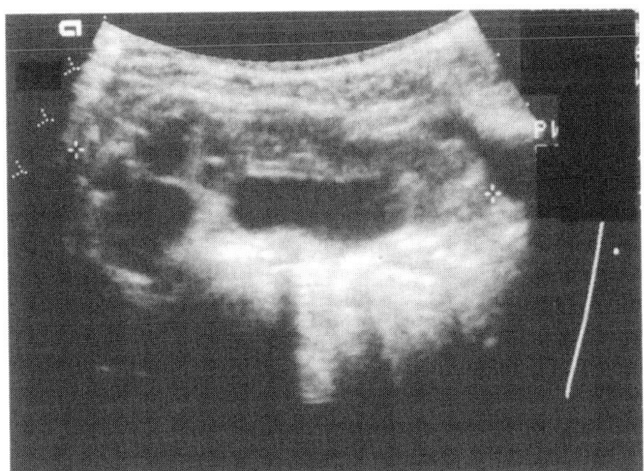

Fig. 54.3. Ultrasound of a newborn female presenting with prenatal hydronephrosis, showing a duplicated right system with a multicystic upper pole system and hydronephrotic lower pole system.

due to Wilms' tumor, mesoblastic nephroma, segmental MCK of a duplex system, and simple renal cysts. MCK may thus be segmental in nature and may be found in segments of duplicated systems (Fig. 54.3), as well as in systems associated with ureteroceles, or even with a contralateral MCK.[11]

It has been discovered recently that there is a high incidence of vesicoureteral reflux in association with MCK. Flack and Bellinger[12] reported a 30% incidence of contralateral reflux in association with MCK. Similarly, Elder *et al.*[13] found a 15% incidence of reflux in the contralateral renal unit, with a mean grade of 3/5 (Fig. 54.4). Considering that this represents reflux into a solitary functioning renal unit, the potential consequences of this reflux may, indeed, be significant. A voiding cystourethrogram (VCUG), therefore, has been recommended in the evaluation of the child with a MCK.

The status of the contralateral kidney deserves further comment. Early reports indicated a high incidence of contralateral renal abnormalities, most commonly hydronephrosis. In 1992, Atyeh *et al.*[14] found that 51% of patients with MCK had an associated abnormality, including reflux, pelviureteric junction obstruction, or a hypoplastic kidney. Data from the US MCK Registry indicated that the contralateral kidney was normal in 73% of cases. More recent reports indicate that multicystic kidney dysplasia, renal agenesis, and ureteropelvic junction obstruction are pathogenetically related,[15] and that combinations of these urological malformations occur in the same individual or in different relatives in the same family.[16]

The cause of MCK remains unknown but it may be related to abnormalities of one or more genes involved in the process of nephrogenesis.[17] It has been suggested that at least some cases may be inherited in an autosomal dominant fashion[18]. Furthermore non-syndromic MCK can occur as part of the spectrum of hereditary dysplasia with autosomal dominant inheritance.[19]

Natural history

US data from the National Multicystic Kidney Registry

There are currently 660 patients registered in the National Multicystic Kidney Registry in the USA. Of the registered cases, 473 (72%) presented by antenatal ultrasound, 97(15%) had a palpable flank mass at presentation, and 25 (4%) presented after evaluation for a urinary tract infection (J. Wacksman, pers. commun.). Males were slightly more commonly afflicted than females (56% vs. 44%).

Contralateral kidney abnormalities were present in 27% of cases, with vesicoureteral reflux seen in approximately 38% and hydronephrosis in the remainder. The majority of those with hydronephrosis involved the renal pelvis only, with one-third involving the ureter as well.

The exact incidence of hypertension in association with MCK has not been determined. Of the 660 patients registered, five had hypertension. Of the registered cases, 234 have undergone nephrectomy, leaving 426 who are being followed. Of those who have their kidneys in place, 5 have hypertension, 15 have had at least a single urinary tract infection, 2 have had hematuria, and 1 had pain. There have been no cases in which a tumor has been identified as having developed. Most of the cases who have been followed are 1 to 5 years from presentation.

With regard to the size of the MCK over time, most evaluations with ultrasound demonstrate a reduction (45%) in the size or no change in size (35%). Of the images, 5% have demonstrated enlargement, while in 14% the renal unit has not been detectable.

European data

Clinical data on the natural history of MCK are available from published series in the British literature and from unpublished data of a cohort of 64 children referred to the Hospital for Sick Children in London between 1988 and 1992. The series will be referred to here as the London, Leeds,[20] Liverpool,[21] and Manchester[22,23] series (Table 54.1).

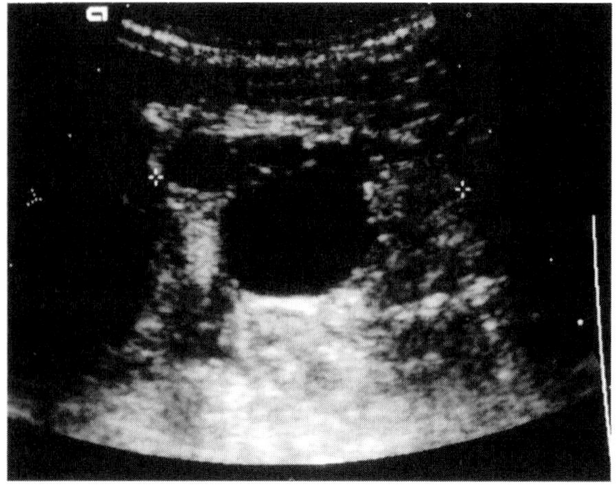
(a)

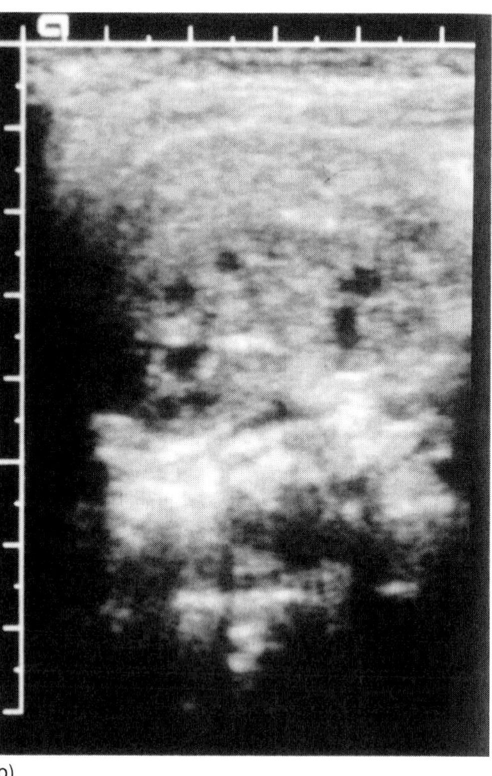
(b)

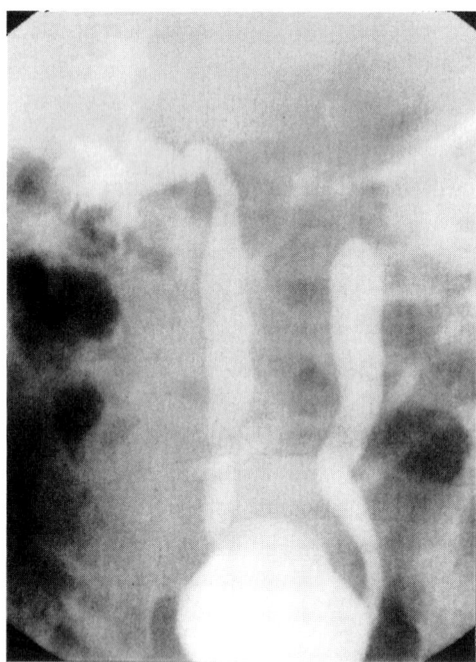
(c)

Fig. 54.4. Newborn female presenting with prenatal hydronephrosis showing: (a) Ultrasound scan, hydronephrotic-type MCK on the left, with no communication between cystic structures (and no functioning on DMSA scan). (b) Ultrasound scan of normal right kidney. (c) MCU, showing bilateral vesicoureteral reflx.

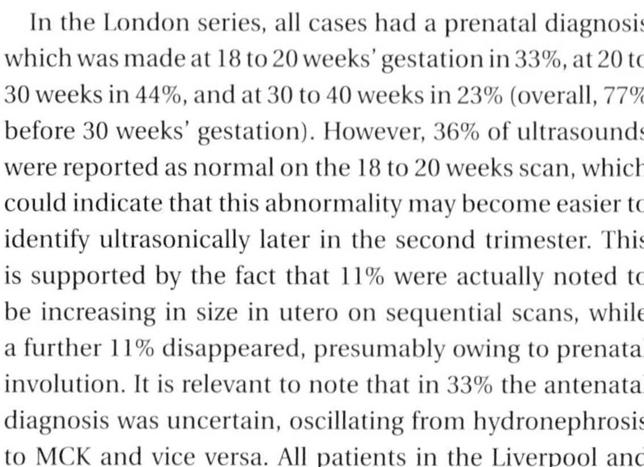

In the London series, all cases had a prenatal diagnosis which was made at 18 to 20 weeks' gestation in 33%, at 20 to 30 weeks in 44%, and at 30 to 40 weeks in 23% (overall, 77% before 30 weeks' gestation). However, 36% of ultrasounds were reported as normal on the 18 to 20 weeks scan, which could indicate that this abnormality may become easier to identify ultrasonically later in the second trimester. This is supported by the fact that 11% were actually noted to be increasing in size in utero on sequential scans, while a further 11% disappeared, presumably owing to prenatal involution. It is relevant to note that in 33% the antenatal diagnosis was uncertain, oscillating from hydronephrosis to MCK and vice versa. All patients in the Liverpool and Manchester series had a prenatal diagnosis with similar findings.

It appears that there is no difference in the prevalence for one sex or for site, and bilateral MCK was diagnosed in only three cases, always prenatally. It is a constant finding in all series that only one-third of the multicystic kidneys were palpable at birth. It is difficult to estimate how many of the prenatally diagnosed palpable kidneys would have been found on routine postnatal examination without the in utero diagnosis. It is realistic to expect that approximately three-quarters of unilateral MCKs remained undiagnosed in the period before prenatal ultrasound diagnosis.

Table 54.1. European data on MCK evolution

Series	Total kidneys	CON	NX	Follow-up	Complete involution		↓	MCK size unchanged	↑	Hypertension
					Pre	Post				
Leeds[20]	22[a]	13	7	1982–87	0	2	6	3	–	0
Liverpool[21]	43[a]	37	5	1979–89	0	10	9	14	0	0
Manchester[22,23]	62	13	49	1982–92	0	4	?	8	?	3
London (unpublished data)	64	51	13	1988–96	6	16	17	20	5	0
Totals	191	114	74							

[a] Leeds:2 bilateral; Liverpool:1 bilateral. CON, conservative management; NX, nephrectomy; pre, prenatal; post, postnatal

Postnatal outcome is demonstrated in Table 54.1. Overall there is data available on 114 patients followed with conservative treatment over a variable period from 5 to 10 years (mean 7). Only in the Liverpool series were 5 patients (13%) eventually lost to follow-up. Prenatal involution was clearly demonstrated in 6 cases in the London series, with 16 further cases involuting postnatally (11 in the first year and five subsequently). Complete involution may be expected in nearly 30%, while a substantial reduction or unchanged size is evident in different proportions (Fig. 54.5). According to the London data, the size of the MCK seems to have an important influence on the possibility of involution. It would seem reasonable to expect that under 5 cm in length all units either disappeared, became smaller, or remain unchanged. If the kidney is 6 cm or greater by the end of the first year, it would be unlikely to involute. Interestingly, over 80% of the MCKs did involute in the London study during the first year. Another important finding was that nearly 8% of the kidneys were enlarging, as observed by other authors.[24,25]

Associated urological abnormalities involved both upper and lower tracts (Table 54.2). As confirmed in other previous studies, there was a significant incidence of vesicoureteral reflux, but this was in most cases low grade and benign with a tendency to spontaneous resolution. Among the contralateral abnormalities, pelviureteric junction obstruction was the most common finding, followed by megaureter. Surgical treatment can be required, and in a few cases the renal function of the solitary kidney was already severely compromised (four cases). A concerning possibility is represented by the association of renal dysplasia contralateral to the MCK, with inevitable progression to renal failure (one case). Lower tract anomalies are mostly represented by bladder or paraureteric diverticula and ureteroceles, which most frequently are ipsilateral to the MCK. Only one patient in the Leeds series with multiple non-urological coexistent anomalies died of a cause unrelated to the MCK at 2 weeks after birth.

None of the children followed conservatively developed malignant change. Three patients in the Manchester series were found to be hypertensive on follow-up, and all became normotensive after nephrectomy.[23] The only urological symptoms (urinary tract infections, renal failure) experienced were always related to a pathological condition elsewhere in the urinary tract rather than to the MCK.

Other reports

In a report by Oliveira *et al.* of 19 patients followed after presenting prenatally with MCDK and confirmed by postnatal evaluation, 13 showed partial involution, 4 complete involution, and 2 an increase in size.[26] A similar study by Kuwertz-Broeking *et al.* reported on the follow-up of 97 patients with MCDK, 82 of which presented prenatally.[27] Of the 75 followed non-operatively, total involution occurred in 25%, reduction in size in 60%, and stable in size in 15%. No cases of malignancy were found. In a recent series of 29 children with prenatally detected MCDK, 52% demonstrated total involution at a median age of 6.5 years.[28]

Eckoldt *et al.* reported on the management of 93 infants prenatally diagnosed with MCDK. Of 37 patients followed non-operatively for an extended period of time, 28 underwent size reduction and 16 complete involution at a mean of 16.2 months.[29]

In a long-term study by Sukthankar and Watson, 52% of patients demonstrated a reduction in size or complete disappearance by 5 years.[30]

The role of nephrectomy

Indications

There is no uniformity of opinion on the role of nephrectomy in the management of MCK. There are a few situations where there is unanimous agreement to remove the kidney.

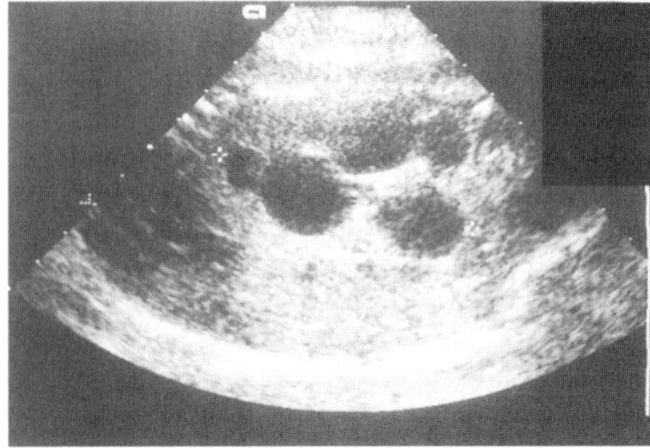

(a)

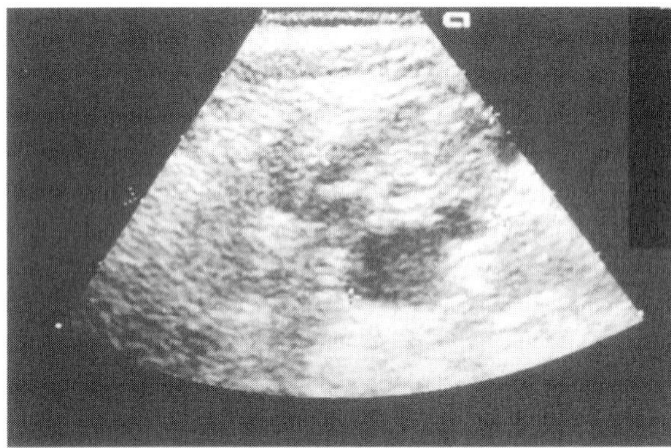

(b)

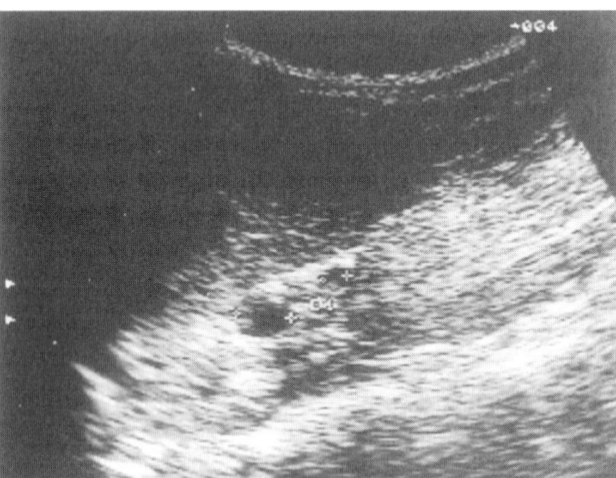

(c)

Fig. 54.5. MCK postnatal involution. (a) Prenatal longitudinal ultrasound scan of a male fetus with unilateral MCK. (b) Ultrasound scan of left MCK at 18 months. (c) Ultrasound scan of left MCK at 36 months.

The presence of a large mass, responsible for compression

Intestinal/respiratory compression

Although percutaneous decompression has been proposed as a temporary relief,[31] nephrectomy is still the preferred option.

To confirm the diagnosis

The sonographic criteria for diagnosing a MCK are now well defined,[32] and the addition of an isotope scan usually confirms the distinction between a non-functioning MCK and a poorly functioning hydronephrotic kidney. On rare occasions it may be critical to establish an unequivocal and early diagnosis of MCK, and if any doubt still remains surgical exploration is indicated.

Increase in volume

In the sonographic follow-up, an increase in volume of a small MCK may indicate a pathological evolution (malignant degeneration, abscess) or a misdiagnosis (cystic nephroma, multilocular cyst).[10] Surgical exploration is mandatory to establish a correct diagnosis.

To relieve symptoms

It seems difficult to argue against the removal of a symptomatic MCK. In practice, pain, hematuria and infection as complications of MCK have been reported only in adults, later in life.[33] Should these symptoms be attributed to MCK, excluding a pathological condition elsewhere in the urinary tract, a nephrectomy is justified. However, such cases perhaps represent a minority in relation to the true incidence of the condition. On the other hand, the presence of hypertension is a clear and absolute indication for surgical treatment.

Concomitant surgical treatment

In the event of concomitant surgery for a urological (or non-urological) problem, removal of the MCK should be considered as part of the program, avoiding a potential subsequent unnecessary procedure.

Poor parental compliance

The decision to maintain an observational approach is based on the assumption that long-term follow-up is required. Although rare or unlikely, the possibility of the development of hypertension or malignant change does exist and it would be incorrect and unethical to withhold this information from parents in the discussion of therapeutic options. In the event of questionable long-term follow-up, nephrectomy should be strongly considered.

Table 54.2. Associated urological anomalies in the European series

	Upper tract		Lower tracts	Other information
Series	Ipsilateral	Contralateral		
Leeds[20]	VUR[a] 1	PUJ 2(S) VUR[a] 2		1 death unrelated causes (duodenal atresia, heart defect)
Liverpool[21]	MCK in ectopic kidney 1	PUJ 1 Megaureter 1		1 aortic coarctation, 1 hip dislocation
Manchester[22,23]	Ureterocele 1 MCK upper pole duplex system 3 VUR[a] 8	Ureterocele 1 Megaureter 1 4PUJ 7 (3S)	Paraureteric diverticula 1 Bladder diverticula 2	1 renal failure (renal dysplasia)
London (unpublished)	Ureterocele 5VUR[a] 2	VUR[a] 10 Renal cyst 1 PUJ 3 (S) Megaureter 2 VUR[a] 10 (1S)	Paraureteric diverticula 2 Bladder diverticula 3	

[a] Leeds:1 bilateral; Manchester: 5 bilateral; London: 2 bilateral. MCK, multicystic kidney; PUJ, pelviureteric junction obstruction; S, surgery; VUR, vesicoureteral reflux.

Nephrectomy technique

While the indications for nephrectomy in MCK continue to be debated, the approach for nephrectomy itself is an additional area of controversy. The traditional approach for nephrectomy of a multicystic kidney is extraperitoneal. This can be accomplished by an anterior muscle-splitting technique or a dorsal lumbotomy technique. Either approach affords a low morbidity and a low complication rate, with hospital stays of 48 hours or less in infants.[13]

Laparoscopic and robotic nephrectomy has been reported by several authors.[34–36] This technique has been reported in infants as well as older children. Each of the reports comments on the superior postoperative course in patients approached laparoscopically, with regard to pain management, length of hospital stay, and cosmetic concerns. Most surgery has been carried out as a day case or with an overnight stay. Operative times are quite variable, from as short as under 1 hour to as long as 5 hours.

One argument against laparoscopic nephrectomy in the pediatric population is the violation of the peritoneal cavity, thus creating potential intraperitoneal complications. Ono *et al.* [37] have advocated a retroperitoneal approach to nephrectomy by dilating the retroperitoneal space, which has been reported in children as well.[38] While this approach avoids potential intraperitoneal complications, it is technically more challenging.

Just because a procedure can be accomplished laparoscopically does not necessarily mean that it should be done that way. There have been no controlled nor randomized studies comparing the laparoscopic approach to a traditional open approach for any of the pediatric laparoscopic procedures. Several factors should be considered. It is obvious that the generic benefits of laparoscopic surgery (i.e., smaller incision and faster recovery) carry somewhat less significance for the very young child, and infants recover from open surgery quite quickly. There is a steep learning curve to laparoscopic surgery, especially in children where the margins for error are smaller in the confined space. Instrumentation, in addition, presents some limitations, although technology is catching up in pediatric laparoscopy. Finally, except in the most able hands, laparoscopic surgical procedures in children require more anesthetic time especially in the younger pediatric patient.

In conclusion, the present authors consider that laparoscopic nephrectomy for MCK is becoming the technique of choice in experienced hands. However, the technology should not change the indications.

The dilemma

Surgeons who routinely advise nephrectomy often cite the potential risk of malignant change and the development of hypertension as the main reasons. The following discussions will therefore focus on an analysis of these two aspects.

Table 54.3. Malignancy related to MCK

Series	Year	Age	Sex	Tumor	Country
Wilms' tumor					
Raffensberger and Aboulseiman[46]	1968	10 m	M	Stage I	USA
Hartman *et al.*[47]	1986	4 yrs	F	Stage II	USA
Oddone *et al.*[48]	1994	17 m	M	Stage I	Italy
Minevich *et al.*[10]	1996	11 m	M	Stage III	USA
De Oliveira *et al.*[49]	1997	18 m	M	Stage II	Brazil
Homsy *et al.*[50]	1997	3 m	F	Stage I	Canada
		5 m	F	Stage II	Canada
Beckwith[41]	1997	23 m	M	Stage II	USA
		46 m	F	Stage I	USA
		6.5yrs	M	Stage IV	USA
		18 m	F	Unknown stage	France
Renal cell carcinoma					
Barret and Wineland[52]	1980	26 yrs	F	Renal cell Ca	USA
Burgler and Hauri[53]	1983	68 yrs	M	Renal cell Ca	Switzerland
Birken *et al.*[54]	1985	15 yrs	F	Renal cell Ca	USA
Shirai *et al.*[55]	1986	33 yrs	F	Renal cell Ca	Japan
Rackley *et al.*[56]	1994	53 yrs	M	Renal cell Ca[a]	USA
Transitional cell carcinoma					
Mingin *et al.*[51]	2000	63 yrs	M	Grade I	USA
Mesothelioma					
Gutter and Hermanek[57]	1957	68 yrs	F	Mesothelioma	Switzerland

[a] Involuted MCK.
(Table adapted from Perez *et al. J. Urol.* 1998; 160:1216.)

Potential for malignant change

It has been demonstrated that the absence of renal tissue determined radiographically does not preclude the presence of residual renal dysplasia.[22,39,40] Involution seems to occur only through reabsorption of cystic fluid, leaving cellular elements, and the potential hazards of neoplastic change remain lifelong.

The incidence of nodular renal blastema in multicystic dysplasia has been reported with a range between 2% and 5%,[41–43] but similar histological specimens have been identified in obstructed kidneys or in dysplastic upper poles of duplex kidneys.[44,45] The clinical significance of this histological finding is unclear, and no correlation has yet been established between nodular renal blastema and the actual development of malignancy. The progression rate of nodular renal blastema into Wilms' tumor has been estimated at approximately one in 100 cases,[41] indicating that nearly 2000 nephrectomies for MCK would be necessary to prevent one Wilms' tumor from occurring.[43]

A review of the literature covering the last 30-year period identified 18 reports of malignancy associated with MCK (Table 54.3). In all 11 pediatric cases there was a nephroblastoma, while in the adults five had a renal cell carcinoma, one a mesothelioma, and one transitional cell carcinoma.[10,41,46–57] From these reports there is evidence of only one case of a renal cell carcinoma in an adult arising in a regressed MCK, with a concomitant orthotopic ureterocele and a blind ending ureter.[56] To date, there have not been any documented cases of MCK in which renal tumors developed in 660 cases followed by the Multicystic Kidney Registry of the Section of Urology of the American Academy of Pediatrics.[58] An analysis by Gordon *et al.*[20] has calculated that an incidence of MCK of 1 in 4300 live births gives a figure of approximately 1000 new cases per annum for the UK and the USA, a theoretical total of nearly 30 000 for the period covered by the literature review. Although this is only a hypothetical figure, it may serve to put into context the actual risk of malignant change. It should be added that the estimated risk of dying from a tumor in a multicystic kidney has to be balanced against the morbidity of nephrectomy and ultimately against the risk of dying from an anesthetic or some other complication of the surgery. Whether or not laparoscopy and robotic technology should alter the paradigm is debatable.

In a comprehensive review Husmann concludes that available literature dictates that the incidence of renal tumors in MCK is so sporadic that the surgical extirpation of dysplastic renal tissue should not be performed solely on the basis of its presence.[59]

Hypertension

Among the justifications for prophylactic nephrectomy, the risk of developing hypertension is probably the one cited most commonly. It is known that there is a link between MCK and hypertension, and there is growing interest in the problem of trying to estimate the magnitude of the risk. Table 54.4 summarizes the reported pediatric cases in the literature of the last 30 years. Gordon and associates undertook a computerized literature search covering a 20-year period and found 9 cases.[20] Of these, 3 had responded to removal of the MCK while 6 had not. The present authors have been able to identify an additional 31 cases reported in the last 10 years, of which 16 definitely responded to nephrectomy.[13,20,23,24,53,60–68]

Webb *et al.*[23] in their report of a case of hypertension in a 14-year-old girl already discharged from follow-up as a result of "disappearance" of the cystic kidney on ultrasound exam, raise the issue of balancing the costs of nephrectomy with a 24-hour hospital stay and one postoperative follow-up visit vs. multiple ultrasound examinations and office visits in the first 5 years of life and annually thereafter.

Emmet and King[68] postulate that the absence of response to nephrectomy does not mean that the hypertension was not caused initially by the MCK. A similar report by Snodgrass *et al.* attributes sustained hypertension after nephrectomy to either damage to the contralateral kidney or other factors such as cardiac hypertrophy.[67] With sustained hypertension, contralateral arteriolar thickening of the "normal" kidney may produce continued hypertension persisting, therefore, even after the removal of the MCK. The published literature on hypertension in childhood, on the other hand, does not seem to identify any case related to MCK, as reported by Taylor *et al.*[69] and Hendren *et al.*[70] in their series of 42 and 22 children, respectively, with "surgical" hypertension.

The role of MCK as a source of hypertension in adult life and the interpretation of the literature on hypertension in adults is much more difficult to evaluate. A few earlier studies have already been analyzed by Gordon *et al.*[20] and their conclusion was that the available evidence does not support the view that MCK poses a significant threat of hypertension later in life or in adult life. We still do not know all the mechanisms by which renal disease induces hypertension. More recently attention has focused on the hypothesis of hyperfiltration damage in solitary kidneys.

The mechanism of hypertension in multicystic dysplasia is still not understood. Multicystic dysplasia results in global kidney aberration affecting nephron development and the vascular tree. Renin and the renin/angiotensin system are central players in hypertension but there is little known about the role of renin in multicystic dysplastic kidneys. It is proposed that renin in the fetal kidney may have a role in vascular development and may modulate the kidney morphogenesis.

Renin localization studies were performed by Konda[71] on non-hypertensive and hypertensive multicystic dysplasia demonstrating increased renin expression. Lapis[72] conversely showed a quantitatively decreased renin in multicystic dysplastic kidneys but a pronounced ectopic renin expression within arterioles and interstitial macrophages was present in hypertensive multicystic dysplastic kidneys (two kidneys) compared to non-hypertensive kidneys (12 kidneys).

With increased sensitivity in the array technology and development of other competing methods, our understanding will hopefully improve in the near future. Further expression profiling analyses of series of multicystic dysplastic and normal kidneys will be helpful in identifying links between renin and other gene families involved in kidney development.

The true incidence of hypertension in children with MCK may be unknown because of the difficulty in determining the blood pressure in a neonate and infant and mostly by the fact that it is not routinely done or reported in these children. As we continue to follow expectantly most of these children, it would be important to include routine blood pressure measurements and possibly to document any form of vascular flow or subsequent changes in the affected kidney. Ideally, whenever possible, additional measurements of plasma renin activity (PRA) and circulating angiotensins (RAS) should be added for all the hypertensive patients. Only in a systematic study may we avoid underestimating the real entity of this potential problem.

Table 54.4. Hypertension related to MCK

Series	Year	*n*	Age	Management	Outcome
Javadpour *et al.*[60]	1970	1	6yrs	Nx	Improved
Burgler and Hauri[53]	1983	1		Nx	Improved
Chen *et al.*[61]	1985	1	1 m	Nx	Improved
Vinocur *et al.*[24]	1988	1	9 yrs	Cons.	NR
Gordon *et al.*[20]	1988	9		Nx	Impr. (3)
Susskind and King[62]	1989	2a	1 m	Nx	Improved
Angermeier *et al.*[63]	1992	1	5 m	Nx	Improved
Wacksman (unpublished data)	1993	5		Nx	? NR
Elder *et al.*[13]	1995	3		Nx	Improved
Andretta *et al.*[64]	1995	1	6 yrs	Nx	Improved
Petterson and Klauber[65]	1996	1		Nx	NR
Webb *et al.*[23]	1997	3	3 m to 14 yrs	Nx	Improved
Rudnik-Schoneborn *et al.*[66]	1998	6b	1 m to 1 yr	Cons(4) Nx(2)	Impr. (2)
Snodgrass[67]	2000	4	1 m to 4 yrs	Nx	Impr. (2)
Oliveira *et al.*[26]	2001	1	1 m	Cons.	Improved

(a) One patient had multiple complications associated with prematurity including intraventricular hemorrhage and the other had ureteropelvic junction obstruction on the contralateral renal unit.

(b) Two patients had cardiovascular anomalies and 1 patient developed hypertension after nephrectomy.

NR = not recorded.

(Table adapted from Oliveira *et al. Pediatr. Nephrol.* 2002; 17:954–958.)

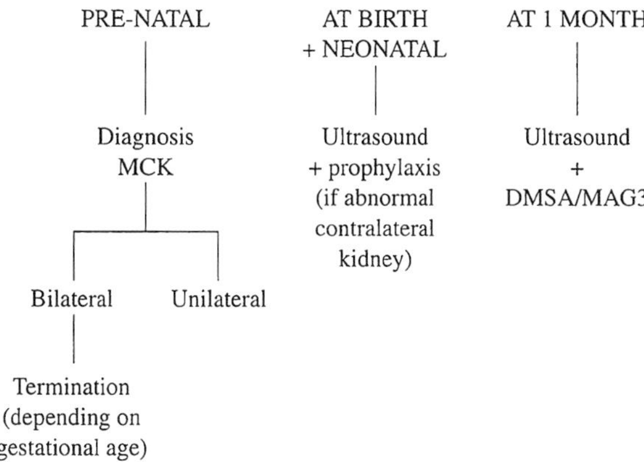

Fig. 54.6. Basic algorithm of current management of MCK.

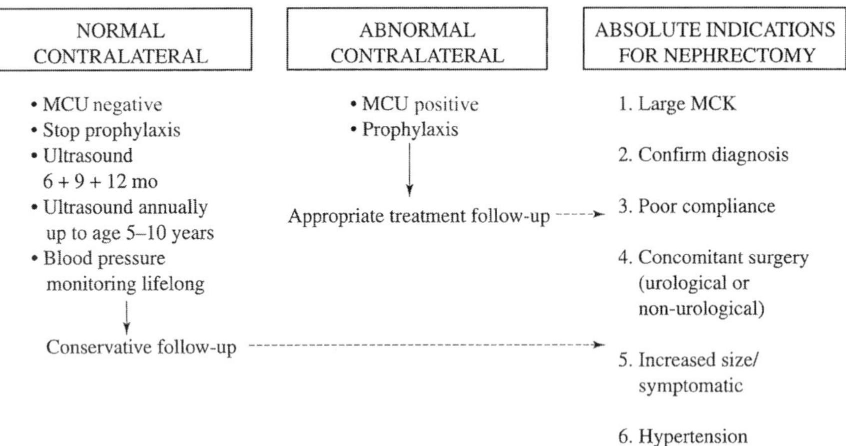

Fig. 54.7. Algorithm for treatment.

The present evidence is that long-term morbidity of MCK is minimal but there is very little data on such long-term outcomes. Undoubtedly, only appropriate long-term studies will eventually confirm this clinical impression.

If one chooses a non-operative approach to management of MCK, one must be assured of adequate follow-up by the family, since the data is not clear on how long follow-up should be undertaken. LaSalle *et al.* reported in a poll of selected insurance companies that only 15% would issue life insurance if a MCK was left *in situ*, while 70% would issue coverage after nephrectomy.[73] While these policies are clearly not based on data, we need to factor these into the care of patients. From an economic standpoint, a cost analysis by Perez *et al.* found that nephrectomy was more cost-effective than ultrasound surveillance if surveillance was performed every 3 months.[74] While the authors acknowledge that the risk of Wilms' tumor in a MCK is low (estimated 0.1%), if one chooses to screen, very frequent ultrasounds should be performed.

Conclusions

It is clear that our understanding of MCK is still incomplete, particularly in terms of the real incidence of its potential complications. The advent of prenatal ultrasound imaging has undoubtedly increased the number of cases with the diagnosis and has presented a potentially new spectrum of patients. The institution of a registry of patients with MCK and a change of attitude was needed to begin to understand better the natural history of this entity.

The authors' current management protocol is summarized by the algorithms in Figs. 54.6 and 54.7.

Neonatal and perinatal evaluation should confirm the diagnosis and carefully identify any contralateral abnormality. Prophylactic antibiotic treatment and MCU screening evaluation should be reserved for those patients whose ultrasound evaluation has clearly demonstrated an abnormal contralateral kidney or any ureteric dilation. The real clinical significance of the vast majority of associated VUR is questionable, being mostly of a low grade and prone to spontaneous resolution. Some clinicians may choose an MCU on all patients with MCK owing to the higher incidence of VUR identified in these patients, but the clinical significance of the low grade of reflux remains to be determined.

Whenever a hydronephrotic solitary kidney is identified (i.e., pelviureteric or vesicoureteric junction obstruction), prompt surgical treatment is indicated to maximize preservation of renal function.

In only a few selected situations does it seem reasonable to offer surgery as a definitive step in the management of an otherwise healthy infant with MCK: with a very large MCK(> 6 cm); when the retained mass appears to be growing; when the diagnosis is in question; when adequate follow-up cannot be assured; and if hypertension or symptoms develop.

Only the future will eventually provide a better understanding of the biology of MCK, its spectrum of occurrence and its developmental origins, as well as its relationship to malignancy. Prophylactic routine nephrectomy is, therefore, unjustified, although it is still very important to recommend lifelong monitoring of blood pressure of all patients with a retained MCK until definitive information on the risk of hypertension becomes available.

Acknowledgment

We would like to acknowledge both Ms. H. K. Dhillon and Dr J. Wacksman for their cooperation in providing unpublished data on MCK patients.

REFERENCES

1. Schwartz, J. An unusual unilateral multicystic kidney in an infant. *J. Urol.* 1926; **35**:259.
2. Spence, H. M. Congenital unilateral multicystic kidney. *J. Urol.* 1955; **74**:693.
3. Pathak, I. G. & Williams, D. I. Multicystic and cystic dysplastic kidneys. *Br. J. Urol.* 1964; **36**:318.
4. Aubertin, G., Cripps, S., Coleman, G. *et al.* Prenatal diagnosis of apparently isolated unilateral multicystic kidney: implications for counselling and management. *Prenat. Diagn.* 2002; **22**:388.
5. Eckoldt, F., Woderich, R., Smith, R. D., & Heling, K. S. Antenatal diagnostic aspect of unilateral multicystic kidney dysplasia-sensitivity, specificity, predictive values, differential diagnoses, associated malformations and consequences. *Fetal Diagn. Ther.* 2004; **19**:163.
6. Felson, B. & Cussen, L. J. The hydronephrotic congenital multicystic disease of the kidney. *Semin. Roentgenol.* 1975; **10**:113.
7. Feldenberg, L. R. & Siegel, N. J. Clinical course and outcome for children with multicystic dysplastic kidneys. *Pediatr. Nephrol.* 2000; **14**:1098–1101.
8. Al-Khaldi, N., Watson, A. R., Zuccollo, J., Twining, P., & Rose, D. H. Outcome of antenatally detected cystic dysplastic kidney disease. *Arch. Dis. Child.* 1994; **70**:520–522.
9. Wacksman, J. Dilemma of the multicystic kidney. *Prob. Urol.* 1990; **4**:574–582.
10. Minevich, E., Wacksman, J., Phipps, L. *et al.* The importance of accurate diagnosis and early close follow-up in patients with suspected multicystic dysplastic kidney. *J. Urol.* 1997; **158**:1301–1304.
11. Agrawal, L., Millard, M. L., Fairhurst, J., & Gilbert, R. D. Bilateral multicystic kidneys – an unusual case. *Pediatr. Nephrol.* 2002; **17**:964.
12. Flack, C. E. & Bellinger, M. F. The multicystic dysplastic kidneys and contralateral vesicoureteral reflux: protection of the solitary kidney. *J. Urol.* 1993; **150**:1873–1874.
13. Elder, J., Kladky, D., & Selzman, A. A. Outpatient nephrectomy for nonfunctioning kidneys. *J. Urol.* 1995; **154**:712–715.
14. Atyeh, B., Husmann, D., & Baum, M. Contralateral renal abnormalities in multicystic dysplastic kidneys disease. *J. Pediatr.* 1992: **121**:65–67.
15. Robson, W. L. M., Rogers, R. C., & Leung, A. K. C. Renal agenesis, multicystic dysplasia, and uretero-pelvic junction obstruction – a common pathogenesis? (letter) *Am. J. Med. Genet.* 1994; **53**:302.
16. Roodhoft, A. M., Birnholz, J. C., & Homes, L. B. Familial natural of congenital absence and severe dysgenesis of both kidneys. *N. Engl. J. Med.* 1984; **310**:1341–1345.
17. Groenen, P. M., Vanderlinden, G., Devriendt, K. *et al.* Rearrangement of the human CDC5L gene by a t(6;19) (p21; q13.1) in a multicystic renal dysplasia. *Genomics* 1998; **49**:218.
18. Srivastava, T., Garola, R. E., & Hellerstein, S. Autosomal dominant inheritance of multicystic dysplastic kidney. *Pediatr. Nephrol.* 1999; **13**:481.
19. Bernstein, J. & Gilbert-Barness, E. Developmental abnormalities of the kidney. In Stenberg, S. S. (ed.) *Diagnostic Surgical Pathology*, 3rd edn. Philadelphia: Lippincott, Williams & Wilkins. 2000: 1685–1700.
20. Gordon, A. C., Thomas, D. F. M., Arthur, R. J. *et al.* Multicystic dysplastic kidney: is nephrectomy still appropriate? *J. Urol.* 1998; **140**:1231–1234.
21. Rickwood, A. M. K., Anderson, P. A. M., & Williams, M. P. L. Multicystic renal dysplasia detected by prenatal ultrasonography: natural history and results of conservative management. *Br. J. Urol.* 1992; **69**:538–540.
22. Gough, D. C. S., Postlewaite, R. J., Lewis, M. A. *et al.* Multicystic renal dysplasia diagnosed in the antenatal period: a note of caution. *Br. J. Urol.* 1995; **76**:244–248.
23. Webb, N. J. A., Lewis, M. A., Bruce, J. *et al.* Unilateral multicystic dysplastic kidney: the case for nephrectomy. *Arch. Dis. Child.* 1997; **76**:31–34.
24. Vinocur, L., Slovis, T. L., Perlmutter, A. *et al.* Follow-up studies of multicystic dysplastic kidneys. *Radiology* 1998; **167**:311–315.
25. Strife, J. L., Souza, A. S., Kirks, D. R. *et al.* Multicystic dysplastic kidney in children:US follow-up. *Radiology* 1993; **186**:785–788.
26. Oliveira, E. A., Diniz, J. S., Vilasboas, A. S., Rabelo, E. A., Silva, J. M., & Filgueiras, M. T. Multicystic dysplastic kidney detected by fetal sonography: conservative management and follow-up. *Pediatr. Surg. Int.* 2001; **17(1)** 54–57.
27. Kuwertz-Broeking, E., Brinkmann, O. A., Von Lengerke, H. J. *et al.* Unilateral multicystic dysplastic kidney: experience in children. *Br. J. Urol. Int.* 2004; **93(3)**:388–392.
28. Belk, R. A., Thomas, D. F., Mueller, R. F., Godbole, P., Markham, A. F., & Weston, M. J. A family study and the natural history of prenatally detected unilateral multicystic dysplastic kidney. *J. Urol.* 2002; **167(2 Pt 1)**:666–669.
29. Eckoldt, F., Woderich, R., Wolke, S., Heling, K. S., Stover, B., & Tennstedt, C. Follow-up of unilatral multicystic kidney dysplasia after prenatal diagnosis. *J. Matern. Fetal Neonatal Med.* 2003; **14(3)**:177–186.
30. Sukthankar, S. & Watson, A. R. Unilateral multicystic dysplastic kidney disease: defining the natural history. Angelia Paediatric Nephrourology Group. *Acta. Paediatr.* 2000; **89(7)**:811–813.
31. Holloway, W. R. & Weinstein, S. H. Percutaneous decompression: treatment for respiratory distress secondary to multicystic dysplastic kidney. *J. Urol.* 1990; **144**:113.
32. Stuck, K. J., Koff, S. A., & Silver, T. M. Ultrasonic features of multicystic dysplastic kidney: expanded diagnostic criteria. *Radiology* 1982; **143**:217.
33. Ambrose, S. S., Gould, R. A., Trulock, T. S. *et al.* Unilateral multicystic renal disease in adults. *J. Urol.* 1990; **128**:366–369.

34. Koyle, M. A., Woo, H. H., & Kavoussi, L. R. Laparoscopic nephrectomy in the first year of life. *J. Pediatr. Surg.* 1993; **28**:693.
35. Erlich, R. M., Gershman, A., Mee, S., & Fuchs, G. Laparoscopic nephrectomy in a child: expanding horizons for laparoscopy in pediatric urology. *J. Endourol.* 1992; **6**:463.
36. Cilento, B. G., Jr. & Peters, C. Laparoscopic and robotic surgery in pediatric urology. In *Pediatric Surgical Procedures*, A. A. Caldamone (ed.), *Atlas Urol. Clin. N. Am.* 2004; **12**:143.
37. Ono, Y., Katoh, N., Kinukana, T. *et al.* Laparoscopic nephrectomy via the retroperitoneal approach. *J. Urol.* 1996; **150**:101–1104.
38. Diamond, D. A., Price, H. M., McDougall, E. M., & Bloom, D. A. Retroperitoneal laparoscopic nephrectomy in children. *J. Urol.* 1995; **153**:1966–1968.
39. Pedicelli, G., Jequier, S. Bowen, A. D. *et al.* Multicystic dysplastic kidneys: spontaneous regression demonstrated with US. *Radiology* 1986; **160**:23.
40. Avni, E. F., Thoua, Y., Lalmand, B. *et al.* Multicystic dysplastic kidney: natural history from *in utero* diagnosis and post-natal follow-up. *J. Urol.* 1987; **138**:1420–1424.
41. Beckwith, J. B. Wilms' tumor and other renal tumors in childhood: an update. *J. Urol.* 1986; **136**:320.
42. Johnson, H. W., Coleman, G. U., & Dimmick, J. E. Wilms' tumorlet, nodular renal blastema and multicystic renal dysplasia: a spectrum. *J. Urol.* 1989; **142**:484–485.
43. Noe, H. N., Marshall, J. H., & Edwards, O. P. Nodular renal blastema in the multicystic kidney. *J. Urol.* 1989; **142**:486–488.
44. Gaddy, C. D., Gibbons, M. D., Gonzales, E. T., Jr. *et al.* Obstructive uropathy, renal dysplasia and nodular renal blastema: is there a relationship to Wilms' tumor? *J. Urol.* 1985, **134**:330.
45. Craver, R., Dimmick, J. E., Johnson, H. W. *et al.* Congenital obstructive uropathy and nodular renal blastema. *J. Urol.* 1986; **136**:305.
46. Raffensperger, J. & Aboulseiman, A. Abdominal masses in children under one year of age. *Surgery* 1968; **63**:514.
47. Hartman, G. E., Smolik, L. M., & Schochat, S. J. The dilemma of the multicystic dysplastic kidney. *Am. J. Dis. Child.* 1986; **140**:925.
48. Oddone, M., Marino, C., Sergi, C. *et al.* Wilms' tumor arising in a multicystic kidney. *Pediatr. Radiat.* 1994; **24**:236.
49. deOliveira-Filho, A. G., Carvalho, M. H., Sbragia-Neto, L. *et al.* Wilms' tumor in a prenatally diagnosed multicystic kidney. *J. Urol.* 1997; **158**:1926–1927.
50. Homsy, Y. Personal communication. In Elder, J., Hladky, D., & Selzman, A. A. Outpatient nephrectomy for nonfunctioning kidneys. *J. Urol.* 1995; **154**:712–715.
51. Mingin, G. C., Gilhooly, P., & Sadeghi-Nejad, H. Transitional cell carcinoma in a multicystic dysplastic kidney. *J. Urol.* 2000; **163**:544.
52. Barrett, D. M. & Wineland, R. E. Renal cell carcinoma in multicystic dysplastic kidney. *Urology* 1980; **15**:152.
53. Bürgler, W. & Hauri, D. Vital complications in multicystic kidney degeneration (multicystic dysplasia). *Urol. Int.* 1983: **38**:251–256.
54. Birken, G., King, D., & Vane, D. Renal cell carcinoma arising in a multicystic dysplastic kidney. *J. Pediatr. Surg.* 1985; **20**:619.
55. Shirai, M., Kitagawa, T., Nakata, H. *et al.* renal cell carcinoma originating from dysplastic kidney. *Acta Path. Jap.* 1986; **36**:1263.
56. Rackley, R. R., Angermeier, K. W., Levin, H. *et al.* Renal cell carcinoma arising in a regressed multicystic dysplastic kidney. *J. Urol.* 1994; **152**:1543–1545.
57. Gutter, W. & Hermanek, P. Maligner Tumor der nierengengend uter dem bilde der Knollenniere (Nierenblastemcystein). *Urol. Int.* 1957; **4**:164.
58. Wacksman, J. Editorial comment. *J. Urol.* 1995; **154**:714.
59. Husmann, D. A. Renal dysplasia: the risks and consequences of leaving dysplastic tissue in situ. *Urology* 1998; **52(4)**:533–536.
60. Javadpour, N., Chelouhy, E., Moncada, L. *et al.* Hypertension in a child caused by a multicystic kidney. *J. Urol.* 1970; **104**:918–921.
61. Chen, Y.-H., Stapleton, B., Roy, S. *et al.* Neonatal hypertension from a unilateral multicystic dysplastic kidney. *J. Urol.* 1985; **133**:664–665.
62. Susskin, M. R., Kim, K. S., & King, L. R. Hypertension and multicystic kidney. *Urology* 1989; **34**:362.
63. Angermeier, K. W., Kay, R., & Levin, H. Hypertension as a complication of multicystic dysplastic kidney. *Urology* 1992; **39**:55.
64. Andretta, E., Aragona, F., Talenti, E., & Passerini Glazel, G. Il rene multicistico. *Urol. Pediatr.* 1995; **1**:31–38.
65. Pettersson, B. A. & Klauber, G. T. Prognosis for children born with multicystic dysplastic kidneys (abstract). *Br. J. Urol.* 1996; **77**(Suppl.1):18.
66. Rudnik-Schöneborn, S., John, U., Deget, F. *et al.* Clinical features of unilateral multicystic renal dysplasia in children. *Eur. J. Pediatr.* 1998; **157**:666–672.
67. Snodgrass, W. T., Wacksman, J., & Homsy, Y. Hypertension associated with multicystic dysplastic kidney in children. *J. Urol.* 2000; **164(2)**:472.
68. Emmert, G. K. & King, L. R. The risk of hypertension is underestimated in the multicystic dysplastic kidney: a personal perspective. *Urology* 1994; **44**:404–405.
69. Taylor, R. C., Azmy, A. F., & Young, D. G. Long-term follow-up of surgical renal hypertension. *J. Pediatr. Surg.* 1997;**22**:228.
70. Hendren, W. H., Kim, S. H., Herrin, J. T. *et al.* Surgically correctable hypertension of renal origin in childhood. *Am. J. Surg.* 1982; **143**:432.
71. Konda, R., Sato, H., Ito, S. *et al.* Renin containing cells are present predominantly in scarred areas but not in dysplastic regions in multicystic dysplastic kidney. *J. Urol.* 2001; **166**:1910.
72. Lapis, H., Doshi, R. H., Watson, M. A. *et al.* Reduced renin expression and altered gene transcript profiles in multicystic dysplastic kidneys. *J. Urol.* 2002; **168(4 Pt 2)**:1816.
73. LaSalle, M. D., Stock, J. A., & Hanna, M. K. Insurability of children with congenital urological anomalies. *J. Urol.* 1997; **158**:1312–1315.
74. Perez, L. M., Naidu, S. I., & Joseph, D. B. Outcome and cost analysis of operative versus nonoperative management of neonatal multicystic dysplastic kidneys. *J. Urol.* 1998; **160**:1207–1211.

55

Urolithiasis

Bartley G. Cilento, Jr,[1] Gerald C. Mingin,[2] and Hiep T. Nguyen[1]

[1]Department of Urology, MA Children's Hospital, Boston,
[2]Department of Urology, Denver Children's Hospital, Denver, CO, USA

Introduction

There is a considerable body of literature dedicated to adult stone disease but very little written about pediatric stone disease. While nephrolithiasis is less prevalent in children, it can be associated with significant morbidity. This chapter will touch upon the pathophysiology, the surgical management, and the current state of evidence base data, particularly long-term outcomes of pediatric stone disease.

Epidemiology

Childhood urolithiasis varies widely around the world both in the composition and location of the stones. For example, it is endemic in the Far East and Turkey where the stones are primarily ammonium uric acid stones. In European countries, the majority of stones found in children are composed of struvite and organic matrix that are frequently the result of urinary tract infections from bacteria containing urease. In the USA, infection-related stones are rare. Stone composition in the USA is mostly calcium-based.

In North America and other developed countries, nephrolithiasis in children has remained stable over the last 20 years. In Europe and the United States, the incidence of stone disease is similar, ranging from 0.13 to 1.0 cases per 1000 hospital admissions.[1,2] The disease always varies geographically within countries. For example, the incidence tends to be higher in the warm climates of the southeastern United States and California.[3] The incidence is also higher in areas with immigrants from countries where stone disease is endemic. The ratio of boys to girls affected by stone disease is 1.2–1.7:1 in the USA and 1.9–3:1 in the UK.[4,5] In these countries the majority of children who form stones are Caucasian, while less than 10% are African American.[2]

In developing countries, stone disease is still endemic, e.g., in countries such as Turkey and parts of North Africa. Forty years ago, 50% of the stones seen in these children were bladder stones, associated with an infectious etiology. Currently, 75%–80% of these children have upper tract stones and 5% appear to be caused by infection.[6] This pattern closely resembles what is seen in North America and in parts of Western Europe, where metabolic disorders are responsible for 50% of stones. This shift in the composition and location of the stone is likely to be due to improved living standards with better health care, and improved nutrition with increased protein consumption.[7] Recent studies suggest a shift in the age of patients presenting with a stone, as well as in the size of the stone. In a retrospective review of 103 patients, children presenting between 1988 and 1995 had a mean age of 13.9 years and an average stone size of 10.7 mm, while those presenting after 1995 had a mean age of 10.9 years, and a stone size of 7.5 mm.[8]

Once a child develops urolithiasis, there is a 6%–54% chance of recurrence within 6 years. Those children identified with a metabolic abnormality have a fivefold chance of recurrence in comparison to those children without an identifiable metabolic abnormality.

In children, the manifestations of stone can be less dramatic than in adults. In terms of presenting symptoms, abdominal pain occurred in 50%, hematuria in 33%, and infection in 11% of children. Urolithiasis was an incidental finding in 15% of children undergoing radiographic imaging.

In the USA, the vast majority of stones are located in the renal pelvis (75%). Ten percent of stones are found in

Pediatric Surgery and Urology: Long-term Outcomes, Mark Stringer, Keith Oldham, Pierre Mouriquand.
Published by Cambridge University Press.

Table 55.1. Metabolic etiology of stones

Calcium lithiasis	
Hypercalciuria (>4 mg/kg per day)	
Normocalcemic (8.7–10.1 mg/dl)	Idiopathic – absorptive, renal leak RTA
Hypercalcemic (>10.1 mg/dl)	Associated with bone resorption – Immobilization, hyperparathyroidism GI hyperabsorption – Vitamin D intoxication – Sarcoidosis – Phosphorus depletion – Hyper- or hypothyroidism – Bartter's syndrome – Malignancy
Hyperoxaluria (>40 mg/1.73 m^2 per day)	Hereditary type I and II Enteric – malabsorption, IBD, bowel resection Dietary (increased oxalate consumption, vitamin C)
Hyperuricosuria (>815 mg/1.73 m^2 per day)	Leukemia, lymphoma Idiopathic, familial Inborn errors of metabolism (glycogen storage disease)
Hypocitraturia (<180 mg/g Cr)	Metabolic acidosis Distal RTA GI disease Potassium depletion
Uric acid lithiasis	
Hyperuricemia (>5.5 mg/dl)	Familial hyperuricemia Blood disorders Inborn errors of metabolism (Lesch–Nyhan syndrome)
Cystine lithiasis (>75 mg/g Cr)	Defect in COLA reabsorption
Misc. inborn errors of metabolism	Xanthinuria Orotic aciduria Adenine phosphoribosyltransferase deficiency

the ureter and another 10% are located within the bladder. Stones larger than 5 mm are unlikely to pass spontaneously. Bladder stones are being found with increasing frequency in patients who have undergone bladder augmentation.

Etiology

Recurrent childhood nephrolithiasis has a number of documented causes, including metabolic abnormalities, infection, structural anomalies, idiopathic, and iatrogenic causes. A metabolic abnormality has been found in more than 50% of children with stones. These metabolic abnormalities include hypercalciuria, hyperoxaluria, hyperuricosuria, hypocitrauria, cystinuria, and renal tubular acidosis (RTA) (Table 55.1).

Hypercalciuria is the most common of the metabolic disorders seen in children. Fifty percent or more of these stones are composed of calcium oxalate or calcium phosphate. The causes of hypercalciuria include idiopathic, reabsorptive, iatrogenic, and granulomatous disease (Table 55.2). Idiopathic hypercalciuria is divided into Type I absorptive (diet independent) with increased calcium absorption on both a normal and increased calcium diet and Type II (diet dependent) with decreased calcium absorption on a low calcium diet. The second type of idiopathic hypercalciuria is renal leak hypercalciuria, where impairment in the tubular reabsorption of calcium results in a subsequent increase in PTH, and 1, 25-OH Vitamin D-mediated calcium absorption.

Primary hyperparathyroidism is caused by an adenoma or hyperplasia of the parathyroid gland. Primary hyperparathyroidism can be sporadic, familial, recessive, or dominant, and is part of the multiple endocrine neoplasia (MEN) syndromes. Hypercalciuria may be due to iatrogenic causes, such as immobilization of children recovering from surgery and the use of calcium wasting diuretics (furosemide).[3] Rarely, hypercalciuria is seen in patients with sarcoidosis.

Another metabolic cause of nephrolithiasis is hyperoxaluria. Primary hyperoxaluria is responsible for 50% of oxalate-related stones.[9] Children have nephrocalcinosis and recurrent stone formation, which will progress to renal insufficiency. Secondary hyperoxaluria occurs in the setting of intestinal malabsorption, resulting in an increase in the colonic permeability of oxalate, as well as less calcium for oxalate binding.

Cystine stones are the least common type of stones in children. Cystinuria is a recessive disorder with an abnormality in the renal and intestinal transport of the dibasic amino acids: cystine, ornithine, lysine, and arginine. Cystine stones may be seen in infancy, where males and females are equally affected.[10] Cystine stones can also be seen in patients with associated metabolic abnormalities (such as hypercalciuria, hyperuricosuria and hypocitraturia), hemophilia, retinitis pigmentosa, muscular dystrophy, trisomy 21, and hereditary pancreatitis.[1,3,10]

Five percent of pediatric stone formers will have a uric acid stone.[1,4,11] Elevated urine uric acid levels are caused by a high purine diet, metabolic errors, myeloproliferative and seizure disorders, hemolysis, and malignancy. Low urine pH or an increased ammonium concentration will cause uric acid stones to precipitate. Increased uric acid

Table 55.2. Major forms of hypercalciuria

Absorptive hypercalciuria

Diet dependent and independent

Increased Ca absorption → Increased serum Ca → ↓PTH, ↓Urine Ca

Renal hypercalciuria

Renal leak

↑ Urine Ca → ↓Serum Ca → ↑ PTH → ↑1,25(OH)$_2$D → ↑ Ca absorption

Primary hyperparathyroidism

Adenoma

↑ PTH → ↑Bone reabsorption → ↑ Serum Ca → ↑ Urine Ca

↑ PTH → ↑ 1,25(OH)$_2$D → ↑ Ca absorption

levels are seen in children with primary gout, Lesch–Nyhan syndrome, glycogen storage disease, pernicious anemia, polycythemia, and renal tubular defects. Drugs such as salicylates, probenicid, phenobarbital, valproic acid, sulfinpyrazone and alcohol are also predisposing factors.[12]

Urinary citrate is a natural inhibitor of stone formation. Hypocitrauria can lead to stone formation and 19%–63% of children diagnosed with a stone have hypocitrauria. Metabolic acidosis can accentuate the problem by leading to a decrease in urine citrate excretion. For example, low citrate levels are seen in distal renal tubular acidosis and in severe dehydration with electrolyte imbalance. Short gut or inflammatory bowel disease, cystic fibrosis, diuretic therapy, and urinary tract infections are also frequent causes of hypocitrauria. A high protein diet and excessive intake of red meat results in an increased acid load and have been shown to decrease urine citrate.[13]

In the USA, infectious stones comprise 24% of total stone formers.[4,11] The majority are boys less than 5 years old with upper tract calculi. Struvite stones are the most common and are due to the urea splitting bacteria such as *Proteus, Klebsiella, Pseudomonas, Providencia*, Enterococci and the non-urea splitting *E. coli*.

Functional obstruction with urinary stasis can predispose children to stone formation. In fact, 30% or more of children with urinary tract stones have a concomitant anatomic abnormality that predisposes to urine stasis. These abnormalities include ureteropelvic and ureterovesical obstruction as well as obstructed megaureter, single system ureterocele, and neuropathic bladder.

Clinical presentation

In children, the manifestations of stone can be less dramatic than in adults. In terms of presenting symptoms, abdominal pain occurred in 50%, hematuria in 33%, and infection in 11% of children with stones. Urolithiasis was an incidental finding in 15% of children undergoing radiographic imaging.

The clinical presentation of a child with nephrolithiasis can vary with age. Hematuria is the most common

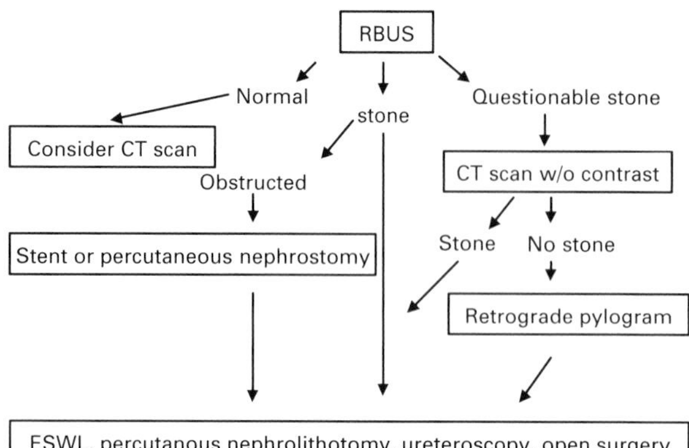

Fig. 55.1. Evaluation for a suspected stone.

presenting sign in children under 5 years old. Gross or microscopic hematuria occurs in 30% to 90% of children with stones, while pain is a more common finding in older children. Unlike in adults, the pain is rarely localized to the flank with radiation to the groin.[12] Children with stones may experience abdominal pain, which can mimic appendicitis or gastroenteritis. Children can also present with infection or other urinary symptoms such as dysuria, frequency, or incontinence. A urinary tract infection may be the only presenting sign of a stone in infants.

Evaluation of a child with a suspected stone

The first step in the evaluation of infants and children with a suspected stone is directed radiologic imaging (Fig. 55.1). The goal of the radiological evaluation is to confirm the diagnosis, assess the stone burden, location, and the degree urinary obstruction. In children, the initial imaging modality of choice is the renal/bladder ultrasound (RBUS) because it is non-invasive. Experienced pediatric ultrasonographers and current imaging technology have dramatically increased the diagnostic accuracy of this modality such that it is uncommon for the authors to need further imaging such as the intravenous pyelogram (IVP) or computerized tomography (CT). Even ureteral stones can be seen with RBUS but are certainly more difficult to visualize than stones located within the kidney. If clinical suspicion is high and the RBUS has not demonstrated a stone, further evaluation with a spiral CT scan (with and without) contrast may be helpful in accessing the stone size, location of the stone, and the amount of kidney function. Because of its high speed and sensitivity, CT scan has eliminated the need for intravenous pyelography. Rarely, a retrograde pyelogram is needed to further clarify the stone position or urinary tract anatomy. In addition to the radiographic studies, a complete blood count (CBC), serum electrolytes, BUN, creatinine, serum calcium, and phosphorus should be obtained to accurately assess the child's condition. The urine should also be cultured for bacteria and analyzed for pH, protein, and white blood cells. The urine should also be examined for stone crystals.

The clinical picture and radiographic findings will determine the treatment approach: observation or surgical intervention. Children should receive narcotics sufficient to relieve pain and be adequately hydrated, usually 1.5 to 2 times maintenance fluid. Urinary tract infections should be treated with antibiotics. Children who are afebrile, have a stone less then 4 mm in size, and have no associated anatomical abnormalities, may be observed. Asymptomatic children with stones greater than 4 mm in size will likely require intervention since these stones are not likely to pass spontaneously. If the child is obstructed, immediate drainage of the affected kidney is required. Uncontrolled pain, nausea, and emesis even in the presence of a small stone are indications for definitive intervention.

Surgical treatment in children with a first-time stone

In children with upper tract stones, extracorporeal shock wave lithotripsy (ESWL) is the preferred first-line therapy particularly for small to moderate calculi (4–10 mm) and no anatomic abnormalities (Fig. 55.2). There are no set guidelines for the use of ESWL in children but it has been shown to be safe and effective. Jayanthi *et al.* reported success with stones up to 1.5 cm in size in children age 17 months to 14 years.[14] Most centers report a stone-free rate between 70% and 80% for medium size stones,[15,16] with even higher stone-free rates using second-generation lithotripters (Table 55.3). Use of ESWL in staghorn or partial staghorn calculi is controversial, with reports of stone-free rates in excess of 70%; however, 50% of these patients required one or more treatments.[17]

The advantages of ESWL in children include its non-invasiveness and infrequent need to place a ureteral stent. Most of the newer ESWL machines use ultrasound localization and thereby avoid exposure to ionizing radiation. Either intravenous sedation and general anesthesia are used during the ESWL procedure and the choice is generally determined by surgeon, anesthesiologist, and institutional preferences. In addition, because of their small size, children have decreased shock wave attenuation, limiting trauma to the surrounding organs. Newer machines like the lithostar, which uses piezoelectric energy to deliver

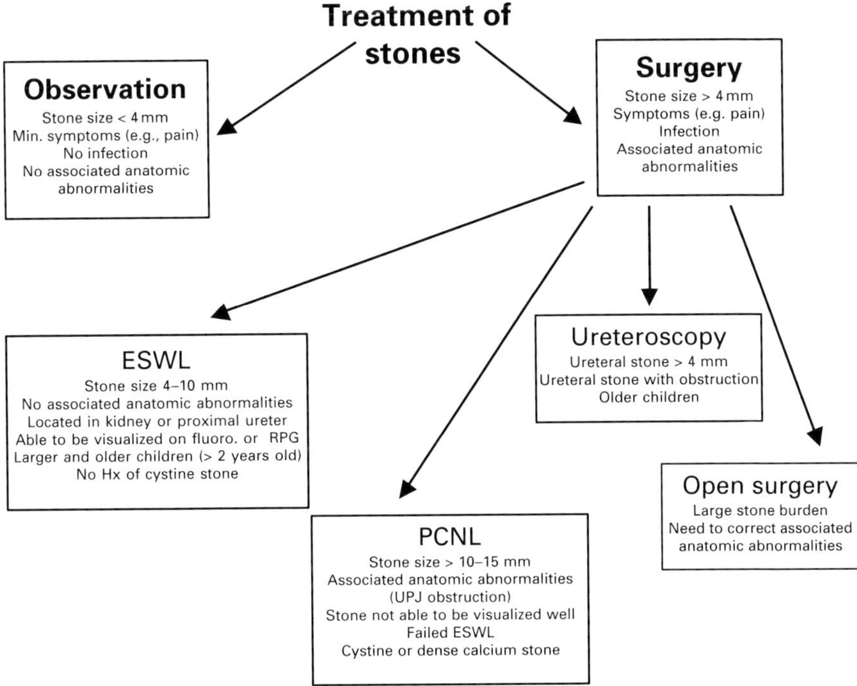

Fig. 55.2. Treatment of pediatric stones.

the shock precisely to a smaller focal zone, minimize damage even further.[17] Long-term studies indicate that ESWL is safe in children. Renal function and linear growth are not affected, and there is no increased risk of hypertension or scarring.[14]

The disadvantages of ESWL include the need for fluoroscopic localization of the stone in some cases, the potential development of urosepsis, steinstrasse (accumulation of multiple stone fragments within the ureter), hematuria, and flank pain. However, these complications occur infrequently with second-generation lithotripters.[18] Another disadvantage is the higher retreatment rate and the number of shocks needed with the second-generation piezoelectric lithotripters. The energy delivered to the stone is actually lower because of the small focal volume, necessitating further treatments when compared to the standard electrohydraulic units.[19]

In children with a large upper tract (1.5 cm) stone, percutaneous nephrolithotomy (PCNL) may be considered. Woodside performed the first pediatric PCNL with a stone free rate of 100% and no complications.[20] Similar series report comparable findings in children of all ages using standard adult techniques (Table 55.3).[21,22] Like ESWL, there are no absolute indications for PCNL. Relative indications include: a large stone burden of 1.5 cm or larger; associated urinary tract anatomical abnormalities; inability to visualize the stone; failed ESWL and evidence of a dense calcium monohydrate or cystine stone. The advantages of PCNL treatment include definitive removal of large stones. The disadvantages of PCNL include renal scarring,[23] a high retreatment rate with the mini-percutanous technique,[24] and higher complication as compared with ESWL. The overall complication rate of PCNL is 4%.[25] However, with appropriate patient selection and the use of laser lithotripsy, retreatment can be minimized.

Distal ureteral stones can be managed with ESWL or ureteroscopy. Children with a ureteral stone of 4 mm or larger that cannot be visualized with ESWL should undergo ureteroscopic stone extraction. The success rate of ureteroscopy varies between 80% and 100%. An EHL or Holmium–Yag probe can be passed through a 6.9 or 7.5 Fr. pediatric ureteroscope. After stone fragmentation, ureteral stents are placed for a period of several days to a week, depending on the amount of manipulation. The stents are then removed cystoscopically. In older children, the stent can be attached to a string, which is brought out through the urethra and removed without a second procedure. Since the incidences of vesicoureteral reflux after ureteroscopy is extremely low,[26] a VCUG is usually not needed after stent removal.

Open stone surgery in children is rarely indicated. A large stone burden that would require multiple endoscopic procedures or the presence of an associated congenital abnormality would be an indication to proceed with open surgery.

Table 55.3. Reported outcomes of pediatric stone therapy

Modality/author	Year	Patients	Outcome – stone free (%)	Retreatment	Follow-up in months
ESWL					
Choong [31]	2000	23	91	13	36
Elsobky [19]	2000	148	86	64	3
Orsola [17]	1999	15	73	36	60
Jayanthi [14]	1999	24	70	NR	1–48
Tekin [32]	1998	59	71	NR	3
Al busaidy [33]	1998	55	87	36	3
Nazli [34]	1998	67	87	42	24
Picramenos [15]	1996	96	82	28	33
Gschwend [35]	1996	27	92	NR	46
Hasanglou [36]	1996	103	63	NR	6
Cranidis [37]	1996	28	55	NR	NR
Van Horn [16]	1995	32	68	NR	67
Myers [38]	1995	238	77	14	3
Longo [39]	1995	70	99	29	3
PCNL					
Choong [31]	2000	30	90	10	36
Sahin [40]	2000	14	100	36	1–16
Badawy [22]	1999	60	83	NR	3–72
Al-Shammari [21]	1998	8	88	12.5	3–6
Jackman [24]	1998	7	85	43	3
Mor [41]	1997	25	92	12	2–66
Kurzrock [42]	1996	8	100	25	5–96
Ureteroscopy					
Van Savage [43]	2000	33	100	0	24
Wollin [44]	1999	19	84	16	.5–12
Jayanthi [14]	1999	12	92	NR	1–48
Al Busaidy [33]	1997	43	94	7	NR
Minevich [45]	1996	7	85	0	NR
Kurzrock [42]	1996	17	100	0	5–96
Smith [46]	1996	11	82	18	.5–22
Scarpa [47]	1995	7	100	0	NR
Shroff [48]	1995	13	77	NR	NR

Consideration should be given to the fact that children tolerate a flank or dorsal lumbotomy incision well. The advantages of open surgery include rapid and effective stone clearance with a single procedure; however, open surgery especially anatrophic nephrolithotomy can be associated with functional renal deterioration.[27]

Evaluation of a child with a recurrent stone

Children with recurrent stones should be thoroughly evaluated in order to identify the etiology of the stone disease and possibly prevent recurrence (Fig 55.3). Twenty to 50% of children with urolithiasis have a family history of stone disease and may point to a metabolic etiology or a tendency toward recurrence.[11] A careful inquiry should be made for a history of metabolic disorders, distal RTA, and malignancy. A review of medications (Table 55.4) such as diuretics, steroids, vitamin D analogues, or chemotherapeutic medications is also important. Whenever possible, a chemical analysis of the stone is essential.

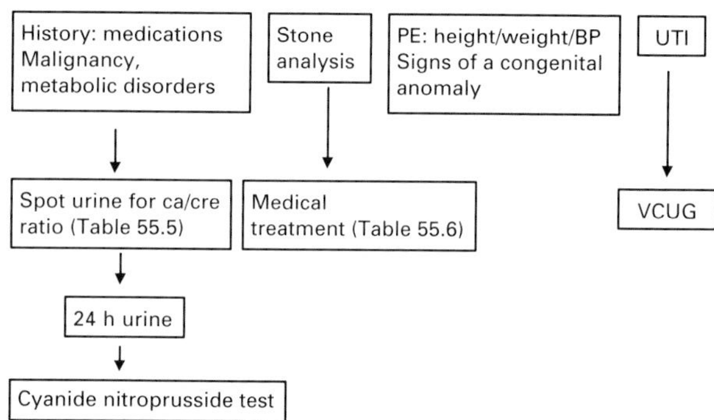

Fig. 55.3. Work-up for a repeat stone former.

The physical examination should assess weight and blood pressure, since these abnormalities may suggest an underlying metabolic, systemic, or anatomic defect. Signs of a congenital anomaly such as myelomeningocele should also be noted. In children with a proven urinary tract infection, a voiding cystourethrography is suggested to rule out associated anatomical abnormalities such as vesicoureteral reflux or posterior urethral valves.

Laboratory studies should include a serum calcium level and spot urine for calcium, uric acid and oxalate level, relative to creatinine (Table 55.5). These are helpful screening tests and for follow-up in younger children, where obtaining multiple samples may prove difficult.[12] If the above results are normal, the work-up is complete. Abnormalities noted on the spot urine test require a 24 h urine collection to characterize the problem better; however, the correlation between the two studies is high. An elevation in calcium, uric acid, or oxalate noted on a 24 h urine collection, can tailor the work-up toward identifying the specific metabolic defect.

The amount of urinary calcium varies with age. In children less than 1 year old, the calcium to creatinine ratio varies between 0.81 and 0.42 (Table 55.5). Hypercalciuria can be confirmed on a 24 h urine collection (≥4 mg/kg per day). It has been shown that preterm and term infants on breast milk have a higher amount of calcium in their urine.[28] If calcium and sodium are both elevated on urine collection, a repeat urine collection after several weeks of

Table 55.4. Medications frequently associated with urolithiasis

Calcium stones	Oxalate stones	Uric acid stones
Acetazolamide	Vitamin C	Probenecid
Calcium channel blockers	Phosphate binding antacids	sulfinpyrazone
Furosemide		
Vitamin D		
Theophylline		
Hyperalimentation		
Triamterene		

Table 55.5. Urinary solute to creatinine ratio

Urinary solute: creatinine ratio	Normal values
Calcium (mg/dl)	
Neonates <34 weeks	<0.81:1
Neonates >34 weeks	<0.42:1
Children	<0.21:1
Oxalate (mg/dl)	
Infants 0–6 months	<0.3:1
Children <4 years	<0.15:1
Children >4 years	<0.1:1
Uric acid (mg/dl)	<0.53
Timed collections	
Calcium (mg/kg per 24 h)	<4
Oxalate	
(mg/1.73 m^2 per 24 h)	<40
(mmol/1.73 m^2 per 24 h)	<0.5
Uric acid (mg/1.73 m^2 per 24 h)	<815
Cystine (mg/24 h)	<20
Citrate (mg/g creatine/24 h)	
Male	>128
Female	>300
Magnesium (mg/kg per 24 h)	1.6

sodium restriction should be obtained. If the urine calcium is still elevated, medical therapy should be instituted.

The amount of urinary oxalate varies with age. The oxalate to creatinine ratio varies from 72 to 147 mol/ml during the first year of life and formula-fed infants normally have higher oxalate excretion. A useful but seldom seen finding associated with hyperoxaluria is nephrocalcinosis (diffuse calcium deposition within the renal parenchyma). Hyperoxaluria should be confirmed on a 24 h urine collection (≥40 mg/1.73 m^2 per day). Hyperoxaluria may be due to intestinal malabsorption or a primary enzyme deficiency. In these cases the patient should be referred to a pediatric gastroenterologist or hepatologist, as the latter can only be diagnosed by a liver biopsy.

In children who have hyperuricuria on a 24 h urine collection (≥815 mg/1.73 m^2 per day), the correct diagnosis depends on evaluation of the serum as well as the urine uric acid concentration. In Lesch–Nyhan syndrome (where there is a complete or partial deficiency of hypoxanthine phosphoribosyltransferase-HPRT) as well as in phosphoribosylpyrophosphate superactivity, uric acid can be elevated in both the plasma and the urine. In patients with low plasma levels of uric acid but a high urinary concentration, renal tubular transport defects such as hereditary renal hypouricemia should be considered in the differential diagnosis. The diaper or the tip of the patient's penis should be inspected for crystal formation, since purine crystals are not very soluble. Once the diagnosis has been confirmed, these children may benefit from medical therapy. Finally, parathyroid hormone (PTH) is rarely elevated and serum levels should be drawn only in children found to have hypercalcemia (≥ 10.1 mg/dl) and hypercalciuria on a 24 h urine collection.

Treatment of recurrent stones

Prevention of recurrent stone treatment involves medical therapy and treatment of any concurrent urinary tract anatomic abnormalities. Medical therapy can be of benefit in a number of disorders (Table 55.6). The type of medical therapy is based on the etiology of the stone and the underlying metabolic disorders. Medical treatment can be instituted for all of the metabolic disorders (Table 55.1).

Children with idiopathic hypercalciuria can be treated with calcium sparing diuretics. Hydrochlorothiazide in liquid form (10 mg/ml) is dosed at 1–2 mg/kg per day. Diuretics work by reducing urine calcium saturation in both renal and absorptive hypercalciuria. Disadvantages of long-term thiazide usage include bone demineralization, increase in serum cholesterol, and low-density lipoproteins

Potassium citrate is useful in treating children with recurrent stone, particularly those with distal renal tubular acidosis or low urinary citrate levels. In older children, Urocit K (Mission, San Antonio Tx) is given at 20 meq three times a day if citrate levels are below 150 mg/g Cr. In children with elevated levels, greater than 150 mg/g Cr the dose can be adjusted to 10 meq in three divided doses. In young children, potassium citrate combined with citric acid can be given in 5 ml doses (1.1 gm potassium citrate/5 ml). Dosing is adjusted according to urine pH and 24 h urine citrate levels. These levels should be obtained within 24 hours of the start of therapy and repeated at 2-month intervals. Finally, idiopathic hypercalciuria refractory to treatment

Table 55.6. Medical treatment of recurrent stones

Stone type	Defect	Treatment
Uric acid	Hyperuricemia Hyperuricosuria	Allopurinol (100 mg tablets): <6 yrs. 150 mg/d >6 yrs. 300 mg/d Potassium citrate: 10–20 meq in three divided doses depending on urine citrate level Dietary restriction of protein
Cystine	Cystinuria	α-MCPG: 15 mg/kg per day in three divided doses (100 mg tablets) Potassium citrate
Struvite	Infection	Complete stone removal
Calcium	Hyperparathyroidism	Parathyroidectomy
	Hypercalciuria	
	Absorptive	Orthophosphates
	Renal leak	HCTZ(1–2 mg/kg per day; 10 mg/ml)
	Immobilization	Weight bearing
	RTA	Potassium citrate
Oxalate	Hyperoxaluria Primary Secondary	Vitamin B_6 and magnesium tablet (25 mg/366 mg) Dietary restriction Magnesium Potassium citrate

may require orthophosphates to reduce urinary calcium saturation and spontaneous nucleation of calcium oxalate.

Medical treatment of hyperuricosuria is most effective with Allopurinol (100 mg tablets, Zyloprim Faro, Bedminster, NJ). It works by reducing uric acid formation, excretion, and saturation as well as inhibiting the nucleation of calcium oxalate crystals. Children under 6 years of age are dosed at 150 mg/day, while older children may take up to 300 mg/day. Dosing is adjusted by monitoring uric acid levels in the urine.

Medical therapy for primary oxaluria is, in most cases, palliative. Pyridoxine (vitamin B 6) will shift glyoxalate to glycolate, decreasing the formation of oxalate. No standard dosage exists for the pediatric population. Pyridoxine comes in a tablet combined with magnesium (25 mg pyridoxine, 366 mg magnesium). Dosing is empirical and urine oxalate levels are monitored. Thiazide diuretics, magnesium, citrate, and phosphate supplements can help by decreasing calcium excretion. However, the disease is invariably progressive. At some point, dialysis will need to be instituted in preparation for kidney transplant (patients with pyridoxine sensitive disease) with or without concurrent liver transplant. Recently, an international registry has been established to follow this cohort of patients which was established at the Mayo Clinic in Rochester, Minnesota.

In children with cystinuria, medical therapy has a proven role. Potassium citrate is used to increase urine pH in combination with 6 mercapto-prionyl-glycine (Thiola), a chelating agent. Thiola is administered at 15 mg/kg day in three divided doses (100 mg tablets). Titrate the dosage to keep urine citrate below 250 mg/g. Penicillamine, another chelating agent, is no longer recommended because of its adverse side effects such as nephritis and aplastic anemia.

Anatomical obstruction as well as neuropathic bladder can lead to stasis of urine and stone formation. Anatomical obstruction, such as ureteropelvic junction, ureterovesicle obstruction, or ureterocele is treated endoscopically or with open surgery. Treatment of the neuropathic bladder involves intermittent catheterization and anticholinergic medications.

Prevention of stones

The single most important aspect in preventing recurrent stone formation is hydration. Increased water intake produces a more dilute urine and lowers the solubility coefficient of the urinary solutes. Dietary modification can also play an important role in prevention. This includes limiting the amount of sodium in the diet, since high sodium intake can lead to inhibition of sodium and calcium absorption in the proximal tubule and along the loop of Henle.[29] A diet high in potassium and potassium supplementation has been shown to reduce hypercalciuria.[30] The mechanism behind this is not well understood but probably relates to phosphate transport and excessive vitamin D synthesis. Reducing protein intake can be helpful since excessive protein can lead to an above average acid load, decreasing urine pH and urine citrate. Finally, every attempt should be made to maintain normal levels of phosphate, citrate, and magnesium, while calcium should never be restricted, as this may lead to decreased bone development.

Current state of evidence-based literature

What do we mean by evidence-based data and how is our evidence classified? Category 1 evidence was data obtained from a metanalysis of randomized controlled trials or randomized controlled trial (RCT). Category 2 evidence was from a well-designed controlled study without randomization. Category 3 evidence was obtained from a well-designed non-experimental descriptive study, such as comparative studies or case-controlled studies. Category 4 evidence was obtained from expert committed reports or opinions.

A full literature search performed independently by the author and a professional medical librarian using the heading of urolithiasis generated 22 591 articles. Limiting the search to "pediatric" (0–18 yrs) generated 4508. When the search was further restricted to 1(a) evidence (meta-analysis) there were none! The search for 1(b) evidence (randomized controlled trial) revealed 55 articles. A search for evidence at Categories 2 and 3 found 198 articles. There were 226 reviews that would be classified as Category 4 evidence.

If one agrees that the best evidence is obtained from RCTs, then it is interesting that only 55 articles can be found in 4508 articles on "pediatric urolithiasis." On further inspection, all but three articles involve children of 13 and older. Nearly all of these articles are composed primarily of adults with some adolescents and are therefore captured in the search under the heading of "child." Taken at face value, the 55 articles fall into four general groups: prevention or recurrence of urolithiasis; comparison of imaging techniques; use of analgesics; and comparison of ESWL techniques.

Health impact and long-term outcomes

The following is a brief synopsis of the evidence based on the categories of evidence described above.

Presentation/prevention/recurrence

Children that present with dysuria, abdominal pain, or a family history of nephrolithiasis should be investigated for hypercalciuria. The lack of hematuria does not exclude the presence of nephrolithiasis or hypercalciuria. Hypercalciuria is common in children and half of children with hypercalciuria have microcalculi (Category 3).[49]

In adults, an increased spot urine sodium potassium ratio (UNa/K) has been associated with urolithiasis. The role of this ratio was studied in children with idiopathic hypercalciuria and found to be elevated as compared to controls (normocalciuric). The elevated UNa/K ratio is accentuated by meals (Category 3).[50]

The role of urinary inhibitors of crystallization such as magnesium, citrate, and glycoaminoglycans have been studied in children with hypercalciuria. In this study, two groups of children with hypercalciuria were compared. One group of children had hypercalciuria alone and the other group had hypercalciuria and hematuria. Both groups had high urinary calcium excretion; however, the significantly lower levels of urinary citrate and glycoaminoglycans appear to account for the increased incidence of urolithiasis in the group with hypercalciuria alone. This suggests that despite the presence of hypercalciuria, the presence of normal levels of urinary inhibitors such as magnesium, citrate, and glycoanimoglycans may be protective (Category 2).[51]

Potassium citrate is thought to increase urinary solubility and possibly prevent further stone recurrence. The role of potassium citrate in stone prevention or stabilization following extracorporeal shock wave lithotripsy (ESWL) was studied in a prospective fashion. Potassium citrate was found to be statistically significant in effectively preventing stone recurrence or stabilizing post ESWL residual stone burden (Category 2).[52]

One prospective study examined the recurrence of nephrolithiasis over 6 years in three treatment groups: diet alone, phosphate therapy, and placebo. Nearly half of all subjects in all three groups remained free of stones during the study period (Category 2).[53]

The role of bladder washout in the prevention of stone formation in pediatric patients following bladder augmentation was studied in a prospective cohort of 30 children with a control group performing clean intermittent catheterization alone. Bladder washout did not significantly reduce the incidence of stone formation in patients with bladder augmentation (Category 3).[54]

Imaging

In randomized prospective fashion, non-contrast enhanced helical computed tomography (CT) was compared with the intravenous urography (IVU)with acute renal colic. The diagnostic accuracy and other attributes were examined. Both studies had a high degree of sensitivity and specificity with the CT being slightly higher. The added advantages of the CT include the identification of alternative diagnoses and a fast, well-tolerated technique without the need for intravenous injection of iodinated contrast. The CT had a higher radiation exposure (Category 3).[55]

Treatment

Non-invasive methods of treating nephrolithiasis by extracorporeal shock wave lithotripsy have been well established in adults. ESWL use has also now been established to be safe and effective in the treatment of renal and ureteral stones. Over a 5-year period, the Siemens Lithostar lithotripter was used to treat 446 pediatric patients with 238 renal stones and 208 ureteral stones. The renal stone-free rate was 68%, residual fragments less than 4 mm was 76.6%, and the retreatment rate was 14.1%. The ureteral stone-free rate was 91.1% and the retreatment rate was 3.5%. Anesthesia was required in 31% of renal and 21% of ureteral procedures. This study demonstrated that the low energy lithotripsy with the Lithostar was safe and effective in children (Category 3).[38]

Over a 5-year period, the effectiveness of the first and second generation lithotripters was studied in 32 children ranging in age from 4 to 18 years old. The two machines were the Dornier HM3 and the Siemen Lithostar. Of patients treated with the HM3, 67% required general anesthesia, while 86% of patients treated with the Siemen required intravenous sedation. When success rates were examined by lithotripter, there was no significant difference between the two machines. Additionally, there was no statistical difference between the two treatment groups with regard to age, stone location, or use of stents. Three patients required adjuvant procedures but none required open or percutaneous procedures (Category 3).[16] Others have documented similar success rates with a variety of other lithotripsy machines.[39]

One unique study investigated the use of ESWL in infants and specially tried to assess the effects on renal parenchyma. Over a 5-year period, 12 children were treated with ESWL for renal or ureteral stones using the Sonolith machine. All children were less that 2 years of age. DMSA scans were obtained prior to EWSL and at least 6 months after being treated with ESWL. Blood pressure was also assessed. The results demonstrated a high treatment success of 84.6% and 100% for first and second treatments, respectively. There were no blood pressure changes or renal scars identified (Category 3).[56]

Safe and successful ureteroscopy has been made possible by the development and introduction of smaller endoscopic equipment. Over a 5-year period in seven children less than 10 years of age, Scapa *et al.* demonstrated the safe and effective use of ureteroscopy in combination with ureterolithotripsy. Both 7 and 4.8 French ureteroscopes were used in conjunction with laser and ballistic lithotripsy. All patients were rendered stone free and no early or late complications were reported (Category 3).[47]

Others have also demonstrated similar success (Category 3).[46,57]

Research opportunities

Hopefully, the reader of this chapter comes to an understanding of the profound lack of published data from adequately powered and well-designed clinical studies regarding all aspects of pediatric urolithiasis. The randomized clinical trial is arguably the gold standard study but it is difficult to conduct and expensive. There are other acceptable methods to acquire meaningful data such as longitudinal cohort studies and well-designed clinical trials without randomization. To date, very few of these studies have been conducted in the field of pediatric urolithiasis. Long-term data (5, 10 or greater years) is equally sparse in any venue ranging from the RCT to retrospective reviews. From a research perspective, the field of pediatric urolithiasis is wide open for anyone to contribute meaningful data with regard to best practices obtained from well-designed clinical trials or long-term data regarding the natural history of pediatric stone disease or effects of intervention and prevention of stone disease.

Research obstacles

There are many obstacles preventing well-designed clinical research in this field. Some of these obstacles are general to clinical research, while others are specific to children and others still are specific to the disease itself. For example, stone disease in children is relatively uncommon making it difficult to accrue a sufficient number of patients to adequately power a clinical trial. This necessitates multi-institutional collaboration that may require national or even international participation. This adds to the complexity and expense of conducting these trials. Funding of research can be a significant obstacle to conducting well-designed research. Even establishment of registries is costly. The upfront cost of designing and establishing a patient registry can approach US $200 000 while the yearly maintenance can be as high as US $100 000.

Conclusions

There is a lack of long-term data and well-designed studies in the field of pediatric urolithiasis. Additionally, there is a lack of clinician-scientists who are: (1) well trained in conducting clinical trials; (2) adequately funded; and (3) have sufficient time to devote to conducting this research. These obstacles are not specific to pediatric urolithiasis but are applicable to most issues regarding pediatric urology. Nevertheless, progress has been made and the pediatric population has benefited from the advances in minimally invasive surgery with stone-free rates continuing to improve with technological advancement. Advances in medical therapy for stone disease have reduced recurrent stone formation but further work is needed. Gene therapy and a further understanding of the pathophysiology of pediatric stone disease may one day lead to the prevention of urolithiasis.

REFERENCES

1. Polinsky, M. S., Kaiser, B. A., Baluarte, H. J., & Gruskin, A. B. Renal stones and hypercalciuria. *Adv. Pediatr*. 1993; **40**:353–384.
2. Noe, H. N., Stapleton, F. B., Jerkins, G. R., & Roy. S. 3rd. Clinical experience with pediatric urolithasis. *J. Urol.* 1983; **129**:1166–1168.
3. Stapleton, F. B. Clinical approach to children with urolithiasis. *Semin. Nephrol*. 1996; **16**:389–397.
4. Choi, H., Snyder, H. M. 3rd., & Duckett, J. Urolithasis in childhood: current Management. *J. Pediatr. Surg*. 1987; **22**:158–164.
5. Milliner, D. Urolithasis in pediatric patients. *Mayo Clin. Proc.* 1993; **68**:241–248.
6. Ozokutan, B. H., Küçükaydin, M., Gündüz, Z., Kabaklioglu, M., Okur, H., & Turan, C. Urolithiasis in childhood. *Pediatr. Surgery International*. 2000; **16**:60–63.
7. Gokdemir, A., Avanoglu, I., & Ulman, I. Pediatric urinary lithasis in Turkey. *Turk. J. Pediatr. Surg*. 1995; **9**:299–303.
8. Miller, O. S., L McAlear, I., Barboroglu, P., & Kaplan, G. W. Pediatric urolithasis: presentation and treatment in the year 2000. Presented at *the Society for Pediatric Urology*. Anaheim CA, 2001.
9. Noe, H. N. & Stapleton, F. B. Pediatric stone disease. In Rous, S, ed. *Stone Disease: Diagnosis and Management*. Orlando, FL: Grune and Stratton; 1987:347–379.
10. Milliner, D. Cystinuria. *Endocrinol. Metab. Clin. North Am.* 1990; **19**:889–907.
11. Gearhart, J. P., Herzberg, G. Z., & Jeffs, R. D. Childhood urolithasis: experience and advances. *Pediatrics* 1991; **87**: 445.
12. Santos-Victoriano, M., Brouhard, B. H., & Cunningham, R. J., 3rd. Renal stone disease in children. *Clin. Pediatr*. 1998; **37**:583–99.
13. Pak, C. Citrate and renal calculi: an update. *Min. Electr. Metab.* 1994; **20**:371–377.
14. Jayanthi, V. R., Arnold, P. M., & Koff, S. A. Strategies for managing upper tract calculi in young children. *J. Urol.* 1999; **162**:1234–1237.
15. Picramenos, D., Deliveliotis, C., Alexopoulou, K., Makrichoritis, C., Kostakopoulos, A., & Dimopoulos, C. Extracorporeal shock wave lithotripsy for renal stones in children. *Urol. Int*. 1996; **56**:86–89.
16. Van Horn, A. C., Hollander, J. B., & Kass, E. J. First and second generation lithotripsy in children: results, comparison and followup. *J. Urol.* 1995; **153**:1969–1971.
17. Orsola, A., Diaz, I., Caffaratti, J., Izquierdo, F., Alberola, J., & Garat, J. M. Staghorn calculi in children: treatment with monotherapy extracorporeal shock wave lithotripsy. *J. Urol.* 1999; **162**:1229–1233.
18. Kroovand, R. H., Harrison, L. H., & McCullough, D. L. Extracorporeal shock wave lithotripsy in childhood. *J. Urol.* 1987; **138**:1106–1108.
19. Elsobky, E. Sheir, K. Z., Madbouly, K., & Mokhtar, A. A. Extracorporeal shock wave lithotripsy in children: experience using two second-generation lithotripters. *BJU Int*. 2000; **86**:851–856.
20. Woodside, J. R., Stevens, G. F., Stark, G. L., Borden, T. A., & Ball, W. S. Percutaneous stone removal in children. *J. Urol.* 1985; **134**:1166–1167.
21. Al-Shammari, A. M., Al-Otaibi, K., Leonard, M. P., & Hosking, D. H. Percutaneous nephrolithotomy in the pediatric population [see comments]. *J. Urol*. 1999; **162**:1721–1724.
22. Badawy, H., Salama, A., Eissa, M., Kotb, E., Moro, H., & Shoukri, I. Percutaneous management of renal calculi: experience with percutaneous nephrolithotomy in 60 children. *J. Urol.* 1999; **162**:1710–1713.
23. Wilson, W. T., Husmann, D. A., Morris, J. S., Miller, G. L., Alexander, M., & Preminger, G. M. A comparison of the bioeffects of four different modes of stone therapy on renal function and morphology. *J. Urol.* 1993; **150**:1267–1270.
24. Jackman, S. V., Hedican, S. P., Peters, C. A., & Docimo, S. Percutaneous nephrolithotomy in infants and preschool age children: experience with a new technique. *Urology*. 1998; **52**:697–701.
25. Stoller, M. I., Wolf, J. S. Jr., & St Lezin, M. A. Estimated blood loss and transfusion rates associated with percutaneous nephrolithotomy. *J. Urol.* 1994; **152**:1997–1981.
26. Thomas, R. Safety and efficacy of pediatric ureteroscopy for the management of calculus disease. *J. Urol.* 1993; **149**:1082.
27. Gough, D. C. & Baillie, C. T. Pediatric anatrophic nephrolithotomy; stone clearance – at what price? *BJU Int*. 2000; **85**:874–878.
28. Hillman, L. S., Chow, W., Salmon, S. S. *et al.* Vitamin D metabolism, mineral homeostasis and bone mineralizationin term infants fed human milk, cow milk-based formula or soy-based formula. *J. Pediatr.* 1988; **112**:864–874.
29. Kleeman, C. R., Bohannan, J., Bernstein, D. *et al.* Effect of variations in sodium intake on calcium excretion in normal humans. *Proc. Soc. Exp. Biol. Med.* 1964; **115**:29–32.
30. Osorio, A. V. & Alon, U. S. The relationship between urinary calcium, sodium, and potassium excretion and the role of potassium in treating idiopathic hypercalciuria. *Pediatrics* 1997; **100**:675–681.
31. Choong, S., Whitfield, H., Duffy, P. *et al.* The management of pediatric urolithiasis. *BJU Int*. 2000; **88**:857–860.
32. Tekin, I., Tekgul, S., Bakkaloglu, M., & Kendi, S. Results of extracorporeal shock wave lithotripsy in children using the Dornier MPL 9000 lithotriptor. *J. Pediatr. Surg.* 1998; **33**:1257–1259.
33. al Busaidy, S. S., Prem, A. R., Medhat, M., Giriraj, D., Gopakumar, P., & Bhat, H. S. Paediatric ureteral calculi: efficacy of primary in situ extracorporeal shock wave lithotripsy. *Br. J. Urol.* 1998; **82**:90–96.
34. Nazali, O., Cal, C., Ozyurt, C. *et al.* Reults of extracorporeal shock wave lithotripsy in the pediatric age group. *Eur. Urol.* 1998; **33**:333–336.

35. Gschwend, J. E., Haag, U., Hollmer, S., Kleinschmidt, K., & Hautmann, R. E. Impact of extracorporeal shock wave lithotripsy in pediatric patients: complications and long-term follow-up. *Urol. Int*. 1996; **54**:241–245.
36. Hasanoglu, E., Buyan, N., Tumer, L., Bozkirli, I., Demirel, F., & Karaoglan, U. Extracorporeal shock wave lithotripsy in children. *Acta Paediatr*. 1996; **85**:377–379.
37. Cranidias, A. I., Karayainis, A. A., Delakas, D. S., Livadas, C. E., & Anezinis, P. E. Cystein stones: the efficacy bof percutaneous shock wave lithotripsy. *Urol. Int.* 1996; **56**:180–183.
38. Myers, D. A., Mobley, T. B., Jenkins, J. M., Grine, W. B., & Jordan, W. R. Pediatric low energy lithotripsy with the lithostar. *J. Urol.* 1995; **153**:453–457.
39. Longo, J. A., Metto, J., N. R. Extracorporeal shock wave lithotripsy in children. *Urology*. 1995; **46**:550–552.
40. Sahin, A., Tekgul, S., Erdem, E., Ekici, S., Hasicek, M., & Kendi, S. Percutaneous nephrolithotomy in older children. *J. Pediatr. Surg.* 2000; **35**:1336–1338.
41. Mor, Y., Elmasry, Y. E., Kellett, M. J., & Duffy, P. G. The role of percutaneous nephrolithotomy in the management of pediatric renal calculi. *J. Urol.* 1997; **158**:1319–1321.
42. Kurzrock, E. A., Huffman, J. L., Hardy, B. E., & Fugelso, P. Endoscopic treatment of pediatric urolithiasis. *J. Pediatr. Surg*. 1996; **31**:1413–1416.
43. Van Savage, J. G., Palanca, L. G., Andersen, R. D., Rao, G. S., & Slaughenhoupt, B. L. Treatment of distal ureteral stones in children: similarities to the American urological association guidelines in adults. *J. Urol.* 2000; **164**:1089–1093.
44. Wollin, T. A., Teichman, J. M., Rogenes, V. J., Razvi, H. A., Denstedt, J. D., & Grasso, M. Holmium:YAG lithotripsy in children [see comments]. *J. Urol.* 1999; **162**:1717–1720.
45. Minevich, E., Rousseau, M. B., Wacksman, J., Lewis, A. G., & Sheldon, C. A. Pediatric ureteroscopy: technique and preliminary results. *J. Pediatr. Surg.* 1997; **32**:571–574.
46. Smith, D. P., Jerkins, G. R., & Noe, H. N. Urethroscopy in small neonates with posterior urethral valves and ureteroscopy in children with ureteral calculi. *Urology* 1996; **47**:908–910.
47. Scarpa, R. M., DeLisa, A., Porru, D., Canetto, A., & Usay, E. Ureterolithotripsy in children. *Urology* 1995; **46**:859–862.
48. Shroff, S. & Watson, G. M. Experience with ureteroscopy in children. *Br. J. Urol.* 1995; **75**:395–400.
49. Polito, C., La Manna, A., Cioce, F., Villani, J., Nappi, B., & Di Toro, R. Clinical presentation and natural course of idiopathic hypercalciuria in children. *Pediatr. Nephrol.* 2000; **15**(3–4):211–214.
50. Polito, C., La Manna, A., Maiello, R., Siciliano, M., & Di Toro, R. Urinary sodium and potassium excretion in idiopathic hypercalciuria in children. *Nephron.* 2002; **91**(1):7–12.
51. Perrone, H. C., Toporovski, J., & Schor, N. Urinary inhibitors of crystallization in hypercalciuric children with hematuria and nephrolithiasis. *Pediatr. Nephrol.* 1996; **10**(4):435–437.
52. Jimenz Verdejo, A., Arrabal Martin, M., Mijan Ortiz, J. L., Hita Rosino, E., Yago, F., & Zuluaga Gomez, A. Effect of potassium citrate in the prophylaxis of urinary lithiasis. *Arch. Esp. Urol.* 2001; **54**(9):1036–1046.
53. Ettinger, B. Recurrence of nephrolithiasis. A six-year prospective study. *Am. J. Med.* 1979; **67**(2):245–248.
54. Brough, R. J., O'Flynn, K. J., Fishwick, J., & Gough, D. C. Bladder washout and stone formation in pediatric enterocystoplasty. *Eur. Urol.* 1998; **33**(5):500–502.
55. Homer, J. A., Davies-Payne, D. L., & Peddinti, B. S. Randomized prospective comparison of non-contrast enhance helical computed tomography and intravenous urography in the diagnosis of acute ureteric colic. *Aust. Radiol.* 2001; **45**(3):285–290.
56. Traxer, O., Lottmann, H., Archambaud, F., Helal, B., & Mercier Pageyral, B. Extracorporeal shock-wave lithotripsy in infants. Study of its repercussions on the renal parenchyma. *Ann. Urol.* 1998; **32**(4):191–196.
57. Delakas, D., Daskalopoulos, G., Metaxari, M., Triantafyllou, T., & Cranidis, A. Management of ureteral stones in pediatric patients. *J. Endourol.* 2001; **15**(7):674–680.

56

Gonadal tumors

J. S. Valla

Department of Pediatric Surgery, Hôpital Lenval, Nice, France

Introduction

Gonadal tumors are rare in children and raise two main questions.[1] First, is the tumor benign or malignant? The risk of malignancy is around 50% in boys and about 10% to 25% in girls (if both solid and cystic lesions are included). For benign tumors, a conservative surgical procedure (tumorectomy with gonadal preservation) should be attempted when possible. Malignant or potentially malignant tumors have an excellent prognosis provided they are properly treated by a surgeon and oncologist – current protocols using platinum and bleomycin are very effective, even for advanced-stage tumors. Second, how is future gonadal function best preserved? Gonadal function can be almost normal after treatment of a unilateral gonadal tumor, but in synchronous or metachronous bilateral tumors, gonadal function may be entirely destroyed. This has two major consequences: a lack of gamete production inducing sterility and a failure of sex hormone production which prevents the progression of natural puberty and the development of secondary sexual characteristics. Hormonal failure can be managed by lifelong hormonal substitution. However, sterility may have major psychological effects.[2] Thus, gonadal function should be preserved if at all possible.[3–5]

Advances in detection, diagnosis, minimally invasive management, and chemotherapy have all required changes in clinical practice, which is aimed at reducing morbidity without compromising oncological treatment.

Excluded from this chapter are the rarer problems of leukemia or lymphoma located in the ovary or testis, rare malignant paratesticular tumors (rhabdomyosarcoma or mesenchymal tumor), and rare soft tissue tumors (fibroma, leiomyoma, hemangioma).

The classification of male and female gonadal tumors share similarities and are considered together (Table 56.1), whilst clinical presentation, treatment, and outcome are discussed separately.

Classification

Gonadal tumors are classified by their putative cell of origin: germ cell, stroma cell (or endocrine cell), and for the ovary, epithelial cell.

Germ cell tumors

Germ cell tumors are the most common type of gonadal tumor in children and adolescents, accounting for 80% of cases. They are divided into subgroups, based on their degree of differentiation and the cellular components involved. The least differentiated are dysgerminoma or seminoma. Dysgerminoma are hormonally biologically inactive, of low grade malignancy, and may express lactate dehydrogenase (LDH-1), a useful serum marker. Embryonic tumors may be differentiated to various extents. Embryonal carcinoma is quite rare in children. Highly differentiated embryonal tumors (mature or immature teratomas) may produce embryonal structures or extraembryonal structures (e.g., yolk sac tumor or endodermal sinus tumor produce alphafetoprotein (AFP) and choriocarcinoma produces human chorionic gonadotrophin (HCG)).

Among the germ cell tumors, teratoma and yolk sac tumor are the most frequent. Only mature teratoma are

Pediatric Surgery and Urology: Long-term Outcomes, Mark Stringer, Keith Oldham, Pierre Mouriquand.
Published by Cambridge University Press. © Cambridge University Press, 2006.

Table 56.1. Ovarian and testicular tumors

	(1) Shared features	
(ii) Histologic origin		
(iii) Tumor markers		
(iv) Good response to chemotherapy		
(v) Good overall prognosis		
(vi) Risk of infertility		
(vii) Risk of bilateral disease		
	(2) Different features	
	Ovary	Testis
Incidence	20 – 50/100 000	0.5 /100 000
Risk of malignancy – Overall rate – Age (peak incidence) – Initial staging	Less than 20% More than 10 years Stage III/IV> 50%	50% Less than 3 years Stage I > 80%
Torsion at presentation	>30%	5%
Histology	30 to 50% non-neoplastic or functional cyst 10 to 15% epithelial tumor Tumor usually heterogeneous – frozen section unreliable	No functional cyst No epithelial tumor Tumor usually homogeneous – frozen section reliable

benign. Dysgerminoma or seminoma are very rare before puberty. The majority of malignant germ cell tumors produce serum markers (AFP and HCG), which are useful when assessing treatment efficacy and detecting potential recurrence. Ovarian malignant tumors are a heterogenous group including yolk sac tumor, choriocarcinoma, immature and mature teratoma; careful pathologic evaluation is important to avoid missing malignant elements in these lesions. This heterogeneity explains why frozen section histology is not reliable during surgery for an ovarian tumor.[6] Malignant testicular tumors are generally pure yolk sac tumors in the infant and mixed tumors (yolk and choriocarcinoma) in the adolescent; frozen section histology can be useful in such cases.

Gonadal stromal tumors

Gonadal stromal tumors (sex cord tumors) are rare in children (5–10% of cases). They arise from stromal components and frequently produce hormones (estrogen or androgen) that may result in clinically apparent changes in the patient. According to the initial cell, two types are distinguished: the granulosa–theca cell tumors and the Sertoli–Leydig cell tumors (arrhenoblastoma). These tumors are usually benign. There is no correlation between hormonal production and potential malignancy.

Epithelial tumors

Epithelial tumors are specific for the ovary and account for 15% of gonadal tumors. They are characteristically benign (serous and mucinous cystadenoma) but are frequently bilateral and spread locally within the pelvis. Some are malignant (serous or mucinous adenocarcinoma). Epithelial ovarian tumors frequently cause elevation of serum levels CA-125 tumor antigen.

Gonadoblastoma

Gonadoblastoma contain both germ cells and stroma cells. They are not a true tumor but rather a pseudotumoral dysgenetic gonad, usually in association with an intersex disorder with a Y-chromosome or evidence of some Y-chromatin. Gonadoblastoma occurs in patients with mixed gonadal dysgenesis, pure gonadal dysgenesis, true hermaphroditism, Turner and Turner-like syndromes, WAGR syndrome, DRASH syndrome, and FRASER syndrome. Gonadoblastoma occur most frequently in post pubertal patients but may be seen in childhood. They are well encapsulated, slow-growing tumors; 40% are bilateral. They are usually asymptomatic but these dysgenetic gonads should be removed prophylactically in infancy or early childhood before malignant transformation occurs (10% to 50% risk).

The classification of ovarian and testicular tumors is summarized in Tables 56.2–56.4. Many of the late clinical sequelae of these tumors are related to their initial treatment and thus this will be briefly considered before discussing long-term outcomes.

Clinical presentation and initial management

Emergency presentations should be considered first, as they can be quite misleading and may compromise the long-term outcome, especially in cases of acute torsion or bleeding of a gonadal tumor. This is a rare presentation in boys but relatively frequent in girls (Table 56.1). In such cases, essential preoperative diagnostic studies should include a plain abdominal radiograph, ultrasound scan and blood samples for AFP and HCG.

Ovarian tumors

In a girl presenting with pelvic pain, an abdominal mass, precocious puberty or virilization, the possibility of an ovarian tumor should be considered.[7–15]

Table 56.2. Gonadal tumors

Gonadal tumors

Yolk sac → Germ cell

Urogenital crest → Mesenchymal cell

Coelomic epithelium → Epithelial cell

Primitive gonad

Dysplasia

Tumor

Primitive germ cell tumor

Marker AFP HCG LDH1

Endocrine stromal tumor

Hormonally active

Epithelial cell tumor

Marker CA 125

Gonadoblastoma

No marker

Table 56.3. Ovarian tumors

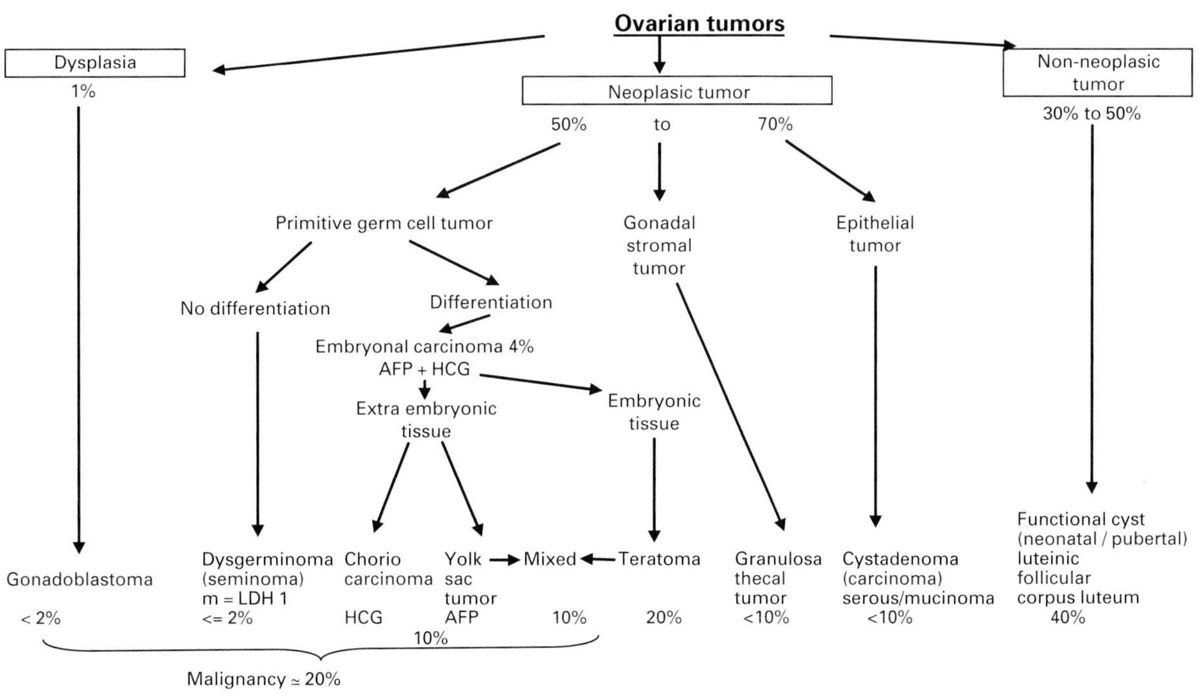

Table 56.4. Testicular tumors

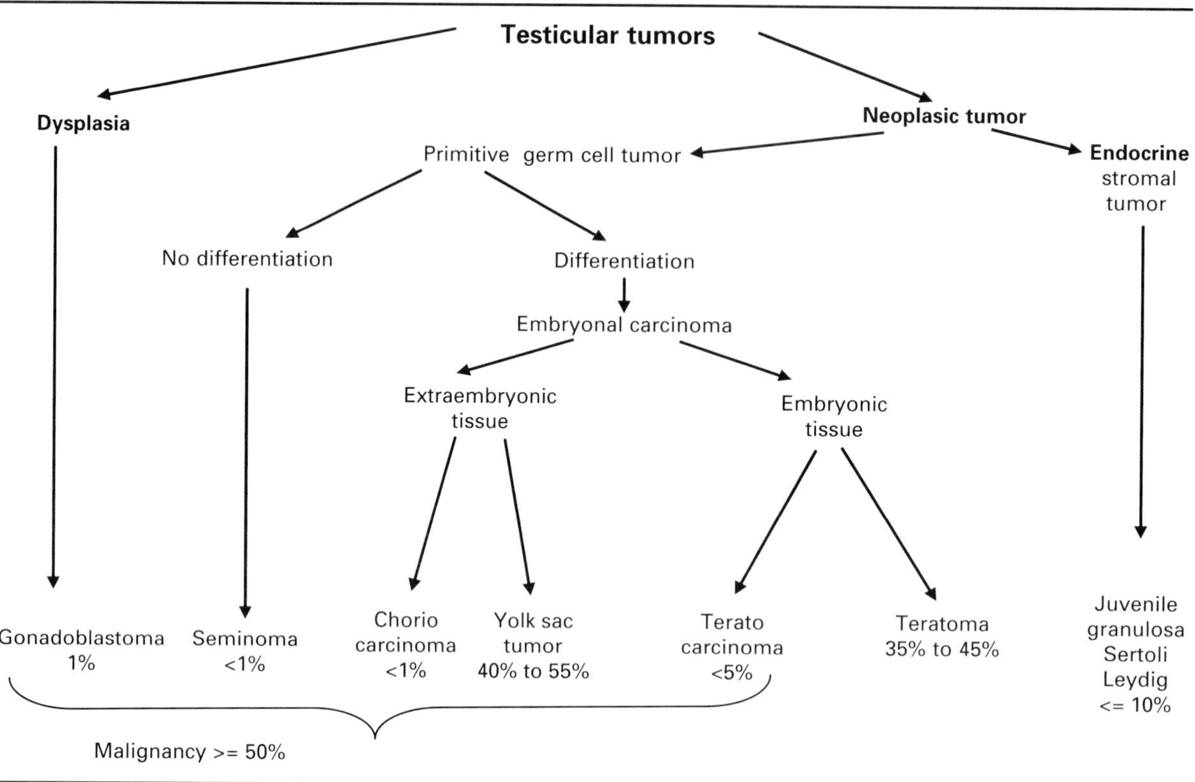

In most cases the benign nature of the tumor is obvious as in pure cystic lesions and in neonatal tumors.

(i) A benign or functional cyst (follicular cyst, corpus luteum cyst, simple cyst) may be discovered antenatally in the fetus during the last trimester of pregnancy, postnatally, or around puberty. They are much more frequently seen now that ultrasound scanning is readily available and they currently represent more than 50% of all ovarian cysts in children and adolescents. These benign cysts may regress spontaneously or may cause complications such as intracystic bleeding and adnexial torsion. Treatment depends on symptoms, the size of the cyst, and the age of the patient: options include simple surveillance, hormonal therapy, percutaneous drainage or surgical enucleation, preferably by laparoscopy.

(ii) Benign mature teratomas (including dermoid cysts, which represent a monophasic teratoma) usually have specific imaging characteristics and tumor markers are within normal limits. They can occur at any age. Classical treatment of children with a mature cystic teratoma includes oophorectomy via a Pfannenstiel incision because of concern about occult germ cell malignancy,[16] potential for recurrence after cystectomy, intraoperative rupture and spillage with the subsequent risk of chemical peritonitis, and adhesion formation. In recent years, following the experience of adult gynecologists,[20–25] laparoscopy has been used in the management of presumed benign ovarian masses in children.[17] Cystectomy can either be performed extraperitoneally after cyst puncture and withdrawal of the ovary outside the abdomen (a laparoscopic-assisted technique) or intraperitoneally using laparoscopic dissection techniques and extraction of the cyst within an endobag. If the cyst is inadvertently ruptured, the site must be irrigated with saline until the lavage is clear.[18] Spillage occurred in 11 cases in one series,[19] but no patient developed peritonitis or fever. Furthermore, this approach does not seem to add any additional risk of recurrence or adhesion formation.[17,18] In order to conserve ovarian tissue, enucleation is performed whenever possible. With a large tumor it may be impossible to preserve any normal ovarian tissue and an oophorectomy is then necessary, conserving the ipsilateral Fallopian tube.[11,17,26–28]

In rare cases, a malignant tumor may be suspected at presentation. For example, an adolescent girl may present with a large (>10 cm) rapidly growing solid tumor associated with elevated tumor markers, signs of local invasion, ascites or metastases. A high level of a tumor marker is sufficient for the diagnosis and is itself a prognostic factor. Usually, preoperative chemotherapy is needed. If the tumor marker level is normal, a laparoscopic or percutaneous biopsy is indicated in order to obtain a precise pathologic diagnosis. Current chemotherapy regimens are effective in treating these tumors. A second surgical evaluation after a complete radiological work-up (CT, MRI, ultrasound) may be needed to confirm complete response to chemotherapy alone. These second-look procedures can be performed via a Pfannenstiel incision (rather than a long midline laparotomy incision) if preceded by laparoscopy to inspect the superior part of the abdomen including the diaphragm.

In other situations, presenting features may be confusing. Ultrasound scans are good at identifying ovarian disorders but cannot reliably distinguish benign from malignant tumours. Solid ovarian masses on ultrasound are more likely to be malignant (30%–40% risk) compared to complex masses (10% risk) or pure cyst (3% risk). The situation may also be unclear when their tumour markers are within normal limits and there is no evidence of metastases since this does not rule out a malignant tumor, especially in prepubertal children. In the retrospective study from van Winter *et al.*[9] of 521 patients with adnexal masses in infancy, childhood or adolescence the frequency of ovarian malignancy was 8%, inversely correlated with patient age. During the last decade of their study, ultrasonography and computed tomography missed no malignancies.

The use of laparoscopy is controversial but can be useful as an initial step, especially in suspected torsion. However, the surgeon must keep in mind the recommendations of the Children's Oncology Group,[29] which stress that the staging used for pediatric ovarian tumors is postoperative (Table 56.5). The guidelines include:

- collection of ascites or peritoneal washings;
- examination of the peritoneal surfaces including the diaphragm with biopsy or excision of any nodules;
- inspection and palpation of the omentum with removal of any adherent or abnormal areas;
- inspection and palpation of the opposite ovary with biopsy of any abnormal areas;
- examination and palpation of lymph nodes in the retroperitoneum with sampling of any firm or enlarged nodes;

Table 56.5. Ovarian germ cell tumors, postsurgical classification

Stage I
– Limited to ovary (ovaries): no evidence of disease beyond the ovaries (except gliomatosis peritonei that did not result in up-staging)
– Peritoneal washings negative
– Tumor markers normal after appropriate half time decline (AFP 5 days, HCG 16 hours)
Stage II
(viii) Microscopic residual or positive lymph nodes (<= 2 cm)
(ix) Peritoneal washings negative
(xx) Tumor marker + or –
Stage III
(xi) Biopsy only or gross residual tumor
(xii) Lymph node involvement > 2 cm
(xiii) Continuous visceral involvement
(xiv) Peritoneal washings +
Stage IV
(xv) Distant metastasis

- complete resection of the tumor-containing ovary with sparing of the Fallopian tube if not involved.

Laparotomy is required for the last two recommendations. The risk of a simultaneous contralateral ovarian tumor varies between 5% and 20% according to the histologic type. Some have suggested a contralateral bivalving biopsy, although this procedure and wedge biopsy both have a risk of hemorrhage, infection, and adhesion formation. Ultrasound is a good predictor of a contralateral ovarian tumor. An intergroup study[29] demonstrated that, in 21 sonographically normal contralateral ovaries, the biopsy was always negative whereas, in 21 sonographically abnormal ovaries, the biopsy was positive in 50%. Hence, preoperative ultrasound and careful inspection of the contralateral ovary at the time of surgery is a safe alternative to systematic contralateral biopsy.

Laparoscopy plays an important role in tumor evaluation. A benign lesion is often cystic, well encapsulated, less than 8 cm in diameter, with a smooth regular surface, and without adhesions to pelvic organs. The laparoscopy is converted to open surgery if the tumor is large, although every effort is made to enucleate the lesion and to preserve normal ovarian parenchyma. A malignant lesion is more often solid with an irregular surface, a thick wall, surrounding adhesions and may be accompanied by ascites and peritoneal deposits. However, some benign teratomas (27% of immature teratomas in one study[30]) are associated with diffusely distributed benign glial tissue (gliomatosis peritonei), which do not require complete removal but only biopsies to confirm the diagnosis. As none of these criteria is absolute and as intraoperative frozen sections are not reliable, especially with large lesions, malignancy should always be suspected initially with ovarian tumors.[6]

Laparoscopy enables the resectability of the tumor to be defined. If it is not resectable (fixed or extensive), a simple laparoscopic biopsy is performed. If it appears to be resectable, a salpingo-phorectomy is usually performed using a classical open approach. Extensive surgery such as bilateral oophorectomy or hysterectomy should not be performed before histologic confirmation. The question of using laparoscopy to remove a resectable suspicious ovarian lesion is still under debate. With accurate preoperative and intraoperative selection, the rate of unexpected malignancy in the large adult series reported by Marana *et al.*[20] was 1.2% and laparoscopic management of these adnexal masses did not adversely impact on prognosis. In another study[31] the risk of unexpected malignancy was 19% but factors predictive of malignancy in adults[32] cannot be directly extrapolated to children. The concept that violating the tumor capsule by laparoscopy or rupturing the tumor intraoperatively results in upstaging of malignant lesions remains valid. The capsule may be ruptured preoperatively or intraoperatively, either accidentally or deliberately during puncture or biopsy. As demonstrated by Templeman *et al.*,[17] the risk of intraoperative rupture is higher with laparoscopy (93% vs. 37%) and in patients managed by cystectomy rather than oophorectomy (92% vs. 15%). In the prospective randomized study reported by Yuen *et al.*[25] in adults the risk of inadvertent rupture was the same with laparotomy or laparoscopy. Billmire *et al.*[29] concluded that the surgeon's assessment of the integrity of the capsule is frequently underestimated and that the survival rate was excellent in girls treated by tumorectomy or initial biopsy and delayed resection. The multicenter study by Cushing *et al.*[30] showed that the presence of capsular rupture had no negative impact on survival in patients presenting with an immature teratoma ± microscopic foci of yolk sac tumor and treated by surgery alone. In summary, the survival rate in recent publications is not affected by deviating from classical clinical surgical guidelines[18] so long as decisions are individualized.

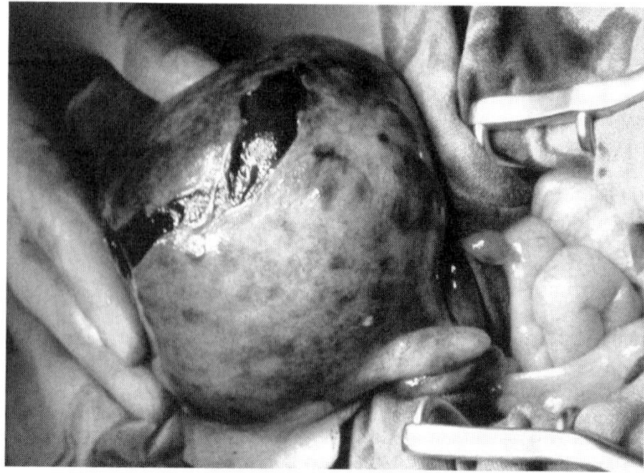

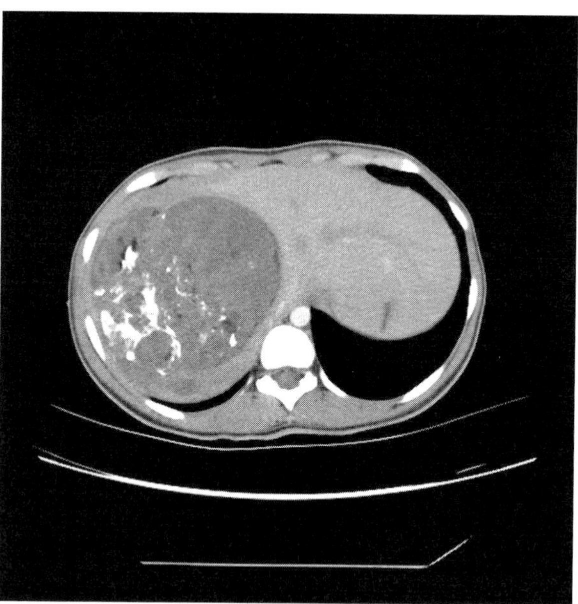

Fig. 56.1. Acute abdomen in a 12-year-old girl. Ultrasound: left heterogeneous ovarian mass 11 × 13 cm. AFP: 123 mg/ml (*N*<10). Photo 1: Pfannenstiel incision in emergency: the torsed tumor is ruptured. Adenexectomy. No preoperative sign of malignancy. Histology: immature teratoma. The patient is lost to follow-up. 27 months later, new hospitalization for right subcostal pain: abdominal X-ray: numerous calcifications in the right liver lobe. AFP: 69400 (see colour plate section). Photo 2: MRI: large hepatic metastasics. There are also numerous enlarged retroperitoneal lymph nodes. After five cures of chemotherapy (cysplastinium ifosfamide, etoposide) the AFP level returns to normal but the hepatic mass remains large (16 cm in diameter). Right hepatectomy. Histology: mature teratoma, other samplings (ascite, lymph node, right ovary): normal. No relapse after 15 years of follow-up. This girl is now the mother of two normal children.

Management of adnexal torsion

One third of ovarian masses are discovered because of torsion and nearly three-quarters of twisted ovaries contain an underlying cystic or solid mass.[33] Preoperative ultrasonography is a poor discriminant of simple ovarian torsion and torsion of an ovarian mass. Similarly, operative findings can be misleading.[3,4] Classical management of ovarian torsion consists of resecting the twisted adnexa to avoid

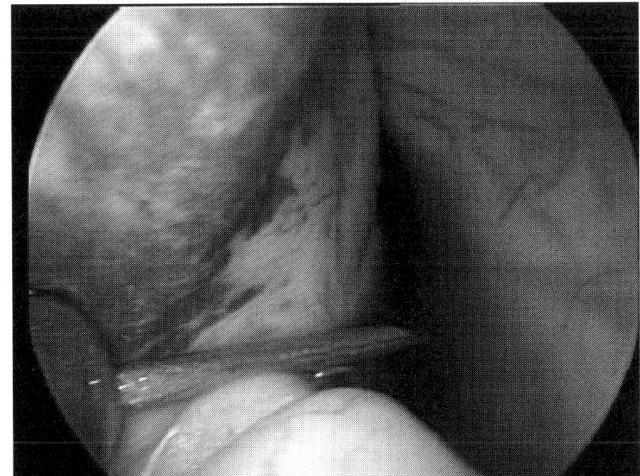

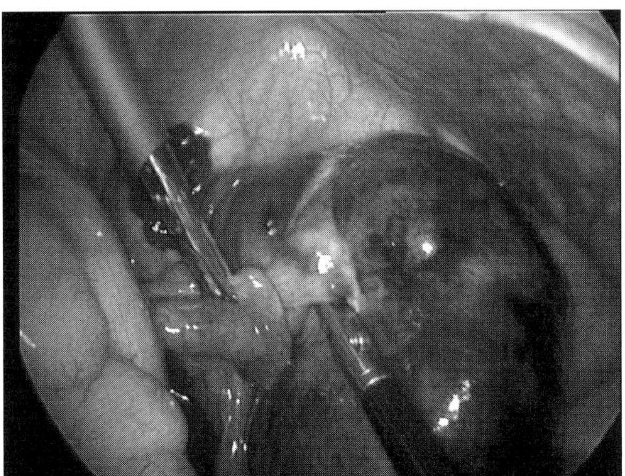

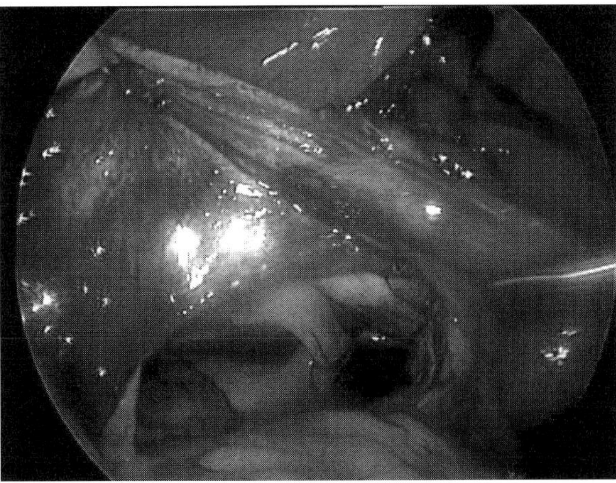

Fig. 56.2. Illustration of new management of adnexal torsion. Acute abdomen in a 13-year-old girl. Ultrasound: torsion of the right adnexa with a 10 cm heterogeneous mass. Marker level: normal: laparoscopy in emergency: view at the beginning. Photo 1: total abdominal exploration (negative in this case) and aspiration of peritoneal ascite in the cul de sac de Douglas (negative cytology). Photo 2: laparoscopic untorsion: after (*cont.*) untorsion the ovarian aspect is much better, allowing immediate laparoscopic cystectomy. Photo 3: cystectomy by stripping technique after puncture of the cyst: extraction in a bag: oophoropexy of the ipsilateral ovary: histology: mucinous cystadenoma (see colour plate section).

the risk of malignant spread on detorsion[2] and to allow complete removal of potential tumor or necrotic ovarian tissue.[3] The theoretical risk of pulmonary embolism has not been reported in children.[35] Solid and cystic ovarian masses have an overall risk of malignancy of around 10% to 20%, whereas only 3% of ovarian torsions contain a malignant tumor (see Fig. 56.1). There were no cases of malignancy in 34 ovarian torsions in several pediatric series.[8,33,35,36] Sommerville *et al.*[37] reported that a benign ovarian neoplasm had a 13-fold increased risk of undergoing adnexal torsion when compared to a malignant neoplasm. All in all, adnexal torsion rarely involves an underlying cancer. One explanation for this is that malignant lesions may cause more inflammation and fibrosis leading to surrounding adhesions. The belief that a grossly black hemorrhagic adnexa is irreversibly damaged is not true: the degree of ischemia is difficult to judge by the surgeon and the time lapse from onset of symptoms to surgery is not a good guide to viability of the ovary. An ovary can be viable despite the absence of arterial or venous blood flow on preoperative Doppler ultrasound scan.[36,38] After detorsion, the most common postoperative symptom is fever. In the longer term, ovarian viability after untwisting, as assessed by ultrasound scan (size of the ovary, presence of follicles), has often been normal in cases reported in the literature.[35,36,39]

Considering the low rate of malignancy, difficulty of assessing ovarian viability and knowing the efficacy of chemotherapy for malignant tumors, treatment recommendations for adnexal torsion have changed. Detorsion is the first step. This may be followed by removal of the cyst if there is prompt recovery of blood flow (see Fig. 56.2) but, in most cases, excision of the cyst may damage the ovary because the tissues are friable and edematous and detorsion alone is preferable. Subsequently, patients with a cystic mass and normal AFP levels should undergo elective ovarian cystectomy 6 to 8 weeks later. Those with a high serum AFP level should be managed by oophrectomy $\pm$ chemotherapy.

The role of oophoropexy is unclear.[40] Fixing the ovaries may prevent recurrent torsion of the same ovary and subsequent torsion of the contralateral ovary. Different techniques of fixation (lateral or medial) have been described.

Table 56.6. Management algorithm for prepubertal ovarian tumors

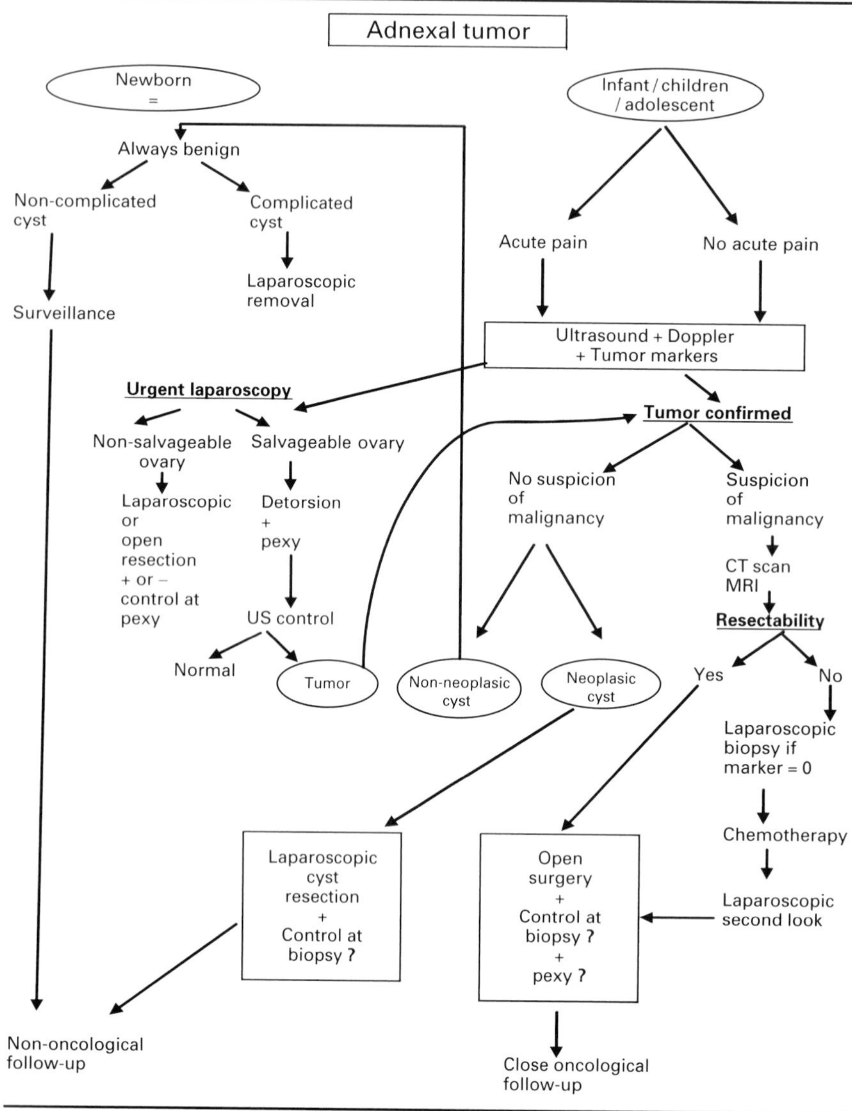

However, oophoropexy may disturb the normal arrangement between the ovary and the Fallopian tube and the morbidity of these procedures has not been clearly reported.[35,36,40,41] Therefore, the author recommends fixing the ipsilateral gonad in cases of ovarian sparing surgery and fixing the contralateral gonad after gonadectomy.

Bilateral synchronous ovarian tumors

The incidence is between 4% and 9%.[8,29] Most are benign and can be treated by gonadal sparing surgery. If there is doubt about possible bilateral malignancy, bilateral biopsies should be performed[42] and not bilateral oophrorectomy.

In summary, for a girl with an ovarian mass and normal tumor markers, the pediatric surgeon should attempt to preserve the ovary by resection of the tumor alone, unless there are obvious signs of cancer. On the rare occasion when the pathologist reports a malignant tumor, three possible options should be considered with the oncologist: close observation, reoperation for surgical staging with or without oophorectomy, and/or chemotherapy (Table 56.6). Late sequelae of these treatments are uncommon.[29]

Testicular tumors

Testicular tumors typically present with a testicular mass, which may be noted by the patient himself or detected during a routine examination. Occasionally, a hydrocele is found and may delay the diagnosis. Alternatively, the patient may present with an acute scrotum from bleeding or torsion or, more rarely, with precocious puberty or gynecomastia. Scrotal ultrasonography should be considered for any boy with a hydrocele and an impalpable testis, or with atypical torsion, or with virilization and no obvious cause.

Blood samples should be taken for tumor markers before any surgery, including emergency cases. Since pediatric testicular tumors are often benign (50% in the French multicenter study,[49]) preoperative evaluation plays a significant role in selecting patients for testis sparing surgery.[50]

Suspected malignancy

In a child over 1 year of age with high AFP levels or diffuse involvement of the testis on ultrasonography, the standard approach is an inguinal orchidectomy.[43–45] After isolating and softly clamping the spermatic cord, the testis is delivered. Once a testicular tumor has been confirmed, the cord is ligated and divided at the internal inguinal ring. The contralateral testis is examined and fixed.[46] If the tumor was biopsied through the scrotum before referral or extracted through the scrotum because of suspected torsion, a hemiscrotal excision is advisable[47,48] because of the risk of tumor seeding. Additional treatments depend on the histology and stage of the primary tumor and tumor markers (Table 56.7).

Suspected benign tumor

This is more likely in the following situations: the neonatal period; when the tumor manifests as an endocrine disorder; and with a micro/multicystic lesion associated with homolateral renal agenesis (highly suggestive of cystic dysplasia of the rete testis).[49,50] In a boy under 6 months of age, sonographic features of a benign cystic tumor are a well-circumscribed, avascular, unilocular lesion with anechoic content. Ultrasound characteristics of an epidermoid cyst include a hypoechoïc mass with a well-defined outline or echogenic rim and an echogenic center caused by multiple acoustic reflections from the keratinous debris. A teratoma has a sonolucent cystic area with intermixed solid portions and is always benign if found before puberty (see Fig. 56.3). These findings, especially if associated with a history of a long-standing, stable lump, allow the surgeon to consider enucleation,[51] which can be performed through an inguinoscrotal incision assisted by frozen section histology.[52] The reliability of frozen section histology is good.[49,53] Whether or not biopsies of surrounding testicular tissue are necessary is debatable. Although the majority of adult testes removed for teratoma contain areas of intratubular germ cell neoplasia, this has not been demonstrated in children and therefore it seems unnecessary to remove adjacent testicular parenchyma in prepubertal teratoma.[49]

Postoperative management, short-term follow-up, and prognosis

Benign tumors

After removal of a benign tumor, the risk of ipsilateral recurrence after enucleation and the risk of developing a contralateral tumor highlight the need for regular gonadal check-ups through puberty and beyond.

Ipsilateral gonadal surveillance

Recurrence of a functional non-neoplastic cyst in an adolescent girl is uncommon. Serial ultrasound scans at various points in the menstrual cycle are recommended. Medical treatment with an antigonadotrophin hormone is indicated for patients with pain and/or a large cyst (> 5 cm). Laparoscopic removal is indicated for acute complications, especially torsion.

With benign tumors, the risk of ipsilateral local recurrence after simple enucleation varies. For mature or immature teratoma (testis and ovary) the recurrence risk in an adult is between 0%[21] and 4%.[54] No cases have been reported in children[8,17] but this may be due to limited follow-up. Long-term follow-up without recurrence after gonadal sparing surgery for a stromal tumor in a boy has been documented.[56] In contrast, a recent report of a large cohort of young women indicated that those with an ovarian cyst have an increased risk of developing ovarian cancer later in life.[57]

Contralateral gonadal surveillance

The risk of subsequently developing a contralateral gonadal tumor is significant (between 5% and 15%). For example, 2 of 44 cases of immature teratoma[30] and 8 of 91 cases in another series.[7] In this latter study, the risk was higher after a malignant tumor (4/19 (21%) cases) than a benign tumor (4/72 (5%) cases). Moreover, it is widely known that women who have undergone excision of one ovary often develop functional cyst(s) in the preserved ovary. The association

Table 56.7. Classification for testicular tumors

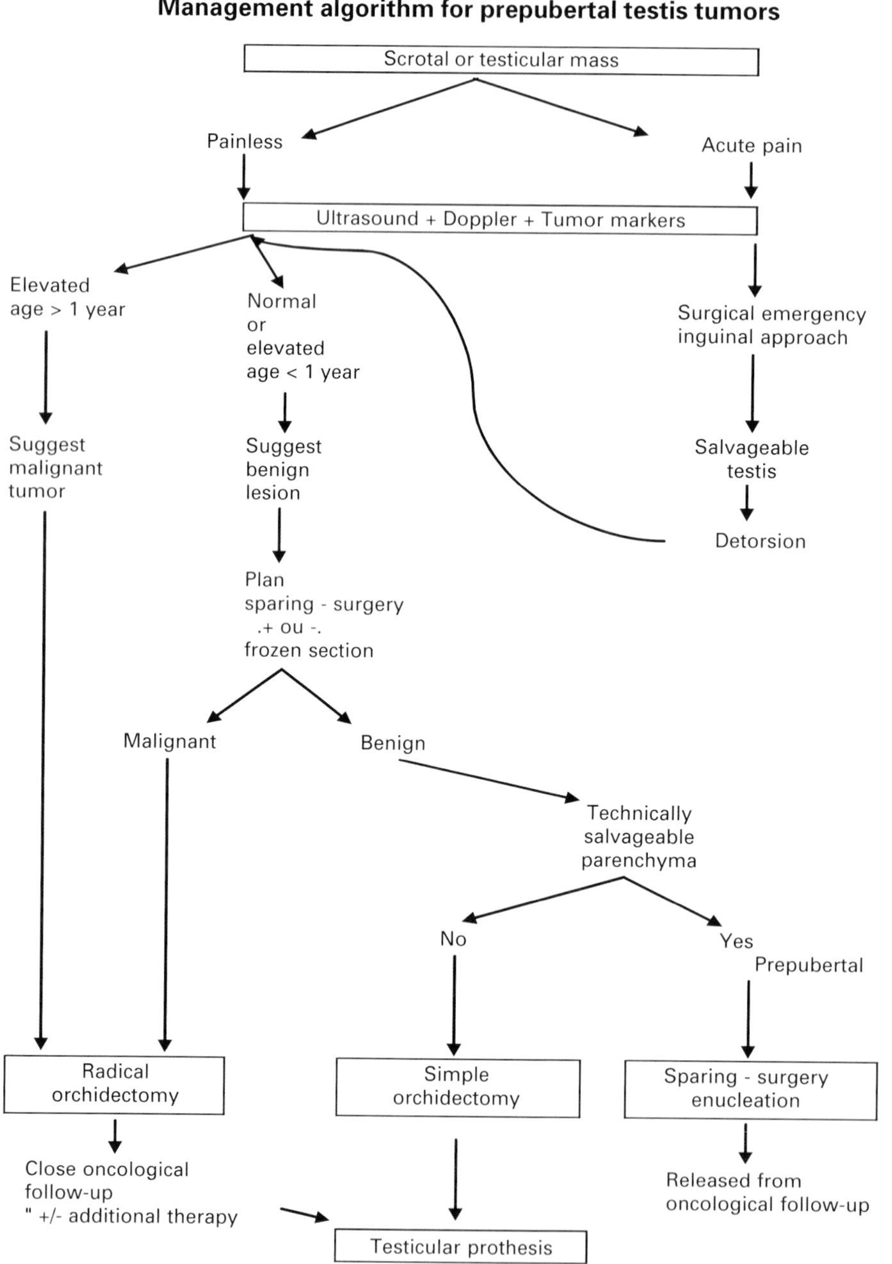

Stage I

(xvi) Limited to testis (normal chest radiograph, normal abdominal CT)

Stage II

(xvii) Confined to testis and retroperitoneal abdominal lymph nodes.

Stage III

(xviii) Supradiaphragmatic nodal disease.

Stage III

(xix) Metastasis

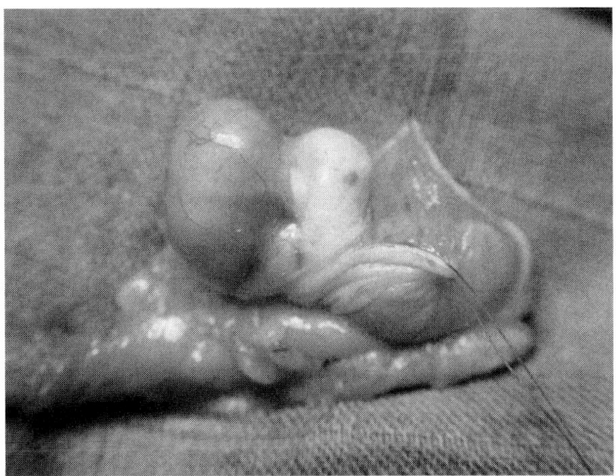

Fig. 56.3. Boy, 6 years old, well-delimited, heterogeneous tumor of the left testis. Tumoral marker at normal level: X-ray showing calcifications: ultrasound heterogeneous aspect. Photo: perioperative view: the cord is clamped; frozen section: mature teratoma. Enucleation with conservative surgery of the testis: microscopic aspect of mature teratoma. Follow-up 8 years. No recurrence.

between a dermoïd ovarian cyst and the future development of a malignant germ cell tumor has been suggested in adult women[42,55] especially in those with bilateral or multiple dermoid cysts, in whom closer surveillance may be advisable.

Another risk in boys with a solitary testis is the possibility of traumatic injury; although contact sport should be permitted, extra protection is recommended.[58]

There is no consensus on follow-up. Testes can be checked by palpation and regular ultrasound scans, ovaries only by ultrasound scan. Annual review seems advisable.

Malignant tumors

Prior to the introduction of chemotherapy in 1975, the mortality from malignant germ cell tumors was close to 100%. A major advance in treatment was the use of platinum-based drugs at the end of the 1970s. Today, the high survival rate with conservative surgery is related to effective chemotherapeutic agents: cisplatin, etoposide, and bleomycin. Previous recommendations for extensive surgical resection of reproductive organs and radical lymph node resection have been successfully abandoned without compromising outcome.[1–3] Today, the survival rate for children with a malignant gonadal tumor is excellent (5% mortality). However, prognosis varies according to tumor stage, tumor marker levels, and histologic findings.

Staging

Accurate staging is mandatory to avoid under or over treatment. In boys, staging relies on appropriate CT imaging. Some patients with lymph nodes between 1 and 2 cm in diameter (stage I) are in fact stage II because these lymph nodes are diseased. However, for stage II patients (with lymph nodes up to 2 cm) the value of chemotherapy is debatable.[45,50] For girls, accurate staging relies on surgery; detailed assessment at the initial laparotomy or laparoscopy is essential. If preoperative staging is insufficient, a laparoscopic second look procedure can be useful. The prognostic value of germ cell tumor staging is less important today as the survival rate is high for all stages. With improved diagnosis, early stage tumors are far more common than before (60%–75%[59,61] compared to 40%–50%[8] historically).

Alphafetoprotein

The initial level of serum AFP is prognostically important. In one retrospective study of 69 children and adults with non-dysgerminomatous ovarian germ cell tumors, an AFP level of 1000 ku/l was associated with a significant higher risk of relapse.[62] In another study, most treatment failures occurred in patients with a very high initial AFP concentration (>15 000 mg/ml).[64]

Malignant ovarian tumors

Malignant non-seminomatous germ cell tumors are treated using different protocols in Europe and the USA. In Europe (SIOP protocol TGM 55 and TGM 90), these tumors are divided into two categories:[1]

- Secreting tumors: if the tumor is localized and has been completely removed (stage I and II) no further therapy is needed. Follow-up includes measurement of serum markers every 2 weeks for 3 months, then monthly for 2 years. An abdominal CT scan is required every 3 months during the first year. Marker levels must return to normal within 3 months of surgery. Chemotherapy is indicated if marker levels remain high or increase again after normalization. Marker levels are the most sensitive index of recurrent tumor. With extensive or incompletely resected tumors (stage III and IV), chemotherapy is mandatory and a surgical second look is recommended. Secreting gonadal germ cell tumors have a much better response to treatment and survival than germ cell tumors arising at other sites.[64] Whatever the stage, the 6-year survival rate in recent series is up to 93%.[29] Choriocarcinomas are less responsive to chemotherapy than other germ cell tumors.
- Non-secreting tumors are rare and usually heterogeneous, e.g., immature teratoma with some foci of yolk

sac tumor. Surgical resection is the primary treatment. Chemotherapy, if needed, is less effective.

In a multicenter study from the USA,[30] secreting and non-secreting ovarian immature teratomas were not considered separately. In this series of 44 cases, the authors concluded that surgery alone was curative for most children and adolescents with tumors of any grade, even when initial AFP levels were elevated or if microscopic foci of yolk sac tumor were present. Capsular rupture, gliomatosis peritonei, or ascites did not have a negative impact on survival. Postoperative chemotherapy was reserved for patients with relapse (only one case in this study). During follow-up, chest radiographs provided no benefit since no metastatic disease was identified.

Most epithelial ovarian tumors in children are benign cystadenoma.[65] Very few are invasive carcinomas which tend to have a poor prognosis when diagnosed at an advanced stage.[65–67] These patients are managed by debulking surgery and triple drug chemotherapy. Intraperitoneal chemotherapy has been used in some cases. The number of pediatric epithelial tumors with borderline malignancy in the literature is too small to formalize treatment and prognosis guidelines. The value of postoperative CA 125 monitoring is debatable.

Pure dysgerminomas spread to retroperitoneal lymph nodes at an early stage. If the tumor is localized, surgery alone is required followed by close clinical and ultrasound surveillance. If there is tumor extension, chemotherapy is preferred to radiotherapy, since this is more likely to preserve fertility even though dysgerminomas are highly radiosensitive.[68] Survival rate is around 100%. These tumors are very rare and the optimal chemotherapy regimen remains unknown. In order to reduce pulmonary damage, several protocols avoid bleomycin.

Gonadal stromal tumors in girls are usually localized granulosa–theca cell tumors. These grow slowly and usually have a favorable outcome. They are treated by conservative surgery alone even after capsular rupture. Precocious puberty and age under 10 years are good prognostic factors. In extensive tumors, the chemotherapy used for germ cell tumors may be effective.

Malignant testicular tumors

Yolk sac tumors, after radical orchidectomy patients with a secreting tumors are closely monitored by serial AFP measurements. With localized tumors (stage I) the relapse rate is 10%–20% during the first 2 years. Patients with scrotal involvement have a significantly higher rate of recurrent disease. All these cases can be treated with chemotherapy.[48] A normal AFP level after 2 years signifies cure but oncologic follow-up must be continued for 5 years. Patients with stage III and IV disease should be treated with platinum-based chemotherapy.[43] Retroperitoneal lymph node dissection carries a significant morbidity (e.g., chylous ascites, failure to ejaculate) even if performed laparoscopically and using a limited unilateral nerve-sparing dissection. Retroperitoneal lymph node dissection has no routine place in the treatment of boys with yolk sac tumor of the testis.[69] It should be reserved for patients with recurrent or persistent retroperitoneal masses following chemotherapy.[50] Chemotherapy should also be considered in patients with a non-secreting tumour in whom early recurrence may be difficult to detect, and in patients with a persistently elevated AFP but normal body CT scan after orchidectomy.[45] The overall survival rate for boys with testicular yolk sac tumor approaches 95% with most deaths occurring within 30 months of presentation. This survival rate is largely due to the high proportion of patients presenting with stage I disease.

Teratomas are cured by surgery alone.[49,70] No relapse has been reported after gonadal sparing surgery but late metastasis has been described in adults. Gonadal stromal testicular tumors are cured by surgery alone but gynecomastia or androgenic changes do not always regress. Aggressive treatment of undifferentiated metastatic stromal tumors is recommended. Table 56.7 shows an algorithm for the surgical management of prepubertal testicular tumors.

Long-term follow-up

Gonadal function

Before puberty, detection of functional gonadal impairment is rarely possible. In girls, normal regular menstrual cycles are likely to be associated with fertility, but not always. Subtle damage may be harder to detect and may present later as infertility and premature menopause. In postpubertal boys, semen analysis is an unreliable method of determining the ability to father a child. Even with abnormal sperm counts, fertility is possible. There are no large series reporting the natural fertility rate of patients operated for benign or malignant gonadal tumors in childhood or early adolescence, although there are many publications in the adult literature focusing on this topic.[61,71–78]

After tumor enucleation without gonadectomy, gonadal function is normal. In one long-term follow-up study of 87 women, conservational ovarian surgery had no significant effect on ovulatory and menstrual function.[79]

After unilateral gonadectomy without chemotherapy, gonadal function is slightly impaired in both sexes. The functional and anatomic contralateral hypertrophy seen in animals has not been demonstrated in humans. Whatever the etiology (torsion, undescended testis, tumor) the fertility of men with a solitary healthy testis is comparable to the normal population.[80,81] What about the fertility of women with a single ovary? Infertility clinic observations indicate that women with a single gonad are more prone to infertility than controls (a 17% increased rate of infertility).[82] However, it is reported that patients who have had an oophorectomy have the same pregnancy rate as the general population. Women with a single ovary have no compensatory mechanism, as the number of primordial follicules is already fixed. The risk of early menopause in this group is debatable.

After unilateral gonadectomy followed by chemotherapy, the effect on future fertility is poorly defined. Chemotherapy has immediate and late adverse effects depending on the type and combination of agents, their dose and frequency. Agents used for germ cell tumors (cisplastin, etoposide, bleomycin) have little effect on gonadal function. For boys, four cycles of cisplatin, vinblastine and bleomycin result in irreversible testicular toxicity in fewer than 20% of cases.[87] Many studies have reported fertility rates after treatment of testicular cancer in adults, including large multicenter studies[73] and case reports.[83–85] If preserving reproductive function is absolutely imperative, some patients may opt for chemotherapy alone leaving the primary tumor in situ; this helps to maintain fertility and no tumor recurrences have thus far been reported.[83,85] The impact of chemotherapy on the adult ovary is similarly low. There are conflicting data regarding the effect of cisplatin on menstruation.[72] Amenorrhea lasting between 2 and 12 months was reported by the majority of patients, although ovulatory cycles were always restored.[74] In many studies, the fertility of women treated by postoperative chemotherapy is not different to that of women who did not require such treatment[61]; this applies to all types of tumor.[60,72,77,78,90] The rate of documented infertility is approximately 10% which matches the rate in the general population.[60]

The impact of chemotherapy also depends on age and sex. Boys are generally thought to be more at risk of infertility than girls. Prepubertal spermatogonia are "at rest" and thus the prepubertal testis is in a "protected state."[89] Similarly, the prepubertal ovary is more resistant to chemotherapy than the active postpubertal ovary, probably because of the large reserve of oocytes. One option in pubertal adolescents is to suppress the hypothalamic–pituitary–gonadal axis with gonadotropin releasing hormone in order to render the gonad quiescent and decrease its germ cell vulnerability to therapy.[4,90] It is unclear whether the use of oral contraceptives during chemotherapy in postmenarchal girls has a protective effect on ovarian function.[61]

Female infertility could also be a consequence of adhesion formation. Laparoscopic surgery induces less adhesions than open surgery. Non-repair of the ovary after cystectomy and/or cystic rupture have been cited as causes of postoperative adhesions. Although no data are available on routine second-look laparoscopy to assess adhesions after laparoscopy, fertility after laparoscopic surgery in women appears to be normal even if the ovary is left open after cystectomy.[23,71,79]

The effect of chemotherapy on the frequency of congenital anomalies in subsequent offspring is debatable. Apart from one report in which four fetuses out of 55 pregnancies were malformed,[61] the literature does not suggest an increased risk of congenital malformations.[72,74]

Assisted reproduction techniques

There are very few clinical situations with pediatric gonadal tumors where infertility is inevitable. Although most patients and their families are prepared to sacrifice fertility, they should be fully informed of the adverse effects of the various treatments including the risk of conservative therapies. Only after fully informed consent can a consensual decision be taken. Assisted reproduction techniques include a wide range of interventions.[81] The simplest is intrauterine insemination (IUI). It is important to spare the uterus for future pregnancy using IUI and donor oocytes in cases of bilateral oophorectomy. The greatest hope, especially for male infertility, comes from a new complex micromanipulation technique in which a single sperm is injected directly into the egg (intracytoplasmic sperm injection [ICSI]). The question is how to obtain and store spermatozoa and/or ova.

The only established option in current clinical practice for preserving male fertility is cryopreservation of spermatozoa in postpubertal adolescents. Sperm can be stored for many years and still retain their viability for ICSI. However, in prepubertal boys the use of sperm precursors is more controversial because of poor results and ethical considerations.[89] The storage of mature ova is not possible at present. To date, attempts to preserve oocytes from unstimulated prepubertal ovaries for future fertilization are more promising. Ovarian preservation in premenarchal girls involves freezing immature oocytes, specifically primordial follicles, which are less vulnerable to the toxic effects of cryopreservation.[90,91] In children with cancer in whom treatment is likely to produce sterility, it is now possible to store germinal tissue to restore fertility either by germ cell transplantation or by in vitro maturation of the harvested germ cell. Grafting the tissue back into the patient seems more physiological, although there is a theoretical risk that malignant cells could also be transferred. An alternative solution is in vitro maturation and ICSI.[92] When and where should germinal tissue be harvested? Because of the risk of subsequent contralateral disease, the best solution might be to take a large biopsy of the contralateral gonad at the time of first surgery. These techniques remain experimental and are only available in a few centers. Ethical aspects are unresolved and standards for best practice in cryopreservation of gonadal tissue in children remain to be defined. Each case selected for gonadal tissue cryopreservation should be the subject of a multidisciplinary discussion. The issue of the effects of ICSI on rates of birth defects requires large long-term studies.

Psychosocial sequelae

There are very few studies that have been conducted to evaluate long-term psychosocial effects of gonadal cancer and its curative treatment during childhood and adolescence.[2] Although the impact of infertility is not easily demonstrated as a parameter of well-being, it is known that women who undergo evaluation and treatment for infertility often experience anger, high levels of anxiety and depression, lowered self-esteem, poor body image, and problems with sexual identity and function.[61] For men, even if 50% are fertile, they still have to cope with changes in body image produced by "disfiguring surgery," a potential source of great concern for an adolescent.[2] Although a testicular prosthesis can improve cosmesis, it is impossible to predict the emotional effect of loss of a testicle on a man. Psychological support should be offered, particularly around puberty.

Secondary malignancies

Second malignancies, particularly leukemia, have been reported in survivors of testicular cancer and ovarian germ cell tumor.

Conclusions

Cure without loss of function should represent the ideal goal for each patient and his/her physician. Surgery continues to play a crucial role in the treatment of gonadal tumors. Benign tumors require only conservative surgery. For ovarian tumors, this represents an excellent indication for laparoscopic surgery. This reduces the morbidity of traditional surgery, especially pain, scarring and peritoneal adhesions. For malignant tumors, the aim of current treatments is to improve survival rates whilst minimizing treatment-induced adverse effects. This goal can only be achieved by close collaboration between pediatric surgeons, oncologists, adult gynecologists, biologists, psychologists, and radiologists. Future progress lies in an improved understanding of tumor biology, better staging of high-risk patients, greater use of laparoscopic techniques, reducing chemotherapy or choosing less gonadotoxic regimens, and improving assisted reproduction techniques. Treatments should be tailored to each individual.

REFERENCES

1. Martelli, H. & Patte, C. Gonadal tumors in children. *Arch. Pédiatr.* 2003; **10**:246–250 (French).
2. Rieker, P. P., Edbrils, D., & Garnick, M. B. Curative testis cancer therapy: psychosocial sequelae. *J. Clin. Oncol.* 1985; **3**:1117–1126
3. Sklar, C. A. & Laquaglia, M. P. The long-term complications of chemotherapy in childhood genitourinary tumors. *Urol. Clin. North Am.* 2000; **27**:563–568.
4. Wallace, W. H. & Thomson, A. B. Preservation of fertility in children treated for cancer. *Arch. Dis. Child.* 2003; **88**:493–496.
5. Lahdenne, P. Late sequelae of gonadal, mediastinal and oral teratoma in childhood. *Acta Paediatr.* 1992; **81**:235–238.
6. Einarsson, J. I., Edwards, C. L., & Zurawin, R. K. Immature ovarian teratoma in adolescent in a case report and review of the litterature. *J. Paediatr. Adolesc. Gynecol.* 2004; **17**:187–189.
7. Brown, M. F., Hebra, A., McGeehin, K., & Ross, A. J. Ovarian masses in children: a review of 91 cases of malignant and benign masses. *J. Pediatr. Surg.* 1993; **28**:930–932.
8. Cass, D. L., Hawkin, S. E., & Brandt, M. L. Surgery for ovarian masses in infants, children and adolescents: 102 consecutives patients treated in a 15 year period. *J. Pediatr. Surg.* 2001; **36**:693–699.
9. van Winter, J. T., Simmons, P. S., & Podratz, K. C. Surgically treated adnexal masses in infancy, childhood and adolescence. *Am J. Obstet. Gynecol.* 1994; **170**:1786–1789.
10. Quint, E. H. & Smith, Y. R. Ovarian surgery in premenarchial girls. *J. Pediatr. Adolesc. Gynecol.* 1999; **12**:27–30.
11. Templeman, C., Fallat, M. E., & Blinchevsky, A. Non-inflammatory ovarian masses in girls and young women. *Obstet. Gynecol.* 2000; **96**:229–233.
12. Lopez Saiz, A., Fernandez, M. S., & Segarra, V. *et al.* Solid ovarian tumors in childhood. *Cir. Pediatr.* 1997; **10**:104–107.
13. Piippo, S., Mustaniemi, L., & Lenko, H. *et al.* Surgery for ovarian masses during childhood and adolescence: a report of 79 cases. *J. Pediatr. Adolesc. Gynecol.* 1999; **12**:223–227.
14. Freud, E., Golinsky, D., Steinberg, R. M. *et al.* Ovarian masses in children. *Clin. Pediatr.* 1999; **38**:573–577.

15. Imai, A., Furui, T., & Tamaya, T. Gyneocologic tumors and symptoms in childhood and adolescence: 10 years experience. *Int. J. Gynecol. Obstet.* 1994; **45**:227–234.
16. Mayer, C., Miller, D. M., & Ehlen, T. G. Peritoneal implantation of squamous cell carcinoma following rupture of a dermoïd cyst during laparoscopic removal. *Gynecol. Oncol.* 2002; **84**:180–183.
17. Templeman, C., Hertwaeck, S. P., Scheetz, J. *et al.* The management of mature cystic teratomas in children and adolescents: a retrospective analysis. *Hum. Reprod.* 2000; **15**:2669–2672.
18. Zanetta, G., Ferrari, L., Mignini-Renzini, M. *et al.* Laparoscopic excision of ovarian dermoïd cyst with controlled intraoperative spillage. *J. Reprod. Med.* 1999; **44**:815–820.
19. Shalev, E., Bustan, M., Romano, S. *et al.* Laparoscopic resection of ovarian benign cystic teratomas: experience with 84 cases. *Hum. Reprod.* 1998; **13**:1810–1812.
20. Marana, R., Muzii, L., Catalano, G. F. *et al.* Laparoscopic excision of adnexal masses. *J. Am. Assoc. Gynecol. Laparosc.* 2004; **11**:162–166.
21. Beiner, M. E., Gotlieb, W. H., Korach, Y. *et al.* Cystectomy for immature teratoma of the ovary. *Gynecol. Oncol.* 2004; **93**:381–384.
22. Howard, F. M. Surgical management of benign cystic teratoma. Laparoscopy us laparotomy. *J. Reprod. Med.* 1995; **40**:495–499.
23. Canis, M., Rabischong, B., Houlle, C. *et al.* Laparoscopic management of adnexal masses: a gold standard? *Curr. Opin Obstet. Gynecol.* 2002; **14**:432–438.
24. Nezhat, C. R., Kalyoncu, S., Nezhat, C. H. *et al.* Laparoscopic management of ovarian dermoid cyst: ten years'experience. *J. Laparoendosc. Surg.* 1999; **3**:179–184.
25. Yuen, P. M., Yu, K. M., Lau, W. C. *et al.* A randomized prospective study of laparoscopy and laparotomy in the management of benign ovarian masses. *Am. J. Obstet. Gynecol.* 1997; **177**:109–114.
26. Lee, K. H., Yeung, C. K., Tam, Y. H. *et al.* The use of laparoscopy in the management of adnexal pathology in children. *Aust. NZ. J. Surg.* 2000; **70**:192–195.
27. Jawad, A. J. & Al Meshari, A. Laparoscopy for ovarian pathologic in infancy and childhood. *Pediatr. Surg. Int.* 1998; **14**:62–65.
28. Nirasawa, Y. & Ito, Y. Reproduction preserving technique for benign cystic teratoma of the ovary. *Pediatr. Surg. Int.* 1995; **10**:126–128.
29. Billmire, D., Vinocur, C., Rescorla, F. *et al.* Outcome and staging evolution in malignant germ cell tumors of the ovary in children and adolescents: an intergroup study. *J. Pediatr. Surg.* 2004; **39**:424–429.
30. Cushing, B., Giller, R., Ablin, A. *et al.* Surgical resection alone is effective treatment for ovarian immature teratoma in children and adolescents: a report of the paediatric oncologic Group and the Children's Cancer Group. *Am. J. Obstet. Gynecol.* 1999; **181**:353–358.
31. Biran, G., Gozan, A., Sagi, R. *et al.* Conversion of laparoscopy to laparotomy due to adnexal malignancy. *Eur. J. Gynecol. Oncol.* 2002; **23**:157–160.
32. Havrilesky, L. J., Peterson, B. L., Dryden, D. K. *et al.* Predictors of clinical out comes in the laparoscopic management of adnexal masses. *Obstet. Gynecol.* 2003; **102**:243–251.
33. Steyaert, H., Meynol, F., & Valla, J. S. Torsion of the adnexa in children: the value of laparoscopy. *Pediatr. Surg. Int.* 1998; **13**:384–387.
34. Heiss, K. F., Zwiren, G. T., & Winn, K. Massive ovarian oedema in the paediatric patient: a rare solid tumor. *J. Pediatr. Surg.* 1994; **29**:1392–1394.
35. Beaunoyer, M., Chapdelaine, J., Bouchard, S., & Ouimet, A. Asynchronous bilateral ovarian torsion. *J. Pediatr. Surg.* 2004; **39**:746–799.
36. Aziz, D., Davis, V., Allen, L., & Langer, J. C. Ovarian torsion in children: is oophorectomy necessary? *J. Pediatr. Surg.* 2004; **39**:750–753.
37. Sommerville, M., Grimes, D. A., Kooning, P. *et al.* Ovarian neoplasm and the risk of adnexal torsion. *Am. J. Obstet. Gynecol.* 1991; **164**:577–578.
38. Templeman, C., Hertweck, S. P., & Fallat, M. E. The clinical course of unresected ovarian torsion. *J. Pediatr. Surg.* 2000; **35**:1385–1387.
39. Oelsner, G., Admon, D., Bider, D. *et al.* Long term follow-up the twisted ischemic adnexa managed by detorsion. *Fertil. Steril.* 1993; **50**:976–979.
40. Nagel, T. C., Sebastian, J., & Malo, J. W. Oophoropexy to prevent sequential or recurrent torsion. *J. Am. Assoc. Gynecol. Laparosc.* 1997; **4**:495–498.
41. Shun, A. Unilateral childhood ovarian loss: an indication for controlateral oophoropexy? *Aust. NZ J. Surg.* 1990; **60**:791–794.
42. Theodore, C., Terrier-Lacombe, M. J., Laplanche, A. *et al.* Bilateral germ cell tumors: 22 year experience at the institute Gustave Roussy. *Br. J. Cancer* 2004; **90**:55–59.
43. Huddart, J.-N., Mann, J.-R., Gornall, P. *et al.* The UK Children's cancer study Group: testicular malignant germ cell tumor 1979–1988. *J. Pediatr. Surg.* 1990; **25**:406–410.
44. Bruce, J. & Gouch, D. C. S. Long term follow up of children with testicular tumors surgical issues. *Br. J. Urol.* 1991; **67**:1429–1433.
45. Ciftci, A. O., Bingol-Kolugu, M., Senocak, M. E. *et al.* Testicular tumors in children. *J. Pediatr. Surg.* 2001; **36**:1796–1801.
46. Mishriki, S. F., Winkle, D. C., & Frank, J. P. Fixation of a simple testis: always, sometimes or never. *Br. J. Urol.* 1992; **69**:311–313.
47. Rogers, D. A., Rao, B. N., Meyer, W. H. *et al.* Indication for hemiscrotectomy in the management of genito urinary tumors in children. *J. Pediatr. Surg.* 1995; **30**:1437–1438.
48. Schlatter, M., Rescorla, F., Giller, R. *et al.* Excellent out come in patients with stade I germ cell tumors of the testis: a study of the Children's Cancer group / Paediatric Oncology group. *J. Pediatr. Surg.* 2003; **38**:319–324.
49. Valla, J.-S. for the Group d'Etude en Urologie Pédiatrique. Testis sparing surgery for benign testicular tumor in children. *J. Urol.* 2001; **165**:2280–2283.

50. Ross, J. H., Rybicki, L., & Kay, R. Clinical behavior and contemporary management algorithm for prepubertal testis tumors: a summary of the prepubertal testis tumor registry. *J. Urol.* 2002; **168**:1675–1679.
51. Shukla, A. R., Woodard, C., Carr, M. C. *et al.* Experience with testis sparing surgery for testicular teratoma. *J. Urol.* 2004; **171**:161–163.
52. Elert, A., Olbert, P., Hegele, A. *et al.* Accuracy of frozen section examination of testicular tumors of uncertain origin. *Eur. Urol.* 2002; **41**:290–293.
53. Steiner, H., Hocil, L., & Manesch, G. C. Frozen section analysis-guided organ-sparing approach in testicular tumor: technique an long term results. *Urology* 2003; **62**:508–513.
54. Anteby, E. Y., Ron, M., Revel, A. *et al.* Germ cell tumor of the ovary avising after dermoïd cyst resection: a long term follow-up study. *Obstet. Gynecol.* 1994; **83**:605–608.
55. Bonazzi, C., Peccatori, F., Colombo *et al.* Pure ovarian immature teratoma a unique and curable disease: 10 years experience of 32 prospectively treated patients. *Obstet. Gynecol.* 1994; **84**:598–604.
56. Konrad, D. & Schoenle, E. J. Ten years follow-up in a boy with Leydig cell tumor after selective surgery. *Horm. Res.* 1999; **51**:96–100.
57. Borgfeldt, C. & Andolf, E. Cancer risk after hospital discharge diagnosis of benign ovarian cyst and endometriosis. *Acta Obstet. Gynecol. Scand.* 2004; **83**:395–400.
58. Mc Aleer, I. M., Kaplan, G. W., & Lo sasso, B. E. Renal and testis injuries in team sports. *J. Urol.* 2002; **168**:1805–1807.
59. Ayhan, A., Celik, H., Taskiran, C. *et al.* Oncologic and reproductive out come after fertility saving surgery in ovarian cancer. *Eur. J. Gynaecol. Oncol.* 2003; **24**:223–232.
60. Low, J. J., Perrin, L. C., Crandon, A. J. *et al.* Conservative surgery to preserve ovarian function in patients with malignant ovarian germ cell tumor. A review of 74 cases. *Cancer.* 2000; **15**:89(2): 391–398.
61. Zanetta, G., Bonazzi, C., Cantu, M. *et al.* Survival and reproductive function after treatment of malignant germ cell ovarian tumors. *J. Clin. Oncol.* 2001; **19**:1015–1020.
62. Mitchell, P. L., Alnasiri, N., A'Hern, R. *et al.* Treatment of non dysgerminomatous ovarian germ cell tumors: an analysis of 69 cases. *Cancer* 1999; **85**:2232–2244.
63. Baranzelli, M. C., Bouffet, E., Quintana, E. *et al.* Non seminomatous ovarian germ cell tumors in children. *Eur. J. Cancer* 2000; **36**:376–383.
64. Bethez, C. A., Mutabagani. K., Hammond, S. *et al.* Non teratomatous germ cell tumors in children. *J. Pediatr. Surg.* 1998; **33**:1122–1127.
65. Morowitz, M., Huff, D., & Von Allmen, D. Epithelial ovarian tumor in children: a retrospective analysis. *J. Pediatr. Surg.* 2003; **38**:331–335.
66. Schilder, J. M., Thomson, A. M., Depriest, P. D. *et al.* Outcome of reproductive age women with stage I A or I C invasive epithelial ovarian cancer treated with fertility sparing therapy. *Gynecol. Oncol.* 2002; **87**:1–7.
67. Shankar, K. R., Wakhlu, A., Kokal, G. K. *et al.* Ovarian adenocarcinoma in premenarchal girl. *J. Pediatr. Surg.* 2001; **36**:511–515.
68. Brewer, M., Gershenson, D. M., Herzog, C. E. *et al.* Outcome and reproductive function after chemotherapy for ovarian dysgerminoma. *J. Clin. Oncol.* 1999; **17**:2670–2674.
69. Grady, R. W., Ross, J. H., & Kay, R. Patterns of metastasis spread in prepubertal yolk sac tumor of the testis. *J. Urol.* 1995; **153**:1259.
70. Gupta, D. K., Kataria, R., & Sharma, M. C. Prepubertal testicular teratomas. *Eur. J. Pediatr. Surg.* 1999; **9**:173–176.
71. Canis, M., Bassil, S., Wattiez, A. *et al.* Fertility following laparoscopic management of benign adnexal cyst. *Hum. Reprod.* 1992; **7**:529–531.
72. Tangir, J., Zelterman, D., Ma, W. *et al.* Reproductive function after conservative surgery and chemotherapy for malignant germ cell tumor of the ovary. *Obstet. Gynecol.* 2003; **101**:251–257.
73. Huyghe, E., Matsuda, T., Daudin, W. *et al.* Fertility after testicular cancer treatments: results of a large multicentric study. *Cancer* 2004; **100**:732–737.
74. Yoshinaka, A., Fukasawa, I., Sakamoto, J. *et al.* The fertility and pregnancy out comes of the patients who under went preservative operation followed by adjuvant chemotherapy for malignant ovarian tumor. *Arch. Gynecol. Obstet.* 2000; **264**:124–127.
75. Mottet, N. & Petit, M. Conservative surgery for testicular tumors. *Progr. Urol.* 2004; **14**:15–18.
76. Heidenreich, A., Weissbach, L., Holtl, W. *et al.* Organ sparing surgery for malignant germ cell tumor of the testis. *J. Urol.* 2001; **166**:2161–2165.
77. Kanazana, K., Suzuki, T., & Sakumoto, K. Treatment of malignant ovarian germ cell tumors with preservation of fertility: reproductive performance after persistant remission. *Am. J. Clin. Oncol.* 2000; **23**:244–248.
78. Camatte, S., Rouzier, R., Boccara-De Keyser, J. *et al.* Prognosis and fertility after conservative treatment for ovarian tumors of limited malignancy: review of 68 cases. *Gynecol. Obstet. Fertil.* 2002; **30**:583–591.
79. Sayegh, R. & Garica, C. R. Ovarian function after conservation ovarian surgery: a long term follow-up study. *Int. J. Gynecol. Obstet.* 1992; **39**:303–309.
80. Woodhead, D. M., Pohl, D. R., & Johnson, D. E. Fertility of patients with solitary testis. *J. Urol.* 1973; **109**:66–67.
81. Bomalaski, D. The pediatric urologist and patient fertility. *Dialog. Pediatr. Urol.* 1999; **22**:11.
82. Lass, A. The fertility potential of women with a simple ovary. *Hum. Reprod. Update* 1999; **5**:546–550.
83. Dieckmann, K. S. A. & Loy, V. Paternity in a patient with testicular seminoma and controlateral testicular intraperitoneal neoplasia. *Int. J. Androl.* 1993; **16**:143–146.
84. Heidenreich, A., Vorreuther, R., Neubauer, S. *et al.* Paternity in patients with bilateral testicular germ cell tumors *Eur. Urol.* 1997; **31**:246–248.

85. Houlgatte, A., Delataille, A., Fournier, R. *et al.* Paternity in a patient with seminoma and carcinoma in situ in a solitary testis treated by partial orchidectomy. *BJU Int.* 1999; **84**:374–375.
86. Ng, R. S. The reproductive imperative: a case report highlighting the possibility of using chemotherapy to conserve the testis in patients with testis cancer. *Clin. Oncol. (R. Coll. Radiol.)* 1997; **9**:334–337.
87. Sawyer, E. J., Oliver, R. T., Tobias, J. S. *et al.* A lesson in the management of testicular cancer in a patient with a solitary testis. *Postgrad. Med. J.* 1999; **75**:481–483.
88. Zanagnolo, V., Sartori, E., Galleri, G. *et al.* Clinical review of 55 cases of malignant ovarian germ cell tumors. *Eur. J. Gynecol. Oncol.* 2004; **25**:315–320.
89. Aslam, I., Fischer, S., Moore, H. *et al.* Fertility preservation of boys undergoing anti-cancer therapy: a review of the existing situation and prospects for the future. *Hum. Reprod.* 2000; **15**:2154–2159.
90. Aubard, Y., Piver, P., Pech, J.-C. *et al.* Ovarian tissue cryopreservation gynaecologic oncology: a review. *Eur. J. Obstet. Gynecol. Reprod. Biol.* 2001; **97**:5–14.
91. Poirot, C., Vacher-Laveau, M. C., Helardot, P. *et al.* Human ovarian tissue cryopreservation: indications and feasibility. *Hum. Reprod.* 2002; **17**:1447–1452.
92. Revel, A., Davis, V. J., & Casper, R. F. Ovarian cortex cryopreservation in paediatric and adolescent medicine. *J. Pediatr. Adolec. Gynecol.* 2000; **13**:95.

Part VI

Oncology

57

Late effects of the treatment of childhood cancer

Mark F. H. Brougham and W. Hamish B. Wallace

Department of Paediatric Haematology and Oncology, Royal Hospital for Sick Children, Edinburgh, UK

Introduction

Survival from childhood cancer has markedly improved over recent decades following major advances in available treatments and supportive care, such that now around 75%–80% of children with cancer will be alive 5 years from diagnosis.[1] The number of long-term survivors is therefore increasing, and it has been estimated that, by the year 2010, about one in 715 of the adult population will have been treated for cancer in childhood.[2] Because of this, the emphasis in the management of childhood cancer has changed, from "cure at any cost" to one in which quality of life after treatment has become increasingly important. Thus, whilst continuing to strive for improved survival, attention must be directed towards minimizing the late effects of treatment.

Adverse late effects of childhood cancer treatment are diverse and include growth impairment, disorders of the endocrine system, infertility, abnormalities of cardiac and pulmonary function, renal and hepatic impairment, second malignancies, and cognitive and psychosocial difficulties. This chapter focuses on these consequences of childhood cancer treatment. Long-term follow-up of these patients is essential, in order that adverse effects are diagnosed early and appropriate counselling and therapeutic intervention instituted. Awareness of the etiology and prevalence of late complications will allow modifications of treatment that will improve the quality of life for long-term survivors of childhood cancer.

Endocrine disorders and growth impairment

Collectively, disorders of the endocrine system represent the commonest long-term complication of cancer treatment, with one study demonstrating endocrine abnormalities in up to 40% of such patients at follow-up.[3] Impairment of growth is also frequently seen following treatment for childhood cancer.[4] Normal growth requires a complex interaction between the skeleton, the endocrine system and the overall health of the child, and thus the etiology of poor growth following childhood cancer is usually multifactorial. Both the disease itself and the treatment, with chemotherapy, radiotherapy or surgery, can contribute to the deleterious effect observed.

Hypothalamic–pituitary dysfunction

The hypothalamic–pituitary axis is central to the control of the endocrine system, and therefore disruption of this axis will have far-reaching consequences. Cranial irradiation is known to cause hypothalamic–pituitary dysfunction,[5] and the resultant hormone deficiency is dependent on the total dose of radiation received and the fractionation schedule.[6]

Growth hormone (GH) secretion is the most radiosensitive of the pituitary hormones, with doses as low as 18Gy resulting in GH deficiency.[7] Subsequently, with increasing radiation dose, deficiencies are seen in gonadotrophin, corticotrophin, and thyrotrophin secretion, commonly in that order.[8]

Pediatric Surgery and Urology: Long-term Outcomes, Mark Stringer, Keith Oldham, Pierre Mouriquand.
Published by Cambridge University Press.

In addition to the dose-dependent effects, hypothalamic–pituitary dysfunction has been demonstrated to become progressively more severe with time after radiation treatment.[8,9] This may, in part, be due to the delayed effects of radiotherapy on the axis as a whole. However, it may also reflect subsequent pituitary dysfunction secondary to earlier hypothalamic damage, as there is increasing evidence that the hypothalamus is more radiosensitive than the pituitary gland.[10]

This latter point has implications with regard to follow-up and investigation of pituitary function. Pituitary function tests currently used rely on pharmacologic provocation tests to detect deficiencies. However, there is evidence to suggest that following radiation damage physiologic secretion of pituitary hormones is impaired, yet peak responses to provocation tests remain normal.[11,12] This impairment, known as neurosecretory dysfunction, can have clinical significance, particularly during the pubertal growth spurt, when increased GH secretion is required.

The prevalence of hypopituitarism may therefore be underestimated by standard provocation tests. However, assessment of physiologic secretion by overnight profiling is difficult in practical terms, and currently remains a research tool. This emphasizes the importance of continued long-term follow-up and clinical vigilance for these patients.

An additional risk factor important in neuroendocrine late effects is the age of the child at the time of radiotherapy. There is evidence to suggest that younger children are more sensitive to radiation-induced damage of the hypothalamic–pituitary axis as compared to older children and adults.[13]

In summary, pituitary deficiencies are likely to be multiple, and manifest rapidly and completely in younger children, those receiving higher radiation doses or where tumors are centrally positioned. By comparison, deficits may be single, evolve more slowly or be qualitative rather than quantitative in nature following irradiation to more distant tumors or after lower cranial doses. This will result in a cohort of survivors who may require hormone replacement therapy as adults, despite not requiring treatment as children.

Growth hormone deficiency

GH deficiency is the commonest endocrine abnormality following cranial irradiation. Short stature after cancer treatment has been well documented, particularly following cranial and craniospinal irradiation,[4] and with treatment received at a younger age.[14] The etiology of short stature following treatment for cancer is multifactorial, as discussed later, but GH deficiency will certainly impair final height.

In addition to effects on height, GH has numerous other physiologic roles. Indeed, deficiency of this hormone has also been implicated in causing a reduced lean body mass and increased fat mass,[15] metabolic abnormalities including an adverse lipid profile and impaired glucose tolerance,[16] a reduction in bone mineral density,[17] and impaired quality of life.[18]

Whilst many other aspects of both treatment and the disease itself play a role in the deleterious effects listed above, GH deficiency is important, and because of this replacement with recombinant growth hormone has been advocated. This treatment has resulted in an improved growth response in children with GH deficiency after cranial irradiation.[19] In addition to the benefits observed in growth, replacement therapy has been demonstrated to reduce fat mass and increase muscle mass, reduce the cardiovascular risk factor profile, increase bone mineral density, and improve quality of life.[20–23]

The treatment of affected children with documented GH deficiency with recombinant GH is therefore now well accepted. Replacement therapy is normally discontinued once attainment of final height has been achieved. However, given the additional benefits of treatment discussed above, continuing therapy into adulthood, at a reduced dose, may also be beneficial.[24]

GH, however, is potentially mitogenic, and therefore concerns have been raised regarding its use in cancer survivors. These concerns include an association with an increased risk of relapse of leukemia and brain tumors,[25] and a recent report suggesting an increased risk of colorectal cancer in adults treated with human pituitary GH prior to 1985.[26] However, several long-term studies of patients treated with physiologic replacement doses of recombinant GH have failed to demonstrate any such increased risk,[27–29] but continued surveillance is essential. Although GH therapy should be commenced early to achieve a maximal response, in view of these concerns most centers do not advocate introducing therapy within the first two years after cancer treatment, as this is the period with the highest relapse rate.

Hypothalamic–pituitary–gonadal axis

Gonadotrophin deficiency

With higher doses of cranial irradiation, damage to the hypothalamic–pituitary axis can also disrupt gonadotrophin secretion. Indeed, patients receiving radiation doses of 35–45 Gy have demonstrated subsequent deficiencies in both Follicle Stimulating Hormone (FSH) and Luteinizing Hormone (LH) secretion.[6] In addition, as with GH, the prevalence of gonadotrophin deficiency increases with time after irradiation.

The clinical sequelae of gonadotrophin deficiency exhibit a broad spectrum of severity, from subclinical abnormalities detectable only by gonadotrophin releasing hormone (GnRH) testing, to a significant reduction in circulating sex hormone levels and delayed puberty. As discussed earlier, the hypothalamus is more radiosensitive than the pituitary gland and therefore the etiology of hypogonadism in these patients following cranial irradiation is hypothalamic GnRH deficiency.[30] In view of this, exogenous GnRH can be used as replacement therapy in order to restore gonadal function and fertility.

Early and precocious puberty

In contrast to the situation described above it appears that, paradoxically, lower doses of cranial irradiation can result in premature activation of the hypothalamic–pituitary–gonadal axis, leading to early or precocious puberty. Precocious puberty is defined as the onset of puberty prior to age 8 years in girls and 9 years in boys, whereas early puberty is categorized as onset between 8 and 10 years in girls and 9 and 11 years in boys. The precise etiology of radiation-induced early puberty is thought to be via disinhibition of cortical influences on the hypothalamus.

Cranial irradiation at doses of around 18–24 Gy has been previously used to prevent recurrent CNS disease in patients with acute lymphoblastic leukemia (ALL). This dose is generally lower than that required for solid tumors of the CNS, and it has subsequently been noted that such treatment is associated with a higher incidence of early and precocious puberty, predominantly affecting girls.[31] Higher doses of cranial irradiation can result in early puberty in both sexes.[32]

Therefore, early puberty as a consequence of cranial irradiation is dose dependent, and the dose threshold of this effect is gender specific. Indeed, following higher doses of irradiation, a patient may enter puberty early but subsequently develop gonadotrophin deficiency as discussed above, thus suggesting differential effects of radiotherapy with time. Treatments to delay puberty in this circumstance should therefore be used with caution.

Entering puberty early results in a premature pubertal growth spurt followed by early epiphysial fusion. As a consequence, final adult height is reduced. If GH deficiency is also present, as discussed earlier, final height is further compromised since peak height velocity is reduced.[33]

In addition to an overall reduction in height, growth in children after treatment is frequently disproportionate in that much of their height loss is secondary to a reduction in sitting height.[34] Spinal growth is important during the latter part of the pubertal growth spurt, and therefore early puberty coincident with undiagnosed GH deficiency clearly has a deleterious effect.

As noted previously, GH replacement therapy is effective in improving final height. In view of the concerns raised above, if the onset of puberty is early, pubertal progression should be suppressed with GnRH analogues. This will delay skeletal fusion, thus maximizing height potential. Combined treatment with growth hormone and a GnRH analogue in this situation improves the height prognosis[35] and final adult height.

It is essential that these patients are followed up after treatment with regard to their growth and puberty. This involves 6-monthly clinical assessment of pubertal status and auxology measurements and, when indicated, biochemical assessment of GH and gonadotrophin secretion, and radiologic assessment of bone age.

Fertility

Whilst cranial irradiation can disrupt the onset of puberty or arrest its progress, the gonads themselves can be directly damaged by radiotherapy involving the spinal or pelvic area or by systemic chemotherapy. This damage may result in subfertility or infertility in both males and females.[36–39]

In males, normal testicular function is dependent on a complex interplay between the Sertoli, Leydig and germ cells. Sertoli cells function to nurture developing germ cells, whereas Leydig cells are responsible for testosterone production. Spermatogenesis involves the proliferation and differentiation of germ cells, and can be impaired by cytotoxic treatment that, by its nature, targets rapidly dividing cells. The adult testis is continually producing mature spermatozoa and is therefore very susceptible to such damage. However, it is clear that gonadotoxic treatment received at any age can lead to subsequent infertility.[37,40] Indeed, there is increasing evidence that the testis demonstrates significant cellular activity before puberty, and that this activity is essential for normal adult testicular function.[41,42] Thus the timing of the gonadotoxic insult in relation to puberty is of less importance than the nature of the insult itself.

In contrast, the female is born with her full complement of eggs, which declines in an exponential fashion to menopause. Both chemotherapy and radiotherapy may accelerate oocyte depletion, leading to truncated fecundity and menopause occurring prematurely.[38,43]

The effects of radiotherapy

The gonads are sensitive to irradiation, and resultant damage depends on the field of treatment, total dose and fractionation schedule.[38,39,44]

In males, radiation doses as low as 0.1–1.2 Gy can result in detectable effects on spermatogenesis, with doses over 4 Gy causing a more permanent detrimental effect.[39,44,45] The somatic cells of the testis are more resistant to radiation-induced damage than the germ cells. Indeed, Leydig cell dysfunction is not observed until doses of around 20 Gy in prepubertal boys and 30 Gy in sexually mature males.[46] Therefore, many patients will produce testosterone and develop normal secondary sexual characteristics, despite severe impairment of spermatogenesis.

In female patients, total body, abdominal or pelvic irradiation will not only cause ovarian damage but may also affect uterine function. As with males, the degree of impairment depends on the radiation dose, field, fractionation schedule and age at the time of treatment.[38,47–49] Depletion of primordial follicles secondary to radiotherapy is proportional to the size of the existing oocyte pool and therefore, for a given dose of radiation, the younger the child at the time of radiotherapy the later the onset of a premature menopause. The human oocyte is very sensitive to radiation, and the LD_{50} (the lethal dose required to kill 50% of the total oocytes) has been estimated to be less than 2 Gy.[50] Based on this model of follicular decline, ovarian ultrasound scanning can indicate the likely age of onset of premature menopause following such treatment.[51]

Irradiation involving the uterus in childhood is associated with an increased incidence of nulliparity, spontaneous miscarriage and intrauterine growth retardation.[48,49,52] The mechanisms underlying these problems remain unclear, but may be secondary to reduced elasticity of the uterine musculature and uterine vascular damage.[49,52] Patients who have received radiation involving the pelvis should be counselled appropriately, and good communication with the obstetrician is essential.

The effects of chemotherapy

Cytotoxic chemotherapy can cause gonadal damage, and the nature and extent of this damage is dependent upon the agent administered, the dose received and the age and sex of the patient.[37,53–55] Although a number of agents have been identified as being gonadotoxic (Table 57.1), including procarbazine, cisplatin, and the alkylating agents such as cyclophosphamide and melphalan, it is important to note that not all chemotherapeutic agents cause permanent gonadal damage. In addition, the relative contribution of each individual drug can be difficult to determine as most treatments are administered as multiagent regimens.

As with radiotherapy involving the testes, the seminiferous epithelium is more sensitive to the detrimental effects of chemotherapy than the somatic cells. Therefore, after receiving gonadotoxic agents, male patients may be rendered oligospermic or azoospermic but testosterone production by the Leydig cells is usually unaffected, and thus secondary sexual characteristics develop normally.[56,57] Following higher cumulative doses of gonadotoxic chemotherapy, Leydig cell dysfunction may also occur.[58]

Table 57.1. Gonadotoxic chemotherapy agents

Alkylating agents	Cyclophosphamide
	Ifosfamide
	Nitrosureas, e.g., carmustine, lamustine
	Chlorambucil
	Melphalan
	Busulphan
Vinca-alkaloids	Vinblastine
Antimetabolites	Cytarabine
Others	Cisplatin
	Procarbazine

Treatment of Hodgkin's disease has involved the use of procarbazine and alkylating agents such as chlorambucil and cyclophosphamide. Whilst this treatment results in excellent survival rates, around 90% of male patients have subsequently developed permanent azoospermia in adulthood.[53,56] In view of this, treatment of this lymphoma has been modified in order to reduce the gonadotoxicity.[59] Whilst procarbazine and alkylating agents are still used, cycles containing these drugs are alternated with cycles containing anthracycline agents which, although potentially cardiotoxic, do not affect spermatogenesis. These "alternating" regimens result in significantly less gonadotoxicity.[60]

In contrast to the effects of radiotherapy, females are, in general, less susceptible to the gonadotoxic effects of the chemotherapeutic agents discussed above. However, ovarian dysfunction following chemotherapy has been described.[61] As with male patients, procarbazine and alkylating agents, as used for the treatment of Hodgkin's disease, are particularly gonadotoxic.[53] The degree of ovarian damage following chemotherapy is also dependent on the age of the patient, with older females being more susceptible to the development of premature ovarian failure.[43] The larger reserve of surviving primordial follicles available after treatment probably explains the relative protection afforded to younger females.

Long-term follow-up is essential for these patients, as premature ovarian failure will result in an early menopause. Byrne *et al.*[62] followed up women treated for cancer before the age of 20 and found that 42% of women treated with radiotherapy and alkylating agent based chemotherapy had reached menopause by the age of 31, compared with 5% of controls. Those patients at risk must be counseled appropriately, not only because their fertile window is substantially reduced, but also with regard to the additional implications of a premature menopause, such as reduced bone mineral density and osteoporosis.

The effects of disease

Although many aspects of cancer treatment may affect fertility, it is important to note that the disease itself may contribute to gonadal dysfunction. Indeed, it has been demonstrated that up to 70% of male patients with Hodgkin's disease assessed before commencing treatment have impaired semen quality.[63] This may also be observed in patients with other malignancies prior to treatment,[64] although perhaps to a lesser extent. In addition to the disease itself, other non-specific conditions commonly observed at presentation, such as fever, anorexia and pain, can impair semen quality.[65]

Similarly, oocytes harvested from female patients prior to cancer therapy are of impaired quality and exhibit an impaired fertilization rate, as compared to those from control females.[66]

These findings will have implications when considering fertility preservation strategies before the commencement of gonadotoxic therapy.

Fertility potential and assessment following cancer treatment

Due to the varied nature of the gonadal insult following chemotherapy or radiotherapy, it can often be very difficult to predict whether a child undergoing cancer treatment will subsequently have impaired fertility. The risk of subfertility can be categorized according to the type of malignancy and its associated treatment (Table 57.2). As noted before, treatment for Hodgkin's disease with alkylating agent based therapy is profoundly gonadotoxic. Conditioning prior to bone marrow transplantation with high dose chemotherapy and total body irradiation (TBI) also carries a substantial risk of gonadotoxicity, as does treatment of metastatic sarcoma. However, current treatment for acute lymphoblastic leukemia (ALL), the commonest malignancy in this age group, represents a relatively low risk of gonadotoxicity.

It is important to note that treatment protocols for malignant disease are continually evolving, in order to improve survival and reduce adverse effects. Whereas treatment for ALL has intensified over the past decade, the management of hepatoblastoma, for example, has become less intensive. In addition, as more is understood about the biology of malignant disease, there is an increasing trend to stratify treatments according to risk of relapse. Therefore, this assessment of risk represents a guide, which needs to be continually reviewed in the light of ongoing research. To complicate matters further, there are reports of patients having received sterilizing treatment who have subsequently demonstrated recovery of spermatogenesis or ovarian function.[67,68] In view of these uncertainties, counselling patients and their families is difficult. Long-term follow-up of these patients must include appropriate discussion and assessment of fertility.

Determining the impact of chemotherapy and radiotherapy on gonadal function currently involves regular clinical assessment of pubertal status, biochemical assessment of gonadotrophins and sex steroids, menstrual history in females and semen analysis in males. However, in prepubertal children, clinical assessment such as this is not possible and biochemical assessment is unreliable because the hypothalamic–pituitary–gonadal axis is relatively quiescent in this age group. Thus it is currently not possible to detect gonadal damage early, due to the lack

Table 57.2. Best assessment of risk of subfertility following current treatment for childhood cancer by disease

Risk of subfertility	Disease/treatment
Low	Acute lymphoblastic leukemia
	Wilms' tumor
	Soft tissue sarcoma: stage 1
	Germ cell tumors (with gonadal preservation and no radiotherapy)
	Retinoblastoma
	Brain tumor: surgery only
	Cranial irradiation $<$24 Gy
Medium	Acute myeloblastic leukemia
	Hepatoblastoma
	Osteosarcoma
	Ewing's sarcoma
	Soft tissue sarcoma
	Neuroblastoma
	Non-Hodgkin's lymphoma
	Hodgkin's disease: "alternating therapy"
	Brain tumor: craniospinal radiotherapy
	Cranial irradiation $>$24 Gy
High	Total body irradiation
	Localised radiotherapy: pelvic/testicular
	Chemotherapy conditioning for bone marrow transplant
	Hodgkin's disease: alkylating agent based therapy
	Soft tissue sarcoma: metastatic

Low risk is assessed as $<$ 20%, high risk as $>$ 80%. Medium risk is difficult to quantify. Males are more susceptible to subfertility following chemotherapy than females, although females may be at risk of premature menopause.

of a sensitive marker of gonadal function in prepubertal children.

There is currently much interest in inhibin B as a potential marker of gonadotoxicity in this age group. Inhibin B is secreted predominantly from Sertoli cells in males and developing antral follicles in females,[69,70] and plays an important role in spermatogenesis and folliculogenesis in adult males and females respectively. There is evidence to suggest that gonadotoxic chemotherapy is associated with a reduction in inhibin B levels.[71] However, this relationship has not been clearly demonstrated in the prepubertal age group,[72] and it remains to be seen if inhibin B will become a useful tool in fertility assessment of these children in the future.

Fertility preservation

Preservation of fertility is dictated by sexual maturity, and currently the only established options are cryopreservation of spermatozoa in the male, and of oocytes in the female, or of embryos in those with a partner. These techniques require time and can be problematic, particularly in the pediatric population.

Sperm banking is not universally practised in pediatric oncology centers, and there are very few suitable "adolescent-friendly" facilities. Following confirmation of a diagnosis of malignancy, cancer therapy is usually commenced as soon as possible. After having received such devastating news regarding the diagnosis, it can often be very difficult for teenagers to then discuss fertility and future children and subsequently go on to produce a semen specimen. Discussions must therefore be dealt with sensitively, and using appropriate language which the patient understands. On the positive side, however, many patients and their families derive benefit from open discussion regarding fertility, particularly as this places emphasis on looking to the future and provides reassurance that curative treatment is the aim.[73] Unfortunately, the semen specimens produced in these circumstances are frequently of poor quality,[74] and this is further compromised by long term cryopreservation.[75] However, all male patients who are able to produce semen should have the opportunity of sperm banking prior to the commencement of cancer treatment.

In post-pubertal females, fertility may be preserved by collection of mature oocytes before gonadotoxic therapy for in vitro fertilization (IVF) and subsequent embryo cryopreservation. This method is only applicable to sexually mature females, and requires a partner or donor sperm for fertilization. For women without a partner, cryopreservation of mature oocytes is an alternative option, but subsequent pregnancy rates are significantly lower as these cells sustain more damage during the freeze–thaw process than do embryos.[76] These techniques also require a period of ovarian hyperstimulation for several weeks, which limits their use in patients with cancer because of the inevitable delay in the commencement of treatment.

These methods of fertility preservation are not applicable to prepubertal children, who represent the majority of pediatric patients requiring gonadotoxic therapy. Strategies for preserving fertility in this patient group are limited, and at present remain entirely experimental.

Although the prepubertal testis does not produce mature spermatozoa, it does contain the diploid stem germ cells from which haploid spermatozoa will ultimately be derived. Therefore, in theory, testicular tissue could be harvested prior to gonadotoxic cancer therapy and cryopreserved. Following cure and on entering adulthood, this tissue could be thawed and used in one of two ways in order to produce offspring. Firstly, the stored germ cells could be reimplanted into the patient's own testes in order to restore natural fertility, a procedure known as germ cell transplantation.[77] Alternatively the stored cells could be matured in vitro until they are able to achieve fertilization using assisted reproduction techniques, such as intracytoplasmic sperm injection (ICSI).

Whilst these techniques have enormous potential, they are associated with a number of problems that must be addressed before their clinical application. Optimal techniques for obtaining the tissue and the subsequent cryopreservation process are uncertain at present. In addition, the procedure for returning the germ cells to the testis for germ cell transplantation has yet to be established.

However, perhaps the most important issue to be addressed with auto-transplantation is that it requires tissue that was removed from a patient with cancer before treatment to be returned to the patient following cure. There is, therefore, a genuine risk of reintroducing malignant cells, with potentially fatal consequences. This is unlikely to occur with malignancies such as Hodgkin's disease, which is often localized at presentation, but the risk would be substantial with hematologic malignancies,[78] where the testes can act as sanctuary sites for leukemic cells. Indeed, any theoretical risk of returning cancer cells following treatment, however small, would not be acceptable.

The technique of maturing stem germ cells in vitro would circumvent this risk. However, although restoration of fertility following in vitro spermatogenesis has been reported,[79] this process has involved maturation of the later stages of spermatogenesis rather than from stem cells. Indeed, it appears unlikely that in vitro maturation of diploid stem cells into haploid spermatozoa will be technically possible in the near future.

An alternative to these techniques in the prepubertal male is hormonal manipulation. Because cytotoxic treatment acts principally on rapidly dividing cells it has been postulated that by rendering the testes quiescent with hormonal treatments, the germ cells will be less susceptible to cytotoxicity. Although this technique, based on suppression of the hypothalamic–pituitary–gonadal axis, has been successful in rodent models treated with chemotherapy and radiotherapy,[80,81] clinical trials have thus far failed to demonstrate any benefit.[82] There may be a number of reasons for the lack of protection afforded to humans, but recent evidence suggests that the proliferation of germ cells in prepubertal primates is actually gonadotrophin independent.[42] Therefore, hormonal manipulation based on suppression of this axis is unlikely to be protective in patients receiving gonadotoxic therapy. Studies are currently in progress in order to identify what factors regulate spermatogonial proliferation, with the hope that these may offer novel targets for testicular protection during cytotoxic therapy.

Although mature oocytes cannot be harvested from prepubertal female patients, ovarian tissue containing germ cells could be removed and stored prior to gonadotoxic therapy. Following cure, this tissue could either be returned to the patient via autotransplantation, or matured in vitro to produce offspring via IVF, in a similar manner as is proposed in male patients at this age.

Ovarian tissue can be removed by either taking multiple biopsies from the ovary, or by performing an oophorectomy. However, perhaps the most promising technique is the harvesting of ovarian cortical strips. This can be done laparoscopically and this tissue is rich in primordial follicles. Autologous transplantation of this tissue would aim to both restore natural fertility and also maintain sex steroid production. The feasibility of this process has been demonstrated in sheep,[83] with both the return of ovarian hormonal activity and the subsequent production of offspring. Following on from such success in animal models, this procedure has been attempted in female patients with ovarian failure.[84,85] A return of sex steroid production has been demonstrated. However, to date, no pregnancies have been reported in patients using such techniques. It is likely that these ovarian grafts will have a limited lifespan.

There remain a number of issues to be clarified before widespread clinical application of these procedures in cancer patients. However, perhaps the greatest concern, as with male patients in whom germ cell transplantation may be considered, is the potential to return malignant cells back to the patient following cure. This is of particular importance in patients with hematologic malignancies,[86] but any theoretical risk, however small, is unacceptable.

Despite the issues that need to be resolved before clinical application of techniques using harvested ovarian tissue, a number of centers have already removed and stored ovarian cortical strips from prepubertal cancer patients. It is hoped that reproductive technology will have advanced sufficiently to allow the appropriate use of this tissue in the future. Opportunities for preserving fertility in these patients must be grasped, even though the potential of these strategies has yet to be fully realized. However, it is equally essential to work within acceptable guidelines and as such a working party from the Royal College of Obstetricians and Gynaecologists in the UK have published a comprehensive document[87] outlining standards of best practice regarding the collection and future use of such tissue.

Offspring of childhood cancer survivors

Whilst these strategies offer real hope of improved fertility prospects for these patients, consideration must be given to subsequent offspring produced. Concerns have been raised that the mutagenic potential of cancer therapy could predispose children of patients who receive such treatment to congenital abnormalities, or even cancer themselves. A large epidemiologic study failed to demonstrate any such link,[88] except in those with familial malignancies. However, these offspring resulted from natural conception, and it remains to be seen if problems may arise from the use of assisted reproduction techniques such as ICSI, whereby the natural selection processes of normal sexual reproduction are circumvented. As nuclear material from a sperm is injected directly into an oocyte, natural mechanisms that prevent either sperm or oocytes with defective DNA from being involved with fertilization are bypassed. Reassuringly in this regard, a recent study demonstrated that sperm from men previously treated for childhood cancer does not carry a greater burden of damaged DNA as compared to age-matched controls.[57] However, long-term surveillance of future offspring is essential.

Ethical and legal issues

Harvesting gonadal tissue for future use is an exciting prospect, but the technology raises a number of important ethical and legal issues. There are concerns regarding the protection of children's reproductive rights, and also about obtaining valid informed consent, both for storage and future use of cryopreserved material. In addition, given the absence of proven therapeutic benefit and the potential risk associated with these procedures, together with the uncertainty of predicting infertility from new chemotherapeutic and reproductive strategies, it is questionable whether such experimentation is justified or ethical in children.[89]

These issues must be addressed so that new techniques are adequately regulated. This will ensure that children with cancer have a realistic and safe prospect for fertility in the future.[90]

Thyroid disorders

Thyroid disorders can occur following treatment for childhood cancer, either via disruption of the hypothalamic–pituitary–thyroid axis or following direct damage to the thyroid gland itself. The abnormalities can be of thyroid function, usually hypothyroidism, or can manifest as thyroid nodules. In addition, there is a small risk of secondary thyroid cancer.[91]

Cranial irradiation can disrupt the hypothalamic–pituitary–thyroid axis, resulting in central hypothyroidism.[8] The incidence of radiation-induced thyroid stimulating hormone (TSH) deficiency is dose dependent[6] and this part of the hypothalamic–pituitary axis appears to be the least vulnerable to radiation damage.[8] In children, disturbances of the hypothalamic–pituitary–thyroid axis are uncommon with doses lower than 40 Gy.[92]

The biochemical diagnosis of central hypothyroidism relies on levels of TSH and thyroid hormone (free T4). However, there is some evidence to suggest that subtle abnormalities of thyrotrophin secretion, not detected in this manner, can be significant enough to have clinical implications. Thus TSH and free T4 may fall within the normal range, yet more detailed investigation of TSH dynamics suggests clinically significant central hypothyroidism.[93] This damage may occur at lower doses of irradiation than that suggested above. The implications of this may be important in deciding thresholds for intervention with thyroxine supplements, and this may be particularly important in the pediatric population as reduced thyroid function may affect growth[94] and physical and intellectual performance. Further investigation is required in order to demonstrate the functional significance of these findings before criteria for clinical intervention are modified. However, this again demonstrates the importance of follow-up and clinical vigilance in these children after treatment.

Thyroid abnormalities may also occur following direct damage to the thyroid gland itself. This is usually secondary to radiotherapy where the neck falls within the radiation field, although chemotherapy can potentiate this radiation-induced damage.[95] Chemotherapy alone rarely affects thyroid function, although damage has been reported following intensive treatment with busulphan and cyclophosphamide,[96] as used for conditioning prior to bone marrow transplantation. Hypothyroidism is the commonest abnormality following direct thyroid damage,[97] and this is usually initially in the form of compensated hypothyroidism with an elevated TSH and normal thyroxine. Despite this, thyroxine replacement may be justified in order to reduce the theoretical risk of thyroid cancer,[98] thought to be secondary to prolonged stimulation of the thyroid gland. Risk factors for developing hypothyroidism in this manner include higher doses of neck irradiation, female sex and older age at diagnosis. The greatest risk is during the first five years following treatment.[97] Hyperthyroidism is less common but can occur following neck irradiation, with those patients receiving higher doses also being at greater risk.[97]

In addition to abnormalities in thyroid function, neoplasms of the thyroid gland, both benign and malignant, are more frequent following irradiation involving the neck.[91,99] The risk of developing thyroid neoplasia increases with higher doses of radiotherapy[100] and with younger age at the time of treatment.[101] In addition, females are at higher risk of developing thyroid cancer.[102]

Benign thyroid nodules include adenomas, focal hyperplasia and colloid nodules. Papillary carcinoma is the commonest thyroid cancer that develops secondary to irradiation,[102] which, if detected early, is associated with a high cure rate. Thus, long-term follow-up of these children must include regular examination of the thyroid gland and some advocate the use of ultrasound as a screening tool.[103]

Hypothalamic–pituitary–adrenal axis

The hypothalamic–pituitary–adrenal axis appears to be relatively radio resistant.[8] Abnormalities in adrenocorticotrophin hormone (ACTH) or cortisol secretion are uncommon after low dose cranial irradiation.[104] However, ACTH deficiency is potentially life-threatening, its symptoms often subtle and it should be considered in patients receiving higher doses of irradiation and in those patients treated for pituitary or closely related tumors.[8] Life-long replacement is necessary and is particularly problematic if posterior pituitary dysfunction is also present, such as after craniopharyngiomas.

As with the assessment of thyroid function, the incidence of abnormalities may be underestimated due to the diagnostic difficulty in evaluating the hypothalamic–pituitary–adrenal axis. In addition, clinical signs of cortisol deficiency can be non-specific and thus the diagnosis may be missed. The insulin tolerance test is regarded as the gold standard but can be problematic, particularly in the pediatric population due to the consequences of severe hypoglycemia. Excessive tiredness in a patient who has received cranial irradiation should warrant testing of the hypothalamic–pituitary–adrenal axis. Hydrocortisone replacement is essential, and increased doses are required during intercurrent illness and surgery.

Growth and bone metabolism following treatment

Endocrine disorders, nutritional problems, reduced physical activity, disturbances in bone and mineral homeostasis, delayed or arrested puberty and psychosocial dysfunction all contribute to problems with growth and bone metabolism. As a consequence children may fail to reach their height potential, and are at risk of reduced bone mineral density leading to osteopenia, osteoporosis and perhaps pathological fractures in later life.[4,105,106]

The effects of radiotherapy

The impact of radiotherapy on the endocrine system, with subsequent effects on growth, has been discussed. However, radiotherapy can also exert a direct effect upon the skeletal system. Spinal growth plays an important role in determining final height, and this may be compromised following radiotherapy involving the spine.[107,108] This includes craniospinal irradiation, total body irradiation and thoracic or abdominal irradiation. Radiotherapy causes permanent disruption of the epiphyses, and the consequence of this on spinal growth results in skeletal disproportion, with a greater reduction in sitting height as compared to leg length. This effect is more pronounced the younger the child is at the time of treatment.[107]

Scoliosis and kyphosis have long been recognized as complications of radiotherapy involving the spine.[109] However, with more modern techniques, in particular the use of megavoltage radiotherapy and symmetrical irradiation of the vertebral bodies, these complications are less frequent,[110] although they may still occur since radiotherapy can cause asymmetry of the paraspinal muscles.

Thus, radiotherapy can have a detrimental effect on spinal growth. Sitting height and spinal curvature should be routinely examined as part of the follow-up for these patients.

The effects of chemotherapy

Chemotherapeutic agents generally target rapidly dividing cells. Because of this they may affect normal growth and bone activity.[105]

Growth has been extensively studied during and after treatment of ALL. Unlike many other cancers, ALL is treated with ongoing chemotherapy of varying intensity over a prolonged period of time. With current protocols in the UK, treatment lasts for at least 2 years, extending up to 3 years in boys. Prior to 1992, cranial radiotherapy, to prevent CNS disease, was part of the management for all children with ALL. This is no longer used routinely and therefore the majority of patients will now receive chemotherapy alone in the treatment of their malignancy.

Growth deceleration has been demonstrated during treatment of ALL, and this effect is most marked during the first year of treatment[111] and in younger children.[112] Obviously many of the longer term studies include children who received radiotherapy in addition to chemotherapy, and as previously noted this will have a detrimental effect on growth. However, studies investigating the role of chemotherapy alone have also demonstrated an impact on growth, although the magnitude of this effect is less marked.[113]

The effect of chemotherapy on the growth of long bones has been demonstrated by measurement of lower leg length during different phases of treatment for ALL.[114] In this study growth of the lower leg was effectively stopped during periods of intensive chemotherapy. With less intensive "maintenance" chemotherapy, growth returned to a rate comparable to that of healthy children and this was followed by a compensatory "catch-up" period of accelerated growth velocity following cessation of treatment.

Thus, catch-up growth does occur but only after chemotherapy is stopped which, as discussed above, may be up to three years after diagnosis. However, there is evidence to suggest that this catch-up growth tends to be complete in patients who receive chemotherapy alone, whereas those who have received radiotherapy still have a suboptimal final height in adulthood.[115]

Bone development is maximal during puberty, and peak bone mass is reached at around 20 years of age.[116] This can be disrupted by childhood cancer and its treatment. Indeed, a reduced bone mineral density (BMD), as measured using DEXA scans, has been demonstrated after treatment for childhood ALL[117] and other malignancies.[106] The etiology of this is likely to be multifactorial and secondary to both the disease itself as well as its treatment.

Various bone markers can be measured in order to assess the impact of chemotherapy on the dynamics of bone turnover and growth. In a prospective study of 22 children with ALL, markers of bone formation, bone resorption, soft tissue turnover and the growth hormone axis were measured.[118] At diagnosis, bone turnover was low, probably secondary to growth hormone resistance associated with the disease itself. During intensive phases of chemotherapy there was further suppression of the markers of bone and soft tissue turnover. However, these markers increased dramatically during periods of less intensive treatment.

Of the chemotherapeutic agents used, steroids and methotrexate have been particularly implicated in playing a pathologic role in bone homeostasis.[118] Steroids cause retardation of bone growth, both directly by decreasing osteoblast activity and turnover, and indirectly by altering calcium homeostasis.[119] Decreased intestinal absorption and increased urinary excretion of calcium causes secondary hyperparathyroidism and consequently, bone resorption. Methotrexate also inhibits bone growth, probably via inhibition of osteoblast proliferation and differentiation, secondary to folate deficiency.[120]

Other factors affecting growth and bone metabolism

As mentioned earlier, the disease itself as well as its treatment can have a detrimental impact on growth and bone metabolism. In leukemia, infiltration and expansion of the bone marrow spaces with leukemic cells may destroy the spongiosa. In addition, the leukemic cells themselves may secrete factors such as osteoblast inhibiting factor and parathyroid hormone related peptide, further contributing to bone loss.[121]

In addition to the direct effects of the disease, other factors in these children are important. Poor nutrition, reduced physical activity and immobilization, prolonged hospitalization and psychosocial factors may all play a role in certain children, although the relative impact of each of these factors is difficult to ascertain.

Therapeutic intervention

Therapeutic intervention of endocrine dysfunction, for example with GH and GnRH analogues, as discussed earlier, may be essential in ensuring adequate growth after treatment for childhood cancer. However, of equal importance is the consideration of the factors discussed above, as these are all part of the long-term management of these children. Optimal nutrition, physical activity and psychosocial support are all vital for these children as they progress through treatment, if later morbidity is to be avoided.

Changes in bone homeostasis may predispose children to osteopenia, premature osteoporosis and possibly pathologic fractures in later life. Assessment of calcium status and BMD at the end of treatment may enable early identification of patients with impaired skeletal development and allow the institution of potential therapies. Nutritional support, ensuring an adequate calcium intake, exercise to optimize body weight and physical fitness, and medical intervention with calcitonin, vitamin D and bisphosphonate treatment may all improve the BMD in these patients.[116,117]

Obesity

Excessive weight gain is a recognized complication of certain childhood malignancies, in particular suprasellar tumors and acute lymphoblastic leukemia.

Obesity is seen frequently in patients with craniopharyngioma, with one recent study demonstrating severe obesity (defined as a body mass index (BMI) greater than 3 standard deviations above the mean) in 44% of patients at follow-up.[122] The etiology of this is likely to be multifactorial, although it appears to be associated with hypothalamic damage.[123]

Obesity is also well documented following treatment of ALL, and a number of risk factors have been postulated. Those children with ALL who received cranial irradiation as part of their treatment have an increased BMI as compared to their peers, and remain at significant risk of becoming overweight in adulthood.[124] GH deficiency is likely to play a role, but other important factors may include damage to areas of the brain that normally control appetite and body composition.

Obesity after treatment for ALL has also been described in patients who have not received cranial irradiation.[125] The etiology of excess weight gain in these patients is likely to be multifactorial, and a number of risk factors have been suggested. Children with ALL are less active than their peers,[126] both during and after treatment, and this appears to be one of the most important factors contributing to the excess weight gain observed. Obesity in this patient group is also more pronounced in girls[127] and is more likely in those who are younger and thinner at diagnosis.[128] In addition, there is also a familial contribution, with a significant number of obese patients having an obese mother.[129] Pulsed steroids are used throughout ALL treatment regimens, causing a significant increase in energy intake and this further contributes to the prevalence of obesity in these children.[130]

Dietetic input is essential in these patients, in order to optimize nutrition and body composition. In addition, the importance of physical activity and a healthy lifestyle must be emphasized.

Cardiovascular and pulmonary morbidity

Cardiovascular disease can occur secondary to childhood cancer treatment, and this may contribute significantly to the late morbidity and mortality of disease-free survivors.[131] Cardiovascular damage is most commonly due to direct damage from radiotherapy and from chemotherapeutic agents, particularly the anthracyclines. However, indirect damage can also occur following insults to other organs.

Radiation-induced damage primarily results from mediastinal irradiation, as used, for example, in certain patients to treat lymphoma. However, patients receiving TBI for BMT conditioning are also susceptible. Coronary artery disease and myocardial infarction can result from such treatment, and the risk of this occurring increases with increasing radiation dose, with those in excess of 30 Gy being particularly problematic.[132] Younger age at the time of irradiation is a further risk factor for subsequent cardiac pathology.[132] Mediastinal radiotherapy appears to induce atheromatous lesions of the proximal carotid arteries but there is no strong evidence that irradiation alters HDL blood lipid levels.

Chemotherapy-induced cardiac damage is particularly associated with anthracyclines, such as doxorubicin and daunorubicin. Subsequent myocardial dysfunction is related to the cumulative dose received,[133] although even relatively low doses can cause adverse cardiac effects, and the likelihood of these occurring increases over time.[134] In addition to dose, younger age at the time of treatment and female gender are further independent risk factors.[135] The mechanism of damage appears to be focal myocyte death with subsequent fibrosis.[131] It is important to note that damage secondary to irradiation has an additive effect to anthracycline-induced cardiotoxicity, and therefore combined treatments should be used with caution.

Assessment of cardiac function primarily involves echocardiography, which should be performed at diagnosis and at regular intervals during and after treatment. However, there is no firm evidence to suggest the appropriate frequency of such assessment. In general, it is recommended that children who have satisfactory left ventricular function and who have received modest cumulative anthracycline doses of less than 250 mg/m^2 should have 3-yearly echocardiogram surveillance. However, this should be increased in patients who have received higher doses or who have had previous cardiac problems. Electrocardiograms should also be performed, as higher anthracycline doses are associated with prolongation of the QT interval.[136] Survivors of childhood cancer who are pregnant and those wishing to partake in competitive sport should have a more detailed cardiologic assessment.

Protection of cardiac function has been attempted by concomitant administration of cardioprotective drugs, such as ICRF-187, with anthracyclines. However, although the risk of developing short-term subclinical cardiotoxicity is reduced by these agents,[137] benefits in the longer term have not yet been established. Treatment of cardiac dysfunction following cancer treatment has involved the use of angiotensin converting enzyme inhibitors such as captopril or enalapril. These agents are, in general, quite safe and are likely to be of benefit, although at present there is little evidence to support this. It is important to encourage appropriate lifestyle changes as required, such as improved diet, smoking cessation and sensible exercise.

Pulmonary function can also be affected by cancer treatment. Radiotherapy can result in restrictive pulmonary disease and reduced compliance. These problems are most commonly seen following thoracic radiation, which may be used in the treatment of lymphoma. TBI will also include the lungs within the treatment field, and this may also cause restrictive defects, although at the doses used pulmonary dysfunction is usually subclinical.[138] The lungs are, in general, less sensitive to the effects of chemotherapy, although both carmustine and bleomycin can cause subsequent pulmonary dysfunction,[139] and this may be potentiated by additional use of radiotherapy.

Follow-up of at-risk patients should include pulmonary function tests. Progressive pulmonary fibrosis is untreatable, other than by lung transplantation, and therefore advice should be given regarding the prevention of further damage from environmental exposure to harmful substances, particularly cigarette smoke.

Renal and hepatic impairment

Acute renal and hepatic dysfunction is commonly observed in children with cancer, both at diagnosis and during treatment. The severity of this toxicity is variable, and occasionally may result in irreversible damage.

The alkylating agents, particularly ifosfamide, and the platinum agents, particularly cisplatin, are the most commonly implicated nephrotoxic drugs.[140,141] Ifosfamide predominantly affects the proximal tubule, resulting in a Fanconi syndrome and causing phosphaturia. The resultant hypophosphatemia may lead to the development of rickets. In addition to tubular dysfunction, glomerular function may also be impaired. Cisplatin predominantly causes glomerular damage, and the extent of this is related to the cumulative dose. Tubular damage secondary to this agent also occurs, and characteristically results in hypomagnesemia, which may persist for many years after chemotherapy is completed. Similarly, radiotherapy may also affect renal function if the kidney is involved in the radiation field. Unfortunately an incomplete understanding of the pathogenesis of nephrotoxicity following cancer treatment has hindered attempts at developing protective strategies.

Assessment of renal function following treatment must include investigation of both glomerular and tubular function, along with regular blood pressure and height and weight measurements.

Although disturbances of liver function are frequently observed during treatment for childhood cancer, chronic liver disease as a consequence of such treatment is rarely seen. Actinomycin D, used for example in the treatment of Wilms' tumour, can cause veno-occlusive disease.[142] In addition, microvascular fatty change and siderosis have been noted in liver biopsies following treatment of ALL, although hepatitis and cirrhosis have not been described.[143] However, after successful treatment of ALL with 6-thioguanine, a small proportion of children have developed an occlusive venopathy and nodular regenerative hyperplasia causing progressive portal hypertension.[144]

Cognitive and psychosocial outcomes

During the course of cancer treatment children can miss substantial amounts of schooling, but a decline in cognitive function is neither a frequent nor inevitable consequence of such treatment.[145] However, cranial irradiation in particular is an important risk factor for subsequent cognitive difficulties, and this risk increases with higher dosage and younger age at the time of treatment. Certain structural brain abnormalities have been described after cranial irradiation, such as reduced volumes of neuronal white matter and temporal lobe calcification.[146] The functional significance of such abnormalities is difficult to determine, but impairment may be associated with vasculopathy, calcification and EEG changes.[146] Follow-up of patients who are at-risk should therefore include a cognitive assessment. The practicalities of performing such assessments can be problematic and, in addition, have significant resource implications. Annual screening using the Wechsler Intelligence Scale for Children (WISC) is appropriate, and if a problem is suspected a more comprehensive assessment of cognition should be performed.

The treatment of childhood cancer is likely to impact on educational, psychologic and social functioning, and thus the effect on overall quality of life may be considerable. Studies addressing these issues are largely observational, and the outcome measures assessed range from formal psychiatric and psychologic assessments, through self-completed questionnaires, to sociodemographic variables such as marriage or employment. Adverse outcomes with regard to these latter variables are, indeed, common findings, although the risk of bias in these studies is high. Overt psychiatric disorders are uncommon, but survivors do seem to be at risk of anxiety, low mood and low self-esteem. Brain tumors and treatment with cranial irradiation are particular risk factors for adverse psychologic and social outcomes. The prevention and management of such adverse sequelae can be difficult, and at present, there are no prospective studies using standardized assessment measures which address potential interventions.

Second primary tumors

Children who have been treated for cancer have an increased risk of developing a second malignancy in later life. In the UK this has been estimated as a 1 in 25 risk of developing a second primary cancer within 25 years of the initial diagnosis, representing approximately a sixfold increased risk.[147] It is likely that this relates both to the carcinogenic effects of chemotherapy and radiotherapy, and to certain genetic factors. A genetic predisposition to developing cancer includes, for example, constitutional mutations of the retinoblastoma gene and of the p53 gene, and many others are being increasingly recognized.

Current knowledge of the longer-term risks of chemotherapy and radiotherapy are based on treatments used many years ago and therefore the longer-term consequences of current therapies are difficult to assess with confidence at present. However, certain cancers, particularly second primary bone cancer and second primary leukemias are associated with previous exposure to radiotherapy and to certain chemotherapeutic agents.

Second primary bone cancer affects about 1 in 100 survivors of childhood cancer by 20 years following the original diagnosis.[148] Bone cancers are the commonest solid second cancers and are mostly osteosarcomas. The increased risk of developing bone tumours in this manner is attributable to radiotherapy and to the alkylating agents.[149]

Second primary leukemia is diagnosed in about 1 in 500 survivors of childhood cancer by 6 years following the original diagnosis.[150] This is around eight times the number expected. Increased cumulative exposure to alkylating agents[151] or epipodophyllotoxins[150] increases the risk of subsequent leukemia. In addition, other topoisomerase II inhibitors, including the anthracyclines, appear leukemogenic.

Radiotherapy is known to cause second tumors within the radiation field. As discussed above these are most commonly osteosarcomas of affected bone. However, other tumors have also been described, such as breast cancer following thoracic irradiation received by female patients with Hodgkin's disease.[152] Indeed, second cancer is the leading cause of death in long-term survivors of this lymphoma. Radiation doses in excess of 40 Gy[151] and younger age at the time of treatment[153] increase the risk of a second malignancy in patients treated for Hodgkin's disease.

Second primary malignancies can be particularly devastating for survivors of childhood cancer and their families. It is hoped that current treatment protocols, and in particular a reduction in the use of radiotherapy, will reduce the incidence of these late sequelae. However, it remains very difficult to assign "safe" doses of these agents, and any reduction in treatment intensity must not compromise survival from the original cancer. This balance may be particularly difficult to achieve in patients with known cancer predisposition syndromes.

Follow-up of childhood cancer survivors

With improving survival rates there is an urgent need for effective long-term follow-up strategies to be developed.[154] At present, there is evidence that wide variation exists in the extent to which survivors of childhood cancer are discharged from hospital follow-up.[155] Uncertainty exists regarding the most appropriate personnel to review these patients, and how frequently they should be seen.

It is clear from the above discussion that the degree and nature of adverse long-term morbidity risk will depend on the underlying malignancy, the type and intensity of the treatment given and the age of the child at the time of treatment. Appropriate follow-up strategies will therefore vary between patients and between treatment groups. At one extreme, there are survivors for whom the benefit of clinical follow-up beyond five years from treatment completion is not established, and for whom annual or 2-yearly postal or telephone contact may be all that is necessary. Such patients would include those treated with surgery alone or low risk chemotherapy (Table 57.3). At the other extreme would be patients who have received radiotherapy (other than low dose cranial irradiation), bone marrow transplantation or megatherapy. Patients in this group should be seen in a medically supervised late effects clinic at least three times per annum until final height is achieved, and at least annually thereafter (Table 57.3).

Multidisciplinary follow-up is vital if adverse late effects are to be anticipated and monitored appropriately. This may involve a variety of personnel including the pediatric oncologist, endocrinologist, neurologist, surgeon, radiation oncologist, clinical psychologist, general practitioner, specialist nurse and social worker.

The development of evidence-based, therapy-based guidelines for follow-up will improve future strategies. Further information will be obtained from national population-based cohort studies and large multi-center clinical studies. Future randomized childhood cancer treatment trials must not only address survival outcomes, but also long-term treatment morbidities.[156]

Conclusions

The successful treatment of childhood cancer is associated with significant morbidity in later life. The major challenge faced by those caring for these children is to sustain the excellent survival rates whilst striving to achieve optimal quality of life.

Adverse late sequelae of cancer treatments are diverse, and vary considerably in severity. Awareness of these complications, with appropriate long-term follow-up and early intervention, is essential in the management of these children. In addition, as follow-up strategies become more standardized, together with centralization of data evaluating late effects of therapy, it is hoped that treatment protocols in the future will be further modified. These modifications will aim to reduce the impact of these late effects without compromising survival, and thus subsequently improve the quality of life for these children as they progress into adulthood.

Table 57.3. Possible levels of follow-up more than 5 years from completion of treatment

Level	Treatment	Method of follow-up	Freq.	Examples
1	– Surgery alone – Low risk chemotherapy	Postal or telephone	1–2 years	– Wilms' stage I/II – LCH (single system) Germ cell tumors (surgery only)
2	– Chemotherapy – Low dose cranial irradiation (<24 Gy)	Nurse or primary care led	1–2 years	– Majority of patients (e.g., ALL in first remission)
3	– Radiotherapy (except above) – Megatherapy	Medically supervised late effects clinic	Annual	– Brain tumors – Post-BMT – Stage 4 patients (any tumor)

LCH = Langerhans' cell histiocytosis, BMT = bone marrow transplant.

REFERENCES

1. Mertens, A. C., Yasui, Y., Neglia, J. P. *et al.* Late mortality experience in five-year survivors of childhood and adolescent cancer: the Childhood Cancer Survivor Study. *J. Clin. Oncol.* 2001;**19**:3163–3172.
2. Scottish Intercollegiate Guidelines Network. Guideline 76: Long term follow up care of survivors of childhood cancer. Edinburgh, 2004.
3. Sklar, C. A. Overview of the effects of cancer therapies: the nature, scale and breadth of the problem. *Acta. Paediatr. Suppl.* 1999; **88**:1–4.
4. Muller, H. L., Klinkhammer-Schalke, M., & Kuhl, J. Final height and weight of long-term survivors of childhood malignancies. *Exp. Clin. Endocrinol. Diabetes* 1998; **106**:135–139.
5. Constine, L. S., Woolf, P. D., Cann, D. *et al.* Hypothalamic-pituitary dysfunction after radiation for brain tumors. *N. Engl. J. Med.* 1993; **328**:87–94.
6. Littley, M. D., Shalet, S. M., Beardwell, C. G., Robinson, E. L., & Sutton, M. L. Radiation-induced hypopituitarism is dose-dependent. *Clin. Endocrinol. (Oxf.)* 1989; **31**:363–373.

7. Brennan, B. M., Rahim, A., Mackie, E. M., Eden, O. B., & Shalet, S. M. Growth hormone status in adults treated for acute lymphoblastic leukaemia in childhood. *Clin. Endocrinol. (Oxf.)* 1998; **48**:777–783.
8. Littley, M. D., Shalet, S. M., Beardwell, C. G., Ahmed, S. R., Applegate, G., & Sutton, M. L. Hypopituitarism following external radiotherapy for pituitary tumours in adults. *Quart. J. Med.* 1989; **70**:145–160.
9. Clayton, P. E. & Shalet, S. M. Dose dependency of time of onset of radiation-induced growth hormone deficiency. *J. Pediatr.* 1991; **118**:226–228.
10. Schmiegelow, M., Lassen, S., Poulsen, H. S. *et al.* Growth hormone response to a growth hormone-releasing hormone stimulation test in a population-based study following cranial irradiation of childhood brain tumors. *Horm. Res.* 2000; **54**:53–59.
11. Bercu, B. B. & Diamond, F. B. Jr. Growth hormone neurosecretory dysfunction. *Clin. Endocrinol. Metab.* 1986; **15**:537–590.
12. Spoudeas, H. A., Hindmarsh, P. C., Matthews, D. R., & Brook, C. G. Evolution of growth hormone neurosecretory disturbance after cranial irradiation for childhood brain tumours: a prospective study. *J. Endocrinol.* 1996; **150**:329–342.
13. Shalet, S. M., Beardwell, C. G., Pearson, D., & Jones, P. H. The effect of varying doses of cerebral irradiation on growth hormone production in childhood. *Clin. Endocrinol. (Oxf.)* 1976; **5**:287–290.
14. Ogilvy-Stuart, A. L. & Shalet, S. M. Growth and puberty after growth hormone treatment after irradiation for brain tumours. *Arch. Dis. Child.* 1995; **73**:141–146.
15. de Boer, H., Blok, G. J., & Van der Veen, E. A. Clinical aspects of growth hormone deficiency in adults. *Endocr. Rev.* 1995; **16**:63–86.
16. Talvensaari, K. & Knip, M. Childhood cancer and later development of the metabolic syndrome. *Ann. Med.* 1997; **29**:353–355.
17. Kaufman, J. M., Taelman, P., Vermeulen, A., & Vandeweghe, M. Bone mineral status in growth hormone-deficient males with isolated and multiple pituitary deficiencies of childhood onset. *J. Clin. Endocrinol. Metab.* 1992; **74**:118–123.
18. Stabler, B. Impact of growth hormone (GH) therapy on quality of life along the lifespan of GH-treated patients. *Horm. Res.* 2001; **56** Suppl 1: 55–58.
19. Vassilopoulou-Sellin, Klein, M. J., Moore, B. D. III, Reid, H. L., Ater, J., & Zietz, H. A. Efficacy of growth hormone replacement therapy in children with organic growth hormone deficiency after cranial irradiation. *Horm. Res.* 1995; **43**:188–193.
20. Murray, R. D., Darzy, K. H., Gleeson, H. K., & Shalet, S. M. GH-deficient survivors of childhood cancer: GH replacement during adult life. *J. Clin. Endocrinol. Metab.* 2002; **87**:129–135.
21. Pfeifer, M., Verhovec, R., & Zizek, B. Growth hormone (GH) and atherosclerosis: changes in morphology and function of major arteries during GH treatment. *Growth Horm. IGF Res.* 1999; **9** Suppl A: 25–30.
22. Longobardi, S., Di Rella, F., Pivonello, R. *et al.* Effects of two years of growth hormone (GH) replacement therapy on bone metabolism and mineral density in childhood and adulthood onset GH deficient patients. *J. Endocrinol. Invest.* 1999; **22**:333–339.
23. Lagrou, K., Xhrouet-Heinrichs, D., Massa, G. *et al.* Quality of life and retrospective perception of the effect of growth hormone treatment in adult patients with childhood growth hormone deficiency. *J. Pediatr. Endocrinol. Metab.* 2001; **14** Suppl 5: 1249–1262.
24. Vahl, N., Juul, A., Jorgensen, J. O., Orskov, H., Skakkebaek, N. E., & Christiansen, J. S. Continuation of growth hormone (GH) replacement in GH-deficient patients during transition from childhood to adulthood: a two-year placebo-controlled study. *J. Clin. Endocrinol. Metab.* 2000; **85**:1874–1881.
25. Watanabe, S., Tsunematsu, Y., Fujimoto, J., & Komiyama, A. Leukaemia in patients treated with growth hormone (letter). *Lancet* 1988; **1**:1159–1160.
26. Swerdlow, A. J., Higgins, C. D., Adlard, P., & Preece, M. A. Risk of cancer in patients treated with human pituitary growth hormone in the UK, 1959–1985: a cohort study. *Lancet* 2002; **360**:273–277.
27. Ogilvy-Stuart, A. L., Ryder, W. D., Gattamaneni, H. R., Clayton, P. E., & Shalet, S. M. Growth hormone and tumour recurrence. *Br. Med. J.* 1992; **304**:1601–1605.
28. Swerdlow, A. J., Reddingius, R. E., Higgins, C. D. *et al.* Growth hormone treatment of children with brain tumors and risk of tumor recurrence. *J. Clin. Endocrinol. Metab.* 2000; **85**:4444–4449.
29. Sklar, C. A., Mertens, A. C., Mitby, P. *et al.* Risk of disease recurrence and second neoplasms in survivors of childhood cancer treated with growth hormone: a report from the Childhood Cancer Survivor Study. *J. Clin. Endocrinol. Metab.* 2002; **87**:3136–3141.
30. Hall, J. E., Martin, K. A., Whitney, H. A., Landy, H., & Crowley, W. F. Jr. Potential for fertility with replacement of hypothalamic gonadotrophin-releasing hormone in long term female survivors of cranial tumors. *J. Clin. Endocrinol. Metab.* 1994; **79**:1166–1172.
31. Leiper, A. D., Stanhope, R., Preece, M. A., Grant, D. B., & Chessells, J. M. Precocious or early puberty and growth failure in girls treated for acute lymphoblastic leukaemia. *Horm. Res.* 1988; **30**:72–76.
32. Ogilvy-Stuart, A. L., Clayton, P. E., & Shalet, S. M. Cranial irradiation and early puberty. *J. Clin. Endocrinol. Metab.* 1994; **78**:1282–1286.
33. Didcock, E., Davies, H. A., Didi, M., Ogilvy-Stuart, A. L., Wales, J. K., & Shalet, S. M. Pubertal growth in young adult survivors of childhood leukaemia. *J. Clin. Oncol.* 1995; **13**:2503–2507.
34. Davies, H. A., Didcock, E., Didi, M., Ogilvy-Stuart, A. L., Wales, J. K., & Shalet, S. M. Disproportionate short stature after cranial irradiation and combination chemotherapy for leukaemia. *Arch. Dis. Child.* 1994; **70**:472–475.
35. Cara, J. F., Kreiter, M. L., & Rosenfield, R. L. Height prognosis of children with true precocious puberty and growth hormone

deficiency: effect of combination therapy with gonadotrophin releasing hormone agonist and growth hormone. *J. Pediatr.* 1992; **120**:709–715.

36. Waring, A. B. & Wallace, W. H. B. Subfertility following treatment for childhood cancer. *Hosp. Med.* 2000; **61**:550–557.
37. Whitehead, E., Shalet, S. M., Jones, P. H., Beardwell, C. G., & Deakin, D. P. Gonadal function after combination chemotherapy for Hodgkin's disease in childhood. *Arch. Dis. Child.* 1982; **57**:287–291.
38. Wallace, W. H., Shalet, S. M., Crowne, E. C., Morris-Jones, P. H., & Gattamaneni, H. R. Ovarian failure following abdominal irradiation in childhood: natural history and prognosis. *Clin. Oncol. (R. Coll. Radiol.)* 1989; **1**:75–79.
39. Speiser, B., Rubin, P., & Casarett, G. Aspermia following lower truncal irradiation in Hodgkin's disease. *Cancer* 1973; **32**:692–698.
40. Relander, T., Cavallin-Stahl, E., Garwicz, S., Olsson, A. M., & Willen, M. Gonadal and sexual function in men treated for childhood cancer. *Med. Pediatr. Oncol.* 2000; **35**:52–63.
41. Chemes, H. E. Infancy is not a quiescent period of testicular development. *Int. J. Androl.* 2001; **24**:2–7.
42. Kelnar, C. J., McKinnell, C., Walker, M. *et al.* Testicular changes during infantile 'quiescence' in the marmoset and their gonadotrophin dependence: a model for investigating susceptibility of the prepubertal human testis to cancer therapy? *Hum. Reprod.* 2002; **17**:1367–1378.
43. Whitehead, E., Shalet, S. M., Blackledge, G., Todd, I., Crowther, D., & Beardwell, C. G. The effect of combination chemotherapy on ovarian function in women treated for Hodgkin's disease. *Cancer* 1983; **52**:988–993.
44. Clifton, D. K. & Bremner, W. J. The effect of testicular x-irradiation on spermatogenesis in man. A comparison with the mouse. *J. Androl.* 1983; **4**:387–392.
45. Centola, G. M., Keller, J. W., Henzler, M., & Rubin, P. Effect of low-dose testicular irradiation on sperm count and fertility in patients with testicular seminoma. *J. Androl.* 1994; **15**:608–613.
46. Shalet, S. M., Tsatsoulis, A., Whitehead, E., Read, G. Vulnerability of the human Leydig cell to radiation damage is dependent upon age. *J. Endocrinol.* 1989; **120**:161–165.
47. Wallace, W. H., Shalet, S. M., Hendry, J. H., Morris-Jones, P. H., & Gattamaneni, H. R. Ovarian failure following abdominal irradiation in childhood: the radiosensitivity of the human oocyte. *Br. J. Radiol.* 1989; **62**:995–998.
48. Sanders, J. E., Hawley, J., Levy, W. *et al.* Pregnancies following high-dose cyclophosphamide with or without high-dose busulfan or total-body irradiation and bone marrow transplantation. *Blood* 1996; **87**:3045–3052.
49. Bath, L. E., Critchley, H. O., Chambers, S. E., Anderson, R. A., Kelnar, C. J., & Wallace, W. H. Ovarian and uterine characteristics after total body irradiation in childhood and adolescence: response to sex steroid replacement. *Br. J. Obstet. Gynaecol.* 1999; **106**:1265–1272.
50. Wallace, W. H. B., Thomson, A. B., & Kelsey, T. W. The radiosensitivity of the human oocyte. *Hum. Reprod.* 2003; **18**:117–121.
51. Wallace, W. H. & Kelsey, T. W. Ovarian reserve and reproductive age may be determined from measurement of ovarian volume by transvaginal sonography. *Hum. Reprod.* 2004; **19**:1612–1617.
52. Critchley, H. O., Wallace, W. H., Shalet, S. M., Mamtora, H., Higginson, J., & Anderson, D. C. Abdominal irradiation in childhood; the potential for pregnancy. *Br. J. Obstet. Gynaecol.* 1992; **99**:392–394.
53. Mackie, E. J., Radford, M., & Shalet, S. M. Gonadal function following chemotherapy for childhood Hodgkin's disease. *Med. Pediatr. Oncol.* 1996; **27**:74–78.
54. Wallace, W. H., Shalet, S. M., Lendon, M., & Morris-Jones, P. H. Male fertility in long-term survivors of childhood acute lymphoblastic leukaemia. *Int. J. Androl.* 1991; **14**:312–319.
55. Wallace, W. H., Shalet, S. M., Crowne, E. C., Morris-Jones, P. H., Gattamaneni, H. R., & Price, D. A. Gonadal dysfunction due to *cis*-platinum. *Med. Pediatr. Oncol.* 1989; **17**:409–413.
56. Kreuser, E. D., Xiros, N., Hetzel, W. D., & Heimpel, H. Reproductive and endocrine gonadal capacity in patients treated with COPP chemotherapy for Hodgkin's disease. *J. Cancer. Res. Clin. Oncol.* 1987; **113**:260–266.
57. Thomson, A. B., Campbell, A. J., Irvine, D. S., Anderson, R. A., Kelnar, C. J. H., & Wallace, W. H. B. Semen quality and spermatozoal DNA integrity in survivors of childhood cancer: a case-control study. *Lancet* 2002; **360**:361–367.
58. Gerl, A., Muhlbayer, D., Hansmann, G., Mraz, W., & Hiddemann, W. The impact of chemotherapy on Leydig cell function in long term survivors of germ cell tumors. *Cancer* 2001; **91**:1297–1303.
59. Thomson, A. B. & Wallace, W. H. Treatment of paediatric Hodgkin's disease: a balance of risks. *Eur. J. Cancer.* 2002; **38**:468–477.
60. Viviani, S., Santoro, A., Ragni, G., Bonfante, V., Bestetti, O., & Bonadonna, G. Gonadal toxicity after combination chemotherapy for Hodgkin's disease. Comparative results of MOPP vs ABVD. *Eur. J. Cancer. Clin. Oncol.* 1985; **21**:601–605.
61. Chiarelli, A. M., Marrett, L. D., & Darlington, G. Early menopause and infertility in females after treatment for childhood cancer diagnosed in 1964–1988 in Ontario, Canada. *Am. J. Epidemiol.* 1999; **150**:245–254.
62. Bryne, J., Fears, T. R., Gail, M. H. *et al.* Early menopause in long-term survivors of cancer during adolescence. *Am. J. Obstet. Gynaecol.* 1992; **166**:788–793.
63. Rueffer, U., Breuer, K., Josting, A. *et al.* Male gonadal dysfunction in patients with Hodgkin's disease prior to treatment. *Ann. Oncol.* 2001; **12**:1307–1311.
64. Hallak, J., Mahran, A., Chae, J., & Agarwal, A. The effects of cryopreservation on semen from men with sarcoma or carcinoma. *J. Assist. Reprod. Genet.* 2000; **17**:218–221.
65. Agarwal, A., Shekarriz, M., Sidhu, R. K., & Thomas, A. J., Jr. Value of clinical diagnosis in predicting the quality of cryopreserved sperm from cancer patients. *J. Urol.* 1996; **155**:934–938.

66. Pal, L., Leykin, L., Schifren, J. L. *et al.* Malignancy may adversely influence the quality and behaviour of oocytes. *Hum. Reprod.* 1998; **13**:1837–1840.
67. Marmor, D. & Duyck, F. Male reproductive potential after MOPP therapy for Hodgkin's disease: a long-term survey. *Andrologia* 1995; **27**:99–106.
68. Nasir, J., Walton, C., Lindow, S. W., & Masson, E. A. Spontaneous recovery of chemotherapy-induced primary ovarian failure: implications for management. *Clin. Endocrinol. (Oxf.)* 1997; **46**:217–219.
69. Anderson, R. A. & Sharpe, R. M. Regulation of inhibin production in the human male and its clinical applications. *Int. J. Androl.* 2000; **23**:136–144.
70. Roberts, V. J., Barth, S., el-Roeiy, A., & Yen, S. S. Expression of inhibin/activin subunits and follistatin messenger ribonucleic acids and proteins in ovarian follicles and the corpus luteum during the human menstrual cycle. *J. Clin. Endocrinol. Metab.* 1993; **77**:1402–1410.
71. Wallace, E. M., Groome, N. P., Riley, S. C., Parker, A. C., & Wu, F. C. Effects of chemotherapy-induced testicular damage on inhibin, gonadotrophin, and testosterone secretion: a prospective longitudinal study. *J. Clin. Endocrinol. Metab.* 1997; **82**:3111–3115.
72. Crofton, P. M., Thomson, A. B., Evans, A. E. M. *et al.* Is inhibin B a potential marker of gonadotoxicity in prepubertal children treated for cancer? *Clin. Endocrinol. (Oxf.)* 2003; **58**:296–301.
73. Wallace, W. H. B. & Thomson, A. B. Preservation of fertility in children treated for cancer. *Arch. Dis. Child.* 2003; **88**:493–496.
74. Postovsky, S., Lightman, A., Aminpour, D., Elhasid, R., Peretz, M., & Arush, M. W. Sperm cryopreservation in adolescents with newly diagnosed cancer. *Med. Pediatr. Oncol.* 2003; **40**:355–359.
75. Hammadeh, M. E., Askari, A. S., Georg, T., Rosenbaum, P., & Schmidt, W. Effect of freeze-thawing procedure on chromatin stability, morphological alteration and membrane integrity of human spermatozoa in fertile and subfertile men. *Int. J. Androl.* 1999; **22**:155–162.
76. Salha, O., Picton, H., Balen, A., & Rutherford, A. Human oocyte cryopreservation. *Hosp. Med.* 2001; **62**:18–24.
77. Brinster, R. L. & Zimmermann, J. W. Spermatogenesis following male germ-cell transplantation. *Proc. Natl. Acad. Sci. USA* 1994; **91**:11298–11302.
78. Jahnukainen, K., Hou, M., Petersen, C., Setchell, B., & Soder, O. Intratesticular transplantation of testicular cells from leukemic rats causes transmission of leukemia. *Cancer. Res.* 2001; **61**:706–710.
79. Tesarik, J., Bahceci, M., Ozcan, C., Greco, E., & Mendoza, C. Restoration of fertility by in-vitro spermatogenesis. *Lancet* 1999; **353**(9152): 555–556.
80. Ward, J. A., Robinson, J., Furr, B. J., Shalet, S. M., & Morris, I. D. Protection of spermatogenesis in rats from the cytotoxic procarbazine by the depot formulation of Zoladex, a gonadotropin-releasing hormone agonist. *Cancer Res.* 1990; **50**:568–574.
81. Kurdoglu, B., Wilson, G., Parchuri, N., Ye, W. S., & Meistrich, M. L. Protection from radiation-induced damage to spermatogenesis by hormone treatment. *Radiat. Res.* 1994; **139**:97–102.
82. Thomson, A. B., Anderson, R. A., Irvine, D. S., Kelnar, C. J., Sharpe, R. M., & Wallace, W. H. Investigation of suppression of the hypothalamic–pituitary–gonadal axis to restore spermatogenesis in azoospermic men treated for childhood cancer. *Hum. Reprod.* 2002; **17**:1715–1723.
83. Gosden, R. G., Baird, D. T., Wade, J. C., & Webb, R. Restoration of fertility to oophorectomized sheep by ovarian autografts stored at −196 degrees C. *Hum. Reprod.* 1994; **9**:597–603.
84. Radford, J. A., Lieberman, B. A., Brison, D. R. *et al.* Orthotopic reimplantation of cryopreserved ovarian cortical strips after high-dose chemotherapy for Hodgkin's lymphoma. *Lancet* 2001; **357**:1172–1175.
85. Oktay, K., Buyuk, E., Rosenwaks, Z., & Rucinski, J. A technique for transplantation of ovarian cortical strips to the forearm. *Fertil. Steril.* 2003; **80**:193–198.
86. Shaw, J. M., Bowles, J., Koopman, P., Wood, E. C., & Trounson, A. O. Fresh and cryopreserved ovarian tissue samples from donors with lymphoma transmit the cancer to graft recipients. *Hum. Reprod.* 1996; **11**:1668–1673.
87. Royal College of Obstetricians and Gynaecologists. Storage of ovarian and prepubertal testicular tissue. Report of a working party. Royal College of Obstetricians and Gynaecologists, London, 2000.
88. Hawkins, M. M., Draper, G. J., & Smith, R. A. Cancer among 1,348 offspring of survivors of childhood cancer. *Int. J. Cancer.* 1989; **43**:975–978.
89. Spoudeas, H. A., Wallace, W. H. B., & Walker, D. Is germ cell harvest and storage justified in minors treated for cancer? (letter) *Br. Med. J.* 2000; **320**:316.
90. Wallace, W. H. & Walker, D. A. Conference consensus statement: ethical and research dilemmas for fertility preservation in children treated for cancer. *Hum. Fertil. (Camb.)* 2001; **4**:69–76.
91. Black, P., Straaten, A., & Gutjahr, P. Secondary thyroid carcinoma after treatment for childhood cancer. *Med. Pediatr. Oncol.* 1998; **31**:91–95.
92. Sklar, C. A., Constine, L. S. Chronic neuroendocrinological sequalae of radiation therapy. *Int. J. Radiat. Oncol. Biol. Phys.* 1995; **31**:1113–1121.
93. Rose, S. R., Lustig, R. H., Pitukcheewanont, P. *et al.* Diagnosis of hidden central hypothyroidism in survivors of childhood cancer. *J. Clin. Endocrinol. Metab.* 1999; **84**:4472–4479.
94. Rose, S. R. Isolated central hypothyroidism in short stature. *Pediatr. Res.* 1995; **38**:967–973.
95. Livesey, E. A. & Brook, C. G. Thyroid dysfunction after radiotherapy and chemotherapy of brain tumours. *Arch. Dis. Child.* 1989; **64**:593–595.
96. Michel, G., Socie, G., Gebhard, F. *et al.* Late effects of allogeneic bone marrow transplantation for children with acute myeloblastic leukaemia in first complete remission: the impact of conditioning regimen without total body

irradiation- a report from the Societe Francaise de Greffe de Moelle. *J. Clin. Oncol.* 1997; **15**:2238–2246.

97. Sklar, C., Whitton, J., Mertens, A. *et al.* Abnormalities of the thyroid in survivors of Hodgkin's disease: data from the Childhood Cancer Survivor Study. *J. Clin. Endocrinol. Metab.* 2000; **85**:3227–3232.
98. Doniach, I., Kingston, J. E., Plowman, P. N., & Malpas, J. S. The association of post-radiation thyroid nodular disease with compensated hypothyroidism. *Br. J. Radiol.* 1987; **60**:1223–1226.
99. Fleming, I. D., Black, T. L., Thompson, E. I., Pratt, C., Rao, B., & Hustu, O. Thyroid dysfunction and neoplasia in children receiving neck irradiation for cancer. *Cancer* 1985; **55**:1190–1194.
100. de Vathaire, F., Hardiman, C., Shamsaldin, A. *et al.* Thyroid carcinomas after irradiation for a first cancer during childhood. *Arch. Intern. Med.* 1999; **159**:2713–2719.
101. Ron, E., Modan, B., Preston, D., Alfandary, E., Stovall, M., & Boice, J. D. Jr. Thyroid neoplasia following low-dose radiation in childhood. *Radiat. Res.* 1989; **120**:516–531.
102. Inskip, P. D. Thyroid cancer after radiotherapy for childhood cancer. *Med. Pediatr. Oncol.* 2001; **36**:568–573.
103. Crom, D. B., Kaste, S. C., Tubergen, D. G., Greenwald, C. A., Sharp, G. B., & Hudson, M. M. Ultrasonography for thyroid screening after head and neck irradiation in childhood cancer survivors. *Med. Pediatr. Oncol.* 1997; **28**:15–21.
104. Crowne, E. C., Wallace, W. H., Gibson, S., Moore, C. M., White, A., & Shalet, S. M. Adrenocorticotrophin and cortisol secretion after low dose cranial irradiation. *Clin. Endocrinol. (Oxf.)* 1993; **39**:297–305.
105. Ogilvy-Stuart, A. L., Shalet, S. M. Effect of chemotherapy on growth. *Acta Paediatr.* Suppl 1995; **411**:52–56.
106. Arikoski, P., Komulainen, J., Riikonen, P., Jurvelin, J. S., Voutilainen, R., & Kroger, H. Reduced bone density at completion of chemotherapy for a malignancy. *Arch. Dis. Child.* 1999; **80**:143–148.
107. Shalet, S. M., Gibson, B., Swindell, R., & Pearson, D. Effect of spinal irradiation on growth. *Arch. Dis. Child.* 1987; **62**:461–464.
108. Wallace, W. H., Shalet, S. M., Morris-Jones, P. H., Swindell, R., & Gattamaneni, H. R. Effect of abdominal irradiation on growth in boys treated for a Wilms' tumor. *Med. Pediatr. Oncol.* 1990; **18**:441–446.
109. Riseborough, E. J., Grabias, S. L., Burton, R. I., & Jaffe, N. Skeletal alterations following irradiation for Wilms' tumor: with particular reference to scoliosis and kyphosis. *J. Bone. Joint. Surg. Am.* 1976; **58**:526–536.
110. Rate, W. R., Butler, M. S., Robertson, W. W., Jr, & D'Angio, G. J. Late orthopedic effects in children with Wilms' tumor treated with abdominal irradiation. *Med. Pediatr. Oncol.* 1991; **19**:265–268.
111. Clayton, P. E., Shalet, S. M., Morris-Jones, P. H., & Price, D. A. Growth in children treated for acute lymphoblastic leukaemia. *Lancet* 1988; **1** (8583): 460–462.
112. Schriock, E. A., Schell, M. J., Carter, M., Hustu, O., & Ochs, J. J. Abnormal growth patterns and adult short stature in 115 long-term survivors of childhood leukaemia. *J. Clin. Oncol.* 1991; **9**:400–405.
113. Sklar, C., Mertens, A., Walter, A. *et al.* Final height after treatment for childhood acute lymphoblastic leukaemia: comparison of no cranial irradiation with 1800 and 2400 centigrays of cranial irradiation. *J. Pediatr.* 1993; **123**:59–64.
114. Ahmed, S. F., Wallace, W. H., Crofton, P. M., Wardhaugh, B., Magowan, R., & Kelnar, C. J. Short-term changes in lower leg length in children treated for acute lymphoblastic leukaemia. *J. Pediatr. Endocrinol. Metab.* 1999; **12**:75–80.
115. Hokken-Koelega, A. C., van Doorn, J. W., Hahlen, K. *et al.* Long-term effects of treatment for acute lymphoblastic leukaemia with and without cranial irradiation on growth and puberty: a comparative study. *Pediatr. Res.* 1993; **33**:577–582.
116. Kroger, H., Kotaniemi, A., Kroger, L., & Alhava, E. Development of bone mass and bone density of the spine and femoral neck- a prospective study of 65 children and adolescents. *Bone. Miner.* 1993; **23**:171–182.
117. Arikoski, P., Komulainen, J., Voutilainen, R. *et al.* Reduced bone mineral density in long-term survivors of childhood acute lymphoblastic leukaemia. *J. Pediatr. Hematol. Oncol.* 1998; **20**:234–240.
118. Crofton, P. M., Ahmed, S. F., Wade, J. C. *et al.* Effects of intensive chemotherapy on bone and collagen turnover and the growth hormone axis in children with acute lymphoblastic leukaemia. *J. Clin. Endocrinol. Metab.* 1998; **83**:3121–3129.
119. Gaynon, P. S. & Lustig, R. H. The use of glucocorticoids in acute lymphoblastic leukaemia of childhood. Molecular, cellular, and clinical considerations. *J. Pediatr. Hematol. Oncol.* 1995; **17**:1–12.
120. Uehara, R., Suzuki, Y., & Ichikawa, Y. Methotrexate (MTX) inhibits osteoblastic differentiation in vitro: possible mechanism of MTX osteopathy. *J. Rheumatol.* 2001; **28**:251–256.
121. Halton, J. M., Atkinson, S. A., Fraher, L. *et al.* Mineral homeostasis and bone mass at diagnosis in children with acute lymphoblastic leukaemia. *J. Pediatr.* 1995; **126**:557–564.
122. Muller, H. L., Bueb, K., Bartels, U. *et al.* Obesity after childhood craniopharyngioma – German multi-center study on pre-operative risk factors and quality of life. *Klin. Padiatr.* 2001; **213**:244–249.
123. de Vile, C. J., Grant, D. B., Hayward, R. D., Kendall, B. E., Neville, B. G., & Stanhope, R. Obesity in childhood craniopharyngioma: relation to post-operative hypothalamic damage shown by magnetic resonance imaging. *J. Clin. Endocrinol. Metab.* 1996; **81**:2734–2737.
124. Sklar, C. A., Mertens, A. C., Walter, A. *et al.* Changes in body mass index and prevalence of overweight in survivors of childhood acute lymphoblastic leukaemia: role of cranial irradiation. *Med. Pediatr. Oncol.* 2000; **35**:91–95.
125. Reilly, J. J., Blacklock, C. J., Dale, E., Donaldson, M., & Gibson, B. E. Resting metabolic rate and obesity in childhood acute lymphoblastic leukaemia. *Int. J. Obes. Relat. Metab. Disord.* 1996; **20**:1130–1132.
126. Reilly, J. J., Ventham, J. C., Ralston, J. M., Donaldson, M., & Gibson, B. Reduced energy expenditure in preobese children

treated for acute lymphoblastic leukaemia. *Pediatr. Res.* 1998; **44**:557–562.

127. Odame, I., Reilly, J. J., Gibson, B. E., & Donaldson, M. D. Patterns of obesity in boys and girls after treatment for acute lymphoblastic leukaemia. *Arch. Dis. Child.* 1994; **71**:147–149.
128. Reilly, J. J., Ventham, J. C., Newell, J., Aitchison, T., Wallace, W. H., & Gibson, B. E. Risk factors for excess weight gain in children treated for acute lymphoblastic leukaemia. *Int. J. Obes. Relat. Metab. Disord.* 2000; **24**; 1537–1541.
129. Shaw, M. P., Bath, L. E., Duff, J., Kelnar, C. J., & Wallace, W. H. Obesity in leukaemia survivors: the familial contribution. *Pediatr. Hematol. Oncol.* 2000; **17**:231–237.
130. Reilly, J. J., Brougham, M., Montgomery, C., Richardson, F., Kelly, A., & Gibson, B. E. Effect of glucocorticoid therapy on energy intake in children treated for acute lymphoblastic leukaemia. *J. Clin. Endocrinol. Metab.* 2001; **86**:3742–3745.
131. Truesdell, S., Schwartz, C. L., Clark, E., & Constine, L. S. Cardiovascular effects of cancer. In Schwartz, C. L., Hobbie, W. L., Constine, L. S., & Ruccione, K. S. (eds) *Survivors of Childhood Cancer*. St Louis Mosby, 1994.
132. Hancock, S. L., Tucker, M. A., & Hoppe, R. T. Factors affecting late mortality from heart disease after treatment of Hodgkin's disease. *J. Am. Med. Assoc.* 1993; **270**:1949–1955.
133. Pihkala, J., Saarinen, U. M., Lundstrom, U. *et al.* Myocardial function in children and adolescents after therapy with anthracyclines and chest irradiation. *Eur. J. Cancer.* 1996; 32A:97–103.
134. Sorensen, K., Levitt, G., Bull, C., Chessells, J., & Sullivan, I. Anthracycline dose in childhood acute lymphoblastic leukemia: issues of early survival versus late cardiotoxicity. *J. Clin. Oncol.* 1997; **15**:61–68.
135. Lipshultz, S. E., Lipsitz, S. R., Mone, S. M. *et al.* Female sex and drug dose as risk factors for late cardiotoxic effects of doxorubicin therapy for childhood cancer. *N. Engl. J. Med.* 1995; **332**:1738–1743.
136. Mladosievicova, B., Foltinova, A., Petrasova, H., & Hulin, I. Late effects of anthracycline therapy in childhood on signal-averaged ECG parameters. *Int. J. Mol. Med.* 2000; **5**:411–414.
137. Wexler, L. H., Andrich, M. P., Venzon, D. *et al.* Randomized trial of the cardioprotective agent ICRF-187 in pediatric sarcoma patients treated with doxorubicin. *J. Clin. Oncol.* 1996; **14**:362–372.
138. Nysom, K., Holm, K., Hesse, B. *et al.* Lung function after allogeneic bone marrow transplantation for leukaemia or lymphoma. *Arch. Dis. Child.* 1996; **74**:432–436.
139. O'Driscoll, B. R., Hasleton, P. S., Taylor, P. M., Poulter, L. W., Gattameneni, H. R., & Woodcock, A. A. Active lung fibrosis up to 17 years after chemotherapy with carmustine (BCNU) in childhood. *N. Engl. J. Med.* 1990; **323**:378–382.
140. Skinner, R., Pearson, A. D., English, M. W. *et al.* Risk factors for ifosfamide nephrotoxicity in children. *Lancet* 1996; **348**:578–580.
141. van Hoff, J., Grier, H. E., Douglass, E. C., & Green, D. M. Etoposide, ifosfamide, and cisplatin therapy for refractory childhood solid tumors. Response and toxicity. *Cancer* 1995; **75**:2966–2970.
142. Barclay, K. L. & Yeong, M. L. Actinomycin D associated hepatic veno-occlusive disease – a report of 2 cases. *Pathology* 1994; **26**:257–260.
143. Halonen, P., Mattila, J., Ruuska, T., Salo, M. K., & Makipernaa, A. Liver histology after current intensified therapy for childhood acute lymphoblastic leukemia: microvesicular fatty change and siderosis are the main findings. *Med. Pediatr. Oncol.* 2003; **40**:148–154.
144. De Bruyne, R., Portmann, B., Samyn, B. *et al.* Chronic liver disease related to 6-thioguanine in children with acute lymphoblastic leukaemia. *J. Hepatol.* 2006; **44**:407–410.
145. Eiser, C. Children and cancer. *Pediatr. Rehabil.* 2002; **5**:187–189.
146. Mulhern, R. K., Reddick, W. E., Palmer, S. L. *et al.* Neurocognitive deficits in medulloblastoma survivors and white matter loss. *Ann. Neurol.* 1999; **46**:834–841.
147. Hawkins, M. M., Draper, G. J., & Kingston, J. E. Incidence of second primary tumours among childhood cancer survivors. *Br. J. Cancer.* 1987; **56**:339–347.
148. Hawkins, M. M., Wilson, L. M., Burton, H. S. *et al.* Radiotherapy, alkylating agents, and risk of bone cancer after childhood cancer. *J. Natl. Cancer. Inst.* 1996; **88**:270–278.
149. Tucker, M. A., D'Angio, G. J., Boice, J. D. Jr. *et al.* Bone sarcomas linked to radiotherapy and chemotherapy in children. *N. Engl. J. Med.* 1987; **317**:588–593.
150. Hawkins, M. M., Wilson, L. M., Stovall, M. A. *et al.* Epipodophyllotoxins, alkylating agents, and radiation and risk of secondary leukaemia after childhood cancer. *Br. Med. J.* 1992; **304**:951–958.
151. Tucker, M. A., Meadows, A. T., Boice, J. D. Jr., *et al.* Leukemia after therapy with alkylating agents for childhood cancer. *J. Natl. Cancer. Inst.* 1987; **78**:459–464.
152. Travis, L. B., Hill, D. A., Dores, G. M. *et al.* Breast cancer following radiotherapy and chemotherapy among young women with Hodgkin disease. *J. Am. Med. Assoc.* 2003; **290**:465–475.
153. Swerdlow, A. J., Barber, J. A., Hudson, G. V. *et al.* Risk of second malignancy after Hodgkin's disease in a collaborative British cohort: the relation to age at treatment. *J. Clin. Oncol.* 2000; **18**:498–509.
154. Wallace, W. H., Blacklay, A., Eiser, C. *et al.* Developing strategies for long term follow up of survivors of childhood cancer. *Br. Med. J.* 2001; **323**:271–274.
155. Taylor, A., Hawkins, M., Griffiths, A. *et al.* Long-term follow-up of survivors of childhood cancer in the UK. *Pediatr. Blood Cancer* 2004; **42**:161–168.
156. Wallace, H. & Green, D. *Late Effects of Childhood Cancer*. Arnold, 2004.

58

Neuroblastoma

Joel Shilyansky

Children's Hospital of Wisconsin, Milwaukee, WI, USA

Introduction

The pathological findings of neuroblastoma, a childhood malignancy of neural crest origin, were initially described by James Homer Wright in 1910.[1] Extracranial neuroblastoma may be found anywhere along the sympathetic axis, including the neck, posterior mediastinum, retroperitoneum, adrenals, and pelvis. The seemingly unpredictable character of neuroblastoma has frustrated physicians for nearly a century. However, data collected over the past 40 years through the large cooperative groups, both in the USA and in Europe, has allowed the stratification of patients into risk groups. The risk of neuroblastoma progression may be predicted, based on the age at presentation, stage of disease, histology, and biological markers. By stratifying patients into risk categories, children with good prognosis receive less intensive therapy, minimizing their morbidity, while children with poor prognosis are treated aggressively, in order to achieve long-term survival.

Presentation

The presentation of neuroblastoma varies with age and stage of disease. Newborns may present with an asymptomatic mass or with paraplegia. Infants may present with skin metastases or abdominal distention secondary to liver metastases and resultant hepatomegaly (stage 4S). Children with early stage (1 or 2) tumors are usually well and present with a mass found by a family member, an examining physician, or noted incidentally on a radiological examination. In contrast, children with advanced disease usually present with a lingering illness lasting 1–3 weeks and a mass found either by family or physician. Occasionally, children may present with lower extremity weakness resulting from impingement of the spinal cord by tumor. Neuroblastoma metastases to the retro-orbital space may present as "raccoon eyes" or bruising around the eyes. Children with neuroblastoma may also develop opsoclonus–myoclonus–ataxia (OMA), an autoimmune syndrome characterized by cerebellar dysfunction. Neuroblastoma is a disease of early childhood with peak incidence between 2 and 4 years of age. Greater than 70% of patients are less than 5 years old at presentation. Neuroblastoma presenting in infancy usually has a good prognosis, while children greater than 12 months old most commonly have advanced disease.

Diagnosis

The diagnosis of neuroblastoma is usually based on characteristic histological findings. While histological diagnosis is generally required, the diagnosis of neuroblastoma is suspected in children with malaise, mediastinal or retroperitoneal mass, and elevated urine catecholamines, vanillylmandelic acid (VMA) or homovanillic acid (HVA). Computed tomography (CT), bone scan and bone marrow biopsy are recommended to establish the diagnosis and to stage neuroblastoma.[2] Metaiodobenzylguanidine (MIBG), which is taken up by 90% of neuroblastomas is increasingly used as a diagnostic modality.

Prognosis

Treatment of children with neuroblastoma is based on risk of disease progression. Age, stage of disease,

Pediatric Surgery and Urology: Long-term Outcomes, Mark Stringer, Keith Oldham, Pierre Mouriquand.
Published by Cambridge University Press.

histopathological classification and biological markers are used to predict prognosis. Patients are grouped into low, intermediate, and poor prognostic groups.

Staging

Several staging schemes for neuroblastoma have been previously devised. In recent years, most institutions have adopted the International Neuroblastoma Staging System (INSS).[3,4] The staging system is based on extent of local disease, as well as regional and distal spread.

Stage 1 disease is localized, does not cross the midline, and is grossly excised. Microscopic residual disease may be present. Non-adherent lymph nodes may not contain tumor, but resected adherent nodes may contain metastases.

Stage 2 disease is either incompletely resected localized tumor without spread to non-adherent ipsilateral lymph nodes (2A), or localized tumor with spread to ipsilateral but not contralateral lymph nodes (2B).

Stage 3 neuroblastoma is unresectable tumor crossing the midline, spread to contralateral lymph nodes or central tumor with bilateral lymph node involvement.

Stage 4 neuroblastoma is associated with dissemination to distant lymph nodes, bone, bone marrow or other organs.

Stage 4S neuroblastoma, initially described by D'Angio, Evans, and Koop in 1971,[5] is unique to children less than 12 months old, who have stage 1 or 2 primary tumor with remote dissemination to liver, skin and/or bone marrow (but not bone). Less than 10% of the bone marrow may be replaced with tumor.

Histopathological classification

The International Neuroblastoma Pathology Classification (INPC), which is based on a classification system devised by Shimada *et al.* in 1984, standardizes the reporting and prognostic evaluation of histological features of neuroblastoma.[6–8] The classification quantifies the degree of cellular differentiation, atypia, mitosis and death. Neuroblastoma is distinguished from ganglioneuroma by stroma-poor appearance. The neuroblastic cells form nests of cells known as Homer Wright rosettes. The differentiation of neuroblastoma is defined based on the proportion of cells exhibiting morphological features of developing ganglion cells. The undifferentiated neuroblastoma cells are small, have a thin or indiscernible rim of cytoplasm, hyperchromatic nuclei with distinct nucleoli and lack neuropil (thin neuritic processes). Increasing frequency of neuroblasts resembling differentiating ganglion cells and the presence of neuropil are associated with increasingly differentiated neuroblastoma. The mitosis–karyorrhexis index (MKI) is defined as the number of tumor cells in mitosis and in process of karyorrhexis (cell death). High MKI correlates with adverse clinical outcome in patients with neuroblastoma.

Biological markers

Genetic markers that predict survival in cancer patients have been sought in recent years. Amplification of the oncogene NMYC, which leads to excess NMYC protein, correlates with the poorly differentiated subtype of neuroblastoma, and is associated with dramatically worse survival in children with neuroblastoma.[9,10] Complexed with Max, NMYC protein inhibits differentiation and promotes proliferation as well as apoptosis, possibly explaining the correlation between NMYC amplification and high MKI. DNA content also correlates with patient prognosis and is used to determine the risk of neuroblastoma progression. Predominantly diploid tumors have a worse prognosis than either aneuploid or hyperdiploid tumors. Additional biological markers are: (1) the neurotrophin receptor Trk-A, which is associated with hyperdiploid DNA content and spontaneous tumor regression, (2) the neurotrophin Trk-B, which is associated with loss of heterozygosity (LOH) at chromosome 14q, gain of chromosome 17q and poor prognosis, as well as (3) LOH at chromosome 1p, which is associated with NMYC amplification and poor prognosis.

Treatment and survival

Currently in North America, the treatment of neuroblastoma is based on the Children's Oncology Group (COG) risk stratification described in Table 58.1.[4] In the past there was great variability in the treatment of children with neuroblastoma and some differences still exist between the approach in North America and in Europe and Australia. COG stratifies patients based on the risk of neuroblastoma progression and mortality, and emphasizes a multidisciplinary approach to treatment. Children are assigned to a low-risk, intermediate-risk or high-risk group based on age, stage, NMYC status, ploidy (DNA content) and histopathological classification (INPC). Initial surgical exploration is performed in nearly all patients in order to establish the diagnosis, obtain tissue for biological characterization, sample regional lymph nodes, and attempt safe resection. Patients with symptomatic involvement of the spinal

Table 58.1. Children's Oncology Group neuroblastoma risk group assignment scheme[a4]

INSS stage	Age	NMYC status	Shimada histology	DNA ploidy	Risk group
I	0–21y	Any	Any	Any	Low
IIA/IIB[b]	<1y	Any	Any	Any	Low
	≥1y	NonAmp	Any	–	Low
	≥1y	Amp	Favorable	–	Low
	≥1y	Amp	Unfavorable	–	High
III[d]	<1y	NonAmp	Any	Any	Intermediate
	<1y	Amp	Any	Any	High
	≥1y	NonAmp	Favorable	–	Intermediate
	≥1y	NonAmp	Unfavorable	–	High
	≥1y	Amp	Any	–	High
IV[d]	<1y	NonAmp	Any	Any	Intermediate
	<1y	Amp	Any	Any	High
	≥1y	Any	Any	–	High
4S[c]	<1y	NonAmp	Favorable	>1	Low
	<1y	NonAmp	Any	=1	Intermediate
	<1y	NonAmp	Unfavorable	Any	Intermediate
	<1y	Amp	Any	Any	High
Biology defined by:	*NMYC* Status: amplified (Amp) vs. non-amplified (NonAmp) Shimada histopathology: favorable vs. unfavorable DNA Ploidy: DNA Index (DI); diploid = 1; hypodiploid tumors (DI < 1) will be treated as hyperdiploid tumors (DI > 1); DI < 1 or > 1 considered favorable; DI = 1 unfavorable.				

[a] Reprinted by permission from COG.
[b] INSS 2A/2B symptomatic patients with spinal cord compression, neurologic deficits, or other symptoms are treated on the low risk neuroblastoma study with immediate chemotherapy for four cycles.
[c] INSS 4S infants with favorable biology and clinical symptoms are treated on the low risk neuroblastoma study with immediate chemotherapy until asymptomatic (2–4 cycles). Clinical symptoms defined as: respiratory distress with or without hepatomegaly or cord compression and neurologic deficit or inferior vena cava compression and renal ischemia; or genitourinary obstruction; or gastrointestinal obstruction and vomiting; or coagulopathy with significant clinical hemorrhage unresponsive to replacement therapy.
[d] INSS 3 or 4 patients with clinical symptoms as above (or if in the investigator's opinion it is in the best interest of the patient) will receive immediate chemotherapy.

cord or with symptomatic 4S disease may be treated with chemotherapy without establishing tissue diagnosis.

Low risk

Low-risk patients are primarily treated with observation (stage 4S) or surgery (stage 1/2). The goal of surgery is to establish the diagnosis of neuroblastoma and to extirpate stage 1 and stage 2 tumors. Chemotherapy is reserved for symptomatic patients with spinal cord compression and stage 4S patients with respiratory compromise secondary to hepatic infiltration. The chemotherapy consists of low dose carboplatin, cyclophosphamide, doxorubicin and etoposide for 6–12 weeks, in order to minimize long-term deleterious effects of the regimen. Children with asymptomatic stage 4S neuroblastoma receiving supportive care only may expect 100% survival. While still investigational, Stage 1 adrenal neuroblastoma without involvement of the spinal canal diagnosed perinatally may be observed without resection or chemotherapy. Children in the low-risk group have greater than 90% expected survival at three years.

Intermediate risk

Intermediate-risk patients are treated with surgery and 12–24 weeks of chemotherapy, using the same regimen as for the low-risk group. The role of surgery is to establish the diagnosis at presentation. Following chemotherapy, surgical resection is recommended. Achieving complete gross or even partial resection correlates with improved survival compared to biopsy alone. However, sacrificing adjacent structures is not recommended since survival of patients undergoing complete and partial resection is equivalent. At 3 years, 70–90% survival is expected for children in the intermediate-risk group.

High risk

High-risk patients are usually not amenable to surgical resection and undergo biopsy followed by aggressive high dose chemotherapy. In addition to the agents described above, ifosfamide and high dose cisplatin are added. Patients responding to chemotherapy undergo surgical exploration and resection of residual primary tumor. Metastatic sites and primary tumor (whether or not resected) undergo irradiation. Patients rendered grossly disease free, may undergo myeloablative therapy and autologous stem cell transplantation. Experimental adjuvant therapy with oral 13-*cis*-retinoic acid and anti-GD2 monoclonal antibody therapy may also be provided.[4] The expected survival for children in the high-risk group is 30% at 3 years. Intensification of the chemotherapy provided, myeloablation and autologous stem cell transplantation, including tandem transplants has increased the incidence of remission and short-term survival to greater than 50%; however, the incidence and severity of hematologic toxicity is also greatly increased.[11–13]

Recurrent neuroblastoma

Recurrent neuroblastoma is treated based on initial risk stratification, patient age, extent of recurrent disease, and tumor biology at the time of recurrence.[4] Local and regional recurrences in children initially classified as low risk are resected with the expectation of long-term survival. If complete resection is not feasible, or recurrent tumor has unfavorable biological characteristics, 12–24 weeks of chemotherapy are added. Older children with unfavorable histology or NMYC amplification require aggressive chemotherapy and possibly myeloablative therapy and stem cell transplantation.[14] Recurrent disease in children initially classified as intermediate-risk is treated with surgery followed by chemotherapy. Neuroblastoma progression, recurrence or metastases, occurring while on chemotherapy or within 3 months of treatment are associated with a poor prognosis, and require aggressive regimens using multidrug chemotherapy, myeloablative therapy and stem cell transplantation. Recurrent neuroblastoma in the high-risk patients carries a poor prognosis. Failure of aggressive chemotherapy, myeloablation and stem cell transplantation to prevent recurrence or disease progression in children initially classified as high-risk warrants phase I or phase II experimental therapy. The outcomes of 31 children with recurrent disease treated at the Hospital for Sick Children in Toronto were retrospectively reviewed.[15] The report suggests that salvage therapy prolongs survival modestly; however, NMYC amplification and early relapse following stem cell transplantation portend a dismal prognosis, with median survival of 2–3 months.

Mass screening

Mass screening for neuroblastoma has been suggested to identify patients with early disease in order to prevent progression. Mass screening however has failed to reduce the incidence of advanced disease and is currently not recommended. The German Neuroblastoma Screening Project investigated the utility of mass screening for neuroblastoma.[16] The study found that screening at 6 months of age did not reduce the frequency of poor prognosis neuroblastoma, did not identify poor prognosis tumors, and did not affect survival. While an increased prevalence of disease was found in the cohort that underwent screening, it was likely due to identification of tumors that would spontaneously undergo maturation and never become clinically apparent. Long-term follow-up of Japanese children treated for neuroblastoma, identified by screening at 1 year of age, demonstrated a recurrence in 6 of 245 patients, 2 deaths related to therapy and only 1 death due to disease.[17] The disease-related death resulted from a tumor with NMYC amplification and unfavorable histology. Failure of mass screening to identify patients in the high-risk group early, suggests that neuroblastomas whose biological characteristics are associated with poor prognosis develop *de novo*, usually later in childhood.

Early morbidity

The COG treatment schema outlined above is based on risk stratification as defined in previous studies. It is designed to reduce neuroblastoma-related mortality and achieve long lasting remission. In addition, this approach aims to minimize treatment-related morbidity, especially in the low and intermediate risk groups. Early morbidity may be categorized as disease and treatment related.[4]

Tumor-related factors

Infants with 4S neuroblastoma can present with respiratory embarrassment, hepatic insufficiency and cardiopulmonary dysfunction due to compression of the inferior vena cava and decreased venous return. Large primary tumors may compress renal vessels leading to hypertension or obstruct the ureters leading to hydronephrosis and renal atrophy. Primary tumors, especially thoracic neuroblastoma, can extend into the spinous foramina, encroach on the spinal canal and cause paralysis, incontinence and altered sensorium. Neuroblastoma may be hormonally active and produce dopamine or epinephrine leading to hypertension.

Treatment-related factors

Surgery

Large retroperitoneal neuroblastomas may encircle the renal vessels, aorta, cava and mesenteric vessels. Early morbidity and mortality from surgical intervention are related principally to bleeding. Excision of large retroperitoneal tumors can put the kidneys at risk. Resection of cervical or upper thoracic tumors may be associated with Horner's syndrome due to disruption of the sympathetic innervation to the head and neck. Laminectomy aimed at resecting neuroblastomas entering the spinal canal can lead to spinal instability and progressive kyphoscoliosis. Resection of pelvic tumors may injure the pelvic parasympathetics or sacral nerve roots, compromising continence and sexual function.

Chemotherapy

Morbidity related to chemotherapy for the treatment of neuroblastoma is nearly universal (Table 58.2). The severity of chemotherapy-related early morbidity is related to the mechanism of action of the drugs and the intensity of the regimen. The majority of early morbidity is related to loss of hematopoietic cell precursors, which leads to immune compromise and increased susceptibility to infections as well as thrombocytopenia and bleeding complications. In most patients the restoration of bone marrow, either spontaneously or by transplantation, leads to eventual recovery. Loss of gastrointestinal mucosal barrier results in compromise of nutrient absorption and barrier function. Renal, neurological and cardiac toxicity may also result from chemotherapy, and may not be reversible.

Radiation therapy

Radiation therapy and chemotherapy have synergistic bone marrow toxicity. Additional morbidity associated with radiation therapy results from direct tissue injury, particularly radiation burns to the skin, microvascular injury to the gastrointestinal tract, pulmonary fibrosis, cardiac dysfunction and developmental delay. Irradiation of bony structures prevents subsequent growth and results in bony deformities.

Table 58.2. Common chemotherapy agents associated with late therapy-related morbidity[a]

Agent/agent class/modality	Affected body system
Anthracyclines	Circulatory (cardiac) Respiratory (pulmonary)
Alkylating agents	Reproductive (gonadal) Second malignant neoplasms
Topoisomerase II inhibitors	Second malignant neoplasms
Platinums	Urinary (renal) Special senses (hearing) Second malignant neoplasms
Corticosteroids	Central nervous system Musculoskeletal (bone and body composition) Musculoskeletal (obesity)
Intrathecal chemotherapy	Central nervous system
Bleomycin	Respiratory (pulmonary)
Methotrexate	Central nervous system
Vincristine	Digestive (dental)
Thioguanine	Digestive (hepatic)

[a] Reprinted by permission from NCI.

Long-term outcome of neuroblastoma treatment

Long-term survivors of neuroblastoma continue to face both tumor and treatment-related complications, and are at an increased risk of early death. The leading causes of death among childhood cancer survivors living at least 5 years after their diagnosis are recurrence, second cancers and cardiac toxicity.[18] Tumor-related factors, such as the site and biological characteristics, and patient-related factors, such as age and comorbidities, dictate the long-term results of neuroblastoma treatment. Additionally, each therapeutic modality, surgery, chemotherapy, radiation therapy, and stem cell transplantation have long-term persistent consequences.

Patient- and disease-related factors

Neuroblastoma in neonates and infants

Neonatal neuroblastoma

Defined as disease presenting in the first 3 months of life, neonatal neuroblastoma may be diagnosed antenatally and has an excellent overall survival.[19–21] Neonates most commonly present with stage I or 4S disease. The United Kingdom Children's Oncology Study Group reported the treatment outcome in 33 neonates. There were three deaths, of which one infant was stillborn, one death resulted from chemotherapy toxicity, and one was unrelated to disease. Four of six (67%) children with intraspinal extension of neuroblastoma had persistent disability, which included paresis, scoliosis, incontinence and abnormal sweating. This incidence is significantly greater than in older children with intraspinal tumor extension (15%). Additionally, kidney infarction as well as chemotherapy-related ototoxicity and learning deficits were encountered. Since neonates are exceptionally vulnerable to morbidity associated with therapy, conservative management aimed at controlling symptoms is associated with improved outcomes. The finding that tumor-related disability present at birth is often not reversible, and the observation that most of these patients present with biologically favorable tumors, justify a conservative surgical approach in neonates.

Infants

Infants less than 1 year of age most commonly present with localized neuroblastoma. Primary gross resection of localized tumors is associated with an excellent chance of survival. However, surgical treatment of neuroblastoma in infants has a 20% complication rate, which includes Horner's, chylous ascites, pleural effusions, scoliosis, renal injury, injury to phrenic nerve, and bowel obstruction.[22] Complications often result from attempted resection of large primary tumors. Primary chemotherapy for stage III neuroblastoma can reduce tumor size in order to achieve resectability and high likelihood of survival. While such an approach may reduce surgical morbidity, chemotherapy-related complications are still substantial in this age group. To determine the efficacy of low dose chemotherapy, 134 localized neuroblastoma patients less than 1 year old, enrolled in the French Society of Pediatric Oncology treatment protocol, were reviewed retrospectively.[23] Eighty-two underwent primary surgical excision. Thirty-nine infants had unresectable tumors (stage III) and no NMYC amplification (intermediate risk group). Low-dose chemotherapy, without anthracyclins, achieved a response allowing surgical resection in 50% of patients. The remaining patients went on to standard chemotherapy and surgery. No deaths or metastases and four local relapses were observed. The local relapses were treated with chemotherapy and surgery leading to remission in each case. The Italian Cooperative Group also reported favorable results (91% overall survival at 5 years) treating unresectable tumors in infants with primary standard chemotherapy regimen followed by resection. Multivariate analysis suggested that only NMYC amplification was an independent predictor of poor outcome.[24] Multimodality therapy, including conservative surgery and chemotherapy, is likely to yield a high rate of survival and decrease morbidity in infants presenting with localized neuroblastoma without NMYC amplification.

4S neuroblastoma

4S neuroblastoma often spontaneously undergoes maturation and involution. Between 70% and 90% survival is expected for children with stage 4S disease. Most deaths occur early as a result of liver infiltration leading to pulmonary insufficiency, compression of the vena cava and renal insufficiency. Thirty-one patients treated over 26 years at the Hospital for Children in London were reviewed retrospectively.[25] Six patients died from progressive disease. Twenty-five patients were alive and 20 had no abnormal clinical findings. Three patients had abnormalities related to their original tumor, including subcutaneous nodules and neurological symptoms secondary to residual mass. Treatment-related abnormalities were found in three patients, including small testes, urethral strictures, musculoskeletal hypoplasia, and Horner's syndrome. Imaging revealed adrenal calcifications suggesting involution of primary tumors. The primary tumor was resected in five patients and persisted in three additional patients. Altered hepatic architecture as suggested by coarse echogenicity, atrophy of the left lobe, and a mass were noted on ultrasound examination. The use of supportive care for asymptomatic infants, and low dose chemotherapy and radiation therapy for infants with respiratory or renal compromise were studied prospectively.[26] Overall and disease-free survival were 92.5% and 86%. Deaths occurred in 7.5% of infants from progressive or unresponsive disease resulting in respiratory embarrassment or disseminated intravascular coagulopathy (DIC), all in children less than 2 months. Although uncommon in children with 4S neuroblastoma, late recurrence resulting in death has been reported.[27] Resection of primary tumor in infants with 4S neuroblastoma was not found to alter local relapse, event-free survival or overall survival in a retrospective review of data from multiple institutions in Italy.[28] Supportive care for asymptomatic patients and low-dose chemotherapy for patients with respiratory, renal, or neurological symptoms appear to achieve high cure rates with low associated morbidity. Only patients with amplified NMYC or local tumor growth despite appropriate chemotherapy may benefit from early surgical intervention.[29] Long-term follow-up is necessary in all patients, since late recurrences, while infrequent, can occur.

Neuroblastoma in adolescents and adults

Neuroblastoma is rare in adolescents and young adults. Thirty patients treated at Memorial Sloan-Kettering were studied retrospectively.[30] None of the tested patients had NMYC amplification but all the tumors available for evaluation had unfavorable Shimada classification. Despite aggressive high-dose chemotherapy, the overall survival was less than 40%. Similar results were reported by the French Society of Pediatric Oncology.[31] Adolescents presenting with stage I/II disease were uniformly cured. Most patients presenting with stage III disease had an indolent but progressive course despite aggressive chemotherapy. Those presenting with stage IV disease had a dismal prognosis.

Advanced neuroblastoma

The majority of children older than 1 year will present with advanced neuroblastoma (stage 3 and 4). For Stage 3 neuroblastoma the long-term results of therapy are predicted by histopathological findings and the presence of NMYC amplification.[32] The role of surgical resection in the treatment of advanced neuroblastoma remains controversial, however. In a retrospective review of patients with stage III neuroblastoma, the pattern of late treatment failures was examined. While local recurrences in the tumor bed and in the lymph nodes outside the initial radiation treatment field were identified, distant spread was also found in each case. The findings suggest that control of metastatic disease, not aggressive surgery or expansion of the radiation field to control local recurrence, is required to improve survival. Nonetheless, complete gross resection of primary tumor, possibly with additional radiation therapy, was suggested in some retrospective studies to be associated with improved survival in children with advanced neuroblastoma.[33,34] A retrospective review of 2251 patients treated in the German Cooperative Neuroblastoma Studies suggested that event-free survival was greater if children older than 1 year presenting with localized neuroblastoma underwent complete or partial resection compared to biopsy alone.[29] Similarly, a correlation between resection of primary tumor and survival was noted in patients with stage IV disease. In a retrospective review, the authors reported approximately 50% survival in 29 patients with advanced (stage 3 and 4) disease and complete gross resection. In a multi-institutional non-controlled, non-randomized prospective study from Spain, a correlation between resection (both complete and incomplete) and survival was noted.[35] Patients who underwent biopsy alone, who did not respond to induction chemotherapy, or who did not undergo resection had shorter disease-free and overall survival. Greater risk of recurrence was noted in patients whose tumors had NMYC amplification. A retrospective review of 141 stage 4 neuroblastoma patients treated at Memorial Sloan Kettering Cancer Center in New York also suggested improved local control and survival in patients who underwent gross tumor resection compared to patients who were not candidates for resection.[36] Taken together, these studies suggest that resection is a marker of favorable biological behavior and response to chemotherapy by the tumor. It is not clear whether resection of primary tumor in patients with advanced neuroblastoma alters survival, as survival is dependent on control of systemic disease. Resection, however, controls symptoms related to local tumor growth. These findings support a conservative approach to primary tumor resection and do not justify sacrificing adjacent or critical structures to achieve a complete gross resection.

Palliation

Surgery and radiation therapy may be used for palliation of local symptoms in patients with advanced neuroblastoma. Enlarging, unresected tumors may have a deleterious effect on patient quality of life due to local tissue compromise. Palliative surgery and radiotherapy for advanced neuroblastoma can reduce the size of a soft tissue mass and provide relief from local discomfort, shrink liver metastases and decrease abdominal distention, relieve respiratory compromise, improve bone pain, and relieve neurological impairment secondary to brain metastases.[37]

Transplantation

Myeloablation and stem cell (or bone marrow) transplantation can achieve remission in patients with advanced neuroblastoma and NMYC amplification. However, such therapy is often complicated by immune compromise, anemia, and bleeding complications due to prolonged hematopoietic insufficiency. The clinical course of 23 patients with neuroblastoma treated with $CD34^+$ cell transplantation in a French multicenter trial was reviewed.[38] Neutropenia and thrombocytopenia resolved a median of 13 and 59 days after transplant. T-cells, especially $CD4^+$ T-cells, were not fully restored for 6 months; B-cells and NK cells were not restored for more than a month. At 1 year, 16 patients were alive and could be evaluated. There were six events of severe sepsis, six severe Varicella Zoster virus infections, and two EBV associated lymphomas. Additionally, individual episodes of CMV infection, HSV infection, and lymphocytic meningitis were documented. Interstitial pneumonitis affected three patients. Thirteen patients (56%) were alive with a median follow-up of 40 months. Of the ten deaths, eight were due to relapse, one was due to severe pneumonitis and one was due to secondary AML, which was found 3 years following transplant. Review of 22 patients treated in accord with the German National Protocol NB90 and NB 97, followed by high-dose chemotherapy, myeloablation (melphalan), CD34$^+$ stem cell transplantation and anti-GD2 immunotherapy, demonstrated 45% disease-free survival with a median follow-up of 55 months.[39] Nine patients died of disease, two have relapsed but were alive, and one died of secondary AML. Review of neuroblastoma patients treated similarly in a Spanish trial suggested improved initial, but not long-term results.[11] Recently, improved short-term survival following tandem and triple transplants was reported in a highly selected group of neuroblastoma patients with poor prognosis.[13] The long-term outcome of such treatment is not yet clear.

Thoracic neuroblastoma

Thoracic neuroblastoma is considered to have a better overall prognosis, but the primary site is not an independent prognostic factor. The overall survival of children with thoracic neuroblastoma in the German Cooperative Study NBL90 was 77%.[40] Complete tumor resection was achieved in 70% of patients either at initial exploration or upon second look examination. Incomplete resection did not impact on survival significantly. Surgical complications were noted in 20% of children. Horner's syndrome, pulmonary complications, chylothorax, and bleeding most commonly complicate attempted resection of thoracic neuroblastoma. In 40% of thoracic neuroblastomas, the tumor extends into the spinal canal. Patients may suffer neurologic compromise either secondary to dumbbell tumors compressing the spinal cord or as a result of attempted resection. Injury to the phrenic and vagus nerves may follow surgical resection or result from tumor compression. Spinal deformities are associated with laminectomy, radiation therapy and paraplegia. Multidisciplinary approach to treatment including conservative surgery and chemotherapy results in the best chances of survival while minimizing long-term morbidity, in patients with thoracic neuroblastoma and in the absence of NMYC amplification.

Pelvic neuroblastoma

Children with localized pelvic neuroblastoma carry a relatively good prognosis, although it is not clear that pelvic location is an independent prognostic factor.[41] Large tumors at presentation, NMYC amplification and nodal spread correlate with worse prognosis. The presence of residual disease does not affect outcome. Children with pelvic neuroblastoma have a high rate of neurological complications. A review of the experience of the French Society of Pediatric Oncology Group demonstrated that 14 patients (30%) presented with neurological impairment, including urinary retention, incontinence, constipation and lower extremity dysasthesia or weakness. Following treatment neurological symptoms resolved in ten children; however, three additional children developed neurological deficits related to surgical intervention. Similar to thoracic tumors, a multidisciplinary conservative approach to treatment of pelvic neuroblastoma is expected to produce long-term survival, while minimizing morbidity.

Intraspinal extension of neuroblastoma

Intraspinal extension of neuroblastoma is common and can lead to significant long-term morbidity secondary to compression of the spinal cord and the nerve roots, or due to bony deformities resulting from radiation therapy and laminectomy. Twenty-six patients treated for symptomatic intraspinal extension of neuroblastoma in two large US children's hospitals were retrospectively reviewed.[42] Fifteen patients were treated with laminectomy. Nine patients, including three with paraplegia, had recovery of neurologic function. Nine of the 15 developed kyphoscoliosis, although most severe deformities were limited to paraplegic patients. Of the eight patients with spinal cord compression treated without laminectomy, only three had recovery of function. Three patients had scoliosis, all with paraplegia. Of note, newborns who presented with paraplegia did not recover neurological function. The French Society of Pediatric Oncology reported a prospective non-randomized study of chemotherapy and selective surgery for intraspinal extension of neuroblastoma.[43] Forty-two patients with intraspinal extension were identified, 27 had neurological symptoms. Patients with rapid onset of neurological symptoms, or with deterioration while on chemotherapy, underwent emergent surgical decompression with complete recovery of the neurological deficit (5/5 children). Patients without symptoms or with stable long-standing deficits were initially treated with chemotherapy. The intraspinal component of the tumor regressed in approximately 50% of patients. Secondary surgical resection was performed in 10 of 19 children. Complete recovery of neurological deficit was documented in 12 patients, partial recovery in three patients and no recovery in four patients. Of note, three of four children with persistent neurological deficit were neonates born with paraplegia, a circumstance where recovery is unlikely. One child had severe cervical kyphoscoliosis requiring surgery and five children had mild scoliosis, which did not require intervention. The study suggests that initial chemotherapy is safe in children with stable long-standing neurological deficits. Restoration of neurological function may be expected in more than half of the children. Urgent surgical resection of intraspinal tumor restored neurological function in children with progression or new onset of neurological deficit. The experience in 22 hospitals in Italy was reviewed retrospectively in order to assess the outcome of treatment for spinal cord compression in 76 children with neuroblastoma.[44] There were 54 long-term survivors, of whom 44% had persistent observable deficits, including scoliosis (33%), anal sphincter dysfunction (28%), paraparesis (14%), and paraplegia (19%). No difference in the incidence of persistent neurological deficits was noted between patients treated with primary laminectomy, radiation therapy or chemotherapy for spinal cord compression. Retrospective review of children with intraspinal extension of neuroblastoma treated by Pediatric Oncology Group (POG) institutions in the US also suggested that chemotherapy effectively treated the intraspinal component of neuroblastoma, either reducing the extent or eliminating the need for laminectomy.[45] Taken together, these studies suggest that judicious selective spinal decompression in children with neuroblastoma may reduce the risk of spinal deformities associated with extensive laminectomies in young children, especially in the cervical region, without compromising neurological recovery. Patients presenting with rapidly progressive neurological symptoms or worsening deficit despite chemotherapy, should be referred for emergent surgical management and most may expect recovery of function.

Opsoclonus–myoclonus–ataxia

The opsoclonus–myoclonus–ataxia syndrome (OMA) is a paraneoplastic neurologic syndrome affecting 2–3% of children with neuroblastoma.[46,47] While children with OMA have higher 5-year survival, they may experience multiple locoregional recurrences and debilitating neurologic impairment, which is likely to be immune mediated. Children with OMA exhibit persistent opsoclonus, characterized by chaotic eye movements, myoclonus, characterized by brief jerking muscle spasms, and ataxia, characterized by unsteady, trembling gait, as well as dysarthria and hypotonia. Motor function, speech and cognition are often severely affected. Treatment with corticosteroids, ACTH, intravenous gamma globulin and chemotherapy produces responses in over 70% of children, but symptoms recur frequently and lead to long-term disability in most cases.[14]

Treatment-related factors

Secondary neoplasm

Increasingly aggressive regimens for the treatment of neuroblastoma have improved survival, but are likely to increase the incidence of secondary malignancies. The use of radiation therapy and chemotherapy correlates most strongly with the risk of secondary malignancy.[32] Imperfect repair of DNA strand damage caused by radiation therapy, especially at the margins of the radiation field, leads to inactivation of tumor suppressor genes and malignant transformation. The risk of malignancy is greater in younger patients, five- to tenfold greater in children less than 5 years old, than in the entire population of cancer survivors. The latent period after radiation therapy is 8–15 years, and children treated with lower doses have a longer latent period. Chemotherapeutic agents can promote DNA breaks, deletions and translocations. The risk of chemotherapy-related malignancies plateaus at 5 years following diagnosis of primary tumor. Chemotherapy and radiation therapy may synergize, increasing the risk of secondary malignancy, particularly in genetically predisposed patients. Patients treated with myeloablation and bone marrow or stem cell transplantation are at a particularly high risk for secondary malignancies due to the intensity of the therapy administered and failure of immune surveillance.

Early development of leukemias and lymphomas in children treated for cancer has been well documented.[48] Secondary leukemias such as AML are associated with radiation therapy and chemotherapy with topoisomerase II inhibitors (epipodophyllotoxins such as etoposide) or alkylating agents, and have a poor prognosis. Epipodophyllotoxin-related leukemias have a short latency period and are characterized by balanced translocations involving chromosome 11q23 or 21q22. Alkylating agents produce unbalanced cytogenetic abnormalities often involving chromosome 5 and 7.

With increasing follow-up, the incidence of secondary solid tumors continues to rise.[49] The true rate of second malignancy following treatment for neuroblastoma is not yet known.[4] Methodology to calculate incidence can affect the estimated risk of second cancer. For example, since the propensity to develop breast cancer rises with age in the general population, the risk data needs to be normalized to the age of patients at the time of the second diagnosis.[50] In a retrospective analysis of 73 neuroblastoma patients listed in the database from the Long Term Survivors Clinic at The National Children's Hospital, 2 (2.7%) had secondary malignancies. This risk is consistent with secondary cancer rate in the overall population of survivors of childhood cancer.[51,52]

Central nervous system (CNS) tumors, soft tissue sarcomas, osteosarcomas, as well as thyroid, parotid gland, and breast carcinomas have been reported in long-term survivors of childhood cancers. Thyroid carcinoma is associated with radiation therapy in childhood with a latent period that may be as long as 30–40 years. Neuroblastoma patients have a fivefold greater incidence of thyroid cancer compared to other childhood cancer survivors, even when controlled for treatment modalities. Breast cancer is the second most common cancer in survivors of neuroblastoma. Incidence of central nervous system (CNS) neoplasms, meningiomas, astrocytomas, gliomas, and sarcomas is increased up to 20-fold and is associated with radiation therapy. Children under 5 years old and bone marrow transplant survivors are at greatest risk for aggressive secondary CNS tumors. Head and neck squamous cell carcinomas are uncommon in children, but have been reported as secondary malignancies. Head and neck irradiation and chemotherapy with alkylating agents have been implicated in their pathogenesis. Soft tissue sarcomas (STS) usually arise in irradiated areas in survivors of childhood cancers with a median latent period of 8 years. Chemotherapy increases the risk of developing STS. The 20-year cumulative risk of STS in patients with neuroblastoma is 1%.[53] STS should be treated as de novo pediatric sarcomas.[54]

Retrospective review of 544 neuroblastoma patients surviving more than 5 years and treated in Britain and France over a 42-year period revealed 13 secondary malignancies, including thyroid carcinoma,[5] breast carcinoma,[3] glioblastoma, osteosarcoma and ALL, a cumulative incidence of 2.2%.[55] The patients reviewed in this study were treated prior to the advent of high intensity chemotherapy and few[11] underwent bone marrow or stem cell transplantation. Long-term survivors most likely had more favorable prognosis and received less therapy. As a result the selection bias may have caused the authors to underestimate the risk of secondary malignancy. Nonetheless, the cumulative risk of secondary malignancy was greater in patients receiving chemotherapy or radiation therapy compared to either the general population or neuroblastoma survivors who did not receive such therapy. In a review of patients treated for neuroblastoma at Memorial Sloan Kettering Cancer Center, the incidence of AML was 7% within 3 years following high dose chemotherapy regimen, and 11% following treatment for recurrence, a significant increase over previous reports.[48,56]

An alternative method for delivering radiation to neuroblastoma in high-risk patients is treatment with ^{131}I-MIBG, which is preferentially concentrated in neuroblastoma tissue. However, thyroid dysfunction in two-thirds of children, despite prophylactic treatment with potassium iodide, suggests that normal tissues are also exposed to radioactivity.[57] Retrospective review of 119 patients treated with ^{131}I-MIBG for neuroblastoma revealed 5 secondary malignancies.[58] The finding was striking since the survival in this group of patients was less than 11% at 15 years. The high frequency of secondary malignancy may be attributed to high stage and consequently high intensity therapy provided to these patients.

A second malignancy is a feared and demoralizing complication of neuroblastoma treatment. The risk of second malignancy is increased with prolonged use and high doses of alkylating agents, topoisomerase II inhibitors and anthracyclins, especially in combination with radiation therapy. Defining the risk of neuroblastoma progression allows reduction in the intensity of therapy for good prognosis patients, decreasing the risk of secondary malignancies without compromising survival. In the poor prognosis group, rapid cytoreduction using shorter high dose chemotherapy regimens combined with surgical resection of residual disease may achieve high rates of remission, yet lead to fewer secondary cancers.[56]

Neuropsychological outcome

Intensive therapy regimens used to treat neuroblastoma can impact greatly on brain development, hearing, social adjustment and academic achievement. The Childhood Cancer Survival Study (CCSS), a multi-institutional collaborative project, compiled a database on a population of 5-year cancer survivors, including 928 neuroblastoma patients, treated in 25 North American institutions.[59] Patients were treated between 1970 and 1986 and questionnaires were completed between 1994 and 2000. The achievement of academic milestones and the need for special education was evaluated.[60] Neuroblastoma patients were more likely to utilize special education (25%) and less likely to complete high school (15%) than their sibling controls. The reasons provided by families for participating in special education were low scores as well as difficulty concentrating and learning. In addition to organic consequences of neuroblastoma treatment, the diagnosis of cancer and the intensive treatment have a significant psychological impact on patients and families, which affects their quality of life. Approximately 12% of long-term childhood cancer survivors suffer from post-traumatic stress syndrome, which is attributed to their disease and contributes to long-term disability.[61–64] To understand the effect of increasingly intensive therapy, the neuropsychological outcome of long-term survivors of extracranial childhood cancers, treated with myeloablation and transplantation at Institut Gustave Roussy, was reviewed.[65] Overall, the performance level was in the normal range with satisfactory professional and academic outcomes. Impaired verbal IQ and reading difficulties were seen in this population, and may be attributed to chemotherapy related deafness as well as prolonged absence from formal schooling. The studies suggest the persistence of significant long-term abnormalities in neuropsychological development and in the ability to achieve academic milestones in a subset of long-term survivors of neuroblastoma. However, provided sufficient resources are available to overcome physical disabilities as well as academic and neuropsychological challenges, long-term neuroblastoma survivors can lead productive fulfilling lives.

Effect of neuroblastoma treatment on fertility

Sexuality and reproductive potential are important concerns to long-term survivors of childhood cancer. The effect of neuroblastoma treatment on sexuality and fertility is difficult to assess because of the young age of patients at presentation. Ovarian failure is commonly found in female patients treated with abdominal radiation or prolonged chemotherapy with alkylating agents.[66,67] Testicular failure can result from pelvic irradiation or intensive chemotherapy with alkylating agents.[25] Additionally, musculoskeletal deformities, postoperative changes and associated illnesses can hinder sexual function, conception or pregnancy.[68–70] Nonetheless, some long-term survivors are sexually active and are able to have children.[69,70]

Health care of cancer survivors

Long-term survivors of neuroblastoma and other childhood cancers have unique health care needs.[4] However, significant deficiencies in the delivery of health care to long-term survivors of childhood cancers have been identified in surveys of patients and physicians.[71,72] A barrier to improving the care of pediatric cancer survivors is the lack of understanding of the health care needs, both on the part of the patients themselves and the primary care providers. In a survey, nearly 90% of all, and 80% of adult survivors of neuroblastoma knew their diagnosis.[73] However, significant deficits existed in the knowledge of basic aspects of the treatment undertaken. Neuroblastoma patients may know less regarding the details of their diagnosis and treatment because they are diagnosed and treated at a very young age. Surveys of adult and adolescent survivors of childhood cancer suggest that self-advocacy training and advanced training of primary care physicians could help address their unique health care needs. Additional access to health care by survivors, as they transition into adulthood, may be limited by socioeconomic status. The development of age independent long-term follow-up clinics may be needed to provide both the education and medical care such patients require. The long-term costs of treating neuroblastoma patients are unknown; however, tools for evaluating the direct treatment costs and the indirect costs to family and community are emerging.[74]

Summary

Data collected through large cooperative groups and increasing understanding of neuroblastoma biology have allowed the stratification of patients based on risk of disease progression and mortality. Patients with poor prognosis should be treated with multimodality high intensity therapy, which may include surgery, chemotherapy, radiation, and stem cell transplantation. Recent studies have suggested that such an approach may finally achieve substantive survival in this group of patients. The trade-off is the likelihood of both short- and long-term morbidity associated with aggressive multimodality regimens. Since mortality and morbidity remain high in this group of patients, novel therapeutic modalities such as immunotherapy, anti-angiogenic therapy and gene therapy need to be developed.[14] It is equally important to identify patients with good prognosis. Patients at low or intermediate risk for neuroblastoma progression and mortality should be treated with less intensive multimodality regimens in order to minimize morbidity. Reduction in the dose or duration of chemotherapy can limit drug toxicity in a proportion of patients, and identify patients who require dose intensification. Primary chemotherapy can reduce the size of the tumor and limit the extent of resection and surgical complications, while achieving a high rate of cure. Long-term survivors of neuroblastoma continue to face the risk of late mortality, recurrence, secondary malignancies, as well as musculoskeletal deformities, neurological deficits and neuropsychological challenges. However, the health care system is ill equipped to provide continuing follow-up for this cohort of patients. Significant deficits are present in the understanding of the needs of long-term survivors both by the care providers and the patients themselves. Difficulties achieving academic milestones, maintaining employment and obtaining health insurance further complicate the delivery of health care to long-term survivors. Despite the many challenges, neuroblastoma patients can expect increased long-term survival and improved quality of life, due to greater insight into neuroblastoma biology and pathophysiology as well as increasing emphasis on controlling long-term morbidity.

REFERENCES

1. Wright, J. H. Neurocytoma or Neuroblastoma; a kind of tumor not generally recognized. *J. Exp. Med.* 1910; **12**:556–561.
2. Brodeur, G. M., Pritchard, J., Berthold, F. *et al.* Revisions of the international criteria for neuroblastoma diagnosis, staging, and response to treatment. *J. Clin. Oncol.* 1993; **11**(8):1466–1477.
3. Ikeda, H., Iehara, T., Tsuchida, Y. *et al.* Experience with international neuroblastoma staging system and pathology classification. *Br. J. Cancer* 2002; **86**(7):1110–1116.
4. PDQ. Neuroblastoma treatment. In www.cancer.gov; 2004.
5. D'Angio, G. J., Evans, A. E., & Koop, C. E. Special pattern of widespread neuroblastoma with a favourable prognosis. *Lancet* 1971; **1**(7708):1046–1049.
6. Shimada, H., Ambros, I. M., Dehner, L. P., Hata, J., Joshi, V. V., & Roald, B. Terminology and morphologic criteria of neuroblastic tumors: recommendations by the International Neuroblastoma Pathology Committee. *Cancer* 1999; **86**(2):349–363.
7. Ambros, I. M., Hata, J., Joshi, V. V. *et al.* Morphologic features of neuroblastoma (Schwannian stroma-poor tumors) in clinically favorable and unfavorable groups. *Cancer* 2002; **94**(5):1574–1583.
8. Shimada, H., Ambros, I. M., Dehner, L. P. *et al.* The International Neuroblastoma Pathology Classification (the Shimada system). *Cancer* 1999; **86**(2):364–372.
9. George, R. E., Variend, S., Cullinane, C. *et al.* Relationship between histopathological features, MYCN amplification, and prognosis: a UKCCSG study. United Kingdom Children Cancer Study Group. *Med. Pediatr. Oncol.* 2001; **36**(1):169–176.
10. Goto, S., Umehara, S., Gerbing, R. B. *et al.* Histopathology (International Neuroblastoma Pathology Classification) and MYCN status in patients with peripheral neuroblastic tumors: a report from the Children's Cancer Group. *Cancer* 2001; **92**(10):2699–2708.
11. Castel, V., Canete, A., Navarro, S. *et al.* Outcome of high-risk neuroblastoma using a dose intensity approach: improvement in initial but not in long-term results. *Med. Pediatr. Oncol.* 2001; **37**(6):537–542.
12. Marcus, K. J., Shamberger, R., Litman, H. *et al.* Primary tumor control in patients with stage 3/4 unfavorable neuroblastoma treated with tandem double autologous stem cell transplants. *J. Pediatr. Hematol. Oncol.* 2003; **25**(12):934–940.
13. Kletzel, M., Katzenstein, H. M., Haut, P. R. *et al.* Treatment of high-risk neuroblastoma with triple-tandem high-dose therapy and stem-cell rescue: results of the Chicago Pilot II Study. *J. Clin. Oncol.* 2002; **20**(9):2284–2292.
14. Weinstein, J. L., Katzenstein, H. M., & Cohn, S. L. Advances in the diagnosis and treatment of neuroblastoma. *Oncologist* 2003; **8**(3):278–292.
15. Lau, L., Tai, D., Weitzman, S., Grant, R., Baruchel, S., & Malkin, D. Factors influencing survival in children with recurrent neuroblastoma. *J. Pediatr. Hematol. Oncol.* 2004; **26**(4):227–32.
16. Schilling, F. H., Spix, C., Berthold, F. *et al.* Neuroblastoma screening at one year of age. *N. Engl. J. Med.* 2002; **346**(14):1047–53.
17. Tajiri, T., Suita, S., Sera, Y. *et al.* Clinical and biologic characteristics for recurring neuroblastoma at mass screening cases in Japan. *Cancer* 2001; **92**(2):349–353.
18. Mertens, A. C., Yasui, Y., Neglia, J. P. *et al.* Late mortality experience in five-year survivors of childhood and adolescent cancer: the Childhood Cancer Survivor Study. *J. Clin. Oncol.* 2001; **19**(13):3163–3172.
19. Sauvat, F., Sarnacki, S., Brisse, H. *et al.* Outcome of suprarenal localized masses diagnosed during the perinatal period: a retrospective multicenter study. *Cancer* 2002; **94**(9):2474–2480.
20. Tsuchida, Y., Ikeda, H., Iehara, T., Toyoda, Y., Kawa, K., & Fukuzawa, M. Neonatal neuroblastoma: incidence and clinical outcome. *Med. Pediatr. Oncol.* 2003; **40**(6):391–393.
21. Moppett, J., Haddadin, I., & Foot, A. B. Neonatal neuroblastoma. *Arch. Dis. Child Fetal Neonatal Ed.* 1999; **81**(2):F134–F137.
22. Ikeda, H., Suzuki, N., Takahashi, A. *et al.* Surgical treatment of neuroblastomas in infants under 12 months of age. *J. Pediatr. Surg.* 1998; **33**(8):1246–1250.
23. Rubie, H., Coze, C., Plantaz, D. *et al.* Localised and unresectable neuroblastoma in infants: excellent outcome with low-dose primary chemotherapy. *Br. J. Cancer.* 2003; **89**(9):1605–1609.
24. Garaventa, A., Boni, L., Lo, Piccolo M. S. *et al.* Localized unresectable neuroblastoma: results of treatment based on clinical prognostic factors. *Ann. Oncol.* 2002; **13**(6):956–964.
25. Levitt, G. A., Platt, K. A., De Byrne, R., Sebire, N., & Owens, C. M. 4S neuroblastoma: the long-term outcome. *Pediatr. Blood Cancer* 2004; **43**(2):120–125.
26. Nickerson, H. J., Matthay, K. K., Seeger, R. C. *et al.* Favorable biology and outcome of stage IV-S neuroblastoma with supportive care or minimal therapy: a Children's Cancer Group study. *J. Clin. Oncol.* 2000; **18**(3):477–486.
27. Kato, K., Ishikawa, K., Toyoda, Y. *et al.* Late recurrence of neuroblastoma stage 4S with unusual clinicopathologic findings. *J. Pediatr. Surg.* 2001; **36**(6):953–955.
28. Guglielmi, M., De Bernardi, B., Rizzo, A. *et al.* Resection of primary tumor at diagnosis in stage IV-S neuroblastoma: does it affect the clinical course? *J. Clin. Oncol.* 1996; **14**(5):1537–1544.
29. von Schweinitz, D., Hero, B., & Berthold, F. The impact of surgical radicality on outcome in childhood neuroblastoma. *Eur. J. Pediatr. Surg.* 2002; **12**(6):402–409.
30. Kushner, B. H., Kramer, K., LaQuaglia, M. P., Modak, S., & Cheung, N. K. Neuroblastoma in adolescents and adults: the Memorial Sloan-Kettering experience. *Med. Pediatr. Oncol.* 2003; **41**(6):508–515.
31. Gaspar, N., Hartmann, O., Munzer, C. *et al.* Neuroblastoma in adolescents. *Cancer* 2003; **98**(2):349–355.

32. Halperin, E. C. Long-term results of therapy for stage C neuroblastoma. *J. Surg. Oncol.* 1996; **63**(3):172–178.
33. Bastian, P. J., Fleischhack, G., Zimmermann, M. *et al.* The role of complete surgical resection in stage IV neuroblastoma. *World J. Urol.* 2004; **22**(4):257–260.
34. Kuroda, T., Saeki, M., Honna, T., Masaki, H., & Tsunematsu, Y. Clinical significance of intensive surgery with intraoperative radiation for advanced neuroblastoma: does it really make sense? *J. Pediatr. Surg.* 2003; **38**(12):1735–1738.
35. Castel, V., Tovar, J. A., Costa, E. *et al.* The role of surgery in stage IV neuroblastoma. *J. Pediatr. Surg.* 2002; **37**(11):1574–1578.
36. La, Quaglia M. P., Kushner, B. H., Su, W. *et al.* The impact of gross total resection on local control and survival in high-risk neuroblastoma. *J. Pediatr. Surg.* 2004; **39**(3):412–417; discussion 412–417.
37. Paulino, A. C. Palliative radiotherapy in children with neuroblastoma. *Pediatr. Hematol. Oncol.* 2003; **20**(2):111–117.
38. Kanold, J., Yakouben, K., Tchirkov, A. *et al.* Long-term results of CD34(+) cell transplantation in children with neuroblastoma. *Med. Pediatr. Oncol.* 2000; **35**(1):1–7.
39. Handgretinger, R., Lang, P., Ihm, K. *et al.* Isolation and transplantation of highly purified autologous peripheral CD34(+) progenitor cells: purging efficacy, hematopoietic reconstitution and long-term outcome in children with high-risk neuroblastoma. *Bone. Marrow Transpl.* 2002; **29**(9):731–736.
40. Haberle, B., Hero, B., Berthold, F., & von Schweinitz, D. Characteristics and outcome of thoracic neuroblastoma. *Eur. J. Pediatr. Surg.* 2002; **12**(3):145–150.
41. Leclair, M. D., Hartmann, O., Heloury, Y. *et al.* Localized pelvic neuroblastoma: excellent survival and low morbidity with tailored therapy – the 10-year experience of the French Society of Pediatric Oncology. *J. Clin. Oncol.* 2004; **22**(9):1689–1695.
42. Hoover, M., Bowman, L. C., Crawford, S. E., Stack, C., Donaldson, J. S., Grayhack, J. J. *et al.* Long-term outcome of patients with intraspinal neuroblastoma. *Med. Pediatr. Oncol.* 1999; **32**(5):353–359.
43. Plantaz, D., Rubie, H., Michon, J. *et al.* The treatment of neuroblastoma with intraspinal extension with chemotherapy followed by surgical removal of residual disease. A prospective study of 42 patients – results of the NBL 90 Study of the French Society of Pediatric Oncology. *Cancer* 1996; **78**(2):311–319.
44. De Bernardi, B., Pianca, C., Pistamiglio, P. *et al.* Neuroblastoma with symptomatic spinal cord compression at diagnosis: treatment and results with 76 cases. *J. Clin. Oncol.* 2001; **19**(1):183–190.
45. Katzenstein, H. M., Kent, P. M., London, W. B., & Cohn, S. L. Treatment and outcome of 83 children with intraspinal neuroblastoma: the Pediatric Oncology Group experience. *J. Clin. Oncol.* 2001; **19**(4):1047–1055.
46. Rudnick, E., Khakoo, Y., Antunes, N. L. *et al.* Opsoclonus–myoclonus–ataxia syndrome in neuroblastoma: clinical outcome and antineuronal antibodies – a report from the Children's Cancer Group Study. *Med. Pediatr. Oncol.* 2001; **36**(6):612–622.
47. Mitchell, W. G., Davalos-Gonzalez, Y., Brumm, V. L. *et al.* Opsoclonus–ataxia caused by childhood neuroblastoma: developmental and neurologic sequelae. *Pediatrics* 2002; **109**(1):86–98.
48. Kushner, B. H., Cheung, N. K., Kramer, K., Heller, G., & Jhanwar, S. C. Neuroblastoma and treatment-related myelodysplasia/leukemia: the Memorial Sloan–Kettering experience and a literature review. *J. Clin. Oncol.* 1998; **16**(12):3880–3889.
49. Vazquez, E., Castellote, A., Piqueras, J. *et al.* Second malignancies in pediatric patients: imaging findings and differential diagnosis. *Radiographics* 2003; **23**(5):1155–1172.
50. Mertens, A. C., Yasui, Y., Liu, Y. *et al.* Pulmonary complications in survivors of childhood and adolescent cancer. A report from the Childhood Cancer Survivor Study. *Cancer* 2002; **95**(11):2431–2441.
51. Neglia, J. P., Friedman, D. L., Yasui, Y. *et al.* Second malignant neoplasms in five-year survivors of childhood cancer: childhood cancer survivor study. *J. Natl. Cancer. Inst.* 2001; **93**(8):618–629.
52. Jenkinson, H. C., Hawkins, M. M., Stiller, C. A., Winter, D. L., Marsden, H. B., & Stevens, M. C. Long-term population-based risks of second malignant neoplasms after childhood cancer in Britain. *Br. J. Cancer* 2004; **91**(11):1905–1910.
53. Menu-Branthomme, A., Rubino, C., Shamsaldin, A. *et al.* Radiation dose, chemotherapy and risk of soft tissue sarcoma after solid tumours during childhood. *Int. J. Cancer* 2004; **110**(1):87–93.
54. Bisogno, G., Sotti, G., Nowicki, Y. *et al.* Soft tissue sarcoma as a second malignant neoplasm in the pediatric age group. *Cancer* 2004; **100**(8):1758–1765.
55. Rubino, C., Adjadj, E., Guerin, S. *et al.* Long-term risk of second malignant neoplasms after neuroblastoma in childhood: role of treatment. *Int. J. Cancer.* 2003; **107**(5):791–796.
56. Kushner, B. H., Kramer, K., LaQuaglia, M. P., Modak, S., Yataghene, K., & Cheung, N. K. Reduction from seven to five cycles of intensive induction chemotherapy in children with high-risk neuroblastoma. *J. Clin. Oncol.* 2004; **22**(24):4888–4892.
57. van Santen, H. M., de Kraker, J., van Eck, B. L., de Vijlder, J. J., & Vulsma, T. Improved radiation protection of the thyroid gland with thyroxine, methimazole, and potassium iodide during diagnostic and therapeutic use of radiolabeled metaiodobenzylguanidine in children with neuroblastoma. *Cancer* 2003; **98**(2):389–396.
58. Garaventa, A., Gambini, C., Villavecchia, G. *et al.* Second malignancies in children with neuroblastoma after combined treatment with 131I-metaiodobenzylguanidine. *Cancer* 2003; **97**(5):1332–1338.
59. Robison, L. L., Mertens, A. C., Boice, J. D. *et al.* Study design and cohort characteristics of the Childhood Cancer Survivor Study: a multi-institutional collaborative project. *Med. Pediatr. Oncol.* 2002; **38**(4):229–239.

60. Mitby, P. A., Robison, L. L., Whitton, J. A. *et al.* Utilization of special education services and educational attainment among long-term survivors of childhood cancer: a report from the Childhood Cancer Survivor Study. *Cancer* 2003; **97**(4):1115–1126.
61. Langeveld, N. E., Grootenhuis, M. A., Voute, P. A., & de Haan, R. J. Posttraumatic stress symptoms in adult survivors of childhood cancer. *Pediatr. Blood Cancer* 2004; **42**(7):604–610.
62. Langeveld, N. E., Grootenhuis, M. A., Voute, P. A., de Haan, R. J., & van den Bos, C. Quality of life, self-esteem and worries in young adult survivors of childhood cancer. *Psychooncology* 2004; **13**(12):867–881.
63. Langeveld, N. E., Grootenhuis, M. A., Voute, P. A., de Haan, R. J., & van den Bos, C. No excess fatigue in young adult survivors of childhood cancer. *Eur. J. Cancer* 2003; **39**(2):204–214.
64. Langeveld, N. E., Ubbink, M. C., Last, B. F., Grootenhuis, M. A., Voute, P. A., & De Haan, R. J. Educational achievement, employment and living situation in long-term young adult survivors of childhood cancer in the Netherlands. *Psychooncology* 2003; **12**(3):213–225.
65. Notteghem, P., Soler, C., Dellatolas, G. *et al.* Neuropsychological outcome in long-term survivors of a childhood extracranial solid tumor who have undergone autologous bone marrow transplantation. *Bone Marrow Transpl.* 2003; **31**(7):599–606.
66. Larsen, E. C., Muller, J., Schmiegelow, K., Rechnitzer, C., & Andersen, A. N. Reduced ovarian function in long-term survivors of radiation- and chemotherapy-treated childhood cancer. *J. Clin. Endocrinol. Metab.* 2003; **88**(11):5307–5314.
67. Larsen, E. C., Muller, J., Rechnitzer, C., Schmiegelow, K., & Andersen, A. N. Diminished ovarian reserve in female childhood cancer survivors with regular menstrual cycles and basal FSH <10 IU/l. *Hum. Reprod.* 2003; **18**(2):417–422.
68. Taylor, A., Hawkins, M., Griffiths, A. *et al.* Long-term follow-up of survivors of childhood cancer in the UK. *Pediatr Blood Cancer* 2004; **42**(2):161–168.
69. Zebrack, B. J., Casillas, J., Nohr, L., Adams, H., & Zeltzer, L. K. Fertility issues for young adult survivors of childhood cancer. *Psychooncology* 2004; **13**(10):689–699.
70. Pinter, A. B., Hock, A., Kajtar, P., & Dober, I. Long-term follow-up of cancer in neonates and infants: a national survey of 142 patients. *Pediatr. Surg. Int.* 2003; **19**(4):233–239.
71. Mertens, A. C., Cotter, K. L., Foster, B. M. *et al.* Improving health care for adult survivors of childhood cancer: recommendations from a delphi panel of health policy experts. *Health Policy* 2004; **69**(2):169–178.
72. Zebrack, B. J., Eshelman, D. A., Hudson, M. M. *et al.* Health care for childhood cancer survivors: insights and perspectives from a Delphi panel of young adult survivors of childhood cancer. *Cancer* 2004; **100**(4):843–850.
73. Kadan-Lottick, N. S., Robison, L. L., Gurney, J. G. *et al.* Childhood cancer survivors' knowledge about their past diagnosis and treatment: Childhood Cancer Survivor Study. *J. Am. Med. Assoc.* 2002; **287**(14):1832–1829.
74. Barr, R. D., Feeny, D., & Furlong, W. Economic evaluation of treatments for cancer in childhood. *Eur. J. Cancer* 2004; **40**(9):1335–1345.

59a

Wilms' tumor: N. American experience

Michael L. Ritchey[1] and Nadeem N. Dhanani[2]

[1]Department of Surgery and Pediatrics, Division of Urology, University of Texas – Houston Medical School, USA
[2]Department of Urology, University of Texas – Houston Medical School, USA

Wilms' tumor therapy

Prior to the modern era of cancer treatment, the only opportunity for cure of Wilms' tumor was complete surgical excision. Wilms' tumor was one of the first pediatric malignancies found to be responsive to systemic chemotherapy. Since the initial report by Farber,[1] there has been a dramatic improvement in survival of children with this tumor. Many of these advances have occurred as a result of collaborative efforts of large pediatric cooperative cancer groups, such as the National Wilms Tumor Study Group (NWTSG) and the International Society of Pediatric Oncology (SIOP), which have been able to enroll large numbers of patients treated in a standardized manner since 1969.[2,3] Now that more than 90% of children with Wilms' tumor can expect cure, these groups are focusing their attention to reducing the intensity of therapy in order to minimize treatment-related toxicity that may adversely affect long-term survival and quality of life. Damage to normal organs and tissues occurs and the effects may not become apparent for many years after treatment.

Tracking the late effects of Wilms' tumor treatment has been an integral part of the NWTSG for many years. Long-term toxicities of treatment are studied in a systematic way among uniform populations of children treated with similar therapies. This has helped to define the long-term adverse effects of treatment in patients alive 5 years or longer after the diagnosis of Wilms' tumor. This review summarizes the experience of the NWTSG treatment of Wilms' tumor, and will examine the short-term and long-term complications of this treatment.

Goals and conclusions of NWTS-1 to NWTS-5

Important findings of the early NWTSG randomized clinical trials, NWTS-1 and NWTS-2 (1969–1978) included: combination chemotherapy was more effective than single agents alone, identification of unfavorable histologic features of Wilms' tumor, and identification of prognostic factors that allowed refinement of the staging system stratifying patients into high risk and low risk treatment groups.[4] It was recognized that the presence of lymph node metastases had an adverse outcome on survival. This underscores the importance of adequate lymph node sampling during the course of removal of a nephroblastoma. Local tumor extension was another important factor identified that increased the risk of tumor relapse. Patients with diffuse tumor spill were therefore considered Stage III and given whole abdominal irradiation. This improved staging system with the ability to stratify patients into different treatment groups was used in the design of subsequent trials to reduce the intensity of therapy for the majority of patients while maintaining overall survival.

The findings of NWTS-3 (1979–1986) validated this approach. Patients with Stage I FH tumors can be treated successfully with an 11 week regimen of vincristine (VCR) and dactinomycin (AMD).[2] The 4-year relapse-free survival was 89%, and the overall survival was 95.6%. Stage II FH patients treated with AMD and VCR without postoperative radiation therapy (XRT) had an equivalent survival, four-year overall survival of 91.1%, to patients who received doxorubicin (DOX) and XRT. The dosage of abdominal irradiation for Stage III FH patients was reduced to 10 Gy. This was shown to be as effective as 20 Gy in preventing

Pediatric Surgery and Urology: Long-term Outcomes, Mark Stringer, Keith Oldham, Pierre Mouriquand.
Published by Cambridge University Press.

abdominal relapse if DOX is added to VCR and AMD. Four-year relapse-free survival for Stage III patients was 82%, and the 4-year overall survival was 90.9%. Patients with Stage IV FH tumors receive abdominal irradiation based on the local tumor stage and also receive 12 Gy to both lungs. The combination of VCR, AMD and DOX produced a 4-year relapse-free survival of 79% and the overall survival was 80.9%. There was no statistically significant improvement in survival when cyclophosphamide was added to the three-drug regimen.

NWTS-4 (1986–1994) compared pulse-intensive chemotherapy regimens employing single doses of AMD and DOX to traditional divided-dose regimens of each drug. In addition, a reduction in treatment duration from 15 months to 6 months was evaluated in children with Stages II to IV favorable histology tumors. The pulse-intensive regimens were found to produce less hematological toxicity than the standard regimens.[5] They were also found to produce significant cost savings.[6] There was no significant difference in 2-year relapse-free survival between patients treated with the pulse intensive regimen (89.4%) and those treated with the traditional divided-dose chemotherapy regimen (90.5%).[7] Comparisons between the short and long treatment regimens found equivalent survival for patients with Stages II to IV favorable histology tumors.[6]

NWTS-5

The most recently closed NWTS-5 study was a single arm therapeutic trial. Patients were not randomized for therapy, but instead biologic features of the tumors were prospectively assessed. The goal of this study was to verify the preliminary findings that loss of heterozygote (LOH) for chromosomes 16q and 1p are useful in identifying patients at increased risk for relapse.[8] The treatment regimens used in NWTS-5 were based on the results of NWTS-4. Children with stage I or II FH, and Stage I anaplastic Wilms' tumor received an 18-week pulse intensive regimen of VCR and AMD. Patients with Stage III FH and Stage II–III focal anaplasia were treated with AMD, VCR and DOX and 10.8 Gy abdominal irradiation. Patients with stage IV FH tumors received abdominal irradiation based on the local tumor stage and 12 Gy to both lungs. A new chemotherapeutic regimen combining VCR, DOX, cyclophosphamide, and etoposide was used in children with Stage II–IV diffuse anaplasia. Final results of the study have not been published.

One unique portion of the NWTS-5 study examined the role of surgery alone for children under 2 years of age with Stage I FH tumors weighing under 550 grams. It was based on preliminary observation of favorable outcomes on small numbers of such patients when postoperative adjuvant therapy had been omitted.[9] This portion of the study was suspended when the number of tumor relapses exceeded the limit allowed by the design of the study and the recommendation was made that all children with stage I tumors receive AMD and VCR. Seventy-five patients were enrolled. The sites of relapse were the lung in five children and the renal bed in three patients. The 2-year disease-free survival rate was 86.5%. The 2-year survival rate of this cohort of patients with small tumors is 100% with a median follow-up of 2.84 years,[10] and extended follow-up continues. Observation of untreated children may yield interesting information on the role of chemotherapy in decreasing the incidence of contralateral relapse in patients with NRs.[10] Three of these children (4%) have developed metachronous contralateral tumors.

Surgical complications

The majority of this chapter will review long-term complications of Wilms' tumor treatment, most of which are related to irradiation and chemotherapeutic agents. However, one should not overlook the morbidity of surgery which can produce both acute and late complications. A review of NWTS-3 patients undergoing primary nephrectomy found a 19% incidence of surgical complications.[11] The most common complications were hemorrhage and small bowel obstruction. The latter occurred most often in the first few months after surgery, but also presented as a late event years after treatment. Survival of patients with complications was similar to patients without complications when stratified by histology and stage. Several risk factors for increased surgical complications were identified including: higher local tumor stage, intravascular extension, *en bloc* resection of other visceral organs and incorrect preoperative diagnosis. En bloc resection of all or parts of adjacent organs to which the tumor is adherent is generally not warranted. If the tumor is found to be unresectable, biopsy of the tumor can be followed by chemotherapy and/or radiation therapy.[12] A more recent review of NWTS-4 patients undergoing primary nephrectomy demonstrated an 11% incidence of surgical complications.[13]

SIOP investigators have reported a lower incidence of surgical complications in patients undergoing nephrectomy after chemotherapy than compared to NWTSG patients undergoing primary nephrectomy.[14] The reduction in tumor size presumably facilitates resection decreasing the complication rate. SIOP and NWTSG investigators are conducting a prospective study comparing surgical complication rates in patients enrolled by the two groups.

Late effects of treatment

As the cure rate of Wilms' tumor patients has risen dramatically, there has been a growing cohort of long-term survivors. Treatment-related morbidity may occur early during therapy or can be silent until decades later during adulthood. Numerous organ systems are subject to the late sequelae of anti-cancer therapy. Clinicians must now become familiar with the spectrum of problems that face these children as they grow into adulthood. Certainly, this has been the impetus to reduce the intensity of treatment in order to prevent or lower the morbidity of multimodal therapy without reducing efficacy. Both NWTSG and SIOP investigators have achieved some success towards this end, but randomized trials will continue to search for new ways to allow the survivors to live more normal and productive lives.

Second malignant neoplasms

Patients with a history of childhood malignancy are at a 10 to 20 times risk of developing a second malignancy compared to age matched controls.[15,16] The risk of a second malignant neoplasm (SMN) after successful treatment of Wilms' tumor is 1.6% 15 years after diagnosis.[16] This is more than eight times the expected incidence. The risk of developing leukemia or lymphoma is greatest in the first 8 years after treatment. The risk of developing a solid tumor continues to increase over time.

A number of risk factors for the development of a SMN after treatment of Wilms' tumor have been identified. Breslow *et al.* showed an increasing risk of SMN with increasing doses of radiation therapy to the renal fossa.[16] Whole abdominal irradiation further increases the risk. Of secondary solid tumors, 73% occurred within the radiation field. All children who developed hepatocellular carcinoma had received flank irradiation.[17] The radiation effects appeared to act multiplicatively on age-specific background rates. If this 10- to 20-fold risk persists, when this at-risk population ages, a large number of irradiated Wilms' tumor survivors may develop another malignancy.

Chemotherapeutic agents that inhibit the activity of topisomerase II, such as anthracyclines (doxorubicin), dactinomycin and the epipodophyllotoxins (etoposide) have been identified as important leukemogens. In a case control study of risk factors for leukemia, increasing dose of doxorubicin was found to be associated with an increasing risk of leukemia as a SMN.[18] Another large study of childhood cancer patients found that treatment with doxorubicin increased the risk of SMN.[19] In patients treated for Wilms' tumor, doxorubicin potentiated the effect of radiation on the development of a SMN. Each 10 Gy of abdominal irradiation was estimated to increase the SMN incidence by 22% if no doxorubicin was included in the initial treatment regimen and by 66% if it was.[16] Treatment of relapse also increased the risk of SMN. The other major class of drugs implicated in chemotherapy-induced second tumors are alkylating agents. In a report from the Late Effects Study Group, 47 of 49 patients who developed a SMN after chemotherapy only received at least one alkylating agent.[20]

Children with Wilms' tumor are also at increased risk for development of a second tumor in the contralateral kidney. The incidence of metachronous tumor is 1.2%.[21] A known risk factor for the development of metachronous tumors is the presence of nephrogenic rests. Beckwith has reported that >90% of patients with metachronous bilateral Wilms' tumor are known to have nephrogenic rests in the initial nephrectomy specimen.[22] While not demonstrated, multiple rests in one kidney usually implies that nephrogenic rests are present in the other kidney.[22] Therefore, this is an extremely important pathologic feature that can identify patients at risk for metachronous Wilms' tumor. The review by Coppes *et al.* found that children <12 months of age diagnosed with Wilms' tumor who also have nephrogenic nests, in particular PL nephrogenic nests, have a markedly increased risk of developing contralateral disease and require frequent and regular surveillance for several years. The fact that contralateral Wilms' tumors do develop in these patients, who usually have been treated with systemic chemotherapeutic agents prior to developing the contralateral tumor, suggests that at least in these children the premalignant nephrogenic rests could not be eradicated by the chemotherapeutic drugs administered.

Reproductive system

Damage to reproductive systems can lead to problems with hormonal dysfunction and/or infertility. Gonadal radiation in males can result in temporary azospermia and hypogonadism.[23] The effect on the testis is dose related, and the prepubertal germ cells also appear to be radiosensitive. In a follow-up of ten men treated for Wilms' tumor in childhood, oligospermia or azoospermia was found in 8.[24] The scatter radiation to the testis was estimated between 2.68 and 9.83 Gy. These patients had received whole abdominal irradiation with exclusion of the testes from the treatment field or shielding with lead. The severity and duration of damage to the testis is dependent on the dose of radiation, treatment field and fractional schedule.[25] Although oligospermia has been reported with doses as low as

0.1–1.2 Gy, complete recovery of spermatogenesis has been shown within 30 months after low-dose single-fraction irradiation with doses as high as 2 to 3 Gy.[26,27] The Leydig cells are more radioresistant than the germ cells, but higher doses can produce damage resulting in inadequate production of testosterone. In these cases, testosterone replacement may be required to prevent delayed sexual maturation and promote potency in adulthood.[28]

Chemotherapeutic agents, particularly alkylating agents can interfere with testicular function. Acute toxicity with germ cell depletion occurs in all age groups. Several experiments have demonstrated that damage to the germ cells may result in permanent oligospermia or azospermia.[29,30] Some long-term studies suggested that prepubertal testes are resistant to chronic toxicity.[31] However, recent studies have indicated that prepubertal testes are not protected from chemotherapy-induced damage.[32,33] One report found that 12 of 19 prepubertal males treated for a variety of solid tumors were sterile as a result of treatment.[33] There were three children with Wilms' tumor, and all had normal sperm counts or testicular biopsies. The most severe toxicities have been noted in patients treated with multiagent regimens for Hodgkin's disease. Vincristine has been implicated as a risk factor for azoospermia. Rautonen *et al.* found a five-fold risk of azoospermia in patients treated with vincristine compared to patients who had not received vincristine.[34] There was a 22% incidence of azoospermia in the Wilms' tumor patients, but all had received subdiaphragmatic irradiation. Leydig cells are not affected to the same degree as germ cells, but Leydig cell failure has been found in patients treated during adolescence or after puberty.

Female Wilms' tumor patients who received abdominal radiation have an increased incidence of ovarian failure.[35] Of 16 women who received whole abdominal irradiation, all had evidence of ovarian failure and 75% were amenorrheic.[36] Stillman *et al.* reported that ovarian failure occurred in 68% of patients whose ovaries were included in the treatment field, and in none of those in whom the ovaries were excluded from the field.[35] As with the testis, the effect on the ovaries is dependent on radiation dose as well as age at time of treatment. A woman's duration of fertility and onset of menopause will directly correlate to the number of primordial follicles present at the time of treatment.[37] Chemotherapy-induced damage to the ovaries is most often associated with alkylating agents. A decrease in the number of follicles is seen in prepubertal girls treated with chemotherapy.[38]

Several studies have addressed the risk of pregnancy in survivors who remain fertile after childhood cancer therapy. Women with prior abdominal radiation have the greatest potential for adverse pregnancy outcomes. In a study of patients treated for Wilms' tumor, an adverse outcome occurred in 3% among non-irradiated women compared to 30% of women who received abdominal irradiation.[39] A more recent report from the NWTSG reviewed 427 pregnancies in survivors of Wilms' tumor treated with or without radiation to the flank or tumor bed.[40] Malposition of the fetus and early or threatened labor were more frequent among irradiated women. Both were more frequent among women who received higher radiation therapy doses. The offspring of the irradiated female patients were more likely to weigh less than 2500 g at birth and to be of less than 36 weeks' gestation, with both being more frequent after higher doses of radiation.

Another issue is whether the offspring of long-term cancer survivors will be normal. A report from the Childhood Cancer Survivor Study found a 3.7% incidence of genetic diseases reported in 4214 children born to cancer survivors.[41] This compared to a 4.1% incidence among 2339 children born to sibling controls. The authors concluded that these preliminary findings provide reassurance that cancer treatments including radiotherapy do not carry much, if any, risk for inherited genetic disease in offspring conceived after exposure. Another report from this group also found no adverse pregnancy outcomes for the partners of male survivors treated with most chemotherapeutic agents.[42]

Renal

Most children treated for Wilms' tumor undergo unilateral nephrectomy as part of the initial treatment. There is risk of dysfunction of the solitary remaining kidney. Impairment of renal function may be related to irradiation, administration of nephrotoxic chemotherapeutic agents, or hyperfiltration of the remaining nephrons. Initially, there is compensatory hypertrophy that develops in this kidney.[43,44] The data is conflicting regarding renal compensatory hypertrophy in patients who receive whole abdominal irradiation. Walker *et al.* found no difference in renal lengths between patients treated with chemotherapy and radiation vs. chemotherapy alone.[43] However, Levitt *et al.* used ultrasound to calculate renal lengths and found that patients receiving radiation had poor compensatory growth.[44]

The kidney is sensitive to the effects of radiation. Radiation doses to the kidney should be limited to 12 to 15 Gy. Mitus and colleagues correlated functional impairment with the renal radiation dose in a review of 100 children treated for Wilms' tumor.[45] The incidence of impaired creatinine clearance was significantly greater for children receiving greater than 12 Gy to the remaining kidney and all cases of overt renal failure occurred in patients who had received more than 23 Gy. Clinical signs of radiation nephritis may occur very acutely or begin months or years after therapy is discontinued.[45] Direct radiation nephrotoxicity is the usual cause with injury to the intrarenal vasculature. However, radiation may cause retroperitoneal fibrosis and secondary ureteral obstruction.

A number of chemotherapeutic agents have been implicated as a cause of nephrotoxicity. In Wilms' tumor patients two agents, ifosfamide in combination with etoposide, have been reported to cause renal damage.[46] Ifosfamide can produce tubular damage resulting in Fanconi's syndrome. The severity ranges from subclinical disease to frank renal failure. This combination was reported in 20% of patients treated for recurrent Wilms' tumor.

There are both experimental and clinical studies that suggest the remaining nephrons, after subtotal nephrectomy, are subject to chronic hyperfiltration that can produce renal dysfunction.[47] Most experimental studies involve a loss of greater than three-quarters of the total renal mass,[47] and the renal lesion that develops is focal glomerulosclerosis. This has been found in adult patients who have more than 50% of their renal mass removed for treatment of renal cell carcinoma.[48] Children with bilateral Wilms' tumor may require removal of more than 50% of the total renal mass and are the group at most risk for the development.[49]

There are several studies that have assessed long-term renal function in children following nephrectomy for Wilms' tumor.[44,50–56] The abnormalities found have included microalbuminuria, proteinuria and a reduced GFR.[44,50–53,57,58] Levitt *et al.* evaluated 53 patients at a mean of 13 years after treatment for Wilms' tumor.[44] None of the patients had developed renal failure. Forty of the 53 patients had received radiation (3–17.2 Gy) to the remaining kidney. Factors found to be associated with renal dysfunction were age <24 months, and radiation doses greater than 12 Gy to the remaining kidney.

However, other investigators have reported absence of these disparities.[54–56] Bailey *et al.* followed 40 patients a median of 8.8 years from time of diagnosis and found that treatment for Wilms' tumor does not have any clinically important nephrotoxic effect in the majority of patients.[59]

The incidence of renal failure following unilateral nephrectomy in 5368 patients reported to NWTSG was less than 0.26%; two-thirds of these had Denys–Drash syndrome-associated nephropathy.[49] Individuals with bilateral tumors had a much higher incidence of renal failure.[49] In patients followed more than 15 years, the incidence of end-stage renal disease is 16.6%, 22.3% and 12.7% for NWTS-1, -2, -3 patients, respectively. The use of cytoreductive chemotherapy prior to surgical resection is now recommended for all children with synchronous bilateral tumors to allow greater renal preservation and avoid renal insufficiency.[60] Another report from the NWTSG noted an increased risk of renal failure in children with Wilms' tumor who also had aniridia or genitourinary abnormalities.[61] The cumulative risk of renal failure at 20 years was 38% for the patients with aniridia.

Cardiac

Cardiac irradiation and the anthracycline chemotherapeutic agents can produce both acute and chronic effects on the heart. These include pericarditis, arrhythmias, heart failure, coronary artery disease, and even death. Radiation-induced cardiac damage is due to fibrosis and endothelial damage to the vessels. The parietal pericardium is most susceptible to damage leading to fibrosis and constrictive pericarditis.[62] The frequency and severity of cardiac damage is dependent on dose and radiation technique used.[63] Risk factors for the development of coronary artery disease have included delivering a higher radiation dose (>40 Gy) than typically used in Wilms' tumor.[64] Isolated radiation-related heart damage is rare in survivors of Wilms' tumor treated using currently accepted techniques.[65]

The combination of cardiac radiation and anthracyclines such as doxorubicin increases the risk for development of cardiac disease following doses of each agent considered safe. Anthracyclines have improved the survival of patients with Stage III and Stage IV Wilms' tumor at the cost of acute and long-term cardiac toxicity. Cardiomyopathy associated with doxorubicin has been recognized for decades. The incidence ranges from 0.4 to 9.0%.[66,67] The onset of cardiac dysfunction may be delayed for many years after anthracycline therapy.[68]

Risk factors for the development of anthracycline include the cumulative anthracycline dose, dose schedule, gender and age at treatment.[66,69,70] The incidence of heart failure is significantly less when the cumulative dose of anthracycline is less than 500 mg/m^2. Since cumulative doses of anthracyclines have been limited, the incidence of congestive heart failure (CHF) is <1% of pediatric patients treated for their initial diagnosis.[71]

A number of studies have documented myocardial dysfunction in asymptomatic patients who received anthracyclines for childhood malignancies despite normal serial cardiac evaluations during and at the completion of therapy.[68,72,73] In a study by Lipshultz *et al.*[72] 65% of survivors of childhood ALL had progressive cardiac abnormalities 6 to 10 years after the completion of doxorubicin therapy. Cases of late onset CHF, symptomatic arrhythmias, and even sudden death are unrelated to the occurrence of CHF during therapy. Sorensen *et al.*[73] reported similar cardiac abnormalities when he studied 97 Wilms' tumor patients treated with a mean cumulative dose of doxorubicin of 300 mg/m^2 at a mean follow-up time of 7.1 years. Twenty five percent of the anthracycline-treated group had cardiac abnormalities. Cardiac radiation was not an independent risk factor for increased afterload or decreased contractility. Wilms' tumor survivors in Sorensen's study treated without anthracyclines had thickened left ventricular walls compared to controls. Both Lipshultz and Sorensen demonstrated that doxorubicin impairs myocardial growth: there is an inappropriate small increase in left ventricular wall thickness in relation to somatic growth in pediatric patients treated with anthracyclines.[72,73]

Green *et al.* evaluated the frequency of and risk factors for the occurrence of CHF in patients entered on NWTS - 1, -2, -3 and -4.[74] The cumulative frequency of congestive heart failure was 4.4% at 20 years after diagnosis among patients treated initially with doxorubicin and 17.4% at 20 years after diagnosis among those treated with doxorubicin for their first or subsequent relapse of Wilms' tumor. The relative risk of CHF was increased in females, by cumulative doxorubicin dose, lung irradiation, and left abdominal irradiation. The authors recommended additional follow-up of those children treated on NWTS-4 to determine if the decrease in doxorubicin dose to 150 mg/m^2 will reduce the risk of CHF.

Serial monitoring of cardiac structure and function has been used to determine safe limits for anthracycline therapy in individual patients. Such monitoring is performed prior to therapy and periodically prior to additional courses of anthracyclines. Since the risk of long-term complications is related to the dose exposure, surveillance schedules may be adapted for individual patients. For example, a prospective study of 184 patients receiving anthracycline revealed that those receiving less than 240 mg/m^2 showed no deterioration of left ventricular end diastolic stress at greater than 10 years from the end of treatment.[75] Although the frequency and extent of surveillance can be modified, monitoring techniques should be continued after drug discontinuation regardless of the presence or absence of cardiac abnormalities during therapy.

Pulmonary

The incidence of radiation-induced pulmonary injury has decreased over time due to improvements in radiotherapy techniques.[76] The incidence and severity of radiation damage to the lungs is related to a number of factors including the volume of lung irradiated, the total dose, the rate of delivery, and the radiation technique used.[77,78] Fractionating radiation doses can significantly reduce pulmonary toxicity. For example, studies have shown that a single dose of 11 Gy to the whole lung can yield as high as 80% mortality, whereas fractionating into 20 doses allows for the delivery of 26.5 Gy with as little as 5% mortality.[79] Radiation pneumonitis is generally first apparent radiographically 8 weeks following lung irradiation, but is most obvious 3 to 4 months following radiotherapy. Although complete resolution of radiation pneumonitis has been suggested, most experience indicates that radiation fibrosis is found to some degree in virtually all patients who receive therapeutic doses of radiotherapy.

Pneumonitis (presumed radiation induced) was reported in 12% of NWTS-3 patients with metastatic pulmonary disease treated with pulmonary irradiation.[80] This was associated with a 25% mortality. Drugs used in the treatment of Wilms' tumor that potentiate pulmonary radiation effects include dactinomycin and adriamycin, agents both commonly used in the treatment of Wilms' tumor.[81,82] The incidence of pneumonitis has been reduced by the reduction in dose of dactinomycin and doxorubicin when given concurrently with radiation.

There are several abnormal reports of pulmonary function in children treated with lung irradiation for metastatic Wilms' tumor.[83–85] These studies all confirm the significant impact radiation has when given during a period of alveolar and chest wall development. All children who receive pulmonary irradiation need careful follow-up. Pulmonary function tests should be performed in all patients with symptoms and in patients who later require general anesthesia.

Liver

The liver may be damaged from both chemotherapy and radiation in Wilms' tumor patients. The liver is included in the abdominal radiation portals for some patients with Wilms' tumor. Although most early reports suggested that hepatic irradiation was the most important factor in hepatic injury, experimental and clinical data implicate both dactinomycin and vincristine, two commonly used agents in the treatment of Wilms' tumor.[86,87] More recent reports have documented the development of hepatotoxicity in the absence of irradiation.[88,89] These patients develop a syndrome resembling hepatic veno-occlusive disease. They present with hepatomegaly, elevation of hepatic enzymes, hyperbiliremia, and ascites. In NWTS-4, the incidence of significant hepatotoxicity ranged from 2.8% to 14.3%.[88] The incidence varied by the dose and schedules of dactinomycin. This suggests a dose-related toxicity. SIOP investigators have noted a similar incidence of hepatotoxicity.[89] Treatment of hepatic veno-occlusive disease is primarily supportive. Chemotherapy does not need to be withheld once the signs have disappeared.

Long-term hepatic dysfunction is uncommon after treatment for Wilms' tumor. Thomas *et al.*[90] reported late hepatic toxicity in 3 of 26 Wilms' tumor patients who had received radiation to at least part of the liver in addition to vincristine and actinomycin D. Secondary hepatocellular carcinoma has also been reported in patients with right-sided Wilms' tumor treated with right upper quadrant irradiation.[17] Longitudinal data regarding hepatic function in long-term survivors of pediatric solid tumors including Wilms' tumor is lacking. Evaluation of liver function should be performed annually in patients at risk of chronic damage including those who have received direct hepatic irradiation.

Musculoskeletal

Radiation interferes with bone growth by causing damage to the chondrocytes and osteoblasts and indirectly by damaging the microvascular supply to the epiphyseal growth plates.[91] Several investigators have suggested that the severity and incidence of scoliosis and other skeletal changes is less since megavoltage radiation therapy has been used to treat Wilms' tumor rather than orthovoltage therapy. Thomas *et al.* reported scoliosis in 53% of Wilms' tumor patients treated with megavoltage irradiation but concluded that the extent of involvement and functional disabilities were minimal compared to Wilms' tumor patients treated with orthovoltage irradiation.[90] Rate *et al.* compared children who were treated with either orthovoltage or megavoltage radiation therapy following nephrectomy for Wilms' tumor.[92] Overall frequency of late orthopedic abnormalities was 84% (26/31). The children who required orthopedic intervention as well as those who had developed scoliotic curves of greater than 20° were treated with orthovoltage irradiation. A report from the NWTSG reported scoliosis in 61% (35/57) of patients treated with megavoltage therapy.[65] Although it is clear that children who did not receive flank irradiation had fewer skeletal abnormalities such as scoliosis and less soft tissue atrophy, the sparing role of megavoltage radiation therapy remains unclear and is therefore subject to longer follow-up.

Short stature may result from the treatment of childhood malignancies secondary to growth hormone deficiency, precocious puberty following cranial irradiation, or from restricted spinal growth following spine irradiation. Probert *et al.* first concluded that spinal irradiation decreased sitting height more than standing height.[93] Wallace *et al.* confirmed these observations in a group of male Wilms' tumor survivors treated with either megavoltage or orthovoltage abdominal radiation therapy.[94] A more recent review of 2778 NWTSG patients found that reduction in stature following radiation therapy to the pediatric spine is dose and age dependent.[95] However, average height deficits observed at maturity for children receiving doses currently recommended by the NWTSG were deemed clinically nonsignificant.

Pediatric patients who have received radiation therapy to any part of the spine are at risk for restricted spine growth and the development of spinal curvature. Careful physical examination and standing anterior/posterior and lateral radiographs of the spine done annually until linear growth has ceased will aid in the early detection of skeletal abnormalities.[96] The measurement of sitting height in addition to standing height is necessary to document the full effect of irradiation on the growing spine.

REFERENCES

1. Farber, S., D'Angio, G., Evans, A., & Mitus, A., Clinical studies of actinomycin D with special reference to Wilms' tumor in children. *Ann. N.Y. Acad. Sci.* 1960; **89**:421–425.
2. D'Angio, G. J., Breslow, N., Beckwith, J. B. *et al.* Treatment of Wilms' tumor: Results of the Third National Wilms' Tumor Study. *Cancer* 1989; **64**:349–360.
3. Tournade, M. F., Com-Nougue, C., Voute, P. A., *et al.* Results of the sixth International Society of Pediatric Oncology Wilms' tumor trial and study: a risk-adapted therapeutic approach in Wilms' tumor. *J. Clin. Oncol.* 1993; **11**:1014–1023.
4. D'Angio, G. J., Evans, A., Breslow, N. *et al.* The treatment of Wilms' tumor: Results of the Second National Wilms' Tumor Study. *Cancer*, 1981, **47**:2302–2311.
5. Green, D., Breslow, N., Beckwith, J. *et al.* A comparison between single dose and divided dose administration of dactinomycin and doxorubicin. A report from the National Wilms Tumor Study Group. *Med. Pediatr. Oncol.* 1996; **27**:218.
6. Green, D. M., Breslow, N. E., Beckwith, J. B. B. *et al.* Effect of duration of treatment on treatment outcomes and cost of treatment for Wilms' tumor: A report from the National Wilms Tumor Study Group. *J. Clin. Oncol.* 1998; **16**:3744–3751.
7. Green, D. M., Breslow, N. E., Beckwith, J. B. *et al.* Comparison between single-dose and divided-dose administration of dactinomycin and doxorubicin for patients with Wilms' tumor: a report from the National Wilms' Tumor Study Group. *J. Clin. Oncol.* 1998; **16**: 237–245.
8. Grundy, P. E., Telzerow, P. E., Breslow, N. *et al.* Loss of heterozygosity for chromosomes 16q and 1p in Wilms' tumor predicts an adverse outcome. *Cancer Res.* 1994; **54**:2331–2333.

9. Green, D. M., Beckwith, J. B., Weeks, D. A. *et al.* The relationship between microsubstaging variables, tumor weight and age at diagnosis of children with stage I/favorable histology Wilms' tumor. A report from the National Wilms Tumor Study. *Cancer* 1994; **74**:1817–1820.
10. Green, D., Breslow, N., Beckwith, J. B. *et al.* Treatment with nephrectomy only for small, stage I/favorable histology Wilms' tumor. A report from the National Wilms Tumor Study Group. *J. Clin. Oncol.* 2001;**19**:3719–3724.
11. Ritchey, M. L., Kelalis, P. P., Breslow, N. *et al.* Surgical complications following nephrectomy for Wilms' tumor: A report of National Wilms' Tumor Study-3. *Surg. Gynecol. Obstet.* 1992; **175**:507–514.
12. Ritchey, M. L., Pringle, K., Breslow, N. *et al.* Management and outcome of inoperable Wilms' tumor. A report of National Wilms' Tumor Study. *Ann. Surg.* 1994; **220**:683–690.
13. Ritchey, M. L., Shamberger, R., Haase, G., Horwitz, J., Bergmann, T., & Breslow, N. Surgical complications after nephrectomy for Wilms' tumor: Report from the the National Wilms Tumor Study Group (NWTSG). *J. Am. Coll. Surg.* 2001; **192**:63–68.
14. Godzinski, J., Tournade, M. F., deKraker, J. *et al.* Surgical complications after postchemotherapy nephrectomy in SIOP-9 Wilms' tumor patients. *Med. Pediatr. Oncol.* 1994; **23**:172.
15. Li, F. P., Yan, J. C., Sallan, S. *et al.* Second neoplasms after Wilms' tumor in childhood. *J. Natl Cancer Inst.* 1983; **71**:1205–1209.
16. Breslow, N. E., Takashima, J. R., Whitton, J. A. *et al.* Second malignant Meoplasms following treatment for Wilms' tumor: A report from the National Wilms' Tumor Study Group. *J. Clin. Oncol.* 1995; **13**:1851–1859.
17. Kovalic, J. J., Thomas, P. R. M., Beckwith, J. B. *et al.* Hepatocellular carcinoma as second malignant neoplasms in successfully treated Wilms' tumor patients. *Cancer* 1991; **67**:342–344.
18. Tucker, M. A., Meadows, A. T., Boice, J. D., Jr. Leukemia after therapy with alkylating agents for childhood cancer. *J. Natl Cancer Inst.* 1987; **78**:459–464.
19. Green, D. M., Zevon, M. A., Reese, P. A. *et al.* Second malignant tumors following treatment during childhood and adolescence for cancer. *Med. Pediatr. Oncol.* 1994, **22**:1–10.
20. Meadows, A. T., Baum, E., Fossati-Bellani, F. *et al.* Second malignant neoplasms in children: an update from the late effects study group. *J. Clin. Oncol.* 1985, **3**:532–538.
21. Coppes, M. J., Arnold, M., Beckwith, J. B., Ritchey, M. L., Green, D. M., & Breslow, N. E. Factors affecting the risk of contralateral Wilms' tumor development. A report from the National Wilms Tumor Study Group. *Cancer* 1999; **85**:1616–1625.
22. Beckwith, J. B. Precursor lesions of Wilms' tumor: clinical and biological implications. *Med. Pediatr. Oncol.* 1993; **21**:158–168.
23. Kinsella, T.J., Trivette, G., Rowland, J. *et al.* Long-term follow-up of testicular function following radiation for early-stage Hodgkin's disease. *J. Clin. Oncol.* 1989, **7**:718–724.
24. Shalet, S. M., Beardwell, C. G., Jacobs, H. S. *et al.* Testicular function following irradiation of the human prepubertal testis. *Clin. Endocrinol.* 1978; **9**:483.
25. Sklar, C. A., Robinson, L. L., Nesbit, M. E. *et al.* Effects of radiation on testicular function in long-term survivors of childhood acute lymphoblastic leukemia: a report from the Children Cancer Study Group. *J. Clin. Oncol.* 1990; **8**:1981–1987.
26. Clifton, D. K. & Bremner, W. J. The effect of testicular X-irradiation on spermatogenesis in man. A comparison with the mouse. *J. Androl.* 1983; **6**:387–392.
27. Rowley, M. J., Leach, D. R. Warner, G. A., & Heller, C. G. Effects of graded ionizing radiation on the human testis. *Radiat. Res.* 1974; **59**:665–678.
28. Sklar, C. Reproductive physiology and treatment-related loss of sex hormone production. *Med. Pediatr. Oncol.* 1999; **33**:2.
29. Heikens, J., Behrendt, H., Adriaanse, R., & Berghout, A. Irreversible gonadal damage in male survivors of pediatric Hodgkin's disease. *Cancer* 1996; **78**(9):2020–2024.
30. Thomson, A. B., Campbell, A. J., Irvine, D. C., Anderson, R. A., Kelnar, C. J., & Wallace, W. H. Semen quality and spermatozoal DNA integrity in survivors of childhood cancer: a case-control study. *Lancet* 2002; **360**(9330):361–367.
31. Lentz, R. D., Berstein, J., Steffens, M. W. *et al.* Postpubertal evaluation of gonadal function following cyclophosphamide therapy before and during puberty. *J. Pediar.* 1977; **91**:385–394.
32. Mustieles, C., Munoz, A., Alonso, M. *et al.* Male gonadal function after chemotherapy in survivors of childhood malignancies. *Med. Pediatr. Oncol.* 1995; **24**:347–351.
33. Aubier, F., Flamant, F., Brauner, R. *et al.* Male gonadal function after chemotherapy for solid tumors in childhood. 1989; **7**:304–309.
34. Rautonen, J., Koskimies, A. I., & Siimes, M. A. Vincristine is associated with the risk of azoospermia in adult male survivors of childhood malignancies. *Eur. J. Cancer* 1992; **28A**:1837–1841.
35. Stillman, R.J., Schinfeld, J.S., Schiff, I. *et al.* Ovarian failure in long term survivors of childhood malignancy. *Am. J. Obstet. Gynecol.* 1987; **139**:62–66.
36. Shalet, S. M., Beardwell, C. G., Morris-Jones, P. H. *et al.* Ovarian failure following abdominal irradiation in childhood. *Br. J. Cancer* 1976; **33**:655.
37. Critchley, H. O., Thompson, A. B., & Wallace, W. H. Ovarian and uterine function and reproductive potential. In Wallace, H. and Green, D., eds. *Late Effects of Childhood Cancer*. Oxford: Oxford University Press, 2004: 226–228.
38. Nicosia, S. V., Matus-Ridley, M., & Meadows, A. T. Gonadal effects of cancer therapy in girls. *Cancer* 1985; **55**:2364–2372.
39. Li, F. P., Gimbrere, K., Gelber, R. D. *et al.* Outcome of pregnancy in survivors of Wilms tumorm. *J. Am. Med. Assoc.* 1987; **257**:216–219.
40. Green, D. M., Peabody, E. M., Nam, B. *et al.* Pregnancy outcome after treatment for Wilms' tumor: a report from the National Wilms Tumor Study Group. *J. Clin. Oncol.* 2002; **20**(10):2506–2513.
41. Boice J. D., Jr., Tawn, E. J., Winther, J. F. *et al.* Genetic effects of radiotherapy for childhood cancer. *Health Phys.* 2003; **85**(1):65–80.
42. Green, D. M., Whitton, J. A., Stovall, M. *et al.* Pregnancy outcome of partners of male survivors of childhood cancer: a report

from the Childhood Cancer Survivor Study. *J. Clin. Oncol.* 2003; **21**(4):716–721.

43. Walker, R. D., Reid, C. F., Richard, G. A. *et al.* Compensatory renal growth and function in postnephrectomized patients with Wilms' tumor. *Urology* 1982; **19**:127–130.
44. Levitt, G. A., Yeomans, E., Dicks Mireaux, C., Breatnach, F., Kingtson, J., & Pritchard, J. Renal size and function after cure of Wilms' tumor. *Br. J. Cancer* 1992; **66**:877–882.
45. Mitus, A., Tefft, M., & Feller, F. X. Long-term follow-up of renal function of 108 children who underwent nephrectomy for malignant disease. *Pediatrics* 1969; **44**:912–921.
46. Miser, J., Krailo, M., & Hammond, G. D. The combination of ifosfamide (IFOS), etoposide (VP16) and MESNA (M): A very active regimen in the treatment of recurrent Wilms' tumor (WT) [abstract]. *Proc. Am. Soc. Clin. Oncol.* 1993; **12**: 417.
47. Provoost, A. P., Baudoin, P., DeKeijzer, M. H. *et al.* The role of nephron loss in the progression of renal failure: experimental evidence. *Am. J. Kidney Dis.* 1991; **17**:27–32.
48. Novick, A. C., Gephardt, G., Guz, B., Steinmuller, D., & Rubbs, R. Long-term follow-up after partial removal of a solitary kidney. *N. Engl. J. Med.* 1991; **325**:1058–1062.
49. Ritchey, M. L., Green, D. M., Thomas, P. *et al.* Renal failure in Wilms' tumor patients: a report from the National Wilms Tumor Study Group. *Med. Pediatr. Oncol.* 1996; **26**:75–80.
50. Bertolone, S. J., Patel, C. C., Harrison, H. L., & Williams, G. Long term renal function in pts. with Wilms' tumor. *Proc. Am. Soc. Clin. Oncol.* 1987; **6**:265, abstract 1040.
51. Baudoin, P., Provoost, A. P., & Molenaar, J. C. Renal function up to 50 years after unilateral nephrectomy in childhood. *Am. J. Kidney Dis.* 1993; **21**:603–611.
52. Robitaille, P., Mongeau, J. G., Lortie, L., & Sinnassamy, P. Long-term follow-up of patients who underwent nephrectomy in childhood. *Lancet* 1985; **1**:1297–1299.
53. de Graaf, S. S. N., van Gent, H., Reitsma-Bierens, W. C. C. *et al.* Renal function after unilateral nephrectomy for Wilms tumour: the influence of radiation therapy. *Eur. J. Cancer* 1996; **32A**:465–469.
54. deToledo, J. S., Galindo, J. R., Melcon, G. C. *et al.* Renal function in long-term survivor of Wilms' tumor. *Med. Pediatr. Oncol.* 1995; **25**:265.
55. Barrera, M., Roy, L. P. & Stevens, M. Long-term follow-up after unilateral nephrectomy and radiotherapy for Wilms' tumor. *Pediatr. Nephrol.* 1989; **3**:430–432.
56. Bhisitkul, D. M., Morgan, E. R., Vozar, M. A., & Langman, C. B. Renal functional reserve in long-term survivors of unilateral Wilms' tumor. *J. Pediatr.* 1990; **118**:698–702.
57. Scully, R. E., Mark, E. J., & McNeely, B. U. Case records of the Massachusetts General Hospital (Case 17–1985). *N. Engl. J. Med.* 1985; **312**:111–1119.
58. Welch, T. R. & McAdams, A. J. Focal glomerulosclerosis as a late sequela of Wilms' tumor. *J. Pediatr.* 1986; **108**:105–109.
59. Bailey, S., Roberts, A., Brock, C. *et al.* Nephrotoxicity in survivors of Wilms' tumours in the North of England. *Br. J. Cancer.* 2002; **87**(10):1092–1098.
60. Ritchey, M. L. & Coppes, M. Management of synchronous bilateral Wilms tumors. *Hematol. Oncol. Clin. N. Am.* 1995; **9**(6):1303–1315.
61. Breslow, N. E., Takashima, J., Ritchey, M. L., Green, D. M., & Strong, L. C. Renal failure in the Denys–Drash and Wilms' tumor-aniridia syndromes. *Cancer Res.* 2000; **60**:4030–4032.
62. Gottdiener, J. S., Maron, B. J., Schooley, R. T., Harley, J. B., Roberts, W. C., & Fauci, A. S. Late cardiac effects of therapeutic mediastinal irradiation. Assessment by echocardiography and radionuclide angiography. *N. Engl. J. Med.* 1983; **308**:569–572.
63. Stewart, J. R. & Fajardo, L. F. Radiation-induced heart disease: an update. *Prog. Cardiovasc. Dis.* 1984; **27**:173–194.
64. Fajardo, L. F. & Stewart, J. R. Radiation-induced heart disease. Human and experimental observations. In Bristow, M. R., ed. *Drug Induced Heart Disease.* Amsterdam: Elsevier, North-Holland Biomedical Press, 1980:241–260.
65. Evans, A. E., Norkool, P., Evans, I. *et al.* Late effects of treatment for Wilms' tumor. A Report from the National Wilms Tumor Study Group. *Cancer* 1991; **67**:331.
66. Von Hoff, D., Layard, M. W., Basa, P. *et al.* Risk factors for doxorubicin-induced congestive heart failure. *Ann. Int. Med.* 1979; **91**:710–717.
67. Gilladoga, A. C., Manuel, C., Tan, C. T. *et al.* The cardiotoxicity of adriamycin and daunomycin in children. *Cancer* 1976; **37**:1070–1078.
68. Steinherz, L., Steinherz, P., & Tan, C. Cardiac failure and dysarhythmias 6–19 years after anthracycline therapy: a series of 15 patients. *Med. Pediatr. Oncol.* 1995; **24**:352–361.
69. Pikkala, J., Saarimen, U. M., Lundstrom, U. *et al.* Myocardial function in children and adolescents after therapy with anthracyclines and chest irradiation. *Eur. J. Can.* 1996; **32A**(1):97–103.
70. Lipshultz, S., Lipsity, S. R., More, S., Goorin, A., & Colan, S. D. Female sex and higher drug dose as risk factors for late cardiotoxic effects of doxorubicin therapy for childhood cancer. *N. Engl. J. Med.* 1995; **332**:1738–1743.
71. Cuthbertson, D. D., Epstein, S. T., Lipshultz, S. E., Goorin, A. M., Epstein, M. L., & Krisher, J. P. Anthracycline cardiotoxicity in children with cancer. *Circulation* 1994; **90**(Suppl): I-50 (abstract).
72. Lipshultz, S., Colan, S., Gelber, R., Pery-Atayade, A., Sallan, S., & Sanders, S. Late cardiac effects of doxorubicin therapy for acute lymphoblastic leukemia in childhood. *N. Eng. J. Med.* 1991; **324**(12): 808–814.
73. Sorensen, K., Levitt, G., Sebay-Montefiore, D., Bull, C., & Sullivan, I. Cardiac function in Wilms' tumor survivors. *J. Clin. Oncol.* 1995; **13**(7):1546–1556.
74. Green, D. M., Grigoriev, Y. A., Nan, B. *et al.* Congestive heart failure after treatment for Wilms' tumor: a report from the National Wilms' Tumor Study group. *J. Clin. Oncol.* 2001; **19**(7):1926–1934.
75. Sorensen, K., Levitt, G. A., Bull, C., Dorup, I., & Sullivan, I. D. Late anthracycline cardiotoxicity after childhood cancer: a prospective longitudinal study. *Cancer* 2003; **97**(8):1991–1998.

76. Villani, F., Viviani, S., Bonfante, V. *et al.* Late pulmonary effects in favorable Stage I and IIA Hodgkin's disease treated with radiotherpy alone. *Am. J. Clin. Oncol.* 2000; **23**:18.
77. Gross, N. J. Pulmonary effects of radiation therapy. *Ann. Int. Med.* 1977; **86**:81–92.
78. Lipshitz, H. I. Radiation changes in the lung. *Semin. Roentgen* 1993; **28**(4):303–320.
79. McDonald, S., Rubin, P., Phillips, T. L., & Marks, L. B. Injury to the lung from cancer therapy: clinical syndromes, measurable endpoints, and potential scoring systems. *Int. J. Radiat. Oncol. Biol. Phys.* 1995; **31**(5):1187–1203
80. Green, D. M., Finklestein, J. Z., Tefft, J. R., & Norkool, P. Diffuse interstitial pneumonitis after pulmonary irradiation for metastatic Wilms Tumor. *Cancer* 1989; **63**:450–453.
81. Phillips, T. L. Efects of chemotherapy and irradiation on normal tissues. *Front. Radiat. Ther. Oncol.* 1992; **26**:45–54.
82. Von der Maase, H. Experimental drug–radiation interactions in critical normal tissues. In Hill, B. T. & Bellamy, S. A., eds. *Antitumor Drug–Radiation Interactions.* Boca Raton FL: CRC Press, 1990:191–205.
83. Wohl, M. E., Griscom, N. T., Traggis, D. G., & Jaffe, N. Effects of therapeutic irradiation delivered in early childhood upon subsequent lung function. *Pediatrics* 1975; **55**(9):507–515.
84. Littman, P., Meadows, A. T., Polgar, G., Borns, P., & Rubin, E. Pulmonary function in survivors of Wilms' tumor. *Cancer* 1976; **37**: 2773–2776.
85. Benoist, M. R., Lemerle, J., Jean, R., Rufin, P., Scheinmann, P., & Paupe, J. Effects on pulmonary function of whole lung irradiation for Wilms' tumour in children. *Thorax* 1982; **37**:175–180.
86. Flentje, M., Weirich, A., Potter, R. *et al.* Hepatotoxicity in irradiated nephroblastoma patients during post operative treatment according to SIOP 9/GPOH. *Radiother. Oncol.* 1994; **31**:222–228.
87. Johnson, F. L. & Balis, F. M. Hepatopathy following irradiation and chemotherapy for Wilms' tumor. *Am. J. Pediatr. Hematol. Oncol.* 1982; **4**:217–221.
88. Green, D. M., Norkool, P., Breslow, N., Finklestein, J., & D'Angio, G. Severe hepatic toxicity after treatment with vincristine and dactinomycin using single dose or divided dose schedules: a report from the National Wilms Tumor Study. *J. Clin. Oncol.* 1990; **8**(9): 1525–1530.
89. Bisogno, G., DeKraker, J., Weirich, A. *et al.* Veno-occlusive disease of the liver in children treated for Wilms' tumor. *Med. Pediatr. Oncol.* 1997; **29**:245–251.
90. Thomas, P. R. M., Griffin, K. D., Fineberg, B. B. *et al.* Late effects of treatment for Wilms' tumor. *Int. J. Radiat. Oncol. Biol. Phys.* 1983; **9**: 651.
91. Rubin, P., Andrews, J. R., Swaim, R., & Gump, H. Radiation induced dysplasia of bone. *Am. J. Roentgenol.* 1959; **82**:206–216.
92. Rate, W. R., Butler, M. S., Robertson, W. W. Jr, & D'Angio, G. J. Late orthopedic effects in children with Wilms' tumor treated with abdominal irradiation. *Med. Pediatr. Oncol.* 1991; **19**:265–268.
93. Probert, J. C., Barker, B. R., & Kaplan, H. S. Growth retardation in children after megavoltage irradiation of the spine. *Cancer* 1973; **32**: 634–639.
94. Wallace, W. H. B., Shalet, S. M., Morris-Jones, P. H., Swindell, R., & Gattamanini, H. R. Effect of abdominal irradiation on growth in boys treated for a Wilms' tumor. *Med. Pediatr. Oncol.* 1990; **18**:441–446.
95. Hogeboom, C. J., Grosser, S. C., Guthrie, K. A., Thomas, P. R., D'Angio, G. J., & Breslow, N. E. Stature loss following treatment for Wilms' tumor. *Med. Pediatr. Oncol.* 2001; **36**:295–304.
96. Green, D. M. The musculoskeletal system. In *Long Term Complications of Treatment for Cancer During Childhood and Adolescence.* Baltimore: Johns Hopkins University Press, 1989, 70–79.

59b

Wilms' tumor: European experience

Patrick G. Duffy, Gill A. Levitt, and Anthony J. Michalski

Department of Paediatric Urology, Great Ormond Street Hospital, London, UK

Wilms' tumor is ideal for studying long-term outcome. Perhaps more than in any other malignancy, the development of Wilms' tumor therapy has exemplified the paired responsibilities of achieving high cure rates but at minimal cost to the patients in terms of late effects. In 1935, only 8% of children with Wilms' tumor survived; the addition of radiotherapy to surgery had improved that figure to 22% by 1954.[1] Currently, the 5-year survival rate is over 90%.[2] This improvement has been achieved by the judicious use of surgery, chemotherapy, and radiotherapy. Real progress only came through collaborative efforts in national and international clinical trials such as the National Wilms' Tumor Studies (NWTS) in the USA, the United Kingdom Wilms' Tumor (UKWT) Studies, and the internationally based International Society of Paediatric Oncology (SIOP). Collaboration was essential as the incidence of Wilms' is only seven cases per million children per annum. Even large individual centers would never have sufficient numbers to mount significant clinical therapeutic trials.

With the mean age at diagnosis being 2–3 years, patient with Wilms' tumor are at risk of developing profound sequelae if their therapy interferes with normal growth and development. Recognition of the late effects of therapy is not new, with the effects of radiotherapy on skeletal growth being described in 1956.[1] However, the excellent 5-year survival rate of more than 80% achieved and maintained over two decades, provides sufficient patient numbers for reliable observation. Many of the survivors are now into adolescence and adult life. Unfortunately, very few longitudinal, multicenter studies on patients treated in a standard manner have been performed, but good single-center studies have been published. In these reports patients may have been treated over various trial periods, and although care must be taken when interpreting the results, the information gained has highlighted adverse effects of treatments and has led to the modification of subsequent protocols.

This chapter aims to show how understanding of the late effects of specific treatments has evolved in the areas of surgery, chemotherapy, and radiotherapy. An overview of the key trials of Wilms' tumor therapy will show how the aim of "cure at least cost" was pursued. A more "holistic" attempt to describe quality of life follows, and a discussion of challenges for the future.

Surgery

In 1887, Jessop described the first successful nephrectomy for Wilms' tumor.[3] Even though surgery alone will cure a maximum of only 25% of patients, resection of the tumor is still central to survival.[4] The early increase in survival rate was related to improved techniques in surgery and anesthesia, as well as to the introduction of radiotherapy, which was described in 1916.[5] In a single British center, survival increased from 0% to greater than 55% between 1944 and 1972.[6,7] The introduction of actinomycin (1956) and vincristine (1963) as "adjuncts" to surgery led to a rapid improvement in outcome.[8,9]

Survival and therapeutic response are determined by histological characteristics and by the stage of the disease at presentation. The role of surgery is therefore threefold: to make an accurate histopathological diagnosis, to establish a postsurgical stage, and to excise the tumor. The surgery for unilateral Wilms' tumor, including inspection of the contralateral kidney, lymph node sampling, and ligation of major renal vessels before mobilization of the tumor, has

Pediatric Surgery and Urology: Long-term Outcomes, Mark Stringer, Keith Oldham, Pierre Mouriquand.
Published by Cambridge University Press.

been well described.[10] However, contemporary accuracy of computerized tomographic (CT) scanning may obviate the need for routine contralateral renal exploration. In a recent United Kingdom Children's Cancer Study Group (UKCCSG) report, CT scanning accurately detected the contralateral lesion in 54/55 bilateral Wilms' tumors with a sensitivity of 98% and 100% specificity.[11] Within the SIOP-9 study, CT scanning was accurate in diagnosing the presence of a malignant tumor (97 Wilms', 5 other tumor) in 105 patients. The three other children had benign tumor at surgery.[12] Many European groups have therefore concluded that CT scanning obviates the need for pretreatment biopsy.

Surgical practice in the UK has traditionally differed from that in mainland Europe. In the UK, nephrectomy has been the initial treatment for the majority of children.[13] In Europe there is a tendency to concentrate on preoperative therapies to reduce surgical morbidity, particularly tumor rupture. Preoperative therapy, however, may lead to treatment of benign lesions and may mask unfavorable histological features,[14] leading theoretically to inadequate chemotherapy after surgery. The first SIOP study demonstrated that preoperative radiotherapy led to a decrease in tumor spillage, and thus improved recurrence-free survival.[15] The fifth SIOP study showed no difference in outcome between chemo/radiotherapy and two-dose chemotherapy.[16] However, SIOP-6, which recommended two-dose chemotherapy in infants older than 6 months, noted that therapy resulted in unacceptable toxicity in this younger age group and recommended a reduced preoperative dose in infants.[17] In the UKCCSG study (UKW3), the aim was to compare primary surgery followed by chemo/radiotherapy with biopsy, chemotherapy and subsequent total or partial nephrectomy in patients with unilateral stage I–III disease. The role of tumor biopsy followed by pre-resection chemotherapy was reviewed in a series of 36 children with advanced Wilms' tumor between 1982 and 1988.[18] These children had metastatic disease (stage IV) or inoperable tumor or tumor in the inferior vena cava. The morbidity of the biopsy was low. The use of chemotherapy resulted in a significant reduction in tumor bulk in 94% of patients. There was complete concordance between histological assessments of the tumor in the biopsy specimen and at subsequent nephrectomy in 26/28 specimens (98%). Tumor spillage at surgery was 29% in patients undergoing primary nephrectomy, compared with 18% in those who received preoperative chemotherapy. In the UKW3 study[19] 12% of renal tumors biopsied were non-Wilms' tumor pathology requiring differing treatment in some. The UKW3 randomized study [20]results reinforce the European rationale for presurgical chemotherapy, finding a decrease in stage III disease in those patients who received preoperative treatment with no difference in overall survival between the two arms.

Bilateral Wilms' tumor (BWT) occurs in 5%–10% of cases and presents an interesting challenge to the surgeon.[21] Most BWTs occur synchronously, tend to be multicentric, and are usually associated with a favorable histological pattern. Conservative surgical treatment of BWT with an initial diagnostic biopsy and chemotherapy before surgery was first recommended in 1966.[22] The standard surgical procedure in the USA had been initial resection of all tumors until NWTS-3 recommended biopsy first with chemotherapy and later surgical resection.[23] The main emphasis is to remove tumor but maintain as much functioning renal tissue as possible. Currently, the most common approach is "core needle" or open biopsy of both tumors followed by chemotherapy, with the major surgery consisting of partial nephrectomies.[24] The overall 10-year survival of 67 children with BWT registered in the SIOP study (1971–80) was 64%. The prognosis was better in those children who had "syndromes" associated with BWT or in those who presented with tumor that would individually have been classified as stage I or II disease.[21] Seventy-one patients with BWT treated between 1980 and 1995 were recently reviewed.[24] Eighty-two percent of these patients were treated with biopsy, chemotherapy and then surgery, while the others received initial resection and chemotherapy. Eighty percent of children received a total nephrectomy, with or without a contralateral procedure consisting of partial nephrectomy, enucleation of tumor, or no surgery. Of the group who received initial chemotherapy, 67% survived with a mean of 45% of their total renal mass. In the group treated with initial surgery, survival was 77% but the mean renal mass was lower at 35%. The overall survival was 69% with a follow-up of 6 years. There was no statistical difference in renal function, but the preservation of renal mass may be significant in the long-term outcome of these patients. Techniques of partial nephrectomy with vascular control, cooling or "bench-surgery" with autotransplantation should enable the surgeon to preserve some function and prolong health without renal supportive therapy.

Preserving renal mass in the management of BWT is clearly an important long-term issue, and the "nephron-sparing" philosophy is under active debate in the management of unilateral Wilms' tumor.[25] Animal studies have documented the potential deleterious effects of renal ablation and the subsequent glomerular hyperfiltration in the remaining renal tissue.[26,27] The presence of hyperfiltration-induced renal injury in normals has been reviewed in an excellent article by Steckler *et al.*,[28] and the authors fail to support the notion that adaptive hyperfiltration in the remaining complete kidney is deleterious to its function. The renal function of 22 children who received unilateral nephrectomy for Wilms' tumor plus abdominal radiation and some form of chemotherapy was studied 5–32 years (average 13.2 ± 1.7) after treatment.[29] None of the patients was in renal failure or treated with antihypertensive drugs. Glomerular filtration rates (GFR) were 82% of those derived from a control group of patients with two normal kidneys. Albumin excretion was not significantly higher in the tumor group than in controls, but the highest value for the albumin excretion in the controls was exceeded by five of the tumor patients. In a subsequent study from the same unit of an unselected group of adults whose kidney was removed in childhood,[30] there was a suggestion of a slow decline in GFR after a more prolonged period of follow-up (7–47 years). Again, however, there was no renal insufficiency or marked increase in blood pressure. The impression of good long-term outcome after unilateral nephrectomies for Wilms' tumor has been supported by other centers with follow-up beyond 10 years'.[31,32]

However, it is not always possible to preserve good renal functioning in patients with Wilms' tumor. Renal transplantation has a role in patients rendered anephric as a result of surgical excision of both kidneys in BWT, or in those with predisposing syndromes, such as Denys–Drash syndrome.[33] Early results, particularly of living related donors, have been satisfactory.[34,35]

Chemotherapy

For treatment of low-stage disease with surgery and chemotherapy, (vincristine alone or in combination with actinomycin D) carries an excellent long-term outlook. Although vincristine may cause peripheral, autonomic or cranial nerve neuropathy[36] with loss of limb power, abnormal sensation, constipation or ptosis, full recovery after finishing treatment usually occurs. The patient group at particular risk is that with a strong family history of hereditary peripheral neuropathies. Vincristine has been documented to unmask and increase the severity of symptoms in patients with a family history of Charcot–Marie–Tooth disease.[37]

Actinomycin is known to cause acute hepatotoxicity. In the first two UK Wilms' tumor studies (UKWT-1 and –2), 1.4% of patients treated with combination chemotherapy without radiation developed a syndrome of hepatopathy and thrombocytopenia. The syndrome occurred early in the course of treatment (within 10 weeks of starting therapy). Although patients had severe thrombocytopenia, all recovered.[38] There have been reports of fatalities in infants. In SIOP[39] 9–10% of patients who were receiving a high weekly dose developed hepatopathy compared with none on the lower dosing (9.4–22.5 μg/kg per wk over 3–5 days, single dose 3.75 μg/kg per wk respectively).[39] No late effects due to the syndrome have been reported.

The anthracyclines are the chemotherapeutic agents that cause the most concern for long-term outcome owing to their potential to cause cardiotoxicity. They were added to treatment regimens in the late 1970s with the immediate benefit of increasing survival in stage III and stage IV disease.[40] Acute heart failure (developing within weeks or months of receiving an anthracycline) was shown to be dose related,[41] and it was hoped that the problem would be solved by reducing the maximum cumulative dose to less than 450 mg m^{-2}. (In the UK protocols the total dose is 360 mg m^{-2} and the maximum dose in the SIOP regimens is 250 mg m^{-2}). In the early 1990s, reports appeared of patients with no previous cardiac history developing cardiac failure many years from diagnosis.[42,43] Further work, including a single study of Wilms' tumor survivors, revealed an incidence of 25%–57% asymptomatic cardiac dysfunction.[44,45] The risk factors identified were high total dose[46] or dose intensity,[44] young age at treatment,[46] and female gender.[46] The incidence of abnormalities was higher in patients with longer follow-up.[47,48] Patients receiving total doses as low as 45–180 mg m^{-2} were not exempt from abnormalities.[45] In Sorensen *et al.*'s[44] detailed echocardiography study on 98 survivors of Wilms' tumor at a mean follow-up of 5 years, 79% were treated in various UK multicenter protocols between 1970 and 1990. They had received a mean total anthracycline dose of 300 mg m^{-2} at doses of either 30 or 40 mg m^{-2} at intervals of 3 or 6 weeks. Some patients received cardiac radiation from lung and/or abdominal fields; both the volume of the heart treated and the maximum total dose to the heart were calculated from the planning films. Cardiac abnormalities were found in 25% of the patients either as increased end-systolic wall stress, (a measure of afterload) and/or decreased contractility. The risk factors identified were the cumulative anthracycline dose and dose intensity. Radiation did not appear to be a risk factor, although three of four patients who had received more then 40 Gy to the heart from combined lung and abdominal field had thin ventricular walls. One of these patients progressed to irreversible heart failure, after estrogen treatment for radiation-induced ovarian failure, and required a cardiac transplant. By contrast, an analysis of cardiac function by echocardiogram and ECG in patients treated on SIOP 9 /GPOH and SIOP 93–01/GPOH with a short mean follow-up of 2.9 years demonstrated abnormalities in 2.5% of patients.[49] At present, the very long-term prognosis for children with asymptomatic cardiac dysfunction is unknown. In a survey of cardiac transplantation in cancer survivors in Great Britain,[50] four of the 16 patients had previously been treated for Wilms' tumor. These patients first presented with cardiac failure 7–11 years after finishing treatment, they all had left-sided tumors (one was bilateral), and in three the treatment included abdominal and/or lung radiation. Patients at particular risk are those with lung metastases and left-sided stage III disease who require radiation with overlapping fields.

Monitoring of cardiac function is important. However, there is disagreement about whether present practice can detect early defects,[51,52] or whether early treatment of asymptomatic abnormalities is appropriate. Simple measurements of fractional shortening (although not optimal in their sensitivity or specificity) do give some information on future cardiac prognosis. Patients in whom cardiac abnormalities have been identified should be counseled particularly regarding exercise, and be carefully watched through pregnancy.[53]

Cyclophosphamide is an alkylating agent that was a component of the multiagent chemotherapy used in the UKW-1 study[54] for treatment of unfavorable and stage IV disease, the recent SIOP Protocol 2001 for high risk histology and the recent National Wilms' Tumor Studies (NWTS) in the USA.

Both the earlier UKWT1 and the recently opened SIOP study prescribe cyclophosphamide up to a maximum total dose of $8\,g/m^2$. No late effects on the bladder or kidneys have been described but fertility may be affected. Further studies will be needed to evaluate fertility as patients mature. Extrapolating from other studies of fertility following cyclophosphamide therapy,[49,55] females who receive doses similar to those used in Wilms' probably maintain normal fertility, but there have been suggestions that the length of their reproductive life may be shortened. The testes are known to be sensitive to alkylating agents, and studies have indicated that oligo- and azoospermia occur in the majority of adults who have received, as children, more than $9\,g\,m^{-2}$ of cyclophosphamide.[56,57]

High dose melphalan with stem cell support is incorporated into Wilms' relapse protocols and will cause sterility in male survivors. Unfortunately, at the present time there is no method of preserving fertility in these prepubertal boys but the rare patient with adolescent/adult Wilms' tumor should be offered sperm preservation.

Ifosfamide was used in SIOP-9 as first-line treatment of stage IV disease and by various other groups in combination for non-responsive or recurrent disease.[58] This alkylating agent is nephrotoxic, causing both tubular (Fanconi's syndrome) and glomerular damage.[59] The risk of developing nephrotoxicity is related to the total cumulative dose of ifosfamide and to patient-related factors such as the presence of a single kidney[60] and young age. Patients with Wilms' are at particular risk. The prognosis of the nephropathy is variable, with some patients no longer needing electrolyte supplementation and others progressing to renal failure. Ifosfamide must therefore, be used with caution; regular monitoring of both glomerular and tubular function throughout treatment and during follow-up is mandatory.[61]

The new SIOP-02 protocol incorporates etoposide and carboplatin for the treatment of high risk disease and as second-line therapy.[62–64] Long-term effects are known for these drugs. In particular, etoposide is associated with an increase in risk of developing secondary leukemia.[65] The poor prognosis of relapsed patients gives little leeway to reduce late effects by avoiding, or reducing the dose of, these effective drugs.

Radiotherapy

The sequelae of radiotherapy are related to a number of technical factors, and anatomical structures vary in their radiation sensitivity. Risk factors for late effects include orthovoltage radiotherapy, high dose (total dose and dose per fraction), large treatment volume, and young age.[66,67] Radiotherapy reduces the growth potential of normal tissues and, therefore, the late effects become more obvious as the child grows. Care must be taken in interpreting long-term follow-up studies where patients may have been treated in the 1960s and 1970s, many with orthovoltage machines, larger fields, and higher doses. Orthovoltage radiotherapy may cause more skeletal long-term problems. Modern radiation fields are tailor-made for each patient and are dependent on the position of the tumor. For example, the radiotherapy field for a patient with a Wilms' tumor of the upper pole of the left kidney would include more of the heart than the field for a patient with a tumor of the lower pole. However, the radiotherapy field for a tumor of the lower pole of either kidney may include the ipsilateral ovary and uterus. Therefore, in order to predict the late effects of radiotherapy, detailed knowledge of all the treatment given is mandatory.

The clinical features of radiotherapy for Wilms' tumor can be divided into effects on the following "systems": musculoskeletal, cardiorespiratory, and intra-abdominal organs (see also Chapter 57).

Musculoskeletal development

The late effects of radiotherapy on the musculoskeletal system are loss of growth potential,[68] spinal deformities,[69] soft tissue hypoplasia,[69] and second tumors.[70]

Spinal radiotherapy causes a change in "body proportions," with significant fall-off in sitting height; this has its maximum effect during puberty when the majority of spinal growth occurs.[71] In Wallace *et al.*'s study[72] of 30 patients treated between 1945 and 1988 who received flank or whole abdominal radiation to a total dose of 20–30 Gy, patients exhibited a decrease in sitting height of 2.4 standard deviation score (SDS), with a median final height of 1.0 SDS below the mean. The degree of loss of height was related to the age at treatment: the estimated loss of height was 10 cm if treated at 1 year of age and 6 cm at 5 years of age. An interesting finding was that megavoltage radiotherapy caused more growth loss than orthovoltage. The later patients were also treated with actinomycin,[66,73] a radiation sensitizer, and this may have increased growth inhibition.

Historically, flank fields resulted in the radiation of only part of the vertebral column (up to the midline), which resulted in marked scoliosis. The treatment of the whole vertebral body has prevented the severe deformities that were reported in patients treated in the 1960s. More recent studies quote occurrence rates of spinal deformities of between 10% and 70%,[68,69,72] the variability in part being due to differences in the method of evaluation (clinical vs. radiological). Scoliosis is the main spinal deformity and the degree of curvature is related to radiation dose.[72] The majority of patients are asymptomatic and require no surgery or bracing.

Soft tissue hypoplasia is particularly apparent if asymmetry is present and so is most obvious in children who have received flank radiation. It rarely causes functional problems, although patients are aware of the deformity and it may affect fashion-conscious individuals. Breast development[74,75] can be affected, with hypoplasia occurring if abdominal irradiation is required for an upper pole tumor. Lung irradiation given at a lower dose (12 Gy vs. more than 29 Gy for abdominal therapy) rarely causes gross breast hypoplasia, but it does affect lactation.[75] Breast implants can be used for cosmetic purposes, but patients must be informed of the risk of breast cancer occurring in previously irradiated tissue and care must be taken to ensure appropriate follow-up.

Cardiorespiratory system

The effects of radiotherapy on the cardiorespiratory system are due to both lung and heart damage. Lung radiation causes damage in two ways: first due to the development of fibrosis of the alveolar septae, which will affect gaseous exchange and lung compliance; and secondly from growth impairment of the lung and chest wall, resulting in reduced lung volume. The severity of these effects is dependent on the age at radiation and radiation dose.[76] Lung infection and the use of concomitant radiosensitizing drugs such as actinomycin may also contribute to respiratory morbidity. Doses used in recent European trials have been relatively low. Patients with pulmonary metastases have received 12 Gy of fractionated whole lung irradiation. In patients with stage III disease, small areas of lung have received higher doses (20–30 Gy) owing to encroachment of the abdominal radiation field on the thorax. Patients who have both pulmonary metastases and stage III abdominal disease have required both whole lung and abdominal radiotherapy. Doses below 15 Gy cause restrictive changes; higher doses also cause a decrease in both lung volume and in gaseous gas exchange.[77] A study from the northwest of England[78] showed that patients who had received doses to their lungs from either whole lung radiation (12–20 Gy), flank or whole abdominal radiation, had no respiratory symptoms but a lower perceived exercise tolerance compared with controls. The risk factors were young age, subsequent lung infection, percentage of lung volume radiated, and the additional use of anthracyclines.

The pathology of radiation-induced cardiotoxicity is distinct from that caused by anthracyclines. Radiation causes damage to the vascular endothelial cells, resulting in vasculitis and subsequent myocyte death and fibrosis, whereas anthracyclines have a direct effect on the myocytes.[79] The two agents are synergistic and reports have shown the additive effect of radiation.[48] Sorensen *et al.*[44] were unable to show a radiation effect if a low total dose or small volume of the heart was radiated.

Intra-abdominal organs

The most important vulnerable intra-abdominal organs affected by radiotherapy are the female reproductive organs. The ovaries and uterus are not shielded from radiation, and so, if within the field, they will receive the maximum dose. The infantile uterus and ovaries are not necessarily in a fixed position but generally lie below the pelvic inlet, so their involvement within abdominal radiotherapy fields is unpredictable.[80] The ovary has a predetermined number of oocytes, which decline in number from birth. Ovarian sensitivity to radiation is age dependent; young women have a 95% chance of permanent sterility with 20 Gy exposure.[81] Studies[82,83] on prepubertal females have shown that patients receiving either hemi-abdominal or whole abdominal radiation with a dose range of 15–30 Gy may have raised follicular stimulating hormone levels (FSH) indicative of suboptimal ovarian function. Wallace *et al.*[84] followed 40 survivors of Wilms' tumor treated from 1940 to 1972 in a single UK center who had received either hemi (flank) or whole abdominal radiation in the dose range 20–30 Gy. Of the 25 patients treated with whole abdominal radiation, 20 had primary ovarian failure, 4 developed premature menopause under the age of 36 years, and one patient had normal ovarian function. Of 14 patients treated with fractionated flank radiation, all but one patient had regular menstrual cycles and appropriate hormone levels; this patient had ovarian failure diagnosed at the age of 12 years, 10 years after tumor diagnosis. The four menopausal patients all conceived but had mid-trimester miscarriages. This may be attributed to ovarian dysfunction, but poor uterine function could be an additional cause. This is supported by Hawkins and Smith's[85] general practitioners' postaestudy investigating pregnancy outcome in British childhood cancer survivors. Patients treated for Wilms' tumor with abdominal irradiation were compared with patients who had no abdominal irradiation. The spontaneous abortion rate was increased in the irradiated group (22% vs. 6%). Live birth outcome was also affected, with the birthweight significantly lower (by a mean of 500 g) compared with the non-irradiated group. A number of reasons have been suggested for these findings, including reduced uterine vascularity and poor uterine elasticity.[86] Studies on patients receiving total body radiation suggest radiotherapy causes a reduction even in the size of the non-pregnant uterus.[87] However, offspring of patients treated with abdominal radiation do not have an increased risk of congenital malformation, suggesting either that germline mutations do not occur or that those mutations that do occur are not compatible with development of the fetus to term.[88]

The testes are not normally within the Wilams' abdominal radiation field but a few older studies have suggested that radiation for Wilms' tumor can cause testicular damage. Shalet *et al.*[89] estimated that the irradiation scatter to testis from abdominal irradiation was in the range 2.7–9.8 Gy. Their study in 1978 of ten men showed that eight had either oligo- or azoospermia and seven had elevated FSH levels. All patients progressed normally through puberty. Whether these concerns about male fertility can be extrapolated to modern-day techniques is questionable and further studies are required.

Radiation of the liver in the doses usually prescribed for Wilms' tumor does not cause clinical problems,[13] but there is a report[90] of veno-occlusive disease occurring in 8% of liver-radiated patients treated on SIOP-9/GPOH protocol. On this regimen, actinomycin is given on a 5-day schedule or at a higher single dose compared with UKW protocols, and this may increase the liver's radiosensitivity.

An increased incidence of diabetes mellitus in association with pancreatic radiation has been suggested,[91] but no large-scale study has verified this observation.

Second neoplasms

Perhaps the most serious concern following radiotherapy is the increased risk of developing a second tumor. Not all second tumors are a serious problem. Osteochondromas, for example, are benign bone tumors associated with radiation of the epiphysis of growing bone. These bone tumors may affect function, become unsightly and cause pain, requiring surgical intervention. An incidence of 6%–20% has been reported,[70,92] and only rarely do these tumors become malignant.[93] These tumors appear in Wilms' patients[94] who have not been irradiated and some of these patients have a family history of multiple exostosis. Recently, a group in Holland[95] have identified one of the gene deletions responsible for "multiple hereditary exostosis." It is on the short arm of chromosome 11. This gene deletion may involve the WT1 gene or may influence its expression and explain the simultaneous occurrence of these rare diseases.

Second malignant neoplasms (SMN) are obviously much more of a concern and have been reported in survivors of Wilms' tumor. Two large population-based studies, one from the Nordic countries[96] and the other from the UK,[97] found a similar cumulative risk of 3% by 20 years from diagnosis, with an increased relative risk of 5–8-fold. The majority of SMN occurred within the radiation field. In the UK series, 6/7 irradiated patients who developed SMN (carcinomas and sarcomas) developed their tumors in irradiated tissues.

Overview of earlier therapeutic trials

Large cooperative trials for Wilms' tumor started in earnest in 1969 with the formation of the NWTS-1 trial in the USA.[98] The first British study, run by the Medical Research Council (MRC), started a year later[99] and the SIOP-1 study in 1971.[15] Since then it is estimated that over 8000 patients have been entered into erative studies worldwide.

Patients with Wilms' tumor are not a homogeneous group. Classifications were required to allow treatment to be based on the perceived "aggressiveness" of the disease. The two factors that influence outcome are the stage of the disease and histology. The initial classification in the NWTS-1 study used "groups," but by NWTS-2 a postsurgical staging system had been devised, classifying patients on the amount of disease remaining following initial surgical excision of the tumor. It is important to realize that these staging systems are not static but change with further analysis of centrally collected data. For example, by the end of the NWTS-2 trial, it became obvious that lymph node involvement carried a poorer prognosis, and so patients with this feature were "up-staged" to stage III; whereas localized spillage of tumor did not signify bad risk, so these patients were "down-staged" to stage II.[40] This process is ongoing and recent data suggest that young children with favorable-histology stage I tumors less than 550 g weight may be a group in whom surgery alone can be considered.[100] The one unfortunate aspect of staging is that classifications are not universally recognized, so that the SIOP staging system differs slightly from that of the NWTS, particularly in the way it classifies lymph node involvement, which is designated stage II in SIOP and stage III in NWTS.

The rate impact of histology on survival has also become clearer. After NWTS-1, tumors were divided into "favorable" and "unfavorable" types[101] it became clear that perhaps this is not the best choice of terminology as patients with "favorable" tumors still die and improvements in therapy have now made some "unfavorable" tumor types eminently treatable. Just as staging is not static, there has also been a continued evolution in the histological classification. For example, one type of unfavorable histology, anaplasia, has been subdivided into focal and diffuse, with focal anaplasia carrying a greatly improved prognosis.[102] Similarly, patients with clear-cell sarcoma have an excellent prognosis if treated on anthracycline-containing regimens,[103] whereas the prognosis for children with rhabdoid tumors remains dismal.[104]

By classifying patients on the basis of stage and histology, various trials have investigated reduction of therapy for patients with "good prognosis" disease and intensification of therapy for bad-risk patients. Patients with favorable-histology stage I tumors initially received radiotherapy after surgery as well as actinomycin, but in NWTS-1 it was shown that radiotherapy did not add a survival advantage.[98] In NWTS-2, these stage 1 patients received vincristine and actinomycin,[40] but in UKW-1 vincristine alone was shown to be as good,[13] and in UKW-2 the duration of vincristine therapy was reduced to 10 weeks. Similarly, in favorable-histology stage II disease there has been a stepwise reduction in therapy, with the MRC-2 trial showing no benefit for the addition of doxorubicin to vincristine and actinomycin[105] NWTS-3 showed that radiotherapy was not necessary,[104] and NWTS-4 reduced the duration of two-drug chemotherapy. Conversely, patients with favorable-histology stage IV disease appear to benefit from at least a year of three-drug chemotherapy and lung irradiation. In UKW-1 these patients were given whole lung irradiation only if their pulmonary metastases had not disappeared 12 weeks into therapy, and the 65% survival at 6 years[13] appeared inferior to the 82% 4-year survival seen in NWTS-3 ($P = 0.04$) patients in whom whole lung radiotherapy was used routinely. There may be other reasons, since in the SIOP studies – in which whole lung irradiation is not used routinely – the results are similar to those of NWTS-3 (84% 4-year survival).[106]

The success of combination chemotherapy has enabled groups to reduce radiotherapy; fewer patients are irradiated and lower doses are used. Abdominal radiation was dropped from the stage II UKW-2 protocol with no significant increase in local relapse rate. SIOP-6 involved a randomization between renal bed radiation or no radiation in stage II node-negative disease, and although there were more local relapses in the non-irradiated group, the disease-free survival was the same.[66] The SIOP regimen of preoperative chemotherapy has reduced abdominal radiation to 25% in Wilms' tumor patients without metastatic disease[66] and this was confirmed in a large randomized study UKW-3 in which the use of preoperative chemotherapy reduced the percentage of patients with stage 3 disease.[20] The doses of lung and abdominal radiation have also been lowered, although not so much as in some NWTS regimens (20 Gy to the flank in UKW-1 to UKW-3, 10 Gy in NWTS), but more patients are irradiated in the NWTS trials.

Health-related quality of life

The clinical morbidity has been discussed above, but what does this mean to the cured patient in terms of quality of life and self-esteem? Does the treatment make them have more problems in adult life from their perspective compared with their peers? No good studies have been undertaken but observations in long-term follow-up suggest that this group has good quality of life with minimal restrictions. A postal study by general practitioners in the UK suggested that 9% of survivors had problems with employment and 10% had difficulties with health insurance. Discrimination has been identified in both the insurance industry and in certain groups of employers; the armed forces, for example will not accept applicants who have undergone nephrectomy. Makipernaa[107] from Finland studied psychosocial functioning in patients with solid tumor

Table 59b.1. Risk of developing clinically relevant late effects from Wilms' tumor therapy

Tumor stage	Wilms' tumor patients with given stage	Late effect	Magnitude of risk of developing late effect
I + favorable histology	30%	Renal	<10%
I + unfavorable histology	16%	Renal	<10%
II	3%	Renal	<10%
III	33%	Renal	<10%
		SMN	<10%
		Musculoskeletal	10–20%
		Cardiac	10–25%
		Female infertility/ fetal loss	10–25%
IV	10%	Renal	<10%
		SMN	<10%
		Musculoskeletal	10–20%
		Respiratory	10–20%
		Cardiac	10–25%
Bilateral	5%	Renal	25–50%

11–28 years after diagnosis and found some emotional psychological problems but many were coping well. These findings were similar to those in a small study conducted in a single UK center.[108]

The sequelae described rarely affect long-term mortality. The population-based study[109] from the UK on late deaths in patients diagnosed between 1979 and 1985 described 15 deaths in 738 survivors, with 9 due to recurrent disease, 3 treatment-related, and one SMN. There were three times the expected number of deaths due to non-neoplastic causes. After 10–15 years there were only four deaths in 489 survivors: one from recurrent tumor resulting in an actuarial percentage of 1.8, and two treatment-related deaths with an actuarial percentage of 1.9.

Table 59b.1 is an attempt to put the risk of late effects into context. In summary, survivors of Wilms' tumor as a group have a good long-term outlook. Radiation causes by far the most detrimental effects based on the present studies, but care must be taken to monitor chemotherapeutic effects, particularly cardiac.

The future of Wilms' tumor therapy

There are obvious areas for further improvement. Rhabdoid tumor and diffuse anaplasia continue to carry a poor prognosis, but numerically these account for only approximately 7% of all Wilms' tumor cases. Patients with recurrent disease still fare poorly, especially if the recurrence is early and follows three-drug chemotherapy and radiotherapy. The use of carboplatin, etoposide, and alkylators such as cyclophosphamide or ifosfamide is being investigated by various national groups.[63,64] The role of high-dose therapy with autologous stem cell or bone marrow rescue is also under review.[110]

However, for the bulk of patients, further improvement in therapy is likely to be difficult. With the 5-year survival in the region of 90%, it is unlikely that there would be much interest in intensifying therapy, thereby adding to the side effects for the 90% of patients cured by current therapy. The treatment of stage I and II disease is comparatively well tolerated and reducing therapy further may jeopardize the excellent current results with no definite gain. It is often difficult to recruit patients to such randomized trials, and the numbers of patients needed to identify small differences in survival is very large.

Perhaps the two areas for continued therapeutic development would be the continued reduction in the use of radiotherapy and a reduction in the potential cardiotoxicity of the anthracyclines. Is there a subgroup of patients with stage IV disease who do not need lung radiotherapy, and how can they be identified? The authors have some data to suggest that patients who were classified as stage III because of microscopic residual disease fare well without radiotherapy.[111] This approach would simply continue a trend in the reduction of the use of radiotherapy in this chemosensitive malignancy. Figure 59b.1 shows how the role of radiotherapy in the treatment of Wilms' tumor has gradually declined and suggests circumstances where its role may decline further in the future.

Changing the method of administration of the anthracyclines to continuous infusion rather than bolus injection may prevent cardiotoxicity, but two recent papers have suggested no benefit, although only moderate dose use of anthracyclines was studied.[112,113] The use of "cardioprotectants" is also under current review.[114]

The expanding knowledge of the molecular genetics of Wilms' tumor has yet to prove useful in management. The WT1 gene on chromosome 11p13 was cloned in 1990,[115,116] but mutations in this gene appear to be surprisingly uncommon in sporadic Wilms' tumors.[117] Loss of heterozygosity studies support the existence of a second Wilms' tumor suppressor gene at 11p15.[118] This genetic locus is also associated with the Weidemann–Beckwith syndrome (in which patients have a predisposition to Wilms' tumor and, less commonly, other pediatric malignancies).[119] There is some evidence to suggest that

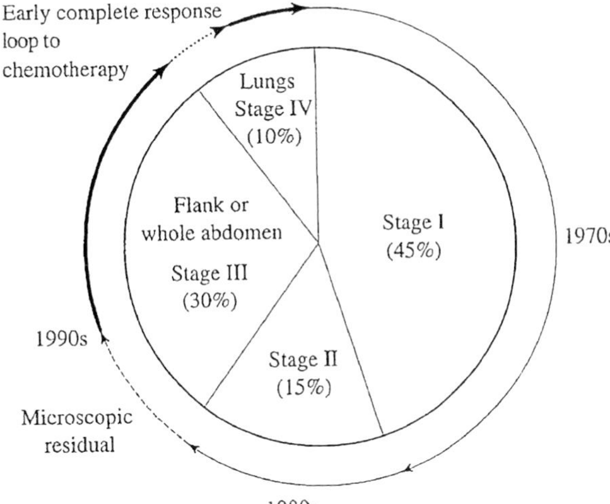

Fig. 59b.1. Schematic representation of the reduction in the use of radiotherapy in Wilms' tumor over time, and the possible instances in which further reduction in the use of this treatment modality may be considered. Each sector corresponds to a particular stage of Wilms' tumor. The proportion of all Wilms' patients classified as that stage is shown as a percentage and is indicated by the size of the sector. The thin solid arrows show the stages in which radiotherapy has been omitted and the dates of the studies. The broken arrows show the possibilities for the reduction of radiotherapy in the future. The thick solid arrows show the circumstances in which the role of radiotherapy is not currently in question. Figure courtesy of Dr J Pritchard.

loss of heterozygosity for chromosome region 16q and 1p may be associated with poor outcome.[120] How should this genetic information be used? In alveolar rhabdomyosarcoma, which can represent a diagnostic challenge using histopathology alone, the presence of the characteristic chromosome translocation between chromosomes 2 and 13 can be useful diagnostically, and its presence denotes a poor prognosis.[121] In neuroblastoma, amplification of the oncogene MYCN is associated with poor outcome and in some cases this information alone can alter therapy.[122] We have yet to define the utility of the molecular changes seen in Wilms' tumor, but potentially they could be used to continue the process of risk stratification that has so successfully directed therapy in other circumstances.

REFERENCES

1. Scott, I. S. Wilms' tumor: its treatment and prognosis. *Br. Med. J.* 1956; **1**:200–203.
2. Green, D. M., Brewslow, N., Beckwith, J. B. *et al.* A comparison between single dose and divided dose administration of dactinomycin and doxorubicin: a report from the National Wilms' Tumor Study Group (abstract). *Proc. Am. Soc. Clin. Oncol.* 1996; **15**:457.
3. Jessop, J. Annotations: extirpation of the kidney. *Lancet* 1877; **i**:889.
4. Lelie, E. M., Mynores, L. S., Draper, G. J., & Gormach, P. D. Natural history and treatment of Wilms' tumors: an analysis of 355 cases occurring in England and Wales 1962–1966. *Br. Med. J.* 1970; **4**:195–200.
5. Friedlander, A. Sarcoma of the kidney treated by the Roentgen X-ray. *Am. J. Dis. Child.* 1916; **XII**:328–330.
6. Williams, I. G. *Tumours of Childhood: a Clinical Treatise.* London: Heinemann, 1972:103–104.
7. Bond, J. V. Prognosis and treatment of Wilms' tumor at Great Ormond Street Hospital for Sick Children. *Cancer* 1975; **36**:102–107.
8. Farber, S., Toch, R., Sear, E. M. *et al.* Advances of chemotherapy in man. In Greenstein, J. P., Haddow (eds), *Advances in Cancer Research.* New York: Academic Press, 1956: A1–A71.
9. Sutow, W. & Thurman, W. G. Vincristine (Leurocristine) sulphate in the treatment of children with metastatic Wilms' tumor. *Paediatrics* 1963; **32**:880–887.
10. Duffy, P. G. Surgical management of Wilms' tumor. In *Rob and Smith's Operative Surgery: Paediatric Surgery,* 5th edn. London: Chapman & Hall, 1995:590–596.
11. Kumar, R., Breatriach, F., & Fitzgerald, R. Is contralateral exploration in Wilms' tumor necessary? Result from UKCCSG Bilateral Wilms' Tumor Study (abstract). 27th SIOP Meeting 1996; **218**:1–30.
12. Weirich, A., Rieden, T., Troger, J. *et al.* Diagnostic value of imaging procedures in nephroblastoma before preoperative chemotherapy: initial results. *Clin. Paediatr.* 1991; **203**(4):251–256.
13. Pritchard, J., Imeson, J., Barnes, J. *et al.* Results of the United Kingdom Children's Cancer Study Group first Wilms' tumor study. *J. Clin. Oncol.* 1995; **13**:124–133.
14. D'Angio, G. J. SIOP and the management of Wilms' tumor. *J. Clin. Oncol.* 1983; **1**:595–596.
15. Lemele, J., Voute, P. A., Toumade, M. F. *et al.* Pre-operative versus post-operative radiotherapy, single versus multiple courses of Actinomycin in the treatment of Wilms' tumors. Preliminary results of a controlled clinical trial by the International Society of Paediatric Oncology [SIOP]. *Cancer* 1976; **38**:647–654.
16. Lemele, J., Voute, P. A., Toumade, M. F. *et al.* Effectiveness of pre-operative chemothearpy in Wilms' tumor: results of an International Society of Paediatric Oncology (SIOP) study. *J. Clin. Oncol.* 1983; **1**:604–610.
17. Coppes, M. J., Tournade, M. F., Lemerle, J. *et al.* Pre-operative care of infants with nephroblastoma: the International Society of Paediatric Oncology Experience. *Cancer* 1992; **69**:2721–2725.
18. Dykes, E. H., Marwaha, R. K., Dicks-Mireaux, C. *et al.* Risks and benefits of percutanous biopsy and primary chemotherapy in advanced Wilms' tumor. *J. Pediatr. Surg.* 1991; **26**:610–612.

19. Vujanic, G. M., Kelsey, A., Mitchell, C. *et al.* The role of biopsy in the diagnosis of renal tumors of childhood: results of the UKCCSG Wilms tumor study 3. *Med. Pediatr. Oncol.* 2003; **40**(1):18–22.
20. Mitchell, C., Shannon, R., Vujanic, G. M. *et al.* The treatment of Wilms' tumor: results of the United Kingdom Children's Cancer Study Group Wilms' Tumor Study. *Br. J. Cancer* **88**(suppl. 1):4.1, S16.
21. Coppes, M. J., de Kraker, J., Van D ykes H. J. M. *et al.* Bilateral Wilms' tumor: long-term survival and some epidemiological features. *J. Clin. Oncol.* 1989; **7**:310–315.
22. Bishop, H. C. & Hope, J. W. Bilateral Wilms' tumor. *J Pediat Surg* 1966; **1**:476–487.
23. Montgomery, B. T., Kelalis, P. P., Blute, M. L. *et al.* Extended follow up of bilateral Wilms' tumor: results of the national Wilms' tumor study. *J. Urol.* 1991; **146**:514–518.
24. Kumar, R., Breatnach, F., & Fitzgerald, R. Bilateral Wilms' tumor: results of the United Kingdom Children's Cancer Group (UKCCSG) (abstract). 27th SIOP Meeting 1996; **219**:1–32.
25. Mclorie, G. A., McKenna, P. H., & Greenberg, M. Reduction in tumor burden allowing partial nephrectomy following preoperative chemotherapy in biopsy proven Wilms' tumor. *J. Urol.* 1991; **146**:589–613.
26. Shimamura, T. & Movision, A. B. Experimental chronic renal insufficiency. *Methods Achieve. Exp. Pathol.* 1966; **1**:455.
27. Hobletter, T. H., Olson, J. L., Rennke, H. G. *et al.* Hyperfiltration in remnant nephrons: a potentially adverse response to renal ablation. *Am. J. Physiol.* 1981; **241**:F85.
28. Steckler, R. E., Riehle, R. A., Jr. Darrocott, Vaughan., J. R. Hyperfiltration-induced renal injury in normal man: myth or reality. *J. Urol.* 1990; **144**:1323–1327.
29. Wikstad, I., Petterson, B. A., & Elinder, S. A comparative study of size and function of the remnant kidney in patients nephrectomised in childhood for Wilms' tumor and hydronephrosis. *Acta. Pediatr. Scand.* 1986; **75**:408–414.
30. Wikstad, I., Celsi, G., Larrson, L. *et al.* Kidney function in adults born with unilateral agenesis or nephrectomised in childhood. *Paediatr. Nephrol.* 1988; **2**:177–182.
31. Makipernaa, A., Kosikimies, O., Jaaskelainen, J. *et al.* Renal growth and function 11–28 years after treatment of Wilms' tumor. *Eur. J. Paediatr.* 1991; **150**:444–447.
32. Bairera, M., Roy, L. P., & Stevens, M. Long-term follow up after unilateral nephrectomy and radiotherapy for Wilms' tumor. *Pediatr. Nephrol.* 1989; **3**:430–432.
33. Jadresic, L., Lake, J., Gordon, I. *et al.* Clinicopathologic review of twelve children with nephropathy, Wilms' tumor and genital abnormalities (Drash sundrome). *J. Pediatr.* 1990; **117**:717–725.
34. Rudin, C., Trompeter, R. S., & Pritchard, J. The role of renal transplantation in the management of bilateral Wilms' tumor (BWT) and of Denys–Drash syndrome (DDS). *Nephrol. Daily. Transpl.* 1998; **13**:1506–1510.
35. Habib, R. Nephrotic syndrome in the 1st year of life. *Pediatr. Nephrol.* 1993; **7**:347–353.
36. Legha, S. S. Vincristine neurotoxicity: pathophysiology and management. *Med. Toxicol.* 1986; **1**:421–427.
37. Graf, W. D., Chance, P. F., Lensch, M. W. *et al.* Severe vincristine neuropathy in Charcot–Marie–Tooth disease type 1A. *Cancer* 1996; **77**:1356.
38. Raine, J., Bowman, A., Wallendszus, K., & Pritchard, J. Hepatopathy thrombocytopenia syndrome; a complication of dactinomycin therapy for Wilms' tumor. Report from the United Kingdom Children's Cancer Study Group. *J. Clin. Oncol.* 1991; **9**:2302–2311.
39. Ludwig, R., Weirich, A., Abel, A. *et al.* Hepatotoxicity in patients treated according to the nephroblastoma trial and study SIOP-9/GPOH. *Med. Pediatr. Oncol.* 1999; **33**(5):462–469.
40. D'Angio, G. J., Evans, A., Breslow, N. *et al.* The treatment of Wilms' tumor: results of the Second National Wilms' Tumor Study. *Cancer* 1981; **47**:2302–2311.
41. Von Hoff., D. D., Rozenewieg, M., Layard, M. *et al.* Daunomycin induced cardiotoxicity in children and adults. *Am. J. Med.* 1977; **62**:200–208.
42. Goorin, A. M., Chauvenet, A. R., & Perez-Atayde, A. R. Initial congestive heart failure six to ten years after doxorubicin chemotherapy for childhood cancer. *J. Pediatr.* 1996; **116**:144–147.
43. Steinherz, L. J., Steinherz, G., & Tan, C. J. Cardiac toxicity 4 to 20 years after completing anthracycline therapy. *J. Am. Med. Assoc.* 1991; **266**:1672–1677.
44. Sorensen, K., Levitt, G., Sebag-Montefiore, D., Bull, C., & Sullivan, I. Cardiac function in Wilms' tumor survivors. *J. Clin. Oncol.* 1995; **13**:1546–1556.
45. Lipshultz, S. E., Colan, S. D., & Gelber, R. D. Late cardiac effects of doxorubicin therapy for acute lymphoblastic leukaemia in children. *N. Engl. J. Med.* 1991; **324**:808–815.
46. Lipshultz, S. E., Lipsitz, S. R., Mone, S. M. *et al.* Female sex and higher drug dose as risk factors for late cardiotoxic effects of doxorubicin therapy for children's cancer. *N. Engl. J. Med.* 1995; **332**:1738–1743.
47. Sorensen, K., Levitt, G. A., Bull, C., Dorup, I., & Sullivan, I. D. Late anthracycline cardiotoxicity after childhood cancer: a prospective longitudinal study. *Cancer* 2003; **97**:1991–1998.
48. Pein, F., Sakiroglu, O., Dahan, M. *et al.* Cardiac abnormalities 15 years and more after adriamycin therapy in 229 childhood survivors of a solid tumor at the Institute Gustave Roussy. *Br. J. Cancer.* 2004; **91**:37–44.
49. Marx, M., Langer, T., Graf, N., Hausdorf, G., Stöhr, W., & Beck, J. D. A multicentre analysis of anthracycline-induced cardiotoxicity in children following treatment according to the nephroblastoma studies SIOP 9/GPOH and SIOP 93-01/GPOH. *Med. Pediatr. Oncol.* 2002, **39**:18–24,
50. Levitt, G. A., Bunch, K., Rogers, C. A., & Whitehead, B. Cardiac transplantation in childhood cancer survivors in Great Britain. *Eur. J. Cancer.* 1996; **32A**:826–830.
51. Steinhertz, L., Graham, T., Hurwitz, R., Sondheimer, H. M., Schwartz, R. G. Guidelines for monitoring of children during anthracycline therapy. Report of the cardiology committee of

the Children's Cancer Study Group. *Paediatrics* 1992; **89**:942–949.

52. Lipshultz, S. E., Sanders, S. P., Colan, S. C., Gorin, A. N., & Sallan, S. S. Monitoring for anthracycline cardiotoxicity. *Paediatrics* 1992; **89**:942–949.
53. Davis, L. E. & Brown, C. E. L. Peripartum heart failure in a patient previously treated with doxorubicin. *Obst. Gyn.* 1988; **71**:506–508.
54. Pritchard, J., Imeson, J., Barnes, J. *et al.* Results of the United Kingdom Children's Cancer Study Group first Wilms' Tumor Study. *J. Clin. Oncol.* 1995; **13**:124–33.
55. Neequaye, J. E., Bryne, J., & Levine, P. H. Menarche and reproduction after treatment for African Burkitt's lymphoma. *Br. Med. J.* 1991; **303**:1033.
56. Kenney, L. B., Lanfer, M. R., Grant, F. D., Grier, H., & Diller, L. High risk of infertility and long term gonadal damage in males treated with high dose cyclophosphamide for sarcoma during childhood. *Cancer* 2001; **91**:613–621.
57. Aubier, F., Oberlin, O., Vathalre, de. F. *et al.* Influence of chemothearpy on male fertility. *Med. Pediat. Oncol.* 1994; **23**:177.
58. Tournade, M. F., Lemerle, J., Brunat-Mentigny, M. *et al.* Ifosfamide is an active drug in Wilms' tumor: a phase II study conducted by the French Society of Pediatric Oncology. *J. Clin. Oncol.* 1998; **6**:793–796.
59. Skinner, R., Pearson, A., Wyllie, R., Coulthard, M., & Craft, A. I. Ifosfamide nephrotoxicity in children: risk factors and the long term outcome. *Med. Pediatr. Oncol.* 1994; **23**:265.
60. Rossi, R., Godde, A., Kleinebrand, M. *et al.* Unilateral nephrectomy and cisplatin as risk factors of ifosfamide induced nephrotoxicity: analysis of 120 patients. *J. Clin. Oncol.* 1994; **12**:159–165.
61. Prasad, V. K., Lewis, I. J., Aparicio, S. A. *et al.* Progressive glomerular toxicity of ifosfamide in children. *Med. Pediatr. Oncol.* 1996; **27**:149–155.
62. Zoubek, A., Kaitar, P., Flucher-Wolfram, B. *et al.* Response of untreated stage IV Wilms' tumor to single dose carboplatin assessed by 'up front' window therapy. *Med. Pediatr. Oncol.* 1995; **25**:8–11.
63. Pein, F., Pinkerton, R., Tournade, M. F. *et al.* Etoposide in relapsed or refractory Wilms' tumor: a phase II study by the French Society of Paediatric Oncology and United Kingdom Children's Cancer Study Group. *J. Clin. Oncol.* 1993; **11**:1478–1481.
64. Pein, F., Tournade, M. F., Zucker, J. M. *et al.* Etoposide and carboplatin, a highly effective combination in relapsed or refractory Wilms' tumor: a phase II study by the French Society of Paediatric Oncology. *J. Clin. Oncol.* 1994; **12**:931–936.
65. Hawkins, M. M., Kinnier Wilson L. M., Stovall, M. A. *et al.* Epidophyllotoxins, Alkylating agents, and radiation and risk of secondary leukaemia after childhood cancer. *Br. Med. J.* 1992; **304**:951–958.
66. Jereb, B., Burgers, M. V., Toumade , M. F. *et al.* Radiotherapy in the SIOP nephroblastoma studies: a review. *Med. Pediatr. Oncol.* 1994; **22**:221–227.
67. D'Angio, G. J., Breslow, N., Beckwith, J. B. *et al.* Treatment of Wilms' tumor. *Cancer* 1989; **64**:349–360.
68. Shalet, S. M., Gibson, B., Swindell, R., & Pearson, D. Effect of spinal irradiation on growth. *Arch. Dis. Child.* 1987; **62**:461–464.
69. Makiprnaa, A., Keikkila, J. T., Merikanto, J., Marttinen, E., & Siimes, M. A. Spinal deformity induced by radiotherapy for solid tumors in childhood: a long term study. *Eur. J. Pediat.* 1993; **152**:197–200.
70. Jaffe, N., Ried, H. L., Cohen, M., McNeese, M. D., & Sullivan, M. P. Radiation induced osteochondroma in long term survivors of childhood cancer. *Int. J. Rad. Oncol. Biol. Phys.* 1983; **9**:665–670.
71. Tanner, J. M. & Whitehouse, R. H. Standards for sitting height and subishial leg length from birth to maturity: *British Children 1978*. Hertford: Castlemead Publications, 1978.
72. Wallace, W. H. B. Shalet, S. M., Moris-Jones, P. H., Swindell, R., & Gattamaneni, H. R. Effect of abdominal irrradiation on growth in boys treated for a Wilms' tumor. *Med. Pediatr. Oncol.* 1990; **18**:441–446.
73. Wallace, W. H. B. & Shalt, S. M. Chemotherapy with Actinomycin D influences the growth of the spine followign abdominal irradiation. *Med. Pediat. Oncol.* 1992; **20**:177.
74. Rosenfield, N. S., Haller, J. O., & Berdon, W. E. Failure of development of the growing breast after radiation therapy. *Pediatr. Radiol.* 1989; **19**:124–127.
75. Rostom, A. Y. & O'Cathail, S. Failure of lactation following radiothearpy for breast cancer. *Lancet* 1986; **1**:163–164.
76. McDonald, S., Rubin, P., Scwartz, C. L. *et al.* (eds). *Pulmonary Effects of Antinoplastic Therapy: Survivors of Childhood Cancer*. New York: Mosby-Yearbook, 1994; 177–195.
77. Attard, Monalto S. P., Kingston, J. E., Eden, O. B., & Plowman, P. N. Late follow up of lung function after whole lung irraidation for Wilms' tumor. *Bri. J. Radiol.* 1992; **65**:1114–1118.
78. Jenney, M. E. M. & Shaw, N. J. Late respiratory effects of treatment for childhood malignancy. *Pediatr. Rev. Commun.* 1994; **8**:17–22.
79. Fajardo, L. J., Bricker, T. J., Green, D. M., & D'Angio, G. J. (eds). *Pathology of Radiation Induced Heart Disease: Cardiac Toxicity after Treatment for Childhood Cancer*. New York: Wiley-Liss, 1993; 7–15.
80. Counsell, R., Bain, G., Williams, M. V., & Dixon, A. K. Artificial radiation menopause; where are the ovaries? *Lin. Oncol.* 1996; **8**:250–253.
81. Torano, A. E., Halperin, E. C., Leventhal, B. G. *et al.* (eds). *The Ovary: Survivors of Childhood Cancer*. Mosby-YearBook, 1994: 213–224.
82. Perrone, L., Sinisi, A. A., Sicuranza, R. *et al.* Prepubertal endocrine follow up in subjects with Wilms' tumor. *Med. Pediatr. Oncol.* 1988; **16**:255–258.
83. Shalet, S. M., Beardwell, C. G., Morris J ones, P. H., Pearson, D., & Orrell, D. H. Ovarian failure following abdominal irradiation in children. *Br. J. Cancer* 1976; **33**:655–658.
84. Wallace, W. H. B., Shalet, S. M., Crowne, E. C., Morris J ones, P. H., & Gattamaneni, H. R. Ovarian failure following

abdominal irradiation in children: natural history and prognosis. *Clin. Oncol.* 1989; **96**:378–380.

85. Hawkins, M. M. & Smith, R. A. Pregnancy outcomes in childhood cancer survivors: probable effect of abdominal irradiation. *Int. J. Cancer* 1989; **43**:399–402.
86. Hawkins, M. M. & Smith, R. A. Pregnancies after childhood cancer. *Br. J. Obst.* 1989; **96**:378–380.
87. Liesner, R. J., Leiper, A. D., Hann, I. M., & Chessells, J. M. Late effects of intensive treatment for acute myeloid leukaemia and myelodysplasia in childhood. *J. Clin. Oncol.* 1994; **12**:916–924.
88. Hawkins, M. M. Is there evidence of a therapy related increase in germ cell mutation among childhood cancer survivors? *J. Natl. Cancer Inst.* 1991; **83**:1643–1650.
89. Shalet, S. M., Beardwell, C. G., Jacobs, H. S., & Pearson, D. Testicular function following irradiation of the human prepubertal testis. *Clin. Endocrinol.* 1978; **9**:483–490.
90. Flentje, M., Weirech, A., Potter, R., & Ludwig, R. Hepatotoxicity in irradiated nephroblastoma patients during postopertive treatment accoing to SIOP9/GPOH. *Radiother. Oncol.* 1994; **31**:222–228. Comment in *Radiother. Oncol.* 1994; **31**:191.
91. Teinturier, C., Tournade, M. F., Cailla-Zucman, S. *et al.* Diabetes mellitus after abdominal radiation therapy (letter). *Lancet* 1995; **346**:633–634. Comment in *Lancet* 1996; **347**:539–540.
92. Lipshitz, H. I. & Cohen, M. A. Radiation induced osteochondromas. *Radiology* 1982; **142**:643–647.
93. Tsuchiva, H., Morikawa, S., & Tomita, K. Osteosarcoma arising from a multiple exostosis lesion; case report. *Japan. J. Clin. Oncol.* 1990; **20**:296–298.
94. Walker, D. A., Dillon, M., Levitt, G. *et al.* Mulitple exotosis (osteochondroma) and Wilms' tumor; a possible association. *Med. Pediatr. Oncol.* 1992; **20**:360–361.
95. Wuyts, W., Van Hul, W., Wauters, J. *et al.* Positional cloning of a gene involved in hereditary multiple exostosis. *Hum. Molec. Genet.* 1996; **5**:1547–1557.
96. Olsen, J. H., Garwicz, Z. S., Hertz, H. *et al.* Second malignant neoplasms after cancer in childhood or adolescence. *Br. Med. J.* 1993; **307**:1030–1036.
97. Hawkins, M. M., Draper, G. J., & Kingston, J. E. Incidence of second primary tumors among childhood cancer survivors. *Br. J. Cancer* 1987; **56**:339–347.
98. D'Angio, G. J., Evans, A. E., Breslow, N. *et al.* The treatment of Wilms' tumuor: results of the National Wilms' Tumor Study. *Cancer* 1976; **38**:633–646.
99. Morris-Jones, P. H., Pearson, D., & Johnson, A. L. Management of nephroblastoma in childhood: clinical study of forms of maintenence chemotherpy. Medical Research Council's Working Party on Embryonal Tumors in Childhood. *Arch. Dis. Child.* 1978; **53**:112–119.
100. Green, D. M., Beckwith, J. B. Weeks, D. A. *et al.* The relationship between microsubstaging variables, age at diagnosis, and tumor weight of children with stage I/favourable histology Wilms' tumor. *Cancer* 1994; **74**:1817–1820.
101. Beckwith, J. B. & Palmer, N. F. Histopathology and prognosis in Wilms' tumor: results from the First National Wilms' Tumor Study. *Cancer* 1978; **41**:1937–1948.
102. Green, D. M., Beckwith, J. B., Breslow, N. E. *et al.* Treatment of children with stages II to IV anaplastic Wilms' tumor: a report from the National Wilms' Tumor Study Group. *J. Clin. Oncol.* 1994; **12**:2126–2131.
103. Green, D. M., Beckwith, J. B., Breslow, N. E. *et al.* Treatment of children with clear cell sarcoma of the kidney: a report from the National Wilms' Tumor Tumor Study Group. *J. Clin. Oncol.* 1994; **12**:2132–2137.
104. D'Angio, G. L., Breslow, N. E., Beckwith, J. B. *et al.* Treatment of Wilms' tumor: results of the third National Wilms' Tumor Study. *Cancer* 1989; **64**:349–360.
105. Morris Jones, P. H., Marsden, H. B., & Pearson, D. The conclusion of the second MRC nephroblastoma study (abstract). Presented at the British Paediatric Association meeting, York, UK, March 1983.
106. de Kraker, J., Lemerle, J., Voute, P. A. *et al.* Wilms' tumor with pulmonary metastases at diagnosis: the significance of primary chemotherapy. *J. Clin. Oncol.* 1990; **8**:1187–1190.
107. Makipernaa, A. Long term quality of life and psychosocial coping after treatment of solid tumors in childhood. *Acta. Paediatr. Scand.* 1989; **78**:728–735.
108. Radford, M. & Evans, S. E. Current lifestyle of young adults treated for cancer in childhood. *Arch. Dis. Child.* 1995; **72**:432–426.
109. Robertson, C. M., Hawkins, M. M., & Kingston, J. E. Late deaths and survival after childhood cancer: implications for cure. *Br. Med. J.* 1994; **309**:162–166.
110. Garaventa, A., Hartmann, O., Bernard J.-L. *et al.* Autologous bone marrow transplantation for paediatric Wilms' tumor: the experience of the European Bone Marrow Transplantation solid tumor registry. *Med. Pediatr. Oncol.* 1994; **22**:11–14.
111. Pachis, A., Pritchard, J., Gaze, M., Levitt, G., & Michalski, A. Radiotherapy omitted in the treatment of selected children under 3 years of age with stage III favorable histology Wilms tumor. *Med. Pediatr. Oncol.* 1998; **31**:150–152.
112. Lipshultz, S. E., Giantris, A. L., Lipsitz, S. R. *et al.* Doxorubicin administration by continuous infusion is not cardioprotective: The Dana-Farber 91–01 Acute Lymphoblastic Leukemia Protocol. *J. Clin. Oncol.* 2002; **20**(6): 1677–1682.
113. Levitt, G. A., Dorup, I., Sorensen, K., & Sullivan, I. Does anthracycline administration by infusion in children affect late cardiotoxicity *Br. J. Haematol.* 2004; **124**(4):463–468.
114. Lipshultz, S. E. Dexrazoxane for protection against cardiotoxic effects of anthracyclines in children. *J. Clin. Oncol.* 1996; **14**:328–331.
115. Call, K. M., Glaser, T., Ito, C. Y. *et al.* Isolation and characterisation of a zinc finger polypeptide gene at the human chromosome 1 Wilms' tumor locus. *Cell* 1990; **60**:509–520.
116. Gessler, M., Poustka, A., Cavenee, W. *et al.* Homozygous deletion in Wilms' tumors of a zinc finger gene identified by chromosome jumping. *Nature* 1990; **343**:774–778.
117. Varanasi, R., Bardeesy, N., Ghahremani, M. *et al.* Fine structure analysis of WT1 gene in sporadic Wilms' tumors. *Proc. Natl. Acad. Sci. USA* 1194; **91**:3554–3558.

118. Reeve, A. E., Sih, S. A., Raiziz, A. M. *et al.* Loss of alleleic heterozygosity at a second locus on chromosome 11 in sporadic Wilms' tumor cells. *Mol. Cell. Biol.* 1989; **9**:1799–1803.
119. Ping, A. J., Reeve, A. E., Law, D. J. *et al.* Genetic linkage of Beckwith–Weidemann syndrome to 11p15. *Am. J. Hum. Genet.* 1989; **44**:720–723.
120. Grundy, P. E., Tezerow, P. E., Breslow, N. E. *et al.* Loss of heterozygosity for chromosomes 16q and 1p in Wilms' tumors predicts an adverse outcome. *Cancer* 1994; **54**:2331–2333.
121. Crist, W., Gehan, E. A., Ragab, A. H. *et al.* The Third Intergroup Rhabdomyosarcoma study. *J. Clin. Oncol.* 1995; **13**:610–630.
122. Brodeur, G. M., Azar, C., Brother, M. *et al.* Neuroblastoma: effect of genetic factors on prognosis and treatment. *Cancer* 1992; **70**:1685–1696.

60

Rhabdomyosarcoma

Dave R. Lal, Charles A. Sklar, and Michael P. LaQuaglia

Department of Surgery and Pediatrics, Memorial Sloan-Kettering Cancer Center, New York, NY, USA

Soft tissue sarcomas are the sixth most common malignancy of childhood, with rhabdomyosarcoma (RMS) by far the most frequent. In the United States, approximately 350 cases of RMS are diagnosed per year. Since 1975, the yearly incidence of RMS has remained stable at approximately 4 per 1 million children younger than 20 years of age.[1]

Over the last 30 years, improved survival and decreased morbidity in treatment of RMS have been accomplished through collaborative clinical trials in both the United States and Europe. In the United States the Intergroup Rhabdomyosarcoma Study Group (IRSG) was established in 1972. Their mission has been to enroll all children diagnosed in North America into randomized prospective clinical trials. This has largely been accomplished with over 80% of North American children diagnosed with RMS enrolled in one of four completed IRSG studies. Since the inception of the IRSG, the overall survival for patients with RMS has improved from about 25% to over 70%. Much of this improvement has been the result of a multidisciplinary approach to rhabdomyosarcoma including surgeons, oncologists, and radiation oncologists. The IRSG (now called the Children's Oncology Group soft tissue sarcoma committee) continues to strive for improved survival with decreasing patient morbidity, and is currently accruing patients for its fifth trial (IRS-V).

Currently, orbital tumors have the best prognosis with a 5-year survival of approximately 95%. The next best outcome was observed in non-bladder/prostate genitourinary tumors that had an overall survival of close to 90%, while bladder/prostate rhabdomyosarcoma had an approximately 80% 5-year survival. Non-orbital head and neck, extremity, and parameningeal primary tumors had survivals of approximately 78%, 75%, and 70% in IRS-III. Patients who present with metastatic disease or who develop recurrence share a dismal prognosis.

The role of extensive surgical resection for rhabdomyosarcoma has become less important with advancements in chemotherapy and radiotherapy. Surgical resection is still advocated when small non-invasive tumors can be completely excised or after clinical response with chemotherapy for extensive tumors. Debilitating or disfiguring surgery is avoided and resorted to when residual disease remains after chemotherapy and radiotherapy or after recurrence of disease managed conservatively. Amputation for extremity rhabdomyosarcomas does not enhance cure and is limited to cases were the lesions are bulky, invasive to the bone or neurovascular structures, or are recurrent. Likewise, radical cystectomy, hysterectomy/vaginectomy, and eye enucleation are reserved for situations in which residual disease remains after chemotherapy and external-beam radiotherapy. The guiding principle of rhabdomyosarcoma surgery is complete tumor resection; however, removal of large amounts of adjacent normal tissue (i.e., muscle group resection, amputation) does not, in itself, affect outcome.

Due to the multidisciplinary approach involving surgery, chemotherapy, and radiotherapy for children with rhabdomyosarcoma, the subsequent short- and long-term consequences of treatment remain vast and diverse. Rhabdomyosarcoma survivors are increasingly living into adulthood and thus require long-term support and follow-up to detect treatment-related sequelae.

Pediatric Surgery and Urology: Long-term Outcomes, Mark Stringer, Keith Oldham, Pierre Mouriquand.
Published by Cambridge University Press.

Radiotherapy

Essential in the treatment of RMS is radiotherapy (RT). Due to the infiltrative character of RMS and sites of origin which often preclude wide surgical excision, local control is enhanced with adjuvant radiotherapy. Clinical data suggest that control of microscopic rhabdomyosarcoma can be accomplished with external beam radiotherapy (EBRT) at doses of 40 Gy, whereas gross deposits require more than 50 Gy for sterilization. Different techniques of radiotherapy delivery and doses have been attempted in an effort to minimize the sequelae of treatment without compromising local control. In IRS-IV, patients with incomplete resection and gross residual tumor were randomized to conventionally fractionated radiotherapy (daily 1.8 Gy for a total dose of 50.4 Gy) vs. hyperfractionated radiotherapy (twice-daily 1.1 Gy for a total dose of 59.4 Gy). No difference in local control or survival was observed. However, the hyperfractionated group suffered from more mucositis, skin reactions, and nausea/vomiting.[2] Wolden *et al.*[3] examined results from IRS I–III, to determine if patients undergoing complete surgical resection (no residual microscopic or gross disease) would benefit from adjuvant RT. With a median follow-up of 12.9 years (IRS-I), 9.1 years (IRS-II), and 4.6 years (IRS-III), patients with embryonal histology did not benefit from addition of RT. Patients with alveolar or undifferentiated RMS treated with RT had significantly improved 10-year failure-free survival (73% vs. 44%) and overall survival (82% vs. 52%) when compared to those not receiving RT. Therefore, conventionally fractionated RT has been instituted in the treatment guidelines of IRS-V for all patients except those with embryonal histology and complete surgical resection.

In an effort to minimize the sequelae of fibrosis, bone marrow irradiation, growth and organ retardation seen after EBRT in children, brachytherapy has been utilized as an alternative. Collateral tissue exposure can be minimized with brachytherapy. Nag *et al.*[4] looked at RMS patients treated with fractionated high dose rate brachytherapy (F-HDR) after chemotherapy and surgery. With a median follow-up of 10 years, patients treated with F-HDR had superb local control (80%) and overall survival (80%). This is comparable to results after conventional EBRT. No evidence of growth suppression was seen in these patients. Long-term complications did include osteonecrosis of the mandible (patient with buccal RMS), vaginal stenosis (vaginal RMS), and periurethral stenosis (vaginal RMS). Of the 20% of patients who developed relapse, 40% were able to be salvaged with surgery, chemotherapy, and EBRT. The authors concluded that F-HDR can be utilized in selected young children with minimal residual disease after surgery, who would be most affected by growth and organ suppression.

Recent advances in RT delivery have led to intensity modulated radiation therapy (IMRT). IMRT modulates the intensity of individual radiation beams, thus allowing for more precise tumor targeting with diminished collateral tissue damage. Combining intensity modulated radiation with three-dimensional target mapping allows for reduced radiation doses to be delivered without altering tumor reduction or increasing local recurrence. Although no long-term data are available on the use of IMRT on children with RMS, it remains a promising treatment modality.

Treatment-related late effects

Cardiac

Delayed cardiotoxicity following treatment for childhood rhabdomyosarcoma is most often due to prior therapy with the anthracycline drugs, doxorubicin and daunomycin.[5] These drugs are associated with the late development of cardiomyopathy, which may be subclinical but can result in cardiac failure and dysrhythmias. Although late cardiac dysfunction is more common following evidence of acute toxicity during anthracycline administration, chronic cardiomyopathy can occur at any time and without prior symptoms or signs.[6,7] Late cardiac dysfunction is associated with higher anthracycline dose, mediastinal irradiation, female sex, and higher rate of drug administration.[7–10]

Steinherz *et al.*[7] reported on the cardiac status of 200 long-term survivors of childhood cancer treated at Memorial Sloan-Kettering Cancer Center. Twenty-three percent manifested abnormal cardiac function on echocardiogram a median of 7 years after completion of anthracycline therapy (median dose 450 mg m^{-2}). An increased incidence of abnormalities was observed with increased cumulative dose, length of follow-up, and in patients treated with chest irradiation.[7] More recently, this group has described late symptoms (6–19 years after therapy) in a series of 15 patients, including three subjects treated for rhabdomyosarcoma.[6] While five of the 15 had required treatment for cardiac symptoms at the end of treatment, ten had no cardiac problems antedating their late decompensation. Four patients died, one from uncontrollable cardiac failure and three suddenly from presumed arrhythmias. One patient underwent a successful heart transplant. Lifestyle factors felt to have contributed to late cardiac decompensation included heavy weight lifting and cocaine and alcohol abuse.[6] Similar results have been reported in a prospective multicenter study from Europe. Langer *et al.*[11] found that 12% of patients treated with doxorubicin developed diminished cardiac function on follow-up echocardiograms. Of these patients, 1.5% required long-term pharmacologic cardiac support. Careful follow-up and long-term surveillance of cardiac function is essential in patients treated with anthracyclines and mediastinal radiotherapy.

Attempts have been made to pharmacologically intervene in patients found to have declining cardiac performance on long-term surveillance. Silber *et al.*[12] recently conducted a double-blind, placebo-controlled study examining the angiotensin-converting enzyme inhibitor enalapril's ability to halt cardiac decline in children exposed to anthracyclines. Although enalapril was found to lower left ventricular end-diastolic wall stress, no improvement was noted in exercise performance or maximal cardiac index. The significance or benefit of reduced wall stress is unknown.

Pulmonary

Late pulmonary dysfunction can be observed following the use of radiation therapy and certain chemotherapeutic agents. Radiation-induced respiratory compromise in adolescents and adults is usually due to direct damage to the pulmonary parenchyma resulting in pulmonary fibrosis, whereas in children the pattern of injury appears to be secondary to impaired growth of both the lung and chest wall.[5] Reductions in lung function have been observed following whole lung radiation doses as low as 12–14 Gy.[13] Children treated with radiation to the lung prior to age 3 years may experience a higher incidence of chronic lung disorders.[14]

The drugs most commonly associated with delayed pulmonary toxicity include bleomycin and carmustine (BCNU).[15,16] While the data in adults suggest that late pulmonary complications are dose dependent, the threshold dose required to cause long-term damage in children for either of these agents is unknown. Furthermore, the use of combination chemotherapy may alter the ability of any single agent to produce delayed effects. Additional agents which may rarely result in pulmonary dysfunction include methotrexate, cyclophosphamide, and busulfan.[5] Pulmonary disease may be exacerbated by factors such as superimposed infections and cigarette smoking.

Kaplan *et al.*[17] have performed pulmonary function tests on a group of 17 survivors of rhabdomyosarcoma treated at Memorial Sloan-Kettering Cancer Center. The subjects were studied a mean of 7 years after diagnosis at a median age of 17 years. All subjects received combination chemotherapy which included bleomycin, methotrexate, and cyclophosphamide. Two of the patients had also received the drug 1,3-*bis* (2-chloroethyl)-1-nitrosourea (BCNU) also called carmustine and an additional two subjects had been treated with radiotherapy to the chest. Although none of the patients complained of any pulmonary symptoms, there was a very high incidence of restrictive ventilatory abnormalities. Total lung capacity was reduced in 87% of subjects, and 70% exhibited a carbon monoxide diffusing capacity below the normal lower limit.[17]

Gastrointestinal tract

Esophagus

Ellenhorn *et al.*[18] reported a series of five patients with treatment-related esophageal strictures. In this group there were two with rhabdomyosarcoma. One 9-year-old girl had an embryonal rhabdomyosarcoma of the oropharynx and soft palate and received multiagent chemotherapy as well as 54 Gy of external beam radiotherapy (36 fractions over 8 weeks). The tumor initially involved the full thickness of the pharyngeal wall along one-third of its circumference. Two years after treatment the patient complained of dysphagia, and barium swallow documented a long cervical esophageal stricture. Flexible esophagoscopy confirmed a tight stricture at the level of the cricopharyngeus muscle and multiple dilatations were required. Finally, the child was managed with home dilatation and was able to take most solid foods.

The second case in this report involved an 8-year-old boy who presented with an embryonal rhabdomyosarcoma of the tracheoesophageal groove. He too received chemotherapy, and 43.5 Gy of external beam radiation to this area (29 fractions over 22 days). At the end of chemotherapy, he developed odynophagia and midscapular pain on coughing. Barium swallow revealed a tight stricture at the level of the aortic arch. Multiple dilatations were required with a total of 15 performed before development of a tracheoesophageal fistula 6 years after initial diagnosis. There was no evidence of tumor recurrence, and a colon esophagoplasty with isolation of the native esophagus was performed. The patient is well 4 years later. Manometric studies performed in both of these patients showed absent or very reduced peristalsis in the esophageal segment that included the stricture. Figure 60.1 shows a patient with an upper esophageal stricture after radiation therapy.

Stomach and small bowel

Chronic enteritis, perforation, and/or fistula formation are all associated with delivery of therapeutic radiation dosages to the bowel.[19–22] Donaldson *et al.*[22] reported the follow-up of 44 children who received whole-abdomen radiation for malignancies, one of which was a retroperitoneal rhabdomyosarcoma. The most common diagnosis was

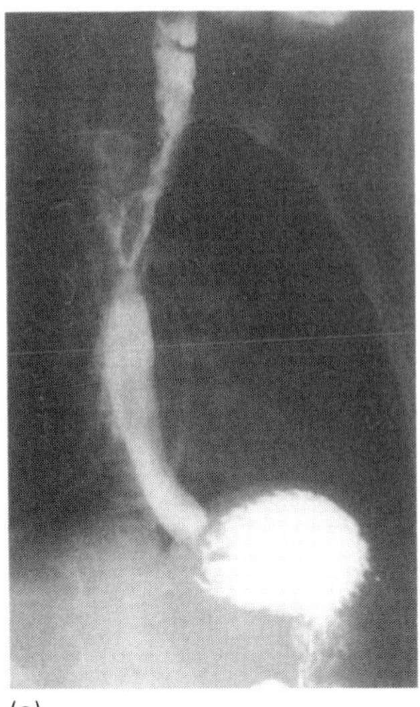
(a)

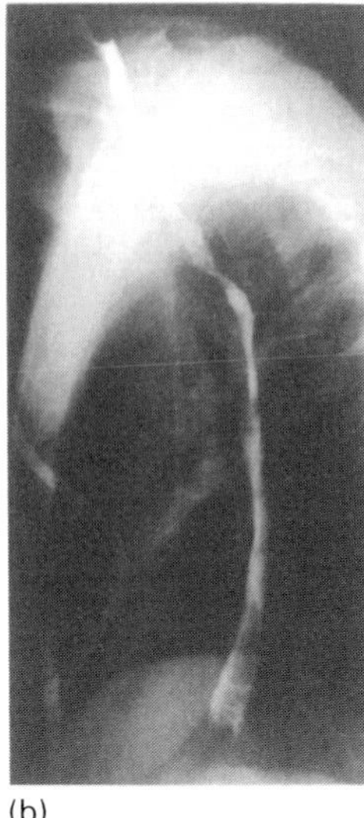
(b)

Fig. 60.1. Barium swallow study, demonstrating an esophageal stricture after radiation therapy for a mediastinal rhabdomyosarcoma. The lateral view also shows the stricture. Colon replacement of the esophagus was eventually required.

abdominal lymphoma followed by Wilms' tumor. They noted that five children (11%) developed an intestinal syndrome after completion of therapy. These patients presented with symptoms and signs of small bowel obstruction. Four of the five patients required laparotomy, which revealed a small bowel obstruction and dense adhesions and fibrosis. Definitive surgical correction was not possible in any of those patients undergoing laparotomy. These patients were subsequently treated with a gluten-free and lactose-reduced diet consisting of 6–12 feedings per day. They were slowly reintroduced to a normal diet and did not suffer progressive symptoms secondary to radiation enteritis. Oya *et al.*,[23] in a histopathological study of radiation enteritis lesions resected because of symptoms, divided the pathological findings into three categories: ulcerative stricture, serosal adhesion, and wall sclerosing. Twenty-one lesions from 19 patients were included in this study and a correlation between the histopathological lesion and the duration of chronic radiation enteritis was made. Patients were divided into two groups consisting of those within 2 years of bowel irradiation ($n = 10$) and those irradiated more than 8 years prior to surgery ($n = 11$). The authors found that ulcerative strictures were much more likely in patients receiving radiation more than 8 years prior to the resection (9/11). In contrast, all cases of serosal adhesion were noted in patients within 2 years of their radiotherapy. Lesions from the patients with longer follow-up were also more likely to be associated with fistulas (2/11), and demonstrate moderate to marked degenerative changes of the vessel wall (8/11). The authors concluded that chronic radiation enteritis results in a progressive injury to the bowel.

Rao *et al.*[19] reported the case of a 3-year-old girl who received 40 Gy of radiation to treat a Wilms' tumor. Fourteen years later she developed a bowel perforation that at laparotomy was located in the jejunum and within the radiation field. Histopathological examination of the resected bowel segment showed severe radiation enteritis. Meric *et al.*[24] recommended the placement of a polyglycolic acid mesh sling at laparotomy to prevent the small bowel from entering the pelvis. This was done to reduce the radiation dose to the small bowel in patients with pelvic malignancies. In their group of eight children the average pelvic radiation dose was 53.5 ± 5.6 Gy. Postoperative imaging studies confirmed that the small bowel remained out of the pelvis in 5/8 patients studied. Mesh disruption occurred in 2–5 months. At a mean follow-up of 20 months there was no evidence of radiation enteritis. Others have formed a sling or pocket of omentum to elevate the small bowel out of the pelvis during radiation therapy to that region.[25,26] Silvain *et al.*[27] studied the long-term outcome of 31 adult patients with severe radiation enteritis who were treated with total parenteral nutrition. Oral feeding could be resumed in only 11 patients (36%) at a median of 40 months. Thirteen patients died from complications of radiation therapy.

Aggressive surgical resections can also lead to short- and long-term abdominal complications. Michalkiewicz *et al.*[28] reported on their experience treating 17 patients after pelvic exenteration for genitourinary rhabdomyosarcoma. Overall, they noted a 76% rate of surgically related postoperative complications. Early complications included fistulae, wound infection, and abscess. Five patients (29%) developed either partial or complete bowel obstructions, four of these developed as late complications, within a median of 8 months after surgery. Adhesiolysis was required in all but one patient.

Gonadal

The therapies employed to treat rhabdomyosarcoma can be associated with clinically significant gonadal damage.[29,30] The extent of gonadal injury sustained appears to be dependent on a variety of factors, including age and pubertal status at the time of treatment,[31,32] dose and fractionation schedule of radiation,[33–35] as well as type and dose of chemotherapy.[31] Additionally, these variables may differ between males and females.

Testicular dysfunction

Male germ cells are extremely sensitive to both radiotherapy and several classes of chemotherapeutic agents.[29,33,36–39] Depletion of the germinal epithelium and infertility are well recognized complications of treatment with alkylating agents (e.g., cyclophosphamide, ifosfamide, the nitrosoureas), drugs frequently employed in the therapy of rhabdomyosarcoma. Toxicity is dose related and more severe when multiple drugs are utilized. While the prepubertal testis may be less vulnerable to injury than the postpubertal testis, oligoazoospermia is well described in young adults who were treated for rhabdomyosarcoma with combination chemotherapy during early childhood.[29,40,41] Chemotherapy induced germ cell dysfunction is often permanent, but instances of recovery many years after treatment have been noted.

Male germ cells are exquisitely sensitive to the effects of ionizing radiation.[31,33] Evidence of injury to the seminiferous tubules in adult men has been observed following single doses as low as 0.15 Gy. The extent of damage and time course to recovery appear dose-dependent. Following fractionated doses of 0.20–1.50 Gy to the adult testicle, recovery of spermatogenesis can occur over a period of 6 months to 2 years.[33] Doses greater than 2 Gy are associated with longstanding azoospermia.[33,38]

Reduced testicular volume and raised plasma concentrations of FSH are the hallmarks of therapy-induced germ cell dysfunction.[37,39] Young adult survivors who manifest both a decrease in testicular size and an elevated FSH level have a high likelihood of impaired sperm production and infertility.[37]

Leydig cells, in contrast to germ cells, are quite resistant to combination chemotherapy and low-dose radiation.[39] Clinically apparent Leydig cell failure requiring testosterone replacement therapy does occur, however, following irradiation of the testes with doses in excess of 20 Gy,[42,43] and has been reported in survivors of pelvic and paratesticular rhabdomyosarcoma.[41,44]

Ovarian dysfunction

Ovaries of prepubertal and pubertal children are generally very resistant to the toxic effects of conventional combination chemotherapy.[26,32,45] Although most young girls will undergo a normal puberty and menarche, some patients, particularly those receiving alkylating agents, will manifest raised levels of gonadotropins for varying periods after treatments.[46] The present authors have recently observed transient episodes of ovarian failure in adolescents receiving high-dose alkylator therapy in the context of autologous bone marrow transplantation. These individuals may require hormone replacement therapy for periods of 1–5 years before recovery takes place. Larsen *et al.*[47] looked at 100 female long-term survivors of pediatric malignancies with a median follow-up of 20 years. All patients were treated with chemotherapy and radiotherapy. Seventeen patients had premature ovarian failure with sustained elevation of FSH and LH requiring long-term hormonal replacement therapy. Patients with normal menstrual cycles were found to have diminished ovarian volume and total antral follicles when compared to normal controls. The authors concluded that although a majority of women regain normal menstruation after treatment for childhood cancer, decreased ovarian follicles may lead to early impairment of fertility. With this in mind, researchers are currently investigating ovarian tissue harvesting and banking as a method to preserve fertility.[48]

Radiation-associated ovarian failure is dose-dependent and the ovaries of younger individuals, with their greater complement of oocytes, are more resistant to damage from irradiation than are the ovaries of older individuals.[32,33,49] Thus, while radiation doses of 6 Gy may be sufficient to produce irreversible ovarian damage in women who have reached 40 years of age,[33] doses in excess of 20 Gy are needed to induce permanent ovarian failure in the majority of females treated during childhood and adolescence.[50–53] Girls treated with pelvic irradiation for a rhabdomyosarcoma are at risk for ovarian failure.[44] It is of interest that the use of both brachytherapy[54] and ovarian transpositions appear to reduce the incidence of ovarian dysfunction in girls requiring radiotherapy for a pelvic/genitourinary rhabdomyosarcoma. Additionally, exposure to alkylating agents and radiation below the diaphragm are both risk factors for a premature menopause.[46]

Pregnancy and offspring

For individuals who retain reproductive function following cancer therapy, the risk of congenital anomalies or cancer in their offspring does not appear to be greater than that of the general population.[55,56] However, women who become pregnant following irradiation of the pelvis are at increased risk of spontaneous abortion, preterm labor, and delivery of low birth weight infants.[57,58]

Retrograde ejaculation and sexual dysfunction after surgery

Jaffe *et al.*[59] and others have pointed out that pelvic lymphadenectomies performed for sarcoma may result in retrograde ejaculation or impotence in males. There are a number of reports that associate retrograde ejaculation and impotence with retroperitoneal lymph node dissection. Nijman *et al.*[60] reported 14 patients who were treated for non-seminomatous testicular tumors with bilateral retroperitoneal lymph node dissections. All patients had normal sexual function preoperatively but antegrade ejaculation was lost completely in 12 after surgery. The other two patients had diminished antegrade ejaculation. In a follow-up study of 101 patients treated with bilateral retroperitoneal lymph node dissection for stage I or II nonseminomatous testicular cancer, antegrade ejaculation was present in only 12 patients.[61] In the remaining 89 patients a "dry ejaculation" was described. In 75 of the patients complaining of dry ejaculation, urine was collected after intercourse or masturbation and analysis suggested retrograde ejaculation in 55 and no evidence of urethral emission in 20. In addition, 17 patients had reduced sexual desire, 12 had difficulty reaching orgasm, and 6 complained of erectile dysfunction.

Takasaki *et al.*[62] correlated the technique of retroperitoneal lymph node dissection with the occurrence of retrograde ejaculation. In this report, 47 patients undergoing retroperitoneal lymph node dissection for testicular cancer were evaluated. Thirty-eight patients had bilateral retroperitoneal lymph node dissections. All 38 suffered from dry ejaculation and, in the 30/38 undergoing examination for seminal emission, no sperm were identified. Retrograde ejaculation was much less common in patients treated with unilateral retroperitoneal lymph node dissection. The exception to this finding was in patients undergoing unilateral dissection who also had a dissection performed at the base of the inferior mesenteric artery. This would have interrupted fibers in the superior hypogastric plexus, explaining the retrograde ejaculations observed in this group. The authors recommend unilateral retroperitoneal lymph node dissection and preservation of the superior hypogastric plexus when possible. In support of this, Kihara *et al.*[63] performed bilateral hypogastric nerve transactions in dogs and seminal emission was measured after manual penile stimulation. All dogs suffered from retrograde ejaculation 1–6 months after transaction, and this was associated with persistent relaxation of the bladder neck. This supports the concept that hypogastric nerve interruption is a physiological determinant of retrograde ejaculation. Tekgul *et al.*[64] treated 32 patients with metastatic testicular germ cell tumors, who had residual disease after chemotherapy, using very limited retroperitoneal lymph node dissections. Essentially, grossly abnormal masses and suspicious adjacent lymph nodes were removed. In this series only one patient developed retrograde ejaculation. Patients undergoing cystectomy or prostatectomy are at higher risk for retrograde ejaculation or even erectile impotence. These ablative procedures may remove the vasa deferentia and seminal vesicles themselves. Also, submucosal infiltration is a hallmark of bladder and bladder/prostate rhabdomyosarcoma. If surgical ablation is required, dissection into the urethra itself may be necessary, with a resultant increase in the type and severity of sexual dysfunction.

Kidneys/bladder/ureters

The kidneys are susceptible to injury by a number of chemotherapeutic agents, including cisplatin, ifosfamide, methotrexate, and to a lesser degree cyclophosphamide.[65–69] Chronic renal failure after chemotherapy can be insidious. Also, urinary diversions that seek to replace a normal bladder with a bowel segment often result in recurrent kidney infections and obstruction that lead to renal failure.

Finally, radiation therapy is nephrotoxic and may result in a diminution of function or renal failure.[70] In one analysis involving Wilms' tumor patients, an impaired creatinine clearance was noted in 28/102 patients (27.4%) after unilateral nephrectomy and abdominal radiation therapy. The creatinine clearance was impaired in 72.7% of patients who received more than 24 Gy, in contrast to 18.5% in those receiving less than 12 Gy. Proteinuria and hypertension may develop as late as 20 years after the initial treatment.

Ureteral strictures secondary to radiation therapy are well known and can occur as late as 20 years after the primary irradiations.[70] This can lead to ureteral obstruction with the necessity of secondary reconstructive procedures, including ureteral re-implantation or urinary diversion. Severe vascular damage and periureteral fibrosis are seen histologically. Ureteral damage is rare after the treatment of childhood malignancies. Most commonly this problem develops when radiation dosages of 45–60 Gy are administered. Ureteral strictures were not reported in an analysis of late effects after the treatment of paratesticular rhabdomyosarcoma in patients enrolled in the Intergroup Rhabdomyosarcoma Studies I and II.[41]

Urinary bladder and urethra

Hemorrhagic cystitis is caused by cyclophosphamide, bladder irradiation, adenovirus, herpes virus infection, and possibly cisplatin and bleomycin.[71–74] Hemorrhagic cystitis develops in approximately 10% of patients receiving pelvic irradiation alone. This increases to 30% when both pelvic radiation therapy and systemic chemotherapy are combined.[70] It results in chronic bladder scarring and contracture. Bladder capacity is reduced and the patient may be susceptible to recurrent infection. This complication, when severe, is very difficult to treat and may require formalin instillation into the bladder or even nephrostomy or cystectomy to control severe bleeding.[72,75] Hemorrhagic cystitis may be chronic, with persistent gross or microscopic hematuria.[76] There have been no prospective studies published of bladder capacity or function after hemorrhagic cystitis.

Irradiation of the bladder can cause chronic bladder dysfunction, fistulas, and urethral strictures. Heyn *et al.*[41] reported two patients from the Intergroup Rhabdomyosarcoma Studies I and II who developed urethral strictures after abdominal radiation for paratesticular rhabdomyosarcoma. Bladder dysfunction after radiotherapy may eventually cause urinary incontinence. A common mechanism is overflow incontinence secondary to a small bladder. Therapy causes a vascular injury that leads to scarring and bladder contracture. This in turn reduces bladder capacity, resulting in incontinence.

Cyclophosphamide is an established bladder carcinogen.[77,78] Travis *et al.*[79] analyzed 6171 2-year survivors of non-Hodgkin's lymphoma and identified 48 patients with secondary cancer of the urinary tract. They found a 4.5-fold increase in the risk of bladder cancer in patients treated with cyclophosphamide. This risk depended on cyclophosphamide dose and was not significantly elevated in patients receiving less than 20 g. The bladder cancer risk was significantly elevated 6-fold for cumulative doses of 20–49 g and 14.5-fold when patients received 50 g or more. Radiotherapy given without cyclophosphamide did not significantly increase the risk of bladder cancer. Also, there was no synergistic effect of combining cyclophosphamide with radiation therapy in producing bladder malignancy.

Bone and soft tissue

Impaired growth of bone and soft tissue are well-described complications of cancer therapy and are observed commonly following high-dose radiation therapy in the young child. Moreover, the radiation effects may be enhanced by the use of specific chemotherapeutic agents such as actinomycin D and adriamycin.[80] The final outcome can be quite severe, with certain patients suffering significant disability, both functional and cosmetic. Complications following doses of radiation in the range of 40–70 Gy have included weakness and limitation of motion of an extremity and hypoplasia of bones and soft tissues leading to deformity and asymmetry.[80,81]

Heyn *et al.*[82] reported that 50% of individuals treated for orbital rhabdomyosarcoma with radiation of 50–60 Gy to the primary site displayed evidence of orbital hypoplasia. The younger the child at the time of irradiation, the greater the degree of bony deformity. Jaffe *et al.*[83] evaluated a group of long-term survivors of childhood head and neck tumors treated with radiation and chemotherapy. They noted a very high incidence of dental and maxillofacial abnormalities, including foreshortening and blunting of roots, delayed tooth development, caries, trismus, and occlusal abnormalities.

Children who receive direct irradiation to the spine can experience varying degrees of growth failure. The ultimate impact on final height will depend on the dose of radiotherapy, the volume irradiated, and the age of the subject at the time of treatment.[84,85] Children receiving treatment to the entire spine prior to age 6 years with doses above 25 Gy are most severely affected. As the spine normally undergoes a period of rapid growth at the time of puberty, the full impact of treatment on spinal growth may not become apparent until the patient reaches adolescence.[86] Radiation-associated growth impairment appears to result primarily from destruction of the growth plates in the spine. In general, this type of injury is not amenable to medical or hormonal treatments.

Short stature secondary to spinal irradiation has been observed in children treated for rhabdomyosarcoma of the head and neck, pelvis, and genitourinary tract.[44,87,88] Hughes *et al.*[87] described persistent and progressive growth impairment in a group of children who received para-aortic irradiation (34–37 Gy) before the onset of puberty. In several instances the loss in growth potential was dramatic (height loss 1.0–3.0 standard deviations). Long-term follow-up of head and neck rhabdomyosarcoma patients treated in Intergroup Rhabdomyosarcoma Studies II and III have found that 48% have failed to maintain their growth velocities.[88]

Second malignant neoplasms

The risk of developing a second malignant neoplasm (SMN) is increased 10–20-fold for survivors of childhood cancer compared with age-matched controls. The incidence of second cancers has been estimated to be in the range 3%–12% during the first 20 years following the initial cancer diagnosis.[5,89] Moreover, the absolute risk increases as the follow-up time increases. Genetic susceptibility and the therapy employed to treat the initial malignancy are the major determinants of subsequent cancer risk.

While the alkylating agents and the epipodophyllotoxins (e.g., etoposide) have been associated with the development of secondary leukemias, primarily non-lymphoblastic leukemias,[89–91] radiation therapy has been linked to secondary solid tumors, principally soft tissue and bone sarcomas.[92] In some studies there has been a dose–response relationship between the risk of developing a second tumor and the dose of radiation. Genetic susceptibility to cancer is increased in a number of conditions, including neurofibromatosis, xeroderma pigmentosum, and the Li–Fraumeni syndrome.[5] Of note, evidence of a genetic

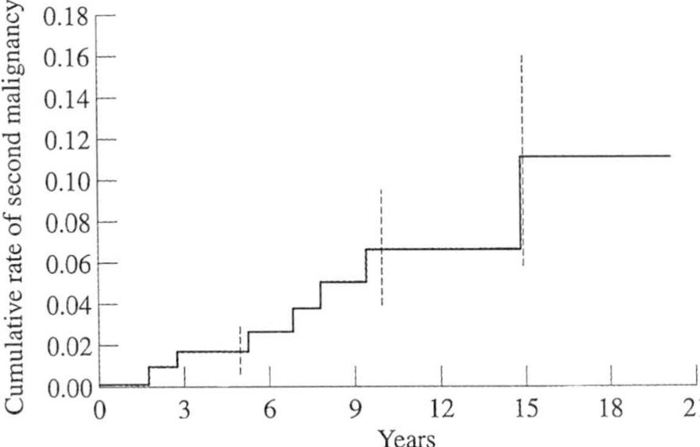

Fig. 60.2. Cumulative rate of second malignant neoplasms after completion of treatment for childhood rhabdomyosarcoma. Standard error bars are shown at 5, 10, and 15 years. From Scaradavou *et al.*[94]

predisposition to cancer may be present in as many as a third of families of children diagnosed with a soft tissue sarcoma.[92]

Two studies have addressed the issue of SMN in survivors of childhood rhabdomyosarcoma. Heyn *et al.*[93] noted 22 SMNs among 1026 patients enrolled in the Intergroup Rhabdomyosarcoma Studies I and II, a cumulative estimated incidence of 1.7% at 10 years. The most common SMNs were bone tumors (nine cases); acute nonlymphoblastic leukemia (ANLL) developed in five cases. A strong association was made between genetic predisposition and development of SMN.[93] More recently, Scaradavou *et al.*[94] have reported on their experience with SMN at Memorial Sloan-Kettering Cancer Center. Among a cohort of 210 newly diagnosed patients with rhabdomyosarcoma, seven patients developed an SMN, including three with ANLL and four with solid tumors. The cumulative estimated incidence of SMN at 10 years was 6% (Fig. 60.2). The risk of as SMN increase in those patients treated with high doses of the chemotherapeutic agents cyclophosphamide and dactinomycin, and in those treated with high-dose (>40 Gy) radiation therapy.[94]

Site-specific late effects

Head and neck

Neuroendocrine dysfunction

Therapeutic external irradiation to the head, nasopharynx, or face that includes the hypothalamic–pituitary axis is known to result in a variety of neuroendocrine disturbances.[95] Hypothalamic–pituitary dysfunction is both dose and time dependent; the higher the dose of radiotherapy and the longer the time interval since treatment, the greater the incidence of any given problem.[96] In general, radiation toxicity is directly proportional to the biologically effective dose, which is determined primarily by the total dose, the dose per fraction, and the duration of treatment.[97,98]

Smaller dose per fraction, as is achieved with hyperfractionation schedules (low-dose fractions given 2–3 times per day) and longer treatment times favor repair of sublethal damage and result in less overall toxicity to most normal tissues.[34,35] The age of the patient at the time of treatment may also be an important variable; children appear more susceptible to radiation damage than do adults.[97]

Growth hormone (GH) deficiency

GH deficiency is the most common anterior pituitary deficit to develop after irradiation of rhabdomyosarcomas of the head and neck.[46,81,82,99] GH deficiency can develop following radiation therapy which exposes the hypothalamic–pituitary region to doses as low as 18–20 Gy.[43,95] The greater the dose of irradiation to the hypothalamic–pituitary unit, the higher the incidence and the shorter the lag time between treatment and the development of GH deficiency.[96] When the dose of radiation to the hypothalamic–pituitary unit exceeds 30 Gy, the majority of subjects will become GH-deficient within 5 years of treatment. Radiation-associated GH deficiency appears to result from damage to the hypothalamus, although at very high doses (>50 Gy) the pituitary gland itself may also be injured directly.[95]

In a study which included seven children treated with radiotherapy for a rhabdomyosarcoma of the face (estimated dose of 25–72 Gy to the hypothalamic–pituitary unit), Bajorunas *et al.*[46] observed biochemical evidence of GH deficiency in six; all the subjects demonstrated impaired linear growth and short stature (height < 10th centile) (Fig. 60.3). Heyn *et al.*,[82] reporting on 50 children with orbital rhabdomyosarcoma treated on the Intergroup Rhabdomyosarcoma Study I, noted a drop of 20 percentiles or more in height in 61% of subjects following combined treatment with radiation and chemotherapy. Unfortunately, since hormonal data were not reported in the latter study, the precise cause of the children's poor linear growth remains uncertain; most likely, however, it was due in large part to impaired GH secretion.

GH deficiency has also been described in pediatric patients treated with only chemotherapy for non-CNS tumors. Rose *et al.*[100] examined their institutional experience with 362 patients with altered growth and development after treatment of pediatric malignancies. Of these,

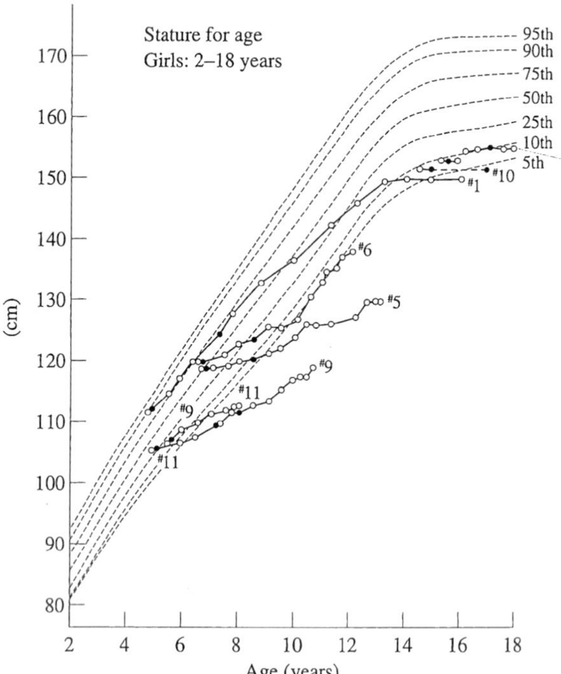

Fig. 60.3. The height histories of girls treated for sarcomas of the head and neck. In each case the first solid circle represents the beginning of therapy and the second solid circle represents the time therapy was stopped. From Bajorunas *et al.*[46]

31 had undergone chemotherapy for non-CNS malignancy and had no history of radiotherapy. Fifteen (48%) were found to be deficient in growth hormone. Other common endocrine abnormalities included central hypothyroidism in 16 (52%) and pubertal abnormalities (including precocious puberty, gonadal failure, and gonadotropin deficiency) in 10 (32%).

Most of the published data concerning the efficacy and safety of GH therapy pertains to children who developed GH deficiency following treatment with high-dose irradiation for tumors of the central nervous system. Although GH treatment may improve final heights in these subjects, the response to treatment has been less than observed in patients with idiopathic GH deficiency.[101,102] Preliminary data suggest that initiating treatment at a younger age and utilizing more contemporary dosing schedules will improve the overall efficacy of GH therapy.

The use of GH in individuals previously treated for a malignancy raises concerns over the risk of tumor recurrence as a result of the growth-enhancing properties of the hormone. To date, there is no evidence that children treated with GH experience an increased rate of relapse of their primary tumor.[103,104] While these data are reassuring, it is important to keep in mind that the published studies involve relatively small numbers of subjects and primarily patients previously treated for a brain tumor. Recently, 361 GH-treated cancer survivors were reported on.[105] No increased risks of primary tumor recurrence or death were found with GH treatment. Furthermore, 39 patients had a primary diagnosis of rhabdomyosarcoma and none experienced disease recurrence after GH-treatment. However, two did go on to develop secondary malignancies (spindle cell sarcoma of the neck and sarcoma of the tongue). Both had initially been treated with alkylating agents and radiotherapy for their original nasopharyngeal rhabdomyosarcoma primary. Statistical analysis failed to show a correlation between GH treatment and increased development of secondary malignancies in the rhabdomyosarcoma group ($P = 0.43$).

Early puberty

Over the past several years it has become apparent that hypothalamic–pituitary irradiation, both at low doses (18–24 Gy) and at higher doses (>35 Gy), is associated with early and precocious puberty.[106–108] For reasons that are unclear, females are affected more often than males. In a study of the authors' patients treated with high-dose irradiation for brain tumors and sarcomas of the orbit and nasopharynx, the estimated probability that a girl would experience the onset of puberty by age 9 years was 42%, compared with 4% in the control population [107] (Fig. 60.4). Age at onset of puberty appears to be directly correlated with age at treatment and indirectly correlated with body mass index.[106–108] The majority of subjects who experience premature sexual maturation have also been found to be GH-deficient.[107] This constellation of hormonal problems may result in premature epiphyseal fusion, an attenuated pubertal growth spurt, and unanticipated adult short stature. The addition of a GNRH agonist to suppress puberty in patients with early puberty may improve final height,[109,110] although the data are preliminary.

Other pituitary abnormalities

Deficiency of the anterior pituitary hormones LH/FSH, TSH, and ACTH appears to occur infrequently and generally following doses above 40 Gy to the hypothalamic–pituitary unit.[46,96,111,112] In two pediatric series following hypothalamic–pituitary irradiation of 40–50 Gy, the incidence of TSH deficiency was under 10% after a mean follow-up of 9–10 years.[113,114] Clinically apparent ACTH deficiency is distinctly uncommon in patients receiving irradiation to the hypothalamus and pituitary under 50 Gy. Nonetheless, evidence of dysregulation of the ACTH–adrenal axis has been observed in individuals with rhabdomyosarcomas of

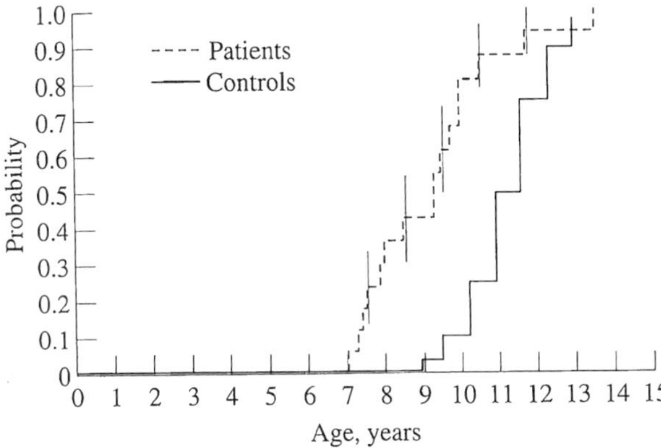

Fig. 60.4. Probability of the onset of puberty at a given age in girls treated with high-dose radiotherapy to the hypothalamus–pituitary unit. From Oberfield *et al.*[107]

the face following irradiation of the hypothalamic–pituitary region with doses in the range 35–55 Gy.[115]

Mild increases in the plasma concentration of prolactin have been observed after hypothalamic–pituitary irradiation with doses greater than 50 Gy, especially among women.[46,111,112] The elevation in prolactin is most likely due to the disruption of hypothalamic centers, which normally exert an inhibitory effect on prolactin secretion.

Primary hypothyroidism is a well-established complication of irradiation to the head and neck. The incidence and severity of thyroid dysfunction appear dose related, with a threshold of approximately 10 Gy when the radiation is administered in conventional daily fractions.[116] Clinically significant thyroid hypofunction is generally seen following irradiation with doses above 20 Gy.[117] While the peak incidence of hypothyroidism occurs 2–4 years following irradiation, new cases have been known to develop as long as 25 years after radiotherapy.[118] Additional cofactors felt to increase the risk of hypothyroidism include younger age at treatment, use of adjuvant chemotherapy, and prior exposure to iodine-containing contrast media (lymphangiography). Bajorunas *et al.*[46] describe several patients who developed increased plasma concentrations of TSH following irradiation of rhabdomyosarcomas of the face and nasopharynx. Estimated doses to the thyroid were in the range of 22–45 Gy.

Irradiation of the thyroid gland is also associated with an increased risk of the development of both benign and malignant thyroid neoplasms (see the earlier discussion of second malignant neoplasms). Contrary to earlier teaching, the risk of malignant neoplasms persists even following high-dose therapeutic radiation. The data of Tucker *et al.*[119] indicate a 50-fold relative risk for thyroid cancer in survivors of childhood cancer, compared with the general population.

Ophthalmological complications

These include cataracts, xerophthalmia, and retinopathy.[81] Chronic conjunctival complications have also been reported.[120] In general these effects are related to radiation treatments to the orbit. Ninety percent of patients receiving orbital radiation therapy will develop cataracts and visual disturbance secondary to lenticular opacification.[82]

In the report by Fromm *et al.*[81] there were 11 radiated eyes in ten patients with total radiation dosages between 8 and 55 Gy and a median follow-up of 6 years. In two patients the involved eye had received 8 and 17 Gy, respectively, and there was no evidence of cataract formation. In the remaining 9 lenses that had received higher doses, 8 developed cataracts while one remained cataract-free. Visual acuity was 20:40 or better with corrective lenses in 10/11 eyes in treated fields. Six of 9 eyes receiving a dose of above 40 Gy developed xerophthalmia which was symptomatic in four patients. Three eyes receiving doses of 40, 43, and 51 Gy, respectively, were found to have asymptomatic retinopathy.

Krebs *et al.*[121] reported the case of a 4.5-year-old treated with 59.5 Gy over 5 weeks for an embryonal rhabdomyosarcoma of the left orbit. Thirteen years after treatment an electroretinogram showed that there were no rod responses and cone responses were 3% of normal. The right eye was normal. The left eye required subsequent enucleation, and electron microscopy showed a significant reduction in the number of photoreceptor cells and collagen sheaths around the retinal vessels.

Otological complications

Otological complications have been rare but may be related to thickening of the tympanic membranes or an increase in the viscosity of the middle ear fluid. Direct eighth cranial nerve toxicity may become more prevalent with the increasing incorporation of cisplatin into sarcoma chemotherapeutic regimens. In the report by Fromm *et al.*[81] there were 19 patients with 27 ears within radiation portals. One patient who received a middle-ear dosage of 54 Gy had a mild sensorineural hearing loss. A second patient, who received a middle-ear dose of 53 Gy, developed a mild to moderate conductive loss due to thickening of the tympanic membrane. Normal hearing was present in 25/27 middle and inner ears included in the radiation fields, with a median follow-up of 6 years.

Table 60.1. Comparison of patients with and without bladder impairment after treatment for bladder or bladder–prostate sarcoma[44]

	Impaired bladder function	Normal bladder function
Patient number	14	38
Median age (range)	2.8 y (3 wk –19 y)	2.7 y (5 mo –17 y)
Partial cystectomy	5	6
Cyclophosphamide dose (ratio receiving >75% of scheduled dose)	9/14	38/38
Number with pelvic irradiation	13	30
Median radiation dose (range)	40 Gy (19.5–50 Gy)	41 Gy (8–60 Gy)

Dental complications

Dental complications have been cited as occurring after radiation therapy for neoplasms of the head and neck. These include root crown defects and radiation caries. Fromm *et al.*[81] reported that 15 head and neck patients in their series had follow-up dental evaluations at a median of 6 years after diagnosis of head and neck sarcoma. Fourteen showed late dental effects, including root foreshortening or agenesis of developing teeth. Crown defects were noted in 9/15 patients and radiation caries in 6 cases. Kielbassa *et al.*[122] recommend root canal obturation with calcium hydroxide rather than removal of carious teeth; these authors suggest that tooth extraction significantly increases the risk of osteoradionecrosis. Others have recommended a 0.12% chlorhexidine rinse as a prophylactic measure.[123]

Salivary gland complications

Salivary gland complications have been associated with head and neck irradiation. In one report, 24 parotid glands in 14 patients had more than 50% of a single gland volume within the radiation field. Nine parotid glands receiving a median dose of 51 Gy had no secretions and all but one of these had doses above 45 Gy. In contrast, secretions were present in 15 glands receiving a median dose of 25 Gy and all but three of these patients had doses below 40 Gy.

Bladder, bladder–prostate, and vagina

In a report from the Intergroup Rhabdomyosarcoma Study, 109 patients with bladder and bladder–prostate sarcoma were followed for between 5 and 15 years.[44] Eighty-six (79%) of these patients had blood urea nitrogen and/or creatinine values reported. Five of these (6%) had abnormalities. This included 3 patients with a slightly elevated blood urea nitrogen, but in these the serum creatinine was not elevated above 1.1 mg dl^{-1}. Another patient was noted 4 years after the initiation of therapy to have a blood urea nitrogen of 15 mmol l^{-1} and serum creatinine of 1.5 mg dl^{-1}. He remained healthy at follow-up 5 years later. A blood urea nitrogen of 26 mmol l^{-1} was recorded in the fifth patient but the serum creatinine was not measured. This patient had an ileal conduit and an associated chronic metabolic acidosis and growth failure. One kidney was removed because of lack of function. Another child, with normal blood parameters, developed hypertension requiring multiple medications for control 9 years after initial diagnosis of sarcoma.

Imaging studies were available in 31 patients, and 16 of these had required urinary diversion as part of their treatment. Ileal conduits (35/55) were the most common technique of urinary diversion in this group, followed by colon conduits (13/55), unspecified conduits (3/55), and continent cecal diversion (1/55). There were also two cases of cutaneous ureterostomies. The imaging studies included: 23 intravenous urograms, six renal scans (isotopic), one renal ultrasound, and one cystogram. Nine patients (of whom six had undergone urinary diversion) had abnormalities. An abnormality on imaging studies of the urinary tract was twice as likely in patients with an ileal conduit. These abnormalities included: seven cases of hydronephrosis, one case of pyelonephritis, and one atrophic kidney. In the 54 patients without urinary diversion there were two cases of unilateral caliectasis and one of pyelonephritis by imaging studies. This compares with five cases of caliectasis and one of renal atrophy found in the 55 patients with ileal conduits.

The proportion of patients with bacteriuria and hematuria was significantly higher with an ileal conduit compared with those with a native bladder. Five of 41 patients with a bladder developed bacteriuria, compared with 16/46 with a urinary diversion. Similarly, the proportion of patients with a bladder who developed hematuria was 9/44, compared with 14/36 of those with a urinary diversion.

Of the 109 bladder and/or prostate sarcoma patients in the Intergroup Rhabdomyosarcoma Study, 54 (50%) retained their bladders. Follow-up data were unavailable on two of these. Thirty-eight of the remaining 52 (73%) were reported by their physicians to have normal bladder function (Table 60.1). However, no formal or uniform

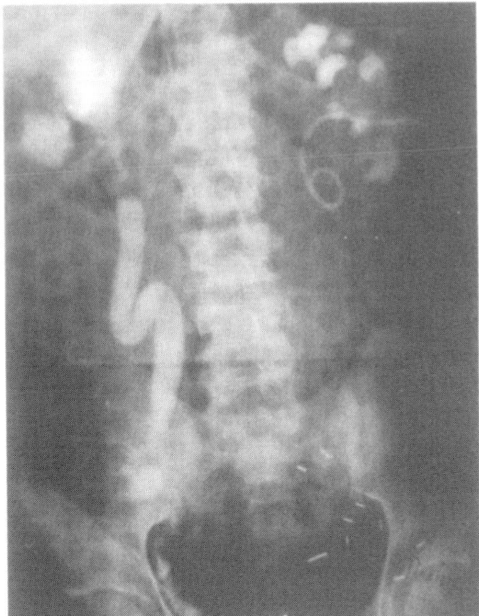

Fig. 60.5. Intraoperative contrast study of an ileal conduit that was done after total cystectomy for bladder rhabdomyosarcoma in infancy. At the time of the study the patient was 15 years of age and had been lost to follow-up for several years. There is severe hydronephrosis of the left kidney (see text).

assessment of bladder function was performed. There were 14 patients who reported bladder dysfunction; 9 suffered incontinence, 4 had frequency and nocturia, and 1 had urinary frequency alone. The median age at diagnosis of these 14 patients was 2.8 years, and 13 received pelvic irradiation. Also, 9 of 14 patients received 75% or more of their scheduled cyclophosphamide dose. Finally, three patients with frequency and one with incontinence were treated with partial cystectomy, as was the only non-irradiated patient in the group.

Figure 60.5 is an intraoperative contrast study of an ileal conduit done after cystectomy for bladder–prostate rhabdomyosarcoma. There has been a previous percutaneous nephrostomy of the left kidney because of a distal ureteral stricture and infection. There is also severe right hydroureteronephrosis. This patient had normal renal function previously but had not returned for follow-up for several years.

Paratesticular rhabdomyosarcoma

Heyn *et al.*[41] reported the late effects of therapy for paratesticular rhabdomyosarcoma in 86 children and adolescents treated on the Intergroup Rhabdomyosarcoma Studies I and II between 1972 and 1984. Patient ages at diagnosis ranged from 10 months to 19 years. Most of these patients had initial retroperitoneal lymph node dissection or sampling. Bowel obstruction occurred in nine patients, loss of normal ejaculatory function in eight cases, development of a hydrocele in five cases, and lymphedema of the leg in five cases. Kidney and bladder function were normal in patients who received radiotherapy to the para-aortic lymph nodes and/or bladder. Four patients who had abdominal radiotherapy had chronic diarrhea, and two developed urethral strictures. Four patients had bone or soft tissue hypoplasia in the field of radiotherapy. One-third of those treated with cyclophosphamide developed hemorrhagic cystitis. Half of these had extended periods of gross hematuria after therapy was discontinued. Testicular size was small in children whose testes were irradiated, and in some who received cyclophosphamide. Tanner staging was normal in 45 patients for whom it was recorded. Elevated follicle-stimulating hormone values or known azoospermia occurred in more than half the patients for whom data were available.

Extremity rhabdomyosarcoma

There has been little written about late effects from the treatment of extremity rhabdomyosarcoma except for the occurrence of secondary neoplasms. Most reports indicate that secondary malignancies develop within, or immediately adjacent to, radiation portals. Newton *et al.*[124] reported that 77% of secondary bone sarcomas arose in irradiated areas, and that rhabdomyosarcoma was among the more frequent primary tumor type. Meadows *et al.*[89] reported that 68% (208/292) of secondary malignant neoplasms developed in tissues that had been exposed to radiation. For patients with soft tissue sarcomas as the first malignancy, the most common secondary tumor was a bone sarcoma, followed by a second soft tissue sarcoma.

Rhabdomyosarcoma of the chest wall

Rhabdomyosarcoma of the chest wall is rare but treatment may result in significant long-term morbidity. Resection of even a single rib and/or denervation of the chest wall may result in scoliosis. DeRosa[125] reported spinal deformity in six pediatric patients after partial chest wall resection. It was stated that scoliosis secondary to chest wall resection in children is progressive, and that the degree of curvature is related to the number of ribs resected. Posterior rib resection was associated with the development of scoliosis while anterior resection was not. It was also noted that the scoliosis is convex toward the normal side, suggesting that the area of resection acts as a tether. Grosfeld *et al.*[126] reported that pulmonary restrictive disease and scoliosis occur with growth in pediatric patients undergoing chest

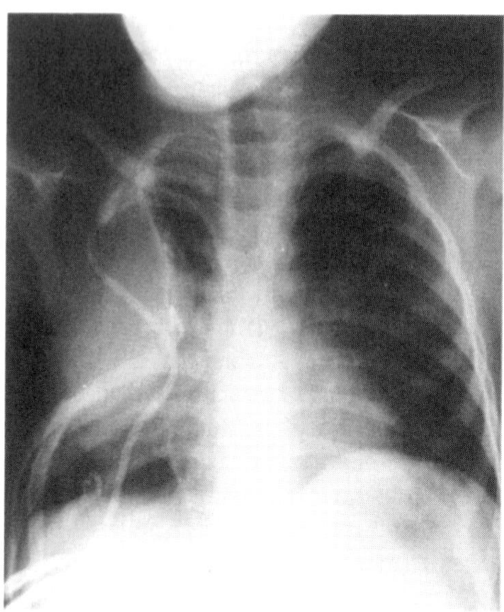

Fig. 60.6. Postoperative plain chest radiograph of a male patient who underwent an extensive chest wall resection for sarcoma.

wall resection. Agadir *et al.*[127] reported that sectioning of the right third, fourth, and fifth intercostal nerves produced scoliosis in young growing New Zealand rabbits within 6 months. The scoliosis was always convex to the left.

Figure 60.6 is a plain chest radiograph of a 5-year-old patient who had undergone an extensive chest wall resection. This defect is likely to produce severe kyphoscoliosis in the future.

Conclusions

Late effects after treatment for childhood rhabdomyosarcoma are myriad and related to the site of the primary tumor as well as the type and intensity of treatment. The present challenge is to discriminate clinically between high- and low-risk rhabdomyosarcoma. Patients with high-risk tumors will still need intensive therapy. However, those with less aggressive neoplasms might be safely treated with a reduced regimen. This should also reduce the number and severity of late treatment effects.

REFERENCES

1. Reis, L., Eisner, M. P., Kosary, C. L. *et al. SEER Cancer Statistic Review, 1975–2000.* Bethesda, MD: National Cancer Institute, 2003.
2. Donaldson, S. S., Meza, J., Breneman, J. C. *et al.* Results from the IRS-IV randomized trial of hyperfractionated radiotherapy in children with rhabdomyosarcoma – a report from the IRSG. *Int. J. Radiat. Oncol. Biol. Phys.* 2001; **51**:718–728.
3. Wolden, S. L., Anderson, J. R., Crist, W. M. *et al.* Indications for radiotherapy and chemotherapy after complete resection in rhabdomyosarcoma: a report from the Intergroup Rhabdomyosarcoma Studies I to III. *J. Clin. Oncol.* 1999; **17**:3468–3475.
4. Nag, S., Tippin, D., & Ruymann, F. B. Long-term morbidity in children treated with fractionated high-dose-rate brachytherapy for soft tissue sarcomas. *J. Pediatr. Hematol. Oncol.* 2003; **25**:448–452.
5. Blatt, J. Copeland, D. R., & Bleyer, W. A. *Late Effects of Childhood Cancer and its Treatment.* Philadelphia: J.B. Lippincott, 1993.
6. Steinherz, L. J., Steinherz, P. G., & Tan, C. Cardiac failure and dysrhythmias 6–19 years after anthracycline therapy: a series of 15 patients. *Med. Pediatr. Oncol.* 1995; **24**:352–361.
7. Steinherz, L. J., Steinherz, P. G., Tan, C. T. *et al.* Cardiac toxicity 4 to 20 years after completing anthracycline therapy. *J. Am. Med. Assoc.* 1991; **266**:1672–1677.
8. Silber, J. H., Jakacki, R. I., Larsen, R. L. *et al.* Increased risk of cardiac dysfunction after anthracyclines in girls. *Med. Pediatr. Oncol.* 1993; **21**:477–479.
9. Lipshultz, S. E., Colan, S. D., Gelber, R. D. *et al.* Late cardiac effects of doxorubicin therapy for acute lymphoblastic leukemia in childhood. *N. Engl. J. Med.* 1991; **324**:808–815.
10. Lipshultz, S. E., Lipsitz, S. R., Mone, S. M. *et al.* Female sex and drug dose as risk factors for late cardiotoxic effects of doxorubicin therapy for childhood cancer. *N. Engl. J. Med.* 1995; **332**:1738–1743.
11. Langer, T., Stohr, W., Bielack, S. *et al.* Late effects surveillance system for sarcoma patients. *Pediatr. Blood Cancer* 2004; **42**:373–379.
12. Silber, J. H., Cnaan, A., Clark, B. J. *et al.* Enalapril to prevent cardiac function decline in long-term survivors of pediatric cancer exposed to anthracyclines. *J. Clin. Oncol.* 2004; **22**:820–828.
13. Littman, P., Meadows, A. T., Polgar, G. *et al.* Pulmonary function in survivors of Wilm's tumor. Patterns of impairment. *Cancer* 1976; **37**:2773–2776.
14. Miller, R. W., Fusner, J. E., Fink, R. J. *et al.* Pulmonary function abnormalities in long-term survivors of childhood cancer. *Med. Pediatr. Oncol.* 1986; **14**:202–207.
15. Eigen, H. & Wyszomierski, D. Bleomycin lung injury in children. Pathophysiology and guidelines for management. *Am. J. Pediatr. Hematol. Oncol.* 1985; **7**:71–78.
16. O'Driscoll, B. R., Hasleton, P. S., Taylor, P. M. *et al.* Active lung fibrosis up to 17 years after chemotherapy with carmustine (BCNU) in childhood. *N. Engl. J. Med.* 1990; **323**:378–382.
17. Kaplan, E., Sklar, C., Wilmott, R. *et al.* Pulmonary function in children treated for rhabdomyosarcoma. *Med. Pediatr. Oncol.* 1996; **27**:79–84.

18. Ellenhorn, J. D., Lambroza, A., Lindsley, K. L. *et al.* Treatment-related esophageal stricture in pediatric patients with cancer. *Cancer* 1993; **71**:4084–4090.
19. Rao, S. P., Anderson, V., Shlasko, E. *et al.* Intestinal perforation 14 years after abdominal irradiation and chemotherapy for Wilms tumor. *J. Pediatr. Hematol. Oncol.* 1996; **18**:187–190.
20. Touboul, E., Balosso, J., Schlienger, M. *et al.* Radiation injury of the small intestine. Radiobiological, radiopathological aspects; risk factors and prevention. *Ann. Chir.* 1996; **50**: 58–71.
21. Bannura, G. Surgical treatment of intestinal complications of pelvic radiotherapy. *Rev. Med. Child.* 1995; **123**:991–996.
22. Donaldson, S. S., Jundt, S., Ricour, C. *et al.* Radiation enteritis in children. A retrospective review, clinicopathologic correlation, and dietary management. *Cancer* 1975; **35**:1167–1178.
23. Oya, M., Yao, T., & Tsuneyoshi, M. Chronic irradiation enteritis: its correlation with the elapsed time interval and morphological changes. *Hum. Pathol.* 1996; **27**:774–781.
24. Meric, F., Hirschl, R. B., Mahboubi, S. *et al.* Prevention of radiation enteritis in children, using a pelvic mesh sling. *J. Pediatr. Surg.* 1994; **29**:917–921.
25. Logmans, A., Trimbos, J. B., & van Lent, M. The omentoplasty: a neglected ally in gynecologic surgery. *Eur. J. Obstet. Gynecol. Reprod. Biol.* 1995; **58**:167–171.
26. Lechner, P. & Cesnik, H. Abdominopelvic omentopexy: preparatory procedure for radiotherapy in rectal cancer. *Dis. Colon Rectum* 1992; **35**:1157–1160.
27. Silvain, C., Besson, I., Ingrand, P. *et al.* Long-term outcome of severe radiation enteritis treated by total parenteral nutrition. *Dig. Dis. Sci.* 1992; **37**:1065–1071.
28. Michalkiewicz, E. L., Rao, B. N., Gross, E. *et al.* Complications of pelvic exenteration in children who have genitourinary rhabdomyosarcoma. *J. Pediatr. Surg.* 1997; **32**:1277–1282.
29. Aubier, F., Flamant, F., Brauner, R. *et al.* Male gonadal function after chemotherapy for solid tumors in childhood. *J. Clin. Oncol.* 1989; **7**:304–309.
30. Damewood, M. D. & Grochow, L. B. Prospects for fertility after chemotherapy or radiation for neoplastic disease. *Fertil. Steril.* 1986; **45**:443–459.
31. Klein, C. E. In Armitage, J. O. & Antman, K. H. (eds). *High Dose Cancer Therapy: Pharmacology, Hematopoietins, Stem Cells.* Baltimore: Williams and Wilkins, 1992; 555–566.
32. Horning, S. J., Hoppe, R. T., Kaplan, H. S. *et al.* Female reproductive potential after treatment for Hodgkin's disease. *N. Engl. J. Med.* 1981; **304**:1377–1382.
33. Lushbaugh, C. C. & Casarett, G. W. The effects of gonadal irradiation in clinical radiation therapy: a review. *Cancer* 1976; **37**:1111–1125.
34. Withers, H. R. Biologic basis for altered fractionation schemes. *Cancer* 1985; **55**:2086–2095.
35. Yahalom J. Strategies for the use of total body irradiation as systemic therapy in leukemia and lymphoma. In Armitage, J. O. & Antman, K. H. (eds). *High Dose Cancer Therapy: Pharmacology, Hematopoietins, Stem Cells.* Baltimore: Williams and Wilkins, 1992; 61–83.
36. Clayton, P. E., Shalet, S. M., Price, D. A. *et al.* Testicular damage after chemotherapy for childhood brain tumors. *J. Pediatr.* 1988; **112**:922–926.
37. Siimes, M. A., Rautonen, J., Makipernaa, A. *et al.* Testicular function in adult males surviving childhood malignancy. *Pediatr. Hematol. Oncol.* 1995; **12**:231–241.
38. Shalet, S. M., Beardwell, C. G., Jacobs, H. S. *et al.* Testicular function following irradiation of the human prepubertal testis. *Clin. Endocrinol. (Oxf.)* 1978; **9**:483–490.
39. Sklar, C. A., Robison, L. L., Nesbit, M. E. *et al.* Effects of radiation on testicular function in long-term survivors of childhood acute lymphoblastic leukemia: a report from the Children Cancer Study Group. *J. Clin. Oncol.* 1990; **8**:1981–1987.
40. Jaffe, N., Sullivan, M. P., Ried, H. *et al.* Male reproductive function in long-term survivors of childhood cancer. *Med. Pediatr. Oncol.* 1988; **16**:241–247.
41. Heyn, R., Raney, R. B., Jr., Hays, D. M. *et al.* Late effects of therapy in patients with paratesticular rhabdomyosarcoma. Intergroup Rhabdomyosarcoma Study Committee. *J. Clin. Oncol.* 1992; **10**:614–623.
42. Leiper, A. D., Grant, D. B., & Chessells, J. M. Gonadal function after testicular radiation for acute lymphoblastic leukaemia. *Arch. Dis. Child.* 1986; **61**:53–56.
43. Rappaport, R. & Brauner, R. Growth and endocrine disorders secondary to cranial irradiation. *Pediatr. Res.* 1989; **25**:561–567.
44. Raney, B., Jr., Heyn, R., Hays, D. M. *et al.* Sequelae of treatment in 109 patients followed for 5 to 15 years after diagnosis of sarcoma of the bladder and prostate. A report from the Intergroup Rhabdomyosarcoma Study Committee. *Cancer* 1993; **71**:2387–2394.
45. Clayton, P. E., Shalet, S. M., Price, D. A. *et al.* Ovarian function following chemotherapy for childhood brain tumours. *Med. Pediatr. Oncol.* 1989; **17**:92–96.
46. Bajorunas, D. R., Ghavimi, F., Jereb, B. *et al.* Endocrine sequelae of antineoplastic therapy in childhood head and neck malignancies. *J. Clin. Endocrinol. Metab.* 1980; **50**:329–335.
47. Larsen, E. C., Muller, J., Schmiegelow, K. *et al.* Reduced ovarian function in long-term survivors of radiation- and chemotherapy-treated childhood cancer. *Obstet. Gynecol. Surv.* 2004; **59**:354–355.
48. Kim, S. S. Ovarian tissue banking for cancer patients. To do or not to do? *Hum. Reprod.* 2003; **18**:1759–1761.
49. Baker, T. G. Radiosensitivity of mammalian oocytes with particular reference to the human female. *Am. J. Obstet. Gynecol.* 1971; **110**:746–761.
50. Stillman, R. J., Schinfeld, J. S., Schiff, I. *et al.* Ovarian failure in long-term survivors of childhood malignancy. *Am. J. Obstet. Gynecol.* 1981; **139**:62–66.
51. Wallace, W. H., Shalet, S. M., Hendry, J. H. *et al.* Ovarian failure following abdominal irradiation in childhood: the radiosensitivity of the human oocyte. *Br. J. Radiol.* 1989; **62**:995–998.
52. Hamre, M. R., Robison, L. L., Nesbit, M. E. *et al.* Effects of radiation on ovarian function in long-term survivors of childhood acute lymphoblastic leukemia: a report from the Childrens Cancer Study Group. *J. Clin. Oncol.* 1987; **5**:1759–1765.

53. Thibaud, E., Ramirez, M., Brauner, R. *et al.* Preservation of ovarian function by ovarian transposition performed before pelvic irradiation during childhood. *J. Pediatr.* 1992; **121**:880–884.
54. Flamant, F., Gerbaulet, A., Nihoul-Fekete, C. *et al.* Long-term sequelae of conservative treatment by surgery, brachytherapy, and chemotherapy for vulval and vaginal rhabdomyosarcoma in children. *J. Clin. Oncol.* 1990; **8**:1847–1853.
55. Green, D. M., Zevon, M. A., Lowrie, G. *et al.* Congenital anomalies in children of patients who received chemotherapy for cancer in childhood and adolescence. *N. Engl. J. Med.* 1991; **325**:141–146.
56. Mulvihill, J. J., Myers, M. H., Connelly, R. R. *et al.* Cancer in offspring of long-term survivors of childhood and adolescent cancer. *Lancet* 1987; **2**:813–817.
57. Li, F. P., Gimbrere, K., Gelber, R. D. *et al.* Outcome of pregnancy in survivors of Wilms' tumor. *J. Am. Med. Assoc.* 1987; **257**:216–219.
58. Hawkins, M. M. & Smith, R. A. Pregnancy outcomes in childhood cancer survivors: probable effects of abdominal irradiation. *Int. J. Cancer* 1989; **43**:399–402.
59. Jaffe, N., McNeese, M., Mayfield, J. K. *et al.* Childhood urologic cancer therapy related sequelae and their impact on management. *Cancer* 1980; **45**:1815–1822.
60. Nijman, J. M., Schraffordt Koops, H., Oldhoff, J. *et al.* Sexual function after bilateral retroperitoneal lymph node dissection for nonseminomatous testicular cancer. *Arch. Androl.* 1987; **18**:255–267.
61. Nijman, J. M., Schraffordt Koops, H., Kremer, J. *et al.* Gonadal function after surgery and chemotherapy in men with stage II and III nonseminomatous testicular tumors. *J. Clin. Oncol.* 1987; **5**:651–656.
62. Takasaki, N., Okada, S., Kawasaki, T. *et al.* Studies on retroperitoneal lymph node dissection concerning postoperative ejaculatory function in patients with testicular cancer. *Hinyokika Kiyo* 1991; **37**:213–219.
63. Kihara, K., Sato, K., Ando, M. *et al.* A mechanism of retrograde ejaculation after bilateral hypogastric nerve transections in the dog. *J. Urol.* 1992; **148**:1307–1309.
64. Tekgul, S., Ozen, H. A., Celebi, I. *et al.* Postchemotherapeutic surgery for metastatic testicular germ cell tumors: results of extended primary chemotherapy and limited surgery. *Urology* 1994; **43**:349–354.
65. Markman, M., Rothman, R., Hakes, T. *et al.* Late effects of cisplatin-based chemotherapy on renal function in patients with ovarian carcinoma. *Gynecol. Oncol.* 1991; **41**:217–219.
66. Hamilton, C. R., Bliss, J. M., & Horwich, A. The late effects of cis-platinum on renal function. *Eur. J. Cancer Clin. Oncol.* 1989; **25**:185–189.
67. Fillastre, J. P., Moulin, B., Godin, M. *et al.* Renal complications of anti-cancer chemotherapy. *Pathol. Biol. (Paris)* 1986; **34**:1013–1028.
68. Skinner, R., Pearson, A. D., English, M. W. *et al.* Risk factors for ifosfamide nephrotoxicity in children. *Lancet* 1996; **348**:578–580.
69. Ashraf, M. S., Brady, J., Breatnach, F. *et al.* Ifosfamide nephrotoxicity in paediatric cancer patients. *Eur. J. Pediatr.* 1994; **153**:90–94.
70. Fichtner, J. & Hohenfellner, R. Damage to the urinary tract secondary to irradiation. *World. J. Urol.* 1995; **13**:240–242.
71. Londergan, T. A. & Walzak, M. P. Hemorrhagic cystitis due to adenovirus infection following bone marrow transplantation. *J. Urol.* 1994; **151**:1013–1014.
72. Dewan, A. K., Mohan, G. M., & Ravi, R. Intravesical formalin for hemorrhagic cystitis following irradiation of cancer of the cervix. *Int. J. Gynaecol. Obstet.* 1993; **42**:131–135.
73. Komiya, I., Nojiri, M., Kuriya, S. *et al.* Hemorrhagic cystitis caused by bleomycin treatment. *Jpn. J. Med.* 1991; **30**:392,
74. Miller, L. J., Chandler, S. W., & Ippoliti, C. M. Treatment of cyclophosphamide-induced hemorrhagic cystitis with prostaglandins. *Ann. Pharmacother.* 1994; **28**:590–594.
75. Zagoria, R. J., Hodge, R. G., Dyer, R. B. *et al.* Percutaneous nephrostomy for treatment of intractable hemorrhagic cystitis. *J. Urol.* 1993; **149**:1449–1451.
76. Talesnik, E., Lagomarsino, E., Gayan, A. *et al.* Chronic hemorrhagic cystitis induced by cyclophosphamide in dermatomyositis refractory to corticosteroid treatment. *Rev. Child. Pediatr.* 1991; **62**:121–124.
77. Fernandes, E. T., Manivel, J. C., Reddy, P. K. *et al.* Cyclophosphamide associated bladder cancer – a highly aggressive disease: analysis of 12 cases. *J. Urol.* 1996; **156**:1931–1933.
78. Talar-Williams, C., Hijazi, Y. M., Walther, M. M. *et al.* Cyclophosphamide-induced cystitis and bladder cancer in patients with Wegener granulomatosis. *Ann. Intern. Med.* 1996; **124**:477–484.
79. Travis, L. B., Curtis, R. E., Glimelius, B. *et al.* Bladder and kidney cancer following cyclophosphamide therapy for non-Hodgkin's lymphoma. *J. Natl. Cancer. Inst.* 1995; **87**:524–530.
80. Tefft, M., Lattin, P. B., Jereb, B. *et al.* Acute and late effects on normal tissues following combined chemo- and radiotherapy for childhood rhabdomyosarcoma and Ewing's sarcoma. *Cancer* 1976; **37**:1201–1217.
81. Fromm, M., Littman, P., Raney, R. B. *et al.* Late effects after treatment of twenty children with soft tissue sarcomas of the head and neck. Experience at a single institution with a review of the literature. *Cancer* 1986; **57**:2070–2076.
82. Heyn, R., Ragab, A., Raney, R. B., Jr. *et al.* Late effects of therapy in orbital rhabdomyosarcoma in children. A report from the Intergroup Rhabdomyosarcoma Study. *Cancer* 1986; **57**:1738–1743.
83. Jaffe, N., Toth, B. B., Hoar, R. E. *et al.* Dental and maxillofacial abnormalities in long-term survivors of childhood cancer: effects of treatment with chemotherapy and radiation to the head and neck. *Pediatrics* 1984; **73**:816–823.
84. Shalet, S. M., Gibson, B., Swindell, R. *et al.* Effect of spinal irradiation on growth. *Arch. Dis. Child.* 1987; **62**:461–464.
85. Papadakis, V., Tan, C., Heller, G. *et al.* Growth and final height after treatment for childhood Hodgkin disease. *J. Pediatr. Hematol. Oncol.* 1996; **18**:272–276.

86. Wallace, W. H., Shalet, S. M., Morris-Jones, P. H. *et al.* Effect of abdominal irradiation on growth in boys treated for a Wilms' tumor. *Med. Pediatr. Oncol.* 1990; **18**:441–446.
87. Hughes, L. L., Baruzzi, M. J., Ribeiro, R. C. *et al.* Paratesticular rhabdomyosarcoma: delayed effects of multimodality therapy and implications for current management. *Cancer* 1994; **73**:476–482.
88. Raney, R. B., Asmar, L., Vassilopoulou-Sellin, R. *et al.* Late complications of therapy in 213 children with localized, nonorbital soft-tissue sarcoma of the head and neck: A descriptive report from the Intergroup Rhabdomyosarcoma Studies (IRS)-II and – III. IRS Group of the Children's Cancer Group and the Pediatric Oncology Group. *Med. Pediatr. Oncol.* 1999; **33**:362–371.
89. Meadows, A. T., Baum, E., Fossati-Bellani, F. *et al.* Second malignant neoplasms in children: an update from the Late Effects Study Group. *J. Clin. Oncol.* 1985; **3**:532–538.
90. Heyn, R., Khan, F., Ensign, L. G. *et al.* Acute myeloid leukemia in patients treated for rhabdomyosarcoma with cyclophosphamide and low-dose etoposide on Intergroup Rhabdomyosarcoma Study III: an interim report. *Med. Pediatr. Oncol.* 1994; **23**:99–106.
91. Tucker, M. A. M. A., Boice J. D., Hoover, R. N., & Fraumeni, J. F. Cancer risk following treatment of childhood cancer. In Boice, J. D., Jr. & Fraumeni, J. F. (eds) *Radiation Carcinogenesis: Epidemiological and Biological Significance*. New York: Raven Press, 1984; 211–224.
92. Hartley, A. L., Birch, J. M., Blair, V. *et al.* Patterns of cancer in the families of children with soft tissue sarcoma. *Cancer* 1993; **72**:923–930.
93. Heyn, R., Haeberlen, V., Newton, W. A. *et al.* Second malignant neoplasms in children treated for rhabdomyosarcoma. Intergroup Rhabdomyosarcoma Study Committee. *J. Clin. Oncol.* 1993; **11**:262–270.
94. Scaradavou, A., Heller, G., Sklar, C. A. *et al.* Second malignant neoplasms in long-term survivors of childhood rhabdomyosarcoma. *Cancer* 1995; **76**:1860–1867.
95. Sklar, C. A. & Constine, L. S. Chronic neuroendocrinological sequelae of radiation therapy. *Int. J. Radiat. Oncol. Biol. Phys.* 1995; **31**:1113–1121.
96. Clayton, P. E. & Shalet, S. M. Dose dependency of time of onset of radiation-induced growth hormone deficiency. *J. Pediatr.* 1991; **118**:226–228.
97. Sklar, C. A. Growth following therapy for childhood cancer. *Cancer Invest.* 1995; **13**:511–516.
98. Ellis, F. Dose, time and fractionation: a clinical hypothesis. *Clin. Radiol.* 1969; **20**:1–7.
99. Richards, G. E., Wara, W. M., Grumbach, M. M. *et al.* Delayed onset of hypopituitarism: sequelae of therapeutic irradiation of central nervous system, eye, and middle ear tumors. *J. Pediatr.* 1976; **89**:553–559.
100. Rose, S. R., Schreiber, R. E., Kearney, N. S. *et al.* Hypothalamic dysfunction after chemotherapy. *J. Pediatr. Endocrinol. Metab.* 2004; **17**:55–66.
101. Sulmont, V., Brauner, R., Fontoura, M. *et al.* Response to growth hormone treatment and final height after cranial or craniospinal irradiation. *Acta. Paediatr. Scand.* 1990; **79**: 542–9.
102. Clayton, P. E., Shalet, S. M., & Price, D. A. Growth response to growth hormone therapy following craniospinal irradiation. *Eur. J. Pediatr.* 1988; **147**:597–601.
103. Ogilvy-Stuart, A. L., Ryder, W. D., Gattamaneni, H. R. *et al.* Growth hormone and tumour recurrence. *BR. Med. J.* 1992; **304**:1601–1605.
104. Moshang, T. Is brain tumor recurrence increased following growth hormone treatment? *Trends Endocrinol. Metab.* 1995; **6**:205–209.
105. Sklar, C. A., Mertens, A. C., Mitby, P. *et al.* Risk of disease recurrence and second neoplasms in survivors of childhood cancer treated with growth hormone: a report from the Childhood Cancer Survivor Study. *J. Clin. Endocrinol. Metab.* 2002; **87**:3136–3141.
106. Leiper, A. D., Stanhope, R., Lau, T. *et al.* The effect of total body irradiation and bone marrow transplantation during childhood and adolescence on growth and endocrine function. *Br. J. Haematol.* 1987; **67**:419–426.
107. Oberfield, S. E., Soranno, D., Nirenberg, A. *et al.* Age at onset of puberty following high-dose central nervous system radiation therapy. *Arch. Pediatr. Adolesc. Med.* 1996; **150**:589–592.
108. Ogilvy-Stuart, A. L., Clayton, P. E., & Shalet, S. M. Cranial irradiation and early puberty. *J. Clin. Endocrinol. Metab.* 1994; **78**:1282–1286.
109. Saggese, G., Cesaretti, G., Andreani, G. *et al.* Combined treatment with growth hormone and gonadotropin-releasing hormone analogues in children with isolated growth hormone deficiency. *Acta. Endocrinol. (Copenh.)* 1992; **127**:307–312.
110. Cara, J. F., Kreiter, M. L., & Rosenfield, R. L. Height prognosis of children with true precocious puberty and growth hormone deficiency: effect of combination therapy with gonadotropin releasing hormone agonist and growth hormone. *J. Pediatr.* 1992; **120**:709–715.
111. Constine, L. S., Woolf, P. D., Cann, D. *et al.* Hypothalamic–pituitary dysfunction after radiation for brain tumors. *N. Engl. J. Med.* 1993; **328**:87–94.
112. Rappaport, R., Brauner, R., Czernichow, P. *et al.* Effect of hypothalamic and pituitary irradiation on pubertal development in children with cranial tumors. *J. Clin. Endocrinol. Metab.* 1982; **54**:1164–1168.
113. Livesey, E. A. & Brook, C. G. Thyroid dysfunction after radiotherapy and chemotherapy of brain tumours. *Arch. Dis. Child.* 1989; **64**:593–595.
114. Oberfield, S. E. & Allen, J. *et al.* Thyroid and gonadal function and growth of long-term survivors of medulloblastoma/PNET. In Green, D. M. & D'Angio, G. J. (eds). *Late Effects of Treatment for Childhood Cancer.* New York: Wiley-Liss, 1992; 55–62.
115. Oberfield, S. E., Nirenberg, A., Allen, J. C. *et al.* Hypothalamic–pituitary–adrenal function following cranial irradiation. *Horm. Res.* 1997; **47**:9–16.

116. Kaplan, M. M., Garnick, M. B., Gelber, R. *et al.* Risk factors for thyroid abnormalities after neck irradiation for childhood cancer. *Am. J. Med.* 1983; **74**:272–280.
117. Devney, R. B., Sklar, C. A., Nesbit, M. E., Jr. *et al.* Serial thyroid function measurements in children with Hodgkin disease. *J. Pediatr.* 1984; **105**:223–227.
118. Hancock, S. L., Cox, R. S., & McDougall, I. R. Thyroid diseases after treatment of Hodgkin's disease. *N. Engl. J. Med.* 1991; **325**:599–605.
119. Tucker, M. A., Jones, P. H., Boice, J. D., Jr. *et al.* Therapeutic radiation at a young age is linked to secondary thyroid cancer. The Late Effects Study Group. *Cancer. Res.* 1991; **51**:2885–2888.
120. Haik, B. G., Jereb, B., Smith, M. E. *et al.* Radiation and chemotherapy of parameningeal rhabdomyosarcoma involving the orbit. *Ophthalmology* 1986; **93**:1001–1009.
121. Krebs, I. P., Krebs, W., Merriam, J. C. *et al.* Radiation retinopathy: electron microscopy of retina and optic nerve. *Histol. Histopathol.* 1992; **7**:101–110.
122. Kielbassa, A. M., Attin, T., Schaller, H. G., & Hellwig, E. Endodontic therapy in a postirradiated child: review of the literature and report of a case. *Quintessence Int.* 1995; **26**:405–411.
123. Simon, A. R. & Roberts, M. W. Management of oral complications associated with cancer therapy in pediatric patients. *ASDC J. Dent. Child.* 1991; **58**:384–389.
124. Newton, W. A., Jr., Meadows, A. T., Shimada, H. *et al.* Bone sarcomas as second malignant neoplasms following childhood cancer. *Cancer* 1991; **67**:193–201.
125. DeRosa, G. P. Progressive scoliosis following chest wall resection in children. *Spine* 1985; **10**:618–622.
126. Grosfeld, J. L., Rescorla, F. J., West, K. W. *et al.* Chest wall resection and reconstruction for malignant conditions in childhood. *J. Pediatr. Surg.* 1988; **23**:667–673.
127. Agadir, M., Sevastik, B., Reinholt, F. P. *et al.* Vascular changes in the chest wall after unilateral resection of the intercostal nerves in the growing rabbit. *J. Orthop. Res.* 1990; **8**:283–290.

61

Liver tumors and resections

Jean de Ville de Goyet and Jean-Bernard Otte

Transplant and Paediatric Surgery, St. Luc University Hospital, Brussels, Belgium

Short- and long-term outcomes of children with malignancies have improved considerably during the last four decades. According to the review by Ries *et al.* (1991), the survival rate for cancer cases diagnosed before 15 years of age has improved from around 50% in the early 1970s to 75% a decade later.[1] This favorable trend has been observed not only in hematologic malignancies but also in many solid tumors such as Wilms' tumor and hepatoblastoma.[2–4] This progress is due to many factors including advances in medical expertise, surgical techniques, and most importantly innovation and refinement of adjuvant chemotherapy.[5–7] With growing numbers of surviving patients, the long-term side effects of chemotherapy are now viewed with increasing concern and may lead us to reconsider therapeutic strategies in the future, possibly promoting further integration of genetic and tumor markers into tailored management protocols.

Children with cancers represent a unique population for studying genetic and environmental mechanisms of cancer etiology, and also genetic factors or tumor markers associated with survival. Identifying mechanisms and/or markers encourages the development of prevention, screening or pre-emptive treatment strategies. However, less is known about children's cancers compared to adults and additional research is necessary; the relatively small number of children with cancer and the lack of co-ordinated studies has led, for too long, to fragmentation and duplication of research effort. Large collaborative trials in pediatric cancer research are a priority.

General aspects of pediatric liver tumors

Mesenchymal hamartoma

Mesenchymal hamartoma of the liver (MHL) is the second most common benign liver tumor in children. Most cases present during the first 2 years of life, with both sexes affected equally.[8,9] MHL is usually multicystic and more commonly reported in the right liver and in small children (Fig. 61.1). They are "tumor-like" but non-neoplastic malformations and composed of mature but disorganized cells indigenous to the liver with some cell types predominating; often they show overgrowth of stroma and presence of malformed bile ducts. These rapidly growing liver tumors may secrete alpha fetoprotein.

Exact etiology is still unknown. A developmental anomaly, biliary obstruction, regional ischemia, and disordered hyperplasia after liver injury have all been implicated in pathogenesis. The observation of aneuploidy in some MHL has led some investigators to suggest they are true neoplasms;[10] this hypothesis is supported by the fact that MHL is derived from mesenchymal and epithelial tissues, as is undifferentiated embryonal sarcoma of the liver (UES). Furthermore, recent cytogenetic studies have shown that 19q translocations can be associated with MHL,[11] and chromosomal abnormalities can be seen in UES.[12,13] Additional observations are also in line with this hypothesis: Lauwer *et al.* (1997) reported cytogenetic and flow cytometric analyses, indicating that there might be a continuum between MHL and UES;[9] a translocation involving 19q13.4 has been identified in MHL and add (19)(q13.4) has been observed in

Pediatric Surgery and Urology: Long-term Outcomes, Mark Stringer, Keith Oldham, Pierre Mouriquand.
Published by Cambridge University Press.

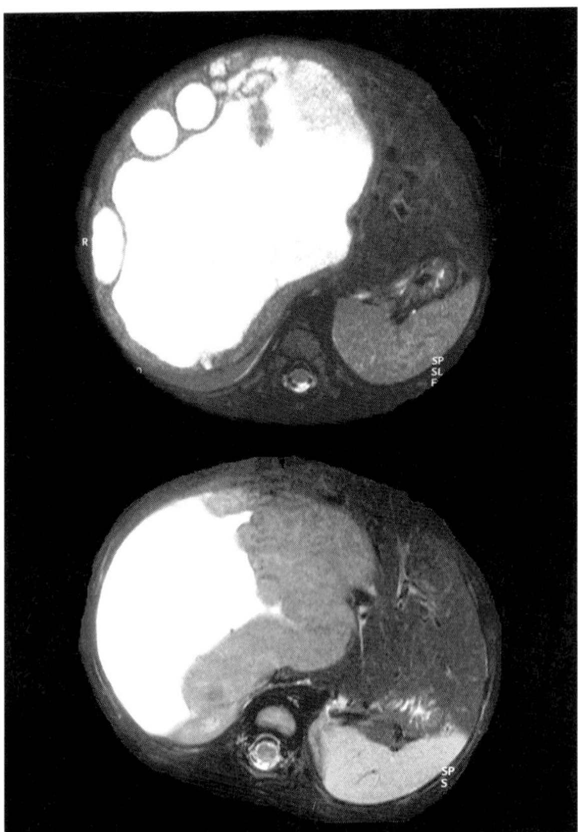

Fig. 61.1. Recurrent mesenchymal hamartoma after previous resection of the cystic components only (hospitalized child with refractory ascites and malnutrition). The solid component of the tumor has grown with time and had to be radically resected for a successful outcome.

UES;[11] there are case reports of UES developing 8 years after incomplete excision of an MHL,[14] of combined UES and MHL,[12,13] and of malignant transformation of MHL.[15,16]

Adenoma

Adenoma accounts for 4%–6% of all benign liver tumors in childhood. In young infants, adenoma develops in otherwise normal liver tissue but in children aged more than 5 years, adenoma is most often associated with an underlying liver disease (e.g., glycogen storage disease type I and III, Fanconi's disease). Adenoma is commonly solitary and only occasionally multiple; polyadenomatosis (>10 lesions) is rare. Histologically, adenomas consist of well-differentiated hepatocytes lacking portal and bile ducts with preservation of the reticulin pattern. Clinically, an adenoma typically presents as a large mass, often associated with pain and fever. Intralesional hemorrhage or rupture with massive intra-abdominal bleeding may occur. The issue of potential malignant transformation into hepatocellular carcinoma remains controversial,[17] although it has been observed in cases of glycogen storage disease-associated adenomas[18] and in polyadenomatosis.[19]

Focal nodular hyperplasia (FNH)

FNH is slightly more frequent in childhood than adenoma and predominates in females. It is exceptional under 1 year of age. It seems to originate from an anomalous arterial supply with or without secondary thrombosis. It may be associated with a variety of conditions including glycogen storage diseases. It usually presents as an asymptomatic mass in an otherwise normal child. It is not premalignant and the risk of bleeding is almost zero. Pathologic examination shows a single, well-circumscribed mass with a characteristic central stellate scar radiating through the tumor. Histologically, it consists of cords of hepatocytes two to three cells thick, without central veins, but with prominent ductular proliferation within fibrous septae; well-formed portal triads are absent. Diagnosis with color Doppler ultrasonography and magnetic resonance imaging (MRI) is straightforward in most cases.

Epithelioid hemangioendothelioma

Hepatic epithelioid hemangioendothelioma is a rare tumor usually seen in adults (female predominance) and is extremely rare in children. It is a low-to-intermediate grade malignancy with slow growth but potential for local recurrence and, with time, distant metastases that also grow relatively slowly. Prolonged survival without treatment[20,21] and even spontaneous resolution has been described. However, the natural history of this tumor is unpredictable[20] and rapid progression may occur. Aggressive tumors are more frequent in children than in adults.

Hepatic epithelioid hemangioendothelioma may be found incidentally but about half of the patients present with upper abdominal pain or discomfort; rarely it presents with jaundice, a Budd–Chiari like syndrome or liver failure. Radiologic features (CT or MRI) vary from a large liver mass to, more often, a diffuse tumor with multiple peripheral hepatic lesions and capsular retraction, peripheral contrast enhancement and evidence of multiple calcifications (Fig. 61.2).[22] The latter type of lesion is believed to be derived from the former unifocal mass. Diagnosis can only be confirmed by histology (preferably a surgical biopsy) which reveals Factor VIII-related-Ag positive cells on immuno-histochemical staining.[21]

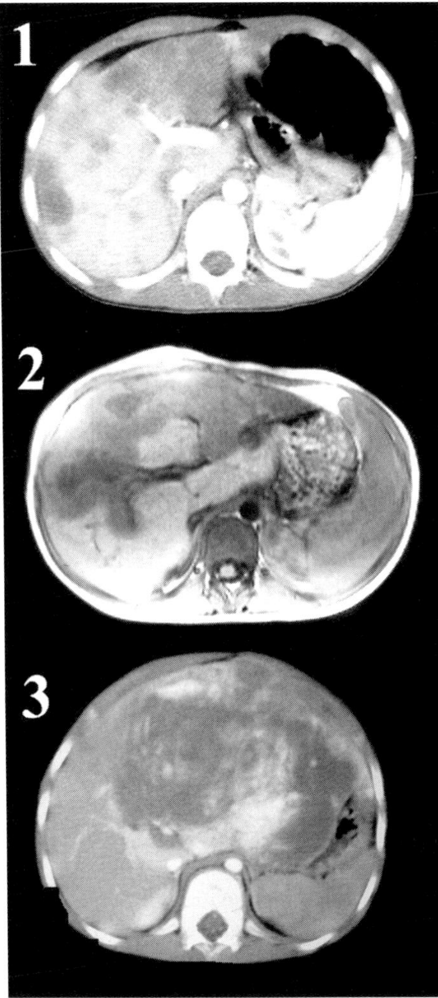

Fig. 61.2. Epithelioid hemangioendotheliomas are usually unresectable at diagnosis (either widespread in the liver or multifocal). Only the third tumor (lower figure) was amenable to surgical resection with *ex situ* surgery, followed by adjuvant chemotherapy (alive and well 3 years later).

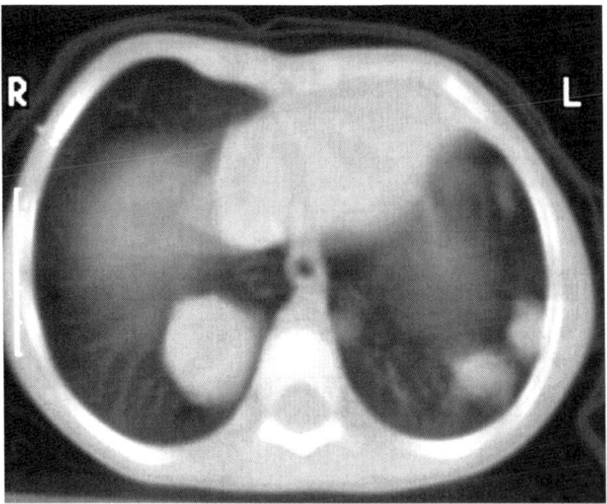

Fig. 61.3. Lung metastases diagnosed 10 months after primary resection of a PRETEXT I hepatoblastoma treated by primary resection without perioperative chemotherapy. Complete cure was obtained by 8 courses of PLADO and surgical resection (alive with no evidence of disease 15 years later).

Hepatoblastoma (HB)

HB is the most frequent pediatric malignant liver tumor with a peak incidence in the first 3 years of life. This embryonic tumor arises from primitive epithelial cells of the fetal liver and typically has a rapid rate of growth. HB is more frequent in boys and usually presents with abdominal distension, a mass, pain and failure to thrive. It can rupture and cause intra-abdominal bleeding. Thrombocytosis is not uncommon. An association with Beckwith–Wiedemann syndrome and hemi-hypertrophy is described; these children should be systematically screened by measuring alpha-fetoprotein and abdominal ultrasonography.[23] HB can also be associated with familial adenomatous polyposis which is related to APC gene mutations.[24]

Alpha-fetoprotein levels are raised in at least 70% of children with HB; when elevated at presentation, this tumor marker is an excellent aid in diagnosis, monitoring response to therapy and, importantly, in the early detection of disease recurrence.[25] A low serum AFP level (<100 ng/ml) at presentation is a poor prognostic factor.[26] HB spreads by vascular invasion, typically to the lungs (Fig. 61.3). Abdominal lymph node involvement is very infrequent.

Histologically, most HBs have an epithelial and a mesenchymal component. The epithelial component can be of fetal or embryonal subtype. Pure fetal histology seems to be more favorable. Macrotrabecular and undifferentiated anaplastic subtypes are uncommon. Whether a diagnostic biopsy is obtained surgically or percutaneously, sampling can be misleading and limits the prognostic value of the initial histology.

Hepatocellular carcinoma (HCC)

Since liver cirrhosis predisposes to neoplasia, HCC is associated with a variety of chronic liver disorders such as chronic hepatitis B and tyrosinemia. In the western world, HCC is much less frequent than HB, hepatitis B being infrequent and tyrosinemia patients being usually managed with the enzyme inhibitor NTBC that gives some, but not complete, protection.

HCC occurs in older children than HB and presents with abdominal distension and a mass; abdominal pain and vomiting are also common. Serum alpha-fetoprotein is elevated in most patients but to lesser extent than in HB. HCC spreads by both lymphatic and vascular invasion. Invasion of hilar, para-aortic and mediastinal lymph nodes is common as well as pulmonary metastases. At the time of diagnosis, the tumor is often extensive and resection is possible in only a minority of cases.

Fibrolamellar HCC is recognized as a distinct clinicopathological variant with a slower growth. A more favorable prognosis was suggested by single center experiences[27] but was not confirmed in a recent multicenter prospective study.[28]

Sarcoma

Sarcoma of the liver (undifferentiated sarcoma) or of the biliary tree (rhabdomyosarcoma) represent the third most common malignant liver tumor type in children. Undifferentiated (mesenchymal or embryonal) sarcomas are heterogenous (solid and cystic) tumors usually seen in older children; spontaneous hemorrhage and/or necrosis may be seen. Rhabdomyosarcoma of the bile ducts arises from major bile ducts in or near the porta hepatis[29] and is seen in younger children. Grossly, it presents as a botryoid, gelatinous mass occluding the lumen of the major bile ducts with dilatation of the intrahepatic bile ducts; the mass can extend into the liver parenchyma.

Clinical presentation of hepatic sarcoma is usually with general deterioration, weight loss and abdominal swelling (sometimes acute from intralesional hemorrhage). Biliary rhabdomyosarcoma usually presents with obstructive jaundice.

Diagnostic imaging

The best initial and least expensive imaging investigation of a child with a liver mass is ultrasonography. It can determine the echogenicity, intrahepatic extent, and relationship of the mass to major venous structures, which is essential for precise surgical staging and assessing resectability. Ultrasound is also helpful for guided biopsy. Differentiation between normal liver tissue and tumor is more accurate with MRI than CT.

In children aged between 6 months and 3 years, a very high serum alpha-fetoprotein and typical imaging appearances are sufficient to diagnose HB. In smaller infants, biopsy is recommended to exclude other tumor types, e.g., mesenchymal hamartoma. In older children, and especially those with modestly raised alpha-fetoprotein levels, HCC must be excluded by histologic examination. Biopsy can be done surgically or, preferably, percutaneously using ultrasound guidance. To prevent tumor seeding, the needle should be advanced through a short depth of normal liver tissue (a portion that will be resected at future surgery).

With modern imaging techniques utilizing appropriate vascular enhancement, there is no longer a place for formal arteriography. Where available, whole-body F-18 fluorodeoxyglucose positron emission tomography (PET-scan) is a very useful additional tool for detecting metastases.[30]

Factors influencing long-term outcome

Stage of disease

Since the extent of disease at diagnosis is variable, and since this directly influences outcome, a reproducible clinical staging system is essential; it facilitates comparison of patients between series, accurate interpretation of data from clinical trials, and should ideally have prognostic value. Different staging systems have been used. The Children's Cancer Study Group in the USA[31] and the Cooperative German Pediatric Liver Tumor Study Group[32] have used a system in which the stage of the disease is determined at the initial surgical intervention, before starting chemotherapy (Table 61.1). In Japan, a modified TNM staging system has been used.[33] These staging systems include information from surgery and are not designed to assess the resectability of a liver tumor at presentation.

The liver tumor study group of the International Society of Pediatric Oncology (SIOPEL) has used, and validated, a grouping system based on the pre-treatment extent of the disease (PRETEXT group) as determined by radiologic findings (Table 61.2 and Fig. 61.4).[26,34] Initially developed for staging the extent of the primary tumor at diagnosis and before therapy, it is now used both at diagnosis and to evaluate response to chemotherapy. PRETEXT stages I to IV (Fig. 61.4) correspond to tumors invading one to four liver sectors, respectively (the liver being divided into four anatomic sectors); the presence of portal vein, hepatic vein and/or vena caval invasion, extrahepatic spread, and metastases are also recorded (Table 61.2). The aim of PRETEXT grouping was to determine whether it would be possible, preoperatively, to identify patients in whom partial hepatectomy could achieve complete tumor resection. This system has been validated in the SIOPEL-1 study where the PRETEXT grouping at presentation was the only significant

Table 61.1. Children's Cancer Study Group staging system

Stage I	Complete resection
Stage II	Resection with microscopic residual disease
Stage III	Resection with gross residual tumor
	– Tumor spill and/or positive lymph nodes
	– Incomplete resection of primary tumor
Stage IV	Distant metastases

Table 61.2. SIOPEL PRETEXT grouping system

(a) Group according to anatomy of tumor (Fig. 61.4)	
Group I	One liver sector
Group II	Two liver sectors
Group III	Three liver sectors
Group IV	All four liver sectors
(b) Additional extension information	
p	portal vein thrombosis or invasion
v	extension into vena cava
e	intra-abdominal extrahepatic disease
m	distant metastases

prognostic parameter in a multivariate analysis.[26] Japanese groups have recently decided to use PRETEXT grouping.

Treatment options

Chemotherapy

Chemotherapy is a cornerstone in the management of malignant liver tumors. Although chemosensitivity varies between patients and tumor types, it is an essential component in the management of such tumors and complementary to radical surgical resection to effect a cure. Major advances and improved success rates have been achieved during the last two decades.

Epithelioid hemangioendothelioma

Hepatic epithelioid hemangioendothelioma was until recently considered unresponsive to chemotherapy and tumor resection was the only management option. However, many of these tumors are multifocal or large and widespread at presentation and partial liver resection is not possible (Fig. 61.2). In such cases, liver transplantation has been proposed as a reasonable option in adults but has not achieved good results in children. The recent observation that Carboplatin and Etoposide seem active against these tumors may offer new hope in the management of this disease. These agents might be used as primary or adjuvant

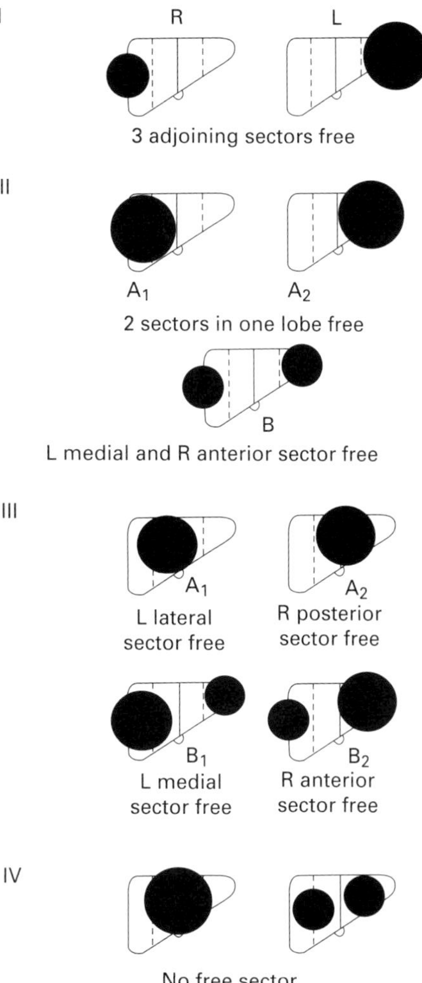

Fig. 61.4. PRETEXT grouping system according to SIOP (Société Internationale d'Oncologie Pédiatrique – International Society of Paediatric Oncology).

(combined with surgery) treatments, or to select and prepare appropriate candidates for liver transplantation.[7]

Hepatoblastoma

The most effective drugs are cisplatin (CDDP), doxorubicin (DOXO) and carboplatin (CARBO).[31,32,35,36] In the United States, primary laparotomy has been a traditional practice with either tumor resection followed (or not[37]) by adjuvant postoperative chemotherapy, or a tumor biopsy followed by chemotherapy and secondary resection.[35,38] Interestingly, other studies in the USA have shown that preoperative chemotherapy can convert an initially unresectable HB to a resectable one.[39,40]

In line with the latter, studies coordinated by the SIOPEL group have concentrated, from the start, on preoperative chemotherapy.[26,36] In SIOPEL-1 (1990–1994), all patients were treated preoperatively with four courses of cisplatin and doxorubicin (PLADO); surgical resection was followed by two further courses.[26] If the tumor was judged unresectable after four courses of chemotherapy, surgery was delayed until after the sixth course. If the tumor remained localized to the liver but still remained unresectable (PRETEXT group IV, or group III tumors in contact with hepatic or portal vein(s) precluding radical excision, or centrally located HB), liver transplantation was recommended as primary surgery (see below). The multivariate analysis of SIOPEL-1 data showed that the PRETEXT category was the only statistically significant prognostic factor for overall 5-year survival.[26] Based on this finding, treatment was stratified in the SIOPEL-2 study (1995–1997) according to the PRETEXT group and the presence of metastases. The aims of the study were to investigate whether intensification of therapy would improve the prognosis of those children with PRETEXT IV disease and/or metastases (defined as "high-risk") and if it would be possible to reduce chemotherapy in those children with PRETEXT group I, II and III disease, defined as "standard-risk".[41] For standard risk HB, treatment was based on CDDP monotherapy and surgery because of concerns about the short- and long-term cardiotoxicity of DOXO. For high risk HB patients, treatment was intensified by adding CARBO to the PLADO regimen. The favorable results of SIOPEL-2 provided the foundation for the SIOPEL-3 study launched in 1998. This is a prospective randomized trial comparing the efficacy of CDDP monotherapy with PLADO as preoperative chemotherapy in standard risk patients. High risk HB patients are treated with three drugs (CARBO, CDDP and DOXO) in a rapidly alternating sequence. The trial is ongoing but current results are encouraging.

In the Cooperative German Pediatric Liver Tumor Study HB-89,[32] patients with HB restricted to one liver lobe underwent primary surgery; larger tumors were initially treated with chemotherapy and resected at second-look surgery. All patients received three drugs (ifosfamide, CDDP and DOXO) either as adjuvant or neoadjuvant therapy. The results obtained in the HB-89 and 94 studies underlined the necessity for preoperative chemotherapy in all HBs that was accepted in the subsequent HB-99 study.[42]

We can conclude that most research groups, with the exception of some in the USA, favor using preoperative chemotherapy, whatever the initial intrahepatic extent of the tumor. Most surgeons agree that preoperative chemotherapy helps to reduce the size of most tumors and to obtain better demarcation between the tumor and surrounding liver. Consequently, tumors are more likely to be completely resected[43] without increasing perioperative morbidity or mortality. It is also speculated that residual microscopic tumor may behave more aggressively under the influence of hepatotrophic factors stimulating liver regeneration if preoperative chemotherapy has not been used.[44]

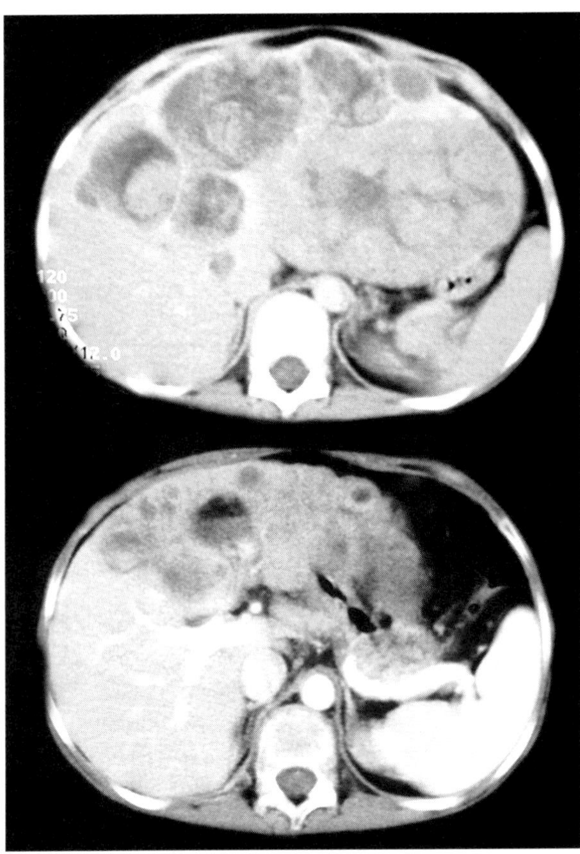

Fig. 61.5. Good response of a hepatocellular carcinoma to chemotherapy, allowing conversion from an unresectable tumor to one treated by successful extended left hepatectomy.

Hepatocellular carcinoma

HCC is often resistant or poorly responsive to chemotherapy. Historically, HCC patients were treated with the same protocols as HB patients. In SIOPEL-1, HCC patients were treated with the same PLADO-based regimen as HB; the event-free survival at 5 years was only 17%. No patient with metastases at presentation survived long term.[45] In SIOPEL-2, treatment was intensified by combining CARBO and PLADO; results were not improved compared with SIOPEL-1, although anecdotally some good responses were observed (Fig. 61.5).

Similarly poor results were obtained in the Cooperative German Pediatric Liver Tumor Studies (either with ifosfamide, CDDP and DOXO (IPA), or with CARBO and etoposide in addition to IPA).[46,47] The American Pediatric Intergroup Hepatoma study compared two regimens (CDDP+VCR+5-FU vs. CDDP+DOXO) in a prospective randomized trial.[48] The 5-year event-free survival was 19% for the entire cohort of 46 children, 8% for unresectable tumors and 0% for metastatic tumors.

Clearly, new treatment strategies are needed for pediatric HCC.[49]

Sarcoma

The prognosis of sarcomas was very poor until the introduction of new improved chemotherapy regimens (e.g., vincristine based protocols). In the European cooperative MMT protocols, the place of radiotherapy (and the risk of late sequelae) has been reduced and a regimen of ifosfamide, vincristine, and actinomycin (IVA) is combined with radical surgery, which may include resection of extrahepatic bile ducts and the hilar plate and vascular reconstruction. Studies are ongoing and results awaited.

Previous experience with MMT protocols has shown that local recurrence can sometimes be managed successfully by further chemotherapy and local surgery. A typical example is shown in Fig. 61.6: a 4-year-old child presented with obstructive jaundice due to an embryonal rhabdomyosarcoma in the left liver involving the left bile ducts. The tumor responded well to three courses of VAC (vincristine, actinomycin and cyclophosphamide) and a full left hepatectomy was performed *en bloc* with the extrahepatic bile ducts and the biliary confluence. Three right segmental bile ducts were drained using a Roux-en-Y loop. Further VAC courses were given postoperatively. Two years later, a local recurrence was diagnosed by ultrasound (node at porta hepatis) and responded well to five courses of chemotherapy (CDDP-VP16). At surgery, a 1 cm residual viable tumor (same histology) was found outside of the liver and radically resected with a small patch of vena cava. Five courses of CDDP-VP16 were given after surgery. The child is alive and in remission 14 years after initial presentation.

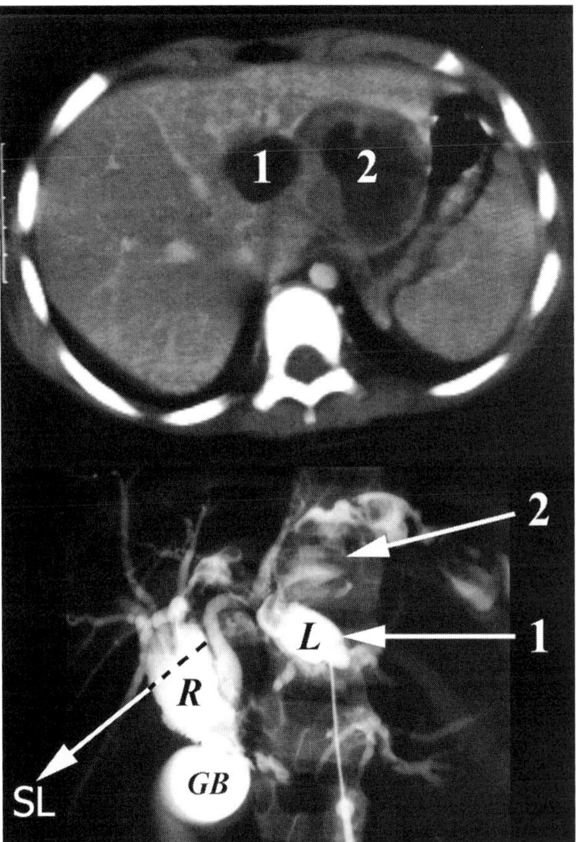

Fig. 61.6. Botryoid type liver sarcoma of the left liver extending along the bile ducts towards the hilar convergence and causing obstructive jaundice. (1: dilated left bile duct (L); 2: botryoid aspect of the tumour; R: right bile ducts; GB: gallbladder; SL: line of division of the right bile duct at radical surgery). (See text for details.)

Hepatic artery chemoembolization (HACE)

Intra-arterial injection of anticancer agents enables smaller doses to be used and increases the local concentration of drugs, thereby reducing systemic side effects whilst the arterial embolization causes ischemic necrosis and shrinkage of the tumor.[50] Experience is very scarce in children since HACE is a much more demanding procedure than conventional chemotherapy: it requires general anesthesia and the skills of an experienced pediatric radiologist, needs repeating every 3–4 weeks depending on efficacy and tolerance, and may lead to liver dysfunction and hepatic artery thrombosis. However, this approach is promising for tumors refractory to usual treatments and possibly in the management of candidates for transplantation.

Although HACE rarely appears to convert a HB or HCC that is unresectable after conventional chemotherapy into a tumor treatable by partial hepatectomy,[51,52] it may turn a patient with a poor response into a good responder, thus allowing transplantation to be considered with a potentially better outcome. This approach has been suggested by a recent report from Pittsburgh in relation to HCC,[53] and was also used recently for epithelioid hemangioendothelioma.[54]

Surgical resection

Benign tumours

A symptomatic single adenoma should be surgically resected, both for relief of symptoms and to prevent hemorrhage into the tumor or malignant transformation to HCC. Adenomas associated with underlying liver disease or polyadenomatosis should be considered for liver transplantation. The Pittsburgh group has reported liver transplantation in six cases of highly symptomatic, unresectable giant adenomas.[55] Asymptomatic, small adenomas should be followed on a regular basis with ultrasonography and serial measurement of serum alpha-fetoprotein.

Focal nodular hyperplasia, when not associated with a high risk of complications, should be left and followed up. Resection can be considered in particular cases, such as a huge median tumor with a high risk of rupture by direct trauma.

Although simple enucleation or marsupialization of large cystic mesenchymal hamartomas were proposed in the past,[8] a proper radical resection is now considered mandatory; recurrence after incomplete excision and malignant transformation are well documented (Fig. 61.1).[16] The operative specimen should include a rim of normal liver parenchyma at the resection margin, as for a malignant tumor.

Malignant tumors

The aim of surgery for a malignant tumor is complete excision, a requirement for cure. Liver resections should be performed along anatomic planes determined by segmental hepatic anatomy. The extent of resection depends on the extent of the tumor but a free margin of around 1 cm or more is advisable for most malignancies; for hepatoblastoma, resection at the tumor margin has been considered acceptable by some groups if a good response to preoperative chemotherapy has been observed.

General technical aspects

The surgical strategy should be based on a sound knowledge of liver anatomy and expertise with the different types of liver resections, including the most extensive ones. Non-anatomical, atypical resections are best avoided, except for particular cases. Young children with no background liver disease can tolerate very extensive liver resections, up to 80% of the liver mass.

Basically, there are five types of resection: left lobectomy (Couinaud segments 2 and 3), left hepatectomy (segments 2 to 4), extended left hepatectomy (left trisegmentectomy, segments 2,3,4,5 and 8), right hepatectomy (segments 5 to 8) and extended right hepatectomy (right trisegmentectomy, segments 4 to 8) (Fig. 61.7). The extent of resection should be planned from preoperative imaging; intraoperative ultrasound is useful to confirm the extent of the tumor and the proximity of major intrahepatic vascular structures.

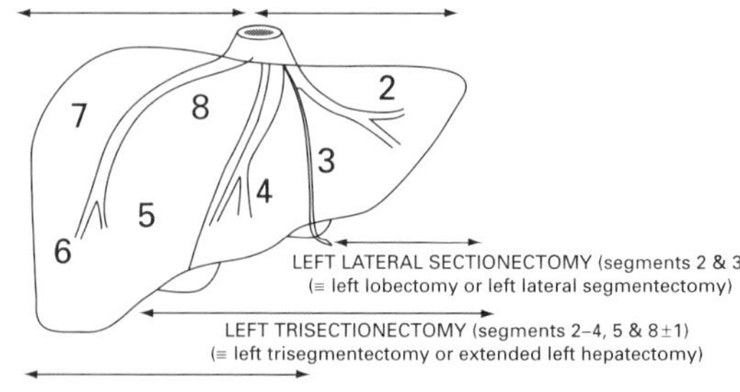

Fig. 61.7. Liver anatomy and types of partial liver resections (reproduced with permission of Stringer 2000).[43]

Precise control of operative bleeding is of paramount importance in decreasing morbidity and limiting the need for blood transfusion, a factor known to be associated with tumor recurrence. To achieve this objective, good surgical exposure through a bilateral subcostal incision with complete mobilization of the liver and control of the liver pedicle and vena cava above and below the liver are standard steps. Appropriate equipment is needed such as an ultrasonic dissector and argon beam coagulator. When a difficult resection is anticipated, temporary clamping of the portal triad (Pringle's maneuver) is advised to minimize blood loss. To further reduce the risk of massive bleeding or air embolism caused by accidental injury to the vena cava or hepatic veins, complete hepatic vascular exclusion combining clamping of the portal triad and occlusion of the vena cava above and below the liver is feasible. Normal liver is remarkably tolerant of up to 60 minutes of warm ischemia.[56]

Special technical aspects

In special cases requiring very extensive resection and/or vascular reconstruction, the patient may have to be put on extracorporeal veno-venous bypass (porto-cavo-jugular) for performing resection on the *in situ* cooled perfused liver. More rarely, the liver can be excised completely for ex-situ resection followed by reimplantation of the remnant segments.[7,57] Since liver transplantation has been validated for unresectable HB, the latter techniques have become obsolete for HB management due to their technical complexity and inherent operative risks; however, they still may have a place for other types of tumor (e.g., HCC).

Extensive lymphadenectomy of the hepatoduodenal ligament is recommended in HCC since lymph node involvement is not uncommon. This contrasts with HB which rarely invades lymph nodes within the liver pedicle. In HB, any extrahepatic intra-abdominal disease should be excised completely, if feasible, at first surgery.

Rhabdomyosarcomas of the biliary tree usually arise from the main bile ducts and therefore a trisegmentectomy with resection of the extrahepatic bile ducts (including the hepatic duct confluence) is usually necessary to achieve radical resection (Fig. 61.6). The bile ducts must be divided flush with the plane of parenchymal section and biliary reconstruction requires a Roux-en-Y loop.

Indications for liver transplantation

Hepatoblastoma

Since the early 1990s, liver transplantation (LTX) has become an integral part of the overall modern management of HB.[3,58–60] Patients with HB showing some response to chemotherapy but whose tumor remains unresectable should nowadays be referred to a transplant centre. LTX is recommended as primary surgery (rather than a futile attempt at partial hepatectomy) for tumors invading all four sectors of the liver (PRETEXT IV) or for those where excision by partial hepatectomy may be incomplete due to close contact with either hepatic vein(s) or portal vein (some PRETEXT III or centrally located tumors). In PRETEXT IV multifocal HB, one sector may apparently clear during chemotherapy; whilst it is tempting to consider that clearance at imaging may correspond to disease-free parenchyma, partial hepatectomy in these cases has been shown to leave viable microscopic residues leading to relapse.[59,61]

Active metastatic disease or extrahepatic tumor deposits *after* chemotherapy are, of course, contraindications to transplantation. However, LTX remains an acceptable option, with good long-term results, for children who present with lung metastases which subsequently clear during chemotherapy.[36] Thoracotomy may be indicated for surgical excision of residual disease if any doubt persists.[4,34,60,62] Macroscopic venous invasion (portal or hepatic veins) is also not an absolute contraindication to transplantation as long as radical excision is possible.[50,60] In contrast, a review of the world experience with LTX confirmed that previous liver resection is an adverse prognostic factor, and that the results are poor in cases of "rescue" transplantation.[60]

In order to prevent the development of tumor resistance to chemotherapy and re-growth, transplantation should not be delayed and should be synchronized with chemotherapy as is conventional surgery.[63] Due to the usual waiting time constraints with cadaveric organs, and despite the use of split liver grafts, a suitable donor organ may not become available and living-related donation is a valuable alternative.[64–66]

There is no evidence that transplant patients should be treated differently from those undergoing radical liver resection with respect to post-surgery chemotherapy. The arguments to give chemotherapy after partial hepatectomy hold true for total hepatectomy and LTX, at least for extrahepatic micrometastases. In our personal experience, we have not observed an increased toxicity from combining chemotherapy with tacrolimus-based immunosuppression. However, a key point is to aim for a low trough level of tacrolimus in order to maintain a reduced level of immunosuppression in cancer patients.[67]

Hepatocellular carcinoma

Experience with LTX in children with these tumors is very limited;[50] guidelines on indications are mainly derived from experience gained with adult patients. The presence of multifocal tumor or underlying liver disease may preclude partial hepatectomy. Patients with an unresectable tumor, either because of intrahepatic extent or underlying cirrhosis, should be assessed for transplant. The Milan criteria have been used to define adults with cirrhosis-associated HCC who are suitable for LTX: no more than three tumors, each no more than 3 cm in size, or a single tumor not more than 5 cm in diameter.[68] When a single tumor is present in an otherwise normal liver, the present cut-off point of 5 cm diameter might be expanded to 6.5 cm[69] or even 7 cm[70] without compromising survival. In any case, macroscopic venous invasion and extrahepatic extension, including lymph node spread and distant metastases, remain absolute contraindications to LTX.

Other tumors

Total hepatectomy and liver transplantation for epithelioid haemangioendothelioma is reported in adults, with five year actuarial survival as high as 71% (disease-free survival = 60%).[71] However, reports of LTX in children with this tumor are anecdotal. Taege *et al.* (1999) reported a successful case[72] but other centers have had bad experiences with rapid recurrence and death. The role of transplantation has been questioned and the place of chemotherapy recently reassessed.[7,72] The use of carboplatin and etoposide and other adjuvant agents should be considered in the future and LTX restricted to children with a good response.[7]

Table 61.3. Cliniques Saint-Luc Brussels experience with hepatoblastoma ($n = 57$) (1978–2003); types of liver resection

(1) Partial hepatectomy	$n = 39$
Left lobectomy	2
Left hepatectomy	1
Left trisegmentectomy	5[a]
Right hepatectomy	12[b]
Right trisegmentectomy	18
Atypical hepatectomy[c]	1
(2) Total hepatectomy and transplantation	$n = 17$
Primary LTX	($n = 13$)
Postmortem donor	2
Live-related donor	11
Rescue LTX	($n = 4$)
Postmortem donor	3
Live-related donor	1
(3) Multiple biopsies (no residual tumor)	$n = 1$

[a]one bench surgery.
[b]one veno-venous bypass and five total vascular exclusion.
[c]segments 1,5,6,7.

Table 61.4. Cliniques Saint-Luc Brussels experience (1978–2003); surgical complications after resection for hepatoblastoma

After partial hepatectomy ($n = 39$)		
Postoperative bleeding requiring surgery	2	Surgical correction
Bile duct stricture	2	Roux-en-Y loop
Bile duct section	1	Roux-en-Y loop
Liver necrosis after ex-situ surgery	1	Rescue transplant
Small bowel obstruction	2	Surgical revision
Portal vein thrombosis	1[a]	Rescue transplant
Budd–Chiari syndrome (late)	1	Rescue transplant
After liver transplantation ($n = 17$)		
Bile leak	1	Surgical revision
Anastomotic stricture	3	Surgical revision
Small bowel obstruction	3	Surgical revision
Portal vein thrombosis	1[a]	Liver failure/death

[a] same patient.

Outcomes

Surgical morbidity and mortality

In experienced surgical units, major intraoperative complications such as severe bleeding, air embolism, and unrecognized bile duct injury are infrequent and operative mortality is very low when there is no underlying liver disease, even after extended hepatectomies. Hepatic regeneration is rapid, despite intensive preoperative chemotherapy, and usually complete within less than 3 months.[73] Liver function rapidly returns to normal without long-term sequelae.

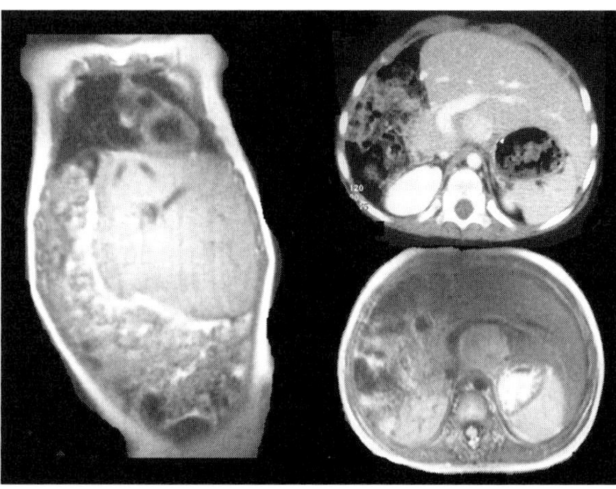

Fig. 61.8. Recurrent hepatoblastoma within the caudate lobe of the liver after previous right hepatectomy and chemotherapy. Successful management by further chemotherapy and re-resection (segment I and IV).

As an example, Table 61.3 summarizes our experience with 57 cases of HB (1978–2003). Of 39 partial hepatectomies, there were 23 right or left trisegmentectomies. Of the latter, three failed for technical reasons and were salvaged by LTX. In one case of *ex situ* left trisegmentectomy, the autograft failed to function adequately and the patient required a split liver transplant. In the second case, a meso-Rex shunt was constructed for bypassing a portal cavernoma before performing a right trisegmentectomy; thrombosis of the bypass required a rescue liver transplant, which failed because extensive thrombosis of the portal system precluded revascularization of the graft. In the third case, right trisegmentectomy was complicated by a Budd–Chiari syndrome due to unrecognized obliteration of the ostium of the left hepatic vein, which recurred despite surgical reanastomosis; a LTX was successfully performed 5 years later. One additional case, a right hepatectomy performed elsewhere for a ruptured HB, was followed by relapse in the left lobe that required a rescue LTX. There were 13 primary transplants, 2 from deceased and 11 from living-related (parent) donors. There was one in-hospital death (1/53 [1.8%]) – the child with extensive portal thrombosis.

Surgical complications are shown in Table 61.4. Postoperative bleeding requiring surgery was encountered in 2 (3.5%) procedures. The incidence of biliary complications was 7.6% (3/39) after partial hepatectomy and 23.5% (4/17)

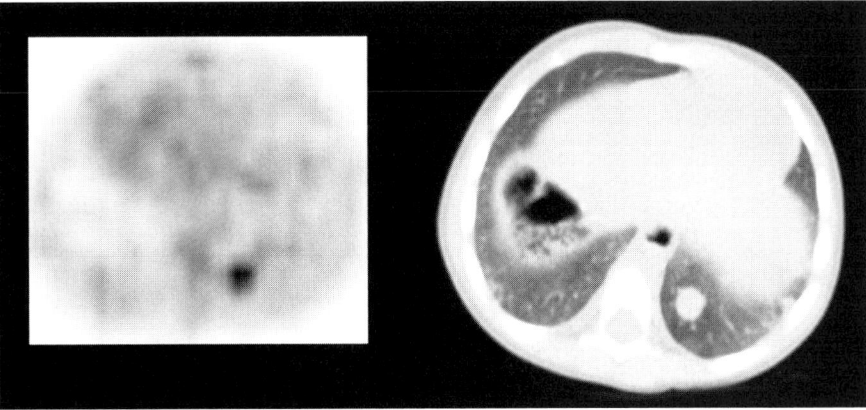

Fig. 61.9. PET-scan detection of a metachronous lung metastasis, in a child with increasing levels of alpha-fetoprotein, 10 months after chemotherapy and liver transplantation. Successful treatment by further chemotherapy and surgical resection of the metastasis.

in liver transplant patients; 2/11(18%) live-related transplants developed an anastomotic biliary stricture which was successfully repaired. In one split liver transplant, an extensive biliary stricture recurred after surgical repair and resulted in acute cholangitis and fatal septic shock 1.5 year post-transplant.

Management of recurrence

Recurrence of a benign tumor may be seen either locally after incomplete resection (true recurrence) (Fig. 61.1), or at other sites in the liver (de novo recurrence) e.g., with adenoma or FNH. Re-resection is usually possible. Recurrence of malignant tumors can be seen within the liver or lymph nodes, or can be extrahepatic and metastatic; the latter is often hopeless, especially when multiple, and usually palliative chemotherapy only is considered. However, when recurrence is confined to the liver, or to very few extrahepatic sites only, and especially when the tumor remains chemosensitive, a combination of surgery and adjuvant chemotherapy can be considered. Although the latter conditions are rarely seen with tumor types other than hepatoblastoma, aggressive management can be considered in selected cases with any tumor type (see above) (Fig. 61.6).

Hepatoblastoma deserves particular mention. The possibility of successfully repeating chemotherapy and surgery for recurrence is shown by the following examples. Figure 61.3 shows a metachronous lung metastasis in a child who had primary surgery (left lobectomy) for a PRETEXT I tumor without chemotherapy. Recurrence was diagnosed 10 months later but he responded well to chemotherapy and surgical resection of residual pulmonary lesions; he is alive and well 15 years later. Figure 61.8 shows a recurrent nodule in the caudate lobe 2 years after right hepatectomy. After chemotherapy, a re-resection of the liver was successfully performed (segments I and IV) and the patient remains well 5 years later. In patients whose alpha-fetoprotein levels return to normal after surgery but increase again at a later date, precise diagnosis of the site of recurrence may be difficult. In these cases, whole body F-18 fluorodeoxyglucose positron emission tomography (PET-scan) may be useful as shown in Fig. 61.9. This child had a mild increase in alpha-fetoprotein 6 months after LTX for HB. Ultrasonographic examination was normal. PET scan showed a single hot spot in the lower left lung, which was confirmed at CT scan and surgery. Histology of the resected nodule confirmed it was the same hepatoblastoma tumor type as the primary tumor and further chemotherapy was given with normalization of the alpha-fetoprotein level.

Long-term disease-free survival

The potential for cure with combined surgical resection and modern chemotherapy is much higher for HB than for HCC. Nowadays, most HB children will survive long term, in contrast to children with HCC or sarcoma, many of whom will get recurrent disease.

Hepatoblastoma

Although individual centers treat relatively small numbers of patients, the best overall survival rates are obtained in experienced units that have liver transplantation in their surgical armamentarium.[58] Some centers have reported their overall experience with HB whilst others have reported their experience with transplanted patients only.

Table 61.5. Hepatoblastoma: survival rates in pediatric series

Reference	Interval	Center	n	Transplant	Survival
(a) Single-center experiences					
Stringer[3]	1981–1993	London, UK	41	2%	67%
Srinivasan[59]	1992–2001	London, UK	13	100%	85%
Pimpalwar[58]	1991–2002	Birmingham, UK	34	41%	91%
Molmenti[81]	1984–2002	Dallas, USA	9	100%	66%
McDiarmid[a]	1984–2001	UCLA, USA	16	100%	75%
Langas[a]	1986–1999	Omaha, USA	10	100%	70%
Gauthier[a]	1985–2004	Paris, France	64	5%	68%
Otte[a]	1978–2003	Brussels, Belgium	53	32%	87%
(b) Multi-center studies					
Sasaki[82]	1991–1999	JPLT-1[b]	134	0%	73%
Schweinitz[32]	<1994	HB-89[c]	72	0%	75%
Fuchs[42]	1994–1998	HB-94[c]	69	3%	77%
Ortega[31]	1989–1992	COG[d]	182	0%	57–69%
Pritchard[36]	1990–1994	SIOPEL-1[e]	154	8%	75%
Perilongo[41]	1995–1998	SIOPEL-2[e]	SR[f]:77	0%	91%
			HR[g]:58	12%	53%

[a]unpublished data, personal communications.
[b]JPLT-1: Japan Study Group for Pediatric Liver Tumors.
[c]HB-89 & HB-94: German Cooperative Pediatric Liver Tumor studies.
[d]COG: Children's Oncology Group,USA.
[e]SIOPEL: Société Internationale d'Oncologie Pédiatrique.
[f]SR: Standard risk.
[g]HR: High risk.

Apart from the SIOPEL group, cooperative study groups have not included transplantation in their strategy. Table 61.5 summarizes relevant reports published during the last decade. It appears that the modern strategy of combining chemotherapy and radical tumor resection enables the majority of children to be cured. The results of treating high-risk HB (involving all four hepatic sectors, and/or presenting with evidence of extrahepatic disease) are still less than satisfactory; better results seem to be achieved when patients are managed within a specialist pediatric center performing both liver and transplant surgery.

In PRETEXT IV tumors (invading all four hepatic sectors) and in multifocal HB, the hope of downstaging the tumor to allow partial hepatectomy is futile. These patients should be referred to a transplant center. In PRETEXT III patients, close proximity of the tumor to the main hepatic veins or main intrahepatic portal branches (centrally located HB) can render it genuinely unresectable without total hepatectomy and LTX. The results of "primary" LTX are significantly better than "rescue" LTX: in the world literature, 82% 6-year survival in the 106 patients receiving a primary LTX versus 30% in the 41 patients receiving a rescue LTX, and in SIOPEL-1, an 85% and 40% 10-year disease-free survival, respectively.[60] Therefore, heroic attempts at partial hepatectomy should be avoided.

Hepatocellular carcinoma

Overall, cure of HCC in children is rarely obtained (Table 61.6), partly because of chemotherapy resistance, and partly because of intra- and extrahepatic spread or venous thrombosis. In the Taipei series,[74] where two-thirds of HCCs were associated with hepatitis B-related cirrhosis, possibilities of resection were limited because of bilateral involvement (63%), portal vein thrombosis (42%), distant metastases (29%), para-aortic lymph node involvement (19%), inferior vena caval thrombi (17%) and hilar invasion (6%). The resectability rate at diagnosis was only 10% with no more than two long-term survivors.

In the SIOPEL-1 study,[45] the extent of pre-treatment intrahepatic disease, as defined by PRETEXT grouping and metastases, was identified as a predictor of overall survival; vascular invasion was a significant negative prognostic factor. SIOPEL-2 included 17 patients who could be analyzed and similarly poor results were obtained despite intensification of chemotherapy; extrahepatic tumor extension and/or vascular invasion were found in 35% of patients. Multifocal tumors prevailed. Metastatic disease was fatal.

The Pittsburgh group has reported the only series of LTX for HCC with a significant number of cases.[50] Overall survival at 5 years was 63%. Vascular invasion, distant metastases, lymph node involvement and tumor size were significant risk factors for recurrence.

Table 61.6. Hepatocellular carcinoma: survival rates in pediatric series

Reference	Interval	Center	*n*	Transplant	Survival
Czaudernan[45]	1990–1994	SIOPEL-1	39	0%	28%
Czaudrnan[a]	1994–1998	SIOPEL-2[b]	17	6%	22%
Von Schweinitz[32]	1989–1993	HB-89[c]	12	0%	33%
Fuchs[42]	1994–1998	HB-94[c]	25	0%	23%
Katzenstein[48]	n.a.	INT-0098[d]	46	0%	19%
Chen[74]	n.a.	Taipei	55[e]	0%	Median, survival 23 months
Reyes[50]	1989–1998	Pittsburgh	17	100%	63%

[a]unpublished data, personal communications.
[b]SIOPEL: Société Internationale d'Oncologie Pédiatrique.
[c]HB-89 & HB-94: German Cooperative Pediatric Liver Tumor Studies.
[d]INT-0098: Paediatric Oncology and Children's Cancer Groups, USA.
[e]68% with cirrhosis.

In conclusion, the outlook for HCC does not seem to have significantly improved over the last decade, with only one-third of cases being amenable to complete resection and cure in a small minority. No improvement can be anticipated without the development of more effective chemotherapy. Whether LTX should be used more liberally remains an open issue but its place will remain limited due to the aggressive nature of this tumor with frequent extrahepatic spread and vascular invasion, both of which remain absolute contraindications.

Long-term effects of adjuvant chemotherapy *(see also Chapter 57)*

The three main drugs currently used to treat pediatric liver malignancies (doxorubicin, cisplatin and carboplatin) all carry long-term toxic side effects on the heart, kidneys and hearing, which are a real concern in children when long-term outcome and quality of life are at issue.

The long-term cardiac toxicity of doxorubicin has been recognized for several years. Steinhertz *et al.* (1995) observed late cardiotoxicity in 15 of 300 patients evaluated 6 to 19 years after anthracycline therapy.[75] Ten of these 15 had no cardiac problems before late decompensation. Conduction abnormalities and dysrhythmias were present in 14 and three died suddenly; one further patient died of uncontrolled cardiac failure. An excess mortality from cardiac disease has been reported 15 years after the diagnosis of malignancies treated with doxorubicin.[76] Heart transplantation has been required in some patients treated years earlier with anthracyclines.[77–79] In recent protocols, measures have been taken to reduce the cardiotoxicity of doxorubicin such as intravenous infusion rather than pulse injection and the use of cardioprotectants.

Nephrotoxicity and ototoxicity are observed with cumulative doses of alkylating agents, less frequently with carboplatin than with cisplatin. Brock *et al.* reported more severe long-term nephrotoxicity in infants than in older children with partial reversibility in the majority of cases during a median follow-up of 2.5 years after treatment.[80] Careful measurement of the glomerular filtration rate by isotope clearance is essential for accurate monitoring of renal status. For patients managed by LTX, careful adjustment of immunosuppression may be necessary in order to avoid cumulative general and renal toxicity.[69] Hypomagnesemia may persist for years after stopping therapy. Ototoxicity increases significantly with the cumulative cisplatin dose and no recovery of hearing was found in affected children followed for a median of 4 years after completion of cisplatin treatment.[80] Careful monitoring of children by an expert audiologist and by serial audiometry throughout treatment with cisplatin is recommended.

With increasing success in the management of children with malignancies, the cohort of long-term survivors is steadily growing. Greater attention will be necessary to prevent secondary problems, late side effects and *de novo* malignancies.

REFERENCES

1. Ries L. A., Hankey B. F., & Miller B. A. *Cancer Statistics. Review 1973–1988.* NIH publication no.91–2789. Bethesda: National Health Institute, 1991.

2. Shafford, E. A. & Pritchard, J. Hepatoblastoma – a bit of a success story? *Eur. J. Cancer* 1994; **30A**:1050–1051.
3. Stringer, M. D., Hennayake, S., Howard, E. R. *et al.* Improved outcome for children with hepatoblastoma. *Br. J. Surg.* 1995; **82**:386–391.
4. Perilongo, G., Brown, J., Shafford, E. *et al.* Hepatoblastoma presenting with lung metastases: treatment results of the first cooperative, prospective study of the International Society of Paediatric Oncology on childhood liver tumors. *Cancer* 2000; **89**:1845–1853.
5. Otte, J. B., Aronson, D., Vraux, H. *et al.* Preoperative chemotherapy major liver resection, and transplantation for primary malignancies in children. *Transpl. Proc.* 1996; **28**:2393–2394.
6. Pimpalwar, A. P., Sharif, K., Ramani, P. *et al.* Strategy for hepatoblastoma management: transplant versus nontransplant surgery. *J. Pediatr. Surg.* 2002; **37**:240–245.
7. Sharif, K., English, M., Ramani, P. *et al.* Management of hepatic epithelioid hemangioendothelioma in children; what option? *Br. J. Cancer* 2004; **90**:1498–1501.
8. Stocker, J. T. & Ishak, K. G. Mesenchymal hamartoma of the liver: report of 30 cases and review of the literature. *Paediatr. Pathol.* 1983; **1**:215–226.
9. Lauwer, Y. G., Grant, L. D., Dnnelly, W. H. *et al.* Hepatic Undifferentiated (embryonal) sarcoma arising in a mesenchymal hamartoma. *Am. J. Surg. Pathol.* 1997; **21**:1248–1254.
10. Otal, T. M., Hendricks, J. B., Pharis, P., & Donnelly, W. H. Mesenchymal hamartoma of the liver. *Cancer* 1994; **74**:1237–1242.
11. Bove, K. E., Blough, R. I., & Soukup, S. Third report of t(19q)(13.4) in mesenchymal hamartoma of liver with comments on link to embryonal sarcoma. *Pediatr. Develop. Pathol.* 1998; **1**:438–442.
12. de Chadarevian, J. P., Pawei, B. R., Faeber, E. N. *et al.* Undifferentiated (embryonal) sarcoma arising in conjuction with mesenchymal hamartoma of the liver. *Modern Pathol.* 1994; **7**:490–494.
13. O'Sullivan, M. J., Swanson, P. E., Knoll, J., Taboada, E. M., & Dehner, L. P. Undifferentiated embryonal sarcoma with unusual features arising within mesenchymal hamartoma of the liver: report of a case and review of the literature. *Pediatr. Dev. Pathol.* 2001; **4**:482–489.
14. Corbally, M. & Spitz, L. Malignant potential of mesenchymal hamartoma. An unrecognized risk. *Pediatr. Surg. Int.* 1992; **7**:321–322.
15. Ramanujam, T. M., Ramesh, J. C., Goh, D. H. *et al.* Malignant transformation of mesenchymal hamartoma of the liver. Case report and review of literature. *J. Pediatr. Surg.* 1999; **34**:1684–1686.
16. Begueret, H., Trouette, Vielh, P. *et al.* Hepatic undifferentiated embryonal sarcoma: malignant evolution of mesenchymal hamartoma? Study of one case with immunohistochemical and flow cytometric emphasis. *J. Hepatol.* 2001; **34**:178–179.
17. Resnick, M. B., Kozakewich, H. P., & Perez-Atayde, A. R. Hepatic adenoma in the pediatric age group. Clinicopathological observations and assessment of cell proliferative activity. *Am. J. Surg. Pathol.* 1995; **19**:1181–1190.
18. Lerut, J. P., Ciccarelli, O., Sempoux, C. *et al.* Glycogenosis storage type I diseases and evolutive adenomatosis: an indication for liver transplantation. *Transpl. Int.* 2003; **16**:879–884.
19. Leese, T., Farges, O., & Bismuth, H. Liver cell adenomas. A 12-year surgical experience from a specialist hepato-biliary unit. *Ann. Surg.* 1988; **208**:558–564.
20. Makhlouf, H. R., Ishak, K. G., & Goodman, S. D. Epithelioid hemangioendothelioma of liver. *Cancer* 1999; **85**:562–582.
21. Uchimura, K., Nakamuta, M., Osoegwa, M. *et al.* Hepatic epithelioid hemangioendothelioma. *J. Clin. Gastroenterol.* 2001; **32**:431–434.
22. Van Beers, B., Roche, A., Mathieu, D. *et al.* Epithelioid hemangioendothelioma of liver. MR and CT finding. *J. Comput. Assist. Tomogr.* 1992; **16**:420–424.
23. Clericuzio, C. L., Chen, E., McNeil, D. E. *et al.* Serum alphafetoprotein screening for hepatoblastoma in children with Beckwith–Wiedemann syndrome or isolated hemihyperplasia. *J. Pediatr.* 2003; **143**:270–272.
24. Thomas, D., Pritchard, J., Davidson, R. *et al.* Familial hepatoblastoma and APC gene mutations: renewed call for molecular research. *Eur. J. Cancer* 2003; **39**:2200–2204.
25. Pritchard, J., da Cunha, A., Cornbleet, M. A., & Carter, C. J. Alpha feta (alpha FP) monitoring of response to adriamycin in hepatoblastoma. *J. Pediatr. Surg.* 1982; **17**:429–430.
26. Brown, J., Perilongo, G., Shafford, E. *et al.* Pretreatment prognostic factors for children with hepatoblastoma – results from the International Society of Paediatric Oncology (SIOP) study SIOPEL 1. *Eur. J. Cancer* 2000; **36**:1418–1425.
27. Hemming, A. W., Langer, B., Sheiner, P., Greig, P. D., & Taylor, B. R. Aggressive surgical management of fibrolamellar hepatocellular carcinoma. *J. Gastrointest. Surg.* 1997; **1**:342–346.
28. Katzenstein, H. M., Krailo, M. D., Malogolowkin, M. H. *et al.* Fibrolamellar hepatocellular carcinoma in children and adolescents. *Cancer* 2003; **97**:2006–2012.
29. Davis, G. L., Kissane, J. M., & Ishak, K. G. Embryonal rhabdomyosarcoma (*Sarcoma botryoides*) of the biliary tree. Report of five cases and a review of the literature. *Cancer* 1969; **24**:333–342.
30. Wudel, L. J., Jr., Delbeke, D., Morris, D. *et al.* The role of [18F]fluorodeoxyglucose positron emission tomography imaging in the evaluation of hepatocellular carcinoma. *Am. Surg.* 2003; **69**:117–124.
31. Ortega, J. A., Douglass, E. C., Feusner, J. H. *et al.* Randomized comparison of cisplatin/vincristine/fluorouracil and cisplatin/continuous infusion doxorubicin for treatment of pediatric hepatoblastoma: a report from the Children's Cancer Group and the Pediatric Oncology Group. *J. Clin. Oncol.* 2000; **18**:2665–2675.
32. von Schweinitz, D., Byrd, D. J., Hecker, H. *et al.* Efficiency and toxicity of ifosfamide, cisplatin and doxorubicin in the treatment of childhood hepatoblastoma. Study Committee of the Cooperative Paediatric Liver Tumour Study HB89 of the German Society for Paediatric Oncology and Haematology. *Eur. J. Cancer* 1997; **33**:1243–1249.

33. Kudo, M., Chung, H., & Osaki, Y. Prognostic staging system for hepatocellular carcinoma (CLIP score): its value and limitations, and a proposal for a new staging system, the Japan Integrated Staging Score (JIS score). *J. Gastroenterol.* 2003; **38**:207–215.
34. Schnater, J. M., Aronson, D. C., Plaschkes, J. *et al.* Surgical view of the treatment of patients with hepatoblastoma: results from the first prospective trial of the International Society of Pediatric Oncology Liver Tumor Study Group. *Cancer* 2002; **94**:1111–1120.
35. Douglass, E. C., Reynolds, M., Finegold, M., Cantor, A. B., & Glicksman, A. Cisplatin, vincristine, and fluorouracil therapy for hepatoblastoma: a Pediatric Oncology Group study. *J. Clin. Oncol.* 1993; **11**:96–99.
36. Pritchard, J., Brown, J., Shafford, E. *et al.* Cisplatin, doxorubicin, and delayed surgery for childhood hepatoblastoma: a successful approach – results of the first prospective study of the International Society of Pediatric Oncology. *J. Clin. Oncol.* 2000; **18**:3819–3828.
37. Finegold, M. J. Chemotherapy for suspected hepatoblastoma without effort at surgical resection is bad practice. *Med. Pediatr. Oncol.* 2002; **39**:484–486.
38. Ortega, J. A., Krailo, M. D., Haas, J. E. *et al.* Effective treatment of unresectable or metastatic hepatoblastoma with cisplatin and continuous infusion doxorubicin chemotherapy: a report from the Childrens Cancer Study Group. *J. Clin. Oncol.* 1991; **9**:2167–2176.
39. Reynolds, M. Conversion of unresectable to resectable hepatoblastoma and long-term follow-up study. *World. J. Surg.* 1995; **19**:814–816.
40. Ehrlich, P. F., Greenberg, M. L., & Filler, R. M. Improved long-term survival with preoperative chemotherapy for hepatoblastoma. *J. Pediatr. Surg.* 1997; **32**:999–1002.
41. Perilongo, G., Shafford, E., Maibach, R. *et al.* Risk-adapted treatment for childhood hepatoblastoma. final report of the second study of the International Society of Paediatric Oncology – SIOPEL 2. *Eur. J. Cancer* 2004; **40**:411–421.
42. Fuchs, J., Rydzynski, J., von Schweinitz, D. *et al.* Pretreatment prognostic factors and treatment results in children with hepatoblastoma: a report from the German Cooperative Pediatric Liver Tumor Study HB 94. *Cancer* 2002; **95**:172–182.
43. Stringer, M. D. Liver tumors. *Semin. Pediatr. Surg.* 2000; **9**:196–208.
44. von Schweinitz, D., Faundez, A., Teichmann, B. *et al.* Hepatocyte growth-factor-scatter factor can stimulate post-operative tumor-cell proliferation in childhood hepatoblastoma. *Int. J. Cancer* 2000; **85**:151–159.
45. Czauderna, P., MacKinlay, G., Perilongo, G. *et al.* Hepatocellular carcinoma in children: results of the first prospective study of the International Society of Pediatric Oncology group. *J. Clin. Oncol.* 2002; **20**:2798–2804.
46. von Schweinitz, D., Burger, D., Bode, U. *et al.* Results of the HB-89 Study in treatment of malignant epithelial liver tumors in childhood and concept of a new HB-94 protocol. *Klin. Padiatr.* 1994; **206**:282–288.
47. von Schweinitz, D., Fuchs, J., & Mildenberger, H. Surgical strategy in pediatric liver malignancies. *Langenbecks Arch. Chir. Suppl Kongressbd.* 1996; **113**:1091–1094.
48. Katzenstein, H. M., Krailo, M. D., Malogolowkin, M. H. *et al.* Hepatocellular carcinoma in children and adolescents: results from the Pediatric Oncology Group and the Children's Cancer Group intergroup study. *J. Clin. Oncol.* 2002; **20**:2789–2797.
49. Bruix, J. & Llovet, J. M. Prognostic prediction and treatment strategy in hepatocellular carcinoma. *Hepatology* 2002; **35**:519–524.
50. Reyes, J. D., Carr, B., Dvorchik, I. *et al.* Liver transplantation and chemotherapy for hepatoblastoma and hepatocellular cancer in childhood and adolescence. *J. Pediatr.* 2000; **136**:795–804.
51. Han, Y. M., Park, H. H., Lee, J. M. *et al.* Effectiveness of preoperative transarterial chemoembolization in presumed inoperable hepatoblastoma. *J. Vasc. Interv. Radiol.* 1999; **10**:1275–1280.
52. Malogolowkin, M. H., Stanley, P., Steele, D. A., & Ortega, J. A. Feasibility and toxicity of chemoembolization for children with liver tumors. *J. Clin. Oncol.* 2000; **18**:1279–1284.
53. Arcement, C. M., Towbin, R. B., Meza, M. P. *et al.* Intrahepatic chemoembolization in unresectable pediatric liver malignancies. *Pediatr. Radiol.* 2000; **30**:779–785.
54. St Peter, S. D., Moss, A. A., Huettl, E. A., Leslie, K. O., & Mulligan, D. C. Chemoembolization followed by orthotopic liver transplant for epithelioid hemangioendothelioma. *Clin. Transpl.* 2003; **17**:549–553.
55. Tepetes, K., Selby, R., Webb, M., Madariaga, J. R., Iwatsuki, S., & Starzl, T. E. Orthotopic liver transplantation for benign hepatic neoplasms. *Arch. Surg.* 1995; **130**:153–156.
56. Huguet, C., Gavelli, A., Chieco, P. A. *et al.* Liver ischemia for hepatic resection: where is the limit? *Surgery* 1992; **111**:251–259.
57. Pichlmayr, R., Grosse, H., Hauss, J. *et al.* Technique and preliminary results of extracorporeal liver surgery (bench procedure) and of surgery on the in situ perfused liver. *Br. J. Surg.* 1990; **77**:21–26.
58. Pimpalwar, A. P., Sharif, K., Ramani, P. *et al.* Strategy for hepatoblastoma management: transplant versus nontransplant surgery. *J. Pediatr. Surg.* 2002; **37**:240–245.
59. Srinivasan, P., McCall, J., Pritchard, J. *et al.* Orthotopic liver transplantation for unresectable hepatoblastoma. *Transplantation* 2002; **74**:652–655.
60. Otte, J. B., Pritchard, J., Aronson, D. C. *et al.* Liver transplantation for hepatoblastoma: results from the International Society of Pediatric Oncology (SIOP) study SIOPEL-1 and review of the world experience. *Pediatr. Blood Cancer* 2004; **42**:74–83.
61. Dall'Igna, P., Cecchetto, G., Toffolutti, T. *et al.* Multifocal hepatoblastoma: is there a place for partial hepatectomy? *Med. Pediatr. Oncol.* 2003; **40**:113–116.
62. Passmore, S. J., Noblett, H. R., Wisheart, J. D., & Mott, M. G. Prolonged survival following multiple thoracotomies for metastatic hepatoblastoma. *Med. Pediatr. Oncol.* 1995; **24**:58–60.
63. von Schweinitz, D., Hecker, H., Harms, D. *et al.* Complete resection before development of drug resistance is essential for

survival from advanced hepatoblastoma – a report from the German Cooperative Pediatric Liver Tumor Study HB-89. *J. Pediatr. Surg.* 1995; **30**:845–852.

64. Otte, J. B. Is it right to develop living related liver transplantation? Do reduced and split livers not suffice to cover the needs? *Transpl. Int.* 1995; **8**:69–73.
65. Dower, N. A., Smith, L. J., Lees, G. *et al.* Experience with aggressive therapy in three children with unresectable malignant liver tumors. *Med. Pediatr. Oncol.* 2000; **34**:132–135.
66. Colombani, P. M., Lau, H., Prabhakaran, K. et al. Cumulative experience with pediatric living related liver transplantation. *J. Pediatr. Surg.* 2000; **35**:9–12.
67. Gehrke, I., Sharif, K., Noujaim, H., de Ville de Goyet, J., McKiernan, P., & Kelly, D. A. Low-tacrolimus serum through levels combined with Daclizumab induction in paediatric liver transplantation; a pilot study. *Pediatr. Transpl.* 2003; **7**:301–305.
68. Mazzaferro, V., Regalia, E., Doci, R. *et al.* Liver transplantation for the treatment of small hepatocellular carcinomas in patients with cirrhosis. *N. Engl. J. Med.* 1996; **334**:693–699.
69. Yao, F. Y., Ferrell, L., Bass, N. M. *et al.* Liver transplantation for hepatocellular carcinoma: expansion of the tumor size limits does not adversely impact survival. *Hepatology* 2001; **33**:1394–1403.
70. Roayaie, S., Frischer, J. S., Emre, S. H. *et al.* Long-term results with multimodal adjuvant therapy and liver transplantation for the treatment of hepatocellular carcinomas larger than 5 centimeters. *Ann. Surg.* 2002; **235**:533–539.
71. Madriaga, J. R., Marino, I. R., Karavias, M. A. *et al.* Long-term results after liver transplantation for primary hepatic Hemangioendothelioma. *Ann. Surg. Oncol.* 1995; **2**:483–487.
72. Taege, C., Holzhausen, H. J., Gunter, G. *et al.* Das Malinge epitheliode haemangioendotheliom der leber. *Pathologie* 1999; **20**:345–350.
73. Wheatley, J. M., Rosenfield, N. S., Berger, L., & LaQuaglia, M. P. Liver regeneration in children after major hepatectomy for malignancy – evaluation using a computer-aided technique of volume measurement. *J. Surg. Res.* 1996; **61**:183–189.
74. Chen, J. C., Chen, C. C., Chen, W. J., Lai, H. S., Hung, W. T., & Lee, P. H. Hepatocellular carcinoma in children: clinical review and comparison with adult cases. *J. Pediatr. Surg.* 1998; **33**:1350–1354.
75. Steinherz, L. J., Steinherz, P. G., & Tan, C. Cardiac failure and dysrhythmias 6–19 years after anthracycline therapy: a series of 15 patients. *Med. Pediatr. Oncol.* 1995; **24**:352–361.
76. Green, D. M., Hyland, A., Chung, C. S., Zevon, M. A., & Hall, B. C. Cancer and cardiac mortality among 15-year survivors of cancer diagnosed during childhood or adolescence. *J. Clin. Oncol.* 1999; **17**:3207–3215.
77. McManus, R. P., & O'Hair, D. P. Pediatric heart transplantation for doxorubicin-induced cardiomyopathy. *J. Heart Lung Transpl.* 1992; **11**:375–376.
78. Luthy, A., Furrer, M., Waser, M. *et al.* Orthotopic heart transplantation: an efficient treatment in a young boy with doxorubicin-induced cardiomyopathy. *J. Heart Lung Transpl.* 1992; **11**:815–816.
79. Dorent, R., Pavie, A., Nataf, P. *et al.* Heart transplantation is a valid therapeutic option for anthracycline cardiomyopathy. *Transpl. Proc.* 1995; **27**:1683.
80. Brock, P. R., Yeomans, E. C., Bellman, S. C., & Pritchard, J. Cisplatin therapy in infants: short and long-term morbidity. *Br. J. Cancer Suppl* 1992; **18**:S36–S40.
81. Molmenti, E. P., Wilkinson, K., Molmenti, H. *et al.* Treatment of unresectable hepatoblastoma with liver transplantation in the pediatric population. *Am. J. Transpl.* 2002; **2**:535–538.
82. Sasaki, F., Matsunaga, T., Iwafuchi, M. *et al.* Outcome of hepatoblastoma treated with the JPLT-1 (Japanese Study Group for Pediatric Liver Tumor) Protocol-1: a report from the Japanese Study Group for Pediatric Liver Tumor. *J. Pediatr. Surg.* 2002; **37**:851–856.

62

Extragonadal germ cell tumors

Christian J. Streck and Andrew M. Davidoff

St. Jude Children's Research Hospital, Memphis, TN, USA

Germ cell tumors (GCTs) are relatively uncommon in childhood, accounting for about 2% to 3% of all neoplasms in patients younger than 15 years.[1] With an annual incidence of approximately 4 per million in this age group, there are about 250 new cases in the United States each year. Germ cell tumors can arise in the gonads or in extragonadal sites, doing so with nearly equal frequency overall. However, extragonadal and testicular tumors predominate in children younger than 3 years, and gonadal tumors predominate in older children. Approximately 30% to 40% of all GCTs are malignant, though the percentage is somewhat higher when considering only extragonadal tumors. Overall, GCTs are more likely to develop in girls than in boys.

Embryogenesis

Germ cell tumors arise from primordial germ cells derived from the embryonic yolk sac endoderm. These primordial germ cells are first recognized in the caudal portion of the yolk sac, near the allantoic stalk, at about the 24th day (2–3 mm embryos). During the 5th and 6th weeks of embryogenesis, these cells migrate along the mesentery of the hindgut toward the genital ridge, which is forming from mesenchyme and mesodermal epithelium.[2] The path of the migrating cells appears to be directed by the interaction of the c-kit ligand, stem cell factor (expressed with an increasing gradient from the yolk sac to the genital ridges), and the c-kit receptor (expressed on the primordial germ cells).[3] During germ cell migration, which ends with the invasion of the genital ridge, the germ cells increase in number by undergoing mitotic division. Neoplastic transformation of these cells is believed to underlie the genesis of GCTs. When this transformation occurs in germ cells that have undergone arrested or aberrant migration to ectopic locations, the ensuing tumor is termed an extragonadal GCT. These cells often come to rest at various sites in or near the midline, such as in the pineal gland or other areas of the brain, the mediastinum, the retroperitoneum, or the sacrococcygeal region. Consequently, these are the most common sites of extragonadal GCTs.

Tumor sites

The most common site of an extragonadal GCT is the presacral/sacrococcygeal region (Table 62.1). The incidence of sacrococcygeal tumors (SCTs) is about 1 in 40 000 infants with three fourths being in female newborns or infants younger than 2 months.[4] Sacrococcygeal tumors in infants are almost always benign, but the probability of malignancy increases with increasing age. More than two thirds of SCTs in infants or children older than 6 months are malignant. Sacrococcygeal teratomas have been classified according to the degree of intrapelvic extension (Fig. 62.1).[4] Type I tumors are predominantly external (47%); Type II are external but with significant intrapelvic extension (35%); Type III are visible externally but with predominant pelvic and intra-abdominal extension (8%); and Type IV are entirely presacral, without external findings (10%). This distinction is important because the type of SCT influences the surgical approach for resection as well as the likelihood of malignancy; the frequency of malignancy is 8% for Type I tumors, 21% for Type II, 34% for Type III, and 38% for Type IV.[4] It may be that the rate of malignancy is higher

Pediatric Surgery and Urology: Long-term Outcomes, Mark Stringer, Keith Oldham, Pierre Mouriquand.
Published by Cambridge University Press.

Table 62.1. Distribution of extragonadal germ cell tumors

Site	% of total	% malignant
Sacrococcygeal	67	20
Intracranial	9	90
Mediastinal	7.5	75
Other	16.5	35

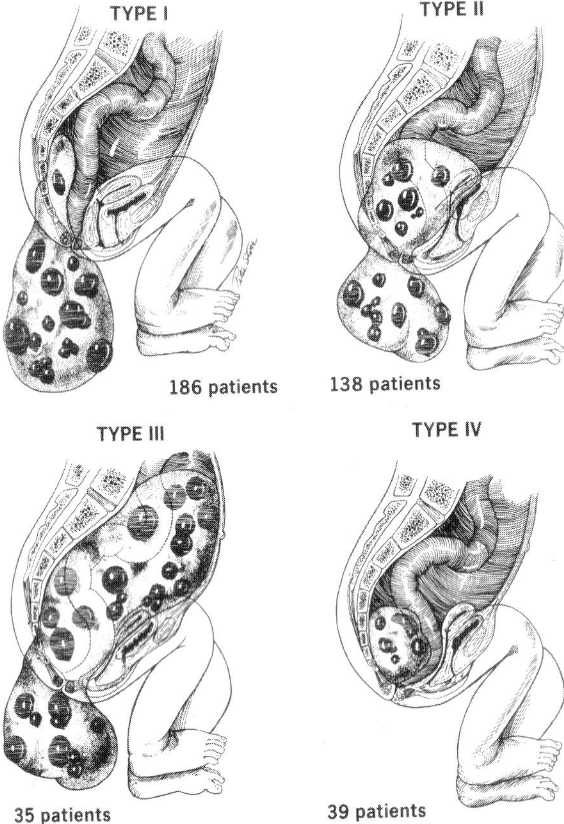

Fig. 62.1. Altman classification for patients with sacrococcygeal teratomas. Reprinted with permission from Young *et al.*[1]

in Type III and IV SCTs because they are less obvious on physical examination, which delays detection and diagnosis. This delay may permit either malignant degeneration or the expansion of a small focus of malignant cells within the tumor mass.

Extragonadal GCTs are also found in the mediastinum, mainly in male adolescents (and adults) who present with chest pain, dyspnea, or cough. In addition, these tumors may be detected incidentally on chest radiographs. Careful examination of the testes is required in these cases, as it is with other apparently extragonadal GCTs in boys, to

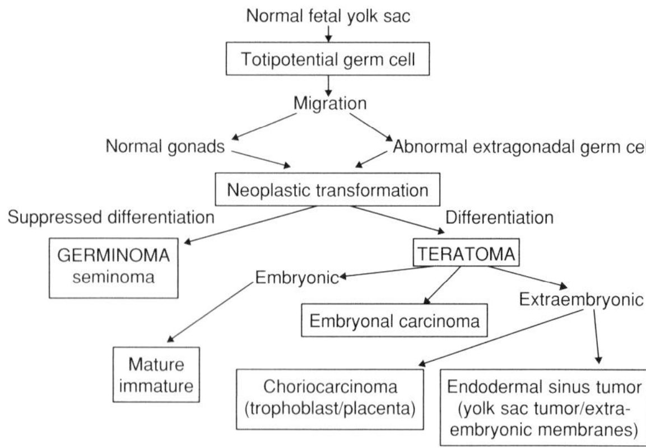

Fig. 62.2. Classification system for germ cell tumors.

be certain that the mediastinal disease is not metastatic disease from a primary gonadal site. Other rare primary sites of extragonadal GCTs include the pineal gland, the retroperitoneum, the omentum, stomach, pancreas, and vagina.

Pathology

Because of the pluripotential nature of germ cells, there is extensive morphologic heterogeneity among GCTs. The type of tumor that develops from the neoplastic transformation of these cells depends, in part, on the degree of differentiation of the germ cell when the transformation occurs. Figure 62.2 describes the histological classification of GCTs.

The term "germinoma" refers to a tumor that arises from the neoplastic transformation of primordial germ cells before any differentiation has occurred. This results in a monophasic tumor that lacks the ability to further differentiate. These tumors are referred to as dysgerminomas when they occur in the ovary and as seminomas when in the testis. Histologically, germinomas appear as sheets or nests of round cells separated by bands of fibrous tissue. The cells have clear, sharply defined cytoplasm and uniform nuclei. This histologic type accounts for 15% of all GCTs in pediatric patients.

Alternatively, neoplastic transformation may occur after the primordial germ cells have undergone variable degrees of differentiation. Teratomas are GCTs that are defined by the presence of all three embryonic layers (endoderm, mesoderm, and ectoderm) and contain tissue foreign to the anatomic site. Teratomas are the most common histologic type of GCT, and 80% are benign. In immature teratomas, one or more of the somatic tissues, usually the neuroepithelial component, has an embryonal appearance. These tumors, although not benign, are usually localized and treated by surgical excision alone. "Metastasizing" immature teratomas are those tumors that likely had small foci of malignant cells that were not detected by routine histopathologic analysis. Malignant teratomas contain one or more malignant germ cell types in addition to well-differentiated tissues.

Malignant GCTs may also have elements that resemble extra-embryonic membranes (endodermal sinus tumor (EST)/yolk sac tumor) or extraembryonic trophoblastic/placental tissue (choriocarcinoma). Histologically, features of EST/yolk sac tumor include tubular and papillary carcinoma with reticulated areas, hyaline bodies that contain α-fetoprotein (AFP), and characteristic Schiller–Duval bodies. Overall, EST is the most common malignant childhood GCT. Histologic features of choriocarcinoma include the finding of cytotrophoblasts and syncytiotrophoblasts arranged in a papillary pattern with marked vascularity and hemorrhage. Choriocarcinoma can arise within the placenta (gestational) or in extraplacental tissues, usually the mediastinum or gonad (non-gestational) of an adolescent, or by transplacental spread in a newborn. Finally, embryonal carcinoma is a GCT composed of multipotential cells capable of differentiating into embryonic or extra-embryonic tumors. These tumors are typically poorly differentiated or anaplastic with extensive necrosis. Like choriocarcinomas, embryonal carcinomas are rare but highly malignant and have a worse prognosis than ESTs.

Staging

The Pediatric Oncology Group/Children's Cancer Group (POG/CCG) staging system for malignant extragonadal GCTs is outlined in Table 62.2. Overall, survival for children with extragonadal GCTs is generally good, with the probability of survival being 90% for children with stage I or II disease and 75% for children with stage III or IV disease. Two serum tumor markers, alpha fetoprotein (AFP) and human chorionic gonadotropin (HCG), are important in the management of GCTs in children. AFP, an important secreted protein in the human fetus, is produced by the embryonic liver, yolk sac, and gastrointestinal tract. It is a very sensitive marker for the presence of EST, and its detection in the serum can be useful when determining if a small malignant component of EST is likely to be part of a predominantly benign-appearing teratoma. The presence of AFP in the serum can also be an early signal for tumor recurrence. Normally, the expression of AFP is fairly high early in the neonatal period and drops to normal, lower levels by 9 months of age.[5] This ontogeny of expression needs to be considered when evaluating AFP levels in infants with GCTs. In addition, benign and malignant conditions of the liver also may be associated with an increased serum AFP level. Human chorionic gonadotropin is secreted by syncytiotrophoblasts and, therefore, is a sensitive marker for choriocarcinoma.

Table 62.2. CCG-POG staging system for malignant extragonadal germ-cell tumors

Stage I	Complete resection at any site; coccygectomy for sacrococcygeal site; negative tumor margins; tumor markers either normal or showing evidence of malignancy.
Stage II	Microscopic residual disease; lymph nodes normal; tumor markers either normal or showing evidence of malignancy.
Stage III	Gross residual disease or biopsy only; retroperitoneal nodes either normal or showing evidence of malignancy; tumor markers normal or showing evidence of malignancy.
Stage IV	Distant metastases, including to the liver.

Treatment

Surgical management

Surgical resection is crucial to the management of most extragonadal GCTs. Sacrococcygeal tumors, the most common extragonadal GCT, usually present at birth as large, external masses. They can even be diagnosed early in gestation (<30 weeks) by prenatal ultrasound, and are often associated with polyhydramnios, larger size, fetal hydrops, and higher perinatal mortality. Planned Cesarean section for tumors >5 cm is currently recommended.[6] For SCTs detected at birth, operative intervention should be undertaken early in the newborn period. Presacral tumors that present later in infancy, often with a greater intra-abdominal component, and those tumors noted at birth but not removed carry a higher risk of malignancy.[4] In a 1998 CCG report of 126 children who had SCTs detected between 1972 and 1994, 32 SCTs (25%) were diagnosed by prenatal ultrasound, 79 (63%) at birth, and 15 (12%) later in infancy. Overall, the SCTs were malignant in 9% of the neonates and in 27% of the infants.[7]

Before large lesions are removed, the degree of pelvic extension should be determined by physical examination and ultrasound or CT scan. If needed, additional tests can include MRI with or without MR angiography. In a 1998 CCG report, operative resection of a SCT was performed in 124 patients; a sacral approach was used in 96 cases (77%) and a combined abdominosacral approach in 28 cases (23%).[7] The external portion of the mass is typically excised using a chevron or inverted "v"-type incision, and circumferential dissection around the capsule is performed. The sacrococcygeal junction is divided with the coccyx being included in the specimen, and the middle sacral vessels being ligated. After the mass has been separated from the rectum and the specimen removed, the levator ani muscles are attached to the presacral fascia with subsequent skin closure. In children with significant pelvic extension of the tumor, laparotomy may be required to mobilize the pelvic portion of the mass, obtain control of the distal aorta and divide the middle sacral artery. In patients with additional risk factors, including prematurity, preoperative rupture, high-output congestive heart failure, hydrops, coagulopathy, and bleeding within the mass, vascular control with the patient in the supine position or staged resection of the abdominal and sacral portion may be beneficial. Despite adverse preoperative factors in some patients, overall operative mortality is generally low.[8] In utero surgery for fetuses <30 weeks' gestational age with hydrops is currently under investigation.[9]

Benign SCTs should be resected completely with close patient follow-up. Similarly, most authors advocate a "watch and wait" approach after complete resection of stage I malignant tumors. In the 1998 CCG study, 2 of 6 stage I SCTs recurred after resection alone; but both were salvaged with additional surgery and cisplatin-based chemotherapy.[7] Similar acceptable results were seen in a recent British study that also used a "watch and wait" approach. All 22 patients in which tumor recurred as EST after surgery and observation, including eight initially treated for a benign teratoma, were cured with chemotherapy. For patients with stage II–IV SCT, platinum-based chemotherapy is required in addition to surgery. In patients with bulky, invasive, or metastatic tumors, an initial biopsy followed by neoadjuvant chemotherapy and delayed resection should be considered to decrease the risk of incomplete resection.

Patients with mediastinal GCTs frequently have large tumors that cause respiratory distress or chest pain. Complete resection remains the recommended treatment for most patients with benign mediastinal teratomas. Historically, prognosis has been very poor for malignant mediastinal GCTs. However, a recent POG/CCG trial showed improved survival after neoadjuvant or adjuvant chemotherapy combined with aggressive surgical resection.[10]

In patients with intracranial GCTs, combination therapy is typically required. Germinomas are the most common on histopathologic analysis, carry a more favorable prognosis, and are typically sensitive to chemotherapy and irradiation. Combined chemotherapy and radiotherapy or surgery with postoperative irradiation for germinoma are both associated with greater than 90% 5-year survival.[11] Mature and immature teratomas should be resected, with adjuvant therapy reserved for recurrences.[12] Intracranial non-germinomatous tumors have a worse prognosis.[12] Aggressive surgical resection in combination with platinum-based chemotherapy and craniospinal irradiation is the current recommendation for this rare subgroup of patients.[13]

Germ cell tumors at other sites are extremely rare. Tumors in the retroperitoneum can be very large, causing significant symptoms despite frequently being benign. Malignant retroperitoneal GCTs are often diffuse with bulky tumor extensions, and neoadjuvant chemotherapy is often required in these patients before tumor resection can be successfully performed.[14] Cervicofacial teratomas are typically benign and may be treated solely by surgery; chemotherapy is reserved for patients with residual tumor or recurrence. There are no reported malignancies in the few patients treated with resection of gastric teratomas. Vaginal GCTs are often malignant ESTs. In a recent Pediatric Intergroup Study, results with neoadjuvant chemotherapy and vagina-preserving surgery were excellent for these tumors that historically have had a poor prognosis.[15]

Chemotherapy

Chemotherapy is also a crucial component in the successful treatment of malignant GCTs. Before the development of modern chemotherapy, the survival rate for patients with malignant GCTs was very poor. Combination chemotherapy introduced by Einhorn *et al.* in the 1970s for testicular cancer, has significantly improved the treatment outcome of children with GCTs.[16] Several groups have reported improved survival using cisplatin-based therapy compared with historical controls. Schropp *et al.* noted that survival was improved from 11% with vincristine, actinomycin, and cyclophosphamide (VAC) before 1978 to 86% after the introduction of a chemotherapy regimen that includes cisplatin, etoposide, and bleomycin (PEB).[8] Davidoff *et al.* reported a similar improvement in survival for children who had ESTs and were treated with PEB after 1985.[17] Several recent studies in the United States and Europe have evaluated the effect of chemotherapy dose and regimen on toxicity, recurrence, and survival in patients with GCTs over the past 20 years. Recent protocols include the German Cooperative Protocols (MAKEI 83/86, 89, 96),[18–22] the United Kingdom Children's Cancer Study Group (UKCCSG GCII),[23–25] the French Society for Pediatric Oncology (TGM 85,90),[26] and the POG/CCG Intergroup Trials (POG 9049/CCG 8882, POG 9048/CCG 8891).[10,14,15,27,28] These studies demonstrate a significant survival benefit in patients with malignant GCTs who were treated with platinum-based chemotherapy. In the most recent Pediatric Intergroup Trial, which included 74 patients with malignant SCTs, all patients with extragonadal malignant GCTs were considered "high-risk" and treated with PEB. Despite the fact that 44 patients (59%) had evidence of metastatic disease at diagnosis, their overall probability of 4-year survival (90%) and event-free survival (EFS) (84%) were both excellent with combined modality therapy for malignant SCTs.[28]

Radiation therapy

In patients with extracranial malignant GCTs, radiation therapy is currently reserved for attempts at salvage in cases with recurrent tumors that cannot be completely resected. Radiation therapy is commonly used, however, in the treatment of intracranial GCTs. Intracranial germinomas are particularly sensitive to radiation therapy although craniospinal irradiation is still frequently used in the treatment of non-germinomatous intracranial malignant GCTs as well.

Outcomes

When considering treatment plans and assessing outcomes for pediatric patients with GCTs, the different sites must be considered separately because the behavior of GCTs in the different sites varies greatly. For example, a recent analysis from the UKCCSG demonstrated a difference in 5-year survival by site in patients with malignant GCTs: testis (>95%), ovary (92.3%), vagina/uterus (>95%), sacrococcyx (87.6%), mediastinum (83.1%), and other sites (87.5%).[25] This can be somewhat problematic, however, because of the rarity of GCTs; the relatively small number of patients with tumors at each site has made statistical analyses difficult. Fortunately, a large, multicenter POG/CCG trial of patients with malignant GCTs has provided several recent analyses of tumors by site. The following discussion focuses primarily on SCTs because they account for the vast majority of extragonadal GCTs. Pertinent evidence-based data regarding tumors at other sites are also provided.

Sacrococcygeal tumors

Preoperative prognostic factors

Several studies have evaluated sex, age, AFP level, and tumor extent as preoperative risk factors for children with SCTs. In 1974, Altman *et al.* reviewed over 400 cases of neonates and infants with SCT; the rate of malignancy was higher with older age at diagnosis (7% of girls and 10% of boys younger than 2 months had malignant SCTs; and 48% of girls and 67% of boys older than 2 months had malignant SCTs) and in lesions with a smaller external component.[4] In a 1998 CCG study, SCTs were malignant in 9% of neonates and 27% of older infants.[7] Of the 15 patients diagnosed in infancy, six had a sacral mass at birth that was not immediately removed, resulting in an average delay in diagnosis of 11 months; two of these six (33%) were malignant. In the POG/CCG trial evaluating patients treated between 1990 and 1996, 74 of 317 (24%) patients had malignant SCTs. Of these, 62 (84%) were girls. Using the Altman classification system, there were 0 type I, 2 type II (3%), 30 type III (40%), and 42 type IV (57%) malignant tumors. The median age at diagnosis of a malignant SCT was 21 months, and the median AFP level was 35 500 ng/ml. No difference in 4-year EFS was seen based on sex, age, AFP level, or stage including the presence of metastasis at diagnosis.[28] In the German Cooperative Protocols, between 1983 and 1995, of 76 patients with malignant SCT, 78% were girls, and median age at diagnosis was 17 months. No difference in 5-year relapse-free survival was seen based on tumor size, local stage/invasion, AFP level, or presence of metastasis at diagnosis. Overall, 5-year survival in patients who received surgery and cisplatin-based chemotherapy was 81% in this study.[18]

In two recent European studies, risk factors were evaluated in patients with malignant GCTs by combining data at all tumor sites. In the UKCCSG GC II trial, 192 patients with malignant GCTs were evaluated between 1989 and 1997, including 37 patients with SCTs. In this analysis, an AFP level higher than 10 000 ng/ml was the strongest prognostic factor; however, no subgroup analysis of AFP levels in patients with SCT was performed.[25] In the French studies (SFOP: TGM 85 and TGM 90), prognostic factors in 152 children treated between 1985 and 1994 with localized malignant GCTs, both gonadal and extragonadal, were analyzed in patients older than 1 year. In this analysis, an AFP level higher than 10 000 ng/ml, stage III disease, and extragonadal primary site were all correlated with a worse prognosis; however, again, no analysis of the subgroup with SCTs was performed.[26] Overall, most recent studies have found less prognostic significance for age, AFP level, and stage in patients with malignant SCTs than in Altman's

1974 report. This finding is most likely secondary to the excellent results currently seen with surgery and platinum-based chemotherapy.

Importance of complete resection

Several studies highlight the importance of complete surgical resection of SCTs, including resection of the coccyx. In 1951, Gross *et al.* noted a 38% recurrence rate of SCTs resected without coccygectomy and a 0% recurrence rate when coccygectomy had been performed.[29] In the German Cooperative Protocols, including patients with benign and malignant SCTs, tumors recurred in 12% of patients with complete tumor resection and in 57% of patients with incomplete resection.[30] A difference in survival rate was also seen with incomplete resection in patients with malignant SCT. Five-year EFS was 92% in patients when resected margins were negative on histopathologic analysis, 69% in patients with microscopic residual disease, and 38% in patients with gross residual tumor.[20] In the POG/CCG analysis of patients with malignant SCTs, 4-year EFS was improved in patients when resection was complete (90%) compared with incomplete or partial resection (77%). However, this finding was not statistically significant, likely due to the effectiveness of adjuvant cisplatin-based chemotherapy.[28]

Tumor histology

Several recent studies have evaluated the relationship between tumor histology and tumor recurrence in survival of patients with SCTs. In most studies, 10% to 25% of specimens contain malignant foci. In the CCG study, SCTs from 124 patients were resected between 1972 and 1994; 69% of tumors were mature teratomas, 20% were immature teratomas, and 11% were ESTs.[7] Similar results were seen in the St. Jude Children's Research 16 Hospital experience, where of 73 (22%) SCTs resected between 1950 and 1990 were malignant.[8] In the German Cooperative Protocols, 76 of 210 SCTs were malignant (36%).[18] The primary malignant subtypes found in SCT specimens are EST and embryonal carcinoma. Interestingly, some regional differences in pathology may exist. In a recent POG/CCG trial of 74 patients with malignant SCTs, 65% of specimens were pure EST, and 35% were embryonal carcinomas.[28] In contrast, in the UKCCSG GC II trial of 37 patients with malignant SCT, 62% of specimens were teratomas with malignant foci and only 38% were pure EST.[25] In most studies, overall 5-year survival is higher than 95% in patients with benign SCT, either mature or immature teratoma, and between 80% and 90% in patients with malignant SCT.[7,27] The impact of malignant histologic subtype on prognosis is unclear because of small sample sizes.

Influence of chemotherapy regimen

Overall survival in patients with GCTs has improved significantly over the last 20 years because of the use of platinum-based chemotherapy.[8,17] Several studies have evaluated the influence of chemotherapy dose and regimen on recurrence and survival in patients treated for malignant GCTs. Because cisplatin has significant side effects including ototoxicity and nephrotoxicity, the optimal dose and the option of substitution with carboplatin are currently being evaluated. A recent POG/CCG trial evaluated the effect of cisplatin dose on patients with malignant GCTs. Patients were randomized to either standard or high-dose cisplatin treatment. Four-year EFS tended to improve in patients with SCTs who received high-dose PEB (89%) compared with those who received standard PEB (78%), but this finding was not statistically significant.[28]

In the UK and France, the substitution of carboplatin has recently been evaluated. Mann *et al.* evaluated carboplatin, etoposide, and bleomycin (JEB) for the treatment of 46 patients with malignant extragonadal GCTs between 1989 and 1995, including 28 patients with SCTs and 8 with mediastinal teratomas (UKCCSG GC II). In comparison with the previous regimen of VAC or PEB (UKCCSG GC I), 5-year survival was improved from 63% to 95% with carboplatin. Furthermore, side effects were significantly decreased. In the UKCCSG GC I trial, renal impairment occurred in 20% and deafness in 37% of patients treated with cisplatin compared with no renal impairment and deafness in only 9% of patients treated with carboplatin in the UKCCSG GC II trial. A different result was seen when carboplatin was used in a French study in which Baranzelli *et al.* demonstrated a significant decrease in efficacy with carboplatin.[26] A decrease in complete response (CR) for first-line treatment from 90% with cisplatin (TGM 85) to 58% with carboplatin (TGM 90) was seen. However, when cisplatin was used as salvage therapy in TGM 90, overall survival was similar between protocols. In the UKCCSG report, the poorer results using carboplatin in the French study were attributed to the lower dose used (400 mg/m^2 in TGM 90 compared with 600 mg/m^2 in the UKCCSG GCII protocol). In the UKCCSG report, the JEB regimen is recommended for initial therapy of malignant GCTs, and more toxic regimens are reserved for patients with recurrent tumors.[24] In a more recent update, including an analysis of survival by site, the probability of 5-year survival in patients treated with this regimen was 87.6% for SCTs and 83.1% for mediastinal GCTs, with an overall survival of 90.9% for all 137 patients (Table 62.3).[25]

Timing of surgery

In patients with bulky or invasive tumors, an important consideration is the timing of chemotherapy and

Table 62.3. Survival for children with malignant sacrococcygeal teratomas

Author (Ref No.)	Number of patients (dates)	Age (mean)	Female	Metastases	Chemotherapy regimen	Neoadjuvant chemotherapy	Follow-up (mean)	Survival
Schropp[38]	9 (1952–1977)	16 mo	62%	78%	VAC	0%	>15 yr	**11%**
Schropp[38]	7 (1978–1992)	16 mo	62%	29%	PB+	0%	54 mo	**86%**
Rescorla[37]	18 (1972–1994)	4 mo	75%	43%	PEB+	0%	91 mo	**89%**
Baranzelli[26]	21 (1985–1994)	NA	72%	0%	PEB JEB	NA	36 mo	**86%**
Gobel[20]	66 (1983–1995)	17 mo	79%	45%	PEB	47%	77 mo	**81%**
Mann[24]	37 (1989–1997)	>12 mo	NA	46%	JEB	23%	53 mo	**88%**
Rescorla[28]	74 (1990–1996)	21 mo	59%	59%	PEB	61%	46 mo	**90%**

NA – Not available.

surgical resection. Gobel *et al.* evaluated the treatment of 66 patients with malignant SCTs using cisplatin chemotherapy and surgery.[20] In children with large tumors or metastatic disease, tumor resection was delayed until after three to four cycles of chemotherapy. In this non-randomized study, resection was delayed in 31 of 66 patients who had predominantly large, invasive tumors. Despite adverse preoperative features, a higher proportion of microscopically complete tumor resections was obtained when resection was delayed (64%) than when resection was performed initially (14%). Although 61% of patients in the delayed surgery group and 31% in the initial resection group had distant metastasis at presentation, 5-year EFS was not statistically different between the two groups (80% delayed vs. 71% primary). Gobel *et al.* suggest that primary resection is appropriate only for patients with small malignant GCTs with no signs of infiltration on radiographs. Side effects from cisplatin were significantly decreased in this trial compared with those reported in the UKCCSG GC I. Grade III/IV renal insufficiency was seen in only 3% of chemotherapy cycles, and hearing loss in only 6% of patients. In the most recent POG/CCG trial of 74 patients with malignant SCT, all patients with extragonadal malignant GCTs were considered "high-risk" and treated with cisplatin-based chemotherapy. In the POG 9049/CCG 8882 trial, resection in patients with lesions involving the rectum, sacrum, or distant metastasis was often delayed until a response to neoadjuvant chemotherapy was seen.[28] Of the 71 patients who underwent resection of malignant SCT, 59% were treated with neoadjuvant therapy and delayed resection. Despite the fact that 63% of patients who underwent delayed resection presented with metastatic disease vs. 23% who underwent initial resection, 4-year EFS was similar between the 2 groups (83% delayed, 90% initial), highlighting the effectiveness of PEB chemotherapy.

Histology of recurrent tumors after resection of benign SCT

After complete resection, neonates with benign SCTs are managed by careful observation, including rectal examination and AFP level monitoring. Most recurrences occur within 2 years, so surveillance should be performed every 3 months for at least 3 years.[31] In the CCG study, disease recurred in 8.6% of patients following resection of a benign teratoma. Overall, disease recurred in 9 of 80 (11%) patients with mature teratoma and in 1 of 24 (4%) patients with immature teratoma. Of these, 78% recurred as EST and 22% as mature teratomas.[7] The importance of thorough histopathological examination is highlighted in a POG/CCG study in which 6 malignant recurrences occurred after resection of "benign" tumors. Retrospective review of the original samples revealed small foci of malignancy in four.[32] In a separate POG/CCG study evaluating patients who had immature GCT at multiple sites treated solely by complete resection, the importance of careful histological evaluation is again highlighted. Malignant foci were missed on histological examination of the original specimens from 23 of 73 (32%) patients. Overall, tumors recurred in 4 of 22 (18%) patients with immature SCTs within 7 months of resection, and in three of these, foci of malignant elements were found when the specimen was re-examined. Fortunately, three of the four patients with recurrent tumors were treated successfully with PEB.[27] Despite recurrence rates between 10% and 22% after resection of benign tumors, and between 10% and 33% for malignant tumors, overall survival is high because of the effectiveness of secondary platinum-based chemotherapy.[7,31]

Treatment of recurrent SCTs

In patients with stage II–IV SCTs, prognosis is significantly worse with recurrence after primary tumor resection. In these patients, neoadjuvant cisplatin-based chemotherapy followed by complete surgical resection offers the best chance of cure. In the French TGM 90 protocol in which carboplatin was given as primary therapy, tumors recurred in 12 patients after resection of malignant SCT; 7 of these patients survived with resection and intensification of therapy using cisplatin.[26] However, treatment of patients with tumors that recur following intensive initial cisplatin-based therapy may be more problematic. In the German Cooperative Protocols, 22 patients were treated for recurrent malignant SCT after surgery and PEB. In 77% of these patients, recurrence was local, and in 14% recurrence was both local and distant, highlighting the importance of complete resection during the initial surgery. In all patients who had tumor recurrence, AFP levels were increased. Median time to recurrence after primary treatment ended was 5.5 months (range 0 to 21 months). In 12 patients (55%), a second complete remission followed preoperative cisplatin-based chemotherapy and resection. In 5 of these 12, tumors recurred a second time, and two patients were cured with another resection. In this study, the most important therapy-related prognostic factor was the completeness of recurrent tumor resection. After treatment of initial recurrence, stable remission was achieved in 71% of patients with complete resection of local recurrence and in only 7% of patients in whom resection was incomplete. Overall, ten patients (45%) survived disease free at 5 years. Gobel *et al.* recommend aggressive therapy for local recurrence of SCTs including preoperative chemotherapy and complete resection. In their analysis, high-dose chemotherapy was not beneficial unless local control was achieved. Furthermore, they recommend irradiation of the surgical site when the tumor is incompletely resected.[20] In an effort to improve local control in patients with recurrent or refractory GCT, a recent phase I/II study evaluating regional deep hyperthermia in 10 patients was performed. A complete response to combined regional deep hyperthermia and cisplatin-based chemotherapy was seen in 50% of patients.[33]

Functional outcomes

Several studies have evaluated functional sequelae after surgical resection of SCTs. Tumors with large presacral components may present later in infancy with lower extremity weakness, constipation, bladder outlet obstruction, and fecal or urinary incontinence, which may be permanent. Furthermore, surgical treatment may play a role in the pathogenesis of functional impairment, highlighting the importance of meticulous surgical technique to preserve pelvic nerves and the anorectal sphincter complex. Malone *et al.* reviewed the functional sequelae of SCT therapy in 27 patients with a mean follow-up of 5 years after resection. Functional impairment was seen in 41% of patients and included urinary and fecal incontinence (15%), chronic constipation (11%), urinary incontinence (7%), and lower extremity weakness (11%). Although fecal incontinence and constipation were managed conservatively in most patients, urinary incontinence often required operative intervention. Functional impairment was seen in 64% of patients with Altman type III and IV tumors and in only 25% of patients with type I and II.[34] Havranek *et al.* performed a similar retrospective review of 25 patients treated for SCT with a mean follow-up of 5.5 years. Fecal soiling was observed in 40% of patients and urinary incontinence in 16%.[35] In contrast to the data from Malone *et al.*, no correlation was seen between functional outcome and tumor histology or Altman type. Boemers *et al.* performed urodynamic studies in 11 patients with a mean follow-up of 5 years. In this small series, abnormal findings including neurogenic bladder–sphincter dysfunction were seen in 82% of patients. Although surgical trauma contributed to impairment in some of these patients, disruption of pelvic floor musculature and tethering of the spinal cord from large presacral tumors also played a role in the functional impairment.[36] Reinberg *et al.* reviewed urologic complications in 29 children treated for SCTs with a mean follow-up of 6.5 years. Urologic complications, including vesicoureteral reflux and neurogenic bladder, were seen in 28% of patients but were not associated with malignancy or recurrence. The incidence of complications was highest with presacral disease (81% of patients with type IV tumors compared with 10% of patients with type I).[37] Rintala *et al.* reviewed long-term (30-year) anorectal function in a case-control study of 26 adults who had been treated for benign SCT in infancy. Fecal continence was reported as good in 88% of patients; however, only 27% had normal bowel habits. No correlation between Altman type and severity of fecal incontinence was seen. In addition, 19% had urinary incontinence. Overall, a significant number of patients had a diminished quality of life as adults from functional sequelae of SCTs.[38] These studies again highlight the importance of meticulous surgical technique and the need for long-term follow-up, including physiological evaluation of anorectal and urinary continence mechanisms in patients treated for SCTs (Table 62.4).

Mediastinal tumors

Preoperative prognostic factors

In a recent POG/CCG trial, sex, age at presentation, and stage were all important prognostic factors in patients with mediastinal GCTs. All tumor-related deaths occurred in older boys with stage III/IV disease.[10] The results of

Table 62.4. Long-term bowel and bladder functional outcomes in patients treated for sacrococcygeal teratoma

Author (Ref No.)	Number of patients	Mean follow-up (years)	Abnormal bowel function	Abnormal bladder function	Association with Altman type
Malone[34]	27	5	26%	22%	Yes
Hvarnek[35]	25	5.5	40%	16%	No
Boemers[36]	11	5	45%	82%	Yes
Reinberg[37]	29	6.5	NA	28%	Yes
Rintala[38]	26	30	73%	38%	No

NA – Not available.

histologic analysis suggested that tumor histology was also an important prognostic factor. In this study, EST was the only malignant element found in girls and boys younger than 5 years. In contrast, mixed malignant GCTs (60%), ESTs (20%), germinomas (16%), and choriocarcinomas (12%) were all seen in older boys, the group with the poorest outcome. The importance of extensive sampling at the time of tumor biopsy and careful pathologic evaluation was highlighted; most tumors (61%) were heterogeneous and contained benign elements.[10] The importance of age at diagnosis as a prognostic factor has also been demonstrated in other studies. In a review of 15 pediatric patients with mediastinal GCTs, all patients with malignant tumors were older than 12 years, while all neonates had immature teratomas.[39] In several other studies in which both pediatric and adult patients with mediastinal GCTs were included, histopathologic analysis provided important prognostic information. In a review of a 30-year experience, Dulmet *et al.* demonstrated the best outcomes are in patients with mature teratoma and in patients younger than 15 years with immature teratoma. Also, although prognosis was worse for mediastinal germinomas than for their testicular counterparts, 5-year survival was 81% in patients with seminomas and 57% in patients with malignant non-seminomatous GCTs.[40]

Timing of surgical resection

In a recent non-randomized POG/CCG trial, initial resection and chemotherapy (PEB) for malignant mediastinal GCTs was compared with neoadjuvant chemotherapy followed by resection. In 14 patients (39%), tumors were amenable to initial resection.[10] The tumor capsule was violated in 79% of these patients. In 18 patients, resection was delayed until at least four cycles of chemotherapy had been completed. In six patients, the tumor remained stable or increased in size, while in the remaining 12 patients, the tumor decreased in size. The tumor capsule was violated in only four (22%) of these patients. In this study, 26 of 36 patients survived with a 4-year overall survival of 71%. All five deaths were in boys older than 15 years with stage III/IV tumors. The authors concluded that neoadjuvant chemotherapy in patients with large tumors compromising the airway or with vascular invasion is a valuable treatment option. Furthermore, in these heterogeneous tumors, failure of the mass to resolve is common and should not preclude aggressive attempts at surgical resection. A non-random association of mediastinal GCTs with hematological malignancies was seen in this study. Three patients (8%) died of a second malignancy within 6 months of diagnosis, one patient with erythrophagocytic syndrome, and two with acute myelogenous leukemia.

Other sites

Preoperative prognostic factors

For intracranial GCTs, histopathologic examination is the most important predictor of outcome. Germinomas and benign teratomas have a much better prognosis than non-germinomatous tumors in the brain.[41] In a recent study evaluating 135 pediatric and adult patients with intracranial GCTs, the 5-year survival rate was 86% for patients with mature teratomas, 80% for germinomas, 67% for immature teratomas, and less than 40% for malignant non-seminomatous GCTs. Germ cell tumors at other sites are extremely rare; thus little data are available for evidence-based recommendations. Vaginal tumors are typically malignant and present as ESTs. These can usually be managed successfully without radical surgery. Retroperitoneal and cervicofacial GCTs are typically benign. There are no reported malignancies in gastric teratomas.

Timing of surgery

The recommended treatment for malignant GCTs at rare sites is similar to that for malignant SCTs. A combination of platinum-based chemotherapy and surgical resection provides the best outcome. In patients with large or invasive tumors, neoadjuvant chemotherapy may improve resectability. In the patients with malignant retroperitoneal

GCTs in the POG 9049/COG 8882 trial, results were excellent with a combination of PEB chemotherapy and surgery. Despite 68% of patients presenting with stage IV tumors, primary resection was performed in 20% of patients and delayed resection was performed after chemotherapy in 52%. An additional 16% of patients were cured with chemotherapy alone. Overall, probability of 6-year EFS was 83%, and 6-year survival was 88% in this group that historically has had poor outcomes.[14] Thirteen patients in the POG/CCG were treated for malignant GCT of the genital region. A complete response was seen in two patients treated with initial resection and in eight of nine (89%) treated with neoadjuvant therapy and resection. In addition, two patients were cured with chemotherapy alone. Tumors recurred in two patients, who both were cured with additional therapy. The 4-year EFS in the patients studied was 76% and 4-year survival was 92%, a significant improvement from previous studies.[15]

Final recommendations

For mature and immature SCTs, complete tumor resection and observation are recommended. Close patient follow-up for at least 3 years is mandatory, because 10% to 20% of benign tumors recur. For stage I malignant SCT, complete resection with close follow-up may also be appropriate. About 33% of malignant stage I SCTs recur, and most patients are adequately treated with re-resection and platinum-based chemotherapy. Patients with stage II–IV malignant SCT may be treated with primary resection if tumors are small and adequate margins can be obtained. Patients with bulky or invasive tumors or patients who have distant metastasis at the time of diagnosis may benefit from neoadjuvant platinum-based chemotherapy and delayed resection. Patients with recurrent malignant SCTs should be treated aggressively with neoadjuvant PEB and complete resection. Radiation therapy may be beneficial for incompletely resected tumors. Regional deep hyperthermia for recurrent or poorly responsive tumors is currently under investigation. Long-term follow-up, including physiological evaluation of anorectal and urinary continence is necessary.

Extragonadal GCTs at other sites are rare. Patients with malignant retroperitoneal and genital GCTs frequently require neoadjuvant chemotherapy followed by surgery. Patients with malignant mediastinal GCTs should be treated with neoadjuvant or adjuvant chemotherapy and complete resection. Patients with mature mediastinal teratomas may be cured solely by tumor resection. Surgical resection in combination with platinum-based chemotherapy and craniospinal irradiation is the current recommendation for patients with malignant intracranial GCTs. Overall survival for patients with malignant extragonadal GCTs has improved significantly over the past two decades with aggressive tumor resection and platinum-based chemotherapy.

REFERENCES

1. Young, J. L., Jr., Ries, L. G., Silverberg, E., Horm, J. W., & Miller, R. W. Cancer incidence, survival, and mortality for children younger than age 15 years. *Cancer* 1986; **58**(2)Suppl.:598–602.
2. Witschi, E. Migration of the germ cells of human embryos from the yolk sac to the primitive gonadal fold. *Contrib. Embryol.* 1948; **32**(69).
3. Strohmeyer, T., Reese, D., Press, M., Ackermann, R., Hartmann, M., & Slamon, D. Expression of the c-kit proto-oncogene and its ligand stem cell factor (SCF) in normal and malignant human testicular tissue. *J. Urol.* 1995; **153**(2):511–515.
4. Altman, R. P., Randolph, J. G., & Lilly, J. R. Sacrococcygeal teratoma: American Academy of Pediatrics Surgical Section Survey-1973. *J. Pediatr. Surg.* 1974; **9**(3):389–398.
5. Wu, J. T., Book, L., & Sudar, K. Serum alpha fetoprotein (AFP) levels in normal infants. *Pediatr. Res.* 1981; **15**(1):50–52.
6. Flake, A. W., Harrison, M. R., Adzick, N. S., Laberge, J. M., & Warsof, S. L. Fetal sacrococcygeal teratoma. *J. Pediatr. Surg.* 1986; **21**(7):563–566.
7. Rescorla, F. J., Sawin, R. S., Coran, A. G., Dillon, P. W., & Azizkhan, R. G. Long-term outcome for infants and children with sacrococcygeal teratoma: a report from the Childrens Cancer Group. *J. Pediatr. Surg.* 1998; **33**(2):171–176.
8. Schropp, K. P., Lobe, T. E., Rao, B. *et al.* Sacrococcygeal teratoma: the experience of four decades. *J. Pediatr. Surg.* 1992; **27**(8):1075–1078.
9. Kamata, S., Imura, K., Kubota, A. *et al.* Operative management for sacrococcygeal teratoma diagnosed in utero. *J. Pediatr. Surg.* 2001; **36**(4):545–548.
10. Billmire, D., Vinocur, C., Rescorla, F. *et al.* Malignant mediastinal germ cell tumors: an intergroup study. *J. Pediatr. Surg.* 2001; **36**(1):18–24.
11. Cho, B. K., Wang, K. C., Nam, D. H. *et al.* Pineal tumors: experience with 48 cases over 10 years. *Childs Nerv. Syst.* 1998; **14**(1–2):53–58.
12. Schild, S. E., Scheithauer, B. W., Haddock, M. G. *et al.* Histologically confirmed pineal tumors and other germ cell tumors of the brain. *Cancer* 1996; **78**(12):2564–2571.
13. Ogawa, K. Toita, T., Nakamura, K. *et al.* Treatment and prognosis of patients with intracranial nongerminomatous malignant germ cell tumors: a multiinstitutional retrospective analysis of 41 patients. *Cancer* 2003; **98**(2):369–376.
14. Billmire, D., Vinocur, C., Rescorla, F. *et al.* Malignant retroperitoneal and abdominal germ cell tumors: an intergroup study. *J. Pediatr. Surg.* 2003; **38**(3):315–318.

15. Rescorla, F., Billmire, D., Vinocur, C. *et al.* The effect of neoadjuvant chemotherapy and surgery in children with malignant germ cell tumors of the genital region: a pediatric intergroup trial. *J. Pediatr. Surg.* 2003; **38**(6):910–912.
16. Einhorn, L. H. & Donohue, J. *Cis*-diamminedichloroplatinum, vinblastine, and bleomycin combination chemotherapy in disseminated testicular cancer. *Ann. Intern. Med.* 1977; **87**(3):293–298.
17. Davidoff, A. M., Hebra, A., Bunin, N., Shochat, S. J., & Schnaufer, L. Endodermal sinus tumor in children. *J. Pediatr. Surg.* 1996; **31**(8):1075–1078.
18. Calaminus, G., Schneider, D. T., Bokkerink, J. P. *et al.* Prognostic value of tumor size, metastases, extension into bone, and increased tumor marker in children with malignant sacrococcygeal germ cell tumors: a prospective evaluation of 71 patients treated in the German cooperative protocols Maligne Keimzelltumoren (MAKEI) 83/86 and MAKEI 89. *J. Clin. Oncol.* 2003; **21**(5):781–786.
19. Gobel, U., Schneider, D. T., Calaminus, G., Haas, R. J., Schmidt, P., & Harms, D. Germ-cell tumors in childhood and adolescence. GPOH MAKEI and the MAHO study groups. *Ann. Oncol.* 2000; **11**(3):263–271.
20. Gobel, U., Schneider, D. T., Calaminus, G. *et al.* Multimodal treatment of malignant sacrococcygeal germ cell tumors: a prospective analysis of 66 patients of the German cooperative protocols MAKEI 83/86 and 89. *J. Clin. Oncol.* 2001; **19**(7):1943–1950.
21. Schneider, D. T., Calaminus, G., Koch, S. *et al.* Epidemiologic analysis of 1,442 children and adolescents registered in the German germ cell tumor protocols. *Pediatr. Blood Cancer* 2004; **42**(2):169–175.
22. Schneider, D. T., Wessalowski, R., Calaminus, G. *et al.* Treatment of recurrent malignant sacrococcygeal germ cell tumors: analysis of 22 patients registered in the German protocols MAKEI 83/86, 89, and 96. *J. Clin. Oncol.* 2001; **19**(7):1951–1960.
23. Huddart, S. N., Mann, J. R., Robinson, K. *et al.* Sacrococcygeal teratomas: the UK Children's Cancer Study Group's experience. I. Neonatal. *Pediatr. Surg. Int.* 2003; **19**(1–2):47–51.
24. Mann, J. R., Raafat, F., Robinson, K. *et al.* UKCCSG's germ cell tumour (GCT) studies: improving outcome for children with malignant extracranial non-gonadal tumours – carboplatin, etoposide, and bleomycin are effective and less toxic than previous regimens. United Kingdom Children's Cancer Study Group. *Med. Pediatr. Oncol.* 1998; **30**(4):217–227.
25. Mann, J. R., Raafat, F., Robinson, K. *et al.* The United Kingdom Children's Cancer Study Group's second germ cell tumor study: carboplatin, etoposide, and bleomycin are effective treatment for children with malignant extracranial germ cell tumors, with acceptable toxicity. *J. Clin. Oncol.* 2000; **18**(22):3809–3818.
26. Baranzelli, M. C., Kramar, A., Bouffet, E. *et al.* Prognostic factors in children with localized malignant nonseminomatous germ cell tumors. *J. Clin. Oncol.* 1999; **17**(4):1212.
27. Marina, N. M., Cushing, B., Giller, R. *et al.* Complete surgical excision is effective treatment for children with immature teratomas with or without malignant elements: a Pediatric Oncology Group/Children's Cancer Group Intergroup Study. *J. Clin. Oncol.* 1999; **17**(7):2137–2143.
28. Rescorla, F., Billmire, D., Stolar, C. *et al.* The effect of cisplatin dose and surgical resection in children with malignant germ cell tumors at the sacrococcygeal region: a pediatric intergroup trial (POG 9049/CCG 8882). *J. Pediatr. Surg.* 2001; **36**(1):12–17.
29. Gross, R. W., Clatworthy, H. W., Jr., & Meeker, I. A., Jr. Sacrococcygeal teratomas in infants and children; a report of 40 cases. *Surg. Gynecol. Obstet.* 1951; **92**(3):341–354.
30. Gobel, U., Calaminus, G., Engert, J. *et al.* Teratomas in infancy and childhood. *Med. Pediatr. Oncol.* 1998; **31**(1):8–15.
31. Bilik, R., Shandling, B., Pope, M., Thorner, P., Weitzman, S., & Ein, S. H. Malignant benign neonatal sacrococcygeal teratoma. *J. Pediatr. Surg.* 1993; **28**(9):1158–1160.
32. Hawkins, E., Issacs, H., Cushing, B., & Rogers, P. Occult malignancy in neonatal sacrococcygeal teratomas. A report from a Combined Pediatric Oncology Group and Children's Cancer Group study. *Am. J. Pediatr. Hematol. Oncol* 1993; **15**(4):406–409.
33. Wessalowski, R., Kruck, H., Pape, H., Kahn, T., Willers, R., & Gobel, U. Hyperthermia for the treatment of patients with malignant germ cell tumors: a phase I/II study in ten children and adolescents with recurrent or refractory tumors. *Cancer* 1998; **82**(4):793–800.
34. Malone, P. S., Spitz, L., Kiely, E. M., Brereton, R. J., Duffy, P. G., & Ransley, P. G. The functional sequelae of sacrococcygeal teratoma. *J. Pediatr. Surg.* 1990; **25**(6):679–680.
35. Havranek, P., Hedlund, H., Rubenson, A. *et al.* Sacrococcygeal teratoma in Sweden between 1978 and 1989: long-term functional results. *J. Pediatr. Surg.* 1992; **27**(7):916–918.
36. Boemers, T. M., van Gool, J. D., de Jong, T. P., & Bax, K. M. Lower urinary tract dysfunction in children with benign sacrococcygeal teratoma. *J. Urol.* 1994; **151**(1):174–176.
37. Reinberg, Y., Long, R., Manivel, J. C., Resnick, J., Simonton, S., & Gonzalez, R. Urological aspects of sacrococcygeal teratoma in children. *J. Urol.* 1993; **150**(3):948–949.
38. Rintala, R., Lahdenne, P., Lindahl, H., Siimes, M., & Heikinheimo, M. Anorectal function in adults operated for a benign sacrococcygeal teratoma. *J. Pediatr. Surg.* 1993; **28**(9):1165–1167.
39. Lakhoo, K., Boyle, M., & Drake, D. P. Mediastinal teratomas: review of 15 pediatric cases. *J. Pediatr. Surg.* 1993; **28**(9):1161–1164.
40. Dulmet, E. M., Macchiarini, P., Suc, B., & Verley, J. M. Germ cell tumors of the mediastinum. A 30-year experience. *Cancer* 1993; **72**(6):1894–1901.
41. Matsutani, M., Sano, K., Takakura, K. *et al.* Primary intracranial germ cell tumors: a clinical analysis of 153 histologically verified cases. *J. Neurosurg.* 1997; **86**(3):446–455.

63

Hemangiomas and vascular malformations

Adam M. Vogel and Steven J. Fishman

Department of Surgery, Children's Hospital, Boston, MA, USA

Introduction

Vascular anomalies consist of a diverse group of blood vessel disorders that typically present in childhood. Historically, the field is clouded by a confusing web of outdated and inappropriate terms that cross-medical disciplines and permeate the literature. For example, a venous malformation is often improperly referred to as a "cavernous hemangioma," and "cystic hygroma" or "lymphangioma" is used to describe a lymphatic malformation. The suffix "oma", when applied to malformations, incorrectly implies a disorder of endothelial proliferation and may overwhelm patients with fears of malignancy. Furthermore, clinicians might be tempted to "treat" these lesions with potent anti-angiogenic medications such as systemic steroids or interferon. Since these venous and lymphatic malformations are congenital, they will not respond to anti-angiogenic therapy. Patients are then placed at unnecessary risk of significant complications and side effects from these potent medications.

This confusion among patients and physicians led the International Society for the Study of Vascular Anomalies to adopt a general, biologic classification scheme (Table 63.1) for vascular anomalies based on physical findings, natural history, and cellular kinetics.[1] In this system, vascular anomalies are described as either malformations or tumors.[2] Vascular tumors exhibit abnormal endothelial cell proliferation while malformations are products of abnormal embryonic vessel development.[3] This schema presents a useful framework for discussing the diagnosis and treatment of vascular anomalies. Although this standard system of nomenclature and classification exists, it is not consistently applied by physicians even in centers with an established vascular anomalies program.

Due to the rarity of these lesions and the long history of nosologic confusion surrounding the field, there is a paucity of well-designed trials investigating various diagnostic and therapeutic modalities. Local and systemic symptoms range from trivial to life-threatening and include disfigurement, pain, bleeding, obstruction, hematologic derangements, endocrine abnormalities, metabolic disorders, pulmonary thromboembolism, and death. Current medical practice is based primarily on anecdotal evidence, case reports, and small case series. Vascular tumor therapy, if necessary at all, focuses on anti-angiogenic pharmacotherapy while symptomatic control and interventional radiologic techniques are initially used to treat malformations. More invasive interventional radiologic procedures and surgical resection are reserved for lesions refractory to medical or less invasive management. Well-designed, prospective, multi-institutional protocols are required to advance the management of these complex anomalies.

Vascular tumors

Vascular tumors are anomalies of abnormal endothelial proliferation.[3] They are almost all histologically benign and follow predictable courses. However, they may be very aggressive in their clinical behavior and sometimes elicit systemic effects. Vascular tumors can be accurately diagnosed and classified based on clinical findings.[1] The overwhelming majority are true hemangiomas of infancy. Less common are congenital hemangioma, Kaposiform

Pediatric Surgery and Urology: Long-term Outcomes, Mark Stringer, Keith Oldham, Pierre Mouriquand.
Published by Cambridge University Press.

Table 63.1. Classification of vascular anomalies

Malformations
Capillary
Lymphatic
Venous
Arteriovenous
Complex combined
Tumors
Hemangioma
Congenital hemangioma
Kaposiform hemangioendothelioma
Tufted angioma
Miscellaneous

hemangioendothelioma, tufted angioma, and rare variants. Imaging studies play a vital role in clarifying and differentiating lesions. The pathogenesis of vascular tumors is rooted in angiogenesis and anti-angiogenic pharmacotherapy has proven to be extremely adept at treating these lesions.[3] Surgery and interventional techniques, therefore, are generally reserved as adjuncts to primary medical therapy.

Infantile hemangiomas

Background

Hemangiomas are the most common tumor of infancy and occur in 4 to 10% of white infants.[4] Hemangiomas are more common in premature infants, Caucasians, and women (3–5:1 female: male ratio).[3,5] Clinically, infantile hemangiomas generally present by 2 weeks of age, although 30 to 50% of cases have an initial sign present at birth consisting of a small pale spot or telangiectatic stain.[3] Sixty percent of lesions are located in the head and neck, 25% are found over the trunk, and 15% are found on the extremities.[1] They usually are solitary and located in the skin. Twenty percent of patients will have multiple cutaneous lesions. These patients have an increased chance of visceral organ (liver, gastrointestinal tract, lung, and brain) involvement. Patients with hemangiomatosis (multiple, small disseminated hemangiomas) should be screened for visceral involvement with ultrasound or magnetic resonance imaging when five or more lesions are present.[6] Tumors involving the superficial dermis present as red and raised (Fig. 63.1), while tumors in the lower dermis, subcutaneous tissue, or muscle may appear bluish with minimally raised skin. These deep hemangiomas may be confused clinically with lymphatic or venous malformations or other tumors. Overall, 90% of hemangiomas can be diagnosed clinically with history and physical examination.[1]

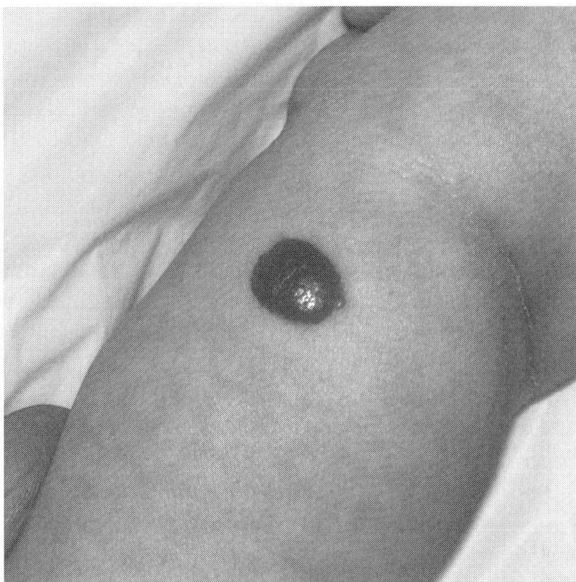

Fig. 63.1. Hemangioma of infancy. A well-circumscribed, elevated, red lesion typical of cutaneous hemangioma of infancy.

Visceral hemangiomas are rare but well defined. Hollow visceral hemangiomas may present with bleeding and symptomatic anemia. The liver is the most common site of visceral involvement. Lesion characteristics vary greatly from small to large and single to multiple; these factors influence the clinical presentation.[7] Large tumors present early in the first few months of life.[8] Single, large tumors are typically diagnosed antenatally and may be associated with a mild to moderate, self-resolving thrombocytopenia. These tumors are more likely rapidly involuting congenital hemangiomas, which are fully grown at birth and involute very rapidly. The thrombocytopenia is not to be confused with the Kasabach–Merritt phenomenon observed with Kaposiform hemangioendothelioma and tufted angioma. Small lesions found in patients with multiple cutaneous lesions may never become symptomatic.

More dangerous hepatic hemangiomas are large tumors with macrovascular shunts between feeding arteries and hepatic veins. These are the variety likely to cause high-output cardiac failure. They are 20% more likely to fail medical management and require transcatheter embolization or operative resection.[8,9] Massive hepatomegaly, causing abdominal compartment syndrome manifested by renal vein and inferior vena cava compression, and restrictive respiratory physiology are potential complications of very large multifocal lesions.[3,8] Hepatic hemangiomas can be visually differentiated from arteriovenous malformations, hepatoblastoma, and metastatic neuroblastoma by radiographic characteristics.[8,10] It is important to differentiate infantile hepatic hemangiomas from adult "cavernous hemangiomas." These lesions differ clinically, biologically, histologically, and radiographically.[3] Adult lesions are more similar to, and should be classified as, hepatic venous malformations.

Hemangiomas may be infrequently associated with other congenital anomalies. They are more common with large, midline lesions. Sternal non-union may be found with cervicothoracic hemangiomas.[11] Lumbosacral lesions may present along with spinal dysraphism such as meningocele or tethered cord.[12] Pelvic and perineal lesions may be associated with urogenital or anorectal anomalies.[13] Finally, craniofacial lesions may be associated with a variety of anomalies such as microphthalmia, cataracts, optic nerve hypoplasia, posterior fossa cystic malformations, hypoplasia or absence of the carotid or vertebral arteries, and malformation of the aortic arch (PHACES syndrome).[14]

Pathophysiology

Infantile hemangiomas have a distinctive life cycle consisting of proliferation (growth during the first year of life), involution (spontaneous, slow regression from one to seven years), and involuted (complete regression).[15] The proliferative phase is characterized by initial (6 to 8 months of age) rapid growth that plateaus by approximately 1 year of age. Involution occurs slowly over several years (one to seven years). Involuting hemangiomas exhibit a fading color and softening of the mass. There is gradual improvement with a return towards "normal" skin character by 10 to 12 years of age. In the involuted phase, 50% of patients have nearly normal skin. Patients with larger tumors may have lax or redundant skin, a yellowish discoloration, or scars in areas with prior ulceration.

The hemangioma life cycle is defined by specific molecular and histologic changes. The proliferative phase is characterized by an upregulation of pro-angiogenic molecules such as vascular endothelial growth factor (VEGF) and fibroblast growth factor (FGF).[15] Matrix metalloproteinases, proteins that assist in the breakdown of extracellular matrix, are up-regulated, facilitating endothelial migration and angiogenesis.[15] These markers can be found in the urine of patients with hemangiomas. Histological examination of the proliferative stage reveals plump, rapidly dividing endothelial cells forming a mass of sinusoidal vascular channels with large feeding arteries and draining veins.[15] Microvessel density increases as shown by mature endothelial cells that stain positively for CD-31, von Willibrand factor, and GLUT-1 (an erythrocyte glucose transporter expressed in infantile hemangioma endothelium).[16–18]

Involuting hemangiomas show down-regulation of pro-angiogenic markers and up-regulation of tissue inhibitors of matrix metalloproteinases.[5] This contributes to the overall suppression of angiogenesis and tumor regression. Histologically, endothelial cells flatten, the vascular channels dilate, and the mass is replaced by fibrofatty stroma with a lobular architecture.[16] The process is characterized by endothelial cell apoptosis. In involuted hemangiomas, the initial mass is replaced completely by fibrofatty tissue with tiny capillaries and mildly dilated draining vessels.

The mechanisms underlying the initiation of hemangioma growth and regression are unknown. As with all disease processes, there is likely a genetic component, although one has yet to be identified.

Imaging

Radiologically, hemangiomas display characteristics that assist in their diagnosis.[19–21] Duplex ultrasound of proliferative hemangiomas shows a dense soft tissue mass with decreased arterial resistance and increased venous flow consistent with fast-flow. MRI of proliferative hemangiomas demonstrates a lobulated mass of intermediate density with T1 spin-echo sequences, moderate hyperintensity of T2 spin-echo, and distinct borders. Flow voids representing fast-flow and vascular shunting can be seen in and around the tumor. Involuting phase studies show a decreased number of flow-voids and vascularity within a lobular and fatty mass. MRI is preferable to CT for diagnosis of hemangioma. Angiography demonstrates homogeneous and centripetal filling of the mass. Radionucleotide imaging with technetium Tc 99m-tagged red blood cells can be used to further locate hemangiomas.[22] Gastrointestinal lesions may require upper and/or lower endoscopy to appropriately delineate the extent of lesions.

Complications

Superficial ulceration, more common in rapidly growing and exophytic tumors, occurs in 5% of patients.[23] Bleeding and pain may also accompany lesions. Additionally, lesion location may compromise function (such as laryngeal hemangioma causing airway obstruction or large liver lesions causing high output congestive heart failure). Lesions involving the eye or eyelid can lead to visual impairment and deprivation amblyopia while lesions of the cornea can cause astigmatic amblyopias.[24] Cosmetic complications, particularly with facial lesions involving the ear, lip and nose can be particularly concerning to patients and their families.

Large hemangiomas can also be associated with hypothroidism.[25] Hemangiomas express type-3-idiothyronine deiodinase, an enzyme that inactivates blood thyroid hormone. A large lesion can alter the balance of the hypothalamic–pituitary–thyroid axis and lead to hypothyroidism. Untreated hypothyroidism in infancy can cause mental retardation. Therefore, patients with large hemangiomas should be screened for hypothyroidism with a measurement of thyroid stimulating hormone. Aggressive treatment in consultation with an endocrinologist should be initiated. The hypothyroidism will resolve as lesions involute.

Treatment and outcomes

Traditionally, most hemangiomas do not require specific treatment. Even the most rapidly growing, aggressive appearing cutaneous lesion will likely spontaneously regress and cause minimal non-cosmetic complications. Indications for treatment include a dangerous location, unusually large size or rapid growth, local complications (ulcerations), or an easily excisable lesion, the residual nature of which would likely require eventual excision. Diligent follow-up is required and serial photography is helpful in documenting how lesions progress over time.

Local wound care is useful for treating ulcerating hemangiomas.[26] Although hydrated petrolatum, viscous lidocaine, topical antibiotics, and hydrocolloid dressings are often effective in minimizing symptoms, surgical excision may be the most practical therapy. Eschars may be sharply debrided and treated with wet-to-dry dressing changes.

Pharmacotherapy targets the inherent angiogenic nature of hemangiomas. Corticosteroids inhibit angiogenesis through multiple mechanisms and are the first line agent of choice. Specifically, they inhibit production of pro-angiogenic molecules such as VEGF, bFGF, prostaglandins, and matrix metalloproteinases. Systemic corticosteroids (prednisone at 2 to 3 mg/kg/day) are effective in treating problematic hemangiomas.[27–29] Occasionally, higher doses may be required. In general, an 80–90% response rate is expected with steroid treatment. Improvement in the color and tension of the mass is generally seen within 10 days. A slow gradual taper is required (approximately every 4 weeks) to avoid rebound growth. Enlargement requires a return to the prior steroid dose with a more gradual taper.[29] Live vaccines are not administered during treatment. Treatment may be complicated by impaired growth and Cushingoid features. Children exhibit catch-up growth when treatment concludes. These complications resolve when the medications are tapered. Rates of infection, myopathy, and osteoporosis are not increased significantly, although they may occur if higher doses are required. Rarely, the presence of hypertension or hypertrophic cardiomyopathy requires discontinuation of the steroid and conversion to an alternate pharmacologic regimen.

Intralesional steroids may be used for local, symptomatic lesions, particularly in patients with facial lesions.[3,30,31] Multiple injections of triamcinolone at 3–5 mg/kg per injection in 6–8 week intervals have a success rate similar to systemic therapy.[3] Subcutaneous atrophy at the injection site is a temporary condition. Blindness following intralesional injection of periorbital hemangiomas has been reported and is thought to result from particle embolization of the retinal vessels through the feeding vessels.[32] Manual compression, therefore, is recommended around the periphery of the lesion during this procedure.

Recombinant interferon alfa 2a or 2b and vincristine are second line agents. These options are indicated only when steroid treatment is contraindicated, fails, or results in intolerable side effects or complications. Interferon is given once daily subcutaneously at a dose of 2–3 million units/m^2 for 3–12 months and works through anti-angiogenic mechanisms.[33–35] The overall success rate is excellent but the response is generally slower than with steroids.[33,36,37] No benefit has been shown for the simultaneous administration of steroids and interferon. Interferon treatment is more likely to be successful when urine angiogenic factors (particularly bFGF) are elevated. Minor complications include fevers during administration, mild transaminase elevation, neutropenia, and anemia. Neutropenia is secondary to demargination and not bone marrow suppression.[38] Spastic diplegia is the most severe complication of interferon therapy and occurs in 5–12% of infants treated.[38–40] The spasticity typically resolves if the drug is discontinued immediately. All children undergoing interferon treatment should be followed by a neurologist. Vincristine, a vinca alkaloid, is increasingly being used as a second line agent in a low dose, high frequency antiangiogenic regimen for patients who do not respond or experience complications from steroid treatment.[41–43] Vincristine may cause constipation and reversible peripheral neuropathy.

Lasers have limited application in the treatment of hemangiomas. In possibly the only prospective, randomized controlled study in the field of vascular anomalies, investigators found that, while treatment with pulsed dye lasers diminishes redness, there was an increase in skin atrophy and hypopigmentation.[44] The authors conclude that laser therapy may not be better than a wait-and-see approach. However, laser treatment may be effective in hastening pain relief in ulcerated lesions and in eradicating the telangiectasias associated with involuted hemangiomas.[30,45] The bare fiber Nd:YAG laser may be utilized intralesionally to debulk obstructing hemangiomas.

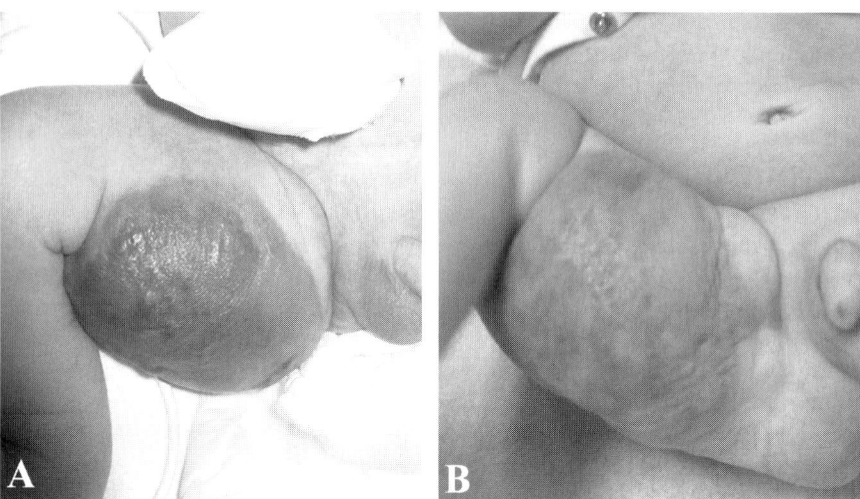

Fig. 63.2. Rapidly involuting congenital hemangioma (RICH). (a) A dome-like lesion typical of RICH in the immediate post-natal period and (b) during rapid involution.

The endoscopic continuous wave carbon dioxide laser has been used unilaterally to treat symptomatic, proliferating hemangiomas in the subglottic area. When combined as an adjunct with steroids, this therapeutic combination has nearly eliminated the need for tracheostomy.[46]

The indications for the surgical resection of infantile hemangiomas are variable. Well localized, bothersome tumors, particularly on the scalp, trunk, and extremities, can be excised with linear primary closure. Similarly, circular excision with purse-string closure minimizes scar and distortion of surrounding tissue.[47] Tumors causing obstructive visual symptoms that do not respond rapidly to medical management may also require excision. Similarly, focal lesions of the gastrointestinal tract may be excised using endoscopic band ligation or open enterectomy. Surgical resection may be contemplated in patients with large lesions that will likely leave lax and disfiguring skin; when the surgical scar would be identical whenever the operation is performed; when it is obvious that resection will occur at some point in the future; and when the scar is easily hidden.[3] Surgical resection of proliferating lesions should be undertaken only in these limited circumstances and with the realization that operations at this early stage may result in increased blood loss, transfusions, and death. In many cases, it is preferable to perform resection at the preschool age to avoid social stigmatization and the development of a poor body image. Involuted hemangiomas are often resected for cosmesis, to excise the residual, unsightly fibrofatty residuum and redundant skin. Excessive scarring may require the use of various plastic reconstructive techniques.

In extreme cases where surgical resection is contraindicated and medical pharmacotherapy is ineffective, angiographic embolization may be required. This treatment should be limited to life threatening lesions in infants with high output congestive heart failure. Arterial catheterization of infants carries significant risks and should only be performed by experienced personnel in specialized centers. Success depends on occluding the macrovascular shunts.

Though surgical resection and even liver transplantation have been utilized in the treatment of hepatic hemangiomas, these therapies should almost never be necessary.[48] It is critical to recognize the heterogeneous clinical manifestations of liver hemangiomas. Many will remain asymptomatic. Others will respond to pharmacotherapy and/or embolization of macrovascular shunts. Only patients with refractory diffuse lesions causing an abdominal compartment syndrome should be evaluated for transplantation.

Congenital hemangiomas

Congenital hemangiomas are hemangiomas that are fully developed at birth. These lesions typically do not exhibit post-natal growth. Rapidly involuting (RICH) and non-involuting (NICH) describe the clinical course of the two types of congenital hemangiomas. RICH typically involute by one year of age. Congenital hemangiomas appear as bulbous hemispherical lesions (Fig. 63.2). They may be dark purple with a pale halo of the skin around the base. Histologically, congenital hemangiomas differ from infantile

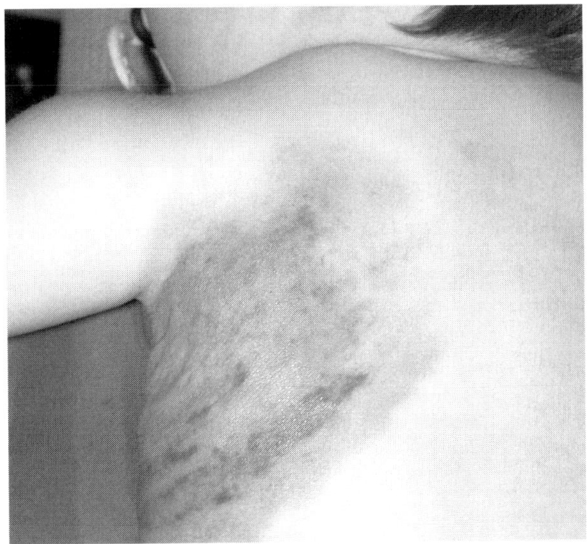

Fig. 63.3. Kaposiform hemangioendothelioma (KHE). An extensive, ecchymotic-appearing cutaneous lesion with ill-defined borders characteristic of KHE.

hemangiomas and likely have a different etiology.[49] For clinically ambiguous lesions, radiographic imaging including MRI and angiography may be required to differentiate congenital lesions from infantile hemangiomas or infantile fibrosarcoma.[50,51] In general, congenital hemangiomas require no treatment.

Kaposiform hemangioendothelioma, tufted angioma, and Kasabach–Merritt phenomenon

Kaposiform hemangioendothelioma (KHE) and tufted angioma (TA) are more aggressive and invasive vascular tumors than infantile hemangiomas. KHE and TA have overlapping clinical and pathological features and likely exist within the same spectrum. These tumors occur equally in males and females, may be diagnosed at birth, and are typically unifocal. TA presents as erythematous macules or plaques and histology shows small tufts of capillaries. Radiologically, TA is plaque-like, nodular, and diffusely enhancing. KHE is a more extensive tumor that presents with red-purple skin discoloration with diffuse ecchymosis (Fig. 63.3). Histopathology shows infiltrating sheets of slender endothelial cells consistent with blood vessel endothelium. MRI demonstrates an enhancing lesion with poorly defined margins that extend across tissue planes. These lesions commonly exhibit Kasabach–Merritt phenomenon with profound thrombocytopenia, petechiae, and bleeding.

Kasabach–Merritt phenomenon (KMP) was first used to describe severe thrombocytopenia, petechiae, and bleeding in association with a "giant hemangioma."[52] Unfortunately, this label is frequently misapplied to thrombocytopenia of any severity that accompanies any "hemangioma". The severe thrombocytopenia, characterized by a platelet count less than 10 000, is seen only with KHE and TA. Decreased fibrinogen levels and an elevated PT and PTT may also be seen. Platelet transfusions are not effective and should be used only with active bleeding. Heparin may stimulate tumor growth and worsen the thrombocytopenia. This phenomenon resolves with treatment of the underlying tumor. Mortality for KHE and TA with KMP is approximately 20%–30%. Treatment with systemic corticosteroids and interferon is effective in about 50% of patients.[3,53–60] Vincristine can also be used for refractory cases. Surgical resection and embolization are reserved for symptomatic tumors refractory to medical management. Most KHE lesions are far too extensive to contemplate resection. Lesions that respond to treatment have a good prognosis, though local musculoskeletal pain syndromes may occur at the site of residual lesions up to decades later.[62] Overall, these tumors proliferate into early childhood and exhibit incomplete involution characterized as a "dormant" vascular tumor.[63]

Vascular malformations

Malformations are dysmorphic lesions with normal endothelial cell turnover and are named for the clinical and histologic appearance of the abnormal channels. They are classified as either slow-flow (capillary malformation, venous malformation, lymphatic malformation) or fast-flow lesions (arteriovenous malformations). Complex combined malformations, typically named with an eponym, such as Klippel–Trenaunay syndrome (capillary-lymphatico-venous malformation) also exist and are often associated with soft tissue and skeletal abnormalities. The vast majority of vascular malformations are sporadic. However, certain hereditary malformations (i.e., HHT, hereditary telangiectasia or Osler–Weber–Rendu) disease hemorrhagic exist and may provide insight into the underlying molecular pathogenesis. Malformations may also present as part of a syndrome in association with other developmental defects.

Vascular endothelial differentiation occurs early in embryogenesis and may play a role in the development of malformations.[64,65] Ephrin signaling describes interactions between membrane bound ligands and receptor tyrosine kinases that appear to control the inherent properties of endothelial cells.[66] These ligands are imprinted and differ among arteries and veins. Specifically, arterial endothelial cells express ephrin-B2 while venous endothelial cells express ephrin-B4. Vascular dysmorphogenesis may be caused by abnormal vascular smooth muscle signaling. Vascular malformations likely result from a combination of defects in endothelial proliferation, apoptosis, cellular differentiation, maturation, and cell–cell interactions.

Diagnosis requires a comprehensive history and physical examination often supplemented with radiographic images. Malformations are congenital and are present at birth. However, lesions may not manifest until expansion during childhood or adulthood. They may be stimulated by puberty, pregnancy, or local trauma. While they may present in any anatomic location, they are fairly equally distributed between the head, trunk, and extremities. Visceral lesions are rare but well described.

Lesions grow in proportion with the child. They affect males and females equally. Treatment may involve cosmetic or laser therapy for cutaneous lesions, and combinations of intralesional sclerotherapy, embolization, and surgical resection for more extensive lesions. It can be very difficult and frustrating to treat vascular malformations because cure is rare and recurrence is common.

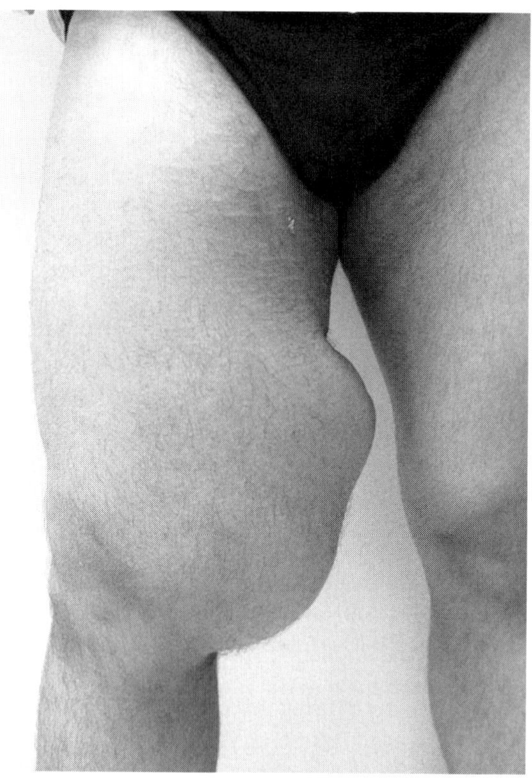

Fig. 63.4. Lymphatic malformation (LM). Right lower extremity LM.

Lymphatic malformations (see also Chapter 7)

Background

Lymphatic malformations (LM) are slow-flow lesions typically noticed at birth or early childhood and may be focal or diffuse. Occasionally they are diagnosed on prenatal imaging studies.[67] LM are sometimes associated with various congenital syndromes including Turner syndrome (45XO), Trisomies 18 and 21, Noonan and Roberts syndromes, and Milroy syndrome, an inherited form of lymphedema. Although typically found in the skin and soft tissues, LM can involve muscle, bone, and rarely internal viscera. Lymphedema is a variant of lymphatic malformation with extensive infiltration of the subcutaneous tissue. Underlying soft tissue and skeletal overgrowth, particularly bony overgrowth of the mandible and facial bones with cervicofacial malformations, can be seen. Antenatal diagnosis is becomming more common. Massive fetal cervicofacial lesions can lead to asphyxiation at delivery and a pre-emptive EXIT (ex-utero intrapartum treatment) with intubation or tracheostomy may be appropriate.[68]

The overlying skin may be normal for deep malformations or may contain vesicles when dermal or subcutaneous structures are involved (Fig. 63.4). Lymphatic malformations are classified as either microcystic, macrocystic, or combined. Histologically, these lesions are composed of vascular spaces filled with eosinophilic, protein-rich fluid.[3] Abnormally formed muscular elements of variable thickness form the channels. Recent evidence suggests that vascular endothelial growth factor receptor 3 (VEGFR3) plays a role in the development of LM.[69–71]

Imaging

Imaging studies can be helpful in confirming the diagnosis of lymphatic malformations.[72] Radiologically, ultrasound demonstrates large cysts in macrocystic lymphatic malformations. MRI with gadolinium contrast is the best means to diagnose lymphatic malformations. All lymphatic malformations are hyperintense on T2-weighted images from their high water content and exhibit fluid–fluid levels from protein and blood layering in macrocysts. With contrast, these lesions exhibit rim or septae enhancement. Contrast lymphangiography, although technically demanding, may be useful for delineating thoracic duct anomalies and chylous leaks.[73]

Complications

Complications of LM include bleeding, infection, and obstruction. External bleeding may be uncomfortable or lead to anemia. Intralesional bleeding and subsequent expansion may be spontaneous or secondary to trauma and can lead to acute or chronic pain. Infections, ranging from superficial cellulitis to systemic sepsis can cause profound morbidity.[74,75] Infections are very difficult to clear and may require prolonged intravenous antibiotic therapy. Poor dental hygiene and bacterial translocation from the gastrointestinal tract may predispose cervicofacial and buttock LM to infection respectively. Lymphatic malformations swell in response to local or distant infection and cause local obstructive symptoms. Deep or organ level lymphatic malformations may present with symptoms related to compressed adjacent structures, such as chylous pleural effusion with thoracic lymphatic malformations or obstructed vision with orbital LM. Patients with gastrointestinal lesions can develop protein-losing enteropathy, chylous ascites, and immunodeficiency. In Gorham–Stout disease, extensive soft tissue and skeletal LM leads to progressive osteoporosis and "disappearing bone disease" with pathologic fractures and vertebral instability.[76]

Treatment and outcomes

Lymphatic malformations are treated with sclerotherapy and/or resection. Indications for treatment include recurrent infections, cosmesis, dysfunction, fluid leakage, and bleeding. Percutaneous aspiration of macrocysts followed by sclerotherapy is a minimally invasive means of treating lymphatic malformations. Commonly used sclerosants include ethanol, sodium tetradecylsulfate, doxycycline, bleomycin, fibrin sealant, OK-432 (killed group A *Streptococcus pyogenes*), and Ethibloc (a mixture of corn protein, alcohol, and contrast media). There are no prospective, randomized, double-blind studies comparing sclerosing agents. Multiple case reports, small case series, and prospective, non-randomized studies have shown that intralesional injection of sclerosant into macrocystic LM results in a durable, long-term cosmetic, functional, and symptomatic benefit.[77–82] In general, microcystic malformations do not demonstrate good response to sclerotherapy.[83] Complex lesions often require multiple treatment sessions. Blistering, skin necrosis, and nerve injury are rare potential local complications. Systemic complications including hemolysis, pulmonary hypertension, cardiac and renal toxicity may occur if an inappropriate volume of sclerosant reaches the systemic circulation. These catastrophic complications can be minimized by proper dosing, adequate control of any lesion-systemic shunts, and sclerosant choice. Despite aggressive intervention, expansion and recurrence is common.

Surgery is the only way to potentially "cure" lymphatic malformations. Unfortunately, as with sclerotherapy, multiple or staged resections may be needed. Complete resection is rarely possible, and recurrence is frequent. Operative complexity parallels lesion complexity as lymphatic malformations have an unforgiving tendency to invade and cross tissue planes. Meticulous dissection is required to avoid injury to surrounding structures. Postoperative management with prolonged closed suction drainage is standard. Postoperative complications include: serous drainage, hematoma, and cellulitis. Ironically, the increased sclerosis and scarring accompanying inflammation from infection may lead to early closure of leaking lymphatics and expedite the removal of postoperative drains. Recurrence rate is about 40% for incomplete resection and 17% after macroscopically complete resection.[84] Failure of resection is due to growth and expansion of unexcised lymphatic channels.

Venous malformations

Background

Venous malformations (VM), often incorrectly termed "cavernous hemangiomas," are the most common type of vascular malformation. They are slow-flow lesions consisting of venous channels that can arise anywhere in the body. They can be localized, multifocal, or diffuse and extensive. VM range from simple varicosities and ectasias to complex channels that can permeate and infiltrate any tissue. Most commonly they are discreet spongy masses. They tend to slowly enlarge with normal growth of the patient, but can dilate and become symptomatic at any time. Growth may be exaggerated during puberty, pregnancy, or traumatic injury. Venous malformations typically consist of sinusoidal vascular spaces with variable communications to adjacent veins. Histology reveals thin walled veins with abnormal smooth muscle architecture detected on smooth muscle actin staining. Genetic errors leading to defective smooth muscle cells in the media of involved vessels have been identified that may, in part, be responsible for these abnormal venous channels. Although the vast majority of lesions are sporadic, an autosomal dominant mutation in the endothelial receptor TIE-2 has been identified in hereditary venous malformations.[85]

Clinically, venous malformations present as soft, bluish, compressible masses that may enlarge with Valsalva maneuver or dependent position. They are most often seen in the skin and subcutaneous tissues (Fig. 63.5). As with other forms of malformations, VM may be associated with local soft tissue overgrowth. Joint and bone involvement may lead to hemarthrosis and pathologic fractures. Phlebothrombosis from stasis may lead to episodes of acute pain and swelling. Pain upon waking in the morning

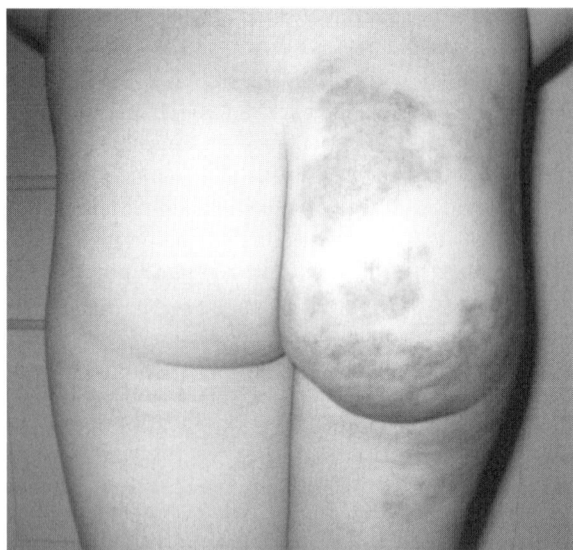

Fig. 63.5. Venous malformation (VM). Right buttock and thigh lesion showing purple–blue subcutaneous mass.

or after vigorous activity is common. Additional symptoms may include local obstructive symptoms, bleeding, or coagulopathy. Stasis of blood in large lesions can lead to a localized intravascular consumptive coagulopathy. Elevated prothrombin times, decreased fibrinogen levels, and elevated D-dimers in the plasma characterize this phenomenon. A mild thrombocytopenia may be present. This thrombocytopenia is different from the marked reduction in platelet count of Kasabach–Merritt phenomenon (2000–10 000 platelets/cm^3) seen with specific vascular tumors

Any part of the gastrointestinal tract may be involved with localized or diffuse venous malformation and may lead to significant bleeding and symptomatic anemia.[86] One characteristic pattern demonstrates diffuse involvement of the left colon, rectum, and adjacent pelvic tissues. Blue rubber bleb nevus syndrome (BRBNS) is a specific disorder of venous malformation with simultaneous multifocal skin and gastrointestinal tract lesions.[87] Skin lesions are typically found on the palms and soles of the feet. Complications include chronic gastrointestinal bleeding, anemia, and intussusception with a malformation serving as the lead point.

Hepatic venous malformations, usually incorrectly termed “hepatic hemangiomas,” present in adulthood, commonly as incidental findings on abdominal imaging studies. Although these lesions tend to be asymptomatic, they may become extremely large. Spontaneous or traumatic rupture is rare, but has been reported and is more likely when the lesion is at the periphery of the liver.

Imaging

Diagnosis is based on clinical appearance and imaging characteristics seen with ultrasound and MRI.[19] Venous malformations appear as slow flow, enlarged vascular channels on Doppler ultrasound. MRI typically shows T2-hyperintense lesions with enhancement of the sponge-like vascular channels. Signal voids may indicate phleboliths or thrombi in the intravascular spaces. Finally, flow-sensitive sequences show the absence of arterial flow.

Treatment and outcomes

Cosmesis, pain, functional loss, and bleeding are indications for treatment of venous malformations. Graded compression stockings can be used for large extremity lesions to decrease the likelihood of expansion over time. Low-dose aspirin may alleviate pain and swelling by preventing the formation of small clots in the malformation. Current treatment consists of sclerotherapy and/or surgical resection. Sclerosing agents (identical to those used to treat LM) cause direct endothelial damage and thrombosis. With sclerotherapy, lesions are accessed by direct puncture and therapeutic agents are injected under fluoroscopy, with compression of venous drainage to prevent systemic administration of the sclerosants.[88,89] Long-term follow-up of 23 patients following sclerotherapy treatment showed improvement in lesion-related symptoms and an improved quality of life.[90] Poor outcome correlated with the extent of the treated malformation. Sclerotherapy is generally contraindicated in gastrointestinal lesions due to the risk of transmural infarction and perforation. Multiple, staged procedures with occasional embolization of large channels may be used for more complex venous malformations. These procedures are best performed by a skilled interventional radiologist with experience treating vascular anomalies.

Like all vascular malformations, venous malformations have a propensity for recurrence after sclerotherapy. Treatment failure is due to angiogenesis and the ingrowth of endothelial cells into the thrombosed malformation leading to recanalization.[91,92] In these patients, treatment outcome is gauged by patient satisfaction from symptomatic improvement.

Surgical resection is reserved for well-localized lesions, but is marked by procedural morbidity and recurrence for complex VM. Preoperative sclerotherapy prior to resection of large lesions is recommended to minimize intraoperative blood loss. Treatment of hepatic venous malformations with formal hepatic resection or enucleation is safe and appropriate for symptoms, high risk of rupture, or to exclude malignancy.[93,94] When possible, enucleation is preferred to minimize potential

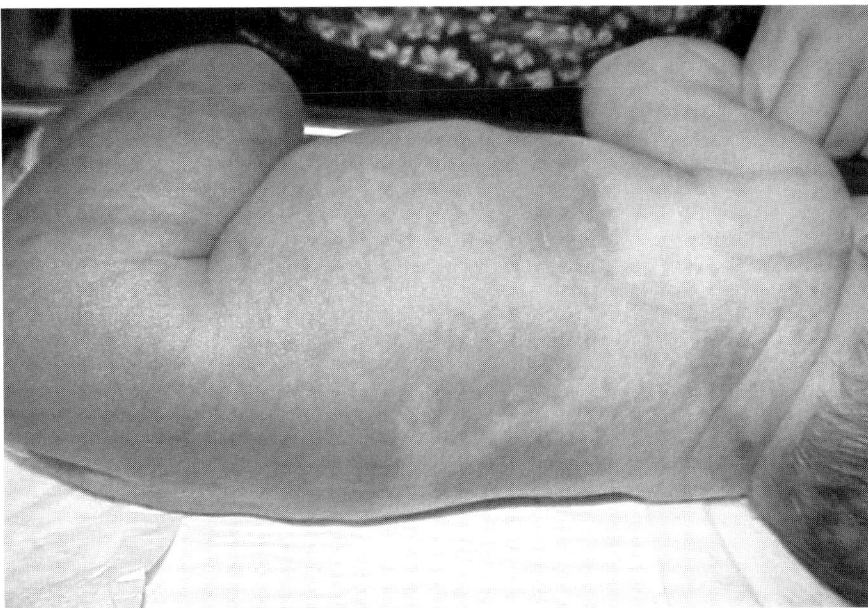

Fig. 63.6. Capillary malformation (CM). Flat, red cutaneous lesion characteristic of CM.

intra-abdominal complications.[93] Gastrointestinal lesions may be ligated or excised.[95] Patients with symptomatic, transfusion-dependent anemia from the chronic bleeding of diffuse colonic lesions may be treated with anorectal mucosectomy and coloanal pull-through with complete, long-term symptomatic relief.[96] This operation ameliorates bleeding by excluding the malformation from the intestinal lumen. Small bowel lesions can be treated by wedge resection and polypectomy rather than segmental excision. Complete surgical excision of all the gastrointestinal lesions of blue rubber bleb nevus syndrome, although tedious, time-consuming, and technically demanding, is a potential modality for treating transfusion-dependent patients.[97] The combination of esophagoduodenoscopy, colonoscopy, and enteroscopy with surgical resection at the time of exploratory laparotomy can provide a satisfying, durable treatment for this difficult disease.

Capillary malformations

Background and diagnosis

Capillary malformations, also known as "port wine stains," present as permanent, flat, red or purple cutaneous lesions (Fig. 63.6). They are most often found on the head and neck, although they can be seen anywhere on the body. They can be localized or extensive and may be associated with hypertrophy of the underlying soft tissue and skeleton. Histologically, dilated capillary-to-venular sized vessels are found in the superficial dermis with minimal innervation. These lesions may darken over time as vessels dilate. CM may appear similar to *nevus flammeus neonatorum* ("angel kiss" or "stork bite"), but will eventually differentiate with its persistence. Cutaneous capillary malformations may also herald an underlying structural abnormality such as a spinal dysraphism associated with a cervical or lumbar skin lesion.[98] Sturge–Weber syndrome describes a facial CM in the ophthalmic trigeminal dermatome associated with ipsilateral ocular and leptomeningeal anomalies.[99] MRI is diagnostic. Leptomeningeal involvement may lead to seizures, hemiplegia, and delayed cognition. Patients are at risk for ocular complications and should be followed by an ophthalmologist.

Treatment and outcomes

Treatment for capillary malformation is elective and usually for cosmesis. The tunable flashlamp pulsed-dye laser allows selective thermolysis to a depth of 1.2 mm and results in significant lightening in some patients.[45,100,101] Studies show that other laser types (argon beam, Nd-YAg, carbon dioxide) are also effective; there is no consensus regarding the best treatment method.[102–105] Overlapping laser spots appear to be more effective than small areas of separation with improved cosmesis without increased scarring.[103] Multiple sessions are frequently required. Timing of treatment is controversial with some practitioners advocating

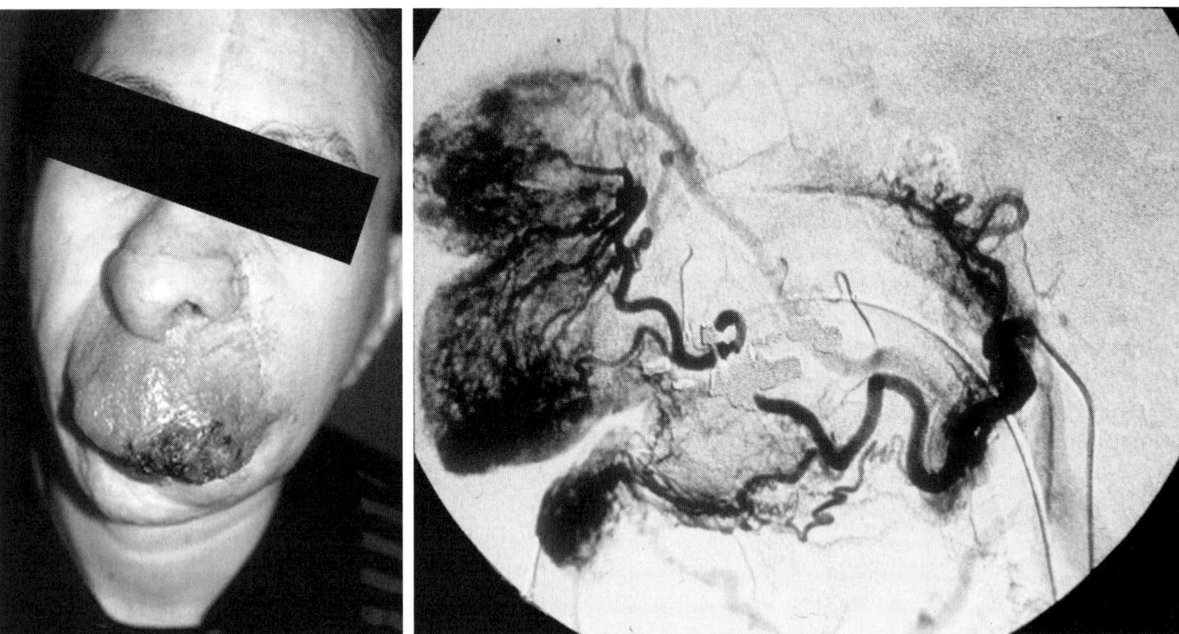

Fig. 63.7. Arteriovenous malformation (AVM). (a) Extensive AVM of the upper and lower lips with ulceration. (b) Angiogram shows large arteriovenous shunts.

treatment beginning in infancy.[104] Concomitant soft tissue and skeletal overgrowth is occasionally treated surgically, as appropriate.

Arteriovenous malformations

Background and diagnosis

Arteriovenous malformations are fast-flow lesions characterized by abnormal shunts between feeding arteries and draining veins and lack an intervening capillary bed. These lesions may be noted at birth but usually appear extremely innocuous. Lesions expand, particularly in response to puberty, pregnancy, or trauma, and may appear as a darkish mass beneath the skin (Fig. 63.7). Local warmth as well as a thrill or a bruit may become apparent over time. Lesions are staged symptomatically ranging from I to IV.[106] Ulceration, bleeding, and pain characterize enlargement. Congestive heart failure may occur if a significant blood volume is shunted through the lesion. These lesions can be confirmed by duplex ultrasound, MRI/MRA, or angiography.

Treatment and outcomes

Treatment options include cautious observation, embolization, or surgical resection. Treatment is traditionally reserved for symptomatic lesions (Stage III or IV) with threatening signs (severe ulceration, ischemic pain, bleeding, or congestive heart failure). Stage I and II lesions are traditionally clinically followed with serial exams, photography, and imaging studies. Angiography with selective arterial or retrograde venous embolization of the nidus may be indicated for palliation when surgery is not possible or resection would result in severe disfigurement.[106] Sclerotherapy, delivered to the malformation nidus with venous and arterial occlusion, may also be attempted. "Cures" have been reported with arterial embolization combined with sclerotherapy, but in general, control or eradication should always be viewed tentatively, since recurrence may become apparent later.[107] Ligation or proximal embolization of feeding vessels should not be performed. This both prohibits future access for nidus embolization and promotes rapid recruitment of adjacent arteries to supply the AVM. Neurologic injury and soft tissue damage are potential complications of intralesional injection procedures. Arterial embolization is commonly employed 24 to 48 hours before surgical resection to minimize bleeding. Preoperative embolization, however, does not decrease the extent of resection. The goal of surgery is complete resection, including the overlying skin, to uninvolved margins. Pretreatment angiograms, MRI, and careful attention to the pattern of bleeding from the wound edges are used to guide the extent of resection. With large resections, tissue transfer techniques and vacuum assist devices may be required for adequate wound closure.

Close follow-up is required to monitor for lesion recurrence.

Combined malformations

Background

Combined slow-flow malformations include Klippel–Trenaunay (KT), Proteus, Maffucci, and Bannayan–Riley–Ruvalcaba syndromes. These disorders are usually associated with skeletal and soft tissue overgrowth. Parkes–Weber syndrome and hereditary hemorrhagic telangiectasia have high flow shunting capacity. Once again, a complex and confusing array of eponyms has been created. Like other malformations, these lesions are best identified and characterized by their anatomic terms.

Klippel–Trenaunay (KT)syndrome

Background

KT is a slow-flow, combined capillary–lymphaticovenous malformation (CLVM) associated with soft tissue and skeletal hypertrophy (Fig. 63.8).[108] This syndrome is always evident at birth and can vary in severity. Lesions may involve the trunk and one or more extremities; however, 95% of lesions involve a lower limb. The macular capillary component is typically patchy over the lateral aspect of the lesions. The lymphatic component may be micro- or macrocystic. Thigh and pelvic lesions tend to be macrocystic while distal extremity and buttock lesions tend to be microcystic. They may be focal or diffuse and pervasive. In many cases, the overlying skin and capillary malformation can become involved with lymphatic vesicles. Venous malformations are also variable. Persistent embryonic veins manifest as dilated, incompetent, anomalous lateral superficial veins. In severe cases, the lower extremity deep venous system is hypoplastic or absent and lower extremity blood flow returns through the abnormal superficial veins. Incompetent valves combined with deep venous anomalies lead to marked superficial varicosities. Thrombophlebitis occurs in 20%–45% of patients with pulmonary emboli in 4%–25% of cases.[109,110] Pelvic involvement with lower extremity lesions may lead to urologic and lower gastrointestinal complications such as infection, obstruction, hematuria, and hematochezia. Similarly, retropleural and posterior mediastinal extension may be seen with upper extremity lesions. Limb hypertrophy appears at birth and progresses over time. Although usually involving the affected limb, overgrowth can occur on any extremity. Unlike other patients with hemihypertrophy syndromes, patients with KT are not at increased risk for Wilms' tumor and screening ultrasounds are not necessary.[111]

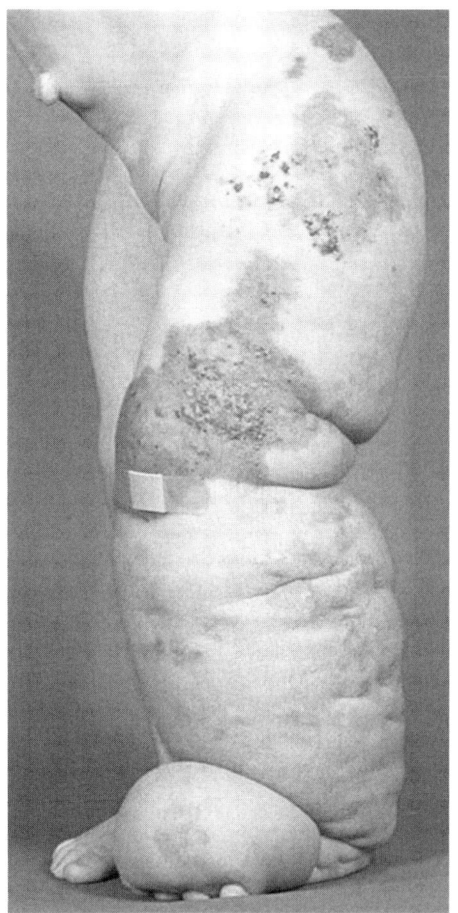

Fig. 63.8. Klippel–Trenaunay syndrome (KT or CLVM). Markedly enlarged left lower extremity with significant soft-tissue and skeletal overgrowth, capillary malformation, and cutaneous lymphatic vesicles characteristic of CLVM.

Imaging

Imaging is often vital in planning diagnosis and treatment. Plain radiography is used to document limb length discrepancies and plan appropriate timing for intervention. MRI delineates lymphatic and venous components as well as hypertrophic adipose tissue.[112] MRV can be used to evaluate the deep venous system. The presence of the marginal vein of Servelle, a subcutaneous embryonic vein along the lateral calf and thigh, is nearly pathognomonic of CLVM. Venography may be used to further assess the venous drainage of the affected extremity. It is important to identify the pattern of venous drainage before proceeding with lower extremity contour resection.

Treatment and outcomes

There is no cure for CLVM. Treatment serves to mitigate symptoms and complications. Compression garments, sclerotherapy, and resection help manage symptoms relating to the lymphatic and venous enlargement. Local vein excision and vein stripping may be employed when a functioning deep venous system is present.[113] Though not widely performed, debulking operations can be of significant benefit in certain situations. Platelet inhibition with low-dose aspirin can be used to prevent pain associated with sludging and thrombosis. Leg length discrepancies are followed by plain radiographs starting at 2 years of age. Shoe lifts are used to minimize limp and prevent back problems. An epiphysiodesis of the distal femoral growth plate, typically around 11 years, may be beneficial to minimize ultimate leg length discrepancy. Selective amputations and contour resections may be used to treat overgrowth that impairs ambulation and the ability to wear shoes. Complications of the vascular malformations include infection, bleeding, weeping, thrombophlebitis and pulmonary embolism.

Parkes–Weber syndrome

Combined fast-flow malformations are rarer than the slow-flow malformations. Parkes–Weber syndrome is a sporadic, combined capillary–arterial–venous malformation that presents at birth with a vascular lesion and extremity overgrowth.[3] Typically, the lower limb contains a pink, macular stain with significantly increased warmth and possibly a bruit. Unlike CLVM, the extremity overgrowth is usually proportional. MRI shows muscular and soft tissue overgrowth with abnormal signal and enhancement. MRA and MRV shows diffuse arterial and venous dilation and contrast angiography demonstrates discrete arteriovenous shunts. Treatment with superselective embolization is reserved for symptomatic lesions (ischemia, pain, high-output congestive heart failure).

Hereditary hemorrhagic telangiectasia

Hereditary hemorrhagic telangiectasia (HHT or Osler–Weber–Rendu disease) is another fast-flow malformation characterized by capillary-venous shunts in the skin, mucus membranes, liver, lungs, and brain that presents in adulthood.[3] Two genes located on chromosome 9 involving transforming growth factor beta have been found to play a role in the disease process. HHT1, encodes a mutated endothelial glycoprotein (endoglin) and HHT2 employs a mutated activin receptor-like kinase.

Rare syndromes

Proteus syndrome is a sporadic and progressive vascular, skeletal, and soft tissue condition defined by linear nevi, lipomas, macrocephaly, and asymmetric limbs.[114] Maffucci syndrome is a sporadic disorder that combines venous malformation with bony exostoses and enchondromas.[3] This syndrome presents in childhood with osseus lesions followed by venous anomalies in bones and subcutaneous tissue. These patients may also develop spindle-cell hemangioendotheliomas that are felt to result from reactive vascular proliferation within a pre-existing venous malformation. Malignant transformation to chondrosarcoma also occurs in 20% to 30% of patients. Finally, Bannayan–Riley–Ruvalcaba syndrome is an autosomal dominant disorder defined by a mutation in PTEN (phosphatase tensin homologue), a tumor suppressor gene on chromosome 10.[115] This lesion is characterized by macrocephaly, multiple lipomas, hamartomatous gastrointestinal polyps, Hashimoto thyroiditis, vascular malformations, and a pigmented macule on the glans penis. The vascular malformation may be of any type and is typically in the skin.

Conclusions

Vascular anomalies have received relatively little focus over the years. Only relatively recently has an effort been made to unify approaches to diagnosis and treatment. Truly scientific outcome analysis is grossly lacking. This presents an opportunity to improve care in this area. The development of multidisciplinary vascular anomaly centers in many institutions has provided resources for patients and physicians.

REFERENCES

1. Finn, M. C., Glowacki, J., & Mullikan, J. B. *et al.* Congenital vascular lesions: clinical application of a new classification. *J. Pediatr. Surg.* 1983; **18**(6):894–900.
2. Mulliken, J. B. & Glowacki, J. Hemangiomas and vascular malformations in infants and children: a classification based on endothelial characteristics. *Plast. Reconstr. Surg.* 1982; **69**(3):412–422.
3. Mulliken, J. B., Fishman, S. J., Burrows, P. E. *et al.* Vascular anomalies. *Curr. Probl. Surg.* 2000; **37**(8):517–584.
4. Holmdahl, K. Cutaneous hemangiomas in premature and mature infants. *Acta Paediatr.* 1955; **44**(4):370–379.
5. Amir, J., Metzker, A., Krikler, R. *et al.* Strawberry hemangioma in preterm infants. *Pediatr. Dermatol.* 1986; **3**(4):331–332.
6. Drolet, B. A., Esterly, N. B., & Frieden, I. J. *et al.* Hemangiomas in children. *N. Engl. J. Med.* 1999; **341**(3):173–181.
7. Boon, L. M., Burrows, P. E., Paltiel, H. J. *et al.* Hepatic vascular anomalies in infancy: a twenty-seven-year experience. *J. Pediatr.* 1996; **129**(3):346–354.
8. Kassarjian, A., Zurakowski, D., Dubois, J. *et al.* Infantile hepatic hemangiomas: clinical and imaging findings and their correlation with therapy. *Am. J. Roentgenol.* 2004; **182**(3):785–795.

9. Chen, C. C., Kong, M. S., Yang, C. P. *et al.* Hepatic hemangioendothelioma in children: analysis of thirteen cases. *Acta Paediatr. Taiwan* 2003; **44**(1):8–13.
10. Kassarjian, A., Dubois, J., & Burrows, P. E. Angiographic classification of hepatic hemangiomas in infants. *Radiology* 2002; **222**(3):693–698.
11. Hersh, J. H., Waterfill, D., Rutledge, J. *et al.* Sternal malformation/vascular dysplasia association. *Am. J. Med. Genet.* 1985; **21**(1):177–186, 201–202.
12. Tubbs, R. S., Wellons, J. C. 3rd, Iskander, B. J. *et al.* Isolated flat capillary midline lumbosacral hemangiomas as indicators of occult spinal dysraphism. *J. Neurosurg. Spine.* 2004; **100**(2):86–89.
13. Bouchard, S., Yazbeck, S., & Lallier, M. Perineal hemangioma, anorectal malformation, and genital anomaly: a new association? *J. Pediatr. Surg.* 1999; **34**(7):1133–1135.
14. Metry, D. W., Dowd, C. F., Barkovich, A. J. *et al.* The many faces of PHACE syndrome. *J. Pediatr.* 2001; **139**(1):117–123.
15. Takahashi, K., Mulliken, J. B., Kozakewich, H. P. *et al.* Cellular markers that distinguish the phases of hemangioma during infancy and childhood. *J. Clin. Invest.* 1994; **93**(6):2357–2364.
16. Gonzalez-Crussi, F. & Reyes-Mugica, M. Cellular hemangiomas ("hemangioendotheliomas") in infants. Light microscopic, immunohistochemical, and ultrastructural observations. *Am. J. Surg. Pathol.* 1991; **15**(8):769–778.
17. Martin-Padura, I., De Castellarnau, C., Uccini, S. *et al.* Expression of VE (vascular endothelial)-cadherin and other endothelial-specific markers in haemangiomas. *J. Pathol.* 1995; **175**(1):51–57.
18. North, P. E., Waner, M., Mizeracki, A. *et al.* GLUT1: a newly discovered immunohistochemical marker for juvenile hemangiomas. *Hum. Pathol.* 2000; **31**(1):11–22.
19. Meyer, J. S., Hoffer, F. A., Barnes, P. D. *et al.* Biological classification of soft-tissue vascular anomalies:MR correlation. *Am. J. Roentgenol.* 1991; **157**(3):559–564.
20. Dubois, J., Patriquin, H. B., Garel, L. *et al.* Soft-tissue hemangiomas in infants and children: diagnosis using Doppler sonography. *Am. J. Roentgenol.* 1998; **171**(1):247–252.
21. Paltiel, H. J., Burrows, P. E., Kozakewich, H. P. *et al.* Soft-tissue vascular anomalies: utility of US for diagnosis. *Radiology* 2000; **214**(3):747–754.
22. Barton, D. J., Miller, J. H., Allwright, S. J. *et al.* Distinguishing soft-tissue hemangiomas from vascular malformations using technetium-labeled red blood cell scintigraphy. *Plast. Reconstr. Surg.* (1992); **89**(1):46–52; discussion 53–5.
23. Margileth, A. M. & Museles, M. Cutaneous hemangiomas in children. Diagnosis and conservative management. *J. Am. Med. Assoc.*, 1965; **194**(5):523–526.
24. Morrell, A. J. & Willshaw, H. E. Normalisation of refractive error after steroid injection for adnexal haemangiomas. *Br. J. Ophthalmol.* 1991; **75**(5):301–305.
25. Huang, S. A., Tu, H. M., Harney, J. W. *et al.* Severe hypothyroidism caused by type 3 iodothyronine deiodinase in infantile hemangiomas. *N. Engl. J. Med.* 2000; **343**(3):185–189.
26. Morelli, J. G., Tan, O. T., Yohn, J. J. *et al.* Treatment of ulcerated hemangiomas infancy. *Arch. Pediatr. Adolesc. Med.* 1994; **148**(10):1104–1105.
27. Sadan, N. & Wolach, B. Treatment of hemangiomas of infants with high doses of prednisone. *J. Pediatr.* 1996; **128**(1):141–146.
28. Boon, L. M., MacDonald, D. M., Mulliken, J. B. *et al.* Complications of systemic corticosteroid therapy for problematic hemangioma. *Plast. Reconstr. Surg.* 1999; **104**(6):1616–1623.
29. Bennett, M. L., Fleischer, A. B., Chamlin, S. L. Jr. *et al.* Oral corticosteroid use is effective for cutaneous hemangiomas: an evidence-based evaluation. *Arch. Dermatol.* 2001; **137**(9):1208–1213.
30. David, L. R., Malek, M. M., & Argenta, L. C. Efficacy of pulse dye laser therapy for the treatment of ulcerated haemangiomas: a review of 78 patients. *Br. J. Plast. Surg.* 2003; **56**(4):317–327.
31. Wang, L. Y., Hung, H. Y., & Lee, K. S. Infantile subglottic hemangioma treated by intralesional steroid injection: report of one case. *Acta Paediatr Taiwan* 2003; **44**(1):35–37.
32. Ruttum, M. S., Abrams, G. W., Harris, G. J. *et al.* Bilateral retinal embolization associated with intralesional corticosteroid injection for capillary hemangioma of infancy. *J. Pediatr. Ophthalmol. Strabismus.* 1993; **30**(1):4–7.
33. Ezekowitz, R. A., Mulliken, J. B., & Folkman J. Interferon alfa-2a therapy for life-threatening hemangiomas of infancy. *N. Engl. J. Med.* 1992; **326**(22):1456–1463.
34. Bauman, N. M., Burke, D. K., Smith, R. J. *et al.* Treatment of massive or life-threatening hemangiomas with recombinant alpha(2a)-interferon. *Otolaryngol. Head Neck Surg.* 1997; **117**(1):99–110.
35. Schiavetti, A., De Pasquale, M. D., DiSalvo, S. *et al.* Recombinant interferon alfa 2a in hepatic hemangiomatosis with congestive heart failure: a case report. *Pediatr. Hematol. Oncol.* 2003; **20**(2):161–165.
36. Hastings, M. M., Milot, J., Barsoum-Homsy, M. *et al.* Recombinant interferon alfa-2b in the treatment of vision-threatening capillary hemangiomas in childhood. *J. Aapos.* 1997; **1**(4):226–230.
37. Deb, G., Donfrancesco, A., Ilari, I. *et al.* Hemangioendothelioma: successful therapy with interferon-alpha: a study in Association with the Italian Pediatric Haematology/Oncology Society (AIEOP). *Med. Pediatr. Oncol.* 2002; **38**(2):118–119.
38. Dubois, J., Hershon, L., Carmant, L. *et al.* Toxicity profile of interferon alfa-2b in children: a prospective evaluation. *J. Pediatr.* 1999; **135**(6):782–785.
39. Deb, G., Jenkner, A., Donfrancesco, A. *et al.* Spastic diplegia and interferon. *J. Pediatr.* 1999; **134**(3):382.
40. Garmendia, G., Miranda, N., Borrosco, S. *et al.* Regression of infancy hemangiomas with recombinant IFN-alpha 2b. *J. Interferon Cytokine Res.* 2001; **21**(1):31–38.
41. Perez Payarols, J., Pardo Masferrer, J., Gomez Bellvert, C. Treatment of life-threatening infantile hemangiomas with vincristine. *N. Engl. J. Med.* 1995; **333**(1):69.

42. Perez, J., Pardo, J., & Gomez, C. Vincristine – an effective treatment of corticoid-resistant life-threatening infantile hemangiomas. *Acta Oncol.* 2002; **41**(2):197–199.
43. Enjolras, O., Breviere, G. M., Roger, G. *et al.* [Vincristine treatment for function- and life-threatening infantile hemangioma]. *Arch. Pediatr.* 2004; **11**(2):99–107.
44. Batta, K., Goodyear, H. M., Moss, C. *et al.* Randomised controlled study of early pulsed dye laser treatment of uncomplicated childhood haemangiomas: results of a 1-year analysis. *Lancet* 2002; **360**(9332):521–7.
45. Gupta, G. & Bilsland, D. A prospective study of the impact of laser treatment on vascular lesions. *Br. J. Dermatol.* 2000; **143**(2):356–359.
46. Sie, K. C., McGill, T., Healy, G. B. *et al.* Subglottic hemangioma: ten years' experience with the carbon dioxide laser. *Ann. Otol. Rhinol. Laryngol.* 1994; **103**(3):167–172.
47. Mulliken, J. B., Rogers, G. F., & Marler, J. J. Circular excision of hemangioma and purse-string closure: the smallest possible scar. *Plast. Reconstr. Surg.* 2002; **109**(5):1544–1554; discussion 1555.
48. Daller, J. A., Bueno, J., Guttierez, J. *et al.* Hepatic hemangioendothelioma: clinical experience and management strategy. *J. Pediatr. Surg.* 1999; **34**(1):98–105; discussion 105–106.
49. Berenguer, B., Mulliken, J. B., Enjolros, O. *et al.* Rapidly involuting congenital hemangioma: clinical and histopathologic features. *Pediatr. Dev. Pathol.* 2003; **6**(6):495–510.
50. Burrows, P. E., Mulliken, J. B., Fellows, K. E. *et al.* Childhood hemangiomas and vascular malformations: angiographic differentiation. *Am. J. Roentgenol.* 1983; **141**(3):483–488.
51. Konez, O., Burrows, P. E., Mulliken, J. B. *et al.* Angiographic features of rapidly involuting congenital hemangioma (RICH). *Pediatr. Radiol.* 2003; **33**(1):15–19.
52. Kasabach, H. H. & Merritt, K. K. Capillary hemangioma with extensive purpura: report of a case. *Am. J. Dis. Child.* 1940; **59**:1063–1070.
53. Enjolras, O., Riche, M. C., Merland, J. J. *et al.* Management of alarming hemangiomas in infancy: a review of 25 cases. *Pediatrics* 1990; **85**(4):491–498.
54. MacArthur, C. J., Senders, C. W., & Katz, J. The use of interferon alfa-2a for life-threatening hemangiomas. *Arch. Otolaryngol. Head Neck Surg.* 1995; **121**(6):690–693.
55. Nako, Y., Fukushima, N., Igarashi, T. *et al.* Successful interferon therapy in a neonate with life-threatening Kasabach–Merritt syndrome. *J. Perinatol.* 1997; **17**(3):244–247.
56. Robenzadeh, A., Don, P. C., & Weinberg, J. Treatment of tufted angioma with interferon alfa: role of bFGF. *Pediatr. Dermatol.* 1998; **15**(6):482.
57. Serafim, A. P., Almeida Junior, L. C., Silva, M. T. *et al.* Kaposiform hemangioendothelioma associated with Kasabach–Merritt syndrome. *J. Pediatr. (Rio J.)* 1998; **74**(4):338–342.
58. Seo, S. K., Suh, J. C., Na, G. Y. *et al.* Kasabach–Merritt syndrome: identification of platelet trapping in a tufted angioma by immunohistochemistry technique using monoclonal antibody to CD61. *Pediatr. Dermatol.* 1999; **16**(5):392–394.
59. Shin, H. Y., Ryu, K. H., & Ahn, H. S. Stepwise multimodal approach in the treatment of Kasabach–Merritt syndrome. *Pediatr. Int.* 2000; **42**(6):620–624.
60. Wananukul, S., Nuchprayoon, I., & Seksarn, P. Treatment of Kasabach-Merritt syndrome: a stepwise regimen of prednisolone, dipyridamole, and interferon. *Int. J. Dermatol.* 2003; **42**(9):741–748.
61. Haisley-Royster, C., Enjolras, O., Frieden, I. J. *et al.* Kasabach–Merritt phenomenon: a retrospective study of treatment with vincristine. *J. Pediatr. Hematol. Oncol.* 2002; **24**(6):459–462.
62. Mac-Moune Lai, F., To, K. F., Choi, P. C. *et al.* Kaposiform hemangioendothelioma: five patients with cutaneous lesion and long follow-up. *Mod. Pathol.* 2001; **14**(11):1087–1092.
63. Enjolras, O., Mulliken, J. B., Wassef, M. *et al.* Residual lesions after Kasabach–Merritt phenomenon in 41 patients. *J. Am. Acad. Dermatol.* 2000; **42**(2 Pt 1):225–235.
64. Folkman, J. & D'Amore, P. A. Blood vessel formation: what is its molecular basis? *Cell* 1996; **87**(7):1153–1155.
65. Vikkula, M., Boon, L. M., Mulliken, J. B. *et al.* Molecular basis of vascular anomalies. *Trends Cardiovasc. Med.* 1998; **8**(7):281–292.
66. Wang, H. U., Chen, Z. F., Anderson, D. J. *et al.* Molecular distinction and angiogenic interaction between embryonic arteries and veins revealed by ephrin-B2 and its receptor Eph-B4. *Cell* 1998; **93**(5):741–753.
67. Marler, J. J., Fishman, S. J., Lipton, J. *et al.* Prenatal diagnosis of vascular anomalies. *J. Pediatr. Surg.* 2002; **37**(3):318–326.
68. Bouchard, S., Johnson, M. P., Flake, A. W. *et al.* The EXIT procedure: experience and outcome in 31 cases. *J. Pediatr. Surg.* 2002; **37**(3):418–426.
69. Dumont, D. J., Fong, G. H., Puri, M. C. *et al.* Vascularization of the mouse embryo: a study of flk-1, tek, tie, and vascular endothelial growth factor expression during development. *Dev. Dyn.* 1995; **203**(1):80–92.
70. Kaipainen, A., Korhonen, J., Mustonen, T. *et al.* Expression of the fms-like tyrosine kinase 4 gene becomes restricted to lymphatic endothelium during development. *Proc. Natl. Acad. Sci. USA* 1995; **92**(8):3566–3570.
71. Jeltsch, M., Kaipainen, A., Joukov, V. *et al.* Hyperplasia of lymphatic vessels in VEGF-C transgenic mice. *Science* 1997; **276**(5317):1423–1425.
72. Burrows, P. E., Laor, T., Paltiel, H. *et al.* Diagnostic imaging in the evaluation of vascular birthmarks. *Dermatol. Clin.* 1998; **16**(3):455–488.
73. Fishman, S. J., Burrows, P. E., Upton, J. *et al.* Life-threatening anomalies of the thoracic duct: anatomic delineation dictates management. *J. Pediatr. Surg.* 2001; **36**(8):1269–1272.
74. Tran Ngoc, N. & Tran Xuan, N. Cystic hygroma in children: a report of 126 cases. *J. Pediatr. Surg.* 1974; **9**(2):191–195.
75. Padwa, B. L., Hayward, P. G., Ferraro, N. F. *et al.* Cervicofacial lymphatic malformation: clinical course, surgical intervention, and pathogenesis of skeletal hypertrophy. *Plast. Reconstr. Surg.* 1995; **95**(6):951–960.

76. Gorham, L. W. & Stout, A. P. Massive osteolysis (acute spontaneous absorption of bone, phantom bone, disappearing bone); its relation to hemangiomatosis. *J. Bone. Joint Surg. Am.* 1955; **37-A**(5):985–1004.

77. Ogita, S., Tsuto, T., Nakamura, K. *et al.* OK-432 therapy in 64 patients with lymphangioma. *J. Pediatr. Surg.* 1994; **29**(6):784–785.

78. Zhong, P. Q., Zhi, F. X., Li, R. *et al.* Long-term results of intratumorous bleomycin-A5 injection for head and neck lymphangioma. *Oral Surg. Oral Med. Oral Pathol. Oral Radiol. Endod.* 1998; **86**(2):139–144.

79. Sung, M. W., Lee, D. W., Kim, D. Y. *et al.* Sclerotherapy with picibanil (OK-432) for congenital lymphatic malformation in the head and neck. *Laryngoscope* 2001; **111**(8):1430–1433.

80. Claesson, G. & Kuylenstierna, R. OK-432 therapy for lymphatic malformation in 32 patients (28 children). *Int. J. Pediatr. Otorhinolaryngol.* 2002; **65**(1):1–6.

81. Giguere, C. M., Bauman, N. M., Sato, Y. *et al.* Treatment of lymphangiomas with OK-432 (Picibanil) sclerotherapy: a prospective multi-institutional trial. *Arch. Otolaryngol. Head Neck Surg.* 2002; **128**(10):1137–1144.

82. Sanlialp, I., Karnak, I., Tanyel, F. C. *et al.* Sclerotherapy for lymphangioma in children. *Int. J. Pediatr. Otorhinolaryngol.* 2003; **67**(7):795–800.

83. Greinwald, J. H., Jr., Burke, D. K., Sato, Y. *et al.* Treatment of lymphangiomas in children: an update of Picibanil (OK-432) sclerotherapy. *Otolaryngol. Head Neck Surg.* 1999; **121**(4):381–387.

84. Alqahtani, A., Nguyen, L. T., Flagiole, H. *et al.* 25 years' experience with lymphangiomas in children. *J. Pediatr. Surg.* 1999; **34**(7):1164–1168.

85. Vikkula, M., Boon, L. M., Carraway, K. L. 3rd. *et al.* Vascular dysmorphogenesis caused by an activating mutation in the receptor tyrosine kinase TIE2. *Cell* 1996; **87**(7):1181–1190.

86. Fishman, S. J., Burrows, P. E., Leichner, A. M. *et al.* Gastrointestinal manifestations of vascular anomalies in childhood: varied etiologies require multiple therapeutic modalities. *J. Pediatr. Surg.* 1998; **33**(7):1163–1167.

87. Oranje, A. P. Blue rubber bleb nevus syndrome. *Pediatr. Dermatol.* 1986; **3**(4):304–310.

88. Gorriz Gomez, E., Carreira Villamor, J. M., Reyes Perez, R. *et al.* Percutaneous treatment of peripheral vascular malformations. *Rev. Clin. Esp.* 1998; **198**(9):565–570.

89. Pappas, D. C., Jr., Persky, M. S., Berenstein, A. *et al.* Evaluation and treatment of head and neck venous vascular malformations. *Ear Nose Throat J.* 1998; **77**(11):914–916, 918–922.

90. Rautio, R., Saarinen, J., Laranne, J. *et al.* Endovascular treatment of venous malformations in extremities: results of sclerotherapy and the quality of life after treatment. *Acta Radiol.* 2004; **45**(4):397–403.

91. Smithers, C. J., Vogel, A. M., Kozakewich, H. P. *et al.* Enhancement of intravascular sclerotherapy by tissue engineering: short term results. *J. Pediatr. Surg.* 2004; **40**(2):412–417.

92. Smithers, C. J., Vogel, A. M., Kozakewich, H. P. *et al.* An injectable tissue-engineered embolus prevents luminal recanalization after vascular sclerotherapy. *J. Pediatr. Surg.* 2005; **40**(6):920–925.

93. Gedaly, R., Pomposelli, J. J., Pomfret, E. A. *et al.* Cavernous hemangioma of the liver: anatomic resection vs. enucleation. *Arch. Surg.* 1999; **134**(4):407–411.

94. Hanazaki, K., Kajikawa, S., Matsushita, A. *et al.* Hepatic resection of giant cavernous hemangioma of the liver. *J. Clin. Gastroenterol.* 1999; **29**(3):257–260.

95. Witte, J. T. Band ligation for colonic bleeding: modification of multiband ligating devices for use with a colonoscope. *Gastrointest. Endosc.* 2000; **52**(6):762–765.

96. Fishman, S. J., Shamberger, R. C., Fox, V. L. *et al.* Endorectal pull-through abates gastrointestinal hemorrhage from colorectal venous malformations. *J. Pediatr. Surg.* 2000; **35**(6):982–984.

97. Fishman, S. J., Smithers, C. J., Folkman, J. *et al.* Blue rubber bleb nevus syndrome: surgical eradication of gastrointestinal bleeding. *Ann. Surg.* 2005; **241**(3):523–528.

98. Enjolras, O. & Mulliken, J. B. The current management of vascular birthmarks. *Pediatr. Dermatol.* 1993; **10**(4):311–313.

99. Enjolras, O., Riche, M. C., & Merland, J. J. Facial port-wine stains and Sturge–Weber syndrome. *Pediatrics* 1985; **76**(1):48–51.

100. Nguyen, C. M., Yohn, J. J., Huff, C. *et al.* Facial port wine stains in childhood: prediction of the rate of improvement as a function of the age of the patient, size and location of the port wine stain and the number of treatments with the pulsed dye (585 nm) laser. *Br. J. Dermatol.* 1998; **138**(5):821–825.

101. Ho, W. S., Ying, S. Y., Chan, P. C. *et al.* Treatment of port wine stains with intense pulsed light: a prospective study. *Dermatol. Surg.* 2004; **30**(6):887–890; discussion 890–891.

102. Tan, O. T., Carney, J. M., Margolis, R. *et al.* Histologic responses of port-wine stains treated by argon, carbon dioxide, and tunable dye lasers. A preliminary report. *Arch. Dermatol.* 1986; **122**(9):1016–1022.

103. Adams, S. J., Swain, C. P., Mills, T. N. *et al.* The effect of wavelength, power and treatment pattern on the outcome of laser treatment of port-wine stains. *Br. J. Dermatol.* 1987; **117**(4):487–494.

104. Tan, O. T., Sherwood, K., Gilchrest, B. A. *et al.* Treatment of children with port-wine stains using the flashlamp-pulsed tunable dye laser. *N. Engl. J. Med.* 1989; **320**(7):416–421.

105. Sheehan-Dare, R. A. & Cotterill, J. A. Copper vapour laser (578 nm) and flashlamp-pumped pulsed tunable dye laser (585 nm) treatment of port wine stains: results of a comparative study using test sites. *Br. J. Dermatol.* 1994; **130**(4):478–482.

106. Kohout, M. P., Hansen, M., Pribaz, J. J. *et al.* Arteriovenous malformations of the head and neck: natural history and management. *Plast. Reconstr. Surg.* 1998; **102**(3):643–654.

107. Yakes, W. F., Rossi, P., Odink, H. *et al.* How I do it. Arteriovenous malformation management. *Cardiovasc. Intervent. Radiol.* 1996; **19**(2):65–71.

108. Mulliken, J. B. & Young, A. E. *Vascular Birthmarks: Hemangiomas and Malformations.* Philadelphia: W.B. Saunders, 1988.
109. Baskerville, P. A., Ackroyd, J. S., Lea Thomas, M. *et al.* The Klippel–Trenaunay syndrome: clinical, radiological and haemodynamic features and management. *Br. J. Surg.* 1985; **72**(3):232–236.
110. Samuel, M. & Spitz, L. Klippel–Trenaunay syndrome: clinical features, complications and management in children. *Br. J. Surg.* 1995; **82**(6):757–761.
111. Greene, A. K., Kieran, M., Burrows, P. E. *et al.* Wilms tumor screening is unnecessary in Klippel–Trenaunay syndrome. *Pediatrics* 2004; **113**(4):e326–e329.
112. Laor, T., Burrows, P. E., & Hoffer, F. A. Magnetic resonance venography of congenital vascular malformations of the extremities. *Pediatr. Radiol.* 1996; **26**(6):371–380.
113. Noel, A. A., Gloviczki, P., Cherry, K. J. *et al.* Surgical treatment of venous malformations in Klippel–Trenaunay syndrome. *J. Vasc. Surg.* 2000; **32**(5):840–847.
114. Biesecker, L. G., Happle, R., Mulliken, J. B. *et al.* Proteus syndrome: diagnostic criteria, differential diagnosis, and patient evaluation. *Am. J. Med. Genet.* 1999; **84**(5):389–395.
115. Cohen, M. M., Jr. Bannayan–Riley–Ruvalcaba syndrome: renaming three formerly recognized syndromes as one etiologic entity. *Am. J. Med. Genet.* 1990; **35**(2):291–292.

Part VII

Transplantation

64

Renal failure and transplantation

Maria H. Alonso, Greg Tiao, and Frederick C. Ryckman

Department of Pediatric General and Thoracic Surgery, Transplantation Division, Cincinnati Children's Hospital Medical Center, OH, USA

Introduction

The management of end-stage renal disease, encompassing the principles of medical management, dialysis, and renal transplantation, formed the early experience with organ failure and replacement. The lessons learned were the basis for the exploding growth of solid organ replacement in children and adults. The care continuum for these patients can be divided into several phases: pretransplant medical management, transplantation, short- and long-term outcome. In this chapter, we will attempt to review the factors affecting success in medical pretransplant management, the transplant procedure, and throughout the short- and long-term follow-up periods. At each stage of care, factors which can determine the likelihood of success may be assigned (age, sex, ethnicity, primary disease, etc.). Some determinants of outcome are variable, that is, they are influenced by choices in care delivery (type of transplant, immunosuppression protocol, experience of transplant center, etc.). As the phases of transplantation are reviewed, we will attempt to identify avenues to improve outcome based on the application of current data.

Information reviewing the management of children with end-stage renal disease has been regularly evaluated and compiled in several large registries, allowing analysis of large cohorts. The United Network for Organ Sharing (UNOS)(www.unos.org) collects information on renal replacement in the United States, the United States Renal Data Systems (www.usrds.org) collects information regarding transplantation in Medicare patients. The North American Pediatric Renal Transplant Cooperative Study (NAPRTCS)(www.NAPRTCS.org), which has collected and analyzed renal transplant data on children since 1987 from the USA, Canada, Mexico, and Costa Rica, has contributed significantly to the overall understanding of outcome factors. Similar contributions from the European experience can be found in the European Dialysis and Transplantation Association Registry (www.EDTA.org). These substantial cooperation reporting organizations have been supplemented by individual center experiences.

Pretransplantation care

Advances in the management of end-stage renal disease and dialysis have greatly improved both the baseline care and transplant preparation for children. End-stage kidney disease is unique for the availability of dialysis as a means of long-term management. Advances in dialysis care and safety have allowed all patients, including infants, to achieve prolonged survival and improved outcomes.

At the present time, peritoneal dialysis is used in 63% of all children with ESRD at some time. Overall, 75% of children undergo some kind of dialysis therapy prior to transplantation, while 25% receive preemptive transplantation (PTx) prior to needing dialysis.[2] Termination of all types of dialysis is primarily due to transplantation (61%). Change in the modality of dialysis in patients on peritoneal dialysis (PD) occurred due to infection in 45% of patients. Overall, infection rates have remained unchanged in the most recent NAPRTCS review, with an annualized rate of 0.80 to 1 episode every 15 months.[3] In contrast, changes from hemodialysis (HD) were most often due to patient or family choice in 45%. The majority of pediatric patients have vascular access through a percutaneous catheter placed in the internal jugular vein.[3]

Pediatric Surgery and Urology: Long-term Outcomes, Mark Stringer, Keith Oldham, Pierre Mouriquand.

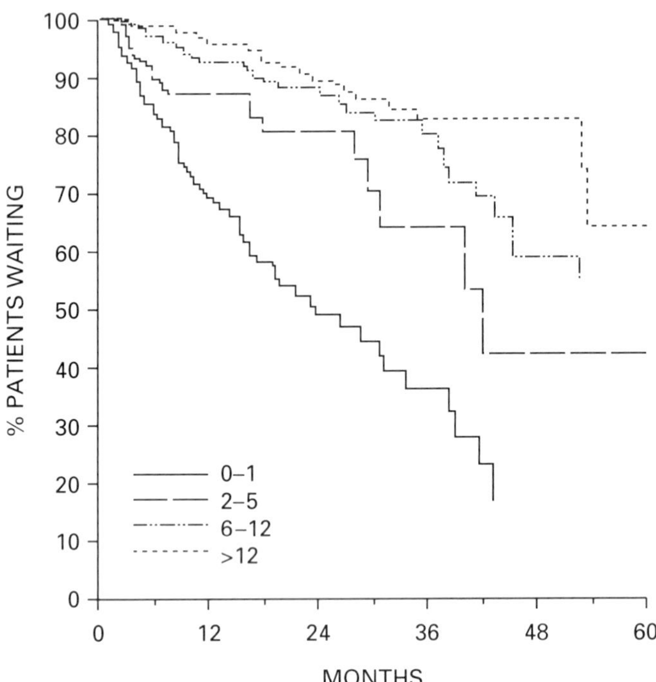

Fig. 64.1. Patient survival, stratified by age at the initiation of dialysis, is shown for the index course of dialysis.[3]

Management on dialysis has improved significantly in recent years. The majority of both HD and PD patients now receive recombinant human erythropoietin (rHuEPO) within 30 days of dialysis institution (88%), and 94% receive this by 2 years. This has led to a significant increase in both the mean and median hematocrit at 6 months of follow-up, presently 32.3% and 33% respectively. 43% of dialysis patients now have hematocrits > 33% after 6 months of therapy. However, this still does not reach the goal of 33–36% in all patients.[3] Further attention to iron deficiency and longer acting rHuEPO preparations may further improve these results. Recombinant human growth hormone use is less common, with 9.4%/8.7% (PD/HD) patients receiving rhGH at the institution of dialysis initially, and 25%/13.8% at 24 months. Treated patients in both the < 6-year-old and > 6-year-old groups showed improved height at 1 year, while both groups of untreated patients showed worsening of their height SDS.

Patient survival, stratified by age at the initiation of dialysis, is shown in Fig. 64.1 for the index course of dialysis. Overall patient survival estimates were 95+/− 0.6%, 90.1 +/− 1.0%, 85.7 +/−1.4% at 12, 24 and 36 months, respectively. Survival estimates are lowest in patients < 12 months of age.[3] The leading specified cause of death was infection (24.5%) cardiopulmonary events were the second leading cause of death at 21.5%.

Transplantation management

Although transplantation has been universally recognized as the treatment of choice for children with end-stage renal disease, the total number of children transplanted per year and the percentage of transplants going to children has changed very little over the past decade. However, there has been a significant shift in the demographics of the transplant population. Although males still represent approximately 60% of recipients, the number of non-white recipients increased from 28% in 1987 to 40% in 2000. The number of living donor (LD) transplants has increased from 42% to 60% with an increasing emphasis on non-related donation during this time. The number of cadaveric donors (CD) less than 10 years of age has decreased from 35% to 10% of all transplants. Cadaveric transplantation in infants < 24 months of age decreased to only 18 cases in 1996–2000. The use of cadaveric donors < 10 years of age has decreased from 35% to 10%, while CDs < 2 years of age decreased from 3.5 to 0.9%. All of these changes evolved from the recognition of variable risk factors and have contributed to improved overall survival.[4]

Factors influencing success – assigned risk

Recipient age

Early data from the NAPRTCS registry demonstrated a significantly worse survival in very young recipients, especially when CD were used. This survival was influenced by both a higher thrombotic risk, and a policy of placing cadaveric donor organs from young donors into young recipients in an ill-conceived attempt to "match" size. Improved technical results, preservation skills, and identification of the increased risk in young donors, all contributed to improving these overall results. The overall 1 year survival of 88% in LD and 78% in CD prior to 1995 has now been improved to 96% in LD and 94% in CD transplants. Infants with allograft survival at 1 year show excellent long-term graft survival, especially in the LD group.[5,6] Adolescents have the lowest long-term graft survival among both LD and CD recipients, for multiple reasons. These include the lowest incidence of complete reversal of rejection for both the first and all rejection episodes.[5] In addition, drug therapy compliance is worst in this group, influencing all aspects of care.

Donor age

One of the most significant differences between adult and pediatric transplant series is the role of living donors in the transplant process. In children, LDs have increased from 42% in 1987 to 60% in 2001. In children, 83% of LDs come from biologic parents, assuring at least a haplotype HLA match.[4] Although CD transplantation has decreased on a national basis, the higher proportion of African-Americans (AA) receiving CDs remains a concern with regard to long-term outcome. The paucity of AA LDs has recently been shown to relate to both unwillingness to donate and a high incidence of comorbid conditions in the donor group.[7] The increased risk of young CD is discussed above.

Sex

Overall, 60% of renal transplants are in males, representing the predominance of congenital obstructive uropathies in this gender group. There are no specific gender-related factors affecting survival independent of diagnosis.

Primary diagnosis

Several primary disease related factors influence transplant results, and are favorably addressed by appropriate pretransplant management. Obstructive uropathies can lead to polyuria or recurrent infection. Proteinuria and the nephrotic syndrome have been associated with increased risk of allograft thrombosis. Hypertension related to many glomerulonephritides can complicate post-transplant management and decrease both patient and allograft function. The distribution of primary diagnosis related to ethnicity also has a significant effect on outcome.

Ethnicity

Consistently decreased survival has been seen in all series in African American recipients. Several factors contribute to poorer outcomes. The most common diagnoses in AA are acquired inflammatory diseases: FSGS (23.2%), obstructive uropathy (15%), renal aplasia/hypoplasia/dysplasia (15%), chronic glomerulonephritis (5%) and systemic lupus erythematosus (SLE) nephritis (4%). In contrast, Caucasian recipients have primarily structural and developmental abnormalities: obstructive uropathy (17%), renal aplasia/hypoplasia/dysplasia (16%), FSGS (9%), reflux nephropathy (6%), and medullary cystic disease (4%). The higher incidence of FSGS and SLE nephritis in the AA group leads to higher rates of recurrence of primary disease and early rejection leading to allograft loss.

Factors influencing success – variable risk subject to influence

Donor source

Although prior reviews have emphasized the improved survival seen in LDs compared to CDs, improved survival in all groups has recently lessened this factor. LD allograft 1-year survival has improved from 91% in the period 1987–1995 to 94% in the years 1996–2000. CD allograft survival has also improved from 81% to 93% during these times. That equal short-term allograft survival is equal for LD and CD recipients is encouraging; however, sufficient data is not available to show similar equivalency in long-term results.

Immunosuppressive protocol

Transplant immunosuppression has evolved substantially over the past decade. Earlier trials included primarily "triple therapy" using cyclosporin, azathioprine or mycophenolate, and glucocorticoids. The evolving use of tacrolimus in place of cyclosporine has increased the efficacy of immunosuppression, but has also increased the incidence of post-transplant diabetes. Induction therapy using anti-CD3 antibodies was shown in earlier NAPRTCS studies to be associated with improved outcomes. Their use of anti-CD3 antibody decreased from 27% to 14% between 1997 and 2000 because of increased interest in the use of IL2 receptor antibodies. The latter are now used in more than 55% of renal transplants. These changes have brought about a related decrease in acute rejection. Increasing recognition of inherent differences in individual immuno responsiveness among recipient subsets has encouraged the development of new protocols. The higher incidence of acute rejection and lower probability for complete reversal of rejection in AA have suggested increased immune responsiveness in this population. Modification of the successful protocols developed for Caucasian and Asian recipients may be necessary to achieve similar success in the AA recipient population. Attention to growth deficiencies has led to increased interest in minimizing steroid use or even steroid free protocols. The shift to chronic rejection as the major reason for graft loss has spurred interest in the use of sirolimus, an anti-proliferative agent, in hopes of decreasing nephrosclerosis. A proliferation of new agents and improved understanding of immune mechanisms make this one of the most fertile areas for future improvement.

Matching

The effect of peak PRA on long-term outcome is difficult to assess due to the limited number of recipients. However, in the United Network for Organ Sharing (UNOS) registry, recipients with a pretransplant peak PRA > 40% demonstrated diminished long-term adjusted survival, with long-term allograft survival decreasing by 8% at 5 years. This effect is not seen in similar adult series, where PRA exerts its negative influence in the first post-transplant year.[8]

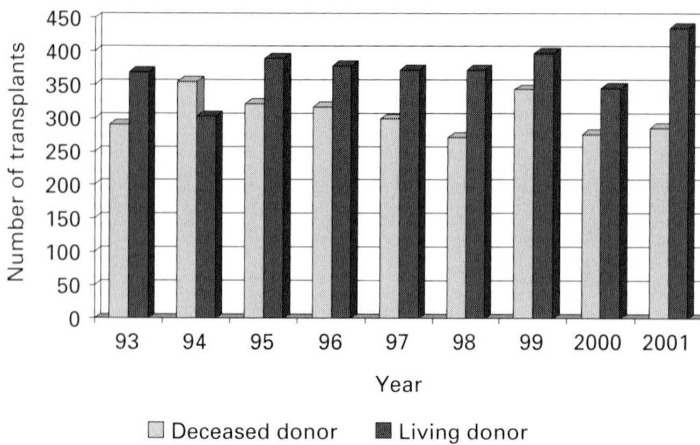

Fig. 64.2. Transplant recipient characteristics, 1993–2002.

Center effect

Center variation was a chief pretransplant factor influencing graft function in the UNOS data analysis. In their review, regardless of the follow-up period or center size, more than 5% of centers exhibited significantly lower or higher adjusted graft survival rates.[8] This could not be explained by the center's volume or the center's emphasis on pediatric vs. adult transplantation. The adjusted 5-year survival ranged from 43% to nearly 100%, suggesting an opportunity to model high success centers and implement protocol-driven improvements in lower achieving centers.

Pre-emptive transplantation

Pre-emptive transplantation (PTx) has increased in recent years, now representing 13% of transplants reported in UNOS and USRDS data, and 24% in the NAPRTCS experience. In all registries, live donor pre-emptive transplant overshadows cadaveric donation by a 2.5–3:1 ratio. Recipients of pre-emptive transplants have significantly improved patient and allograft survival.[4] This advantage appears to be primarily seen in the live donor recipients, compared to the peritoneal and hemodialysis groups of patients. In the cadaveric donor group, pre-emptive transplantation was not associated with improved outcome compared to the peritoneal dialysis group. Similar studies by Mahmoud *et al.*[9] support this conclusion, whereas other smaller studies have shown no significant differences following preemptive transplantation.[2]

Mode of dialysis

In their recent review, NAPRTCS showed similar patient survival rates among the peritoneal dialysis, hemodialysis and pre-emptive transplantation groups. Pretransplant dialysis modality (peritoneal dialysis vs. hemodialysis) did not affect the overall graft survival rates. However, graft survival was improved in children who underwent pre-emptive transplantation, primarily in the live donor recipients.[2] Vascular thrombosis appears to be more common following peritoneal dialysis. This association is hypothesized to be related to a hypercoagulable state that is multifactorial related to albumen loss in the peritoneal dialysis fluid, imbalance between procoagulant and fibrinolytic proteins, and altered lipid metabolism.[2]

Donor options for kidney transplantation

Selection of the appropriate donor source for transplantation is a decision for the transplant team and the family to consider together. A related, immediate family member donor kidney has the advantage of a low likelihood of postoperative delayed graft function and also an improved histologic match that may lead to fewer rejection episodes and extended organ function. At present, 60% of children receive a living donor kidney.[5] The major concern of living donation is the risk and morbidity to potential donors. Although mortality is very low, estimated at 0.03%, possible morbidity related to wound complications, perioperative work restrictions, and long-term concerns related to hypertension and future kidney disease must be openly discussed with all potential donors on several occasions prior to proceeding with this significant step to help a relative in need of care.[10] This increasing influence of living donation in pediatric renal transplantation is illustrated in Fig. 64.2.

Living donor nephrectomy employing minimally invasive surgical techniques has been shown to yield allografts for transplant that yield equal success rates when compared to open donor nephrectomy. The potential improvement in postoperative pain, faster work and lifestyle rehabilitation, and shorter possible hospital stay have all combined to encourage living donor availability. Multiple centers have now documented the safety and success of this procedure. However, the health-related contraindications to living donation for laparoscopic and open donation are identical. Therefore, the selection of donors should be undertaken independent of the possibility for minimally invasive donor nephrectomy.

Cadaver kidneys are used in the remaining 40% of pediatric renal transplants at present. Inability to control donor factors and the need to establish a negative antibody crossmatch make surgical planning more difficult with cadaveric donors. However, children are advantaged in the matching system because of their age. Because of the special considerations afforded in pediatric end-stage renal disease patients, children receive additional points in the allocation system. This is stratified by age: 1 to 5 years, 6 to 10 years and 11 to 17 years. This advantage extends further in that there is a time imposed from the time of listing to transplant. If transplant is not done within 6 to 18 months after listing, reassignment to a position higher on the list is done by the UNOS allocation system. This system has contributed significantly to improvement in graft survival rates for children and to decreased waiting times while listed.[11] These advantages in access must be balanced against the health history of the donor, stability and predictability of renal function for the donor organ, and the size/age of both the donor and the recipient.

Post-transplant phase

With improvements in the immunologic and technical aspects of transplantation, the primary risks for allograft failure have changed in contemporary practice. Chronic rejection is now the leading cause of allograft failure, causing 32% of all primary allograft loss. Acute rejection remains the second most common cause (15%). The third most frequent cause is vascular thrombosis, occurring in 12% of primary allografts, and the fourth is recurrent disease (5.9%).[4] A similar profile exists for subsequent allograft failures as well. Overall, 10% of graft loss is caused by non-transplant-related patient death with a functioning allograft in place.

Short-term outcome

Factors affecting patient survival

Pediatric kidney transplantation has shown marked improvement over the years with reduced morbidity and increased graft survival. Patients transplanted since 1995 have 4-year survival rates of 96% for both living donor (LD) and cadaver recipients(CD).[5] Overall, adjusted one and five year patient and allograft survival from the UNOS OPTN / SRTR Registry Annual Report is detailed in Fig. 64.3 (A – patient, B – allograft). Infection, cardiovascular disease and malignancy account for 34%, 15% and 12% of the current patient mortality respectively.[5] Infection continues to be the most frequent cause of death in pediatric kidney transplant recipients. The development of more potent immunosuppressive agents has led to a decrease in acute rejection rates with an associated increase in both early and late infections (Fig. 64.4).[1,5] Infectious death rates related to viral infections as compared to infection of bacterial origin have remained stable.[1]

In the general pediatric population, cardiovascular disease as a cause of death is rare, accounting for less than 1.4 deaths per 100 000 population between the ages of 1 and 14 years.[4] Cardiovascular disease as a cause of death in children with end-stage renal disease is 1000-fold more common, contributing to 25% of pediatric end-stage renal disease deaths.[4] However, USRDS data demonstrate that, in spite of the increased risk of dyslipidemia and hypertension associated with immunosuppression, the risk of death from cardiovascular disease is lower in transplanted children compared to those on dialysis.[12]

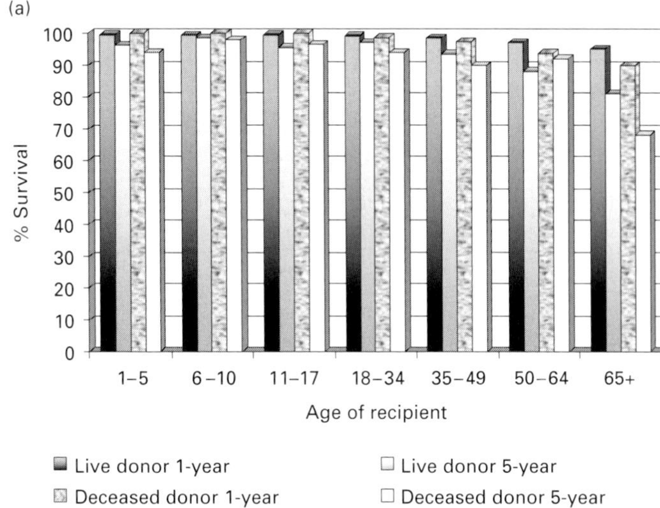

Fig. 64.3(a). Adjusted 1- and 5-year patient survival by recipient age.

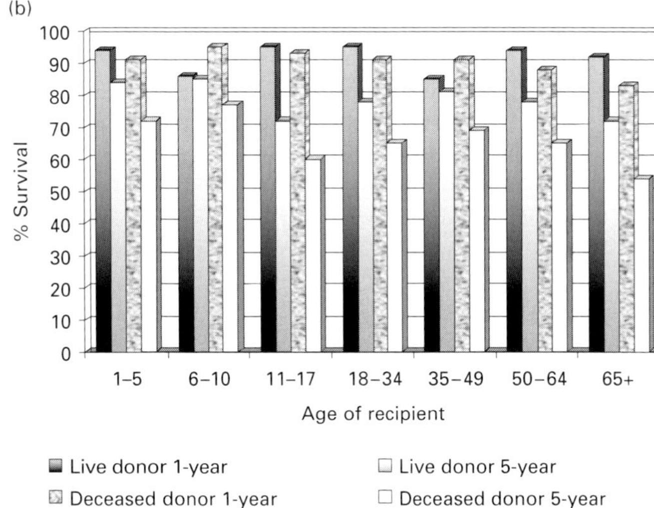

Fig. 64.3(b). Adjusted 1- and 5-year graft survival by recipient age.

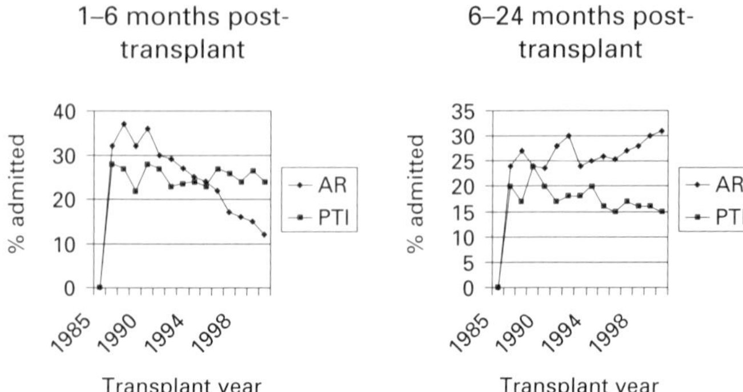

Fig. 64.4. Fall in percent admissions for acute rejection (AR) vs. the increase in admissions for post-transplant infection (PTI)[1].

Table 64.1. Relative risk factors for U.S pediatric renal allograft loss from chronic rejection

	RR increase	p-value	95% CI
First AR	2.9	<0.001	2.0–4.3
>2 AR	4.2	<0.001	3.3–5.3
Late initial AR(>365 days)	2.2	<0.001	1.7–2.9
CD source	1.4	0.002	1.1–1.7
African-American	1.6	<0.001	1.2–2.0
Day 30 CsA dose <5 mg/kg	1.4	0.003	1.1–1.8
Prior transplant	1.5	0.004	1.1–1.9

Risk factors

AR-acute rejection, CD-cadaveric donor, CsA-cyclosporine A, RR-relative risk[14]

Mortality associated with malignancy in pediatric recipients is most commonly secondary to post-transplant lymphoproliferative disease (PTLD). PTLD has been reported to have a prevalence of 1.6% but this may be an underestimate. In more modern cohorts the prevalence may be as high as 10% of transplanted children.[13]

Factors affecting patient morbidity

Acute rejection

With contemporary improvements in immunosuppressive agents, the probability of acute rejection has diminished and the time to the first episode of rejection has lengthened. The 1-year risk of acute rejection has decreased from 57% in live donor recipients and 70% in cadaveric donor graft in 1987 to 32% (LD) and 36% (CD) in the most recent reporting period.[4,5] Risk factors for increased probability of acute rejection continue to be African American race, increasing DR HLA mismatch and lack of induction therapy.[5] Also, current approaches to rejection treatment show improved likelihood of rejection reversal, with complete reversal now achieved in 65% of rejection episodes.[4,5] The frequency of complete reversal decreases with increasing number of rejections, increased recipient age when the time of first rejection episode is greater than 1 year after transplant.[5]

Chronic rejection

Improvements in post-transplant management have made chronic rejection the leading cause of graft loss, now accounting for over 30% of all renal allograft loss.[4,5,14] Over 90% of children losing their transplanted kidney to chronic rejection had at least one prior acute rejection episode, compared to an incidence of only 53% for those who did not lose their grafts to chronic rejection.[14] Similar correlation can be demonstrated for multiple episodes of rejection, 71% and 24%, respectively; and late (> 1 year) initial rejection, 18% and 9%, respectively.[14] Table 64.1 shows the relative risk factors for graft loss from chronic rejection: > 2 episodes of acute rejection and late initial acute rejection being the most significant.[14]

Recurrent disease

Recurrence of the original kidney disease contributes to 6% of allograft losses. The most significant of these in the pediatric population is focal segmental glomerulosclerosis (FSGS). The primary presentation of this disease process often is progressive, steroid-resistant nephrotic syndrome. Primary treatment success is limited and progression to end-stage renal disease occurs in many patients. Despite a variety of treatment regimens, the incidence of patients developing end-stage renal disease and requiring transplantation has not changed.[15] Following renal transplantation, FSGS has been reported to recur in 20% to 50% of patients.[5] Reported risk factors for recurrence include rapid progression from the onset of disease to end-stage renal disease, younger age, mesangial proliferation, and Caucasian race.[15,16] Children with FSGS also have worsened short-term allograft survival rates with twice the rate of primary non-function and early post-transplant acute tubular necrosis. Furthermore, transplanted children do not see the graft survival benefits usually associated with living donor grafts.[4]

Many therapeutic regimes have been examined for FSGS, including high dose cyclosporine, pulse glucocorticoids, cyclophosphamide, plasmapheresis and immunoadsorption with protein A columns. Some single center studies have shown decreased frequency and severity of FSGS recurrence with higher plasma cyclosporine levels; however, other studies have shown no benefit.[4,17]

Some long-lasting remissions have been seen with oral cyclophosphamide therapy.[18] Several reports have documented short-term clinical responses with decreased proteinuria after plasmaphoresis, but these reports do not demonstrate long-term benefits.[17,18] At present, no single intervention has demonstrated reliable success in preventing post-transplant FSGS recurrence.

Hemolytic uremic syndrome (HUS) is the most common cause of acute renal failure in children, accounting for almost 5% of pediatric kidney transplants.[4,5] Classic HUS is associated with *E. coli* 0157:H7 infection, usually causing significant diarrhea. Atypical HUS is not associated with diarrhea and has multiple etiologies including other infection, pregnancy, oral contraception, cyclosporine and familial inheritance. Children with atypical HUS are particularly at risk for end stage renal disease and have up to a 50% recurrence rate after transplantation.[19] However, NAPRTCS data document recurrent HUS in only 8.2% of 68 renal transplanted patients with classical HUS as the primary disease.[5,20]

Infectious complications

Several factors have been shown to increase risk for the development of infectious complications: younger age at transplant, more recent year of transplant, and continued use of antimicrobial prophylaxis at month 6 post-transplant.[1] Female gender is a risk factor for bacterial infections and cadaver donor source is a similar risk factor for viral infections.[1] The use of polyclonal antibody for induction immunosuppression therapy beginning on day 0/1 was also predictive of increased hospitalization rates for infection.[1] Although the percentage of fungal infections has not risen, hospitalization for fungal infection was associated with an increased risk of graft loss.[1]

Infections with agents in the herpesvirus family, especially cytomegalovirus (CMV), varicella zoster virus (VZV), and Epstein–Barr virus (EBV), pose significant risks for patients after renal transplantation. Those who develop their first exposure leading to a primary infection after transplantation are at greater risk for morbidity and mortality. Appropriate use of antiviral medications for prophylaxis and treatment, specifically ganciclovir, has diminished the incidence and morbidity of CMV infections. With rapid recognition of exposure and disease, significant VZV complications can be avoided with the use of varicella zoster immune globulin and acyclovir. Epstein–Barr virus related lymphoproliferative disease is a major complication in pediatric transplantation. Most young children are EBV naïve and experience their first exposure after transplantation or secondary to transplantation with an EBV positive donor organ.

Thrombotic complications

The third leading cause of allograft failure in children is vascular thrombosis, with a rate of 11.6% in the NAPRTCS registry.[5] The same registry also shows that centers with a higher annual transplant volume and therefore more overall experience, report fewer episodes of vascular complications with rates in the range of 2%–6%.[21] Several groups of recipients are at increased risk for developing vascular thrombosis. These are children who are maintained on peritoneal dialysis, recipients less than 2 years of age, recipients whose cadaver donor is less than 5 years of age, recipients of cadaver donors with a cold ischemia time greater than 24 hours, and children who are being retransplanted.[2,4]

Ureteral complications

Ureteral complications can occur at any time after kidney transplantation, but most occur within the first 2 years. These complications are rarely the cause of graft loss although many pediatric recipients have underlying lower urinary tract abnormalities. Urinary leakage occurs in 4 to 4.5% of recipients and ureteral obstruction occurs in up to 3.8% of recipients.[22,23] There does not appear to be a difference in the rate of urologic complications among the different types of ureteral reconstruction: extravesical with or without a stent, and primary ureteroureterostomy.[22–24] Finally, renal transplantation into a dysfunctional lower urinary tract produced a 35% rate of urinary tract complications but no statistical difference in graft survival. Renal allograft survival in those with a normal lower urinary tract is 83% compared to 69% graft survival rate in the dysfunctional lower tract group in one report.[25]

Retransplantation

Graft survival rates for second and subsequent transplants are lower than for the primary kidney transplant. NAPRTCS data show that recipients with prior transplantation have a 28% incidence of delayed graft function vs. 16% for recipients of a primary transplant.[26] Chronic rejection is the leading cause of graft loss in primary transplants with a 32% incidence. Chronic rejection is likely to occur in subsequent transplants at a similar rate, 33%.[5,26] For cadaveric grafts, the relative risk increase for graft failure with a prior kidney transplant is 1.32, an increase similar to that graft loss risk seen in African-Americans.[27]

Long-term outcome

Neurocognitive development

Neurocognitive growth is one of the most critical and unique events of infancy and childhood. The ability to achieve normal development is also a sensitive marker of adequacy of care in children with renal failure. Intensive intervention is often necessary in the pretransplant and post-transplant phases of care to achieve optimal growth and development. Historically, infants with chronic renal disease have had evidence of poor neurocognitive development, manifest as acquired microcephaly, mental and motor developmental deficits, poor school achievement, and delayed separation and maturation during adolescence.[4]

Previous reports have suggested that poor cognitive outcome could be attributed to inadequate nutrition and exposure to aluminum as a phosphate binder.[28] Because half of postnatal brain growth takes place in the first year of life, injury or insult from uremia at this critical developmental stage may be associated with irreversible neurologic and developmental damage. Recently, several reports documenting neurodevelopmental outcomes of children who developed end-stage renal disease in infancy have shown that aggressive nutritional support, the elimination of aluminum as a phosphate binder, effective dialysis and subsequent transplantation all combined to achieve a favorable developmental outcome.[28,29] In selected patients, serial head circumference standard deviation scores improved or remained constant from the initiation of dialysis through the post-transplant period. General mental development was felt to be appropriate in 73%–79% of the patients. When measured, mean IQ scores were 87, and 79% of children tested performed within the average to low average range. Eighty to 94% of these children attended normal schools; however, 13 to 20% required special education classes.[29,30] Psychological outcomes, however, may be less favorable than expected. Over half of the study patients demonstrated emotional and behavioral difficulties when compared to a normal population. Areas of primary concern frequently related to peer relationship difficulties, conduct problems, and hyperactivity behaviors. Although the development of these psychological abnormalities are not the result of single events, the limited opportunities to socialize as a healthy child and to develop appropriate peer relationships, as well as the stress generated within affected families are thought to be significant contributors.[29] The length of time or frequency of admission to the hospital did not correlate with these behavioral abnormalities, suggesting it is more likely the lifestyle effects of chronic childhood illness that are most important.[31]

One would expect that children who have congenital forms of renal disease and onset of renal failure in early childhood would not perform as well on neuropsychological functioning tests as children with later acquired renal failure. Several factors would anticipate this result including: (1) longer exposure to organ failure in infancy; (2) an extended period of poor nutrition and chronic medication need; and (3) earlier exposure to relevant neurotoxins with deleterious impact on the developing nervous system. In addition, patients with acquired disease may have established basic educational fundamentals prior to the development of uremia. When these factors were analyzed by Crocker *et al.*, they found that children with congenital abnormalities leading to end-stage renal disease had significantly more difficulty integrating non-verbal information and long-term memory. In addition, those patients were found to have significantly worse fine motor coordination than those with later onset of acquired renal failure. However, there was no difference between groups with regard to IQ, academic scores, behavior profile, or expressive vocabulary. Furthermore, there was no difference in global self-worth score or self-esteem.[32] The explanations for these observations remain speculative.

Growth

Despite significant improvements in pretransplant management, many children undergoing renal transplantation have significant growth abnormalities. The use of recombinant human growth hormone (rhGH) in single center and multicenter trials consistently led to significant improvements in height velocity and height standard deviation scores.[33] However, despite improvements in renal function following transplantation, many allograft recipient children do not experience improvements in growth status.[4] Patients with severe growth failure prior to transplant have a greater likelihood of experiencing some catch-up growth, and children transplanted at less than 5 years of age also show significant improvement. Older children and adolescents experience no acceleration in height velocity and have persistently low height SD scores. Multiple factors contribute to these observations, but post-transplant immunosuppression and the use of steroids appear to contribute heavily. Other factors include allograft dysfunction, decreased GH/insulin-like growth factor axis function, and renal tubular acidosis. Evidence that alternate day steroid immunosuppression protocols have improved growth velocity without increasing the risk of rejection has been developed in recent years.[34] However, fewer than 30% of patients in the NAPRTCS registry currently receive alternate day steroid therapy. Complete steroid withdrawal, or steroid-free immunosuppressive protocols using IL2r antibody and Sirolimus for induction, all hold hope for decreasing the morbidity of steroids in the future. Building on the success of rhGH therapy pre-transplant, recent open label studies and controlled trials have demonstrated the safety and efficacy of rhGH post-transplant. Improved height velocity and SD scores were achieved without increasing the incidence of acute or chronic rejection.[4] However, patients in these trials who had a history of acute rejection were at higher risk for further episodes of acute rejection with rhGH therapy. As a result of these successes, children transplanted prior to puberty today often achieve normal final adult height.[35,36]

Immunosuppressive-related complications

Post-transplant lymphoproliferative disease (PTLD)

PTLD in renal transplant patients has not historically presented with the same incidence or likelihood of progression that has been noted in other solid organ transplant recipients. However, renewed interest in transplantation of younger children and pre-emptive transplantation, seronegativity for Epstein–Barr virus (EBV) in transplant recipients may increase. In addition, the renewed interest in induction immunotherapy and the use of more potent immunosuppressive agents such as tacrolimus may predispose to higher PTLD risk. In a recent review by NAPRTCS, the overall incidence of PTLD was 1.2%. Although this reflects an overall case rate of 298/100 000 years of post-transplant follow-up, the incidence has increased from 254/100 000 between 1987 and 1991 to 395/100 000 between 1992 to 1996. In addition, the median time to development of PTLD during these sampling frames decreased from a median of 356 days to 190 days. Because of the limited long-term follow-up in the more recent transplant group, the actual incidence of PTLD may be underestimated in this review.[13] Similar to other solid organ transplant experience, and the NAPRTCS database, 66% of children with PTLD were EBV seronegative prior to transplantation, 44% had evidence of previous or concurrent CMV infection.

De novo malignancy

The risk of developing *de novo* malignancy in children undergoing transplantation is becoming an increasingly important concern. *De novo* malignancies in adult recipients of renal transplantation occur with an incidence six to seven times higher than in the general population. This cumulative incidence varies from 2.6% to 19.4% on long-term follow-up, with non-melanoma skin cancers being the most frequent malignancy seen. Although the experience with patients undergoing transplantation in the pediatric age group is less extensive, similar malignancy types and trends have been found. The most common malignancy reported in past pediatric renal allograft recipients was skin cancer (57%). Squamous cell carcinoma of the skin was more common than basal cell carcinoma, with a ratio of 7:3. Non-Hodgkin's lymphoma represents approximately 25% of malignancies and occurred earlier during the follow-up course than expected in the normal population. Potent immunosuppressive regimes and early Epstein–Barr virus infection appear to contribute to this premature onset. These findings suggest a standardized risk (S. R.) of 222 for skin cancer and 46 for non-Hodgkin's lymphoma.[37] As long-term survival increases, surveillance will be more necessary to treat this unintended consequence of immunosuppression.

Chronic rejection

Chronic rejection has become the most common cause of renal allograft loss in recent studies.[38] Although the incidence of acute rejection has decreased secondary to improved initial immunosuppressive protocols, the mechanism of chronic rejection is less well elucidated and potentially beneficial preventive protocols do not presently exist. Non-immunological factors most likely contribute as well.

Factors contributing to the development of chronic renal allograft rejection have been analyzed in a recent NAPRTCS review of patients transplanted prior to 1995 compared to 2777 children transplanted between 1995 and 2000. In past similar reviews, acute rejection, multiple rejections and late acute rejections were risk factors for future graft failure from chronic rejection.[14] This recent large experience confirmed the results of single center adult and European studies where acute rejection was a significant risk for the development of late chronic rejection.[39] When subjected to multivariate analysis and a proportional hazards model, late onset initial acute rejection episodes increased the risk of chronic rejection induced graft failure 3.6-fold, while a second acute rejection episode resulted in further increase of 4.2-fold. When adjusted for acute rejection episodes, cadaveric donor recipients, African-American patients, and patients with more than one transplant were more likely to develop graft failure from chronic rejection. The nature of the primary disease leading to transplantation was not a factor in chronic rejection development.[38,39] This study showed that the relative risk of future chronic rejection in recently transplanted patients was significantly lower ($RR = 0.66$, $P = 0.005$) because of their decreased acute rejection risk.

Health-related quality of life

Health-related quality of life (HRQL) assessment includes multiple issues examined from the patient's perspective, including physical, psychological, and social functioning as well as overall well-being. It is increasingly possible to evaluate diseased age-specific as well as generic HRQL in clinical trials as subjective measures of patients' state of health.

As significant quantitative improvements in patient and renal allograft survival have been achieved, HRQL assessment has become a validated outcome measurement in all areas of transplantation. As a major goal of transplantation is to achieve maximum quality and quantity of life while minimizing the effects of primary renal disease, evaluating these subjective and objective goals is highly relevant in the evaluation of long-term success. However, no single methodology is ideal for measurement of health-related quality of life under all circumstances.

A significant factor in kidney transplant recipient HRQL is the potential adverse effects of immunosuppressive agents. Studies by both Shield and Reimer have shown better physical state and appearance in renal transplant patients receiving Tacrolimus and or cyclosporin.[40] Reasons for these observations apparently include a lower incidence of diabetes, decreased gingival hyperplasia and less hirsutism. In addition, rejection episodes were associated with poorer HRQL scores. Improvements in HRQL were seen after cyclosporin withdrawal.

Although the criteria vary, most studies demonstrate good or excellent HRQL after kidney transplantation. Of 57 long-term survivors of kidney transplantation aged 12 to 38 years studied by Morel *et al.*, 91% rated their health as good to excellent, and 90% were satisfied with their lives.[41] The majority (91%) were satisfied with their ability to perform at work, school, or home; however, 76% were satisfied with their personal relationships. In a similar study, Apajasalo *et al.* found that the overall perceived HRQL for adult and adolescent patients was similarly good.[42] Transplanted adolescents are more optimistic than a reference population. This high HRQL score has also been noted in adolescent populations with other chronic diseases such as myopathy or cystic fibrosis, and may be related to a radical change of adolescent life values imposed by the circumstances of acute and chronic illness.[43] The HRQL of preadolescence transplant patients, however, was significantly lower than for controls, especially in areas related to school and hobbies, friendships, and physical appearance.

Despite this high level of overall satisfaction, several significant issues have been identified among long-term survivors. Academic performance and reintegration into school activities post-transplant represent significant problems for some children. School re-entry is complicated by alterations in physical appearance and heightened self-awareness, especially in adolescence. In a recent review of school performance by NAPRTCS., significantly more transplant recipients did not participate in regular or special classroom learning when compared to controls (30% vs. 9%).[44] There was also a trend toward more behavioral problems (11% vs. 3%) and learning disabilities (24% vs. 13%) in transplant patients compared to sibling controls.[45]

The effects of uremia on the rapidly developing neurologic system during infancy is a significant concern. Satisfactory elementary school performance in children with infant onset uremia who have undergone successful transplantation has been seen; however, special assistance is often necessary: 76% at 10 full-time regular classrooms while 10 and 14%, respectively, require part-time or full-time special assistance. Maths and reading remedial assistance was required in nearly 50% of transplanted children in full-time or part-time regular classrooms. Overall, 21% of post-transplant children were diagnosed with behavioral problems such as aggression, anxiety, depression, or Attention Deficit Disorder. The prevalence of Attention Deficit Disorder was 14%, compared to 3% in a similar general population.[45]

Long-term outcome in renal transplant recipients who underwent transplantation as children between 1967 and 1999 was recently reviewed by Bartosh *et al.*[46] Immunosuppressive complications were common. Nearly half of all respondents were severely short and 27% were obese. More than half of the patients were maintained on antihypertensive medications, hypercholesterolemia was present in 32% and 2% of responding survivors had experienced a marked real myocardial infarction. Hypercholesterolemia has been reported in 51% of long-term pediatric kidney transplant survivors and up to 78% of adult transplant recipients.[47,48] As cardiovascular mortality accounts for nearly half of all deaths among adult patients with functioning renal transplants, this risk among these young transplant recipients is concerning. Hyperparathyroidism, hypertension, abnormal vascular calcification, and altered calcium and phosphorus metabolism contribute to their early and increased risk of coronary artery disease.

In addition to these cardiovascular issues, bone and joint disease and fractures were reported by a majority of these patients, including a disproportionately high incidence of joint symptoms in females, perhaps related to estrogen influence. Cataracts have also been identified in 28 to 56% of long-term pediatric transplant recipients surviving to adulthood.[46] In addition, patients frequently rank decreased sexual interest or ability as common (greater than 60%) and a significant factor in life satisfaction. "Normal" sexual relationships were identified in 42% of adult survivors of pediatric renal transplantation, with unsatisfactory sexual assessment as common in women as in men.[41]

Despite these significant health issues, most renal transplant recipients report their HRQL as good, and describe themselves as being just as or more content than others.

These results correspond to findings in other areas of chronic disease. It appears that the point of reference for standards in life is shifted, meaning that the normal population cannot serve as the only point of comparison for the patient's satisfaction in life.[46]

Health-related quality of life in living donors following renal transplantation

Because of the increasing use of living donation in pediatric transplantation, long-term quality of life assessment among donors assumes evermore importance. There is near consensus that donors have an improved sense of well-being and a boost in self-esteem following organ donation. This perception in donors is independent of the duration of time since donation. The vast majority view the donor experience as a positive one and would readily donate again if possible. A small number (approximately 4%) would not donate again and regret their decision to do so. Overall, relatives other than first-degree and donors whose recipient died within 1 year of transplant were more likely to say they would not donate again. Female donors and those who had perioperative complications were more likely to feel that the donor experience was extremely stressful.[49] When the donor experience was contrasted with the recipient and other third-party family members' view, unique differences were appreciated. All three parties agreed that the donation experience was generally satisfactory and the relationship between the recipient and donor improved after transplantation. However, both recipients and other third-party individuals underestimated the prevalence of donor concerns. Third parties more accurately identified actual donor concerns compared to recipients, perhaps related to limitations in free communication between recipients and prospective donors. Recipients overestimated donor pain and other recovery concerns. Directly addressing these discrepancies may further improve donor acceptance.[50]

Conclusions

Advancements in the management of pediatric end-stage renal disease have led to increasingly successful short- and long-term renal transplant patient and graft survival. Due to the extensive efforts of many organizations, specific factors influencing pre- and postoperative success have been identified and stratified. Future improvements will be based on the ability to modify protocols and address risk factors to successfully bring the advantages of renal transplantation to all individuals with end-stage renal disease. Significant efforts to expand the donor organ pool will be necessary to meet the expanding needs of this population.

REFERENCES

1. Dharnidharka, V. R., Stablein, D. M., & Harmon, W. E. Post-transplant infections now exceed acute rejection as cause for hospitalization: a report of the NAPRTCS. *Am. J. Transpl.* 2004; **4**(3):384–389.
2. Vats, A. N., Donaldson, L., Fine, R. N., & Chavers, B. M. Pretransplant dialysis status and outcome of renal transplantation in North American children: a NAPRTCS Study. North American Pediatric Renal Transplant Cooperative Study. *Transplantation* 2000; **69**(7):1414–1419.
3. Neu, A. M., Ho, P. L., McDonald, R. A., Warady, B. A. Chronic dialysis in children and adolescents. The 2001 NAPRTCS Annual Report. *Pediatr. Nephrol.* 2002; **17**(8):656–663.
4. Benfield, M. R. Current status of kidney transplant: update 2003. *Pediatr. Clin. North Am.* 2003; **50**(6):1301–1334.
5. Benfield, M. R., McDonald, R. A., Bartosh, S. *et al.* Changing trends in pediatric transplantation: 2001 Annual Report of the North American Pediatric Renal Transplant Cooperative Study. *Pediatr. Transpl.* 2003; **7**(4):321–335.
6. Ojogho, O., Sahney, S., Cutler, D. *et al.* Superior long-term results of renal transplantation in children under 5 years of age. *Am. Surg.* 2002; **68**(12):1115–1119.
7. Hidalgo, G., Tejani, C., Clayton, R. *et al.* Factors limiting the rate of living-related kidney donation to children in an inner city setting. *Pediatr. Transpl.* 2001; **5**(6):419–424.
8. Gjertson, D. W. & Cecka, J. M. Determinants of long-term survival of pediatric kidney grafts reported to the United Network for Organ Sharing kidney transplant registry. *Pediatr. Transpl.* 2001; **5**(1):5–15.
9. Mahmoud, A., Said, M. H., Dawahra, M. *et al.* Outcome of preemptive renal transplantation and pretransplantation dialysis in children. *Pediatr. Nephrol.* 1997; **11**(5):537–541.
10. Najarian, J. S., Chavers, B. M., McHugh, L. E., & Matas, A. J. 20 years or more of follow-up of living kidney donors. *Lancet* 1992; **340**(8823):807–810.
11. OPTN/SRTR Annual Report. 2003.
12. Parekh, R. S., Carroll, C. E., Wolfe, R. A., & Port, F. K. Cardiovascular mortality in children and young adults with end-stage kidney disease. *J. Pediatr.* 2002; **141**(2):191–197.
13. Dharnidharka, V. R., Sullivan, E. K., Stablein, D. M. *et al.* Risk factors for posttransplant lymphoproliferative disorder (PTLD) in pediatric kidney transplantation: a report of the North American Pediatric Renal Transplant Cooperative Study (NAPRTCS). *Transplantation* 2001; **71**(8):1065–1068.
14. Tejani, A. & Sullivan, E. K. The impact of acute rejection on chronic rejection: a report of the North American Pediatric Renal Transplant Cooperative Study. *Pediatr. Transpl.* 2000; **4**(2):107–111.

15. Benfield, M. R., McDonald, R., Sullivan, E. K. *et al.* The 1997 Annual Renal Transplantation in Children Report of the North American Pediatric Renal Transplant Cooperative Study (NAPRTCS). *Pediatr. Transpl.* 1999; **3**(2):152–167.
16. Cheong, H. I., Han, H. W., Park, H. W. *et al.* Early recurrent nephrotic syndrome after renal transplantation in children with focal segmental glomerulosclerosis. *Nephrol. Dial. Transpl.* 2000; **15**(1):78–81.
17. Marcen, R., Navarro, J. F., Mampaso, F. *et al.* Recurrence of focal-segmental glomerulosclerosis in kidney transplant patients on ciclosporin. *Nephron* 1994; **68**(4):497–499.
18. Dall'Amico, R., Ghiggeri, G., Carraro, M. *et al.* Prediction and treatment of recurrent focal segmental glomerulosclerosis after renal transplantation in children. *Am. J. Kidney Dis.* 1999; **34**(6):1048–1055.
19. Siegler, R. L. Hemolytic uremic syndrome in children. *Curr. Opin. Pediatr.* 1995; **7**(2):159–163.
20. Quan, A., Sullivan, E. K., & Alexander, S. R. Recurrence of hemolytic uremic syndrome after renal transplantation in children: a report of the North American Pediatric Renal Transplant Cooperative Study. *Transplantation* 2001; **72**(4):742–745.
21. Schurman, S. J., Stablein, D. M., Perlman, S. A., & Warady, B. A. Center volume effects in pediatric renal transplantation. A report of the North American Pediatric Renal Transplant Cooperative Study. *Pediatr. Nephrol.* 1999; **13**(5):373–378.
22. Nuininga, J. E., Feitz, W. F., van Dael, K. C. *et al.* Urological complications in pediatric renal transplantation. *Eur. Urol.* 2001; **39**(5):598–602.
23. Lapointe, S. P., Charbit, M., Jan, D. *et al.* Urological complications after renal transplantation using ureteroureteral anastomosis in children. *J. Urol.* 2001; **166**(3):1046–1048.
24. Khauli, R. Modified extravesical ureteral reimplantation and routine stenting in kidney transplantation. *Transpl. Int.* 2002; **15**(8):411–414.
25. Luke, P. P., Herz, D. B., Bellinger, M. F. *et al.* Long-term results of pediatric renal transplantation into a dysfunctional lower urinary tract. *Transplantation* 2003; **76**(11):1578–1582.
26. Tejani, A. H., Sullivan, E. K., Alexander, S. R. *et al.* Predictive factors for delayed graft function (DGF) and its impact on renal graft survival in children: a report of the North American Pediatric Renal Transplant Cooperative Study (NAPRTCS). *Pediatr. Transpl.* 1999; **3**(4):293–300.
27. Seikaly, M., Ho, P. L., Emmett, L., & Tejani, A. The 12th Annual Report of the North American Pediatric Renal Transplant Cooperative Study: renal transplantation from 1987 through 1998. *Pediatr. Transpl.* 2001; **5**(3):215–231.
28. Warady, B. A., Belden, B., & Kohaut, E. Neurodevelopmental outcome of children initiating peritoneal dialysis in early infancy. *Pediatr. Nephrol.* 1999; **13**(9):759–765.
29. Qvist, E., Pihko, H., Fagerudd, P. *et al.* Neurodevelopmental outcome in high-risk patients after renal transplantation in early childhood. *Pediatr. Transpl.* 2002; **6**(1):53–62.
30. Ehrich, J. H., Rizzoni, G., Broyer, M. *et al.* Rehabilitation of young adults during renal replacement therapy in Europe. 2. Schooling, employment, and social situation. *Nephrol. Dial. Transpl.* 1992; **7**(7):579–586.
31. Madden, S. J., Ledermann, S. E., Guerrero-Blanco, M. *et al.* Cognitive and psychosocial outcome of infants dialysed in infancy. *Child Care Health Dev.* 2003; **29**(1):55–61.
32. Crocker, J. F., Acott, P. D., Carter, J. E. *et al.* Neuropsychological outcome in children with acquired or congenital renal disease. *Pediatr. Nephrol.* 2002; **17**(11):908–912.
33. Fine, R. N., Kohaut, E., Brown, D. *et al.* Long-term treatment of growth retarded children with chronic renal insufficiency, with recombinant human growth hormone. *Kidney Int.* 1996; **49**(3):781–785.
34. Jabs, K., Sullivan, E. K., Avner, E. D., & Harmon, W. E. Alternate-day steroid dosing improves growth without adversely affecting graft survival or long-term graft function. A report of the North American Pediatric Renal Transplant Cooperative Study. *Transplantation* 1996; **61**(1):31–36.
35. Fine, R. N., Ho, M., & Tejani, A. The contribution of renal transplantation to final adult height: a report of the North American Pediatric Renal Transplant Cooperative Study (NAPRTCS). *Pediatr. Nephrol.* 2001; **16**(12):951–956.
36. Fine, R. N., Stablein, D., Cohen, A. H. *et al.* Recombinant human growth hormone post-renal transplantation in children: a randomized controlled study of the NAPRTCS. *Kidney Int.* 2002; **62**(2):688–696.
37. Coutinho, H. M., Groothoff, J. W., Offringa, M. *et al.* De novo malignancy after paediatric renal replacement therapy. *Arch. Dis. Child.* 2001; **85**(6):478–483.
38. Tejani, A., Ho, P. L., Emmett, L., & Stablein, D. M. Reduction in acute rejections decreases chronic rejection graft failure in children: a report of the North American Pediatric Renal Transplant Cooperative Study (NAPRTCS). *Am. J. Transpl.* 2002; **2**(2):142–7.
39. Guyot, C., Nguyen, J. M., Cochat, P. *et al.* Risk factors for chronic rejection in pediatric renal allograft recipients. *Pediatr. Nephrol.* 1996; **10**(6):723–727.
40. Fiebiger, W., Mitterbauer, C., & Oberbauer, R. Health-related quality of life outcomes after kidney transplantation. *Health Qual. Life Outcomes* 2004; **2**(1):2.
41. Morel, P., Almond, P. S., Matas, A. J. *et al.* Long-term quality of life after kidney transplantation in childhood. *Transplantation* 1991; **52**(1):47–53.
42. Apajasalo, M., Rautonen, J., Sintonen, H., & Holmberg, C. Health-related quality of life after organ transplantation in childhood. *Pediatr. Transpl.* 1997; **1**(2):130–137.
43. Manificat, S., Dazord, A., Cochat, P. *et al.* Quality of life of children and adolescents after kidney or liver transplantation: child, parents and caregiver's point of view. *Pediatr. Transpl.* 2003; **7**(3):228–235.
44. Smith, J. M. & McDonald, R. A. Progress in renal transplantation for children. *Adv. Ren. Replace. Ther.* 2000; **7**(2):158–171.
45. Davis, I. D. Pediatric renal transplantation: back to school issues. *Transpl. Proc.* 1999; **31**(4A):61S–62S.
46. Bartosh, S. M., Leverson, G., Robillard, D., & Sollinger, H. W. Long-term outcomes in pediatric renal transplant recipients

who survive into adulthood. *Transplantation* 2003; **76**(8):1195–1200.
47. Sharma, A. K., Myers, T. A., Hunninghake, D. B. *et al.* Hyperlipidemia in long-term survivors of pediatric renal transplantation. *Clin. Transpl.* 1994; **8**(3 Pt 1):252–257.
48. Appel, G. Lipid abnormalities in renal disease. *Kidney Int.* 1991; **39**(1):169–183.
49. Johnson, E. M., Anderson, J. K., Jacobs, C. *et al.* Long-term follow-up of living kidney donors: quality of life after donation. *Transplantation* 1999; **67**(5):717–721.
50. Burroughs, T. E., Waterman, A. D., & Hong, B. A. One organ donation, three perspectives: experiences of donors, recipients, and third parties with living kidney donation. *Prog. Transpl.* 2003; **13**(2):142–150.

65

Liver transplantation

Paolo Muiesan and Nigel D. Heaton

Liver Transplant Surgical Services, Institute of Liver Studies, King's College Hospital, London, UK

Historical aspects

Over the past 40 years, orthotopic liver transplantation (OLT) has evolved from an experimental procedure to a routine treatment of end-stage liver failure in children. The first attempt at pediatric liver transplantation by Thomas Starzl in 1963[1] was not successful but 4 years later he reported the first survivor. These early liver transplants were in high-risk recipients and hemorrhage, coagulopathy, and poor graft function resulted in significant intraoperative and early postoperative mortality. Prednisolone and azathioprine were the primary immunosuppressive drugs but some regimens included combinations of cyclophosphamide, antilymphocyte globulin, splenectomy, total body irradiation, and thymectomy. Despite advances in surgical techniques, 1-year survival after liver transplantation remained poor and by 1978 was only 30%.

The introduction of the immunosuppressant, cyclosporin, into clinical practice in 1979 transformed the outcome after OLT. Cyclosporin acts by blocking lymphocyte production of interleukin-2 and other cytokines thereby reducing the incidence and severity of acute cellular rejection. The combination of cyclosporin and corticosteroids resulted in a marked increase in graft and patient survival and reduced the need for long-term use of high dose steroids with their attendant side effects. The National Institute of Health consensus conference in 1983 concluded that liver transplantation for end-stage liver disease deserved broad application as a therapeutic option rather than an experimental procedure.[2]

The development of newer immunosuppressive drugs, refinements in operative techniques, improved organ preservation and donor management and advances in anesthetic and intensive care have contributed further to improvements in recipient survival. University of Wisconsin (UW) preservative solution became available for clinical use in 1988 and extended cold preservation of the liver graft for up to 20 hours. The success of liver transplantation has led to a broadening of the indications for treatment and increasing demand resulting in a shortage of size matched donor organs for children. Consequently, surgical techniques have been developed in which adult livers are cut down to fit small children; these have increased the potential pool of donors and reduced waiting list mortality. Earlier referral, improved pretransplant nutritional management, and increasing experience in managing postoperative and immunosuppression-related complications have also helped to improve outcomes. The current 1-year survival of children undergoing liver transplantation for chronic liver disease is 85–95%, with the majority of recipients enjoying a good quality of life.

Indications and contraindications

Indications

Any child with a life-threatening liver disorder should be considered for liver transplantation. The indications can be summarized as follows.

Chronic liver disease

Liver transplantation should be considered in any child with end-stage liver disease and a predicted survival

Pediatric Surgery and Urology: Long-term Outcomes, Mark Stringer, Keith Oldham, Pierre Mouriquand.

of less than 1 year. Poor synthetic function (abnormal clotting, low serum albumin, ascites); disordered metabolism (jaundice, encephalopathy, loss of muscle mass, osteoporosis); portal hypertension (variceal bleeding, ascites); lethargy, and intractable pruritus may all be indications for transplantation.[3] Extrahepatic manifestations of liver disease such as hepatopulmonary syndrome or pulmonary hypertension may also be indications for transplantation even in the presence of adequate liver function.

The timing of transplantation is important. Too early jeopardizes the child's life unnecessarily. Too late and the chances of success are reduced. There are a number of factors including the etiology of the underlying liver disease, age, quality of life, severe growth retardation, increased hepatic artery resistance index, and past medical/surgical history, which have been suggested as guides to the timing of transplantation. Biliary atresia is the most common indication, accounting for approximately half of all cases. It is now accepted that a single attempt at portoenterostomy is worthwhile but if it fails, liver transplantation is indicated. Inborn errors of metabolism resulting in cirrhosis, including Wilson's disease and alpha-1-antitrypsin deficiency, constitute the second most common indication. Approximately 100 children are transplanted each year in the United Kingdom for a variety of disorders listed in Table 65.1.

Table 65.1. Indications for pediatric liver transplantation

Cholestatic diseases	
Biliary atresia	
Sclerosing cholangitis	
Alagille's syndrome	
Familial cholestasis	
Metabolic diseases	
Byler's disease	
Wilson's disease	
Alpha-1-antitrypsin deficiency	
Crigler-Najjar type I	
Glycogen storage disease types I, III, and IV	
Tyrosinemia	
Miscellaneous	
Chronic active hepatitis	
Acute liver failure	
Neonatal hepatitis	
Tumors	
Budd–Chiari syndrome	
Congenital hepatic fibrosis	
Acute liver failure	
Viral hepatitis	– Seronegative
	– Hepatitis A
	– Hepatitis B
Wilson's disease	
Congenital hemochromatosis	
Drug/toxin induced	– Paracetamol (acetaminophen) toxicity
	– Halothane
	– Carbamazepine
	– Antituberculous drugs
	– Amanita phalloides poisoning

Acute liver failure

Acute liver failure is a rare but severe illness associated with a significant mortality. A variety of causes have been identified (Table 65.1). The commonest cause is cryptogenic which may be associated with subsequent bone marrow failure. Paracetamol (acetaminophen) toxicity and, more recently, ecstasy in adolescents are less common causes. Viruses, antituberculous drugs, non-steroidal anti-inflammatory agents, and antiepileptic drugs are other recognized causes. Direct toxic injury can occur with Amanita phalloides poisoning. Other potential causes include Wilson's disease, tyrosinemia type 1, autoimmune hepatitis, and congenital hemochromatosis. Hemophagocytosis must be excluded prior to listing for transplantation.

The prognostic indicators and criteria for listing for liver transplantation in children with acute liver are not as clearly defined as in the adult population.[4] Poor prognosis is predicted by the presence of encephalopathy, severe metabolic acidosis, cardiovascular instability, a rapidly shrinking liver, and the presence of renal failure.[5] Most importantly, an international normalized ratio (INR) greater than 4 carries a mortality of more than 80% without transplantation.

Contraindications

These continue to evolve as surgical and medical expertise improves. Absolute contraindications to transplantation are few, but include overwhelming bacterial, fungal, or viral sepsis outside the liver, severe cardiovascular disease, extrahepatic malignancy, and certain inherited diseases with multisystem involvement, such as respiratory chain disorders. HIV positivity is not a contraindication because of the efficacy of the highly active antiretroviral therapy. Previous contraindications including portal vein thrombosis, congenital anomalies such as absence of the inferior vena cava, and previous extensive abdominal surgery are no longer considered a bar to liver transplantation.

Psychosocial issues may complicate candidacy for transplantation particularly if there are problems with non-compliance.

Operative techniques

Donor liver procurement

Liver grafts come from living donors, cadaveric heart beating (brainstem dead) donors, or non-heart-beating donors. Causes of brainstem death include head injury, spontaneous intracranial bleed, anoxia, meningitis, or primary brain tumor. Non-heart beating donor (NHBD) livers have rarely been used in children, since worldwide experience is still limited. Our early experience in seven children with livers from controlled NHBD is promising with 100% graft and patient survival, albeit with relatively short follow-up. There are few absolute contraindications to organ donation: malignancy (excluding primary cerebral tumors); active systemic infection; hepatitis B, C and HIV infection; chronic liver disease; and prion infections such as Jakob–Creutzfeldt disease.

There are no selection criteria which will guarantee good graft function. Risk factors which increase the risk of graft dysfunction or non-function include age over 50 years, prolonged cardiac or respiratory arrest, use of vasopressors, intensive care stay of greater than 5 days, particularly in the absence of enteral feeding and fatty infiltration of the liver. For NHBD livers, a warm ischemic time of more than 30 minutes should be avoided and cold ischemia should be kept as short as possible. The most reliable method of assessing a potential liver graft is examination by an experienced transplant surgeon. Abnormalities of routine liver function tests do not by themselves predict graft function and survival.[6]

Donors should have satisfactory liver function tests and negative virology for hepatitis A, B, C, and HIV. Cytomegalovirus (CMV) antibodies are also tested. The majority of cadaveric donor livers are removed as part of a multiorgan retrieval.[3] The procedure for non-heart beating donation is a modification of the super rapid technique described by Casavilla *et al.*[7]

Orthotopic liver replacement

The recipient hepatectomy may be more difficult in children who have undergone previous surgery such as a Kasai portoenterostomy because of the presence of adhesions and portal hypertension. The abdomen is opened through a bilateral subcostal muscle cutting incision using diathermy. Occasionally, it is extended vertically in the midline to the xiphoid process for further exposure. Following division of adhesions, the porta hepatis is dissected to ligate and divide the common bile duct or previous Roux-en-Y loop and common hepatic artery. The portal vein is skeletonized and liver mobilization is then completed. Vascular clamps are placed on the portal vein and inferior vena cava above and below the liver, which is then excised.

The supra- and infrahepatic vena cava are anastomosed using a continuous or interrupted everting suture to ensure endothelial apposition. Residual preservative solution is flushed from the graft. The portal vein is anastomosed and following reperfusion of the liver, the gallbladder is removed. The donor hepatic artery is anastomosed to the recipient common hepatic artery using fine interrupted sutures. If the native artery is small or has a poor flow, an infrarenal donor iliac conduit may be used to re-arterialize the graft (Fig. 65.1). Splenic artery ligation has also been used to improve hepatic arterial inflow without apparent complication.

Biliary drainage is established either by primary end-to-end anastomosis of the bile duct using interrupted 6/0 PDS sutures or by Roux-en-Y hepaticojejunostomy. After securing hemostasis, one or two tube drains are inserted and the abdomen is closed with absorbable sutures.

Liver reduction techniques

Liver reduction techniques were developed to expand the donor pool available for pediatric transplantation.[8] Reduction techniques are based on the segmental anatomy of the liver and can be used to produce three basic types of liver graft of differing size. The left lateral segment (Fig. 65.2) (segments II and III), comprises 25 to 30% of the whole liver and allows a size reduction from donor to recipient of up to 10:1. Use of a left lobe (segments I–IV), provides a size reduction of 3:1 and the right lobe (segments V–VIII), of 1.5:1.

The liver reduction can be performed in one of two ways: as a bench procedure with the liver immersed in cold (4 °C) UW solution (ex situ) or performing the division at the time of donor surgery (in situ). In using the right or left lobe of the liver, the parenchymal transection is along the principal plane slightly to the left or right of the middle hepatic vein, respectively. The structures of the portal triad can be transected within the parenchyma. The donor vena cava is left with the index lobe and the residual liver is discarded. After division, the cut surface is tested for leaks by perfusing the portal vein, hepatic artery and bile duct and these are oversewn. Right or left lobes are implanted in a similar fashion to a whole graft. Transplantation of the left lateral segment involves resecting the recipient's native liver off the inferior vena cava which is left in situ and the graft is *piggybacked* onto the cava by anastomosing the donor left hepatic vein to a common orifice of the recipient hepatic veins (Fig. 65.3). These techniques have significantly

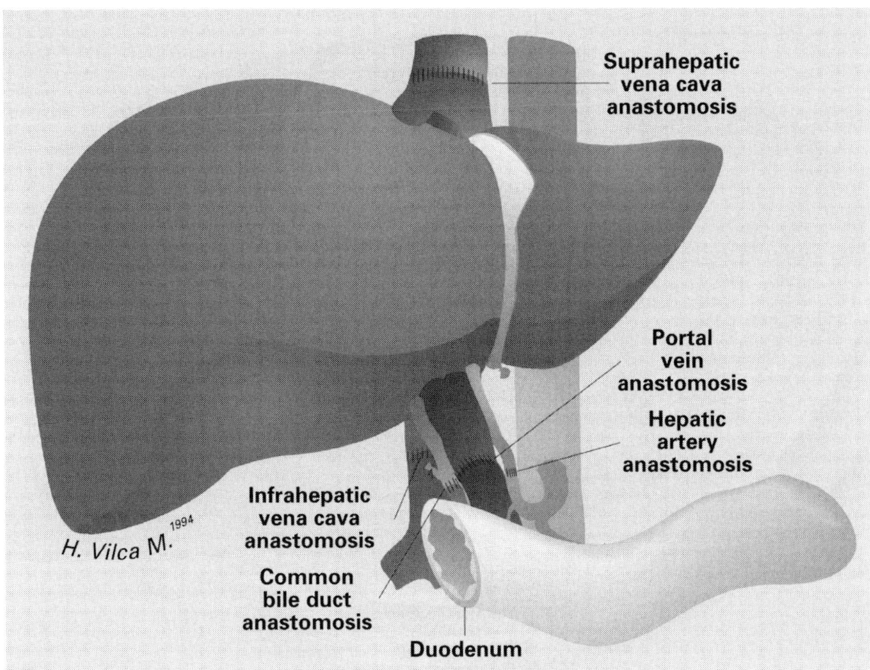

Fig. 65.1. Standard orthotopic liver replacement showing the anastomoses that have to be performed.

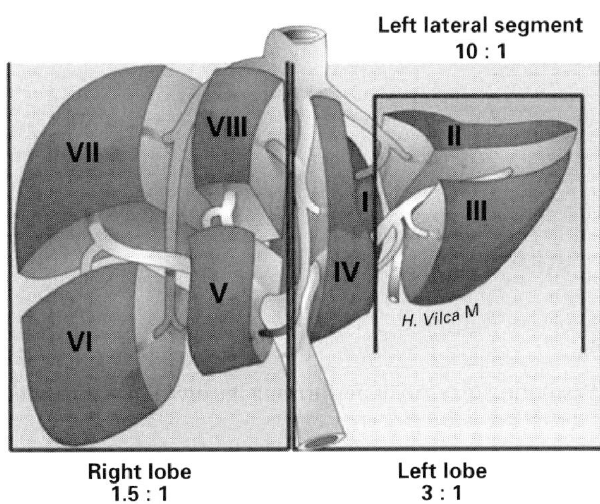

Fig. 65.2. Segmental nature of the liver, showing segments II and III which together comprise the left lateral segment graft.

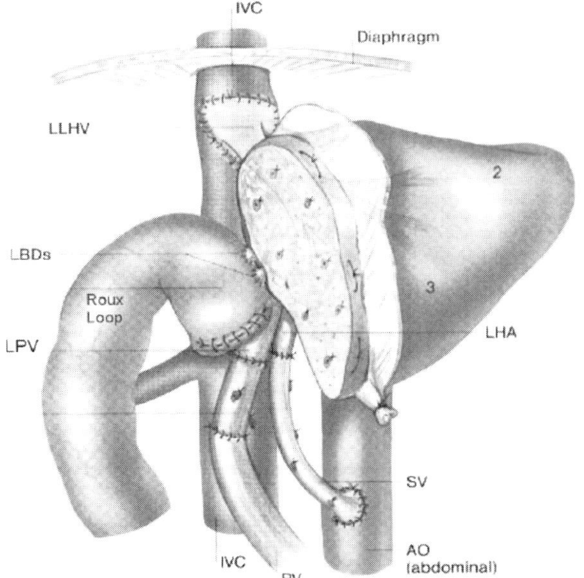

Fig. 65.3. Left lateral segment transplant piggybacked onto the native inferior vena cava.

reduced transplant waiting times for small children but, in recent years, liver reduction has been progressively abandoned in favor of liver splitting to maximize the liver donor pool.

Split liver transplantation

Familiarity with the techniques of liver reduction led to liver splitting, which provides two grafts, a left lateral segment for a child and a right lobe for an adult (Fig. 65.4). The first attempt at splitting a liver ex situ was by Pichlmayr in 1988; the left lateral segment was transplanted into a 2-year-old child who died 4 months later but the right lobe recipient

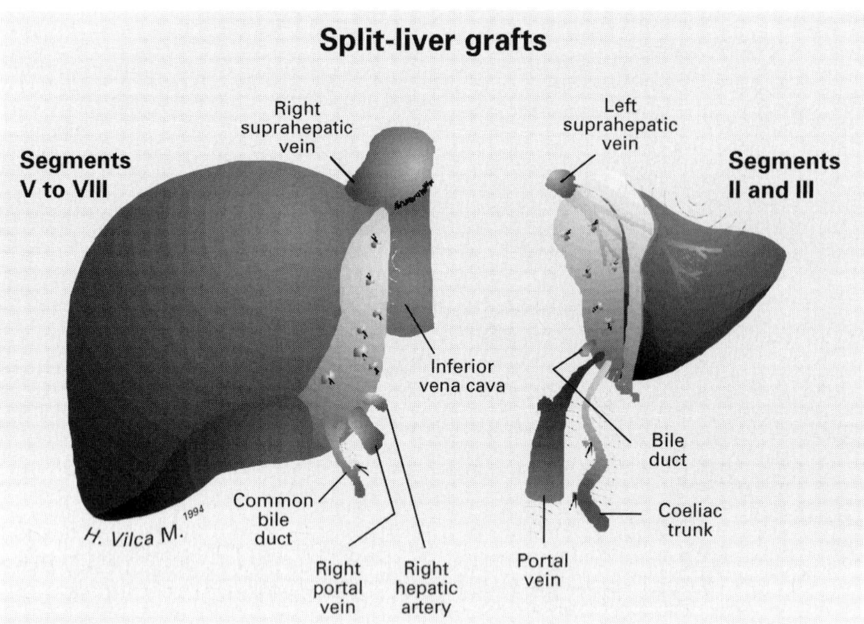

Fig. 65.4. Split liver transplantation to show the two grafts with segment IV discarded.

has survived for more than 15 years. Approximately 90% of livers have favorable vascular and biliary anatomy for splitting. The results of 80 pediatric split liver transplants in our unit showed a 93% patient and 89% graft actuarial survival at 1 year and outcome continues to improve.[9] Centers performing in situ splitting have published comparable outcomes. In situ splitting helps the logistics of organ sharing and also secures cut surface hemostasis at retrieval, but requires a more experienced surgical team and a longer donor operation. Early attempts at split liver transplantation were met with numerous vascular and biliary complications but, with increasing surgical expertise, the morbidity and mortality approaches that obtained with whole liver transplantation.

Living donor liver transplantation

Living donor liver transplantation (LDLT) was first performed in Brazil by Raia *et al.*[10] The technique was popularized in Japan and Chicago to overcome a shortage of pediatric grafts in the late 1980s.[11,12] The left lateral segment of the liver and its associated blood vessels are removed from a parent and transplanted into their child. In countries such as Japan, which until recently had no brainstem death legislation, LDLT has been the only way of performing transplantation. Over 2000 left lateral segment LDLT have been performed with a donor mortality of approximately 0.2%. The reported morbidity of 5% includes bile leak, hemorrhage, splenectomy, small bowel obstruction, incisional hernia, deep vein thrombosis, and pulmonary embolism.

One advantage of LDLT is that it can be performed as an elective procedure thus avoiding prolonged waiting times. The donor is carefully assessed to ensure size and blood group compatibility as well as fitness for surgery.

The live donor's left lateral segment is removed through a bilateral subcostal incision. The left lobe of the liver is mobilized and the left hepatic vein and left portal triad structures are isolated. The liver parenchyma is divided to the right of the falciform ligament and vascular and biliary radicles are ligated. The bile duct and blood vessels are transected after the parenchymal dissection is completed and the liver graft is then perfused with cold UW solution. Subsequent implantation is identical to that for the cadaveric left lateral segmental graft.

Living donor liver grafts have excellent early graft function and the recipient's hospital stay is shorter than after a cadaveric transplant. The incidence of acute rejection is no different from cadaveric grafts, but chronic rejection appears to be less common and it has been suggested that tolerance is more likely in this group of transplant recipients. Reported 1-year patient survival ranges from

Table 65.2. Audit of the Royal College of Surgeons of England: data on early survival after liver transplantation in children at King's College Hospital

		3 months	1 year
Elective transplantation	**289**	95.1%	93.6%
Urgent transplantation	**63**	82.5%	80.9%
Retransplantation	**44**	86.4%	77%

90% to 100%.[13] Whilst LDLT is an alternative for families, it should represent a second-line option in countries where cadaveric split liver grafts are available. Pediatric LDLT also offers a solution for some critically ill children with acute liver failure or decompensated chronic liver disease when the window of opportunity for transplantation is small.[14,15]

The first year after liver transplantation

Survival and early mortality

Overall survival after liver transplantation has improved progressively. One-year survival in 1982 was 35%[16] but it had improved dramatically to 85% by 1991. The majority of deaths occur within the first 3 months. Shaw *et al.* reported that 43% of their pediatric deaths after OLT occurred within 1 month[17], and Busuttil *et al.* 86% within 5 months.[18] During the late 1980s, mortality on the waiting list for liver transplantation was as high as 25% in some centers as a result of the shortage of size-matched donors.[19] The introduction of reduced, split and living related liver transplantation led to a significant and sustained fall in waiting list deaths to approximately 4%.[20] The data from King's College Hospital regarding early survival after liver transplantation in children are shown in Table 65.2.

Infection is the single most important cause of early mortality accounting for approximately 60% of all deaths.[21,22] Surgical complications such as hepatic artery thrombosis and primary graft dysfunction, together with recipient age and size, and status at transplantation all have an impact on early survival. In contrast to adults, pretransplant nutritional status appears to have a lesser impact on survival.[23] Transplantation for acute liver failure is associated with a mortality of approximately 20% within the first 3 months of transplantation. Although results are improving, survival after emergency transplantation in small children and infants is slightly less than in older children (Figs 65.5 and 65.6).

Complications

Primary non-function (PNF)

Primary non-function occurs in fewer than 5% of pediatric liver transplants (range 0%–16%).[24] The incidence is lower after living donor and split liver transplantation probably because of donor selection, graft quality and short cold ischemic time which tend to minimize reperfusion injury.[25] The only treatment for PNF is emergency retransplantation which, despite improvements in care, has at least a 50% mortality.[26] A variety of factors tend to contribute to PNF including the nature and mode of donor death, length of donor stay on intensive care, organ preservation and retrieval techniques, and technical or immunologic complications in the recipient.

Early graft function is assessed by hemodynamic stability of the patient, early production of bile, correction of lactic acidosis, normal blood glucose levels and improvement in coagulopathy. Daily laboratory monitoring of INR, liver function tests (particularly aspartate transaminase (AST) levels) and serum creatinine is essential. Signs of poor graft function include hemodynamic instability requiring inotrope support, persistent or increasing acidosis and bleeding due to coagulopathy. An INR greater than 4 and first day AST levels of greater than 2000 IU/l reflect major parenchymal injury, but even levels of more than 5000 IU/l may settle and be associated with good long-term graft function. From 48 hours post-transplant, daily halving of the serum AST levels indicates recovery from preservation and reperfusion injuries. The arterial ketone body ratio has been used to predict graft recovery in children. Early graft dysfunction, with a ratio of more than 1 within 40 hours of reperfusion, is associated with a good outcome.[27] Recently, indocyanine green pulse oximetry has been used to assist in monitoring graft function.

Postoperative bleeding

Postoperative bleeding occurs in less than 5% of patients and its incidence has steadily decreased in recent years. Risk factors for bleeding include poor graft function, pre- and post-transplant renal failure, high intraoperative blood loss and hemodiafiltration. Correction of coagulopathy or thrombocytopenia will often lead to hemostasis. Bleeding from the cut surface of a segmental graft may be a sign of venous outflow obstruction. In over 50% of cases explored for postoperative hemorrhage no specific bleeding point is identified.

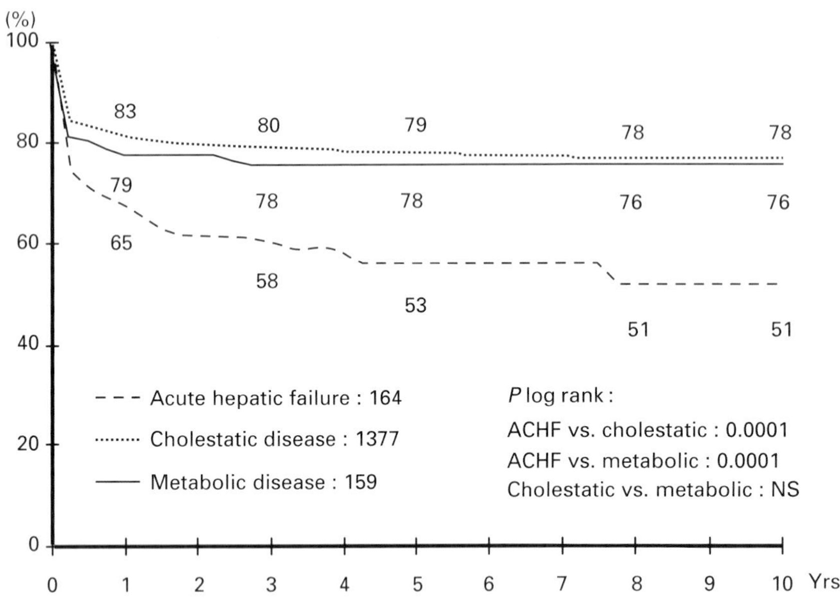

Fig. 65.5. ELTR data (1988–2002) for survival of children <2 years according to the first indication.

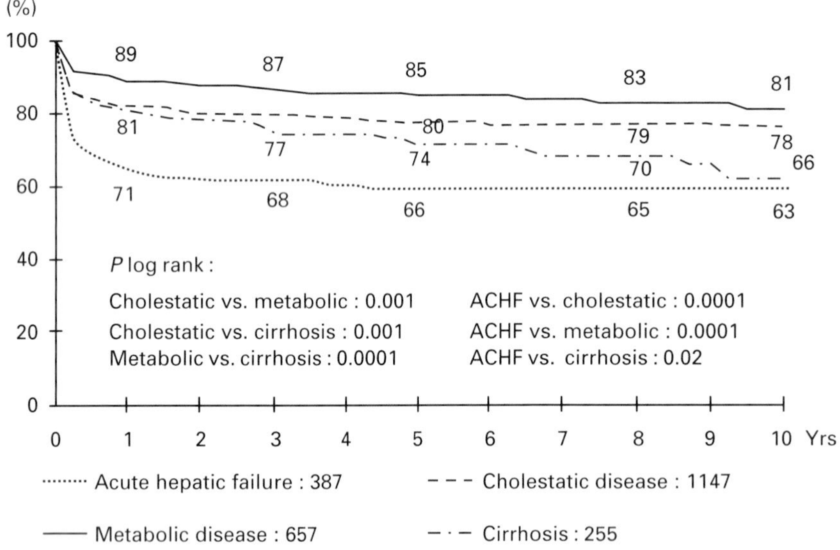

Fig. 65.6. ELTR data (1988–2002) for survival of children ≥ 2 years according to the main indication.

Vascular

Hepatic artery thrombosis

Hepatic artery thrombosis (HAT) is the most serious technical complication as the transplanted liver is initially critically dependent on an intact arterial inflow. The reported incidence is approximately 3% in adults and 7–8% in children.[28,29] It may present insidiously, with fever, cholangitis or with a biliary leak, stricture or abscess formation. In 'missed' cases it may give rise to hepatic necrosis progressing rapidly to death in the absence of retransplantation.

The diagnosis may be suspected on routine Doppler ultrasonography if the hepatic artery is not visualized or if the arterial waveform is abnormal. Confirmation of the diagnosis is by conventional arteriography or CT angiography.[30] Using a selective policy of retransplantation, revascularization, and conservative treatment, more than 80% of children survive HAT. The cautious use of fibrinolytics via interventional radiology or at the time of surgical thrombectomy may improve revascularization rates of those cases that are detected early. Approximately 40% of children with HAT survive without needing retransplantation due to the development of a satisfactory collateral supply to the graft. This collateral arterialization seems to be more effective in segmental as opposed to whole liver grafts, and when a Roux loop has been used for biliary drainage. The administration of hyperbaric oxygen has been used to try and salvage the graft but without much success.[28]

Risk factors for HAT include small vessel size particularly with whole grafts, faulty placement of sutures, intimal dissection and inappropriate angulation at the anastomotic site.[31] Medical factors associated with increased risk include an underlying prothrombotic disorder, elevated hematocrit, severe acute rejection and prolonged cold preservation.

Late hepatic artery thrombosis may present several years after transplantation. These may represent missed cases where collateralization has been rapid or mistaken for a damped signal and the intrahepatic arterial supply has reconstituted. Late presentation is often subtle with mild liver dysfunction, biliary stricture, recurrent low-grade cholangitis, bacteremia or evidence of centrilobular hepatocyte fallout on liver biopsy. The majority are managed successfully by conservative means, but whether these grafts will function satisfactorily in the very long term is unknown. Late hepatic artery thrombosis may have a more aggressive course with the development of intrahepatic biliary necrosis requiring retransplantation; a procoagulant defect such as antiphospholipid syndrome should be excluded in these cases.[32]

Hepatic artery stenosis has been reported in 5% to 10% of transplants and successful management has been reported with angioplasty. Some cases continue to have cholangitis or graft dysfunction and eventually come to retransplantation.

Portal vein thrombosis/stenosis and portal hypertension
Portal vein thrombosis is an uncommon complication after adult liver transplantation (with an incidence of less than 2%), but may occur in up to 33% of high-risk pediatric liver transplant recipients.[33] Risk factors include a hypoplastic portal vein, the use of whole liver grafts, hemoconcentration, hypercoagulability, severe acute rejection and elective splenectomy after transplantation. The manifestations of early portal vein thrombosis include a prolonged INR, a persistent metabolic acidosis and, in severe cases, a rise in the AST. Urgent re-exploration and revision of the portal vein anastomosis will usually rescue the graft. Systemic fibrinolysis has been used to treat recurrent thrombosis.

Late portal vein complications are increasingly recognized and reported in children. Presentation is with clinical features of portal hypertension, particularly variceal hemorrhage, ascites and increasing splenomegaly. The underlying cause may be technical or due to other factors such as late rejection or biliary sepsis. The risks of early and late portal vein thrombosis and stenosis after living donor transplantation are higher than after segmental cadaveric graft transplantation (up to 4% of cases).[34] The short length of the living donor left portal vein is probably a contributory factor; this may become stretched after regeneration and remodeling of the graft. Use of cryopreserved donor iliac or femoral vein substantially increases the risk of late thrombosis (up to 50%).[35]

Spleen size is often a good guide to the continuing presence or development of portal hypertension post-transplant. A low platelet count and mild prolongation of the INR are indirect indicators of portal hypertension. Provided liver function is otherwise satisfactory then graft and patient survival, at least over 5 years, is excellent. The majority of children develop venous collaterals that sustain the graft. Different strategies have been used to deal with portal vein stenosis including percutaneous angioplasty with or without stenting. Late portal vein thrombosis can be managed with beta-blockers and endoscopic treatment of esophageal varices. If gastrointestinal bleeding recurs a distal splenorenal shunt can be performed. Alternatively, in cases with a patent intrahepatic portal system the Rex shunt (mesenterico-left portal bypass) can effectively cure the problem by restoring normal portal inflow to the graft.[36] Any procoagulant disorder must be identified beforehand so that appropriate prophylactic anticoagulation is given postoperatively.

A further cause of recurrent late portal hypertension is the development of nodular regenerative hyperplasia (NRH). Previously, NRH was considered a complication of long-term azathioprine administration[37] but in children it is most commonly associated with portal or hepatic vein complications and prothrombotic disorders. The typical appearance is that of multiple hyperplastic parenchymal nodules similar to those seen in cirrhosis, but without perinodular fibrosis. Affected children present approximately 5 years after transplantation with ascites, edema and bleeding esophageal varices. Although the gamma glutamyltranspeptidase (γGT) and alkaline phosphatase may be elevated, liver function tests are often normal. Histology may show features of venous outflow obstruction. Those with symptomatic portal hypertension should be considered for a portosystemic shunt, such as a distal splenorenal or mesocaval shunt. A good outcome without major graft dysfunction has been reported in the short to medium term but there is a small subgroup of children who develop progressive graft failure and require retransplantation.

Caval obstruction

Caval complications are uncommon and usually due to technical problems. Suprahepatic caval stenosis presents with lower trunk and leg edema and signs of portal hypertension with ascites, renal impairment, liver dysfunction and splenomegaly. Doppler ultrasound and cavography with pressure measurements will confirm a significant gradient across the stenosis. Percutaneous venoplasty or stenting may lead to dramatic resolution as seen in one of our children when the sudden restoration of venous return precipitated acute cardiac failure. When stenting is required, care must be taken to position the stent so that it does not interfere with potential future surgery. Late complications are infrequent but their incidence appears to be increased with the use of the piggyback technique both in the setting of reduced and whole grafts, and particularly after retransplantation.[35] We have also seen late caval obstruction from probable torsion at the level of the caval anastomosis after graft remodeling.

Biliary

Traditionally, biliary complications have been the Achilles heel of liver transplantation with a high incidence in pediatric recipients (5%–30%); the overall incidence is about 10%. In addition to an anastomotic bile leak or stricture segmental grafts are also at risk of a bile leak from their cut surface. Better knowledge of segmental vascular and biliary anatomy enabling preservation of ductal blood supply and meticulous identification and closure of biliary radicles on the cut surface have contributed to a significant reduction in the incidence of biliary complications. Despite this, biliary complications have been reported in up to one-third of children after living related left lateral segment liver transplantation.[38] Little difference has been reported in the biliary complication rate after duct-to-duct anastomosis (with or without a T-tube) and hepaticojejunostomy.[39] Hepatic artery thrombosis should be excluded as a potential cause in all biliary complications.

An early postoperative bile leak may be from the biliary anastomosis, the cut surface of a partial graft, from an unrecognized segmental bile duct, or from the site of insertion of a T-tube. Patients present with fever and/or mild graft dysfunction which, if unrecognized, progresses to biliary peritonitis. Endoscopic or percutaneous cholangiography and biliary stenting usually leads to resolution, thereby avoiding the need for surgical reconstruction in the majority of cases.

Anastomotic biliary strictures occur in 5%–10% of patients, usually within 12 months of transplant, and present with cholangitis or liver dysfunction. Late bile duct strictures are occasionally recognized often in the presence of remarkably normal liver function tests. The γGT remains the most sensitive indicator of bile duct complications. Hepatic artery thrombosis may be the cause of up to 25% of all biliary complications and should be specifically excluded. Ultrasonography will usually reveal dilated proximal bile ducts. Early cases respond to dilatation and stenting. Anastomotic strictures presenting more than 6 months after transplant tend to recur after dilatation and invariably require surgical revision.

Non-anastomotic biliary strictures are relatively rare and tend to present late, often more than a year after transplantation. Intraductal stones and bile casts can be seen within the damaged ducts and cause recurrent cholangitis. An ischemic cholangiopathy has been reported after hepatic artery thrombosis, prolonged cold ischemia and transplantation with grafts from ABO incompatible and non-heart beating donors. Although some patients can be managed conservatively, most will need to be retransplanted.

The use of a T-tube after duct-to-duct anastomosis has been associated with complications in up to 20% of cases including bile leakage from the insertion site and obstruction. Leaks have been reported even when T-tube removal is delayed for 6 months post-transplant. Early recognition of a bile leak after T-tube removal and endoscopic stenting avoids the need for surgery. Other potential T-tube problems include dislodgment, obstruction and foreign body reaction with secondary cholangitis. T-tube removal under prophylactic antibiotic cover in these cases leads to resolution.

Complications of Roux loop hepaticojejunostomy occur in approximately 5% of cases and include bile leak or stricture. Surgical revision is usually required although early cases may respond to percutaneous transhepatic dilatation. Occasionally, a child presents several years after transplantation with recurrent low-grade cholangitis. The hepaticojejunostomy drains satisfactorily at cholangiography but there may be evidence of Roux loop obstruction or reflux. DISIDA scanning is particularly useful in determining whether there is hold up in the flow of bile and the site of obstruction. Surgical revision of the Roux loop and the use of anti-reflux techniques, when indicated, are often curative.

Bowel and wound complications

Bowel perforation is a well-recognized complication of OLT, occurring in about 6% of cases. Contributory factors include previous surgery, steroid therapy, viral infection, malnutrition and lymphoproliferative disease. The incidence is higher in children who have undergone transplantation for biliary atresia after previous portoenterostomy.[40,41] The incidence of reperforation is also high but with prompt treatment there are no long-term sequelae. The incidence of symptomatic postoperative adhesions appears to be no greater than after other types of abdominal surgery. Unlike adults, incisional hernias are rare in children. Late muscle closure (at 1 year) is needed for the occasional child whose abdomen is closed by suturing the skin alone or in whom a silastic mesh is used.

Acute rejection

Acute rejection is seen in more than 50% of children. There are two forms, hyperacute and acute rejection. Hyperacute rejection is antibody mediated, occurs within hours of the transplant, and leads to early graft loss. It is rare after liver transplantation. Acute rejection is T-cell mediated and tends to occur between 5 and 14 days post-transplant. It is uncommon after 1 month unless immunosuppression levels are inadequate. Acute rejection may be relatively asymptomatic and only suspected by elevation of plasma AST, bilirubin, alkaline phosphatase and γGT. Typical symptoms include fever, malaise and loss of appetite. Suspected acute rejection should be confirmed by needle liver biopsy, which shows a mixed portal inflammatory cell infiltrate, subendothelial inflammation of portal and hepatic veins and bile duct inflammation. Doppler ultrasound should be used to exclude hepatic artery thrombosis or biliary complications.

The level of immunosuppression influences the incidence of acute rejection. Lower rates of rejection can be achieved with higher levels of immunosuppression but the risk of infective complications increases. During the last decade a variety of immunosuppressive protocols have been used for induction, maintenance, and treatment of acute rejection. Triple therapy using cyclosporin, azathioprine, and prednisolone has given way to tacrolimus and prednisolone in our institution. Steroids are tapered and, if appropriate, withdrawn by 3 months. Rejection is treated with pulsed steroids and, if severe, an IL-2 blocker and mycophenolate mofetil are added. For mild episodes an increased level of calcineurin inhibitor may suffice. For severe rejection unresponsive to steroids and IL-2 blockade, OKT3 may be considered. We have rarely needed to use this powerful immunosuppressant, which is associated with significant infective complications. Graft loss from acute rejection is rare after liver transplantation.

Chronic rejection

Chronic rejection has become a less common cause of graft loss during the past 10 years. The incidence of chronic rejection after pediatric liver transplantation has decreased from 10% to less than 5%.[13] The Pittsburgh group has noted its absence in children receiving tacrolimus, provided baseline immunosuppression is maintained.[42] In an early series from our institution over half of all retransplants were performed for chronic rejection but, more recently, the proportion was down to 26%.[9] A North American multicenter study of 91 children with chronic rejection converted to tacrolimus showed a 70% response rate; responders were more likely to have been converted within 3 months of transplantation and have a serum bilirubin of less than 10 mg/dl.[43] Risk factors for chronic rejection include previous episodes of chronic rejection, recipients non-indigenous to the donor population, CMV infection, HLA match/mismatch, and positive lymphocytotoxic cross-matching.[44] Chronic rejection can occur as early as 6 weeks after OLT but typically develops within 1 year of transplant. It has been reported 10 years later, possibly because of intermittent compliance. Clinical presentation is with jaundice and pruritus (which often appears first). There is usually marked cholestasis with only mild to moderate elevation of serum transaminases. Hepatic synthetic function is usually well preserved. Histologic appearances are of a cellular infiltrate of lymphocytes, macrophages, and plasma cells within the portal tracts. T-cells and neutrophils surround the bile ducts with subsequent ductal necrosis. Bile duct loss or ductopenia, is usually confined to interlobular ducts. Rescue strategies for chronic rejection continue to evolve as new immunosuppressants become available. Currently, mycophenolate mofetil is used in patients developing chronic rejection on tacrolimus immunosuppression. Sirolimus and anti-IL-2 receptor monoclonal antibodies have also been used with some success.[45] In adults with severe jaundice, the molecular adsorbent recirculating system (MARS) has produced significant reductions in serum bilirubin, urea and creatinine levels which provides temporary support until an organ becomes available. Retransplantation is the only realistic option when rescue therapy fails.[46]

Infection

Infectious complications are among the most significant causes of morbidity and mortality in the first 3 months post-transplant. Risk factors include poor graft function, prolonged intensive care unit stay, ventilator dependence, gut perforation, retransplantation and the use of anti-lymphocyte antibodies to treat rejection.[47,48] Young children may experience more severe infections with certain viral (e.g., respiratory syncytial virus) and bacterial (e.g., coagulase-negative staphylococcus) pathogens than the mild infections sustained by adult recipients. In contrast, certain pathogens such as *Cryptococcus neoformans* rarely cause infection before adulthood. Age is also an important factor governing clinical expression of infection with CMV and Epstein–Barr virus (EBV). Young patients are less likely to have been exposed to these viruses and are therefore susceptible to primary infections, which tend to be more severe than viral reactivation. Bacteria account for the majority of infections within the first two weeks, fungal sepsis is seen from the second week onwards and viral infections tend to occur later.

Bacterial

Chest infection is the commonest cause of sepsis, particularly in the first week after transplant. Gram-positive organisms from venous access lines are also an important cause of sepsis during this period and lines should be changed every 5 days. Gram-negative sepsis has become less common with the use of prophylactic antibiotics during and after OLT. The presence of gram-negative organisms and *Candida* in peritoneal fluid postoperatively is indicative of a bowel or biliary leak. Increasing problems are being encountered with antibiotic resistant organisms such as methicillin-resistant *Staphylococcus aureus* (MRSA), *Klebsiella* and *Enterococcus*. Cholangitis, intra-abdominal abscess, and wound infection tend to present after the first 2 weeks because clinical signs may be masked by immunosuppressive drugs.

Fungal

Liver transplant recipients are at risk of fungal sepsis because of immunosuppression, invasive monitoring, and multiple courses of antibiotics with resultant changes in gut flora. Fungal sepsis is common in children with acute liver failure and routine prophylaxis is mandatory. Other risk factors for fungal infection after liver transplantation include retransplantation, graft dysfunction, hepatic artery thrombosis, bowel perforation, and reintubation. Most fungal sepsis is from *Candida* species but infections with *Aspergillus*, *Mucormycosis*, *Coccidioidomycosis* or *Cryptococcus* can occur and are associated with a high mortality. Fungal sepsis should be suspected in any transplant recipient with a fever and high white blood count in the presence of broad-spectrum antibiotic therapy. Fluconazole is well tolerated as prophylaxis and therapy with few acute toxic side effects and is an effective drug for *Candida* infections. Liposomal amphotericin is the mainstay of treatment for invasive aspergillosis but itraconazole is also effective. Voriconazole is an option for treating infection with some *Candida* species resistant to fluconazole. Since the azole drugs are metabolized by the hepatic cytochrome P-450 system, a variety of interactions can occur with other medications, e.g., the metabolism of cyclosporin, sirolimus, and tacrolimus are inhibited, resulting in increased serum concentrations and potential drug toxicity. Caspofungin is effective in vitro against *Candida* sp. (including azole-resistant isolates) and *Aspergillus* sp. and reduces peak serum tacrolimus levels by approximately 20% to 25%.

Viral

Viral infections which include Herpes simplex and zoster, CMV, EBV, and Adenovirus are all potential causes of early and late infection, often associated with over-immunosuppression. Adenovirus pneumonitis and hepatitis and disseminated CMV disease are particularly severe and associated with a poor outcome. The incidence of CMV disease has declined as immunosuppressive regimens have improved and prophylaxis for high-risk recipients (CMV-negative recipient receiving a CMV-positive donor) has become routine. Children are at increased risk because most are CMV negative prior to transplantation and primary CMV infection occurs in over 70%. The reported mortality was 7% prior to the introduction of Ganciclovir.[49] Reactivation of CMV occurs in up to 60% of children and can also be fatal. Treatment with Ganciclovir has dramatically transformed the course and prognosis of CMV infection. Without prophylaxis, the peak incidence of disease is around 28–38 days post-transplant.[50] Over-immunosuppressed patients and those receiving antilymphocyte antibodies such as OKT3 for severe graft rejection are at greater risk of CMV disease.[51] Late CMV disease is characterized by malaise, fever, leukopenia, thrombocytopenia, and arthralgia but it may cause hepatitis, enteritis, or pneumonitis. CMV chorioretinitis is of particular concern because it signals a failing immune system and a poor prognosis; symptoms include decreased visual acuity, photophobia, scotomata, floaters, redness, or pain. Other rare late CMV manifestations include myocarditis, vasculitis, and encephalomyelitis. Prophylaxis can delay or prevent the development of CMV infection.[52]

EBV infection is common in childhood and characterized by latency, liver involvement, and the potential for reactivation. The clinical features in a normal host include lymphadenopathy, pharyngitis, tonsillitis, hepatitis, and splenomegaly, which may be more severe in the immunocompromised patient, with an increased risk of atypical lymphocyte transformation and proliferation.

The potential for EBV-driven lymphoproliferative disease after liver transplantation is a concern (see below). Primary EBV infection or reactivation can be a cause of graft dysfunction.[53]

Both CMV and EBV infections tend to occur within the first 6 months after transplantation but should always be considered as a potential cause of late graft dysfunction. Adenovirus infection may cause acute hepatitis or necrotizing pneumonitis in the early post-transplant period. Serotypes 1, 2, and 5 are most commonly implicated; type 5 is responsible for the development of hepatitis that carries a mortality of up to 45%.[54]

Human herpes virus-6 (HHV-6) and human herpes virus-7 (HHV-7) are ubiquitous in humans and cause exanthema subitum, a benign disease seen in infancy. They remain latent after primary infection, but are able to reactivate in immunocompromised patients. HHV-6 infection occurs in 20%–30% of solid organ transplant recipients, 2–3 weeks after the procedure. Clinical problems ascribed to this virus include fever, skin rash, pneumonia, bone marrow suppression, encephalitis, and rejection. There are few studies on HHV-7 infection in organ transplant recipients but it may act as a cofactor for CMV disease.[55]

The significance of parvovirus B19 infection in pediatric solid organ transplant patients is unclear. The overall prevalence of parvovirus B19 infection is about 1%–2% during the first year post-transplant. Most commonly, it causes anemia, but leukopenia and thrombocytopenia have also been observed. Rare cases of hepatic dysfunction, myocarditis, vasculitis, and respiratory failure have been reported. Whereas serology is of limited value in the early post-transplant period, a search for parvovirus B19 DNA is worthwhile in transplant patients with unexplained anemia. Specific antiviral therapy is not available but intravenous immunoglobulin produces a rapid improvement in most cases. Although relatively rare, severe complications of parvovirus B19 infection in the transplant patient can generally be avoided by early diagnosis and treatment.[56]

Influenza A and B are common viral pathogens associated with upper and lower respiratory tract infections. They typically occur in winter, and in any given year, one strain of either virus predominates. Immunosuppressed patients should receive the inactivated influenza vaccine annually. Respiratory syncytial virus is a common cause of lower respiratory tract infection in young children. It seldom causes life-threatening complications in the transplant recipient except if it occurs within the first few weeks; nebulized ribavirin can be given in severe cases.

Late infections

Late opportunistic bacterial infections including legionellosis, nocardiosis and tuberculosis may occur, particularly in children who have received heavier immunosuppression or who have been transplanted for acute liver failure. Children from ethnic minorities may be at increased risk of developing tuberculosis. The risk of mycobacterial infection is 1%–2% with onset between one month and 5 years after transplantation. Many cases are due to atypical mycobacteria, which can cause skin, lymph node, pulmonary or miliary disease. This possibility should be considered in children with an unusual or unresolving chest infection.

Atypical pneumonia due to *Pneumocystis carinii* presents with fever, a dry cough and hypoxia. Children with poor graft function, high levels of immunosuppression and chronic rejection are more vulnerable but late infection is occasionally seen in the absence of these risk factors. Treatment is with high dose trimethoprim/sulphamethoxazole.

Central nervous system infection with Toxoplasmosis is rare but should be considered in any child with evidence of seroconversion and neurologic signs. Reduction in immunosuppression and treatment with pyrimethamine/sulfadiazine or high dose penicillin usually leads to resolution.

Endoscopy and intestinal biopsy are recommended for pediatric transplant patients who present with chronic diarrhea of unknown etiology to exclude cryptosporidiosis. Again, this is associated with more intense immunosuppression.[57]

Immunization

Immunization regimens for diphtheria, tetanus, and pertussis remain the same. Live vaccines should be avoided. Oral polio vaccine should not be given to patients or close family members because of the risk of viral transmission; inactivated polio vaccine is safe. Measles, mumps, and rubella (MMR) vaccine is not routinely given, although the risks of the disease may outweigh the risks of immunization. Immunizations such as hepatitis B should be given before transplantation when possible. *Haemophilus influenzae* B vaccination should be given to children under 5 years of age or to those with defective splenic function. The latter should also be immunized against pneumococcal infection in addition to receiving daily prophylactic penicillin. Immunosuppressed children exposed to chickenpox should be given zoster immunoglobulin and aciclovir if they are varicella antibdy negative.

Immunosuppressive problems and side effects

Children appear to require more immunosuppression than adults in the first year after liver transplant. The recipient and their family exchange the problems of liver disease for those of immunosuppression. Currently, recipients

Table 65.3. Side effects of cyclosporin and tacrolimus

Cyclosporin	Tacrolimus
Hypertension	Hypertension
Nephrotoxicity	Nephrotoxicity
Neurotoxicity	Neurotoxicity
Hirsutism	Insomnia
Gingival hyperplasia	Pruritus
Diabetes mellitus	Diabetes mellitus
	Anorexia

Table 65.4. Drug interactions with cyclosporin

Increased concentration	Decreased concentration	Increased nephrotoxicity
Danazol	Carbamazepine	Amphotericin –B
Diltiazem	Phenobarbitone	Aminoglycosides
Erythromycin	Phenytoin	Vancomycin
Ketoconazole	Rifampicin	NSAIDs
Metoclopramide	Isoniazid	
Methyltestosterone		
Nicardipine		
Norethisterone		
Verapamil		
Cimetidine		

Table 65.5. Drug interactions with tacrolimus

1. **Potential inhibitors of tacrolimus metabolism resulting in increased levels**:

Cimetidine	Doxycycline	Ketoconazole
Cyclosporin	Erythromycin	Nicardipine
Danazol	Fluconazole	Voriconazole
Itraconazole	Verapamil	

2. **Potential inducers of tacrolimus metabolism resulting in decreased levels**:

Carbamazepine	Isoniazid	Phenytoin
Corticosteroids	Phenobarbital	Rifampicin

3. **Potential additive/synergistic nephrotoxicity**:
   Aminoglycosides: Gentamicin, Tobramycin, Streptomycin, Amikacin
   Netilmycin
   Amphotericin B
   Cisplatin
   Cyclosporin
   Vancomycin
4. **Potential hyperkalemia**:
   Potassium supplements
   Spironolactone
   Amiloride
5. **Possible additive/synergistic neurotoxicity**:
   Aciclovir
   Ciprofloxacin
   Ganciclovir
   Imipenem
   Norfloxacin

and their families are counseled that immunosuppression is lifelong but there is considerable research into the possibility of inducing host tolerance to the graft and subsequent withdrawal of long-term immunosuppression.

Long-term surveillance after liver transplantation is necessary to identify and prevent complications of immunosuppressive therapy. Major side effects associated with cyclosporin and tacrolimus are listed in Table 65.3. Both drugs share similar side effects but cyclosporin is associated with more hypertension, hirsutism, and gingival hyperplasia, whereas tacrolimus is associated with increased neurotoxicity, diabetes mellitus, pruritus, and insomnia. Tacrolimus allows earlier and more aggressive steroid withdrawal during the first year after transplant in most children, thus helping to preserve growth potential. Other advantages of tacrolimus include a reduced incidence of rejection and an absence of cosmetic side effects. OKT-3 is now rarely used for induction and treatment of rejection because of its profound immunosuppression-related side effects. In contrast, anti IL-2 receptor monoclonal antibodies are increasingly used to supplement immunosuppression in the early postoperative period, particularly when renal function is impaired or if there is steroid-resistant rejection.

There are numerous potential drug interactions in patients taking cyclosporin or tacrolimus that may result in significant changes in blood concentrations. Some of these are shown in Tables 65.4 and 65.5.

Renal

Renal insufficiency is perhaps the most significant long-term complication. Children have a lower incidence of renal dysfunction before and after transplantation than adults. Some children have renal impairment prior to liver transplantation from disorders such as hereditary tyrosinemia type I associated with Fanconi's syndrome, congenital cystic disease of the kidneys, and Alagille's syndrome. Intrinsic glomerular abnormalities occur commonly in association with liver cirrhosis regardless of the etiology of the liver disease. Hepatorenal syndrome associated with severe liver dysfunction is reversed by successful liver transplantation but may be associated with subsequent susceptibility to renal injury.

Clinical evaluation of renal function in children with advanced liver disease is not always straightforward. High levels of serum bilirubin (greater than 200–500 μmol/l) can interfere with the measurement of serum creatinine.[58] In addition, serum creatinine levels may be falsely low in wasted, malnourished children and creatinine clearance may not accurately reflect renal function in children with advanced liver disease. The circulating blood volume of children awaiting liver transplantation must be carefully monitored since a reduction in the effective plasma volume may result in a rapid decline in renal function. Diuretics or paracentesis must be used cautiously in children with large volume ascites. Diarrhea, infection, or sepsis may further compromise renal function and gastrointestinal bleeding must be treated promptly. Nephrotoxic antibiotics and non-steroidal anti-inflammatory drugs should be avoided if possible.

Acute tubular necrosis, particularly of ischemic origin, is responsible for almost half of the cases of acute renal failure post-transplant. Aminoglycosides and volume depletion account for most of the remainder, although early graft function is important in maintaining renal function. Long-term nephrotoxicity is almost exclusively secondary to immunosuppression with calcineurin inhibitors (CNIs). The toxicity of these agents is mediated by renal vasoconstriction. Chronic arteriolar changes are associated with interstitial abnormalities, which are often segmental in distribution. Glomerular filtration appears to stabilize in most patients despite progressive pathologic changes because of compensatory hypertrophy of undamaged glomeruli.

Children appear to suffer a progressive decrease in their GFR which falls by 20%–50% in more than half the cases 2 to 4 years after liver transplantation. The issue of progressive injury is particularly important since children have a cumulative exposure to CNIs over several decades. Both tacrolimus and cyclosporin have similar nephrotoxic properties but liver allograft function in particular affects the plasma levels of tacrolimus. Poor graft function increases the plasma level of tacrolimus and the risk of nephrotoxicity.[59] Initially, tacrolimus was considered to be more nephrotoxic than cyclosporin but subsequent studies using lower tacrolimus trough levels have shown that both drugs have similar nephrotoxicity after liver transplantation.[60] In acute renal insufficiency, dose reductions of cyclosporin or tacrolimus lead to improved renal function. Contrary to some statements, chronic renal impairment may also improve after reducing the dose of CNIs many years after transplant.

Table 65.6. Side-effects of mycophenolate mofetil and sirolimus

Mycophenolate mofetil	Sirolimus
Diarrhea, constipation	Dyslipidemia
Nausea, vomiting	Hypertension
Leucopenia	Acne
Headache	Rash
Convulsions	Anemia, thrombocytopenia
Edema	Joint pain
Dyspnea	Diarrhea

At present, there are no non-nephrotoxic drugs that can completely replace CNIs in the early post-transplant period. Drugs which act synergistically with CNIs, thereby allowing their dose to be reduced, include anti-IL-2 monoclonal antibodies, mycophenolate mofetil (MMF), and sirolimus. These drugs offer an effective calcineurin inhibitor-sparing strategy both early and late after transplantation. MMF and sirolimus are utilized in the longer term; their side effects are listed in Table 65.6. In selected cases, they may even allow CNI withdrawal. Currently, C2 levels are recommended to monitor cyclosporin therapy and 12-hour trough levels for tacrolimus. If there is evidence of renal impairment at 3 months or 1 year post-transplant then, unless CNIs are reduced or withdrawn, the recipient is likely to develop end-stage renal disease within 5 years. The avoidance of renal impairment remains the most important aspect of life long management of children after liver transplantation.

Hypertension

Between 50% and 80% of adult patients develop systemic hypertension after liver transplantation (defined as systolic blood pressure >150 mmHg and diastolic blood pressure >90 mm Hg).[61] The number of children with chronic hypertension appears to be lower but this still represents a significant long-term problem that may also contribute to the development of renal impairment. Onset of hypertension is early, often within weeks of starting CNIs and steroids. Up to 87% of children require antihypertensive therapy during their initial hospital stay and 50% may still need treatment at the time of discharge.[62] Hypertension may persist despite reducing the dose of steroids and CNI. The incidence of hypertension appears to decline during the first year post-transplant and, by the end of the first year, only 6% of children remain on antihypertensive treatment. However, this increases to 10% by the end of the second year and 16% after 3 years as a consequence of ongoing CNI nephrotoxicity.[63] Cyclosporin-induced hypertension results in a loss of the nocturnal fall in blood pressure and has been associated with nocturnal headaches and a reversal of day/night sodium excretion patterns.[64] Left ventricular hypertrophy may develop in these patients.[65] Cyclosporin-induced hypertension does not always progress but may nevertheless cause organ damage particularly in children who were normotensive pretransplant.[66] Low magnesium levels may contribute to hypertension but adrenergic mechanisms do not appear to play a role as sympathetic tone is decreased after transplant. Cyclosporin appears to have a direct effect on the endothelium as well as impairing sodium excretion which causes an increase in intravascular volume. Tacrolimus also induces hypertension but the incidence may be lower than with cyclosporin. This may in part be related to the reduced steroid requirement with tacrolimus. Patients with hypertension converted from cyclosporin to tacrolimus for steroid-resistant acute rejection were more easily controlled after conversion and many could be weaned off antihypertensives.[67]

The optimum therapy of post-transplant hypertension has yet to be defined. First-line treatment includes dietary sodium restriction and, where possible, a reduction in the dose of steroids and CNI. Thereafter, calcium-blocking agents are used. These induce smooth muscle vasodilatation and inhibit the potent vasoconstrictive effects of endothelin.[68] They may also provide a degree of renal protection. Some calcium-antagonists (e.g., verapamil and diltiazem) can increase CNI levels and should be used with caution. Other antihypertensive agents, particularly beta-blockers, are effective but can potentiate hyperlipidemia. Angiotensin converting enzyme inhibitors are less effective and potentiate CNI induced hyperkalemia; they should be avoided if there is renal impairment. Approximately one-third of transplant recipients are controlled with a calcium channel blocker such as nifedipine or with the beta- and alpha-1-adrenergic antagonist labetalol. A further third require the addition of a second agent. Side effects such as edema, headache, fatigue and postural intolerance may limit compliance.[69]

Hyperlipidemia

Problems of raised triglyceride and cholesterol levels were first reported in renal transplant recipients.[70] The situation is complex after liver transplantation. Lipoproteins are synthesized in the liver and transport triglycerides and cholesterol in the plasma. Disorders of lipoprotein metabolism in the donor may therefore be passed on to the recipient. Donors with primary hypercholesterolemia should not be used. After liver transplantation, hyperlipidemias have been found in 40%–50% of patients, although these tend to be less severe than after heart or kidney transplantation. Steroid therapy has been implicated but the role of cyclosporin and tacrolimus is unclear. The use of low dose steroids may reduce the likelihood of this complication.

Treatment includes dietary changes and the use of lipid lowering agents.[71] Sirolimus has been used in pediatric recipients and increases in blood cholesterol and triglycerides have been controlled with statins.[72] Whether the combined risks of hypertension and hyperlipidemia will increase the future risk of cardiovascular disease is not known.

Oral complications

Gingival hyperplasia occurs in a significant number of children receiving cyclosporin and also in some patients treated with nifedipine. Gingival changes develop during the first 2–6 months after starting cyclosporin and reach a plateau at about 1 year. Gingival overgrowth begins with gum enlargement between the teeth but can extend to cover portions of the tooth crown and interfere with chewing and speech. The increase in gingival mass is due to a connective tissue response by fibroblasts resulting in the production of an amorphous ground substance containing a high level of glycosaminoglycans. The presence of dental plaque pretransplant appears to predispose to gingival hyperplasia.

Meticulous oral hygiene and dental care should be established before liver transplantation and continued afterwards. If gingival hyperplasia becomes established, dental hygiene is important to avoid recurrent bacteremia and septicemia. All dental procedures post-transplant must be covered with prophylactic antibiotics (e.g., amoxicillin). Surgical removal of the hyperplastic tissue or switching to tacrolimus has been the mainstay of therapy. Recently, Azithromycin has been found to be beneficial in some children after renal transplantation.

Hair growth

A common side effect of cyclosporin is hypertrichosis. Hair growth is induced by both topical and oral cyclosporin. Oral tacrolimus does not have this side effect. Young girls find the excess hair growth distressing and they can be converted to tacrolimus. Failure to do this may lead to non-compliance. Topical tacrolimus can stimulate hair growth probably as a result of direct stimulation of hair follicles.[73]

Warts

Warts are common in children after liver transplantation. The frequency of warts in transplant recipients is three times that seen in normal children.[74] It is likely that suppression of cell-mediated, and to a lesser extent, humoral immunity predisposes to the development of warts. DNA extracted from wart scrapings shows that the types of human papilloma virus present are the same as those in the general population.[74] Ingelfinger *et al.* found that, in 18 of 49 pediatric renal transplant recipients treated for warts, only five had them successfully eradicated.[75] Acitretin, a second-generation retinoid, has proved effective in some cases.[76]

Neurologic and psychiatric disorders

Neurologic complications in the early post-transplant period include seizures, central pontine myelinolysis, strokes, delirium, and other forms of organic brain disorder. Some of these complications can have significant long-term sequelae. Almost one-third of liver transplant recipients will develop a transient organic brain disorder. Risk factors include preoperative encephalopathy, lengthy surgery, volume and electrolyte shifts, the use of immunosuppressants and opiates, graft dysfunction, fever, and infection.[77] Symptoms include seizures, blindness, aphasia, paresthesiae, neuropathy, delusions, and agitation; coma, status epilepticus, and neurologic death are rare. Antipsychotic agents such as haloperidol or droperidol, combined with benzodiazepines that do not have active metabolites (e.g., lorazepam or clonazepam) are effective in controlling acute symptoms but should be used alongside measures to correct any underlying precipitants.

Most children will experience some degree of neurotoxicity from CNIs. Tremor is common and responds to dose reduction and correction of magnesium levels. Headache, paresthesiae, and insomnia can be particularly troublesome; headache is associated with high blood levels and also responds to dose reduction or taking the medication with food which blunts its absorption profile. Although CNI neurotoxicity is generally observed as an early postoperative problem, it has also been reported months after transplantation.[78] Tacrolimus appears to be associated with more severe neurotoxicity than cyclosporin[79,80] and this may be exacerbated by hypomagnesemia.

Seizures

Cyclosporin and tacrolimus are both associated with seizures, particularly in the first 2 weeks after transplantation.[81] Hypomagnesemia and hypocalcemia may precipitate seizures,[82] as may other drugs such as ganciclovir. Central nervous system lesions may be evident in some patients with seizures, including diffuse white matter changes, microinfarcts, central pontine myelolinolysis, and edema. Seizure activity may persist in the long term.

Headache

Liver transplant recipients taking CNIs may complain of a severe symmetrical headache.[83] Headaches typically develop in the early postoperative period and can be associated with other symptoms such as scotomata, photophobia and nausea. Headache may also be a feature of more severe neurologic manifestations such as transient cortical blindness. This initially presents with headache and seizure with bilateral occipital edema on magnetic resonance scan; the blindness and edema resolve after cessation of CNI. Isolated visual hallucinations have been reported with cyclosporin, ganciclovir and many antibiotics.[84]

Mood disorders

Several case reports have described both manic and depressive states in the post-transplant patient after initiating CNI therapy and high dose steroids. Depressive disorders and psychotic states have also been attributed to other drugs such as aciclovir,[85] and to sleep deprivation and stress reactions following liver transplantation.

Post-transplant malignancies

Immunosuppression-related tumors are a major concern in children after liver transplantation.[86,87] Several mechanisms are implicated in the development of post-transplant malignancies: the inability of a suppressed immune system to destroy malignant cells; abnormal stimulation by the graft or blood products leading to lymphoproliferative disease; direct DNA damage from drugs such as azathioprine and CNIs; and the oncogenic potential of viral infections such as EBV (lymphoproliferative disease), herpes and papilloma viruses (carcinoma of skin, lips, and perineum) and CMV (Kaposi sarcoma). Liver transplant recipients seem to have a different pattern of susceptibility to malignancy compared to renal transplant recipients. This may reflect differences in the degree and type of immunosuppression and the longer follow-up of renal patients. The commonest malignancies after renal transplantation in adults include Kaposi's sarcoma (after a mean of 22 months), lymphoma (32 months), skin tumors (69 months), and carcinoma of the vulva and perineum (113 months). The long-term risk of adenocarcinoma of the lung, colon, breast, or prostate does not seem to be increased.[88] After liver transplantation in children, the most common tumors (over 50%) are lymphoproliferative disorders; the incidence of these is approximately 4%–6%. Smooth muscle tumors have been reported several years after transplantation in young children. These occur more often in children who have had a post-transplant lymphoproliferative disorder (PTLD) and they may contain clonal EBV, suggesting that the virus had a role in their development.[89] Clinical response to immunosuppression withdrawal has been reported.[90]

Long-term surveillance and prevention of post-transplant malignancies are essential. The level of immunosuppressive therapy should be kept as low as possible but sufficient to maintain good graft function. Early CMV disease should ideally be avoided. Exposure to ultraviolet radiation is a well-recognized risk factor for the development of skin cancers, particular squamous cell carcinoma. Children must avoid excessively exposure to sunlight, particularly those with fair skins, and advice about the use of effective sunscreens is mandatory.

Lymphoproliferative disorders

Despite different pre-emptive strategies, PTLD continues to affect 5%–15% of children after liver transplantation. The incidence in high-risk groups such as children receiving combined liver and small bowel grafts may be as high as 30%.[91] There is convincing evidence that PTLD is associated with Epstein–Barr virus (EBV) infection. This virus has a tropism for B-lymphocytes and oropharyngeal epithelial cells. Not only does it cause infectious mononucleosis but it can also promote the development of oral leukoplakia, lymphoproliferative diseases (in immunosuppressed individuals), Burkitt's lymphoma, Hodgkin's disease, T-cell lymphoma, and nasopharyngeal carcinoma.

EBV enters and infects the B-lymphocyte, stimulating the cell to produce a large number of viral particles that are then released. In the latent infection phase, the EBV genome is episomal (extrachromosomal) with low copy amplification and no production of infectious viral particles. After production of several copies of the EBV genome, some EBV DNA may become integrated into the host DNA of B-lymphocytes; this process may be enhanced by mitogens that provide growth stimulatory signals to B-lymphocytes. However, most EBV DNA exists in the episomal form. EBV persists in this latent form for the lifespan of the host cell. After primary infection EBV seroconversion occurs early in life in nearly 50% of the population. A second peak of seroconversion occurs in the second decade of life. Cellular immunity is also important in the regulation of EBV infected lymphocytes in immunosuppressed hosts. Defective cellular immunity induced by immunosuppressive therapy may explain the proliferation of EBV-infected B-lymphocytes, which leads to malignant transformation.

The incidence of PTLD in children is higher because of the lack of viral exposure prior to transplantation.[92] The risk of PTLD may be as high as 2.8% per year resulting in a cumulative risk of approximately 20% at 7 years.[93] Primary EBV infection after pediatric liver transplantation is a much greater risk factor for the development of PTLD than viral reactivation.[93,94] Other risk factors for PTLD include young age at the time of transplant, the type of transplant, and the type and intensity of immunosuppression. It has been suggested that OKT3 and tacrolimus are associated with a higher risk, particularly in young children.

The majority of post-transplant lymphomas are non-Hodgkin's lymphomas and most of these are B-cell tumors. T-cell lymphomas account for 14% and null cells for less than 1%. In most patients with central nervous system involvement, lesions are confined to the brain, whereas in cases of cerebral lymphoma in the general population other organs are usually involved. Another remarkable feature of lymphomas in transplant recipients is that there is either macroscopic or microscopic evidence of allograft involvement in 18% of cases.

PTLD presents with three different clinical patterns: a solid tumor, diffuse parenchymal infiltration, or enlargement of native lymphoid tissue. Solid tumors are indistinguishable from lymphoma at a macroscopic level but their appearance is often modified when they occur in the gastrointestinal tract; ulcerating mucosal lesions may progress to frank perforation and symptoms of an acute abdomen. The microscopic appearance of PTLD is that of a diffuse proliferation of lymphoid cells that can be characterized according to the degree of lymphocyte heterogeneity. In one series of 91 patients, 54% had monoclonal lesions, 25% polyclonal, and 20% were combined.[95]

Clinical presentation is often non-specific and tissue biopsy is necessary to establish the diagnosis. The presence of fever, often chaotic and without obvious cause, anemia and positive fecal occult blood loss should raise suspicion of EBV infection or PTLD. Recognition of PTLD by the pathologist is crucial because the atypical lymphoid proliferation may present in the transplant allograft and needs to be differentiated from acute cellular rejection. The latter requires heightened immunosuppression whereas a diagnosis of PTLD demands less immunosuppression. Moreover, acute graft rejection is a common side effect of PTLD management. EBV viral load determination by quantitative polymerase chain reaction of peripheral blood samples is so far the only predictive marker for PTLD prevention and treatment monitoring, although it is limited by a lack of specificity. Antiviral drugs and CMV-immunoglobulin may have a limited role in preventing PTLD.

Because PTLD results from functional over-immunosuppression, initial management is by reducing immunosuppression. Antiviral agents, interferon and chemotherapy also have a role in treating this disorder. Chemotherapy regimens have included CHOP

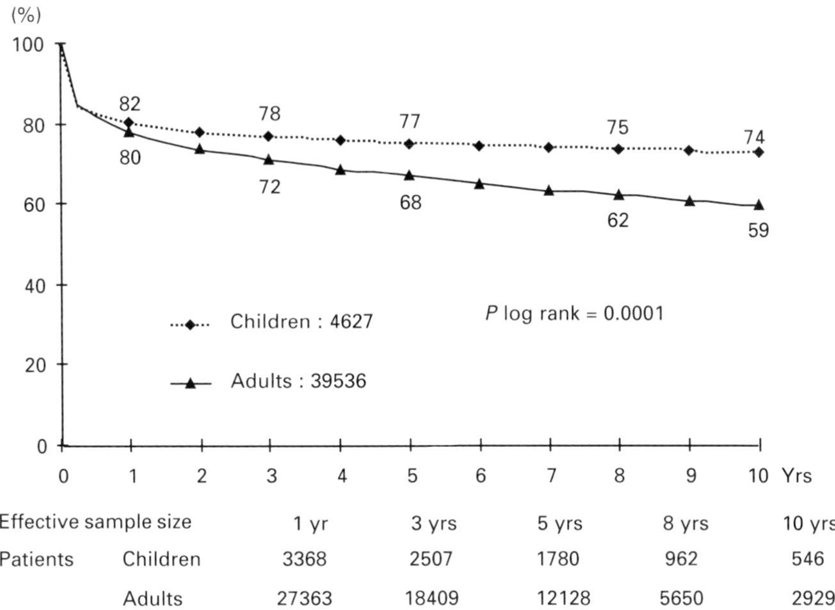

Effective sample size		1 yr	3 yrs	5 yrs	8 yrs	10 yrs
Patients	Children	3368	2507	1780	962	546
	Adults	27363	18409	12128	5650	2929

Fig. 65.7. ELTR data (1988–2002) for patient survival according to recipient age.

(cytoxan, hydroxydoxorubicin, oncovin, prednisone), COMP (cytoxan, oncovin, methotrexate, prednisone) and ProMACECytaBOM (procarbazine, methotrexate, adriamycin, cytoxan, etoposide, ARA-C, bleomycin, oncovin, methotrexate) but only occasional patients respond. PTLD is less responsive to chemotherapy than lymphomas in "normal" hosts. Currently, there is no standardized approach to the evaluation and treatment of PTLD. Recently, a new therapeutic approach based on anti-B-cell immunotherapy has been used with success in adults and children with B-cell PTLD.[96] Rituximab, an anti-CD20 antibody, when combined with withdrawal of CNI therapy, has resulted in a decreased EBV titre and disappearance of tumor but longer term outcomes are needed. However, late rejection is a possibility and immunosuppression needs to be reintroduced rapidly in such cases to prevent lethal chronic liver graft rejection.[97] Future progress in antiviral therapy and gene therapy may provide new approaches.[98]

Late mortality

There are few reports of the long-term outcome and causes of late mortality after liver transplantation in children but survival is generally better than in adults (Fig. 65.7).[99] Jain *et al.* reported an actuarial patient survival of 64.4% at 20 years in a cohort of 808 children.[100] The 10-year actuarial patient survival was significantly better with tacrolimus (82.9%) than with cyclosporin (61%); most of the difference in mortality emerged within 3 months of OLT. However, these findings are not solely related to differences in immunosuppression and are likely to reflect many advances in pediatric liver transplantation in the tacrolimus era. European Liver Transplant Registry (ELTR) data have shown no difference in the actuarial survival of recipients transplanted under 2 years of age compared to older children (Fig. 65.8).

The majority of reports analyzing late mortality after OLT in children relate to cyclosporin-based immunosuppression. Fridell *et al.* reviewed 577 pediatric recipients and found that the commonest cause of death (60%) after the first year was infection.[22] PTLD and recurrence of primary liver disease each accounted for 12.5% of late deaths. The largest study to date in the cyclosporin era was by Sudan *et al.*, who reported an actuarial survival of 65.4% at 10 years in a cohort of 263 children transplanted between 1985 and 1995.[101] In the 212 children who survived more than one year, actuarial survival at 10 years was 84% (mean follow-up 5.3 years). The majority of late deaths were due to graft failure (9 cases) secondary to chronic rejection (4), late biliary complications (3) and recurrent disease (2). A further eight deaths (35%) were due to infection: five were in previously healthy children who developed sudden, overwhelming sepsis at home, two children died of sepsis after percutaneous cholangiography, and one after appendicectomy. Two of these eight children had undergone splenectomy

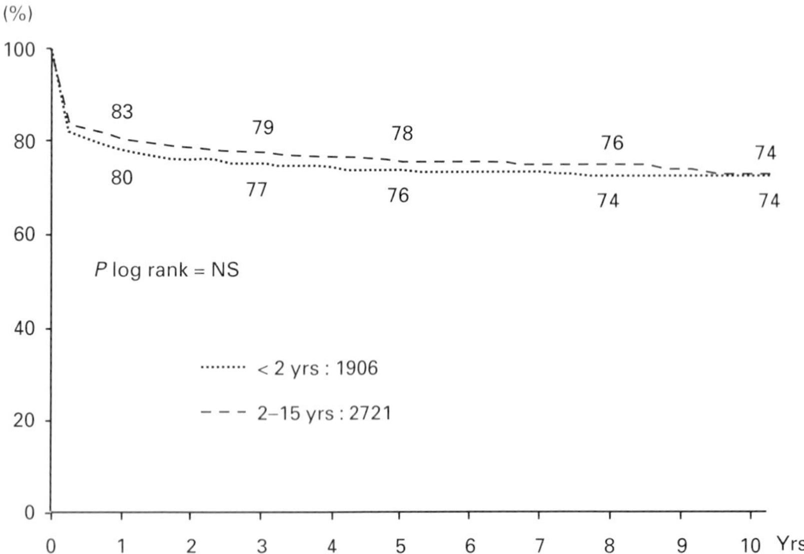

Fig. 65.8. ELTR data (1988–2002) for patient survival according to recipient age of child.

around the time of liver transplant. Similar deaths have been observed in our own series and percutaneous cholangiography appears to be a particular risk even in a previously well child. Transplanted children should receive prophylactic antibiotics for all invasive procedures including endoscopy, dental care, cholangiography, and liver biopsy. Children who develop a fever should receive antibiotics routinely and there is an argument for parents keeping a supply of antibiotics at home for such circumstances. Most deaths from sepsis occurred in the second and third year after transplantation.

Non-compliance was the other important cause of late death (17%) and was the leading cause between 10 and 17 years of age. Since the majority of children undergoing liver transplantation are less than 5 years of age the problem of non-compliance during adolescence is certain to increase. New strategies have to be developed to ensure that these patients continue to take their immunosuppression. There was only one late death from PTLD (most occurred in the first year after OLT). In the study by Sudan *et al.*, there were no differences in long-term survival related to age at transplantation, sex, etiology of underlying disease, or immunosuppressive regimen.[101]

In summary, infections are the most significant cause of late death after pediatric liver transplantation. PTLD has become less common. Deaths from chronic rejection have been greatly reduced by tacrolimus-based immunosuppression and the availability of other drugs such as mycophenolate mofetil. Non-compliance is gradually assuming a greater importance, especially in adolescents, and is rapidly becoming the most important cause of late death.

The causes of late death in children are very different from those observed in adults where about 50% of all late deaths are graft-related,[98] recurrent primary disease being responsible for most. Cardiovascular events and de novo malignancy are the causes of most non-graft related deaths.[102]

Late graft dysfunction

Late graft dysfunction characterized by abnormal liver function tests rather than portal hypertension has been evaluated by liver biopsy. The most frequent cause is acute/chronic rejection, often secondary to non-compliance.[103] Findings of a non-specific hepatitis are also common. Some of these children have features compatible with autoimmune hepatitis including the development of autoantibodies. This de novo or post-transplant autoimmune hepatitis responds to steroids and azathioprine or mycophenolate based immunosuppression, but may progress to fibrosis and retransplantation.[104] Late viral infection due to CMV, EBV, and hepatitis B or C should be excluded. Other late causes of graft dysfunction include biliary stricture, either anastomotic or non-anastomotic, hepatic artery thrombosis, nodular regenerative hyperplasia, lymphoproliferative disease and atypical infections.

Retransplantation

Results of retransplantation have been consistently worse than those of primary transplant. Retransplantation rates have been decreasing in recent years. Deshspande *et al.* have reviewed the short- and long-term outcomes of 50 children who were retransplanted in our institution during an 11-year period and found a rate of 16% between 1990 and 1995 and 9% after 1995.[105] Early retransplantation was most often performed for HAT, which accounted for more than 50% of cases, and for graft dysfunction. The most common reasons for late retransplantation, performed after the first month, were chronic rejection and late vascular and biliary complications. In this cohort of 50 patients, 9 (18%) underwent transplantation for a third time.

In our series, patient and graft survival rates 1 year after retransplantation were 71.7% and 65.6%, respectively. However, since 1995 patient survival has approached that seen after primary transplantation. Results depend on whether the retransplant is urgent or elective. Patient survival of 82% was reported after elective retransplant versus 46% for urgent cases. Patient and graft survival are consistently lower in patients undergoing urgent or early retransplantation; most of these children have acute insults such as PNF or HAT and many have multisystem failure and sepsis.[106,107] Retransplantation for recurrence of underlying liver disease is an infrequent indication in children. Although retransplantation improves overall survival rates, an individual patient's chances of survival decline by up to 20% after the first retransplant and the gap widens with each successive attempt.

Nutrition and growth

Poor nutritional status is associated with a higher post-transplant mortality and morbidity in cirrhotic patients.[108,109] Children commonly suffer from malnutrition prior to transplant and their recovery can be promoted by pre- and postoperative nutritional support.

Impaired growth and short stature have a negative effect on psychosocial development in children. Growth failure must be recognized and limited as much as possible in pediatric transplant candidates. Children with end-stage liver disease have impaired growth from poor nutritional intake and altered absorption and metabolism, which deteriorates further with complications such as cholangitis and ascites. Inadequate protein and calorie intake manifests as poor weight gain, decreased fat stores, and muscle wasting. It is often difficult to maintain adequate nutritional support because of fluid restriction. Even when sufficient calories are delivered, lean body mass may not increase because of alterations in energy metabolism and resistance to growth hormone (both endogenous growth hormone and synthetic recombinant human growth hormone [rhGH]).[110]

Almost all pediatric transplant recipients with chronic liver disease are growth retarded but can expect some catch-up growth after OLT.[111] Within the first year after transplant, children under 2 years of age achieve growth equal to that of an age-matched population; older children show improved growth but remain growth retarded. Residual growth deficits are frequently erased during the prepubertal growth spurt. Children transplanted for biliary atresia or alpha-1-antitrypsin deficiency demonstrate greater growth gains than those transplanted for chronic hepatitis or acute liver failure. Boys tend to be less growth retarded than girls at the time of transplant and grow better afterwards. Delaying transplantation in older children impedes their potential growth.[112]

Causes for delayed linear growth in children after transplant include high dose steroid therapy, poor graft function, and the need for multiple operations.[113] Sarna *et al.*[114] found that growth acceleration did not occur in patients with chronic rejection or impaired graft function. Data accumulated during the long-term follow-up of children after renal transplantation show that whilst growth retardation may improve,[115] it may be limited by poor graft function and/or endocrine abnormalities.[116] Corticosteroids, particularly when given in large doses for extended periods, are probably the most important cause of growth retardation and delay of skeletal maturation.[117]

Pre-transplant management

Careful nutritional assessment will identify children in need of specialist support. End-stage liver disease may make accurate assessment difficult since body weight may be falsely distorted by hepatosplenomegaly or ascites. By itself, body weight is therefore an unreliable measure of nutritional status and lean body mass.[118] Height measurement can help to identify those children with chronic malnutrition (decreased height for age). Mid-arm circumference and skin-fold thickness are indices of skeletal muscle mass and body fat reserves.[119] Micronutrients can be measured biochemically.

Nutritional therapy aims to provide adequate calories, protein, vitamins, minerals, fluid, and electrolytes without aggravating symptoms of end-stage liver disease, such as encephalopathy or ascites.[120] The degree of nutritional support is variable but generally caloric intake is increased to 130% of the recommended daily allowance by adding glucose polymers, MCT oil, and essential fatty acids. Overnight nasogastric feeds may be required to ensure an adequate intake.[121] Some oral intake should continue to maintain feeding skills. Iron and vitamin deficiencies should be corrected. Proteins rich in branched chain amino acids are given in moderation in compensated cirrhotics; protein restriction may be necessary if there is encephalopathy.

Post-transplant management

Immediately after transplantation, surgical stress and corticosteroids contribute to a catabolic state. During this phase, early enteral tube feeding is advisable. Although a gastric and colonic ileus may be present soon after transplantation, nasojejunal feeding is usually well tolerated, even in the absence of bowel sounds. Enteral feeding is preferable to parenteral nutrition; it is associated with lower infection rates, a decreased metabolic response to stress, fewer technical and metabolic problems, and enhanced visceral protein synthesis at a much lower cost.[122–125] Post-transplant complications (e.g., biliary, rejection, renal, and wound) will delay nutritional rehabilitation. Children should progress to normal oral feeding as soon as possible after liver transplantation. Early satiety and taste disturbances from medication are common complaints. Tube feeding should be continued until patients are able to consistently consume at least two-thirds of their estimated requirements.

Successful liver transplantation reverses the growth disturbances caused by chronic liver disease.[126] The most severely affected parameters, mid-arm circumference and skin-fold thickness, recover most rapidly. Children with the most severe growth retardation before transplant show the greatest catch-up growth afterwards,[127] particularly if steroids are used sparingly.[128] Improved nutritional status is associated with increased muscle bulk and subsequent gains in motor scores. Tacrolimus seems to provide a long-term advantage in this respect over cyclosporin-based immunosuppression. Despite adequate nutrition, children with Alagille's syndrome continue to have impaired growth after liver transplantation.[129]

Quality of life

Now that the majority of pediatric liver transplant centers achieve 1-year patient survival rates of 90% or more for children with chronic liver disease, greater attention has been given to quality of life issues. Quality of life is subjective and difficult to measure, especially in children, although some attempts have been made. An early study, prior to the introduction of cyclosporin, of 44 children surviving more than one year after liver transplant, showed that most of the survivors were able to return to school. Quality of life for this cohort ranged from "poor to superior."[130] Quality of life after liver transplantation continues to be partly dependent on good graft function and an absence of complications. Good liver and kidney function after transplantation result in the resolution of ascites, jaundice and pruritus. Metabolic bone disease steadily improves. For example, children who are unable to walk before transplantation because of rickets are able to do so independently within a year.[131]

Survival curves for pediatric liver transplantation tend to plateau after one year and the majority of survivors have relatively few hospital admissions. Prior to the introduction of cyclosporin patients spent 39% of the first year and 5% of subsequent years in hospital. Under cyclosporin immunosuppression, patients spend an average of 8 days (2.3%) in hospital each year. The commonest reason for admission is viral infection, which accounts for nearly 20% of cases. Other admissions are largely due to transplant-related complications.

What about the longer-term drug burden? From about 3 months after OLT, many children only need to take cyclosporin or tacrolimus, with or without prednisolone; the dose of CNIs is gradually reduced to minimize potential toxicity. Antihypertensive agents are the next most common long-term medication.

Neurodevelopmental outcome

Successful liver transplantation affects not only life expectancy and physical growth but also mental and psychosocial development. Zitelli *et al.* found that the majority of children awaiting liver transplantation had gross motor delay, which was more prevalent in preschool children.[132] One year after liver transplantation there was a significant improvement, most marked in children under 2 years of age. In this study, 51% of children were in age-appropriate schools, 26% were a grade below and only 9% required special education. One surprising finding was the high incidence of enuresis, which was nearly four times greater than expected, but the reason for this was unknown. Wayman *et al.*[133] looked at neurodevelopmental function in children transplanted for biliary atresia. At 1 year after transplant, 25% were developing normally, 40% showed delayed psychomotor development, and 35% had delays in both psychomotor and mental development. Infants were at greatest risk of being delayed, especially in the development of expressive language and in independent walking. Development was most significantly impaired if liver transplantation had been performed before 6 months of age.

These studies suggest liver transplantation contributes to improved cognitive function but, in the short term, social and psychomotor development remain delayed.

Psychosocial function

The earliest study on the impact of liver transplantation on psychosocial function was by Zitelli and coworkers.[132] Prior to liver transplantation, parents reported that their children were overly dependent and demanding but 1 year after surgery behavior had improved except for an increase in defiance and aggression. A further problem was abnormal school separation behavior before transplant – parents kept children away from school because they were judged to be too sick or because of parental anxiety. This behavior continued after the transplant, although to a lesser extent. Parents worried that the child would be vulnerable to infection.

School career is an important indicator of psychosocial adjustment. Studies have shown that all eligible children attended school, but between 16 and 45% were one or two grades behind and 9–30% required special education.[132,134–136] Stone *et al.* investigated the long-term psychological adjustment of 20 children followed-up for 5–10 years after liver transplantation.[135] They found that all were in school, and 70% were in an age-appropriate grade. Eighty percent of children participated in organized sport and 85% in extracurricular activities. Most children had reasonably normal family function.[137] The most detailed study of psychosocial adjustment after pediatric liver transplantation was by Tornqvist *et al.*, who investigated 146 children who had been transplanted 2–12 years previously.[134] Children aged 8 to 13 years perceived themselves as being less competent athletically and girls also regarded themselves as being less well behaved and having less scholastic ability. Younger children (4 to 11 years) were considered by their parents as having more problems than healthy children particularly with respect to poor attention and concentration. Increased problems were experienced in adolescents, possibly due to a deeper realization of the consequences of liver transplantation on their future and differences between themselves and their peers.

While many positive aspects of psychosocial function have been noted in children after liver transplantation, problems in school attendance, participation in social activities, and the ability to cope with everyday stress, suggest that these children experience psychosocial difficulties. These may manifest with behavioral problems, depression, anxiety, and reduced self-esteem. These findings support the need for psychological support and intervention in pediatric liver transplant recipients. Although parents tend to view themselves as more relaxed and able to discipline their child more consistently after the transplant, many families find it difficult to adjust. The family hierarchy has invariably been organized around an ill child and rearrangements after successful transplantation may cause major disruption. The child has been used to taking a disproportionate amount of the parents' time and attention often to the detriment of other siblings. Parents remain anxious about their child's prognosis and have persistent long-term concerns about rejection, side-effects of treatment, becoming overprotective, and continuing medical and "social" expenses. Parents who previously devoted most of their energy to the care of a chronically ill child may have abandoned their professional life and find their role within the family with a "well" child more difficult.[138] Penn *et al.* found that children with biliary atresia had limited sibling and peer group interactions and were extremely dependent on their parents but, after successful liver transplantation and with appropriate family support, they interacted freely and more appropriately.[139] Children who were less well adjusted preoperatively developed extreme dependency on the ward environment or severely adverse reactions to hospitalization.[139] Despite these family pressures, the divorce rate among parents of transplanted children appears to be no greater than that reported in families with healthy children.

Conclusions

Long-term survival after liver transplantation can now be anticipated in more than 80% of children. Early surgical and medical obstacles have been successfully negotiated, but the physical, psychological, and social problems engendered by successful transplantation are only beginning to be understood. We still have little idea of the life expectancy of these children and the problems they face as adults. The goal remains donor specific tolerance to enable transplantation without long-term immunosuppression. The quality of life enjoyed by transplant recipients and their families requires further study. We must be alert to the problems of drug compliance, particularly during adolescence and we must continue to strive to ensure that our patients receive the support and education they deserve so that they may fulfil their potential.

REFERENCES

1. Starzl, T. E., Marchioro, T. L., Von Kaulla, K. *et al.* Homotransplantation of the liver in humans. *Surg. Gynecol. Obstet.* 1963; **117**:659–676.

2. National Institutes of Health Consensus Development Conference Statement: Liver Transplantation. June 20–23, 1983. *Hepatology* 1984; **4** (suppl): 107S–110S.
3. Williams, R., Portmann, B., & Tan, K. C. *The Practice of Liver Transplantation*. Edinburgh: Churchill Livingstone, 1995.
4. O'Grady, J. G., Alexander, G. J., Hayllar, K. M., & Williams, R. Early indicators of prognosis in fulminant hepatic failure. *Gastroenterology* 1989; **97**:439–445.
5. Corbally, M. T., Rela, M., Heaton, N. D. *et al.* Orthotopic liver transplantation for acute hepatic failure in children. *Transpl. Int.* 1994; **7**:S104–S107.
6. Starzl, T. E., Demetris, A. J., & Van Thiel, D. Liver transplantation (1). *N. Engl. J. Med.* 1989; **321**:1014–1022.
7. Casavilla, A., Ramirez, C., Shapiro, R. *et al.* Experience with liver and kidney allografts from non-heart-beating donors. *Transplantation* 1995; **59**:197–203.
8. Bismuth, H. & Houssin, D. Reduced size orthotopic liver graft in hepatic transplantation in children. *Surgery* 1984; **95**:367–370.
9. Deshpande, R. R., Bowles, M. J., Vilca-Melendez, H. *et al.* Results of split liver transplantation in children. *Ann. Surg.* 2002; **236**:248–253.
10. Raia, S., Nery, J. R., & Mies, S. Liver transplantation from live donors. *Lancet* 1989; **2**(8661):497.
11. Broelsch, C. E., Whitington, P. F., Emond, J. C. *et al.* Liver transplantation in children from living related donors. Surgical techniques and results. *Ann. Surg.* 1991; **214**:428–439.
12. Ozawa, K., Vemoto, S., Tanaka, K. *et al.* An appraisal of pediatric liver transplantation from living relatives. *Ann. Surg.* 1992; **216**:547–553.
13. Reding, R., de Goyet, J. de V., Delbeke, I. *et al.* Pediatric liver transplantation with cadaveric or living related donors: comparative results in 90 elective recipients of primary grafts. *J. Pediatr.* 1999; **134**:280–286.
14. Liu, C. L., Fan, S. T., Lo, C. M. *et al.* Live donor liver transplantation for fulminant hepatic failure in children. *Liver. Transpl.* 2003; **9**:1185–1190.
15. Broering, D. C., Mueller, L., Ganschow, R. *et al.* Is there still a need for living-related liver transplantation in children? *Ann. Surg.* 2001; **234**:713–721.
16. Kilpe, V. E., Krakauer, H., & Wren, R. E. An analysis of liver transplant experience from 37 transplant centers as reported to Medicare. *Transplantation* 1993; **56**:554–561.
17. Shaw, B. W. Jr, Wood, R. P., Stratta, R. J., Pillen, T. J., & Langnas, A. N. Stratifying the causes of death in liver transplant recipients. An approach to improving survival. *Arch. Surg.* 1989; **124**:895–900.
18. Busuttil, R. W., Seu, P., Millis, J. M. *et al.* Liver transplantation in children. *Ann. Surg.* 1991; **213**:48–57.
19. Otte, J. B., de Ville de Goyet, J., Sokal, E. *et al.* Size reduction of the donor liver is a safe way to alleviate the shortage of size-matched organs in pediatric liver transplantation. *Ann. Surg.* 1990; **211**:146–157.
20. Broelsch, C. E., Emond, J. C., Thistlethwaite, J. R. *et al.* Liver transplantation, including the concept of reduced-size liver transplants in children. *Ann. Surg.* 1988; **208**:410–420.
21. Andrews, W. S., Wanek, E., Fyock, B., Gray, S., & Benser, M. Pediatric liver transplantation: a 3-year experience. *J. Pediatr. Surg.* 1989; **24**:77–82.
22. Fridell, J. A., Jain, A., Reyes, J. *et al.* Causes of mortality beyond 1 year after primary pediatric liver transplant under tacrolimus. *Transplantation* 2002; **74**:1721–1724.
23. Shaw, B. W. Jr., Wood, R. P., Stratta, R. J., Pillen, T. J., & Langnas, A. N. Stratifying the causes of death in liver transplant recipients. An approach to improving survival. *Arch. Surg.* 1989; **24**:895–900.
24. Bilik, R., Yellen, M., & Superina, R. A. Surgical complications in children after liver transplantation. *J. Pediatr. Surg.* 1992; **27**:1371–1375.
25. Farmer, D. G., Yersiz, H., Ghobrial, R. M. *et al.* Early graft function after pediatric liver transplantation: comparison between in situ split liver grafts and living-related liver grafts. *Transplantation* 2001; **72**:1795–1802.
26. Sieders, E., Peeters, P. M., TenVergert, E. M. *et al.* Graft loss after pediatric liver transplantation. *Ann. Surg.* 2002; **235**:125–132.
27. Egawa, H., Shaked, A., Konishi, Y. *et al.* Arterial ketone body ratio in pediatric liver transplantation. *Transplantation* 1993; **55**:522–526.
28. Mazariegos, G. V., O'Toole, K., Mieles, L. A. *et al.* Hyperbaric oxygen therapy for hepatic artery thrombosis after liver transplantation in children. *Liver. Transpl. Surg.* 1999; **5**:429–436.
29. Stringer, M. D., Marshall, M. M., Muiesan, P. *et al.* Survival and outcome after hepatic artery thrombosis complicating pediatric liver transplantation. *J. Pediatr. Surg.* 2001; **36**:888–891.
30. Cheng, Y. F., Chen, C. L., Huang, T. L. *et al.* 3D CT angiography for detection of vascular complications in pediatric liver transplantation. *Liver Transpl.* 2004; **10**:248–252.
31. Rela, M., Muiesan, P., Bhatnagar, V. *et al.* Hepatic artery thrombosis after liver transplantation in children under 5 years of age. *Transplantation* 1996; **61**:1355–1357.
32. Valente, J. F., Alonso, M. H., Weber, F. L., & Hanto, D. W. Late hepatic artery thrombosis in liver allograft recipients is associated with intrahepatic biliary necrosis. *Transplantation* 1996; **61**:61–65.
33. Langnas, A. N., Marujo, W., Stratta, R. J., Wood, R. P., & Shaw, B. W. Jr. Vascular complications after orthotopic liver transplantation. *Am. J. Surg.* 1991; **161**:76–82.
34. Millis, J. M., Seaman, D. S., Piper, J. B. *et al.* Portal vein thrombosis and stenosis in pediatric liver transplantation. *Transplantation* 1996; **62**:748–754.
35. Buell, J. F., Funaki, B., Cronin, D. C. *et al.* Long-term venous complications after full-size and segmental pediatric liver transplantation. *Ann. Surg.* 2002; **236**:658–666.
36. de Ville de Goyet, J., Clapuyt, P., & Otte, J. B. Extrahilar mesenterico-left portal shunt to relieve extrahepatic portal hypertension after partial liver transplant. *Transplantation* 1992; **53**:231–232.
37. Gane, E., Portmann, B., Saxena, R. *et al.* Nodular regenerative hyperplasia of the liver graft after liver transplantation. *Hepatology* 1994; **20**:88–94.

38. Kling, K., Lau, H., & Colombani, P. Biliary complications of living related pediatric liver transplant patients. *Pediatr. Transpl.* 2004; **8**:178–184.
39. Bhatnagar, V., Dhawan, A., Haider, C. *et al.* The incidence and management of biliary complications following liver transplantation in children. *Transpl. Int.* 1995; **8**:388–391.
40. Shaked, A., Vargas, J., Csete, M. E. *et al.* Diagnosis and treatment of bowel perforation following pediatric orthotopic liver transplantation. *Arch. Surg.* 1993; **128**:994–998.
41. Vilca Melendez, H., Vougas, V., Muiesan, P. *et al.* Bowel perforation after paediatric orthotopic liver transplantation. *Transpl. Int.* 1998; **11**:301–304.
42. Jain, A., Mazariegos, G., Pokharna, R. *et al.* The absence of chronic rejection in pediatric primary liver transplant patients who are maintained on tacrolimus-based immunosuppression: a long-term analysis. *Transplantation* 2003; **75**:1020–1025.
43. Sher, L. S., Cosenza, C. A., Michel, J. *et al.* Efficacy of tacrolimus as rescue therapy for chronic rejection in orthotopic liver transplantation: a report of the U.S. *Multicenter Liver Study Group. Transplantation* 1997; **64**:258–263.
44. Klintmalm, G. B., Nery, J. R., Husberg, B. S., Gonwa, T. A., & Tillery, G. W. Rejection in liver transplantation. *Hepatology* 1989; **10**:978–985.
45. Aw, M. M., Taylor, R. M., Verma, A. *et al.* Basiliximab (Simulect) for the treatment of steroid-resistant rejection in pediatric liver transpland recipients: a preliminary experience. *Transplantation* 2003; **75**:796–799.
46. Cho, J. H., Bhatnagar, V., Andreani, P. *et al.* Chronic rejection in paediatric liver transplantation. *Transpl. Proc.* 1997; **29**:4520–4533.
47. Deen, J. L. & Blumberg, D. A. Infectious disease considerations in pediatric organ transplantation. *Semin. Pediatr. Surg.* 1993; **2**:218–234.
48. Rubin, R. H. Prevention of infection in the liver transplant recipient. *Liver Transpl. Surg.* 1996; **2**(5 Suppl 1):89–98.
49. Mellon, A., Shepherd, R. W., Faoagali, J. L. *et al.* Cytomegalovirus infection after liver transplantation in children. *J. Gastroenterol. Hepatol.* 1993; **8**:540–544.
50. Wiesner, R. H., Marin, E., Porayko, M. K. *et al.* Advances in the diagnosis, treatment, and prevention of cytomegalovirus infection after liver transplantation. *Gastroenterol. Clin. North Am.* 1993; **22**:351–366.
51. Stratta, R. J., Shaefer, M. S., Markin, T. S. *et al.* Cytomegalovirus infection and disease after liver transplantation: an overview. *Dig. Dis. Sci.* 1992; **37**:673–688.
52. Martin, M., Manez, R., Linden, P. *et al.* A prospective randomized trial comparing sequential ganciclovir-high dose acyclovir to high dose acyclovir for prevention of cytomegalovirus disease in adult liver transplant recipients. *Transplantation* 1994; **58**:779–785.
53. Langnas, A. N., Markin, R. S., Inagaki, M. *et al.* Epstein–Barr virus hepatitis after liver transplantation. *Am. J. Gastroenterol.* 1994; **89**:1066–1070.
54. Michaels, M. G., Green, M., Wald, E. R., & Starzl, T. E. Adenovirus infection in pediatric liver transplant recipients. *J. Infect. Dis.* 1992; **165**:170–174.
55. Green, M. Viral infections and pediatric liver transplantation. *Pediatr. Transpl.* 2002; **6**:20–24.
56. Broliden, K. Parvovirus B19 infection in pediatric solid-organ and bone marrow transplantation. *Pediatr. Transpl.* 2001; **5**:320–330.
57. Gerber, D. A., Green, M., Jaffe, R., Greenberg, D., Mazariegos, G., & Reyes, J. Cryptosporidial infections after solid organ transplantation in children. *Pediatr. Transpl.* 2000; **4**:50–55.
58. Halstead, A. C. & Nanji, A. A. Artificial lowering the serum creatinine levels in the presence of hyperbilirubinemia. *J. Am. Med. Assoc.* 1984; **251**:38–39.
59. Abu Elmagd, K., Fung, J. J., Alessiani, M. *et al.* The effect of graft function on FK 506 plasma levels, dosages and renal function, with particular reference to the liver. *Transplantation* 1991; **52**:71–77.
60. Platz, K. P., Meuller, A. R., & Blumhardt, G. Nephrotoxicity following orthotopic liver transplantation. *Transplantation* 1994; **58**:170–178.
61. Myers, B. D., Ross, J., Newton, L. *et al.* Cyclosporine-associated chronic nephropathy. *N. Engl. J. Med.* 1984; **311**:699.
62. Hiatt, J. R., Ament, M. E., Berquist, W. E. *et al.* Pediatric liver transplantation at UCLA. *Transpl. Proc.* 1987; **19**:3282.
63. McDiarmid, S. V., Ettenger, R. B., Hawkins, R. A. *et al.* The impairment of true glomerular filtration rate in long-term cyclosporine treated pediatric allograft recipients. *Transplantation* 1990; **49**:81–85.
64. Thompson, M. E., Shapiro, A. P., Johnsen, A. M. *et al.* The contrasting effects of cyclosporin-A and azathioprine on arterial blood pressure and renal function following cardiac transplantation. *Int. J. Cardiol.* 1986; **11**:219–229.
65. Weidle, P. J. & Vlasses, P. H. Systemic hypertension associated with cyclosporin. A review. *Drug Intel. Clin. Pharm.* 1988; **22**:443–450.
66. Textor, S. C. De novo hypertension after liver transplantation. Clinical conference. *Am. J. Hypertens.* 1993; **22**:257–267.
67. Egawa, H., Esquivel, C. O., So, S. K. *et al.* FK 506 conversion therapy in paediatric liver transplantation. *Transplantation* 1994; **57**:1169–1173.
68. Epstein, M. Calcium antagonists and renal protection. *Kidney Int.* 1992; **41**:S66–S72.
69. Textor, S. C., Schwartz, L., Augustine, J. *et al.* Hypertension after transplantation; Hemodynamic and renal effects of labetalol and nifedipine monotherapy. (Abstr.) *Am. J. Hypertens.* 1992; **5**:8A.
70. Ghosh, P., Evans, D. B., Tomlinson, S. A., & Calne, R. Y. Plasma lipids following renal transplantation. *Transplantation* 1973; **15**:521–523.
71. Kobashigawa, J. A., Katznelson, S., Laks, H. *et al.* Effect of pravastatin on outcomes after cardiac transplantation. *N. Engl. J. Med.* 1995; **333**:621–627.
72. Sindhi, R. Sirolimus in pediatric transplant recipients. *Transpl. Proc.* 2003; **35**(3 Suppl.):113S–114S.

73. Yamamoto, S. & Kato, R. Hair growth-stimulating effects of cyclosporin A and tacrolimus, potent immunosuppressants. *Skin. Pharmacol.* 1994; **7**:101–104.
74. Dyall-Smith, D., Trowell, H., & Dyall-Smith, M. L. Benign human papillomavirus infection in renal transplant recipients. *J. Am. Acad. Dermatol.* 1989; **21**:167–179.
75. Ingelfinger, J. R., Grupe, W. E., Topor, M., & Levey, R. H. Warts in a pediatric renal transplant population. *Int. J. Dermatol.* 1991; **30**:785–789.
76. Yuan, Z. F., Davis, A., Macdonald, K., & Bailey, R. R. Use of acitretin for the skin complications in renal transplant recipients. *N. Z. Med. J.* 1995; **108**:255–256.
77. Plevak, D. J., Southorn, P. A., Narr, B. J. *et al.* Intensive care unit experience in the Mayo liver transplant program: the first 100 cases. *Mayo Clin. Proc.* 1989; **64**:433–445.
78. De Bruijn, K. M., Klompmaker, I. J., Sloof, M. J. H. *et al.* Cyclosporin neurotoxicity late after liver transplantation. *Transplantation* 1989; **47**:575–576.
79. European FK506 Multicentre Liver Study Group. Randomised trial comparing tacrolimus (FK506) and cyclosporin in prevention of liver allograft rejection. *Lancet* 1994; **344**:423–428.
80. US Multicentre FK506 Liver Study Group A comparison of tacrolimus (FK506) and cyclosporine for immunosuppression in liver transplantation. *N. Engl. J. Med.* 1994; **331**:1110–1115.
81. Lopez, O. L., Estol, C., Colina, I., Quirogga, J., Imvertarza, O. C., & Van Thiel, D. H. Neurological complications after liver retransplantation. *Hepatology* 1992; **16**:162–166.
82. Bennett, M. W. R., Webster, N. R., & Sadek, S. A. Alterations in plasma magnesium concentrations during liver transplantation. *Transplantation* 1993; **56**:859–861.
83. Adams, D. H., Gunson, B., Honigsberger, L. *et al.* Neurological complications following liver transplantation. *Lancet* 1987; **1**:949–951.
84. Noll, R. B. & Kulkarni, R. Complex visual hallucinations and cyclosporin. *Arch. Neurol.* 1984; **41**:329–330.
85. Di Martini, A., Pajer, K., Trzepacz, P., Fung, J., Starzi, T., & Tringali, R. Psychiatric morbidity in liver transplant patients. *Transpl. Proc.* 1991; **23**:3179–3180.
86. Penn, I. The changing patterns of posttransplant malignancies. *Transpl. Proc.* 1991; **23**:1101–1103.
87. Penn, I. Cancers complicating organ transplantation. (Editorial) *N. Engl. J. Med.* 1990; **323**:1767–1769.
88. Penn, I. Why do immunosuppressed patients develop cancer? *Crit. Rev. Oncogen.* 1989; **1**:27–52.
89. Lee, E. S., Locker, J., Nalesnik, M. *et al.* The association of Epstein-Barr virus with smooth-muscle tumors occurring after organ transplantation. *N. Engl. J. Med.* 1995; **332**: 19–25.
90. Brichard, B., Smets, F., Sokal, E. *et al.* Unusual evolution of an Epstein–Barr virus-associated leiomyosarcoma occurring after liver transplantation. *Pediatr. Transpl.* 2001; **5**:365–369.
91. Jain, A., Nalesnik, M., Reyes, J. *et al.* Posttransplant lymphoproliferative disorders in liver transplantation: a 20-year experience. *Ann. Surg.* 2002; **236**:429–436.
92. Morgan, G. & Superina, R. A. Lymphoproliferative disease after pediatric liver transplantation. *J. Pediatr. Surg.* 1994; **29**:1192–1196.
93. Malatack, J. F., Gartner, J. C., Urbach, A. H., & Zitelli, B. J. Orthotopic liver transplantation, Epstein–Barr virus, cyclosporine, and lymphoproliferative disease: a growing concern. *J. Pediatr.* 1991; **118**:667–675.
94. Ho, M., Miller, G., Atchinson, R. W. *et al.* Epstein–Barr virus infections and DNA hybridization studies in posttransplantation lymphoma and lymphoproliferative lesions: the role of primary infection. *J. Infect. Dis.* 1985; **152**:876–886.
95. Cohen, J. Epstein–Barr virus lymphoproliferative disease associated with acquired immunodeficiency. *Medicine* 1991; **70**:137–160.
96. Oertel, S. H., Anagnostopoulos, I., Bechstein, W. O. *et al.* Treatment of posttransplant lymphoproliferative disorder with the anti-CD20 monoclonal antibody rituximab alone in an adult after liver transplantation: a new drug in therapy of patients with posttransplant lymphoproliferative disorder after solid organ transplantation? *Transplantation* 2000; **69**:430–432.
97. Serinet, M. O., Jacquemin, E., Habes, D., Debray, D., Fabre, M., & Bernard, O. Anti-CD20 monoclonal antibody (Rituximab) treatment for Epstein–Barr virus-associated, B-cell lymphoproliferative disease in pediatric liver transplant recipients. *J. Pediatr. Gastroenterol. Nutr.* 2002; **34**:389–393.
98. Benkerrou, M., Durandy, A., & Fischer, A. Therapy for transplant-related lymphoproliferative diseases. *Hematol. Oncol. Clin. North Am.* 1993; **7**:467–475.
99. Abu-Elmagd, K., Bronsther, O., Jain, A. *et al.* Recent advances in hepatic transplantation at the University of Pittsburgh. *Clin. Transpl.* 1993; 137–152.
100. Jain, A., Mazariegos, G., Kashyap, R. *et al.* Pediatric liver transplantation in 808 consecutive children: 20-years experience from a single center. *Transpl. Proc.* 2002; **34**:1955–1957.
101. Sudan, D. L., Shaw, B. W. Jr, & Langnas, A. N. Causes of late mortality in pediatric liver transplant recipients. *Ann. Surg.* 1998; **227**:289–295.
102. Vogt, D. P., Henderson, J. M., Carey, W. D., Barnes, D. The long-term survival and causes of death in patients who survive at least 1 year after liver transplantation. *Surgery* 2002; **132**:775–780.
103. McDiarmid, S., Busuttil, R. W., Goss, J. *et al.* Causes of late graft dysfunction, retransplantation (RE-TX) and death after pediatric (OLT) orthotopic liver transplantation. (Abstract). *Liver Transpl. Surg.* 1997; **30**:1397.
104. Kerkar, N., Hadzic, N., Davies, E. T. *et al.* De-novo autoimmune hepatitis after liver transplantation. *Lancet* 1998; **35**:409–413.
105. Deshpande, R. R., Rela, M., Girlanda, R. *et al.* Long-term outcome of liver retransplantation in children. *Transplantation* 2002; **74**:1124–1130.
106. Shaw, B. W., Gordon, R. D., Iwatsuki, S. *et al.* Hepatic transplantation. *Transpl. Proc.* 1985; **17**:264–271.
107. Esquivel, C. O., Koneru, B., Todo, S. *et al.* Is multiple organ failure a contraindication for liver transplantation in children? *Transpl. Proc.* 1987; **19** (Suppl. 3): 47–48.

108. Muller, M. J., Lautz, H. U., Plogmann, B., Burger, M., Korber, J., & Schmidt, F. W. Energy expenditure and substrate oxidation in patients with cirrhosis: The impact of cause, clinical staging and nutritional state. *Hepatology* 1992; **15**:782–794.
109. Pikul, J., Sharpe, M. D., Lowndes, R., & Chent, C. N. Degree of preoperative malnutrition is predictive of postoperative morbidity and mortality in liver transplant recipients. *Transplantation* 1994; **57**:469–472.
110. Bucuvalas, J. C., Cutlield, W., Horn, J., & Balistreri, W. F. Resistance to the growth promoting and metabolic effects of GH in children with chronic liver disease. *J. Pediatr.* 1990; **117**:397–402.
111. Becht, M. B., Pedersen, S. H., Ryckman, F. C., & Balistreri, W. F. Growth and nutritional management of pediatric patients after orthotopic liver transplantation. *Gastroenterol. Clin. North Am.* 1993; **22**:367–380.
112. Renz, J. F., de Roos, M., Rosenthal, P. *et al.* Posttransplantation growth in pediatric liver recipients. *Liver Transpl.* 2001; **7**:1040–1055.
113. Urbach, A. H., Gartner, J. C., & Malatac, J. J. Linear growth following pediatric liver transplantation. *Am. J. Dis. Child.* 1987; **141**:547–549.
114. Sarna, S., Sipila, I., Jaianko, H., Laine, J., & Holmberg, C. Factors affecting growth after pediatric liver transplantation. *Transpl. Proc.* 1994; **26**:161–164.
115. Van Diemen-Steenvoorde, R. & Donckerwoicke, R. A. *et al.* Growth and sexual maturation in children after kidney transplantation. *Acta Paediatr. Scand.* Suppl. 1988; **343**:109–117.
116. Holt, R. I., Baker, A. J., & Miell, J. P. The pathogenesis of growth failure in pediatric liver disease. *J. Hepatol.* 1997; **27**:413–423.
117. Wehrenberg, W. B., Janowski, B. A., Piedring, A. W., Cullier, F., & Jones, K. L. Giucocorticoids: potent inhibitors and stimulators of growth hormone secretion. *Endocrinology* 1990; **126**:3200–3203.
118. Hehir, D. J., Jenkins, R. L., & Bistrian, B. R. Nutrition in patients undergoing orthotopic liver transplant. *J. Parenter. Enteral. Nutr.* 1985; **9**:695–700.
119. Ryckman, F. R., Fisher, R. A., Pedersen, S. H., & Balistreri, W. F. Liver transplantation in children. *Semin. Pediatr. Surg.* 1992; **1**:162–172.
120. Munoz, S. J. Nutritional therapies in liver disease. *Semin. Liver Dis.* 1991; **11**:278–291.
121. Moreno, L. A., Gottrand, F., Hoden, S. *et al.* Improvement of nutritional status in cholestatic children with supplemental nocturnal enteral nutrition. *J. Pediatr. Gastroenterol. Nutr.* 1991; **12**:213–216.
122. Zaloga, G. P. & MacGregor, D. A. What to consider when choosing enteral or parenteral nutrition: is the guideline still "if the gut works, use it"? *J. Crit. Ill* 1990; **5**:1180–1200.
123. Bower, R. H., Talamini, M. A., Sax, H. C., Hamilton, F., & Fischer, J. E. Postoperative enteral versus parenteral nutrition: a randomized controlled trial. *Arch. Surg.* 1986; **121**:1040–1045.
124. Kudsk, K. A., Croce, M. A., Fabian, T. C. *et al.* Enteral versus parenteral feeding: effects on septic morbidity after blunt and penetrating abdominal trauma. *Ann. Surg.* 1992; **215**:503–513.
125. Moore, F. A., Feliciano, D. V., Andrassy, R. J. *et al.* Early enteral feeding compared with parenteral reduces postoperative septic complications: The results of a meta-analysis. *Ann. Surg.* 1992; **216**:172–183.
126. Chin, S. E., Shepherd, R. W., Thomas, B. J. *et al.* The nature of malnutrition in children with end-stage liver disease awaiting orthotopic liver transplantation. *Am. J. Clin. Nutr.* 1992; **56**:164–168.
127. Holt, R. I., Broide, E., Buchanan, C. R. *et al.* Orthotopic liver transplantation reverses the adverse nutritional changes of end-stage liver disease in children. *Am. J. Clin. Nutr.* 1997; **65**:534–542.
128. Spolidoro, J. V., Berquist, W. E., & Pehiivanoglu, E. Growth acceleration in children after orthotopic liver transplantation. *J. Pediatr.* 1988; 112:41–44.
129. Bucuvalas, J. C., Horn, J. A., Carisson, L. *et al.* Growth hormone insensitivity associated with elevated circulating growth hormone binding protein in children with Alagille Syndrome and short stature. *J. Clin. Endocrinol. Metabol.* 1994; **76**:1477–1482.
130. Starzl, T. E., Koep, L. J., Schroter, G. P. J. *et al.* The quality of life after liver transplantation. *Transpl. Proc.* 1979; **11**:252–256.
131. Zitelli, B. J., Miller, J. W., Gartner, J. C. *et al.* Changes in lifestyle after liver transplantation. *Pediatrics* 1988; **82**:173–180.
132. Zitelli, B. J., Gartner, J. C., Malatack, J. J. *et al.* Pediatric liver transplantation: patient evaluation and selection, infectious complications, and life-style after transplantation. *Transpl. Proc.* 1987; **4**:3309–3316.
133. Wayman, K. I., Cox, K. L., & Esquivel, C. O. Neurodevelopmental outcome of young children with extrahepatic biliary atresia 1 year after liver transplantation. *J. Pediatr.* 1997; **131**:894–898.
134. Tornqvist, J., Van Broeck, N., Finkenauer, C. *et al.* Long-term psychosocial adjustment following pediatric liver transplantation. *Pediatr. Transpl.* 1999; **3**:115–125.
135. Stone, R. D., Beasley, P. J., Treacy, S. J. *et al.* Children and families can achieve normal psychological adjustment and a good quality of life following pediatric liver transplantation: a long-term study. *Transpl. Proc.* 1997; **29**:1571–1572.
136. Zamberlan, K. E. Quality of life in school-age children following liver transplantation. *Maternal–Child Nurs. J.* 1992; **20**:167–229.
137. Schulz, K. H., Hofmann, K., Sander, S. *et al.* Comparison of quality of life and family stress in families of children with living-related liver transplants versus families of children who received a cadaveric liver. *Transpl. Proc.* 2001; **33**:1496–1497.
138. Gold, L. M., Kirkpatrick, B. S., Fricker, F. J., & Zitelli, B. J. Psychosocial issues in pediatric organ transplantation. The parent's perspective. *Pediatrics* 1986; **77**:738–744.
139. Penn, I., Bunch, D., Olenik, D. *et al.* Psychiatric experience with patients receiving renal and hepatic transplants. *Semin. Psychiatry* 1971; **3**:133–144.

66

Intestinal and multivisceral transplantation

Jorge Reyes and Geoffrey Bond

Children's Hospital of Pittsburgh, PA, USA

Introduction

Visceral transplantation is the accepted standard of care for patients in end-stage organ failure. It is well established in kidney, liver, and cardiac failure. Recently pancreas and lung transplantation have also become routine, although infrequently performed in the pediatric population. Although one of the first organs to be transplanted as an *en-bloc* procedure with the liver, the intestine has been a notoriously difficult organ to successfully transplant. Early results were universally poor, and it wasn't until the development and use of tacrolimus in 1990 that the procedure could be performed with reasonable expectation of success. Even so, initial outcomes were marginal with many programs performing only a handful of cases before terminating their experience. A few centers persevered, and with ongoing experience and continued development have greatly advanced the field. It has evolved in every aspect, technically and medically, but this is true in particular with respect to advances in immunosuppression protocols. Currently, the outcomes are approaching that achieved in other types of organ transplantation, and it has become the accepted standard of care for patients with irreversible intestinal failure who are failing parenteral nutrition.

Historical perspective

Clinical organ transplantation dates back to 1960 with the first successful kidney transplantation.[1] Successes followed in liver,[2] pancreas,[3] heart[4] and lung.[5] On the contrary, the early experience with intestinal transplantation, either alone or with other organ combinations, both in humans and research animals, was universally poor. Even into the 1980s, successful human intestinal transplantation was rare and mostly short lived.[7–10] The longest current surviving intestinal transplant patient is a recipient of a cadaveric isolated intestinal transplant in Paris in 1989 under cyclosporin immunosuppression.[11]

The large mass of lymphoid tissue associated with the mesentery of the intestine and within the gut itself predisposed the recipient to episodes of rejection that were more difficult to control. In addition to immunological hurdles, significant technical and infectious complications made management difficult. It was not until 1990 with the clinical use of the new and more effective immunosuppressant tacrolimus, that intestinal transplantation could be routinely performed with any reasonable notion of success.[12]

Over the next decade, intestinal transplantation became dependent on the art of balancing treatment of rejection with increasingly potent immunosuppression protocols whilst monitoring and treating infectious and other related complications caused by these very protocols. At the same time, surgical and medical advances, combined with ever increasing experience, allowed for advancement and expansion in the field.

Although short-term patient and graft survival have markedly improved, now approaching that possible with other organ transplants, emphasis on long-term outcomes and the effort to avoid complications related to immunosuppression has led to the development of novel "tolerogenic" protocols at several centers. Using lymphocyte-depleting induction therapy and steroid-free, low dose monotherapy postoperatively, these protocols place patients on dosing regimens never before used in intestinal recipients. This is diametrically opposed

Pediatric Surgery and Urology: Long-term Outcomes, Mark Stringer, Keith Oldham, Pierre Mouriquand.
Published by Cambridge University Press.

Table 66.1. Primary indication for pediatric intestinal transplantation

Gastroschisis	22%
Volvulus	19%
Necrotizing enterocolitis	13%
Pseudo-obstruction	10%
Intestinal atresia	9%
Hirschsprung's disease	8%
Microvillus inclusion disease	7%
Miscellaneous	12%

Modified from the International Intestinal Transplant Registry 2003.

Table 66.2. Primary indication for adult intestinal transplantation

Ischemia	24%
Crohn's disease	15%
Trauma	11%
Desmoid/Gardner's	13%
Motility disorders	9%
Volvulus	7%
Short gut (other)	7%
Miscellaneous	14%

Modified from the International Intestinal Transplant Registry 2003.

to the increasingly potent immunosuppression protocols employed previously. It is expected that moderation of immunosuppression will have profound long-term benefits to the recipients, especially in the pediatric population.

Indications for intestinal transplantation

Intestinal failure can be defined as the inability of a patient to maintain nutritional and fluid/electrolyte balance without intravenous support. In the pediatric population, intestinal failure also prevents normal growth and development. When this situation becomes irreversible, the patient is committed to indefinite parenteral nutrition and fluid support. The majority of patients with intestinal failure have an anatomically short gut, resulting from either congenitally deficient or shortened intestine from an acquired condition. Etiologies in children and adults are typically different (Tables 66.1 and 66.2). In children many of the conditions are congenital, such as intestinal atresia, volvulus or gastroschisis.[13] In others, the condition is acquired, such as necrotizing enterocolitis, or trauma. In a small proportion, the cause of intestinal failure is functional. This can be due to dysmotility syndromes, such as intestinal pseudo-obstruction or Hirschsprung's disease, or functional abnormalities of the intestinal mucosa, such as microvillus inclusion disease or enteropathies. In rare circumstances, benign tumors, such as inflammatory pseudotumor and desmoid tumor associated with familial polyposis/Gardner's syndrome necessitate intestinal resection and subsequent short gut.

The initial treatment of intestinal failure necessitates intravenous nutritional support via a central line. Parenteral nutrition has become a lifesaving therapy over the last 30 years; however, its use and delivery is not without complications.[12,14] Short gut management issues encompass related problems, including liver failure and line related complications, such as sepsis and venous thrombosis. Parenteral nutrition-related liver disease is more prevalent in the pediatric population, especially in neonates, than in adults. Onset of liver disease in the circumstance of short bowel syndrome heralds imminent demise of the patient. Hence, although the intestine itself is not a vital organ, the therapy to overcome its deficiency can create life-threatening complications. As a result of this, intestinal transplantation was developed to restore physiological function of the gastrointestinal tract and remove the need for venous access and parenteral nutrition.

Types of intestinal transplant and implantation techniques

The experimental and clinical basis of intestinal and multivisceral transplantation is based on the early canine work by Lillehei[15] and Starzl,[6] and human trials in 1987. Early human results for malignancy related multivisceral transplantation were discouraging due to tumor recurrence.[16,17] However, this experience helped establish the principles of *en-bloc* organ recovery and organ replacement. Subsequent technical modifications[12,18] limited the organs transplanted to only those required (intestine and liver). Technical considerations produced further changes,[19,20] to preserve the hepatobiliary and duodenal complex for composite liver and intestine allografts. To allow for maximal organ utilization, and with new understanding of the blood flow to the abdominal visceral organs, procurement of abdominal organs in isolation or *en-bloc* became established. In particular, it was shown that liver, pancreas and intestine could be procured as separate and fully functioning entities suitable for transplantation.[21]

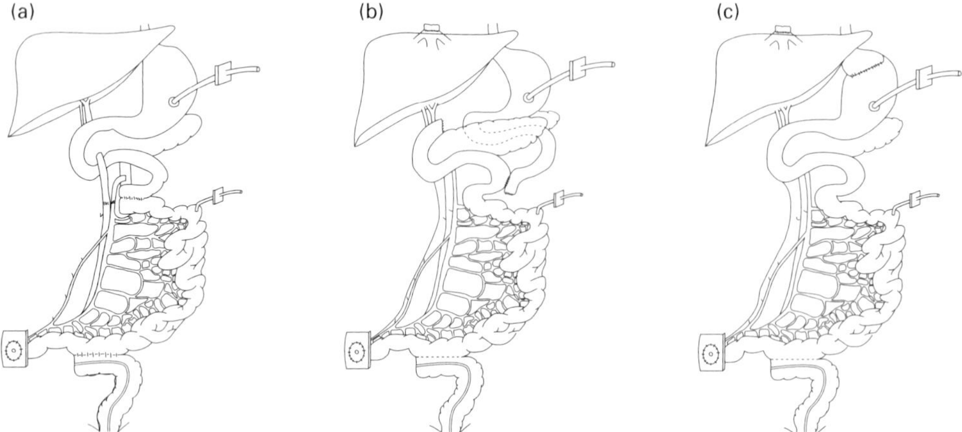

Fig. 66.1. (a) Isolated intestinal transplant – allograft jejunum anastomosed to native jejunum. Allograft ileum anastomosed to native colon. Terminal allograft ileum brought out as ileostomy. G-tube (gastrostomy) and J-tube (feeding jejunostomy) shown. Arterial inflow via aortic conduit to allograft SMA. Venous outflow from allograft SMV to native SMV (can also drain into IVC).
(b) Liver intestine transplant – native stomach, duodenum, pancreas, and proximal jejunum retained, drained to the intestinal allograft via native jejunum/allograft jejunum anastomosis. Arterial inflow via aortic vascular graft. Venous outflow via donor suprahepatic cava to recipient cava.
(c) Full multivisceral transplant – entire GI tract and liver replaced with remaining cuff of native cardia anastomosed to donor stomach. (With a modified multivisceral transplant, the native liver is utilized, and the native duodenum and pancreas remains. Pancreatico-biliary secretions are drained to the transplanted allograft via a native jejunum to donor jejunum anastomosis.)

Some of the earliest intestinal transplants were intestinal segments procured from live donors.[22] Results were poor, as was typical of the time, and this form of procurement remains controversial and uncommon today, as reflected in the International Intestinal Registry[23] in which less than 4% of intestinal grafts come from live donors.

There are three basic types of intestinal transplants; transplantation in isolation, in combination with the liver, or as a multivisceral graft (Fig. 66.1). However, as the operation has become more individualized to the patients needs, numerous variations and techniques have been developed. Donor and recipient operative details have been described in detail.[24] Donors should be ABO identical (worse outcomes if not), otherwise young, fit and healthy (minimal cardiovascular risk factors), and hemodynamically stable on minimal inotropic agents. Careful donor selection and a meticulous procurement operation are vital to subsequent successful transplantation.

Isolated intestinal transplant

In this operation the entire cadaveric small intestine (jejunum and ileum) from the ligament of Treitz to the ileocecal valve is procured. In the majority of cases, it is transplanted in its entirety. Recently, due to limited availability of size-matched organs especially in very small children, allograft reduction has been utilized.

For the most part, arterial inflow is via a vascular conduit (donor iliac or carotid artery) anastomosed from the recipient aorta to the donor superior mesenteric artery (SMA). Occasionally, where an adequate recipient SMA is available, arterial flow can be established via this route, with or without an arterial interposition extension graft.

Venous outflow is via the donor superior mesenteric vein (SMV). It can be anastomosed to either the recipient SMV (portal flow) or inferior vena cava (systemic flow) directly or utilizing a venous extension graft (iliac or jugular/subclavian vein). The decision is based on technical factors as well as the assessment of recipient liver disease and portal hypertension. The choice of outflow (portal vs. systemic circulation) appears to have no bearing on outcome.[25]

Enteric anastomoses to restore gastrointestinal continuity are dependent on the remnant native intestinal tract. The proximal anastomosis is typically to the remaining native jejunum or duodenum in a side-to-side or end-to-side fashion. If there is remnant colon or rectum, or rarely native distal ileum, a distal anastomosis is made to this. If there is insufficient or dysfunctional lower gastrointestinal tract (as in pseudo-obstruction), or none at all, an end ileostomy is brought out. In all cases, a temporary ileostomy is made, primarily for monitoring purposes. This can be done as either a Brooks type ileostomy, or a loop ileostomy just proximal to the lower ileocolic anastomosis. In the former, the ileocolic anastomosis is made and a short segment of terminal ileal allograft brought out to the skin and a stoma made (that segment is often referred to as the "chimney" component).

A minority of centers persist in transplanting a segment of colon with the intestinal allograft. Others reported increased infectious complications from its use.[26] As fluid losses could be managed with pharmacological agents and it did not perform an essential role, they abandoned its use.

Liver/intestine transplant

Combined liver and intestinal transplant replaces both the failing native liver and provides intestinal function. Initially, the organs were transplanted as separate entities. This necessitated the formation of an intestinal roux-en-Y loop, creating functional loss of some transplanted intestine, as well as producing other biliary and vascular complications. To overcome this, the duodenum and pancreatic head were preserved to maintain hepatobiliary continuity,[20] and arterial inflow was maximized via a Carrel patch containing the entire celiac artery and SMA axis. This technique also allowed for improved utilization of very small donor organs and is the basis for contemporary liver/intestine transplants. Initially, the pancreas was resected distal to the SMA and oversewn. More recently the whole pancreas has been included in the allograft bloc to avoid pancreatic leaks and provide supplemental pancreatic endocrine function.

The donor organs (liver, duodenum, pancreas, and intestine) are recovered *en-bloc* complete with the entire descending thoracic aorta. The arterial inflow is via the donor thoracic aorta, which is divided and anastomosed separately to the recipient abdominal aorta and the donor Carrel patch of celiac artery and SMA. Once the organs are brought into the field, a simple donor to donor aortic anastomosis is performed. Venous outflow for the entire organ bloc is via the donor liver hepatic vein/caval confluence to the native hepatic vein/caval confluence.

A portosystemic shunt to drain venous blood from the native stomach, duodenum, pancreas, spleen and proximal jejunum is made between the native portal vein and IVC. This can later be taken down and redirected to the transplanted portal vein; however, no benefit from this maneuver has been identified.[27] Enteric continuity is established via the terminal portion of the proximal native intestine (duodenum or jejunum) and proximal allograft jejunum (side to side or end to side). The distal allograft ileum is either brought out as an end ileostomy or anastomosed to the remaining distal gastrointestinal tract as described above for an isolated intestinal graft.

Multivisceral transplant

Full multivisceral transplant

This technique provides for transplantation of all abdominal intraperitoneal components, excluding remnant colon. This transplant includes the stomach, duodenum, pancreas, intestine and liver. The donor procedure is similar to a liver/intestine transplant, with the stomach and left gastric artery being retained. Recipient stomach (except a small cuff of cardia), duodenum, pancreas, spleen, remaining proximal gut and liver are excised. Native colon is preserved as pathologically and clinically indicated.

Arterial inflow is via the donor thoracic aorta to either the supraceliac or infrarenal recipient aorta. Venous outflow for the entire bloc is via the hepatic vein/caval complex as described above. Proximal gastrointestinal continuity is restored via a gastro-gastric anastomosis. In some centers an esophagogastric or esophagoesophageal anastomosis is performed. Pyloroplasty is necessary consequent to vagal denervation from the donor procedure. The distal intestine is managed as described above.

Modified multivisceral transplant (MMV)

In this procedure, the entire donor gastrointestinal tract is transplanted except that the donor liver can be transplanted into another patient as the recipient liver is viable. This can be achieved by either complete excision of the native stomach, duodenum, pancreas, spleen and intestine (as for familial polyposis/desmoid tumor) or by excision of the stomach and intestine whilst retaining the hepaticoduodenopancreatic complex (as possible in pseudo-obstruction). The donor operation is similar to that described previously, except that the liver allograft is removed and transplanted into another recipient. The hepatic artery is divided distal to the takeoff of the splenic artery to keep the left gastric and splenic artery with the multivisceral allograft. It is not essential to keep the gastroduodenal artery with the MMV bloc. An aberrant left hepatic artery arising from the left gastric artery usually precludes a MMV allograft as the liver allograft takes priority with vascular supply. The portal vein is divided above the junction of SMV and splenic vein, allowing appropriate length for the liver allograft.

Arterial inflow is as described for a full multivisceral allograft. Venous outflow is via the donor portal vein to the recipient portal vein, replacing the previous portal inflow to the liver, or via the SMV if the native pancreaticoduodenal complex is retained. Enteric reconstruction is as described for a full multivisceral transplant. When the entire gastrointestinal tract has been excised, the bile duct is divided as a matter of course. Initially, biliary reconstruction was achieved with a roux-en-Y choledochojejunal anastomosis, but this resulted in functional intestinal allograft loss. A recently described innovation utilizes the procurement of part of the donor bile duct to allow for primary duct to duct anastomosis in suitable sized recipients.

Other variations of intestinal transplant

In uncommon circumstances where intestinal failure and pancreatic complications coexist, such as cystic fibrosis and insulin-dependent diabetes, simultaneous en-bloc pancreas and intestine transplant has been performed. This can be achieved like a modified multivisceral transplant with the stomach excised, utilizing the Carrel patch technique. If the celiac axis is not available, the splenic artery can be divided and a donor arterial Y-graft is used to supply blood flow to the splenic artery and SMA, as is done with an isolated pancreatic allograft.

In pseudo-obstruction, there is controversy as to whether there is a need to replace the stomach, as is done with a MMV transplant. An alternative is to perform an isolated intestinal transplant with gastrojejunal drainage. Recently one center has included the donor spleen with the transplant in an attempt to promote chimerism. The concept here is similar to that of donor bone marrow augmentation which has been utilized by a few centers.[28–30] However, results from this procedure have not led to any significant improvements and the use of the spleen remains controversial.

Live donation

As mentioned, some of the earliest intestinal transplant grafts were procured from live donors. Conceptually there are benefits from an organizational point of view and timing of the case; however, except for identical twins there appears to be minimal immunological benefit. Cold ischemic time may well be reduced, presumably leading to decreased ischemia-reperfusion injury, but no data are currently available to show that this is clinically significant. As well, there is little problem in obtaining isolated intestine from a cadaveric donor, negating concern of time spent on the waiting list. Outcomes to date have not been any better than for cadaveric donors. Live donor intestinal allografts performed during the early experience all failed, mostly due to chronic rejection.

Patient evaluation/selection criteria

It is advisable that all patients with intestinal failure be considered for intestinal transplantation. Unfortunately, many physicians are, unaware of recent successes and advancements in intestinal transplantation. Therefore, patients are delayed in referral and may develop terminal complications of parenteral nutrition (end-stage liver failure or near complete loss of venous access). Timely evaluation allows for adequate assessment of patient needs.

Patient evaluation involves a multidisciplinary team of health professionals. Evaluation can be an extensive process and frequently requires admission to hospital. Initial assessment includes transplant surgeons, pediatric surgeons, gastroenterologists and nutritionists, transplant co-ordinators, and psychosocial/ fiscal experts. Further evaluation may require expertise in the fields of radiology (especially interventional radiology), cardiopulmonary medicine, hematology, and other areas.

In some patients, modifications in parenteral and enteral nutrition may allow for adaptation that can avert or delay transplantation. In others, surgical corrective and reconstructive techniques can be employed to avoid transplantation. The aim of evaluation is to determine whether a patient requires intestinal transplantation, and then determine the type of transplant required. It is then imperative to determine if they are medically fit and surgically able to undergo transplantation (devoid of major cardiac, pulmonary or central nervous system disorders).

As of October 2000 in the United States, the federal government (Medicare Program)[31] has accepted intestinal transplantation as the standard of care for patients with end-stage intestinal failure who are failing parenteral nutrition. Criteria include parenteral nutrition associated liver failure, loss of venous access (thrombosis of three or more of the six major veins), and recurrent hospital admissions for life-threatening venous access-related infections. These criteria have been widely used for intestinal transplantation, although some centers have recently proposed earlier transplantation in circumstances where it appears intestinal transplantation is either inevitable or the patient would otherwise benefit from intestinal transplantation.[32]

Once irreversible intestinal failure occurs, and complications from parenteral nutrition become evident, the evaluation process tries to determine what type of transplant is required. Is it possible to perform an isolated intestinal transplant, or will a composite allograft including the liver be required? Various factors are assessed, including degree of hyperbilirubinemia, splenomegaly, portal hypertensive gastropathy/gastric varices, and thrombocytopenia.

Persistently elevated serum bilirubin is associated with a high mortality risk and the patient should be considered for transplantation.[33] Routine clinical abnormalities seen in liver disease, such as ascites and encephalopathy, may not be evident in the patient with short gut syndrome.[34] Nutritionally, these patients may not appear deplete due to the use of parenteral nutrition. The ultimate assessment includes liver biopsy, most safely performed via a transjugular route at the time of venous assessment; however, even this may not always be conclusive. In the face of a normal liver biopsy and other normal liver parameters, the decision not to replace the liver is straightforward. Likewise, when cirrhosis and major liver dysfunction is present, a composite allograft is required. When the evaluation falls somewhere in-between, the decision becomes less clear. For maximal organ utilization and other patient-derived factors, it is preferable not to replace the liver unless essential; however, an isolated intestinal graft may fail if the liver does not have sufficient reserve. In this circumstance, experience and good judgment is vital if the optimal decision is to be made.

It is important to determine venous patency to establish candidacy for transplantation, urgency of transplantation (near loss of all access), and possible anesthetic/surgical access during the operative and postoperative period. This can be performed by ultrasound, although venograms are both more sensitive and specific.

Other contentious issues include the type of intestinal transplantation in patients with pseudo-obstruction, as disease extent is variable. In particular, does the stomach need replacement, and can a part of the native colon or rectum be retained for distal reconstruction? In part, these questions can be assessed by motility and manometric studies, although even these may not be definitive. Functional and radiological assessment of the entire gastrointestinal tract is important.[35] An alternative is to perform an isolated intestinal transplant with gastrojejunal bypass. Especially in functional conditions, one also has to be aware of a patient possibly presenting with Munchausen's disease, or Munchausen's by proxy in the pediatric population.

Contraindications to intestinal transplantation

Contraindications to intestinal transplantation are similar to those routinely established in other forms of transplantation and include recent malignancy (within 5 years), uncontrolled infection, including HIV, significant cardiac and/or respiratory disease and neurological dysfunction. Some of these have become less absolute in recent years, and individual factors are taken into consideration. Bacterial infection of a venous catheter for example is not a contraindication if recognized and under treatment. There are no specific age or weight restrictions, although it is difficult to obtain size matched organs for children weighing less than 5 kg.

Post-transplant management

Early

Intestinal transplant recipients, especially those requiring concurrent liver transplantation, are some of the most challenging and difficult patients to manage in any field of medicine. These patients, who are often extremely sick with multiple system dysfunction prior to the transplant, then undergo the complex stress of having multiple organs removed and new (albeit better but foreign) ones transplanted. Management involves all body systems, in particular cardiopulmonary support, renal/fluid management and infectious disease prophylaxis and treatment, as well as manipulation of the immune system. Understandably, initial patient care is in the intensive care unit (ICU). Length of ICU stay is longer with the composite allografts consequent to their pre-morbid liver disease and complications related to this. Patients remain intubated and ventilated until neurologically recovered, hemodynamically stable and able to breathe on their own. Much of the initial management revolves around proper fluid balance without compromising pulmonary function. Due to low albumin levels, SPA (concentrated salt-poor albumin) is often required, in addition to diuretics, such as furosemide. Manipulation of the parenteral nutrition, including reducing the protein content to assist in lowering the serum BUN may be required. Judicious use of lipids is necessary, especially if postoperative pancreatitis is present. In recent pediatric cases, parenteral nutrition is avoided and the patient managed with intravenous fluids using early enteral feeding via jejunostomy.

Immunologically these patients are challenging, especially during early management, whilst the interaction between recipient and donor immune system is established. With current tolerogenic protocols using a lymphocyte depleting agent, this is even more pronounced. Fevers are routine, and may be immunological in origin, similar to a serum sickness reaction. However, this is often a diagnosis of exclusion, as infectious causes must be ruled out. Graft versus host reaction with skin rashes may also be seen and must be differentiated from drug reactions. Skin biopsy and chimeric blood studies assist in determining subsequent management.

Once transferred from the ICU, the patient progresses with further recovery and rehabilitation. This involves both physical therapy, but also nutritional rehabilitation, as typically the recipient has been unable to eat properly for some period of time. Major issues include fluid and electrolyte balance, pain management and introducing new medications. It is not uncommon for the patient to require further surgeries. Once medically and surgically fit, the patient can be discharged to some local outpatient setting for follow-up in the clinic, or occasionally transferred to a dedicated rehabilitation unit depending on the degree of disability.

Intermediate

The first 6 to 12 months after an intestinal or multivisceral transplant are still challenging. Recipients and their caregivers are required to stay in the local area for the first month or two after discharge until a stable state is achieved. Early readmissions to the hospital are common. When clinically stable, older patients have to learn to cope for themselves, and become less reliant on caregivers. Caregivers also have to undergo change, returning independence to the recipient and resuming their pre-illness roles, which may be challenging. For pediatric patients, the goal is to regain health, become stronger and develop. Often there is a catch-up growth phase, as the recipient has been sick for an extended period.

During this period, close monitoring of the graft and patient is carried out. The intensity of follow-up becomes less frequent in a stable recipient. Issues include nutritional status, appropriate growth and development, fluid and electrolyte management, monitoring of the graft for rejection, compliance with medications, immunosuppressive changes and monitoring for infectious complications.

Late

Intensity of follow-up lessens with time, however vigilance is still required. Close communication between the recipient/caregivers and local medical facilities with the transplant team is essential for optimal outcomes, as most facilities have little experience with intestinal transplant recipients. Issues include potential complications from chronic immunosuppression, including renal dysfunction, diabetes, hypertension, and infectious complications. Episodes of acute cellular rejection can still occur, especially when the immune system is activated during a period of incidental viral infection. More worrisome is chronic rejection, occurring more frequently in the isolated intestinal allografts. Although a point of controversy, many centers believe the liver provides a protective effect to the intestinal allograft, accounting for the lower incidence of chronic intestinal rejection in the composite allografts.[29]

Monitoring

The development of techniques to monitor the allograft and recipient for complications, and the experience gained in managing these issues over the last decade has added immeasurably to the markedly improved clinical outcomes. Although the transplant itself is of vital importance, it is the post-transplant management that really dictates the eventual outcome, both short and long term. Centers with larger experiences have been shown to have significantly improved results.[23] The ability to recognize potential or actual complications early, and manage them before they become life or allograft threatening, distinguishes the more successful centers.

Allograft rejection and function

As with all transplant recipients, monitoring of the allograft function and the interaction with the recipient is essential for both short- and long-term outcomes to be successful. Unlike other solid organs, the symptoms and signs of intestinal rejection may be vague and non-specific. As yet, there is no readily available biochemical marker for intestinal allograft rejection, such as serum transaminases for the liver, amylase, lipase and blood sugar control for the pancreas, and creatinine for the kidney. Serum citrulline levels are being investigated, but this is unlikely to impact on current practice.[36,37] Hence, routine surveillance with ileoscopies and allograft biopsies are essential. The zoom video endoscope provides greater visual detail, but has yet to replace the need for biopsies to diagnose all grades of rejection. Biopsies are initially performed twice weekly for the first 4 – 6 weeks after transplant. These can be performed less frequently once a stable state has been achieved. When concern with rejection is present (fever, nausea, vomiting, diarrhea, blood through the stoma, abdominal pain and distension), more urgent ileoscopy and biopsy is indicated to discriminate rejection from infectious enteritides. Histopathological examination using established criteria for diagnosing rejection[38,39] is the gold standard. Rejection can be classified as none, indeterminate, mild, moderate, or severe. Depending on the histopathology, modification of the immunosuppressive therapy is undertaken. The aim is to provide the clinician with information to help establish appropriate dosing levels, avoiding overimmunosuppression, but also to prevent rejection of the allograft before significant damage has occurred.

With the development of recent tolerogenic protocols, some of the histopathological appearances of the allograft have been altered. This may be due in part to the absence of steroids, as increased eosinophilia and neutrophilic infiltrates are present. These findings may reflect an altered pathway to rejection, a possibility which is currently being investigated. Interestingly, histopathological immune activation is particularly observed now in patients undergoing immunosuppression weaning. It is often difficult, especially at the onset, to determine what is an acceptable level of activation, or if the process will become destructive and result in rejection of the allograft. Monitoring of immunological factors, including evaluation of mixed lymphocyte reactions and the Cylex immune cell function assay, may assist in determining which patients can successfully be weaned on their immunosuppressants. However, regular surveillance biopsies, especially during the time of decreasing dosing, are essential for the safety of patient and allograft.

Infectious complications

The ability to monitor for opportunistic infections, such as cytomegalovirus (CMV) and Epstein–Barr virus (EBV), has led to significant improvements in patient outcomes. It has allowed pre-emptive therapy to be instituted once a rising blood antigen level is identified. Previously, these infections caused significant morbidity and mortality, but with contemporary molecular monitoring techniques, the patient can be treated before clinical disease is evident. CT scans of the sinuses and chest are important tools to investigate possible fungal infections, especially *Aspergillus* which previously carried a high mortality rate. The serum galactomannan assay, may be helpful in detecting *Aspergillus* infections earlier rather than waiting for culture results. Prophylactic and aggressive antifungal therapy has decreased mortality related to this entity. It is important at times of augmented immunosuppression (treatment of rejection), that these infections are closely monitored, as this is the time when the patient is at particular risk.

Nutritional and fluid/electrolyte status

Nutritional and fluid and electrolyte status can be monitored both physically and with laboratory investigations. Weight gain or loss, once corrected for hydration, is an important indicator of adequate graft function. Likewise, peripheral edema may reflect poor nutritional status and hypoalbuminemia. This can be confirmed with laboratory findings. Dehydration, clinically and confirmed by a rising BUN and creatinine, may reflect either poor intake due to nausea or vomiting, or high stomal output. This prompts further investigations, to rule out rejection (acute and chronic) from other causes.

Patient and graft survival

The intestine has been the last solid organ to be transplanted successfully. Early experience was poor with only one long-term survivor from the period prior to 1990. Since then, with the use of tacrolimus and numerous other advances, survival has continually improved almost on a yearly basis. In the early experience, many patients were in hospital at the time of transplantation. Data from the International Intestinal Transplant Registry[23] revealed a poorer outcome for this group of patients compared to those who were at home prior to the transplant. This is understandable, as it reflects a sicker population of patients undergoing transplantation. However, over the last decade a higher proportion of patients are coming to transplantation from home, perhaps reflecting better pre-transplant management, but also probably more appropriate earlier referral. As the results have improved and the specialty becomes better known and recognized, patients are being referred in a more timely manner, giving them a greater chance of getting to transplantation and a successful outcome, and lessening the risk of dying on the waiting list.

Patient and graft survival in the early experience was relatively poor, with 1- and 5-year survival rates of less than 65% and 45%, respectively. A self-imposed moratorium was instituted at Pittsburgh in 1995 due to these poor results, while an assessment of that early experience was made.[26] A number of items were identified, including inferior results with the use of the colon due to infectious complications. Changes included exclusion of the colon, use of CMV negative donors for CMV negative isolated intestinal recipients, close monitoring for infectious complications, and modifications in immunosuppression such as donor bone marrow augmentation, induction agents and additional immunosuppressants. Since that time, cumulative experience in Pittsburgh and elsewhere has led to advances in every aspect of the transplant. The field has progressed from a perceived experimental entity to a viable clinical entity, now recognized as the standard of care for patients with intestinal failure who are failing parenteral nutrition.

It is the sum of continual modifications and advancements in many areas that have led to the improved outcomes. An analysis of the entire pediatric intestinal experience at Pittsburgh now reveals the patient and graft survival to be 81% and 78%, respectively, at 1 year, 62% and 56% respectively at 5 years, and 35% and 29%, respectively, at 10 years. Each year the analysis improves as current recipient survival becomes better. Analysis of survival by "eras" using the different immunosuppression protocols reveals a marked improvement over time, with current patient and graft survival of 97% and 89% at one and almost 3 years, respectively. This compares favorably with most other types of organ transplants. Similar improvements in results are also seen in the other major centers with experience in intestinal transplantation, with most now having 1 year patient survival greater than 90%.

Intestinal rejection and modifications in immunosuppression protocols

The most vexing complication facing intestinal and multivisceral transplantation is the intestine's propensity to reject. This has been recognized from the very early days of transplantation. The advent of tacrolimus allowed for the procedure to be performed more routinely; however, the incidence of acute cellular rejection was greater than 80%. Severe rejection occurred in up to 30%–40% of patients, necessitating the use of very potent immunosuppressive therapy with Muromonab-CD3 (OKT3, a monoclonal antibody) and additional immunosuppressants. Although most rejection episodes could be controlled, this high level of immunosuppression placed the recipients at significant risk of developing opportunistic infections. In fact, many of the early patients died of infectious complications, directly related to the high levels of immunosuppression required to prevent allograft rejection.

The story of the improved successes in intestinal transplantation is related principally to the advancements and modifications in immunosuppressive therapy. Revised management protocols were established with the advent of new immunosuppressants and with experience gained in other types of organ transplants. A third immunosuppressive agent, such as azathioprine, mycophenolate mofetil and more recently sirolimus has been added to the baseline tacrolimus and steroid regimen. Induction agents, such as cyclophosphamide and an interleukin-2 blocker (such as daclizumab) were also added. However, these strategies relied on combinations of even more potent immunosuppressants to control the rejection episodes, albeit with better understanding and management practices to minimize and monitor for the complications. Other modifications, such as the use of donor bone marrow augmentation to try to improve allograft acceptance, failed to significantly decrease the rates of acute or chronic rejection. Manipulation of the donor allograft was also attempted, for example lymphocyte depleting agents (OKT3) were given to the donor, or irradiation of the intestinal allograft was done ex-vivo prior to implantation. The latter effort yielded an incidence of acute rejection previously unseen (14%) in the Pittsburgh adult intestinal experience, but this still utilizes a high dose immunosuppression protocol.

Since 2001 a few centers have initiated tolerogenic protocols in an attempt to decrease long-term immunosuppression requirements. Pre-conditioning induction therapy is done with either anti-thymocyte globulin (Thymoglobulin) or Alemtuzumab (Campath-1 H) given to the recipient immediately pre- and post-transplantation. The patients are then treated with tacrolimus monotherapy, and steroids are only instituted for biopsy proven rejection. The acute rejection rate in pediatric recipients has dropped to approximately 45%. Then, if at 60 – 90 days post-transplantation the recipient is stable with no recent rejection episodes, the dose of tacrolimus is reduced, from twice a day, to once a day, to every other day and then down as low as 2–3 times a week. Interestingly, many patients have rejection in the early post-transplant experience but are still able to wean successfully. During this weaning period close monitoring of the allograft is essential to detect any rejection as early as possible. Rejection occurs in approximately 25% of the weaning patients, and if caught early, can usually be reversed with treatment, returning to the dosing schedule prior to the rejection episode. To date, no grafts have been lost during the weaning process in the Pittsburgh pediatric experience. More than 60% of the pediatric patients undergoing the tolerogenic preconditioning protocol are on monotherapy, with the majority on spaced doses, as little as twice a week. It is expected that the lack of steroids and the lower tacrolimus dosing will have substantial long-term benefit. However, it is too early to determine long-term graft function and the incidence of chronic rejection.

Chronic rejection, and other changes in the mesentery that may be immunologically based, such as mesenteric sclerosis, are issues that persist in the long-term evaluation of intestinal transplant recipients, especially those with isolated intestinal transplants. Many centers believe an allograft liver provides a protective immunological effect. The rate of chronic rejection of the intestinal allograft is low in the composite allografts, but continues to increase with time post-transplantation in the isolated intestinal recipients. Hopefully, the new protocols may change this outlook.

Graft vs. host disease and chimerism

In transplant immunology, the two-way paradigm of donor and recipient cell migration forms the basis of the concept for allograft acceptance.[40] Graft versus host disease (GVHD) was one of the most worrisome entities with intestinal and multivisceral transplantation. Due to the large amount of lymphoid tissue being transplanted, it was feared GVHD would be a common lethal complication. In reality, GVHD has not been common, the incidence being 5%–8%.[41] It is seen more frequently in the pediatric population. Presentation includes a skin rash, often localized to the palms and interdigit spaces, and ulceration of the tongue, oropharynx and native intestinal tract. Peripheral chimerism studies, analyzing the percentage of donor cells in the recipient's peripheral circulation, often reveal micro- (<1%) or macro-chimerism, even if no symptoms or signs of GVHD are present. Recently, with the new tolerogenic protocols, there have been more rashes observed, consistent with immunological activity but not completely diagnostic for true GVHD. This has been called "graft vs. host reaction," and frequently the peripheral chimerism analysis shows significant cellular chimerism. Often this rash settles of its own or with minimal modification of the immunosuppressants. Treatment for GVHD includes steroid bolus therapy and changes in maintenance dosing. Management of the tacrolimus dosing is controversial, but in the majority of patients the dose and subsequent blood levels have been decreased with good result. It is hoped that these patients with high chimeric loads that can establish symbiosis between recipient and graft may in fact be the group which will become completely tolerant, or at least can be more easily weaned to lower and irregular doses.

Management of infectious issues

Even with the newer immunosuppression protocols, monitoring for and treatment of infectious complications is paramount in intestinal transplant patients. Bacterial, viral, fungal and other opportunistic infections are all a concern. Given the nature of the operation, wound infections are surprisingly uncommon. Intra-abdominal fluid collections are frequent, even with the insertion of multiple drains at the time of transplantation. These may be hematomas from postoperative oozing due to the large raw operative surfaces; they may be serous or chylous in nature resulting from divided lymphatics that become evident after beginning enteral feeds. These collections are at risk for infection, and they may require drainage (operatively or by interventional radiology). The arterial conduit is at risk for rupture or developing pseudo-aneurysm from a local infection, especially with fungal and resistant bacterial infections. Resistant strains of microorganisms are a major concern, and this is attributed to the broad spectrum antibiotic therapies utilized in the treatment of these patients. Pneumonias are common postoperatively and aggressive respiratory care and early weaning from the ventilator is desirable. Venous line infections should always be considered and the line removed or changed wherever possible. Translocation of pathogens from the GI tract is a concern, and this is frequently seen at times of rejection due to mucosal injury. It is now recognized that in addition to antibiotic therapy, increased immunosuppression to treat the rejection is required. Translocation may also occur at times of endoscopic procedures if considerable manipulation and air insufflation is utilized. This is less frequent with experience in these procedures.

In general, children are at risk for common viral infections, and this is even more so after transplantation. Risks include respiratory syncytial virus, parainfluenza virus, adenovirus and other less common gastrointestinal infections. In addition, herpetic infections, primary or recurrent need to be considered. Antiviral therapy is usually reserved for invasive disease or for patients who are very ill from the infection. Both early diagnosis and the use of new antiviral agents have played a role in improved outcomes with these infections.

Opportunistic viral infections include cytomegalovirus (CMV) and Epstein–Barr virus (EBV). Previously these infections led to significant morbidity and mortality. The incidence of CMV disease in recipients peaked at 56% in the 1990s, but currently occurs in only 5% of the recipients. It is more common in those at high risk from organ CMV mismatch (donor positive to recipient negative). The cause for the reduction in risk is multifactorial. One key lesson learned is to avoid high risk CMV mismatched isolated intestinal allografts, although this is not practical in composite allografts. More importantly, with current surveillance techniques (pp-65 antigenemia), increasing viremic load can frequently be identified prior to the onset of clinical disease. Clinical symptoms and signs may well be non-specific, including fever, malaise and ulceration seen in the allograft or changes on a chest X-ray. CMV inclusion bodies can be identified on biopsy, and stains for CMV are available to confirm the diagnosis. Treatment consists of cautious lowering of immunosuppression (but not enough to induce rejection), antiviral therapy with ganciclovir and cytogam (CMV specific hyperimmunoglobulin) and continued monitoring. Aggressive prophylactic therapy, especially with moderate to high risk recipients has also lessened the impact of this disease over time.

EBV may lead to post-transplant lymphoproliferative disease (PTLD).[42] PTLD is primarily a pediatric complication seen previously in up to 44% of the intestinal transplant recipients, but infrequently seen in the adult population. The incidence of PTLD is now decreasing, and is present in only 3% of recent recipients. Symptoms and signs can be vague, with lymphadenopathy and abdominal masses being the most important physical findings.

CT scan may show adenopathy which can also be used as a marker of disease resolution, especially in the non-EBV derived PTLD. Treatment is similar to that for CMV, with cautious reduction of immunosuppression, antiviral therapy and cytogam. Other possible therapies include Rituximab, interferon and chemotheraputic agents. Routine surveillance via serum EBV-PCR has allowed for early pre-emptive therapy as with CMV. Prophylactic therapy has also assisted in decreasing the impact of this disease. EBV was previously fatal in 45% of affected patients, but now this is an infrequent occurrence.[43]

Fungal infections always need to be considered, especially in patients who are receiving high dose immunosuppression (such as during a rejection episode), with indwelling venous lines, intestinal rejection or leaks, or receiving broad spectrum antibacterial therapy. Fluconazole (Diflucan) is mostly avoided because of its hepatotoxic effect and its adverse interaction with tacrolimus (increasing its level). Liposomal amphotericin, Caspofungin and Voriconazole are preferred therapeutic agents in these transplant patients, depending on the nature of the infection. The spectrum ranges from the relatively common varieties of Candida, to *Torulopsis glabrata* and even Aspergillus. Less common is Scetosporia, which is often lethal. Atypical infections, including mycobacteria, legionella, and amoebe must also be considered, especially with a rapidly worsening clinical picture. In patients with an isolated intestinal transplant, it has been recognized that it may be preferable to remove the allograft (to be able to stop the immunosuppression) and retransplant the patient when fully recovered, rather than add further immunosuppression and place the recipient at risk of death from infection. This management strategy has contributed to an overall improvement in patient survival.

Allograft function

The vast majority of intestinal and multivisceral transplant recipients are nutritionally independent after transplantation. Greater than 96% of recipients are able to be removed from parenteral nutrition (PN). Previously, recipients had the PN resumed immediately after transplantation and were weaned off over time. Recently, the majority of pediatric recipients have not returned to PN after transplantation, and quickly progress to oral intake and tube feeds. Many children, especially infants who have never fed before, have oral aversion, and training is required before complete transition to the oral route is established.

Even though therapeutic agents (Imodium, tincture of opium, levsin, adding fiber to the feeds) are utilized to modify the amount of stool output, a few patients require supplemental intravenous fluids to control fluid and electrolyte balance. This is seen when patients are recovering from episodes of severe rejection with high output, and early on with some who have required partial bowel reductions for size issues. In this latter group, further investigations are underway to identify the optimal location and maximum allowable resection length.

Quality of life

The intestine is not normally considered a life-saving organ, but its importance should not be overlooked. There are patients who are running out of venous access, sustaining repeated life-threatening infections, or developing liver failure in which an intestinal transplant will reverse the decline. Apart from strict medical indications, there are definite quality of life issues. Most take for granted the ability to eat and drink. In contrast, parenteral nutrition is time consuming and life-style limiting for patient and caregiver. As well, the majority of patients with intestinal failure have issues with pain management and narcotic dependency, which can be overcome with transplantation. Although transplantation is not without its own complications and medical issues, studies on post-transplant recipients reveal marked satisfaction with the procedure. More than 80% of patients place themselves in the 90th percentile or above on the modified Karnovsky scale, essentially near normal. A successful intestinal transplant can truly give the patient a life they never knew or had forgotten was possible.

Future directions

As results continue to improve and as greater experience is obtained, there is no doubt the demand for intestinal and multivisceral transplantation will continue to grow. No longer is it considered experimental. Greater understanding of the complex immunology related to the intestinal allograft, and the delicate balancing of donor and host immune reactions will allow for further refinements in immunosuppression management. If this can be achieved, allowing for reductions in the complication rate, then intestinal transplants will be performed more widely. However, these patients continue to be the most challenging of all visceral organ transplants. Countries that have never before performed intestinal transplants and centers in other countries where it is already performed, are currently assessing the need to expand into this field. To achieve successful transplantation with good long-term outcomes requires knowledge, skill and dedication from a well coordinated team.

REFERENCES

1. Merrill, J., Murray, J., Harrison, H. *et al.* Successful homotransplantations of the kidney between non-identical twins. *N. Engl. J. Med.* 1960; **262**:1251–1260.
2. Starzl, T., Groth, C., Brettschneider, L. *et al.* Orthotopic homotransplantation of the human liver. *Ann. Surg.* 1968; **1680**:392–415.
3. Kelly, W., Lillehei, R., Merkel, F. *et al.* Allotransplantation of the pancreas and duodenum along with the kidney in diabetic nephropathy. *Surgery* 1967; **61**:827–837.
4. Barnard, C. What we have learned about heart transplants. *Thorac. Cardiovasc. Surg.* 1968; **56**:457–468.
5. Derom, F., Barbier, F., Ringoir, S. *et al.* Ten-month survival after lung homotransplantation in man. *J. Thorac. Cardiovasc. Surg.* 1971; **61**:827–837.
6. Starzl, T. E. & Kaupp, H. Mass homotransplantation of abdominal organs in dogs. *Surg. Forum* 1960; **11**:28–30.
7. Starzl, T., Rowe, M., Todo, S. *et al.* Transplantation of multiple abdominal viscera. *J. Am. Med. Assoc.* 1989; **261**:1449–1458.
8. Grant, D., Wall, W., Mineualt, R. *et al.* Successful small bowel/liver transplantation. *Lancet* 1990; **335**:181–184.
9. Margreiter, R., Konigsrainer, A., Schmid, T. *et al.* Successful multivisceral transplantation. *Transpl. Proc.* 1992; **24**:1226–1227.
10. Deltz, E., Schroeder, P., Gerbhard, H. *et al.* Successful clinical small bowel transplantation: report of a case. *Clin. Transpl.* 1989; **21**:89–91.
11. Goulet, O., Revillon, Y., Brousse, N. *et al.* Successful small bowel transplantation in an infant. *Transplantation* 1992; **53**:940–943.
12. Bueno, J., Ohwada, S., Kocoshis, S. *et al.* Factors impacting the survival of children with intestinal failure referred for intestinal transplantation. *J. Pedatr. Surg.* 1999; **34**:27–33.
13. Kauffman, S., Atkinson, J., Bianchi, A. *et al.* Indications for pediatric intestinal transplantation. *Pediatr. Transpl.* 2001; **5**:80–87.
14. Cavicchi, M., Beau, P., Crenn, P. *et al.* Prevalence of liver disease and contributing factors in patients receiving home parenteral nutrition for permanent intestinal failure. *Ann. Int. Med.* 2000; **132**:525.
15. Lillehei, R., Goott, B., Miller, F. The physiological response of the small bowel of the dog to ischemia including prolonged in vitro preservation of the bowel with successful replacement and survival. *Ann. Surg.* 1959; **150**:543–561.
16. Starzl, T. E., Todo, S., Tzakis, A. *et al.* Abdominal organ cluster transplantation for the treatment of upper abdominal malignancies. *Ann. Surg.* 1989; **210**:374–386.
17. Starzl, T., Todo, S., Tzakis, A. *et al.* The many faces of multivisceral transplantation. *Surg. Gynecol. Obstet.* 1991; **172**:335–344.
18. Sindhi, R., Fox, I., Heffron, T. *et al.* Procurement and preparation of human isolated small intestinal grafts for transplantation. *Transplantation* 2000; **60**:680–687.
19. Bueno, J., Abu-Elmagd, K., Mazariegos, G. *et al.* Composite liver-small bowel allografts with preservation of donor duodenum and hepatic biliary system in children. *J. Pediatr. Surg.* 2000; **35**:291–295.
20. Sudan, D., Iyer, K., Deroover, A. *et al.* A new technique for combined liver-small intestinal transplantation. *Transplantation* 2001; **72**:1846–1848.
21. Abu-Elmagd, K., Fung, J., Bueno, J. *et al.* Logistics and techniques for procurement of intestinal, pancreatic, and hepatic grafts from the same donor. *Ann. Surg.* 2000; **232**:680–697.
22. Fortner, J., Sichuk, G., Litwin, S., & Beattie, E. Immunological responses to an intestinal allograft with HLA-identical donor-recipients. *Transplantation* 1972; **14**:531–535.
23. Grant, D., Abu-Elmagd, K., Reyes, J. *et al.* Report on the intestine transplant registry: A new era has dawned. *Ann. Surg.* 2004; in press.
24. Abu-Elmagd, K., Reyes, J., Bond, G. *et al.* Clinical intestinal transplantation: A decade of experience at a single center. *Ann. Surg.* 2001; **234**(3):404–417.
25. Berney, T., Kato, T., Nishida, S. *et al.* Portal versus systemic drainage of small bowel allografts: Comparative assessment of survival, function, rejection, and bacterial translocation. *J. Am. Coll. Surg.* 2002; **195**(6):804–813
26. Todo, S., Reyes, J., Furukawa, H. *et al.* Outcome analysis of 71 clinical intestinal transplantations. *Ann. Surg.* 1995; **222**:270–282.
27. Kato, T., Tzakis, A., Selvaggi, G., & Madariaga, J. Surgical techniques used in intestinal transplantation. *Curr. Opin. Org. Transpl.* 2004; **9**(2):207–213.
28. Gruessner, R., Uckun, F., Pirenne, J. *et al.* Recipient preconditioning and donor-specific bone marrow infusion in a pig model of total bowel transplantation. *Transplantation* 1997; **63**:12–20.
29. Abu-Elmagd, K., Reyes, J., Todo, S. *et al.* Clinical intestinal transplantation: New persoectives and immunologic considerations. *J. Am. Coll. Surg.* 1998; **186**(5):512–527.
30. Reyes, J., McGhee, W., Mazariegos, G. *et al.* Thymoglobulin in the management of steroid resistant acute cellular rejection in children. *Transplantation* 2002; **74**:419.
31. Medicare coverage policy "Intestinal,combined liver and intestinal and multivisceral transplantation" (CAG-00036) *Decision memorandum*, dated October 4, 2000.
32. Schuster, B., Bond, G., Martin, L. *et al.* Acute irreversible intestinal failure and early intestinal transplantation: Indications and Survival outcomes. *Transpl Suppl.* 2004; **78**(2):23.
33. Beath, S., Booth, I., & Murphy, M. Nutritional care in candidates for small bowel transplantation. *Archi. Dis. Child.* 1995; **73**:348.
34. Fryer, J., Pellar, S., Ormond, D. *et al.* Mortality in candidates waiting for combined liver-intestine transplants exceeds that for other candidates waiting for liver transplants. *Liver Transpl.* 2003; **9**(7):748–753.
35. Sigurdsson, L., Reyes, J., Kocoshis, S. *et al.* Intestinal transplantation in children with chronic intestinal pseudo-obstruction. *Gut* 1999; **45**:570–574.

36. Pappas, P., Saudubray, J., Tzakis, A. *et al.* Serum citrulline and rejection in small bowel transplantation: a preliminary report. *Transplantation* 2001; **72**:1212.
37. Pappas, P., Tzakis, A., Saudubray, J. *et al.* Trends in serum citrulline and acute rejection among recipients of small bowel transplants. *Transpl. Proc.* 2004; **36**(2):345–347.
38. Ruiz, P., Bagni, A., Brown, R. *et al.* Histological criteria for the identification of acute cellular rejection in human small bowel allografts: results of the pathology workshop at the VIII International Small Bowel Transplant Symposium. *Transpl. Proc.* 2004; **36**(2):335–337.
39. Wu, T., Abu-Elmagd, K., Bond, G. *et al.* A Schema for histologic grading of small intestine allograft acute rejection. *Transplantation* 2003; **75**(8):1241–1248.
40. Starzl, T. & Zinkernagel, R. Transplantation tolerance from a historical perspective. *Nat Revi.* 2001; **1**(3):233–239
41. Mazariegos, G., Abu-Elmagd, K., Jaffe, R. *et al.* Graft versus host disease in intestinal transplantation. *Am. J. Transpl.* 2004; **4**:1459–1465.
42. Reyes, J., Green, M., Bueno, J. *et al.* Epstein–Barr virus associated post-transplant lymphoproliferative disease after intestinal transplantation. *Transpl. Proc.* 1996; **28**:2768–2769.
43. Green, M., Reyes, J., Webber, S., & Rowe, D. The role of antiviral and immunoglobulin therapy in the prevention of Epstein-Barr virus infection and post-transplant lymphoproliferative disease following solid organ transplantation. *Transpl. Infect. Dis.* 2001; **3**:97–103.

67

Heart and lung transplantation

Thomas Spray and Stephanie M. P. Fuller

Heart, Lung and Heart Transplant Services, Children's Hospital of Philadelphia, PA, USA

Introduction

Thoracic organ transplantation is an important treatment option in children with acquired or congenital cardiopulmonary disease. In recent years, there has been considerable improvement in early outcomes following thoracic organ transplantation in children and 1-year survival is similar now to that in adults. Approximately 250 pediatric heart transplants and 60 lung transplants are performed annually in the United States. Thoracic organ transplantation in neonates and infants has been limited by donor availability, and the number of thoracic organ transplants performed each year in children has plateaued. Complications such as acute and chronic rejection, graft coronary artery disease (CAD) or bronchiolitis obliterans, as well as those of immunosuppression, pose serious threats to the long-term success of thoracic organ transplantation in children. Despite these potential impediments, life expectancy and quality of life for patients following transplantation exceed that for patients with end-stage cardiopulmonary disease who are managed medically. This chapter focuses on the clinical aspects of heart and lung transplantation in infants and children including indications, preoperative evaluation, postoperative course and management, complications and long-term outcomes.

Indications

Heart transplantation

As published by the Registry for the International Society for Heart and Lung Transplantation (ISHLT) in the Seventh Official Report in May 2004, the number of pediatric heart transplants has remained relatively constant over the last 10 years (Fig. 67.1). The most common indication for heart transplantation in the neonatal population remains complex congenital heart disease for which no reasonable corrective or palliative surgical therapy is available. The most prevalent diagnosis is cardiomyopathy in the older infant through adolescent population (Figs. 67.2, 67.3 and 67.4).[1]

The most frequent indication for neonatal heart transplantation is hypoplastic left heart syndrome (HLHS), a group of defects characterized by aortic or mitral atresia/stenosis with a diminutive left ventricle. Historically, shifts in management practices resulting from initial poor outcomes with a staged palliative approach to HLHS led some centers to consider orthotopic heart transplantation as the primary treatment for this anomaly. However, as transplant waiting lists have become increasingly long, most institutions now perform stage I reconstruction (Norwood or Sano procedure) to help stabilize the patient followed by a completion Fontan repair at a later age. With improvement in early survival from such repair, the majority of cardiac centers continue to prefer staged reconstruction and reserve primary transplantation for those patients with unusually high risk, including aortic atresia or severe tricuspid regurgitation, or re-operative transplantation for those patients with cardiac failure after the Norwood or Fontan operations.

Other forms of congenital heart disease that have been treated with cardiac transplantation in infancy include unbalanced atrioventricular canal, pulmonary atresia/intact ventricular septum with a right ventricular dependent coronary circulation, truncus arteriosus, double-outlet right ventricle, Ebstein's anomaly, and transposition of the great arteries. Of note, congenital

Pediatric Surgery and Urology: Long-term Outcomes, Mark Stringer, Keith Oldham, Pierre Mouriquand.
Published by Cambridge University Press. © Cambridge University Press, 2006.

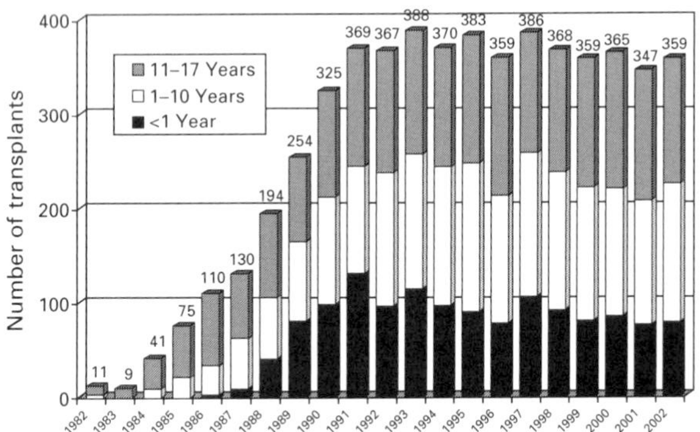

Fig. 67.1. Age distribution of pediatric heart recipients by year of transplant done from January 1996 to June 2003. (International Society of Heart and Lung Transplantation, 2004 from *The Journal of Heart and Lung Transplantation* 2004, 23:8.)

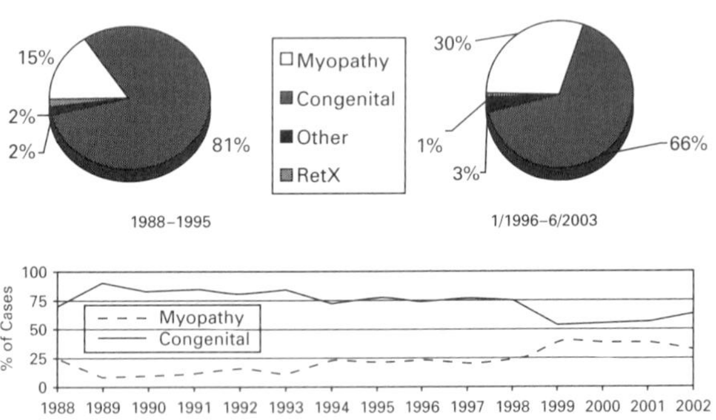

Fig. 67.2. Diagnoses for pediatric heart transplant recipients (age <1 year). ReTX = re-transplantation. (International Society of Heart and Lung Transplantation, 2004, as above.)

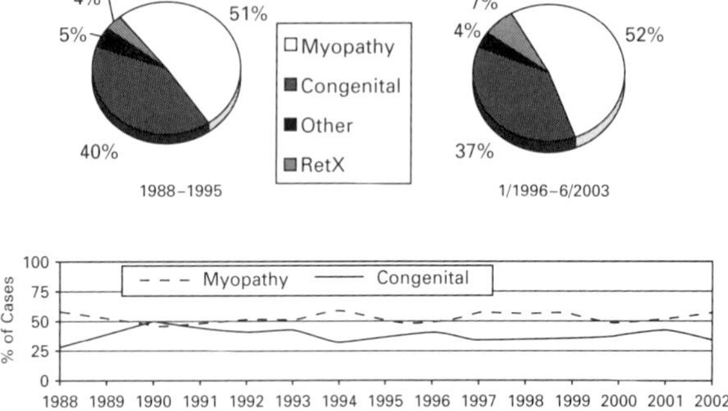

Fig. 67.3. Diagnoses for pediatric heart transplant recipients (age 1 to 10 years). ReTX = re-transplantation. (International Society of Heart and Lung Transplantation, 2004, as above.)

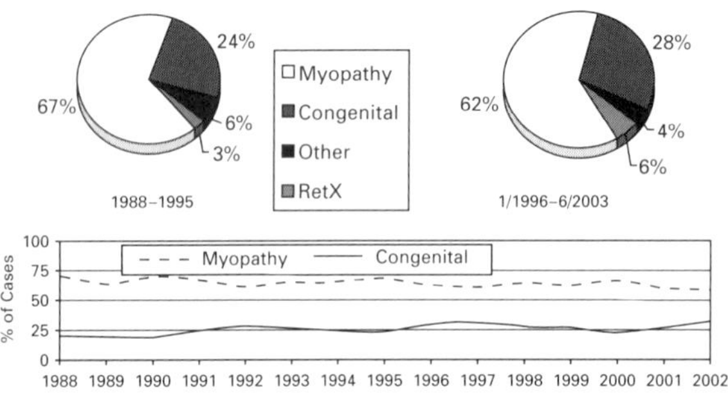

Fig. 67.4. Diagnoses for pediatric heart transplant recipients (age 11 to 17 years). ReTX = re-transplantation. (International Society of Heart and Lung Transplantation, 2004, as above.)

cardiomyopathy is a rare indication for heart transplantation in infancy. Essentially any infant who has undergone previous corrective or palliative procedures for congenital heart disease yet who exhibits residual or progressive cardiac dysfunction may ultimately require transplantation. In these cases, postoperative cardiac dysfunction is often related to atrioventricular or semilunar valvar insufficiency that eventually results in a dilated cardiomyopathy. Multiple previous palliative procedures do not therefore preclude successful transplantation[2] and approximately 30%–45% of pediatric transplants are performed after repair or palliation of congenital disease.

Idiopathic dilated cardiomyopathy is the most common indication for pediatric cardiac transplantation after infancy (greater than 1 year of age). Viral, familial and hypertrophic cardiomyopathies may also require cardiac transplantation but less commonly. Indications for transplantation in these patients relate to symptoms of chronic congestive heart failure limiting activity and uncontrollable arrhythmias unresponsive to medications. The timing of transplantation in these children is unclear, as some patients may improve with medical therapy; however, mortality for idiopathic dilated cardiomyopathy is highest in the first year after diagnosis and, as suggested, is mainly determined by the degree of left ventricular failure. Indicators of poor outcome include elevated left ventricular end-diastolic pressure, left ventricular ejection fraction of less than 20%, sustained ventricular arrhythmia and a family history of cardiomyopathy.[3,4] Cardiomyopathy attributable to inflammation or intermittent arrhythmia tends to have a more favorable outcome, and these patients should be supported as long as possible before transplantation to allow for the possibility of spontaneous recovery. Other less common indications for cardiac transplantation are doxorubicin-induced cardiotoxicity from chemotherapy for malignancy and obstructive cardiac tumors such as fibromas and rhabdomyomas that are not amenable to surgical resection.

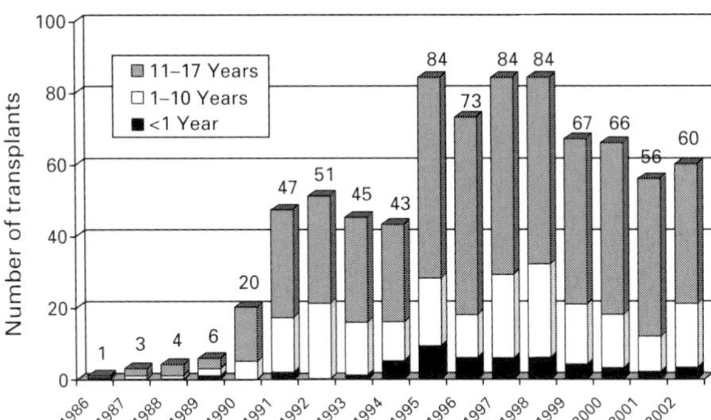

Fig. 67.5. Age distribution of pediatric lung recipients by year of transplant. Age distribution for pediatric lung recipients (transplants from January 1996 to June 2003). (International Society of Heart and Lung Transplantation, 2004, as above.)

Lung transplantation

The ISHLT reported in 2004 that the number of lung transplants peaked at approximately 80 per year in the late 1990s and has remained relatively stable at approximately 60 a year for the past 4 years (Fig. 67.5). Indications for lung transplantation in infancy include pulmonary hypertension (primary and secondary), congenital heart disease, bronchopulmonary dysplasia, congenital surfactant deficiency, congenital diaphragmatic hernia, and pulmonary vein stenosis whereas the majority of older children have either cystic fibrosis or pulmonary hypertension (Table 67.1). [1]

Primary pulmonary hypertension usually affects young adults, but some patients present early in life and may be severely symptomatic. Indications for transplant include NYHA Class IV symptoms, cardiac index <2.3 L/min per m^2, right atrial pressure >10 mm Hg or pulmonary vascular resistance >20 Wood's units.[5] Patients with pulmonary hypertension due to cardiac defects (Eisenmenger's syndrome) commonly reach adulthood before severe symptoms develop, but some develop end-stage disease in childhood. Children with pulmonary hypertension, especially those with pulmonary vein stenosis, are at an increased risk of sudden death.

Although most patients with cystic fibrosis survive until adulthood before pulmonary function deteriorates sufficiently to require transplantation, a small number progress rapidly and require transplantation as children. Children with cystic fibrosis should be considered for lung transplant when they have progressive hypercapnea ($PaCO_2$ of greater than 50 mmHg) or oxygen dependence (FEV_1 of less than 30% with PaO_2 of less than 55 mm Hg), worsening exercise tolerance, increasing frequency of hospitalizations for infectious episodes, or poor weight gain despite adequate nutritional supplementation.[6] At this point, 2-year mortality is more than 50%.

Although single-lung transplantation is rarely performed in children, bilateral operation is indicated for septic lung disease, such as cystic fibrosis, to minimize the risk of contamination in the transplanted lungs, and is generally recommended for children with pulmonary hypertension. When single-lung transplantation is performed in patients with pulmonary hypertension, the donor lung is shunted most of the cardiac output and the increased flow may be poorly tolerated. Some patients with congenital heart disease and pulmonary hypertension may undergo bilateral lung transplantation with simultaneous cardiac repair, rather than combined heart–lung transplantation.[7]

Table 67.1. Indications for transplant for pediatric lung transplants (transplants from January 1991 to June 2003)

Diagnosis	Age <1 year	Age 1–10 years
Cystic fibrosis		66 (35.9%)
PPH	7 (14.3%)	25 (13.6%)
Congenital heart disease	23 (46.9%)	20 (10.9%)
IPF		13 (7.1%)
Pulmonary vascular disease	6 (12.2%)	6 (3.0%)
Re-Tx: non-OB	3 (6.1%)	8 (4.3%)
Re-Tx: OB		11 (6.0%)
OB (non-Re-Tx)		7 (3.8%)
Bronchiectasis		2 (1.1%)
COPD/emphysema		2 (1.1%)
Other	10 (20.0%)	24 (13.0%)

COPD, chronic obstructive pulmonary disease; IPF, idiopathic pulmonary fibrosis; OB, obliterative bronchiolitis; PPH, primary pulmonary hypertension; re-Tx, re-transplantation.
(From *J. Heart Lung Transpl.* 2004;23:944.)

Heart–lung transplantation

Less than 20 heart–lung transplantations are performed annually in the United States, likely attributable to improved outcomes in lung-only transplants. The combined procedure is recommended for patients with pulmonary hypertension or pulmonary parenchymal disease in conjunction with poor cardiac function, significant valvular pathology, or complex uncorrectable congenital heart disease such as Eisenmenger's syndrome. Heart–lung transplantation rather than bilateral lung transplantation has been used occasionally for patients with cystic fibrosis.

Table 67.2. Evaluation of candidates for heart transplantation

History and physical examination
Blood type
Panel reactive antibody
Complete blood count with differential
Chemistry panel with electrolytes
Liver function tests
Lipid profile
Serological examination for antibodies to varicella, CMV, EBV, herpes simplex, measles, hepatitis A to D, HIV and toxoplasmosis
Chest radiograph
Chest computed tomography
Pulmonary function tests
Cardiology evaluation with electrocardiogram, echocardiogram, MUGA scan – ventricular ejection fraction, cardiac catheterization, exercise stress test
Consultation with pediatric cardiologist, transplant coordinator, infectious disease specialist, pulmonologist, nutritionist, psychiatrist, social worker, dentist

* CMV-cytomegalovirus; EBV-Epstein–Barr virus; HIV-human immunodeficiency virus; MUGA-multiple uptake gated acquisition.

In these cases, the heart from the recipients can be used for subsequent transplantation into another patient, known as the "domino" procedure. Currently, most centers perform lung transplantation only for patients with pulmonary disease and normal cardiac function.

Contraindications to thoracic transplantation

Contraindications to thoracic organ transplantation include active collagen–vascular disease, poorly controlled diabetes mellitus, untreated malignancy, unmanageable hepatic or renal failure, bacterial infection outside of the respiratory tract, multiple congenital anomalies, severe chromosomal abnormalities, neurological dysfunction which precludes a meaningful quality of life or recovery, a history of poor medical compliance, and a lack of family support. Pulmonary infection, particularly in cystic fibrosis patients, is not a contraindication to lung transplantation, unless the organisms are resistant to all antibiotics. Many of the standard exclusion criteria in adult transplant programs – such as mechanical ventilation, previous thoracotomy and steroid therapy – are not applicable to children. In fact, many infants with parenchymal lung disease who are referred for lung transplantation are ventilator dependent until an organ becomes available. Cyanotic patients who have undergone previous thoracotomy for palliative procedures must be evaluated carefully by angiogram prior to transplantation as they are at significant risk of hemorrhage from the chest wall which results from collateral vessels that form in response to the need for increased pulmonary blood flow.

Preoperative evaluation

The pretransplantation evaluation is a multidisciplinary screening process that serves as the key to successful organ transplantation (Table 67.2). Potential recipients undergo a thorough physical and psychosocial evaluation, carefully examining cardiac, pulmonary, neurologic, renal, infectious, and socioeconomic systems. The presence of an adequate family support system is of paramount importance to survival postoperatively. Parents must demonstrate the ability and resources to comply with the complex medical regimens required and to cope with the potential for long or frequent hospitalizations even years after transplantation. As part of this multidisciplinary evaluation, patients undergo screening laboratory tests, including a viral serology panel (e.g., human immunodeficiency virus, cytomegalovirus (CMV), human Epstein–Barr virus, hepatitis).

Cardiac evaluation is performed mainly by echocardiography and cardiac catheterization in which the anatomy of systemic and pulmonary venous connections of the heart and lungs are precisely identified. Important hemodynamic data are obtained at cardiac catheterization and used to screen candidates including the systemic cardiac output and the pulmonary vascular resistance (PVR), both indexed to the patient's body area. These numbers become significant as the major contraindication to transplantation is fixed pulmonary hypertension, unresponsive to pulmonary vasodilators. Patients with elevated PVR (greater than 4 to 6 Wood units) are tested with pulmonary vasodilators, including sodium nitroprusside, oxygen (FIO_2 100%), and inhaled nitric oxide to establish whether the pulmonary vascular bed is reactive. In general, the presence of a fixed PVR in excess of 6 to 8 Wood units is a contraindication to orthotopic heart transplantation as the donor heart is unable to tolerate right-sided dilation caused by high pulmonary resistance. These patients, however, would be considered for heart–lung transplantation. Patients who demonstrate improvement with vasodilators may be transplanted with a survival rate comparable to that in patients with normal resistance.[2] Although patients with fixed pulmonary hypertension have been successfully transplanted, they have a much higher mortality rate, usually because of postoperative right ventricular failure. Other contraindications to cardiac transplantation include multiple non-cardiac congenital anomalies, active malignancy, infection, severe metabolic disease (i.e., diabetes mellitus), multiple organ failure, multiple congenital anomalies and the lack of an adequate family support system in addition to socioeconomic factors that lead to non-compliance with drug regimens and follow-up care.

Children listed for thoracic transplantation should be closely monitored until their transplantation, either as outpatients if their condition permits, or while hospitalized. Good nutritional status should be maintained and supplementation such as tube feedings or TPN used as needed. A close watch for infectious complications is important and any subtle indications of infection should be thoroughly investigated. Major infections require patients to have their transplantation status put on hold until they are treated adequately. Anticongestive therapy should be optimized, using digoxin, diuretics and afterload reduction with captopril or other angiotensin-converting enzyme inhibitors. If heart failure worsens, hospitalization may be required for inotropic support with dobutamine or phosphodiesterase inhibitors such as milrinone. Long-term therapy may require the placement of an intravenous access device such as a broviac catheter. The use of extracorporeal membrane oxygenation (ECMO) as a bridge to cardiac transplantation in critically ill children has been limited, mostly to children with postcardiotomy ventricular failure. In general, results have been poor although several studies show survival rates ranging from 45% to 73% for using ECMO as a bridge to cardiac transplantation.[8,9] Older children and adolescents have excellent survival using long-term ventricular assist devices (VADs) as a bridge to transplantation although size restrictions limit their use in the infant population.

The neonate referred for cardiac transplantation requires several other unique considerations. Infants with complex congenital heart disease such as HLHS are commonly confined to a neonatal intensive care unit (ICU), and are usually maintained on a continuous infusion of prostaglandin E1 to prevent closure of the ductus arteriosus if there is duct-dependent physiology. Implantation of expandable stents in the ductus may allow discontinuation of prostaglandin during waiting. Balloon atrial septostomy with or without stenting may be helpful if there is a restrictive patent foramen ovale to improve mixing of saturated and desaturated blood, and to decompress the left atrium. Other important issues are the maintenance of adequate nutritional support, avoidance of renal and metabolic complications, and the prompt and thorough treatment of any infectious complications, especially line sepsis, in these fragile infants. Common neonatal problems such as seizures, necrotizing enterocolitis and intraventricular hemorrhage are also seen in these patients. At the minimum, 10% to 20% of infants die while awaiting a donor heart. As mentioned earlier, initial palliative procedures such as the Norwood procedure for HLHS or Blalock-Taussig shunt for lesions with ductal-dependent pulmonary blood flow can be performed in the face of a prolonged wait for a donor.

The United Network for Organ Sharing (UNOS) determines organ allocation in the United States. In January 2005, UNOS revised their classification for pediatric patients awaiting thoracic organ transplantation in order to benefit pediatric patients, particularly those aged 12–18 years. For lung transplant, the allocation system is based on the seriousness of the patient's medical condition, need for transplant and likelihood of success after transplantation. Factors used to determine necessity and assess survivability include need for ventilatory support or mechanical circulatory support, age, NYHA functional status class, exercise capacity, presence of diabetes or renal failure and many others. Status 1A applies to patients requiring ventilatory or mechanical circulatory support (i.e., LVAD, ECMO or balloon pump), multiple- or high-dose inotropes, infants younger than 6 months of age with pulmonary pressures greater than 50% of systemic levels, or any patient with a life expectancy of less than 14 days without a heart transplant, such as those with life-threatening arrhythmia. Status 1B applies to patients requiring single-dose inotropic support or infants less than 6 months of age who have significant failure to thrive (less than the fifth percentile for weight and/or height, or loss of 1.5 standard deviations of expected growth). All other patients with less acuity are classified as status 2. A patient's status may change depending on changes in clinical condition, or the patient may be temporarily placed on hold (status 7) due to an infectious, malignant or other complication, and later be reactivated. As of 2005, within each heart/lung status, an organ retrieved from an adolescent (ages 11–18) organ donor will be allocated to a pediatric candidate prior to allocation to an adult. Candidates in the 12–18 age range are given priority for lung transplantation based on the above-mentioned transplant benefit measures whereas children aged 0–11 years are prioritized according to waiting time.

Donor evaluation and organ procurement

Criteria for an ideal cardiac organ donor are as follows: meets requirements for brain death, consent from next of kin, ABO compatibility in older children, weight compatibility (one to three times that of the recipient), normal echocardiogram, age younger than 35 years, and normal heart by visual inspection at the time of harvest. A history of cardiopulmonary resuscitation is not an absolute contraindication to cardiac donation for pediatric recipients. Ideally, donors for lung transplant would have no history of chest wall trauma, no history of lung disease and a period of mechanical ventilation less than 1 week. A smoking history is not an absolute contraindication. Donor radiographs should be free of infiltrates or other lesions and bronchoscopic assessment should be performed. All potential donors are evaluated carefully for cause of death including the presence of chest trauma, need for cardiopulmonary resuscitation and cardiac function prior to death. For neonates, most donors have suffered sudden infant death syndrome or birth asphyxia whereas older donors are victims of violence and car accidents.

The shortage of suitable organ donors, especially for neonatal recipients, has led to many attempts at expanding the donor pool. Hearts from donors with moderately impaired ventricular function by echocardiogram (left ventricular shortening fraction greater than 25% without major wall motion abnormalities) have been successfully transplanted in infant recipients.[10] Donor-to-recipient weight ratios of up to 4:1 have been used in infants. Tamisier and colleagues demonstrated that the higher the PVR, the larger the donor heart is needed for a successful transplant and hearts with PVRs thought to be in excess of normal can also be used.[11] Although ideal donor time is from 2 to 4 hours, ischemic times have been successfully extended beyond 9 hours. Deviations from the "ideal" donor criteria should be individualized and although the use of a marginal donor for a dying infant on ECMO may be justified, the use of the same heart for a child who is stable as an outpatient might not.

ABO-incompatible transplantation has been introduced as a method to decrease recipient waiting times and associated waiting list mortality.[12] Because neonates do not have the ability to produce antibodies to T-cell antigens, including major blood group antigens, ABO-incompatibility becomes a negligible complication. ABO-incompatible transplantation has been infrequently used in the United States and the age at which it is no longer feasible is still not clearly defined. For lung transplantation, donor and recipient human leukocyte antigen (HLA) matching is not required but ABO compatibility is essential.

In lung transplantation, living donor assessment must be both psychosocial and physiologic. Evaluation includes room air arterial blood gas analysis, spirometry, echocardiography, ventilation/perfusion scan, chest X-ray and computed tomography of the chest to exclude pathology.

Good donor management is a vital part of successful organ transplantation. The main goals are maintenance of normothermia, euvolemia, adequate tissue perfusion, and prevention of infection. Often, donors with poor cardiac function on initial evaluation will respond to volume loading and low-dose inotropic support with a significant improvement in function following heart retrieval, usually as a part of a multiorgan retrieval procedure. All donors are screened for viruses that might cause serious infection in the immunocompromised host such as CMV, EBV, HIV, hepatitis and Toxoplasma. Presence of antibodies to CMV, EBV and Toxoplasma is not a contraindication to transplant but helps to guide post-transplantation therapy.

There are four major goals in the procurement of the donor heart: (1) to work effectively with the other teams to ensure optimal condition of each recovered organ; (2) to evaluate the hemodynamic status of the patient and the gross function of the heart and lungs by inspection; (3) to use an effective cardioplegia and venting procedure that maximizes preservation of the heart; and (4) to expertly remove the heart and adjoining vascular connections to ensure optimal anatomy for implantation. Procurement is performed via a median sternotomy. Donor blood is obtained for viral titers and retrospective HLA-typing. The initial dissection separates the aorta from the main pulmonary artery to allow cross clamping. Careful inspection of the heart is performed. The patient is systemically heparinized. Procurement commences when the aorta is cross-clamped. Cardioplegia solution is infused through the aortic root and the heart is vented via the right atrial appendage or superior vena cava for the right side and the superior pulmonary vein or left atrial appendage for the left side. The superior vena cava is dissected free of its pericardial attachments up to the innominate vein and the azygos vein is ligated and divided. The pericardial reflections around the right superior pulmonary vein and the inferior vena cava are sharply divided. The cardiectomy begins with inferior vena cava transection, followed by right and left pulmonary vein transection at the pericardial reflection. The main pulmonary artery is then divided. The posterior pericardial attachments are divided and the superior vena cava is divided. Lastly, the aorta is transected at the level of the innominate artery or more distally if the aorta is needed for the recipient. The donor heart is immersed in cold (4 °C), sterile saline and then triple-bagged in a sterile manner for transport. In general, cold ischemia time should be limited to a maximum of 4 to 5 hours.

Lungs are typically harvested simultaneously with the heart. The inferior pulmonary ligament is incised. With the lungs maintained gently inflated, the pulmonary artery is infused with two preservative solutions and iced saline slush is applied to the lungs. The main pulmonary artery is divided at its bifurcation, and the pulmonary veins are detached from the heart with a preserved cuff of left atrium. The lungs are freed once the trachea is divided just above the carina. The most common pediatric lung transplant procedure performed is the bilateral sequential transplant. In the case of a single lung transplant, the donor bronchi are then divided at their origin with a stapling device to leave the airway to both lungs sealed during transport.

In the case of a living donor lobectomy, the right lower lobe is typically used as the graft for the right lung in the recipient and the left lower lobe from a different donor is the left lung graft. Donor lobectomy is performed through a standard posterolateral thoracotomy.

In the case of heart–lung transplantation, the heart and lungs are removed en bloc.

Postoperative management

The recipient is returned from the operating room to an isolation room in the ICU. Mechanical ventilation is weaned as rapidly as possible. Antibiotics are continued until all monitoring lines and chest tubes have been removed. Some level of inotropic support is required in virtually all heart transplant recipients. Isoproterenol is often an ideal choice because of the pulmonary vasodilatory effects as well as inotropic and chronotropic effects as many patients have a slower than optimal heart rate initially. This transient sinus node dysfunction is rarely permanent. Dobutamine and dopamine, especially at "renal dose," are also frequently used to augment ventricular contractility. Epinephrine and norepinephrine are usually reserved for poor graft function. Sodium nitroprusside infusion or phosphodiesterase inhibitors are used for afterload reduction in the early postoperative period. Right ventricular dysfunction due to pulmonary hypertension may respond to phosphodiesterase inhibitors such as milrinone. Inhaled nitric oxide has been shown to be an effective selective pulmonary vasodilator with few systemic side effects and is useful in cardiac transplant recipients with pulmonary hypertension.

Transplant immunosuppression

The prevention and treatment of rejection is dependent upon the use of a combination of immunosuppressive agents. Standard triple-drug immunosuppression therapy consisting of prednisone, cyclosporine and azathioprine has been successfully used in pediatric cardiac transplant recipients and remains the most common regimen.[13] The induction and maintenance doses of medications used for immunosuppression at the Children's Hospital of Philadelphia are listed in Table 67.3. Because of the adverse effects of corticosteroids, withdrawal from prednisone is usually attempted at 6 months post-transplantation. Up to 80% of recipients may be successfully weaned from steroids; only one-fourth of these patients have an episode of rejection in the first 6 months after discontinuing the prednisone.[14] Adverse effects of steroid therapy include a Cushingoid appearance, hypertension, growth retardation, osteoporosis, and diabetes mellitus.

Survival after thoracic organ transplantation improved significantly with the introduction of cyclosporine therapy. However, there are significant side effects, including hypertension, renal dysfunction, hirsuitism, and gingival hyperplasia. Gingival hyperplasia can be a problem in infants and may impair or prevent eruption of primary teeth.

Tacrolimus (formerly called FK-506) has been shown[15] to be an effective immunosuppressive agent in children, and its usage has increased over the last 5 years with approximately 40% of all pediatric cardiac transplant patients receiving it for maintenance immunosuppression 1 year after transplantation in the place of cyclosporine.[1] Overall, patients on tacrolimus appear to have a lower incidence of rejection. In addition, the incidence of hypertension, hirsuitism, and gingival hyperplasia is reduced with FK-506 compared with cyclosporin, but adverse effects include anemia, renal toxicity and chronic diarrhea.

Side effects of azathioprine therapy, such as bone marrow depression, have precipitated the use of mycophenolate mofetil (MMF) in its place. MMF is well tolerated with few side effects and has been shown in large clinical trials to have benefits in improved survival and decreased treated rejection episodes.[16] An increasing number of centers recommend the use of induction immunosuppression in pediatric cardiac recipients with close to 40% of patients now receiving either a polyclonal anti-T-cell preparation, OKT3 (a murine monoclonal CD3 antibody), or an interleukin-2 receptor antibody immediately following transplantation. However, there have been no significant differences in the average number of rejection episodes in those patients treated for rejection regardless of the type of induction agent used.[1] In addition, OKT3 has been associated with an increased incidence of post-transplant lymphoproliferative disease (PTLD).

Infection prophylaxis includes oral nystatin for fungal prophylaxis and oral trimethoprim-sulfamethoxazole three times per week. Pentamidine inhalation treatment is an effective alternative to trimethoprim-sulfamethoxazole for *Pneumocystis carinii* prophylaxis if bone marrow suppression is a problem. Routine CMV prophylaxis is not used in cardiac transplant recipients at our institution.

Table 67.3. Heart transplantation immunosuppression regimen at the Children's Hospital of Philadephia

Drug	Dosage
Azathioprine/Mycophenolate mofetil (MMF)	2 mg/kg IV given in the operating room before transplantation. Then 2 mg/kg IV given once daily for 5 d (neonates), 7 d (infants), or 9 d (adolescents)
	Change over to MMF 120 mg/kg per day IV given twice daily (target level 2.5–3.0) after the azathioprine course is completed
	Change over to MMF orally as intestinal function returns.
Cyclosporine	0.02 mg/kg per hr IV infusion beginning in the operating room, before transplantation. Then 0.02 mg/kg/h IV infusion for 24 h (target level 100)
	Change over to ATG (rabbit antithymocyte globulin) on postoperative day 3 and give 1.5 mg/kg IV once daily for 3 d (neonates), 5 d(infants), or 7 d(adolescents)
	Change back to cyclosporine orally after ATG course is completed to maintain target levels of approximately 125 in neonates and 150–175 in older children by discharge. Dosing should be carefully adjusted over the next 2 months to achieve levels of 125–150 in neonates, 175–200 in infants, 250 in 6- to 12-year-olds, and 250–300 in adolescents.
Solumedrol	10–15 mg/kg IV given in the operating room, before transplantation. Then 3 mg/kg IV twice daily for three doses.

IV-Intravenous.

Early complications

Acute rejection and infection are the most common early complications after cardiac transplantation. Nearly 60% to 75% of patients have at least one episode of rejection, and it should be expected that about one-third will have an episode in the first 3 months, 50% within the first year post-transplantation.[17] Some studies suggest that infants may be less prone to rejection than older children. Rejection surveillance is based on clinical evaluation, echocardiography and endomyocardial or bronchoscopic biopsy. Clinical assessment includes changes in a patient's activity or appetite. Atrial or ventricular ectopy including tachycardia is suspicious for rejection and mandate evaluation. Echocardiography is particularly useful in neonates in whom biopsy is technically difficult and carries significant risk due to patient size. Echocardiographic evaluation is typically performed weekly for the first month and then monthly for the first year post-transplant. Echocardiography-guided transjugular endomyocardial biopsy has been shown to be an effective means of monitoring pediatric transplant recipients for rejection and remains the gold standard for detection of rejection.[18] An aggressive approach has been adopted at the Children's Hospital of Philadelphia for rejection surveillance with routine endomyocardial biopsy weekly for the first month following transplant, every second week for the second month, and then once monthly for the remainder of the first year. Subsequent biopsies are obtained twice annually, and at any time point after if rejection is clinically suspected. Most biopsies are performed on an outpatient basis. For lung transplant recipients, fluoroscopic guided transbronchial biopsy is performed at 1, 4, 8, and 12 weeks post-transplant and at subsequent 3 month intervals thereafter for the first year and annually thereafter. Heart–lung recipients are at risk for individual or simultaneous rejection of both organs. Lung rejection is more common and simultaneous rejection is rare. Both organs must be routinely biopsied. The international grading system for cardiac transplant rejection is shown in Table 67.4.

Episodes of acute rejection for either thoracic organ are usually treated with a 3-day course of intravenous methylprednisolone (10 mg per kg). OKT3 and antithymocyte globulin are reserved for an incomplete response or rejection refractory to steroids. Response is confirmed by follow-up biopsy 1 to 2 weeks after treatment.

Although infectious complications are common in cardiac transplant recipients, infection-related deaths do not appear to be. Bacterial infections are most common in the early post-transplantation period, when immunosuppression is most intense, but can also occur late after transplantation and usually respond to proper antibiotic therapy. In lung transplant patients, most infections originate in the transplanted lungs and occur in approximately 25% of all patients (usually those with cystic fibrosis). Of viral infections, CMV appears to be the most common and is treated with intravenous ganciclovir. Viral respiratory infections usually occur with a frequency similar to that in normal children and appear to be well tolerated by the recipient of either heart or lung transplants. Exceptions include

Table 67.4. International Society for Heart and Lung Transplantation categories of acute rejection

Grade 0	No evidence of cellular rejection
Grade 1A	Focal perivascular or interstitial infiltrate without myocyte injury
Grade 1B	Multifocal or diffuse sparse infiltrate without myocyte injury
Grade 2	Single focus of dense infiltrate with myocyte injury
Grade 3A	Multifocal dense infiltrates with myocyte injury
Grade 3B	Diffuse, dense infiltrates with myocyte injury
Grade 4	Diffuse and extensive polymorphous infiltrate with myocyte injury – may have hemorrhage, edema and microvascular invasion

From Rodriguez, E. R. *J. Heart Lung Transpl.* 2003; **22**:3.

adenovirus, parainfluenza and varicella. Epstein–Barr virus is uncommon but concerning after transplantation due to its association with post-transplantation lymphoproliferative disease. Fungal infections occur rarely but can be fatal, particularly aspergillosis in lung transplant patients

Surgical complications of lung transplant specifically include anastomotic complications (breakdown or stricture), persistent postoperative bleeding, or vocal cord and/or hemidiaphragm paralysis, and gastric emptying abnormalities. Although typically presenting late, anastomotic complications include stenoses of the bronchial anastomosis, the pulmonary artery or vein. Bronchial stricture is usually treated by bronchoscopic dilatation. In rare and severe cases, silicone or covered metallic stents have been used to maintain patency.

Aside from rejection and infection, the immediate postoperative complications after heart and/or lung transplantation are hypertension, seizures, renal dysfunction and diabetes. Nearly 10% of infant heart transplant recipients require perioperative peritoneal dialysis. Among neonates, 10% to 15% require phenobarbital therapy for postoperative seizures which may result from the use of circulatory arrest in these patients[19] and the use of cyclosporin or tacrolimus immunosuppression.

Late complications

The primary late complications seen in pediatric cardiac transplant recipients are chronic rejection, post-transplantation lymphoproliferative disease (PTLD) or transplant coronary artery disease (TCAD). These manifestations of chronic rejection may account for up to 40% of deaths after cardiac transplantation.[1]

PTLD presents similar to mononucleosis with reactive lymph nodes, polyclonal lymphoproliferation and monoclonal B-cell lymphoma and is most commonly found in the oropharynx and gastrointestinal tracts. It is currently treated with reduction in immunosuppressants, acyclovir and chemo/radiotherapy.

The onset of graft TCAD has a prevalence of 10% to 15% and may be suggested by symptoms of congestive heart failure in recipients. It is the leading cause of late death in cardiac transplant recipients. Echocardiograms are performed routinely during follow-up visits of heart transplant recipients and worsening ventricular function is a sign of graft CAD. The new onset of arrhythmias after transplantation, especially ventricular, may also be an indication of underlying CAD.[20] CAD may also be found on routine follow-up catheterization or intracoronary ultrasound, without any prior suggestion of disease. A number of etiologies have been implicated in the development of graft CAD, including chronic cellular rejection, hyperlipidemia, vascular rejection, and CMV infection. Unlike in adult cardiac transplant recipients, CAD appears to develop in pediatric patients relatively early after transplantation, with one series demonstrating an incidence of 35% by 2 years after transplantation.[21]

A review of 815 pediatric transplantation patients found nearly 8% to have significant CAD by angiogram or autopsy findings.[20] The mean time post-transplantation to diagnosis was 2.2 years, with one patient having significant CAD 2 months after transplantation. Conventional therapies for coronary artery disease such as percutaneous transluminal angioplasty and coronary artery bypass grafting are of little use in treating TCAD. Retransplantation appears to be the only viable option for these patients, although the results in general are not encouraging, with 1- and 3-year survival rates of 71% and 47%, respectively, and with CAD developing in the second grafts in 20% of retransplantation patients.[22] However, the Loma Linda group has reported a significantly better retransplantation experience in infants who were first transplanted at less than six months of age.[10] In this group, a 10-year actuarial survival of 91% was observed following retransplantation, potentially related to this center's early adoption of a steroid-free immunosuppressive regime. In addition, medical therapy targeted at cholesterol and lipid-lowering therapies are currently under investigation.[23]

The primary long-term complication of lung transplantation is an end-stage process similar to that of TCAD in heart transplantation known as bronchiolitis obliterans (OB). Although associated with multiple episodes of acute rejection, airway ischemia and airway denervation, it is most likely a manifestation of chronic rejection. It

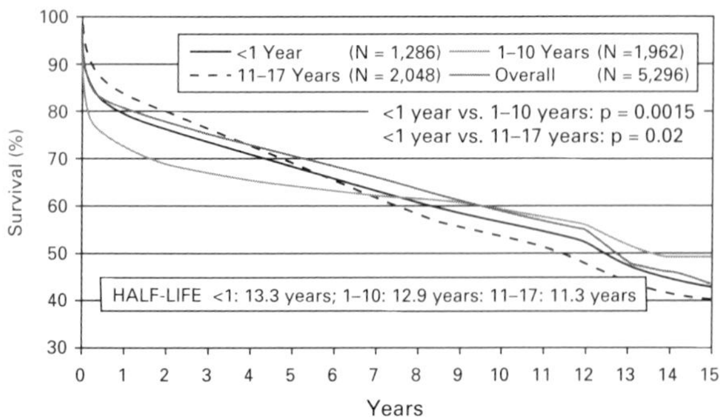

Fig. 67.6. Pediatric heart transplantation Kaplan-Meier survival (January 1982 to June 2002). (International Society of Heart and Lung Transplantation, 2004, as above.)

is diagnosed by a persistent decline in pulmonary function tests (>20% decline in FEV_1) in the absence of infection or rejection. The standard treatment is an increase in immunosuppression, although the response is poor. Retransplantation for patients with end-stage OB remains controversial.

Outcome following thoracic organ transplantation

Heart transplantation

Results from the Registry of the International Society for Heart and Lung Transplantation reveal a perioperative mortality rate higher for infants than for older children (Fig. 67.6).[1,24] Despite the much greater early mortality, however, the half-life of 13.3 years is longer than that of the childhood or adolescent survivors. For the childhood age group of 1 to 10 years, the half-life was 17.5 years versus 13.7 years for the adolescent age group, thus conferring on the younger patients a significant survival advantage. Averaged over 15 years, the infant recipient would have an approximate 2%-per-year risk of mortality whereas for older children it remains approximately 4%, indicating a long-term survival advantage for the younger cardiac transplant recipient. The most predictive risk factors for 1-year mortality in the pediatric population remain congenital heart disease, retransplant, donor age, pulmonary artery systolic pressure >35 mm Hg, the need for mechanical ventilation and hospitalization while awaiting transplant. Amongst the most significant risk factors for 5-year mortality are dialysis, congenital diagnosis and female gender. Causes of death include CAD, acute rejection, lymphoma, graft failure and infection. Additional risk factors for mortality in the registry data were repeat transplantation, pre-transplantation mechanical support, transplantation for congenital heart disease, longer graft ischemia time, and low center transplant volume. Prevalent post-transplant morbidities for survivors include hypertension (45%), renal dysfunction (5.4%), hyperlipidemia (9.9%) and diabetes (3.2%).[1]

The largest group of infant cardiac transplant recipients reported in the literature is from Loma Linda, where 233 heart transplantations in infants younger than 6 months of age have been performed.[10] Nearly 65% of these were for HLHS, and the rest were for other complex congenital anomalies (29%) or cardiomyopathy or tumor (8%). The operative (30-day) survival rate was 89%, with the primary causes of mortality primary graft failure, technical problems, pneumonia or acute rejection. The overall 1-year survival was 84%, with a 5- and 10-year actuarial survival rate of 73% and 68%, respectively. In addition, those patients transplanted at less than 30 days of age had a significantly better outcome compared with older infants with an actuarial survival rate of 80% and 77% at 5 and 10 years, potentially related to improved immune tolerance in the younger subgroup.

Razzouk *et al.*[25] reported intermediate term results for cardiac transplantation used as primary therapy for HLHS. Between 1985 and 1995, 176 infants with HLHS were listed for transplantation, but 34 died before organs became available. Transplantation was performed in 142 patients at a median age of 29 days. Survival was 91% at 30 days, 84% at 1 year and 70% at 5 years. Graft coronary artery disease developed in 8 patients. Rejection was the primary cause of late death.

St. Louis Children's Hospital reported an infant survival of 94%, similar to that of Loma Linda, after 45 infant heart transplants.[24] HLHS was the indication for transplant in well over half of these infants.

A recent multicenter report analyzed 191 heart transplants performed on patients between 1 and 18 years of age.[26] Actuarial survival at 1 month was 93%. One-year and 2-year survival rates were 82% and 81%, respectively. Hazard function analysis demonstrated that the highest risk for death was in the first 2 weeks after transplantation with a single declining phase. Rejection was the most common cause of recipient death (29%), followed by early graft failure (19%), infection (16%) and sudden death (13%). Multivariate analysis showed risk factors for death after transplant to be preoperative mechanical support, non-identical ABO blood types between donor and recipient, and younger age of recipient (< 5 years).

The Stanford series [27] includes 72 patients less than 18 years of age who underwent heart transplant since 1977. Only 25% of these recipients were under 1 year of age, with a mean age at operation of 9 years. The indication for transplantation in almost two-thirds of recipients was cardiomyopathy unrelated to congenital heart disease. The operative survival was 87.5%, with early deaths primarily due to right ventricular failure from pulmonary hypertension, or acute rejection. There were 20 late deaths, 24% due to rejection, and 17% due to graft vasculopathy. Actuarial survival rates at 1, 5, and 10 years were 75%, 60%, and 50%, respectively. No survival difference between age groups was found in this series.

More recently, in January 2005, Groetzner *et al.* released data on 50 transplants performed over a 15-year period starting in 1988. Perioperative mortality was 6% due to primary graft failure with a 12% late mortality mainly attributable to acute rejection. Actuarial 1, 5, and 10 year survival was 86%, 86% and 80%, respectively, with no difference in outcome between those patients with congenital heart disease and dilated cardiomyopathy. Survival was notably improved after 1995 with a 92% 5-year survival for these children. Freedom from acute rejection was attributed to the introduction of mycophenolate mofetil.

Aside from survival, it has been demonstrated that transplanted hearts in children appear to grow normally and the left ventricle increases muscle mass to maintain the normal left ventricular mass–volume ratio over time.[28] Exercise testing in older heart transplant recipients has shown peak heart rate and oxygen consumption to be consistently two-thirds of that predicted.[29] Somatic growth appears to be normal in infants after heart transplantation, and neurological development generally preserved, although some neurologic abnormalities may be seen in up to 20% of neonatal recipients on long-term follow-up.[1]

Lung transplantation

The 2004 report of the ISHLT documented approximately 60 procedures for 2002. Sixty-seven percent of the recipients were adolescents while the majority of donor organs are from adults. The designated changes in organ allocation previously described have been made in an effort to increase donor availability to pediatric recipients. Congenital heart disease and pulmonary hypertension were the most common indications in children under 5 years of age. Cystic fibrosis was the most common indication in older children, while primary pulmonary hypertension accounted for 20% of patients in both age groups. For those patients with primary pulmonary hypertension, actuarial 1-year survival was 60%–70% with better survival following bilateral transplantation as opposed to single lung transplantation, thus conferring a significant survival benefit

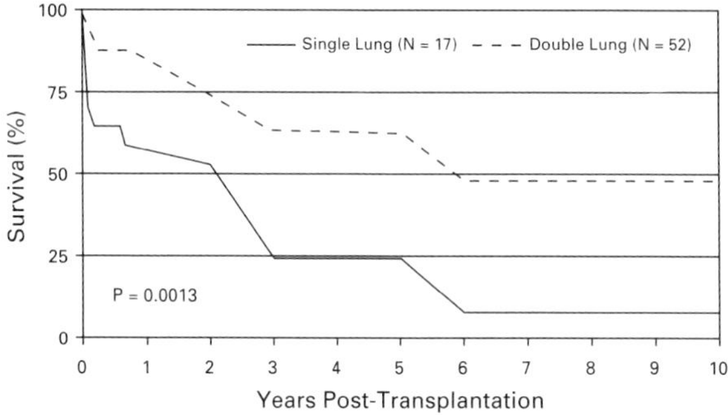

Fig. 67.7. Pediatric lung transplantation Kaplan-Meier survival by procedure-type, diagnosis of PPH (transplants from January 1990 to June 2002). (International Society of Heart and Lung Transplantation, 2004, as above.)

(Fig. 67.7). However, 5-year survival post lung transplant still averages under 50%.

Per the ISHLT database, the leading early (less than 1 year) causes of death after lung transplantation between 1992 and June 2003 were graft failure and infection. Between 1 and 3 years post-transplant, bronchiolitis obliterans surpassed both as the leading cause of death. Complications include hypertension (which was present in 71% of patients 5 years post-transplant) and mild to moderate renal dysfunction. Fortunately, functional status remained good in late survivors after pediatric lung transplantation with greater than 80% of patients reporting no activity limitation at 1, 3 and 5 years of follow-up.

Early data from the 1996 St. Louis Lung Transplant Registry reported a 1-year survival of 60%, a 2-year survival of 57% and a 3-year survival of 48% for the 191 pediatric lung transplant patients under 16 years of age.[30] Cystic fibrosis patients appeared to have a better survival (70% at one year and 62% at 2 years) than did pulmonary hypertension patients (62% at 1 year and 56% at 2 years). Recipients with pulmonary hypertension receiving bilateral lungs had a slightly higher survival than single-lung recipients: 66% vs. 58% at 1 year, and 60% vs. 52% at 2 years.

In 2002, Mendeloff *et al.* from St. Louis reported results consisting of 207 isolated transplants occurring in 190 children over a 10-year period.[31] Thirty-two patients were less than 1 year of age, 22 were 1 to 5 years of age, 32 were 5 to 10 years of age, and 121 were 10 to 18 years old with cystic fibrosis as the primary diagnosis. Survival was 77% at 1 year, 62% at 3 years and 55% at 5 years. There was no difference in survival according to primary diagnosis or age at time of transplantation. While the most common cause of early death was graft failure, bronchiolitis obliterans was by far the most common cause of late death. The average onset of time to development of bronchiolitis obliterans is 679 days and risk factors identified leading to the development of bronchiolitis obliterans were age older than 3 years, more than two episodes of acute rejection, and organ ischemic time of longer than 180 minutes.[31]

A combined report from St. Louis Children's Hospital and the Children's Hospital of Philadelphia reviewed lung transplantation in 17 patients under 2 years of age.[32] Hospital survival was 71%, with one late death due to overwhelming gastroenteritis. Operative deaths were due to hemorrhage, and three early deaths were secondary to viral pneumonitis.

Bridges *et al.*[5] reported a follow-up of 20 patients (mean age 6.3 years) who underwent lung transplantation for pulmonary hypertension. Congenital heart defects were present in 19, and all were in New York Heart Association (NYHA) class IV at the time of transplantation. Three patients were on ECMO support and 3 were mechanically ventilated prior to transplantation. Cardiac repair was performed in 19 patients at the time of transplantation. Hospital survival was 70% (14/20). Hemorrhage related to previous thoracic operations contributed to 3/6 hospital deaths. There were 3 late deaths, all related to bronchiolitis obliterans. Ten of the 11 late survivors were NYHA class I at a mean follow-up of 18 months.

A recent report from the Children's Hospital of Philadelphia concentrated on "high-risk" characteristics in ten children undergoing lung transplantation.[33] These characteristics included previous thoracic operations, high dose steroid therapy, preoperative ventilator dependence with or without tracheostomy, preoperative ECMO support, need for cardiac repair, and previous lung transplantation. Actuarial 1-year survival and 1-year freedom from death or retransplantation were 86% and 70%, respectively. This series demonstrates that standard exclusion criteria utilized for adult transplant recipients are not generally applicable to the pediatric population and so the decision to proceed with transplantation must be individualized.

Lobar transplantation from either cadaveric or living donors has been advocated to increase organ availability. Starnes *et al.*[34] reported lobar transplantation in 25 pediatric recipients. Fourteen patients received bilateral lower lobes from living donors, and cadaveric lobes were used in eleven patients. There was no difference in rejection or pulmonary function tests 12 months postoperatively. However, at 24 months those patients who received living lobes had greater FEV1 than those who received cadaveric lungs. Interestingly, after two years, bronchiolitis obliterans was found in no living donor lungs and in 86% of the cadaveric lungs possibly reflecting the short ischemic times in living donor transplants. There were no donor deaths, and donor morbidity was limited to prolonged air leaks.

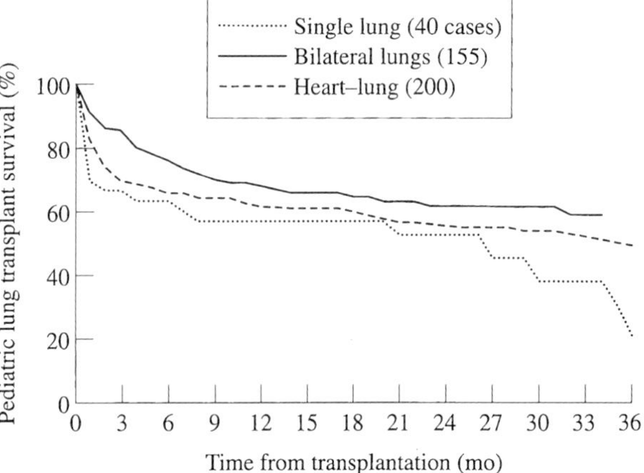

Fig. 67.8. Actuarial survival following pediatric lung and heart–lung transplantation (from Hosenpud, J. D. *et al. J. Heart Lung Transpt.* 1996; **15**: 65–71).

Wider application of this technique awaits further evaluation as the growth potential of lobes from mature donors is of some concern. The absence of bronchiolitis obliterans in the living lobe recipients is indicative of successful long-term outcome. In a larger series published by the same authors in 2004[35] examining both adult and pediatric populations, infection was the predominant cause of death with bronchiolitis obliterans accountable for only 12.7% of late deaths.

Heart–lung transplantation

The ISHLT Registry in 1996 reported 200 heart–lung transplants in children since 1982. As the use of lung transplantation has increased, the number of heart–lung transplants performed each year has decreased dramatically. Fewer than ten heart–lung transplants were performed in children in 1995 (Fig. 67.8). The ISHLT Registry reported an operative survival of nearly 85% for pediatric heart–lung transplant recipients, with a 1-year and 2-year survival of 62% and 55%, respectively (Fig. 67.9). Independent risk factors for mortality within the first year after transplant included year of surgery (prior to 1991), preoperative ventilator dependence, and graft ischemic time.

Conte *et al.*[36] reported the Stanford experience with pediatric heart–lung transplantation in 1996. A total of 19 heart–lung transplants were performed in 17 patients, at a median age of 10 years. Most of the transplants were performed for pulmonary vascular disease secondary to congenital heart disease. The 30-day operative mortality rate was 5.2%, and 88% of the recipients were discharged from the hospital. Multiorgan system failure was the most common cause of early death. The mean follow-up was 29 months, and

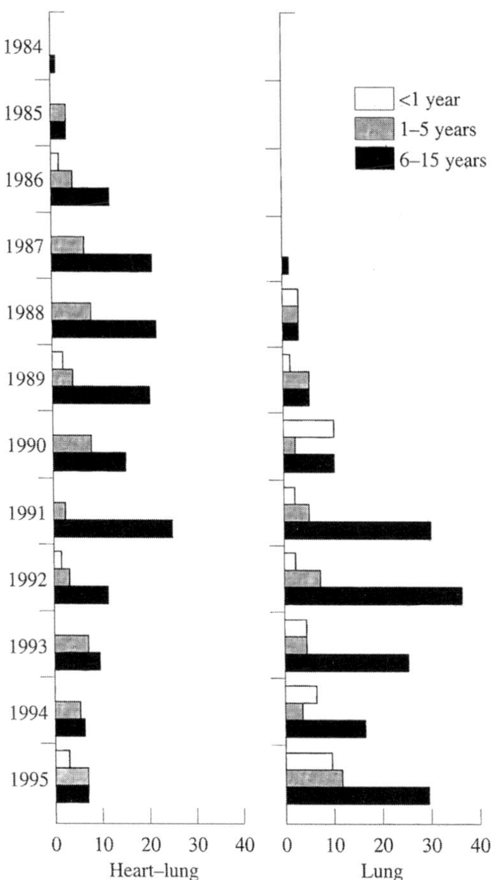

Fig. 67.9. Numbers of children undergoing lung abd heart–lung transplantations each year (from Hosenpud J. D. *et al. J. Heart Lung Transpl.* 1996; **15**: 665–674).

actuarial survival rates at 1, 3, and 5 years after transplant were 67%, 51% and 41%, respectively. Actuarial survival for the hospital survivors was 82%, 62% and 51% at 1, 3 and 5 years, respectively. Bronchiolitis obliterans developed in 32% of all recipients, and was the cause of nearly half of the deaths following heart–lung transplantation, and two-thirds of the late deaths. Isolated lung rejection occurred frequently (in 73% of recipients), with isolated heart rejection occurring less frequently. Simultaneous heart and lung rejection were even less common. Graft coronary artery disease was the cause of late death in only one patient.

Madden *et al.*[37] reported results with 303 consecutive patients after heart–lung transplantation from Harefield Hospital and the National Heart and Lung Institution in London. Half of the recipients had pulmonary vascular disease while the remainder had parenchymal lung disease, mainly cystic fibrosis. The operative (30-day) mortality rate was approximately 30%. The most frequent causes of early death were multiple organ system failure, bleeding and infections. Actuarial survival rates at 1 and 2 years after transplantation were 61% and 51%, respectively. Late deaths were most commonly due to bronchiolitis obliterans, bacterial infection, or CMV infection.

Whitehead *et al.*[38] reported results of heart-lung transplantation for cystic fibrosis in children. Of 76 patients who were listed for transplantation between 1988 and 1993, 36 patients died waiting, and 25 underwent operation. Actuarial survival rates were 67% at 1 year, 61% at 2 years, and 54% at 3 years. Three patients developed tracheal anastomotic stenosis. Bronchiolitis obliterans developed in 52% of the survivors, and other complications included diabetes mellitus and hypertension.

Growth and development

Most children are able to return to school and to other age-appropriate activities following thoracic organ transplantation. Growth and neurodevelopmental outcome, however, remain major concerns. Prolonged steroid therapy is the likely source of any significant growth retardation. Many centers attempt to withdraw steroids within 6 months of operation in cardiac transplant patients, if possible, or to avoid maintenance steroids entirely. Backer *et al.*[27] reported normal growth and development in 16 survivors of neonatal heart transplantation. In this study, patients tended to retain their initial percentile on growth charts, and no patient had neurological impairment or developmental delay as assessed by Denver Developmental Screening Testing. Baum *et al.*[39] documented normal linear growth in a group of 20 infants at a follow-up of 3–7 years following transplantation and normal growth at a mean of 3 years' follow-up was documented in 10/13 children transplanted at Stanford at a mean age of 5 years.[40] There was proportional growth of the heart in these patients and no evidence of anastomotic obstruction.

A recent study from St. Louis Children's Hospital evaluated somatic growth in 26 children who underwent transplantation for HLHS at a mean age of 27 days.[41] Height and weight were in the normal range throughout the follow-up period. However, there was a late trend towards smaller height and weight. Interestingly, no difference in somatic growth was seen when children in whom steroid therapy was discontinued were compared with those maintained on low-dose steroids.

Many investigators have documented normal growth of the transplanted heart in children. Hearts from oversized donors are frequently used for pediatric heart transplantation (200% of bodyweight or greater). Echocardiographic studies have shown that the ratio of left ventricular mass to bodyweight is increased immediately after transplantation. In the first month following operation, the ratio normalizes and remains normal during further growth, suggesting adaptation to the smaller size of the recipient.

Few data are available concerning growth following lung transplantation in children. Bridges *et al.*[32] reported normal linear growth velocity in 11 survivors, but children tended to be small for their age. Body weight for three of the survivors was less than the 3rd percentile for age, and 5 were shorter than the 3rd percentile for age.

The assessment of lung growth is more difficult. Routine measurements of pulmonary function tests may reflect either an increase in the average volume of each alveolar unit or an increase in the number of alveoli or available surface area for gas exchange. It is noted that an increase in lung volume and gas exchange proportionate to somatic growth occurs in infants and children.[42]

Cognitive function appears to be in the normal range in most children following thoracic organ transplantation, although scores on developmental tests may be lower than in controls. Cardiac transplantation in infants with HLHS may require the use of a period of deep hypothermic circulatory arrest that could lead to adverse neurodevelopmental sequelae. The Bayley Scales of Infant Development were used to assess neurodevelopmental outcome in 48 infants who underwent transplantation before 6 months of age.[39] Scores were in the normal range in 32 children and abnormal or suspect in the remaining 16 patients. The incidence of behavioral problems may be increased in the children, but it is difficult to separate the effects of chronic illness and repeated hospitalizations from any specific effects of transplantation.

Exercise capacity is improved following transplantation, although maximal exercise capacity is decreased compared with normals.[43] Following heart and heart–lung transplantations, the heart is denervated, and thus the ability to augment cardiac output during exercise and an increase in heart rate is attenuated. Peak minute ventilation during exercise is decreased following lung and heart–lung transplantations.

Conclusions

Despite further improvements in surgical technique, immunosuppression, perioperative management, and rejection surveillance, long-term results with pediatric heart and lung transplantation have shown little change over recent years, with a 15-year survival rate of approximately 50%. Chronic rejection, graft CAD, bronchiolitis obliterans and the long-term effects of steroids on growth continue to cloud the development of cardiac and lung transplantation as the primary treatment of complex congenital heart disease. However, for many children with end-stage cardiomyopathy and structural heart disease not amenable to corrective surgery, transplantation is the only option. Future areas of research interest include the use of xenografts, ABO incompatible transplants, permanent mechanical support and widening the bridge to transplant with smaller and more adaptable pediatric assist devices.

REFERENCES

1. Boucek, M. M., Edwards, L. B., Keck, B. M. *et al.* The Registry of the International Society for Heart and Lung Transplantation: Seventh Official Pediatric Report – 2004. *J. Heart and Lung Transpl.* 2004; **23**:933.
2. Cooper, M. M., Fuzesi, L., Addonizio, L. I. *et al.* Pediatric heart transplantation after operations involving the pulmonary arteries. *J. Thorac. Cardiovasc. Surg.* 1991; **102**:386.
3. Lewis, A. B. Prognostic value of echocardiography in children with idiopathic dilated cardiomyopathy. *Am. Heart J.* 1994; **128**:133.
4. Wiles, H. B., McArthur, P. D., Taylor, A. B. *et al.* Prognostic features of children with idiopathic dilated cardiomyopathy. *Am. J. Cardiol.* 1991; **68**:1372–1376.
5. Bridges, N. D., Mallory, G. B., Jr, Huddleston, C. B. *et al.* Lung transplantation in children and young adults with cardiovascular disease. *Ann. Thorac. Surg.* 1995; **59**:813.
6. Kerem, E., Reisman, J., Corey, M. *et al.* Prediction of mortality in patients with cystic fibrosis. *N. Engl. J. Med.* 1992; **326**:1187.
7. Shaddy, R. E., Bullock, E. A., Morwessel, N. J. *et al.* Murine monoclonal CD3 antibody (OKT3)-based early rejection prophylaxis in pediatric heart transplantation. *J. Heart and Lung Transpl.* 1993; **12**:434–439.
8. del Nido, P. J., Armitage, J. M., Fricker, F. J. *et al.* Extracorporeal membrane oxygenation support as a bridge to pediatric heart transplantation. *Circulation* 1994; **90**(2):11–66.
9. Kirshborn, P. M., Bridges, N. D., Myung, R. J. *et al.* Use of extracorporeal membrane oxygenation in pediatric thoracic organ transplantation. *J. Thorac. Cardiovasc. Surg.* 2002; **123**(1):130–136.
10. Fortuna, K. S., Chinnock, R. E., Bailey, L. L. *et al.* Heart transplantation among 233 infants during the first six months of life: the Loma Linda experience. *Clin. Transpl.* 1999:263–272.
11. Tamisier, D., Vouhe, P., Le Bidois, J. *et al.* Donor–recipient size matching in pediatric heart transplantation; a word of caution about small grafts. *J. Heart Lung Transpl.* 1996; **15**:190–195.
12. West, L. J., Pollock-Barziv, S. M., Dipchand, A. I. *et al.* ABO-incompatible heart transplantation in infants. *N. Engl. J. Med.* 2001; **344**(11):793.
13. Canter, C. E., Soffitz, J. E., Moorehead, S. *et al.* Early results after pediatric cardiac transplantation with triple immunosuppression therapy. *Am. J. Cardiol.* 1993; **71**:971.

14. Canter, C. E., Moorehead, S., Soffitz, J. E. *et al.* Steroid withdrawal in the pediatric heart transplant recipient initially treated with triple immunosuppression. *J. Heart Lung Transpl.* 1994; **13**:74.
15. Swenson, J. M., Fricker, F. J., & Armitage, J. M. Immunosuppression switch in pediatric heart transplant recipients: cyclosporine to FK506. *J. Am. Coll. Cardiol.* 1995; **25**(5):1183.
16. Kobashigawa, J. A. Mycophenolate mofetil in cardiac transplantation. *Curr. Opin. Cardiol.* 1998; **13**(2):117–121.
17. Braunlin, E. A., Canter, C. E., Olivari, M. T. *et al.* Rejection and infection after pediatric cardiac transplantation. *Ann. Thorac. Surg.* 1990; **49**:385.
18. Canter, C. E., Appleton, R. S., Soffitz, J. E. *et al.* Surveillance for rejection by echocardiographically guided endomyocardial biopsy in the infant heart transplant recipient. *Circulation* 1991; **84**(Suppl III) 111–310.
19. Bailey, L. L., Gundry, S. R., Razzouk, A. J. *et al.* Bless the babies: one hundred fifiteen late survivors of heart transplantation in the first year of life. *J. Thorac. Cardiovasc. Surg.* 1993; **105**:805.
20. Pahl, E., Zalos, V. R., Ficker, F. I. *et al.* Posttransplant coronary artery disease in children: a multicenter national survey. *Circulation* 1994; **9**(2):11–56.
21. Braulin, E. A., Hunter, D. W., Canter, C. E. *et al.* Coronary artery disease in pediatric cardiac transplant recipients receiving triple-drug immunosuppression. *Circulation* 1991; **84**(Suppl III):111–303.
22. Michler, R. E., Edward, N. M., Hsu, D. *et al.* Pediatric retransplantation, *J. Heart Lung Transpl.* 1993; **12**:5319.
23. Seipelt, I. M., Crawford, S. E., Rodgers, S. *et al.* Hypercholesterolemia is common after pediatric heart transplantation: initial experience with pravastatin. *J. Heart Lung Transpl.* 2004; **23**(3):317–322.
24. Spray, T. L. Transplantation of the heart and lungs in children. *Am. Rev. Med.* 1994; **45**:139–148.
25. Razzouk, A. J., Chinnock, R. E., Gundry, S. R. *et al.* Transplantation as primary treatment for hypoplastic left heart syndrome: intermediate-term results. *Ann. Thorac. Surg.* 1996; **62**:1–8.
26. Shaddy, R. E., Naftel, D. C., Kirklin, J. K. *et al.* Outcome of cardiac transplantation in children: survival in a contemporary multi-institutional experience. *Circulation* 1996; **94**(Suppl):II69–II73.
27. Backer, C. L., Zales, V. R., Harrison, H. L. *et al.* Intermediate term results of infant orthotopic cardiac transplantation from two centers. *J. Thorac. Cardiovasc. Surg.* 1991; **101**:826–832.
28. Zales, V. R., Wright, K. L., Pahl, E. *et al.* Normal left ventricular muscle mass and mass/volume ratio after pediatric cardiac transplantation. *Circulation* 1994; **90**(2):11–61.
29. Nixon, P. A., Fricker, F. J., Noyes, B. E. *et al.* Exercise testing in pediatric heart, heart–lung and lung recipients. *Chest* 1995; **107**:1328.
30. Cooper, J. D. 1996 Report of the St Louis International Lung Transplant Registry.
31. Huddleston, C. B., Bloch, J. B., Sweet, S. C. *et al.* Lung transplantation in children. *Ann. Surg.* 2002; **236**(3):270–276.
32. Bridges, N. D., Mallory, G. B., Jr, Huddleston, C. B. *et al.* Lung transplantation in infancy and early childhood. *J. Heart Lung Transpl.* 1996; **15**:895–902.
33. Koutlas, T. C., Bridges, N. D., Gaynor, J. W. *et al.* Pediatric lung transplantation: are there surgical contraindications? *Transplantation* 1997; **63**:269–274.
34. Starnes, V. A., Barr, N. L., & Cohen, R. G. Lobar transplantation. *J. Thorac. Cardiovasc. Surg.* 1994; **108**:403–411.
35. Starnes, V. A., Bowdish, M. E., Woo, M. S. *et al.* A decade of living lobar lung transplantation: recipient outcomes. *J. Thorac. Cardiovasc. Surg.* 2004; **127**:115–122.
36. Conte, J. V., Robbins, R. C., Reishenspurner, H. *et al.* Pediatric heart–lung transplantation: intermediate-term results. *J. Heart Lung Transpl.* 1996; **15**:692–699.
37. Madden, B., Radley-Smith, R., Hodson, M. *et al.* Medium term results of heart and lung transplantation. *J. Heart Lung Transpl.* 1992; **11**:S241–S243.
38. Whitehead, B. F., Rees, P. G., Sorensen, K. *et al.* Results of heart–lung transplantation in children with cystic fibrosis. *Eur. J. Cardiothorac. Surg.* 1995; **9**:1–6.
39. Baum, M., Chinnock, R., Ashwal, S. *et al.* Growth and neurodevelopmental outcome of infants undergoing heart transplantation. *J. Heart Lung Transpl.* 1993; **12**:S211–S217.
40. Bernstein, D., Kolla, S., Miner, M. *et al.* Cardiac growth in pediatric heart transplantation. *Circulation* 1992; **85**:1433–1439.
41. Hirsch, R., Huddleston, C. V., Mednedloff, E. N. *et al.* Infant and donor organ growth after heart transplantation in neonates with hypoplastic left heart syndrome. *J. Heart Lung Transpl.* 1996; **15**:1093–1100.
42. Sweet, S. C. Pediatric lung transplantation: update 2003. *Pediatr. Clin. N. Am.* 2003; **50**:1393–1417.
43. Nixon, P. A., Fricker, F. J., Noyes, B. E. *et al.* Exercise testing in pediatric heart, heart–lung and lung recipients. *Chest* 1995; **107**:1328.

Part VIII

Trauma

68

Introduction, scoring, and trauma management systems

Peter F. Ehrlich

University of Michigan Department of Pediatric Surgery, C.S. Mott Children's Hospital, Ann Arbor, MI, USA

Introduction

Trauma is the leading cause of morbidity and mortality in children under the age of 19 year.[1] In the United States approximately 10 million non-fatal injuries occur each year with 500 000 hospital admissions due to injury. It is estimated that there are 21 000 deaths a year with 50 000 permanent injuries. While absolute numbers may be different, the enormity of unintentional injury in North America and Europe is very similar. The predominant mechanism of injury is blunt, with motor vehicle crashes accounting for over 50% of all etiologies.[1,2] One of the most eloquent reports that underscores the burden that injury has on society was published by Trunkey in 1983. In this article he highlights the magnitude of injury as compared to cancer and heart disease, the importance for research, prevention and surgical care of the injured patient.[3]

The problem of injury has been recognized by the pediatric surgical community for many years. It would be ideal to have all injured children treated at specific children's hospitals with verified and designated trauma programs and to have effective trauma systems in each reagion.; however, the reality is that only 2%–3% of pediatric injuries are treated in this fashion in North America.[4] In conjunction with the adult trauma community, efforts have been undertaken to improve care of injured children through understanding patterns and severity of injuries (trauma scoring systems) and by promoting regionalization of care through pediatric trauma systems. The focus of this chapter is twofold: first to review the strengths and weaknesses of pediatric trauma scoring measures used to evaluate outcomes in trauma care; second to describe and evaluate what impact regionalization, verification and designation of trauma systems has on injury-related morbidity and mortality in children.

Trauma scoring systems

Introduction

Trauma scoring systems form an integral component of the trauma care structure. Many scoring systems have been described in the literature and understanding the differences between each can be confusing. To further complicate matters, most trauma scoring systems for pediatric care are derived from adult data. Some of the most commonly utilized scoring systems will be discussed.

Trauma scoring systems serve two specific functions. The first is to help determine where best an injured patient should be treated. These scores help "triage" the injured child and therefore help determine the risk of requiring a trauma center to care for the injury. The best known and most widely used is the Glasgow Coma Scale. The second quantifies the "severity of the illness" (SOI) or the risk of mortality or severity of injuries. These are typically determined retrospectively and serve as markers for quality assurance, benchmarking and research; particularly for health services and outcome studies. Triage scores can also form a component of a severity of injury tool. For example, the Glasgow Coma Scale is used both as a triage tool and in outcome models. Scoring systems use a variety of variables to construct their models. These include the diagnosis (International Classification of Diseases (ICD-9-CM)), demographic, anatomic, physiologic and laboratory

Pediatric Surgery and Urology: Long-term Outcomes, Mark Stringer, Keith Oldham, Pierre Mouriquand.

Table 68.1. Glasgow Coma Scale adult and pediatric variables[7]

Best Response	Adult GCS	Pediatric GCS	Score
Eye	No eye opening	No eye opening	1
	Eye opening to pain	Eye opening to pain	2
	Opening to verbal command	Eye opening to speech	3
	Open spontaneously	Open spontaneously	4
Verbal	No verbal response	No vocal response	1
	Incomprehensible	Inconsolable, agitated	2
	Inappropriate	Inconsistently consolable, moaning	3
	Confused conversation	Cries but is consolable, inappropriate interactions	4
	Orientated	Smiles, orientated to sounds, follows objects, interacts	5
Motor	No motor response	No motor response	1
	Extension to pain	Extension to pain	2
	Flexion to pain	Flexion to pain	3
	Withdrawal from pain	Withdrawal from pain	4
	Localizing pain	Localizing pain	5
	Obeys commands	Obeys commands	6

variables. Triage scoring systems tend to have few data points to assess, are simple to use and fast – thus they are designed to help make quick decisions. Alternatively the SOI scoring systems have many variables and are more cumbersome and are frequently computer generated.

Methodology

A detailed statistical summary of the theorems behind each scoring system is beyond the scope of this chapter; however, an excellent review can be found in a recent article by Marcin and Pollack.[5] Nevertheless certain common principles deserve attention. Scoring systems must be valid and reliable. Valid scoring systems must reflect a clinical problem and reflect the outcome you want to measure. For example as the score changes, so should the risk of a good or poor outcome. Reliability is a measure of consistency between observations both intra- and interobserver. Therefore a scoring system which can only be utilized by a few highly experienced health care professionals is less reliable and has decreased utility. The relative weights of various components are typically derived from logistic regression models depending on whether a variable is continuous, dichotomous or categorical. Understanding the sensitivity, specificity, positive and negative predictive values of scoring systems are also essential for effective use of each tool. For example. it is important to know the risk of a triage score either under or over predicting the need for specialized care. These measures are usually determined through evaluation from independent databases and investigators.

Triage scores: where best is the injured child treated?

An ideal triage scoring system would have: few data points, be easy to apply, have limited subjective assessments, have a high sensitivity and specificity. Unfortunately no triage score accomplishes all of these tasks. Each measure does have strengths and limitations. For example, studies have shown that assessments made in the field by paramedics are less accurate and reliable for pediatric trauma patients as compared to adults.[6] Alternatively, comparisons between adult and pediatric trauma triage scores have not shown that a pediatric specific trauma score provides a significant advantage over the original adult measure. Finally, it should be noted that trauma scores themselves should only be part of the triage assessment of the injured child, not the only factor in the decision process.

Glasgow Coma Scale

In 1974 Teasdale and Jennett first introduced the Glasgow Coma Scale. Since then it has become the most widely used triage tool for measuring unconsciousness and for triaging trauma patients.[7] A lower score reflects a lower level of consciousness and therefore for an injured patient a potentially a more serious head injury. Scores can range from 3 to a maximum of 15 (normal). The GCS measures three specific components of consciousness (eye movement, verbal and motor responses) with scores given to the best response. A GCS of 13–14 is considered a mild head injury, 9–12 moderate and 8 or lower is a severe insult. Adaptations to the GCS for the pediatric population have occurred and a "Pediatric Glasgow Coma Scale" is widely utilized (Table 68.1).

Studies examining the reliability and variability of the GCS demonstrate that the GCS is more variable in the intubated, very young non-verbal children.[8] GCS scores determined in the field are less predictive of outcome than those generated at a hospital.[9] When each individual

Table 68.2. Revised trauma score [12]

Clinical	Parameter	Score
Respiratory rate	10–24	4
	25–24	3
	>35	2
	<10	1
	0	0
Systolic blood pressure	>90	4
	70–89	3
	50–69	2
	<50	1
	0	0
Glasgow Coma Scale	14–15	4
	11–13	3
	8–10	2
	5–7	1
	3–4	0

component of the GCS is evaluated, the motor component is the strongest predictor of outcome.

Revised Trauma Score

The revised trauma score (RTS) is a physiologic based triage score (Table 68.2). The RTS was derived from two earlier versions of a triage scores, the Triage Index and Trauma Score.[10–12] There are three variables- respiratory rate, systolic blood pressure and GCS. The RTS is the sum of each multiplied by a weighted coefficient.

$$\text{RTS} = 0.9368(\text{GCS}) + 0.7326\ (\text{SBP}) + 0.22908(\text{RR value})$$

[GCS = Glasgow Coma Scale; SBP = systolic blood pressure; RR = respiratory rate]

These variables were determined to correlate statistically with survival/mortality. A higher RTS is associated with a better chance of survival. An injured patient with a RTS score of 11 or less is recommended to be treated at a designated trauma center. Eichelberger established and developed pediatric coefficients for the RTS and compared it to, and validated it in, the pediatric population.[13] The RTS is also recommended as one of the triage tools in the American College of Surgeons trauma guidelines "Resources for the Optimal Care of the Injured Patient".[14]

Prehospital Index

The Prehospital Index was proposed as a triage score in 1986 and validated prospectively in 1987.[15,16] It has five components: four physiologic variables (systolic blood pressure, pulse, respirations, and consciousness) and one mechanism score (penetrating chest or abdominal injury). Scores range from 0 to 24 with a low score reflecting a less severe injury. Scores greater then 3 are thought to require a designated trauma center for care. The Prehospital Index is cumbersome and offers no distinct advantage over other scoring systems and therefore is not widely utilized.

Table 68.3. Pediatric trauma score[18]

Clinical	Parameter	Score
Weight (kg)	>20	2
	10–19	1
	<10	−1
Airway	Normal	2
	Maintainable	1
	Unmaintainable	−1
Systolic blood pressure	>90	2
	50–89	1
	<50	−1
Central nervous system	Awake	2
	Obtunded or loss of consciousness	1
	Coma or decerebrate	−1
Open wound	None	2
	Minor	1
	Major or penetrating	−1
Skeletal	None	2
	Closed fracture	1
	Open or multiple fractures	−1

Triage trauma rule

This is the simplest of all the scoring elements.[17] No calculations are required and only three elements are needed (systolic blood pressure less then 85, GCS motor response less then 5 and potential penetrating injury to head or trunk). The simplicity of this score is very attractive. In retrospective analysis using the Oregon Trauma system entry criteria, however, the sensitivity and specificity were low with a significant number of "under-triaged" patients, thus limiting its utility.

Alert, Verbal Painful Unresponsive (APVU)

This is a simple scale that assigns a patient's condition as: Alert, Verbal, Painful or Unresponsive. No numerical scores are given but an injured child with a P or U should be taken to the designated trauma center. Subjective interpretation is inherent in this score and it is best used as a component of the triage process, especially for children where the age and development of the child will impact the response. There is a significant risk of under triaging patients utilizing this score.

Pediatric trauma score (PTS)

The pediatric trauma score was first introduced in the literature by Tepas in 1987.[18,19] Its design was thought to be more reflective of pediatric injuries (Table 68.3). There

Table 68.4. Age-specific pediatric trauma score.[21] Age-specific variables are stratified by degree of severity and coded values (0–3) are assigned to each variable. The integer scores are then summed (maximum score is 12)

GCS	SBP	Pulse	RR	Score
1–15	Normal	Normal	Normal	3
1–13	Mild to moderate hypotension (SBP<−2SD)	Tachycardia (pulse>mean + SD)	Tachypnea (RR>mean + SD)	2
4–9	Severe hypotension (SBP<−3SD)	Bradycardia (pulse>mean − SD)	Hypoventilation (RR<mean −SD)	1
3	0	0	0 or intubated	0

SBP, systolic blood pressure; RR, respiratory rate.

are six variables comprising both physiologic and injury attributes. A number score is totaled with a score of 8 or less considered a marker for children requiring care at a designated trauma center. A limitation of the PTS is that some variables are subjectively scored, particularly the CNS assessment and therefore there is a risk of inter- and intra-rater variability. Furthermore, the PTS has been compared to the RTS with surprisingly few apparent differences or inherent advantages.[18–20]

Age-specific PTS

The most recent proposed triage score is the age-specific PTS (Table 68.4).[21] First described by Potoka *et al.* in 2001, the main addition is the use of age-specific physiologic variables. To date, a single study suggests that it is better then traditional adult scores, therefore the clinical utility as a triage score remains to be defined. This is, however, a pediatric-specific tool which addresses areas where other adult scores become less accurate (extremes of age), but long-term data is lacking.

Severity of injury (SOI) and probability of survival scores (Ps)

In contrast to the triage scores, SOI or probability of survival scores are complex and include a wider variety of variables (e.g., diagnostic codes and demographic data) often incorporating all or some of the components of a triage score.

Abbreviated injury scale (AIS)

$$\text{AIS Score} = \sum(\text{AIS body region 1–9})$$

The abbreviated injury scale emerged from the automotive industry in 1969.[22,23] It was designed initially as an epidemiological tool to describe motor vehicle crashes but has been adapted to all types of trauma.[22,23] Revised and updated several times over the years the most recent version is the AIS-90 in 1998.[23] The score evaluates nine body regions. A scale from 1 to 6 is used to define injuries (1= minor; 2 moderate; 3 = serious; 4 = severe; 5 = critical; 6 = maximal). The underlying premise is the relationship of the injury as a threat to life. A body region with a score of six is considered a non-survivable injury. The scores are determined retrospectively based primarily on ICD-9 codes. There is a significant amount of expertise required to assign these ratings; therefore inter- and intrarater variability is a problem. To help limit this phenomenon, software has been developed to convert the ICD 9 codes directly to an AIS score. Nevertheless ICD 9 coding is inherently variable.[24,25]

Injury severity score

$$\text{ISS} = (\text{AIS body region 1})^2 + (\text{AIS body region 2})^2 + (\text{AIS body region 3})^2$$

The ISS is one of the most widely utilized scoring systems in the trauma literature. It correlates well with several important trauma outcomes such as mortality and duration of hospitalization. Developed in 1974, the ISS is a method of characterizing the multiplied injured trauma patient.[26,27] The ISS is based on the AIS body region framework. The ISS uses six anatomic regions: head, face, chest, abdomen, extremities or pelvic girdle, and external injuries. The ISS exponentially transforms the AIS to account for the relationship of the AIS score to the risk of mortality. The top three AIS scores are squared and added together to derive the ISS. Values range from 0 to 75, an AIS score of 6 automatically assigns a score of 75. Two modifications have been reported to the ISS score. The first, the modified ISS (MISS), was based on the AIS-80 to account for pediatric trauma patients and the fact that the head is injured more often than other body parts. The MISS uses GCS to replace the AIS for head region score and only evaluates four of the six AIS regions (face–neck, chest, abdomen: pelvis, pelvis–extremities). The three most severely injured regions are squared and added together. The second modification is the new ISS. Rather than using body regions, it sums and squares the three most severe injuries. However, evaluation of both the MISS and the new ISS has not shown advantages over the standard ISS. Therefore, in many centers and registries, AIS 90 still remains the standard severity of injury scoring system.

Survival probability-trauma score and injury severity score (TRISS)

TRISS is not a score but a method of predicting mortality. It was first proposed in the literature in 1987 and combines the physiologic variables in the RTS with the anatomic severity of injury scores generated by the ISS.[28] The final result is that P_s or probability of survival is generated.

$$P_s = 1 / (1 + e^{-b})$$

e = is the base of the natural log 2.72183

$b = b_o + b_1(RTS) + b_2(ISS) + b_3(\text{age factor})$

Age factor 0 for those less than 55 and 1 for greater

b_0, b_1, b_2, b_3 are blunt and penetrating trauma coefficients for adult[28] and pediatric populations.[13]

TRISS is the most widely used predictor of survival in the trauma literature. As with other statistical processes, limitations exist. These are specifically noted in patients over 54 years of age (extremes of age), and with trauma patients whose ISS is greater than 25. In fact, some authors suggest because of the TRISS deficiency that this method of calculating survival probabilities should be abandoned completely, particularly in urban centers.[29,30]

Application of the TRISS results (W and Z scores): A common application of the TRISS and P_s is to compare practice-based outcomes to population-based outcomes. Typically, this comparison is to a group of national norms that were identified in the Major Trauma Outcome Study.[31] The MTOS is a data set derived from 160 000 hospitalized patients at 139 centers between 1982 and 1989. Children comprised 11% of this population. From 80 544 adult patients in this data set, regression coefficients for predicting mortality were derived based on the revised trauma score and ISS (TRISS methodology). A single data set can be compared to the MTOS. A "Z score" is generated, whereby:

$$Z = (A - E)/S$$

A = actual outcomes

E = expected outcomes

$E = \sum Pi$

S is a scale factor that accounts for statistical variation

$S = \sqrt{\sum Pi(1-Pi)}$

Pi is the TRISS survival probability for ith patient. Z norms should be between 1.96 and –1.96. If the Z statistic is greater than 1.96, survival is better than the MTOS norms, and if it is less than –1.96, actual survival is less than MTOS norms.

A probability slope (PRE) is calculated using the RTS vs. ISS. A P_s50 slope can be calculated which represents a 0.50 probability of survival (based on MTOS data). Survivors above this line and deaths below this line represent statistically unexpected outcomes.

W scores

W is used when the Z score is found to be significant. W measures the statistical differences between the actual (A) and expected (E) survivors in a patient group. Sample size plays an important role in delineating the clinical significance of the difference between actual and expected number of survivors[32],

$$W = A = E/(N/100)$$

A and E are same as in the Z

N = number of children analyzed

W is the number of survivors, more or less, that would be expected per 100 children.

Both the W and Z scores are limited by the same factors that limit TRISS data.

A severity characterization of trauma (ASCOT)

ASCOT is an attempt to revise and fix the limitations found utilizing TRISS methodology (severely injured patients and extremes of age).[33] ASCOT incorporates a modification of AIS entitled "the Anatomic Profile" and uses individual components of the RTS (not totaled). Furthermore it excludes those patients with either very severe or nonserious injuries (maximum AIS < 2 and RTS > 0; AIS of 6 and RTS $= 0$). The Anatomic Profile categorizes the AIS scores $>$ 2 into three groups: head, brain spinal cord injuries; thorax or neck injuries; and all other serious injuries). A comparison of ASCOT vs. TRISS with a pediatric population did not provide more reliable or accurate scoring over the TRISS.

Pediatric age-adjusted TRISS

This is a recent tool used to describe mortality, which applies the pediatric specific age-adjusted PTS and may be a more promising predictor of mortality. However, at present, data are limited and it has not been validated by other investigators.[34]

The multitude of scoring systems reflect the reality that no one approach addresses all aspects of pediatric trauma accurately or provides the necessary tools to answer all research questions. Many suffer from inherent inaccuracies of coding (discharge diagnoses, ICD 9, death certificates). Physiologic variables generally seem to outperform anatomic variables in these systems, but experience is required to code these. Finally, certain elements of the

Table 68.5. American College of Surgeons: criteria for trauma system development[14]

1. State authority to designate, certify, identify or categorize trauma center
2. Existence of a formal process to designate or otherwise identify trauma centers
3. Use of the ACS standards to designate/identify trauma centers
4. Inclusion of onsite verification during the designation /identification process and use of out of area surveyors
5. Authority to limit the number of trauma centers based on the need for trauma services
6. Existence of a process for monitoring trauma center performance
7. Statewide coverage of a trauma system

laboratory data have been shown to be a strong predictor of mortality, yet these variables are not included in the prediction models.

Pediatric trauma systems

Historical development

In North America, widespread efforts to improve trauma care began in the 1960s and 1970s.[3,35–37] Pediatric trauma systems did not develop in isolation but in concert with adult care. Trauma care was advanced with the military experiences of treating injured soldiers in both the Korean and Vietnam wars. In addition, a report by Howard *et al.* highlighted the enormity of the injury problem and stressed its significance as a neglected public health problem.[38] Furthermore a series of "preventable death studies" were published which provided fodder for community and political support of coordinated care for injured patients. Funding for emergency medical services first became available in 1966 with the National Highway Safety Act and further support followed with the Emergency Medical Services System Act in 1973.[37] However at present, funding for trauma care still lags far behind other medical diseases. In 1968 Cook County Hospital in Chicago (adult) and Kings County Hospital in Brooklyn (pediatric) were recognized as the first specialized centers for civilian trauma care in the United States. In 1969, the University of Maryland and the Maryland State police developed a coordinated transport system for injured patients, to preferentially take them to a hospital with specific interest in caring for injured patients.[39,40] Illinois is credited as the first state to develop a comprehensive statewide trauma system including categorization of trauma hospitals, establishment of a communication system and a trauma registry.[41] In 1984 the Department of Health and Human Services in conjunction with the National Highway Traffic Safety Administration began the Emergency Medical Services for Children Program in the US. This funding has been a critical resource for developing programs and research to improve systems for emergency services for children.

A great effort to improve trauma care in North America has been the programs developed through the American College of Surgeons Committee on Trauma (ACSCOT). This has been accomplished through publication of standards for trauma systems, educational courses for healthcare professionals and verification programs to ensure published standards are met. In 1976, the first version of the *Optimal Resources for Care of Seriously Injured* was released.[14] This publication described criteria for levels of trauma centers (I–III), resource requirements for pre-hospital care through discharge, as well as specific pediatric needs. It remains a dynamic and important document. Eight criteria for trauma system development were defined and have become accepted benchmarks for trauma care (Table 68.5). The fourth version of this publication is currently in use and has been re-titled *Resources for the Optimal Care of Injured Patient*. In 1986 the ACSCOT established its consultation and verification program to ensure that these standards are being met. At present in North America there are 150 verified level I centers with 13–15 being pediatric level I centers. As of 2000, 43 states in the US had some regional or local trauma system, 23 states had complete state coverage, but only 5 met all criteria published by the ACSCOT.[42]

Another valuable contribution by the ACSCOT is the Advanced Trauma Life Support Course (ATLS). First released in 1979, it is now taught all over the world (most recently in China).[43] The first pediatric chapter was introduced in 1983. Although initially designed for surgeons, a wide variety of healthcare professionals involved in trauma care participate today. The ATLS course provides a common language, framework and approach to injured patients that allows for health care professionals to communicate with each other to optimize and prioritize care. Regular recertification is mandated to keep physicians current with new advances in trauma management. Similar to other ACSCOT programs the ATLS course is constantly evolving with the seventh edition to be released shortly.

Components of trauma systems

Death due to injury classically happens in one of three distinct time frames. The first peak occurs at the time of injury, the second within the first few hours after trauma, and the third peak late due to complications from the injuries sustained at the time of impact. Almost 70% of all deaths occur at the time of injury. As trauma systems approach injured patients, recognition of these patterns is necessary. Thus a trauma system is not simply an isolated hospital that cares for injured patients, but a broad coalition of participants that includes an integrated approach to trauma, including prevention, prehospital care, and hospital care through to rehabilitation.[44,45]

A primary step in developing an effective trauma system is a needs assessment of the community that it serves. For example, rural trauma systems are different from urban settings. They each have different mortality rates, injury patterns, geography, available resources and expertise.[46,47] Community responsibility and involvement (particularly with injury prevention) are essential for political support and funding. Studies support the concept that community injury prevention programs play a substantial role in reducing morbidity and mortality.[48,49]

A second important consideration in developing a regional trauma system is to understand that all facilities have a role in treating injured patients. A tiered (e.g., Level I–IV) approach with hospitals designated to care for various complexity of injured patients is essential. Level I hospitals are tertiary/quaternary centers with level II and III centers having fewer capabilities and resources. Level IV hospitals are distinct because of their remote nature (rural trauma). A list of recommendations for what is required for each level of care can be found in the ACSCOT publication *Resources for the Optimal Care of the Injured Patient*: 1999.[14] A requirement within this tiered system is a central communication (central command) structure and a well-developed triage system so that the most severely injured patients go first to the appropriately designated hospital. In addition, a trauma registry system is essential for outcomes analysis and quality assurance programs.

A third point is that a trauma system is not an isolated surgical program but a multidisciplinary team of physicians, nurses, technicians and allied health professions. A large trauma program will use a significant percentage of hospital resources for everything from the blood bank to social work. Regular meetings of all stakeholders are needed to problem solve and respond to changing injury patterns and community needs.

Trauma system effectiveness

The cost, administration and clinical effort to maintain a state, regional or hospital trauma system is substantial. Research efforts have examined how and if a trauma system make a difference. In 1998 a conference (Skamania, Washington) focusing just on trauma system effectiveness was held to examine the published data on these questions. A comprehensive review was published in the *Journal of Trauma*.[50] The primary end point in most studies was a reduction in mortality. Three levels of data were reviewed; these included panel reviews, institutional or practice-based studies and population-based studies. Several considerations must be remembered when reviewing these studies. First, there has been a natural reduction in hospital mortality in many medical disorders, including trauma. In addition, results are influenced by how many patients with minor injuries are included in the evaluation.

Practiced-based and population-based studies

Practiced-based studies are registry-based reviews and frequently compare institutional results to the Major Trauma Outcome Study (MTOS) data. The MTOS data set is described in a previous section. Jurkovich did a systematic review of published literature assessing trauma systems effectiveness by using registry-based data.[51] Eight of 11 articles reviewed provided comparable data and consistently demonstrated a 15 to 20% reduction in the risk of death for similar patients in centers that were part of a trauma system when compared to MTOS norms. The limitations of the MTOS study were described earlier. Trauma registries would be strengthened by including both prehospital and postdischarge trauma deaths, standardizing trauma registry inclusion criteria and developing national reference norms for trauma outcomes.

Evaluating mortality through practice-based/registry studies provides only an institutional perspective on outcomes. No insight into the overall mortality of a region served by the trauma system can be inferred. In addition, for level 1 centers, mortality may actually increase or remain unchanged after institution of a regional trauma system. This may be a result of several factors, notably the volume of patients with higher ISS and therefore lower probability of survival may come to the center as a consequence of improved triage.

Population-based studies tend to provide a larger or regional prospective. Population-based studies also provide insight into how a trauma system alters the patterns of care for injured children. Nathens *et al.* compared regions with trauma center to those without, based on 1995 mortality data.[49] In this study of 22 states with trauma systems there was a 9% lower crude injury mortality rate than for those without. When MVC-related mortality was evaluated separately, there were 17% fewer deaths. After controlling for age, state speed laws, restraint laws, and population distribution, there remained a 9% reduction in MVC-related mortality rate in states with a trauma system. Rural states had higher mortality rates as did those states with higher speed limits. Those who benefited the most from regional coordination of care were children 14 years old and younger. A second study focused solely on motor vehicle crashes using a cross-sectional time-series analysis of crash mortality data from 1979 to 1995.[52] Ten years following trauma system implementation, mortality due to traffic crashes began to decline; about 15 years following trauma system implementation, mortality was reduced by 8% (95% confidence interval [CI], 3%–12%) after adjusting for trends in crash mortality, age, and the introduction of traffic safety laws. Implementation of primary enforcement of restraint laws and laws deterring driving while intoxicated resulted in reductions in crash mortality of 13% and 5%. The impact of trauma systems development however is not immediate, as mortaility reduction became significant after 10 years of development. This finding is consistent with the maturation of trauma triage protocols, interhospital transfer agreements, organization of trauma centers and quality assurance efforts.

In addition to altering mortality rates, trauma systems appear to alter the pattern of death in a region.[48] In 1987, Oregon implemented a statewide pediatric trauma system that was fully functioning by the early 1990s. Hulka *et al.* evaluated pediatric trauma in Oregon (30 of 36 counties are rural) to determine the influence of a state wide trauma system on pediatric hospitalization and outcome.[48] Prior to development of regional trauma networks the factors associated with pediatric traumatic death in Oregon included younger age, and severe head, chest and abdominal injuries; thus the small, more severely injured child was at greater risk. Following implementation of the regional networks these risk factors changed to include only severe head injuries. This is the same major risk factor as is found in urban centers.

A study from Rogers demonstrated excellent trauma outcomes without a formal trauma system.[53] In this specific instance, prior educational efforts and collaborative efforts by a primary center may have yielded a de facto system, although not formally designated or verified. Many of the important elements recommended by the American College of Surgeons were in fact functioning.

After development of a trauma system and center, patient volumes generally increase.[45] Studies have looked at whether increased volumes produce better outcomes.[54,55] Cooper was unable to document an inverse relationship between hospital volume and inpatient mortality rate for trauma centers in New York State and concluded that volume criteria should not be considered as an indicator of the quality of trauma care.[54] In a study by Nathens, trauma mortality in high volume centers was only lower in a subset of seriously injured patients (penetrating abdominal trauma in shock and coma).[55] This data has not been replicated in pediatric studies. What does appear to be important is that centers which meet prespecified standards tend to have better outcomes. Osler showed that ACS-verified pediatric centers have significantly higher survival rates than do unverified pediatric centers.[56] Potoka demonstrated that centers with certification for care of children had better pediatric outcomes than those with verification only as an adult trauma center.[57] Survival for head, spleen, and liver injuries was significantly better at Level 1 pediatric trauma centers compared with adult trauma centers with added qualification for children. In addition, children who sustained moderate or severe head injuries were more likely to undergo neurosurgical intervention and have a better outcome when treated at a pediatric trauma center. Severely injured children (Injury Severity Score > 15) with head, spleen, or liver injuries had the best overall outcome when treated at pediatric trauma centers. These differences in outcome may be attributable to the approach to operative and non-operative management of head, liver, and spleen injuries.[57]

Mortality is an important clinical end point. However the development of a regional trauma system (regional and within a hospital) provides results and benefits in other areas as well. Richardson *et al.* examined the effect of trauma center verification in a rural center and its role within a regional trauma network.[58] Their study concluded that regional trauma networks enhance appropriate transfer patterns for patients requiring higher levels of care. Therefore, if a regional trauma system is effective, the most seriously injured patients should be transferred to the center with the best ability to give definitive care. If this does not occur, the care that children receive at a non-trauma center may be suboptimal. Ehrlich *et al.* reported on the impact that American College of Surgeons (ACS) verification had on a developing trauma center.[44,45] The end points were changes in clinical standards and these were monitored through monthly performance improvement audits. Both qualitative and quantitative changes occurred in clinical indicators that reflect trauma care competencies from prehospital through to discharge. Consequently, performance improvement audits can generate quantitative data indicating the percentage of patients who meet specific criteria. Specifically, emergency department trauma patient evaluation (including radiology) and disposition out of the emergency department (<120 minutes) was markedly reduced in this study. Enhanced nursing documentation correlated with improved clinical care. Examples included early acquisition of head CAT scans in neurological injured patients; intensive care unit and overall hospital length of stay decreased; increase in institutional morale with recognition of trauma excellence within the hospital; resurgence of the trauma research programs (60 IRB approved projects); and increased funds to the trauma program for capital expenditures. However, there are other approaches in addition to the ACS program that improve trauma care. For example, in a study by Simons *et al.* from British Columbia, Canada, similar quantitative and qualitative improvements in trauma care delivery were noted after developing a trauma center program.[59]

Summary

How does our present understanding of long-term outcomes with trauma influence contemporary practice?

The major learning point derived from examination of long-term outcomes of pediatric trauma care is recognition that injury is best treated within a coordinated system. This is particularly important for rural regions. All team members including areas of injury prevention, prehospital care through to rehabilitation have vital roles. Trauma is a multisystem disease and must be treated as such. This approach combined with public injury prevention policies has reduced mortality by 10%–15% in Western countries. Regional centers which are designated and verified have significantly better outcomes for treating injured children than those who do not maintain that status. The ATLS training program and ACS standards provide one framework and should be considered as a basis for any regional trauma system. Finally, the continued observation that the majority of children who die following injury do so at the scene, points out the need for effective injury prevention programs to further reduce the pediatric disease burden from injury.

What are the current controversies in light of long-term outcomes?

A major area of controversy for pediatric trauma systems will be the roles of prehospital intervention and the involved prehospital personnel. Two different philosophies currently govern development of prehospital care systems. The first is characterized by a "stay and stabilize" approach using advanced life support (ALS) techniques at the scene. The second is the "scoop and run" or basic life support approach in which rapid transport and minimal field care is provided.

The former model is best demonstrated by the system of trauma care system in Germany. Trauma care in Germany is the most comprehensive and advanced in Europe. A ground system of physician-staffed ambulances is supported by a network of physician-staffed air service all over Germany.[60] The air group system is centrally coordinated. German studies have supported the efficacy of physician response teams with advanced field intervention. Schmidt compared trauma patients with equivalent ISS patients transported by helicopter in Germany vs. the United States. In Germany, patients were treated by a trauma surgeon and paramedic in the field, in the United Stated they were not. The German patients had more advanced interventions and a decrease in early mortality and better outcomes compared to the MTOS.[61] This study has not been replicated.

The rationale behind advanced field care is to stabilize an injured patient and prevent clinical deterioration until definitive care can be administered. These advanced interventions (e.g., intravenous placement, pneumatic antishock garments, endotracheal intubation, etc.) may increase the time at the scene and likely delay transfer to definitive care. Furthermore, very few of these interventions have been studied, and those that have been evaluated have shown no benefit to patient survival. In fact, in some instances morbidity and mortality may be increased.[62–66]

Recently, Liberman *et al.* examined the issue of advanced interventions ("scoop and run" vs. "stay and stabilize") in the prehospital environment in a 5-year observational study from three different cities.[65] In one city, BLS support personnel provided prehospital care only, in another this was done by providers trained in ALS, and in a third by ALS-physicians. The mortality rates across multiple variables (i.e., major but survivable trauma) were highest in the ALS physician group and lowest in the BLS providers. The authors concluded that in "urban centers with Level 1 trauma centers, there was no benefit in having on-site ALS for the prehospital management of trauma patients."

A pediatric specific issue is airway control in the field, specifically comparing prehospital endotracheal intubation (ETI) to prehospital bag valve masking (BVM). Airway control is a primary tenet of trauma care and proper ETI is recognized as a definitive method to achieve airway control. However, endotracheal intubation in children can be a difficult skill to acquire and maintain in comparison to BVM. Gausche *et al.*, in conjunction with the US Department of Health and Human Services, conducted a prospective randomized controlled trial comparing ETI to BVM in Los Angeles 1994–1997.[64] This study had an educational arm for prehospital providers as well as a randomized treatment component. It took 2 years and 614 six-hour courses to train the prehospital providers. The results of this urban-based study found no difference in survival or neurological outcomes between the groups whose airway was managed by BVM compared to ETI. ETI was associated with a higher complication rate. Examination of a small subset of the patients in the Gausche report suggested that ETI did help children who had sustained severe head injuries, but not at a statistically significant level. Cooper *et al.*, using a larger data set from the National Pediatric Trauma Registry, retrospectively examined survival of severely head-injured children who were managed initially by BVM or ETI.[62] In this registry-based study, no survival advantage or disadvantage was noted between the BVM group and the ETI group. Another large series demonstrated that over 90% of children could be adequately ventilated by BVM and multiple attempts at ETI were associated with significant complications.[46]

Conclusions

Trauma care is a continuum from injury prevention, prehospital, hospital and rehabilitation care. The integration of a multisystem approach to the injured child has and continues be an important element to reduce morbidity and mortality form injury. Trauma scoring systems help triage patients based on injury characteristics to ensure that the most seriously injury child is treated at the facility that has the best capabilities. Severity of injury scores allow for benchmarking and health services research. Finally evidence supports that injured children strongly benefit from the advent of regional trauma systems and verifications programs.

REFERENCES

1. Baker, S. P., O'Neil, B., Ginburg, M. J., & Li, G. *The Injury Fact Book*. 2nd edn. New York: Oxford University Press Inc, 1992.
2. Department of Rehabiliatation Medicine. *Biannual Report of the National Pediatric Trauma Registry*. Department of Rehabiliatation Medicine, ed. Tufts University/ New England Medical Center, 1995.
3. Trunkey, D. D. Trauma. *Sci. Am.* 1983; **249**:28–45.
4. Knudson, M. M., Shagoury, C., & Lewis, F. R. Can adult trauma surgeons care for injured children. *J. Trauma* 1992; **32**:130–137.
5. Marcin, J. P. & Pollack, M. M. Triage scoring systems, severity of illness measures, and mortality prediction models in pediatric trauma. *Crit. Care. Med.* 2002; **30**[11(suppl.)]:S457–S467.
6. Engum, S. A., Mitchell, M. K., Scherer, L. R. *et al.* Prehospital triage in the injured pediatric patient. *J. Pediatr. Surg.* 2000; **35**:82–87.
7. Teasdale, G. & Jennett, B. Assessment of coma and impaired consciousness: a practical scale. *Lancet* 1974; **2**:81–84.
8. Ross, S. E., Leipold, L. S., & Terregino, C. Efficacy of the motor component of the Glasgow Coma Scale in trauma triage. *J. Trauma* 1998: **45**;42–44.
9. Meredith, W., Rutledge, R., Hansen, A. R. *et al.* Field triage of trauma patients based upon the ability to follow commands: a study in 29,573 injured patients. *J. Trauma* 1995; **38**[1]:129–135.
10. Champion, H. R., Sacco, W. J., & Hannan, D. S. Assessment of injury severity: the triage index. *Crit. Care Med.* 1980; **8**:201–208.
11. Champion, H. R., Sacco, W. J., & Carnazzo, A. J. The trauma score. *Crit. Care Med.* 1981; **9**:623–629.
12. Champion, H. R., Sacco, W. J., Copes, W. S. *et al.* A revision of the Trauma Score. *J. Trauma* 1989; **29**:623–629.
13. Eichelberger, M. R., Champion, H. R., Sacco, W. J. *et al.* Pediatric coefficients for TRISS analysis. *J. Trauma* 1993; **34**:319–322.
14. Committee on Trauma. American College of Surgeons. *Resources for Optimal Care of the Injured Patient*: 3rd edn., 1999.
15. Koehler, J. J., Baer, L. J., Malafa, S. A. *et al.* Prehospital Index: a scoring system for field triage of trauma victims. *Ann. Emerg. Med.* 1986; **15**:178–182.
16. Koehler, J. J., Malafa, S. A., Hillesland, J. *et al.* A multicenter validation of the prehospital index. *Ann. Emerg. Med.* 1987; **16**:380–385.
17. Baxt, W. G., Jones, G., & Fortlage, D. The trauma triage rule: a new, resource-based approach to the prehospital identification of major trauma victims. *Ann. Emerg. Med.* 1990; **19**:1401–1406.
18. Tepas, J. J. 3rd, Mollitt, D. L., Talbert, J. L., & Bryant, M. The pediatric trauma score as a predictor of injury severity in the injured child. *J. Pediatr. Surg.* 1987; **22**:14–18.
19. Tepas, J. J. 3rd, Ramenofsky, M. L., Mollitt, D. L. *et al.* The Pediatric Trauma Score as a predictor of injury severity: an objective assessment. *J. Trauma* 1988; **28**:425–429.
20. Nayduch, D. A., Moylan, J., Rutledge, R. *et al.* Comparison of the ability of adult and pediatric trauma scores to predict pediatric outcome following major trauma. *J. Trauma* 1991; **31**:452–457.
21. Potoka, D. A., Schall, L. C., & Ford, H. R. Development of a novel age-specific pediatric trauma score. *J. Pediatr. Surg.* 2001; **36**:106–112.
22. Rating the severity of tissue damage. I. The abbreviated scale. *J. Am. Med. Assoc.* 1971; **215**:277–280.
23. Association for the Advancement of Automotive Medicine. *The Abbreviated Injury Scale*, 1990.
24. MacKenzie, E. J., Shapiro, S., & Eastham, J. N. Jr. The Abbreviated Injury Scale and Injury Severity Score. Levels of inter- and intrarater reliability. *Med. Care* 1985; **23**:823–835.
25. MacKenzie, E. J., Steinwachs, D. M., & Shankar, B. Classifying trauma severity based on hospital discharge diagnoses. Validation of an ICD-9CM to AIS-85 conversion table. *Med. Care* 1989; **27**:412–422.
26. Baker, S. P., O'Neill, B., Haddon, W. Jr. *et al.* The injury severity score: a method for describing patients with multiple injuries and evaluating emergency care. *J. Trauma* 1974; **14**:187–196.
27. Baker, S. P. & O'Neill, B. The injury severity score: an update. *J. Trauma* 1976; **16**:882–885.
28. Boyd, C. R., Tolson, M. A., & Copes, W. S. Evaluating trauma care: the TRISS method. Trauma Score and the Injury Severity Score. *J. Trauma* 1987; **27**:370–378.
29. Cayten, C. G., Stahl, W. M., Murphy, J. G. *et al.* Limitations of the TRISS method for interhospital comparisons: a multihospital study. *J. Trauma* 1991; **31**:471–481.
30. Demetriades, D., Chan, L. S., Velmahos, G. *et al.* TRISS methodology in trauma: the need for alternative. *Br. J. Surg.* 1998; **85**:379–384.

31. Champion, H. R., Copes, W. S., Sacco, W. J. *et al.* The Major Trauma Outcome Study: establishing national norms for trauma care. *J. Trauma* 1990; **30**:1356–1365.
32. Taylor, M. S., Sacco, W. J., & Champion, H. R. On the power of a method for comparing survival of trauma patients to a standard survival curve. *Com. Bio. Med.* 1986; **16**:1–6.
33. Champion, H. R., Copes, W. S., Sacco, W. J. *et al.* A new characterization of injury severity. *J. Trauma* 1990; **30**:539–545.
34. Schall, L. C., Potoka, D. A., & Ford, H. R. A new method for estimating probability of survival in pediatric patients using revised TRISS methodology based on age-adjusted weights. *J. Trauma* 2002; **52**:235–241.
35. Morrison, W., Wright, J. L., & Paidas, C. N. Pediatric trauma systems. *Crit. Care Med.* 2002; **30**(11 (suppl.)):S448–S456.
36. Haller, J. A. Life-threatening injuries in children: what have we learned and what are the challenges? *Bull. Am. Coll. Surg.* 1995; **80**:8–18.
37. Mullins, R. J. A historical perspective of trauma system development in the United States. *J. Trauma* 1999; **47**[3 suppl]:S8–S14.
38. Howard, J. M. Accidental death and disability: the neglected disease of modern society. Washington DC, National Committee of Trauma and Committee of Shock National Academy of Sciences/National Research Council. 1966.
39. Cowley, R. A., Hudson, F., Scanlan, E. *et al.* An economical and proved helicopter program for transporting the emergency critically ill and injured patient in Maryland. *J. Trauma* 1973; **13**:1029–1038.
40. Cowley, R. A. & Scanlan, E. University trauma center: operation, design and staffing. *Am. Surg.* 1979; **45**:79–85.
41. Boyd, D. R., Dunea, M. M., & Flashner, B. A. The Illinois plan for a statewide system of trauma centers. *J. Trauma* 1973; **13**:24–31.
42. Bass, R. R., Gainer, P. S., & Carlini, A. R. Update on trauma system development in the United States. *J. Trauma* 1999; **47**[3 suppl]:S16–S21.
43. American College of Surgeons Committe on Trauma. *Advanced Life Support for Doctors.* Sixth edn. Chicago: American College of Surgeons, 1997.
44. Ehrlich, P. F., Ortega, J., & Mucha, P. Jr. The need for a statewide trauma system. *W. V. Med. J.* 2001; **98**:66–68.
45. Ehrlich, P. F., Rockwell, S., Mucha, P. Jr, & Kincaid, S. American College of Surgeons, Committee on Trauma Verification Review: does it really make a difference? *J. Trauma* 2002; **53**:811–816.
46. Ehrlich, P. F., Helmkamp, J. C., Seidman, P. A. *et al.* Endotracheal intubation in rural pediatric patients. *J. Pediatr. Surg.* 2004; **39**:1376–1380.
47. Rodgers, F. B., Shackford, S. R., Osler, T. M., Vane, D. W., & Davis, J. Rural trauma: the challenge for the next decade. *J. Trauma* 1999; **47**:802–818.
48. Hulka, F., Mullins, R. J., Mann, N. C. *et al.* Influence of a statewide trauma system on pediatric hospitalization and outcome. *J. Trauma* 1997; **42**:514–519.
49. Nathens, A. B., Jurkovich, G. J., Rivara, F. P., & Maier, R. V. Effectiveness of state trauma systems in reducing injury-related mortality: a national evaluation. *J. Trauma* 2000; **48**:25–30.
50. Mullins, R. J. & Mann, N. C. Introduction to the academic symposium to evaluate evidence regarding the efficacy of trauma systems. *J. Trauma* 1999; **47**[3 suppl]:S3–S7.
51. Jurkovich, G. J. & Mock, C. Systematic review of trauma system effectiveness based on registry comparisons. *J. Trauma* 1999; **47**[3 suppl]:S46–S55.
52. Nathens, A. B., Jurkovich, G. J., Cummings, P. *et al.* The effect of organized systems of trauma care on motor vehicle crash mortality. *J. Am. Med. Assoc.* 2000; **283**[15]:1990–1994.
53. Rodgers, F. B., Osler, T. M., Shackford, S. R., Martin, F., & Healey, M. Population-based study of hospital trauma care in a rural state without a formal trauma system. *J. Trauma* 2001; **50**:409–413.
54. Cooper, A., Hannan, E. L., Bessey, P. Q. *et al.* An examination of the volume–mortality relationship for New York State trauma centers. *J. Trauma* 2000; **48**:16–23.
55. Nathens, A. B., Jurkovich, G. J., Maier, R. V. *et al.* Relationship between trauma center volume and outcomes. *J. Am. Med. Assoc.* 2001; **285**:1164–1171.
56. Osler, T. M., Vane, D. W., Tepas, J. J. *et al.* Survival following trauma in children: do pediatric trauma centers have better survival rates. *J. Trauma* 2001; **50**:96–101.
57. Potoka, D. A., Schall, L. C., Gardner, M. J. *et al.* Impact of pediatric trauma centers on mortality in a statewide system. *J. Trauma* 2000; **49**:237–245.
58. Richardson, J. D., Cross, T., Lee, D., & Polk, H. C., Jr. Impact of Level III verification on trauma admissions and transfer: comparisons of two rural hospitals. *J. Trauma* 1997; **42**:498–503.
59. Simons, R., Eliopoulos, V., Laflamme, D., & Brown, D. R. Impact on process of trauma care delivery 1 year after the introduction of a trauma program in a provincial trauma center. *J. Trauma* 1999; **46**:811–815.
60. Westhoff, J., Hildebrand, F., Grotz, M. *et al.* Trauma care in Germany. *Injury* 2003; **34**:674–683.
61. Schmidt, U., Frame, S. B., Nerlich, M. L. *et al.* On-scene helicopter transport of patients with multiple injuries – comparison of a German and an American system. *J. Trauma* 1992; **33**:548–555.
62. Cooper, A., DiScala, C., Foltin, G., & Tunik, M. Prehospital endotracheal intubation for severe head injury in children; a reappraisal. *Semin. Pediatr. Surg.* 2001; **10**:3–6.
63. Demetriades, D., Chan, L., Cornwell, E., & Belzberg, H. Paramedic vs private transportation of trauma patients. Effect on outcome. *Arch. Surg.* 1996; **131**:133–138.
64. Gausche, M., Lewis, R. J., Stratton, S. J., & Haynes, B. E. Effect of out-of- hospital pediatric endotracheal intubation on survival and neurologic outcome. *J. Am. Med. Assoc.* 2000; **283**:783–790.
65. Liberman, M., Mulder, D., Lavoie, A., Denis, R. Multicenter Canadian study of prehospital trauma care. *Ann. Surg.* 2000; **237**:153–160.
66. Mattox, K. L., Pepe, P. E., Bickell, W. H., & Mangelsdorff, A. D. Prospective randomized evaluation of antishock MAST in post-traumatic hypotension. *J. Trauma* 1986; **26**:779–786.

69

Prognosis and recovery of pediatric head injury

P. David Adelson[1], Neil Buxton[2] and Richard Appleton[3]

[1]Department of Pediatric Neurosurgery, Children's Hospital of Pittsburgh and the University of Pittsburgh, Pittsburgh, Pennsylvania, USA
[2]Department of Paediatric Neurosurgery, Royal Liverpool Children's Hospital, Liverpool, UK
[3]The Roald Dahl EEG Unit, Department of Paediatric Neurology, Royal Liverpool Children's Hospital, Liverpool, UK

Introduction

Trauma remains a significant societal and public health problem in the world, especially in children. It is the leading cause of death and disability accounting for over 50% of the deaths in the pediatric population.[1,2] Head trauma occurs in the majority of these cases and is a major factor affecting both mortality and outcome.[3,4] There are frequent long-term cognitive, motor and behavioral dysfunctions in severely injured children,[5] even in those children who have suffered mild or moderate head injuries.[6] However, determining the prognosis and outcome following head injury in children has been difficult. Recently, much has been learned about how children respond acutely to traumatic brain injury but relatively little is known about the differences in long-term outcome and prognosis in the different age ranges and among individuals.

In reviewing the prognosis and recovery potential of children following brain injury, several aspects of childhood impact on the developing brain that are unique and which must be taken into consideration. It is critical to try and understand the effect that a brain injury has during the different stages of brain development. In addition, the degree of neuroplasticity from birth and early brain growth to the final mature adult brain will also alter the final prognosis. Lastly, the impact of an intervention may differ at different stages of maturation. By defining the different physiologic and secondary injury responses of children to different types of injury, the impact of that injury on recovery, and the capacity to regain or attain normal function, improved treatment (surgical, pharmacological and psychological) can then be designed and implemented to optimize the final functional outcome.

In this chapter, discussion will focus on the different mechanisms and types of injury seen in children, and their relationship to injury recovery, and the effects that age and development may have on the potential for recovery from traumatic brain injury.

Epidemiology and mechanisms of injury

In the United States there are approximately 100–200 000 new head injuries in children (up to 18 years old) each year, with an estimated population incidence of 193–367 /100,000.[2] Patients under the age of 20 years make up the majority of victims of traumatic brain injury.[7] In children, there are two peak periods of incidence, the first in early childhood (less than 5 years of age) and the second in mid-to-late adolescence (e.g., up to 15–16 years old).[7,8] Up to the age of 5 years, the incidence in males and females is equal but after the age of 5, there is a higher incidence of head injury amongst males, with a ratio of approximately 2–4:1.[3,6–10] Socioeconomic factors can also affect the rate of head injuries in all ages with the highest rate of injuries reported among the lower socioeconomic classes.[8,11] Ten to 15% of children hospitalized with head trauma each year will have suffered a severe head injury and of these, 1/3 to 1/2 will die. In addition, many of the children who survive their injury will manifest permanent deficits.[12]

The majority of fatal head injuries in adults are secondary to motor vehicle collisions.[13,14] Similar to adults, most children with fatal head trauma are injured in much the same way. Other non-fatal causes of head injury include: motor vehicle collisions, falls, bicycle injuries, pedestrian accidents, assault, and penetrating injuries with the majority being motor vehicle or motor vehicle-related injuries.[3] The

Pediatric Surgery and Urology: Long-term Outcomes, Mark Stringer, Keith Oldham, Pierre Mouriquand.
Published by Cambridge University Press.

proportion of motor vehicle and motor vehicle-related collisions increase with increasing age: 20% in the 0–4 year range but up to 66% in teenagers.[10] The injuries related to motor vehicles also account for the higher proportion of fatal injuries among all children. In one study, motor vehicle collisions due to pedestrian or cyclist injuries accounted for 50% of the injuries in children under the age of 14 years.[3]

Amongst infants, toddlers, and young children, the major causes of head trauma are pedestrian–motor vehicle accidents, cycle–motor vehicle accidents, falls, child abuse, and sports-related injuries with assaults and motor vehicle accidents representing the major causes of injury in infants and preschool children.[10] Falls and assaults resulted in approximately 20% of traumatic brain injuries in one study, but almost 2/3 were in the 0–4 year range.[10] Later in childhood, including adolescence, the leading causes of trauma become similar to adults and include motor vehicle accidents, sports, and recreational activities.[8]

Child abuse tends to predominate in very young children (less than 4 years of age) and may even be the major cause of severe brain injury in this group.[15] In babies and infants who are shaken vigorously, the injuries tend to be multiple and diffuse, differing from the single impact insults seen in motor vehicle or sports injuries. As a result, there may be differences in outcome, though this has not yet been studied in detail. Child abuse reporting together with mortality caused by child assault have increased over the past few years.[14] This recent rise in reported mortality is probably due to multiple reasons and may be both real and apparent. Physicians are much more aware of this mechanism of injury in young children, and as a result, they are better able to identify suspicious "falls" and report them to investigatory services. Previously, many reports noted fatalities due to falls from less than 3 feet.[16] It is now clear that fatality from falls from low heights or distances are rare and most likely reflect inaccurate reporting. Second, in many developed countries there are laws requiring reporting of suspected child abuse and, as a result, physicians who were previously uncomfortable in breaching the doctor–patient/family relationship and confidentiality, are now duty bound to report any concerns. This legal support of the child relieves the physician of responsibility of being the major factor in the legal decision making, and keeps the interaction on a patient–physician level. Finally, the hospital and its supportive services have become much more of an advocate for the child and, as a result, services are available to help families of abused children to counsel and treat rather than remove the child permanently from the home. In this way, further injury and possibly death can be avoided.

Mortality

The overall mortality related to head trauma in children is less than in adults.[3] There are multiple factors that contribute to overall mortality following traumatic brain injury, particularly in children. These include: mechanism of injury, the age of the child at time of injury, the severity of the injury, and the extent of the secondary injury.[3] The majority of deaths following severe head injury in children are caused by either the severity of the initial impact or the development of secondary complications that may be both cerebral and non-cerebral (e.g., respiratory) in nature.

Mechanisms of head injuries

As previously stated, mortality following head injury often depends on the primary mechanism of injury as well as the severity of that injury. Traumatic brain injuries can be grouped into different categories depending on the mechanism of injury including focal versus diffuse, closed vs. penetrating, and primary vs. secondary. Focal injuries such as an intracerebral contusion or hemorrhage, or a mass lesion such as a subdural or epidural hematoma are most often caused by a single impact in a linear vector and are much less common in children (20%) than in adults (40%).[4,10,17] Hematomas are more often due to falls in children and to motor vehicle accidents in adults.[10] Children more commonly exhibit a diffuse injury with generalized swelling and resultant intracranial hypertension.[4,18] The histopathologic findings of a diffuse, primary injury include: diffuse axonal injury or shearing, brain laceration, and vascular injury. These injuries can also result from linear deceleration injury but are most often caused by rotational acceleration/deceleration forces.

Closed head injuries usually arise from external forces applied to the head and neck which are transmitted to the skull and brain. The disruptive effect on tissue is caused either directly by the force of impact and transmittal of the energy to, and within susceptible structures (e.g., cortex, cortical veins entering the dural venous sinuses, etc.), or indirectly by hematoma formation and compression of the cerebral cortex. A penetrating injury results in a direct disruption of the brain parenchyma by a projectile (missile) or foreign object. This can cause either focal or diffuse injury depending on the amount of tissue or vasculature disrupted. The extent of injury is a function of the velocity and mass of the penetrating object and the transmitted kinetic energy. The amount of kinetic energy increases logarithmically the higher the velocity of a missile. Therefore, tissue damage from a high velocity impact may be much more diffuse than could simply be explained by the track of a bullet.

Focal, diffuse, closed head, and penetrating injuries are all considered primary mechanisms of injury and the damage occurs at the time of impact. Each of these primary mechanisms of injury can potentially elicit a secondary response from the brain as a reaction to that injury. The secondary response is a series of related biochemical and physiologic events within the brain which often leads to diffuse swelling and further tissue damage and neuronal loss. Aldrich *et al.*[19] reported a strong association between diffuse brain swelling and either hypoxia or early hypotension, and commented that these factors may play a particular role in the pathogenesis of diffuse swelling. Children may be more vulnerable to suffering a hypoxic or hypotensive episode following head trauma and as a result may be more likely develop diffuse brain swelling.

Vascular disruption due to the injury can cause ischemia and subsequent infarction that is independent from an intracranial mass lesion such as intracerebral hematoma. Mass effect or shift in a localized area may have diffuse effects, particularly if these lead to decreased perfusion of the basal structures or brainstem. Uncal herniation may lead to direct vascular and brainstem compression and death if not treated appropriately.

Secondary effects of the primary injury can also include loss of cerebral autoregulation, breakdown of the blood–brain barrier, diffuse brain swelling, intracellular and extracellular edema, diffuse and focal edema and ischemic brain injury.[20] Multiple factors are believed to contribute to secondary injury and specifically hypoxic/ischemic injury, intracranial hypertension, loss of homeostatis and hypotension and vasospasm.[7] These pathophysiologic responses affect the primarily injured but viable tissue during a vulnerable period of recovery. They occur at a time when insults may contribute to further injury and worsened mortality and morbidity. The variability of injury, age susceptibility of cerebral insult and resulting neuropathology all impact mortality. The very young developing brain may be particularly susceptible to extensive damage. During the period of development, the immature brain may be anatomically more vulnerable to shearing, or to dysautoregulation of cerebral perfusion after injury.[6] Adults more commonly suffer from intracranial hemorrhage or intracerebral hematomas, whereas children tend to develop diffuse cerebral swelling more commonly. Diffuse cerebral edema occurs in 17%–44% of children with severe head injuries[10,12,18,21,22] Poor outcomes are seen more commonly with frontal rather than extra-frontal hematomas in children,[17] and are probably due to a higher association with parenchymal injuries. Epidural hematomas less frequently complicate skull fractures in children (40% incidence) when compared to adults (61% incidence). Frontal epidural hematomas are often associated with parenchymal injuries in both adults and children.[17] Good outcomes in this series were seen in 83% of children ($<$ 15 years old) compared to only 56% of adults ($\geq$ 15 years old).[17]

Effects of age

Annegers[9] reported that 10 per 100 000 children will die each year from head injury. Kraus *et al.*[8] evaluated the difference between the overall mortality in children and those with severe injury. He reported that the overall mortality rate was 5% in children following all degrees of head injury, but 59% of children died if they had severe traumatic brain injury. Seventeen percent of all head injuries were considered severe or moderately severe. Importantly these data did not include patients who were not taken to the hospital due to death at the injury (accident) scene.

Jennett *et al.*[23] reported a mortality rate in the under 20-year-old age group of 29%. Gross *et al.*[3] had a case fatality rate in children of 33% compared with 48% in patients who were older than 15 years. Walker *et al.*[4] reported an overall mortality incidence of 25% in his series of pediatric head injury, but it was twice as common in patients who had multiple trauma compared to those with isolated head injury (32% vs. 17% respectively). In the patients with an isolated head injury, intracranial hypertension, a Glasgow Coma Score (GCS) of 3–4, and apnea were cited as the major factors associated with mortality. In the patients who died with head injury in conjunction with multiple trauma, almost 90% had associated hypoxia, hypercarbia, and/or systemic hypotension.[4] The development of diffuse brain swelling has a variable effect on outcome in the literature, with mortality rates of 12–53% when it occurs in children.[18,19,24,25,18] The mortality rate from epidural hematomas is lower (3–10%) than for a diffuse type injury.[17,26] Overall, focal mass lesions have a wide variance in reported mortality, ranging from 6 to 33%[19,27] Finally most studies have shown that the majority of head injury related deaths occur within the first week of admission.[7,10]

Overall, children survive severe traumatic brain injury more often than adults.[7,10,12] However, if one stratifies the pediatric population by age, there is a clear difference in mortality between young, middle, and older children. Younger children (less than 4 years of age) and mid-to-late teenagers have a higher mortality compared to school-age children.[6,7,10] The reason for this difference may be due to the differing mechanisms of injury that occur in early childhood and adolescence compared to young school-age children. Children in the younger age group tend to have mechanisms of injury that result in diffuse injuries and may also suffer multiple insults. Adolescents and older children in contrast tend to have high impact injuries secondary to motor vehicle collisions and missile injuries.[7] Both are associated with higher mortality than the types of head injuries that occur during the middle childhood years. These children tend to have more focal injuries due to a higher percentage of falls, sports-related injuries, and bicycling accidents.[7] As a result, the true mortality for the mechanism of injury at each age has not been accurately assessed.

Effect of initial severity

In adults, the GCS has historically been an indicator of the severity of injury and prognosis.[28] The motor sub-score of the GCS upon presentation and following resuscitation appears to have a close relationship with the final functional recovery.[29,30] For children beyond 4 years of age, the GCS assessment appears valid since the expected elicited responses are age appropriate. Although the GCS has been modified for younger children to make it age appropriate, its validity for this age group remains uncertain. This is because the verbal and eye sub-scores are not easily assessed in this age group even though mortality in the young child is increased with a lower GCS. Consequently the motor sub-score alone is still regarded as being more indicative of the severity of injury, even though good outcomes and recovery may still be seen following very low initial motor scores in young children. In one series of children and adults with epidural hematomas and a low GCS, poor outcome was seen in only 16% of children compared to 31% of adults.[17] Others have seen similar outcomes for all types of injuries,[3] and in a study by Walker *et al.*,[4] a low GCS was a major factor in determining mortality in children with isolated head injuries.

Pupillary and brainstem dysfunction are other features in the initial assessment that may be helpful in determining prognosis. Brainstem dysfunction in particular usually indicates a severe central injury and will typically result in a poor or very poor outcome.[13] Patients with pupillary dysfunction or altered oculovestibular reflexes have been shown to have a worse prognosis both in adults[31] and children.[4] Abnormal reactions to light as well as a distorted shape of the pupil are much more reliable indications of brainstem involvement.

Morbidity

As a group, children are more likely to have a good recovery than patients 15 years or older.[3] However, this finding is based on the gross functional Glasgow Outcome Score and does not test true functional differences between groups. The final functional outcome of children at different ages often depends on the functional aspects of the brain at the time of injury and the stage of neural development. Many of the functions of the developing brain are specifically directed at acquiring new information and interpreting incoming stimuli.[10] Disruption or damage to these centers at this stage may impact on the acquisition of new and higher functions by not permitting the normal processing of new information. In the adult brain, cognitive recovery is a process of reacquiring already learned information. As a result, evaluation of the neurobehavioral outcome in children must consider not only the mechanism of injury and severity of injury of the injury, but the developmental maturity or critical period of development of the brain at the time of injury. This will determine not only the ability to retain what has already been learned, but the ability to process new information in the future.

It is important to consider that often following head injury, and particularly severe injury, all aspects of neurologic and neuropsychologic function can be affected. These include declines in intellect (full scale and performance IQ), attention/concentration dysfunction, memory disorders (spatial and verbal), language dysfunctions (syntax, location, linguistic ability), visual motor skills, achievement and academic performance, and motor function.[22,32] Emotional behavioral changes and even exaggeration of pre-existing behavioral problems are frequently seen following severe head injury in children, and may be magnified in the post-traumatic recovery period.[10,33] Additional morbidity includes post-traumatic seizures, speech and gait abnormalities, hearing and visual changes, and cranial nerve dysfunction.[8] Few children (10–16%) are left in vegetative states following traumatic brain injury.[10,34] A similar proportion (approximately 20%) attain a good or only rarely a "normal" outcome after severe injury.[10]

Effect of age

In addition to mechanism of injury, age plays a major role in determining the long-term functional outcome after severe brain injury. The majority of patients will have a dramatic recovery in cognitive function in the first 12 months following their head injury.[13,35,36] It should also be emphasized that patients with mild and moderate injuries will often show some impairment in academic and non-academic achievement and, for this reason, patients should be reviewed at 6 months and one year after injury to ensure that they have maintained their academic abilities and performance.[36] Similar to the mortality statistics, injury early in childhood (infancy) can result in a worse outcome compared to older children.[35–37] In a study by Koskiniemi *et al.*,[37] preschool age children (7 years or less) were evaluated after suffering a severe traumatic brain injury to determine their long-term ability to recover school and work performance. Over half (59%) were able to return to school and 78% of these children were able to perform normally in school. Long-term follow-up, though, showed that only 21% of these children had the capability of working full-time outside the home, even if they had been able to attend and graduate from a normal school. Further analysis revealed that none of the children with a severe injury before the age of 4 years were able to work independently outside a structured environment while 29% of those patients aged 4 and above were able to work outside the home. Some have commented that 2 years of age is a critical age with regard to functional outcome,[6,10] whilst others have noted that 4 years may be the watershed for predicting long-term outcome.[37] Raimondi[38] showed that infants who were less than one year of age had a poorer recovery than toddlers (e.g., 1–4 years old) and Bagnato and Mayes[24] showed that children with a prenatal injury had a better recovery than post-natal injury, though mechanisms of injury differed and it is difficult to make comparisons. Ewing-Cobbs *et al.*[39] noted that children aged less than 31 months had reduced language skills compared to those children aged 31–64 months old. Infants and preschool children were also significantly more impaired than older children in this study.

Effect of severity and long-term coma state on outcome

Severity of injury also has a major impact on the final outcome and often the length of coma is a measure of the severity of injury. Multiple studies have shown that the extent and length of coma and post-traumatic amnesia correlated with intellectual and psychological outcome, where the longer the length of coma, the worse the outcome.[35,40,41] Coma lasting under 24 hours was rarely associated with permanent neurological or neuropsychological sequelae[3,6,10,15] and the eventual recovery of motor and cognitive function was proportional to the duration of coma.[24] Brink *et al.*[35] showed these proportional differences in intellectual outcome correlated closely with duration of coma. The average length of coma for those returning to baseline was 1.7 weeks, for lowered intelligence 3 weeks, for moderately impaired, 8 weeks, and severely impaired, 11 weeks. In this study, only 24% returned to normal school classes. In another study, 56% of patients who spent less than one week in coma were able to work, while only 13% of those patients who had been unconscious for more than one week were able to work full time.[37] Less than 10% of children were left in a vegetative state with clearly a very poor long-term outcome. Pagni *et al.*[33] showed that only 10% of children who had a mean duration of coma of approximately 6 weeks had normal neurologic function at follow-up.

Intelligence and memory function after head injury

Intellectual dysfunction, as measured by intelligence quotient (IQ) has been well-documented following severe traumatic brain injury.[10,15,29,42,43] There are significant differences between these studies regarding which scale it affected the most. In particular, a larger decrement in full and performance scale IQ over verbal IQ has been reported and performance scale IQ scores were lower compared to full scale IQ in some patients.[15,29,42] Verbal IQ was seen to return to within normal ranges in some studies,[32,43] whilst others have demonstrated persistent deficits in verbal performance.[15,29,42] In another study, verbal IQ was lower than performance IQ, but performance IQ recovered the most by 9 months after the injury.[43] Although recovery was observed in some of the patients with severe injuries, there was still a 20% difference in IQ between these patients and those with mild head injuries.[15] It is clear that following severe head injury, intellectual impairment may be significant and persistent.

This observation has been frequently confirmed and importantly it has also been shown that even a normal post-traumatic IQ does not necessarily imply any long-term sequelae.[44] These investigators found that childhood cognitive deficits were similar to those seen in adults and, again importantly, there was no evidence that children recover better or more fully, than adults with similarly severe injuries.[44]

It is worth noting that the least amount of information regarding intellectual impairment has been reported in patients with mild head injury, who comprise the majority of patients with traumatic brain injury. In general though, children with mild head injuries have a good recovery and rarely have long-term sequelae – although it must again be emphasized that this may simply reflect an under-recognition of more subtle cognitive and attentional deficits. In contrast, children with severe injuries often have extensive impairments.[43] In preschool age children, the majority will have major severe disabilities in intellectual function in long-term follow-up after severe head injury.[6]

In one study of long-term follow-up of preschool age children with severe traumatic brain injuries, 30% had a below normal IQ when tested in adulthood. The mean IQ for these patients was only 85, indicating function at the lower end of the normal range.[37] In a study by Brink *et al.*[35] intellectual impairment was more pronounced in the younger age group with only 14% of children aged less than 8 years having an IQ > 84, in contrast to 52% of children aged 8 years and older. The severity of the injury is clearly related to impaired IQ and impaired acquisition and retention of visuospatial memory.[45] Even with a normal IQ, impaired retrieval of information is common.[7] Older children and adolescents with traumatic brain injury consistently performed better than did children < 8 years on verbal learning and delayed recall tasks.[45]

Memory dysfunction is one of the most common cognitive deficits following severe head injury in children.[32] Verbal memory and the storage and retrieval of words is often lost after significant injury, but tends to recover (although not always completely) in mild and moderate head injuries. It is often persistent on long-term follow-up following severe injuries. Verbal recognition is frequently impaired as non-verbal or spatial memory (in particular remembering shapes) may be. This is often a particular problem in the younger child.[45,46] Klonoff *et al.*[29] noted that non-verbal memory was worse in children who were less than 9 years of age when injured, and the deficit persisted for up to 3 years following the head injury. Patients older than 9 years of age at injury often experienced persistent problems in these areas of memory function for at least one year following their injury. A traumatic brain injury during early childhood is believed to have a direct and often irreversible impact on the ability to process information, as well on adaptive functioning and overall cognitive dysfunction.[29,35,37]

Most patients in the initial post-traumatic period, irrespective of the severity of the head injury will manifest persistent difficulties of attention and concentration, and speed of information processing.[47] Following the initial acute stage, mild and, to a lesser extent, the moderately head-injured patients recover quickly from these deficits. Children with severe injury often continue to have an inability to maintain their concentration both in short- and long-term follow-up studies.[47] Many of these patients are eventually diagnosed with attention deficit disorders, which is often further compounded by impulsivity and disinhibition, common sequelae of frontal lobe dysfunction. It is this group that has been treated chronically with medication (including stimulants) to try and ameliorate these persistent attentional and processing difficulties.

Speech and language

Following traumatic brain injury, dysphasia or mutism is common, although usually transient. The most common speech disorders following severe injury include expressive dysphasia, impaired repetition, decreased length and syntactically complex sentences, and dysarthria,[35,39] Patients with mild or moderate brain injuries may also show difficulties with naming objects, fluency, repetition and written language. Fortunately most of these difficulties only rarely persist by 1 year after mild to moderate head injury. The greater deficit occurs in those with severe head injuries and will have a significant impact on communication and language in approximately two-thirds of the patients.[10] In one study comparing the degree of language dysfunction,[39] the greatest impact was noted in the earlier developmental groups (< 31 months of age). The younger children were noted to have deficits in both receptive and expressive language while those patients who were older (up to mid-adolescence) had difficulty with comprehension or written expression. Levin *et al.*[45] noted decreased verbal fluency, which appeared to be closely correlated with abnormalities on magnetic resonance imaging. Abnormalities within the deeper (white–grey interface) rather than more superficial dorsilateral areas of the frontal lobes tend to be more commonly associated with difficulties in verbal fluency.

Motor function

Motor deficits frequently complicate traumatic brain injury. The extent of these deficits is dependent on the location and mechanism of the injury as well as the age at the time of injury. These same factors are also important in determining the final functional outcome. Some have found that there is a more complete recovery of intellectual function than of motor function in some severely injured children,[39] although others have reported minimal permanent motor impairment.[29] Plasticity in the young brain is greater than that of the more mature child or adult, and motor deficits tend to progressively recover during the first 6–12 months following head injury. Deficits in fine motor movements are the most common persistent sequelae, even up to one year after injury,[6,29] and these deficits can involve the limbs, face, and motor speech.[29,39] In one report, the two most common sequelae following severe head injury were spasticity and ataxia.[35] Even in preschool children, in whom plasticity is maximal and potential for recovery greatest, many had incapacitating neurological deficits including hemi- or tetraparesis, ataxia, dyskinesias, and cranial nerve deficits at long-term follow-up, even into adulthood.[29,37,39] Of severely injured patients in these series, only 28% or less had deficits categorized as mild and not incapacitating. In contrast, Mahoney *et al.*[6] reported that only 9% of head injured children had permanent motor deficits, but these patients had a mean duration of coma of only 15.5 days. Others have also noted that motor dysfunction appears to be directly related to length of coma.[35,48] Severity of injury is also proportional to the extent of motor slowing on motor speed performance testing.[32,43]

Some have attributed the differences in motor and intellectual recovery to the anatomical differences of the tissue subsisting their function. Generally, motor function is regarded as more topographic and subcortical, whereas intellectual function tends to be more associative.[31,39] It is hypothesized that the topographic organization is less flexible or "plastic" for functional or structural reorganization, although this may be somewhat simplistic. Cognitive functions, in contrast, being associative between cortical areas may show increased flexibility due to greater synaptic/connective plasticity.[10] In addition, severely head-injured children perform significantly slower on motor and intellectual tests requiring speed, and in particular highly speeded performance tests.[49]

Such impairments do show some improvement over time, but the rate of improvement slows with time especially for moderate and severe head-injured children. The most rapid improvement occurs in the first year after injury.[50]

For improvement to occur and to be maintained, however, Beaulieu[51] contends that the training and involvement of family members in rehabilitation techniques is essential for a successful outcome. This rehabilitation should be implemented as soon as possible after injury.

Epilepsy

The majority of children who have a head injury do not experience a seizure. The overall risk of epilepsy developing after a head injury is approximately 5%, but it is slightly higher (up to almost 10%) in children under 5 years of age.[52] Not surprisingly, the more severe the head injury, the greater the risk of developing late, post-traumatic epilepsy. In the severe injury group, the overall incidence may be as high as 9 or 10%.[53–55] A number of factors are associated with this increased risk including: early seizures[53] (seizures occurring in the first week after the head injury), depressed skull fracture, a missile injury (causing focal cerebral damage, particularly if of high velocity), intracerebral hematoma, prolonged (> 24 hrs) post-traumatic amnesia and, probably, a genetic predisposition to epilepsy. Early post-traumatic seizures are associated with a 20%–25% probability of late epilepsy. This risk increases to 40% if there has also been an intracerebral hemorrhage and can be up to 60% if most of the above risk factors are present. Approximately 20% of children with late seizures will experience their initial seizure in the first month following the head injury, with over half of late seizures occurring within the first year. However, late post-traumatic epilepsy may still develop up to 5 or even 10 years after the head injury. The majority of late post-traumatic epileptic seizures are generalized, although these are likely to be secondarily generalized following an initial partial (focal) seizure that is not witnessed or recognized as a seizure. Although many children continue to experience occasional infrequent seizures when receiving antiepileptic medication, a significant number will become seizure-free for at least 12 months whilst receiving antiepileptic medication. Finally, in most children (and, subsequently as adults), the epilepsy will not remit spontaneously and antiepileptic medication may be required for many years, if not the duration of their life.

Behavioral problems

Behavioral and mood changes are common following both moderate and severe traumatic brain injury. These are manifest by increased irritability, temper/rage outbursts and impulsivity, aggressive behavior, hyperactivity, and problems with interpersonal social adaption. This commonly results in secondary (and usually major), impairment of and problems with family dynamics. Consequently, this contributes to the overall public health and economic burden of traumatic brain injury. In the mild to moderate brain-injured child, these changes may resolve,[56] although this is not invariable. This is in contrast to those who have suffered a severe head injury, where these behavioral problems are often both persistent and magnified. In the younger age groups, hyperactivity, tantrums, aggressive or destructive behavior, and impulsiveness tend to predominate. In older children, poor judgment, euphoria, and depression were more commonly observed.[35] In one study, 94% of children had personality and behavioral aberrations as a result of their head injury.[57] In many studies, over 50% of children with severe head injuries will continue to have impulsivity, hyperactivity, and learning difficulties even up to one year after injury.[35,43,46] Emanuelson *et al.*[58] reported that none of the children in this review were able to adjust to normal life after the trauma due to disabling behavioral and personality disturbances. Bagnato and Mayes showed that traumatically injured infants and pre-schoolers often had deficits in self-regulatory functions and that these functions were the least affected by intervention.[24]

The majority of patients will have a dramatic recovery in motor and cognitive function in the first 12 months following head injury.[13,39] It should be noted that even patients with mild and moderate injuries can have academic and achievement performance declines, and for this reason they are often followed at 6 months and one year after injury to ensure that they have maintained their academic abilities and performance.[13] Children who return with new deficits or further exacerbation of cognitive difficulties that were premorbid, require evaluations to define their deficiencies and determine an appropriate treatment plan.[5,37] The goal of rehabilitation following severe brain injury in children is the recovery of lost functions and the reattainment of the ability to gain new functions. Because of the high rate of disability amongst young children following brain injury, it is necessary to further define the age specific neurobehavioral sequelae in order to develop appropriate rehabilitative strategies.[10,35] Generally, age specific treatment plans are lacking due to the previous pooling of data for wide age ranges of children.[59] Intensive interdisciplinary, early intervention treatment programs have been shown to enhance the development and behavioral functioning of young children with brain injuries.[24,35,60] Long-term studies have shown continued improvement up to 3 years after injury.[10,35] Using a program consisting of an integrated therapy team that concentrated on physical and communication problems in the first year, and higher level language, perceptual and cognitive deficits in the second and third year in children, Boyer and Edwards showed continued and measurable recovery up to at least 3 years following injury.[10] Future interventions and rehabilitative programs will need to consider not only the acute period of recovery but the effects of early rehabilitation on the later recovery potentials.

Conclusions

As a group, children tend to have a better outcome than adults following moderate or severe head injuries. Many factors influence this prognosis in the pediatric population. Similar to adults, the mechanism of injury, the severity of the injury as measured by the GCS, other injuries, secondary injury, and brainstem involvement, all have an impact on, and are directly related to, the final outcome. Age at the time of the head injury is an additional important factor and perhaps somewhat surprisingly, very young and preschool children have worse outcomes in terms of both mortality and long-term morbidity (motor, cognitive, and behavioral difficulties) than older children and teenagers. The majority of children will continue to dramatically improve motor and cognitive function during the first 12 months after injury. Long-term studies have now shown that improvement can continue even longer. Outcomes can be improved with reduction in mortality and severe neurological sequelae by preventing either the initial injury or reducing/minimizing any secondary cerebral and hemodynamic insults. Better age at injury outcome measures are needed to better understand the differences and the effects that injury has on the pediatric brain.

Lastly, numerous preventative measures have been, and continue to be, introduced to reduce the risk of head injuries. These include appropriately fitted and properly used car seats, the wearing of cycle helmets (compulsory in only a few countries), traffic-calming measures, educational programs such as ThinkFirst, and, perhaps most importantly, the reduction of severe socio-economic deprivation. Additional measures including programmes to reduce violence in the home and to reduce sports injuries are also likely to have a major impact in either reducing or preventing the original head injury.

REFERENCES

1. Guyer, B. & Ellers, B. Childhood injuries in the United States. Mortality, morbidity, and cost. *Am. J. Dis. Child.* 1990; **144**:649–652.
2. Wegman, W. E. Annual summary of vital statistics – 1981. *Pediatrics* 1982; **75**:835–843.
3. Gross, C. R., Wolf, C., Kunitz, S. C. *et al.* Pilot Traumatic Coma Data Bank: a profile of head injuries in children. In Dacey, R. G., Jr. *et al.* (eds.): *Trauma of the Central Nervous System.* New York: Raven Press, 1985:19–26.
4. Walker, M. L., Mayer, T. A., Storrs, B. B. *et al.* Pediatric head injury – factors which influence outcome. *Concepts Pediatr. Neurosurg.* 1985; **6**:84–97.
5. Oddy, M., Coughlan, T., Tyerman, A. *et al.* Social adjustment after closed head injury. A further follw-up seven years after injury. *J. Neurol., Neurosurg., Psychiatry* 1985; **48**:564–568.
6. Mahoney, W. J., D'Souza, B. J., Haller, A. *et al.* Long-term outcome of children with severe head trauma and prolonged coma. *Pediatrics* 1983; **71**(5):756–762.
7. Luerssen, T. G., Klauber, M. R., & Marshall, L. F. Outcome from head injury related to patient's age. A longitudinal prospective study of adult and pediatric head injury. *J. Neurosurg.* 1988; **68**:409–416.
8. Kraus, J. F., Fife, D., & Conroy, C. Pediatric brain injuries: the nature, clinical course, and early outcomes in a defined United States' population. *Pediatrics* 1987; **79**(4):501–507.
9. Annegers, F. The epidemiology of head trauma in children. In Shapiro, I. (ed.) *Pediatric Head Trauma.* New York: Futura Publishing Co., 1983.

10. Boyer, M. G. & Edwards, P. Outcome 1 to 3 years after severe traumatic brain injury in children and adolescents. *Injury* 1991; **22**(4):315–320.
11. Demellweek, C., Baldwin, T., Appleton, R., & Al-Kharusi, A. A prospective study and review of pre-morbid characteristics in children with traumatic brain injury. *Pediatr. Rehab.* 2002; **5**:81–89.
12. Bruce, D. A., Raphaely, R. C., Goldberg, A. I. *et al.* Pathophysiology, treatment and outcome following severe head injury in children. *Child's Brain* 1979; **5**:174–191.
13. Choi, S. C., Barnes, T. Y., Bullock, R. *et al.* Temporal profile of outcomes in severe head injury. *J. Neurosurg.* 1994; **81**:169–173.
14. Christoffel, K. K. Violent death and injury in US children and adolescents. *Am. J. Dis. Child.* 1990; **144**:697–706.
15. Duhaime, A. C., Alario, A. J., Lewander, W. J. *et al.* Head injury in very young children: Mechanism, injury types, and ophthalmologic findings in 100 patients younger than 2 years of age. *Pediatrics* 1992; **90**:179–185.
16. Hendrick, E. B., Harwood-Harsh, D. C. F., & Hudson, A. R. Head injuries in children: a survey of 4,465 consecutive cases at the Hospital for Sick Children, Toronto, Canada. *Clin. Neurosurg.* 1964; **11**:46–64.
17. Mohanty, A., Kolluri, V. R. S., Subbakrishna, D. K. *et al.* Prognosis of extradural haematomas in children. *Pediatr. Neurosurg.* 1995; **23**:57–63.
18. Bruce, D. A., Schut, L., Bruno, L. A. *et al.* Outcome following severe head injuries in children. *J. Neurosurg*. 1978; **48**:679–688.
19. Aldrich, E. F., Eisenberg, H. M., Saydjari, C. *et al.* Diffuse brain swelling in severely head-injured children A report from the NIH Traumatic Coma Data Bank. *J. Neurosurg.* 1992; **76**:450–454.
20. Graham, D. I., Ford, I., & Adams, J. H. Fatal head injury in children. *J. Clin. Pathol.* 1989; **42**:18–22.
21. Berger, M. S., Pitts, L. H., Lovely, M. *et al.* Outcome from severe head injury in children and adolescents. *J. Neurosurg.* 1985; **62**:194–199.
22. Johnston, R. B. & Mellits, E. D. Pediatric coma: prognosis and outcome. *Develop. Med. Child. Neurol.* 1980; **22**:3–12.
23. Jennett, B., Teasdale, G., Braakman, R. *et al.* Prognosis of patients with severe head injury. *Neurosurgery* 1979; **4**(4):283–289.
24. Bagnato, S. J. & Mayes, S. D. Patterns of developmental and behavioral progress for young brain-injured children during interdisciplinary intervention. *Develop. Neuropsychol* 1986; **2**(3):213–240.
25. Bruce, D. A., Alavi, A., Bilaniuk, L. T. *et al.* Diffuse cerebral swelling following head injuries in children: the syndrome of "malignant brain edema". *J. Neurosurg.* 1981; **54**:170–178.
26. Moura dos Santos, A. L., Plese, J. P. P., Ciquini, O., Jr. *et al.* Extradural haematomas in children. *Paediatr. Neurosurg.* 1994; **21**:50–54.
27. Alberico, A. M., Ward, J. D., Choi, S. C. *et al.* Outcome after severe head injury. Relationship to mass lesions, diffuse injury, and ICP course in pediatric and adult patients. *J. Neurosurg.* 1987; **67**:648–656.
28. Becker, D. P., Miller, J. D., Word, J. D. *et al.* The outcome from severe head injury with early diagnosis and intensive management. *J. Neurosurg.* 1982; **56**:26–32.
29. Klonoff, H., Low, M. D., & Clark, C. Head injuries in children: a prospective five year follow-up. *J. Neurol. Neurosurg. Psychiatry* 1977; **40**:1211–1219.
30. Kumar, R., West, C. G. H., Quirke, C. *et al.* Do children with severe head injury benefit from intensive care? *Child's Nerv. Syst.* 1991; **7**:299–304.
31. Young, B., Rapp, R. P., Norton, J. A. *et al.* Early prediction of outcome in head-injured patients. *J. Neurosurg.* 1981; **54**:300–303.
32. Levin, H. S., High, W. M., Jr., Ewing-Cobbs, L. *et al.* Memory functioning during the first year after closed head injury in children and adolescents. *Neurosurgery* 1988; **22**:1043–1052.
33. Pagni, C. A., Signoroni, G., Crotti, F. *et al.* Severe traumatic coma in infancy and childhood: results after surgery and resuscitation. *J. Neurosurg. Sci.* 1975; **19**:120–128.
34. Levin, H. S., Aldrich, E. F., Saydjari, C. *et al.* Severe head injury in children: experience of the Traumatic Coma Data Bank. *Neurosurgery* 1992; **31**(3):435–444.
35. Brink, J. D., Garrett, A. L., Hale, W. R. *et al.* Recovery of motor and intellectual function in children sustaining severe head injuries. *Develop. Med. Child. Neurol.* 1970; **12**:565–571.
36. Levin, H. S., Eisenberg, H. M., Wigg, N. R. *et al.* Memory and intellectual ability after head injury in children and adolescents. *Neurosurgery* 1982; **11**:668–673.
37. Koskiniemi, M., Kyykka, T., Nybo, T. *et al.* Long-term outcome after severe brain injury in preschoolers is worse than expected. *Arch. Pediatr. Adolesc. Med.* 1995; **149**:249–254.
38. Raimondi, A. J. & Hirschauer, J. Head injury in the infant and toddler. *Child's Brain* 1984; **11**:12–35.
39. Ewing-Cobbs, L., Miner, M. E., Fletcher, J. M. *et al.* Intellectual, motor, and language sequelae following closed head injury in infants and preschoolers. *J. Pediatr. Psychol.* 1989; **14**(4):531–547.
40. Brooks, N., McKinlay, W., Symington, E. *et al.* Return to work within the first seven years of severe head injury. *Brain Injury* 1987; **1**:5–19.
41. Heiskanen, O. & Kaste, M. Late prognosis of severe brain injury in children. *Develop. Med. Child. Neurol.* 1974; **16**:11–14.
42. Jaffe, K. M., Fay, G. C., Polissar, N. L. *et al.* Severity of pediatric traumatic brain injury and early neurobehavioral outcome: a cohort study. *Arch. Phys. Med. Rehabil.* 1992; **73**:540–547.
43. Knights, R. M., Ivan, L. P., Ventureyra, E. C. G., *et al.* The effects of head injury in children on neuropsychological and behavioral functioning. *Brain Injury* 1991; **5**(4):339–351.
44. Laurent-Vannier, A., Brugel, D. G., & De Agostini, M. Rehabilitation of brain injured children. *Childs Nerv. Syst.* 2000; **16**(10–11):760–764.
45. Levin, H. S., Culhane, K. A., Fletcher, J. M. *et al.* Dissociation between delayed alternation and memory after pediatric head

injury: relationship to MRI findings. *J. Child. Neurol.* 1994; **9**:81–89.

46. Chadwick, O., Rutter, M., & Brown, G. A prospective study of children. IV. Specific cognitive deficits. *J. Clin. Neuropsych.* 1981; **3**:101–120.
47. Stuss, D. T., Ely, P., Hugenholtz, H. *et al.* Subtle neuropsychological deficits in patients with good recovery after closed head injury. *Neurosurgery* 1985; **17**:41–47.
48. Winogron, H. W., Knights, R. M., & Bawden, H. N.. Neuropsychological deficits following head injury in children. *J. Clin. Neuropsych.* 1984; **6**:269–286.
49. Bawden, H. N., Knights, R. M., & Winogron, H. W. Speeded performance following head injury in children. *J. Clin. Exp. Neuropsychol.* 1985; **7**(1):39–54.
50. Jaffe, K. M., Polissar, N. L., Fay, G. C., & Liao, S. Recovery trends over three years following pediatric traumatic brain injury. *Arch. phys. Med. Rehabil.* 1995; **76**(1):17–26.
51. Beaulieu, C. L. Rehabilitation and outcome following pediatric traumatic brain injury. *Surg. Clin. North. Am.* 2002; **82**(2):393–408.
52. Jennett, B. Trauma as a cause of epilepsy in childhood. *Dev. Med. Child. Neurol.* 1973; **15**:56–62.
53. Appleton, R. E. & Demellweek, C. Post-traumatic epilepsy in children requiring inpatient rehabilitation following head injury. *J. Neurol. Neurosurg. Psychiatry* 2002; **72**:669–672.
54. Hahn, Y. S., Fuchs, S., Flannery, A. M. *et al.* Factors influencing post-traumatic seizures in children. *Neurosurgery* 1988; **22**:864–867.
55. Lewis, R., Yee, L., Inkelis, S. *et al.* Clinical predictors of post-traumatic seizures in children with head trauma. *Ann. Emerg. Med.* 1993; **22**:1114–1118.
56. Rutter, M., Chadwick, O., & Shaffer, D. Head injury. In Rutter, M. (ed). *Developmental Neuropsychiatry.* New York: Guilford Press, 1983; 83–111.
57. Dillon, H. & Leopold, R. L. Children and post-concussion syndrome *J. Am. Med. Assoc.* 1961; **175**:86–92.
58. Emanuelson, I., Von Wendt, L., Lundalv, E. *et al.* Rehabilitation and follow up of children with severe traumatic brain injury. *Childs Nerv Syst*. 1996; **12**:460–465.
59. Levin, H. S. Neurobehavioral recovery. *J. Neurotrauma* 1992; **9**:S359–373.
60. Bagnato, S. J. & Neisworth, J. T. Neurodevelopmental outcomes of early brain injury: a follow-up of fourteen case studies. *TECSE* 1989; **9**(1):72–89.

Truncal trauma

Steven Stylianos and Michael G. Vitale

Columbia University College of Physicians & Surgeons and Children's Hospital of New York-Presbyterian, NY, USA

In the early 1900s, an American surgeon named Ernest Amory Codman introduced the concept of "the end result idea" to encourage scrutiny of patient outcomes in hospitalized patients. Codman suggested that this approach be used to compare hospitals and surgeons and thus the era of benchmarking began. Controversy ensued as "the end result idea" threatened to shift focus from a system based on the privileges of seniority to a more objective one. Prompted by Codman's idea, the American College of Surgeons (ACS) developed a committee called the Standardization of Hospitals in the late 1920s that ultimately became the Joint Commission for the Accreditation of Hospitals.[1] Let's jump ahead 60 years to the reports of Wennberg who reported remarkable differences in the rate of carotid endarterectomies, tonsillectomies, and hysterectomies in various geographic regions.[2,3] These early reports ushered in the era of evidence-based medicine, defined as the integration of the current best evidence with clinical expertise and patient preferences used in making decisions regarding care. Trauma research focusing on outcome studies and evidence-based methodology is in its early stages and will be reviewed below.

Trauma systems

Optimal pediatric trauma care: pediatric vs. adult trauma centers

The debate regarding the optimal setting for pediatric trauma care delivery has existed for more than two decades and is unresolved at present. The Major Trauma Outcome Study and TRISS methodology have been used in several studies to highlight care of the pediatric trauma victim in adult trauma centers. These studies usually describe the experience at a single center and rely solely on mortality and Z statistics which fall short in defining efficacy. The expectation that pediatric trauma centers (PTC) would have better results than adult trauma centers (ATC) caring for injured children seems logical, but it may be argued that the overall volume seen at an ATC could more than offset the advantage of a dedicated PTC.

Potoka *et al.* analyzed more than 13 000 injured children from the Pennsylvania Trauma Outcome Study and used mortality as the major outcome variable to compare care at two regional PTC vs. 24 adult trauma centers (ATC). Four patients treated at PTC and ATC had similar injury severity as determined by median Injury Severity Score (ISS), mean Revised Trauma Score, and Glasgow Coma Scale. Overall, survival was significantly better at PTC and ATC with added pediatric qualifications compared with ATC without added qualifications. Survival for head, spleen, and liver injuries was significantly better at PTC compared with all ATC regardless of added pediatric qualifications. Children who sustained moderate or severe head injuries were more likely to undergo neurosurgical intervention and have a better outcome when treated at PTC. Despite similar injury severity, significantly more children underwent surgical exploration for spleen and liver injury at ATC.

Contrary data were reported in a recent review of more than 53 000 pediatric trauma patients from the National Pediatric Trauma Registry (NPTR) treated at 22 pediatric trauma centers and 31 adult trauma centers.[5] Although pediatric trauma centers had higher overall survival rates than adult trauma centers, this difference disappeared when the analysis was controlled for Injury Severity Score, Pediatric Trauma Score, age, mechanism, and ACS

Pediatric Surgery and Urology: Long-term Outcomes, Mark Stringer, Keith Oldham, Pierre Mouriquand.

verification status. The logistic regression model used differed from the analysis of the previous study.

The optimal allocation of recourses within PTC was the subject of a recent review by Doolin *et al.*[6] Fifty-nine PTC that contributed more than 40 000 patients to phase II of the NPTR responded to a survey examining resources. Outcomes measured included PICU and overall length of stay, mortality, time in ED, and long-term impairment. The data indicated that an in-house attending surgeon reduced the amount of time a mildly injured patient (ISS<16) spent in the ED, as did the presence of a separate pediatric ED, and in-house pediatric emergency physician. An in-house attending surgeon reduced the mortality rate in older (>7 years) and severely injured (ISS > 36) patients. As the demand for cost-effective and efficient care increases, components of a health care delivery such as pediatric trauma care will be under great scrutiny. More detailed analysis will be necessary to define optimal care of injured children throughout the full spectrum of institutions.

Optimal pediatric trauma care: pediatric vs. adult trauma surgeons

The controversy over the optimal setting for the delivery of care for injured children is magnified further when individual cohorts of trauma surgeons are compared. Two recent studies examined the outcome of children with blunt splenic injury treated by pediatric surgeons compared to adult surgeons. Keller and Vane reported 817 children (142 from the Vermont registry and 675 from the NPTR) and found that the operative intervention rate was 21% by pediatric surgeons and 52% by adult surgeons ($P < 0.05$).[7] The difference remained statistically significant when controlled for injury severity and age. The overall splenectomy rate was nearly doubled in children treated by adult surgeons (24% vs. 13%, $P < 0.05$). Both transfusion requirement and hospital cost were lower for patient management non-operatively. Mooney *et al.* reported 126 children with splenic injury from New Hampshire Uniform Hospital Discharge Data Sets.[8] The large majority of patients (84%) were treated by adult surgeons at general hospitals. Crude splenectomy rates were 5.5% at the children's hospitals compared to 32.4% at general hospitals. The authors concluded that the overwhelming majority of splenectomies and splenorrhaphies could have been avoided if general hospitals treated children with splenic injury in the same manner as the children's hospitals. Further analysis has revealed a significant reduction in operative treatment of children with blunt spleen injury if the treating surgeon had pediatric surgical training.[9]

Table 70.1. Rate of operative treatment in children with blunt spleen injury

	General hospital	Children's hospital	General hospital with children's unit
No operation	2487 (82%)	356 (97%)	1062 (88%)
Yes operation	539 (**18%**)*	11 (**3%**)[a]	140 (**12%**)[a]

[a]Chi-Square $P < 0.001$.

To compare how children were managed across all hospitals, Guice *et al.* used the Agency for Healthcare Research and Quality's 2000 KID dataset, a nationwide sample of pediatric (age < 20) discharges from the Hospital Cost Utilization Project's State Inpatient Databases.[10] This database contains information reflecting approximately 7.3 million discharges. Records were selected (1) based upon emergency or urgent hospital admission; (2) by splenic injury diagnosis codes; (3) by splenic operation codes; (4) by E-Codes indicating vehicular accident; and (5) were excluded for other abdominal operations. Selected records were weighted to estimate a national sample of children with isolated blunt splenic injury. Data were analyzed by whether patients underwent operation on the spleen (Table 70.1). Hospitals were stratified to reflect either children's hospitals, general hospitals, or children's units with general hospitals, defined by the National Association of Children's Hospitals and Related Institutions (NACHRI). No significant difference among groups was found for deaths, suggesting comparable case severity. Obvious conclusions are that the rate of splenic operation in injured children is significantly different when comparing treatment at children's hospitals vs. non-children's hospitals. Broader application of non-operative management consensus guidelines for blunt splenic injury is indicated.

Assessing pediatric functional outcomes

As the leading cause of death and disability in children, pediatric trauma accounts for some 11 million hospitalizations, 100 000 permanent disabilities, and 15 000 childhood deaths every year in the United States. While children more often survive significant polytrauma than adults, long-term morbidity is all too common. Four children are left with permanent disability for every trauma related mortality.[11] This statistic highlights the need to assess long-term functional status and quality of life in this population. The direct costs alone for childhood injury exceed 8 billion dollars per year in the United States. While it is impossible to accurately quantify the indirect costs to families and to society in general, it is clear that they are staggering. Given this, the area of pediatric trauma represents perhaps the greatest public health challenge in pediatric health care today. Efforts must be focused to better understand the ways in which we can both decrease the frequency of pediatric injury and optimize the outcomes of those injured.

While we have indeed made great strides in our ability to care for injured children, we have made much less progress in our ability to assess the broadly defined long-term outcomes of these injuries. Data which meet the methodological rigor supporting Class I standards of care in pediatric trauma are very difficult to obtain. Admittedly, clinical research in the setting of pediatric trauma, including the assessment of pediatric health status and quality of life, has numerous intrinsic difficulties. Any functional assessment in children must be performed in a developmental context. Key aspects of quality of life such as physical, emotional, and social function rapidly evolve as the child ages. Measures of health status for this population must allow for comparison to age-adjusted normative values. Despite these difficulties, rigorous patient-oriented clinical research, focusing on issues germane to the injured child, is a prerequisite for the timely evolution of clinical practice in this area. Fortunately, new clinical research methodologies present exciting opportunities to explore issues related to these outcomes.

Functional status and quality of life assessment in a pediatric population

While children are more likely to survive traumatic injury, many endure significant problems in physical function and overall health. Aitken *et al.* recently reviewed the experience of the National Pediatric Trauma Registry (NPTR) and found that, even when excluding head injuries, 14.5% children captured in this 6-year study had persistent disabilities.[11a] The ability to quantify deficits in functional status and health related quality of life is germane to the assessment of injured children.

Fortunately, measures to assess functional status and quality of life in children have recently become widely available. The Child Health Questionnaire (CHQ) is perhaps the best-validated measure for the assessment of general health status in children.[12] Akin to the Short Form-36 (SF-36) which has been widely used in the adult literature, the CHQ consists of a short questionnaire which is quantifiable and generates multiple domains which span the spectrum of physical, psychosocial, and social health in injured children. Age-adjusted normative values are available and offer the prospect of comparison of health status after trauma in children, for whom premorbid scores are not available. The Pediatric Orthopedic Society of North America has developed another health status questionnaire, which also exhibits good validity and reliability across a range of pediatric musculoskeletal conditions.[13]

Much less has been documented concerning the long-term outcomes of injured children. In a review of the literature in this area published in 1997, Van der Sluis *et al.*[14] identified only seven studies that focused on the "long term" (the maximum follow-up in this group was 2.4 years) outcome of injured children and concluded that there was a "dearth of outcome studies on severely injured children." The authors went on to collect information regarding functional status (as measured by the Functional Independence Measure, the FIM) and Quality of Life (as measured by the Short Form-36) at an average of 9 years after injury on a cohort of children who sustained significant polytrauma. Despite the fact that 42% of these patients had some degree of resultant cognitive impairments, SF-36 scores were generally satisfactory. On the other hand, Wesson *et al.*[15] found that pediatric trauma had profound effects on the physical and psychological health of children and their families at 12 month follow-up. Among children who experienced major trauma, 71% had persistent physical limitations, 41% had behavioral disturbances and many children exhibited a decrease in academic performance. Another study by the same author showed that 88% of children surviving severe injuries had functional limitations at discharge with 54% still having limitations at 6-month follow-up.[16] Valadka *et al.*[17] recently published the results of a retrospective study, which assessed health status of children via a telephone interview at a minimum of one year after significant trauma. At a minimum follow-up 6 years after injury, half of injured children were found to have long-term sequelae. Thus, the available body of literature suggests that a large percentage of children who sustain significant trauma have persistent functional limitations and disability, despite modern improvements in patient care.

Injury-specific outcomes

While liver and spleen injuries are the most common blunt abdominal injuries in children, long-term sequelae are few. Increasing application of specific consensus guidelines based on injury severity has resulted in conformity in patient management, improved utilization of resources, and validation of guideline safety (Table 70.2). Significant reduction of ICU stay, hospital stay, follow-up imaging and length of activity restriction has been achieved without adverse short-term sequelae when compared to our retrospective database.[18–20]

Table 70.2. Consensus guidelines for resource utilization in children with isolated spleen or liver injury

CT grade	I	II	III	IV
ICU days	None	None	None	1 day
Hospital stay	2 days	3 days	4 days	5 days
Predischarge imaging	None	None	None	None
Postdischarge imaging	None	None	None	None
Activity restriction[a]	3 weeks	4 weeks	5 weeks	6 weeks

[a] Return to **full-contact, competitive sports** (i.e., football, wrestling, hockey, lacrosse, mountain climbing, etc.) should be at the discretion of the individual pediatric trauma surgeon. The proposed guidelines for return to unrestricted activity include "normal" age-appropriate activities.

Routine follow-up imaging studies have identified pseudocysts and pseudoaneurysms following splenic injury.[21,22] Splenic pseudoaneurysms often cause no symptoms and appear to resolve with time. The true incidence of self-limited, post-traumatic splenic pseudoaneurysms is unknown, as routine follow-up imaging after successful non-operative treatment has been largely abandoned. Once identified, the actual risk of splenic pseudoaneurysm rupture is also unclear. Angiographic embolization techniques can successfully treat these lesions obviating the need for open surgery and loss of splenic parenchyma. Splenic pseudocysts can achieve enormous size, leading to pain, gastrointestinal disturbance or other local symptoms. Simple percutaneous aspiration is associated with a high recurrence rate. Laparoscopic excision and marsupialization is highly effective.

Renal trauma

The kidney is the most commonly injured organ in the urogenital system and children appear to be more susceptible to major renal trauma than adults.[23] Several unique anatomic aspects contribute to this observation including: less cushioning from perirenal fat, weaker abdominal musculature, and a less well ossified thoracic cage. The child's kidney also occupies a proportionally larger space in the retroperitoneum than does an adult kidney. In addition, the pediatric kidney may retain fetal lobulations, permitting easier parenchymal disruption.

Pre-existing or congenital renal abnormalities, such as hydronephrosis, tumors, or abnormal position, may predispose the kidney to trauma despite relatively mild traumatic forces. Historically, the incidence of congenital abnormalities in injured kidneys has been reported to vary from 1% to 21%. More recent reviews have narrowed the range to less than 10%.[24,25] Renal abnormalities, particularly hydronephrotic kidneys, may be first diagnosed after minor blunt abdominal trauma. Most often, these patients present with hematuria following blunt trauma.

Treatment of renal injury

Minor renal injuries constitute the majority of blunt renal injuries and usually resolve without incident. The management of major renal parenchymal lacerations, although accounting for only 10% to 15% of all renal trauma patients, is currently controversial. Surgery is not mandatory if there is hemodynamic stability and many major blunt renal injuries may be managed conservatively.[26–32] When necessary, the goals of surgical renal exploration are to either definitively treat major renal injuries with preservation of renal parenchyma when possible, or to thoroughly evaluate a suspected renal vascular injury. Two recent series of major renal injuries in children reported operative treatment in 31% and 37%.[27,28]

Long-term outcomes are measured by the amount of functioning renal parenchyma. The incidence of kidney loss (nephrectomy or atrophy) in children following severe renal parenchymal or renal vascular injury ranges between 20% and 60%.[27,28,30] This wide range reflects differences in follow-up strategies including CT and radionuclide scintigraphy. Hypertension in the early post-trauma period is uncommon. Hypertension may develop in the ensuing months and in most instances requires no further treatment other than medical management. Occasionally, delayed nephrectomy is indicated for persistent hypertension.

Pancreas

Recently, two major children's centers (Toronto and San Diego) reported their experience with divergent methods of managing blunt traumatic pancreatic injuries in a series of reports.[33–37] Canty and coworkers (San Diego) reported 18 patients with major pancreatic injuries over a 14-year period.[33–35] The most frequent mechanism of injury was car or bike crashes. Sixteen of the 18 patients had CT scan on admission. Of these, 11 suggested injury and in five the injury was not recognized or not visualized. Distal pancreatectomy was performed for eight patients (44%). In five of six patients, with either proximal duct injuries or injuries missed on initial CT scan, pseudocysts developed. In two other children who had minimal initial symptoms, and no admission CT scan performed, pseudocysts also occurred.

Of these seven pseudocysts, two resolved and five were treated by cystogastrostomy. The remaining two patients, more recently treated, received ERCP with duct stenting with resolution of symptoms and complete healing. They concluded that distal injuries should be treated with distal pancreatectomy; proximal injury with observation; pseudocysts with observation or cystogastrostomy, and acute ERCP management with stent placement was safe and effective. They also concluded that CT scanning is suggestive but not always diagnostic for the type and location of pancreatic injury.

The experience summarized in two reports from Toronto is markedly different.[36,37] In the first brief report, two patients with documented pancreatic duct disruption (by ERCP or cathetergram) had complete duct healing without operative intervention.[36] This was followed by a retrospective report of 35 consecutive children treated over 10 years (1987–1996).[37] Twenty-three had early diagnosis (< 24 hours), while in 12 diagnosis was delayed (2–14 days). Twenty eight children were treated non-operatively; the remaining seven had operations for other causes. In the 28 cases not surgically treated, CT scan was diagnostic, revealing five patterns of injury: contusion, stellate fragmentation, partial fracture, complete transection and pseudocyst. In these 28 patients, pseudocysts occurred in 10 (36%), average time for initiation of oral feeds was 15 days, and mean hospital stay for all patients treated non-operatively was 21 days. In comparing the San Diego (aggressive operative intervention) to the Toronto protocols (predominately non-operative treatment), the striking differences in these series are: the 100% diagnostic sensitivity of CT scanning in Toronto vs. 69% in San Diego and the 44% operative rate in San Diego vs. 0% in Toronto. A subsequent study from Toronto provided follow-up data on 10 patients with duct transections from the earlier report, and complete follow-up was available in nine.[37] In these children four (44%) developed pseudocysts, with three percutaneously drained. Mean hospital stay was 24 days. All recovered. Follow-up CT scan in eight of nine patients revealed atrophy of the distal pancreas in six and completely normal glands in two. There was no exocrine or endocrine dysfunction with a mean of 47 months of follow-up. The authors conclude that following non-operative management of pancreatic blunt trauma, atrophy (distal) or recanalization occurs in all cases with no long-term morbidity.

Published reports from centers in Dallas and Seattle favor early distal pancreatectomy for transection to the left of the spine to shorten hospital stay.[38,39] However, long-term sequelae of adhesive intestinal obstruction and endocrine and exocrine dysfunction were not assessed. Other reports document the efficacy of early ERCP intervention for diagnosis and treatment with ductal stenting, the use of somatostatin to decrease pancreatic secretions and promote healing, and MRCP as a diagnostic tool.[40–44] However, further study of these modalities is clearly indicated.

Of note, a large single-center experience from Chiba, Japan reported non-operative management in 19 of 20 children with documented pancreatic injury (nine contusions, six lacerations and five main duct disruptions).[45] In all cases recovery was complete without surgery. Their experience with pseudocyst formation and treatment and overall outcome virtually mirrors the Toronto report.

In summary, we believe that the available literature and our experience supports the following approach: (1) early spiral CT with oral and IV contrast in all patients who, by history, physical or mechanism of injury may have blunt trauma to the pancreas; (2) documentation of injuries and early ERCP to provide duct stenting in selected cases; (3) non-operative management with NPO and TPN; and (4) expectant management of pseudocyst formation; percutaneous drainage for symptomatic, infected, or enlarging pseudocyst. However, the optimal approach to diagnosis and management of these patients is a point of ongoing controversy.

Pelvic fracture

Pediatric pelvic fractures can have an immense effect on the health of affected children. Mortality is less common than in adults with one recent study reporting a 5% overall mortality rate among 722 pediatric patients with pelvic fractures reported in the NPTR, compared to a 17% mortality rate among similar injuries in an adult population.[46] However, associated injuries, including abdominal, genitourinary and head trauma, are commonplace in both adults and children.[47,48]

There is a paucity of data regarding long-term outcomes including functional status and quality of life after pediatric pelvic fracture. In a review of 17 children under 12 years of age who sustained unstable pelvic ring fractures, Schwarz *et al.* found that bony asymmetry and malposition resulted in low back pain and functional impairment.[49] On the other hand, in a retrospective review of 54 children at a mean follow-up of 11 years, Rieger *et al.* found that long-term disability was rare and related to severe pelvic ring disruptions, acetabular fractures or concomitant injuries.[50] Noting that little is known about functional outcome in pelvic fractures in children, Upperman *et al.* reviewed the functional independence measure (FIM), which is part of many pediatric trauma registries, for a group of children who sustained pelvic fracture.[51] They found that a majority of children have significant limitations in locomotion and transfers at discharge.

The relative lack of data describing long-term outcomes in this area has led to significant controversy regarding the appropriate treatment of these uncommon but potentially devastating injuries. Some orthopedic surgeons have opted for a non-operative approach, even to unstable injuries, citing the potential for remodeling inherent in the immature skeleton.[52,53] On the other hand, others have opted towards surgical intervention.[49,54]

The American Pediatric Surgical Association Outcomes and Clinical Trials Centers began a study to evaluate the spectrum of pelvic fractures, and examine variability in clinical management, morbidity and functional outcomes utilizing a multi-center pediatric hospital network. Data was collected retrospectively on 240 children from 20 institutions.[55] Seventy percent had associated injuries, including 8.5% with bladder or urethral injuries. Only 21% required transfusion. Twenty-three percent had unstable fractures, and these were more likely to require transfusion, and have a longer LOS. Only 10% had operative intervention. The median time for ambulating with assistance and without assistance was 3 and 4 days, respectively, but significantly longer in patients with unstable fractures or associated injuries. Functional independence measurement (FIM) scores at discharge were available in 56/240 patients, and demonstrated significant disability at discharge. Seventy percent were discharged home, 9.5% home with nursing care, and 15.5% to rehabilitation or nursing facilities. Overall mortality was 5.5%. It was concluded that isolated pelvic fractures in children are associated with minimal in-hospital morbidity. There appears to be significant variability in orthopedic management of the fracture, and it is not clear whether this impacts outcome. FIM scores after discharge and other long-term follow-up data is scarce. This led to a prospective study examining functional status and quality of life 6 months after discharge following pelvic fracture.[56] Preliminary findings indicate that children with pelvic fractures improve their functional ability at 6 months after injury.

Generally speaking, treatment recommendations over the last decade have evolved towards more aggressive surgical treatment for childhood pelvic fractures in an attempt to improve anatomical reduction of the pediatric pelvis.[57] Nevertheless, there remains substantial variability in the orthopedic management of pediatric pelvic fractures. This variability reflects clinical uncertainty and demands rigorous, patient-based clinical research in this area comparing various treatment strategies and improved information regarding long-term, broadly defined outcomes of pediatric pelvic fracture. Further research is necessary to elucidate the intermediate and long-term outcomes of children with specific pelvic injuries and to help guide the appropriate indications for surgical intervention in this area.

Table 70.3. Life expectancy of children with spinal cord injury surviving at least 1 year postinjury

Current age	No SCI	Paraplegia	Tetraplegia	Ventilator dependent
5	71.6	59.5	52.6	39.4
10	66.6	54.6	47.6	34.9
15	61.7	49.8	43	30.4

Life expectancy in years. SCI = spinal cord injury.
Modified from Vogel, L. C. and Anderson, C. J. *Spinal Cord Med.* 2003; **26**:193–203.

Spinal cord injuries

Spinal cord injuries in childhood are uncommon, but devastating. Of 11 000 persons who suffer a spinal cord injury each year in the United States, approximately 1000 are aged 15 years or less. Nearly half of these children suffer a complete spinal cord injury with little prospect for significant improvement. Children surviving the first month after a spinal cord injury have an average life span of 60 years when paraplegic, and 52 years when tetraplegic (Table 70.3). The majority of children with spinal cord injuries complete high school, attend college and are ultimately employed.[58]

Significant recovery of motor function may occur over the first 3 months after injury. Further motor recovery, at a slower pace, may be noted over the next 6 months, with smaller improvements in functional recovery documented up to 2 years after injury.[59] The recovery of motor function occurs more rapidly with incomplete spinal cord injuries and is more likely to occur in younger patients. Despite this recovery, a motor examination performed 1 month following injury may be prognostic of ultimate recovery. The presence of even 1/5 strength in a muscle group 1 month after injury is associated with a 97% chance of recovery of antigravity strength (3/5) in that muscle group by 1 year after injury. In contrast, muscle groups with no strength (0/5) at one month have only a 10% chance of achieving antigravity strength by 1 year after injury.

A number of late effects of spinal cord injury, as well as a number of medical complications may adversely affect ultimate functional outcome.

Scoliosis is common following spinal cord injury in children, and its severity is increased by younger age at onset, complete lesions vs. incomplete, and paraplegia vs. tetraplegia.[60] Kyphosis also commonly occurs, and has been associated with an increased risk of syringomyelia when greater than 15 degrees. Whether associated with kyphosis or not, post-traumatic syringomyelia may occur in 25% of paraplegic patients, and may lead to progressive neurological deterioration. Progressive non-cystic tethering of the spinal cord has also been reported, and may lead to a similar neurological deterioration.[61] It is hoped that this late deterioration may be prevented with more aggressive spine stabilization.

Children with spinal cord injuries are at significantly increased risk of low-energy orthopedic injuries compared to patients without spinal cord injury. These fractures most commonly occur in the lower extremities. The femur is 32 times more likely to be fractured in a patient with a spinal cord injury.[62]

Urinary tract complications are common in children with a spinal cord injury. Shortly following injury, the majority of children are placed on a clean, intermittent catheterization schedule, which results in a lower urinary tract infection rate than an indwelling catheter.[63] The use of prophylactic antibiotics is controversial, and was not recommended by a recent national consensus panel. Renal calculi, typically struvite calculi, develop in a small percentage of children. Stones occur more frequently in children with complete spinal cord injuries, vesico-ureteral reflux, and permanent indwelling catheters.

Unlike other pediatric injury victims, children with a spinal cord injury are at risk for the development of venous thromboembolism (VTE) and pulmonary embolism. VTE develops in children with a spinal cord injury at the same rate as adults, in approximately 10% of patients.[64] The period of greatest risk is in the first 2 weeks after injury and persists for 8 to 12 weeks. Long-term sequelae of VTE in children with a spinal cord injury includes postphlebitic syndrome, which occurs in approximately 3% of children.[65]

Children with a spinal cord injury return quickly to school, a mean of 10 days following discharge from rehabilitation for paraplegic children and 62 days for tetraplegic children.[66] Educational performance among children with a spinal cord injury is excellent. In one study, most patients graduated from high school and pursued higher education. Many schools modified their curricula to accommodate the needs of the children, most of whom had teacher aides.

The prognosis may seem bleak for children with a high cervical spinal cord injury who leave the hospital ventilator-dependent. However, Oo *et al.* found that, of 107 adult patients who were ventilator dependent upon discharge, 21% subsequently recovered adequate diaphragmatic function to allow them to be weaned from the ventilator.[67] Many of these patients required more than a year to recover sufficient diaphragmatic strength to not require ventilator support.

Bowel problems are common following spinal cord injury. Goetz studied 88 children with spinal cord injuries and found that 68% reported that their bowel habits interfered with school and other activities and resulted in dissatisfaction.[68] Most patients require the long-term use of oral and/or rectal medications for bowel control. Krogh reported that up to 75% of patients report at least a few episodes of fecal incontinence per month, and that nearly 1/3 felt that their bowel problems were more burdensome than their sexual or urologic dysfunction.[69]

Issues such as these contribute to dissatisfaction with the quality of life after spinal cord injury. Using standardized measures of quality of life, Kannisto found that patients with a spinal cord injury scored significantly lower than the population sample. Not surprisingly, patients with spinal cord injury placed greater significance upon the measures for mental functioning, communicating and social participation.[70] Gorman examined the psychological health of 86 children who suffered a spinal cord injury prior to 16 years of age, and found that self-esteem, depression and self-perception were lower than average, regardless of the age or level of injury.[71]

REFERENCES

1. Fabian, T. C. Evidence-based medicine in trauma care: whither goest thou? *J. Trauma* 1999; **47**:225–232.
2. McPherson, K., Wennberg, J. E., Hovind, O. B., & Clifford, P. Small-area variations in the use of common surgical procedures: an international comparison of New England, England, and Norway. *N. Engl. J. Med.* 1982; **307**:1310–1304.
3. Wennberg, D. E., Lucas, F. L., Birkmeyer, J. D., *et al.* Variation in carotid endarterctomy mortality in the Medicare population: trial hospitals, volume, and patient characteristics. *J. Am. Med. Assoc.* 1998; **279**:1278–1281.
4. Potoka, D. A., Schall, L. C., Gardner, M. J. *et al.* Impact of pediatric centers on mortality in a statewide system. *J. Trauma* 2000; **49**:237–245.
5. Osler, T. M., Vane, D. W., Tepas, J. J., *et al.* Do pediatric trauma centers have better survival rates than adult trauma centers? An examination of the National Pediatric Trauma Registry. *J. Trauma* 2001; **50**:96–101.
6. Doolin, E. J., Browne, A. M., & DiScala, C. Pediatric trauma center criteria: an outcome analysis. *J. Pediatr. Surg.* 1999; **34**:885–890.
7. Keller, M. S. & Vane, D. W. Management of pediatric blunt splenic injury: comparison of pediatric and adult trauma surgeons. *J. Pediatr. Surg.* 1995; **30**:221–225.
8. Mooney, D. P., Birkmeyer, N. J. O., Udell, J. V. *et al.* Variation in the management of pediatric splenic injuries in New Hampshire. *J. Pediatr. Surg.* 1998; **33**:1076–1080.

9. Mooney, D. P. & Forbes, P. W. Variation in the management of pediatric splenic injuries in New England. *J. Trauma* 2004; **56**:328–333.
10. Guice, K. S. Unpublished communication.
11. Nakayama, D. K., Copes, W. S., & Sacco, W. Differences in truama care among pediatric and nonpediatric trauma centers. *J. Pediatr. Surg.* 1992; **27**(4):427–431.
11a. Aitken, M. E., Tilford, J. M., Barrett, K. W. *et al.* Health Status of children after admission for injury. *Pediatrics* 2002; **110**(2 pt 1):337–342.
12. Landgraf, J. M., Maunsell, E., Speechley, K. N. *et al.* Canadian–French, German and UK versions of the Child Health Questionnaire: methodology and preliminary item scaling results. *Qual. Life Res.* 1998; **7**(5):433–445.
13. Daltroy, L. H., Liang, M. H., Fossel, A. H. *et al.* The POSNA pediatric musculoskeletal functional health questionnaire: report on reliability, validity, and sensitivity to change. Pediatric Outcomes Instrument Development Group. Pediatric Orthopaedic Society of North America. *J. Pediatr Orthop.* 1998; **18**(5):561–571.
14. van der Sluis, C. K., Kingma J., Eisma, W. H., & ten Duis, H. J. Pediatric polytrauma: short-term and long-term outcomes. *J. Trauma* 1997; **43**(3):501–506.
15. Wesson, D. E., Scorpio, R. J., Spence, L. J. *et al.* The physical, psychological, and socioeconomic costs of pediatric trauma. *J. Trauma* 1992; **33**(2):252–255; discussion 255–257.
16. Wesson, D. & Hu, X. The real incidence of pediatric trauma. *Semin. Pediatr. Surg.* 1995; **4**(2):83–87.
17. Valadka, S., Poenaru, D., & Dueck, A. Long-term disability after trauma in children. *J. Pediatr. Surg.* 2000; **35**(5):684–687.
18. Stylianos, S. and the APSA Trauma Committee. Evidence-based guidelines for resource utilization in children with isolated spleen or liver injury. *J. Pediatr. Surg.* 2000; **35**:64–169.
19. Stylianos, S. and the APSA Trauma Study Group. Prospective validation of evidence-based guidelines for resource utilization in children with isolated spleen or liver injury. *J. Pediatr. Surg.* 2002; **37**:453–456.
20. Leinwand, M. J., Atkinson, C. C., & Mooney, D. P. Application of the APSA evidence-based guidelines for isolated liver or spleen injuries: a single institution experience. *J. Pediatr. Surg.* 2004; **39**:487–490.
21. Norotsky, M. C., Rogers, F. B., Shackford, S. R. Delayed presentation of splenic artery pseudoaneurysms following blunt abdominal trauma: case reports. *J. Trauma* 1995; **38**:444–447.
22. Lovvorn, H. N. Nonoperative management of splenic trauma in children: failure, complications, and pseudoaneurysms. Unpublished communication.
23. Brown, S. L., Elder, J. S., & Spirank, J. P. Are pediatric patients more susceptible to major renal injury from blunt trauma? A comparative study. *J. Urol.* 1998; **160**:134–138.
24. Choprs, P., St. Vil, D., & Yazbeck. S. Blunt renal trauma: blessing in disguise. *J. Pediatr. Surg.* 2002; **37**:779–782.
25. McAleer, I. M., Kaplan, G. W., & LoSasso, B. E. Congenital urinary tract anomalies in pediatric renal trauma patients. *J. Urol.* 2002; **168**:1808–1810.
26. Smith, E. M., Elder, J. S., & Spirnak, J. P. Major blunt renal trauma in the pediatric population: is a nonoperative approach indicated? *J. Urol.* 1993; **149**:546–548.
27. Delarue, A., Merrot, T., Fahkro, A. *et al.* Major renal injuries in children: the renal incidence of kidney loss. *J. Pediatr. Surg.* 2002; **37**:1446–1450.
28. Margenthaler, J. A., Weber, T. R., & Keller, M. S. Blunt renal trauma in children: Experience with conservative management at a pediatric trauma center. *J. Trauma* 2002; **52**:928–932.
29. Bass, D. H., Semple, P. L., & Cywes, S. Investigation and management of blunt renal injuries in children: a review of 11 years' experience. *J. Pediatr. Surg.* 1991; **26**:196–200.
30. Abdalati, H., Bulas, D. I., Majd, M. *et al.* Blunt renal trauma in children: healing of renal injuries and recommendations for imaging follow-up. *Pediatr. Radiol.* 1994; **24**:573–576.
31. Patrick, D. A., Bensard, D. D., Moore, E. E. *et al.* Nonoperative management of solid organ injuries in children results in decreased blood utilization. *J. Pediatr. Surg.* 1999; **34**:1695–1699.
32. Baumann, L., Greenfield, S. P., Aker, J. *et al.* Nonoperative management of major blunt renal trauma in children: in hospital morbidity and long-term followup. *J. Urol.* 1992; **148**:691–693.
33. Jobst, M. A., Canty, T. G. Sr., & Lynch, F.P. Management of pancreatic injury in pediatric blunt abdominal trauma. *J. Pediatr. Surg.* 1999; **34**:818–824.
34. Canty, J. G. Sr. & Weinman, D. Treatment of pancreatic duct disruption in children by an endoscopically placed stent. *J. Pediatr. Surg.* 2001; **36**:345–348.
35. Canty, T. G. Sr. & Weinman, D. Management of major pancreatic duct injuries in children. *J. Trauma* 2001; **50**:1001–1007.
36. Shilyansky, J., Sen, L. M., Kreller, M. *et al.* Nonoperative management of pancreatic injuries in children. *J. Pediatr. Surg.* 1998; **33**:343–345.
37. Wales, P. W., Shuckett, B., & Kim, P. C. Longterm outcome of non-operative management of complete traumatic pancreatic transection in children. *J. Pediatr. Surg.* 2001; **36**:823–827.
38. Meier, D. R., Coln, C. D., Hicks, B. A., & Guzzetta, P. C. Early operation in patients with pancreas transsection. *J. Pediatr. Surg.* 2001: **36**:341–344.
39. McGahren, E.D., Magnuson, D., Schauer, R. T., & Tapper, D. Management of transection of the pancreas in children. *Aust. N. Z. J. Surg.* 1995; **65**:242–246.
40. Rescorla, F. J., Plumkey, D. A., Sherman, S., Scherer, L. R. 3rd, West, K.W., & Grosfeld, J.L. The efficacy of early ERCP in pediatric pancreatic trauma. *J. Pediatr. Surg.* 1995; **30**:336–340.
41. Harrell, D. J., Vitale, G. C., & Larson, G. M. Selective role for endoscopic retrograde cholangiopancreatography in abdominal trauma. *Surg. Endosc* 1998; **12**:400–404.
42. Kim, H. S., Lee, D. K., Kim, I. W. *et al.* The role of retrograde pancreatography in the treatment of traumatic pancreatic duct injury. *Gastrointest. Endocs.* 2001; **54**:45–55.
43. Boman-Vermeeren, J. M., Vermeeren-Walters, G., Broos, P., & Eggermont, E. Somatastatin in the treatment of a pancreatic

pseudocyst in a child. *J. Pediatr. Gastroenterol. Nutr.* 1996; **23**:422–425.

44. Soto, J. A., Alvarez, O., Munera, F., Yepes, N. L., Sepulveda, M. E., & Perez, J. M. Traumatic Disruption of the pancreatic duct; diagnosis with MR Pancreatography. *Am. J. Roentgenol.* 2001; **176**:175–178.
45. Kouchi, K., Tanabe, M., Yoshida, H. *et al.* Nonoperative management of blunt pancreatic injury in children. *J. Pediatr. Surg.* 1999; **34**:1736–1738.
46. Ismail, N., Bellemare, J. F., Mollitt, D. L. *et al.* Death from pelvic fracture: children are different. *J. Pediatr. Surg.* 1996; **31**(1):82–85.
47. Mosheiff, R., Suchar, A., Porat, S. *et al.* The "Crushed open pelvis" in children. *Injury* 1999; **30 Suppl 2**:B14–B18.
48. Garvin, K. L., McCarthy, R. E., Barnes, C. L. *et al.* Pediatric pelvic ring fractures. *J. Pediatr. Orthop.* 1990; **10**(5):577–582.
49. Schwarz, N., Posch, E., Mayr, J. *et al.* Long-term results of unstable pelvic ring fractures in children. *Injury* 1998; **29**(6):431–433.
50. Rieger, H. & Burg, E. Fractures of the pelvis in children. *Clin. Orthop. Rel. Res.* 1997; **336**:226–239.
51. Upperman, J. S., Gardner, M., Gaines, B. *et al.* Early functional outcome in children with pelvic fractures. *J. Pediatr. Surg.* 2000; **35**(6):1002–1005.
52. Lane-O'Kelly, A., Fogarty, E., & Dowling, F. The pelvic fracture in childhood: a report supporting nonoperative management [see comments]. *Injury* 1995; **26**(5):327–329.
53. Pohlemann, T. & Williams, W. W. The pelvic fracture in childhood: a report supporting nonoperative management [letter; comment]. *Injury* 1995; **26**(10):708–709.
54. Van den Bosch, E. W., Van der Kleyn, R., Hogervosst, M. *et al.* Functional outcome of internal fixation for pelvic ring fractures. *J. Trauma* 1999; **47**(2):365–371.
55. Winthrop, A. L., Krishnan, A., Stylianos, S. *et al.* The spectrum of pediatric pelvic fractures: a multi-center study. *J. Trauma* 2005; **58**:468–474.
56. Signorino, P. R., Densmore, J., Winthrop, A. *et al.* Pediatric pelvic injury: Functional outcome at 6 month follow-up. *J. Pediatr. Surg.* 2005; **40**:107–113.
57. Korovessis, Baikousis, A., Stamatakis, M. *et al.* Medium and long term results of open reduction and internal fixation for unstable pelvic ring fractures. *Orthopedics* 2000; **23**(11):1165–1171.
58. Dudgeon, B. J., Massagali, T. L., & Ross, B. W. Educational participation of children with spinal cord injury. *Am. J. Occup. Ther.* 1997; **51**(7):553–561.
59. Ditunno, J. F., Jr., Stover, S. L., Freed, M. M. *et al.* Motor recovery of the upper extremities in traumatic quadriplegia: a multicenter study. *Arch. Phys. Med. Rehabil.* 1990; **73**(5):431–436.
60. Bergstrom, E. M., Short, D. J., Frankel, H. L. *et al.* The effect of childhood spinal cord injury on skeletal development: a retrospective study. *Spinal Cord* 1999; **37**(12):838–846.
61. Falci, S. P., Lammertse, D. P., Best, L. *et al.* Surgical treatment of posttraumatic cystic and tethered spinal cords. *J. Spinal Cord Med.* 1999; **22**(3):173–181.
62. Vestergaard, P., Krogh, K., Rejnmark, L. *et al.* Fracture rates and risk factors for fractures in patients with spinal cord injury. *Spinal Cord* 1998; **36**(11):790–796.
63. Cass, A. S., Luxenberg, M., Gleich, P. *et al.* Clean intermittent catheterization in the management of the neurogenic bladder in children. *J. Urol.* 1984; **132**(3):526–528.
64. Radecki, R. T. & Gaebler-Spira, D. Deep vein thrombosis in the disabled pediatric population. *Arch. Phys. Med. Rehabil.* 1994; **75**(3):248–250.
65. David, M. & Andrew, M. Venous thromboembolic complications in children [see comments]. *J. Pediatr.* 1993; **123**(3):337–346.
66. Sandford, P. R., Falk-Palec, D. J., & Spears, K. Return to school after spinal cord injury. *Arch. Physi. Med. Rehabil.* 1999; **80**(8):885–888.
67. Oo, T., Watt, J. W., Soni, B. M. *et al.* Delayed diaphragm recovery in 12 patients after high cervical spinal cord injury. A retrospective review of the diaphragm status of 107 patients ventilated after acute spinal cord injury. *Spinal Cord* 1999; **37**(2):117–122.
68. Goetz, L. L., Hurvitz, E. A., Nelson, V. S. *et al.* Bowel management in children and adolescents with spinal cord injury. *J. Spinal Cord Med.* 1998; **21**(4):335–341.
69. Krogh, K., Nielsen, J., Djurhuus, J. C. *et al.* Colorectal function in patients with spinal cord lesions. *Dis. Colon Rectum* 1997; **40**(10):1233–1239.
70. Kannisto, M. & Sintonen, H. Later health-related quality of life in adults who have sustained spinal cord injury in childhood. *Spinal Cord* 1997; **35**(11):747–751.
71. Gorman, C., Kennedy, P., & Hamilton, L. R. Alterations in self-perceptions following childhood onset of spinal cord injury. *Spinal Cord* 1998; **36**(3):181–185.

Part IX

Miscellaneous

71

Vascular access

A. Martin Barrett[1] and Roly Squire[2]

[1]Royal Victoria Infirmary, Newcastle upon Tyne, UK
[2]St. James's University Hospital and Leeds General Infirmary, Leeds, UK

Introduction

The intravascular administration of drugs has a long history, dating back to at least the seventeenth century, when William Harvey defined vascular anatomy (*Exercitatio Anatomica De Motu Cordis et Sanguinis*). However, early techniques were crude, relying on natural materials such as quill and bladder. A significant advance occurred in 1853, when Alexander Wood employed the recently developed needle and syringe to give intravenous medications. Contemporary practice is based on these early developments, but it is only in the last 50 years that progressive refinements of equipment and technique have allowed the routine use of vascular access through various routes. In 1952 Aubaniac introduced a technique for central venous catheterization,[1] and bravely stated "elle est strictement sans danger". Many subsequent publications have demonstrated the overconfidence of this pronouncement but, at the same time, reviews of the various procedures have shown that vascular access can be performed effectively with a high degree of safety. In the UK, the National Institute for Clinical Excellence (NICE) has issued guidance which recommends the use of ultrasound guidance for percutaneous cannulation of the internal jugular veins in all patients over 3 kg.[2] Table 71.1 outlines the range of vascular access procedures currently in common usage. Unfortunately, there are very little data on long-term outcomes. In particular, there are no long-term longitudinal cohort studies in children. Our current knowledge is therefore based on extrapolation from published short- to mid-term data.

Complications of vascular access

The most serious problems caused by vascular access are due to the presence of an intravascular foreign body. Other complications relate to the techniques used to insert and access the catheter, the size of the catheter in relation to the size and age of the patient,[3] the mode of delivery of drugs or infusions, and the composition of the infusate. Table 71.2 lists the most common complications of vascular access, all of which may have an impact on long-term outcomes. These are now considered in more detail.

Infection

The commonest complication related to long-term vascular access is that of infection. *There is no generally agreed definition of catheter-related sepsis.* Depending on the criteria used, infection can occur in as many as 40% of cases. The commonest organisms are gram-positive (78%–96%), followed by gram-negative (4%–20%), and then fungal (3%).[4] A number of reports have suggested lower rates of catheter-related sepsis associated with the use of implantable ports. Whilst line sepsis is usually an indication for removal of temporary access catheters, indwelling devices are often precious, and it is therefore currently common practice to attempt to salvage the line with antibiotic therapy. Approximately two-thirds of such episodes can be treated without catheter removal providing they are not fungal in origin.[5,6] Catheter sepsis is often associated with intravascular

Pediatric Surgery and Urology: Long-term Outcomes, Mark Stringer, Keith Oldham, Pierre Mouriquand.
Published by Cambridge University Press.

Table 71.1. Common indications for vascular access and routes of administration

	Procedure	Indications
Short term	Peripheral venous	Fluid and drug administration
	Peripheral arterial	Monitoring
		Sampling
	Central venous	Hemodialysis
		Parenteral nutrition
		ECMO
	PICC	Parenteral nutrition
	Central arterial	Radiologic procedures
		ECMO
		Cardiovascular monitoring
		Cardiac output measurement
	Intraosseus	Resuscitation
Long term	Central venous	Parenteral nutrition
		Cytotoxic chemotherapy
		Hemodialysis
		Prolonged antibiotic therapy
		Regular transfusion
		Coagulation products
		Immunoglobulin infusion
		Bone marrow transplantation
		Stem cell harvest
	Central arterial	Regional chemotherapy

PICC: peripherally inserted central venous catheter.
ECMO: extra corporeal membrane oxygenation.

Table 71.2. Common complications of vascular access

Infection	
Thrombosis/thromboembolism	
Extravasation/migration	
Malposition/displacement	
Vascular stenosis	
Catheter fracture and embolization	
Surgical injury:	nerve
	lymphatic
	vascular
	pleura
Poor cosmesis	

or pericatheter thrombosis,[7] and line malfunction often precedes clinical signs of infection or thrombosis.

Factors that predispose to catheter sepsis include immunosuppression, antibiotic therapy, short bowel syndrome, infection elsewhere, poor catheter care, length of time the catheter is in situ, presence of a fibrin sheath,[8] and length of hospitalization. The administration of total parenteral nutrition in association with chemotherapy more than doubles the infection risk for central venous catheters (CVCs). There is some evidence to suggest that the use of single-shot antibiotic prophylaxis at the time of catheter insertion reduces the risk of subsequent infection.

Whilst little long-term morbidity would be expected in survivors of simple line infections, in a small proportion of patients complications of the bacteremia may have long-term implications; these include renal failure, brain abscess, and endocarditis.

Thrombosis

Thrombosis, and especially thromboembolic phenomena, are assuming greater importance as an expanding cohort of children have CVCs for longer periods of time. Data from the Canadian Childhood Thrombophilia Registry have shown that central venous lines are the leading risk factor for venous thromboembolic disease in childhood and infancy.[9] The Registry has also reported a mortality of nearly 4% directly related to central venous line thrombosis, as well as a significant recurrent thrombosis rate.[10] If catheter care is suboptimal, the likelihood of thrombus occluding the lumen increases. Regular flushing of catheters is essential; flushing with a mixture of heparin and urokinase[11] may be the most effective method of preventing clot formation. Catheter-related thrombosis can also be reduced by inserting heparin-bonded catheters and this may also reduce sepsis rates. Once a clot has formed treatment with urokinase, by bolus or infusion, often successfully unblocks the lumen. In the authors' experience, 80% of pediatric hemodialysis catheters contain clot fragments despite these precautions (M. Coulthard, personal communication, 1996). Newer recombinant thrombolytic agents such as alteplase[12] may have a role in the prevention and treatment of these clots.

There is a greater risk of intravascular thrombosis with catheters in the inferior vena cava as compared with the superior vena cava.[13] Silicone catheters appear to be associated with a higher incidence of thrombosis than polyurethane catheters, resulting in more frequent late obstruction. There is also some evidence that parenteral nutrition predisposes to catheter thrombosis.[14] Fortunately, clinical thrombosis in premature infants, currently the largest population receiving parenteral nutrition, is rare.[15] However, long-term survivors may have a degree of cardiopulmonary compromise consequent on catheter thromboembolism, which will not become apparent for many years. In some groups of patients (e.g., diabetics, thalassemics, children receiving long-term TPN) concurrent treatment with low molecular weight heparin or warfarin has been recommended.[16,17]

Extravasation and catheter migration

There are several different ways in which fluid extravasation can complicate vascular access. The severity of this complication depends on the toxicity of the infusate and the site of the leakage. Peripheral venous catheters frequently "tissue" – indeed this is a common signal to indicate the need for a new cannula. Extravasation from central lines is much rarer, occurring in about 1% of neonatal CVCs.[18] Infusions liable to cause significant local tissue damage are generally not given via peripheral venous catheters but, unfortunately, this is not always the case. Extravasation from either central or peripheral catheters can cause significant short- and long-term morbidity. Infusion into subcutaneous tissues may cause tissue necrosis, particularly if the infusate contains calcium, bicarbonate, or toxic drugs such as chemotherapy agents or thiopentone.[19] Immediate subcutaneous irrigation with saline or hyaluronidase has been shown to reduce the amount of tissue damage,[20,21] and the addition of an intralesional steroid injection may help further. Other local measures, such as cooling the area, or topical dimethylsulfoxide, may also ameliorate the injury. Liposuction has been used to remove necrotic tissue in an attempt to preserve overlying skin. Occasionally, specific antidotes are available. Unfortunately, despite its common usage, elevation of the affected area is probably of limited value.[22]

Extravasation from CVCs may result in direct leakage through the vessel wall causing cardiac tamponade, hydrothorax, or even peritonitis. Catheters inserted from the left side of the neck have an increased risk of damaging the right wall of the superior vena cava. Infusates may also track back along the fibrin sheath, which surrounds the intravascular portion of the catheter. Migration of the tip of the catheter results in the infusate reaching unexpected places such as the bronchus or even the spinal canal. If a catheter tip within the superior vena cava migrates into the azygos vein, it may result in catheter blockage and venous thrombosis. Migration into the vertebral veins can cause brachial neuropathy.

Fracture of the external part of a CVC in the absence of external physical abuse is now rare since most catheters have a reinforced section for use with the clamp. However, up to 14% of lines still suffer a split or fracture during their life. This is often as a result of a distal obstruction and the high intraluminal pressures exerted in trying to unblock the line. Although fractures in the external portion of a CVC can be easily repaired, they do expose the patient to risks from infection or skin injury from leakage of toxic fluid.

Important measures can be taken to prevent extravasation. Toxic agents should not be infused into central catheters without first checking that blood can be aspirated through the line, or into peripheral catheters that have not first been tested with a benign solution such as 0.9% saline. Dislodgement of the access needle from a subcutaneous port during infusion of cytotoxic therapy poses a particular hazard. These needles must be secured well, and the child carefully observed for signs of discomfort. A policy of regular examination of all catheter and cannula sites should at least minimize any damage caused by extravasation.

The long-term outcome after an extravasation episode will depend on the amount of tissue lost, and the site of the injury. Minimization of the extent of the necrosis means that currently the majority of these injuries heal fully with no long-term sequelae.[20] However, skin grafting is sometimes required and scarring from these injuries can be particularly damaging over joint surfaces, resulting in long-term disability. Unusual problems such as diaphragmatic paralysis have been reported. Even if function is normal, the scar will be there for life, and cosmetic complications of treatment can be surprisingly disruptive to the normal social development of a child.

Malposition or dislodgement

Dislodgement from a previously satisfactory position is mainly restricted to external central venous catheters. However, the definition of what constitutes a "satisfactory position" is a matter of debate. Some clinicians believe the catheter tip must be in the right atrium whereas others suggest that fewer problems occur with catheter tips in the superior vena cava. A survey of catheter tip positions in the United Kingdom suggested that 21% were positioned in the superior vena cava, 11% at the junction between the cava and atrium, and 62% in the right atrium.[23] Catheters placed via the superior vena cava, with the catheter tip located low in the right atrium, are liable to migrate through the tricuspid or even pulmonary valves, possibly producing tricuspid incompetence, ventricular dysrhythmias or impedance of pulmonary blood flow (particularly if thrombus formation occurs). Line tips left too high in the superior vena cava are more likely to malfunction, or even become dislodged completely from the venous system resulting in extravasation. Lines can also be unintentionally advanced into inappropriate veins at the time of insertion, for example into an anomalous pulmonary vein, an internal mammary vein or the azygos vein.[24]

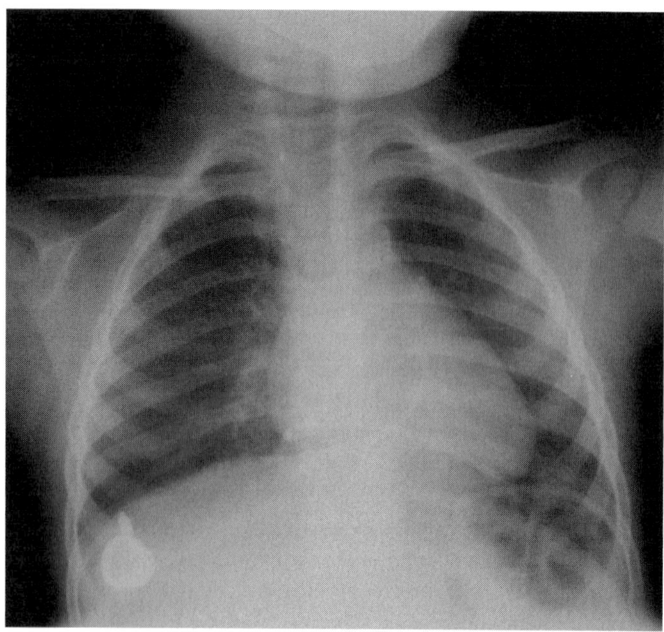

(a)

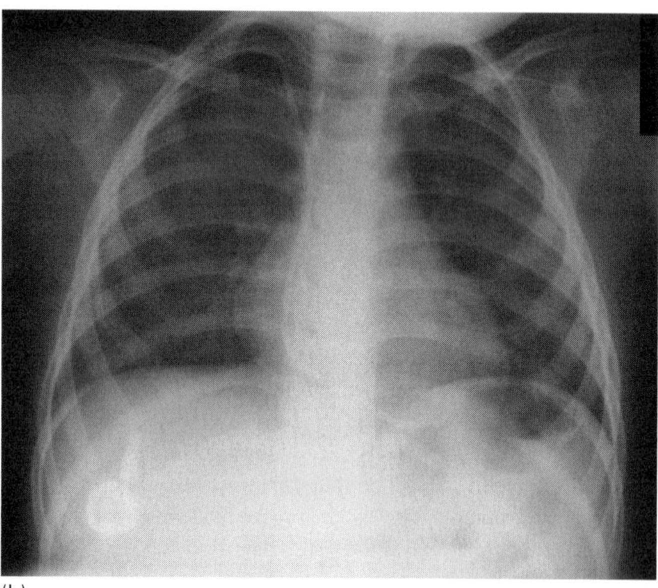

(b)

Fig. 71.1. These radiographs show two examples of totally implantable venous access devices complicated by line fracture. Both lines have broken at the junction with the port, a common site of fracture. The other common site of fracture is where the catheter crosses the clavicle (or first rib with subclavian lines).
(a) The fractured line in this patient had migrated into the right atrium and ventricle and was successfully removed by an interventional radiologist
(b) The fractured line in this patient was adherent to its subcutaneous fibrin sheath and was removed without difficulty

A United Kingdom Children's Cancer Study Group (UKCCSG) prospective audit of 824 CVCs used in pediatric oncology patients showed that the need for a perioperative platelet transfusion, the use of multilumen external CVCs, the absence of an exit site suture, and patient age under 2 years were all associated with a higher risk of early dislodgement of the catheter.[25] Two-thirds of dislodgements occurred in the first seven weeks after insertion. Good line fixation is clearly important in preventing this complication. A variety of garments can be used to keep the external portion of the catheter shielded from prying fingers. These measures help to minimize complications related to dislodgement.

Vascular stenosis

Stenosis in association with vascular access has most commonly been reported in patients undergoing hemodialysis (see below). However, vascular narrowing is likely in many patients where vessels have been used for vascular access. Fortunately, this seems to be of little long-term clinical significance. Occasionally, asymptomatic narrowing is important because it prevents the vein being recannulated in patients who are dependent on long-term central venous access. With careful surgery it is often possible to maintain patency of veins such as the internal jugular even after open insertion of a long-term CVC. One of the authors has confirmed an 80% patency rate when the vein is used for a second time.[26] Some veins do become occluded as a result of cannulation, and this can result in inadequate venous drainage producing such problems as the "superior vena cava syndrome." Generally, the effects of this resolve spontaneously as collateral veins enlarge once the CVC has been removed.

Catheter fracture resulting in foreign body embolism

There are numerous anecdotal reports of catheter fragment embolism into the right side of the heart, pulmonary arteries or lung (Fig. 71.1). Fracture of a CVC distal to the retaining cuff is most likely to occur at the time of line removal, though it can occur at any time as a result of stress on the catheter as it crosses bony prominences. One of the authors has experience of this complication occurring at the site of a purse-string suture being placed around the catheter central to the cuff. Fortunately, catheter embolism is not usually fatal. Percutaneous retrieval of catheter fragments is successful in more than 90% of cases, with minimal adverse effects.[27] A recent report suggested that in some cases retained catheter fragments could be left in situ without risk, at least in the medium term.[28]

Table 71.3. Rare complications of vascular access

Infected retained cuff
Inability to remove catheter
Adverse reaction to catheter material
Vocal cord paralysis
Horner's syndrome
Superior vena caval syndrome
Cervical oropharyngeal edema
Hypoacusia
Chest pain
Back pain
Iliac artery aneurysm
Pseudotumor cerebri
Aortoatrial fistula
Arteriovenous fistula
Air embolism
Meningitis
Discitis: disc prolapse
Glomerulonephritis
Enteral formula infusion

Surgical injury

At the time of central line insertion there is a risk of damage to adjacent structures, such as arteries, nerves, lymphatics and the lung. The use of superficial veins such as the external jugular, cephalic, and long saphenous may minimize this risk, and help to preserve patency of larger central veins.

Rare complications

There are a large number of case reports highlighting unusual problems that can occur as a result of vascular access. Although many of these are reported in adult patients there is clearly the potential for them to occur in all age groups. Table 71.3 lists some examples.

Long-term outcomes

Vascular access for chemotherapy

A great deal is already known about the causes of early line complications, but there are little data on long-term outcomes. Much of the current literature is in the form of retrospective analyses and many of the published findings need to be confirmed by prospective studies. However, more than 70% of children with malignant disease are now long-term survivors, and members of this ever-expanding cohort are being monitored regularly in long-term follow-up clinics. Late effects related to vascular access are not being reported, despite the occasional extravasation incident occurring during therapy. This is clearly encouraging, but needs validation.

Vascular access for parenteral nutrition

Nutritional support was the first indication for long-term central venous access in children, and remains one of the commonest indications for central line insertion. In premature infants peripherally inserted central catheters (PICCs) predominate, and these appear to have minimal long-term sequelae. PICCs can occasionally be difficult to remove, risking line fracture and embolization, but there are no reports of late problems as a result of this.

Direct central venous cannulation via the jugular vein has also been studied in neonates. One long-term follow-up study of neonates who had developed jugular thrombi from central venous catheterization showed that almost 25% still had partial or complete obstruction to jugular blood flow at a mean age of 4 years.[29] However, this was clinically insignificant.

In short gut syndrome cuffed external central venous catheters such as Hickman(R) or Broviac(R) catheters are frequently used. These catheters are prone to the same range of complications as other CVCs. Moukarzel *et al.*[30] reported on the outcome of 27 children receiving parenteral nutrition (PN) through CVCs for more than 5 years, with good success. Line infection occurred on average every 884 days, and was the commonest reason for line removal and replacement. The frequency of infection may be particularly important in this group of children since it may accelerate the development of liver failure, a critical complication with regard to prognosis. Candida infection may occur in 5% of patients receiving PN via a central line;[31] administration of broad-spectrum antibiotics being a particular risk factor. Fungal sepsis is difficult and often impossible to eradicate without line removal. Concomitant neutropenia or steroid use is associated with an increased mortality.

Recent reports have highlighted the particular risk of thrombus formation and thromboembolism in these children. Pulmonary embolism was thought to be a rare complication of long-term PN, but anecdotal reports of this complication have since been followed by studies screening cohorts of children on home PN.[32,33] Dollery *et al.* studied 34 children on long-term PN and reported a 26% 5-year mortality from thrombotic events; only 53% of patients were free from any evidence of thromboembolism. It is uncertain as to whether interventions such as periodically

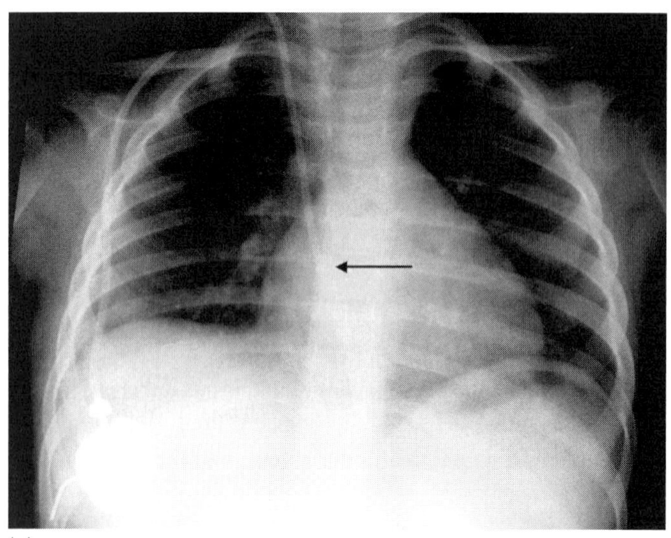
(a)

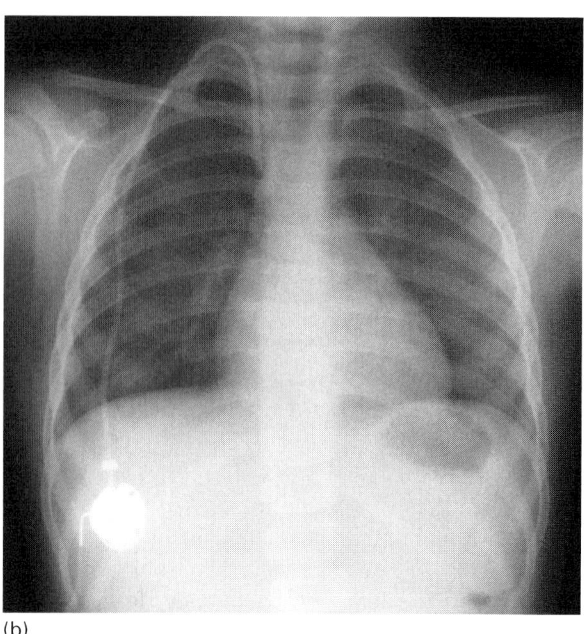
(b)

Fig. 71.2. Catheter tip migration with growth of the child. This 2-year-old girl had a port inserted with the catheter tip in the right atrium (a) but 26 months later when the line was malfunctioning, a radiograph showed that the catheter tip was high in the superior vena cava.

changing the catheter or the regular infusion of thrombolytic agents will reduce this risk.

In addition to the risk of sudden, unexpected, late death from pulmonary embolism, some children on long-term PN suffer respiratory symptoms thought to be due to catheter-related microemboli. The resultant compromise of cardiopulmonary function may preclude potentially life-saving transplant procedures.[34]

Despite these problems home PN monitored by a specialist support team can be provided safely over many years.[34,35]

Vascular access in cystic fibrosis

In the mid 1980s totally implantable venous access devices (ports) were introduced as a convenient route for intermittent antibiotic therapy in children with cystic fibrosis (CF), and subsequent experience confirmed their advantages.[36] Initial reports mainly related to Port-a-cath[(R)] systems, but recently there has been a trend towards smaller more discreet devices, such as the P.A.S. port[(R)]. These systems can remain in place for many years, and in some cases the access device can outlast the patient. However, removal is sometimes necessary, and it is reasonable to suppose that all of these devices have a finite life dictated by the nature of their material, and influenced by the number of needle punctures. With the growing number of children who have had a single port for more than 5 years, a picture of long-term function is emerging, which is generally encouraging. In early published data the overall complication rate was 1 in 1483 catheter days, infection occurring at a rate of 1 in 5929 days, while mechanical complications occurred in 1 in 1976 days.[37] Unpublished data from one of the authors' institution relate to 43 implantable access devices in children with CF (E. Moya, personal communication, 1997). These ports had been in place for between 9 and 77 months (median 24 months). Ten had to be removed due to complications: six for blockage, three for infection and one for line fracture. Nearly half of the devices gave problems in sampling blood, and some had become temporarily blocked requiring thrombolytic therapy. However, most of the catheters were of great value for a prolonged period. Even a port which had been in place for over 6 years had been accessed fewer than 100 times, well within the limit recommended by the manufacturer.

There are some specific late complications that should be highlighted in these children. First, catheter disconnection and embolization was observed in early reports; the catheter was usually retrieved without major complications and no fatal outcome was reported. Although this is not a common complication, this type of event may be seen more frequently as catheters currently in place for more than 5 years approach their recommended life expectancy.

Second, children with CF and implantable access devices appear to be prone to candidemia. Late fungal infections have been reported,[38] the risk probably being directly related to the length of time the catheter is in place. Certain risk factors predispose to candidemia, including severe background respiratory deficiency, acute respiratory exacerbation, malnutrition, repeated and frequent broad-spectrum antibiotic therapy, parenteral nutrition, and diabetes mellitus. Fungal infection in these patients is an indication for system removal in order to reduce mortality and morbidity,[6] and a low threshold for suspecting candidemia in these patients is advised.

A third major long-term risk is thrombosis. Superior vena caval thrombosis was associated with 3 of 22 catheters in the series reported by Sola *et al.*,[37] who consequently recommended aspirin prophylaxis in these patients. The risk of this complication may be reduced by good catheter care and appropriate placement. It should be remembered, however, that, if a catheter is to remain in situ for many years in a growing child, the position of the tip will inevitably change in relation to the heart and major vessels (Fig. 71.2). There are no data to indicate if there is a role for prophylactic revision in these children to ensure longer and safer function, but presumably with continued close follow-up of these children these issues will be addressed. There have been no randomized studies looking at the prevention and management of these complications or the long-term outcomes of children with CF and totally implantable venous access devices.[39]

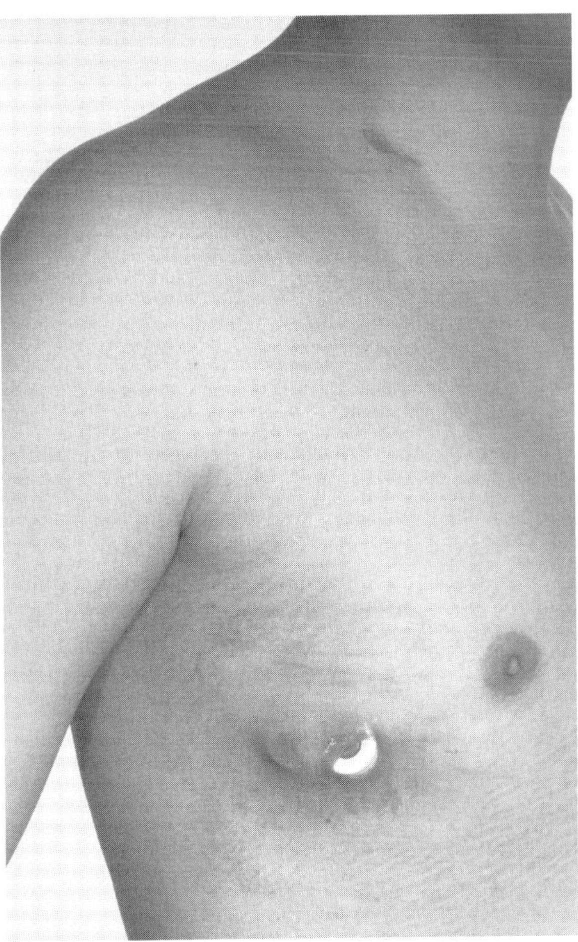

Fig. 71.3. Erosion of a totally implantable venous access device through the skin. Erosion may signify low-grade infection but, in this case, cultures were sterile.

Vascular access for coagulopathies and other indications

Long-term vascular access is being used increasingly for a number of less common indications, such as for factor VIII administration in hemophiliacs, and regular blood transfusion in children with thalassemia. For these children requiring only intermittent venous access, subcutaneous ports are ideal. Arteriovenous fistulae are an alternative in selected cases.[40] Ports are also generally preferred for similar reasons in the small group of patients with inborn errors of metabolism in whom venous access, usually in a crisis, is either difficult or impossible. These children are generally otherwise healthy, with normal immunity, and they tolerate long-term venous access well.[41] In such cases ports are reported to have an average lifespan of approximately 2 years, although many will remain functional for much longer. Repeated use tends to eventually result in erosion of the skin overlying the port (Fig. 71.3); this is more liable to become a problem after about 5 years of continued use, with many ports likely to need revision within 7 years.[42,43] However, many hemophilic children need just one port to help them through a difficult period (e.g., from infancy to early childhood) following which they can successfully use peripheral cannulas. Most port removals in this population are for catheter-related sepsis, with infection occurring at a rate of approximately 0.7 per 1000 days.[44] Ports are sometimes removed because of malfunction due to catheter tip migration (as the child grows), pain from the needle access site after repeated use, and thrombus formation.

Patients with chronic immunodeficiency states are most commonly managed with external central venous catheters since their treatment regimens are so intensive. These lines are prone to the same complications as those seen in patients with malignancy who become immunosuppressed as a result of their disease and chemotherapy.

Vascular access for dialysis

Temporary vascular access is commonly required to manage acute renal failure in children. Chronic renal failure is preferentially managed by ambulatory peritoneal dialysis and subsequent renal transplant, but a few children are maintained on hemodialysis. Arteriovenous fistulae are often less successful in children than in adults, and so long-term central venous access is sometimes required.

Infection and thrombosis are the most common complications,[45] although in small children the size of the lumen and the difficulty in maintaining the position of a hemodialysis catheter for long periods may result in poor blood flow during dialysis.

Late complications are evident from the adult rather than the pediatric literature. The predominant long-term problem is central venous stenosis, which restricts the function of subsequently fashioned fistulae. Stenoses develop after 10% of catheter insertions into the internal jugular vein,[46] and can occur after just one week of dialysis. Stenosis is probably more likely if the hemodialysis catheter has been infected. Stenosis may cause the arm to be swollen, but the main problem is that it predisposes to subsequent fistula thrombosis.[47]

Arterial cannulation

Peripheral arterial cannulation is a standard component of intensive care in the management of very sick children and is used for both invasive monitoring and blood sampling. Central arterial catheterization is relatively common in sick newborns via the umbilical arterial route, and is also used in radiologic procedures, usually via the femoral route. Complications of arterial cannulation and catheterization are listed in Table 71.4. The most important complication relating to long-term outcome is irreversible distal ischemia. After radial artery cannulation the incidence of hand or forearm ischemia in neonates is probably less than 5%.[48] Only a small proportion of these children will go on to develop a significant long-term deficit, although severe ischemia necessitating amputation has been described after radial artery cannulation.[49]

After neonatal umbilical artery catheterization the incidence of aortic thrombosis as determined by Doppler ultrasound may be as high as 15%.[50] One large study demonstrated that catheter tips placed in the abdominal aorta caused more peripheral vascular problems than those in the thoracic aorta.[51] Rarely, thrombosis can necessitate lower limb amputation, and malpositioned catheters can cause massive infarction of pelvic and perineal tissues.[52]

Table 71.4. Complications of arterial cannulation

Ischemia	– thrombosis
	– embolism
	– spasm
	– catheter occlusion
Aneurysm	
Pseudoaneurysm	
Coarctation	
Bleeding	
Compartment syndrome	
Endocarditis	

Long-term sequelae of ischemia caused by arterial cannulation can be greatly reduced by rapid intervention. If the catheter is malpositioned, then immediate withdrawal or adjustment is indicated. Cannulas in distal vessels such as the radial artery are generally also best removed if any signs of ischemia develop. Correctly positioned central arterial catheters suspected of causing thrombosis may be retained initially for administration of thrombolytic therapy.[53] If the ischemia persists, then early surgical intervention is advisable.[54]

Careful placement of arterial cannulas/catheters reduces complications. Cannulas which do not completely occlude the arterial lumen should be selected. Ideally, peripheral arteries with adequate collateral flow, as demonstrated by a combination of digital pressure and Doppler flow studies, should be chosen. It is clear that arterial cannulation carries a risk of long-term morbidity and this should be borne in mind when considering the indication for the procedure. The incidence of severe disability or loss of limb is small, but the implications of even one case are enormous. These risks need to be fully discussed with parents, and clinicians must respond rapidly to these complications. Any adverse outcome is liable to have medicolegal implications, with high compensation costs.

Intraosseus infusion

Insertion of an intraosseus needle is now a standard technique when gaining emergency vascular access in children. There are no reports of the long-term follow-up of patients successfully resuscitated in this way, and true complication rates are currently unknown. However, the technique is usually tolerated well, provided it is used for short periods.

After intraosseus infusion, a compartment syndrome can occur requiring emergency decompression.[55] With immediate fasciotomy a good result can be expected, but this condition is easy to overlook in a sick child, and, if neglected, can result in a severe ischemic myopathy. Cases of massive distal tissue necrosis have been reported.[56]

Clearly long-term studies are needed, but when performing intraosseus infusion it should be remembered that there is a small but significant risk to the limb in the long term, ranging from cutaneous scarring to marked loss of function, and possibly even amputation.

Extracorporeal membrane oxygenation (ECMO)

Since Bartlett reported early successes using ECMO in 1982, a large cohort of children has emerged who have had large bore catheters inserted into their neck vessels, frequently both the right internal jugular vein and right common carotid artery. Neurologic complications may occur in as many as 24% of infants undergoing ECMO, two-thirds of whom may be long-term survivors.[57] The use of venovenous ECMO in some centers has halved the short-term neurologic complications, but the long-term implications are not clear. Since gross neurologic outcome following ECMO is comparable to that following conventional therapy, the influence of the vascular access procedure by itself may in fact be small.[58] However, concern about the potential role of carotid occlusion in the development of cerebral infarction has been commented upon by many authors, and there may be a case for arterial reconstruction after decannulation in order to improve cerebral blood flow.[59] Newer cannula materials and methods of insertion may further minimize morbidity.[60]

REFERENCES

1. Aubaniac, R. L'injection intraveneuse sous-claviculaire. *Presse Med.* 1952; **60**:1456.
2. National Institute for Clinical Excellence. Final Appraisal Determination. Ultrasound locating devices for placing central venous catheters. NICE guidelines – Aug.2002. www.nice.org.uk.
3. Janik, J. E., Conlon, S. J., & Janik, J. S. Percutaneous central access in patients younger than 5 years: size does matter. *J. Pediatr. Surg.* 2004; **39**:1252–1256.
4. Karthaus, M., Doellmann, T., Klimasch, T. *et al.* Central venous catheter infections in patients with acute leukaemia. *Chemotherapy* 2002; **48**:154–157.
5. Raad, I., Davies, S., Khan, A. *et al.* Impact of central venous catheter removal on the recurrence of catheter-related coagulase negative staphylococcal bacteremia. *Infect. Control Hosp. Epidemiol.* 1992; **13**:215–221.
6. Eppes, S. C., Troutman, J. L. & Gutman, L. T. Outcome of treatment of candidemia in children whose central catheters were removed or retained. *Pediatr. Infect. Dis. J.* 1989; **8**:99–104.
7. Raad, I. I., Luna, M., Khalil, S. A. *et al.* The relationship between the thrombotic and infectious complications of central venous catheters. *J. Am. Med. Assoc.* 1994; **271**:1014–1016.
8. Mehall, J. A., Saltzman, D. A., Jackson, R. J. *et al.* Fibrin sheath enhances central venous catheter infection. *Crit. Care Med.* 2002; **30**:908–912.
9. Massicote, P., Dix, D., Monagle, P. *et al.* Central venous catheter-related thrombus in children: analysis of the Canadian Registry of Thromboembolic Complications. *J. Pediatr.* 1998; **133**:770–776.
10. Monagle, P., Adams, M., Mahoney, M. *et al.* Outcome of paediatric thromboembolic disease. A report from the Canadian Childhood Thrombophilia Registry. *Pediatr. Res.* 2000; **47**:763–766.
11. Dillon, P. W., Jones, R., Bagnall-Reeb, H. A. *et al.* Prophylactic urokinase in the management of long-term venous access devices in children: a Children's Oncology Group study. *J. Clin. Oncol.* 2004; **22**:2718–2723.
12. Terrill, K. R., Lemons, R. S. & Goldsby, R. E. Safety, dose and timing of releplase in treating occluded central venous catheters in children with cancer. *J. Pediatr. Haematol. Oncol.* 2003; **25**:864–867.
13. Pippus, K. G., Giacomantonio, J. M., Gillis, D. A. *et al.* Thrombotic complications of saphenous central venous lines. *J. Pediatr. Surg.* 1994; **29**:1218–1219.
14. Ross, P. Jr., Ehrenkranz, R., Kleinman, C. S. *et al.* Thrombus associated with central venous catheters in infants and children. *J. Pediatr. Surg.* 1989; **24**:253–256.
15. Alkalay, A. L., Mazkereth, R., Santulli, T. Jr. *et al.* Central venous line thrombosis in premature infants: a case management and literature review. *Am. J. Perinatol.* 1993; **10**:323–326.
16. Newall, F., Barnes, C., Savoia, H. *et al.* Warfarin therapy in children who require long-term total parenteral nutrition. *Pediatrics* 2003; **112**:e386.
17. Worly, J. M., Fortenberry, J. D., Hansen, I. *et al.* Deep venous thrombosis in children with diabetic ketoacidosis and femoral central venous catheters. *Pediatrics* 2004; **113**:e57–e60.
18. Keeney, S. E. & Richardson, C. J. Extravascular extravasation of fluid as a complication of central venous lines in the neonate. *J. Perinatol.* 1995; **15**:284–288.
19. Kassner, E. Evaluation and treatment of chemotherapy extravasation injuries. *J. Pediatr. Oncol. Nursing* 2000; **17**:135–148.
20. Gault, D. T. Extravasation injuries. *Br. J. Plast. Surg.* 1993; **46**:91–96.
21. Davies, J., Gault, D., & Buchdahl, R. Preventing the scars of neonatal intensive care. *Arch. Dis. Child.* 1994; **70**:F50–F51.
22. Yucha, B., Hasting-Tolsma, M., & Szevenji, N. M. Effect of elevation on intravenous extravasation. *J. Intraven. Nursing* 1994; **17**:231–234.
23. Tweddle, D. A., Windebank, K. P., Barrett, A. M. *et al.* Central venous catheter usage in UKCCSG oncology centres. *Arch. Dis. Child.* 1997; **77**:58–59.

24. Lee, A. C., Patel, J. V., Picton, S. V. *et al.* Internal thoracic vein cannulation as a complication of central venous catheter insertion. *Med. Pediatr. Oncol.* 2003; **40**:195–196.
25. Barrett, A. M., Imeson, J., Leese, D. *et al.* Factors influencing early failure of central venous catheters in children with cancer. *J. Pediatr. Surg.* 2004; **39**:1520–1523.
26. Willetts, I. E., Ayodeji, M., Ramsden, W. H. *et al.* Venous patency after open central venous cannulation. *Pediatr. Surg. Int.* 2000; **16**:411–413.
27. Angel, C. Y., Brenot, P., Rion, J. Y. *et al.* Extraction des corps estrangers intra-vasculaires. *Presse Med.* 1995; **24**:665–670.
28. Jones, S. A. & Giacomantonio, M. A complication associated with central line removal in the pediatric population: retained fixed catheter fragments. *J. Pediatr. Surg.* 2003; **38**: 594–596.
29. Rand, T., Kohlhauser, C., Popow, C. *et al.* Sonographic detection of internal jugular vein thrombosis after central venous catheterization in the newborn period. *Pediatr. Radiol.* 1994; **24**:577–580.
30. Moukarzel, A. A., Haddad, I., Ament, M. E. *et al.* 230 patient years of experience with home long-term parenteral nutrition: natural history and life of central venous catheters. *J. Pediatr. Surg.* 1994; **29**:1323–1327.
31. Stratov, I., Gottlieb, T., Bradbury, R. *et al.* Candidaemia in an Australian teaching hospital: relationship to central line and TPN use. *J. Infect.* 1998; **36**:203–207.
32. Dollery, C. M., Sullivan, I. D., Bauraind, O. *et al.* Thrombosis and embolism in long-term central venous access for parenteral nutrition. *Lancet* 1994; **344**:1043–1045.
33. Pollard, A. J., Sreeram, N., Wright, J. G. *et al.* ECG and echocardiographic diagnosis of pulmonary thromboembolism associated with central venous lines. *Arch. Dis. Child.* 1995; **73**:147–150.
34. Wesley, J. R. Efficiency and safety of total parenteral nutrition in pediatric patients. *Mayo Clin. Proc.* 1992; **67**:671–675.
35. Shiba, E., Kanbasyashi, J., Sahon, M. *et al.* Septic pulmonary emboli after prolonged use of central venous catheter for parenteral nutrition. *Eur. J. Surg.* 1992; **158**:59–61.
36. Essex-Cater, A., Gilbert, J., Robinson, T. *et al.* Totally implantable venous access systems in paediatric practice. *Arch. Dis. Child.* 1989; **64**:119–123.
37. Sola, J. E., Stone, M. M., Wise, B. *et al.* Atypical thrombotic and septic complications of totally implantable venous access devices in patients with cystic fibrosis. *Pediatr. Pulmonol.* 1992; **14**:239–242.
38. Horn, C. K. & Conway, S. P. Candidaemia therefore risk factors in patients with cystic fibrosis who have totally implantable vascular access systems. *J. Infect.* 1993; **26**:127–132.
39. A-Rahman, A. & Spencer, D. Totally implantable venous access devices for cystic fibrosis. *Cochrane Database Syst. Rev.* 2003; **3**:CD004111.
40. Santagostino, E., Gringeri, A., Berardinelli, L. *et al.* Long-term safety and feasibility of arteriovenous fistulae as vascular accesses in children with haemophilia: a prospective study. *Br. J. Haematol.* 2003; **123**:502–506.
41. Wesenberg, F., Flaaten, H., & Janssen, C. W. Jr. Central venous catheter with subcutaneous injection port (Port-A-Cath): 8 years clinical follow up with children. *Pediatr. Hematol. Oncol.* 1993; **10**:233–239.
42. Girvan, D. P., de Verber, L. L., Inwood, M. J. *et al.* Subcutaneous infusion ports in the paediatric patient with haemophilia. *J. Pediatr. Surg.* 1994; **29**:1220–1223.
43. McMahon, C., Smith, J., & Khair, K. *et al.* Central venous access devices in children with congenital coagulation disorders: complications and long-term outcome. *Br. J. Haematol.* 2000; **110**:461–468
44. Leisner, R. J., Vora, A. J., Hann, I. M. *et al.* Use of central venous catheters in children with severe congenital coagulopathy. *Br. J. Haematol.* 1995; **91**:203–207.
45. Bambauer, R., Inniger, R., Pirrung, K. J. *et al.* Complications and side effects associated with large-bore catheters in the subclavian and internal jugular veins. *Artif. Organs* 1994; **18**:318–321.
46. Schillinger, F., Schillinger, D., Montagnac, R. *et al.* Stenosis veinuses centrales en hemodialyse: etude angiographique comparative des acces soud-claviers et jugulaires internes. *Nephrologie* 1994; **15**:129–131.
47. Kovalik, E. C., Newman, G. E., Suhooki, P. *et al.* Correction of central venous stenosis: use of angioplasty and vascular wall stents. *Kidney Int.* 1994; **45**:1177–1181.
48. Hack, W. W. M., Vos, A., & Okken, A. Incidence of forearm and hand ischaemia related to radial artery cannulation in newborn infants. *Intens. Care Med.* 1990; **16**:50–53.
49. Bright, E., Baines, D. B., French, B. G. *et al.* Upper limb amputation following radial artery cannulation. *Anaesth. Intens. Care* 1993; **21**:351–353.
50. Berger, C., Dwand, C., Francoise, M. *et al.* Surveillance echographique ud cathetrisine arterial umbilical chez le noueau-ne. *Arch. Pediatr.* 1994; **1**:998–1003.
51. Anonymous. Relationship of intraventricular hemorrhage or death with the level of umbilical artery catheter placement: a multicenter randomized clinical trial. Umbilical Artery Catheter Trial Group. *Pediatrics* 1992; **90**:881–887.
52. Cumming, W. A. & Burkfield, D. J. Accidental catheterization of internal iliac branches: a serious complication of umbilical artery catheterization. *J. Perinatol.* 1994; **14**:304–309.
53. Kirk, C. R., & Qureshi, S. A. Microvascular surgery to preserve a preterm infant's ischaemic arm (letter). *Br. Med. J.* 1988; **297**:1198.
54. Davison, P. M. & Scully, L. Microvascular surgery to preserve a preterm infant's ischaemic arm. *Br. Med. J.* 1988; **297**:788.
55. Vidal, R., Kissoon, N. & Gayle, M. Compartment syndrome following intraosseus infusion. *Pediatrics* 1993; **91**:1201–1202.
56. Simmons, C. M., Johnson, N. E., & Perkin, R. M. *et al.* Intraosseus extravasation complication reports. *Ann. Emerg. Med.* 1994; **23**:363–366.
57. Stolar, C. J. H., Snedecor, S. M., & Bartlett, R. H. Extracorporeal membrane oxygenation and neonatal respiratory failure:

experience from the Extracorporial Life Support Organisation. *J. Pediatr. Surg.* 1991; **26**:563–571.

58. Page, J., Frisk, V., & White, H. Developemental outcome of infants treated with extra corporeal membrane oxygenation (ECMO) in the neonatal period: is the evidence all in? *Paediatr. Perinatal. Epidemiol.* 1994; **8**:123–139.

59. Levy, M. S., Shore, A. C., & Fauza, D. *et al.* Fate of the reconstructed carotid artery after extracorporeal membrane oxygenation. *J. Pediatr. Surg.* 1995; **30**:1046–1049.

60. Somme, S. & Liu, D. C. New trends in extracorporeal membrane oxygenation in newborn pulmonary diseases. *Artif. Organs.* 2001; **25**:633–637

72

Myelomeningocele and hydrocephalus

Bruce A. Kaufman

Medical College of Wisconsin and Children's Hospital of Wisconsin, Milwaukee, Wisconsin, USA

Introduction

The "long-term" care and complications related to the population of hydrocephalic and myelomeningocele patients have been infrequently considered. Effective treatment, and even survival, for these patients began in the late 1950s, and was not widespread until the mid 1970s. The first effective hydrocephalic shunt was introduced in 1955.[1] Routine treatment of all myelomeningocele patients did not begin until the late 1970s, after repudiation of "selection" criteria.[2] Only now is the oldest generation of patients approaching their 40s, and the largest cohort of patients is barely into the young adult years. There has been little work published on the long-term medical and care issues for these patients.

It is clear in the care of these patients that the natural history of their disease does not include a decline in function. Caregivers and patients must recognize that a loss of function is either a new problem, such as the development of a syrinx leading to scoliosis, or the morbid sequela of a potentially treatable event, such as an infection leading to brain injury. There is some overlap between these two groups of patients. The majority of myelomeningocele patients also have hydrocephalus, and require management of the problems associated with hydrocephalus in addition to the unique issues involved with myelodysplasia.

This monograph will briefly review the pertinent pathology and initial treatment of these conditions. The more typical problems associated with each diagnosis will be discussed. The evolving longer-term issues affecting these patients will be highlighted.

Hydrocephalus: anatomy and initial treatment

Cerebrospinal fluid (CSF) is produced within the lateral cerebral ventricles and the III and IV ventricles. The normal flow of fluid is from the lateral ventricles through the Foramen of Monro into the III ventricle, down the Aqueduct of Sylvius to the IV ventricle, and then out through medial and lateral foramen into the cranial and spinal subarachnoid spaces. The CSF is absorbed directly into the venous system, mostly through the Pacchionian granulations along the superior sagittal sinus. The daily volume of CSF production can be as much as 400 ml, even in small infants.

Abnormal accumulation of CSF, and the concomitant increase in intracranial pressure (ICP) are the pathological condition of hydrocephalus. Hydrocephalus can be due to either poor absorption of the CSF or some form of outflow obstruction. Absorption is most frequently impaired after intracranial hemorrhage, such as after subarachnoid hemorrhage or intraventricular hemorrhage. It is presumed that the blood breakdown products interfere with the venous absorption pathways, likely in a non-reversible fashion. Obstruction usually occurs at strategic locations in the CSF circulation pathway where a small mass can obstruct the flow, such as at the Foramen of Monro or at the cerebral aqueduct. Infections of the central nervous system (CNS) can impair absorption and create such blockage, usually from scarring.

The treatment of hydrocephalus in all forms is diversion of the CSF – shunting the fluid to another location where it can be absorbed. In the most common forms of shunting, CSF is obtained from the lateral ventricles (or sometimes

Pediatric Surgery and Urology: Long-term Outcomes, Mark Stringer, Keith Oldham, Pierre Mouriquand.

from the lumbar CSF space) and diverted to the venous system or peritoneal cavity. The typical shunt system (tubing and valves) is made from silastic but may have metal components. It is composed of three parts: a proximal catheter (source of the CSF), a flow-regulating valve, and a distal catheter. Occasionally, the CSF can be internally diverted around an obstruction, for example, through a fenestration of the ventricle into an extracerebral subarachnoid space. The most common internal diversion is the IIIrd ventriculostomy, where a hole is created in the floor of the III ventricle providing alternative drainage into the suprasellar subarachnoid space.

Myelomeningocele: anatomy and initial treatment

Patients with myelomeningoceles have been described as having the greatest collection of malformations and derivative problems that are compatible with life (D. McLone, pers. commun.). The open spinal defect is obvious at birth, and requires prompt closure to prevent infection. In addition, nearly 90% of these patients will develop hydrocephalus within a short time after birth and require treatment. Less obvious but equally important are the problems associated with the associated malformations of the brain itself.

The Chiari II malformation is the most significant of these associated CNS abnormalities. Its primary manifestation is at the cranio-cervical junction, with compression of the neural structures and herniation of the brainstem into the cervical canal. In contemporary practice, the Chiari II malformation is responsible for much of the early morbidity and many of the deaths in this population. As the patients become older, cognitive difficulties become more apparent. The perceptual and processing problems these patients manifest affect both their school performance and their ability to care for themselves.

The initial priority for a child with a myelomeningocele is closure of the spinal defect. This is normally undertaken within days of birth. The surgical objectives are to disconnect the spinal cord from its attachment to the skin, and then cover the neural tissue and canal with the dural and skin flaps. Effective closure prevents leakage of CSF and secondary infection of the CNS. Hydrocephalus, if not present at birth, will begin to develop within days of the spinal defect closure. Shunting is ultimately required to control the hydrocephalus in 70–90% of the patients.[3,4]

Long-term complications

For patients with hydrocephalus, shunt malfunction is the most common and important ongoing problem. Associated with shunted hydrocephalus are the issues of device infection, difficulty or failure to diagnose a shunt malfunction, and the mechanical and diagnostic problems associated with very small, slit-like ventricles. Patients with long-standing shunts will also have headaches, and the various etiologies other than shunt malfunction must be correctly deciphered. Eventual independence from the shunt has been a conceptual possibility since the beginning of shunt treatment, and is an often-raised goal of patients and families. However, achieving this goal remains unlikely at present (see below: Hydrocephalus: shunt dependence). Myelomeningocele patients have additional problems including learning disabilities, decline in their ability to ambulate (independent of loss of motor function), and loss of various spinal cord functions from tethering. Both hydrocephalic and myelomeningocele patients are now beginning to experience problems associated with transitioning their care from typical pediatric-based facilities and caregivers to providers who deal primarily with adults.

Mortality

The initial success in treating both of these conditions must be tempered by the reality that they remain potentially lethal throughout life. The high initial mortality rate associated with myelomeningocele patients born before 1974 has been greatly reduced through the application of early surgical closure techniques, antibiotics, and effective and improved imaging.[5,6] Myelomeningocele patients continue to have a mortality risk in the first few years of life that ranges from 11% to 18% in published reports.[2,7,8] This risk is primarily related to malformations of the brainstem that are untreatable, and the complications of the Chiari II malformation often manifested by respiratory insufficiency and possibly aspiration.

There is also ongoing mortality in these patients related principally to shunt malfunctions and increased ICP. Most published reports have a death rate of 7%–18%, with most of this occurring in the first years of life.[7–12] A population-based study in one region in Alabama identified cumulative deaths related to hydrocephalus and found that, within 15 months of shunting, their hydrocephalus patients had a 3% mortality rate, and the myelomeningocele patients had a nearly 7% mortality rate.[9] More importantly, nearly half of these patients were found to have had symptoms of increased ICP for at least 24 hours, if not for several weeks prior to death. These and other reported deaths in hydrocephalic patients suggest that shunt malfunction was present and potentially preventable with appropriate evaluation and treatment.[13]

To summarize, it should be understood that hydrocephalus is a long-term illness, and that even with effective shunting treatment, subsequent deterioration can and does happen. The deterioration can be rapid, and delay in diagnosis of even a few days can result in death. It is also a fallacy to believe that older children and adults have fewer malfunctions of their shunts. This commonly held belief may actually reflect failure to diagnose shunt malfunctions or lack of awareness of shunt malfunction manifestations by the caregivers.

Hydrocephalus: shunt infection and malfunction

The two major morbidities associated with a CSF shunt are infection of the device and occlusion requiring revision.[14] Infection is the most frequent complication of shunt surgery, with a reported operative risk varying from less than 1% to greater than 10%.[7,11,15,16] Nearly 80% of shunt infections occur within 6 months of surgery on the shunt, suggesting that the source of infection is perioperative contamination. Later infections are usually associated with a distant source of bacteremia, such as an abscess, or with perforation of a viscus or erosion of the shunt through the skin.[15]

Erosion of the shunt through the bowel can present as an acute abdomen or may be clinically quite innocuous. A shunt tap will demonstrate CSF flow and proximal function of the shunt. Evidence of bacterial contamination of the proximal CSF may or may not be present. Imaging of the abdomen rarely demonstrates a point of bowel entry, and the utility of imaging is limited to defining the presence of an abscess.

Treatment of bowel perforation by shunt tubing begins with simple removal of the tubing from the abdomen with external drainage, usually through a skin incision at the costal margin (where it is easy to isolate the tubing). There is no indication for an immediate laparotomy. Even with manual inspection of the bowel, the entry point is often impossible to identify. Nearly all patients demonstrate improvement in their condition and symptoms within 12 hours of catheter removal, and it is rare for the perforation to be a source of ongoing soilage of the peritoneal cavity.

The treatment of shunt infections, regardless of etiology, usually requires the removal of all shunt components, continued CSF drainage using an externalized ventriculostomy, and appropriate antibiotics for a number of days (defined by the organism and rapidity with which the infection clears from the CSF). The shunt is internalized when the CSF is sterilized, and the device can usually be returned to the abdomen even if there had been frank peritonitis.[15] The greatest risk to the patient from a shunt infection is failure to clear the infection from the CNS, and subsequent decline in intellectual function.[16]

The incidence of reported shunt occlusion or malfunction is dependent on the duration of follow-up. The overall risk appears to be in the range of 10% per year.[8] Most reviews report a revision rate of 50–64% in the first year after placement, but this includes a 5–15% shunt infection rate.[7,8,11,17] However, many patients will have years without a shunt revision, with 35%–45% of patients having no revisions for more than 10 years.[7,11] Most shunt malfunctions are due to obstruction of the proximal catheter or valve.

Evaluation of the shunt for malfunction has traditionally included CT imaging of the ventricular system to look for an increase in size. However, it is clear that there can be a substantial elevation in ICP with no change in size of the ventricles on CT.[18,19] Other evaluation techniques include plain radiographs of the shunt ("shunt series" or "survey") to look for disconnections between components. Most shunt systems have a reservoir that can be accessed percutaneously to determine proximal patency and directly measure the ICP. Flow through the shunt can be assessed with the injection of radioisotope tracers ("nuclear shuntogram").[14]

Correction of any shunt occlusion requires surgery, with its attendant risks of infection. Revision of a proximal catheter occlusion also has risk of intracranial hemorrhage as any tissue caught in the catheter is torn on catheter removal. Intraventricular hemorrhage in this setting can be catastrophic, with severe brain injury and the need for extended external ventricular drainage. Coagulating any tissue within the shunt catheter prior to removal can minimize this risk. This can be done using a metal stylet or a small Bugbee wire.[14]

With longer durations of implantation, it is now clear that the non-metallic shunt materials are altered by the intracorporeal environment in which they reside. The silastic material is degraded and calcification of the tissues around the tubing occurs.[20–23] In addition, the microstructure of the tubing is altered, resulting in increased brittleness and a tendency to fracture.[20] The patient may complain of pain or a pulling sensation where the tubing is calcified. Local areas of calcification and scarring are not necessarily contiguous and the induced differential mobility in these areas can lead to stretching and fracture or disconnection of the tubing from connections causing shunt malfunction. Elective revision is reserved for those patients with severe pain, since the tubing is adherent along an extended tract making removal difficult. Although the tubing may be removed, the calcified track will remain behind and may continue to cause local symptoms.

Ventricular shunts may be placed with the distal catheter in the vascular system. These vascular shunts offer the potential for a number of unique complications over time.[14] These include thrombosis, embolization, and shunt nephritis. Providers should routinely evaluate for evidence of these events. A thrombus that forms on the distal end of a shunt may propagate retrograde, possibly to the superior vena cava, potentially causing venous obstruction and symptomatic superior vena cava syndrome. Emboli from these catheters can lodge anywhere in the pulmonary artery distribution, and recurrent embolization may go undetected until pulmonary hypertension or cor pulmonale develops. Autopsy studies in the past have shown that nearly half of the patients with ventriculo-atrial shunting had some degree of thrombus formation or evidence of pulmonary emboli. Doppler ultrasound of the heart and superior vena cava can be used to diagnose thrombosis. In contemporary practice, this is an accurate, non-invasive tool and is the best available technique for screening purposes. If a shunt-related thrombus develops, catheter withdrawal can usually be done without complication.

Shunt nephritis is an infrequent result of chronic infection of a vascular CSF shunt.[10,24–28] Symptoms or signs of infection always precede the renal dysfunction, although those signs may be subtle. The causative organisms are typically staphylococcal species, especially coagulase-negative forms, but diphtheroid species have also been associated with the syndrome. The pathogenesis seems similar to that seen with subacute bacterial endocarditis. Patients with a vascular CSF shunt should have routine evaluation of renal function including urinalysis. An increase in urinary protein or erythrocytosis in a patient with an intravascular shunt should not be disregarded as a mere urological problem. Failure to detect this condition can lead to permanent renal failure.[27] Treatment of the underlying shunt infection usually, but not always, leads to resolution of the renal dysfunction.

Hydrocephalus: headaches

Most caregivers assume that any headache in a patient with a shunt is related to shunt occlusion. However, not all headaches are a sign of shunt obstruction or failure.[19] Headaches that are related to shunting but not due to obstruction include excessive drainage of CSF through the shunt or intermittent obstructions. Headaches not related to the shunt or ICP elevation may occur as well.

The geometry and design of a shunt system may cause siphoning of CSF with "overdrainage" resulting in very low intracranial pressure. The resulting headache is similar in character and cause to that seen after a spinal tap. The treatment for shunt overdrainage may be as simple as upgrading the valve pressure, or possibly the addition of an antisiphoning device.

Intermittent blockage of the shunt usually involves the proximal catheter residing in very small ventricles. The classic example of this problem would be the "slit ventricle syndrome," defined as short duration headaches (10–90 minutes), in the presence of small slit-like ventricles, with very slow flow through the valve system.[19] The intermittent obstruction occurs as the small ventricles collapse around the proximal catheter and block the inlet. This remains occluded until the pressure rises (causing headache) and the ventricles enlarge enough to re-establish flow. Treatment is to increase the valve resistance or add antisiphoning components to the system to reduce the flow out of the ventricles, and maintain the size and volume that keeps the shunt unobstructed.

Patients with shunts can have headaches unrelated to changes in ICP, including migraine or tension headaches. These types of headaches should respond to the same treatments used in the non-hydrocephalic population. Given the consequences of missing a shunt malfunction, however, these are diagnoses best reached after demonstrating appropriate functioning of the shunt.

Evaluation of headache in a shunted patient should include appropriate studies to establish adequate functioning of the shunt system. The clinician may use any number of evaluations looking for disconnection of the shunt (shunt radiographs), enlargement of the ventricles (CT or MR imaging), or flow through the shunt (shunt tap or shuntogram). Implantation of an intracranial pressure monitor may be useful if headaches persist in the face of studies that suggest adequate shunt function. Changes in ICP can then be directly correlated with the headaches.

Hydrocephalus: shunt dependence

A patient's lifelong need for an implanted CSF shunt has never been completely defined. In one study, 6% of patients were considered "independent" of the shunt but the follow-up duration was very short.[13] Some physicians and surgeons have held the belief that patients "once shunted, always shunted," while others have entertained the possibility that some shunted individuals might be "weaned" from the shunt. There are patients with known disconnections of their shunt who appear to be doing well from a clinical perspective.

Rekate *et al.* have attempted to identify patients who could be "weaned" from their shunt.[29] When their shunt was removed, nearly a third of the group of non-communicating hydrocephalic patients (including myelomeningocele patients) died or suffered severe and irreversible deterioration.[29] Unfortunately, the timing of deterioration was not predictable, varying from 12 hours to

5 years after disconnection. When the shunt was removed from patients with communicating hydrocephalus, the ICP increased but without the severe sequelae seen in the non-communicating group.[29] In addition, this author has personally observed patients with disconnected and presumed non-functional shunts who do well for several years. However, many presented later with symptoms of increasing ICP or with the finding of increasing ventricular size on serial CT examinations. The risks of shunt removal are significant and it does not appear to be a reasonable goal to pursue.

It has long been recognized that there are physical changes in the skull and brain associated with prolonged shunting.[30] Ventricular shunting can lead to collapse and fusion of the cerebral aqueduct, effectively turning a communicating form of hydrocephalus into an obstructive form.[31] These patients would thus be at risk for sudden or serious problems if their shunt were disconnected. Most patients will develop a scar tract along the shunt tubing, and this tract may offer a conduit for some CSF flow in the absence of shunt tubing. Eventually, most of these tracts will contract and close, causing problems for a patient still dependent on that flow. Since these patients cannot be easily identified, all patients with shunt disconnections must be carefully observed using serial clinical and radiographic examinations. A nuclear shuntogram to assess flow through the tract can be used to identify patients who should undergo revision of the disconnection.

There has been a recent resurgence in enthusiasm for and use of IIIrd ventriculostomy. One concept has been that the patient treated with a ventriculostomy will not require shunt, and becomes "cured" of the need for CSF diversion. Unfortunately, Kaplan–Meier survival analysis of IIIrd ventriculotomy function suggests that they fail nearly as frequently and in the same time interval, as typical shunts. Nearly 50% are non-functional after 2–3 years.[32] In addition, there have been a number of sudden deaths in patients treated with III ventriculostomy (J. Drake, personal communication). It is not clear if these were in truly asymptomatic patients, or if the patients and families had been ignoring symptoms of increased ICP.

Patients treated with a III ventriculostomy must be treated and followed as if they had a shunt. In fact, they have an internal shunt, which has a failure and complication rate similar to the standard shunts. These patients must be encouraged to seek attention for the same symptoms of increased intracranial pressure as any other shunted patient.

Myelomeningocele: intellectual impairment

A large proportion of patients with myelomeningocele have some degree of intellectual impairment, often not identified until they have entered schooling. Only 35%–60% of all these patients are in age appropriate school classes, and in some reports, 45% have identifiable school problems.[7,8,13,34] It was originally believed that all of these individuals had significant intellectual impairment.[6] However, it is now clear that this population has a typical "bell-shaped" distribution of intellectual abilities.[35] It is important to recognize that there are actually quite a few extremely intelligent individuals in this population. Untreated hydrocephalus and the sequelae of infection likely account for much of the earlier data suggesting that the entire group was impaired. Shunt malfunctions and infections can be directly associated with impairment of intelligence, likely through direct brain injury.[7,35]

Neuropsychological studies demonstrate that most myelomeningocele patients have some degree of cognitive or intellectual dysfunction, with more pronounced difficulties in performance IQ as opposed to verbal IQ.[33,35,36] In particular, they have poor visual perception, visual spatial abilities, and construction skills. These individuals also have some difficulty with some aspects of learning and memory. In general, they have intact language abilities including basic reading and spelling. This results in adequate basic academic performance, but their deficiencies become more apparent as they advance in school, due to their problems with reading comprehension, written expression, and mathematical skills.

Myelomeningocele: ambulation

One of the most important functions for myelomeningocele patients is the ability to ambulate independently. The goal is of course to achieve the greatest degree of function, and then to maintain it throughout life. Use of Caesarean section has been reported in one retrospective review to be associated with better motor function in the newborn (compared to vaginal delivery), leading many obstetricians to routinely recommend this method of delivery for the diagnosis of an open spinal defect.[37] However, it has not been proven that the long-term functional results in these patients are improved or whether the increased risk to the mother is justified by this approach.

The ability to ambulate as a child, without or with an orthosis – the "community ambulator" is directly correlated with level of motor function present in the child. The presence of an L4 motor level (movement across the knee) generally allows for long-term ambulation. In late follow-up, 50–60% of myelomeningocele patients can be community ambulators.[2,8] Patients with function limited to the L3 level are often able to ambulate as children, but as they grow, the energy expenditure required to move a larger body leads them to use a wheelchair. It is very important to understand that this is not a loss of function, but a choice related to ease of function. Similarly, if these patients become obese, and most myelomeningocele patients are at risk of inappropriate weight gain, they are more likely to become nonambulatory.[8]

Myelomeningocele: tethering

The greatest threat to the function of myelomeningocele patients is "tethering" of the spinal cord and an associated loss of function, at any age. Clinically significant tethering occurs in 15% of the myelomeningocele population.[8] The process is more technically a "retethering" of the cord, since the spinal cord is tethered at birth by its connection to the skin. After myelomeningocele closure there is a physical reattachment to surrounding structures by scarring at the closure site.

On imaging, nearly all myelomeningocele patients will appear to be tethered, with the low lying conus medullaris in direct contact with the scar.[38] Therefore, the relevant diagnosis of tethering is made on clinical grounds; however, the evaluation of tethering should include magnetic resonance imaging to look for associated structural pathology. Associated findings include: dermoid cyst, syringomyelia, and other dysraphism such as diastematomyelia.

Tethering is defined by progressive decline in neurological function detected on clinical examination.[39] There can be a loss of motor function, generally seen as changes in gait or muscle tone. There may be a change in bowel or bladder function or habits, with loss of continence, urinary dribbling or leaking between catheterizations. Local pain in the back at the repair site, or extending into the buttocks and down the leg (not necessarily in a radicular distribution) is very common. The onset of these problems is quite variable, occurring in as little as 9 months or many years after closure.[38,40,41] Interestingly, the pathophysiology of tethering is not clear. Physical traction and vascular compromise of the cord have been postulated.[39] However, tethering is not worse in or limited to patients with high-level or extensive myelomeningocele repairs, as even patients with low sacral lesions can experience a loss of function.[42] Surgical treatment requires careful disconnection of the neural tissue from the surrounding scar. Extensive arachnoiditis or the presence of functional neural tissue buried within scar may prevent complete untethering.

The results of surgical release for cord tethering vary with the presenting symptom.[40] Pain is almost always relieved. Decreased motor function will improve in most patients, and remain stable in the others.[39,41] Unfortunately, urological dysfunction only improves in about one-third of these symptomatic patients.

Tethering can occur at any time, and is not directly related to periods of somatic growth. Patients therefore must have ongoing and thorough evaluations of their function by neurosurgeons, orthopedic surgeons, and urologists. It is most important to understand that loss of function is not part of the natural history of myelomeningocele, and any new or progressive deficits must be considered to be pathological change.

Transitioning care

A major dilemma now facing the aging hydrocephalic and myelomeningocele populations is the need to transition their health care to providers who are willing and able to treat adults. Whether the need is shunt related or functional, failure to obtain appropriate care results in greater morbidity and possibly mortality for these patients. This is not a new issue as it was recognized in the 1980s, but little has been done to address the need and we now have increasing numbers of these patients reaching adulthood.[43]

Unfortunately, there are no clear models for such transitioning. Even in children, there is great variability in how and where care is provided. As infants and children, these patients benefited from the development of various pediatric subspecialty services, including Pediatric Neurosurgery. These pediatric subspecialists brought attention to the ongoing care of hydrocephalic patients, and developed comprehensive and coordinated care systems for the myelomeningocele patients. Multidisciplinary clinics were a common method used to meet these needs. In these settings, there was frequently one individual or group that functioned as the coordinator of the complex care provided to the patient.

In the United States, federal and state programs have failed to adapt to permit the transition from these care settings to adult settings. Some of this is driven by high costs for these complex patients, but there are also problems with the care providers. Many physicians who care for adults are unwilling to see patients with these diagnoses. They often lack the breadth and depth of knowledge or experience with these diagnoses. It is typical that a pediatric neurosurgeon's practice would have approximately 40% of patients with hydrocephalus, and 10%–20% with myelodysplasia, while an adult practice may not include cranial procedures or shunting.

There are other systems issues. For example, the adult model of care rarely includes a multidisciplinary clinic setting. If there is no "coordinator of care" for these patients, then significant lapses in care occur. A late follow-up study of myelomeningocele patients who had been cared for in a multidisciplinary clinic that was discontinued showed severe morbidity.[44] There were instances of patients suffering from organ failure or receiving amputations, all of which were preventable complications. The majority of these patients also failed to obtain routine but needed care, despite the continuing availability of all relevant specialty services outside of the multidisciplinary setting.

In some situations there are statutory or institutional policies that restrict appropriate care.[45] For example, continued care of adults may be forbidden in children's facilities or programs, precluding the use of existing systems. Insurance may change as the patient ceases to be dependent or fails to gain employment, and policy limitations may no longer pay for the breadth of services the patient and family have come to expect.[44,45] Another major issue in the United States is simply that many providers are no longer delivering specific components of care needed by these patients because of unattractive reimbursement policies.

The patients and families may also be deficient in the skills needed to work with the new system into which they are thrust. They may be unable to understand the new system and its limitations. They may be unable to communicate their condition and the associated needs. If a patient does not understand her/his diagnosis or know the symptoms associated with problems, then they will fail to participate in their own care. Unfortunately, in one survey of young patients with hydrocephalus, 57% were unable to discuss or explain their disability. (Hydrocephalus Association, patient pamphlet on transitioning care:www.hydrocephalus.org). Fifty percent did not know the name of their medications or the reason for each medication.

The "transitioning" from child-oriented to adult-directed care must become the normal experience. Physicians, patients and families must be active in the process. There is no one best way to transition from care delivered to pediatric patients in pediatric oriented facilities. Ideally, a health care continuum will be designed and appropriately financed to deliver the special care needed for these patients. Undoubtably, a variety of systems can work, some are likely to be unique to local circumstances. Ongoing attention is being directed to this problem, but clearly the planning should begin well in advance of the need.[45]

Conclusions

Patients with hydrocephalus or myelomeningocele should not have deterioration in their clinical status; it is not a natural or expected component of their disease process. Caregivers must recognize the sometimes subtle presentation of problems associated with these conditions. Increased life expectancy as a result of improvements in care for these patients has created a need for specialized care in the adult years. Planning for the transition of care to adult providers and systems must begin early, and must be tailored to the resources available in each region.

REFERENCES

1. Nulsen, F. E. & Spitz, E. B. Treatment of hydrocephalus by direct shunt from ventricle to jugular vein. *Surg. Forum*, 1951; **2**:399–403.
2. McLone, D. G. Results of treatment of children born with a myelomeningocele. *Clin. Neurosurg.* 1983; **30**:407–412.
3. Kaufman, B. A. Congenital intraspinal anomalies: spinal dysraphism-embryology, pathology, and treatment, in Bridwell, K. H. & Dewald, R. L. (eds.), *The Textbook of Spinal Surgery*, 2nd edn, vol. 1 Philadelphia:Lippincott-Raven, 1997a:365–400.
4. Rolle, U. & Grafe, G. About the rate of shunt complications in patients with hydrocephalus and myelomeningocele. *Eur. J. Pediatr. Surg.* 1999; **9**(Suppl. I):51–52.
5. Dillon, C. M., Davis, B. E., Duguay, S., Seidel, K. D., & Shurtleff, D. B. longevity of patients born with myelomeningocele. *Eur. J. Pediatr. Surg.* 2000; **10**(Suppl. I):33–34.
6. Lorber, J. Results of treatment of myelomeningocele: an analysis of 524 unselected cases with special references to possible selection for treatment. *Dev. Med. Child Neurol.* 1971; **13**:279–303.
7. Casey, A. T. H., Kimmings, E. J., Kleinlugtebeld, A. D., Taylor, W. A. S., Harkness, W. F., & Hayward, R. D. The long-term outlook for hydrocephalus in childhood. A ten-year cohort study of 155 patients. *Pediatr. Neurosurg.* 1997; **27**:63–70.
8. Steinbok, P., Irvine, B., Cochrane, D. D., & Irwin, B. J. Long-term outcome and complications of children born with meningomyelocele. *Child's Nerv. Syst.* 1992; **8**:92–96.
9. Iskandar, B. J., Tubbs, S., Mapstone, T. B., Grabb, P. A., Bartolucci, A. A., & Oakes, W. J. Deaths in shunted hydrocephalic children in the 1990s. *Pediatr. Neurosurg.* 1998; **28**:173–176.
10. Keucher, T. R. & Mealey, J. Long-term results after ventriculoatrial and ventriculoperitoneal shunting for infantile hydrocephalus. *J. Neurosurg.* 1979; **50**:179–186.
11. Tuli, S., Drake, J., & Lamberti-Pasculli, M. Long-term outcome of hydrocephalus management in myelomeningoceles. *Child's Nerv. Syst.* 2003; **19**:286–291.
12. Vernet, O., Campiche, R., & de Tribolet, N. Long-term results after ventriculoatrial shunting in children. *Child's Nerv. Syst.* 1993; **9**:253–255.
13. Sgouros, S., Malluci, C., Walsh, A. R., & Hockley, A. D. Long-term complications of hydrocephalus. *Pediatr. Neurosurg.* 1995; **23**:127–132.

14. Kaufman, B. A. Management of complications of shunting, in McLone, D. G. (ed.), *Pediatric Neurosurgery: Surgery of the Developing Nervous System*, 4th edn, Philadelphia: W.B. Saunders, 2001:529–547.
15. Kaufman, B. A. Infections of cerebrospinal fluid shunts, in Scheld, W. M., Whitley, R. J., & Durack, D. T. (eds.), *Infections of the Central Nervous System*, 2nd edn, vol. 1 Philadelphia: Lippincott-Raven, 1997:555–577.
16. Mirzai, H., Ersahin, Y., Mutluer, S., & Kayahan, A. Outcome of patients with myelomeningocele – The Ege University experience. *Child's Nerv. Syst.* 1998; **14**:120–123.
17. Genitori, L., van Calenbergh, F., Lena, G., & Choux, M. Mechanical and functional complications in shunts. A series of 1298 children and 2967 operations. *Child's Nerv. Syst.* 1993; **9**:355.
18. Engel, M., Carmel, P. W., & Chutorian, A. M. Increased intraventricular pressure without ventriculomegaly in children with shunts: "normal volume" hydrocephalus. *Neurosurgery* 1979; **5**:549–552.
19. Rekate, H. L. Classification of slit-ventricle syndromes using intracranial pressure monitoring. *Pediatr. Neurosurg.* 1993; **19**:15–20.
20. Boch, A. L., Hermelin, E., Sainte-Rose, C., & Sgouros, S. Mechanical dysfunction of ventriculopertioneal shunts caused by calcification of the silicone rubber catheter. *J. Neurosurg.* 1998; **88**:975–982.
21. Del Bigio, M. R. Biological reactions to cerebrospinal fluid shunt devices: a review of the cellular pathology. *Neurosurgery* 1998; **42**:319–326.
22. Echizenya, K., Satoh, M., Murai, H., Ueno, H., Abe, H., & Komai, T. Mineralization and biodegradation of CSF shunting systems. *J. Neurosurg.* **67**:584–591.
23. Yamamoto, S., Ohno, K., Aoyagi, M., Ichinose, S., & Hirakawa, K. Calcific deposits on degraded shunt catheters: long-term follow-up of VP shunts and late complications in three cases. *Child's Nerv. Syst.* 2002; **18**:19–25.
24. Finney, H. L. & Roberts, T. S. Nephritis secondary to chronic cerebrospinal fluid-vascular shunt infection: "shunt nephritis". *Child's Brain* 1980; **6**:189–193.
25. James, H. E. Infections associated with cerebrospinal fluid prosthetic devices, in Sugarman, B. & Young, E. J. (eds.), *Infections Associated with Prosthetic Devices*, 1st edn. Chicago: CRC Press, 23–42.
26. Kontny, U., Hofling, B., Gutjahr, P., Voth, D., Schwarz, M., & Schmitt, H. J. CSF shunt infections in children. *Infection* 1993; **21**:89–92.
27. Samtleben, W., Bauriedel, G., Bosch, T., Goetz, C., Klare, B., & Gurland, H. J. Renal complications of infected ventriculoatrial shunts. *Artificial Organs* 1993; **17**:695–701.
28. Schoenbaum, S. C., Gardner, P., & Shillito, J. Infections of cerebrospinal fluid shunts: epidemiology, clinical manifestations, and therapy. *J. Infect. Dis.* 1975; **131**:543–552.
29. Rekate, H. L., Nulsen, F. E., Mack, H. L., & Morrison, G. Establishing the diagnosis of shunt independence. *Monographs in Neural Sci.* 1982; **8**:223–226.
30. Kaufman, B., Weiss, M. H., Young, H. F., & Nulsen, F. E. The effects of prolonged cerebrospinal fluid shunting on the skull and brain *J. Neurosurg.* 1973; **38**:288–297.
31. Foltz, E. L. & Shurtleff, D. B. Conversion of communicating hydrocephalus to stenosis or occlusion of the aqueduct during ventricular shunt. *J. Neurosurg.* 1965; **24**:520–529.
32. Tuli, S., Alshail, E., & Drake, J. Third ventriculostomy versus cerebrospinal fluid shunt as a first procedure in pediatric hydrocephalus. *Pediatr. Neurosurg.* 1999; **30**:11–15.
33. Yeates, K. O., Enrile, B. G., Loss, N., & Blumenstein, E. Verbal learning and memory in children with myelomeningocele.. *J. Pediatr. Psychol.* 1995; **20**:801–815.
34. Yeates, K. O., Loss, N., Colvin, A. N., & Enrile, B. G. Do children with myelomeningocele and hydrocephalus display nonverbal learning disabilities? An empirical approach to classification. *J. Int. Neuropsychol. Soc.* 2003; **9**:653–662.
35. Wills, K. E. Neuropsychological functioning in children with spina bifida and/or hydrocephalus. *J. Clin. Child Psychol.* 1993; **22**:247–265.
36. Fletcher, J. M., Dennis, M. F., & Northrup, H. Hydrocephalus, in Yeates, K. O., Ris, M. D., & Taylor, H. G. (eds.) *Pediatric Neuropsychology: Research, Theory, and Practice*, New York: Guilford Press, 2000; 25–46.
37. Luthy, D. A., Wardinsky, T., Shurtleff, D. B. *et al.* Cesarean section before the onset of labor and subsequent motor function in infants with meningomyelocele diagnosed antenatally. *N. Engl. J. Med.* 1991; **324**:662–666.
38. Caldarelli, M., Di Rocco, C., Colosimo, C., Fariello, G., & Di Gennaro, M. Surgical treatment of late neurological deterioration in children with myelodysplasia. *Acta Neurochir. (Wien)* 1995; **137**:199–206.
39. Kaufman, B. A. Neural tube defects. *Pediatr. Clin. North Am.* 2004; **51**:389–419.
40. Sarwark, J. F., Weber, D. T., Gabrieli, A. P., McLone, D. G., & Dias L. Tethered cord syndrome in low motor level children with myelomeningocele. *Pediatr. Neurosurg.* 1996; **25**:295–301.
41. Schoenmakers, M. A. G. C., Gooskens, R. H. J. M., Gulmans, V. A. M. *et al.* Long-term outcome of neurosurgical untethering on neurosegmental motor and ambulation levels. *Dev. Med. Child Neurol.* 2003; **45**:551–555.
42. Brinker, M. R., Rosenfeld, S. R., Feiwell, E. *et al.* Myelomeningocele at the sacral level. Long-term outcomes in adults. *J. Bone Joint Surg. (Am.)* 1994; **76A**:1293–1300.
43. Blum, R. W. Introduction. *Pediatrics* 2002; **110**:1301–1303.
44. Kaufman, B. A., Terbrock, A., Winters, N., Ito, J., Klosterman, A., & Park, T. S. Disbanding a multidisciplinary clinic: effects on the health care of myelomeningocele patients. *Pediatr. Neurosurg.* 1994; **21**:36–44.
45. Reiss, J. & Gibson, R. Health care transition: destinations unknown. *Pediatrics* 2002; **110**:1307–1314.

73

Outcomes after maternal–fetal surgery

Preeti Malladi, Karl Sylvester, and Craig T. Albanese

Lucile Packard Children's Hospital at Stanford Medical Center, Department of Surgery, Division of Pediatric Surgery, CA, USA

Until the 1980s, physicians had few options for parents of fetuses with congenital malformations; essentially, these were to terminate the pregnancy or continue and possibly modify the timing and/or method of delivery. Rapid advances in prenatal imaging and diagnosis over the last 20 years, coupled with increased understanding of the natural history of many fetal anomalies, has led to the identification of the fetus as a patient and to the burgeoning field of fetal surgery. An increasing number of selected fetal anomalies are amenable to prenatal intervention (Table 73.1), yet it has been difficult to demonstrate efficacy with regard to improved outcomes. With the exception of myelomeningocele and twin–twin transfusion syndrome, anomalies amenable to fetal repair yield only 2–5 cases per year at the busiest fetal treatment centers. Thus, the dearth of patient volume has dictated that outcome assessment be done over a long time often using historical controls. Also, anomalies in which no prenatal treatment reliably results in fetal death (e.g., lung lesion producing hydrops) cannot be ethically "randomized" for prospective study. Randomized prospective trials have been done for several "high" volume anomalies. To date, there are two completed randomized trials for congenital diaphragmatic hernia, and there are ongoing prospective randomized trials for myelomeningocele and twin–twin transfusion syndrome, each of which is illustrated below.

Risks and benefits

Assessing risks and benefits in fetal surgery is a complex task. Both the fetus and the mother must be considered. For the fetus, surgical treatment historically has been limited to predictably lethal conditions; so that the benefit of possible survival clearly outweighed the risk of intervention. Now that fetal therapy is addressing non-lethal conditions (e.g., myelomeningocele), benefits to the fetus, including morbidity and quality of life, must be balanced against the natural history of each disease process in the context of evolving current standard postnatal treatment.

The paramount consideration in fetal surgery is evaluating maternal risk and benefit. On the one hand, without antenatal treatment, the pregnant woman faces little health risk beyond that of pregnancy. With antenatal treatment, the pregnant woman incurs discomfort and morbidity directly proportional to the level of invasiveness of the procedure, as well as the prospect of fetal loss due to the procedure. In addition, the psychosocial impact of making a decision about performing antenatal treatment and accepting the outcome is a factor not easily quantified. The obvious benefit is the possibility of saving the life of her child and having a child less burdened by chronic disability.

The maternal risk of amniocentesis, chorionic villous sampling, percutaneous umbilical blood sampling, and sonographically guided aspiration of fetal fluids (blood, ascites, pleural fluid, urine) is negligible, whereas the fetal loss rate is 1% to 3% for each.[1] More extensive sonographically guided percutaneous procedures such as shunt placements, fetoscopic procedures, and open fetal surgery carry more profound risks to the mother. These risks can be categorized into perioperative, short-term, and long-term risks. There have been no reported maternal deaths during or after fetal surgery. Short-term morbidities include bleeding, wound infection, amniotic fluid leak, oligohydramnios, amniotic band formation, chorioamnionitis,

Pediatric Surgery and Urology: Long-term Outcomes, Mark Stringer, Keith Oldham, Pierre Mouriquand.
Published by Cambridge University Press.

Table 73.1. Summary of applications of fetal surgery

Defect	Effect on development			Open	Minimal access
Lethal					
Placental vascular anomalies	Vascular steal through placenta	->	Fetal hydrops/demise	Fetectomy	Photocoagulation of chorangiopagus
Twin–twin transfusion syndrome (TTTS)			Surviving twin with severe morbidity	Fetectomy	
Twin reversed arterial perfusion syndrome (TRAP)	Normal co-twin heart pumps for both twins		High output cardiac failure Hydrops		Selective reduction via umbilical cord ligation or radiofrequency needle
Obstructive uropathy	Hydronephrosis Lung hypoplasia	->	Renal failure Pulmonary failure	Vesicostomy	Vesicoamniotic shunt Valve ablation
Congenital diaphragmatic hernia	Lung hypoplasia	->	Pulmonary failure	Complete repair Temporary tracheal occlusion	Temporary tracheal occlusion (PLUG)
Cystic adenomatoid malformation/sequestration	Lung hypoplasia or hydrops	->	Respiratory insufficiency Fetal hydrops/demise	Pulmonary lobectomy	Radiofrequency ablation
Sacrococcygeal teratoma	High-output heart failure	->	Fetal hydrops/demise	Debulk Complete resection	Laser vascular occlusion Radiofrequency ablation
Complete heart block	Low output failure	->	Fetal hydrops/demise	Pacemaker	Pacemaker
Pulmonary/aortic stenosis	Ventricular hypertrophy	->	Heart failure Single ventricle physiology	Valvuloplasty	Catheter valvuloplasty
Pericardial teratoma	Heart failure	->	Fetal hydrops/demise	Resection	
Ebstein's anomaly	Heart failure Pulmonary hypoplasia	->	Fetal hydrops/demise Pulmonary failure	Valve repair and atrial reduction	
Congenital high airway obstruction syndrome	Overdistention by lung fluid	->	Fetal hydrops/demise	Tracheostomy EXIT strategy	Tracheostomy
Obstructive hydrocephalus	Hydrocephalus	->	Brain damage	Ventriculoamniotic shunt Ventriculoperitoneal shunt*	Ventriculoamniotic shunt
Non-lethal					
Myelomeningocele	Chiari formation Exposed spinal cord Hydrocephalus	->	Paralysis Neurogenic bladder/bowel Orthopedic anomalies	Repair	Repair
Tension hydrothorax	Lung hypoplasia	->	Respiratory failure		Serial thoracenteses Thoracoamniotic shunt
Cleft lip/palate	Facial defect	->	Persistent deformity	Repair	Repair
Previable premature rupture of membranes	Pre-term labor	->	Fetal demise Fetal/maternal infection		Amniopatch Amniograft Amnioexchange
Gastroschisis	Bowel exteriorization	->	Bowel perivisceritis Prolonged ileus		
Amniotic bands	Limb/digit/umbilical cord constriction	->	Limb/digit deformity or amputation Fetal demise (cord occlusion)		Laser separation of bands
Other					
Stem cell/enzyme defects	Hemoglobinopathy Immunodeficiency storage diseases	->	Anemia Infection Neurological impairment		Stem cell transplants Gene therapy
Chronic fetal vascular access					Vascular access*
Predictable organ failure	Hypoplastic heart, kidney, lung	->	Neonatal heart, kidney, lung failure		Cell transplant to induce tolerance for postnatal organ transplant
Tissue engineering	Bladder exstrophy	->	Urinary tract dysfunction		Videoscopic cell harvest*

* Not yet performed in humans.

placental abruption, preterm labor, premature rupture of membranes, complications of tocolytic therapy (e.g., pulmonary edema), deep venous thrombosis, and pulmonary embolism. In one retrospective review of 50 open fetal surgery cases during the development of these procedures at University of California, San Francisco (prior to 1994),[2,3] maternal bleeding during open fetal surgery was approximately 455 ml, ranging from 150 ml to 1400 ml. Six patients required blood transfusions. Significant bleeding is rare during fetoscopic or percutaneous cases. Premature rupture of membranes (PROM) is an extremely common complication of fetal surgery and the most common fetoscopic complication.[4] Perinatal loss rates are as high as 50% due to the sequelae of PROM.[5] In fetoscopic cases, single port procedures have a 6%–10% rate of PROM[6] and multiple port cases have a 40%–60% rate.[7,8]

Preterm labor (PTL) occurs to varying degrees after all fetal surgical procedures, and the morbidity to the pregnant woman is primarily related to PTL and its treatment. PTL may be due to PROM, changes in uterine volume, infection, hormonal changes, and stress.[9] Treatment includes a variety of tocolytics.

Long-term outcomes focus on the ability to conceive and carry a pregnancy in the future. Fetal therapy does not seem to affect fertility[10] as reported by Farrell *et al.* In this study, 32 of 35 mothers who attempted to conceive after fetal surgery were successful, with 31 live births resulting. Two of the women unable to conceive had a strong previous history of infertility, and the third had been trying for only 6 months. When the hysterotomy is not made in the lower uterine segment (which includes virtually all mid-gestation hysterotomies), the index and all subsequent pregnancies cannot sustain labor and must be delivered via Cesarean section because of the 12% risk of uterine rupture. In Farrell's study, two mothers who labored against medical advice had uterine scar dehiscence without adverse sequelae. Although not noted in this study, there is an increased risk of placenta previa and placenta accreta in future pregnancies in those who have undergone previous Cesarean delivery.

Congenital diaphragmatic hernia

Congenital diaphragmatic hernia (CDH) is a condition that develops when there is normal failure of fusion of the four embryonic structures which form the diaphragm: the septum transversum, the pleuroperitoneal membranes, dorsal mesentery of the esophagus, and the body wall.[11] Abdominal viscera herniate through the defect into the thoracic cavity. If the abdominal organs intermittently move in and out of the thorax, there is usually little negative impact on thoracic structures; but if viscera such as the liver get trapped in the thorax, compression of the lungs can stunt pulmonary development and possibly displace the heart and vessels. This leads to pulmonary hypoplasia, pulmonary hypertension and postnatal respiratory failure.

CDH affects approximately 1 in 3500 live births.[12] The clinical course for neonates ranges from exceedingly good with postnatal care, to death despite maximal interventions (e.g., extracorporeal membrane oxygenation (ECMO) support, inhaled nitric oxide therapy). Historically, the reported mortality for neonates diagnosed with CDH at birth has been 30%–50%,[13] and the reported mortality for those diagnosed antenatally has been up to 88%[14,15] despite the most sophisticated postnatal support. Although this has been a point of controversy, this difference has been referred to as the "hidden mortality,"[15] and reflects fetal death in utero or shortly after birth. Fetuses with the poorest outcomes may be risk stratified by prenatal ultrasound identifying left lobe of the liver herniation (liver-up)[16] or a low lung-to-head ratio (LHR – length times width of right lung divided by the head circumference).[17,18] Fetuses with "liver-up" CDH have a 43% survival vs. 93% in those with "liver-down" CDH. Liver-down fetuses with LHRs less than 1 have 100% mortality; between 1 and 1.4 have 60% mortality; and greater than 1.4 have zero mortality. Some have argued that new non-surgical therapies have improved survival for CDH infants, but Stege *et al.*[19] contend that reported increases in survival for CDH over the 1990s have been due to selection bias and that newer therapies such as ECMO, high-frequency oscillatory ventilation, and inhaled nitric oxide have had no significant effect on the mortality of approximately 62%. They state that the only significant correlation with survival of live births has been with rate of elective termination and inversely with additional anomalies. Recent advancements in ventilatory care have improved these statistics in some studies. Bagolan *et al.*[20] reviewed 70 high-risk CDH infants who were prenatally diagnosed or had respiratory distress at birth between1996 and 2001. From 1996 to 1999, infants were treated with inhaled nitric oxide and high frequency oxygen ventilation with a survival rate of 47%–50%. Starting in 2000, some of these patients were treated with "gentle" ventilation and permissive hypercarbia and had a survival of up to 90%. Another study reported a survival rate of 75.8% with permissive hypercapnea and spontaneous respiration as the respiratory strategy.[21]

Beginning in the 1980s, poor postnatal survival rates and a desire to reduce the "hidden mortality," led surgeons at the University of California, San Francisco (UCSF) to attempt to repair diaphragmatic hernias in utero to prevent the subsequent detrimental effects on fetal lung

Table 73.2. Congenital diaphragmatic hernia: open complete fetal repair experience[26–28]

Case	Gest. age at operation (weeks)	Gest. age at delivery (weeks)	Survival	Cause of death
1	27		A	Probably cardiac arrest after hepatic blood loss, bradycardia, poor monitoring
2	27		A	Kinking of umbilical vein
3	24	34	C	Died postop after postnatal repair, persistent pulmonary hypoplasia
4	21		A	Hypovolemia with umbilical cord compression?
5	26	31	C	Endotracheal tube dislodgement and respiratory failure
6	27	28	C	Intestinal obstruction, perforation, sepsis
7	24.5	32	**E**	
8	25		A	Kinked umbilical vein
9	25		B	Umbilical distortion, liver ischemia
10	25	32	**E**	
11	24		A	"Battledore" placenta
12	24	28	**E**	
13	24	26	C	Pulmonary hypoplasia, small disruption in diaphragm
14	23		A	Kinked umbilical vein
15	28		B	
				?Distorted umbilical vein
16	25		A	Sinus venosus cut
17	24.5		A	Uterine contractions
18	25.5	34	**E**	
19	25.5		B	Bradycardia?
20	25.5	28	C	Pre-term labor, poor uterine blood flow
21	25	34	**E**	
22	25	33	**E**	
23	25	32	**E**	
24	25	29	C	Withdrawal of support

A = Died intraoperatively.
B = Died in utero but not intra-operatively.
C = Died within 30 days of birth.
D = Died after 30 days old.
E = Long-term survival.

development. Experimental results in sheep and primates showed improvement in lung growth, pulmonary function, and neonatal survival.[22–25] Although the open surgical repair (i.e., hysterotomy, partial fetal delivery and repair of the diaphragmatic defect) was demonstrated to be feasible in humans,[26–28] there were many factors which limited its usefulness. These included the global issues for open fetal surgery, preterm labor and maternal morbidity, as well as CDH-specific issues such as compromise of the umbilical circulation upon reduction of the liver into the abdominal cavity (of course, an issue not relevant to repairs after birth).

In 1997, Harrison *et al.*[29] reported the results of a prospective, National Institutes of Health (NIH)-funded trial comparing open repair to standard postnatal care (which included ECMO, when indicated). Four fetuses with isolated left-sided CDH, significant lung volume reduction, and no liver herniation underwent prenatal repair, and seven were repaired after birth. There was no difference in survival (75% vs. 86%, respectively). Therefore, they concluded that fetuses with prenatally diagnosed CDH without liver herniation, should be treated with standard postnatal care. Yet, the severe CDH fetuses with liver herniation and low LHR needed alternative methods of treatment. Table 73.2 summarizes the initial experience with open repair of CDH in human fetuses.

Returning to the laboratory, the UCSF group searched for ways to exploit the observation that fetal lungs externally drained of fluid do not grow, whereas prevention of the efflux of fluid from the lungs via tracheal obstruction promotes lung growth.[30–32] This principle, applied to animal models of CDH, resulted in functionally robust lungs in liver-up and liver-down fetuses and reduced herniated viscera.[33–39] Subsequently, several methods of reversible tracheal occlusion were devised and applied in humans. The initial human experience at UCSF with tracheal occlusion (PLUG technique – "plug the lung until it grows")[40] involved open surgery (Table 73.3) with placement of an intratracheal plug or external tracheal clips. These devices

Table 73.3. Congenital diaphragmatic hernia: open fetal tracheal occlusion (UCSF experience)[40]

Case	Gest. age at diagnosis (weeks)	Gest. age at operation (weeks)	Gest. age at delivery (weeks)	Survival	Cause of death	Other
1	23	27	30	E		Foam plug
2	18	27	31	C	Plug not occlusive, pulmonary hypoplasia	Foam plug
3	18	25	29	B	Umbilical cord accident	Hemoclip
4	20	25	28	C	Intracranial hemorrhage, support withdrawn	Hemoclip
5	20	27	27	B	Tocolytic failure, IUFD	Aneurysm clip
6	20	27	34	D	Plug not occlusive, death at 4 mo	Aneurysm clip
7	19	26	29	D	Bowel necrosis at 4 mo	Hemoclip
8	18	27	32	D	CNS damage at 4 mo, support withdrawn	Hemoclip
9	23	26	27	B	Hydrops from rapid, excessive lung growth	Hemoclip
10	21	29	30	C	Ipsilateral sequestration	Hemoclip
11	20	30	33	C	Tetrasomy 12p, death at 4 hr	Hemoclip
12	21	30	31	C	No biologic response to occlusion, death at 1 hr	Hemoclip
13	26	30	33	C	No biologic response to occlusion, death at 30 hr	Hemoclip

A = Died intraoperatively.
B = Died in utero but not intraoperatively.
C = Died within 30 days of birth.
D = Died after 30 days old.
E = Long-term survival.

were removed at the time of birth using the EXIT (Ex Utero intrapartum treatment) strategy. The EXIT strategy[41] differs from a Cesarean delivery in that the uterus is opened with a hemostatic stapler and only the fetal head and upper torso are delivered while the baby is still on placental support. A bronchoscope is passed into the trachea, the occlusive device is removed, the trachea is repaired if necessary, an endotracheal is placed, and bag ventilation is instituted before the umbilical cord is cut. Initially, eight fetuses underwent tracheal occlusion. The first occlusion device was an internal foam plug, which produced the desired result on the lung, but was associated with tracheomalacia. In the second case, a smaller plug was used to avoid tracheal injury, but it failed to produce lung enlargement, probably due to leak around the plug. To resolve these problems, an external clip technique was developed using aneurysm clips (two cases) and subsequently hemoclips (four cases), which were easily removed.

Flake *et al.*[42] at the Children's Hospital of Pennsylvania (CHOP) reported their experience with open fetal tracheal occlusion with hemoclips (Table 73.4). From 1995 to 1999, 15 fetuses underwent open temporary tracheal occlusion. These fetuses had isolated, severe right- and left-sided CDH with low LHR. Five (33%) fetuses survived long term, and of these, three had severe neurological deficits. Lung growth was variable but those occluded early (before 26 weeks' gestation) showed more consistent lung growth. This group observed that, even in the fetuses with dramatic lung growth, lung function seemed impaired postnatally. They attributed this to prematurity, to the detrimental effect on the number and function of Type II pneumocytes by tracheal occlusion,[43–45] and possibly to altered lymphatic drainage secondary to increased fetal intrathoracic pressure impairing lung fluid clearance after birth.

The open tracheal occlusion procedures were performed by hysterotomy and therefore were complicated by the ever present specter of preterm labor and delivery. Surgeons continued to investigate ways to minimize the trauma to the uterus. To that end, video-assisted fetal endoscopy (FETENDO) was developed.[46–48] This technique utilized a maternal laparotomy and three access ports. Under ultrasound guidance, the fetal neck is fixed in extension with a chin stay-suture and the tracheal midline is identified with the placement of a suture on a T-fastener. A perfusion pump circulates warmed irrigation fluid and suction via the hysteroscope. The trachea is dissected and occluded with two titanium clips.

Table 73.4. Congenital diaphragmatic hernia: open fetal tracheal occlusion (CHOP experience)[42]

Enrolment and selection	
Total number of cases	15
Right-sided liver herniation	2
Left-sided liver herniation	13
Maternal morbidity	
Early preterm labor (POD 2, 5)	2
Complicated post-op course	3
	(1) Readmission for tocolysis
	(2) Pulmonary edema and ventilation
	Vaginal bleeding and possible chorioamnionitis
	(3) Uterine irritability and cervical change
	Bedrest, preterm labor
Lung growth after fetal tracheal occlusion	
Late tracheal occlusion (27–28 wks) with clear lung growth	3/7
Early tracheal occlusion (25–26 wks) with clear lung growth	5/6
Survival	
Right sided/left sided	2/3 (total 5 (33%))
ECMO required	4 (1 survived)
LHR (left-sided lesion only)	0.73
Average hospitalization for survivors	76 days
Average hospitalization for deaths	18 days
Causes of death	(1) Early preterm labor 2
	(2) Atrial perforation with central line 1
	(3) Inadequate lung growth, inability to be resuscitated 1
	(4) Multisystem organ failure 6
Long-term survival	
Tracheal stenosis	0
Severe neurologic deficits	3
Recurrent pneumonia	2

LHR = Lung–head ratio.
POD = Postoperative day.
ECMO = Extracorporeal membrane oxygenation.

A comparison of the FETENDO technique with open tracheal occlusion and standard postnatal care was reported in 1998 in a retrospective study by the UCSF group.[7] From 1994 to 1997, the initial eight fetuses and an additional five fetuses (four of which were conversions from fetoscopy) underwent open tracheal occlusion. Thirteen underwent standard postnatal care, and eight were treated with fetoscopic tracheal occlusion. The results were very promising for FETENDO with a 75% survival rate compared to 38% with standard postnatal care and 15% with open surgery. Seven out of the eight FETENDO fetuses demonstrated good lung physiologic response to the occlusion; whereas only 5 of the 13 open fetuses had evidence of lung growth.

In July 2003,[49] UCSF reported progress with the FETENDO technique and discussed 11 additional fetoscopic cases (Table 73.5), making a total of 19 fetuses treated with FETENDO clips between 1996 and 1999. They reported a 68% survival 90 days after delivery with an 86% survival for fetuses with LHR > 1 and 63% for LHR < 1. One fetus died in utero on postoperative day two. Regarding obstetrical complications, six mothers suffered from pulmonary edema (none required postoperative mechanical ventilation), 12 developed chorioamniotic membrane separation, and 12 had premature rupture of membranes. There was procedure-specific fetal morbidity in the form of vocal cord paresis/paralysis, tracheomalacia, and tracheal stenosis in five patients. Although the early attempts at endoluminal plugging encountered problems with tracheomalacia and leak, this concept was revisited. The evolution of the endoluminal approach involved a gelfoam plug, an expanding umbrella, and finally a detachable balloon.[39,50,51] In May, 2001, UCSF reported two cases of CDH treated by a fetoscopically placed detachable balloon.[52] Maternal

Table 73.5. Congenital diaphragmatic hernia: FETENDO clip experience[7,49]

Case	Gest. age at Diagnosis (weeks)	Gest. age at operation (weeks)	Gest. age at delivery (weeks)	Survival	Cause of death	Other
1	23	30	33	C	Multiple pterygium syndrome, support withdrawn	
2	16	30	31	E		
3	21	30	33	E		Vocal cord paresis, tracheostomy Died at 11 mo, tracheostomy dislodgement
4	19	28	35	E		Vocal cord paresis, tracheostomy
5	20	29	35	C	No biologic response to occlusion	
6	19	27	31	E		Laceration, repair at EXIT
7	18	28	29	E		
8	19	27	32	E		
9	23	29	32	E		Died at 9 mo, meningitis
10	24	28	31	C	No biologic response to occlusion	
11	20	26	30	E		Vocal cord paresis, tracheostomy Died at 15 mo, tracheostomy dislodgement
12	16	25	26	B	Fetal demise	
13	19	26	27	C	Pneumonia, sepsis, pulmonary hemorrhage, ischemic bowel	
14	21	26	30	C	During CDH repair	
15	24	27	32	E		Laceration, repair at EXIT
16	21	26	33	E		
17	17	25	29	E		Vocal cord paresis, tracheostomy, malacia with multiple stents
18	17	26	31	E		Malacia with multiple stents Cotton procedure
19	17	26	32	E		

A = Died intraoperatively.
B = Died in utero but not intraoperatively.
C = Died within 30 days of birth.
D = Died after 30 days old.
E = Long-term survival.
EXIT = Ex utero intrapartum treatment.

laparotomy was still performed, but only a single 5 mm trocar was used. Hydrodissection with a newly developed continuous perfusion fetoscope allowed for access to the fetal mouth and trachea, and a detachable balloon loaded on a catheter was placed in the trachea via the side port of the hysteroscope. It was inflated to optimize the seal but at a low pressure designed to avoid tracheal ischemia. Both fetuses survived and did well without any airway-related problems.

Before this technique could be widely disseminated, the UCSF group embarked on an NIH-sponsored prospective, randomized trial to compare fetoscopic tracheal occlusion (balloon) with optimal contemporary postnatal care. In November 2003, the results of that trial were reported (Table 73.6).[53] Women with fetuses between 22 and 27 weeks' gestation with severe left-sided CDH (liver herniation and LHR<1.4) were randomized. After the enrolment of 24 women, an interim analysis demonstrated no difference in 90-day survival between groups (77% vs. 73% for postnatal care and tracheal occlusion, respectively). This was an unexpectedly high survival in the postnatal care group. It was determined that it would not be feasible to accrue enough patients to show a difference in mortality between groups and the study was terminated. All women in both groups who desired further pregnancies were able to conceive and carry to term healthy babies. There was a significant difference in gestational age at delivery for the fetuses in the tracheal occlusion group (mean of 31 weeks' gestation) vs. 37 weeks for the postnatal care group. This result combined with the survival statistics suggested that the benefits of lung development with tracheal occlusion may be offset by the risks to the fetus resulting from prematurity.

Table 73.6. Congenital diaphragmatic hernia: FETENDO balloon versus postnatal care randomized trial data[53]

Parameter (%)	Standard care (N=13)	Tracheal occlusion (N=11)
Maternal age	28.5 +/− 5.7	29.5 +/− 5.6
Fetal sex (% male)	9 (69%)	8 (73%)
Gestational age at randomization	25.4 +/− 1.3	24.5 +/− 1.6
LHR	0.96 +/− 0.20	0.97 +/− 0.14
Maternal wound infection	0	1 (9%)
Preterm labor	4 (31%)	8 (73%)
PROM	3 (23%)	11 (100%)
Time from tracheal occlusion to PROM		24.8 +/− 14.8
Time from PROM to delivery	<1	9.5 +/− 8.5
Placental abruption	1 (8%)	3 (27%)
Mode of delivery EXIT / vaginal / Cesarean section	0 / 12 (92%) / 1 (8%)	11 (100%) / 0 / 0
Gestational age at delivery	37 +/− 1.5	30.8 +/− 2.0
Birthweight	3.03 +/− 0.48	1.49 +/− 0.36
Survival LHR < 0.79	0/0	0/1
Survival LHR 0.79 – 1.06	8/11 (73%)	5/7 (71%)
Survival LHR 1.07 – 1.39	2/2 (100%)	3/3 (100%)
Age at CDH repair	6.7 +/− 2.2	5.7 +/− 2.3
Prosthetic patch CDH repair	10/11 (91%)	11/11 (100%)
Age at successful extubation	35.3 +/− 20.5	38.8 +/− 15.5
Age at hospital discharge	62.1 +/− 28.7	59.6 +/− 17.9
Supplemental oxygen at discharge	4/9 (44%)	4/8 (50%)
Age at full enteral feeding	27.2 +/− 10.5	31.9 +/− 11.9
Fundoplication	8/11 (73%)	7/11 (64%)
Gastrostomy tube	3/10 (30%)	1/9 (11%)
Tube feeding at discharge	5/9 (55%)	4/8 (50%)
Antireflux meds at discharge	8/9 (89%)	7/8 (88%)
Weight gain at discharge	680 +/− 490	570 +/− 540

LHR = Lung–head ratio.
PROM = Premature rupture of membranes.
CDH = Congenital diaphragmatic hernia.
EXIT = Ex utero intrapartum treatment.

Another significant finding was the direct correlation of LHR to mortality. The hazard ratio for death associated with an LHR > 0.9 to an LHR = 0.9 was 0.13.

The results of this study have generated additional questions. The optimal timing and duration of fetal tracheal occlusion in humans are unknown. Developments in endoscopic instrumentation may improve the preterm labor rates with fetoscopy and therefore eliminate some of the morbidity of prematurity. Finally, fetuses with LHR < 0.9 still have a very poor prognosis. Therefore, the Eurofetus group is developing plans for a randomized controlled trial targeting this particular subset of CDH fetuses.[53] The unexpectedly high survival with standard care may be evidence of the advancement in perinatal care concurrent with advances in surgical treatment. The "trial effect" may also be a contributing factor since every aspect of care was optimized in this tertiary care setting. These results may not be applicable in a more general setting.

Thoracic lesions

A highly select group of patients with congenital cystic adenomatoid malformation (CCAM) and bronchopulmonary sequestration (BPS) are candidates for antenatal therapy. Depending on the nature of the lesion (cystic vs. solid), its physiologic effect, and the gestational age, there are several treatment options. These include placement of a thoracoamniotic shunt, thoracentesis, cyst aspiration, or open fetal surgery with mass resection. CCAM is a rare condition characterized by an overgrowth of terminal respiratory bronchioles forming cysts.[54] BPS is characterized by lung tissue with no connection to the tracheobronchial tree that is supplied by an anomalous systemic artery.[55] These masses, if large, can cause lung compression and hypoplasia, mediastinal shift and cardiovascular compromise, polyhydramnios, hydrops, and death. The prognosis is excellent in the absence of severe fetal distress characterized by hydrops.[56] These two conditions can be difficult to distinguish via prenatal ultrasound, although the identification of a systemic arterial blood supply is pathognomonic for BPS.[57] In addition, ultrafast fetal MRI can help differentiate these lesions. Other conditions that can be confused with these include CDH, thoracic lymphangioma, enteric cyst, neurenteric cyst, pericardial cyst, mediastinal cystic teratoma, bronchial atresia or stenosis, neuroblastoma, congenital lobar emphysema, and hemangioma.[58] CCAMs have a variable natural history. Up to 40% are associated with hydrops due to a mass effect and up to 15% regress during gestation. BPS usually does not cause a mass effect. It can, however, cause a tension hydrothorax. Up to 68% of BPS regress during gestation.[55,58] In order to select fetuses that may be at risk for hydrops and thus be possible candidates for fetal intervention, Adzick[54] devised a measurement called the cystic adenomatoid volume ratio (CVR), which is a sonographic measurement of the CCAM volume divided by head circumference. Crombleholme *et al.*[59] demonstrated that a CVR of greater than 1.6 denotes about a 75% risk of developing hydrops. These fetuses require serial sonographic monitoring and intervention if hydrops develops.

Several therapeutic interventions for these fetuses have been attempted. CCAMs with large cysts may be treated with cyst aspiration instead of open resection. The efficacy of cyst aspiration has been limited due to rapid reaccumulation of fluid.[60] This technique may be used as a temporizing measure prior to shunting, resection, or early delivery. Chronic cyst decompression for unilocular cysts with thoracoamniotic shunting has met with some success. Clark *et al.*[61] described the first case of CCAM treated with thoracoamniotic shunting. The hydrops resolved and the baby was delivered 3 weeks after shunting without evidence of pulmonary hypoplasia. Several other successful thoracoamniotic shunt placements have been reported.[62–64] Adzick *et al.*[65] described nine fetuses with CCAM and hydrops that were treated with shunts. The masses had a 61% reduction in volume, 100% resolution of hydrops, and an 11% mortality rate. This group[66] also described two fetuses with BPS that suffered from tension hydrothorax and resultant hydrops. Shunting resolved the hydrops, and the fetuses survived through delivery.

Massive multicystic or predominantly solid CCAM lesions may require open fetal surgery with resection. The technique involves the creation of a hemostatic hysterotomy, exposure of the head and torso of the fetus, and a thoracotomy at the fifth intercostal space. The appropriate pulmonary lobe(s) are resected, and the thoracotomy is closed. Adzick *et al.*[67] report 22 cases of fetal lobectomy for these lesions. All cases were fetuses with large multicystic lesions and hydrops. Of these, 50% survived with hydrops resolution in 1 to 2 weeks, return of mediastinum to midline in 3 weeks, and follow-up normal developmental testing. The deaths were due to a variety of issues including unresolved maternal "mirror syndrome" necessitating early delivery, fetal bradycardia, intra-operative uncontrolled uterine contractions, and chorioamnionitis. One-half of the deaths occurred from bradycardia immediately after delivery of the mass from the chest. This was probably due to abrupt cardiac decompression and hemodynamic collapse. Maternal morbidity in this series included one wound seroma, one wound infection, two blood transfusions, two cases of mild pulmonary edema, one case of chorioamnionitis, and one patient with uterine wound dehiscence. Thirteen mothers have had subsequent pregnancies with normal Cesarean section deliveries.

Future directions for the antenatal treatment of thoracic lesions include minimal access techniques. Bruner *et al.*[68] describe the ultrasound-guided percutaneous application of a Nd:YAG laser through an 18-gauge needle to debulk a CCAM in a 23-week gestation fetus with hydrops. The treatment was performed twice, 1 week apart, but hydrops worsened and fetal death occurred. This technique may not have the accuracy or the adequate debulking ability to successfully treat these lesions. Medical management with a course of maternal betamethasone may help resolve hydrops and CCAM growth as demonstrated in three cases at UCSF.[69]

Twin–twin transfusion syndrome

Twin–twin transfusion syndrome (TTTS) is a complication of a monochorionic pregnancy. Twenty to 30% of all twins are monochorionic, and approximately 10% of these suffer from varying degrees of TTTS.[70] This phenomenon can occur in twin pregnancies but can occur in higher-order multiple gestation pregnancies as well. In diamniotic pregnancies, it is defined by the presence of polyhydramnios (maximum vertical pocket (MVP) greater than 8 cm) in the recipient twin's sac and oligohydramnios (MVP less than 2 cm) in the donor or "stuck" twin's sac.[71] The syndrome results from imbalance in blood flow between the twins due to abnormal placental vascular communications. The donor twin typically suffers from growth retardation and progressive renal failure, whereas

Table 73.7. Twin–twin transfusion syndrome staging [73]

Stage I	−BDT
Stage II	−BDT
	−CAD
Stage III	−BDT
	+CAD
Stage IV	Hydrops
Stage V	In utero demise

BDT = Urine visible in bladder of donor twin by ultrasound.
CAD = Critically abnormal Doppler studies.

the recipient twin experiences high output cardiac failure and hydrops, possibly in utero demise. Expectant management results in 80% to 100% mortality of both twins.[70,72]

Quintero *et al.*[73] described a staging system to risk stratify these twins based on a retrospective analysis (Table 73.7). The absence of urine in the donor twin bladder after 60 minutes of ultrasonographic observation, coupled with critically abnormal Doppler studies in either twin (e.g., absent or reversed end-diastolic velocity in the umbilical artery, pulsatile umbilical venous flow, or reversed flow in the ductus venosus) are poor prognostic indicators. Hydrops in either twin, indicative of cardiac failure, is an extremely poor prognostic indicator, and finally death of either twin is usually followed by death of the other or the delivery of an extremely compromised (usually neurological compromise) twin. This group's 1999 study demonstrated a statistically significant difference in survival rates by stage, but another study by Taylor *et al.*[74] reports that prognosis correlated with a change in stage rather than the stage on presentation.

Treatment strategies for TTTS have included expectant management, serial amniocenteses (amnioreduction), laser therapy, umbilical cord occlusion, and septostomy. Expectant management results in less than 20% survival.[75] One may argue for a role of expectant management in stage I disease late in gestation.

Serial amniocentesis of the polyhydramniotic sac to reduce the amniotic fluid volume has been shown to prolong pregnancy and improve survival by an unknown mechanism.[75–78] This procedure has an overall success rate of 66% (at least one twin survival) with a risk of neurological impairment of 15%.[71] A recent study by Johnsen *et al.*[79] examined 24 pregnancies with TTTS between 1993 and 1999. Seventy-nine percent of pregnancies had at least one fetus survive with 50% of both fetuses surviving. The mean gestational age was 34.6 weeks.

In 1990, De Lia *et al.*[80] demonstrated the feasibility of using Nd-YAG laser photocoagulation as a treatment modality for TTTS. In this technique, all placental vessels crossing the intertwin membrane are photocoagulated using fetoscopy. By 1995,[81,82] this group had shown a 53% survival rate (28/53) with this technque. Ville *et al.*[6] used photocoagulation in a study of 132 pregnancies and demonstrated a 55% overall fetal survival rate, a 73% survival rate of at least one twin, and a 4.2% incidence of adverse neurologic sequelae after 1 year.

In a 1999 retrospective study by Hecher *et al.*[83] 73 of the patients treated with laser therapy were compared to 43 patients treated with amniocentesis. The two groups had similar survival rates (61% vs. 51%), but the laser group had a greater number of pregnancies with 1 or more survivors (79% vs. 60%), fewer spontaneous intrauterine deaths (3% vs. 19%), a lower incidence of brain abnormalities (6% vs. 18%), and a longer interval between intervention and delivery (90 vs. 72 days) and, therefore, higher birthweights (1750 g vs. 1145 g). The next year, the same group[84] reported a 68% survival rate with an 81% survival rate of one of the twins and a 42% survival rate of both twins in a series of 200 pregnancies.

In 1998, Quintero *et al.*[85] introduced the concept of selective laser photocoagulation of communicating vessels (S-LPCV) vs. non-selective laser photocoagulation (NS-LPCV). In this technique, not all vessels crossing the intertwin membrane are targeted. This group argued that, because of the amniotic fluid imbalance, the intertwin membrane is pushed towards the placental territory of the donor twin. Therefore, coagulating all vessels crossing this anatomic boundary will not only interrupt the communicating vessels, but will also target some of the donor twin's critical vessels not involved in TTTS. In the selective technique, only unpaired vessels are targeted. Arteriovenous communications are identified by noting that the terminal end of one artery does not have a corresponding returning vein to the same fetus but, rather, returns to the other fetus. Also, arterio–arterio and venous–venous communications are identified by following these vessels from one fetus to the other. In 2000, the group published data[86] comparing the two approaches. There were 18 pregnancies in the NS-LPCV group and 74 in the S-LPCV group. Survival of at least one twin was higher in the S-LPCV group (83% vs. 61%) since there was a lower rate of intrauterine demise of both fetuses (5.6% vs. 22%). There were more hydropic fetuses in the NS-LPCV group (27% vs. 5.4%). Feldstein *et al.*[87] describe a similar but "super selective" technique denoted the "SELECT" procedure[88] (sonographically evaluated, laser endoscopic coagulation for twins) where a TTTS pregnancy, unresponsive to serial amniocenteses, was successfully treated by identifying by color and spectral Doppler and fetoscopy the single offending arteriovenous anastomosis. Only this putative anastomosis was laser coagulated.

One anatomic variation, which could hamper the visualization of the vessels is an anteriorly placed placenta. A few groups have studied this issue and have developed techniques that reliably address it. Quintero *et al.*[89] maintain a percutaneous approach and describe using a flexible endoscope or a rigid endoscope and a side-firing laser fiber through a second port. DePrest *et al.*[90,91] describe an alternative approach using a minilaparotomy, a curved fiberscope, and a flexible cannula. These studies showed similar survival rates to posterior placentas, but the operating time was approximately 25% longer.

Prospective, randomized clinical trials are currently under way in Europe and in the United States to compare the efficacy of amnioreduction and laser photocoagulation. The inclusion criteria for the multicenter United States trial include monochorionic diamniotic pregnancies diagnosed with TTTS prior to 22 weeks' gestation, oligohydramnios in the donor twin and polyhydramnios in the recipient twin, decompressed bladder in the donor (stages II–V), and no structural abnormalities or known CNS abnormality by MRI. Patients will be randomized to either aggressive serial amnioreduction or selective fetoscopic laser photocoagulation before 24 weeks' gestation and stratified by pregnancies presenting prior to 20 weeks' and after 20 weeks' gestation. The pregnancies will be followed with ultrasound, MRI, and echocardiography. The primary outcome measure is 30-day survival after delivery (with no treatment failure), and secondary measures include neonatal comorbidities, imaging data, placental examination, long-term maternal morbidities, and long-term neurodevelopmental assessment. This trial differs from the European trial in the use of selective laser photocoagulation (vs. nonselective in Europe), and in the rigorous assessment of long-term developmental outcomes. Patient recruitment began in March 2002.

One of the options for a TTTS pregnancy is umbilical cord occlusion, but this is usually reserved for the severe case in which fetal death of one twin is likely. When one twin dies, hypotension in the dying twin causes an acute transfusion from the healthy twin into the dying one and the resultant hypotension in the remaining twin usually causes death or neurologic damage.[92] The goal of umbilical cord occlusion is to eliminate the blood exchange between the two fetuses by ligating[93,94] or cauterizing[95,96] the umbilical cord of the terminal twin. This can limit the acute transfusion event, although some transfusion can occur through other anomalous connections. In a recent study by Taylor *et al.*,[96] bipolar cord coagulation was performed on 15 stage III and IV TTTS pregnancies with a survival rate of 93%. This is marginally higher than the single survivor rate (85%) for laser coagulation of vessels for stage III/IV.[86] The overall survival is 46% compared to 57%.[86,96] Quintero reports a survival rate of 76% with no incidence of cerebral palsy with umbilical cord ligation.[71]

Septostomy was first described by Saade in 1995[97] as a method to equalize volumes in each fetal sac and minimize the number of invasive procedures. The technique used a needle to puncture the intertwin membrane, allowing fluid to accumulate around the oligohydramnios fetus. The same group showed in 1998 that septostomy is associated with a survival rate of 83% (20/24), comparable to more invasive methods. Johnson *et al.*[98] compared amnioreduction to septostomy and demonstrated a similar overall survival rate (78%). These groups suggest that septostomy may provide similar benefit as amnioreduction with fewer numbers of procedures, more room for the "stuck fetus," and possibly older age at delivery. Some believe that the problems with septostomy make it a poor treatment option. Quintero *et al.*[71] demonstrated that there is no pressure differential between the two sacs;[99,100] thus obviating the need for eliminating the membrane. He states that septostomy can result in the following outcomes: a pseudomonoamniotic state fraught with the problems of cord entanglement and fetal demise; it can limit the ability to monitor the disease progress since amniotic fluid volume will not reflect urinary function; and finally, this will make future laser therapy more difficult because of interference from the floating divided membrane. A randomized multicentered trial is being considered to compare these options.[101]

Twin reversed arterial perfusion and twins discordant for a lethal anomaly

Twin reversed arterial perfusion (TRAP) is a rare complication of monozygotic twin pregnancy and occurs in approximately 1% of these pregnancies.[102] The TRAP sequence is the most severe form of twin–twin transfusion syndrome. A normal (pump) twin provides circulation for itself and for an abnormally developing acardiac (perfused) twin. The acardiac twin is not connected to the placenta but, rather, directly to the umbilical cord of the pump twin. The acardiac twin is perfused by the normal twin, pumping in a reversed direction into the acardiac twin. The pump twin is at risk for developing high output cardiac failure, hydrops and death.[103] The mortality for the acardiac twin is 100% and 35%–55% for the pump twin.[104–106] One prognostic indicator is the twin: weight ratio (weight of the acardiac twin expressed as a percentage of the weight of the other twin). Moore *et al.*[106] noted that in 49 TRAP pregnancies, a 70% ratio predicted a 90% preterm delivery rate, 40% polyhydramnios rate, and 30% congestive heart failure rate in the pump twin.

Table 73.8. Outcomes of vascular occlusion techniques for fetuses with twin–twin transfusion syndrome, twin reversed arterial perfusion, and those discordant for lethal anomaly[103,124,129]

Technique	Procedures	Gestational age at procedure (weeks)	Success of occlusion	PROM	Total loss	Gestational age at delivery (weeks)
Embolization	22	24 (18–27)	17 (77%)	2 (9%)	7 (32%)	34^{24-39}
Ligation	24	22 (17–26)	21 (88%)	7 (39%)	9 (35%)	30^{24-37}
Monopolar coagulation	13	20 (16–24)	11 (85%)[a]	1 (8%)	4 (31%)	36^{32-42}
Bipolar coagulation	108	21 (13–28)	108 (100%)	21 (21%)	19 (18%)	33^{24-41}
Radiofrequency ablation	16	20 (17–24)	15 (94%)	3 (19%)	2 (13%)	38^{24-40}

PROM = premature rupture of membranes.
[a]The two failures required a second occlusion.

Interventions for TRAP that have been described include termination of pregnancy, expectant management with early delivery, treatment of polyhydramnios with indomethacin,[107] treatment of heart failure with digoxin,[103,108] and early delivery of the abnormal twin by hysterotomy (termed sectio parvo).[109–111] All of these options have significant risks to the mother and the normal fetus. Currently, the treatment goals for TRAP sequence, discordant anomalies and stage V TTTS is selective reduction of the acardiac, anomalous, or hydropic cotwin. Depending on the placental anatomy, this can be done via umbilical cord embolization, ligation, ultrasonic transection, laser coagulation, or thermal coagulation using monopolar, bipolar and radiofrequency (RF) energy.

Agents used in embolization have ranged from fibrin and thrombogenic coils to ethanol and gels.[112–116] Embolization, however, has high failure rates (23%) and pregnancy loss rates (32%).[103] It is contraindicated in monochorionic pregnancies.

In 1994, Quintero described the first successful endoscopically guided suture ligation of the cord of an acardiac twin. The mother had an uncomplicated birth of a normal twin at 36 weeks.[117] In 1998, DeProst *et al.*[8] reviewed 23 cases of cord ligation which had a survival rate of 73%, but a high risk of premature rupture of membranes (PROM) (40%).

Laser photocoagulation of the cord is performed fetoscopically.[118–120] The root of the anomalous twin's umbilical cord is targeted with an Nd:YAG laser. Lewi *et al.*[121] reported described consecutive series of 50 cases. Forty-six percent of the cases failed and were completed with bipolar coagulation. They noted a 75% survival rate and a persistent PROM rate of 25%. Moldenhauer *et al.*[103] describe two successful cases of laser coagulation through a 16-gauge needle under ultrasound guidance.

Because of the high failure rate of photocoagulation, thermal coagulation has been attempted. A monopolar technique was first performed and reported for four cases by Rodeck *et al.*[122] In this technique, a sonographically guided wire is placed into, or adjacent to, the lumen of the aorta. Three of the cases had good outcomes. In one case the blood flow was reduced not terminated. The acardiac twin stopped growing after 2 weeks, and the hydrops of the pump twin improved. The mother suffered from pre-eclampsia and the baby was delivered at 32 weeks' gestation with hyaline membrane disease and developmental delay. Rodeck *et al.* contend that the sonographically guided needle and wire are safer and less expensive than other techniques and targeting the aorta versus the umbilical cord is relatively easy. It can also be performed early in gestation.[122–124]

Bipolar coagulation in 108 cases was reported with excellent success (100%), but with a high rate of PROM (20%) in a recent multicenter review.[103] This procedure is performed under ultrasound guidance using a bipolar cautery device through an endoscopic trocar. The umbilical cord is grasped, thermal energy applied, and cessation of blood flow is confirmed by Doppler.

Bipolar energy via a single trocar has been used to transect the umbilical cord.[125–127] The quickest and simplest method for selective reduction in these cases is the use of RF energy.[127–129] Using sonographic guidance, a no. 14-gauge needle is percutaneously placed at the base of the umbilical cord. Energy is applied and blood flow ceases within five minutes. This needle can be placed through an anterior placenta without complication. Tsao *et al.*[129] described 13 TRAP cases treated with RF ablation. Twelve of the 13 delivered a healthy twin, and one was prematurely delivered and died subsequently.

Tan and Sepulveda[130] reviewed treatment of acardiac twins through 2002. They identified 75 cases treated with minimally invasive techniques and divided these into two treatment modality groups: umbilical cord occlusion and intrafetal ablation. Cord occlusion included embolization, ligation, laser coagulation, and monopolar and bipolar thermocoagulation. Intrafetal ablation included alcohol, monopolar thermocoagulation, interstitial laser photocoagulation, and radiofrequency ablation. The overall twin survival rate was 76%. Comparing intrafetal ablation to umbilical cord occlusion, they found lower technical failure rates (13% vs. 35%), lower rate of premature delivery or rupture of membranes (23% vs. 58%), higher median gestational age at delivery (37 vs. 32 wks), and a longer interval between treatment and delivery (16 vs. 19.5 wks) with the intrafetal ablation techniques. This group, therefore, claims that the treatment of choice for TRAP should utilize intrafetal ablation. A summary of experience with vascular occlusion techniques is listed in Table 73.8.

Some monochorionic twin pregnancies are complicated by one twin that is discordant for a lethal anomaly, that is, one has an anomaly likely to result in in utero demise. Usually, there is no placental anomaly. However, if the abnormal twin dies in utero, the normal cotwin may be impaired or die due to a hemodynamic "unloading" into the dead cotwin. Many of the aforementioned techniques can be used to selectively terminate the discordant cotwin (Table 73.8). Radiofrequency ablation appears to hold the most promise for treating this anomaly.

Obstructive uropathy

Lower urinary tract obstruction (LUTO) in the fetus can lead to irreversible renal damage from renal dysplasia and to lung hypoplasia from oligo- or anhydramnios.[131] Oligohydramnios is associated with face and limb deformities, and bladder distention can lead to abdominal muscle deficiency. Congenital obstructive abnormalities of the urinary tract occur in 1% of pregnancies, but only 1 out of 500 pregnancies have severe urologic malformations.[132] The most common causes of LUTO in males are posterior urethral valves and urethral atresia. Females typically have developmental abnormalities associated with syndromes (e.g., cloacal anomaly) that are not amenable to antenatal treatment.[132] Neonates with early gestation, completely obstructing posterior urethral valves have a 45% mortality rate[133] mostly due to pulmonary hypoplasia. Early oligohydramnios (<22 weeks' gestation) has a mortality rate as high as 95%.[134]

The clinical picture of fetal LUTO was reproduced experimentally in a sheep model by Harrison *et al.*,[135] where ligation of the fetal lamb urachus and urethra in utero produced bilateral hydronephrosis and severe pulmonary hypoplasia with high perinatal mortality. The same group was able to ameliorate these effects by relieving the obstruction with suprapubic cutaneous cystostomies.[136] These experiments suggested that the fetus with early and severe obstructive uropathy may be salvageable.

In 1982, Harrison *et al.*[137,138] reported the first human clinical experience with antenatal surgical intervention. Of 26 pregnancies with hydronephrosis, nine underwent antenatal interventions. Three were diagnosed by percutaneous vesicoamniotic shunting to have poor renal function and were aborted. Four had percutaneous vesicoamniotic shunts successfully placed. Only one underwent open fetal surgery with the creation of bilateral ureterostomies. Three of the five unaborted fetuses died postnatally and two survived. Of those that died, one had multiple anomalies whereas the two others had irreversible kidney damage. With five out of nine fetuses having renal failure, this experience illustrated the need for better diagnosis and identification of fetuses that could benefit from prenatal intervention.

In 1994, Johnson *et al.*[139] reported 24 cases of fetal obstructive uropathy and proposed an algorithm for identifying fetuses for antenatal treatment (Fig. 73.1). The steps include (1) a detailed ultrasound exam identifying the signs of LUTO and also screening for other structural abnormalities; (2) fetal karyotype analysis; and (3) three serial fetal bladder aspirations (over 3 to 5 days) with analysis of fetal urinary electrolytes and protein to assess kidney function (Table 73.9). The third aspiration is believed to most accurately reflect fetal renal function. Candidates for fetal surgery need to have a normal male karyotype, no other lethal anomalies, a favorable urinalysis, and favorable-appearing kidneys by ultrasound (i.e., no evidence of corticomedullary dysplasia or cystic changes).

Current treatment therapies for LUTO include percutaneous sonographically guided vesicoamniotic shunt placement and direct valve ablation via fetal cystoscopy. In early surgical experience, open fetal therapy was performed but was abandoned due to the advent of percutaneously placed shunts which resulted in less morbidity to mother and fetus than the open hysterotomy approach.[140] Only five cases of open fetal surgery for obstructive uropathy have been published (Table 73.10). One patient was treated with bilateral ureterostomies, and the others were treated with cutaneous vesicostomies. Two survived (40%) with one having end-stage renal disease. Preterm labor occurred in all. Four out of the five had restoration of amniotic fluid volume and there were no perioperative deaths.

Subsequently, there have been a number of larger series examining clinical experience with vesicoamniotic shunts. Vesicoamniotic shunting is performed percutaneously with ultrasound guidance. A pigtail shunt is placed

Table 73.9. Favorable levels of fetal urinary electrolytes and protein [139]

Electrolyte	Cutoff
Sodium	< 100 mg/dl
Chloride	< 90 mmol/l
Calcium	< 8 mg/dl
Osmolality	< 200 mOsm/l
B_2-Microglobulin	< 4 mg/l
Total protein	< 40 mg/dl

between the bladder and the amniotic cavity to temporarily divert urine and to relieve the obstruction and the oligohydramnios. The initial double-J catheter used was subsequently replaced by a double pigtail catheter by Rodeck *et al.*[141]

The first large series was reported by Elder *et al.*[142] reviewing all cases of antenatal intervention for fetal obstructive uropathy through the end of 1985. Of the 57 interventions (from bladder aspirations to vesicostomies), 21 were technically successful placements of vesicoamniotic shunts, 10 were unsuccessful. The complications included shunt migration or poor drainage (11) and shunt extrusion into the peritoneal cavity (2). Of the nine patients with oligohydramnios treated by shunt, only two survived, three were terminated and four died. Forty-five percent of fetuses reviewed had complications (although not all of these had shunt placement).

In 1986, the report of the International Fetal Registry was published.[143] It described 73 placements of catheter shunts for fetal obstructive uropathy with a 41% survival rate (48% if elective terminations not included) and a 4.1% procedure-related mortality rate. The majority of deaths were perinatal due to pulmonary hypoplasia. Although this was encouraging and demonstrated feasibility, efficacy could not be established due to the selection bias in this cohort.

In 1990, Crombleholme *et al.*[144] presented 19 cases of vesicoamniotic shunting. This was formed to restore amniotic fluid levels and prevent pulmonary hypoplasia in nine out of 17 (53%) fetuses with oligohydramnios. Overall survival for shunted fetuses was 58% (11/19). The report

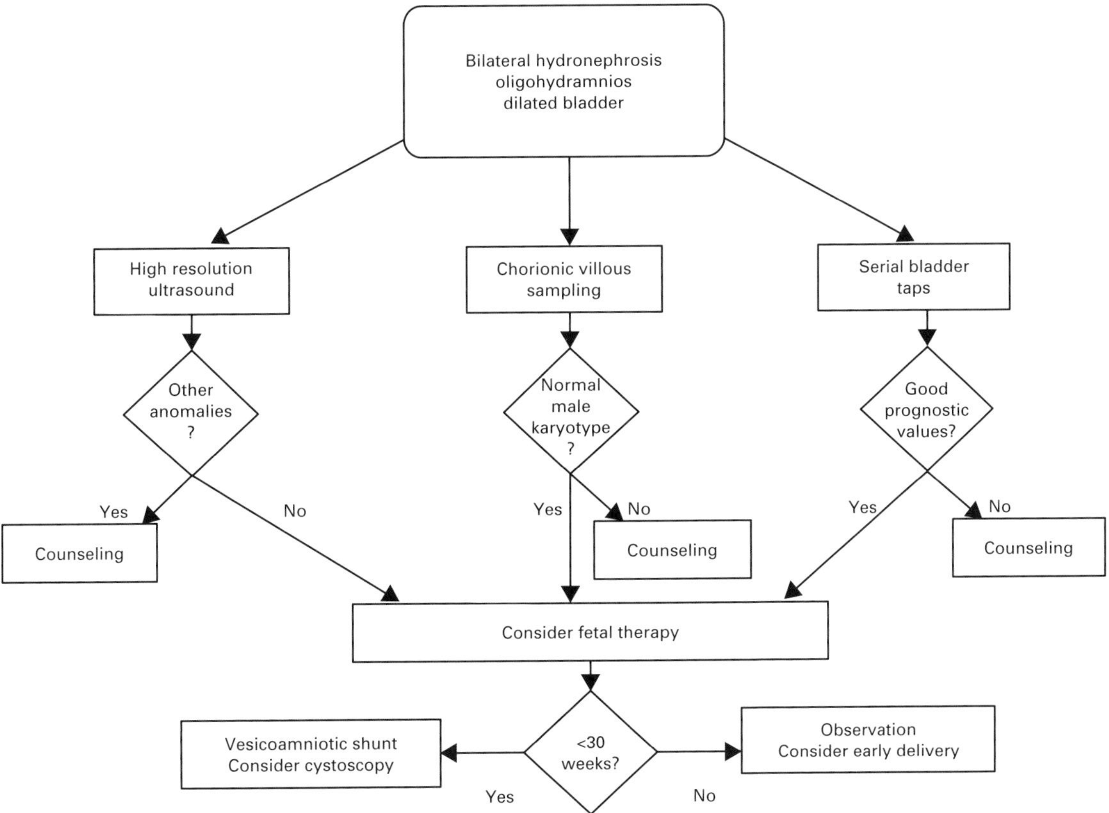

Fig. 73.1. Management algorithm for fetal obstructive uropathy.[139]

Table 73.10. Open fetal surgery for obstructive uropathy[138,292,293]

Case	Gest. age at diagnosis (weeks)	Gest. age at operation (weeks)	Resolution of oligohydramnios	PROM / PTL	Gest. age at delivery (weeks)	Survival	Cause of death	Other
1	20	21	N	N/Y	35	D	Pulmonary hypoplasia	Bilateral ureterostomies, renal dysplasia
2	22	24	Y	N/Y	34	E		Vesicostomy, ESRD −>transplant list
3	22	23	Y	Y/Y	33	D	GI pseudo-obstruction, septicemia	Microileum and microcolon requiring diversion
4	16	18	Y	Y/Y	32	E		Neurogenic bladder dysfunction, normal creatinine
5	20	22	Y	N/Y	32	C	Pulmonary hypoplasia	Renal dysplasia, urethral atresia

C = Died within 30 days of birth.
D = Died after 30 days old.
E = Long-term survival.
Y = Yes.
N = No.
ESRD = End-stage renal disease.

divided the cases into those with good and poor prognosis according to the prenatal diagnostic evaluation. In the poor prognosis group, 3/10 survived with shunting and 0/14 survived without. In the good prognosis group, 8/9 survived with shunting, and 5/7 survived without.

In 1993, Lipitz *et al.*[145] examined a series of 25 fetuses with LUTO, 14 of whom underwent vesicoamniotic shunting. Of these 14 fetuses, two were electively terminated, one died in utero, five died in the newborn period, and six survived (43%). Five out of the six survivors had evidence of renal damage. Three out of 11 (27%) survived without a shunt, with two having evidence of renal damage. Although the numbers in this study were small, these data suggest shunting is worthwhile, although there was one procedure-related death.

In 1996, Freedman *et al.*[146] reviewed 55 cases of fetal obstructive uropathy. Of these 28 were shunted with an overall survival of 61%. Of the poor prognosis fetuses, 50% of those shunted survived, whereas none of the non-shunted survived. Of the good prognosis fetuses, 64% of those shunted survived, and 45% of the non-shunted survived. Of the 13 fetuses with posterior urethral valves, 6/9 (67%) of those shunted survived (vs. 0/4 (0%) non-shunted). Of 9 prune-belly fetuses, 5/5 (100%) of shunted survived (vs. 1/4 (25%) of non-shunted). None of the 11 fetuses with urethral atresia survived.

Coplen[147] reviewed these five large series and noted that even with 169 successful shunt placements, 15 others were unsuccessful or had serious complications including three severe maternal infections and seven procedure-related intrauterine deaths. Other complications included catheter obstruction, migration, and fetal injury. Failure to restore amniotic fluid levels met with 100% mortality, and 40% of survivors still suffered from end-stage renal disease.

In 1999, Freedman *et al.*[148] looked at the long-term outcomes of children who underwent antenatal intervention for LUTO (Table 73.11). Of 34 patients who underwent vesicoamniotic shunting from 1987 to 1996 at the Children's Hospital of Michigan, 17 survived, but three were lost to follow-up. The 14 available survivors evaluated had a range of diagnoses, with most having prune-belly syndrome or posterior urethral valves; 43% had normal renal function, but 36% required renal transplantation. Some suffered multiple urinary tract infections postnatally that may have worsened baseline renal function. The authors concluded that antenatal intervention for children with severe obstructions resulted in outcomes similar to children with less severe disease diagnosed postnatally. These children had normal cognitive abilities, participated in normal activities, but had required special medical and surgical care throughout childhood.

This same group compiled data on their complications with vesicoamniotic shunts.[149] They compared 31 fetuses who underwent shunt placement to 31 who did not. Forty-eight percent of the shunted fetuses suffered from mechanical complications: 35% had migration out of the bladder; 23% developed urinary ascites (three from

Table 73.11. Long-term outcomes for children after vesicoamniotic shunting[148,150]

		Number	%
Total Number of children studied		20	100
Diagnoses			
	Prune belly	8	40
	Posterior urethral valves	8	40
	Urethral atresia	2	10
	Vesicoureteral reflux	1	10
	Megacystitis	1	10
Renal function			
	ESRD with transplant	7	35
	Renal insufficiency	4	20
	Normal function	9	43
Voiding function			
	Incontinent	3	15
	Continent	12	60
	Not toilet trained yet	5	25
Urinary tract infections			
	< 3 in last year	10	50
	> 6 in last year	4	20
	Prophylactic antibiotics	10	50
Growth			
	Height < 25%	14	70
	Height < 50%	9	45
	Weight < 25%	8	40
Respiratory function			
	Asthma	2	10
	Chronic bronchitis / frequent respiratory tract infections	4	20
Development			
	Developmental delay	2	10
	Speech therapy	3	15
	Physical therapy	1	5
Total surgeries performed on these children		62	
	Bladder augmentation	5	25
	Renal transplant	7	35

ESRD = End-stage renal disease.

intraperitoneal shunt migration and four from bladder fistula); three had bowel herniation at the insertion site. Preterm delivery occurred in 71% of cases: 32% had PROM; 6% had chorioamnionitis; 6% had died in utero. There were no periprocedure deaths. Of the 16 non-shunted and non-aborted fetuses, 50% had preterm delivery due to PROM (13%), chorioamnionitis (13%), and in utero death (25%).

In 2001, McLorie *et al.*[150] described the experience at Mt. Sinai Hospital and the Hospital for Sick Children in Toronto from 1989 to 1998. Of 89 fetuses with obstructive uropathy, nine underwent vesicoamniotic shunting. One fetus was electively terminated after shunting, and two with poor prognostic urinalysis died shortly after birth from pulmonary disease; 6/8 (75%) survived. Two out of six (33%) had renal failure, and 3/6 (50%) had bladder dysfunction requiring augmentation (one still requiring intermittent catheterizations). The authors encountered a few complications including shunt migration with need for reinsertion and bladder prolapse in a fetus with prune belly syndrome. These long-term outcomes and those from Freedman *et al.*[148] are included in Table 73.11.

In 2001, the UCSF compiled their data on 14 patients with posterior urethral valves (PUV) treated prenatally[151]

Table 73.12. Fetal therapy for posterior urethral valves – UCSF experience 1981–1999[151]

Case (units)	Gest. age at electrolyte (weeks)	Na mEq./l	Cl mEq./l	Osmolarity Osm	Gest. age at operation (weeks)	Technique	Survival	Cause of death	Serum Cr (age > 12 m) 7 mg/dl	Renal transplant?
1	20	98	84	210	20	CU	C	PTL, resp failure		
2	18	95	82	205	18	BM	**E**		0.5	N
3	24	88	83	202	24	BM	**E**		2.2	Y
4	25	52	39	119	25	ABL	**E**		1.4	N
5	22	87	70	179	22	ABL VAS	C	PTL, resp failure		
6	18	95	77	194	24	VAS	C	PTL, resp failure		
7	19	90	74	193	18	VAS	B	Terminated		
8	19	93	89	189	19	VAS	C	PTL, resp failure		
9	19	93	66	175	19	VAS	**E**		1.0	N
10	24	85	70	170	24	VAS	**E**		3.1	List
11	24	81	64	170	24	VAS	**E**		3.3	Y
12	25	92	81	103	25	VAS	**E**		2.0	N
13	28	73	72	172	28	VAS	C	PTL, resp failure		
14	30	70	68	158	30	VAS	**E**		0.5	N

CU = cutaneous ureterostomy, VAS = vesicoamniotic shunt, BM = bladder marsupialization, ABL = *in utero* valve ablation, PTL = pre-term labor and delivery.

A = Died intraoperatively.
B = Died in utero but not intraoperatively.
C = Died within 30 days of birth.
D = Died after 30 days old.
E = Long-term survival.
Y = Yes.
N = No.

(Table 73.12). All had favorable urine electrolytes and only two had sonographic evidence of renal dysfunction. Interventions included cutaneous ureterostomies (1), bladder marsupialization (2), laser ablation of valves (2), and placement of vesicoamniotic shunts (9). Overall mortality was 43% (six fetuses). Five of the surviving eight (63%) have chronic renal disease and five have required urinary diversion due to poor urinary drainage. One has required an augmentation cystoplasty. Three have exhibited uninhibited bladder contractions, but normal bladder compliance and no vesicoureteral reflux. Two have decreased bladder emptying. These cases strikingly illustrate, again, current inability to accurately identify fetuses with reversible renal disease. Sixty-three percent of survivors in this series had chronic renal disease which is a higher rate than estimated to occur in prenatally diagnosed, postnatally treated PUV.[152] This may indicate that prenatal treatment improved lung development and decreased perinatal mortality from lung hypoplasia, but did not prevent renal disease. Therefore, more babies survived the immediate perinatal period only to be faced with chronic renal disease. The investigators suggested that the poor results may be due to diagnosis and treatment that is already too late to prevent irreparable disease. Also, the screening criteria for salvageable renal function are controversial. Since four of five children with renal disease had no evidence by ultrasound of their renal disease, we cannot reliably determine renal salvageability. Fetal urinary electrolytes were also considered to be only somewhat reliable since all fetuses in this study had "good" urine electrolytes. They concluded that this study did not support the ability of prenatal intervention to salvage renal function for posterior urethral valves, but that improvements in minimally invasive techniques and tocolysis may improve outcomes in the future.

The clinical outcomes of vesicoamniotic shunting for fetal obstructive uropathy demonstrate that there are some significant limitations. Although shunting does diminish the incidence of lung hypoplasia and perinatal death for patients with oligohydramnios, shunting has a high rate of complications including shunt migration and shunt obstruction. It is only a temporizing measure, and the fetus requires another procedure(s) for definitive treatment. Finally, many survivors still suffer from renal damage and bladder dysfunction. Since the bladder does not experience the developmentally important normal emptying and filling cycle, it shrinks and develops poor compliance.[131] This "valve bladder" has decreased residual capacity, which has led to some of the PUV children requiring bladder augmentation after birth. Postnatally this contributes to urinary tract infections which can worsen renal function.[131]

A new approach to the treatment of obstructive uropathy utilizing cystoscopy appears promising. Quintero *et al.*[153] described the first case of fetal cystoscopy and fulguration of posterior urethral valves in 1995. The 19-week gestation fetus was diagnosed with LUTO by ultrasound. Using an ultrafine fiberoptic endoscope, fetal percutaneous cystoscopy was performed. The valves were electrocoagulated, and the distal urethra was immediately visualized. At 31 weeks' gestation, the mother developed preterm labor and gave birth to a baby boy. His urethra was patent as evidenced by spontaneous urine emission at birth, but he died 4 days later with pulmonary hypoplasia. This case demonstrated that posterior urethral valves can be treated in utero.

Variations on this technique have developed. Quintero *et al.* examined the use of fetoscopically guided cystotomy in two cases where safe percutaneous vesicoamniotic shunt placement was not possible.[154] Hofmann *et al.*[155] described a fetoscopic approach in the antegrade placement of a transurethral stent, which may avoid possible urethral and sphincter damage from laser ablation. Quintero *et al.*[156] used cystoscopy to guide a laser incision of a ureterocele causing bladder outlet obstruction and oligohydramnios. The right kidney was dysplastic by ultrasound. The oligohydramnios resolved. At birth, the right kidney was nonfunctional, but the left kidney's function was preserved.

As minimally invasive techniques evolve, patient selection should be continually revisited and current algorithms revised. For example, asymmetric renal injury is currently not accurately assessed. The assumption of stable "normal" fetal urine composition is also inaccurate because it actually varies with gestational age.[157] In addition, uniformly recognized outcomes measures need to be adopted in order to better assess efficacy of these treatments. Freedman *et al.*[149] contend that rates of gross survival, postnatal survival, and shunted survival, as well as nadir serum creatinine levels at 1 year are important parameters to use for comparison.

Sacrococcygeal teratoma

Sacrococcygeal teratoma (SCT) is a tumor arising from extragonadal germ cells in proximity to the sacrum (see Chapter 62). It occurs with a frequency of approximately 1 out of 35 000 to 40 000 live births, and is four times more common in females.[158] Ninety per cent of SCTs are benign.[159] Neonates with SCT usually have an excellent prognosis after resection, but the fetus diagnosed with a large, rapidly growing, solid, vascular SCT is at high risk for hydrops, placentomegaly, and high-output cardiac failure with subsequent, rapid fetal demise due to "vascular steal" from high blood flow through tumor.[160] Other complications include tumor rupture, preterm labor, and dystocia.[161–163] Additionally, pregnant women may develop a hyperdynamic "mirror syndrome" similar to preeclampsia that mimics the fetal condition.

The goal of fetal intervention is to interrupt the high flow circulation through the tumor. Historically, this was accomplished by open hysterotomy with tumor debulking or complete resection. In 1989, the first case attempted was reported by Langer *et al.*[164] The 22-week gestation fetus had a large SCT, hydrops, and placentomegaly. The tumor was debulked and its major blood supply interrupted successfully, but the fetus was delivered prematurely at 26 weeks and died from pulmonary immaturity. The first successful case was reported by Adzick *et al.*[165] A 25-week gestation fetus underwent successful resection with a resolution of hydrops. The fetus was delivered at 29 weeks, underwent resection of the remaining tumor mass and coccyx, and did well. In 2000, a unique case was described of an SCT fetus whose rectal atresia was discovered at the time of surgery. The SCT was resected, and a pull-through anorectoplasty and a bilateral ureterostomy performed. The fetus survived and delivered at 31 weeks (prompted by chorioamnionitis), but died several days postnatally from iatrogenic atrial rupture from a central venous catheter. The experience at UCSF and CHOP[164–169] has demonstrated the feasibility of open surgery (Table 73.13), but it continues to be limited by the problems inherent in open hysterotomy surgery.

Potentially promising, less invasive approaches have been attempted to minimize these complications. In the context of predominantly cystic, avascular tumors, cyst aspiration to reduce uterine irritability or maternal discomfort has been used with some success.[167] Cyst aspiration at

Table 73.13. Sacrococcygeal teratoma: open fetal resection experience[164–169]

Case	Gest. age at operation (weeks)	Gest. age at delivery (weeks)	Survival	Cause of death
1	24	26	C	Pulmonary immaturity
2	27	28	C	Air embolus
3	24	–	A	Intraoperative death
4	27	31	C	Iatrogenic atrial rupture
5	24	34	**E**	
6	23	28	**E**	
7	25	29	**E**	

A = Died intraoperatively.
B = Died in utero but not intraoperatively.
C = Died within 30 days of birth.
D = Died after 30 days old.
E = Long-term survival.

Table 73.14. Sacrococcygeal teratoma: radiofrequency ablation experience [175]

Case	Gest. age at operation (weeks)	Gest. age at delivery (weeks)	Outcome
1	20	20	Died (in utero) – hemorrhage into tumor
2	21	28	Alive: perineal necrosis
3	19	31	Alive: gluteal necrosis
4	22	25	Died postnatally: hemorrhage into tumor

or near delivery has helped prevent tumor rupture[167] and even allowed for a vaginal delivery.[170] Some groups have placed cyst–amniotic shunts to alleviate obstructive uropathy due to the tumor's mass effect.[171,172] These are not the cases that lead to a vascular steal and hydrops, but are associated with preterm labor and dystocia.

For large and predominantly solid, highly vascular tumors in fetuses with impending heart failure, minimally invasive approaches have been attempted, including tumor embolization, balloon occlusion, sclerosis, endoscopic snaring of the tumor neck, laser ablation, thermocoagulation, and radio-frequency ablation. Tumor embolization, balloon occlusion, sclerosis, and endoscopic snaring have been attempted without success.[168]

Hecher *et al.*[173] described the successful use of a fetoscopically guided Nd:YAG laser to reduce blood flow to the tumor in a 20-week gestation fetus with polyhydramnios, but no hydrops. Three weeks after surgery, there was bleeding into the cystic portion of the tumor requiring intrauterine blood transfusion and repeat laser coagulation. Yet, the maternal morbidity was minimal, and the baby was successfully delivered at 37 weeks and underwent surgical treatment. This fetus, however, did not meet standard criteria for fetal intervention (i.e., hydrops) so the survival may or may not have been related to the therapy. Lam *et al.*[174] attempted thermocoagulation of the tumor neck of one fetus with fetal death on postoperative day two. The cause of death was not evident, but may have been due to microbubbles from thermocoagulation, hyperkalemia from tissue necrosis, or hyperthermia from hemolysis.

Paek *et al.*[175] attempted percutaneous coagulation using radiofrequency ablation of the tumors in four fetuses (Table 73.14). Two fetuses died due to hemorrhage after ablation of a large percentage of the tumors. The other two fetuses survived with delivery at 28 and 31 weeks after having only the tumor necks ablated. There was minimal maternal morbidity but the neonates had gluteal and perineal necrosis requiring additional reconstruction operations. Ibrahim *et al.*[176] reported the long-term sequelae of a newborn (case no.3, Table 73.14) after radiofrequency ablation of an SCT. The child was born at 31 weeks' gestation with a large soft-tissue defect over the left hip, exposure of the dislocated hip, and loss of sciatic nerve function. These experiences reflect the inherent risks using current techniques and equipment.

Myelomeningocele

Myelomeningocele, or "spina bifida," is a devastating birth defect affecting five children per ten thousand live births, or approximately 1500 infants per year in the United States[177] at a cost of approximately $200 000 000 annually.[178] It is the most common congenital malformation of the central nervous system. Although typically nonlethal, this neural tube defect may result in a spectrum of morbidity including somatosensory loss, paresis, neurogenic sphincter dysfunction of bowel and bladder, musculoskeletal deformities, sexual dysfunction, Arnold–Chiari malformation, hydrocephalus, and impaired mental development. Eighty-five percent of patients require lifelong cerebrospinal fluid decompression, with mortality in the first two decades of life approaching 30%, primarily due to shunt complications.[179]

The clinical effects of a myelomeningocele are believed to result from a two-"hit" theory: a defect in neurulation which causes the neural tube defect and myelodysplasia (this step is complete by the fourth week of gestation); and subsequent exposure of the spinal cord to the intrauterine environment causing chronic chemical and mechanical trauma.[180]

Experimental data suggest that fetal therapy focusing on alleviating the traumatic insult to the spinal cord may be of benefit. A variety of animal experiments involving mice, rat, rabbit, sheep, pig, and monkey have been employed.[181–184] These experiments showed that surgical creation of spinal dysraphism replicates the neurologic sequelae of myelomeningocele and immediate surgical repair allows for normal development. In addition, experiments by Paek *et al.*[185] in sheep demonstrates that hindbrain herniation may be prevented with in utero repair. Fetoscopic repair in sheep by Copeland *et al.* showed that a minimally invasive approach may be feasible.[186]

Since the risks to the mother and fetus were originally believed to outweigh the potential benefit of open repair, a minimally invasive approach was first attempted. Four fetoscopic repairs were attempted at Vanderbilt University Medical Center (VUMC).[187] The technique involved a maternal laparotomy, placement of three uterine ports,

Table 73.15. Outcome of fetoscopic repair of myelomeningocele [187]

Gestational age at procedure (weeks)	Lesion (US)	Technique	Gestational age at delivery/ outcome (weeks)
VUMC			
22 3/7	L4-S3, mild VM, AC	maternal STSG, fibrin glue	35 wk 1 d / Planned c-section, lesion covered by thin translucent membrane, neonatal closure and VPS, mild somatosensory deficit at 30 mos
23 6/7	L3-S2, mild VM, AC, bil talipes	maternal STSG, fibrin glue	24 wk 5 d / Amnionitis, death in delivery room, lesion uncovered, graft not attached
22 4/7	T12-S5, mild VM, AC	maternal STSG, fibrin glue, absorbable sutures	28 wk 1d / Disruption of membranes, pre-term labor, c-section, lesion covered with thin translucent membrane, neonatal closure and VPS, mild somatosensory deficit at 6 mos
24 3/7	T12-S3, hemivertebra L-3, mild VM, AC, bil talipes	maternal STSG, fibrin glue, absorbable sutures	24 wk 3 d / Intraoperative uterine contractions, placental abruption, intraoperative demise
UCSF			
25	L2-S1, unilat VM, AC	1 layer w/ Alloderm patch with suture, converted to open to control placental bleeding	35 wk / Planned c-section, patch partially pulled away from fetal skin, neonatal closure and VPS, somatosensory level to L4 by 1 yr
24	L3-S, AC, bil talipes	2-layer closure	31 wk / Spontaneous rupture of membranes, c-section, lesion with some CSF leak, neonatal repair and VPS, somatosensory level to L4, re-presented at 1 mo with urosepsis with eventual demise
19	L3-S1, AC, bil talipes	Converted to open due to difficulty with fetal positioning, 3-layer closure using chorioamnion patch, fetal ankle dislocation and laceration repaired, fetal bradycardia treated with epinephrine	21 wk / Premature rupture of membranes and spontaneous abortion of non-viable fetus

GA = gestational age, US = ultrasound, L = lumbar, S = sacral, VM = ventriculomegaly, AC = Arnold–Chiari II malformation, VPS = ventriculoperitoneal shunt, STSG = split thickness skin graft.

aspiration of the amniotic fluid, and replacement with CO_2 for the duration of the procedure. A maternal skin graft was then fixed over the neural tube defect with fibrin glue and, in two cases, also sutures. The uterine cavity was refilled with either amniotic fluid or sterile saline. One fetus died intraoperatively from preterm labor. One died a few weeks later after preterm labor from amnionitis. The other two delivered near term, but the skin graft could not be identified and the defect was essentially unrepaired.

The UCSF group reported three attempts at fetoscopic repair.[188] In one case, an alloderm patch was placed fetoscopically, but the case was converted to open due to placental bleeding. At delivery, the patch was partially disrupted. The baby required re-repair and a VP shunt. In the second case, the defect was repaired with a two-layer closure. The mother delivered pre-term due to spontaneous rupture of membranes, and the baby required re-repair and VP shunt due to CSF leak. The baby later died from urosepsis. The third case was converted to open due to an anterior placenta. The fetus, however, was spontaneously aborted 2 weeks later. Table 73.15 summarizes the experience in human fetoscopic repair of myelomeningocele.

The fetoscopic approach to meningomyelocele repair was then abandoned and open repair was, again, contemplated. Advances in tocolysis and other means of management, coupled with the fact that the meningomyelocele fetus is otherwise healthy, apparently diminished the risks to mother and fetus. The first open repairs were done in 1997 and, in 2000, Bruner *et al.*[189] compared the

Table 73.16. Outcomes after open repair for fetal myelomeningocele

	Conventional treatment	Intrauterine repair	Conclusion
Total shunt-dependent hydrocephalus[193]	162/189 (85.7%)	56/104 (53.9%)	Significant difference at all levels
Thoracic lesions	35/35 (100%)	4/5 (80%)	
Lumbar lesions	100/114 (87.7%)	49/84 (58.3%)	
Sacral lesions	27/40 (67.5%)	4/15 (26.7%)	
Moderate to severe hindbrain herniation	50%	4%	Significant difference
Reversal of pre-existing hindbrain herniation	0%	8/9 with moderate to severe hindbrain herniation. After repair, 5/9 with NO hindbrain herniation and 4/9 with mild herniation	Significant reversal of hindbrain herniation
Lower extremity function[191]	Average radiographic level – L4 (N=40) Average neurologic level – L4	Average radiographic level – L4/L5 (N = 37) Average neurologic level – L5	No significant difference
Urodynamic profile[192]			No significant difference to published postnatal results
Decreased bladder compliance	18% – 70%	26% (N=25)	
Reflux		17%	
Uninhibited contractions		13%	
Hypotonia		43%	
Decreased capacity		34%	
Leak point pressure > 40 cm H_2O		82%	
Detrusor-sphincter dyssynergia		13%	

initial endoscopic cases to the initial open cases. They concluded that the hysterotomy approach was technically superior because of shorter operating times, no fetal mortality, shorter neonatal hospital stay, and a suggestion of better functional outcomes.

Since 1997, nearly 200 open repairs have been performed. The open repairs have followed the standard technique of laparotomy, hysterotomy, neurosurgical dissection, three-layer closure with or without lumbar–peritoneal shunt placement, and occasionally amnion patch placement. Sutton *et al.*[190] provide MRI evidence that hindbrain herniation is improved by intrauterine repair, but this does not prove that there is an improvement in neurologic symptoms or a reduced incidence of hydrocephalus. Other studies report that lower extremity and bladder function are not improved with intrauterine repair over conventional postnatal therapy.[191,192] Recently, in a large retrospective review, Tulipan *et al.*[193] compared all intrauterine meningomyelocele repairs performed at VUMC and CHOP from 1997 until 2000 with conventionally treated patients from 1983 to 2000. The study indicated that fetuses repaired before 25 weeks' gestation have a 50% reduction in the need for ventriculoperitoneal shunts compared to historical controls. The clinical outcomes of open repair are summarized in Table 73.16. Even with the apparent decrease in VP shunt rates, the fetal and maternal morbidity (11%) and fetal mortality (4%) are still significant for the treatment of a non-lethal disease.[194] As minimally invasive techniques and instrumentation improve, these techniques will be revisited for myelomeningocele treatment. Currently, robot-assisted endoscopic repair of skin defects has been shown to be feasible in animal studies.[195] Another innovative treatment may be amnioexchange: exchange of meconium-stained amniotic fluid with a fluid replacement. This has been shown to minimize damage to exposed intestine in animal gastroschisis models and has shown some efficacy in the few human cases.[196,197] Olguner *et al.*[198] demonstrated that damage to the neural tissue was greatly minimized in a chick model of myelomeningocele.

A randomized, prospective trial with three participating centers, Vanderbilt University Medical Center, CHOP, and UCSF, has been underway since 2002 in an effort to definitively compare fetal myelomeningocele repair. The primary outcome variable is the need for a ventriculoperitoneal shunt at one year of age. The results are pending as is future discussion regarding the overall risk–benefit question.

Tension hydrothorax

Tension hydrothorax is an uncommon fetal lesion, which occurs in approximately 1 out of 15 000 pregnancies.[199] It has a male predominance and is typically right-sided.[200] It is caused primarily by focal leakage of lymph or secondarily associated with hydrops or certain anatomic abnormalities. Congenital hydrothorax has a 57% to 100% perinatal mortality.[141] The main cause of death is pulmonary hypoplasia secondary to extrinsic compression.[201] Intrauterine death is usually caused by fetal hydrops due to mediastinal shift with compression of the heart and/or the vena cavae. Fetuses with hydrothorax that exhibit hydrops have a 76% mortality vs. a 25% mortality if present without hydrops.[202]

Intrauterine therapy has focused on ameliorating lung compression, preventing or reversing hydrops, and improving postnatal pulmonary function. For effusions that are large and/or increasing in size, therapies have included percutaneous ultrasound-guided thoracenteses and thoracoamniotic shunts. The first cases of fetal intervention for pleural effusion were published in 1982. In 1992, Weber and Philipson[203] conducted a review of 124 cases of fetal pleural effusions. They noted that poor outcomes were significantly associated with three risk factors: < 32 weeks' gestational age at delivery, presence of hydrops, and no antenatal therapy. They reported a mortality rate of 50% with no antenatal therapy, 42% with thoracentesis alone, and 22% with thoracoamniotic shunting.

In1993, Hagay *et al.*[204] reviewed all published cases of fetal pleural effusion without hydrops at initial diagnosis. Of the 82 cases reviewed, 54 fetuses did not undergo antenatal intervention and the mortality rate in this group was 37%. Fetuses with any prenatal intervention had a comparable mortality rate of 33%. In 1997, Wilkins-Haug and Doubilet[205] studied the treatment of unilateral pleural effusions. Both hydropic and non-hydropic fetuses had good outcomes with thoracoamniotic shunting. Those treated conservatively (all without hydrops) resulted in death in three out of ten.

In 1998, Aubard *et al.*[202] reviewed 204 cases of primary fetal hydrothorax. The mortality rates with and without antenatal treatment were 57% and 78%, respectively. Those fetuses with hydrops had a 23.5% chance of survival with no treatment, a 10% survival with thoracentesis only, and a 66.6% survival with shunting. Without hydrops, fetuses had a 21.3% survival without treatment, a 60% survival with thoracentesis, and a 100% survival with shunting. Based on their findings, Aubard *et al.* recommended a management algorithm for treatment of congenital hydrothorax. Since most pleural effusions rapidly reaccumulate after aspiration, the invesitigators recommended thoracentesis only in a fetus with acute signs of distress, in late gestation fetuses (>32 weeks), or in fetuses just prior to birth to optimize postnatal respiratory function. They recommend that a shunt be placed for fetuses that progressively deteriorate and are less than 32 weeks' gestation, or have failed thoracentesis. Aubard *et al.* noted complications associated with thoracoamniotic shunts, including shunt failure (11/80) and catheter migration/obstruction (10/80).

Congenital heart defects

Treatment of complex congenital heart defects (CHD) and arrhythmias is an exciting and promising new frontier in fetal surgery. CHDs are the most common congenital malformations in humans, affecting 8 in 1000 live births. Twenty percent of perinatal mortality from congenital malformations[206]and half of the deaths in childhood caused by malformations are due to CHD.[207,208] Many CHD are successfully treated postnatally with good long-term outcomes. Unfortunately, some are impossible to correct at the time of birth and surgery is only palliative. These CHDs are potential targets for in utero treatment. Particular attention has been paid to severe aortic and pulmonary valve obstructions, both of which can lead to severe dysfunction and malformation of the affected ventricle. The theoretical basis for fetal therapy is the concept that treating the obstruction early enough in the disease process will prevent secondary myocardial hypoplasia. Several studies describe progression of hypoplasia due to valvular stenosis.[209,210]

Current standards for screening of CHD allow the majority of serious fetal CHD to go undetected. The standard "four-chamber" view by echocardiography, even with additional views of the outflow tracts, identifies only gross structural abnormalities such as hypoplasia or vessel defects.[211] Only real-time pulse-wave and color Doppler evaluation can detect valve stenosis and the degree of obstruction prior to the evolution of hypoplasia,[212] and these are not used routinely in screening.

Another barrier to in utero intervention is access to the fetus. Innovative animal research has been performed to develop methods of fetal access. Cardiac bypass has been studied in fetal sheep[213,214] and has been shown to be feasible after surmounting issues related to perturbation of the placental circulation. Endoscopic techniques and advanced intra-amniotic imaging have been developed by Kohl *et al.* to perform balloon valvuloplasties in sheep through umbilical vessel access.[215–218]

In human fetuses, the most common fetoscopic procedures for cardiac intervention have been ultrasound-guided balloon valvuloplasty in cases of severe aortic stenosis and pulmomary stenosis. In these cases, a needle is advanced percutaneously with ultrasound guidance through the maternal abdomen, into the amniotic sac and then through the fetal chest wall. It is placed into the obstructed ventricle, and then a coronary artery balloon catheter is advanced over a guidewire. Maxwell *et al.*[219] reported the first two balloon valvuloplasties in humans. A decade later, a total of 12 cases of aortic balloon valvuloplasties were performed and reviewed by Kohl *et al.*[220] The outcomes of this initial clinical experience were poor. The mean gestational age at detection was 25.7 weeks and at the time of intervention, 29.2 weeks' gestation. Success was defined by echocardiographic relief of obstruction following the procedure. Seven fetuses (all without atresia) had successful valvuloplasties although only one survived. Of the five technical failures, only one survived with postnatal surgery. There was no preterm labor. The authors attributed the poor results primarily to the severity of cases, technical problems, high postnatal mortality, and complications ranging from fetal bradycardia and bleeding, to difficulties with catheter introduction and withdrawal. The child who survived after successful valvuloplasty was doing very well at age four with a valve gradient of 20 mmHg, trace mitral and aortic regurgitation, and an ejection fraction of 55%.[221]

Recently, two cases of pulmonary valvuloplasty were reported by Tulzer *et al.*[222] Both fetuses (28 and 30 weeks' gestation) had severe pulmonary valve obstruction (one stenotic and the other atretic) and imminent hydrops. Both demonstrated more favorable results immediately postoperatively with improved hemodynamics demonstrated by resolution of pericardial effusions and improved RV function. Both delivered near term gestation and required postnatal valvuloplasties and placement of systemic-to-pulmonary arterial shunts. All published balloon-valvuloplasties are summarized in Table 73.17.

At the 2004 meeting of the Society of Maternal–Fetal Medicine, 15 unpublished cases of aortic balloon valvuloplasties were presented by a group from the Brigham and Women's Hospital and Children's Hospital of Boston.[223] All were treated prior to 28 weeks' gestation. The group's technical success rate was 66% (10/15) with a combined laparoscopic/percutaneous approach (9/11) being more successful than a solely percutaneous approach (1/4). The only maternal complication was pulmonary edema requiring diuretics and supplemental oxygen. Given the relatively low risk to the mother and the apparently low risk of preterm labor, fetal balloon valvuloplasties may become more efficacious with better patient selection and improved technical methods.

Another target for in utero intervention is the pericardial teratoma. Pericardial teratomas are extremely rare neoplasms. They are typically large and multicystic with associated pericardial effusions. They frequently cause cardiorespiratory failure due to tamponade or obstruction to blood flow.[224] There have been multiple reports of fetal pericardiocentesis to stabilize fetuses at high risk for tamponade.[224–228] There has been one reported attempt of in utero resection of a pericardial teratoma.[229] A 24-week gestation hydropic fetus underwent open fetal surgery for teratoma resection. The tumor was removed, but the hydrops did not resolve. Three weeks later, the mother experienced severe pre-eclampsia which was deemed maternal mirror syndrome. Therefore, emergency C-section was performed, but the baby died immediately after birth.

Fetal cardiac arrhythmias have also been treated by in utero therapy. Fetuses with complete heart block have been treated unsuccessfully with ventricular pacemaker placement, both by open approach and by catheter approach.[2,230,231] Maternal dexamethasone treatment has been shown to have some efficacy in fetuses with complete heart block.[232]

Ex utero intrapartum treatment (EXIT)

Ex utero intrapartum treatment strategy, or EXIT, was originally designed for the controlled removal of the tracheal occlusion device placed for antenatal treatment of congenital diaphragmatic hernia. It is an ingenious technique, which allows surgeons to obtain fetal airway control while the baby is still on placental support or "maternal–fetal bypass" thus avoiding uncontrolled delivery room intubations of the newborn. It is a typically coordinated event involving pediatric surgery, obstetrics, radiology, neonatology, anesthesia and nursing. The baby is "half" delivered through a hysterotomy. Uterine relaxation is sustained with inhalational anesthetics and intravenous tocolytics; thus uteroplacental blood flow and gas exchange is maintained. The main risk to the mother is intraoperative hemorrhage. The risk of uterine bleeding due to atony is reduced by the use of hemostatic uterine staplers as well as by infusion of oxytocin and decrease of inhalational anesthetics prior to umbilical cord ligation. Risk of placental hemorrhage is reduced by accurate placental identification with ultrasound and intraoperative amnioreduction if polyhydramnios obscures visualization.

The use of the EXIT procedure has expanded to a variety of conditions (Table 73.18) including: reversal of tracheal occlusion after CDH treatment; airway management of fetuses with neck masses, congenital high airway obstruction (CHAOS) and certain thoracic lesions; and as a

Table 73.17. Fetal balloon valvuloplasties[220,222]

Case	Diagnosis	Gest. age at diagnosis (weeks)	Gest. age at operation (weeks)	Gest. age at delivery (weeks)	Technical success	Survival	Cause of death	Other
1	AV stenosis	30	31	34	Y	C	LV dysfunction	Balloon rupture Intermittent bradycardias
2	AV stenosis	32	33	38	Y	**E**		Balloon rupture Intermittent bradycardias
3	AV stenosis	30	30	35	Y	C	LV dysfunction	Balloon rupture Intermittent bradycardias
4	AV stenosis	29	32	32	Y	A	Sustained bradycardia	Balloon rupture Intermittent bradycardias. Hemopericardium
5	AV stenosis	21	30	30	N	**E**		Balloon rupture Intermittent bradycardias
6	AV stenosis	24	26	37	Y	C	Postnatal post-op	
7	AV stenosis	26	28	38	Y	C	Postnatal post-op	
8	AV stenosis	27	27	38	Y	C	Postnatal intra-op	Balloon rupture
9	AV atresia	22	28	28	N	A	Hemothorax	Intermittent bradycardias Hemothorax
10	AV atresia	20	29	30	N	A	Chorioamnionitis	Intermittent bradycardias
11	AV stenosis with PV stenosis	24	27	27	N	A	Sustained bradycardia	Sustained bradycardia
12	AV stenosis with PV atresia	24	28	28	N	A	Sustained bradycardia	Sustained bradycardia Hemopericardium
13	PV atresia		28	38	Y	**E**		
14	PV stenosis		30	35	Y	**E**		

A = Died intraoperatively.
B = Died in utero but not intraoperatively.
C = Died within 30 days of birth.
D = Died after 30 days old.
E = Long-term survival.
AV = Aortic valve.
PV = Pulmonic valve.
LV = Left ventricle.

Table 73.18. Applications of the EXIT strategy

Lesion
Reversal of tracheal occlusion for CDH
Intrinsic laryngotracheal anomalies resulting in congenital high airway obstruction – laryngeal web/atresia/cyst/stenosis; tracheal stenosis/atresia
Extrinsic airway compression – cervical teratoma/lymphangioma
Epignathus
Severe hydrops from a cystic adenomatoid malformation of the lung
Bilateral tension hydrothorax
Unilateral pulmonary agenesis
EXIT to ECMO in fetus with CDH and congenital heart disease
EXIT to separation for thoracoomphalopagus twins
Delivery of twins with potentially obstructing neck lesion

transition from birth to ECMO or from birth to separation for conjoined twins. The EXIT strategy has been performed for up to 2.5 hours[233] during which time procedures such as bronchoscopy, laryngoscopy, tracheostomy, arterial and venous access, administration of surfactant, resection of neck or lung masses, and cannulation for ECMO can be performed.

In the original application for EXIT, the tracheal occlusion from antenatal treatment of CDH was reversed. Initially, CDH was treated with external clip application; therefore, these clips were removed through neck dissection along with any necessary tracheal repair during EXIT. Also, bronchoscopy was performed and surfactant was administered. For fetuses who were treated with occlusive balloons, EXIT bronchoscopy was used to pierce and suction out the tracheal balloon.

Fetuses with neck masses are ideal candidates for the EXIT strategy in order to manage potential airway obstruction. Common types are cervical teratoma and lymphangioma. Mackenzie *et al.*[234] state that tracheal deviation observed by fetal MRI, especially in association with polyhydramnios, is a strong indicator of airway compromise and an absolute indicator for the EXIT procedure. Normal delivery of these fetuses can result in over 20% mortality due to upper airway obstruction.[235] Over 30 EXIT procedures have been reported for neck masses with a survival rate in excess of 90%.[236] In one case, both intubation and tracheostomy placement proved impossible, so the mass was resected with subsequent tracheostomy placement, remaining on placental support 2.5 hours.[237]

Congenital high airway obstruction syndrome (CHAOS) is a condition marked by enlarged, echogenic lungs, dilated tracheobronchial tree, flattened diaphragm, and fetal ascites with possible hydrops. It is caused by complete or near-complete obstruction of the fetal airway. There have been six cases of successful tracheostomy during EXIT for this rare condition reported in the literature.[233,238–242] The concept of fetoscopic tracheostomy has been proposed to decompress the lungs, and resolve mediastinal compression and resulting hydrops; however, chronic lung fluid drainage through a tracheostomy may result in pulmonary hypoplasia.[243]

Rare thoracic abnormalities have been managed via EXIT. The drainage of large bilateral pleural effusions has been performed during EXIT with subsequent lung expansion and improved ability to ventilate.[244] Another fetus with a large congenital cystic adenomatoid malformation was unable to be ventilated after intubation during EXIT; therefore, resection was successfully performed in 66 minutes on placental support with immediately improved ventilation. The EXIT procedure allowed a third fetus with unilateral pulmonary agenesis to be intubated and stabilized for subsequent esophageal atresia repair and reconstruction of a stenotic bronchus.[245]

EXIT can be used as a transition to ECMO. Bouchard *et al.*[245] describe a case of a fetus which would certainly require ECMO after birth. The fetus had CDH with an LHR of 1.15 and tetralogy of Fallot. An EXIT procedure was performed on delivery during which ECMO cannulas were placed and ECMO support was initiated while the neonate was on placental support. The newborn avoided acidosis or hypoxemia during the 90-minute procedure. Michel *et al.*[246] describe another case in which EXIT was used to transition to ECMO for a fetus with pulmonary hypoplasia and airway obstruction due to a large pulmonary arterio-venous malformation. The mother did well, but after the cardiac anomalies were repaired, the neonate had hemodynamic instability and non-survivable pulmonary hypoplasia; therefore, ECMO was withdrawn.

Mackenzie *et al.*[247] describe a case of thoracoomphalopagus in which the EXIT procedure was used to transition to emergency operative separation at birth. Twin A had a four-chambered heart, and twin B had a rudimentary heart with complete heart block. Twin A was in compensated heart failure with a probable arterial connection to twin B. Because of the high likelihood of cardiovascular decompensation of twin A at birth off of placental support, an EXIT-to-separation strategy was devised. EXIT was performed at 34 weeks with controlled placement of support lines and echocardiographic localization of the arterial feeding vessel. The twins were, then, immediately taken to the operating room for separation. Twin B died immediately after ligation of the feeding vessel. Twin A survived and was doing well at 14 months of age.

One relevant case of epignathus, or oropharyngeal teratoma, has been reported in the literature.[248] Prenatal ultrasound revealed a large, growing oropharyngeal mass and increasing polyhydramnios. Preterm labor required emergent Cesarean section with EXIT at which time a tracheostomy was performed. The large mass was later resected, and the neonate eventually tolerated oral feedings. The infant's cleft palate was scheduled for repair at 10 months.

Bouchard *et al.*[245] reported 31 EXIT procedures performed at CHOP from 1996 to 2001. Indications included reversal of tracheal occlusion (13), fetal neck mass (13), EXIT-to-ECMO (1), for resection of congenital cystic adenomatoid malformation (1), unilateral pulmonary agenesis (1), EXIT-to-separation for conjoined twins (1), and CHAOS (1). The average duration of uteroplacental support was 30.3 ± 14.7 minutes. Estimated maternal blood loss was 848.3 ± 574.1 ml.

In a recent retrospective series, Hirose *et al.*[233] described 52 EXIT procedures performed between 1993 and 2003 at UCSF. Forty-five were performed for reversal of tracheal occlusion for CDH. Of these, 30 had clips removed with two requiring tracheal repair, and 15 underwent bronchoscopy and tracheal balloon removal. Five of the EXIT procedures were performed for airway management of fetuses with neck masses. Three of these underwent tracheostomy, one had endotracheal intubation and one had a successful resection of the mass. The final two neonates had tracheostomies performed for CHAOS. Time on placental support was 45 ± 25 minutes and survival was 52% (all deaths were in CDH patients). The average maternal blood loss was 970 ± 510 ml.

Concerning maternal morbidity, Noah *et al.*[249] demonstrated that there was equivalent blood loss and hospital stay for mothers undergoing EXIT vs. normal Cesarean section; however, women who underwent the EXIT procedure had a higher incidence of wound complications and endometritis (Table 73.19).

Table 73.19. Maternal outcomes of EXIT strategy[249]

Short-term maternal outcomes	EXIT ($N = 34$)	Cesarean section ($N = 52$)
Estimated blood loss	1104 ml	883 ml
Average postoperative infection	8 (24%)	6 (12%)
Hematocrit change	5.3%	4.6%
Wound complications	5 (15%)	1 (2%)
Endometritis	5 (15%)	1 (2%)
Length of hospital stay	3.5 days	3.5 days
Surgical operating time	110 minutes	57 minutes
Fetal operating time	24.2 minutes	2.6 minutes

Premature rupture of membranes

One of the complications associated with the innovations in fetal surgery is premature rupture of membranes (PROM). Iatrogenic PROM occurs with a frequency of approximately 1.2% after amniocentesis, 3%–5% after diagnostic fetoscopy, and 5%–8% after operative fetoscopy.[250] The perinatal mortality of iatrogenic and spontaneous PROM managed expectantly is 60%.[251,252]

Based on the concept of a blood patch for treatment of spinal headache following lumbar puncture by Gormley in 1960,[253] Quintero *et al.* successfully treated iatrogenic PROM with an intra-amniotic injection of platelets and cryoprecipitate (the "amniopatch").[254] The initial patient had been leaking amniotic fluid beginning the fourth postoperative day after fetoscopic umbilical cord ligation. She was expectantly managed for three weeks with continued leakage and reduction of amniotic fluid on ultrasound. One unit of platelets and one unit of cryoprecipitate were administered under ultrasound guidance. The leak stopped and the pregnancy continued with delivery at term. Another group reported success using whole blood to treat PROM in a patient after genetic amniocentesis.[255]

In 2003, Quintero *et al.*[250] reported a series of 28 patients treated with amniopatch. Patients with iatrogenic PROM between 16 and 18 weeks' gestation without evidence of infection were placed on bedrest and antibiotics for 1 week. If there was no spontaneous sealing of the membranes, autologous (if possible) platelets followed by cryoprecipitate were administered via amniocentesis into the largest amniotic fluid pocket. Initially, one unit of each was administered, but subsequently one half unit of platelets was given with good results. The platelet quantity was reduced because some of the early fetal deaths were probably due to activation of a large number of platelets. Eleven had a large membrane detachment but no detectable leak, while the remaining seventeen had a gross leak. Amniocentesis was responsible for PROM in 10 (36%) patients. The average gestational age at delivery was 33.4 weeks. Membrane sealing occurred in 19 patients (67.9%). The published amniopatch experience is outlined in Table 73.20.

The same group[250] attempted to use the technique on women with spontaneous PROM. The first 12 patients did not respond to the treatment and continued to leak. To learn more about the membranes in spontaneous PROM, four women were studied endoscopically while undergoing the amniopatch procedure. These cases indicated that the membrane defect is usually located over the internal cervical os, vs. other sites with iatrogenic PROM. The membrane defect became larger and the edges became more

Table 73.20. Amniopatch experience for premature rupture of membranes[250,255,296,297]

Case	Procedure	Gestational age (weeks) at PROM	Gestational age (weeks) at amniopatch	Gestational age (weeks) at delivery	Outcome	Membrane sealed? / comment
1	TRAP, operative fetoscopy	17.9	20.5	37.9	Alive and well	Yes
2	AMA, genetic amniocentesis	16.3	16.5	37	Normal delivery and neonate	Yes / Used maternal whole blood
3	TTTS, operative fetoscopy	17.1	18.1	22.0	Miscarriage, incompetent cervix	Yes
4	TTTS, operative fetoscopy	21.3	21.3	33.7	Double alive and well	Yes
5	AMA, genetic amniocentesis	16.1	17.1	35.6	Alive and well	Yes
6	AMA, genetic amniocentesis	15.4	16.4	18.9	IUFD, probably from too large infusion of platelets	1st No, 2nd Yes
7	Genetic amniocentesis	17.1	20.6	32	Induction pre-eclampsia, uneventful neonatal course	Yes / Used platelets and fibrin glue
8	TTTS, therapeutic amniocentesis	22.1	23.1	29.6	Double neonatal demise	Yes
9	Bladder obstruction	18.7	19.7	19.4	IUFD, bladder obstruction	No
10	TTTS, operative fetoscopy	16.1	17.1	33.3	Double alive and well	Yes
11	TTTS, operative fetoscopy	18.3	19.3	34.1	Double alive and well	Yes
12	TTTS, therapeutic amniocentesis	17.9	18.9	24.0	One IUFD, one alive and well	No
13	TTTS, operative fetoscopy	26.1	27.1	33.9	Double alive and well	Yes
14	TTTS, operative fetoscopy	16.9	17.9	20.6	TOP	No
15	Selective IUGR, operative fetoscopy	19.6	20.6	31.9	Double alive and well	No
16	TTTS, operative fetoscopy	20.0	21.0	34.1	Double alive and well	Yes
17	Amniotic bands, operative fetoscopy	23.3	24.3	29.1	Alive and well, surgery for residual bands	No
18	AMA, genetic amniocentesis	15.6	16.6	37.5	Alive and well	Yes
19	TTTS, operative fetoscopy	18.0	19.0	21.0	Miscarriage	No
20	Anencephaly acrania, operative fetoscopy	16.7	17.7	33.6	Alive with cardiac malformation of newborn	Yes
21	TTTS, operative fetoscopy	18.4	19.4	31.1	Double alive and well	Yes
22	Teratoma, operative fetoscopy	27.7	28.7	28.6	Alive, surgery for rectum necrosis	No
23	TTTS, therapeutic amniocentesis	22.2	23.2	30.6	One alive, died of meningitis two wks after discharge from hospital	Yes
24	AMA, CVS transvaginal	13.1	14.1	38.6	Alive and well	Yes
25	AMA, genetic amniocentesis	20.1	21.1	21.1	Miscarriage	No
26	AMA, genetic amniocentesis	17.6	18.6	18	TOP, trisomy 18	Yes
27	TTTS, therapeutic amniocentesis	22.1	23.1	34.9	One alive and well	Yes
28	LUTO, operative fetoscopy	20.9	21.9	21.7	TOP	No
29	TTTS, operative fetoscopy	21.9	22.9	36.0	Both twins alive and well	Yes
30	AMA, genetic amniocentesis	19.3	20.3	41.0	Alive and well	Yes
31	TRAP, operative fetoscopy	17.2	18.5	30.5	C-section, chorioamnionitis, uneventful neonatal course except *E. coli* sepsis	Yes
32	TTTS, operative fetoscopy	22	23	30	IUFD 1 twin, elective c-section, uneventful neonatal course	Yes

AMA advanced maternal age, TTTS twin–twin transfusion syndrome, TRAP twin reversed arterial perfusion, CVS chorionic villous sampling, LUTO lower urinary tract obstruction, IUFD intrauterine fetal demise, TOP voluntary termination of pregnancy, GA gestational age.

Table 73.21. Experience with fetoscopic release of amniotic bands[263,264]

GA	Lesion (US)	Technique	GA at delivery / Outcome
22	Bil cleft lip, bands to face and left arm, left forearm edema, arterial blood flow ok	Initially two ports but due to bleeding second port removed, scissors used under ultrasound guidance	39 wk / Bil cleft lip, craniofacial cleft, right microphthalmia, left arm – minimal scarring, radial paresis and mild hypoplasia
23*	Band constricting left ankle, distal edema, minimal blood flow	Two ports>one port due to bleeding, scissors attempted – no success, YAG laser	34.5 wk / PROM at 31 wks, z-plasties of amniotic band remnants, expected full functional recovery of foot
23	Circumferential band around left wrist, distal edema, compromised blood flow via single artery	600-micron endostat with Nd–YAG laser	33 wk / Normal blood flow to left wrist but persistent lymphedema. Viable hand but limited range of motion secondary to scarring from reconstruction for lymphedema.
20	Circumferential band around right wrist, distal edema, compromised perfusion. Intraoperative findings also included bands around right calf and right thigh.	400-micron endostat with Nd–YAG laser	Atrophic, malformed, viable right hand – later amputated for prosthesis. Normal right lower extremity.

GA gestational age, US ultrasound, Nd–YAG neodymium–yttrium aluminum gamet, PROM premature rupture of membranes.

rolled and less sharp with more time between PROM and intervention. It is suggested that intervention may be more successful in the early stages of spontaneous PROM.

In vitro and in vivo experiments with rabbits and sheep demonstrated the feasibility of using an Nd:YAG laser to weld a Biosis patch over the amniotic membrane defect.[256,257] The first human spontaneous PROM repair with this method was described in 2002.[258] PROM occurred at 16.5 weeks' gestation, and severe oligohydramnios was documented 2 weeks later. The fetus had a normal karyotype so the "amniograft" procedure with the Biosis graft was performed. The patient did not leak for two weeks, but then had a recurrent leak. This was managed expectantly and the baby was delivered at 32 weeks by Cesarean section.

Amniotic band syndrome

Estimates of the incidence of amniotic band syndrome vary widely: ranging from 1 in 1200 to 1 in 15 000 live births per year.[259] This syndrome is characterized by a collection of acquired or congenital malformations involving the limbs, craniofacial region, and trunk resulting from fibrous bands attached to the fetus, which cause constriction and deformation. These bands are thought to arise from rupture of the amnion and can result in digit or limb amputations, facial clefting, and even death. Umbilical cord compromise by amniotic bands arising after uterine instrumentation can be fatal and these may be targeted for intrauterine release.[260] Data from a sheep model of amniotic band syndrome suggest that fetoscopic release of these bands may prevent limb deformities.[261,262]

The published human experience with amniotic band release is limited to four cases at present (Table 73.21). Quintero *et al.* performed the first fetoscopic releases of amniotic bands in two patients.[263] The first fetus was 21 weeks' gestation with evidence on ultrasound of a band constricting her left upper extremity with abnormal deviation and distal edema. She was considered at risk of arm amputation. The fetus had bilateral cleft lip and normal karyotype. It was planned to cut the band with scissors under fetoscopic guidance. However, uterine bleeding led to the conclusion to remove the second port, and ultrasound guidance was used thereafter. Band release resulted in immediate improvement in the angulation of the arm and the edema improved over time. The second case involved a fetus with a band constricting the ankle. A YAG laser fiber was used to disrupt the band. There was marked improvement to the foot. It developed normally and full functional recovery was expected.

In 2003, Keswani *et al.* attempted fetoscopic release of amniotic bands on two patients with isolated limb constrictions.[264] One fetus had a circumferential band involving the right wrist and this was released with an Nd–YAG laser. The wrist recovered normal blood flow and proved viable but suffered from secondary lymphedema. The second case involved bands to the right upper and lower extremities, both released with laser. Both extremities were viable at birth, but the upper extremity was atrophic and subsequently amputated for prosthesis compatibility.

Fetal surgery has previously been a treatment option only in otherwise lethal conditions. These cases indicate that there may be a role for fetoscopic amniotic band release for limb salvage. The potential risks to the fetus and mother need to be carefully considered before undertaking this procedure.

Gastroschisis

Gastroschisis is a condition affecting apparently 1 out of 10 000 live births.[265] It is a condition in which the bowel resides outside of the abdominal cavity, herniated through a paraumbilical defect. After delivery, the bowel is surgically replaced into the abdomen, at once if possible or over time if necessary. The survival rate is generally about 90%, but at least 25% of these babies suffer from perivisceritis. These infants, typically, have a prolonged stay in the NICU and hospital averaging 20 and 80 days respectively with a delay to enteral feeding of 25 days.[266]

Study of animal models of gastroschisis has led to the understanding that gastrointestinal waste in the amniotic fluid can contribute to the intestinal inflammatory lesions of the fetus with gastroschisis.[267] In 1998, Aktug *et al.*[268,269] demonstrated that exchanging the amniotic fluid with saline or saline plus dextrose decreased intestinal lesions in a chick gastroschisis model. Improvement was also seen with amnioexchange in a lamb model.[270]

The first case of human amnioexchange was reported in 1998 by Aktug *et al.*[196] Four amnioexchanges were performed by an ultrasound-guided percutaneous approach for a fetus with a gastroschisis. After delivery, the baby's abdomen was primarily closed with low intra-abdominal pressure. Feeding was initiated by day 5, and discharge was on day 8.

Luton *et al.*[197] compared ten fetuses who underwent amnioinfusion with ten who did not. Their data suggest that amnioinfusion decreased the inflammation of the bowel and allowed for immediate and easier primary closure of the defect. The treated babies required fewer days of ventilation, hospitalization and earlier initiation of enteral feeds. These differences were not statistically significant, but suggest a trend that may or may not be substantiated as more cases are performed.

Chronic fetal vascular access

As fetal surgery advances, the need for vascular access to the fetus becomes more dominant. The ability to obtain blood samples, have continuous pH monitoring and administer medication, fluids, and blood is vital for the fetal surgical patient. This avenue of access may be used to treat non-surgical disease as well. In the future, parenteral nutrition may improve intrauterine growth retardation,[271] antibiotics may help treat infection, and stem cells can be delivered for transplantation.[272]

Lemery *et al.*[273] in 1995 described a technique of ultrasound-guided umbilical vein catheterization in four pregnant baboons. Although all four catheterizations were successful in this report, three fetuses died immediately due to fetal intra-amniotic hemorrhage. However, the group was able to obtain daily blood samples from the remaining fetus without occlusion of umbilical vessels or hemorrhage. This study demonstrated the feasibility of obtaining chronic vascular access of the fetus. Hedrick *et al.*[274] demonstrated successful fetoscopically guided catheterization of placental vessels through an extra-amniotic approach in six third trimester rhesus monkeys and 18 second trimester sheep. All were successfully cannulated (artery and vein), and only one primate fetus died postoperatively. All of the remaining catheters were functional. More recently, Paek *et al.*[275] studied the long-term safety of chronic fetal vascular access in four pregnant sheep. A midline laparotomy with mini uterine incision was performed and a catheter was placed in a placental vessel, tunneled under the mother's skin, and attached to a subcutaneous port. The pregnancies were allowed to go to term. All four access ports remained functional throughout the pregnancies. The lambs were delivered vaginally without complications.

Gene therapy

Genetic interventions, whether gene based or cell based, offer the prospect of exciting new areas for fetal therapy. The human genome project, advances in DNA micro-array technology, and new methods for obtaining fetal DNA, together offer the potential to diagnose virtually all human genetic disease prior to birth. In utero treatment is becoming an option and antenatal treatment of genetic diseases has a number of potential advantages over postnatal therapy. The cells of the fetus are highly proliferative; within the developing fetus, large numbers of stem cells migrate and differentiate into a variety of tissues; the small size of the fetus allows for more cells/vector per kg dosages; and, finally, but perhaps most importantly, the developing fetal immune system may be trained to accept the new cells/genes as "self."[276]

Some congenital diseases that may be amenable to in utero stem cell transplantation are those that have been treated by bone marrow transplants postnatally. These include hemoglobinopathies, immunodeficiency diseases, inborn errors of metabolism such as mucopolysaccharidoses, and other hematopoietic diseases.[277] To date, there have been over 40 in utero stem cell transfers in humans for the treatment of immunodeficiency disorders. Only treatment of x-linked severe combined immunodeficiency syndrome has been successful, but in this area results are comparable to postnatal bone marrow transplant. In these fetuses, multiple intraperitoneal injections of CD34 enriched paternal bone marrow created split chimerism and full reconstitution of T-lymphocytes. This success points to the feasibility of the treatment, but highlights the need for a survival advantage of the donor cells in order for successful engraftment and treatment of disease.[278–280] Since the ability to produce hematopoietic chimeras has been demonstrated, another interesting avenue for further study is the prenatal induction of tolerance for postnatal transplantation.[281]

In contrast, gene transfer therapy still requires much more study both in vitro and in vivo before clinical application. Issues include what type of vector to use to optimize transduction, how to administer the vector, how to target the appropriate tissue, how to sustain gene expression, and how to avoid the potential problems with transfection such as germline incorporation and insertional mutagenesis.[276]

Cleft lip

Cleft lip and palate occur in 1 out of 700 live births.[282] These conditions are traditionally repaired postnatally but significant life-long scar can result from the lip repair. An in utero treatment of cleft lip is appealing because of the ability of early gestation fetal skin to heal with minimal to no scarring compared to postnatal skin.

Small and large animal models have been developed that demonstrate scarless healing after in utero repair.[283] Some have argued that immediate repair of a surgically created cleft in these models is not realistic. Therefore, Hedrick *et al.*[284] demonstrated that in utero repair delayed for 2 weeks can result in scarless healing. Congenital models of clefting in goats have also been developed and used to study in utero repair.[285–287] Estes *et al.*[288] demonstrated the feasibility of endoscopic repair of fetal cleft lips in lambs. Others have developed microclips that allow for faster fetoscopic repair.[289,290] Some argue that a multilayered open repair is superior to endoscopic techniques when evaluating cosmetic and functional outcomes.[291] As advancements are made in the prevention of maternal and fetal morbidity with prenatal surgery, antenatal cleft lip repair may be applied to humans but is presently not an option.

REFERENCES

1. Hogge, W., Schonberg, S., & Golbus, M. S. Chorionic villous sampling: experience of the first 1000 cases. *Am. J. Obstet. Gynecol.*, 1986; **154**:1249.
2. Harrison, M. R. Fetal Surgery. *West. J. Med.*, 1993; **159**:341–349.
3. Longaker, M., Golbus, M., & Filly, R. A. Maternal outcome after open fetal surgery. *J. Am. Med. Assoc.*, 1991; **265**:737–741.
4. DeProst, J. A. & Gratacos, E. Obstetrical endoscopy. *Curr. Opin. Obstet. Gynecol.* 1999; **11**(2):195–203.
5. Adzick, N. S. & Harrison, M. R. Fetal surgical therapy. *Lancet* 1994; **343**(8902):897–902.
6. Ville, Y., Hecher, K., & Gagnon, A. Endoscopic laser coagulation in the management of severe twin-to-twin transfusion syndrome. *Br. J. Obstet. Gynaecol.* 1998; **105**:446–453.
7. Harrison, M. R., Mychaliska, G. B., Albanese, C. T. *et al.* Correction of congenital diaphragmatic hernia in utero IX: fetuses with poor prognosis (liver herniation and low lung-to-head ratio) can be saved by fetoscopic temporary tracheal occlusion. *J. Pediatr. Surg.* 1998; **33**(7):1017–1022; discussion 1022–1023.
8. DeProst, J., Evrard, V., & Vanballer, P. Experience with fetoscopic cord ligation. *Eur. J. Obstet. Gynecol.* 1998; **81**:157–164.
9. Dennes, W. & Bennett, P. Preterm labor: the Achilles heel of fetal intervention. In Harrison, M. R. (Ed.) The Unborn Patient: the Art and Science of Fetal Therapy, Philadelphia; W.B. Saunders, 2001:171–181.
10. Farrell, J., Albanese, C. T., & Kilpatrick, S. J. Maternal fertility is unaffected after fetal surgery. *Fetal. Diagn. Ther.* 1999; **14**:190–192.
11. Wenstrom, K. D. Fetal surgery for congenital diaphragmatic hernia. *N. Engl. J. Med.* 2003; **349**(20):1887–1888.
12. Langham, M. R., Jr., Kays, D. W., Ledbetter, D. J. *et al.* Congenital diaphragmatic hernia. Epidemiology and outcome. *Clin. Perinatol.* 1996; **23**(4):671–688.
13. Wilcox, D. T. Irish, M. S., Holm, B. A., & Glick, P. L. Prenatal diagnosis of congenital diaphragmatic hernia with predictors of mortality. *Clin. Perinatol.* 1996; **23**(4):701–709.
14. Adzick, N. S., Harrison, M. R., & Glick, P. L. Diaphragmatic Hernia in the fetus: prenatal diagnosis and outcome in 49 fetuses. *J. Pediatr. Surg.* 1985; **20**:357–361.
15. Harrison, M. R., Adzick, N. S., Estes, J. M., & Howell, L. J. A prospective study of the outcome for fetuses with diaphragmatic hernia. *J. Am. Med. Assoc.*, 1994; **271**:382–384.
16. Albanese, C. T., Lopoo, J., & Goldstein, R. B. Fetal liver position and perinatal outcome for congenital diaphragmatic hernia. *Prenat. Diagn.* 1998; **18**:1138–1142.
17. Lipshutz, G. S., Albanese, C. T., & Feldstein, V. Prospective analysis of lung-to-head ratio predicts survival for patients with prenatally diagnosed congenital diaphragmatic hernia. *J. Pediatr. Surg.* 1997; **32**:1634–1636.
18. Metkus, A. P., Filly, R. A., Stringer, M. D. *et al.* Sonographic predictors of survival in fetal diaphragmatic hernia. *J. Pediatr. Surg.* 1996; **31**:148–152.
19. Stege, G., Fenton, A., & Jaffray, B. Nihilism in the 1990s: the true mortality of congenital diaphragmatic hernia. *Pediatrics* 2003; **112(3** Pt 1):532–535.
20. Bagolan, P. Casaccia, G., Creseenzi, F. *et al.* Impact of a current treatment protocol on outcome of high-risk congenital diaphragmatic hernia. *J. Pediatr. Surg.* 2004; **39**(3):313–318; discussion 313–318.

21. Boloker, J., Bateman, D. A., Wung, J. T., & Stolar, C. J. Congenital diaphragmatic hernia in 120 infants treated consecutively with permissive hypercapnea/spontaneous respiration/elective repair. *J. Pediatr. Surg.* 2002; **37**(3):357–366.
22. Harrison, M. R., Jester, J. A., & Ross, N. A. Correction of congenital diaphragmatic hernia in utero.I. The model: intrathoracic balloon produces fatal pulmonary hypoplasia. *Surgery* 1980; **88**:174.
23. Harrison, M. R., Bressack, M. A., & Churg, A. M. Correction of congenital diaphragmatic hernia in utero II. Simulated correction permits fetal lung growth with survival at birth. *Surgery* 1980; **88**:260.
24. Harrison, M. R., Ross, N. A., & de Lorimier, A. A. Correction of congenital diaphragmatic hernia in utero. III. Development of a successful surgical technique using abdominoplasty to avoid compromise of umbilical blood flow. *J. Pediatr. Surg.* 1981; **16**(6):934–942.
25. Adzick, N. S., Outwater, K. M., Harrison, M. R. *et al.* Correction of congenital diaphragmatic hernia in utero. IV. An early gestational fetal lamb model for pulmonary vascular morphometric analysis. *J. Pediatr. Surg.* 1985; **20**(6):673–80.
26. Harrison, M. R., Adzick, N. S., & Longaker, M. T. Successful repair in utero of a fetal diaphragmatic hernia after removal of the herniated viscera from the chest. *N. Engl. J. Med.* 1990; **322**:1582.
27. Harrison, M. R., Langer, J. C., Adzick, N. S. Correction of congenital diaphragmatic hernia in utero, V. Initial clinical experience. *J. Pediatr. Surg.* 1990; **25**(1):47–55; discussion 56–7.
28. Harrison, M. R., Adzick, N. S., & Flake, A. W. Correction of congential diaphragmatic hernia in utero. VI. Hard-earned lessons. *J. Pediatr. Surg.* 1993; **28**:1411.
29. Harrison, M. R., Adzick, N. S., & Bullard, K. M. *et al.* Correction of congenital diaphragmatic hernia in utero VII: a prospective trial. *J. Pediatr. Surg.* 1997; **32**(11):1637–1642.
30. Alcorn, D., Adamson, T. M., Lambert, T. F. *et al.* Morphological effects of chronic tracheal ligation and drainage in the fetal lamb lung. *J. Anat.* 1977; **123**(3):649–660.
31. Carmel, J. A., Friedman, F., & Adams, F. H. Fetal tracheal ligation and lung development. *Am. J. Dis. Child.* 1965; **109**:452–456.
32. Adzick, N. S., Harrison, M. R., Glick, P. L., Villa, R. L., & Finkbeiner, W. Experimental pulmonary hypoplasia and oligohydramnios: relative contributions of lung fluid and fetal breathing movements. *J. Pediatr. Surg.* 1984; **19**(6):658–665.
33. Nardo, L., Hooper, S. B., & Harding, R. Lung hypoplasia can be reversed by short-term obstruction of the trachea in fetal sheep. *Pediatr. Res.* 1995; **38**(5):690–696.
34. Bealer, J. F., Skarsgard, E. D., Hedrick, M. H. *et al.* The 'PLUG' odyssey: adventures in experimental fetal tracheal occlusion. *J. Pediatr. Surg.* 1995; **30**(2):361–364; discussion 364–365.
35. Beierle, E. A., Langham, M. R. Jr., & Cassin, S. In utero lung growth of fetal sheep with diaphragmatic hernia and tracheal stenosis. *J. Pediatr. Surg.* 1996; **31**(1):141–146; discussion 146–147.
36. DiFiore, J. W., Fauza, D. O., Slavin, R. *et al.* Experimental fetal tracheal ligation reverses the structural and physiological effects of pulmonary hypoplasia in congenital diaphragmatic hernia. *J. Pediatr. Surg.* 1994; **29**(2):248–256; discussion 256–257.
37. Hedrick, M. H. Estes, J. M., Sullivan, K. M. *et al.* Plug the lung until it grows (PLUG): a new method to treat congenital diaphragmatic hernia in utero. *J. Pediatr. Surg.* 1994; **29**(5):612–617.
38. Wilson, J. M., DiFiore, J. W., & Peters, C. A. Experimental fetal tracheal ligation prevents the pulmonary hypoplasia associated with fetal nephrectomy: possible application for congenital diaphragmatic hernia. *J. Pediatr. Surg.* 1993; **28**(11):1433–1439; discussion 1439–1440.
39. Luks, F. I., Gilchrist, B. F., Jackson, B. T., & Piasecki, G. J. *et al.* Endoscopic tracheal obstruction with an expanding device in a fetal lamb model: preliminary considerations. *Fetal Diagn. Ther.* 1996; **11**(1):67–71.
40. Harrison, M. R., Adzick, N. S., Flake, A. W. *et al.* Correction of congenital diaphragmatic hernia in utero VIII: Response of the hypoplastic lung to tracheal occlusion. *J. Pediatr. Surg.* 1996; **31**(10):1339–1348.
41. Mychaliska, G. B., Bealer, J. F., Graf, J. L. *et al.* Operating on placental support: the ex utero intrapartum treatment procedure. *J. Pediatr. Surg.* 1997; **32**(2):227–230; discussion 230–231.
42. Flake, A. W., Crombleholme, T. M., Johnson, M. P., Howell, I. J., & Adzick, N. S. Treatment of severe congenital diaphragmatic hernia by fetal tracheal occlusion: clinical experience with fifteen cases. *Am. J. Obstet. Gynecol.* 2000; **183**(5):1059–1066.
43. Benachi, A., Chailley-Heu, B., Delezoide, A. L. *et al.* Lung growth and maturation after tracheal occlusion in diaphragmatic hernia. *Am. J. Respir. Crit. Care Med.* 1998; **157**(3 Pt 1):921–927.
44. Bin, Saddiq, W., Piedboeuf, B., Laberge, J. M. *et al.* The effects of tracheal occlusion and release on type II pneumocytes in fetal lambs. *J. Pediatr. Surg.* 1997; **32**(6):834–838.
45. O'Toole, S. J., Karamanoukian, H. L., Irish, M. S. *et al.* Tracheal ligation: the dark side of in utero congenital diaphragmatic hernia treatment. *J. Pediatr. Surg.* 1997; **32**(3):407–410.
46. Skarsgard, E., Meuli, M., Van der Wall, K. J. *et al.* Fetal endoscopic tracheal occlusion ('Fetendo-PLUG') for congenital diaphragmatic hernia. *J. Pediatr. Surg.* 1996; **31**(10):1335–1338.
47. VanderWall, K. J., Skarsgard, E. D., Filly, R. A. *et al.* Fetendo-clip: a fetal endoscopic tracheal clip procedure in a human fetus. *J. Pediatr. Surg.* 1997; **32**(7):970–972.
48. Albanese, C. T., Jennings, R. W., Filly, R. A. *et al.* Endoscopic fetal tracheal occlusion: evolution of techniques. *Pediatr. Endosurg. Innovative Techniques* 1998; **2**:47–53.
49. Harrison, M. R., Sydorak, R. M., Farrell, J. A. *et al.* Fetoscopic temporary tracheal occlusion for congenital diaphragmatic hernia: prelude to a randomized, controlled trial. *J. Pediatr. Surg.* 2003; **38**(7):1012–1020.

50. DeProst, J., Evrard, V., & Van Ballaer, P. P. Tracheoscopic endoluminal plugging using an inflatable device in the fetal lamb model. *Eur. J. Obstet. Gynecol.* 1998; **81**:165–169.
51. Chiba, T., Albanese, C. T., Farmer, D. L. *et al.* Balloon tracheal occlusion for congenitaL diaphragmatic hernia: experimental studies. *J. Pediatr. Surg.* 2000; **35**(11):1566–1570.
52. Harrison, M. R., Albanese, C. T., Hawgood, S. B. *et al.* Fetoscopic temporary tracheal occlusion by means of detachable balloon for congenital diaphragmatic hernia. *Am. J. Obstet. Gynecol.* 2001; **185**(3):730–733.
53. Harrison, M. R., Keller, R. L., Hawgood, S. B. *et al.* A randomized trial of fetal endoscopic tracheal occlusion for severe fetal congenital diaphragmatic hernia. *N. Engl. J. Med.* 2003; **349**(20):1916–1924.
54. Adzick, N. S. The fetus with a lung mass. In Harrison, M. R. (Ed.) *The Unborn Patient: the Art And Science of Fetal Therapy*, Philadelphia: W.B. Saunders Company, 2001:287–296.
55. Adzick, N. S. Management of fetal lung lesions. *Clin. Perinatol.* 2003; **30**(3):481–492.
56. Davenport, M., Warne, S. A., Cacciaguerra, H. *et al.* Current outcome of antenally diagnosed cystic lung disease. *J. Pediatr. Surg.* 2004; **39**(4):549–556.
57. Quinn, T. M., Hubbard, A. M., & Adzick, N. S. Prenatal magnetic resonance imaging enhances prenatal diagnosis. *J. Pediatr. Surg.* 1998; **33**:312–316.
58. Tsao, K., Albanese, C. T., & Harrison, M. R. Prenatal therapy for thoracic and mediastinal lesions. *World. J. Surg.* 2003; **27**(1):77–83.
59. Crombleholme, T. M., Coleman, B., Hedrick, H. *et al.* Cystic adenomatoid malformation volume ratio predicts outcome in prenatally diagnosed cystic adenomatoid malformation of the lung. *J. Pediatr. Surg.* 2002; **37**(3):331–338.
60. Chao, A. & Monoson, R. F. Neonatal death despite fetal therapy for cystic adenomatoid malformation. A case report. *J. Reprod. Med.* 1990; **35**(6):655–657.
61. Clark, S. L.Vitale, D. J., Minton, S. D. *et al.* Successful fetal therapy for cystic adenomatoid malformation associated with second-trimester hydrops. *Am. J. Obstet. Gynecol.* 1987; **157**(2):294–5.
62. Thorpe-Beeston, J. G. & Nicolaides, K. H. Cystic adenomatoid malformation of the lung: prenatal diagnosis and outcome. *Prenat. Diagn.* 1994; **14**(8):677–688.
63. Dommergues, M., Louis-Sylvestre, C., Mandelbrot, L. *et al.* Congenital adenomatoid malformation of the lung: when is active fetal therapy indicated? *Am. J. Obstet. Gynecol.* 1997; **177**(4):953–958.
64. Bernaschek, G., Deutinger, J., Hansmann, M. *et al.* Feto-amniotic shunting – report of the experience of four European centres. *Prenat. Diagn.* 1994; **14**(9):821–833.
65. Baxter, J. K., Johnson, M. P., & Woilson, R. D. Thoracoamniotic shunts: pregnancy outcome for congenital cystic adenomatoid malformation and pleural effusion. *Am. J. Obstet. Gynecol.* 1998; **185**:S245.
66. Adzick, N. S., Harrison, M. R., Crombleholme, T. M. *et al.* Fetal lung lesions: management and outcome. *Am. J. Obstet. Gynecol.* 1998; **179**(4):884–889.
67. Adzick, N. S., Flake, A. W., & Crombleholme, T. M. Management of congenital lung lesions. *Semin. Pediatr. Surg.* 2003; **12**(1):10–16.
68. Bruner, J. P., Jarnagin, B. K., & Reinisch, L. Percutaneous laser ablation of fetal congenital cystic adenomatoid malformation: too little, too late? *Fetal Diagn. Ther.* 2000; **15**(6):359–363.
69. Tsao, K., Hawgood, S., Vu, L. *et al.* Resolution of hydrops fetalis in congenital cystic adenomatoid malformation after prenatal steroid therapy. *J. Pediatr. Surg.* 2003; **38**(3):508–510.
70. Machin, G. & Keith, L. Can twin-to-twin transfusion syndrome be explained, and how is it treated? *Clin. Obstet. Gynecol.* 1998; **41**:104–113.
71. Quintero, R. Twin–twin transfusion syndrome. *Clin. Perinatol.* 2003; **30**:591–600.
72. Weir, P., Rattern, G., & Beischner, N. Acute polyhydramnios: a complication of monozygous twin transfusion syndrome. *Br. J. Obstet. Gynaecol.* 1979; **86**:849–853.
73. Quintero, R., Morales, W., & Allen, M. Staging of twin–twin transfusion syndrome. *J. Perinatol.* 1999; **8**:550–555.
74. Taylor, M., Govendor, L., & Jolly, M. Validation of Quintero staging system for twin–twin transfusion syndrome. *Obstet. Gynecol.* 2002; **100** (6):1257–1265.
75. Saunders, N., Snijders, R., & Nicolaides, K. Therapeutic amniocentesis in twin–twin transfusion syndrome appearing in the second trimester of pregnancy. *Am. J. Obstet. Gynecol.* 1992; **166**:820–824.
76. Roberts, D., Neilson, J. P., & Weindling, A. M. Interventions for the treatment of twin–twin transfusion syndrome. *Cochrane Database Syst. Rev.*, **2001**(1):CD002073.
77. Trespidi, L., Boschetto, C., & Caravelli, E. Serial amniocentesis in the management of twin–twin transfusion syndrome: when is it valuable? *Fetal Diagn. Ther.* 1997; **12**:15–20.
78. Urig, M. A., Clewell, W. H., & Elliott, J. P. twin–twin transfusion syndrome. *Am. J. Obstet. Gynecol.* 1990; **163**(5 Pt 1):1522–1526.
79. Johnsen, S. L., Albrechtsen, S., & Pirhonen, J. Twin–twin transfusion syndrome treated with serial amniocenteses. *Acta Obstet. Gynecol. Scand.* 2004; **83**(4):326–329.
80. De, Lia, J., Cruikshank, D., & Keye, W. Fetoscopic neodymium:YAG laser occlusion of placental vessels in severe twin–twin transfusion syndrome. *Obstet. Gynecol.* 1990; **75** (6): 1046–1053.
81. De, Lia, J., Kuhlman, R., & Harstad, T. Twin–twin transfusion syndrome treated by fetoscopic neodymium:YAG laser occlusion of chorioangiopagus. *Am. J. Obstet. Gynecol.* 1993; **168**:308.
82. De, Lia, J., Kuhlman, R., & Harstad, T. Fetoscopic laser ablation of placental vessels in severe previable twin–twin transfusion syndrome. *Am. J. Obstet. Gynecol.* 1995; **172**:1202–1208.
83. Hecher, K., Plath, H., & Brezenger, T. Endoscopic laser surgery versus serial amniocentesis in the treatment of severe

twin–twin transfusion syndrome. *Am. J. Obstet. Gynecol.* 1999; **180**:717–724.

84. Hecher, K., Diehl, W., & Zikulnig, L. Endoscopic laser coagulation of placental anastomoses in 200 pregnancies with severe midtrimester twin-to-twin transfusion syndrome. *Eur. J. Obstet. Gynecol.* 2000; **92**:135–139.
85. Quintero, R., Morales, W., & Mendoza, G. Selective photocoagulation of placental vessels in twin–twin transfusions syndrome: evolution of a surgical technique. *Obstet. Gynecol.* 1998; **53**:s97–s103.
86. Quintero, R., Comas, C., & Bornick, P. Selective versus non-selective laser photocoagulation of placental vessels in twin–twin transfusion syndrome. *Ultrasound Obstet. Gynecol.* 2000; **16**:230–236.
87. Feldstein, V., Machin, G., & Albanese, C. T. Twin–twin transfusion syndrome: the Select procedure. *Fetal Diagn. Ther.* 2000; **15**:257–261.
88. Farmer, D. & Hirose, S. Fetal intervention for complications of monochorionic twinning. *World J. Surg.* 2003; **27**:103–107.
89. Quintero, R., Bornick, P., & Allen, M. Selective laser photocoagulation of communicating vessels in severe twin–twin transfusion syndrome in women with an anterior placenta. *Obstet. Gynecol.* 2001; **97**:477–481.
90. DeProst, J., Van Schoubroeck, D., & Evrard, V. Fetoscopic Nd:YAG laser coagulation for twin–twin transfusion syndrome in cases of anterior placenta. *J. Am. Assoc. Gynecol. Laparosc.* 1996; **3**:s9.
91. DeProst, J., Van Schoubroeck, D., & Van Ballaer, P. Alternative technique for Nd:YAG laser coagulation in twin-to-twin transfusion syndrome with anterior placenta. *Ultrasound Obstet. Gynecol.* 1998; **11**:347–352.
92. De, Lia, J., Fisk, N., Hecher, K. *et al.* Twin-to-twin transfusion syndrome – debates on the etiology, natural history and management. *Ultrasound Obstet. Gynecol.* 2000; **16**(3):210–213.
93. Lemery, D., Vanlieferinghen, P., & Gasq, M. Fetal umbilical cord ligation under ultrasound guidance. *Ultrasound Obstet. Gynecol.* 1994; **4**:399–401.
94. Quintero, R., Romero, R., & Reich, H. In utero percutaneous umbilical cord ligation in the management of complicated monochorionic multiple gestations. *Ultrasound Obstet. Gynecol.* 1996; **8**:16–22.
95. DeProst, J., Audibert, F., & Van Schoubroeck, D. Bipolar coagulation of the umbilical cord in complicated monochorionic twin pregnancy. *Am. J. Obstet. Gynecol.* 2000; **182**:340–345.
96. Taylor, M., Shalev, E., & Tanawattanacharoen, S. Ultrasound guided umbilical cord occlusion using bipolar diathermy for stage III/IV twin–twin transfusion syndrome. *Prenat. Diagn.*, 2002; **22**:70–76.
97. Saade, G., Olson, G., & Belfort, M. Amniotomy: a new approach to the 'stuck twin' syndrome. *Am. J. Obstet. Gynecol.* 1995; **172**:429.
98. Johnson, J., Rossi, K., & R. O'Shaughnessy Amnioreduction versus septostomy in twin–twin transfusion syndrome. *Am. J. Obstet. Gynecol.* 2001; **185**(5):1044–1047.
99. Quintero, R., Quintero, L., & Morales, W. Amniotic fluid pressures in severe twin–twin transfusion syndrome. *Prenat. Neonat. Med.* 1998; **3**:607–610.
100. Hartung, J., Chaoui, R., & Bollman, R. Amniotic fluid pressure in both cavities of twin-to-twin transfusion syndrome: a vote against septostomy. *Fetal Diagn. Ther.* 2000; **15**(2):79–82.
101. Lewi, L., Schoubroeck, D., & Gratacos, E. Monochorionic diamniotic twins: complications and management options. *Curr. Opin. Obstet. Gynecol.* 2003; **15**(2):177–194.
102. Napolitani, F. & Schreiber, I. The acardiac monster: a review of world literature and presentation of 2 cases. *Am. J. Obstet. Gynecol.* 1960; **80**:582–587.
103. Moldenhauer, J., Gilbert, M., & Johnson, A. Vascular occlusion in the management of complicated multifetal pregnancies. *Clin. Perinatol.* 2003; **30**:601–621.
104. Van Allen, M., Smith, D., & Shepard, T. Twin reversed arterial perfusion sequence: a study of 14 twin pregnancies with acardius. *Semin. Perinatol.* 1993; **7**:285–293.
105. Healey, M. Acardia: predictive risk factors for the co-twin's survival. *Teratology* 1994; **50**:205–213.
106. Moore, T., Gale, S., & Bernirschke, K. Perinatal outcome of forty-nine pregnancies complicated by acardiac twinning. *Am. J. Obstet. Gynecol.* 1990; **163**:907–912.
107. Ash, K., Harman, C., & Gritter, H. TRAP sequence – successful outcome with indomethacin treatment. *Obstet. Gynecol.* 1990; **76**:960–962.
108. Simpson, P., Trudinger, B., & Walker, A. The intra-uterine treatment of fetal cardiac failure in a twin pregnancy with an Acardiac, acephalic monster. *Am. J. Obstet. Gynecol.* 1983; **147**:842–845.
109. Fries, M., Goldberg, J. D., & Golbus, M. S. Treatment of acardiac–acephalus twin gestations by hysterotomy and selective delivery. *Obstet. Gynecol.* 1992; **79**:601–604.
110. Robie, G., Payne, G., & Morgan, M. Selective delivery of an acardiac, acephalic twin. *N. Engl. J. Med.* 1989; **320**:512–513.
111. Ginsberg, N., Applebaum, M., & Rabin, S. Term birth after midtrimester hysterotomy and selective delivery of an acardiac twin. *Am. J. Obstet. Gynecol.* 1992; **167**:33–37.
112. Hamada, H., Okane, M., & Koresawa, M. Fetal therapy in utero by blockage of the umbilical blood flow of acardiac monster in twin pregnancy. *Nippon Sanka Fujinka Gakkai Zasshi* 1989; **41**:1803–1809.
113. Roberts, R., Shah, D., & Jeanty, P. Twin, acardiac, ultrasound-guided embolization. *Fetus* 1991; **1**(3):5–10.
114. Porreco, R., Barton, S., & Haverkamp, A. Occlusion of umbilical artery in acardiac, acephalic twin. *Lancet* 1991; **337**:326–327.
115. Holzgreve, W., Tercanli, S., Krings, W., & Schuierer, G. A simpler technique for umbilical-cord blockade of an acardiac twin. *N. Engl. J. Med.* 1994; **331**(1):56–57.
116. Donner, C., Shehabi, S., Thomas, D. *et al.* Selective feticide by embolization in twin–twin transfusion syndrome. A report of two cases. *J. Reprod. Med.* 1997; **42**(11):747–50.

117. Quintero, R., Reich, H., & Puder, K. Brief report: umbilical-cord ligation of an acardiac twin by fetoscopy at 19 weeks of gestation. *N. Engl. J. Med.* 1994; **330**:469–471.
118. Ville, Y., Hyett, J. A., Vandenbussche, F. P., & Nicolaides, K. H. Endoscopic laser coagulation of umbilical cord vessels in twin reversed arterial perfusion sequence. *Ultrasound Obstet. Gynecol.* 1994; **4**(5):396–398.
119. Hecher, K., Reinhold, U., Gbur, K., & Hackeloer, B. J. Interruption of umbilical blood flow in an acardiac twin by endoscopic laser coagulation. *Geburtshilfe Frauenheilkd.* 1996; **56**(2):97–100.
120. Hecher, K., Hackeloer, B., & Ville, Y. Umbilical cord coagulation by operative microendoscopy at 16 weeks gestation in an acardiac twin. *Ultrasound Obstet. Gynecol.* 1997; **10**:130–132.
121. Lewi, L., Gratacos, E., & Van Schoubroeck, D. Consecutive cord coagulations in monochorionic mulitplets. *Am. J. Obstet. Gynecol.* 2003; **187**:S61.
122. Rodeck, C., Deans, A., & Jauniaux, E. Thermocoagulation for the early treatment of pregnancy with an acardiac twin. *N. Engl. J. Med.* 1998; **339**:1293–1295.
123. Chang, P. J., Liou, J. D., Hsieh, C. C., Chao, A. S., & Soong, Y. K. Monopolar thermocoagulation in the management of acardiac twins. *Fetal Diagn. Ther.* 2004; **19**(3):271–274.
124. Holmes, A., Jauniaux, E., & Rodeck, C. Monopolar thermocoagulation in acardiac twinning. *Bjog* 2001; **108**(9):1000–1002.
125. Lopoo, J. B. Paek, B. W., Maichin, G. A. *et al.* Cord ultrasonic transection procedure for selective termination of a monochorionic twin. *Fetal Diagn. Ther.* 2000; **15**(3):177–179.
126. Bermudez, C., Tejada, P., Gonzales, F. *et al.* Umbilical cord transection in twin-reverse arterial perfusion syndrome with the use of a coaxial bipolar electrode (Versapoint). *J. Matern. Fetal. Neonat. Med.* 2003; **14**(4):277–278.
127. Sydorak, R. M. Feldstein, V., Machin, G. *et al.* Fetoscopic treatment for discordant twins. *J. Pediatr. Surg.* 2002; **37**(12):1736–1739.
128. Shevell, T., Malone, F. D., Weintraub, J. *et al.* Radiofrequency ablation in a monochorionic twin discordant for fetal anomalies. *Am. J. Obstet. Gynecol.* 2004; **190**(2):575–576.
129. Tsao, K., Feldstein, V. A., Albanese, C. T. *et al.* Selective reduction of acardiac twin by radiofrequency ablation. *Am. J. Obstet. Gynecol.* 2002; **187**(3):635–640.
130. Tan, T. Y. & Sepulveda, W. Acardiac twin: a systematic review of minimally invasive treatment modalities. *Ultrasound Obstet. Gynecol.* 2003; **22**(4):409–419.
131. Kumar, S. & Fisk, N. M. Distal urinary obstruction. *Clin. Perinatol.* 2003; **30**(3):507–519.
132. Johnson, M. Fetal obstructive uropathies. In Harrison, M. R., Adzick, N. S., & Evans, M. I. (Eds.) *The Unborn Patient: Prenatal Diagnosis and Treatment*, Philadelphia: Saunders, 2001:259–286.
133. Nakayama, D. K., Harrison, M. R., & de Lorimier, A. A. Prognosis of posterior urethral valves presenting at birth. *J. Pediatr. Surg.* 1986; **21**(1):43–45.
134. Mahony, B. S., Callen, P. W., & Filly, R. A. Fetal urethral obstruction: US evaluation. *Radiology* 1985; **157**:221–224.
135. Harrison, M. R., Ross, N., Noall, R., & de Lorimier, A. A. *et al.* Correction of congenital hydronephrosis in utero. I. The model: fetal urethral obstruction produces hydronephrosis and pulmonary hypoplasia in fetal lambs. *J. Pediatr. Surg.* 1983; **18**(3):247–256.
136. Harrison, M. R., Naikayama, D. K., Noall, R., & Lorimier, A. A. *et al.* Correction of congenital hydronephrosis in utero II. Decompression reverses the effects of obstruction on the fetal lung and urinary tract. *J. Pediatr. Surg.* 1982; **17**(6):965–974.
137. Harrison, M. R., Golbus, M. S., Filly, R. A. *et al.* Management of the fetus with congenital hydronephrosis. *J. Pediatr. Surg.* 1982; **17**(6):728–742.
138. Harrison, M. R., Golbus, M. S., Filly, R. A. *et al.* Fetal surgery for congenital hydronephrosis. *N. Engl. J. Med.* 1982; **306**(10):591–593.
139. Johnson, M., Bukowski, T., & Reitleman, C. In utero surgical treatment of fetal obstructive uropathy: a new comprehensive approach to identify appropriate candidates for vesicoamniotic shunt therapy. *Am. J. Obstet. Gynecol.* 1994; **170**(1770–1779).
140. Coplen, D. E., Hare, J. Y., Zderic, S. A. *et al.* 10-year experience with prenatal intervention for hydronephrosis. *J. Urol.* 1996; **156**(3):1142–1145.
141. Rodeck, C. H., Fisk, N. M., Fraser, D. I., & Nicolini, U. Long-term in utero drainage of fetal hydrothorax. *N. Engl. J. Med.* 1988; **319**(17):1135–1138.
142. Elder, J. S., Duckett, J. W. Jr., & Snyder, H. M. Intervention for fetal obstructive uropathy: has it been effective? *Lancet* 1987; **2**(8566):1007–1010.
143. Manning, F. A., Harrison, M. R., & Rodeck, C. Catheter shunts for fetal hydronephrosis and hydrocephalus. Report of the International Fetal Surgery Registry. *N. Engl. J. Med.* 1986; **315**(5):336–340.
144. Crombleholme, T. M., Harrison, M. R., Globus, M. S. *et al.* Fetal intervention in obstructive uropathy: prognostic indicators and efficacy of intervention. *Am. J. Obstet. Gynecol.* 1990; **162**(5):1239–1244.
145. Lipitz, S., Robson, S. C., Ryan, G., Haeusler, M. C., & Rodeck, C. H. Management and outcome of obstructive uropathy in twin pregnancies. *Br. J. Obstet. Gynaecol.* 1993; **100**(9):879–880.
146. Freedman, A. L., Bukowski, T. P., Smith, C. A. *et al.* Fetal therapy for obstructive uropathy: diagnosis specific outcomes [corrected]. *J. Urol.* 1996; **156**(2 Pt 2):720–723; discussion 723–724.
147. Coplen, D. Prenatal intervention for hydronephrosis. *J. Urol.* 1997; **157**:2270–2277.
148. Freedman, A., Johnson, M., & Smith, C. Long-term outcome in children after antenatal intervention for obstructive uropathies. *Lancet* 1999; **354**:374–377.
149. Freedman, A. L., Johnson, M. P., & Gonzalez, R. Fetal therapy for obstructive uropathy: past, present, future? *Pediatr. Nephrol.* 2000; **14**(2):167–176.
150. McLorie, G., Farhat, W., Khoury, A., Geary, D., & Ryan, G. Outcome analysis of vesicoamniotic shunting in a comprehensive population. *J. Urol.* 2001; **166**(3):1036–1040.

151. Holmes, N., Harrison, M. R., & Baskin, L. Fetal surgery for posterior urethral valves: long term postnatal outcomes. *Pediatrics* 2001; **108**:E7.

152. Smith, G. H., Canning, D. A., Schulman, S. L. *et al.* The long-term outcome of posterior urethral valves treated with primary valve ablation. *J. Urol.* 1996; **155**:1730–1734.

153. Quintero, R., Hume, R., & Smith, C. Percutaneous fetal cytoscopy and endoscopic fulguration of posterior urethral valves. *Am. J. Obstet. Gynecol.* 1995; **172**:206–209.

154. Quintero, R. A., Morales, W. J., Allen, M. H. *et al.* Fetal hydrolaparoscopy and endoscopic cystotomy in complicated cases of lower urinary tract obstruction. *Am. J. Obstet. Gynecol.* 2000; **183**(2):324–330; discussion 330–333.

155. Hofmann, R., Becker, T., Meyer-Wittkopf, M. *et al.* Fetoscopic placement of a transurethral stent for intrauterine obstructive uropathy. *J. Urol.* 2004; **171**(1):384–386.

156. Quintero, R. A., Homsy, Y., Bornick, P. W., Allen, M., & Johnson, P. K. In-utero treatment of fetal bladder-outlet obstruction by a ureterocele. *Lancet* 2001; **357**(9272):1947–1948.

157. Nicolini, U., Fisk, N. M., Rodeck, C. H., & Beacham, J. Fetal urine biochemistry: an index of renal maturation and dysfunction. *Br. J. Obstet. Gynaecol.* 1992; **99**(1):46–50.

158. Altman, R., Randolph, J., & Lilly, J. Sacrococcygeal teratoma. The American Academy of Pediatrics Surgical Section Survey 1973. *J. Pediatr. Surg.* 1974; **9**:389–398.

159. Rescorla, F., Sawin, R., & Coran, A. Long-term outcome for infants with sacrococcygeal teratoma: a report from the Children's Cancer Group. *J. Pediatr. Surg.* 1998; **33**:171–176.

160. Bond, S., Harrison, M. R., & Schmidt, K. Death due to high output cardfiac failure in fetal sacrococcygeal teratoma. *J. Pediatr. Surg.* 1990; **25**:1287–1291.

161. Flake, A., Harrison, M. R., & Adzick, N. S. Fetal sacrococcygeal teratoma. *J. Pediatr. Surg.* 1986; **21**:563–566.

162. Musci, M., Clark, M. & Ayres, R. Management of dystocia caused by a large sacrococcygeal teratoma. *Obstet. Gynecol.*, 1983: **62**:10s–12s.

163. Gross, S., Benzie, R., & Sermer, M. Sacrococcygeal teratoma: prenatal diagnosis and management. *Am. J. Obstet. Gynecol.* 1987; **156**:393–396.

164. Langer, J. C., Harrison, M. R., Schmidt, K. G. *et al.* Fetal hydrops and death from sacrococcygeal teratoma: rationale for fetal surgery. *Am. J. Obstet. Gynecol.* 1989; **160**(5 Pt 1):1145–1150.

165. Adzick, N. S., Crombleholme, T. M., & Morgan, M. A. A rapidly growing fetal teratoma. *Lancet* 1997; **349**:538.

166. Graf, J. L. & Albanese, C. T. Fetal sacrococcygeal teratoma. *World J. Surg.* 2003; **27**:84–86.

167. Hedrick, H., Flake, A. W., & Crombleholme, T. Sacrococcygeal teratoma: prenatal assessment, fetal intervention, and outcome. *J. Pediatr. Surg.* 2004; **39**(3):430–438, discussion 430–438.

168. Graf, J. L., Albanese, C. T., Jennings, R. W., Farrell, J. A., & Harrison, M. R. Successful fetal sacrococcygeal teratoma resection in a hydropic fetus. *J. Pediatr. Surge.* 2000; **35**(10):1489–1491.

169. Chiba, T., Albanese, C. T., Jennings, R. W. *et al.* In utero repair of rectal atresia after complete resection of a sacrococcygeal teratoma. *Fetal Diagn. Ther.* 2000; **15**(3):187–190.

170. Kay, S., Khalife, S., & LaBerge, J. Prenatal percutaneous needle drainage of cystic sacrococcygeal teratoma. *J. Pediatr. Surg.* 1999; **34**:1148–1151.

171. Garcia, A., Morgan, W., & Bruner, J. In utero decompression of cystic grade IV sacrococcygeal teratoma. *Fetal. Diagn. Ther.* 1998; **13**:305–308.

172. Jouannic, J., Dommergues, M., & Auber, F. Successful intrauterine shunting of a sacrococcygeal teratoma causing fetal bladder obstruction. *Prenat. Diagn.* 2001; **21**:824–826.

173. Hecher, K. & Hackeloer, B. Intrauterine endoscopic laser surgery for fetal sacrococcygeal teratoma. *Lancet* 1996; **347**:470.

174. Lam, Y., Tang, M., & S. TW Thermocoagulation of fetal sacrococcygeal teratoma. *Prenat. Diagn.* 2002; **22**:99–101.

175. Paek, B., Jennings, R. W., & Harrison, M. R. Radiofrequency ablation of human fetal sacrococcygeal teratoma. *Am. J. Obstet. Gynecol.* 2001; **184**:503–507.

176. Ibrahim, D., Ho, E., & Scherl, S. Newborn with an open posterior hip dislocation and sciatic nerve injury after intrauterine radiofrequency ablation of a sacrococcygeal teratoma. *J. Pediatr. Surg.* 2003; **38**(2):248–250.

177. Lary, J. & Edmonds, L. Prevalence of spina bifida at birth – United States, 1983–1990: a comparison of two surveillance systems. *Morb. Mortal. Wkly Rep.* 1996; **45**:15–26.

178. Goodman, R. Economic burden of spina bifida – United States, 1980–1990. *Morb. Mortal. Wkly Rep.* 1989; **38**:264–267.

179. Hirose, S., Farmer, D. L., & Albanese, C. Fetal surgery for meningomyelocele. *Curr. Opin. Obstet. Gynecol.* 1997; **10**:316–320.

180. Heffez, D., Aryanpur, J., Hutchins, G. M., & Freeman, J. M. The paralysis associated with myelomeningocele: Clinical and experimental data implicating a preventable spinal cord injury. *Neurosurgery* 1990; **26**:987–992.

181. Inagaki, T., Schoenwolf, G., & Walker, M. Experimental model: change in the posterior fossa with surgically induced spina bifida aperta in mouse. *Pediatr. Neurosurg.* 1997; **26**:185–189.

182. Heffez, D., Aryanpour, J., & Rotellini, N. Intrauterine repair of experimentally created dysraphism. *Neurosurgery* 1993; **32**:1005–1010.

183. Housley, H. T., Graf, J., & Lipshutz, G. S. Creation of myelomeningocele in the fetal rabbit. *Fetal. Diagn. Ther.* 1995; **15**:275–279.

184. Meuli, M., Meuli-Simmen, C., & Hutchins G. In utero surgery rescues neurologic function at birth in sheep with spina bifida. *Nat. Med.* 1995; **1**:342–347.

185. Paek, B., Farmer, D., & Wilklinson, C. C. Hindbrain herniation develops in surgically created myelomeningocele but is absent after repair in fetal lambs. *Am. J. Obstet. Gynecol.* 2000; **183**:1119–1123.

186. Copeland, Bruner, M., J. & Richards, W. A model for in utero endoscopic treatment of myelomeningocele. *Neurosurgery* 1993; **33**:542–544.

187. Bruner, J., Richards, W. & Tulipan, N. Endoscopic coverage of fetal myleomeningocele in utero. *Am. J. Obstet. Gynecol.* 1999; **180**:153–158.
188. Farmer, D. L., Von Koch, C. S., Peacock, W. J. *et al.* In utero repair of myelomeningocele: experimental pathophysiology, initial clinical experience, and outcomes. *Arch. Surg.* 2003; **138**(8):872–878.
189. Bruner, J., Tulipan, N., & Richards, W. In utero repair of myelomeningocele: a comparison of endoscopy and hystertomy. *Fetal Diagn. Ther.* 2000; **15**:83–88.
190. Sutton, L., Adzick, N. S., & Bilaniuk, L. Improvement in hindbrain herniation demonstrated by serial fetal magnetic resonance imaging following fetal surgery for myelomeningocele. *J. Am. Med. Assoc.*, 1999; **282**:1826–1831.
191. Tubbs, R. S., Chambers, M. R., Smyth, M. D. *et al.* Late gestational intrauterine myelomeningocele repair does not improve lower extremity function. *Pediatr. Neurosurg.* 2003; **38**(3):128–132.
192. Holzbeierlein, J., Pope, J. C. IV, Adams, M. C. *et al.* The urodynamic profile of myelodysplasia in childhood with spinal closure during gestation. *J. Urol.* 2000; **164**(4):1336–1339.
193. Tulipan, N., Sutton, L. N., Bruner, J. P. *et al.* The effect of intrauterine myelomeningocele repair on the incidence of shunt-dependent hydrocephalus. *Pediatr. Neurosurg.* 2003; **38**(1):27–33.
194. Tulipan, N. Intrauterine myelomeningocele repair. *Clin. Perinatol.* 2003; **30**(3):521–530.
195. Aaronson, O. S., Tulipan, N. B., Cywes, R. *et al.* Robot-assisted endoscopic intrauterine myelomeningocele repair: a feasibility study. *Pediatr. Neurosurg.* 2002; **36**(2):85–89.
196. Aktug, T., Demir, N., Akgur, F. M., & Olguner, M. *et al.* Pretreatment of gastroschisis with transabdominal amniotic fluid exchange. *Obstet. Gynecol.* 1998; **91**(5 Pt 2):821–823.
197. Luton, D., de Legausie, P., & Guibourdenche, J. *et al.* Effect of amnioinfusion on the outcome of prenatally diagnosed gastroschisis. *Fetal Diagn. Ther.* 1999; **14**(3):152–155.
198. Olguner, M., Akgur, F. M., Ozdemir, T. *et al.* Amniotic fluid exchange for the prevention of neural tissue damage in myelomeningocele: an alternative minimally invasive method to open in utero surgery. *Pediatr. Neurosurg.* 2000; **33**(5):252–256.
199. Longaker, M. T., Laberge, J., & Dansereau, J. Primary fetal hydrothorax: natural history and management. *J. Pediatr. Surg.* 1989; **24**:573–576.
200. Chernick, V. & Reed, M. H. Pneumothorax and chylothorax in the neonatal period. *J. Pediatr.* 1970; **76**(4):624–632.
201. Castillo, R. A., Devoe, L. D., Falls, G. *et al.* Pleural effusions and pulmonary hypoplasia. *Am. J. Obstet. Gynecol.* 1987; **157**(5):1252–1255.
202. Aubard, Y., Derouineau, I., Aubard, V. *et al.* Primary fetal hydrothorax: a literature review and proposed antenatal clinical strategy. *Fetal Diagn. Ther.* 1998; **13**(6):325–333.
203. Weber, A. & Philipson, E. Fetal pleural effusion: a review and meta-anlysis for prognostic indicators. *Obstet. Gynecol.* 1992; **79**:281–286.
204. Hagay, Z., Reece, A., Roberts, A., & Hobbins, J. C. Isolated fetal pleural effusion: a prenatal management dilemma. *Obstet. Gynecol.*, 1993; **81**(1):147–152.
205. Wilkins-Haug, L. E. & Doubilet, P. Successful thoracoamniotic shunting and review of the literature in unilateral pleural effusion with hydrops. *J. Ultrasound. Med.* 1997; **16**(2):153–160.
206. Young, I. D. & Clarke, M. Lethal malformations and perinatal mortality: a 10 year review with comparison of ethnic differences. *Br. Med. J. (Clin. Res. Ed.)*, 1987; **295**(6590):89–91.
207. Keith, J., Rowe, R., & Vlad, P. *Heart Disease in Infancy and Childhood.* 3rd edn. New York: Macmillan Publishing Co., 1978.
208. Yagel, S., Weissman, A., Rotstein, Z. *et al.* Congenital heart defects: natural course and in utero development. *Circulation* 1997; **96**:550–555.
209. Simpson, J. M. & Sharland, G. K. Natural history and outcome of aortic stenosis diagnosed prenatally. *Heart* 1997; **77**(3):205–210.
210. McCaffrey, F. M. & Sherman, F. S. Prenatal diagnosis of severe aortic stenosis. *Pediatr. Cardiol.* 1997; **18**(4):276–281.
211. Carvalho, J. S., Marrides, E., Shinebourne, E. A. *et al.* Improving the effectiveness of routine prenatal screening for major congenital heart defects. *Heart* 2002; **88**(4):387–391.
212. Tworetzky, W. & Marshall, A. Balloon valvuloplasty for congenital heart disease in the fetus. *Clin. Perinatol.* 2003; **30**:541–550.
213. Reddy, V., Liddicoat, J., & Klein, J. Fetal cardiac bypass using an in-line axial flow pump to minimize extracorporeal surface and avoid priming volume. *Ann. Thorac. Surg.* 1996; **62**:393–400.
214. Reddy, V., Liddicoat, J. R., Klein, J. R. *et al.* Long-term fetal outcome after fetal cardiac bypass: Fetal survival to full term and organ abnormalities. *J. Cardiovasc. Surg.* 1996; **111**:536–544.
215. Kohl, T., Szabo, Z., & Suda, K. Fetoscopic and open transumbilical fetal cardiac catheterization in sheep. *Circulation* 1997; **95**:1048–1053.
216. Kohl, T., Kirchhof, P., & Gogarten, W. Fetoscopic and open transumbilical fetal cardiac catheterization in sheep. *Circulation* 1999; **100**:772–776.
217. Kohl, T., Strumper, D., & Witteler, R. Fetoscopic direct fetal cardiac access in sheep: an important experimental milestone along the route to human fetal cardiac intervention. *Circulation* 2000; **102**:1602–1604.
218. Kohl, T., Hartlage, M. G., Westphal, M. *et al.* Intra-amniotic multimodal fetal echocardiography in sheep: a novel imaging approach during fetoscopic interventions and for assessment of high-risk pregnancies in which conventional imaging methods fail. *Ultrasound Med. Biol.* 2002; **28**(6):731–736.
219. Maxwell, D., Allan, L., & Tynan, M. Balloon dilation of the aortic vlave in the fetus. A report of two cases. *Br. Heart J.* 1991; **65**:256–258.
220. Kohl, T., Sharland, G., Allan, L. D. *et al.* World experience of percutaneous ultrasound-guided balloon valvuloplasty in human fetuses with severe aortic valve obstruction. *Am. J. Cardiol.* 2000; **85**:1230–1233.

221. Allan, L., Maxwell, D. J., Carminati, M., & Tynan, M. J. Survival after fetal aortic balloon valvuloplasty. *Ultrasound Obstet. Gynecol.* 1995; **5**:90–91.
222. Tulzer, G. Arzt, W., Franklin, R. C. *et al.* Fetal pulmonary valvuloplasty fro critical pulmonary stenosis or atresia with intact septum. *Lancet* 2002; **360**:1567–1568.
223. Wilkins-Houg, L. Experience with fetal aortic valvotomies. In Society of Maternal Fetal Medicine. New Orleans, LA., 2004.
224. Benatar, A., Vaughan, J., Nicolini, U. *et al.* Prenatal pericardiocentesis. Its role in the mangement of intrapericardial teratoma. *Obstet. Gynecol.* 1992; **79**:856–859.
225. Sklansky, M., Greenberg, M., Lucas, V., & Gruslin-Giroux, A. Intrapericardial teratoma in a twin fetus: diagnosis and management. *Obstet. Gynecol.* 1997; **89**:807–809.
226. Bruch, S. W., Adzick, N. S., Reiss, R., & Harrison, M. R. Prenatal therapy for pericardial teratomas. *J. Pediatr. Surg.* 1997; **32**(7):1113–1115.
227. Fujimori, K., Honda, S., Akatsu, H. *et al.* Prenatal diagnosis of intrapericardial teratoma: a case report. *J. Obstet. Gynaecol. Res.* 1999; **25**(2):133–136.
228. Sepulveda, W., Gomez, E., & Gutierrez, J. Intrapericardial teratoma. *Ultrasound Obstet. Gynecol.* 2000; **15**(6):547–548.
229. Sydorak, R., Kelly, J., & Feklstein, V. A. *et al.* Prenatal resection of a fetal pericardial teratoma. *Fetal Diagn. Ther.* 2002; **17**:281–285.
230. Carpenter, R., Strasburger, J. F., Garson, A. Jr. *et al.* Fetal ventricular pacing for hydrops secondary to complete atrioventricular block. *J. Am. Coll. Cardiol.* 1986; **8**:1434–1436.
231. Walkinshaw, S., Welch, C. R., McCormack, J., & Walsh, K. In utero pacing for fetal congenital heart block. *Fetal Diagn. Ther.* 1994; **9**:183–185.
232. Rosenthal, D., Druzin, M., Chin, C., & Dubin, A. A new therapeutic approach to the fetus with congenital complete heart block: preemptive, targeted therapy with dexamethasone. *Obstet. Gynecol.* 1998; **92**(4 Pt 2):689–691.
233. Hirose, S., Farmer, D. L., Lee, H. *et al.* The ex utero intrapartum treatment procedure: looking back at the EXIT. *J. Pediatr. Surg.* 2004; **39**(3):375–380; discussion 375–380.
234. MacKenzie, T. C., Crombleholme, T. M., & Flake, A. W. The ex-utero intrapartum treatment. *Curr. Opin. Pediatr.* 2002; **14**(4):453–458.
235. Tanaka, M., Sato, S., Naito, H., & Nakayama, H. Anaesthetic management of a neonate with prenatally diagnosed cervical tumour and upper airway obstruction. *Can. J. Anaesth.* 1994; **41**(3):236–240.
236. Hirose, S. & Harrison, M. R. The ex utero intrapartum treatment (EXIT) procedure. *Semin. Neonatol.* 2003; **8**(3):207–214.
237. Hirose, S., Sydorak, R. M., Tsao, K. *et al.* Spectrum of intrapartum management strategies for giant fetal cervical teratoma. *J. Pediatr. Surg.* 2003; **38**:446–450.
238. DeCou, J. M., Jones, D. C., Jacobs, H. D., & Touloukian, R. J. Successful ex utero intrapartum treatment (EXIT) procedure for congenital high airway obstruction syndrome (CHAOS) owing to laryngeal atresia. *J. Pediatr. Surg.* 1998; **33**(10):1563–1565.
239. Crombleholme, T. M., Sylvester, K., Flake, A. W., & Adzick, N. S. Salvage of a fetus with congenital high airway obstruction syndrome by ex utero intrapartum treatment (EXIT) procedure. *Fetal Diagn. Ther.* 2000; **15**(5):280–282.
240. Bui, T. H., Grunewald, C., & Frenckner, B. *et al.* Successful EXIT (ex utero intrapartum treatment) procedure in a fetus diagnosed prenatally with congenital high-airway obstruction syndrome due to laryngeal atresia. *Eur. J. Pediatr. Surg.* 2000; **10**(5):328–333.
241. Paek, B. W., Callen, P. W., & Kitterman, J. *et al.* Successful fetal intervention for congenital high airway obstruction syndrome. *Fetal Diagn. Ther.* 2002; **17**(5):272–276.
242. Kanamori, Y., Kitano, Y., & Hashizume, K. *et al.* A case of laryngeal atresia (congenital high airway obstruction syndrome) with chromosome 5p deletion syndrome rescued by ex utero intrapartum treatment. *J. Pediatr. Surg.* 2004; **39**(1):E25–E28.
243. Fewell, J. E., Hislop, A. A., Kitterman, J. A., & Johnson, P. Effect of tracheostomy on lung development in fetal lambs. *J. Appl. Physiol.* 1983; **55**(4):1103–1108.
244. Prontera, W., Jaeggi, E. T., Pfizenmaier, M., Tassaux, D., & Pfister, R. E. Ex utero intrapartum treatment (EXIT) of severe fetal hydrothorax. *Arch. Dis. Child Fetal Neonat. Ed.* 2002; **86**(1):F58–F60.
245. Bouchard, S., Johnson, M. P., & Flake, A. W. *et al.* The EXIT procedure: experience and outcome in 31 cases. *J. Pediatr. Surg.* 2002; **37**(3):418–426.
246. Michel, T. C., Rosenberg, A. L., & Polley, L. S. *EXIT to ECMO. Anesthesiology* 2002; **97**(1):267–268.
247. Mackenzie, T. C., Crombleholme, T. M., & Johnson, M. P. *et al.* The natural history of prenatally diagnosed conjoined twins. *J. Pediatr. Surg.* 2002; **37**(3):303–309.
248. Izadi, K., Smith, M., & Askari, M. *et al.* A patient with an epignathus: management of a large oropharyngeal teratoma in a newborn. *J. Craniofac. Surg.* 2003; **14**(4):468–472.
249. Noah, M., Norton, M. E., & Sandberg, P. *et al.* Short term maternal outcomes that are associated with the EXIT procedure, as compared to cesarean delivery. *Am. J. Obstet. Gynecol.* 2002; **186**:773–777.
250. Quintero, R. Treatment of previable premature rupture of membranes. *Clin. Perinatol.* 2003; **30**:573–589.
251. Bengtson, J. M., Van Marter, L. J., & Barss, V. A. *et al.* Pregnancy outcome after premature rupture of the membranes at or before 26 weeks' gestation. *Obstet. Gynecol.* 1989; **73**(6):921–927.
252. Beydoun, S. N. & Yasin, S. Y. Premature rupture of the membranes before 28 weeks: conservative management. *Am. J. Obstet. Gynecol.* 1986; **155**(3):471–479.
253. Gormley, J. Treatment of postspinal headache. *Anesthesiology* 1960; **21**:565–566.
254. Quintero, L., Romero, R., Dzieczkowski, J. *et al.* Sealing of ruptured amniotic membranes with intra-amniotic platelet-cryoprecipitate plug. *Lancet* 1996; **347**:1117.
255. Senor, T., Ozalp, S., Hassa, H. *et al.* Maternal blood clot patch therapy: a model for postamniocentesis amniorrhea. *Am. J. Obstet. Gynecol.* 1997; **177**:1535–1536.

256. Quintero, R., Mendoza, G., & Allen, M. In-vivo laser welding of collagen-based graft material to the amnion in a rabbit model of ruptured membranes. *Prenat. Neonat. Med.* 1999; **4**:453–456.
257. Quintero, R. A. Treatment of previable premature ruptured membranes. *Clin. Perinatol.* 2003; **30**(3):573–589.
258. Quintero, R., Moralez, W. J., & Bornick P. W. *et al.* Surgical treatment of spontaneous rupture of membranes: the amniograft – first experience. *Am. J. Obstet. Gynecol.* 2002; **186**:155–157.
259. Seeds, J., Cefalo, R., & Herbert, W. Amniotic band syndrome. *Am. J. Obstet. Gynecol.* 1982; **144**:243–248.
260. Graf, J., Bealer, J., & Gibbs, D. Chorioamniotic membrane separation: a potentially lethal finding. *Fetal Diagn. Ther.* 1997; **12**:81–84.
261. Crombleholme, T., Dirkes, K., & Whitney, T. Amniotic band syndrome in fetal lambs I: Fetoscopic release and morphometric outcome. *J. Pediatr. Surg.* 1995; **30**:974–978.
262. Strauss, A., Hasbargen, U., & Paek, B. Intra-uterine fetal demise caused by amniotic band syndrome after standard amniocentesis. *Fetal. Diagn. Ther.* 2000; **15**:4–7.
263. Quintero, R., Morales, W., & Phillips, J. In utero lysis of amniotic bands. *Ultrasound Obstet. Gynecol.* 1997; **10**:316–320.
264. Keswani, S., Johnson, M., & Adzick, S. In utero limb salvage: Fetoscopic release of amniotic bands for threatened limb amputation. *J. Pediatr. Surg.* 2003; **38**:848–851.
265. Luton, D., Guibourdenche, J., & Vuillard, E. *et al.* Prenatal management of gastroschisis: the place of the amnioexchange procedure. *Clin. Perinatol.* 2003; **30**(3):551–572, viii.
266. Luton, D., Lagausie, P., & Guibourdenche, J. *et al.* Prognostic factors of prenatally diagnosed gastroschisis. *Fetal Diagn. Ther.* 1997; **12**(1):7–14.
267. Olguner, M., Akgur, F. M., Api, A. *et al.* The effects of intraamniotic human neonatal urine and meconium on the intestines of the chick embryo with gastroschisis. *J. Pediatr. Surg.* 2000; **35**(3):458–461.
268. Aktug, T., Ucan, B., Olguner, M. *et al.* Amnio-allantoic fluid exchange for prevention of intestinal damage in gastroschisis II: Effects of exchange performed by using two different solutions. *Eur. J. Pediatr. Surg.* 1998; **8**(5):308–311.
269. Aktug, T., Ucan, B., & Olguner, M. *et al.* Amnio-allantoic fluid exchange for the prevention of intestinal damage in gastroschisis. III: Determination of the waste products removed by exchange. *Eur. J. Pediatr. Surg.* 1998; **8**(6):326–328.
270. Luton, D., de Lagausie, P., & Guibourdenche, J. *et al.* Influence of amnioinfusion in a model of in utero created gastroschisis in the pregnant ewe. *Fetal Diagn. Ther.* 2000; **15**(4):224–228.
271. Harding, J., Lui, L., & Evans, P. *et al.* Intrauterine feeding of the growth retarded fetus: can we help? *Early. Hum. Dev.* 1992; **29**(1–3):193–197.
272. Peranteau, W. H., Hayashi, S., & Kim, H. B. *et al.* In utero hematopoietic cell transplantation: what are the important questions? *Fetal Diagn. Ther.* 2004; **19**(1):9–12.
273. Lemery, D. J., Santolaya-Forgacs, J., & Wilson, L., Jr. *et al.* A nonhuman primate model for the in utero chronic catheterization of the umbilical vein. A preliminary report. *Fetal Diagn. Ther.* 1995; **10**(5):326–332.
274. Hedrick, M. H., Jennings, R. W., & MacGillivray, T. E. *et al.* Chronic fetal vascular access. *Lancet* 1993; **342**(8879):1086–1087.
275. Paek, B. W., Lopoo, J. B., & Jennings, R. W. *et al.* Safety of chronic fetal vascular access in the sheep model. *Fetal Diagn. Ther.* 2001; **16**(2):98–100.
276. Flake, A. W. Genetic therapies for the fetus. *Clin. Obstet. Gynecol.* 2002; **45**(3):684–696; discussion 730–732.
277. Flake, A. W. The fetus with a hematopoietic stem cell defect: In Harrison, M. R. (Ed.) *The Unborn Patient: The Art and Science of Fetal Therapy.* Philadelphia: W.B. Saunders Company, 2001:591–603.
278. Flake, A. W. & Zanjani, E. D. In utero hematopoietic stem cell transplantation. A status report. *J. Am. Med. Assoc.* 1997; **278**(11):932–937.
279. Jones, D. R., Bui, T. H., Anderson, E. M. *et al.* In utero haematopoietic stem cell transplantation: current perspectives and future potential. *Bone Marrow Transpl.* 1996; **18**(5):831–837.
280. Flake, A. W., Roncarlo, M.-G., & Puck, J. Treatment of X-linked severe combined immunodeficiency by in utero transplantation of paternal bone marrow. *N. Engl. J. Med.* 1996; **335**:1806–1810.
281. Albanese, C. T. & Barcena, A. Ontogeny of the fetal immune system: implications for fetal tolerance induction and postnatal transplantation In Harrison, M. R. (Ed.) *The Unborn Patient: The Art and Science of Fetal Therapy.* Philadelphia: W.B. Saunders Company, 2001:605–615.
282. Danzer, E., Sydorak, R., & Harrison, M. R. Minimal access fetal surgery. *Eur. J. Obstet. Gynecol. Reprod. Biol.* 2003; **108**:3–13.
283. Longaker, M. T. The fetus with cleft lip/palate and craniofacial anomalies. In Harrison, M. R. (ed.) *The Unborn Patient: The Art and Science of Fetal Therapy,* 3rd edn. Philadelphia: W.B. Saunders Company, 2001.
284. Hedrick, M. H., Rice, H. E., & Vander Wall, K. J. *et al.* Delayed in utero repair of surgically created fetal cleft lip and palate. *Plast. Reconstr. Surg.* 1996; **97**(5):900–905; discussion 906–907.
285. Weinzweig, J., Panter, K. E., & Pantaloni, M. *et al.* The fetal cleft palate: I. Characterization of a congenital model. *Plast. Reconstr. Surg.* 1999; **103**(2):419–428.
286. Weinzweig, J., Panter, K. E., & Pantaloni, M. *et al.* The fetal cleft palate: II. Scarless healing after in utero repair of a congenital model. *Plast. Reconstr. Surg.* 1999; **104**(5):1356–1364.
287. Weinzweig, J., Panter, K. E., & Spangenberger, A. *et al.* The fetal cleft palate: III. Ultrastructural and functional analysis of palatal development following in utero repair of the congenital model. *Plast. Reconstr. Surg.* 2002; **109**(7):2355–2362.

288. Estes, J. M., Whitby, D. J., & Lorenz, H. P. *et al.* Endoscopic creation and repair of fetal cleft lip. *Plast. Reconstr. Surg.* 1992; **90**(5):743–746; discussion 747–749.
289. Evans, M. L., Oberg, K. C., & Kirsch, W. *et al.* Intrauterine repair of cleft lip-like defects in lambs with a novel microclip. *J. Craniofac. Surg.* 1995; **6**(2):126–131.
290. Oberg, K. C., Evans, M. L., Nguyen, T. *et al.* Intrauterine repair of surgically created defects in mice (lip incision model) with a microclip: preamble to endoscopic intrauterine surgery. *Cleft Palate Craniofac. J.* 1995; **32**(2):129–137.
291. Stelnicki, E. J., Van der Wall, K., Hoffman, W. Y. *et al.* Adverse outcomes following endoscopic repair of a fetal cleft lip using an ovine model. *Cleft Palate Craniofac. J.* 1998; **35**(5):425–429.

74

Conjoined twins

Lewis Spitz

Department of Paediatric Surgery, Institute of Child Health and Great Ormond Street Hospital, London, UK

Historical aspects

Mankind has been fascinated by abnormal births since antiquity. Descriptions of conjoined twins date back to the ancient Egyptians, but the earliest recorded case is that of the "Biddenden maids" born in Kent in 1100. Mary and Eliza Chulkhurst were joined at the hips and shoulders and lived together for 34 years when Mary suddenly became ill and died. She refused to be separated from her dead sister saying "As we came together we will also go together" and died 6 hours later.[1]

Geoffrey Saint Hilaire cited an example of girls born in 1495 joined at the forehead causing them to stand face to face: "when one walked forward, the other was compelled to walk backward." They lived until the age of 10 years, and when one died an unsuccessful attempt was made at separation.[2]

Ambroise Paré[3] reported on a 40-year-old man in Paris in 1530, who carried a parasite without a head which hung a pendant from his belly. Batholinus described the history of Lazarus-Joannes Bapista Colloredo, born in Genoa in 1617 who exhibited himself all over Europe. An imperfectly developed twin comprising one thigh, hands, body, arms and a well-formed head hung from his epigastrium. These are two examples of asymmetrical conjoined twins.

The Isle–Brewer xiphopagus twins, Priscilla and Aquila, were born in 1680 and were joined from the "navel up to a point just beneath the nipples." The twins were visited daily by hundreds of people keen to view "the monstrous work of Nature and admire so great a piece of curiosity." They died some time during that year.[4]

The first successful separation of conjoined twins was reported by Koenig in 1689. Elizabeth and Catherine Mayerin were born in Basel on 24 November 1689. A surgeon, Johannes Fatio, was consulted and "the following day, in the presence of a galaxy of medical men he proceeded to separate the xypho-omphalopagus twins." Fatio was able to isolate the umbilical vessels and follow them to the navel, where he tied them separately. He then transfixed and tied the bridge between the two infants with a silken cord, and cut the isthmus. "The ligature fell off on the ninth postoperative day and both children recovered." Koenig, a young physician, was present as a spectator during the operation; he published the case using Fatio's illustrations but never mentioned his name![5]

Helen and Judith, the Hungarian sisters born in 1701 in Szony, are an early example of pygopagus conjoined twins. They were objects of great curiosity until, at the age of 9 years, they were placed in a convent where they died aged 22 years. They were joined back-to-back in the lumbar region and had "all their parts separate except for the anus which was present between the right thigh of Helen and the left of Judith and a single vagina."[6]

The most celebrated conjoined twins are Chang and Eng born in Thailand (formerly known as Siam, hence the popular term "Siamese twins") in 1811. They were joined at the umbilicus by a short band which gradually stretched until they were eventually able to stand side-by-side. Their father was a fisherman and the family lived on a floating house on the Mekong river where they became famous swimmers. Their peculiar movement in the water attracted the attention of Robert Hunter, a Scottish merchant, and finally led to their leaving their country in search of fortune. They lived in North Carolina for many years where they married sisters and fathered 21 children between them. Physiologically and psychologically they were totally different. Chang

Pediatric Surgery and Urology: Long-term Outcomes, Mark Stringer, Keith Oldham, Pierre Mouriquand.
Published by Cambridge University Press.

was smaller and more feeble. What Chang liked to eat, Eng detested. Eng was good-natured, Chang cross and irritable. They often quarrelled and not infrequently came to blows. Chang drank heavily – at times getting drunk; but Eng was unaffected. They lived to the age of 63 years and died in 1874.[7]

The latter two case histories illustrate that conjoined twins can have totally different physical and psychological characteristics. This phenomenon has been recognized on a number of occasions in the series treated at Great Ormond Street Hospital, London. They also demonstrate that conjoined twins can survive together for many years. This poses the ethical problem of whether separation should always be recommended. If there is a significant risk to separation, perhaps it would be advisable to allow the twins to exist in the joined state.

By 1990, there were over 600 publications on conjoined twins and 167 attempts at separation.[8] In 1996, Spencer[9] was able to review 1200 cases from the literature over the past century.

Incidence and etiology

The frequency of conjoined twins has been estimated at 1 set per 50 000 births, but since about 60% are stillborn, the true incidence is 1 in 200 000 live births. With the widespread use of routine antenatal ultrasound scanning, especially in the developed countries, and the likely rise in elective terminations, the incidence of live born conjoined twins will inevitably decrease even further. Female twins predominate in a ratio of 3:1.

The most widely held view is that conjoined twins develop from a single fertilized ovum that fails to undergo complete division of the embryonic disc around the 15–17th day of gestation.[10,11] Spencer[9] contests this fission theory and proposes, as an alternative, fusion of the developing parts in a uniovular embryo as a more acceptable embryologic basis for the condition. It is postulated that, at the very beginning, a single embryonic cell mass divides completely into two individual twin cell masses. At an early stage, these two embryos abut and fuse involving only a few or alternatively many cells, the number of which determines the extent of union.

Classification

Conjoined twins are classified according to the most prominent site of connection, plus the Greek term for fixed, "pagus." The most practical classification from the surgical point of view is that of Cywes *et al.* (Table 74.1).[12]

Table 74.1. Classification of conjoined twins[12]

I. Symmetrical and equally developed twins:
- (A) each component complete
  - (a) thoracopagus
  - (b) omphalopagus
  - (c) pygopagus
  - (d) ischiopagus
  - (e) craniopagus
- (B) each component less than an entire individual
  - (a) duplication of the cranial end of the body
    - (i) monocephalus diproscagus – single head with duplication of the features of the face
    - (ii) dicephalus – two distinct heads with separate necks and one body (recently retermed *parapagus*)
  - (b) duplication in the caudal region – pygus
  - (c) duplication of both cranial and caudal regions

II. Asymmetrical or unequal conjoined twins (heteropagus):
- Parasite attached to the visible surface of the autosite
- Parasite attached to the back on sacrococcygeal region
- Parasite developed within the autosite (fetus-in-fetu)

Table 74.2. Embryologic classification of conjoined twins (with % incidence)

Ventral 87%		
Rostral	Cephalopagus	11%
	Thoracopagus	19%
	Omphalopagus	18%
Caudal	Ischiopagus	11%
Lateral	Parapagus	28%
Dorsal 13%		
Craniopagus	5%	
Rachipagus	2%	
Pygopagus	6%	

An alternative classification based on embryologic factors has been proposed by Spencer (Table 74.2).[13]

The various types of symmetrical conjoined twins, their incidence and the frequency with which organs are shared in each category are shown in Table 74.3.

Prenatal diagnosis

The diagnosis of conjoined twins should be considered in any twin pregnancy that has a single placenta and no visible separating amniotic membrane. Polyhydramnios occurs in as many as 50% of conjoined twin pregnancies compared with 10% of normal twins and 2% of singleton pregnancies.

Prenatal ultrasonography is capable of diagnosing conjoined twin pregnancies as early as 12 weeks' gestation.[14]

Table 74.3.

Type of fusion	Incidence	Shared structures	
Thoracopagus	40%	Liver	100%
		Pericardium	90%
		Heart	75%
		Upper intestine	50%
		Biliary tree	25%
Omphalopagus	33%	Liver	80%
		Terminal ileum and colon	33%
Pygopagus	19%	Sacrum and coccyx	100%
		Lower GI tract	25%
		Genitourinary tract (ureters often cross)	15%
Ischiopagus	6%	Pelvic bones	100%
		Lower GI tract	70%
		Genitourinary	50%
Craniopagus	2%	Skull, venous sinuses and meninges	100%
		Cerebral cortex	37%

The sonographic findings in conjoined twins include inseparable fetal bodies and skin contours, an unchanging relative position of the fetuses, both fetal heads persistently at the same level, and a single umbilical cord containing more than three vessels.[15] Detailed scanning at around 20 weeks' gestation will define with reasonable accuracy the extent of the conjoined area and provide an assessment of which viscera are shared. Fetal echocardiography is particularly important since twins with a shared heart have an extremely poor prognosis and termination of the pregnancy is invariably recommended. Computerised tomography (CT) and magnetic resonance imaging (MRI) have been performed antenatally,[16] but once the decision has been made to proceed with the pregnancy, these investigations can be carried out with greater accuracy after delivery.[17] An additional advantage of prenatal diagnosis is that the time, place and mode of delivery can be planned.[15] In all instances, the delivery should take place at, or close to, the surgical unit where separation will be performed. Delivery must always be by Cesarean section at 36–38 weeks' gestation.[18]

Postnatal management

Following initial resuscitation, the early postnatal management comprises stabilization followed by detailed physical examination and specialized investigations to determine as accurately as possible the precise anatomy of the union and to define any associated anomalies, particularly cardiac malformations. A single QRS complex on electrocardiography is an ominous sign of cardiac fusion.[19] Further more detailed investigations will include echocardiography and/or angiography. At this early stage it is important to decide whether separation is feasible. Alternatively, a decision on no surgical treatment should be made positively and nature allowed to take its course.

Management after birth can take one of three courses:

1. *Non-operative management* is indicated when there is complex cardiac union without the possibility of reconstructing even a single functioning heart or where there is extensive cerebral fusion. Parents faced with the prospect of severe deformity of the twins may refuse consent to proceed to separation. In seven of our cases, six had complex cardiac fusion and the parents of one set with extensive parapagus fusion (with a normal triplet in the gestation) refused surgery. All seven twins died within a short period.
2. *Emergency separation* is necessary when one twin is dead or dying and threatening the survival of the other, where there is a correctable anomaly incompatible with survival if left untreated, or where serious damage has occurred to the connecting bridge or area of fusion.

   Emergency separation was necessary in seven of our sets of conjoined twins. Prenatal assessment failed to confirm the diagnosis in an omphalopagus set who were born by vaginal delivery. Following rupture of the shared exomphalos, the united liver split causing massive hemorrhage resulting in the immediate death of one twin. An emergency procedure was undertaken to salvage the surviving twin who died at the end of the procedure. In two sets of thoracopagus twins, cardiac instability prompted urgent separation on day 3 and day 8 of life, respectively. In the first set, one girl, currently 15 years old, survives but her twin died at 6 weeks of age from pulmonary atresia. In the second set, one twin had a unilocular heart and died at separation; the remaining twin survived the surgical procedure but succumbed to a cot death at 6 weeks of age. Emergency separation at 16 h of age was attempted but failed in a set of thoracopagus twins with a conjoined heart and an associated congenital diaphragmatic hernia. Separation was performed on omphalopagus twin girls in whom prenatal volvulus of the conjoined intestine had occurred. The affected intestine had become necrotic and perforated while the proximal and distal small bowel had sealed leaving atresias. Both twins survived, albeit with foreshortened intestines which required many months for adaptation to occur. Omphalopagus twins were diagnosed at 18 weeks' gestation. They were delivered by

Cesarean section at 38 weeks'. One twin suffered severe respiratory distress requiring mechanical ventilation. He failed to respond to intensive resuscitation and died during transfer. The conjoined area was compressed digitally and emergency separation of the surviving male infant was performed successfully. One set of parapagus conjoined twins had three lungs. One of the twins had a severe congenital cardiac malformation (AV canal). Shortly after birth they developed intractable severe pulmonary hypertension. The twin with the cardiac anomaly was critical and was jeopardizing the survival of her sibling. One twin died intraoperatively and the other within a few hours of separation.

The survival rate for emergency separation was 4 out of 14 infants (28%). However, survival was not expected in four sets, including two with cardiac connections, one of the omphalopagus twins with hypoplastic lungs and the pair of parapagus twins with severe persistent pulmonary hypertension.

3. *Planned separation* – if the twins are stable and healthy at birth, they should be allowed to thrive and feed normally. This provides time to carry out a range of investigations aimed at defining as accurately as possible the extent of the shared organs. It also allows time to apply methods to assist with primary closure of the defects left following separation such as tissue expansion, cultured keratocytes, skin flaps etc. The operative procedure can be carefully planned with the involvement of the relevant staff (e.g., theater, intensive care, ward).

   The optimum age at separation is 2–3 months, but this will be dependent on the age at which the twins are referred.

The range of investigations is determined by the site and extent of union.[20] Evaluation may include plain and contrast radiography, ultrasonography, echocardiography, CT and MRI scanning with intravenous contrast enhancement, radionuclide scanning, and angiography. Magnetic resonance imaging and helical CT have emerged as the most valuable investigations as a three-dimensional image can be constructed around the site of union giving accurate information essential to the planned separation. Tc^{99}-labelled iminodiacetic acid (HIDA/DISIDA) is extremely useful in assessing the hepatobiliary systems and DMSA (dimercaptosuccinic acid) and DTPA (diethylene triamine penta-acetic acid) scanning for renal anatomy and urinary excretory function, respectively.

Skin cover

It is important to estimate the likely extent of skin deficiency following separation and to plan a contingency programme. If one twin is deemed unsalvageable, the definitive incision should be planned to include sufficient skin to achieve primary closure of the surviving twin. A myocutaneous flap derived from the common fused posterior limb of an ischiopagus tripus twin should provide enough tissue to enable primary closure of both twins. Alternative means of providing additional skin cover include the use of preoperative tissue expanders[21,22] (subcutaneous or intraperitoneal), artificial pneumoperitoneum, or the use of meshed allogenic skin and autologous cultured keratinocytes.[23] Should one twin unexpectedly succumb in the early postoperative period, split-skin grafts may be taken soon after death to provide a useful source of skin cover for the surviving twin.

Specialist colleagues such as pediatric urologists, cardiac, orthopedic and plastic surgeons, must be involved at an early stage in the planning process. Prior to the actual procedure it is important to hold planning conferences to define responsibilities.[24] The hospital press liaison officer should be kept informed of progress but no information need be released until separation has been achieved.

Anesthesia

Anesthesia involves two completely separate teams with all members being clearly aware for which twin they are responsible. All drugs and intravenous fluids administered are calculated on a total weight basis with half being delivered to each twin. Because of the cross-circulation, drugs given intravenously may have an unpredictable effect and particular care must be taken to administer drugs such as opioids incrementally.[25] Endotracheal intubation should be via the nose for added security during repositioning (especially when separation has been achieved and the infants are moved to individual theatres or at least to separate operation tables), and for continuation of respiratory support postoperatively. Full arterial and central venous monitoring is essential and, in addition, ECG, pulse oximetry, capnography and urine output must be carefully monitored. Regular blood gas analyses are undertaken during the procedure. Adequate venous access is crucial as brisk hemorrhage necessitating rapid large volume transfusion may occur. Cardiovascular monitoring is particularly important since, with relative changes in position of the two infants, significant shifts in blood volume may occur.[26]

The operative procedure

Technical details of the operative procedure are dictated by the anatomy of union and by the extent of sharing of organs and structures.[27] In thoracopagus, the liver is invariably shared. In 90% of cases there is a common pericardium, which can be separated to provide an individual pericardial sac for each twin. Major myocardial connections are present in 75% of cases and only a few attempts have been made at separation with sacrifice of one twin, but no long-term survivors have been reported. The upper gastrointestinal tract is common in 50% of cases and the biliary system shared in 25%. In omphalopagus, the liver is shared in 80% of cases and in 33% the intestines join at the level of a Meckel's diverticulum; the common terminal ileum and colon have a dual blood supply. The lower intestinal tract is common in both pygopagus and ischiopagus and the genitourinary tract is shared in 15% of the former and 50% of the latter. It is not uncommon for the ureters in these situations to cross over from one twin and enter the contralateral bladder. The high mortality rate associated with craniopagus is almost entirely due to cerebral fusion, which is also responsible for the neurodevelopmental sequelae in survivors.

Blood loss may be a major intraoperative problem, especially when there is pelvic bony fusion. Blood loss occurring during division of the liver should be minimized by using ultrasonic dissection, meticulously ligating major connecting vessels and coagulating minor vessels, and by applying fibrin glue to the raw surface, which reduces postoperative ooze of blood and leakage of bile. Despite every attempt to define as accurately as possible all anatomical connections prior to surgery, "unexpected events" are frequently encountered during the operation. Examples in our experience include abnormal vascular communications, and previously unidentified intestinal and genitourinary anomalies. The surgical team should be aware of these variations in anatomy and be prepared to vary the operative procedure accordingly.

If, despite all possible maneuvers, primary closure of the residual defect proves impossible, it will be necessary to insert prosthetic material (polypropylene mesh, silicone sheet, Goretex[R]) as a temporary measure. The insertion of a prosthetic patch to close the abdomen is preferable to "closure under tension," which may embarrass respiration or inhibit venous return.

Postoperative management

Postoperatively, the surviving infant(s) are extremely fragile. All intraoperative monitoring must be continued postoperatively in the intensive care unit and, because of the prolonged duration of surgery, the infants are electively paralyzed and mechanically ventilated for a variable period of time. Meticulous attention should be directed at monitoring fluid and electrolyte balance and, in particular, avoiding overhydration which may precipitate cardiovascular instability. Sepsis is a major cause of mortality and morbidity and strict infectious precautions must be exercised, particularly when large skin defects are present.[25] Late, unexpected deaths following separation are unfortunately not uncommon.[26,28]

Table 74.4. Percentage survival rates[8]

	Overall	Both surviving	One survivor	Both died	One sacrificed
Thoracopagus	45–75[a]	27	32	32	9
Omphalopagus	70	49	35	14	2
Ischiopagus	82	69	12	14	5
Craniopagus	50	29	26	32	13
Pygopagus	75	60	33	7	–

[a] The survival rate for thoracopagus improved from 45% overall to 75% in the years 1980–1986.

Table 74.5a. Conjoined twins: the Great Ormond Street series. Separation not attempted ($n = 7$)

Year	Type	Sex	Major problem	Associated anomalies
1986	Thoracopagus	F	Cardiac fusion	Pulmonary valve atresia, Esophageal atresia
1989	Thoracopagus	F	Cardiac fusion	Exomphalos
1994	Thoracopagus	F	Cardiac fusion	
1996	Parapagus	F	Extent of union	(Triplet)
1999	Thoracopagus	F	Cardiac fusion	
2002	Thoracopagus	F	Cardiac fusion	
2003	Thoracopagus	F	Cardiac fusion	

Results

Hoyle[8] analyzed all reports on attempts at separation of conjoined twins up to 1987. Of over 600 publications in the literature, 167 attempts at separation had been carried out and reported. It is clear that many additional attempts at separation, most of which were probably unsuccessful, were not documented. The percentage survival rates for the various types of conjoined twins documented by Hoyle is shown in Table 74.4.

The outcome of the 25 cases managed by the team at Great Ormond Street Hospital, London, are shown in Tables 74.5a–c.[29–31] Two sets of twins were fully investigated and

Table 74.5b. Conjoined twins: the Great Ormond Street series. Emergency separation ($n = 7$)

Year	Type	Sex	Age (days)	Shared organs	Associated anomalies	Outcome
1985	Thoracopagus	F	3	Pericardium, diaphragm, liver, bile duct, small bowel	Pulmonary valve atresia	1 alive & well 1 died @ 6 wks
1993	Omphalopagus	F	1	Liver, small bowel, cloacal anomaly	Exomphalos (ruptured)	Both died
1995	Thoracopagus	M	8	Cardiac (atrial), liver	Unilocular heart, absent hepatic vein	1 early death 1 died @ 6 wks
1997	Thoracopagus	F	1	Cardiac fusion, liver	Unilocular heart, congenital diaphragmatic hernia	Both died
1998	Omphalopagus	F	2	Liver, midgut	Exomphalos, volvulus, atresia	Both alive
1999	Omphalopagus	M	1	Bowel, bladder	Imperforate anus, hypoplastic lungs	1 alive, 1 dead
2000	Parapagus	F	1	Lung, diaphragm, aorta, liver, intestine	Atrioventricular canal defect, persistent pulmonary hypertension	Both died

Table 74.5c. Conjoined twins: the Great Ormond Street series. Planned separation ($n = 9$)

Year	Type	Sex	Age	Shared organs	Associated anomalies	Outcome
1968	Craniopagus	F	2 m	Sagittal sinus	–	1 alive, 1 died at 6 m
1987	Ischiopagus	M	8 m	Liver, distal GI, genitalia	Anorectal malformation	Alive and well
1992	Parapagus	F	3 y	Pericardium, diaphragm, liver, distal GI, genitourinary	Renal agenesis	1 alive, 1 died at 3 d
1993	Parapagus	M	10 m	Pericardium, liver, distal GI, genitourinary	Anorectal malformation	1 alive, 1 died at 6 m
1994	Thoracopagus	F	3 m	Pericardium, liver, bile duct, small bowel	Exomphalos	Alive and well
1997	Omphalopagus	F	3 m	Liver	–	Alive and well
2001	Pygopagus	F	2 m	Spinal cord	Anorectal malformation	Alive and well
2002	Ischiopagus	F	2 m	Pelvis, exstrophy	Anorectal malformation	Alive and well
2003	Omphalopagus	F	6 w	Liver	–	Alive and well

scheduled for separation but elected to go elsewhere for surgery.

Prenatal diagnosis is now common and prospective parents need to be fully and carefully counseled about all possible outcomes. Elective termination of pregnancy will invariably be recommended for thoracopagus twins with conjoined hearts. In craniopagus twins, the likelihood of major neurodevelopmental disabilities needs to be discussed. The probability of successful separation of thoraco- and omphalopagus twins with separate hearts is high enough (75% in recent years) to advise continuation of the pregnancy. The almost inevitable anorectal and genitourinary deformities in ischio- and pygopagus twins need to be carefully considered by the parent(s) before a decision is made to proceed with the pregnancy.

There have been no reported long-term survivors in conjoined twins with a shared heart. Attempted separation under these circumstances is doomed to failure. The only instance in which one twin in our series was deliberately sacrificed was in a thoracopagus conjoined twin with atrial connection. The non-viable twin had a unilocular heart. The surviving twin appeared to be making good progress but unexpectedly died 6 weeks postoperatively. At necropsy, he was found to have bronchopneumonia. In all other instances where planned separation was performed, the intention was to give both twins an equal chance of survival. It is generally accepted that following separation the twins are extremely fragile. There was one unexpected sudden death in one of our patients and a similar outcome occurred following successful separation of a craniopagus

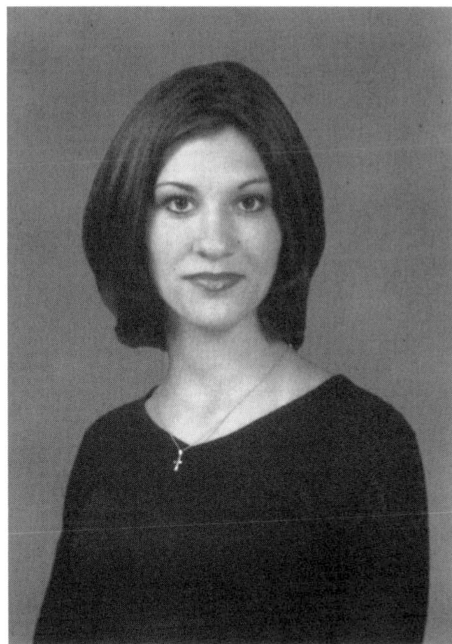

Fig. 74.1. Surviving 18-year-old girl following separation of thoracopagus twins at 3 days of age.

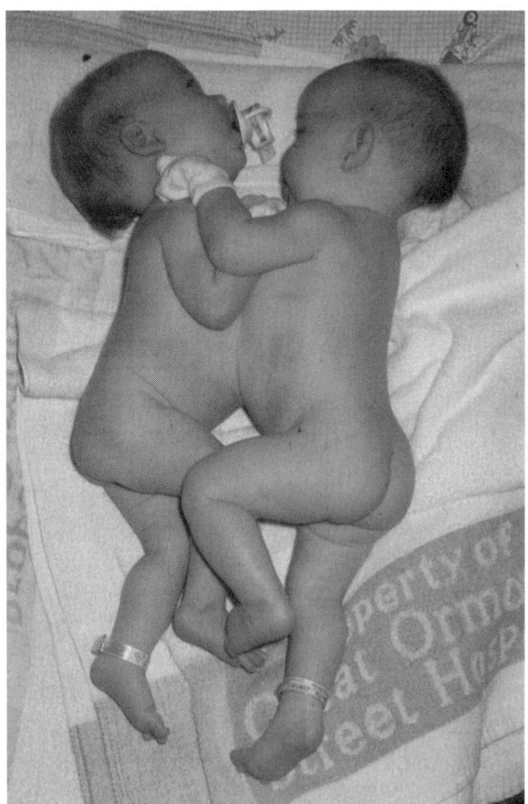

Fig. 74.2. Thoracopagus twins, both of whom survived.

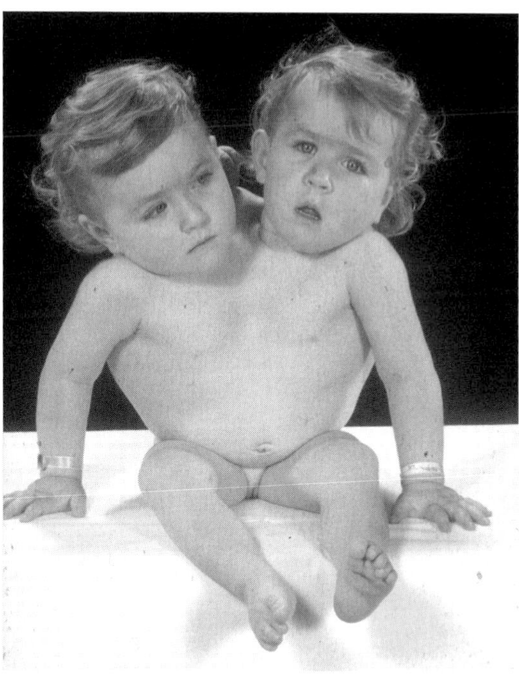

Fig. 74.3. Parapagus twins at 3 years of age.

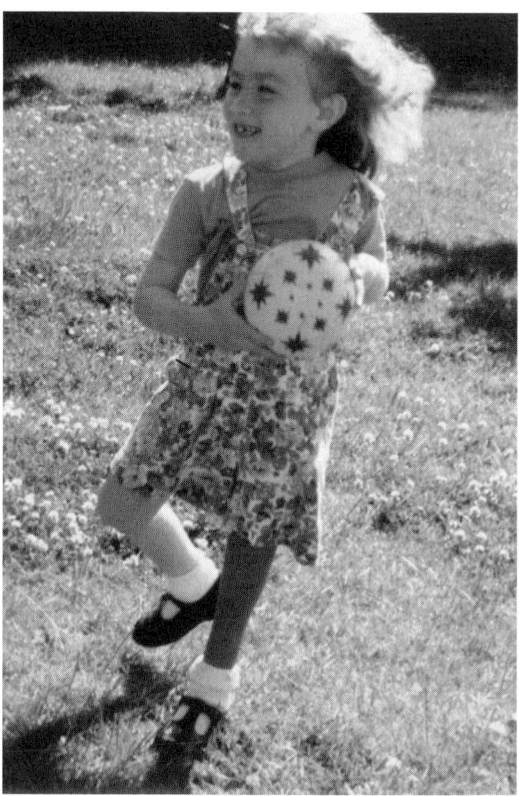

Fig. 74.4. Surviving twin following separation of parapagus twins, aged 7 years, wearing a prosthesis.

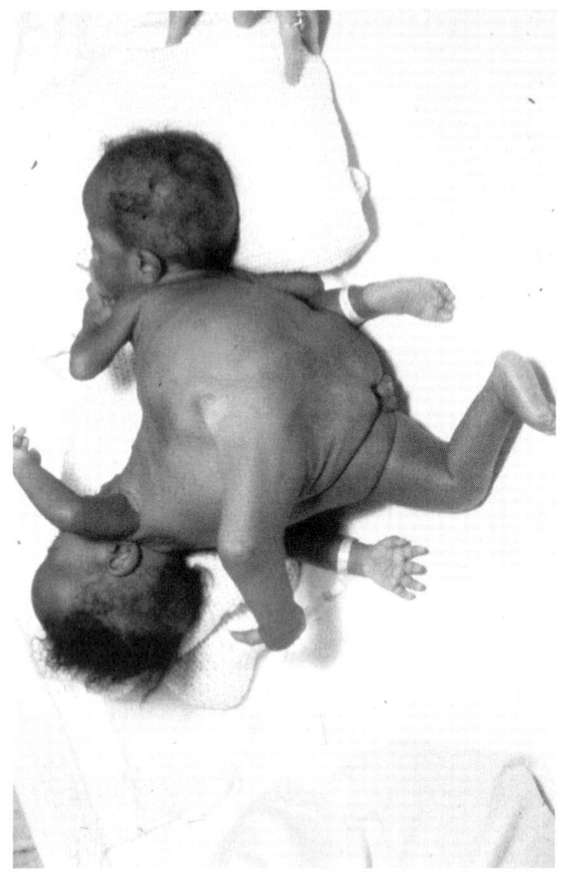

Fig. 74.5. Ischiopagus twins aged 4 months.

Table 74.6. Outcome of separation of conjoined twins in three major series[29,36,37]

Series	No.	No operation	Emergency separation survivors (%)	Planned separation survivors (%)
O'Neill (USA)	18	5	5 sets 1 (10%)	8 sets 13 (81%)
Cywes (S Africa)	14	4	5 sets 2 (20%)	5 sets 8 (80%)
Spitz & Kiely (UK)	22	6	7 sets 4 (29%)	9 sets 15 (83%)

twin in the author's previous experience. Late deaths have also been reported in other series including three deaths in the series from Cywes *et al.* (1997),[36] two of which occurred after thoracopagus separation, and one following separation of an omphalopagus set of conjoined twins.

Long-term follow-up

Depending on the nature and extent of union, after separation the surviving twin(s) may have minimal (Fig. 74.1) or major residual handicap. Separation of thoracopagus (Fig. 74.2) and omphalopagus leave extensive, unsightly scars and defects, particularly involving the sternum. Ischiopagus conjoined twins will almost invariably remain with major genitourinary and anorectal deformities, as well as having only a single lower limb (Figs. 74.3–74.6).[32] They may have a permanent intestinal stoma and be incontinent of urine requiring either intermittent catheterization or urinary diversion.[29,30,33] In addition, major vertebral deformities will invariably result in scoliosis and the need for corrective spinal surgery.[34] The limb deficit will require a complex prosthesis which will need to be renewed every few years during growth.[31] Hematometrocolpos has been documented as a late complication following separation of ischiopagus conjoined twins.[35]

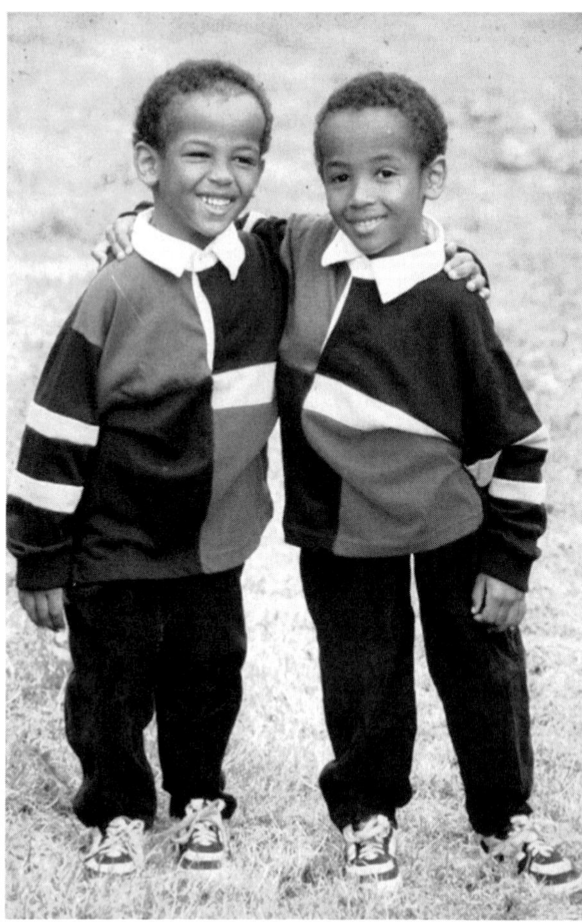

Fig. 74.6. Both surviving twins aged 6 years.

Psychological problems need to be carefully monitored and appropriate therapeutic strategies adopted. Particularly difficult examples include residual genital deformities

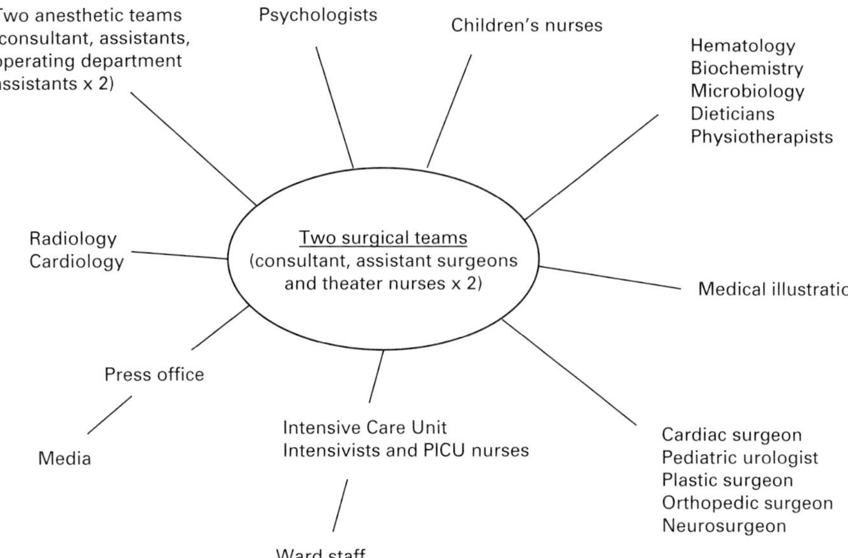

Fig. 74.7. The team of specialists in the separation of conjoined twins.

in ischiopagus twins with shared genitalia and where one twin is assigned the anorectum and the other the genitourinary system.

The outcome in three major series in the literature is shown in Table 74.6,[29,36,37] while Fig.74.7 shows the team of specialists involved in this type of surgery.

REFERENCES

1. Bondeson, J. The Biddenden Maids: a curious chapter in the history of conjoined twins. *J. Roy. Soc. Med.* 1992; **85**:217–221.
2. Geoffrey St. Hilaire, I. *Histoire general et particulaiere des anomalies de l'organisation chez l'homme et les animaux*. Paris (1832–1837).
3. Pare, A. *Complete Works*. First French edn. Translated into English by Thomas Johnson 1678.
4. Bondeson, J. The Isle–Brewers conjoined twins of 1680. *J. Roy. Soc. Med.* 1993; **86**:106–109.
5. Rickham, P. P. The dawn of paediatric surgery: Johannes Fatio (1649–1691) – his life, his work and his horrible end. *Prog. Pediatr. Surg.* 1986; **20**:94–105.
6. Broman, L., quoted in *Normale und abnorme Entwicklung des Menschen*. Weisbaden, 1911, p. 680.
7. Luckhardt, A. B. Report of the autopsy of the Siamese twins together with other interesting information covering their life. A sketch of the life of Chang and Eng. *Surg. Gynecol. Obstet.* 1941; **72**:116–125.
8. Hoyle, R. M. Surgical separation of conjoined twins. *Surg. Gynecol. Obstet.* 1990; **170**:549–562.
9. Spencer, R. Conjoined twins: theoretical embryological basis. *Teratology* 1992: **45**:591–602.
10. Zimmerman, A. A. Embryologic and anatomic considerations of conjoined twins. *Birth. Defects.* Original Article Series 1967; **111**:18–27.
11. Jones, K. L. In Jones, K. L. (ed.) *Smith's Recognizable Patterns of Human Malformation*, 2nd edn., Philadelphia: W.B. Saunders, 1988:594–595.
12. Cywes, S., Davies, M. R. Q., & Rode, H. Conjoined twins – the Red Cross War Memorial Children's Hospital experience. *S. Afr. J. Surg.* 1982; **20**:105–118.
13. Spencer, R. Theoretical and analytical embryology of conjoined twins. Part I: Embryogenesis. *Clin. Anat.* 2000; **13**:36–53.
14. Schmidt, W., Hebarling, D., & Kubli, F. Antepartum ultrasonographic diagnosis of conjoined twins in early pregnany. *Am. J. Obstet. Gyncecol.* 1981; **139**:961–963.
15. Barth, R. A., Filly, R. A., Goldberg, J. D., Moore, P., & Silverman, N. H. Conjoined twins: prenatal diagnosis and assessment of associated malformations. *Radiology* 1990; **177**:201–207.
16. Turner, R. J., Hankins, G. D. V., Weinreb, J. C. *et al.* Magnetic resonance imaging and ultrasonography in the antenatal evaluation of conjoined twins. *Am. J. Obstet. Gynecol.* 1986; **155**:645–649.
17. Fitzgerald, E. J., Toi, A., & Cochlin, D. L. Conjoined twins. Antenatal ultrasound diagnosis and a review of the literature. *Br. J. Radiol.* 1985; **58**:1053–1056.
18. Rudolph, A. J., Michaels, J. P., & Nichols, B. L. Obstetric management of conjoined twins. *Birth Defects*. Original Article Series 1967; Vol. III: 28–37.
19. Leachman, R. D., Latson, J. R., Kohler, C. M., & McNamara, D. G. Cardiovascular evaluation of conjoined twins. *Birth. Defects.* Original Article Series 1967; Vol. III:81–89.
20. Kingston, C. A., McHugh, K., Kumaradevan, J., Kield, E. M., & Spitz, L. Imaging in the preoperative assessment of conjoined twins. *Radiographics* 2001; **21**(5):1187–1208.

21. Zuker, R. M., Filler, R. M., & Lalla, R. Intraabdominal tissue expansion: an adjunct in the separation of conjoined twins. *J. Pediatr. Surg.* 1986; **21**:1198–2000.
22. Spitz, L., Capps, S. N. J., & Kiely, E. M. Xipho-omphalo-ischiopagus tripus conjoined twins: successful separation following abdominal wall expansion. *J. Pediatr. Surg.* 1991; **26**:26–29.
23. Spitz, L., Stringer, M. D., Kiely, E. M., Ransley, P. G., & Smith, P. Separation of branchio-thoraco-omphalo-ischiopagus bipus conjoined twins. *J. Pediatr. Surg.* 1994; **21**:1198–2000.
24. Clemessy, J. L., Brusset, M. C., Frot, C. M., Mayer, M. N., Nihoul-Fekete, C., & Barrier, G. Anaesthetic management for ischiopagus tetrapus conjoined twins separation. *Paediatr. Anaesth.* 1996; **6**:160–162.
25. Keats, A. S., Cave, P. E., Slataper, E. L., & Moore, R. A. Conjoined twins – a review of anaesthetic management for separating operations. *Birth Defects* Original Series 1967; Vol. III:81–89.
26. Diaz, J. H. & Furman, E. B. Perioperative management of conjoined twins. *Anesthesiology* 1987; **76**:965–973.
27. Kiesewetter, W. B. Surgery on conjoined (Siamese) twins. *Surgery* 1996; **59**:860–871.
28. O'Neill, J. A., Holcomb, G. W., Schnaufer, L. *et al.* Surgical experience with thirteen conjoined twins. *Ann. Surg.* 1985; **208**:299–312.
29. Spitz, L. & Kiely, E. M. Experience in the management of conjoined twins. *Br. J. Surg.* 2002; **89**:1188–1192.
30. Spitz, L. Surgery for conjoined twins (Hunterian Lecture). *Ann. R. Coll. Surg. Engl.* 2003; **85**:230–235.
31. Spitz, L. & Kiely, E. M. Conjoined twins. *J. Am. Med. Assoc.* 2003; **289**:1307–1310.
32. Hoyle, R. M. & Thomas, C. G. Twenty-three year follow-up of separated ischio-pagus tetrapus conjoined twins. *Ann. Surg.* 1988; **210**:673–679.
33. Shapiro, E., Fair, W. R., Ternberg, J. L., Siegel, M. J., Bell, M. J., & Manley, C. B. Ischiopagus tetrapus twins: urological aspects of separation and 10-year follow up. *J. Urol.* 1991; **145**:120–125.
34. Albert, M. C., Drummond, D. S., O'Niell, J. A., & Watts, H. The orthopedic management of conjoined twins: a review of 13 cases and report of 4 cases. *J. Pediatr. Orthop.* 1992; **2**:300–307.
35. Beller, U., Quagliarello, J., de, Haro, H. L., & Orderica, S. Hematometra-hematocolpos: a late complication of successful separation of conjoined twins. *Surgery* 1988; **103**:704–705.
36. Cywes, S., Millar, A. J. W., Rode, H., & Brown, R. A. Conjoined twins – the Cape Town experience. *Pediatr. Surg. Int.* 1997; **12**:234–238.
37. O'Neill, J. A. Conjoined twins. In O'Neill, J. A., Rowe, M., Grosfeld, J. L., Fonkalsrud, E. W., & Coran, A. G. (eds.) *Pediatric Surgery.* Vol 2. 5th edn. St. Louis, Mo; Mosby-Year Book Inc, 1998:1925–1938.

Index

Note: page numbers in *italics* refer to figures and tables.
'Plate' refers to illustration numbers in the Plates section.

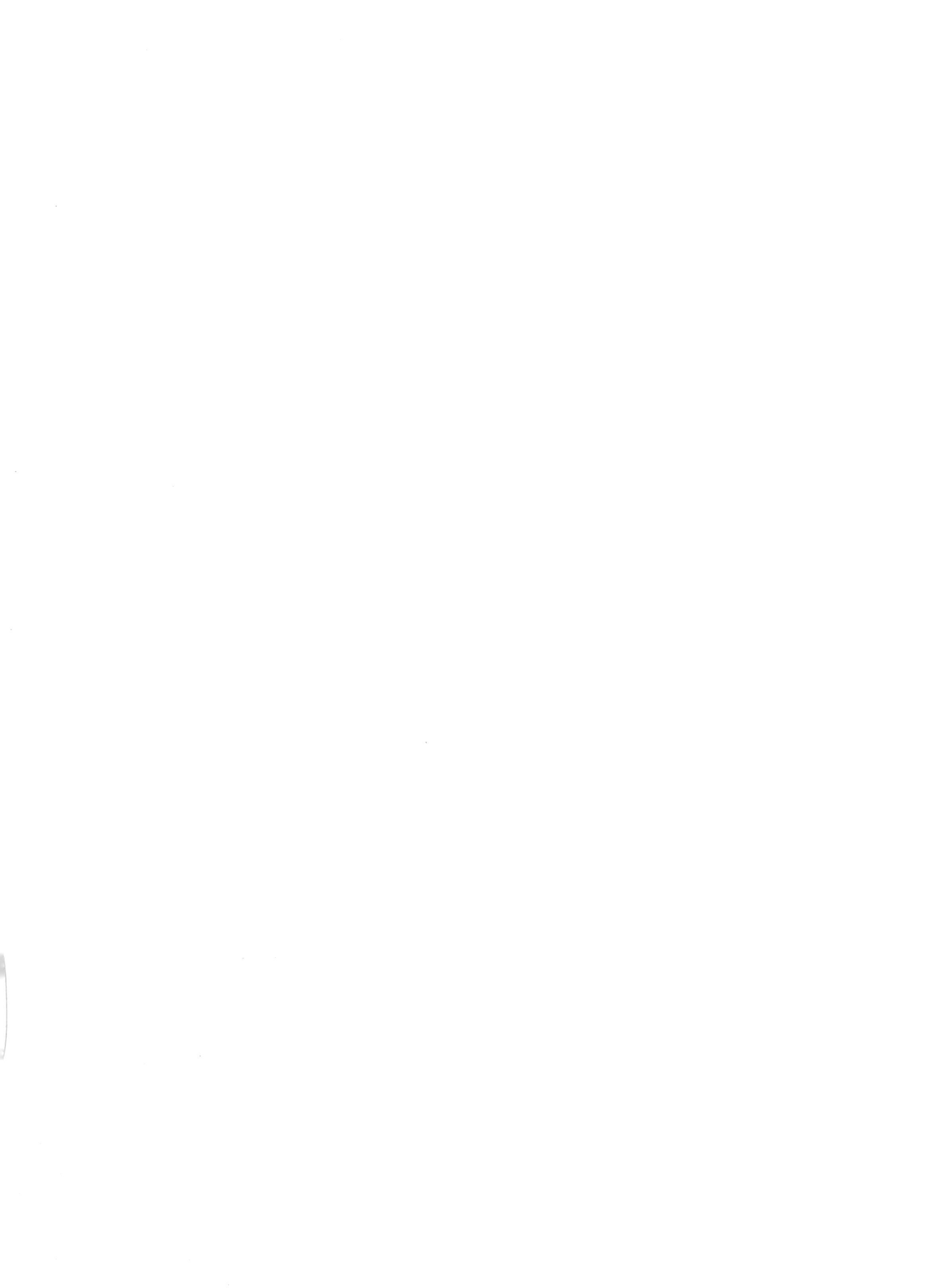